WITHDRAWN
HEALTH LIBRARY AT COUNTY

CONTENTS IN BRIEF

RG 951.

KT-477-177

LIBRARY
USE
ONLY

FIFTH EDITION

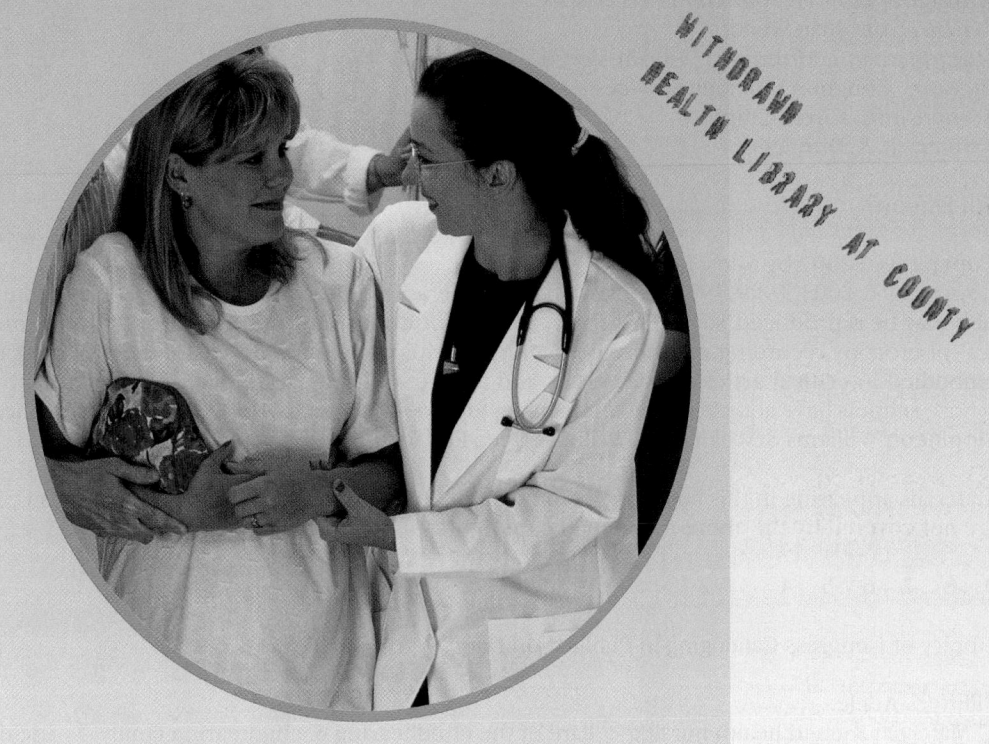

WITHDRAWN
HEALTH LIBRARY AT COUNTY

Maternal & Child Health Nursing
Care of the Childbearing & Childrearing Family

Adele Pillitteri, PhD, RN, PNP
Associate Professor
University of Southern California
Los Angeles, California
Former Director, Neonatal Nurse Practitioner Program
State University of New York at Buffalo
Buffalo, New York

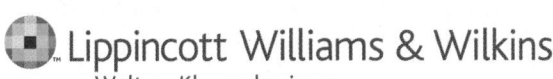 Lippincott Williams & Wilkins
a Wolters Kluwer business

Philadelphia · Baltimore · New York · London
Buenos Aires · Hong Kong · Sydney · Tokyo

Senior Acquisitions Editor: Elizabeth Nieginski
Development Editors: Alison Darrow, Melanie Cann
Editorial Assistant: Betsy Gentzler
Senior Production Editor: Tom Gibbons
Senior Production Manager: Helen Ewan
Managing Editor/Production: Erika Kors
Art Director: Joan Wendt
Manufacturing Manager: William Alberti
Indexer: Coughlin Indexing Services
Compositor: Circle Graphics
Printer: R. R. Donnelley

5th Edition

Copyright © 2007 by Adele Pillitteri.
Copyright © 2003, 1999, 1995, 1992 by Adele Pillitteri. All rights reserved. This book is protected by copyright. No part of it may be reproduced, stored in a retrieval system, or transmitted, in any form or by any means—electronic, mechanical, photocopy, recording, or otherwise—without prior written permission of the publisher, except for brief quotations embodied in critical articles and reviews and testing and evaluation materials provided by publisher to instructors whose schools have adopted its accompanying textbook. Printed in the United States of America. For information write Lippincott Williams & Wilkins, 530 Walnut Street, Philadelphia PA 19106.

Materials appearing in this book prepared by individuals as part of their official duties as U.S. Government employees are not covered by the above-mentioned copyright.

9 8 7 6 5 4 3 2

Library of Congress Cataloging-in-Publication Data

Pillitteri, Adele.
  Maternal & child health nursing : care of the childbearing & childrearing family / Adele
Pillitteri. — 5th ed.
        p. ; cm.
  Includes bibliographical references and index.
  ISBN 0-7817-7776-3 (cloth : alk. paper)
  1. Maternity nursing. 2. Pediatric nursing.
  [DNLM: 1. Maternal-Child Nursing. 2. Family Health. WY 157.3 P641m 2007] I. Title.
II. Title: Maternal and child health nursing.
RG951.P637 2007
618.2'0231—dc22

2005029299

    Care has been taken to confirm the accuracy of the information presented and to describe generally accepted practices. However, the authors, editors, and publisher are not responsible for errors or omissions or for any consequences from application of the information in this book and make no warranty, express or implied, with respect to the content of the publication.
    The authors, editors, and publisher have exerted every effort to ensure that drug selection and dosage set forth in this text are in accordance with the current recommendations and practice at the time of publication. However, in view of ongoing research, changes in government regulations, and the constant flow of information relating to drug therapy and drug reactions, the reader is urged to check the package insert for each drug for any change in indications and dosage and for added warnings and precautions. This is particularly important when the recommended agent is a new or infrequently employed drug.
    Some drugs and medical devices presented in this publication have Food and Drug Administration (FDA) clearance for limited use in restricted research settings. It is the responsibility of the health care provider to ascertain the FDA status of each drug or device planned for use in his or her clinical practice.

Library Education & Resource Centre
University Hospitals of North Midlands Trust
County Hospital
Weston Road
Stafford
ST16 3SA

Health Library
Clinical Education Centre
University Hospital of
North Staffordshire
Newcastle Road
Stoke-on-Trent ST4 6QG

To my husband Joseph and my family: Rusty, Dawn, Bill, Heather,

J.J., Lauren, Thomas, and Lynn

with love

This book is due for return on or before the last date shown below.

R E V I E W E R S

Kim Abel, RN, BS
Nursing Instructor
Illinois Valley Community College
Oglesby, Illinois

Karen Booth, RN, BSN, Med, MSN
Professor of Nursing
Owens Community College
Toledo, Ohio

Beverly June Davis Bye, MS, EdD (c), Med, RN, CRNP, FNE-A, CES
Clinical Assistant Professor, Family Nurse Practitioner
Towson University
Towson, Maryland

Ernestine Hunter Cuellar, RN, PhD (c), APRN, BC
Associate Professor
The University of Texas Medical Branch at Galveston
Galveston, Texas

Frances Anne Freitas, MSN, RNC
Assistant Professor
Kent State University—Ashtabula Campus
Ashtabula, Ohio

Robyn C. Leo, RN, MS
Assistant Professor Maternal/Child Nursing
Worcester State College
Worcester, Massachusetts

Janet Pinkelman, MSN, RNC
Instructor of Nursing
Owens Community College
Toledo, Ohio

Glenda L. Smith, DSN, RNC, NNP, APRN, BC, PNP
Assistant Professor of Nursing
University of Texas Health Science Center at Houston
Houston, Texas

Mary Thibault, RN, MSN, Med
Professor
Owens Community College
Toledo, Ohio

P R E F A C E

Maternal-newborn and child health nursing are expanding areas as a result of the broadening scope of practice within the nursing profession and the recognized need for better preventive and restorative care in these areas. The importance of this need is reflected in the fact that many of the year 2010 health goals for the nation focus on these areas of nursing.

At the same time that the information in these areas of nursing is increasing, less time is available in nursing programs to teach it. Students experience difficulty reading all of the material contained in two separate textbooks.

Maternal and Child Health Nursing: Care of the Childbearing and Childrearing Family, Fifth Edition, is written with this challenge in mind. It views maternal-newborn and child health care not as two separate disciplines but as a continuum of knowledge. It is designed to present the content of the two disciplines comprehensively but not redundantly. It is based on a philosophy of nursing care that respects clients as individuals, yet views them as part of families and society.

The book is designed for undergraduate student use in either a combined course in maternal-newborn and child health or for a curriculum in which these courses are taught separately. It provides a comprehensive, in-depth discussion of the many facets of maternal and child health nursing, while promoting a sensitive, holistic outlook on nursing practice. As such, the book will also be useful for practicing nurses or graduate students who are interested in reviewing or expanding their knowledge in these areas.

Basic themes that are integrated into this text include the experience of wellness and illness as family-centered events, the perception of pregnancy and childbirth as periods of wellness in the life of a woman, and the importance of knowing normal child development in the planning of nursing care. Also included are themes reflective of changes in health care delivery and the importance of meeting the needs of a culturally diverse population.

THE CHANGING HEALTH CARE SCENE

Managed care has drastically changed the health care delivery system, increasing the role of the nurse from a minor to a major player. It has made understanding multidisciplinary approaches to care greater than ever before. An increasingly multicultural population is reflected among both nurses and their clients, necessitating fine-tuning of culturally sensitive care. In order that nurses can be prepared for this new level of responsibility, educational changes have to keep pace with this health care reform.

New nursing curricula that are in keeping with this spirit of change emphasize expected outcomes, a greater focus on communication, therapeutic interventions, critical thinking, and nursing process.

Nursing issues that grow out of the current climate of change include the following:

- **The importance of health teaching with families as a cornerstone of nursing responsibility:** The teaching role of the nurse has greater significance in the new health care milieu as the emphasis on preventive care and short stays in the acute care setting create the need for families to be better educated in their own care. Focus on Family Teaching displays throughout the text address this issue.
- **An emphasis on National Health Goals:** As a way to focus care and research, National Health Goals have gained wider attention at a time when there is a greater need than ever to be wise in the choice of how dollars are spent. Students can familiarize themselves with these goals by referring to the Focus on National Health Goals displays that appear throughout the book.
- **The importance of individualizing care according to sociocultural uniqueness:** This is a reflection of both greater cultural sensitivity and an increasingly diverse population of caregivers and care recipients. Greater emphasis is being placed on the implications of multiple sociocultural factors in terms of how they affect a patient's response. Focus on Diversity of Care displays throughout the text show how cultural factors can be given consideration in the planning of care.
- **Changing areas of practice:** The variety of new care settings, as well as the diversity of roles in which nurses can practice, is reflected both in the proliferation of community-based nursing facilities and also in the increase in the numbers of nurse-midwives and pediatric and neonatal nurse practitioners. This new edition places emphasis on the specific needs of clients related to the various health care settings in which they find themselves today. Focus on Evidence-Based Practice boxes expand this area.
- **Nursing process:** The nursing process format found throughout this text provides a strong theoretical underpinning for this important concept and is designed to help a student understand how to use the nursing process in clinical practice.

ORGANIZATION OF THE TEXT

Maternal and Child Health Nursing follows the family from the pregnancy period, through labor, delivery, and the postpartal period; it then follows the child in the family from birth through adolescence. Coverage includes ambulatory and in-patient care and focuses on primary as well as secondary and tertiary care.

The book is organized in nine units:

Unit I provides an introduction to maternal and child health nursing. A framework for practice is presented, as well as current trends and the importance of considering childbearing and childrearing within a family context.

Unit II examines the nursing role in preparing families for childbearing and childrearing. Reproductive and sexual health, reproductive life planning, and the concerns of the infertile family are discussed.

Unit III presents the nursing role in caring for the pregnant family. Care of the family during pregnancy and of the growing fetus is discussed. Separate chapters address the role of the nurse when a woman has a pre-existing illness, develops a complication of pregnancy, has a special need, or will be cared for at home during pregnancy. Additional chapters detail the role of the nurse as a genetic counselor and an advocate for fetal health.

Unit IV addresses the nursing role in caring for a family during labor and birth. Separate chapters detail the labor process, the role of the nurse in providing comfort during labor, the nursing role when a woman develops a complication of labor and birth, and cesarean birth.

Unit V describes the nursing role in caring for a family during the postpartal period. Separate chapters discuss the care of a woman and her family, the newborn, and the changing role when a complication for either a woman or her newborn develops.

Unit VI discusses the nursing role in health promotion during childhood. The chapters in this unit cover principles of growth and development and care of the child from infancy through adolescence, including child health assessment and communication and health teaching with children and families.

Unit VII presents the nursing role in supporting the health of children and their families. The effects of illness on children and their families, diagnostic and therapeutic procedures, medication administration, and pain management are addressed, with respect to care of the child and family in hospital, home, and ambulatory settings.

Unit VIII examines the nursing role in restoring and maintaining the health of children and families when illness occurs. Disorders are presented according to body systems so that students have a ready orientation for locating content.

Unit IX discusses the nursing role in restoring and maintaining the mental health of children and families. Separate chapters discuss the role of the nurse when intimate partner or child abuse or mental, long-term, or fatal illness is present.

PEDAGOGIC FEATURES

Each chapter in the text is organized to provide a complete learning experience for the student. Numerous pedagogic features are included to help a student understand and increase retention. Important elements include the following:

- **Chapter Objectives:** Learning objectives are included at the beginning of each chapter to identify outcomes expected after the material in the chapter has been mastered.
- **Key Terms:** Terms that would be new to a student are listed at the beginning of each chapter in a ready reference list. When the terms first appear in the text, they are shown in boldface type and then defined. Definitions appear again in the Glossary.

- **Chapter-Opening Case Studies:** Short scenarios appear at the beginning of each chapter. These vignettes are designed to help students appreciate that nursing care is always individualized and provide a taste of what is to come in the chapter. At the end of the chapter, Critical Thinking questions related to the scenario bring the chapter full circle.
- **Tables and Displays:** Numerous tables and displays summarize important information and provide detail on some topics so that a student has a ready reference.
- **Checkpoint Questions:** Throughout the text, multiple-choice Checkpoint Questions appear to help readers check progress and comprehension. They ask readers to use the knowledge just gained in the last few pages, helping them retain this information. Answers are supplied at the end of the book.
- **"What If" Questions:** "What If" (critical-thinking) questions also appear periodically throughout the text. These ask readers to apply the information just acquired in an "actual" situation. Readers must process the information and apply it to the new situation, thus maximizing learning and emphasizing critical thinking.
- **Key Points:** A review of important points is highlighted at the end of each chapter, to help students monitor their own comprehension.
- **Critical Thinking Exercises:** To involve a student in the decision-making realities of the clinical setting, several thought-provoking questions are posed at the end of each chapter. They could also serve as a basis for conference or class discussion.
- **References and Suggested Readings:** These provide a student with the information needed to do more in-depth reading of the sources noted in the text, as well as other relevant articles on the topics included in the chapter.
- **Appendices:** Appendices provide a quick reference to laboratory values, growth charts, vital sign parameters, nutrition pyramids, and drugs safe for use during lactation.

ANCILLARY PACKAGE

A complete learning and teaching package includes the following:

- **Free Interactive Self-Study CD-ROM:** Found on the inside front cover of each book, this free CD contains **300 multiple-choice NCLEX-style questions** to challenge the student's comprehension and application of the material in the textbook. Feedback is provided for each answer. Also included are samples from our forthcoming **video** series, *Lippincott's Maternity Nursing Video Series* and *Lippincott's Pediatric Nursing Video Series.*
- **Instructor's Resource CD-ROM:** The perfect complement to classroom teaching strategies, this resource contains useful lecture points, discussion questions, and assignments for each chapter (as well as the answers to the critical thinking exercises that appear in

the text). Also included is a **computerized test bank,** containing more than 1000 multiple-choice NCLEX-style questions; an **image bank** containing art from the text; and **PowerPoint presentations** for every chapter.

- **Study Guide:** This companion to the text challenges the student's retention of key concepts and encourages crit-

ical thinking and application of information to actual nursing situations.

- **Connection Website:** Students and teachers can find additional resources to enhance learning at http://connection.lww.com.

Adele Pillitteri, PhD, RN, PNP

Nursing Process Overview: Each chapter begins with a review of nursing process in which specific suggestions, such as examples of nursing diagnoses and outcome criteria helpful to modifying care in the area under discussion, are presented. These reviews are designed to improve students' preparation in clinical areas so they can focus their care planning and apply principles to practice.

Nursing Process Overview

For a Woman With a Labor or Birth Complication

● *Assessment*

One of the major assessments used to detect deviations from normal in labor and birth is fetal and uterine monitoring. Working with such apparatus involves explaining its importance to parents, winning their cooperation, and using judgment in reading the various patterns. Typically, monitoring women in labor entails problems not found in other high-risk areas such as an intensive care unit (ICU). In an ICU, the person being monitored has been admitted to the unit because he or she is seriously ill. The person lies still to prevent artifacts on the tracing. However, a woman in labor, who is well except for the complication of labor, may be less accepting of technologic or pharmacologic intervention. She moves about rather than lying still, because she is in pain. Her movement causes artifacts on tracings, requiring frequent adjustment of equipment to achieve a clear tracing. Understanding that this is a normal consequence of labor is essential for effective assessment and continued care.

- **Nursing Diagnoses and Related Interventions:** A consistent format highlights the nursing diagnoses and related interventions throughout the text. A special heading draws the students' attention to these sections where individual nursing diagnoses and outcome evaluation are detailed for the major conditions and disorders discussed.

NURSING DIAGNOSES AND RELATED INTERVENTIONS FOR DYSFUNCTIONAL LABOR

It is impossible to prevent all dysfunctional labor, just as it is impossible to predict the functioning of any woman's hormonal system or individual response to labor. However, a number of nursing interventions can contribute to the progression of normal labor and help change a dysfunctional labor to a functional one.

Nursing Diagnosis: Fatigue and anxiety related to prolonged labor

- **Nursing Outcomes and Nursing Interventions:** These boxes highlight appropriate outcomes and inter-

ventions using terminology identified by the Nursing Outcomes Classification and Nursing Interventions Classification (NOC and NIC).

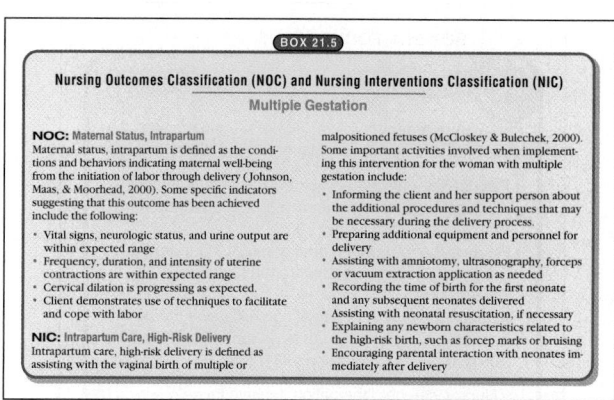

- **Focus On Nursing Care Planning: Multidisciplinary Care Maps:** Because nurses rarely work in isolation, but rather as a member of a health care team or unit, Multidisciplinary Care Maps written for specific clients are included throughout the text to demonstrate the use of the nursing process, provide examples of critical thinking, and clarify nursing care for specific client needs. Multidisciplinary care maps not only demonstrate nursing process but also accentuate the increasingly important role of the nurse as a coordinator of client care.

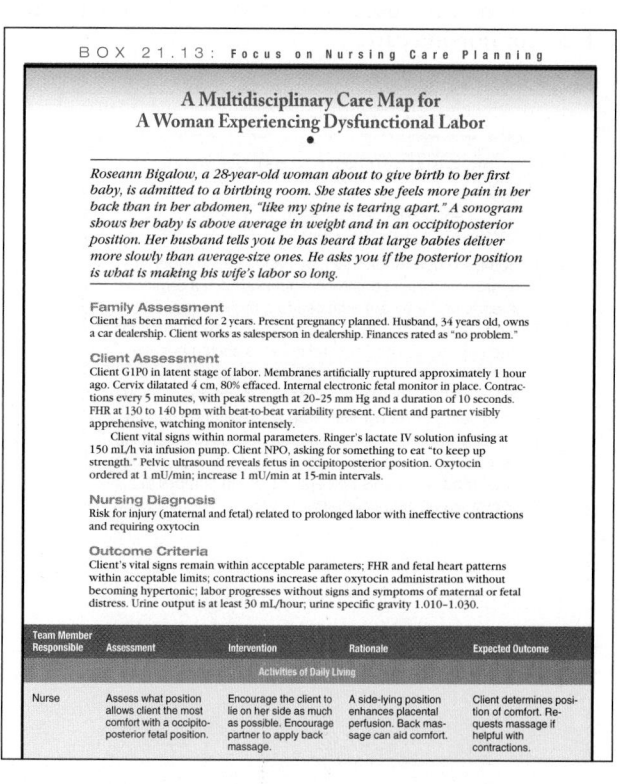

- **Focus on National Health Goals:** To emphasize the nursing role in accomplishing the health care goals of our nation, these displays state specific ways in which maternal and child health nursing can provide better outcomes for both mother and child. They help the student to appreciate the importance of national health planning and the influence that nurses can have in creating a healthier nation.

BOX 21.1 FOCUS ON . . .

NATIONAL HEALTH GOALS

A number of National Health Goals speak directly to complications of labor (DHHS, 2000).

- Reduce the number of cesarean births among low-risk women to no more than 15 per 100 births, from a baseline of 18 per 100.
- Reduce the maternal mortality rate to no more than 3.3 per 100,000 live births, from a baseline of 7.1 per 100,000.
- Reduce the rate of maternal complications during hospitalized labor and birth to no more than 24 per 100 births, from a baseline of 31.2 per 100 births.

Nurses can help the nation achieve these goals by helping identify women in labor who are developing a complication; by assisting with cesarean births and uterine monitoring; and by being alert to the preliminary symptoms of uterine rupture, which accounts for a substantial number of maternal deaths during labor. Further nursing research is needed to explore whether breech and occipitoposterior positions can be effectively prevented by position changes during pregnancy.

- **Focus on Evidence-Based Practice:** These displays summarize research on topics related to maternal and child health nursing. They appear throughout the text to accentuate the use of evidence-based practice as the basis for nursing care.

BOX 21.3 FOCUS ON . . .

EVIDENCE-BASED PRACTICE

Do some women perceive labor contractions better than others?

Some women report that they have been in labor for hours when their contractions finally reach a 5-minute interval and they are admitted to a birthing unit; others report a much shorter time interval before contractions become regular and spaced close to each other. To see if the reason for these different types of history could be that some women perceive uterine contractions better or earlier than others, researchers tested 7,808 women with singleton pregnancies to determine how many uterine contractions they perceived during a set period. Women's perceptions of the number of contractions that occurred were then compared with

- **Focus on Communication:** This feature presents case examples of less effective communication and more effective communication, illustrating for the student how an awareness of communication can improve the patient's understanding and positively impact outcomes.

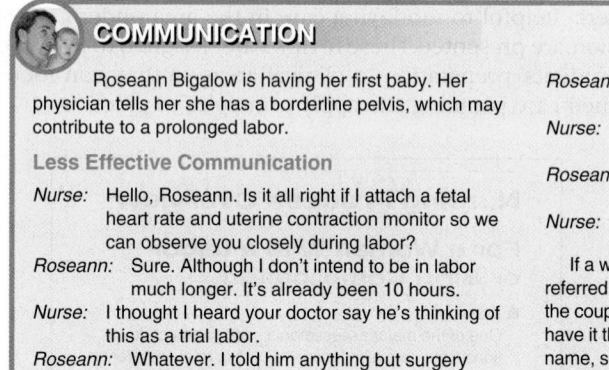

BOX 21.7 FOCUS ON . . .

COMMUNICATION

Roseann Bigalow is having her first baby. Her physician tells her she has a borderline pelvis, which may contribute to a prolonged labor.

Less Effective Communication

Nurse: Hello, Roseann. Is it all right if I attach a fetal heart rate and uterine contraction monitor so we can observe you closely during labor?

Roseann: Sure. Although I don't intend to be in labor much longer. It's already been 10 hours.

Nurse: I thought I heard your doctor say he's thinking of this as a trial labor.

Roseann: Whatever. I told him anything but surgery would be all right.

Nurse: I'm glad you have a positive outlook. That always makes labor seem to go faster.

More Effective Communication

Nurse: Hello, Roseann. Is it all right if I attach a fetal heart rate and uterine contraction monitor so we can observe you closely during labor?

- **Focus on Diversity of Care:** These displays serve to broaden the student's perspective on the many specific cultural influences that can affect the goals and interventions that nurses provide in the maternal and child health setting. They stress the need for nursing care to be modified to meet individualized needs.

BOX 18.4 FOCUS ON . . .

DIVERSITY OF CARE

For most health care providers in the United States, a placenta has little importance or meaning after its work of oxygenation is done and it is delivered. For many women, however, the placenta has continuing importance. For this reason, women may ask if they can take it home with them. In a number of Asian and Native American cultures, women bury the placenta to ensure that the child will continue to be healthy. In some parts of China, the placenta is cooked and eaten to ensure the continued health of the mother. Be certain when supplying placentas to women that you respect standard precautions and hospital policy.

- **Focus on Family Teaching:** These boxes present detailed health teaching information for the family, emphasizing the importance of a partnership between nurses and clients in the management of health and illness.

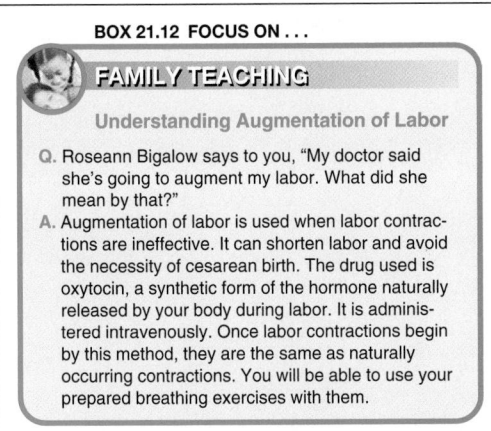

BOX 21.12 FOCUS ON . . .

FAMILY TEACHING

Understanding Augmentation of Labor

Q. Roseann Bigalow says to you, "My doctor said she's going to augment my labor. What did she mean by that?"

A. Augmentation of labor is used when labor contractions are ineffective. It can shorten labor and avoid the necessity of cesarean birth. The drug used is oxytocin, a synthetic form of the hormone naturally released by your body during labor. It is administered intravenously. Once labor contractions begin by this method, they are the same as naturally occurring contractions. You will be able to use your prepared breathing exercises with them.

- **Focus on Pharmacology:** These boxes provide quick reference for medications that are commonly used for the health problems described in the text. They give the drug name (brand and generic, if applicable), dosage, pregnancy category, side effects, and nursing implications.

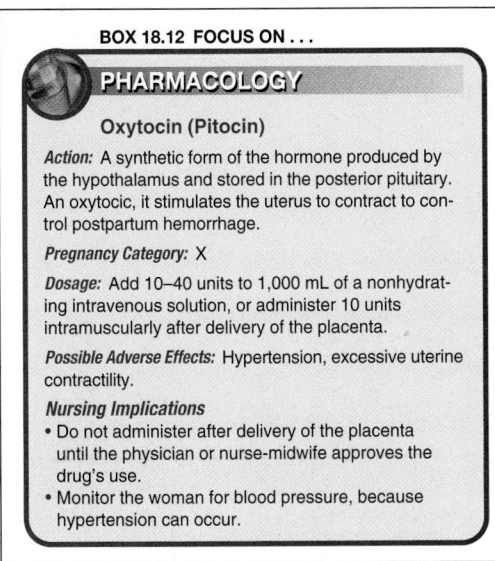

BOX 18.12 FOCUS ON . . .

PHARMACOLOGY

Oxytocin (Pitocin)

Action: A synthetic form of the hormone produced by the hypothalamus and stored in the posterior pituitary. An oxytocic, it stimulates the uterus to contract to control postpartum hemorrhage.

Pregnancy Category: X

Dosage: Add 10–40 units to 1,000 mL of a nonhydrating intravenous solution, or administer 10 units intramuscularly after delivery of the placenta.

Possible Adverse Effects: Hypertension, excessive uterine contractility.

Nursing Implications
- Do not administer after delivery of the placenta until the physician or nurse-midwife approves the drug's use.
- Monitor the woman for blood pressure, because hypertension can occur.

- **Nursing Procedures:** Techniques of procedures specific to maternal and child health care are boxed in an easy-to-follow two-column format, often enhanced with color figures.

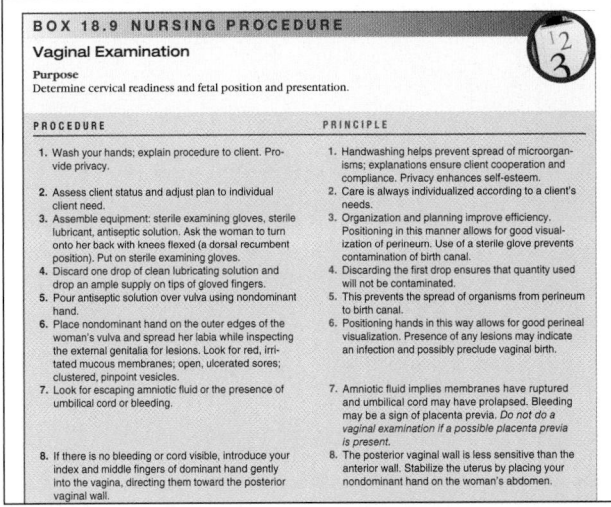

BOX 18.9 NURSING PROCEDURE

Vaginal Examination

Purpose
Determine cervical readiness and fetal position and presentation.

PROCEDURE	PRINCIPLE
1. Wash your hands; explain procedure to client. Provide privacy.	1. Handwashing helps prevent spread of microorganisms; explanations ensure client cooperation and compliance. Privacy enhances self-esteem.
2. Assess client status and adjust plan to individual client need.	2. Care is always individualized according to a client's needs.
3. Assemble equipment: sterile examining gloves, sterile lubricant, antiseptic solution. Ask the woman to turn onto her back with knees flexed (a dorsal recumbent position). Put on sterile examining gloves.	3. Organization and planning improve efficiency. Positioning in this manner allows for good visualization of perineum. Use of a sterile glove prevents contamination of birth canal.
4. Discard one drop of clean lubricating solution and drop an ample supply on tips of gloved fingers.	4. Discarding the first drop ensures that quantity used will not be contaminated.
5. Pour antiseptic solution over vulva using nondominant hand.	5. This prevents the spread of organisms from perineum to birth canal.
6. Place nondominant hand on the outer edges of the woman's vulva and spread her labia while inspecting the external genitalia for lesions. Look for red, irritated mucous membranes; open, ulcerated sores; clustered, pinpoint vesicles.	6. Positioning hands in this way allows for good perineal visualization. Presence of any lesions may indicate an infection and possibly preclude vaginal birth.
7. Look for escaping amniotic fluid or the presence of umbilical cord or bleeding.	7. Amniotic fluid implies membranes have ruptured and umbilical cord may have prolapsed. Bleeding may be a sign of placenta previa. *Do not do a vaginal examination if a possible placenta previa is present.*
8. If there is no bleeding or cord visible, introduce your index and middle fingers of dominant hand gently into the vagina, directing them toward the posterior vaginal wall.	8. The posterior vaginal wall is less sensitive than the anterior wall. Stabilize the uterus by placing your nondominant hand on the woman's abdomen.

- **Assessment:** These visual guides provide head-to-toe assessment information for overall health status or specific disorders or conditions.

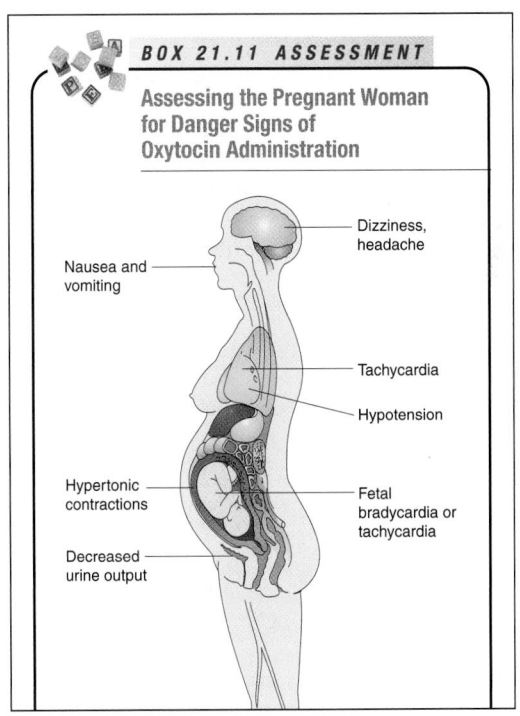

BOX 21.11 ASSESSMENT

Assessing the Pregnant Woman for Danger Signs of Oxytocin Administration

Dizziness, headache
Nausea and vomiting
Tachycardia
Hypotension
Hypertonic contractions
Fetal bradycardia or tachycardia
Decreased urine output

ACKNOWLEDGMENTS

I would like to express my sincere appreciation to Alison Darrow, Developmental Editor; Melanie Cann, Senior Developmental Editor; Elizabeth Nieginski, Senior Acquisitions Editor; Helen Ewan, Senior Production Manager; Tom Gibbons, Senior Production Editor; Joan Wendt, Art Director; and all the members of the Production Services Group involved with this text for their assistance and guidance throughout the project.

A.P.

CONTENTS

UNIT VII

The Nursing Role in Supporting the Health of Ill Children and Their Families 1065

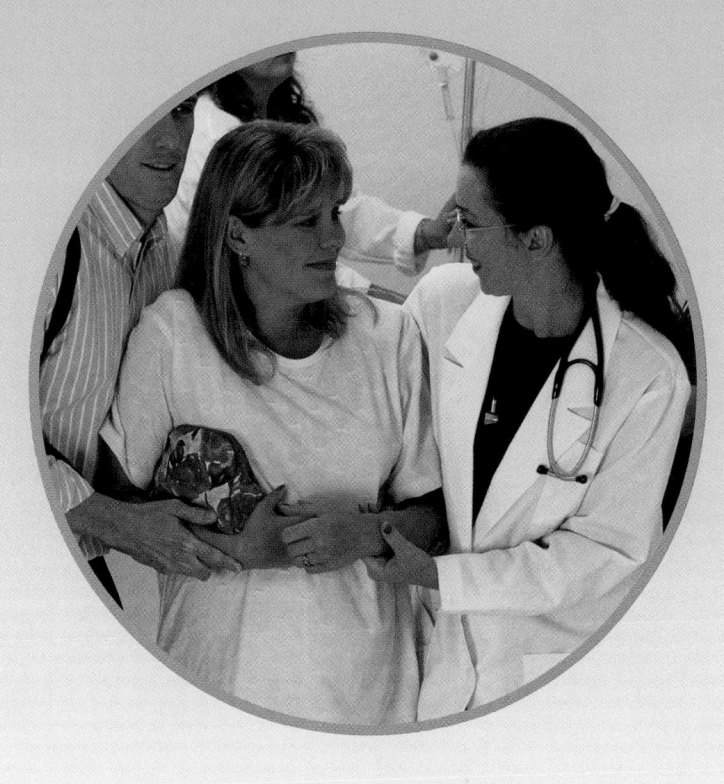

UNIT ONE

Maternal and Child Health Nursing Practice

•

CHAPTER 1

A Framework for Maternal and Child Health Nursing

Key Terms

clinical nurse specialist
evidence-based practice
family nurse practitioner
fertility rate
maternal and child health
    nursing
mortality rate
neonatal nurse practitioner
neonate
nurse-midwife
nursing research
pediatric nurse practitioner
puerperium
scope of practice
women's health nurse
    practitioner

Objectives

After mastering the contents of this chapter, you should be able to:

1. Identify the goals and philosophy of maternal and child health nursing.
2. Describe the evolution, scope, and professional roles for nurses in maternal and child health nursing.
3. Define common statistical terms used in the field, such as infant and maternal mortality.
4. Discuss the implications of the common standards of maternal and child health nursing and the health goals for the nation for maternal and child health nursing.
5. Discuss the interplay of nursing process, evidence-based practice, and nursing theory as they relate to the future of maternal and child health nursing practice.
6. Use critical thinking to identify areas of care that could benefit from additional research or application of evidence-based practice.
7. Apply concepts of family-centered care to maternal and child health nursing.
8. Integrate knowledge of trends in maternal and child health care with the nursing process to achieve quality maternal and child health nursing care.

Anna Chung is a premature neonate who must be transported to a regional center for care about 30 miles from your local hospital. Her parents, Melissa and Robert, have many concerns. They don't want to be so far from their daughter, and they don't know how they will pay for her special care. Also, Melissa, 37 years old, believes she is too old to leave the hospital so soon after having a cesarean birth. She recalls staying in the hospital much longer after having her first child, Micko, now 6 years old.

This chapter discusses standards and philosophies of maternal-child health care and how these standards and philosophies affect care.

What are some health care issues evident in this scenario? How has modern cost containment changed this scenario?

What is the nursing role here?

After you've studied this chapter, access the accompanying website. Read the patient scenario and answer the questions to further sharpen your skills, grow more familiar with RN-CLEX types of questions, and reward yourself with how much you have learned.

The care of childbearing and childrearing families is a major focus of nursing practice, because to have healthy adults you must have healthy children. To have healthy children, it is important to promote the health of the childbearing woman and her family from the time before children are born until they reach adulthood. Both preconceptual and prenatal care are essential contributions to the health of a woman and fetus and to a family's emotional preparation for childbearing and childrearing. As children grow, families need continued health supervision and support. As children reach maturity and plan for their families, a new cycle begins and new support becomes necessary. The nurse's role in all these phases focuses on promoting healthy growth and development of the child and family in health and in illness.

Although the field of nursing typically divides its concerns for families during childbearing and childrearing into two separate entities, maternity care and child health care, the full scope of nursing practice in this area is not two separate entities, but one: maternal and child health nursing (Fig. 1.1).

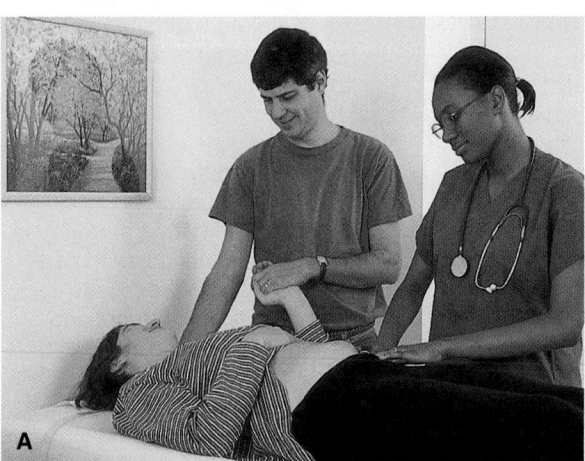

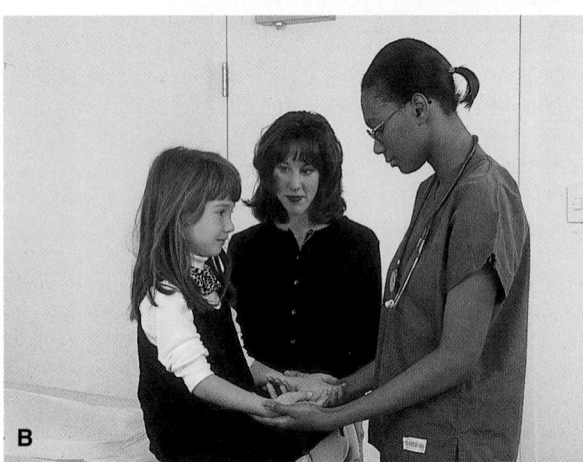

FIGURE 1.1 Maternal and child health nursing includes care of the pregnant woman, child, and family. (**A**) During a prenatal visit, a maternal child health nurse assesses that a pregnant woman's uterus is expanding normally. (**B**) During a health maintenance visit, a maternal child health nurse assesses a child's growth and development. (© Barbara Proud.)

GOALS AND PHILOSOPHIES OF MATERNAL AND CHILD HEALTH NURSING

The primary goal of **maternal and child health nursing** care can be stated simply as the promotion and maintenance of optimal family health to ensure cycles of optimal childbearing and childrearing. Major philosophical assumptions about maternal and child health nursing are listed in Box 1.1. The goals of maternal and child health nursing care are necessarily broad because the scope of practice is so broad. The range of practice includes

- Preconceptual health care
- Care of women during three trimesters of pregnancy and the **puerperium** (the 6 weeks after childbirth, sometimes termed the fourth trimester of pregnancy)
- Care of children during the perinatal period (6 weeks before conception to 6 weeks after birth)
- Care of children from birth through adolescence
- Care in settings as varied as the birthing room, the pediatric intensive care unit, and the home

In all settings and types of care, keeping the family at the center of care delivery is an essential goal. Maternal and

---

BOX 1.1

Philosophy of Maternal and Child Health Nursing

- Maternal and child health nursing is family-centered; assessment data must include a family and individual assessment.
- Maternal and child health nursing is community-centered; the health of families depends on and influences the health of communities.
- Maternal and child health nursing is research-oriented, because research is the means whereby critical knowledge increases.
- Both nursing theory and evidence-based practice provide a foundation for nursing care.
- A maternal and child health nurse serves as an advocate to protect the rights of all family members, including the fetus.
- Maternal and child health nursing includes a high degree of independent nursing functions, because teaching and counseling are so frequently required.
- Promoting health is an important nursing role, because this protects the health of the next generation.
- Pregnancy or childhood illness can be stressful and can alter family life in both subtle and extensive ways.
- Personal, cultural, and religious attitudes and beliefs influence the meaning of illness and its impact on the family. Circumstances such as illness or pregnancy are meaningful only in the context of a total life.
- Maternal and child health nursing is a challenging role for a nurse and is a major factor in promoting high-level wellness in families.

child health nursing is always family-centered; the family is considered the primary unit of care. The level of family functioning affects the health status of individuals, because if the family's level of functioning is low, the emotional, physical, and social health and potential of individuals in that family can be adversely affected. A healthy family, on the other hand, establishes an environment conducive to growth and health-promoting behaviors that sustain family members during crises. Similarly, the health of an individual and his or her ability to function strongly influences the health of family members and overall family functioning. For these reasons, a family-centered approach enables nurses to better understand individuals and, in turn, to provide holistic care. Box 1.2 provides a summary of key measures for the delivery of family-centered maternal and child health care.

STANDARDS OF MATERNAL AND CHILD HEALTH NURSING PRACTICE

The importance a society places on human life can best be measured by the concern it places on its most vulnerable members—its elderly, disadvantaged, and youngest citizens. To promote consistency and ensure quality nursing care and outcomes in these areas, specialty organiza-

tions develop guidelines for care in their specific areas of nursing practice. In maternal-child health, standards have been developed by the Division of Maternal-Child Health Nursing Practice of the American Nurses Association in collaboration with the Society of Pediatric Nurses. These are shown in Box 1.3.

The Association of Women's Health, Obstetric, and Neonatal Nurses (AWHONN) has developed similar standards for the nursing care of women and newborns. These are summarized in Box 1.4.

A FRAMEWORK FOR MATERNAL AND CHILD HEALTH NURSING CARE

Maternal and child health nursing can be visualized within a framework in which nurses, using nursing process, nursing theory, and evidence-based practice, care for families during childbearing and childrearing years through four phases of health care:

- Health promotion
- Health maintenance
- Health restoration
- Health rehabilitation

Examples of these phases of health care as they relate to maternal and child health are shown in Table 1.1.

The Nursing Process

Nursing care, at its best, is designed and implemented in a thorough manner, using an organized series of steps, to ensure quality and consistency of care (Carpenito, 2004). The nursing process, a proven form of problem solving based on the scientific method, serves as the basis for assessing, making a nursing diagnosis, planning, organizing, and evaluating care. That the nursing process is applicable to all health care settings, from the prenatal clinic to the pediatric intensive care unit, is proof that the method is broad enough to serve as the basis for all nursing care.

Because nurses rarely work in isolation, but rather as a member of a health care team or unit, Multidisciplinary Care Maps are included throughout the text to demonstrate the use of the nursing process for selected clients, provide examples of critical thinking, and clarify nursing care for specific client needs. Multidisciplinary care maps rather than nursing care plans are shown, because they not only demonstrate the nursing process but accentuate the increasingly important role of the nurse as a coordinator of client care.

In addition, selected chapters also identify specific nursing outcomes using the terminology presented in the Nursing Outcomes Classification (NOC) and nursing activities using the terminology presented in the Nursing Interventions Classification (NIC) developed by the Iowa Intervention Project (Johnson et al., 2000; McCloskey & Bulechek, 2000).

Evidence-Based Practice

Evidence-based practice involves the use of research or controlled investigation of a problem in conjunction with

---

BOX 1.2

Common Measures to Ensure Family-Centered Maternal and Child Health Care

Principle
- The family is the basic unit of society.
- Families represent racial, ethnic, cultural, and socioeconomic diversity.
- Children grow both individually and as part of a family.

Nursing Interventions
- Consider the family as a whole as well as its individual members.
- Encourage families to reach out to their community so that family members are not isolated from their community or from each other.
- Encourage family bonding through rooming-in in both maternal and child health hospital settings.
- Participate in early hospital discharge programs to reunite families as soon as possible.
- Encourage family and sibling visits in the hospital to promote family contacts.
- Assess families for strengths as well as specific needs or challenges.
- Respect diversity in families as a unique quality of that family.
- Encourage families to give care to a newborn or ill child.
- Include developmental stimulation in nursing care.
- Share or initiate information on health planning with family members so that care is family-oriented.

BOX 1.3

American Nurses Association/Society of Pediatric Nurses Standards of Care and Professional Performance

Standards of Care

Comprehensive pediatric nursing care focuses on helping children and their families and communities achieve their optimum health potentials. This is best achieved within the framework of family-centered care and the nursing process, including primary, secondary, and tertiary care coordinated across health care and community settings.

Standard I: Assessment
The pediatric nurse collects patient health data.

Standard II: Diagnosis
The pediatric nurse analyzes the assessment data in determining diagnoses.

Standard III: Outcome Identification
The pediatric nurse identifies expected outcomes individualized to the child and the family.

Standard IV: Planning
The pediatric nurse develops a plan of care that prescribes interventions to obtain expected outcomes.

Standard V: Implementation
The pediatric nurse implements the interventions identified in the plan of care.

Standard VI: Evaluation
The pediatric nurse evaluates the child's and family's progress toward attainment of outcomes.

Standards of Professional Performance

Standard I: Quality of Care
The pediatric nurse systematically evaluates the quality and effectiveness of pediatric nursing practice.

Standard II: Performance Appraisal
The pediatric nurse evaluates his or her own nursing practice in relation to professional practice standards and relevant statutes and regulations.

Standard III: Education
The pediatric nurse acquires and maintains current knowledge and competency in pediatric nursing practice.

Standard IV: Collegiality
The pediatric nurse interacts with and contributes to the professional development of peers, colleagues, and other health care providers.

Standard V: Ethics
The pediatric nurse's assessment, actions, and recommendations on behalf of children and their families are determined in an ethical manner.

Standard VI: Collaboration
The pediatric nurse collaborates with the child, family, and other health care providers in providing client care.

Standard VII: Research
The pediatric nurse contributes to nursing and pediatric health care through the use of research methods and findings.

Standard VIII: Resource Utilization
The pediatric nurse considers factors related to safety, effectiveness, and cost in planning and delivering patient care.

American Nurses Association and Society of Pediatric Nurses. (2003). *Scope and standards of pediatric clinical practice.* Washington, D.C.: American Nurses Publishing House.

clinical expertise as a foundation for action. Bodies of professional knowledge grow and expand to the extent that people in that profession plan and carry out research. **Nursing research,** the controlled investigation of problems that have implications for nursing practice, provides evidence for practice, upon which the foundation of nursing grows, expands, and improves. In addition, evidence-based practice provides the justification for implementing activities for outcome achievement, ultimately resulting in improved and cost-effective patient care.

A classic example of how the results of nursing research can influence nursing practice is the application of the research carried out by Rubin (1963) on a mother's approach to her newborn. Before the publication of this study, nurses assumed that a woman who did not immediately hold and cuddle her infant at birth was a "cold" or unfeeling mother. After observing a multitude of new mothers, Rubin concluded that attachment is not a spontaneous procedure;

rather, it more commonly begins with only fingertip touching. Armed with Rubin's findings and integrating these findings into practice, nurses became better able to differentiate healthy from unhealthy bonding behavior in postpartum women and their newborns. Women following this step-by-step pattern of attachment were no longer recognized as unfeeling, but normal. By documenting these normal parameters, nurses can identify women who do not follow such a pattern, and interventions can be planned and instituted to help these mothers gain a stronger attachment to their new infants. Additional nursing research in this area (discussed in Chapter 22) has provided further substantiation about the importance of this original investigation.

Evidence-based practice requires ongoing research to substantiate current actions as well as to provide guidelines for future actions. Some examples of current questions that warrant nursing investigation in the area of maternal and child health nursing include the following:

BOX 1.4

Association of Women's Health, Obstetric, and Neonatal Nurses Standards and Guidelines

Standards of Professional Performance

Standard I: Quality of Care
The nurse systematically evaluates the quality and effectiveness of nursing practice.

Standard II: Performance Appraisal
The nurse evaluates his/her own nursing practice in relation to professional practice standards and relevant statutes and regulations.

Standard III: Education
The nurse acquires and maintains current knowledge in nursing practice.

Standard IV: Collegiality
The nurse contributes to the professional development of peers, colleagues, and others.

Standard V: Ethics
The nurse's decisions and actions on behalf of patients are determined in an ethical manner.

Standard VI: Collaboration
The nurse collaborates with the patient, significant others, and health care providers in providing patient care.

Standard VII: Research
The nurse uses research findings in practice.

Standard VIII: Resource Utilization
The nurse considers factors related to safety, effectiveness, and cost in planning and delivering patient care.

Standard IX: Practice Environment
The nurse contributes to the environment of care delivery within the practice settings.

Standard X: Accountability
The nurse is professionally and legally accountable for his/her practice. The professional registered nurse may delegate to and supervise qualified personnel who provide patient care.

Association of Women's Health, Obstetric, and Neonatal Nurses. (1998). *Standards for the nursing care of women and newborns* (5th ed.). Washington, D.C.: Author.

- What is the most effective stimulus to encourage women to come for prenatal care or parents to bring children for health maintenance care?
- How can nurses be instrumental in fostering diversity in care?
- What are the special needs of women who are discharged from a hospital or birthing center within a short time after childbirth? Of children, after ambulatory surgery?
- How much self-care should young children be expected (or encouraged) to provide during an illness?
- What is the effect of market-driven health care on the quality of nursing care?
- What active measures can nurses take to reduce the incidence of child or intimate partner abuse?
- How can nurses best help families cope with the stress of long-term health care?
- What are the long-term effects of violence on families, and how can nurses help modify these effects?
- How can nurses be active in helping prevent violence in communities?

TABLE 1.1

Definitions and Examples of Phases of Health Care

Term	Definition	Examples
Health promotion	Educating clients to be aware of good health through teaching and role modeling	Teaching women the importance of rubella immunization before pregnancy; teaching children the importance of safer sex practices
Health maintenance	Intervening to maintain health when risk of illness is present	Encouraging women to come for prenatal care; teaching parents the importance of safeguarding their home by childproofing it against poisoning
Health restoration	Promptly diagnosing and treating illness using interventions that will return client to wellness most rapidly	Caring for a woman during a complication of pregnancy or a child during an acute illness
Health rehabilitation	Preventing further complications from an illness; bringing ill client back to optimal state of wellness or helping client to accept inevitable death	Encouraging a woman with gestational trophoblastic disease to continue therapy or a child with a renal transplant to continue to take necessary medications

- What do maternal-child health nurses need to know about alternative therapies such as herbal remedies to keep their practices current?

The answers to these and other questions provided by research help to bolster a foundation for specific actions and activities that have the potential to improve maternal and child health care. The Focus on Evidence-Based Practice boxes included in chapters throughout the text contain summaries of current maternal and child health research studies and are designed to assist you in developing a questioning attitude regarding current nursing practice and in thinking of ways to incorporate research findings into care.

Nursing Theory

One of the requirements of a profession (together with other critical determinants, such as member-set standards, monitoring of practice quality, and participation in research) is that the concentration of a discipline's knowledge flows from a base of established theory.

Nursing theorists offer helpful ways to view clients so that nursing activities can best meet client needs—for example, by seeing a pregnant woman not simply as a physical form but as a dynamic force with important psychosocial needs, or by viewing children as extensions or active members of a family as well as independent beings. Only with this broad theoretical focus can nurses appreciate the significant effect on a family of a child's illness or of the introduction of a new member.

Another issue most nursing theorists address is how nurses should be viewed or what the goals of nursing care should be. At one time, the goal of nursing care could have been stated as "Providing care and comfort to injured and ill people." Most nurses today would perceive this view as a limited one, because they are equipped to do preventive care as well. Extensive changes in the scope of maternal and child health nursing have occurred as health promotion, or keeping parents and children well, has become a greater priority.

A third issue addressed by nurse theorists concerns the activities of nursing care: as goals become broader, so do activities. For example, when the primary goal of nursing was considered to be caring for ill people, nursing actions were limited to bathing, feeding, and providing comfort. Currently, with health promotion as a major nursing goal, teaching, counseling, supporting, and advocacy are also common roles. In addition, with new technologies available, nurses are caring for clients who are sicker than ever before. Because care of women during pregnancy and of children during their developing years helps protect not only current health but also the health of the next generation, maternal-child health nurses fill these expanded roles to a unique and special degree.

Table 1.2 summarizes the tenets of a number of common nursing theorists and suggests ways in which they could be applied to maternal-child health care through the situation of one child. The third column of the table ("Emphasis of Care") demonstrates that although the theoretical bases of these approaches to nursing care differ, the result of any one of them is to provide a higher level of care. These different theories, therefore, do not contradict but rather complement each other in the planning and implementation of holistic nursing care.

Checkpoint Question 1

Suppose Melissa Chung asks you whether maternal child health nursing is a profession. What qualifies an activity as a profession?

a. Members supervise other people.
b. Members use a distinct body of knowledge.
c. Members enjoy good working conditions.
d. Members receive relatively high pay.

MATERNAL AND CHILD HEALTH NURSING TODAY

At the beginning of the 20th century, the infant mortality rate in the United States (i.e., the number of infants per 1,000 births who die during the first year of life) was greater than 100 per 1,000. In response to efforts to lower this rate, health care shifted from a treatment focus to a preventive one, dramatically changing the scope of maternal and child health nursing. Research on the benefits of early prenatal care led to the first major national effort to provide prenatal care to all pregnant women through prenatal nursing services (home visits) and clinics. Today, thanks to these and other community health measures (such as efforts to encourage breast-feeding, increased immunization, and injury prevention), as well as many technological advances, the U.S. infant mortality rate has fallen to 6.9 per 1,000 (National Center for Health Statistics [NCHS], 2005).

Medical technology has contributed to a number of important advances in maternal and child health: childhood diseases such as measles and poliomyelitis are almost eradicated through immunization; specific genes responsible for many inherited diseases have been identified; stem cell therapy may make it possible in the next few years to replace diseased cells with new growth cells; new fertility drugs and techniques allow more couples than ever before to conceive; and the ability to delay preterm birth and improve life for premature infants has grown dramatically. In addition, a growing trend toward health care consumerism, or self-care, has made many childbearing and childrearing families active participants in their own health monitoring and care. Health care consumerism has also moved care from hospitals to community sites and from long-term hospital stays to overnight surgical and ambulatory settings.

Even in light of these changes, much more still needs to be done. National health care goals established in 2000 for the year 2010 continue to stress the importance of maternal and child health to overall community health (Department of Health and Human Services [DHHS], 2000). Although health care may be more advanced, it is still not accessible to everyone. These and other social changes and trends have expanded the roles of nurses in maternal and child health care and, at the same time, have made the delivery

TABLE 1.2

Summary of Nursing Theories

Terry is a 7-year-old girl who is hospitalized because her right arm was severely injured in an automobile accident. There is a high probability she will never have full use of the arm again. Terry's mother is concerned because Terry showed promise in art. Previously happy and active in Girl Scouts, Terry has spent most of every day since the accident sitting in her hospital bed silently watching television.

Theorist	Major Concepts of Theory	Emphasis of Care
Patricia Benner	Nursing is a caring relationship. Nurses grow from novice to expert as they practice in clinical settings.	Assess Terry as a whole. An expert nurse is able to do this intuitively from knowledge gained from practice.
Dorothy Johnson	A person comprises subsystems that must remain in balance for optimal functioning. Any actual or potential threat to this system balance is a nursing concern.	Assess the effect of lack of arm function on Terry as a whole; modify care to maintain function to all systems, not just musculoskeletal.
Imogene King	Nursing is a process of action, reaction, interaction, and transaction; needs are identified based on client's social system, perceptions, and health; the role of the nurse is to help the client achieve goal attainment.	Discuss with Terry the way she views herself and illness. She views herself as a well child, active in Girl Scouts and school; structure care to help her meet these perceptions.
Madeleine Leininger	The essence of nursing is care. To provide trans-cultural care, the nurse focuses on the study and analysis of different cultures with respect to caring behavior.	Assess Terry's family for beliefs about healing. Incorporate these into care.
Florence Nightingale	The role of the nurse is viewed as changing or structuring elements of the environment such as ventilation, temperature, odors, noise, and light to put the client into the best opportunity for recovery.	Turn Terry's bed into the sunlight; provide adequate covers for warmth; leave her comfortable with electronic games to occupy her time.
Betty Neuman	A person is an open system that interacts with the environment; nursing is aimed at reducing stressors through primary, secondary, and tertiary prevention.	Assess for stressors such as loss of self-esteem and derive ways to prevent further loss such as praising her for combing her own hair.
Dorothea Orem	The focus of nursing is on the individual; clients are assessed in terms of ability to complete self-care. Care given may be wholly compensatory (client has no role); partly compensatory (client participates in care); or supportive-educational (client performs own care).	Arrange overbed table so Terry can feed herself; urge her to participate in care by doing as much for herself as she can.
Ida Jean Orlando	The focus of the nurse is interaction with the client; effectiveness of care depends on the client's behavior and the nurse's reaction to that behavior. The client should define his or her own needs.	Ask Terry what she feels is her main need. Terry says that returning to school is what she wants most. Stress activities that allow her to maintain contact with school, such as doing homework or telephoning friends.
Rosemarie Rizzo Parse	Nursing is a human science. Health is a lived experience. Man-living-health as a single unit guides practice.	Ask Terry what being sick means to her. Allow her to participate in care decisions based on her response.
Hildegard Peplau	The promotion of health is viewed as the forward movement of the personality; this is accomplished through an interpersonal process that includes orientation, identification, exploitation, and resolution.	Plan care together with Terry. Encourage her to speak of school and accomplishments in Girl Scouts to retain self-esteem.
Martha Rogers	The purpose of nursing is to move the client toward optimal health; the nurse should view the client as whole and constantly changing and help people to interact in the best way possible with the environment.	Help Terry to make use of her left side as much as possible so that she returns to school and to her previous level of functioning as soon as possible.
Sister Callista Roy	The role of the nurse is to aid clients to adapt to the change caused by illness; levels of adaptation depend on the degree of environmental change and state of coping ability; full adaptation includes physiologic interdependence.	Assess Terry's ability to use her left hand to replace her right-hand functions, which are now lost; direct nursing care toward replacing deficit with other factors, self-concept, role function, and skills.

of quality maternal and child health nursing care a continuing challenge.

National Health Goals

In 1979, the U.S. Public Health Service first initiated the formulation of health care objectives. Health care goals were reestablished in 2000, to be completed in 2010 (DHHS, 2000). Many of these objectives directly involve maternal and child health care, because improving the health of this young age group will have such long-term effects. The nation's priority goals (leading health indicators) are shown in Box 1.5. Goals specific for each content area are highlighted in later chapters. National health goals are intended to help everyone more easily understand the importance of health promotion and disease prevention and to encourage wide participation in improving health in the next decade. Maternal and child health nurses need to be familiar with these goals, because nurses play a vital role in helping the nation achieve these objectives through both practice and research. The goals also serve as the basis for grant funding and financing of evidence-based practice.

Trends in the Maternal and Child Health Nursing Population

The maternal and child population is constantly changing because of changes in social structure, variations in family lifestyle, and changing patterns of illness. Table 1.3 summarizes some of the social changes that have occurred over the past 20 to 30 years that have altered health care priorities for maternal and child health nurses. Today, client advocacy, a philosophy of cost containment, an increased focus on health education, and new nursing roles are ways in which nurses have adapted to these changes.

Measuring Maternal and Child Health

Measuring maternal and child health is not as simple as defining a client as ill or well. Individual clients and health care practitioners may have different perspectives on illness and wellness. For example, some children with chronic but controllable asthma think of themselves as well; others with the same degree of involvement consider themselves ill. Although pregnancy is generally considered a well state, some women think of themselves as ill during this period. A more objective view of health is provided by national health statistics.

A number of statistical terms are used to express the outcome of pregnancies and births and to describe maternal child health (Box 1.6). Statistics for these terms require accurate collection and analysis so that the nation's health can be described accurately. Such statistics are useful for comparisons among states and for planning of future health care needs.

Birth Rate

The birth rate in the United States has gradually decreased over the past 10 years to 13.9 per 1,000 population at present (NCHS, 2005) (Fig. 1.2). Currently, the average family in the United States has 1.2 children. Boys are born more often than girls, at a rate of 1,050 boys to every 1,000 girls (NCHS, 2005). Births to teenaged mothers are steadily declining, and those to women older than 40 years of age are steadily increasing.

Fertility Rate

The term **fertility rate** reflects what proportion of women who could have babies are having them. The fertility rate is currently at 64.8%, a healthy reproductive rate for a country (NCHS, 2005).

Fetal Death Rate

Fetal death is defined as the death in utero of a child (fetus) weighing 500 g or more, roughly the weight of a fetus of 20 weeks' or more gestation. Fetal deaths may occur because of maternal factors (e.g., maternal disease, premature cervical dilation, maternal malnutrition) or fetal factors (e.g., fetal disease, chromosome abnormality, poor placental attachment). Many fetal deaths occur for reasons unknown. The fetal death rate is important in evaluating the health of a nation because it reflects the overall quality of maternal health and prenatal care. The emphasis on both preconceptual and prenatal care has helped to reduce this rate from a number as high as 18% in 1950 to 6.4% at present (NCHS, 2005).

Neonatal Death Rate

The first 28 days of life are known as the neonatal period, and an infant during this time is known as a **neonate.** The neonatal death rate reflects not only the quality of care available to women during pregnancy and childbirth but also the quality of care available to infants during the first month of life.

The leading causes of infant mortality during the first 4 weeks of life are prematurity (early gestational age), low birthweight (less than 2,500 g), and congenital anomalies. Approximately 80% of infants who die within 48 hours after birth weigh less than 2,500 g (5.5 lb). The proportion of infants born with low birthweight is about 7% of all births. This number rises slightly each year as better prenatal care allows infants who would have died in utero (fetal death) to be born and survive (Martin et al., 2005).

Perinatal Death Rate

The perinatal period is defined in a number of ways. Statistically, the period is defined as the time beginning when the fetus reaches 500 g (about week 20 of pregnancy) and ending about 4 to 6 weeks after birth. The perinatal death rate is the sum of the fetal and neonatal rates.

Maternal Mortality Rate

The **maternal mortality rate** is the number of maternal deaths that occur as a direct result of the reproductive process per 100,00 live births. Early in the 20th century, this rate in the United States reached levels as high as 600

BOX 1.5 FOCUS ON . . .

11

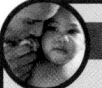

NATIONAL HEALTH GOALS

Leading Health Indicators

Physical Activity

Regular physical activity throughout life is important for maintaining a healthy body, enhancing psychologic well-being, and preventing premature death. The objectives selected to measure progress in this area are:

- Increase the proportion of adolescents who engage in vigorous physical activity that promotes cardiorespiratory fitness 3 or more days per week for 20 or more minutes per occasion.
- Increase the proportion of adults who engage regularly, preferably daily, in moderate physical activity for at least 30 minutes per day.

Overweight and Obesity

Overweight and obesity are major contributors to many preventable causes of death. The objectives selected to measure progress in this area are:

- Reduce the proportion of children and adolescents who are overweight or obese.
- Reduce the proportion of adults who are obese.

Tobacco Use

Cigarette smoking is the single most preventable cause of disease and death in the United States. Smoking results in more deaths each year in the United States than AIDS, alcohol, cocaine, heroin, homicide, suicide, motor vehicle crashes, and fires—combined. The objectives selected to measure progress in this area are:

- Reduce cigarette smoking by adolescents.
- Reduce cigarette smoking by adults.

Substance Abuse

Alcohol and illicit drug use are associated with many of this country's most serious problems, including violence, injury, and HIV infection. The objectives selected to measure progress in this area are:

- Increase the proportion of adolescents not using alcohol or any illicit drugs during the past 30 days.
- Reduce the proportion of adults using any illicit drug during the past 30 days.
- Reduce the proportion of adults engaging in binge drinking of alcoholic beverages during the past month.

Responsible Sexual Behavior

Unintended pregnancies and sexually transmitted diseases (STDs), including infection with the human immunodeficiency virus that causes AIDS, can result from unprotected sexual behavior. The objectives selected to measure progress in this area are:

- Increase the proportion of adolescents who abstain from sexual intercourse or use condoms if currently sexually active.
- Increase the proportion of sexually active persons who use condoms.

Mental Health

Approximately 20% of the U.S. population is affected by mental illness during a given year; no one is immune. Of all mental illnesses, depression is the most common disorder. More than 19 million adults in the United States suffer from depression. Major depression is the leading cause of disability and is the cause of more than two thirds of suicides each year. The objective selected to measure progress in this area is:

- Increase the proportion of adults with recognized depression who receive treatment.

Injury and Violence

More than 400 Americans die each day from injuries, due primarily to motor vehicle crashes, firearms, poisonings, suffocation, falls, fires, and drowning. The risk of injury is so great that most persons sustain a significant injury at some time during their lives. The objectives selected to measure progress in this area are:

- Reduce deaths caused by motor vehicle crashes.
- Reduce homicides.

Environmental Quality

An estimated 25% of preventable illnesses worldwide can be attributed to poor environmental quality. In the United States, air pollution alone is estimated to be associated with 50,000 premature deaths and an estimated $40 billion to $50 billion in health-related costs annually. The objectives selected to measure progress in this area are:

- Reduce the proportion of persons exposed to air that does not meet the U.S. Environmental Protection Agency's health-based standards for ozone.
- Reduce the proportion of nonsmokers exposed to environmental tobacco smoke.

Immunization

Vaccines are among the greatest public health achievements of the 20th century. Immunizations can prevent disability and death from infectious diseases for individuals and can help control the spread of infections within communities. The objectives selected to measure progress in this area are:

- Increase the proportion of young children who receive all vaccines that have been recommended for universal administration for at least 5 years.
- Increase the proportion of noninstitutionalized adults who are vaccinated annually against influenza and ever vaccinated against pneumococcal disease.

Access to Health Care

Strong predictors of access to quality health care include having health insurance, a higher income level, and a regular primary care provider or other source of ongoing health care. Use of clinical preventive services, such as early prenatal care, can serve as indicators of access to quality health care services. The objectives selected to measure progress in this area are:

- Increase the proportion of persons with health insurance.
- Increase the proportion of persons who have a specific source of ongoing care.
- Increase the proportion of pregnant women who begin prenatal care in the first trimester of pregnancy.

Department of Health and Human Services. (2000). Leading health indicators. *Healthy People 2010.* Washington, D.C.: DHHS.

TABLE 1.3

Trends in Maternal and Child Health Care and Implications for Nurses

Trend	Implications for Nursing
Families are smaller than in previous decades.	Fewer family members are present as support in a time of crisis. Nurses must fulfill this role more than ever before.
Single parents are increasing in number.	A single parent may have fewer financial resources; this is more likely if the parent is a woman. Nurses need to inform parents of care options and to provide a backup opinion when needed.
An increasing number of women work outside the home.	Health care must be scheduled at times a working parent can bring a child for care. Problems of latch-key children and the selection of child care centers need to be discussed.
Families are more mobile than previously; there is an increase in the number of homeless women and children.	Good interviewing is necessary with mobile families so a health database can be established; education for health monitoring is important.
Abuse is more common than ever before.	Screening for child or intimate partner abuse should be included in family contacts. Be aware of the legal responsibilities for reporting abuse.
Families are more health-conscious than previously.	Families are ripe for health education; providing this can be a major nursing role.
Health care must respect cost containment.	Comprehensive care is necessary in primary care settings because referral to specialists may no longer be an option.

per 100,000 live births. It is still that high in developing countries. In the United States at present, the maternal mortality rate has declined to a low of 6.5 per 100,000 live births (NCHS, 2005) (Fig. 1.3). This dramatic decrease can be attributed to improved preconceptual, prenatal, labor and birth, and postpartum care, such as the following:

BOX 1.6

Statistical Terms Used to Report Maternal and Child Health

Birth rate: The number of births per 1,000 population.

Fertility rate: The number of pregnancies per 1,000 women of childbearing age.

Fetal death rate: The number of fetal deaths (over 500 g) per 1,000 live births.

Neonatal death rate: The number of deaths per 1,000 live births occurring at birth or in the first 28 days of life.

Perinatal death rate: The number of deaths of fetuses more than 500 g and in the first 28 days of life per 1,000 live births.

Maternal mortality rate: The number of maternal deaths per 100,000 live births that occur as a direct result of the reproductive process.

Infant mortality rate: The number of deaths per 1,000 live births occurring at birth or in the first 12 months of life.

Childhood mortality rate: The number of deaths per 1,000 population in children, 1 to 14 years of age.

- Greater detection of disorders such as ectopic pregnancy or placenta previa and prevention of related complications through the use of ultrasound
- Increased control of complications associated with hypertension of pregnancy
- Decreased use of anesthesia with childbirth

For most of the 20th century, uterine hemorrhage and infection were the leading causes of death during pregnancy and childbirth. This has changed because of the increased ability to prevent or control hemorrhage and infection, and now hypertensive disorders are the leading causes of death in childbirth. Pregnancy-induced hypertension adds to preexisting hypertensive disorders, especially in older women. Nurses who are alert to the signs and symptoms of hypertension are invaluable guardians of the health of pregnant and postpartum women.

Infant Mortality Rate

The infant mortality rate of a country is an index of its general health, because it measures the quality of pregnancy care, nutrition, and sanitation as well as infant health. This rate is the traditional standard used to compare the state of national health care with that of previous years or of other countries.

Thanks to health care advances and improvements in child care, the infant mortality rate in the United States has been steadily declining in recent years; it has reached a record low of 6.9 per 1,000 population (NCHS, 2005). Unfortunately, infant mortality is not equal for all people. African-American infants, for example, have a mortality rate of almost 15% (NCHS, 2005). This difference in African-American and white infant deaths is thought to be related to the higher proportion of births to young African-American

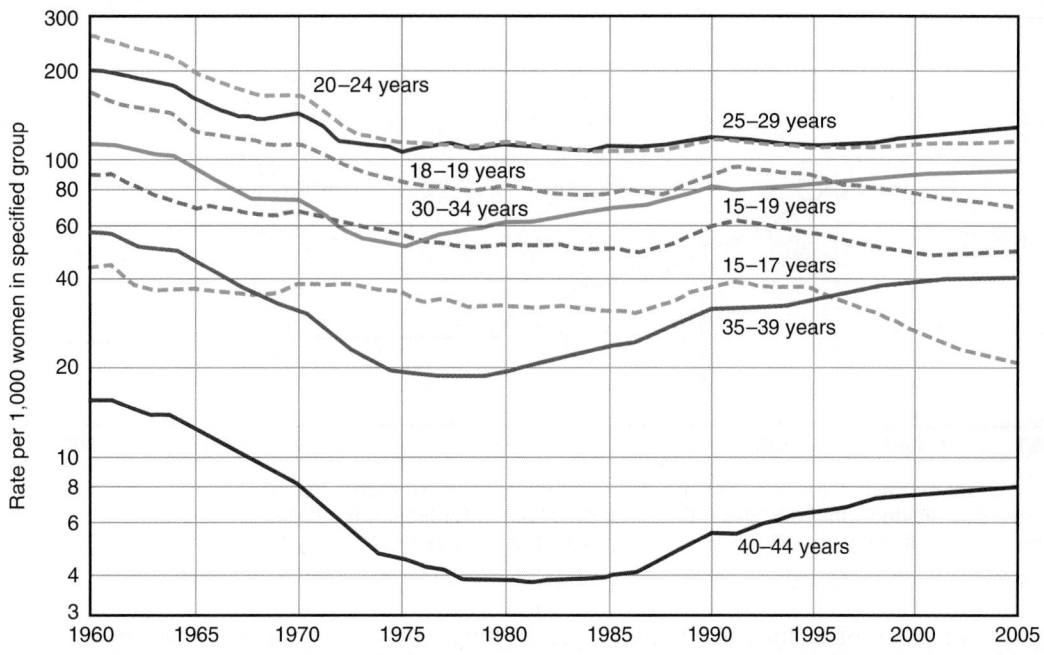

NOTE: Rates are plotted on a log scale.

FIGURE 1.2 Birth rates by age of mother: United States, 1960–2004. (National Center for Health Statistics. [2004]. Births, marriages, divorces and deaths. *National Vital Statistics Report, 49*(1), 6.)

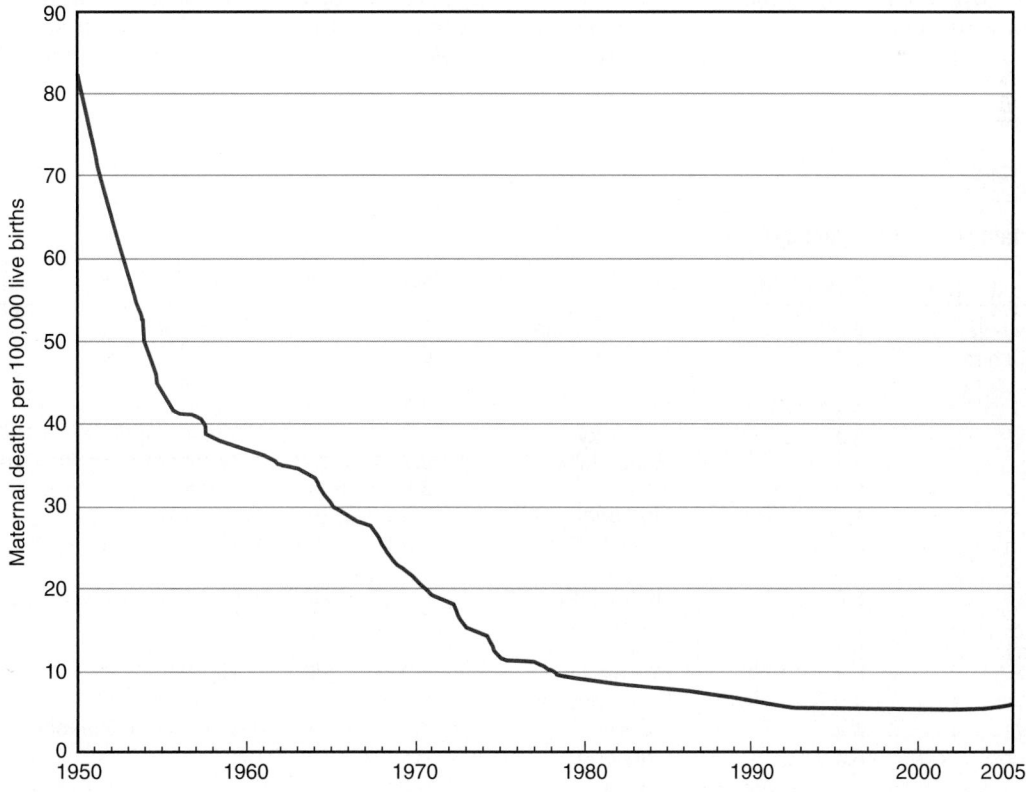

FIGURE 1.3 Maternal mortality rates, 2004. (National Center for Health Statistics. [2004]. *National Vital Statistics Report, 50*(1), 3.)

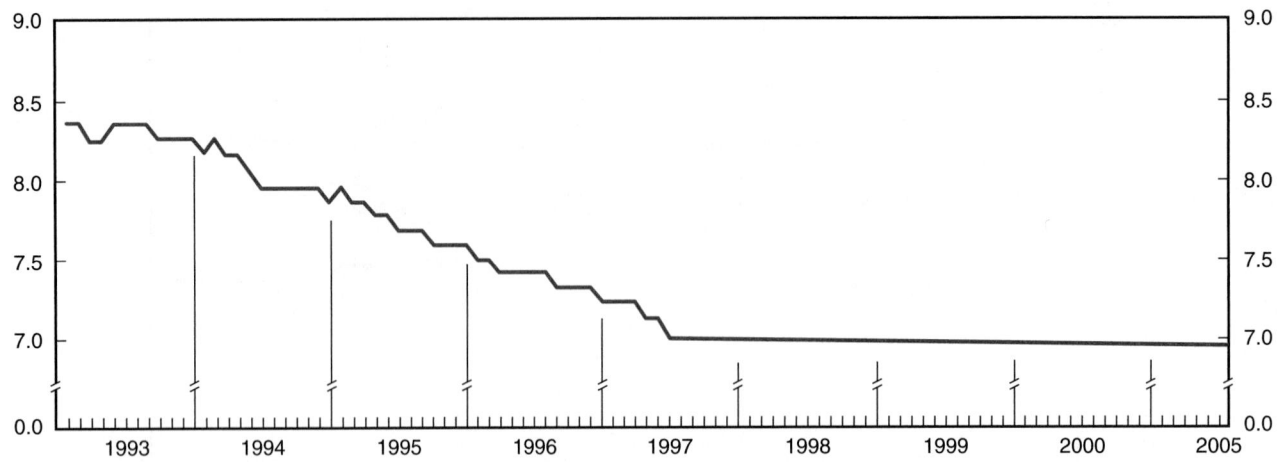

FIGURE 1.4 Infant mortality rates per 1,000 live births for successive 12-month periods ending with month indicated: United States, 2004. (National Center for Health Statistics. [2004]. Births, marriages, divorce and deaths. *National Vital Statistics Report, 50*(1), 2.)

mothers, unequal provision of health care, and the higher percentage of low-birthweight babies born to African-American women: 12%, compared with approximately 5% for white and Asian women (NCHS, 2005). Despite this negative trend, the overall steady drop in total infant mortality is encouraging (Martin et al., 2005) (Fig. 1.4).

The infant mortality rate also varies greatly from state to state within the United States (Table 1.4). For example, in the District of Columbia, the area with the highest infant mortality, the rate is more than two times that in Massachusetts, the state with the lowest rate.

Table 1.5 shows the ranking of the United States compared with other developed countries. One would expect that a country such as the United States, which has one of

the highest gross national products in the world and is known for its technological capabilities, would have the lowest infant mortality rate. However, in 2000, the U.S. infant mortality rate was higher than that of 27 other countries (United Nations, 2000).

One factor that may contribute to national differences in infant mortality is the type of health care available. In Sweden, for example, a comprehensive health care program provides free maternal and child health care to all residents. Women who attend prenatal clinics early in pregnancy receive a monetary award; this almost guarantees that all women will come for prenatal care. Many people believe that a guaranteed health care system such as this would lead to lower infant mortality in the United States.

TABLE 1.4

Infant Mortality Rates per 1,000 by State

State	Rate	State	Rate	State	Rate
Massachusetts	4.8	South Dakota	6.4	Missouri	7.7
New Hampshire	4.9	Wyoming	6.5	Ohio	7.7
Maine	5.1	Idaho	6.6	Illinois	7.8
Utah	5.3	Arizona	6.7	North Dakota	7.8
California	5.4	Kentucky	6.7	West Virginia	7.9
Minnesota	5.5	Rhode Island	6.7	Oklahoma	8.0
Oregon	5.5	Alaska	6.8	Michigan	8.1
Texas	5.5	Montana	6.9	Arkansas	8.3
Washington	5.5	Wisconsin	6.9	North Carolina	8.4
Iowa	5.8	Kansas	7.0	Georgia	8.7
Colorado	6.0	Nebraska	7.0	South Carolina	9.0
Nevada	6.0	Florida	7.2	Tennessee	9.0
New Jersey	6.1	Hawaii	7.2	Alabama	9.3
New York	6.1	Virginia	7.2	Delaware	9.6
Vermont	6.2	Pennsylvania	7.3	Louisiana	9.8
Connecticut	6.4	Indiana	7.7	District of Columbia	11.4
New Mexico	6.4	Maryland	7.7		

National Center for Health Statistics. (2005). *Trends in the health of Americans.* Hyattsville, MD: NCHS.

TABLE 1.5

Infant Mortality Rate (Deaths per 1,000 Live Births) for Selected Countries, 2000

COUNTRY	Girls	Boys
1. Japan	3	4
2. Sweden	3	4
3. Finland	4	4
4. Hong Kong SAR	4	4
5. Austria	4	5
6. Belgium	4	5
7. Germany	4	5
8. Iceland	4	5
9. Netherlands	4	5
10. Norway	4	5
11. Singapore	4	5
12. Switzerland	4	5
13. Czech Republic	5	5
14. Denmark	5	5
15. France	5	5
16. Australia	5	6
17. Canada	5	6
18. Italy	5	6
19. Slovenia	5	6
20. Spain	5	6
21. United Kingdom	5	6
22. Ireland	6	6
23. Israel	6	6
24. Luxembourg	6	6
25. New Zealand	6	6
26. Greece	6	7
27. Portugal	6	7
28. United States	7	7

United Nations Statistics Division. (2000). Infant mortality. *The world's women 2000: Trends and statistics.* New York: Author.

Fortunately, the proportion of pregnant women who receive prenatal care in the United States is increasing (about 80% now begin care in the first trimester). Early prenatal care is important, because it identifies potential risks and allows preventive strategies to help reduce complications of pregnancy. The United States also differs from other countries in the increased number of infants born to adolescent mothers (30% of infants are born to mothers younger than 20 years of age). Because teenage pregnancy leads to increased premature births, this may result in infants being born who are not as well prepared as others to face extrauterine life.

The main causes of early infant death in the United States are problems that occur at birth or shortly thereafter. Prematurity, low birthweight, congenital anomalies, sudden infant death syndrome, and respiratory distress syndrome are major causes. Although other factors that contribute to sudden infant death syndrome are yet to be determined, the recommendation to place infants on their back or side to sleep, made by the American Academy of Pediatrics in 1992, has led to an almost 50% decrease in its incidence (Daley, 2004).

Before antibiotics and formula sterilization practices became available, gastrointestinal disease was a leading cause of infant death. By advocating breast-feeding and teaching mothers strict adherence to good sanitary practices, health care practitioners can help ensure that gastrointestinal infection does not again become a major factor in infant mortality.

Checkpoint Question 2

Nursing is changing because social change affects care. Which of the following is a trend that is occurring in nursing because of social change?

a. So many children are treated in ambulatory units that nurses are hardly needed.
b. Immunizations are no longer needed for infectious diseases.
c. The use of skilled technology has made nursing care more complex.
d. Pregnant women are so healthy today that they rarely need prenatal care.

Childhood Mortality Rate

Like the infant mortality rate, the childhood mortality rate in the United States is also declining. In 1980, for example, the mortality rate was about 6.4% for children aged 1 to 4 years and 3.1% for children aged 4 to 14 years; today, it is 3.0% and 1.8%, respectively (NCHS, 2005). The risk of death in the first year of life is higher than that in any other year before age 55. Children in the prepubescent period (age 5 to 14 years) have the lowest mortality rate of any child age group (NCHS, 2005).

The most frequent causes of childhood death are shown in Box 1.7. Motor vehicle accidents remain the leading cause of death in children, although many of these accidents are largely preventable through education about the value of car seats and seat belt use, the dangers of drinking/drug abuse and driving, and the importance of pedestrian safety.

A particularly disturbing mortality statistic is the high incidence of suicide in the 15-to-24-year-old age group (more girls than boys attempt suicide, but boys are more successful). Although school-age children and adolescents may not voice feelings of depression or anger during a health care visit, such underlying feelings may actually be a primary concern. Nurses who are alert to cues of depression or anger can be helpful in detecting these emotions and lowering the risk of suicide. The high incidence of homicide (1.5% in school-age children and 20% in adolescents) and an increase in the number of adolescents infected with human immunodeficiency virus (HIV) are also growing concerns.

Childhood Morbidity Rate

Health problems commonly occurring in large proportions of children today include respiratory disorders (including asthma and tuberculosis), gastrointestinal disturbances, and consequences of injuries. As more immunizations become available, fewer children in the United States are affected by common childhood communicable diseases. For instance, the incidence of poliomyelitis (once a major killer

BOX 1.7

Major Causes of Death in Childhood

Under 1 Year
Congenital malformations, chromosomal
    abnormalities
Disorders related to short gestation age and low
    birthweight
Sudden infant death syndrome
Newborn affected by maternal complications of
    pregnancy
Newborn affected by complications of placenta,
    cord, or membranes
Unintentional injuries
Respiratory distress of newborn
Bacterial sepsis of newborn
Diseases of the circulatory system
Intrauterine hypoxia and birth asphyxia

1–4 Years
Unintentional injuries
Congenital malformations, chromosomal abnormalities
Homicide
Malignant neoplasms
Diseases of the heart
Influenza and pneumonia
Septicemia
Chronic lower respiratory tract diseases

Disorders originating in the perinatal period
Benign neoplasms

5–14 Years
Unintentional injuries
Malignant neoplasms
Congenital malformations, chromosomal abnormalities
Homicide
Suicide
Diseases of the heart
Chronic lower respiratory tract diseases
Septicemia
Cerebrovascular accident
Influenza and pneumonia

15–24 Years
Unintentional injuries
Homicide
Suicide
Malignant neoplasm
Diseases of the heart
Congenital malformations, chromosomal abnormalities
Chronic lower respiratory tract diseases
Human immunodeficiency virus (HIV) disease
Diabetes mellitus
Cerebrovascular diseases

National Center for Health Statistics. (2005). *Trends in the health of Americans.* Hyattsville, MD: NCHS.

of children) is now extremely low (almost zero), because almost all children in the United States are immunized against it (NCHS, 2005). Measles flared in incidence in the early 1990s but now is scheduled as a disease to be completely eradicated by 2010. It is important that this happen, because measles encephalitis can be as destructive and lethal as poliomyelitis. Continued education about the benefits of immunization against rubella (German measles) is also needed, because if a woman contracts this form of measles during pregnancy, her infant may be born with severe congenital anomalies.

Although the decline in the overall incidence of preventable childhood diseases is encouraging, as many as 50% of children younger than 4 years of age in some communities are still not fully immunized (NCHS, 2005). There is a potential for childhood infectious diseases to increase again if immunization is not maintained as a high national priority.

The advent of HIV disease has changed care considerations in all areas of nursing, but it has particular implications for maternal and child health nursing. Childbearing women and sexually active teenagers are at risk for becoming infected with HIV through sexual contact or exposure to blood and blood products; in addition, infected women may transmit the virus to a fetus during pregnancy through placental exchange. To help prevent the spread of HIV, adolescents and young adults must be educated about safer sexual practices. Standard precautions must be strictly followed in maternal and child health

nursing, as in other areas of nursing practice, to safeguard health care providers and other clients.

Other infectious diseases that are increasing in incidence include syphilis, genital herpes, hepatitis A and B, and tuberculosis. The rise in cases of syphilis and genital herpes probably stems from an increase in nonmonogamous sexual relationships and lack of safer sex practices. The increase in hepatitis B is due largely to drug abuse and the use of infected injection equipment. One reason for the increase in hepatitis A is shared diaper-changing facilities in day care centers. Tuberculosis, once considered close to eradication, has experienced a resurgence, occurring today at approximately the same rate as measles in young adults. One form occurs as an opportunistic disease in HIV-positive persons and is particularly resistant to the usual therapy (Burgos et al., 2003).

Trends in Health Care Environment

The settings for maternal and child health care are changing to better meet the needs of increasingly well-informed and vocal consumers.

Cost Containment

Cost containment refers to systems of health care delivery that focus on reducing the cost of health care by closely monitoring the cost of personnel, use and brands of supplies, length of hospital stays, number of procedures carried out, and number of referrals requested (Schwartz, 2003).

Before the philosophy of cost containment became prominent, health care insurance paid separately for each procedure or piece of equipment the client received. Under managed care, the agency receives a certain sum of money for the client's care, no matter how many supplies, procedures, or personnel are used in care. In a managed care environment, helping to curtail cost is an important nursing function. Suggestions such as using generic-brand supplies, never breaking into kits of supplies to remove a single item, and urging the use of disposable supplies so that less personnel time will be spent on cleaning and sterilizing are welcome, cost-effective suggestions.

Cost containment has had dramatic effects on health care, most noticeably in limiting the number of hospital days and changing the roles of personnel. Before managed care, women stayed in a hospital for 3 or 4 days after childbirth; today, they rarely stay longer than 48 hours. Before managed care, nurses completed all care procedures for patients, no matter how small or unskilled the task. With managed care, ancillary personnel (e.g., unlicensed assistive personnel) perform many tasks under the supervision of the nurse. This system is designed to move the registered nurse (RN) to a higher level of function, because it makes the RN accountable for a fuller range of services to patients. It accentuates point-of-service care. It also increases the accountability and responsibility of RNs to delegate tasks appropriately. As a result of managed care, the new advanced-practice role of case manager has been created.

It is important to know the legal aspects of delegation, as identified in individual state nursing practice acts, because some laws address specific tasks and activities that RNs may or may not delegate in that state. Accountability for completion and quality of the task remains with the nurse, so the nurse is responsible for knowing that the condition of the patient and the skill level of the assistive person are conducive to safe delegation. There are four rules to follow when delegating:

- Right task for the situation
- Right person to complete the task
- Right communication concerning what is to be done
- Right feedback or evaluation that the task was completed

Examples of delegation responsibility that can occur in maternal and child health are highlighted in the Multidisciplinary Care Maps located throughout this text.

When managed care was introduced, it was viewed as a system that could lead to poor-quality nursing care because it limits the number of supplies and time available for care. In settings where it works well, however, it has increased opportunities for nurses because it rewards creativity.

Alternative Settings and Styles for Health Care

The last 100 years has seen several major shifts in settings for maternity care. At the turn of the 19th century, most births took place in the home, with only the very poor or ill giving birth in "lying-in" hospitals. By 1940, about 40% of live births occurred in hospitals, and today the figure has risen to 98% (DHHS, 2005). Today, a less dramatic but no less important trend is occurring: an increasing number of families are once more choosing childbirth at home or in alternative birth settings rather than hospitals. These alternative settings provide families with increased control of the birth experience and options for birth surroundings unavailable in hospitals. One strength of this movement is its encouragement of family involvement in birth. It also increases nursing responsibility for assessment and professional judgment and provides expanded roles for nurse practitioners, such as the nurse-midwife. Of all births in the United States, 5% currently are attended by midwives rather than physicians (Martin et al., 2005).

Hospitals have responded to consumers' demand for a more natural childbirth environment by refitting labor and delivery suites as birthing rooms, often called labor-delivery-recovery (LDR) or labor-delivery-recovery-postpartum (LDRP) rooms. Partners, family members, and other support people may remain in the room, which is designed to be a homelike environment, and participate in the childbirth experience (Fig. 1.5). Couplet care—care for both the mother and newborn by the primary nurse—is encouraged after the births. LDRP rooms promote a holistic, family-centered approach to maternal and child health care and are appealing to many families who might otherwise have opted against a hospital birth. However, LDRPs are not without fault. It has been argued that they are less private for laboring families, tend to be less relaxing for postpartum families, and make it difficult for nurses to manage the needs of women both in labor and after birth. Many hospitals are continuing to search for the best labor, delivery, and postpartum options. Whether childbirth takes place at home, in a birthing center, or in a hospital, the goal is to keep it as natural as possible while ensuring the protection that experienced nurse-midwives or physicians can provide.

Health care settings for children are also changing. Clients' homes, community centers, ambulatory clinics, well-baby clinics, schools, and group homes are some settings in which comprehensive health care may be administered. In these settings, a nurse may provide immunizations, screenings, health and safety education, counseling, crisis

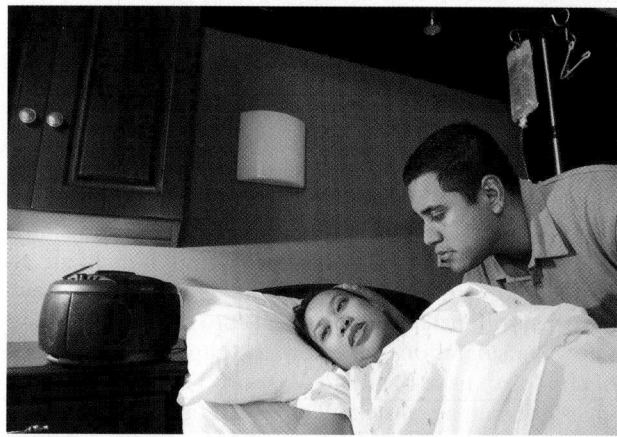

FIGURE 1.5 A couple, soon to be parents, share a close moment in a birthing room.

intervention for teens, parenting classes, and care of the ill child and family. Community-based care can provide cost-effective health promotion, disease prevention, and patient care to a large number of children and families in an environment that is familiar to them.

Strengthening the Ambulatory Care System

The ambulatory care system continues to broaden its base. More and more people who might otherwise have been admitted to a hospital are now being cared for in ambulatory clinics or at home. This option has proved especially important in the care of sick children and women who are experiencing a pregnancy complication or who want early discharge after childbirth. Separating a child from his or her family during an illness has been shown to be potentially harmful to the child's development, so any effort to reduce the incidence of separation should have a positive effect (see Chapter 35). Avoiding long hospital stays for women during pregnancy is also a preferable method of care, because it helps to maintain family contact.

What if... Melissa Chung has to remain in the hospital after the birth of her new baby while her baby is transported to a regional center for care? How could you help her keep in touch with her new baby?

Shortening Hospital Stays

More and more hospitals perform children's surgeries such as tonsillectomy or umbilical or inguinal hernia repair without requiring an overnight stay. Early on the morning of surgery, the parent and child arrive at the hospital, and the child receives a preoperative physical examination and medication. After surgery, the child is sent to a recovery room and then to a short-term observation unit. If the child is doing well and shows no complications by about 4 hours after surgery, he or she can be discharged. Similarly, women who have begun preterm labor stay in the hospital while labor is halted and then are allowed to return home on medication with continued monitoring. The routine hospital stay for mothers and newborns after an uncomplicated birth is now 2 days or less.

Short-term hospital stays require intensive health teaching by the nursing staff and follow-up by home care or community health nurses. Parents must be taught to watch for danger signs in the child without being frightened. A woman with a complication of pregnancy must be taught to watch for signs that warrant immediate attention. New parents must be taught about their newborn's nutritional needs, umbilical cord care, bathing, and safety considerations, all before the euphoria and fatigue of childbirth have begun to wear off. This type of teaching is difficult, because it includes not only imparting the facts of self-care but also providing support and reassurance that the client or parents are capable of this level of care.

Including the Family in Health Care

Most hospitals have developed policies that minimize the effects of separation from parents when children must be admitted for extended stays. Open visiting hours allow parents to visit as much as possible and sleep overnight in a bed next to their child. Parents also are allowed and encouraged to do as much for the child as they wish during a hospital stay, such as feeding and bathing the child or administering oral medicine. Most of a parent's time, however, is spent simply being close by to provide a comfortable, secure influence on the child. For the same reasons, parents on a maternity unit are encouraged to room-in and give total care to their well newborn (Box 1.8).

Because parents are so important to their child's hospital experience and overall well-being, family-centered nursing is vital. Therefore, the nurse's client load will not be just four children, for example, but four children plus four sets of parents; not just a single newborn, but his or her two parents as well.

Increase in the Number of Intensive Care Units

Over the past 20 years, care of infants and children has become extremely technical. It is generally assumed that newborns with a term birthweight (more than 2,500 g or 5.5 lb) will thrive at birth. However, many infants are born each year with birthweights lower than 2,500 g or who are ill at birth and do not thrive. Such infants are regularly transferred to a neonatal intensive care unit (NICU) or in-

---

BOX 1.8 FOCUS ON . . .

EVIDENCE-BASED PRACTICE

What are the ingredients of effective family-centered care?

Working on the premise that family-centered care is best achieved when a mutually beneficial partnership exists between health care providers and families, nurse researchers attempted to identify health care practices that promote or limit a family-centered philosophy. For the study, 34 women (mostly African-American) who were using maternity services at a large urban hospital were interviewed as to what they liked or didn't like about their maternity care. The results revealed two important perceived barriers to family-centered maternity care: problems among health caregivers in coordinating services and lack of patient access to services. Factors that aided effective care were prompt response to high-risk patients and the availability of health-related support outside the hospital. The authors concluded that each childbearing woman and her family should be treated, in clinical situations, as if they were extraordinary. In this way, practitioners can alter routines that cause the woman and her family to lose individualized care.

Source: Gramling, L., Hickman, K., & Bennett, S. (2004). What makes a good family-centered partnership between women and their practitioners? A qualitative study. *Birth, 31*(1), 43–48.

tensive care nursery (ICN). Children who are undergoing cardiac surgery or recovering from near-drownings or multiinjury accidents are cared for in a pediatric intensive care unit (PICU). Intensive care at this early point in life is one of the most costly types of hospitalization. Expenses of $1,000 a day, or $20,000 to $100,000 for a total hospital stay, are not rare for care during a high-risk pregnancy or care for a high-risk infant. As the number of these settings increases, the opportunities for advanced-practice nurses also increase.

Regionalization of Intensive Care

To avoid duplication of care sites, it is an accepted practice for communities to establish centralized maternal or pediatric health services. Such planning creates one site that is properly staffed and equipped for potential problems. For example, ill newborns may be transported to a central high-risk nursery for care. High-risk pregnant women and ill children may be cared for in a regional setting equipped with specialized resources for the diagnosis and treatment of specific health problems. When a newborn, older child, or parent is hospitalized in a regional center, the family members who have been left behind need a great deal of support. They may feel they have "lost" their infant, child, or parent unless health care personnel keep them abreast of the ill family member's progress by means of phone calls and snapshots and encourage the family to visit as soon as possible.

When regionalization concepts of newborn care first became accepted, transporting the ill or premature newborn to the regional care facility was the method of choice (Fig. 1.6). Today, however, if it is known in advance that a child may be born with a life-threatening condition, it may be safer to transport the mother to the regional center during pregnancy, because the uterus has advantages as a transport incubator that far exceed those of any commercial incubator yet designed.

An important argument against regionalization for pediatric care is that children will feel homesick in strange settings, overwhelmed by the number of sick children they see, and frightened because they are miles from home. An important argument against regionalization of maternal care is that being away from her community and support network places a great deal of stress on the pregnant woman and her family and limits her own doctor's participation in her care. These are important considerations. Because nurses more than any other health care group set the tone for hospitals, they are responsible for ensuring that clients and families feel as welcome in the regional centers as they would have been in a small hospital. Staffing should be adequate to allow sufficient time for nurses to comfort frightened children and prepare them for new experiences or to support the pregnant woman and her family. Documenting the importance of such actions allows them to be incorporated in critical pathways and preserves the importance of the nurse's role.

Increased Reliance on Comprehensive Care Settings

Comprehensive health care is designed to meet all of a child's needs in one setting. In the past, care of children

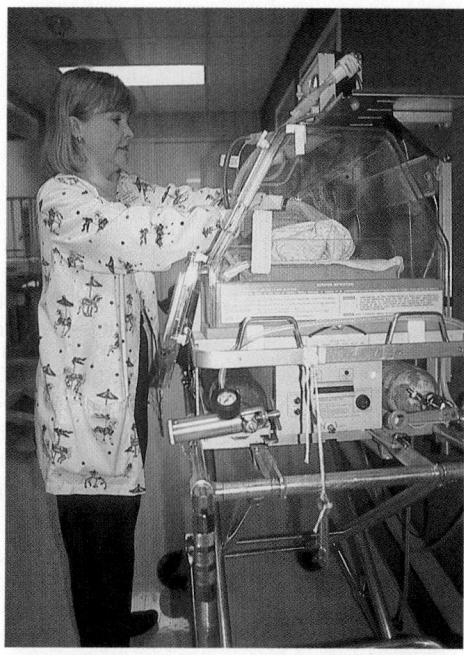

FIGURE 1.6 A nurse prepares an infant transport incubator to move a premature infant to a regional hospital. Helping with safe movement of pregnant women and ill newborns to regional centers is an important nursing responsibility. (© Caroline Brown, RNC, MS, DEd.)

tended to be specialized. For example, a child born with an illness (e.g., myelomeningocele, cerebral palsy) might have been followed by a team of specialists for each facet of the problem. Such a team might include a neurologist, a physical therapist, an occupational therapist, a psychologist for intelligence quotient testing, a speech therapist, an orthopedic surgeon, and finally, a special education teacher. The parents might need to find a special dentist who accepts clients with multiple disabilities. Each specialist would look at only one area of the child's needs rather than the whole child's development. Without extra guidance, parents would find themselves lost in a maze of visits to different health care personnel. If they were not receiving financial support for their child's care, they might not have been able to afford all the necessary services at one time. It might have been difficult to decide which of the child's problems needed to be treated immediately and which could be left untreated without worsening and developing into a permanent disability. Although specialists are still important to a child's care, a trusted primary care provider to help parents coordinate these specialized services is essential in today's managed care environment. In many settings, this primary care provider, who follows the child through all phases of care, is an advanced-practice nurse such as a family nurse practitioner, pediatric nurse practitioner, or a women's health nurse practitioner. Nurses can be helpful in seeing that both parents and children have all their needs met by a primary health care provider in this way. The family must become empowered to seek out a family-centered setting that will be best for their health (Box 1.9).

BOX 1.9 FOCUS ON . . .

FAMILY TEACHING

Tips for Selecting a Health Care Setting

Q. Melissa Chung, the patient you met at the beginning of the chapter, asks you, "With so many health care choices and settings available, how do we know which one to choose?"

A. When selecting a health care setting, use the following as a guide to help you decide what is best for your family:

- Can it be reached easily? (Going for preventive care when well or for care when ill should not be a chore.)
- Will the staff provide continuity of care so you'll always see the same primary care provider if possible?
- Does the physical setup of the facility provide for a sense of privacy, yet a sense that health care providers share pertinent information so you do not have to repeat your history at each visit?
- Is the cost of care and the number of referrals to specialists explained clearly?
- Are preventive care and health education stressed (keeping well is as important as recovering from illness)?
- Do health care providers respect your opinion and ask for your input on health care decisions?
- Do health care providers show a personal interest in you?
- Is health education done at your learning level?
- Is the facility accessible to handicapped individuals?

Increased Use of Alternative Treatment Modalities

There is a growing tendency for families to consult providers of alternative forms of therapy, such as acupuncture or therapeutic touch, in addition to, or instead of, traditional health care providers. Nurses have an increasing obligation to be aware of complementary or alternative therapies, which have the potential to either enhance or detract from the effectiveness of traditional therapy (Fletcher & Clarke, 2004; Weier & Beal, 2004).

In addition, health care providers who are unaware of the existence of some alternative forms of therapy may lose an important opportunity to capitalize on the positive features of that particular therapy. For instance, it would be important to know that an adolescent who is about to undergo a painful procedure is experienced at meditation, because asking the adolescent if she wants to meditate before the procedure could help her relax. Not only could this decrease the child's discomfort, but it could also offer her a feeling of control over a difficult situation. People are using an increasing number of herbal remedies, so asking about these at health assessment is important to prevent drug interactions. Ginger, for example, is frequently taken during pregnancy to relieve morning sickness (Senyak et al., 2005).

Increased Reliance on Home Care

Early hospital discharge has resulted in the return home of many women and children before they are fully ready to care for themselves. Ill children and women with complications of pregnancy may choose to remain at home for care rather than be hospitalized. This has created a "second system" of care requiring many additional care providers (Asensio et al., 2005). Nurses are instrumental in assessing women and children on hospital discharge to help plan the best type of continuing care, devise and modify procedures for home care, and sustain clients' morale and interest in health care during such situations as home monitoring to prevent premature labor. Because home care is a unique and expanding area in maternal and child health nursing, it is discussed in relation to maternal care in Chapter 16 and in relation to children in Chapter 35.

Increased Use of Technology

The use of technology is increasing in all health care settings. The field of assisted reproduction (e.g., in vitro fertilization), with the possibility of stem cell research, is forging new pathways (Jain et al., 2004). Charting by computer, seeking information on the Internet, and monitoring fetal heart rates by Doppler ultrasonography are other examples. In addition to learning these technologies, maternal and child health nurses must be able to explain their use and their advantages to clients. Otherwise, clients may find new technologies more frightening than helpful to them.

Health Care Concerns and Attitudes

The 1980s brought about considerable change in the health care system. As we progress through the 21st century, there are likely to be even more changes as the United States actively works toward effective health goals and improved health care for all citizens. These steps can create new concerns.

Increasing Concern Regarding Health Care Costs

The advent of managed care has concentrated efforts on reducing the cost of health care. This has direct implications for maternal and child health nursing, because nurses must become more cost-conscious about supplies and services. Lack of financial ability to pay and health care provider's insensitivity to cultural values are major reasons why women do not obtain prenatal care. A woman may fear that changing jobs or not working during pregnancy may lead to loss of insurance coverage, thereby reducing her ability to pay for services. As a result, she may continue to work long hours or in unfit conditions during pregnancy. Nurses are challenged to help reduce costs while maintaining quality care so that prenatal care remains available.

Increasing Emphasis on Preventive Care

A generally accepted theory is that it is better to keep individuals well than to restore health after they have become ill. Counseling parents on ways to keep their homes safe for children is an important form of illness prevention in maternal and child health nursing. Research supporting the facts that accidents are still a major cause of death in children and that women still do not receive preconceptual or prenatal care are testaments to the need for much more anticipatory guidance in this area.

Increasing Emphasis on Family-Centered Care

Health promotion with families during pregnancy or child-rearing is a family-centered event, because teaching health awareness and good health habits is accomplished chiefly by role modeling. Illness in a child is automatically a family-centered event. Parents may need to adjust work schedules to allow one of them to stay with the ill child; siblings may have to sacrifice an activity such as a birthday party or having a parent watch their school play; and family finances may have to be readjusted to pay for hospital and medical bills. When a mother is pregnant, family roles or activities may have to change to safeguard her health. A family may feel drawn together by the fright and concern of an acute illness. On the other hand, if an illness becomes chronic, it may pull a family apart or destroy it.

By adopting a view of pregnancy, childbirth, or illness as a family event, nurses are well equipped to provide family-centered care. Nurses can be instrumental in including family members in events from which they were once totally excluded, such as an unplanned cesarean birth. They can help child health care to be family-centered by consulting with family members about a plan of care and providing clear health teaching so that family members can monitor their own care (Fig. 1.7). Nurses play an active role in both teaching health promotion and sustaining families through a child's illness.

In recent years, the U.S. government has recognized that the care of individual family members is a family-centered event. The Family Medical Leave Act of 1993 is a federal law that requires employers with 50 or more employees to provide a minimum of 12 weeks of unpaid, job-protected leave to employees under four circumstances crucial to family life:

- Birth of the employee's child
- Adoption or foster placement of a child with the employee
- Need for the employee to care for a parent, spouse, or child with a serious health condition
- Inability of the employee to perform his or her functions because of a serious health condition

A serious health condition is defined as "an illness, injury, impairment, or physical or mental condition involving such circumstances as inpatient care or incapacity requiring 3 workdays' absence" (U.S. Department of Labor, 1995). Specifically mentioned in the law is any period of incapacity due to pregnancy or for prenatal care with or without treatment. Illness must be documented by a health care provider. Nurse practitioners and nurse-midwives are specifically listed as those who can document a health condition.

Increasing Concern for the Quality of Life

In the past, health care of women and children was focused on maintaining physical health. More recently, however, a growing awareness that quality of life is as important as physical health has expanded the scope of health care to include the assessment of psychosocial facets of life in such areas as self-esteem and independence. Good interviewing skills are necessary to elicit this information at health care visits. Nurses can help obtain such information and also plan ways to improve quality of life in the areas the client considers most important.

One way in which quality of life is being improved for children with chronic illness is the national mandate to allow them to attend regular schools, guaranteeing entrance despite severe illness or use of medical equipment such as a ventilator (Public Law 99-452). Nurses serving as school nurses or consultants to schools play important roles in making these efforts possible.

Increasing Awareness of the Individuality of Clients

Maternal and child clients today do not fit readily into any set category. Varying family structures, cultural backgrounds, socioeconomic levels, and individual circumstances lead to unique and diverse clients. Some women having children are younger than ever before, and an increasing number of women are experiencing their first pregnancies after the age of 35 (Carolan, 2003). Many women are having children outside of marriage. Gay and lesbian couples are also beginning to raise families, conceiving children through artificial insemination or adoption. As a result of advances in research and therapy, women who were once unable to have children, such as those with cystic fibrosis, are now able to manage a full-term pregnancy. Individuals with cognitive and physical challenges are also establishing families and rearing children.

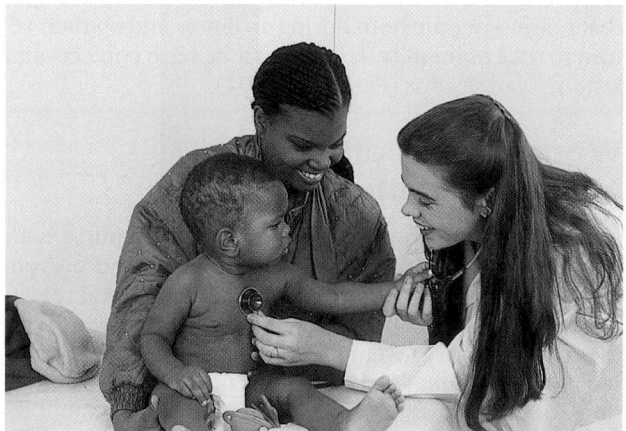

FIGURE 1.7 A nurse involves the mother in a physical exam to promote family-centered care. (© Barbara Proud.)

Many families who have come from foreign countries enter the U.S. health care system for the first time during a pregnancy or with a sick child. This requires a greater sensitivity on the part of health care providers to the socio-cultural aspects of care. As the level of violence in the world increases, more and more families are exposed to living in violent communities. The incidence of abused children and pregnant women is also increasing. All of these concerns require increased nursing attention.

Empowerment of Health Care Consumers

In part because of the influence of market-driven care and a strengthened focus on health promotion and disease prevention, individuals and families have recently begun to take increased responsibility for their own health. This begins with learning preventive measures to stay well. For some families, it means following a more nutritious diet and planning regular exercise; for others, it can mean an entire change in lifestyle. When a family member is ill, empowerment means learning more about the illness, participating in the treatment plan, and preventing the illness from returning. Families are very interested in participating in decision making regarding their childbearing options. Parents want to accompany their ill children into the hospital for overnight stays. They are eager for information about their child's health and want to contribute to the decision-making process. They may question treatments or care plans that they believe are not in their child's best interest. If health care providers do not provide answers to a client's questions or are insensitive to needs, many health care consumers are willing to take their business to another health care setting.

Nurses can promote empowerment of parents and children by respecting their views and concerns, addressing clients by name, and regarding parents as important participants in their own or their child's health, keeping them informed and helping them to make decisions about care. Although a nurse may have seen 25 clients already in a particular day, he or she can make each client feel as important as the first by showing a warm manner and keen interest. Family Teaching displays are presented throughout this text to provide insight into ways in which nurses can help empower families.

What if... In the past, children with pneumonia were always hospitalized. What if Melissa Chung demands that her 6-year-old, diagnosed with pneumonia, be hospitalized, even though it is your clinic's policy to have such children cared for at home by their parents? Would you advocate for hospitalization or not?

ADVANCED-PRACTICE ROLES FOR NURSES IN MATERNAL AND CHILD HEALTH

As trends in maternal and child health care change, so do the roles of maternal and child health nurses. All maternal and child health nurses function in a variety of settings as caregivers, client advocates, researchers, case managers, and educators.

Many nurses with a specified number of years of direct patient care, clinical expertise, and validated completion of pertinent continuing education programs are certified in their specialty. In addition, maternal and child health nurses function in a variety of advanced-practice roles.

Clinical Nurse Specialists

Clinical nurse specialists are nurses prepared at the master's-degree level who are capable of acting as consultants in their area of expertise, as well as serving as role models, researchers, and teachers of quality nursing care. Examples of areas of specialization are neonatal, maternal, child, and adolescent health care; childbirth education; and lactation consultation.

Consider, for example, how a child health clinical specialist might intervene to help in the care of a 4-year-old child with diabetes mellitus who has been admitted to the hospital. The child is difficult to care for because he is so fearful of hospitalization and perplexed because his parents are having difficulty accepting his diagnosis. A clinical nurse specialist could be instrumental in helping a primary nurse organize care and in meeting with the parents to help them accept what is happening. Neonatal nurse specialists manage the care of infants at birth and in intensive care settings; they provide home follow-up care to ensure the newborn remains well. Childbirth educators teach families about normal birth and how to prepare for labor and birth. Lactation consultants educate women about breast-feeding and support them while they learn how to do this well themselves.

Case Manager

A case manager is a graduate-level nurse who supervises a group of patients from the time they enter a health care setting until they are discharged from the setting, or, in a seamless care system, into their homes as well, monitoring the effectiveness, cost, and satisfaction of their health care. Case management can be a vastly satisfying nursing role, because if the health care setting is "seamless," or one that follows people both during an illness and on their return to the community, it involves long-term contacts and lasting relationships (Peterson, 2004).

Women's Health Nurse Practitioner

A **women's health nurse practitioner** is a nurse with advanced study in the promotion of health and prevention of illness in women. Such a nurse plays a vital role in educating women about their bodies and sharing with them methods to prevent illness; in addition, they care for women with illnesses such as sexually transmitted infections, offering information and counseling them about reproductive life planning. They play a large role in helping women remain well so that they can enter a pregnancy in good health and maintain their health throughout life.

Family Nurse Practitioner

A **family nurse practitioner** (FNP) is an advanced-practice role that provides health care not only to women but to total families. In conjunction with a physician, an FNP can provide prenatal care for a woman with an uncomplicated pregnancy. The FNP takes the health and pregnancy history, performs physical and obstetric examinations, orders appropriate diagnostic and laboratory tests, and plans continued care throughout the pregnancy and for the family afterward. FNPs then monitor the family indefinitely to promote health and optimal family functioning.

Neonatal Nurse Practitioner

A **neonatal nurse practitioner** (NNP) is an advanced-practice role for nurses who are skilled in the care of newborns, both well and ill. NNPs may work in level 1, level 2, or level 3 newborn nurseries; neonatal follow-up clinics or physician groups. They also transport ill infants to different care settings. The NNP's responsibilities include managing and carrying out patient care in an intensive care unit, conducting normal newborn assessments and physical examinations, and providing high-risk follow-up discharge planning (Bissell, 2004).

Pediatric Nurse Practitioner

A **pediatric nurse practitioner** (PNP) is a nurse prepared with extensive skills in physical assessment, interviewing, and well-child counseling and care. In this role, a nurse interviews parents as part of an extensive health history and performs a physical assessment of the child (Fig. 1.8). If the nurse's diagnosis is that the child is well, he or she discusses with the parents any childrearing concerns mentioned in the interview, gives any immunizations needed, offers necessary anticipatory guidance (based on the plan of care), and arranges a return appointment for the next well-child checkup. The nurse has served as a primary health caregiver or as the sole health care person the parents and child see at that visit.

If the PNP determines that a child has a common illness (e.g., iron deficiency anemia), he or she orders the necessary laboratory tests and prescribes appropriate drugs for therapy. If the PNP determines that the child has a major illness (e.g., congenital subluxated hip, kidney disease, heart disease), he or she consults with an associated pediatrician; together, they decide what further care is necessary. Nurse practitioners may also work in inpatient or specialty settings providing continuity of care to hospitalized children. As school nurse practitioners, they provide care to all children in a given community or school setting.

Nurse-Midwife

Throughout history, the **nurse-midwife,** an individual educated in the two disciplines of nursing and midwifery and licensed according to the requirements of the American College of Nurse-Midwives (ACNM), has played an important role in assisting women with pregnancy and childbearing. Either independently or in association with an obstetrician, the nurse-midwife assumes full responsibility for the care and management of women with uncomplicated pregnancies. Nurse-midwives play a large role in making birth an unforgettable family event as well as helping to ensure a healthy outcome for both mother and child (Dawley, 2003) (Fig. 1.9).

LEGAL CONSIDERATIONS OF MATERNAL-CHILD PRACTICE

Legal concerns arise in all areas of health care. Maternal and child health nursing carries some legal concerns that extend above and beyond other areas of nursing, because care is often given to an "unseen client"—the fetus—or to clients who are not of legal age for giving consent for medical procedures. In addition, labor and birth of a neonate are considered "normal" events, so the risks for a lawsuit are greater when problems arise. Nurses are legally responsible for protecting the rights of their clients, including confidentiality, and are accountable for the quality of their individual nursing care and that of other health care team members. In a society in which child abuse is of national concern, nurses are becoming increasingly responsible for identifying and reporting incidents of suspected abuse in children.

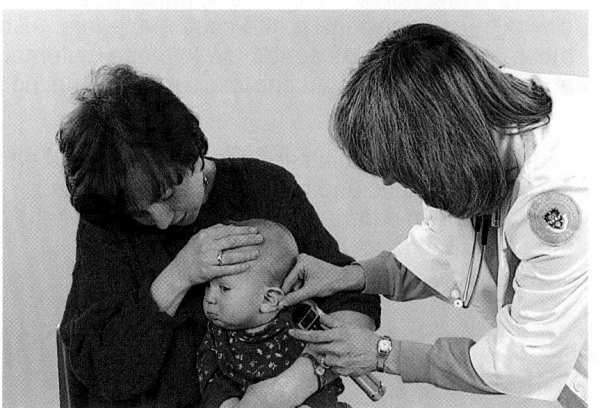

FIGURE 1.8 A pediatric nurse practitioner examines a one-year-old child. (© Barbara Proud.)

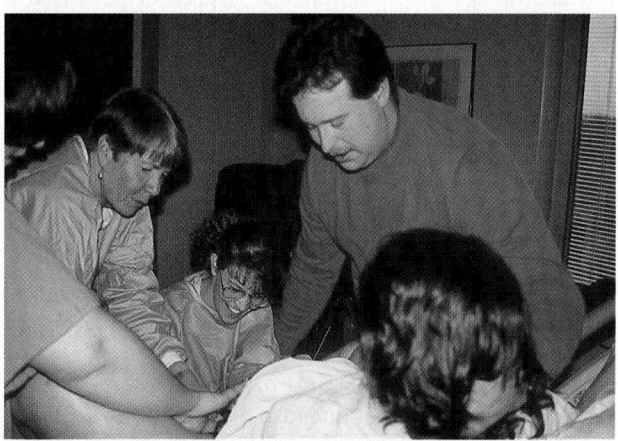

FIGURE 1.9 A nurse-midwife plays an important role in ensuring a safe and satisfying birth. (© Caroline Brown, RNC, MS, DEd.)

Understanding the **scope of practice** (the range of services and care that may be provided by a nurse based on state requirements) and standards of care can help nurses practice within appropriate legal parameters.

Documentation is essential in protecting a nurse and justifying his or her actions. This concern is long-lasting, because children who feel they were wronged by health care personnel can bring a lawsuit at the time they reach legal age. This means that a nursing note written today may need to be defended as many as 21 years into the future. Nurses need to be conscientious about obtaining informed consent for invasive procedures and determining that pregnant women are aware of any risk to the fetus associated with a procedure or test. In divorced or blended families (those in which two adults with children from previous relationships now live together), it is important to establish who has the right to give consent for health care. Personal liability insurance is strongly recommended for all nurses, so that they do not incur great financial losses during a malpractice or professional negligence suit.

If a nurse knows that the care provided by another practitioner was inappropriate or insufficient, he or she is legally responsible for reporting the incident. Failure to do so can lead to a charge of negligence or breach of duty.

The specific legal ramifications of procedures or care are discussed in later chapters that describe procedures or treatment modalities.

ETHICAL CONSIDERATIONS OF PRACTICE

Ethical issues are increasing in frequency in health care today. Some of the most difficult decisions in health care settings are those that involve children and their families. The following are just a few of the major potential conflicts:

- Conception issues, especially those related to in vitro fertilization, embryo transfer, ownership of frozen oocytes or sperm, cloning, stem cell research, and surrogate mothers
- Abortion, particularly partial-birth abortions
- Fetal rights versus rights of the mother
- Use of fetal tissue for research
- Resuscitation (for how long should it be continued?)
- The number of procedures or degree of pain that a child should be asked to endure to achieve a degree of better health
- The balance between modern technology and quality of life

Legal and ethical aspects of issues are often intertwined, which makes the decision-making process complex. Because maternal and child health nursing is so strongly family-centered, it is common to encounter some situations in which the interests of one family member are in conflict with those of another. It is not unusual for the values of a client not to match those of a health care provider. For example, if a pregnancy causes a woman to develop a serious illness, the family must make a decision either to terminate the pregnancy and lose the child or to keep the pregnancy and work to support the mother through the crisis. If the fetus is also at risk from the illness, the decision may be easier to make; however, the circumstances usually are not clearcut, and the decisions that need to be made are difficult. These and other issues are bound to emerge during the course of practice. Nurses can help clients who are facing such difficult decisions by providing factual information and supportive listening and by helping the family clarify their values.

The Pregnant Woman's Bill of Rights and the United Nations Declaration of Rights of the Child (see Appendix A) provide guidelines for determining the rights of clients in regard to health care.

Checkpoint Question 3

The best description of the FNP role is

a. To give bedside care to critically ill family members.
b. To supervise the health of children up to age 18 years.
c. To provide health supervision for families.
d. To supervise women during pregnancy.

Key Points

Standards of maternal and child health nursing practice have been formulated by the American Nurses Association, the Society of Pediatric Nurses, and AWHONN to serve as guidelines for practice.

Nursing theory and use of evidence-based practice are methods by which maternal and child health nursing expands and improves.

The most meaningful and important measure of maternal and child health is the infant mortality rate. It is the number of deaths among infants from birth to 1 year of age per 1,000 live births. This rate is declining steadily, but in the United States it is still higher than in 27 other nations.

Trends in maternal and child health nursing include changes in the settings of care, increased concern about health care costs, improved preventive care, and family-centered care.

Advanced-practice roles in maternal and child health nursing include women's health, family, neonatal, and pediatric nurse practitioners; nurse-midwives; clinical nurse specialists; and case managers. All of these expanded roles contribute to make maternal and child health care an important area of nursing and health care.

Maternal and child health care has both legal and ethical considerations and responsibilities over and above those in other areas of practice because of the role of the fetus and child.

Critical Thinking Exercises

1. How might family-centered care help the Chung family, described in the beginning of the chapter? How can you explain recent changes in health care so that

Melissa might understand why her hospital stay is so much shorter this time? How can you empower the family so that they feel more in control of what is happening to them?

2. Mrs. Chung says she has trouble paying for health care. Other countries throughout the world have a health care delivery system based not on profit but on provision of care for all citizens through a tax-supported program. The infant mortality rate in many of these countries is lower than in the United States. What are some reasons that might contribute to these lower rates?

3. The age at which women are having babies is increasing. For many women such as Melissa Chung, this age is now 35 years or older.
   a. How do you anticipate that this trend will change health care in the future?
   b. Are there special services that should be provided for such women?
   c. How will this trend influence childrearing in the future?

4. Examine the National Health Goals related to maternal, newborn, and child health. Most government-sponsored money for nursing research is allotted based on these goals. What would be a possible research topic to explore, pertinent to these goals, that would be applicable to the Chung family and would also advance evidence-based practice?

References

American Nurses Association and Society of Pediatric Nurses. (2003). *Scope and standards of pediatric clinical practice.* Washington, D.C.: Authors.

Arsenio, O., et al. (2005). Home intravenous antibiotics for cystic fibrosis. *Cochrane Library (Oxford) (1)* (CD001917).

Association of Women's Health, Obstetric, and Neonatal Nurses. (1998). *Standards for the nursing care of women and newborns* (5th ed.). Washington, D.C.: Author.

Bissell, G. (2004). The phenomenon of high-level nursing practice within neonatal units: Who does it? *Journal of Neonatal Nursing, 10*(1), 21-25.

Burgos, M., et al. (2003). Effect of drug resistance on the generation of secondary cases of tuberculosis. *Journal of Infectious Diseases, 188*(12), 1878-1884.

Carolan, M. (2003). The graying of the obstetric population: Implications for the older mother. *JOGNN: Journal of Obstetric, Gynecologic, and Neonatal Nursing, 32*(1), 19-27.

Carpenito, L. J. (2004). *Handbook of nursing diagnosis* (10th ed.). Philadelphia: Lippincott Williams & Wilkins.

Daley, K. C. (2004). Update on sudden infant death syndrome. *Current Opinion in Pediatrics, 16*(2), 227-232.

Dawley, K. (2003). Origins of nurse-midwifery in the United States and its expansion in the 1940s. *Journal of Midwifery and Women's Health, 48*(2), 86-95.

Department of Health and Human Services (2000). *Healthy people 2010.* Washington, D.C.: DHHS.

Department of Health and Human Services (2004). Births, marriages, divorces, and deaths for 2000. *Monthly Vital Statistics Report, 49*(12), 1.

Fletcher, P. C., & Clarke, J. (2004). The use of complementary and alternative medicine among pediatric patients. *Cancer Nursing, 27*(2), 93-99.

Gramling, L., Hickman, K., & Bennett, S. (2004). What makes a good family-centered partnership between women and their practitioners? *Birth, 31*(1):43-48.

Jain, T., Missmer, S. A., & Hornstein, M. D. (2004). Trends in embryo-transfer practice and in outcomes of the use of assisted reproductive technology in the United States. *New England Journal of Medicine, 350*(16), 1639-1645.

Johnson, M., Maas, M., & Moorhead, S. (2000). *Nursing outcomes classification* (2nd ed.). St. Louis: Mosby.

Martin, J. A., et al. (2005). Annual summary of vital statistics. *Pediatrics, 115*(3), 619-634.

McCloskey, J., & Bulechek, G. (2000). *Nursing interventions classification* (3rd ed.). St. Louis: Mosby.

National Center for Health Statistics. (2005). *Trends in the health of Americans.* Hyattsville, MD: NCHS.

Peterson, V. (2004). When quality management meets case management. *Case Management, 9*(2), 108-109.

Rubin, R. (1963). Maternal touch. *Nursing Outlook, 11,* 828-829.

Schwartz, P. A. (2003). Contemporary view of the effect of managed care on the ethics in perinatal medicine. *Clinics in Perinatology, 30*(1), 167-180.

Senyak, S., et al. (2005). Trends in alternative medicine: What's hot. *Alternative Medicine, 1*(73), 76-81.

United Nations Statistics Division. (2000). *The world's women 2000: Trends and statistics.* New York: Author.

U.S. Department of Labor. (1995). Family Medical Leave Act. *Federal Register, 60*(4), 2179.

Weier, K. M., & Beal, M. W. (2004). Complementary therapies as adjuncts in the treatment of postpartum depression. *Journal of Midwifery and Women's Health, 49*(2), 96-104.

Suggested Readings

Ahluwalia, I. B., et al. (2003). Who is breast-feeding? Recent trends from the Pregnancy Risk Assessment and Monitoring System. *Journal of Pediatrics, 142*(5), 486-491.

Callister, L. C. (2003). Toward evidence-based practice: U.S. trends in obstetric procedures, 1990-2000. *MCN: American Journal of Maternal/Child Nursing, 28*(1), 52.

Foster, J. (2004). Fatherhood and the meaning of children: An ethnographic study among Puerto Rican partners of adolescent mothers. *Journal of Midwifery and Women's Health, 49*(2), 118-125.

Kitchener, M., et al. (2005). Medicaid and community-based services: National program trends. *Health Affairs, 24*(1), 206-212.

Nelms, B. C. (2004). The joy of pediatrics: Working with children. *Journal of Pediatric Health Care, 18*(2), 55-56.

Oxtoby, K. (2003). Men in nursing. *Nursing Times, 99*(32), 20-23.

Poole, J. H., & Long, J. (2004). Maternal mortality: A review of current trends. *Critical Care Nursing Clinics of North America, 16*(2), 227-230.

Porreco, R. P., et al. (2005). Expectation of pregnancy outcome among mature women. *American Journal of Obstetrics and Gynecology, 192*(1), 38-41.

Simpson, K. R., & Atterbury, J. (2003). Trends and issues in labor induction in the United States: Implications for clinical practice. *JOGNN: Journal of Obstetric, Gynecologic, and Neonatal Nursing, 32*(6), 767-779.

Turner, P. K. (2004). Mainstreaming alternative medicine: Doing midwifery at the intersection. *Qualitative Health Research, 14*(5), 644-662.

CHAPTER 2

The Childbearing and Childrearing Family and Community

Key Terms

community
ecomap
family
family nursing
family of orientation
family of procreation
family theory
genogram

Objectives

After mastering the contents of this chapter, you should be able to:

1. Describe family structure, function, and family roles.
2. Assess a family for structure and healthy function.
3. Formulate nursing diagnoses related to family health.
4. Develop expected outcomes to help a family achieve optimal health.
5. Plan health teaching strategies, such as helping a family modify its lifestyle to adjust to a pregnancy or accommodate an ill child.
6. Implement nursing care, such as teaching a family more effective wellness behaviors.
7. Evaluate outcome criteria for achievement and effectiveness of nursing care to be certain that expected outcomes have been achieved.
8. Identify National Health Goals related to the family and specific ways that nurses can help the nation achieve these goals.
9. Identify areas of care related to family nursing that could benefit from additional nursing research or the application of evidence-based practice.
10. Use critical thinking to analyze additional ways that nursing care can be more family-centered or that maternal-child health care can better include family members.
11. Integrate knowledge of family nursing with nursing process to promote quality maternal and child health nursing care.

Marlo Hanovan is a 32-year-old bookkeeper. She has a 10-year-old child, Carey, from a first marriage. She is pregnant now with her second child, from her current husband, Stone. Carey has been sick since birth with cystic fibrosis. He needs long-term respiratory therapy, although he attends the local grade school. Stone, Marlo's present husband, has a 2-year-old son, Brian. Stone is currently unemployed because of an accident at work a year ago. He has some income from selling woodworking products at craft shows. Mrs. Hanovan states that on many weeks she is forced to choose between health care and groceries.

The previous chapter discussed the philosophy of maternal and child health nursing and the many roles that nurses fulfill in this area. This chapter adds information about families and communities that can help to ensure a healthy outcome for families. This is important information, because inadequate parenting due to a dysfunctional family structure or a lack of community resources can contribute to poor pregnancy outcomes and poor child-rearing practices.

Is the Hanovan family a well family?

After you've studied this chapter, access the accompanying website. Read the patient scenario and answer the questions to further sharpen your skills, grow more familiar with RN-CLEX types of questions, and reward yourself with how much you have learned.

No social group has the potential to provide the same level of support and long-lasting emotional ties as one's own family. Maintaining healthy family life is so important to the health and welfare of the nation that several National Health Goals speak directly to maintaining healthy family and community life (Box 2.1). Because the family has such an influence on the individual, nursing care that considers the family, not the individual (**family nursing**), has become a focus of modern nursing practice. **Family theory** details a set of perspectives from the family's point of view that can help nurses address the important health issues of the child-bearing and child-rearing family.

For instance, for a family to adjust to a new family member, the family's structure and roles must be flexible enough to adjust to the changes that pregnancy and a newborn will bring. An ill family member or one who is going through a difficult developmental period, such as adolescence, can put a tremendous strain on a family. The roles individuals assume in the family and their ability to adjust to new roles can influence a family's perception of a child's illness, as well as the family's ability to adjust to these situations and work through to a positive family outcome. Because families do not live in isolation, the family's ability to thrive in a community and gain strength from the community is equally important. For this reason, the modern concept of maternal and child health nursing is not limited to assessing individuals or individual circumstances, but rather examines them from a family and community standpoint.

Family and community-centered maternal and child health nursing considers the strengths, vulnerabilities, and patterns of family and community function to support families during childbirth and childrearing and to

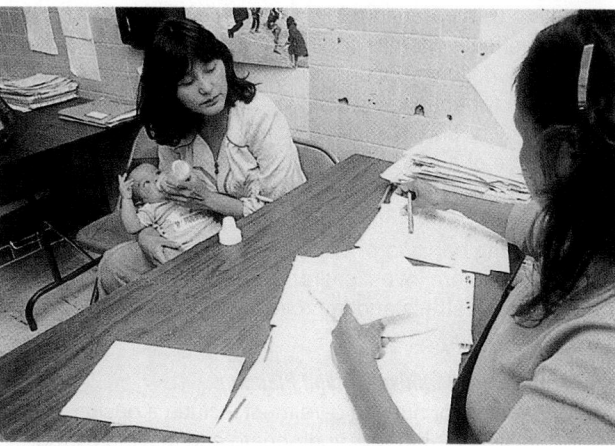

FIGURE 2.1 Community health nurses can be instrumental in helping a new parent gain access to area programs to improve child care.

encourage healthy coping mechanisms in families facing a crisis. Health assessment and intervention planning should include consideration of the family's social, emotional, spiritual, and financial resources, as well as the physical and emotional condition of the home and the community (Fig. 2.1).

Nursing Process Overview

For Promotion of Family Health

● *Assessment*
Family/community assessment provides information to a family on the ability to remain well or the meaning of a current health situation, as well as the emotional support an individual family member can expect from other family members or the community. This is vital to understanding what a pregnancy or childhood illness means to different members of the family, especially if not all members are in agreement. Family structure and function both need to be considered.

● *Nursing Diagnosis*
Nursing diagnoses used in connection with families and communities generally relate to the family's ability to handle stress and to provide a positive environment for individual growth and development. Examples include the following:

- Parental role conflict related to prolonged separation from child during long hospital stay
- Interrupted family processes related to emergency hospital admission of oldest child
- Impaired parenting related to unplanned pregnancy
- Ineffective family coping related to inability to adjust to mother's illness during pregnancy
- Readiness for enhanced family coping related to improved perceptions of child's capabilities
- Health-seeking behaviors related to birth of first child

"Impaired parenting" and "parental role conflict" are diagnoses that suggest that parents need additional

---

BOX 2.1 FOCUS ON . . .

NATIONAL HEALTH GOALS

A number of National Health Goals speak directly to achieving healthy family and community life. The following goals are representative of these:

- Lower the current baseline of 25.2 children per 1,000 younger than age 18 who are maltreated.
- Reduce physical abuse directed at women by male partners to no more than 27 per 1,000 couples from a current baseline of 30 per 1,000 couples.
- Eliminate the prevalence of blood lead levels exceeding 10 µg/dL in children aged 1 month to 6 years from a baseline of 4.4% (DHHS, 2000).

Nurses can help to see that goals such as these for healthier family living are met by assessing families and their environment to identify families at risk, assisting with counseling or further testing, and maintaining contact with families to ensure that long-term measures for care can be instituted. Intimate partner violence is further discussed in Chapter 14 and child abuse in Chapter 55; lead poisoning from excessive lead in the environment is discussed in Chapter 52.

help with parenting. The first family coping diagnosis ("ineffective family coping") indicates that a family is not functioning at an optimal level; the second ("readiness for enhanced family coping") is used for a well family or one that is exhibiting enhanced growth because of a specific event, such as the sudden diagnosis of illness in a child or an unplanned pregnancy. "Readiness for enhanced parenting" and "health-seeking behaviors" are diagnoses that apply to families who are investigating more effective ways to manage stress and improve family/community functioning.

- **Outcome Identification and Planning**
  Planning for nursing care must include a design that is family-centered and appropriate and desired by the majority of family members; otherwise, family members may have difficulty following the plan. The plan must also consider the community. For example, it is not helpful to suggest that a family take regular walks together to encourage shared decision making and improve family communication if walking in their neighborhood is unsafe; participation in a family gym class at a local YMCA might be more practical in this instance.

- **Implementation**
  A plan for improving family/community health should flow smoothly if family members have agreed on it out of support for one another. It may be necessary in some instances to encourage family members to agree on a plan or to abide by a chosen plan. Otherwise, they may expend needless energy carrying out an activity that is counterproductive or in direct opposition to their major goal.

- **Outcome Evaluation**
  Evaluation should reveal not only that a goal was achieved but also that the family feels more cohesive after working together toward the goal. If evaluation does not reveal these two factors, reassessment is necessary to determine whether further interventions are required. Examples of expected outcomes that might be established include the following:

  - Family members state they are adapting well to the presence of a newborn.
  - Mother states she feels prepared to manage home care of her ill child.
  - Father states he has arranged the family finances to accommodate new health care expenses for the family.

THE FAMILY

How well a family works together and how well it can organize itself against potential threats depend on its structure (who its members are) and its function (the activities or roles family members carry out). Recognizing different family structures allows health care providers to focus on family-centered care or provide a family-friendly environment for care (Franck & Callery, 2004).

Defining the Concept of Family

A **family** is defined by the U.S. Census Bureau (2005) as "a group of people related by blood, marriage, or adoption living together." This definition is workable for gathering comparative statistics but is limited when assessing a family for its health concerns or the support people available, because some families are made up of unrelated couples, and at certain points in life not all family members may live together. Allender and Spradley (2004) defined the family in a much broader context as "two or more people who live in the same household (usually), share a common emotional bond, and perform certain interrelated social tasks." This is a better definition for health care providers, because it addresses the broad range of types of families that health care providers encounter.

Family Types

Many types of families exist, and family types change over time as they are affected by birth, work, death, divorce, and the growth of family members. For the purposes of assessing families in maternal and child health nursing, two basic family types can be described:

- **Family of orientation** (the family one is born into; or oneself, mother, father, and siblings, if any)
- **Family of procreation** (a family one establishes; or oneself, spouse or significant other, and children)

More specific descriptions of family types vary greatly depending on family roles, generational issues, means of family support, and sociocultural influences. Almost all families, regardless of type, share common activities.

The Dyad Family

A dyad family consists of two people living together, usually a woman and a man, without children. Many single young adults live together as a dyad in shared apartments, dormitories, or homes for companionship and financial security while completing school or beginning their careers. Dyad families are generally viewed as temporary arrangements, but if the couple chooses child-free living, this can also be a lifetime arrangement.

The Nuclear Family

The traditional nuclear family structure is composed of a husband, wife, and children. It is the most common structure seen worldwide and throughout history. Today, however, the number of nuclear families in the United States has declined to about 50% of families due to the increase in divorce, single parenthood, and remarriage and the greater acceptance of alternative lifestyles. Increasing in incidence is the single-headed family (from 10% of all families in 1960 to almost 32% today) (National Center for Health Statistics [NCHS], 2005). An advantage of a nuclear family is its ability to provide support to family members, because, with its small size, people feel genuine affection for each other. In a time of crisis, this same characteristic may become a challenge to a family (i.e., there are few family members to share the burden and offer support). This makes helping nuclear families locate and reach out to support people during a crisis an important nursing responsibility.

The Cohabitation Family

Cohabitation families are composed of heterosexual couples who live together like a nuclear family but remain unmarried. Although such a relationship may be temporary, it may also be as long-lasting and as meaningful as a more traditional alliance and therefore offer as much psychological comfort and financial security as a marriage. Long-term cohabitation unions are growing in number because of the pressure to adhere to a monogamous relationship to avoid contracting a sexually transmitted infection, and also because of a more widespread acceptance of cohabitation by society. Because cohabitation unions simulate nuclear families, the strengths and challenges of these families are the same as those of nuclear unions.

The Extended (Multigenerational) Family

The extended family includes not only the nuclear family but also other family members such as grandmothers, grandfathers, aunts, uncles, cousins, and grandchildren. An advantage of such a family is that it contains more people to serve as resources during crises and provides more role models for behavior or values. A possible disadvantage of an extended family is that family resources, both financial and psychological, must be stretched to accommodate all members. When assessing such families, remember that because of the many members present, a parent's strongest support person may not be a spouse or intimate partner, and a child's primary caregiver may not be his or her mother or father. The grandmother or an aunt or another sibling, for example, may provide the largest amount of support or child care, even though spouses and the child's parents are also present every day.

The Single-Parent Family

In as many as 50% to 60% of families with school-age children today, only one parent lives in the home. Of those families, 17% have a man as the single parent (NCHS, 2005). This increase in single-parent families is a result of both the high rate of divorce and the increasingly common practice of women raising children outside marriage. A health problem in a single-parent family is almost always compounded: if the parent is ill, there is no back-up person for child care. In addition, if a child is ill, there is no close support person to give reassurance or a second opinion on whether the child's health is worsening or improving.

Low income is often an additional problem encountered by single-parent families, because the parent is most often a woman and women's incomes are lower than men's by about 24% (Benokraitus, 2005). Single parents also may have difficulty with role modeling or clearly identifying their role in the family (i.e., they must provide duplicate roles, or financial support as well as child care). Trying to fulfill several central roles in this way is not only time-consuming but also mentally and physically exhausting and, in many instances, not rewarded. Such a parent may develop low self-esteem (if a spouse left or if the other pa-

rent refuses to help with child support). Single-parent fathers may have difficulty with home management or child care if they had little experience with these roles before the separation. Such feelings can interfere with decision making and can impede daily functioning.

A single-parent family has the advantage of offering a child a special parent–child relationship and increased opportunities for self-reliance and independence. If there has been a divorce, one parent may have been given legal custody of the children, or both parents may have joint custody. Either way, both parents often participate in decision making. At a time of illness, both may visit the ill child and be eager to receive reports of the child's progress. Identifying who is the custodial parent is especially important when consent forms for care are signed.

The Blended Family

In a blended family, or a remarriage or reconstituted family, a divorced or widowed person with children marries someone who also has children. Advantages of blended families include increased security and resources for the new family. Another benefit is that the children of blended families are exposed to different ways of life and may become more adaptable to new situations.

Childrearing problems may arise in this type of family from rivalry among the children for the attention of a parent or from competition with the stepparent for the love of the biologic parent. In addition, each spouse may encounter difficulties in helping rear the other's children. Often stepparents believe they are thrust into a limited or challenged role of authority. Children may not welcome a stepparent because they have not yet resolved their feelings about the separation of their biologic parents (through either divorce or death); the stepparent may differ from the biologic parent, particularly in terms of discipline and caregiving; or they may believe that the stepparent threatens their relationship with their biologic parent. They may have heard so many stories about evil stepparents that they come to the new family prejudiced against their new parent. They may also become distressed at seeing their other biologic parent move into another home and become a stepparent to other children.

Although financial difficulties usually lessen in this type of family, finances can be severely limited, especially if one or both parents are obligated to pay child support for children from a previous marriage while supporting the children of the current marriage. If there is economic disparity between the biologic parents, conflicts and distorted expectations can occur. Nurses can be instrumental in offering emotional support to members of a remarriage family until the adjustments for mutual living have been made.

The Communal Family

Communes comprise groups of people who have chosen to live together as an extended family. Their relationship to each other is motivated by social or religious values rather than kinship (Benokraitus, 2005). Members often fulfill few traditional family roles. The values of commune members may be more oriented toward freedom and free choice than those of a traditional family. Some communes are described as cults or comprise a group of people who follow a charismatic leader. Adolescents, because they are in the process of determining what values to adopt for their future life, may find this type of commune particularly appealing.

People living in a commune may not wish to follow traditional health care regimens, preferring instead to use complementary or alternative therapies (health care may be seen as an established system that they are rejecting). On the other hand, people who reject traditional values may be the most creative people in a community, the most interested in participating in their own care and ripe for health teaching and learning.

The Gay or Lesbian Family

In homosexual unions, individuals of the same sex live together as partners for companionship, financial security, and sexual fulfillment. Such a relationship offers support in times of crisis comparable to that offered by a nuclear or cohabitation family. Some lesbian and gay families include children from previous heterosexual marriages or through the use of artificial insemination, adoption, or surrogate motherhood. Laws governing homosexual partners can affect health care if they limit health insurance coverage. Lack of understanding by health care providers of the strength and richness of these unions can further impede health care (Bevaqua, 2004).

Checkpoint Question 1

The Hanovan family was a single-parent one before Mrs. Hanovan remarried. What is a common concern of single-parent families?

a. Too many people give advice.
b. Finances are inadequate.
c. Children miss many days of school.
d. Children don't know any other family like theirs.

The Foster Family

Children whose parents can no longer care for them may be placed in a foster or substitute home by a child protection agency (Kapp and Vela, 2004). Foster parents may or may not have children of their own. They receive remuneration for their care and concern for the foster child. Foster home placement is theoretically temporary until children can be returned to their own parents. If return is impossible or is not imminent, children may be raised to adulthood in foster care. Such children may experience almost constant insecurity, concerned that soon they will have to move again. In addition, they may have some emotional difficulties related to the reason they were removed from their original home.

When caring for children from foster homes, it is important to determine who has legal responsibility to sign for health care for the child (a foster parent may or may not have this responsibility). Most foster parents are as concerned with health care as biologic parents and can be depended on to follow health care instructions conscientiously.

The Adoptive Family

Families of a great many types (nuclear, extended, single-parent, gay and lesbian) adopt children today. No matter what the family structure, adopting brings a number of challenges to the adopting parents and the child, as well as to any other children in the family (McCarthy et al., 2003).

Methods of Adoption

Agency Adoption. In traditional agency adoption, a couple usually contacts an agency by first attending an informational meeting. If the couple decides to apply to the agency, they are then put on a waiting list for processing. A process that includes extensive interviewing and a home visit by an agency social worker determines whether the couple can be relied on to provide a safe and nurturing environment for an adopted child. Once approved by the agency, the couple is placed on a second waiting list. When a child has been located for them, the agency notifies the couple. Depending on the area of the country and the couple's particular requests, this may take anywhere from less than a year to 5 or 6 years. There are children in every state who are waiting for adoption and can be placed almost immediately into adopting homes, but most of these children are older and have lived with many foster families or have gone back and forth between the homes of their birth parents and foster care. Many others have special health care needs, are of a different ethnic or cultural background from the prospective adoptive parents, or are learning challenged. Although this is not an option that is appealing for every couple, adoption of such children can be a very rewarding experience for the right couple and will achieve a family for them.

Historically, there was little or no communication between the woman placing her baby for adoption and the adopting couple. In the past, this was seen as an advantage because the birth mother could then not interfere in the new couple's lives. Today, the disadvantage of this arrangement for the child is being realized: should a child want to learn his or her birth family's name or medical history or location, this information was not available. This has led to "open adoption" procedures, in which the identity of neither the birth mother nor the adoptive parents is kept secret, allowing as much interaction as desired between the two sets of parents (Rushton, 2003).

International Adoption. International adoption can often provide a baby in less time than a traditional agency adoption, but there may be unanswered questions about prenatal health care or the birth parent's background with this method. In addition, countries that are willing to permit abandoned or orphaned children to be adopted internationally are often economically disadvantaged or war-torn, meaning the child's health or development may have suffered. War conditions may allow children to be released from the country one day but not the next. This means that couples who are waiting for an international adoption must be ready at a moment's notice to travel to the foreign country or to a neutral location to pick up their child or to give up the adoption because political reforms have stopped the release of children.

A home visit from a local agency and a significant amount of paperwork and communication with the international

creased focus on health promotion and maintenance have added to the increased responsibilities for families to monitor their own health.

Because of consumer awareness, nurses have an increased responsibility to include parents and children in health care decisions. Using the nursing process for planning helps to accomplish this, because the goal-setting step encourages patient participation. Health teaching, such as reducing smoking in the home or increasing the fiber content in meals, becomes more effective if the learners are interested in improving their health.

Increased Abuse in Families

An alarming statistic is that incidence and reports of domestic abuse (both child and intimate partner) is increasing yearly. This is apparently related to both an increased stress level in the population as a whole and better reporting of abuse. Detecting abuse begins with the awareness that it does occur. Careful screening at family contacts reveals this. Abuse is covered in Chapter 55.

ASSESSMENT OF FAMILY STRUCTURE AND FUNCTION

Family health can be assessed on a variety of levels and in varying degrees of detail. The type of family data collected and the method of collection should match the way in which the assessment data will be used.

General characteristics of family type and functioning can be assessed using observation and general history questions (Table 2.1). If more detailed information about family environment and roles is required, use of an assessment tool specifically developed for that purpose is most effective.

The Well Family

Assessment of psychosocial family wellness requires measurement of how the family relates and interacts as a unit, including communication patterns, bonding, roles and role relationships, division of tasks and activities, governance of the family structure, decision-making and problem-solving, and leadership within the family unit. Assessment also looks at how the family relates to the outside community.

The **genogram,** a diagram that details family structure, provides information about the family's history and the roles of various family members over time, usually through several generations (Fig. 2.2). The genogram provides a basis for discussion and analysis of family interaction.

The Family APGAR (Smilkstein, 1978) is a screening tool of the family environment (Fig. 2.3). A family APGAR form is administered to each family member, and their scores are compared. The tool is easy to use and can complement the history.

TABLE 2.1

Family Assessment

Area of Assessment	Questions to Ask
Type of family	Who lives in the home? Is the family nuclear, extended, or other?
Family finances	Are finances adequate? Is money divided evenly among family members?
Safety	Is the home safe from fire or unintentional injuries (are smoke alarms present and police and fire numbers posted?)
Health	Does the family eat a nutritious diet? Do they receive adequate sleep? Are immunizations current? Is there a balance between work and recreation? Can they cope with problems adequately?
Emotional support	
Within family	Do members eat together or spend an equal amount of time with each other daily? Do they band together to defend each other from outsiders?
Outside family	Is the family active in community organizations or activities? Do they visit (or are they visited by) friends and relatives? Can the family name one outside person they can always rely on for help in a time of crisis?
Family roles	
Nurturing figure	Who is the primary caregiver to children or any physically or cognitively challenged member?
Provider	Who brings in the bulk of the family's income?
Decision-maker	Who makes decisions, particularly in the area of lifestyle and leisure time?
Financial manager	Who supervises the family finances (pays the bills, provides for future savings?)
Problem-solver	Who does the family depend on to provide the solution for problems?
Health manager	Who ensures that family members keep health appointments, immunizations are kept current, and preventive care such as a mammogram for the mother is scheduled?
Gatekeeper	Who determines what information will be released from the family or what new information can be introduced?

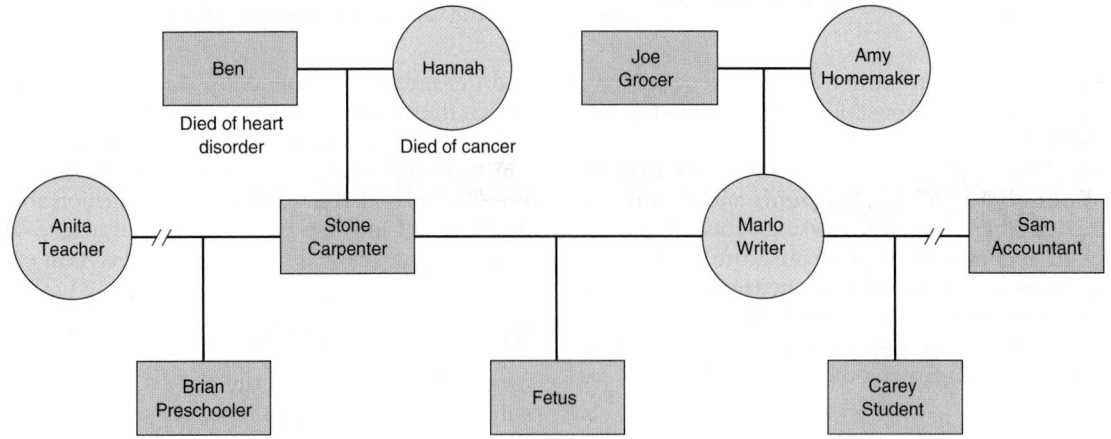

FIGURE 2.2 A Hanovan family genogram showing three generations. Males are shown by squares, females by circles.

The Family APGAR Questionnaire

	Almost always	Some of the time	Hardly ever
I am satisfied with the help that I receive from my family* when something is troubling me.	_____	_____	_____
I am satisfied with the way my family discusses items of common interest and shares problem solving with me.	_____	_____	_____
I find that my family accepts my wishes to take on new activities or make changes in my lifestyle.	_____	_____	_____
I am satisfied with the way my family expresses affection and responds to my feelings such as anger, sorrow and love.	_____	_____	_____
I am satisfied with the way my family and I spend time together.	_____	_____	_____

SCORING

Scoring: The patient checks one of three choices, which are scored as follows: 2 points for "Almost always," 1 point for "Some of the time" and 0 for "Hardly ever." The scores for each of the five questions are then totaled. A score of 7 to 10 suggests a highly functional family. A score of 4 to 6 suggests a moderately dysfunctional family. A score of 0 to 3 suggests a severely dysfunctional family.

WHAT IS MEASURED

Adaptation	How resources are shared, or the member's satisfaction with the assistance received when family resources are needed.
Partnership	How decisions are shared, or the member's satisfaction with mutuality in family communication and problem solving.
Growth	How nurturing is shared, or the member's satisfaction with the freedom available within the family to change roles and attain physical and emotional growth or maturation.
Affection	How emotional experiences are shared, or the member's satisfaction with the intimacy and emotional interaction within the family.
Resolve	How time* is shared, or the member's satisfaction with the time commitment that has been made to the family by its members.

*Besides sharing time, family members usually have a commitment to share space and money. Because of its primacy, time was the only item included in the Family APGAR; however, the nurse who is concerned with family function will enlarge understanding of the family's resolve by inquiring about family member's satisfaction with shared space and money.

FIGURE 2.3 The Family Apgar Questionnaire. (Smilkstein, G. [1978]. The Family APGAR, *Journal of Family Practice, 6,* 1231.)

The Family in Crisis

Nursing assessment of the family often occurs when the family is in crisis. The way families react to a crisis depends largely on the particular crisis, their past experiences with problem-solving, their perception of the event (whether they can clearly see what is the problem), and the resources available to them to help solve the problem. McCubbin and colleagues (2000) suggested that assessing these factors is vital to predicting the probable extent of the crisis for the family. A crisis can change a family's perceptions and the resources available to them, so renewed assessment is necessary to see how the family is weathering the impact (a double ABCX model of assessment; Fig. 2.4).

To use this model, first assess what is the stressor (an event or transition that has the potential to influence the family's dynamics) that is affecting the family. A house fire would be an example. Next, assess the family's perception of the stressor. If the family states, for example, that they had adequate insurance so everything can be replaced, the stressor may have little effect, but if they feel overwhelmed by the loss of their home and possessions, it is causing a major effect. The third step is to evaluate the resources available to the family, both internal and external. What is the family type? What are their challenges? Do they have friends who can help replace their possessions? Do they belong to a church or temple that will help? Every family makes some kind of adjustment to a problem. This adjustment and the resulting changed perception of the event by the family lead to a need for further assessment.

This model is a useful one for family assessment, because it does not assume that just because a stressor happens, an automatic outcome will occur. It respects the individuality of families, an important factor to remember in family assessment.

Listing a family's strengths and coping abilities as well as its possible challenges helps in planning care; in addition, this process actually strengthens the family as it brings out insights and better prepares family members to cope with the current level of stress and the difficult decisions that may be ahead. Box 2.8 provides practical suggestions to help families enduring periods of stress.

THE FAMILY AS PART OF A COMMUNITY

Community can be defined in many ways, but it is generally accepted to refer to a limited geographic area in which the residents relate to and interact among themselves. When asked what community they are from, people may mention an entire city, a school district, a geographic district ("the East Side"), a street name ("Pine Street area"), or a natural marking ("the Lower Creek area").

Because the health of individuals is influenced by the health of their community, it is important to become acquainted with the community in which you practice. If you are caring for a client or family from a community unknown to you, then assess that community to see if there are aspects about it that contributed to an illness (and therefore need to be corrected) and to determine whether the person will be able to return to the community without extra help and counseling after recovering from an illness (Fig. 2.5).

Community assessment consists of examining the various systems that are present in almost all communities to see whether they are functioning adequately. Knowing the individual aspects of families or community can help you understand why some people reach the illness level they do before they come for health care (e.g., a woman living alone in a city has no transportation available to her until her husband comes home from work, so she cannot

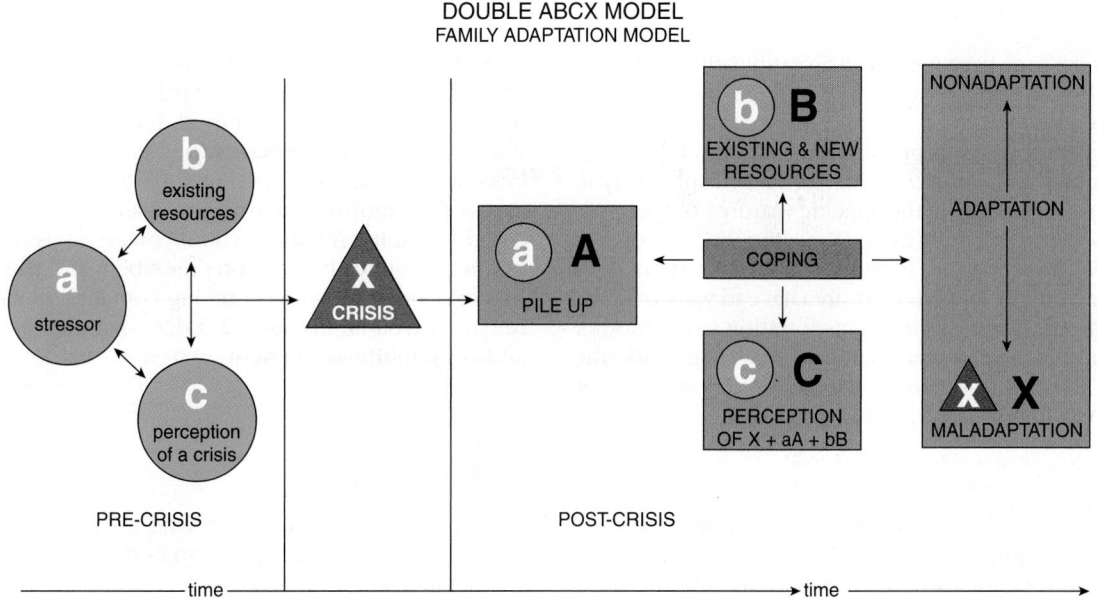

DOUBLE ABCX MODEL
FAMILY ADAPTATION MODEL

FIGURE 2.4 The ABCX System for Family Assessment. (McCubbin, H. I., Thompson, E. A., Thompson, A. L. & Futrell, J. A. [2000]. *The dynamics of resilient families.* Thousand Oaks, CA: Sage Publications.)

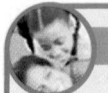

BOX 2.8 FOCUS ON . . .

FAMILY TEACHING

Tips for Reducing Family Stress

Q. Suppose Mr. Hanovan tells you he is worried because the tension level in his family is growing. He asks you, "How can my family better manage stress?"

A. Managing stress calls for interventions specific to each family, but some general suggestions are:

1. Recognize that stress levels differ from person to person. Because one person is not upset by some condition does not mean that another person will not be annoyed or upset. On the other hand, if a situation does not annoy a person, that person should not feel that he or she has to react to it just because someone else does.
2. Learn to change those things you cannot accept and accept those things you cannot change. Trial and error is often required to determine the difference.
3. Often a total change is unnecessary; a simple modification will be ample to make the difference.
4. State your personal reactions to stress. Almost nothing limits the extent of a threat more than being able to describe it accurately.
5. Reach out for support. People under stress are often so involved in their problems that they do not realize that people around them want to help. Sometimes the people closest to the person feeling stress are under a similar threat and so are no longer able to offer support. When this happens, the person must call on second- or third-level support people (family or community) for help.
6. Reach out to give support when others are being threatened. Survival is a collaborative function of social groups; a favor offered now can be called in when you are in need at a later date.
7. Face a situation as honestly as possible. As a rule, knowing the exact nature of a threat is less stressful than a "something-is-out-there" feeling. On the other hand, do not feel compelled to face intense threats, such as a serious complication of pregnancy or a fatal illness in a child, until you have had time to mobilize your defenses, or you may be overwhelmed.
8. Do not rush decisions or make final adaptive outcomes to a stressful situation. As a rule, major decisions should be delayed at least 6 weeks after an event; 6 months is even better.
9. Anticipate life events and plan for them to the extent possible. Anticipatory guidance will not totally prepare you for a coming event but will at least serve notice that distress over the situation is normal.
10. Remember that unintentional injuries increase when people are under stress. A person worrying about a complication of pregnancy, for example, is more apt to have an automobile accident than a person who is stress-free. Children are more apt to poison themselves when the family is under stress.
11. Action feels good during stress because doing something brings a sense of control over feelings of helplessness and disorganization. Action often is so satisfying that people do things such as write threatening letters or shout harmful remarks that they later regret. Channel your energy into therapeutic action (such as going for a long walk) instead.

come for daytime prenatal care; a 5-year-old child develops measles because there are no free immunization services in the community).

It is easier for you to prepare a woman or child for return to a community after childbirth or a hospital stay if, for example, you know the specific features of the community where the family lives. (Does the Pine Street area have well or city water? How many flights of stairs does someone from the Stevens Plaza area have to walk to reach an apartment? Is there public transportation so the mother can return for her 2-week and 6-week visits with the baby?) Table 2.2 summarizes areas of community assessment to use in discharge planning.

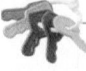

What if... your assessment of one child who is ready for hospital discharge shows that his family has multiple connections with the community, but the assessment of Carey and the Hanovan family shows only the hospital as a connection? Which family might need more discharge planning?

A second aspect of community assessment is to determine the health problems in particular communities and the relationship of the family to the community. This is done by means of an **ecomap,** a diagram of family and community relationships (Fig. 2.6). Such a map helps to assess the emotional support available to a family from the community. A family whom you assess as having few connecting lines between its members and the community may need increased nursing contact and support to remain a well family. Box 2.9 demonstrates both family and community assessment.

Key Points

A family is a group of people who share a common emotional bond and perform certain interrelated social tasks.

Common types of families include nuclear, extended, single-parent, blended, cohabitation, single alliance, gay and lesbian, foster, and adopted families.

Team Member Responsible	Assessment	Intervention	Rationale	Expected Outcome
Psychosocial/Spiritual/Emotional Needs				
Nurse	Help each family member identify the area of his or her greatest stress.	Help family members reduce stress by teaching better problem-solving techniques.	Identifying problems is the first step in effective problem solving.	Family members identify the greatest stressors in their family life and potential means to decrease stress.
Nurse	Assess stress-reducing measures currently being used.	Help family members develop strategies such as better time management to assist each other in meeting priority needs.	Use of therapeutic measures assists in clarifying the family needs and expectations and also helps reduce stress.	Family members say that they are using strategies such as time management to better meet priorities.
Discharge Planning				
Nurse	Meet with family to identify areas of needed support. Encourage family members to verbalize needs and feelings.	Help family identify a common activity enjoyed by all members that can be used to encourage family bonding. Encourage weekly participation in this activity.	Working together on a common task can foster group interaction, communication, trust, and bonding.	Family members say that they all participate in at least one enjoyable home activity by 2 months.
Nurse/Case Manager	Assess home rule and delegation of responsibilities.	Encourage joint cooperation in household tasks so client doesn't feel so isolated when home alone.	Joint ownership of household tasks encourages a sense of family.	Family members demonstrate they have a family schedule that evens out tasks and involves all members.
Nurse/Case Manager	Assess what resources are available in the Hanovans' community, such as the Cystic Fibrosis Foundation, that could be used as support resources.	Meet with family to see if members are interested in using any identified community organizations as resources.	Community resources provide additional support in areas of need.	Family members say that they have attended at least one Parents of Cystic Fibrosis Children meeting by 3 months' time.

Dreachslin, J. L., & Curtis, E. F. (2004). Study of factors affecting the career advancement of women and racially/ethnically diverse individuals in healthcare management. *Journal of Health Administration Education, 21*(4), 441–484.

Duvall, E. M., & Miller, B. (1990). *Marriage and family development.* Philadelphia: J. B. Lippincott.

Franck, L. S., & Callery, P. (2004). Re-thinking family-centered care across the continuum of children's healthcare. *Child: Care, Health and Development, 30*(3), 265–277.

Johnson, M., Maas, M., & Moorhead, S. (2000). *Nursing outcomes classification* (2nd ed.). St. Louis: Mosby.

Kapp, S. A., & Vela, R. H. (2004). The unheard client: Assessing the satisfaction of parents of children in foster care. *Child and Family Social Work, 9*(2), 197–206.

McCarthy, G., Janeway, J., & Geddes, A. (2003). The impact of emotional and behavioural problems on the lives of children growing up in the care system. *Adoption and Fostering, 27*(3), 14–19.

McCloskey, J., & Bulechek, G. (2000). *Nursing interventions classification* (3rd ed.). St. Louis: Mosby.

McCubbin, H. I., et al. (2000). *The dynamics of resilient families.* Thousand Oaks, CA: Sage Publications.

Menke, E. M. (2005). Children's experiences of being without a place to call home: What the research tells us. *Nursing Science Quarterly, 18*(1), 59–65.

Mezey, G., et al. (2005). Domestic violence, lifetime trauma and psychological health of childbearing women. *BJOG: An International Journal of Obstetrics and Gynecology, 112*(2), 197–201.

National Center for Health Statistics. (2005). *National Vital Statistics Reports 53*(17), 9.

Rojjanasrirat, W. (2004). Working women's breast-feeding experiences. *MCN: American Journal of Maternal/Child Nursing 29*(4), 222–229.

Rushton, A. (2003). Support for adoptive families: A review of current evidence on problems, needs and effectiveness. *Adoption and Fostering, 27*(3), 41–50.

Smilkstein, G. (1978). The family APGAR. *Journal of Family Practice, 6,* 1231.

Spencer, N. J. (2005). Disentangling the effects of different components of socioeconomic status on health in early childhood. *Journal of Epidemiology and Community Health, 59*(1), 2.

Trossman, S. (2004). No easy answers: Addressing the needs of undocumented immigrants. *American Nurse, 36*(6), 1–4.

United States Census Bureau. (2005). *Statistical abstract of the United States.* Washington, D.C.: U.S. Department of Commerce.

Wood, J. J., Repetti, R. L., & Roesch, S. C. (2004). Divorce and children's adjustment problems at home and school: The role of depressive/withdrawn parenting. *Child Psychiatry and Human Development, 35*(2), 121–142.

ABC XYZ Suggested Readings

Baumann, S. L., Dyches, T. T., & Braddick, M. (2005). Being a sibling. *Nursing Science Quarterly, 18*(1), 51–58.

Coren, E., & Barlow, J. (2005). Individual and group-based parenting programmes for improving psychosocial outcomes for teenage parents and their children. *Cochrane Library (Oxford) (1)* (CD002964).

Forbes, H., & Dziegielewski, S. F. (2003). Issues facing adoptive mothers of children with special needs. *Journal of Social Work, 3*(3), 301–320.

Griffin, T. (2003). Facing challenges to family-centered care: Anger in the clinical setting. *Pediatric Nursing, 29*(3), 212–214.

Holm, K. E., Patterson, J. M., & Gurney, J. G. (2003). Parental involvement and family-centered care in the diagnostic and treatment phases of childhood cancer: Results from a qualitative study. *Journal of Pediatric Oncology Nursing, 20*(6), 301–313.

Hughes, P. C., & Dickson, F. C. (2005). Communication, marital satisfaction, and religious orientation in interfaith marriages. *Journal of Family Communication, 5*(1), 25–41.

Litrownik, A. J., et al. (2003). Long-term follow-up of young children placed in foster care: Subsequent placements and exposure to family violence. *Journal of Family Violence, 18*(1), 19–28.

Mesich, H. M. (2005). Mother-infant co-sleeping: Understanding the debate and maximizing infant safety. *MCN: American Journal of Maternal/Child Nursing, 30*(1), 30–39.

Ochieng, B. M. (2003). Minority ethnic families and family-centered care. *Journal of Child Health Care, 7*(2), 123–132.

Zoritch, B., Roberts, I., & Oakley, A. (2005). Day care for preschool children. *Cochrane Library (Oxford) (1)* (CD000564).

CHAPTER 3

Sociocultural Aspects of Maternal and Child Health Nursing

Key Terms

acculturation
assimilation
cultural values
culture
ethnicity
ethnocentrism
mores
norms
pain threshold
pain tolerance
stereotyping
taboos
transcultural nursing

Objectives

After mastering the contents of this chapter, you should be able to:

1. Describe ways that sociocultural influences affect maternal and child health nursing care.
2. Assess a family for sociocultural influences that might influence the way it responds to childbearing and childrearing.
3. Formulate nursing diagnoses related to culturally appropriate aspects of nursing care.
4. Develop outcomes to assist families who have specific cultural needs to thrive in their community.
5. Plan and implement nursing care that respects the sociocultural needs and wishes of families.
6. Evaluate expected outcomes for achievement and effectiveness of care.
7. Identify National Health Goals related to sociocultural considerations that nurses can help the nation achieve.
8. Identify areas of care related to sociocultural considerations that could benefit from additional nursing research or application of evidence-based practice.
9. Use critical thinking to analyze how the sociocultural aspects of care affect family functioning and develop ways to make nursing care more family-centered.
10. Integrate sociocultural aspects of care with nursing process to achieve quality maternal and child health nursing care.

*M*aria Rodriques is a 12-year-old child who is hospitalized for surgical repair of a broken tibia, which was broken when she rode her bicycle into a busy street. She has a cast on her right leg and will be on bed rest for 3 days, then gradually allowed to learn crutch walking.

In planning care for her, you assume that because her culture is Hispanic, her family orientation will be male-dominant, her time focus will be on the present rather than the future, and her nutrition preferences will be Mexican American. Based on this, you consult with Maria's father regarding the major aspects of her care. You concentrate on talking mainly about her current problem (bed rest) rather than future care at home. You speak to the dietitian about avoiding milk, because lactase deficiency is present in many Mexican Americans.

You are surprised to hear Maria tell you on the second day of her hospital stay that she feels like a second-class person because her father has been asked for more input about her care than she has. She says she is particularly concerned that bone healing will not take place because she has had no milk to drink. She doesn't feel bed rest is a problem but is more concerned about being able to play soccer by next month.

Previous chapters described the standards and philosophy of maternal and child health nursing and family structure and function. This chapter adds information on how to care for families from diverse cultures. This is important information, because it both enriches care and helps protect the health of both women and children.

What went wrong with Maria's care?
If you had actually planned care in this way, of what would you have been guilty?
What would have been a better approach for determining this child's cultural preferences?

After you've studied this chapter, access the accompanying website. Read the patient scenario and answer the questions to further sharpen your skills, grow more familiar with RN-CLEX types of questions, and reward yourself with how much you have learned.

t is important to assess sociocultural status, ethnicity, and cultural beliefs of families and clients to understand why people take the type of preventive health measures that they do or seek a particular type of care for illness. Such factors can strongly influence their actions (Flowers, 2004).

Ethnicity refers to the cultural group into which a person was born, although the term is sometimes used in a narrower context to mean only race. **Culture** is a view of the world and a set of traditions that a specific social group uses and transmits to the next generation. **Cultural values** are preferred ways of acting based on those traditions. The way people react to health care is a cultural value.

Cultural values differ from nation to nation because they often arise from environmental conditions (for instance, in a country where water is scarce, daily bathing is not valued; in a country where meat is scarce, ethnic recipes use little meat). The usual values of a group are termed **mores** or **norms.** Expecting women to come for prenatal care and parents to bring children for immunizations are examples of norms in the United States, but these are not beliefs worldwide. Actions that are not acceptable to a culture are called **taboos.** Three taboos that are universal are murder, incest, and cannibalism. Issues such as abortion and robbery are controversial because these are taboos only to some people, not all people.

Cultural values strongly influence the manner in which people plan for childbearing and childrearing, as well as the way they respond to health and illness. In a culture in which men are the authority figures, for example, it might be the father rather than the mother who expects to answer questions about an ill child. If you are from a culture in which women usually provide all child care, you might find it annoying to hear a man taking over these responses at a health interview. If you have been culturally influenced to believe that stoic behavior is the "proper" response to pain, you may be impatient with a woman who has been influenced to believe that expressing discomfort during childbirth is "proper." Nurses need to be mindful to include all cultural groups in nursing research samples, so that more can be learned about cultural preferences in relation to nursing interventions and care.

Cultural differences occur across not only different ethnic backgrounds but also different lifestyles. Adolescents, urban youth, the hearing-challenged, and gays or lesbians have separate cultures from the mainstream. A parent who has been deaf since birth, for example, expects her deaf culture to be respected by having health care professionals attempt to communicate with her in her language. A lesbian mother could become irritated if she is asked, "Where is your husband?" as if, of course, everyone has one.

The United States is a country of such varied cultural groups and socioeconomic conditions that you are likely to see a wide range of behaviors exhibited (Fig. 3.1). Given the cultural mix, almost any behavior can be considered appropriate for some individuals at some time and place. Nursing care that is guided by cultural aspects and respects individual differences is termed **transcultural nursing** (Leininger, 2003).

Stereotyping means expecting a person to act in a characteristic way without regard to his or her individual traits It is generally derogatory in nature. Statements such as, "Men never diaper babies well," or "Japanese

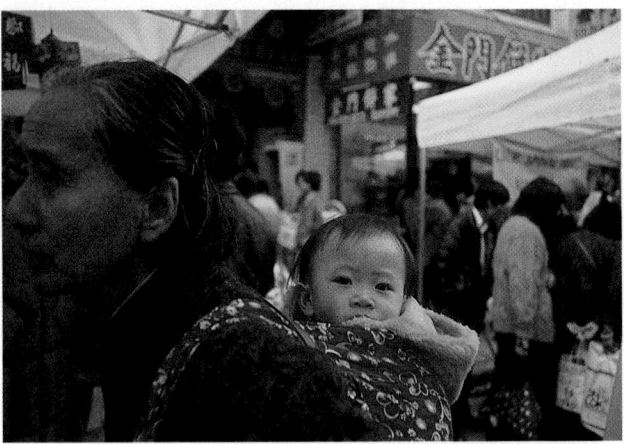

FIGURE 3.1 Various cultural preferences are evident in childrearing. In some cultures, extended family members such as grandparents take an active role in caring for children. Learning about different ways is important in care planning. (© Kathy Sloane.)

women are never assertive," are examples of stereotyping. Stereotyping occurs largely because of lack of exposure to enough people in a particular group and, consequently, a lack of understanding of the wide range of differences among people. In the examples given, the first speaker, having seen one man change diapers poorly, assumes that this represents the entire male population. The second example demonstrates lack of knowledge of a changing culture. If this person were exposed to more Japanese women, she or he certainly would find that the statement is not true. Stereotyping prevents you from planning care that is appropriate, individualized, and valued.

On the other hand, it is important not to ignore cultural characteristics, because most people are proud of their cultural heritage. It is possible to acknowledge and celebrate a client's culture without stereotyping by admiring the way in which he or she expresses cultural characteristics. Culture influences health so much that several National Health Goals have been established in reference to sociocultural aspects of care (Box 3.1).

Nursing Process Overview

That Respects Sociocultural Aspects of Care

● *Assessment*
Assessment of sociocultural factors is important to be certain that care is planned based not on predetermined assumptions but on the actual preferences of a family. To do this, each client must be assessed as an individual, not merely as one of a group. Note the cultural characteristics of the client that differ from the cultural expectations of the setting in which care is being provided, so that potential conflicts can be acknowledged and culturally competent care can be planned. Learn as much as you can about different cultures by reading about or talking to members of as many different ethnic groups as possible. Specific areas to assess,

BOX 3.1 FOCUS ON . . .

NATIONAL HEALTH GOALS

A number of National Health Goals are concerned with health practices that may be influenced by cultural factors:

- Increase the proportion of pregnant women who receive early and adequate prenatal care from a baseline of 74% to a target of 90%.
- Increase the proportion of mothers who breast-feed their babies in the early postpartum period from a baseline of 64% to a target of 75%, and increase the number who continue to breast-feed until their babies are 6 months of age from a baseline of 29% to a target of 50%.
- Increase the proportion of healthy full-term infants who are put down to sleep on their backs from a baseline of 35% to a target of 70%.
- Increase the proportion of young children who receive all vaccines that have been recommended for universal administration from a baseline of 73% to a target of 80% (DHHS, 2000).

Nurses can help the nation achieve these goals by designing prenatal and childcare services that take into account the cultural diversity in our country and by promoting the nutritional and immunologic advantages of breast-feeding in a culturally sensitive manner. Additional nursing research is needed on ways to make prenatal care and child health services more appealing to culturally diverse populations and on the educational methods that best reach people whose English is limited.

along with important findings in these areas, are shown in Table 3.1.

Assessing the culture of a community is as important as assessing individual families, because families are intrinsically joined to their community. An important area to assess is whether the family matches the dominant culture in the community. This is important because the type of foods stocked in supermarkets, the type of entertainment events that are planned, and the values and history that are stressed in schools and work settings are all influenced by the dominant culture.

Communities age, the same as families do. When homes are first built, many families tend to be young adults with children. Over the years, these families "settle in" to middle age, and later the homes are filled with families at retirement.

Older adults may find it difficult to relate if they move into a "young" community. A family who moves into a retirement-age community with young children may feel equally out of place. In all instances, a family that is of a culture other than the dominant one may have strong ties within the family but may have difficulty making strong, effective relationships in the community; this causes it to be more isolated than it would like to be. Community assessment is further discussed in Chapter 2.

● *Nursing Diagnosis*

Several nursing diagnoses speak to the consequences of ignoring cultural preferences in care:

- Powerlessness related to expectations of care not being respected
- Powerlessness related to sociocultural isolation
- Impaired verbal communication related to limited English proficiency
- Nutrition, less than body requirements, related to unmet cultural food preferences
- Anxiety related to a cultural preference for not bathing while ill
- Fear related to inability to buy food due to poor economic status

● *Outcome Identification and Planning*

Planning needs to be very specific for the family and the circumstances involved, because sociocultural preferences tend to be very personal. Care may begin with in-service education for health care providers who are unfamiliar with a particular cultural practice and its importance to the specific family involved. It may include arranging for variations in policy, such as the length of family visiting hours, types of food served, or type of child care provided. Such planning is beneficial because it can make health care more acceptable to a child or family and can also motivate providers to examine policies and question the rationale behind them.

● *Implementation*

Appreciate that cultural values are ingrained and usually very difficult to change (in yourself and in others). An example of implementing care might be making arrangements for a new Native American mother to take home the placenta if that is important to her, or planning home care for a Chinese-American child whose family believes in herbal medicine. It might be establishing a network of health care agency personnel or personnel from a nearby university or importing firm to serve as interpreters. It might be educating a child, family, or community about the reason for a hospital practice. Do not feel that you and the health care agency are always the ones who must adapt; a particular situation may call for both sides to adjust (cultural negotiation).

● *Outcome Evaluation*

Assessing whether expected outcomes have been met should reveal that a family's sociocultural preferences were considered and respected during care. If this was not achieved, procedures may need to be modified until this can be realized. Examples of expected outcomes that might be established include the following:

- Parents list three ways they are attempting to preserve cultural traditions in their children.
- Child states she no longer feels socially isolated because of cultural differences.
- Family members state they have learned to substitute easily purchased foods for traditional foods unavailable in local stores in order to obtain adequate nutrition.
- Child with severe hearing impairment writes that he feels communication with ambulatory care staff has been adequate.

TABLE 3.1

Assessing for Cultural Values

Area of Assessment	Questions to Ask or Observations to Make
Ethnicity	What country or race is the family from?
Communication	What's the main language used in the home?
Touch	Does the family typically touch each other? Do they use intimate or conversational space?
Time	Is being on time important? Is the family planning for the future?
Occupation	Is work important to the family? Do they plan leisure time or leave it unstructured?
Pain	Does the family express pain or remain stoic in the face of it? What do they believe relieves pain best?
Family structure	Is the family nuclear? Extended? Single-parent? Are family roles clear? Can an individual name a family member he/she would call on for support in a crisis?
Male and female roles	Is the family male or female dominant?
Religion	What is the family's religion? Do they actively practice their religion?
Health beliefs	What does the family believe about health? What do they believe causes illness? Makes illness better? Do they use alternative therapies or established practices?
Nutrition	Does the family eat an ethnic diet? Are the foods they enjoy available in their community?
Community	Is the predominant culture in the community the same as the family's? Can they name a neighbor they could call on in a crisis? Is the community a "young," a "settled-in," or a "retired" one? Is the culture one of immigration or stability?

SOCIOCULTURAL DIFFERENCES AND THEIR IMPLICATIONS FOR MATERNAL AND CHILD HEALTH NURSING

Respecting sociocultural values is particularly important in maternal and child health care, because childbearing and childrearing are times in life that are surrounded by many cultural traditions (Lawlor et al., 2005). Nurses can better provide multicultural care by understanding cultural concepts and sociocultural influences on families (Box 3.2).

Changing Cultural Concepts

Until recently, the United States was viewed as a giant cultural "melting pot," wherein all new arrivals gave up their native country's traditions and values and became "Americans." **Acculturation** refers to the loss of ethnic traditions. Cultural **assimilation** means that people have adopted the values of the dominant culture.

In the past, many Americans were intolerant of any behavior that was not like that of middle-class Americans, because they believed that the American way (which actually was the northern European way) was the "best" way. This belief that one's own culture is superior to all others is referred to as **ethnocentrism.** Ethnocentrism can lead to prejudice, because the feelings and ways of other cultures cannot be understood or appreciated without the philosophy that the world is large enough to accommodate a diversity of ideas and behaviors and that there is probably no "best" way to accomplish anything.

Traditionally, people whose cultures differ most drastically from the dominant culture suffer the greatest amount of rejection, because they are least able to assimilate. Over years of familiarity, mutual cultural assimilation does occur. As an example, when many Italians moved into American communities in the early 1900s, the average Italian family learned to speak English and the average American family learned to cook spaghetti with Italian sauce.

Today, many people question the idea that America ever was a melting pot; instead, the preferred concept is that of a "salad bowl," in which cultural traditions and values are tossed together, but with all their crispness and flavor retained, to make a perfect mix. Retaining ethnic traditions strengthens and enriches family life. It provides security to younger family members to realize that they are one of a continuing line of people who have a past and will have a future (Fig. 3.2) (Box 3.3).

Cultural competence, the integration of cultural elements to enhance communication and work effectively with people, is a goal worth achieving (Edwards, 2003). Numerous levels of cultural intolerance or acceptance persist, because many people continue to hold different beliefs along the cultural competence continuum (Fig. 3.3).

When planning nursing care, try to not only respect people's cultural differences but also help people share their cultural beliefs with health care providers, so that their beliefs can be considered and respected. As a nurse, you will have the opportunity to meet many people who hold cultural values different from your own. Throughout this text, Diversity of Care boxes feature specific cultural preferences as they relate to health care or nursing. Women are often the "keepers of the culture" or the

BOX 3.2 FOCUS ON . . .

EVIDENCE-BASED PRACTICE

Can cultural sensitivity education for nurses increase the satisfaction of culturally diverse patients?

To answer this question, nurse researchers assigned 114 health care providers (nurses and home care workers) and 133 patients (from two community agencies and one hospital) to either an experimental group, in which they received education in cultural sensitivity, or a control group, in which no cultural sensitivity education was given. Changes in people's attitudes were evaluated by a number of questionnaires. The results revealed that education in cultural sensitivity increased openmindedness and cultural awareness, improved understanding of multiculturalism, and augmented health care providers' ability to communicate with people from other cultures. After 1 year, patients (mostly of European and British origin) who received care from the providers in the experimental group showed improvement in using social resources and in overall functional capacity. The researchers concluded that cultural sensitivity education not only can improve knowledge and attitudes among health care providers but also yields positive health outcomes for their patients, without increasing health cost expenditures.

This is an important study for nurses because it suggests that change toward a more culturally sensitive health care system is possible if health care providers are willing to invest time and study in reducing the disparities that occur because of sociocultural influences.

Source: Majumdar, B., et al. (2004). Effects of cultural sensitivity training on health care provider attitudes and patient outcomes. *Journal of Nursing Scholarship, 36*(2), 161–166.

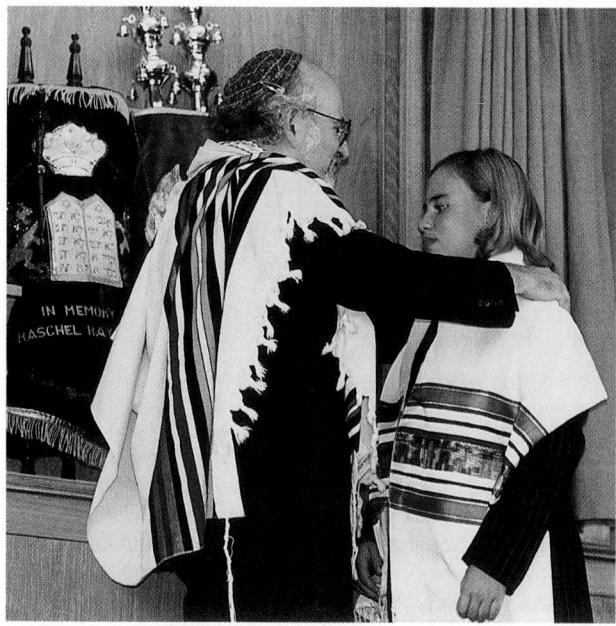

FIGURE 3.2 Cultural traditions offer a sense of security to children. (© Caroline Brown, RNC, MS, DEd.)

BOX 3.3 FOCUS ON . . .

FAMILY TEACHING

Preserving Cultural Heritage

Q. Mrs. Rodriques asks you, "How can I help my family preserve our cultural heritage?"

A. Preserving your individual heritage when living in another culture calls for creative planning. Some suggestions for doing this include the following:

- Plan an "ethnic night" once a week when only ethnic food is served. Encourage children to invite friends for the meal and discuss the traditions behind the various foods.
- If a foreign language is part of your traditions, reserve one night a week when family members speak only the native language.
- Choose books for children that are written by authors from your culture or that advantageously describe the culture. Read them together.
- Monitor television for programs that focus on your culture. Watch them with your children.
- As bedtime stories or "talk time," talk to your children about your childhood and traditions and values that differ from those of other families.
- Celebrate holidays in the traditional manner. Including cultural influences in holiday celebrations adds a rich ingredient and feeling of security to these occasions.

people most influential in passing on cultural traditions from one generation to another.

Checkpoint Question 1

Maria Rodriques is the 12-year-old student you met at the beginning of the chapter. Which statement by her is the best example of ethnocentrism?

a. My school, Stevens Park, is the best in the city.
b. Many schools in my city have good soccer teams.
c. Children from many cultures attend my school.
d. I want to go to a public, not a private college.

Techniques of Sociocultural Assessment

When assessing families as to whether there are socioeconomic or cultural influences that will make special considerations of care necessary, several categories of information related to the structure (composition) and function (roles and actions) of a family need to be examined.

Communication Patterns

Communication patterns (not only what people say, but also how they say it) are determined by culture and are

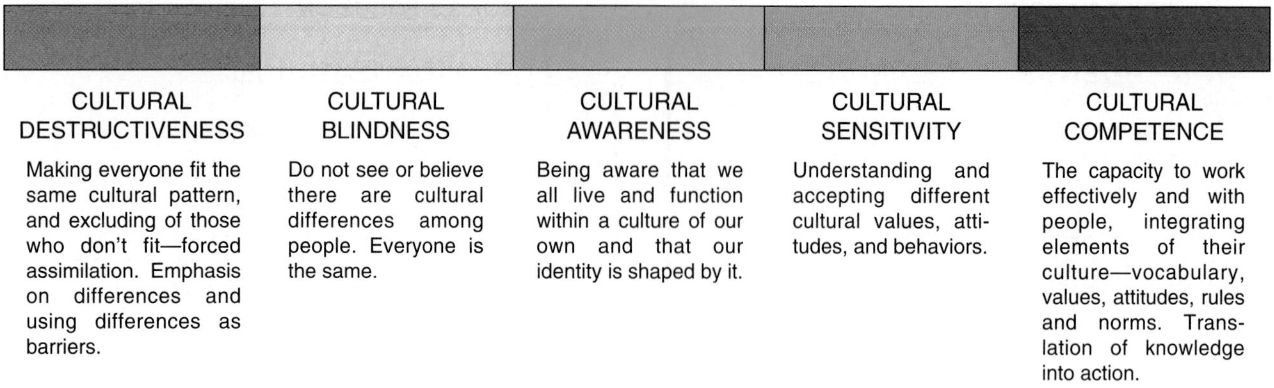

CULTURAL DESTRUCTIVENESS	CULTURAL BLINDNESS	CULTURAL AWARENESS	CULTURAL SENSITIVITY	CULTURAL COMPETENCE
Making everyone fit the same cultural pattern, and excluding of those who don't fit—forced assimilation. Emphasis on differences and using differences as barriers.	Do not see or believe there are cultural differences among people. Everyone is the same.	Being aware that we all live and function within a culture of our own and that our identity is shaped by it.	Understanding and accepting different cultural values, attitudes, and behaviors.	The capacity to work effectively and with people, integrating elements of their culture—vocabulary, values, attitudes, rules and norms. Translation of knowledge into action.

FIGURE 3.3 Cultural competence continuum. (Courtesy of the National Council of La Raza.)

increasingly important during times of stress. People who ordinarily associate only with members of their own culture, and therefore always speak their native language, may have great difficulty detailing a health history in English to a health care provider. Language barriers can be particularly significant for people who must give health histories when they or their child is ill, because their ability to cope and to express themselves in English may be at a low point. Even if people are able to converse well in English at work or in stores, they may not be able to recall the English words for symptoms such as nausea or dizziness, because these are not words that are commonly used. Unless you appear receptive, this person might omit mentioning a symptom rather than try to pantomime it or describe it in a different way.

Children who are embarrassed or bashful about speaking another language may simply not talk, and their needs may go unmet. As a general rule, it is unfair to ask children to interpret for their parents. If a child is frequently asked to interpret for his or her parents, he or she may be forced to miss days of school. Translating also can place a child in situations that require adult judgment (Jacobs, 2004). In some cultures, it might be unacceptable for a younger person to serve as an interpreter for an older person, because this shifts authority (Box 3.4).

The terms "Hispanic" and "Latina" or "Latino" refer to people who identify with a Spanish culture. There are about 16 million documented persons of Mexican, Puerto Rican, Cuban, or other Spanish-speaking origin in the United States. When added to the number of Spanish-speaking people who are undocumented or living illegally in the country, this group numbers close to 25 million, or about 12% of the total U.S. population (U.S. Census Bureau, 2004). Health care providers and Hispanic communities are encouraged to work together to bridge communication gaps by both helping community members who are not English proficient to learn more English and health care providers who are not Spanish proficient to learn to communicate better in Spanish.

Communication problems arise not only from foreign languages but also from dialects within a country. Something as simple as a New Englander's adding an "r" sound to the end of words (e.g., "idear" instead of "idea") may make an explanation difficult to follow. The slow cadence of a person from the South may seem strange to someone

BOX 3.4 FOCUS ON . . .

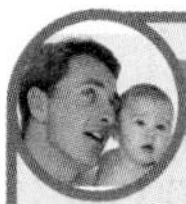

COMMUNICATION

Anna Rodriques brings her 4-year-old son, Pedro, to your pediatric clinic because she thinks he has an ear infection. She has brought a neighbor as an interpreter.

Less Effective Communication

Nurse: What's the reason you're here today?
Neighbor: She thinks her son has an ear infection.
Nurse: Is he pulling or tugging at it?
Neighbor: Not that I've seen.
Nurse: Does he have any pain?
Neighbor: She hasn't said anything about that.
Nurse: Well, I'll take his temperature, but I doubt it's an infection.

More Effective Communication

Nurse: What's the reason you're here today?
Neighbor: She thinks her son has an ear infection.
Nurse: Ask if he has been pulling or tugging at it.
Neighbor: I haven't seen him doing that.
Nurse: Would you ask if his mother has?

[The neighbor addresses Anna and then reports back.]

Neighbor: She says he's been pulling at it all morning.
Nurse: Ask Pedro if he has any pain.

[The neighbor addresses the child and then reports back.]

Neighbor: He says yes.
Nurse: Those are symptoms of an ear infection, all right.

Effectively using an interpreter adds additional responsibility to history taking. The nurse in the first scenario asked her first question of the mother but then directed all other questions to the interpreter. This means she secured a secondary history. When using an interpreter, be certain that the interpreter is "interpreting," not giving the history.

who is used to the rapid speech pattern of residents of New York City. Inner-city residents often speak a dialect unique to them. To care for such clients, it is important to learn their dialect's cadence and common words without attempting to use them yourself, unless that is your dialect. Trying to speak in a dialect not your own could be misinterpreted as mockery.

Touch is a form of communication. Whether people greet one another with hugs and kisses or do not touch each other at all is culturally determined. Not all people like to be touched or even to shake hands. For instance, some Asian Americans feel that rumpling the hair or palpating fontanelles is an intrusive gesture because they believe the head is the seat of the body's spirit and should not be touched (Liamputtong & Naksook, 2003).

Whether people look at one another when talking is also culturally determined. Chinese Americans, for example, may not make eye contact during a conversation. This social custom shows respect for the position of the health care professional and is a compliment, not an avoidance issue.

Be certain that cultural variations are respected in written as well as oral communications. In many instances, written communication is even more problematic than oral communication: many people can speak a second language but cannot write or read it. Using short, easy sentences and being certain not to use words with double meanings are important techniques (Box 3.5).

Use of Conversational Space

People of different cultures use the space around them differently. In the Western world, physical examinations are conducted in a very tight (intimate) space, because palpation is a part of the examination. Conversation, on the other hand, is usually held at a distance of between 18 inches and 4 feet. Business is most often conducted at a 4-foot distance. People from Eastern cultures may not be comfortable in this same space. Being aware that use of space is culturally determined helps you to respect the use of space for clients.

Respect for modesty is a way to respect close space. Be aware that women from some Middle Eastern cultures adhere to a level of modesty exceeding what you may be used to.

Time Orientation

The cultural pattern in the United States is geared toward punctuality regarding appointments. "Time is money" is an often-quoted axiom. Other cultures may not have this concern for time. They may have, instead, a concept that time is to be enjoyed. For such a person, there is no such thing as wasted time. In some South Asian cultures, being late for appointments is a sign of respect (giving the person you are meeting time to organize and be prepared for your arrival). Women who do not have a strict time orientation may view as strange the hospital's practice of feeding infants at designated times (e.g., 10 AM, 2 PM). People who are not accustomed to adhering to schedules in this way may have difficulty following a strict medical regimen. If they are told, for example, to give a child a medication at 8 AM, noon, and 6 PM daily and to return for another appointment at 2 PM in a week's time, you may have to stress that the medication should be taken three times a day, not necessarily at the specific times, but that returning for a checkup at a set time is important because the physician is in the health care facility only at that time.

Another way that time orientation differs is in whether a culture concentrates on the past, the present, or the future. The dominant U.S. culture is oriented to the present and future. People are expected not only to take care of themselves at the present moment but also to make plans for the future. Other cultures are oriented toward the past: they carefully preserve traditions, allowing only the slightest changes or variations in practices. Others are oriented toward the present; saving money for college (a future-oriented action) may not be a high priority in these cultures. If a family's orientation is for the present or the past, members may have difficulty accepting a long-term rehabilitation plan (e.g., by 6 months after an accident a boy will be walking with crutches, but it will be a full year before he will be fully ambulatory again). They may need to be motivated by present indications of progress (e.g., this afternoon the child will be allowed to sit up for the first time; this evening he can begin to have periods of time without oxygen).

The Amish are an example of a past-oriented culture: they adhere to time-honored traditions that do not include technologic advances such as immunizations. Some Native Americans also hold a past orientation. People from lower socioeconomic groups tend to be more present-oriented than those in middle or higher socioeconomic groups because of the struggle just to get through each day. People with strong religious convictions may be future-oriented

---

BOX 3.5

Improving Health Care When Clients Have Limited English Proficiency

Mrs. Rodriques' English proficiency is limited. What are some tips for working with families when communication is potentially blocked this way?

1. Many people can speak a second language better than they can read it. Assess the client's reading level and rewrite information at an easier reading level if necessary.
2. Ask an interpreter to translate material into the family's primary language.
3. Be certain that rooms in your health care agency, such as bathrooms, are labeled with international symbols.
4. Learn a few phrases, such as "Good morning" or "This won't hurt," from other languages, and use them in interactions with clients.
5. Use hand gestures or draw a figure, if need be, to communicate better. Imparting health information is what is important for safe care, not worrying how you look.
6. When using an interpreter, do not ignore the person seeking health care in preference to the interpreter.

(looking forward to a future existence better than their present one). Knowledge of these time orientations helps to plan effective care.

Work Orientation

The predominant culture in the United States stresses that everyone should be employed productively (called the Protestant work ethic) and that work should be a pleasure and valued in itself (as important as the product of the work). Other cultures do not value work in itself but see it as only a means to an end (you work to get money or food, not satisfaction). A woman with this latter orientation might be more distressed to learn that bed rest during pregnancy will interfere with her ability to continue a hobby (going to baseball games) than with her occupation (teaching). Do not interpret this behavior as lazy or unproductive; it is merely a cultural or individual variation.

Family Orientation

Family structure and the roles of family members may be culturally determined. In most cultures, the nuclear family (mother, father, and children) is most common. In other cultures, extended families (nuclear family plus grandparents, aunts, uncles, and cousins) and single-parent families (single parent and child) may be more common. Information about a family may be carefully guarded and not given freely at health care visits, as a way of keeping the family intact and unique (and as a reflection of mistrust for health care providers). When caring for children, however, be certain to identify a child's primary caregiver before giving health care instructions. Identifying the family decision-maker is also important, because this role can vary greatly from family to family.

Male and Female Roles

In most cultures, the man is the dominant figure. In such a culture, if approval for hospital admission or therapy is needed, the man is the one to give this approval. In a culture in which men are very dominant and women are extremely passive, a woman may be unable to offer an opinion of her own health or embarrassed to submit to a physical examination, especially from a male physician or nurse practitioner, unless a female nurse is also present. The incidence of intimate partner violence may be higher in male-dominant cultures. In an extremely male-dominated family, a woman's pregnancy may have resulted not from a mutual decision but from sexual relations she felt she could not refuse.

In contrast, in some cultures, the woman may be the dominant person in the family. The oldest woman in the home would be the one to give consent for treatment or hospital admission.

It is important to evaluate male and female roles in this way, because knowing the identity of the dominant person in the household also helps you to understand the impact of the illness on the family. If a woman is the family's dominant person and can no longer make her usual decisions because she is ill during pregnancy, for example, the entire family may be thrown into confusion. If the woman is a nondominant member, you may have to act as an advocate for her rights with a more dominant person.

In most hospitals today, the nursing staff expects the father to play an active role during labor and during a child's hospital stay. However, a man who does not maintain this role expectation or custom may be uncomfortable participating in labor or playing with a child. Awareness that male roles differ from country to country can help you find a middle ground for male participation in labor and child care.

What if... Mr. Rodriques says he wants no role in labor when his wife has her new baby? Would you encourage him to time contractions (a typical role for fathers) or allow him to sit quietly in a corner of the room, as he prefers?

Religion

Religion is culturally determined, although there are wide variations in what religions people practice. Because religion guides a person's overall life philosophy, it influences how he or she feels about health and illness, birth and death. Knowing what religion a family practices helps you locate a support person when needed, because this differs according to religion. It helps you in planning care because many nutritional practices, such as whether the family eats meat, can be dictated by religious beliefs. It also can have important implications for decision making during a difficult pregnancy or for childhood terminal care.

Health Beliefs

Health beliefs are not universal. Most people are familiar with the current controversy about whether male circumcision is necessary, for example. More surprising to most people is a belief that female circumcision (amputation of the clitoris and perhaps a portion of the vulva) is thought to be necessary in some cultures (Campbell, 2004).

It is generally assumed in the United States that illness is caused by documented factors such as bacteria, viruses, or trauma. In other cultures, however, illness may be viewed primarily as a punishment from God or an evil spirit, or as the work of a person who wishes harm to the sick person. An example of this is a belief among some Hispanics that an evil eye (*mal ojo*) can cause illness. People who believe that their own sins caused an illness may not be highly motivated to take medication or other measures to get well again (such a woman, when ill during a pregnancy, does not believe that a spoonful of penicillin will cure her). People from some cultures may receive more comfort from a spiritualist or "witch doctor" than from their physician or nurse practitioner. They may believe it is necessary to suffer pain to be rid of the illness. People with this belief might be reluctant to ask for pain medication. Understanding different beliefs allows you to understand cultural differences and to work out mutual goals, even when the patient's views are not those you would choose for yourself or for a member of your family (Box 3.6).

A Multidisciplinary Care Map for
A Child Needing Sociocultural Care

•

Maria Rodriques is a 12-year-old child who is hospitalized following surgical repair of a broken tibia, which was broken when she rode her bicycle into a busy street. She has a cast on her right leg and will be on bed rest for 3 days, then gradually allowed to learn crutch walking.

Family Assessment

Maria lives with her mother, Anna, her father, Carlos, and a 4-year-old brother, Pedro. She attends a local grade school and enjoys playing video games and reading Harry Potter books.

Client Assessment

Temperature, 99.4°F; pulse, 96 beats/min; respirations, 24/min. Observed lying on side, gritting teeth as if in pain. Hands clenched and eyes tearing. When asked if she has pain, she quietly states, "No. I'm okay." Father overheard saying to her, "We're proud you're so brave."

Cast on right leg dry and intact. Toes warm to touch. Intravenous fluid infusing without difficulty at keep-vein-open rate. Oral intake primarily tea and soup. Client's mother states, "She needs 'hot' foods to get better. Don't you have anything hotter?"

Nursing Diagnosis

Pain related to tissue trauma of surgery, with cultural belief to not voice pain.

Outcome Criteria

Client accepts pain medication when offered; nonverbal expressions of pain are minimal to absent. Begins to eat and manage self-care.

Team Member Responsible	Assessment	Intervention	Rationale	Expected Outcome
Self-Care Activities				
Nurse/ Physical Therapist	Assess what self-care activities child feels ready to begin.	Plan a program of self-care that is possible within constraints of limited ambulation.	Ability to complete self-care can add to self-esteem and supply physiologic benefits.	Client feeds self, is out of bed, and completes hygiene measures at 12-year-old level.
Consultations				
Nurse	Assess whether pain relief is adequate and determine what child feels will relieve pain.	Consult with pain management team to establish a total pain relief plan for client.	Optimal health care is often a collaborative practice.	Child states that pain management team plan is acceptable to her.
Procedures/Medications				
Nurse	Assess for both verbal and nonverbal indicators of pain.	Offer pain medication as prescribed before pain becomes acute.	Offering medications relieves the client of the need to ask for relief when her belief is that she should not express pain. It also allows the child to have some choice and control in her care.	Child's chart documents that pain medication was offered every 4 hours throughout hospital stay.

(continued)

Team Member Responsible	Assessment	Intervention	Rationale	Expected Outcome
Nutrition				
Nurse/ Nutritionist	Assess whether the child has food preferences that are not being met by hospital service.	Encourage the family to bring in foods from home that meet their cultural preferences, because food can be comforting.	Allowing the family to bring in foods demonstrates respect for their culture and increases the child's sense of security and being cared for.	Client increases nutrient intake by including foods brought from home.
Patient/Family Education				
Nurse	Assess the child's knowledge of broken bones and of why trauma leads to pain.	Explain the physiology of pain to family members as a way of explaining why the client is experiencing it.	Explanations help a child of this age understand what is happening, to minimize fear.	Client describes what pain is and acknowledges that she will have some until healing is complete and that asking for something to relieve it is expected and acceptable.
Spiritual/Psychosocial/Emotional Needs				
Nurse	Assess whether child has unmet needs other than pain relief.	Explain to child that you want to help, but that she needs to verbally express her needs to enable you to do so.	Children may imagine that health care providers are all-knowing.	Child agrees to participate in expressing the presence of other factors, such as loneliness or fear.
Discharge Planning				
Nurse	Assess with child what modifications she will need to make in her daily routine to adjust to cast.	Discuss with parents that their child may need modifications in daily routine to return to school.	Well-informed parents are able to make informed decisions.	Child says that she attends school daily because of modifications in usual lifestyle.

Women's concept of whether pregnancy is a time of wellness or illness differs in various cultures. Most American women visit health care facilities early in pregnancy, follow prenatal directives, and, at birth, allow a health care provider to supervise the birth. In other cultures, pregnancy and childbearing are considered such natural processes that a health care provider is unnecessary. The woman knows the special rules and taboos she must follow to ensure a safe birth and a healthy child, and she is an active participant in labor and birth. She may plan to breast-feed until the next child is born, or for as long as 1 to 5 years. Unless differences such as these are respected, it is difficult to plan prenatal care that meets an individual woman's needs.

The type of health care provider chosen is yet another trait that is not uniform across cultures. The health care delivery system in Mexico, for example, is less structured than the one in the United States. There are few physicians for the total population. Many drugs are available without prescription; therefore, a local pharmacist rather than a physician may serve as the main health care resource for many families. Families may first seek help for illness from a trusted family member. Such a member is termed *el que sabe* (the one who knows). During an illness, this person's approval of therapy is crucial; if it is not given, the ill person cannot comply with therapy. Outside the family structure are *yerberos* (herbalists), who grow and instruct people in the use of herbs or cures. Another advice source is a *curandero,* or one who heals by the use of herbs or diet. Others healers are *espiritualistos,* who can treat supernaturally caused illnesses, and *brujos,* who not only revoke evil spells but also turn them around onto others. *Parteras* are midwives who care for women during pregnancy and birth. For many people, turning to a *yerbero* or *curandero* is preferable to professional health care because these people do not charge a fee but only accept donations or an exchange of goods or services. Also, relating health problems to them is not difficult because there is no language problem (Page, 2004).

The type of therapy people choose to restore health is also dependent on culture. When one person wakes up with an upper respiratory infection, for example, he or she may immediately call a health care provider for a formal prescription. Another person with the same symptoms would first try an herbal or "natural" self-help method (Kemper and Barnes, 2003). Be aware when taking health histories how many people today are relying on complementary or alternative therapies and ask about these.

Checkpoint Question 2

While she is in the hospital, Maria Rodriques makes the following statements. Which is the best example of stereotyping?

a. My doctor is funny; he tells jokes and makes me laugh.
b. I'm glad I'm Mexican because all Mexicans are smart.
c. I'm sure my leg will heal quickly; I'm overall healthy.
d. I like Mexican food, although not if it tastes too spicy.

Nutrition Practices

Foods and their methods of preparation are strongly culturally related (Lee et al., 2005). In many instances, hospitalized children cannot find on the menu any foods that appeal to them because of cultural preferences. A Japanese diet, for example, includes many vegetables such as bean sprouts, broccoli, mushrooms, water chestnuts, and alfalfa. Children with this preference tire very quickly of the corn and peas common to a middle-class American diet. Fortunately, in most instances, a child's family can provide food that is appealing culturally and is still within prescribed dietary limitations (Fig. 3.4).

When counseling a woman about good nutrition during pregnancy, remember that respect for culturally preferred foods is important. People from some cultures, for example, tend to eat much less meat than those from other cultures. Adequate protein can be ingested, however, by mixing sources of incomplete protein such as beans and rice. Some women may omit various foods during pregnancy because they believe a particular food will mark a baby (e.g., strawberries cause birthmarks, raisins cause

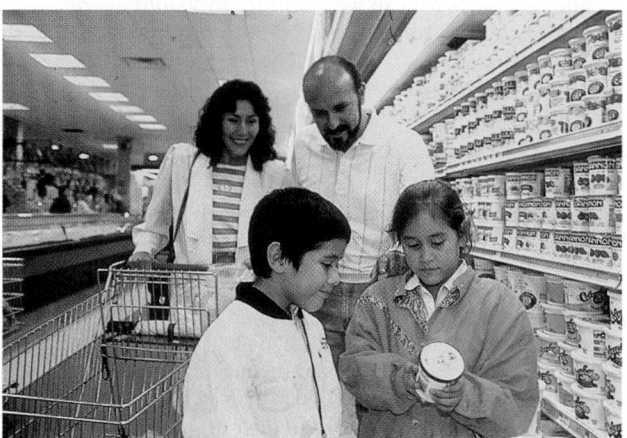

FIGURE 3.4 Families differ as to what food selections they prefer because of sociocultural preferences. (© Photo Researchers/Jeffrey Greenberg.)

brown spots), or they believe that it is necessary to eat "hot" or "cold" foods to ensure fetal growth. Pregnancy is usually considered a "hot" condition, so it may be difficult for a woman who is trying to eat only "cold" foods to agree to increase her intake of meat, usually considered a hot food. Asian women may believe in a similar pattern of required balances (yin and yang).

Be aware of what is available in your health care agency's local food stores. Women who cannot buy the foods you recommend in their own neighborhood may not eat well because of the inconvenience involved in shopping elsewhere.

A trait that is ethnically determined is lactose intolerance. This is the absence of lactase, the enzyme that breaks down the sugar (lactose) in milk so it can be used by the body. People with lactose intolerance (including many Asians and blacks) develop diarrhea and stomach cramps if they drink milk because of lactase deficiency (Gremse, 2003).

Pain Responses

A person's response to pain is both individually and culturally determined (Callister, 2003). Although people may all have the same threshold sensation (the amount of stimulus that results in pain), their **pain threshold** (the point at which the individual reports that a stimulus is painful) and **pain tolerance** (the point at which an individual withdraws from a stimulus) vary greatly.

A person's culture dictates attitudes toward pain and the proper response to pain. One woman in labor might report labor contractions as "agonizing" and scream each time she feels one, whereas a woman in the room next to her, experiencing the same degree of pain, might report her pain as tolerable and barely change her facial expression with contractions.

Caring for a person having pain can be problematic when the caregiver's concept of "proper" responses to pain differs from the patient's. Because there are so many possible responses to pain, it is important to assess each person individually.

Six strategies to help recognize cultural influences on pain management are (1) use an assessment tool, such as a 1 to 10 scale, to assist in measuring pain; (2) appreciate that people do not always express pain in the same way; (3) appreciate that people do not all communicate their level of pain in the same way; (4) recognize that communication of pain may not even be acceptable within a culture; (5) appreciate that the meaning of pain varies among cultures; and (6) develop an awareness of your personal values and beliefs that may affect how you respond to people in pain (Davidhizar & Giger, 2004).

Further assessment of pain and its meaning to people is discussed in Chapters 19 and 38.

What if... the Rodriques family tells you that they believe the accident that caused Maria's broken leg was "God's will," not Maria's fault? Would it be appropriate to educate Maria about street safety, or would doing so interfere with the family's cultural beliefs?

Key Points

Culture is an organized structure that guides behavior into acceptable ways for that group. Usual customs are termed mores or norms. Actions that are not acceptable to a culture are taboos.

Each culture differs to some degree from every other. Most people are proud of these differences or cultural traits.

Culture is transmitted by both formal and informal ways from generation to generation.

Although cultural concepts adapt from time to time, they tend to remain constant.

Cultural practices arise from environmental conditions.

There is wide variation within a culture concerning values and actions, because individuals make up the group and individually express their cultural heritage.

People bring cultural values and beliefs to nursing interactions, and these affect nursing and health care.

Cultural aspects that are important to assess are communication patterns; use of conversational space; response to pain; time, work, and family orientation; and social organization, including nutrition, family roles, and health beliefs.

Critical Thinking Exercises

1. Maria Rodriques is the 12-year-old child you met at the beginning of the chapter. What went wrong with her care? If you had actually planned care in this way, of what would you have been guilty? What would have been a better approach for determining this family's cultural preferences? Supposing Maria is present-oriented: how would you approach discussions of a long-term rehabilitation program for her?

2. When you talk to Mrs. Rodriques, you realize that she is pregnant but hasn't gone for prenatal care. She states that before coming to the clinic she wants to visit a *yerbero* who will both predict her child's sex and guarantee a safe birth. Would recommending that she have a sonogram (which also could predict the fetal sex) be likely to be as satisfying for her?

3. Maria enjoys vegetarian enchiladas. Suppose the dietitian in your health care agency says it's too expensive to serve ethnic foods. What could you suggest from a typical hospital menu that would best meet Maria's food preferences?

4. Examine the National Health Goals related to sociocultural aspects of health care. Most government-sponsored money for nursing research is allotted based on these goals. What would be a possible research topic to explore pertinent to these goals that would be applicable to the Rodriques family and also advance evidence-based practice?

References

Callister, L. C., et al. (2003). The pain of childbirth: Perceptions of culturally diverse women. *Pain Management Nursing, 4*(4), 145-154.

Campbell, C. C. (2004). Care of women with female circumcision. *Journal of Midwifery and Women's Health, 49*(4), 364-365.

Department of Health and Human Services. (2000). *Healthy people 2010*. Washington, D.C.: DHHS.

Davidhizar, R., & Giger, J. N. (2004). A review of the literature on care of clients in pain who are culturally diverse. *International Nursing Review, 51*(1), 47-55.

Edwards, K. (2003). Increasing cultural competence and decreasing disparities in health. *Journal of Cultural Diversity, 10*(4), 111-112.

Flowers, D. L. (2004). Culturally competent nursing care: A challenge for the 21st century. *Critical Care Nurse, 24*(4), 48-52.

Gremse, D. A., et al. (2003). Abdominal pain associated with lactose ingestion in children with lactose intolerance. *Clinical Pediatrics, 42*(4), 341-345.

Jacobs, E. A., et al. (2004). Overcoming language barriers in health care: Costs and benefits of interpreter services. *American Journal of Public Health, 94*(5), 866-869.

Kemper, K. J., & Barnes, L. (2003). Considering culture, complementary medicine, and spirituality in pediatrics. *Clinical Pediatrics, 42*(3), 205-208.

Lawlor, D. A., et al. (2005). Association between childhood and adulthood socioeconomic position and pregnancy induced hypertension. *Journal of Epidemiology and Community Health, 59*(1), 49-55.

Lee, S., Hoerr, S. L., & Schiffman, R. F. (2005). Screening for infants' and toddlers' dietary quality through maternal diet. *MCN: American Journal of Maternal/Child Nursing, 30*(1), 60-66.

Leininger, M. (2003). Founder's focus: Transcultural nursing care makes a big outcome difference. *Journal of Transcultural Nursing, 14*(2), 157-158.

Liamputtong, P., & Naksook, C. (2003). Perceptions and experiences of motherhood, health and the husband's role among Thai women in Australia. *Midwifery, 19*(1), 27-36.

Majumdar, B., et al. (2004). Effects of cultural sensitivity training on health care provider attitudes and patient outcomes. *Journal of Nursing Scholarship, 36*(2), 161-166.

Page, R. L. (2004). Positive pregnancy outcomes in Mexican immigrants: What can we learn? *JOGNN: Journal of Obstetric, Gynecologic, and Neonatal Nursing, 33*(6), 783-790.

U.S. Census Bureau. (2004). *Population projection program*. Washington, D.C.: Population Division.

Suggested Readings

Flores, G. (2004). Culture, ethnicity, and linguistic issues in pediatric care: Urgent priorities and unanswered questions. *Ambulatory Pediatrics, 4*(4), 276-282.

Foster, J. (2004). Fatherhood and the meaning of children: An ethnographic study among Puerto Rican partners of adolescent mothers. *Journal of Midwifery and Women's Health, 49*(2), 118-125.

Garcia, E. A., et al. (2004). A comparison of the influence of hospital-trained, ad hoc, and telephone interpreters on perceived satisfaction of limited English-proficient parents presenting to a pediatric emergency department. *Pediatric Emergency Care, 20*(6), 373–378.

Kim-Godwin, Y. S. (2003). Postpartum beliefs and practices among non-Western cultures. *MCN: American Journal of Maternal Child Nursing, 28*(2), 74–78.

Krowchuk, H. V., & Moore, M. L. (2004). Should learning Spanish be strongly encouraged in the undergraduate nursing curriculum? *MCN: American Journal of Maternal/ Child Nursing, 29*(4), 218–219.

Lewallen, L. P. (2004). Healthy behaviors and sources of health information among low-income pregnant women. *Public Health Nursing 21*(3), 200–206.

McEvoy, M. (2003). Culture and spirituality as an integrated concept in pediatric care. *MCN: American Journal of Maternal Child Nursing, 28*(1), 39–43.

Roberts, K. S. (2003). Providing culturally sensitive care to the childbearing Islamic family. *Advances in Neonatal Care, 3*(5), 250–255.

Shuzman, E. (2003). Facing stillbirth or neonatal death: Providing culturally appropriate care for Jewish families. *AWHONN Lifelines, 7*(6), 537–543.

Webb, E., & Sergison, M. (2003). Evaluation of cultural competence and antiracism training in childhealth services. *Archives of Disease in Childhood, 88*(4), 291–294.

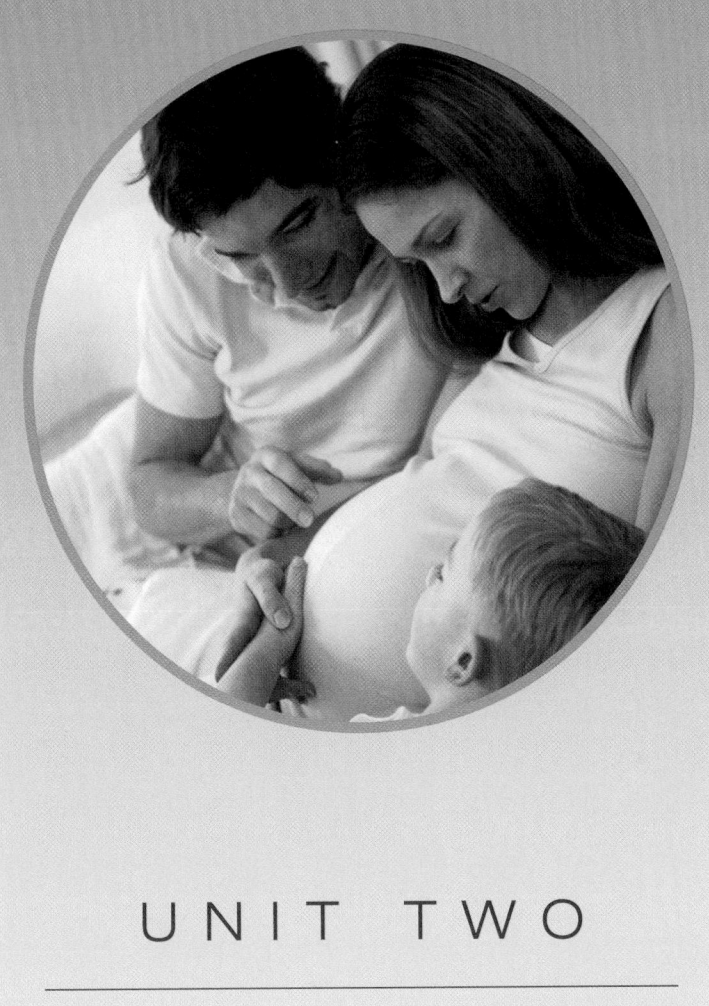

UNIT TWO

The Nursing Role in Preparing Families for Childbearing and Childrearing

CHAPTER 4

Reproductive and Sexual Health

Key Terms

adrenarche
andrology
anteflexion
anteversion
aspermia
bicornuate
  uterus
biologic
  gender
culdoscopy
cystocele
dyspareunia
erectile
  dysfunction
gender
  identity
gender role
gonad
gynecology

gynecomastia
laparoscopy
lesbian
menarche
menopause
menorrhagia
metrorrhagia
oocyte
premature
  ejaculation
rectocele
retroflexion
retroversion
thelarche
transsexual
transvestite
vaginismus
voyeurism

Objectives

After mastering the contents of this chapter, you should be able to:

1. Describe anatomy and physiology pertinent for reproductive and sexual health.
2. Assess a couple for anatomic and physiologic readiness for childbearing, biologic gender, gender role, and gender identity.
3. Formulate nursing diagnoses related to reproductive and sexual health.
4. Identify appropriate outcomes for reproductive and sexual health education.
5. Plan nursing care related to anatomic and physiologic readiness for childbearing or sexual health, such as helping adolescents discuss concerns in these areas.
6. Implement nursing care related to reproductive and sexual health, such as educating about menstruation.
7. Evaluate expected outcomes for achievement and effectiveness of care.
8. Identify National Health Goals related to reproductive health and sexuality that nurses can help the nation achieve.
9. Identify areas of care in relation to reproductive and sexual health that could benefit from additional nursing research or application of evidence-based practice.
10. Use critical thinking to analyze ways in which clients' reproductive and sexual health can be improved for healthier childbearing and adult health within a family-centered framework.
11. Integrate knowledge of reproductive health and sexuality with nursing process to achieve quality maternal and child health nursing care.

*S*uzanne and Kevin Matthews, a young adult couple, 12 weeks pregnant, come to your antepartal clinic *for a routine visit. Suzanne, in tears, states, "My husband doesn't seem interested in me anymore. We haven't had sex since I became pregnant." Kevin states, "I'm afraid I'll hurt the baby."*

Previous chapters presented the scope of maternal and child health and how the structure and function of families can have an impact on health. This chapter adds information about how to educate children, women, and their partners about anatomy, physiology, and sexuality to your knowledge base.

How would you counsel Suzanne and Kevin Matthews?

After you've studied this chapter, access the accompanying website. Read the patient scenario and answer the questions to further sharpen your skills, grow more familiar with RN-CLEX types of questions, and reward yourself with how much you have learned.

Whether people are planning on childbearing or not, everyone is wiser by being familiar with reproductive anatomy and physiology and his or her own body's reproductive and sexual health. Women and their partners who are planning for childbearing may be especially curious about reproductive physiology and the changes a pregnant woman will undergo, so this is an opportune time to educate both partners about reproductive and gynecologic health.

In addition, sexuality is a major area of concern for adolescents and individuals or families of childbearing age. The nurse who cares for childbearing or childrearing families may be asked a variety of detailed questions, such as this one about sexuality.

Although the general public is becoming increasingly sophisticated about their bodies, misunderstandings about sexuality, conception (preventing or promoting), and childbearing still abound. For instance, many young adults want to know what is considered a "normal" sexual response or the "normal" expected frequency for sexual relations. A general rule of thumb in answering this question is that normal sexual behavior includes any act mutually satisfying to both sexual partners. Actual frequency and type of sexual activity vary widely.

One of the biggest contributions nurses can make is to encourage clients to ask questions about sexual and reproductive functioning. With this attitude, problems of sexuality and reproduction are brought out into the open and made as resolvable as other health concerns or problems.

Nurses who can clearly explain the physical and emotional changes of puberty to the adolescent, the physiologic changes of pregnancy to a young adult couple, or the expected changes of menopause to a middle-aged woman provide much-needed health teaching information. A number of National Health Goals that speak directly to improving reproductive or sexual health are shown in the Box 4.1.

Nursing Process Overview

For Promotion of Reproductive and Sexual Health

● *Assessment*

Problems of sexuality or reproductive health may not be evident on first meeting a client, because it may be difficult for that person to bring up the topic until he or she feels more secure. Good follow-through and planning are important, because a person may find the courage to discuss a problem once but then be unable to do so again. If the problem is ignored or forgotten through a change in caregivers, it may never be addressed again.

Any change in physical appearance (such as happens with puberty or with pregnancy) can intensify or create a sexual or reproductive concern. The person with a sexually transmitted infection (STI), excessive weight loss or gain, a disfiguring scar from surgery or an accident, hair loss such as occurs with chemotherapy, surgery or inflammation or infection of reproductive organs, chronic fatigue or pain, spinal cord injury, or the

BOX 4.1 FOCUS ON . . .

NATIONAL HEALTH GOALS

A number of National Health Goals speak directly to reproductive and sexual health:

- Reduce the proportion of adolescents who have engaged in sexual intercourse to no more than 15% by age 15, from a baseline rate of 27% of girls and 33% of boys.
- Increase to at least 50% the proportion of sexually active, unmarried people who used a condom at last sexual intercourse, from a baseline rate of 19%.
- Reduce deaths from cancer of the uterine cervix to no more than 1.3 per 100,000 women, from a baseline rate of 2.8 per 100,000.
- Reduce breast cancer deaths to no more than 20.6 per 100,000 women, from a baseline rate of 23 per 100,000 (DHHS, 2000).

Nurses can help the nation achieve these goals by educating adolescents about abstinence and refusal skills, safer sex practices, and the need to participate in screening activities such as breast mammography or testicular self-examination.

presence of a retention catheter needs to be assessed for problems regarding his or her sexual role as well as other important areas of reproductive functioning.

Assessing sexuality may not be appropriate as a routine part of every health assessment. However, it should be included when appropriate, such as when discussing adolescent development or before providing reproductive life planning information, during pregnancy, or after childbirth. At other times, it is wise to listen for verbal or nonverbal clues that suggest a person wants to discuss a sexual or reproductive concern. These clues are often subtle: "I guess marriage isn't for everyone"; "I'm not the woman I used to be"; "Are there ever funny effects from this medicine I'm taking?" Telling a seemingly inappropriate sexual joke may be yet another clue. Nonverbal clues may include extreme modesty or obvious embarrassment in response to a question about voiding or perineal pain or stitches.

Assessment in the area of reproductive health begins with interviewing clients to determine what they know about the reproductive process and STIs. Any concerns they might have about their own reproductive functioning or safer sex practices should be explored. This area of health interviewing takes practice and the conviction that exploring sexual health is as important as exploring less emotionally involved areas of health, such as dietary intake or activity level. The 14-year-old girl who is not yet menstruating, for instance, may be anxious about that fact but may be reluctant to say so unless asked directly. A statement such as the following invites discussion: "Although many of your friends at school may be menstruating, it's not at all uncommon for some girls not to begin their periods until age 15 or 16. How do you feel about not yet having

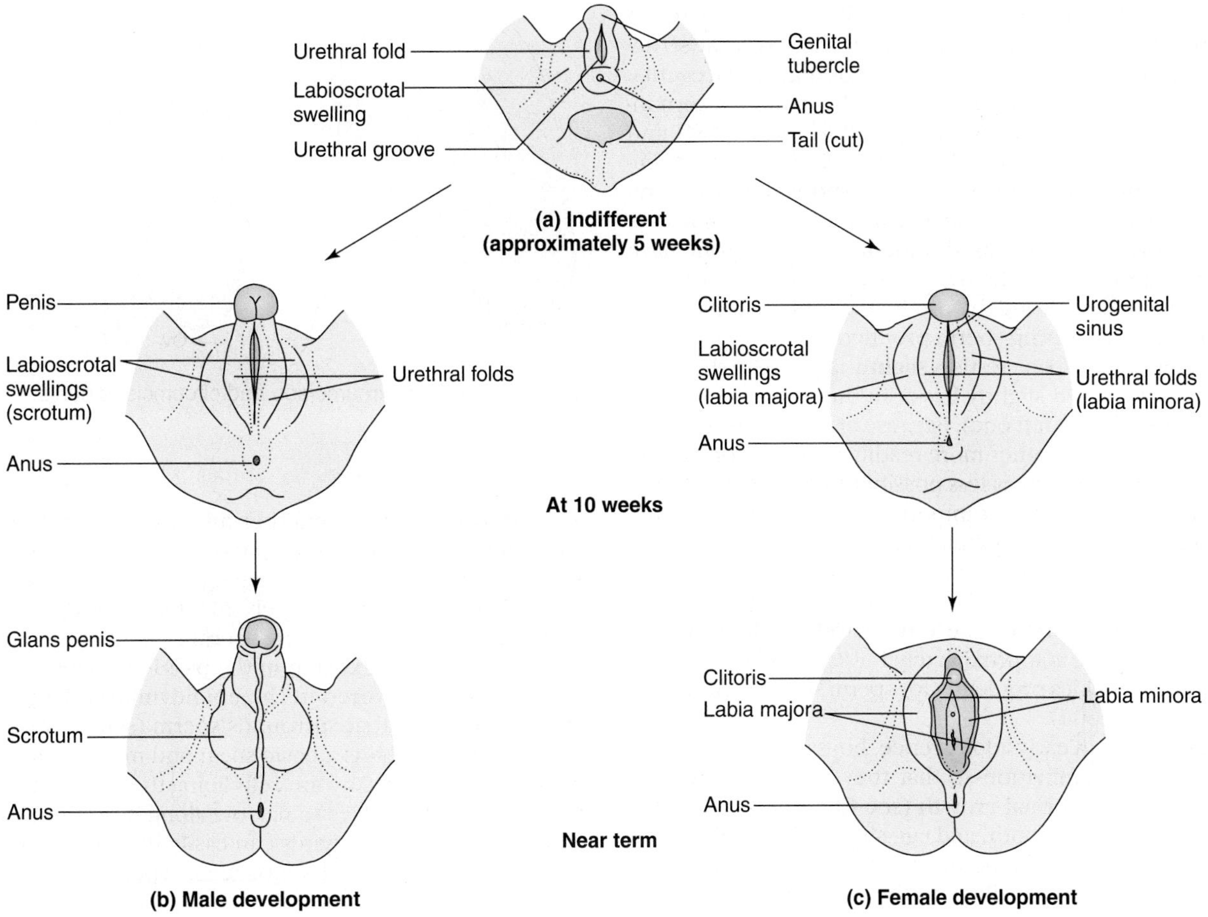

Urethral fold

Labioscrotal swelling

Urethral groove

Genital tubercle

Anus

Tail (cut)

(a) Indifferent (approximately 5 weeks)

Penis

Labioscrotal swellings (scrotum)

Anus

Urethral folds

Clitoris

Labioscrotal swellings (labia majora)

Anus

Urogenital sinus

Urethral folds (labia minora)

At 10 weeks

Glans penis

Scrotum

Anus

Clitoris

Labia majora

Anus

Labia minora

Near term

(b) Male development

(c) Female development

FIGURE 4.1 (continued)

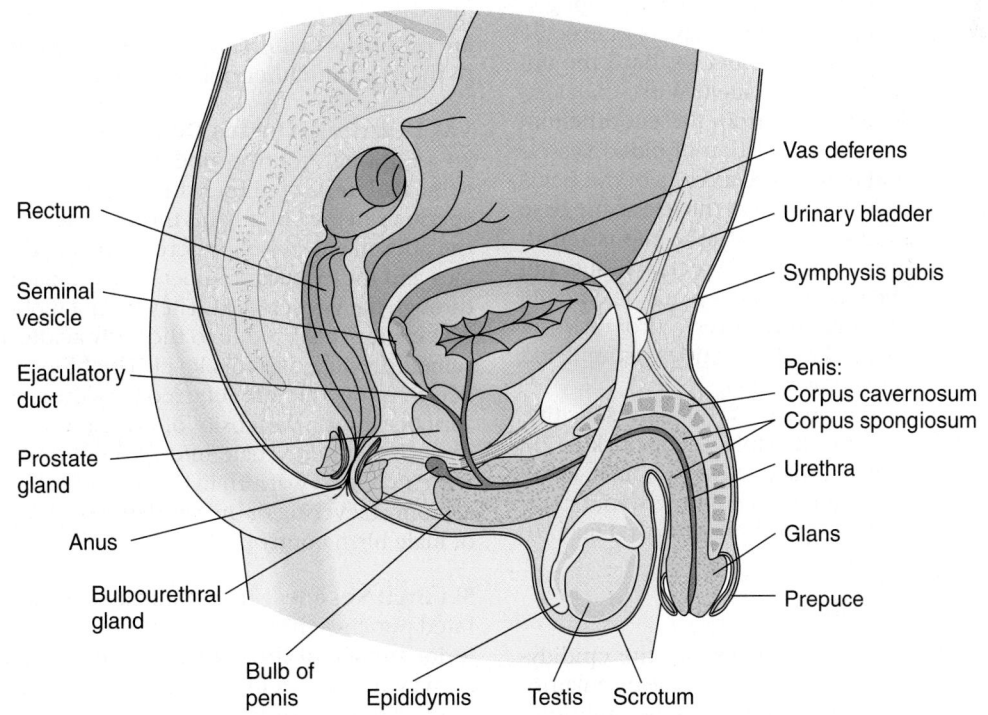

Rectum

Seminal vesicle

Ejaculatory duct

Prostate gland

Anus

Bulbourethral gland

Bulb of penis

Epididymis

Testis

Scrotum

Vas deferens

Urinary bladder

Symphysis pubis

Penis:
Corpus cavernosum
Corpus spongiosum

Urethra

Glans

Prepuce

FIGURE 4.2 Male internal and external reproductive organs.

Spermatozoa are produced in the testes and reach maturity, surrounded by semen, in the external structures through a complex sequence of regulatory events. First, the hypothalamus releases GnRH, which in turn influences the anterior pituitary gland to release FSH and LH. FSH is then responsible for the release of androgen-binding protein (ABP), and LH is responsible for the release of testosterone. ABP binding of testosterone promotes sperm formation. Increased amounts of testosterone have a feedback effect on the hypothalamus and anterior pituitary gland, decreasing the production of FSH and LH and ultimately decreasing sperm production.

In most males, one testis is slightly larger than the other and is suspended slightly lower in the scrotum than the other (usually the left one). Because of this, the testes tend to slide past each other more readily on sitting or muscular activity, and there is less possibility of trauma to them. Most body structures of importance are more protected than are the testes (for example, the heart, kidneys, and lungs are surrounded by ribs of hard bone). Spermatozoa do not survive at a temperature as high as that of the body. However, the location of the testes outside the body, where the temperature is approximately 1°F lower than body temperature, provides protection for sperm survival (McCance & Huether, 2004).

Beginning in early adolescence, boys need to learn testicular self-examination so that they can detect tenderness or any abnormal growth (see Chapter 33). Normal testes feel firm, smooth, and egg-shaped. The epididymis (the tube that carries sperm away from the testes) can be palpated as a firm swelling on the superior aspect of the testes. Caution boys not to mistake this structure for an abnormal growth.

Penis. The penis is composed of three cylindrical masses of erectile tissue in the penis shaft: two termed the corpus cavernosa, and a third termed the corpus spongiosum. The urethra passes through these layers of erectile tissue, so the penis serves as the outlet for both the urinary and the reproductive tracts in men. With sexual excitement, nitric oxide is released from the endothelium of blood vessels. This results in dilation of blood vessels and an increase in blood flow to the arteries of the penis (engorgement). The ischiocavernosus muscle at the base of the penis then contracts, trapping both venous and arterial blood in the three sections of erectile tissue and leading to distention and erection of the penis. The penile artery, a branch of the pudendal artery, provides the blood supply for the penis. Penile erection is stimulated by parasympathetic nerve innervation.

At the distal end of the organ is a bulging, sensitive ridge of tissue, the glans. A retractable casing of skin, the prepuce, protects the nerve-sensitive glans at birth. Many infants in the United States undergo circumcision, or surgical removal of the prepuce, shortly after birth (Fig. 4.3).

Male Internal Structures

The male internal reproductive organs are the epididymis, the vas deferens, the seminal vesicles, the ejaculatory ducts, the prostate gland, the urethra, and the bulbourethral glands (see Fig. 4.2).

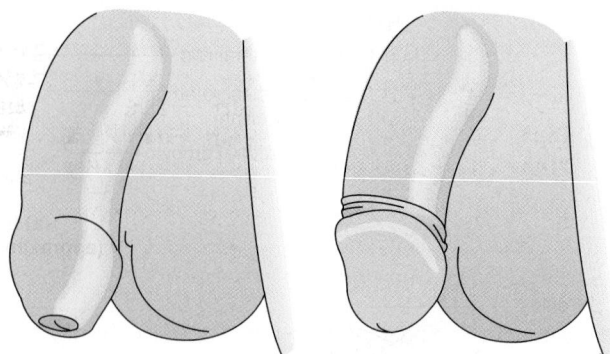

FIGURE 4.3 Uncircumcised and circumcised penis.

Epididymis. The seminiferous tubule of each testis leads to a tightly coiled tube, the epididymis. Because each epididymis is so tightly coiled, its length is extremely deceptive: it is actually approximately 20 ft long. The epididymis is responsible for conducting sperm from the testis to the vas deferens, the next step in the passage to the outside. Some sperm are stored in the epididymis, and a part of the alkaline fluid that surrounds sperm (semen, or seminal fluid that contains a basic sugar and mucin, a form of protein) is produced by the cells lining the epididymis. Because the epididymis is so narrow along its entire length, infection of the epididymis can easily lead to scarring of the lumen that prohibits passage of sperm beyond the scarred point.

Sperm are immobile and incapable of fertilization as they pass or are stored at the epididymis level. It takes at least 12 to 20 days for them to travel the length of the epididymis, and a total of 64 days for them to reach maturity. This is one reason that **aspermia** (absence of sperm) and oligospermia (fewer than 20 million sperm per milliliter) are problems that do not appear to respond immediately to therapy but rather only after 2 months.

Vas Deferens (Ductus Deferens). The vas deferens is an additional hollow tube surrounded by arteries and veins and protected by a thick fibrous coating. It carries sperm from the epididymis through the inguinal canal into the abdominal cavity, where it ends at the seminal vesicles and the ejaculatory ducts. Sperm mature as they pass through the vas deferens. They are not mobile at this point, however, probably due to the fairly acidic medium of the semen produced at this level. The blood vessels and vas deferens together are referred to as the spermatic cord. A varicocele, or a varicosity of the internal spermatic vein, can contribute to male infertility by causing congestion with increased warmth in the testes (Johnson, 2003). Vasectomy (severing of the vas deferens) is a popular means of male birth control.

Seminal Vesicles. The seminal vesicles are two convoluted pouches that lie along the lower portion of the posterior surface of the bladder and empty into the urethra by way of the ejaculatory ducts. These glands secrete a viscous portion of the semen, which has a high content of a basic sugar, protein, and prostaglandins and is alkaline. Sperm become increasingly motile with this added fluid, because it surrounds them with nutrients and a more favorable pH.

Ejaculatory Ducts. The two ejaculatory ducts pass through the prostate gland and join the seminal vesicles to the urethra.

Prostate Gland. The prostate is a chestnut-sized gland that lies just below the bladder. The urethra passes through the center of it, like the hole in a doughnut. The prostate gland secretes a thin, alkaline fluid. When added to the secretion from the seminal vesicles and the accompanying sperm from the epididymis, this alkaline fluid further protects sperm from being immobilized by the naturally low pH level of the urethra. In middle life, many men develop hypertrophy of the prostate. This swelling interferes with both fertility and urination. It can be relieved by medical therapy or surgery.

Bulbourethral Glands. Two bulbourethral or Cowper's glands lie beside the prostate gland and empty by short ducts into the urethra. Like the prostate gland and seminal vesicles, they secrete an alkaline fluid that helps counteract the acid secretion of the urethra and ensure the safe passage of spermatozoa. Semen, therefore, is derived from the prostate gland (60%), the seminal vesicles (30%), the epididymis (5%), and the bulbourethral glands (5%).

Urethra. The urethra is a hollow tube leading from the base of the bladder, which, after passing through the prostate gland, continues to the outside through the shaft and glans of the penis. It is approximately 8 in (18 to 20 cm) long. Like other urinary tract structures, it is lined with mucous membrane.

Checkpoint Question 2

Suppose Kevin Matthews tells you that he is considering a vasectomy after the birth of his new child. Vasectomy is incision of which organ?

a. The testes
b. The vas deferens
c. The epididymis
d. The scrotum

Female Reproductive System

The female reproductive system, like the male system, has both external and internal components.

Female External Structures

The structures that form the female external genitalia are termed the vulva (from the Latin word for covering) and are illustrated in Figure 4.4.

Mons Veneris. The mons veneris is a pad of adipose tissue located over the symphysis pubis, the pubic bone joint. It is covered by a triangle of coarse, curly hairs. The purpose of the mons veneris is to protect the junction of the pubic bone from trauma.

Labia Minora. Just posterior to the mons veneris spread two hairless folds of connective tissue, the labia minora. Before menarche, these folds are fairly small; by childbearing age, they are firm and full; after menopause, they atrophy and again become much smaller. Normally the folds of the labia minora are pink; the internal surface is

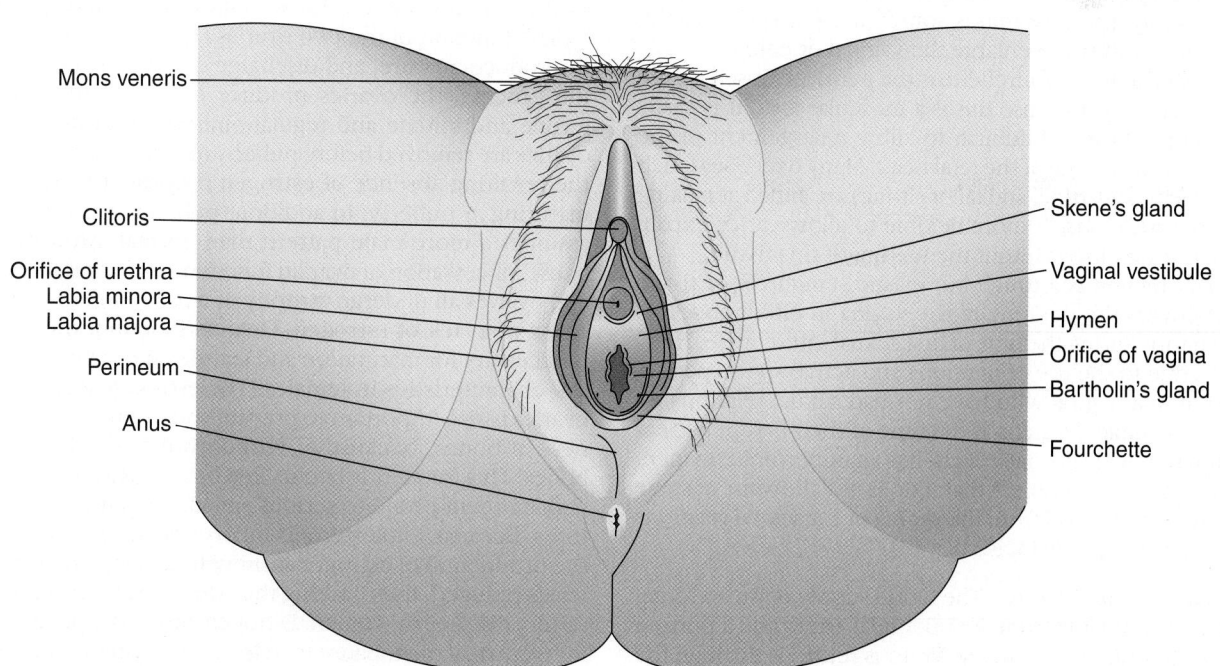

FIGURE 4.4 Female external genitalia.

covered with mucous membrane, and the external surface with skin. The area is abundant with sebaceous glands, so localized sebaceous cysts may occur here.

Labia Majora. The labia majora are two folds of adipose tissue covered by loose connective tissue and epithelium; they are positioned lateral to the labia minora. Covered by pubic hair, the labia majora serve as protection for the external genitalia and the distal urethra and vagina. They are fused anteriorly but separated posteriorly. Trauma to the area, such as occurs from childbirth or rape, can lead to extensive edema formation because of the looseness of the connective tissue base.

Other External Organs. The vestibule is the flattened, smooth surface inside the labia. The openings to the bladder (the urethra) and the uterus (the vagina) both arise from the vestibule. The clitoris is a small (approximately 1 to 2 cm), rounded organ of erectile tissue at the forward junction of the labia minora. It is covered by a fold of skin, the prepuce. The clitoris is sensitive to touch and temperature and is the center of sexual arousal and orgasm in the female. Arterial blood supply for the clitoris is plentiful. When the ischiocavernosus muscle surrounding it contracts with sexual arousal, the venous outflow for the clitoris is blocked, leading to clitoral erection.

Two Skene's glands (paraurethral glands) are located just lateral to the urinary meatus, one on each side. The ducts open into the urethra. Bartholin's glands (vulvo-vaginal glands) are located just lateral to the vaginal opening on both sides. Their ducts open into the distal vagina. Secretions from both of these glands help to lubricate the external genitalia during coitus. The alkaline pH of their secretions helps to improve sperm survival in the vagina. Both Skene's glands and Bartholin's glands may become infected and produce a discharge and local pain.

The fourchette is the ridge of tissue formed by the posterior joining of the two labia minora and the labia majora. This is the structure that is sometimes cut (episiotomy) during childbirth to enlarge the vaginal opening.

Posterior to the fourchette is the perineal muscle or the perineal body. Because this is a muscular area, it is easily stretched during childbirth to allow enlargement of the vagina and passage of the fetal head. Many exercises (such as Kegel's, squatting, and tailor-sitting) are aimed at making the perineal muscle more flexible to allow easier expansion during birth without the tearing of this tissue.

The hymen is a tough but elastic semicircle of tissue that covers the opening to the vagina in childhood. It is often torn during the time of first sexual intercourse. However, due to the use of tampons and active sports participation, many girls who have not had sexual relations do not have intact hymens at the time of their first pelvic examination. Occasionally, a girl has an imperforate hymen, or a hymen so complete that it does not allow for passage of menstrual blood from the vagina or for sexual relations until it is surgically incised.

Vulvar Blood Supply. The blood supply of the external genitalia is mainly from the pudendal artery and a portion of the inferior rectus artery. Venous return is through the pudendal vein. Pressure on this vein by the fetal head can cause extensive back-pressure and development of vari-cosities (distended veins) in the labia majora. Because of the rich blood supply, trauma to the area, such as occurs from pressure during childbirth, can cause large hematomas. This ready blood supply also contributes to the rapid healing of any tears in the area after childbirth (McCance & Huether, 2004).

Vulvar Nerve Supply. The anterior portion of the vulva derives its nerve supply from the ilioinguinal and genito-femoral nerves (L1 level). The posterior portions of the vulva and vagina are supplied by the pudendal nerve (S3 level). Such a rich nerve supply makes the area extremely sensitive to touch, pressure, pain, and temperature. Anesthesia for childbirth may be administered locally to block the pudendal nerve; this eliminates pain sensation at the perineum during birth. Normal stretching of the perineum with childbirth causes temporary loss of sensation in the area.

Female Internal Structures

Female internal reproductive organs (Fig. 4.5) are the ovaries, the fallopian tubes, the uterus, and the vagina.

Ovaries. The ovaries are approximately 4 cm long by 2 cm in diameter and approximately 1.5 cm thick, or the size and shape of almonds. They are grayish-white and appear pitted, or with minute indentations on the surface. An unruptured, glistening, clear, fluid-filled graafian follicle (an ovum about to be discharged) or a miniature yellow corpus luteum (the structure left after the ovum has been discharged) often can be observed on the surface of an ovary.

Ovaries are located close to and on both sides of the uterus in the lower abdomen. It is difficult to locate them by abdominal palpation because they are situated so low in the abdomen. If an abnormality is present, such as an enlarging ovarian cyst, the resulting tenderness may be evident on lower-left or lower-right abdominal palpation.

The function of the two ovaries (the female gonads) is to produce, mature, and discharge ova (the egg cells). In the process, the ovaries produce estrogen and progesterone and initiate and regulate menstrual cycles. If the ovaries are removed before puberty (or are nonfunctional), the resulting absence of estrogen prevents breasts from maturing at puberty; in addition, pubic hair distribution assumes a more male pattern than normal. After menopause, or cessation of ovarian function, the uterus, breasts, and ovaries all undergo atrophy or a reduction in size because of a lack of estrogen. Ovarian function, therefore, is necessary for maturation and maintenance of secondary sex characteristics in females. The estrogen secreted by ovaries is also important to prevent osteoporosis, or weakness of bones, because of withdrawal of calcium from bones. This frequently occurs in women after menopause, making them prone to serious spinal, hip, and wrist fractures. Because cholesterol is incorporated into estrogen, the production of estrogen is thought to keep cholesterol levels reduced, thus limiting the effects of atherosclerosis (artery disease) in women. Estrogen used to be prescribed for women at menopause to help prevent osteoporosis and cardiovascular disease. However, this type of long-term estrogen supplementation may contribute to breast can-

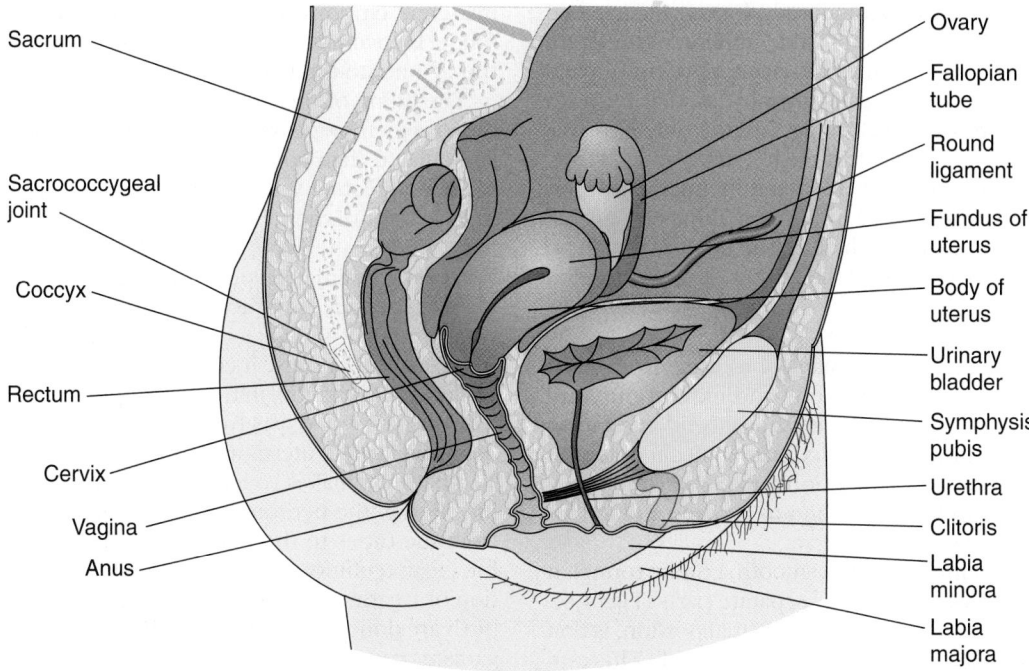

FIGURE 4.5 Female internal reproductive organs.

cer, so it is no longer routinely recommended (Speroff & Fritz, 2005).

The ovaries are held suspended and in close contact with the ends of the fallopian tubes by three strong supporting ligaments attached to the uterus or the pelvic wall. They are unique among pelvic structures in that they are not covered by a layer of peritoneum. Because they are not encased in this way, ova can escape from them and enter the uterus by way of the fallopian tubes. Because they are suspended in position rather than being firmly fixed in place, an abnormal tumor or cyst growing on them can enlarge to a size easily twice that of the organ before pressure on surrounding organs or the ovarian blood supply leads to symptoms of compression. This is the reason that ovarian cancer continues to be one of the leading causes of death from cancer in women (i.e., the tumor grows without symptoms for an extended period).

Ovaries are formed with three principal divisions:

1. A protective layer of surface epithelium
2. The cortex, which is filled with the ovarian and graafian follicles. Here the immature (primordial) follicles mature into ova and produce large amounts of estrogen and progesterone.
3. The central medulla, which contains the nerves, blood vessels, lymphatic tissue, and some smooth muscle tissue

Division of Reproductive Cells (Gametes). At birth, each ovary contains approximately 2 million immature ova (oocytes), which were formed during the first 5 months of intrauterine life. Although these cells have the unique ability to produce a new individual, they basically contain the usual cell components: a cell membrane, an area of clear cytoplasm, and a nucleus containing chromosomes.

The oocytes differ from all other body cells in the number of chromosomes they contain in the nucleus. The nu-

cleus of all other human body cells contains 46 chromosomes, consisting of 22 pairs of autosomes (paired matching chromosomes) and one pair of sex chromosomes (two X sex chromosomes in the female, an X and a Y sex chromosome in the male). Reproductive cells (both ova and spermatozoa) have only half the usual number of chromosomes, so that, when they combine (fertilization), the new individual formed from them will have the normal number, 46 chromosomes. If both the ova and the spermatozoa carried the full complement of chromosomes, a new individual formed from them would have twice the normal amount of chromosome material. There is a difference in the way reproductive cells divide that causes this change in chromosome number.

Cells in the body, such as skin cells, undergo cell division by mitosis, or daughter cell division. In this type of division, all the chromosomes are duplicated in each new cell just before cell division, giving every new cell the same number of chromosomes as the original parent cell. Oocytes divide in intrauterine life by one mitotic division. Division activity then appears to halt until at least puberty, when a second type of cell division, meiosis (cell reduction division), occurs. In the male, this reduction division occurs just before the spermatozoa mature. In the female, it occurs just before ovulation. After this reduction division, an ovum has 22 autosomes and an X sex chromosome, whereas a spermatozoon has 22 autosomes and either an X or a Y sex chromosome. A new individual formed from the union of an ovum and an X-carrying spermatozoon will be female (an XX chromosome pattern); an individual formed from the union of an ovum and a Y-carrying spermatozoon will be male (an XY chromosome pattern).

Maturation of Oocytes. Each oocyte lies in the ovary surrounded by a protective sac, or thin layer of cells, called a follicle. The structure in this underdeveloped state is called a primordial follicle. Between 5 and 7 million of these are first formed in utero. The majority never develop beyond the primitive state and actually atrophy, so that by birth only 2 million are present. By age 7 years, only approximately 500,000 are present in each ovary; by 22 years, there are approximately 300,000; and by menopause, or the end of the fertile period in females, none are left (all have either matured or atrophied). "The point at which no functioning oocytes remain in the ovaries" is one definition of menopause.

Fallopian Tubes. The fallopian tubes arise from each upper corner of the uterine body and extend outward and backward until each opens at its distal end, next to an ovary. Fallopian tubes are approximately 10 cm in length in a mature woman. Their function is to convey the ovum from the ovaries to the uterus and to provide a place for fertilization of the ovum by sperm.

Although a fallopian tube is a smooth, hollow tunnel, it is anatomically divided into four separate parts (Fig. 4.6). The most proximal division, the interstitial portion, is that part of the tube that lies within the uterine wall. This portion is only about 1 cm in length; the lumen of the tube is only 1 mm in diameter at this point. The isthmus is the next distal portion. Like the interstitial tube, it is extremely narrow. This segment is approximately 2 cm in length. This is the portion of the tube that is cut or sealed in a tubal ligation, or tubal sterilization procedure. The ampulla is the third and also the longest portion of the tube. It is approximately 5 cm in length. It is in this ampullar portion that fertilization of an ovum usually occurs. The infundibular portion is the most distal segment of the tube. It is approx-

imately 2 cm long and is funnel-shaped. The rim of the funnel is covered by fimbria (small hairs) that help to guide the ovum into the fallopian tube.

The lining of the entire fallopian tube is composed of mucous membrane, which contains both mucus-secreting and ciliated (hair-covered) cells. Beneath the mucous lining is connective tissue and a circular muscle layer. The muscle layer of the tube produces peristaltic motions that help conduct the ovum the length of the tube. This migration of the ovum is aided by the action of the ciliated lining and the mucus, which acts as a lubricant. The mucus produced may also act as a source of nourishment for the fertilized egg, because it contains protein, water, and salts.

Because the fallopian tubes are open at their distal ends, a direct pathway exists from the external organs, through the vagina to the uterus and tubes, and to the peritoneum. This pathway makes conception possible. It can also lead to infection of the peritoneum (peritonitis) if disease spreads from the tubes to the peritoneum. For this reason, careful, clean technique must be used during pelvic examination or treatment. Vaginal examinations during labor and birth are done with sterile technique to ensure that no organisms can enter.

Uterus. The uterus is a hollow, muscular, pear-shaped organ located in the lower pelvis, posterior to the bladder and anterior to the rectum. During childhood, it is approximately the size of an olive, and its proportions are reversed from what they are later on (i.e., the cervix is the largest portion of the organ). When a girl reaches approximately 8 years of age, an increase in the size of the uterus begins. An adolescent is 17 years old before the uterus reaches its adult size. This may be a contributing factor to the low-

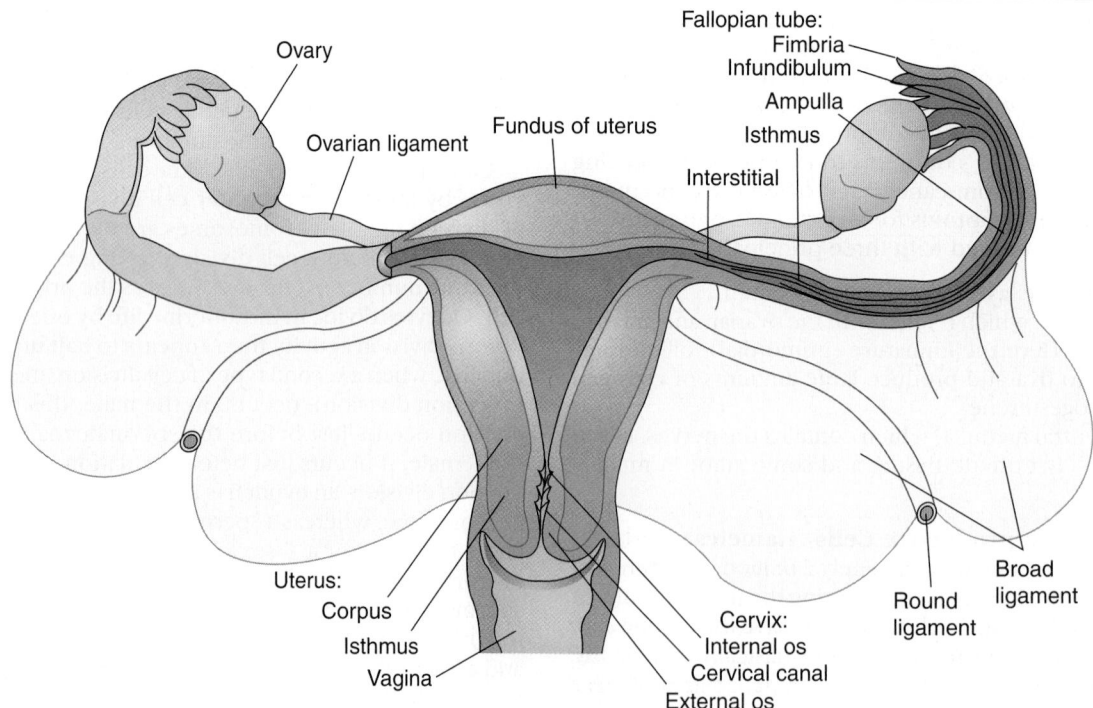

FIGURE 4.6 Anterior view of female reproductive organs showing relationship of fallopian tubes and body of the uterus.

birthweight babies typically born to adolescents younger than this age.

With maturity, a uterus is approximately 5 to 7 cm long, 5 cm wide, and, in its widest upper part, 2.5 cm deep. In a nonpregnant state, it weighs approximately 60 g. The function of the uterus is to receive the ovum from the fallopian tube; provide a place for implantation and nourishment during fetal growth; furnish protection to a growing fetus; and, at maturity of the fetus, expel it from a woman's body.

After a pregnancy, the uterus never returns to its nonpregnant size. In a woman who has borne a child, uterine dimensions are approximately 9 cm long, 6 cm wide, 3 cm thick, and 80 g in weight.

Anatomically, the uterus consists of three divisions: the body or corpus, the isthmus, and the cervix. The body of the uterus is the uppermost part and forms the bulk of the organ. The lining of the cavity is continuous with that of the fallopian tubes, which enter at its upper aspects (the cornua). The portion of the uterus between the points of attachment of the fallopian tubes is termed the fundus. During pregnancy, the body of the uterus is the portion of the structure that expands to contain the growing fetus. The fundus is the portion that can be palpated abdominally to determine the amount of uterine growth occurring during pregnancy, to measure the force of uterine contractions during labor, and to assess that the uterus is returning to its nonpregnant state after childbirth.

The isthmus of the uterus is a short segment between the body and the cervix. In the nonpregnant uterus, it is only 1 to 2 mm in length. During pregnancy, this portion also enlarges greatly to aid in accommodating the growing fetus. It is the portion of the uterus that is most commonly cut when a fetus is born by a cesarean birth.

The cervix is the lowest portion of the uterus. It represents approximately one third of the total uterus size and is approximately 2 to 5 cm long. Approximately half of it lies above the vagina and half extends into the vagina. A central cavity is termed the cervical canal. The opening of the canal at the junction of the cervix and isthmus is the internal cervical os; the distal opening to the vagina is the external cervical os. The level of the external os is at the level of the ischial spines (an important relationship in estimating the level of the fetus in the birth canal).

Uterine and Cervical Coats. The uterine wall consists of three separate coats or layers of tissue: an inner one of mucous membrane (the endometrium), a middle one of muscle fibers (the myometrium), and an outer one of connective tissue (the perimetrium).

The endometrium layer of the uterus is the one that is important for menstrual function. It is formed by two layers of cells. The layer closest to the uterine wall, the basal layer, is not influenced by hormones. In contrast, the inner glandular layer is greatly influenced by both estrogen and progesterone. It grows and becomes so thick and responsive each month under the influence of estrogen and progesterone that it is capable of supporting a pregnancy. If pregnancy does not occur, this is the layer that is shed as the menstrual flow.

The mucous membrane lining of the cervix is termed the endocervix. The endocervix, continuous with the endo-metrium, is also affected by hormones, but changes are manifested in a more subtle way. The cells of the cervical lining secrete mucus to provide a lubricated surface so that spermatozoa can readily pass through the cervix; the efficiency of this lubrication increases or wanes depending on hormone stimulation. At the point in the menstrual cycle when estrogen production is at its peak, as much as 700 mL of mucus per day is produced; at the point that estrogen is very low, only a few milliliters is produced. Because mucus is alkaline, it helps to decrease the acidity of the upper vagina, aiding in sperm survival. During pregnancy, the endocervix becomes plugged with mucus, forming a seal to keep out ascending infections.

The lower surface of the cervix and the lower third of the cervical canal are lined not with mucous membrane but with stratified squamous epithelium, similar to that lining the vagina. Locating the point at which this tissue changes from epithelium to mucous membrane is important when obtaining a Papanicolaou smear (a test for cervical cancer), because this tissue interface is most often the origin of cervical cancer.

The myometrium, or muscle layer of the uterus, is composed of three interwoven layers of smooth muscle, the fibers of which are arranged in longitudinal, transverse, and oblique directions. This network offers extreme strength to the organ. The myometrium serves the important function of constricting the tubal junctions and preventing regurgitation of menstrual blood into the tubes. It also holds the internal cervical os closed during pregnancy to prevent a preterm birth. When the uterus contracts at the end of pregnancy to expel the fetus, equal pressure is exerted at all points throughout the cavity because of its unique arrangement of muscle fibers. After childbirth, this interlacing network of fibers is able to constrict the blood vessels coursing through the layers, thereby limiting the loss of blood in the woman. Myomas, or benign uterine tumors, arise from the myometrium.

The perimetrium, or the outermost layer of the uterus, serves the purpose of adding strength and support to the structure.

Uterine Blood Supply. The large descending abdominal aorta divides to form two iliac arteries; main divisions of the iliac arteries are the hypogastric arteries (Fig. 4.7). These further divide to form the uterine arteries and supply the uterus. Because the uterine blood supply is not far removed from the aorta, it is copious and adequate to supply the growing needs of a fetus. As an additional safeguard, after supplying the ovary with blood, the ovarian artery (a direct subdivision of the aorta) joins the uterine artery as a fail-safe system to ensure that the uterus will have an adequate blood supply. The blood vessels that supply the cells and lining of the uterus are tortuous against the sides of the uterine body in nonpregnant women. As a uterus enlarges with pregnancy, the vessels "unwind" and so can stretch to maintain an adequate blood supply as the organ enlarges. The uterine veins follow the same twisting course as the arteries; they empty into the internal iliac veins.

An important organ relationship to be aware of is the association of uterine vessels and the ureters. The ureters from the kidneys pass directly in back of the ovarian vessels, near the fallopian tubes. As shown in Figure 4.7, they

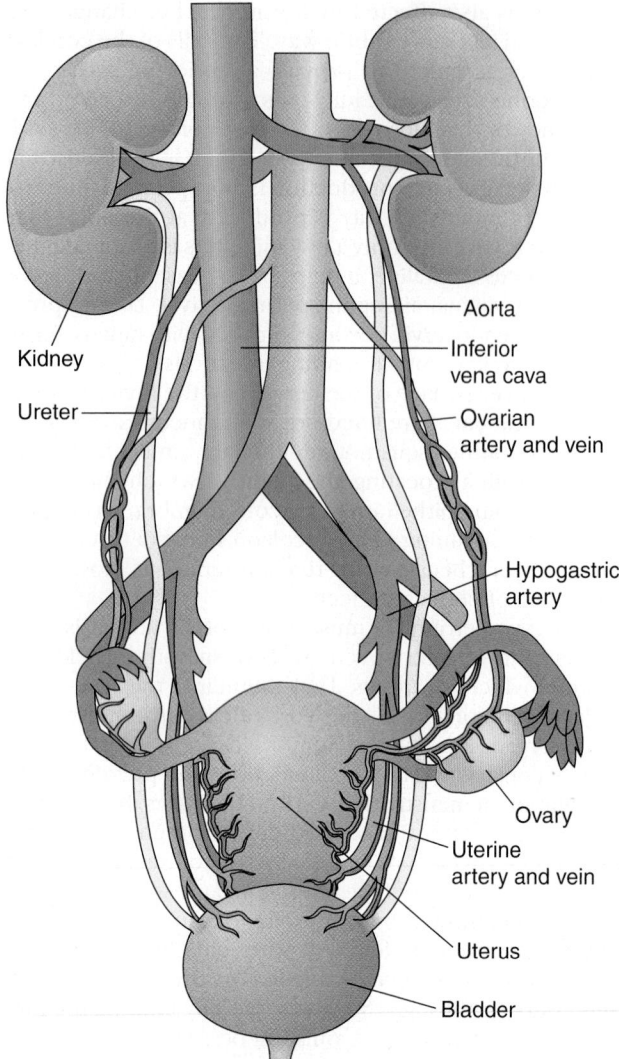

FIGURE 4.7 Blood supply to the uterus.

cross just beneath the uterine vessels before they enter the bladder. This close anatomic relationship has implications in procedures such as tubal ligation, cesarean birth, and hysterectomy (removal of the uterus), because a ureter may be injured by a clamp if bleeding is controlled by clamping of the uterine or ovarian vessels.

What if... Suzanne Matthews decides to have a tubal ligation (clamping of the fallopian tubes) after the birth of her baby? Why is observing women for urine output after uterine or fallopian tube surgery of this kind always a critical assessment?

Uterine Nerve Supply. The uterus is supplied by both efferent (motor) and afferent (sensory) nerves. The efferent nerves arise from the T5 through T10 spinal ganglia. The afferent nerves join the hypogastric plexus and enter the spinal column at T11 and T12. The fact that sensory innervation from the uterus registers lower in the spinal

column than does motor control has implications in controlling pain in labor. An anesthetic solution can be injected near the spinal column to stop the pain of uterine contractions at the T11 and T12 levels without stopping motor control or contractions (registered higher, at the T5 to T10 level). This is the principle of epidural anesthesia (see Chapter 19).

Uterine Supports. The uterus is suspended in the pelvic cavity by a number of ligaments that also help support the bladder and further supported by a combination of fascia and muscle. Because it is not fixed, the uterus is free to enlarge without discomfort during pregnancy. If its ligaments become overstretched during pregnancy, they may not support the bladder well afterward, and the bladder can then herniate into the anterior vagina (a **cystocele**). A **rectocele** (Fig. 4.8) may develop in the same way if the rectum pouches toward the vaginal wall (De and Wilson, 2004).

A fold of peritoneum behind the uterus is the posterior ligament. This forms a pouch (Douglas' cul-de-sac) between the rectum and uterus. Because this is the lowest point of the pelvis, any fluid such as blood in the pelvis tends to collect in this space. The space can be examined for the presence of fluid or blood such as might occur with a ruptured tubal pregnancy by inserting a culdoscope through the posterior vaginal wall (**culdoscopy**) or a laparoscope through the abdominal wall (**laparoscopy**).

The broad ligaments are two folds of peritoneum that cover the uterus front and back and extend to the pelvic sides. The round ligaments are two fibrous, muscular cords that pass from the body of the uterus near the attachments of the fallopian tubes, through the broad ligaments and into the inguinal canal, inserting into the fascia of the vulva. The round ligaments act as "stays" to steady the uterus. If a pregnant woman moves quickly, she may pull one of these ligaments. This causes a quick, sharp pain of frightening intensity in one of her lower abdominal quadrants that can be mistaken for labor pain.

Uterine Deviations. A number of uterine deviations (shape and position) may interfere with fertility or pregnancy. In the fetus, the uterus first forms with a septum or a fibrous division, longitudinally separating it into two portions. As the fetus matures, this septum dissolves, so that typically at birth no remnant of the division remains. In some women, the septum never atrophies, and so the uterus remains as two separate compartments. In others, half of the septum is still present. Still other women have oddly shaped "horns" at the junction of the fallopian tubes, termed a **bicornuate uterus.** Any of these malformations may decrease the ability to conceive or to carry a pregnancy to term. Some variations of uterine formation are shown in Figure 4.9. The specific effects of these deviations on fertility and pregnancy are discussed in later chapters.

Ordinarily, the body of the uterus is tipped slightly forward. Positional deviations of the uterus that may occur include the following:

- **Anteversion,** a condition in which the fundus is tipped forward
- **Retroversion,** a condition in which the fundus is tipped back

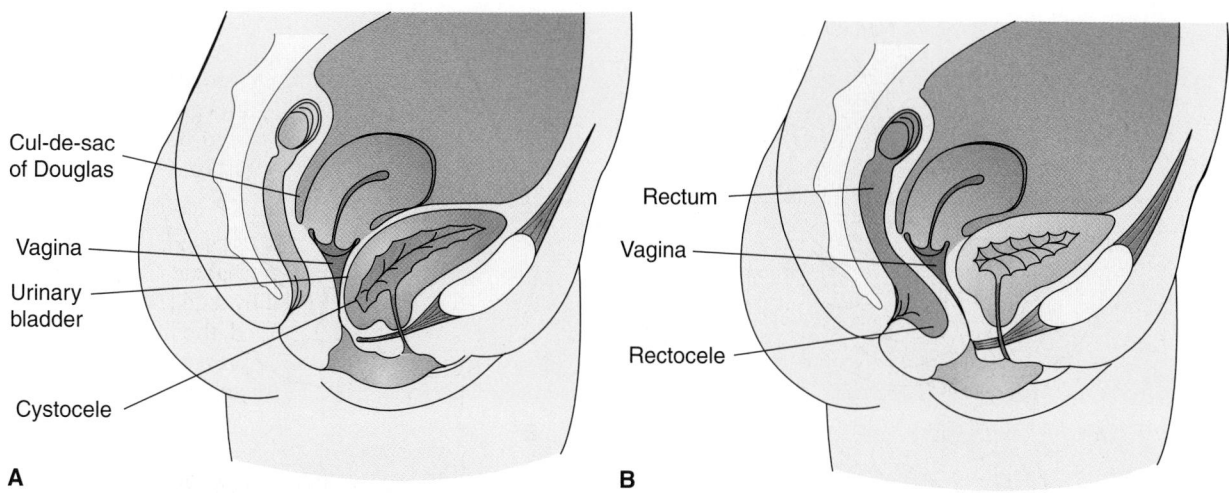

FIGURE 4.8 (A) Cystocele. The bladder has herniated into the anterior wall of the vagina. **(B)** Rectocele. The posterior of the vagina is herniated.

- **Anteflexion,** a condition in which the body of the uterus is bent sharply forward at the junction with the cervix
- **Retroflexion,** a condition in which the body is bent sharply back just above the cervix

Minor variations of these positions usually cause no reproductive problems. Extreme abnormal flexion or version positions may interfere with fertility, because they may block the deposition or migration of sperm (Johnson, 2003). Examples of these abnormal uterine positions are shown in Figure 4.10.

Vagina. The vagina is a hollow, musculomembranous canal located posterior to the bladder and anterior to the rectum. It extends from the cervix of the uterus to the external vulva. Its function is to act as the organ of intercourse and to convey sperm to the cervix so that sperm can meet with the ovum in the fallopian tube. With childbirth, it expands to serve as the birth canal.

When a woman is lying on her back, as she does for a pelvic examination, the course of the vagina is inward and downward. Because of this downward slant and the angle of the uterine cervix, the length of the anterior wall of the vagina is approximately 6 to 7 cm; the posterior wall is 8 to 9 cm. At the cervical end of the structure, there are recesses on all sides of the cervix, termed fornices. Behind the cervix is the posterior fornix; at the front, the anterior fornix; and at the sides, the lateral fornices. The posterior fornix serves as a place for the pooling of semen after coitus; this allows a large number of sperm to remain close to the cervix and encourages sperm migration into the cervix.

The vaginal wall is so thin at the fornices that the bladder can be palpated through the anterior fornix, the ovaries through the lateral fornices, and the rectum through the posterior fornix. The vagina is lined with stratified squamous epithelium similar to that covering the cervix. It has a middle connective tissue layer and a strong muscular wall.

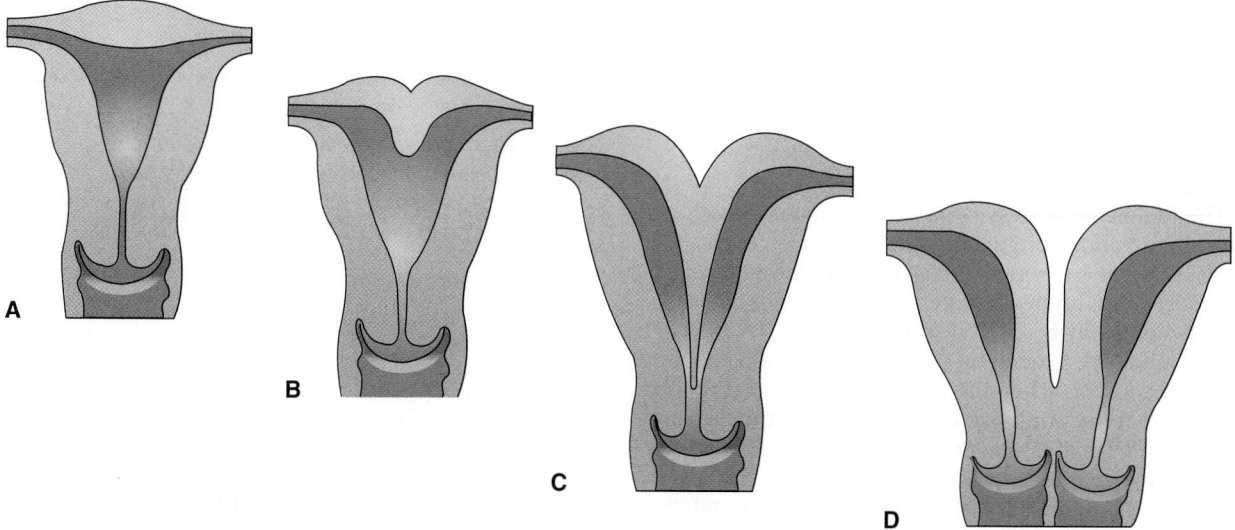

FIGURE 4.9 (A) Normal uterus. **(B)** Bicornuate uterus. **(C)** Septum dividing uterus. **(D)** Double uterus. Abnormal shapes of uterus allow less placenta implantation space.

Normal position

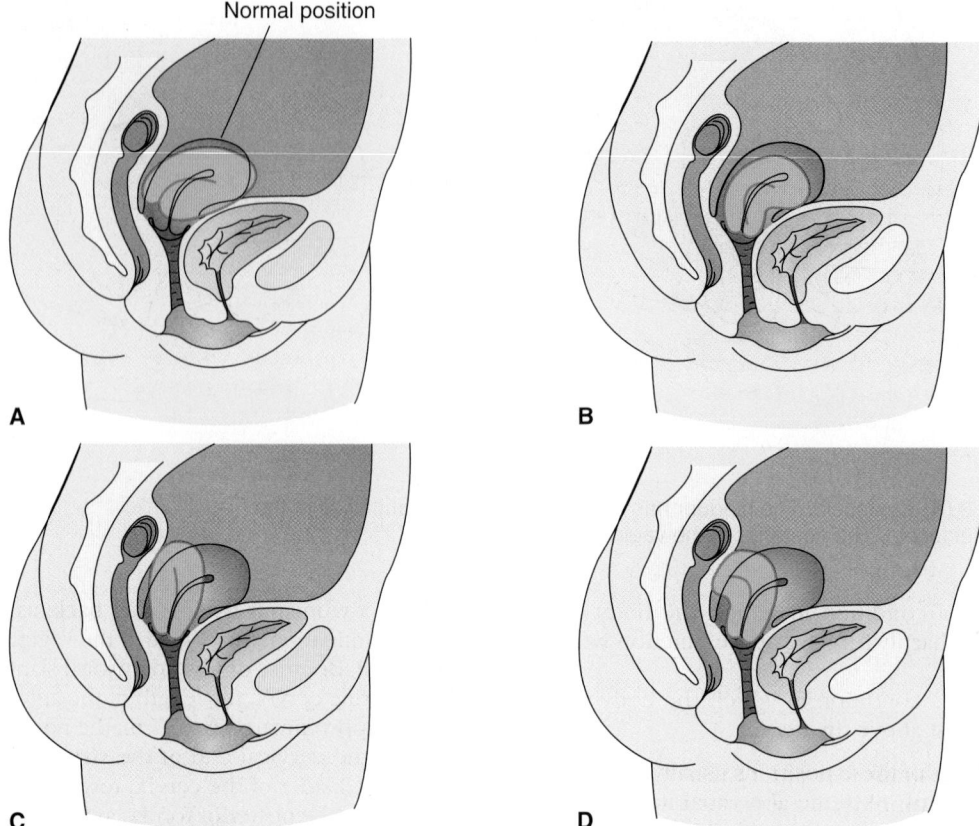

FIGURE 4.10 Uterine flexion and version. (**A**) Anteversion. (**B**) Anteflexion. (**C**) Retroversion. (**D**) Retroflexion.

Normally, the walls contain many folds or rugae and lie in close approximation to each other. These folds make the vagina very elastic and able to expand at the end of pregnancy to allow a full-term baby to pass through without tearing. A circular muscle, the bulbocavernosus, at the external opening of the vagina acts as a voluntary sphincter. Women preparing for childbirth are advised to relax and tense this external vaginal sphincter muscle a set number of times each day to make it more supple for birth and to help maintain tone after birth (Kegel's exercises).

The blood supply to the vagina is furnished by the vaginal artery, a branch of the internal iliac artery. Vaginal tears at childbirth tend to bleed profusely because of this rich blood supply. The same rich blood supply is also the reason that any vaginal trauma at birth heals rapidly.

The vagina has both sympathetic and parasympathetic nerve innervations originating at the S1 to S3 levels. The vagina is not an extremely sensitive organ, however. Sexual excitement, often attributed to vaginal stimulation, is influenced mainly by clitoral stimulation.

The mucus produced by the vaginal lining has a rich glycogen content. When this glycogen is broken down by the lactose-fermenting bacteria that frequent the vagina (Döderlein's bacillus), lactic acid is formed. This makes the usual pH of the vagina acid, a condition detrimental to the growth of pathologic bacteria, so that even though the vagina connects directly to the external surface, infection is not usually present. Under normal circumstances, women should be instructed not to use vaginal douches or sprays

as a daily hygiene measure, because they may clean away the natural acid medium of the vagina, inviting vaginal infections. After menopause, the pH of the vagina becomes closer to 7.5 or slightly alkaline, a reason that vulvovaginitis infections occur more frequently in women in this age group.

Checkpoint Question 3

On physical examination, Suzanne Matthews is found to have a cystocele. A cystocele is:

a. A sebaceous cyst arising from a vulvar fold.
b. Protrusion of the intestine into the vagina.
c. Prolapse of the uterus and cervix into the vagina.
d. Herniation of the bladder into the vaginal wall.

Breasts

The mammary glands, or breasts, form from ectodermic tissue early in utero. They remain in a halted stage of development until a rise in estrogen at puberty produces a marked increase in their size. The size increase consists mainly of connective tissue plus deposition of fat. The glandular tissue of the breasts, necessary for successful breast-feeding, remains undeveloped until a first pregnancy begins. Boys may notice a temporary increase in breast size at puberty, termed **gynecomastia.** If boys are not prepared that this is a normal change of puberty, they may be concerned that they are developing abnormally. The change is most evident in obese boys (Wise et al., 2005).

Breasts are located anterior to the pectoral muscle (Fig. 4.11), and in many women breast tissue extends well into the axilla. Breast self-examinations apparently are not effective in detecting early breast lesions and are no longer recommended (Kosters and Gotzsche, 2004). Women should have a yearly breast examination done by a health care professional, however. When health care providers palpate for breast health this way, they should always include the axillary region in the examination, or some breast tissue will be missed. Milk glands of the breasts are divided by connective tissue partitions into approximately 20 lobes. All of the glands in each lobe produce milk by acinar cells and deliver it to the nipple via a lactiferous duct. The nipple has approximately 20 small openings through which milk is secreted. An ampulla portion of the duct, located just posterior to the nipple, serves as a reservoir for milk before breast-feeding.

A nipple is composed of smooth muscle that is capable of erection on manual or sucking stimulation. On stimulation, it transmits sensations to the posterior pituitary gland to release oxytocin. Oxytocin acts to constrict milk gland cells and push milk forward into the ducts that lead to the nipple. The nipple is surrounded by a darkly pigmented area of epithelium approximately 4 cm in diameter, termed the areola; the areola appears rough on the surface because it contains many sebaceous glands, called Montgomery's tubercles.

The blood supply to the breasts is profuse; it is supplied by thoracic branches of the axillary, internal mammary, and intercostal arteries. This effective blood supply is important in bringing nutrients to the milk glands and makes possible a plentiful supply of milk for breast-feeding. However, it also aids in the metastasis of breast cancer if this is not discovered early by breast examination or mammography (McCance & Huether, 2004).

Pelvis

The pelvis serves both to support and protect the reproductive and other pelvic organs. It is a bony ring formed by four united bones: the two innominate (flaring hip) bones, which form the anterior and lateral portion of the ring, and the coccyx and sacrum, which form the posterior aspect (Fig. 4.12).

Each innominate bone is divided into three parts: ilium, ischium, and pubis. The ilium forms the upper and lateral portion. The flaring superior border of this bone is what forms the prominence of the hip (the crest of the ilium). The ischium is the inferior portion. At the lowest portion of the ischium are two projections: the ischial tuberosities. This is the portion of bone on which a person sits. These projections are important markers used to determine lower pelvic width. The ischial spines are small projections that extend from the lateral aspects into the pelvic cavity. They mark the midpoint of the pelvis. The pubis is the anterior portion of the innominate bone. The symphysis pubis is the junction of the innominate bones at the front of the pelvis.

The sacrum forms the upper posterior portion of the pelvic ring. There is a marked anterior projection of this bone at the point where it touches the lower lumbar vertebrae (the sacral prominence). This is a landmark to identify when securing pelvic measurements.

The coccyx, just below the sacrum, is composed of five very small bones fused together. Although it is stiff, there is a degree of movement possible in the joint between the sacrum and the coccyx (the sacrococcygeal joint). This movement is important because it permits the coccyx to be pressed backward, allowing more room for the fetal head as it passes through the bony pelvic ring at birth.

For obstetric purposes, the pelvis is further divided into the false pelvis (the superior half) and the true pelvis (the inferior half) (Fig. 4.13). The false pelvis supports the uterus during the late months of pregnancy and aids in directing the fetus into the true pelvis for birth. The false pelvis is divided from the true pelvis only by an imaginary

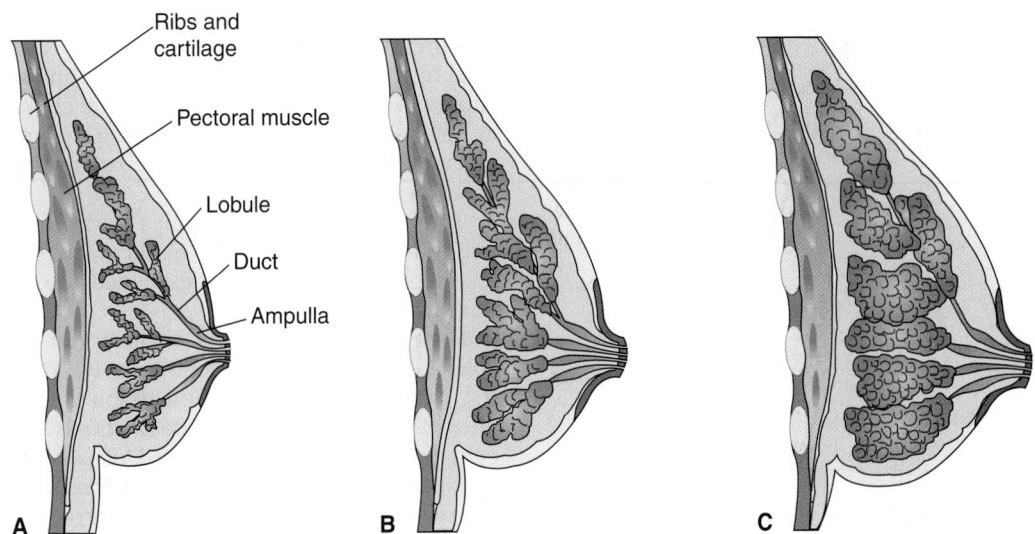

FIGURE 4.11 Anatomy of the breast. (**A**) Nonpregnant. (**B**) Pregnant. (**C**) During lactation.

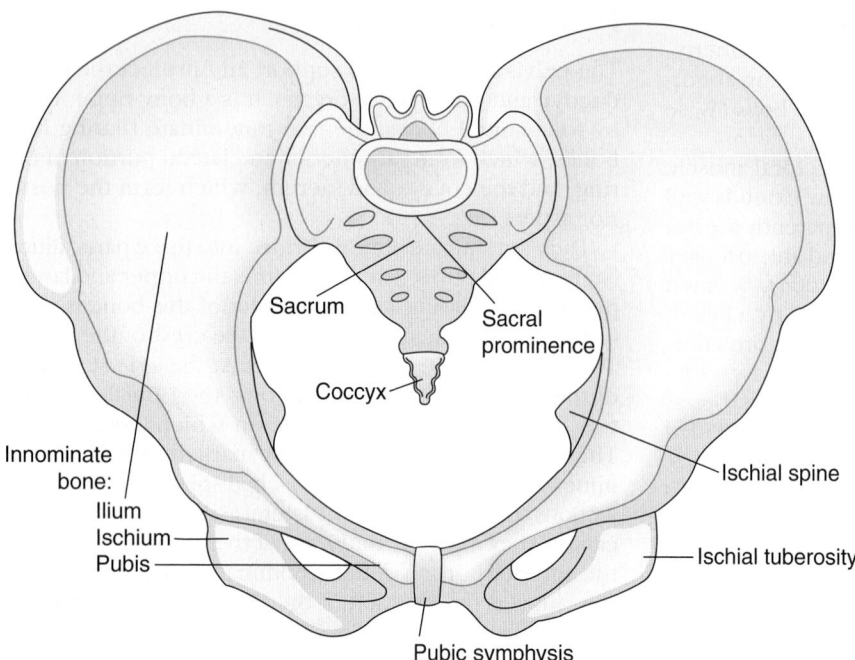

Sacrum

Sacral prominence

Coccyx

Ischial spine

Innominate bone:
Ilium
Ischium
Pubis

Ischial tuberosity

Pubic symphysis

FIGURE 4.12 Structure of the pelvis.

line, the linea terminalis. This imaginary line is drawn from the sacral prominence at the back of the pelvis to the superior aspect of the symphysis pubis at the front of the pelvis. The area above the line is the false pelvis, and that below it is the true pelvis.

Other important terms in relation to the pelvis are the inlet, the pelvic cavity, and the outlet. The inlet is the en-

False pelvis

True pelvis

Linea terminalis (pelvic inlet)

Diagonal conjugate

Ischial spine

Coccyx

Pelvic outlet

Ischial tuberosity

Symphysis pubis

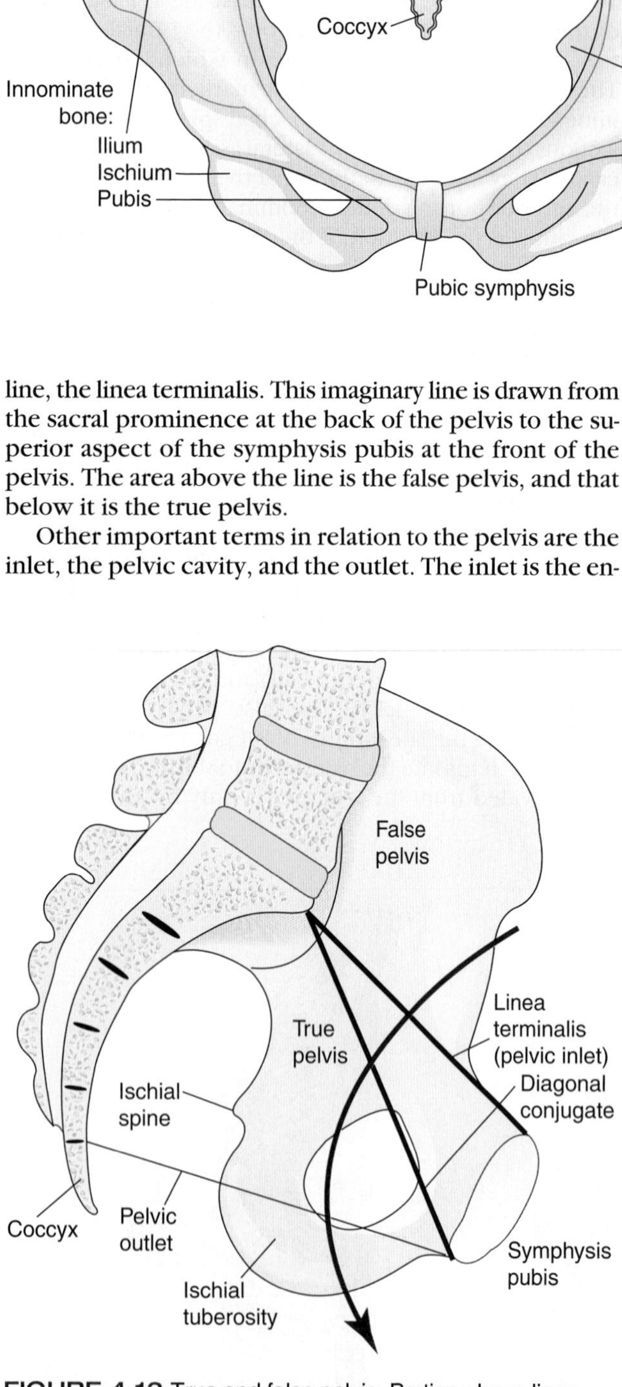

FIGURE 4.13 True and false pelvis. Portion above linea terminalis is false pelvis; portion below is true pelvis. *Arrow* shows "stovepipe" curve that the fetus must follow to be born.

trance to the true pelvis, or the upper ring of bone through which the fetus must pass to be born vaginally. It is at the level of the linea terminalis or is marked by the sacral prominence in the back, the ilium on the sides, and the superior aspect of the symphysis pubis in the front. If one looks down at the pelvic inlet, the passageway at this point appears heart-shaped because of the jutting sacral prominence. It is wider transversely (sideways) than in the anteroposterior dimension.

The outlet is the inferior portion of the pelvis, or that portion bounded in the back by the coccyx, on the sides by the ischial tuberosities, and in the front by the inferior aspect of the symphysis pubis. In contrast to the inlet of the pelvis, the greatest diameter of the outlet is its anteroposterior diameter.

The pelvic cavity is the space between the inlet and the outlet. This space is not a straight but a curved passage. The curve slows and controls the speed of birth and therefore reduces sudden pressure changes in the fetal head, which might rupture cerebral arteries. The snugness of the cavity compresses the chest of the fetus as he or she passes through, helping to expel lung fluid and mucus and thereby better prepare the lungs for good aeration at birth.

The level of the ischial spines marks the midplane or midpoint of the pelvis. This marker is used to assess the level to which the fetus has descended into the birth canal during labor.

For a baby to be delivered vaginally, he or she must be able to pass through the inlet, the cavity, and the outlet of the pelvic bone. This is not a problem for the average fetus; it may be a problem if the mother is a young adolescent girl who has not yet achieved full pelvic growth (girls younger than age 14 years are most prone to this difficulty) or a woman who has had a pelvic injury (e.g., from an automobile accident). Different pelvic types and an assessment of pelvic size are discussed in detail in Chapter 10.

MENSTRUATION

A menstrual cycle (also termed a female reproductive cycle) can be defined as episodic uterine bleeding in response to cyclic hormonal changes. It is the process that allows for conception and implantation of a new life. The purpose of a menstrual cycle is to bring an ovum to maturity and renew a uterine tissue bed that will be responsible for its growth should it be fertilized. Menarche, the first menstrual period in girls, may occur as early as age 8 or 9 or as late as age 17 and still be within normal limits. Because menarche may occur as early as 9 years of age, it is good to include health teaching information on menstruation to both girls and their parents as early as fourth grade as part of routine care. It is a poor introduction to sexuality and womanhood for a girl to begin menstruation unwarned and unprepared for the important internal function it represents.

The length of menstrual cycles differs from woman to woman, but the accepted average length is 28 days (from the beginning of one menstrual flow to the beginning of the next). However, it is not unusual for cycles to be as short as 23 days or as long as 35 days. The length of the average menstrual flow (termed menses) is 4 to 6 days, although women may have periods as short as 2 days or as long as 7 days (Speroff & Fritz, 2005).

Because there is such variation in length, frequency, and amount of menstrual flow and such variation in the onset of menarche, many women have questions about what is considered normal. Contact with health care personnel during a yearly health examination or prenatal visit is often their first opportunity to ask questions they have had for some time. Table 4.1 summarizes the normal characteristics of menstruation for quick reference.

Physiology of Menstruation

Four body structures are involved in the physiology of the menstrual cycle: the hypothalamus, the pituitary gland, the ovaries, and the uterus. For a menstrual cycle to be complete, all four structures must contribute their part; inactivity of any part results in an incomplete or ineffective cycle (Fig. 4.14).

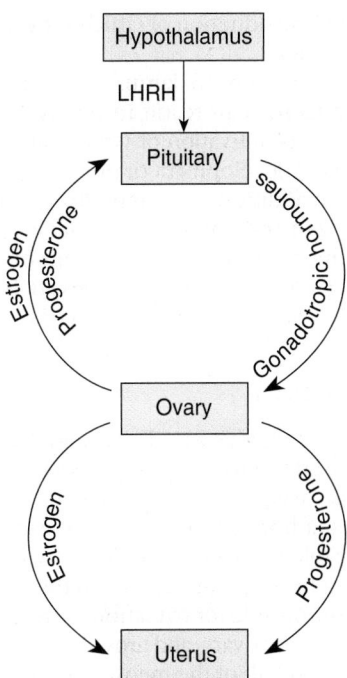

FIGURE 4.14 The interaction of pituitary-uterine-ovarian functions in a menstrual cycle.

Hypothalamus

The release of GnRH (also called luteinizing hormone-releasing hormone, or LHRH) by the hypothalamus initiates the menstrual cycle. When the level of estrogen (produced by the ovaries) rises, release of the hormone is repressed, and menstrual cycles do not occur. During childhood, the hypothalamus is apparently so sensitive to the small amount of estrogen produced by the adrenal glands that release of the hormone is suppressed. Beginning with puberty, the hypothalamus becomes less sensitive to estrogen feedback; this results in the initiation every month in females of the hormone GnRH. GnRH is transmitted from the hypothalamus to the anterior pituitary gland and signals the gland to begin producing the gonadotropic hormones FSH

TABLE 4.1

Characteristics of Normal Menstrual Cycles

Characteristic	Description
Beginning (menarche)	Average age at onset, 11–13 years; average range, 9–17 years
Interval between cycles	Average, 28 days; cycles of 23–35 days not unusual
Duration of menstrual flow	Average flow, 2–7 days; ranges of 1–9 days not abnormal
Amount of menstrual flow	Difficult to estimate; average 30–80 mL per menstrual period; saturating pad or tampon in less than an hour is heavy bleeding
Color of menstrual flow	Dark red; a combination of blood, mucus, and endometrial cells
Odor	Similar to that of marigolds

and LH. Because production of GnRH is cyclic, menstrual periods also cycle.

Diseases of the hypothalamus causing deficiency of this releasing factor can result in delayed puberty. Diseases causing early activation of GnRH can lead to abnormally early sexual development or precocious puberty (see Chapter 47). In addition to the inhibitory feedback mechanism of estrogen and progesterone that halts production of the releasing factor for the remainder of each month, high levels of pituitary-based hormones such as prolactin, FSH, or LH can also inhibit production of GnRH.

Pituitary Gland

Under the influence of GnRH, the anterior lobe of the pituitary gland (the adenohypophysis) produces two hormones that act on the ovaries to further influence the menstrual cycle: (1) FSH, a hormone that is active early in the cycle and is responsible for maturation of the ovum, and (2) LH, a hormone that becomes most active at the midpoint of the cycle and is responsible for ovulation, or release of the mature egg cell from the ovary, and growth of the uterine lining during the second half of the menstrual cycle.

Ovary

FSH and LH are called gonadotropic hormones because they cause growth (trophy) in the gonads (ovaries). Every month during the fertile period of a woman's life (from menarche to menopause), one of the ovary's primordial follicles is activated by FSH to begin to grow and mature. As it grows, its cells produce a clear fluid (follicular fluid) that contains a high content of estrogen (mainly estradiol) and some progesterone. As it reaches its maximum size, it is propelled toward the surface of the ovary. At full maturity, it is visible on the surface of the ovary as a clear water blister approximately 0.25 to 0.5 inches across. At this stage of maturation, the small ovum (barely visible to the naked eye, approximately the size of a printed period), with its surrounding follicle membrane and fluid, is termed a graafian follicle.

By day 14 before the end of a menstrual cycle (the midpoint of a typical 28-day cycle), the ovum has divided by mitotic division into two separate bodies: a primary oocyte, which contains the bulk of the cytoplasm, and a secondary oocyte, which contains so little cytoplasm that it is not functional. The structure also has accomplished its meiotic division, reducing its number of chromosomes to the haploid (having only one member of a pair) number of 23.

After an upsurge of LH from the pituitary, prostaglandins are released and the graafian follicle ruptures. The ovum is set free from the surface of the ovary, a process termed ovulation. It is swept into the open end of a fallopian tube. It is important to teach women that ovulation occurs on approximately the 14th day before the onset of the next cycle. Because ovulation happens at the midpoint of a 28-day cycle, many women think incorrectly that the midpoint of their cycle is their day of ovulation. If the cycle is only 20 days long, however, their day of ovulation would be day 6, not the 10th or middle day. If a cycle is 44 days long, ovulation would occur on day 30, not day 22.

After the ovum and the follicular fluid have been discharged from the ovary, the cells of the follicle remain in the form of a hollow, empty pit. The FSH has done its work at this point and now decreases in amount. The second pituitary hormone, LH, continues to rise in amount and acts on the follicle cells of the ovary. This influence causes the follicle cells to begin to produce lutein, a bright-yellow fluid, instead of follicular fluid. Lutein is high in progesterone and contains some estrogen, whereas the follicular fluid is high in estrogen with some progesterone. This yellow fluid fills the empty follicle, which is then termed a corpus luteum (yellow body).

The basal body temperature of a woman drops slightly (by 0.5° to 1°F) just before the day of ovulation, because of the extremely low level of progesterone that is present at that time. It rises by 1°F on the day after ovulation, because of the concentration of progesterone (which is thermogenic) that is present at that time. The woman's temperature remains at this level until approximately day 24 of the menstrual cycle, when the progesterone level again decreases (McCance & Huether, 2004).

If conception (fertilization by a spermatozoon) occurs as the ovum proceeds down a fallopian tube and the fertilized ovum implants on the endometrium of the uterus, the corpus luteum remains throughout the major portion of the pregnancy (approximately 16 to 20 weeks). If conception does not occur, the unfertilized ovum atrophies after 4 or 5 days, and the corpus luteum (called a "false" corpus luteum) remains for only 8 to 10 days. As the corpus luteum regresses, it is gradually replaced by white fibrous tissue, and the resulting structure is termed a corpus albicans (white body). Figure 4.15 shows the times when ovarian hormones are secreted at peak levels during a typical 28-day menstrual cycle.

Uterus

Stimulation from the hormones produced by the ovaries causes specific monthly effects on the uterus. Figure 4.15 illustrates the uterine changes that occur during the menstrual cycle. These changes are detailed in the following paragraphs.

First Phase of Menstrual Cycle (Proliferative). Immediately after a menstrual flow (which occurs during the first 4 or 5 days of a cycle), the endometrium, or lining of the uterus, is very thin, approximately one cell layer in depth. As the ovary begins to produce estrogen (in the follicular fluid, under the direction of the pituitary FSH), the endometrium begins to proliferate. This growth is very rapid and increases the thickness of the endometrium approximately eightfold. This increase continues for the first half of the menstrual cycle (from approximately day 5 to day 14). This half of a menstrual cycle is termed interchangeably the proliferative, estrogenic, follicular, or postmenstrual phase.

Second Phase of Menstrual Cycle (Secretory). After ovulation, the formation of progesterone in the corpus luteum (under the direction of LH) causes the glands of the uterine endometrium to become corkscrew or twisted in appearance and dilated with quantities of glycogen (an elementary sugar) and mucin (a protein). The capillaries

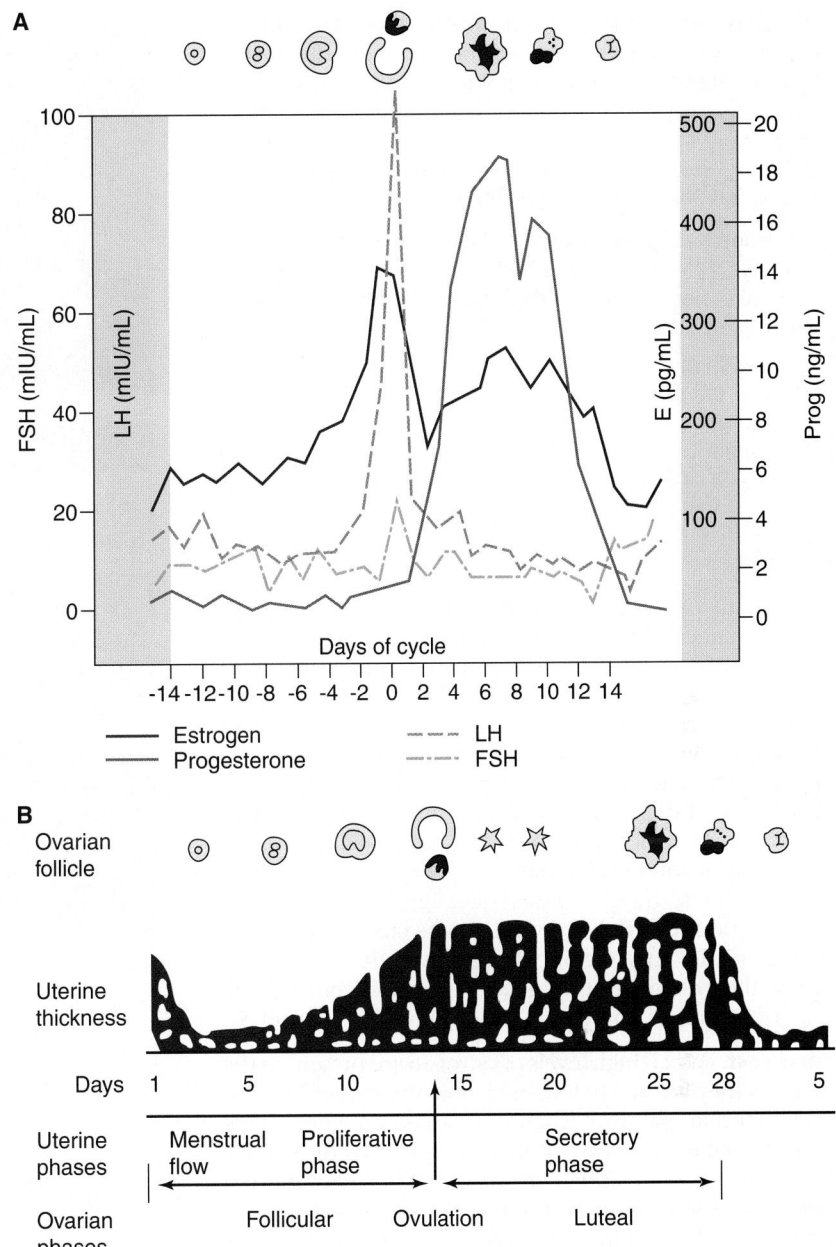

FIGURE 4.15 (**A**) Plasma hormone concentrations in the normal female reproductive cycle. (**B**) Ovarian events and uterine changes during the menstrual cycle.

of the endometrium increase in amount until the lining takes on the appearance of rich, spongy velvet. This second phase of the menstrual cycle is termed the progestational, luteal, premenstrual, or secretory phase.

Third Phase of Menstrual Cycle (Ischemic). If fertilization does not occur, the corpus luteum in the ovary begins to regress after 8 to 10 days. As it regresses, the production of progesterone and estrogen decreases. With the withdrawal of progesterone stimulation, the endometrium of the uterus begins to degenerate (at approximately day 24 or day 25 of the cycle). The capillaries rupture, with minute hemorrhages, and the endometrium sloughs off.

Menses: The Final Phase of a Menstrual Cycle. The following products are discharged from the uterus as the menstrual flow or menses:

- Blood from the ruptured capillaries
- Mucin from the glands
- Fragments of endometrial tissue
- The microscopic, atrophied, and unfertilized ovum

Menses is actually the end of an arbitrarily defined menstrual cycle. Because it is the only external marker of the cycle, however, the first day of menstrual flow is used to mark the beginning day of a new menstrual cycle.

Contrary to common belief, a menstrual flow contains only approximately 30 to 80 mL of blood; if it seems like more, it is because of the accompanying mucus and endometrial shreds. The iron loss in a typical menstrual flow is approximately 11 mg. This is enough loss that many women need to take a daily iron supplement to prevent iron depletion during their menstruating years.

In women who are going through menopause, menses may typically consist of a few days of spotting before a heavy flow, or a heavy flow followed by a few days of spotting, because progesterone withdrawal is more sluggish or tends to "staircase" rather than withdraw smoothly.

Checkpoint Question 4

Suzanne Matthews typically has a menstrual cycle of 34 days. She tells you she had coitus on days 8, 10, 15, and 20 of her last cycle. Which is the day on which she most likely conceived?

a. The 8th day
b. The 10th day
c. Day 15
d. Day 20

Cervix

The mucus of the uterine cervix, as well as the uterine body, changes each month during the menstrual cycle. During the first half of the cycle, when hormone secretion from the ovary is low, cervical mucus is thick and scant. Sperm survival in this type of mucus is poor. At the time of ovulation, when the estrogen level is high, cervical mucus becomes thin and copious. Sperm penetration and survival at the time of ovulation in this thin mucus are excellent. As progesterone becomes the major influencing hormone during the second half of the cycle, cervical mucus again becomes thick and sperm survival is again poor.

Education regarding cervical mucus changes can help women plan coitus to coincide with ovulation, so as to increase their chances of pregnancy, or avoid coitus at the time of ovulation, to prevent pregnancy (see Chapter 5).

Fern Test. When high levels of estrogen are present in the body, as they are just before ovulation, the cervical mucus forms fernlike patterns when it is placed on a glass slide and allowed to dry. The patterns are caused by the crystallization of sodium chloride on mucus fibers. This pattern is known as arborization or ferning (Fig. 4.16). When progesterone is the dominant hormone, as it is just after ovulation, when the luteal phase of the menstrual cycle is beginning, a fern pattern is no longer discernible. Cervical mucus can be examined at midcycle to detect whether ferning or a high estrogen surge is present. Women who do not ovulate continue to show the fern pattern throughout the menstrual cycle (i.e., progesterone levels never become dominant), or they never demonstrate it because their estrogen levels never rise.

Spinnbarkeit Test. At the height of estrogen secretion, the cervical mucus not only becomes thin and watery, but it also can be stretched into long strands. This stretchability is in contrast to its thick, viscous state when progesterone is the dominant hormone. Performing this test, known as spinnbarkeit, at the midpoint of a menstrual cycle is another way to demonstrate that high levels of estrogen are being produced and, by implication, that ovulation is about to occur. A woman can do this herself by stretching a mucus sample between thumb and finger, or it can be tested in an examining room by smearing a cer-

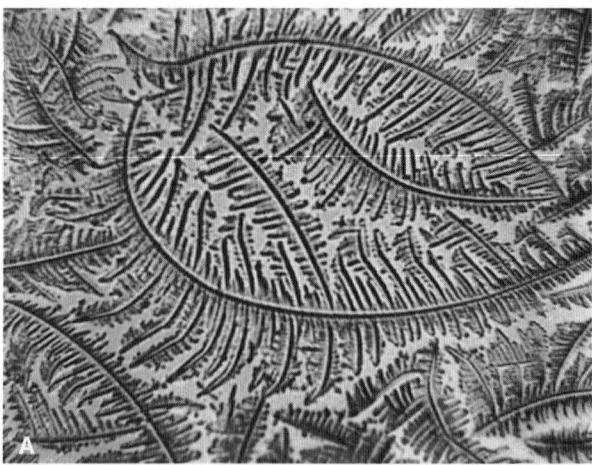

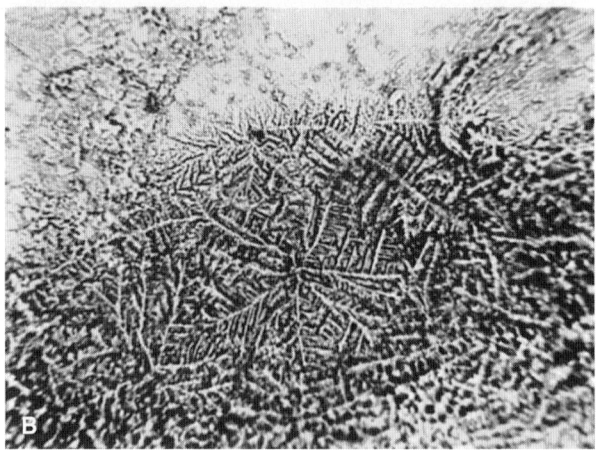

FIGURE 4.16 (A) A ferning pattern of cervical mucus occurs with high estrogen levels. **(B)** Incomplete ferning during secretory phase of cycle. (From Scott, J. R. [1990]. *Danforth's obstetrics and gynecology* [6th ed.]. Philadelphia: J. B. Lippincott.)

vical mucus specimen on a slide and stretching the mucus between the slide and cover slip (Fig. 4.17).

Education for Menstruation

Education about menstruation is an important component of comprehensive sexuality education (Kalman, 2003). Many myths about menstruation still exist, such as that women should not get a permanent during menses; that they should not plant vegetables because the vegetables will die; or that they should not eat sour foods because this will cause cramping. Early preparation for menstruation to dispel these myths is important to a girl's concept of herself as a woman, because it teaches her to trust her body or to think of menstruation as a mark of pride or growing up rather than a burden. Education regarding menstruation is equally important for boys so they can appreciate the cyclic process that a woman's reproductive system activates and can be active participants in helping plan or prevent the conception of children (Howard et al., 2004).

Girls who are well prepared for menstruation and view it as a positive happening are more likely to cope with menstrual discomforts and pain effectively, which means

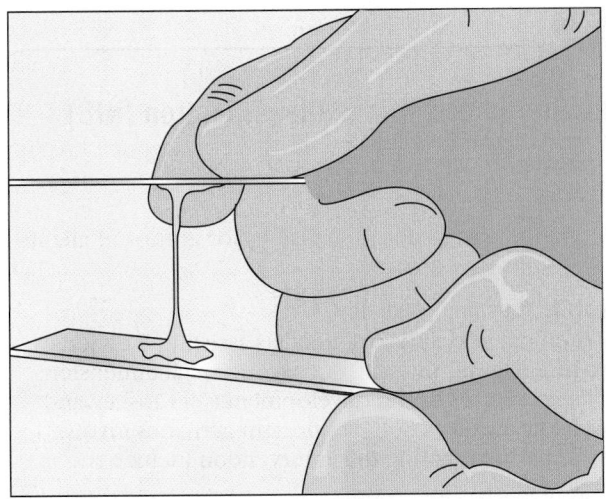

FIGURE 4.17 Spinnbarkeit is the property of cervical mucus to stretch a distance before breaking.

fewer missed school days than among those who view menstruation as an ill time. Important teaching points for girls at menarche regarding menstruation are summarized in Table 4.2. Menstrual disorders, including dysmenorrhea (painful menstruation), **menorrhagia** (abnormally heavy menstrual flows), **metrorrhagia** (bleeding between menstrual periods), menstrual migraines, and premenstrual dysphoric syndrome, are discussed in Chapter 47 with other reproductive system disorders.

Menopause

Menopause is the cessation of menstrual cycles. The postmenopausal period is the time of life after menopause. Perimenopausal is a term used to denote the period during which menopausal changes are occurring (Cedars & Evans, 2003). The age range at which menopause occurs is wide, between approximately 40 and 55 years. Both the age of menarche and the age of menopause tend to be familial (if menarche occurred early in a mother, it will probably occur early in her daughter; if menopause began early in a mother, it may begin early in her daughter). The earlier the age of menarche, the earlier menopause tends to occur. Women need health teaching to learn the normal parameters of menopause so that they may continue to monitor their own health during this time.

Women often refer to this period as a "change of life," because it marks the end of their ability to bear children and the beginning of a new phase of life. This role change can produce stress, especially if falling estrogen levels result in "hot flashes" or osteoporosis (bone loss) (Nachtigall & Nachtigall, 2004). Through health teaching, nurses can help a woman appreciate that loss of uterine function may make almost no change in her life and, for a woman with dysmenorrhea (painful menstruation) or with no desire for more children, it may be a welcome change.

SEXUALITY AND SEXUAL IDENTITY

Sexuality is a multidimensional phenomenon that includes feelings, attitudes, and actions. It has both biologic and cultural components. It encompasses and gives direction to a person's physical, emotional, social, and intellectual responses throughout life. Each person is born a sexual being, and his or her gender identity and gender role behavior evolve from and usually conform to the societal expectations within that person's culture. Nurses can play a major role in promoting sexual health through education and discussion. Box 4.3 highlights appropriate outcomes and interventions using the terminology identified by the Nursing Outcomes Classification (NOC) and Nursing Interventions Classification (NIC).

TABLE 4.2

Teaching About Menstrual Health

Area of Concern	Teaching Points
Exercise	It's good to continue moderate exercise during menses for a general sense of well-being. Sustained excessive exercise, such as professional athletes maintain, can cause amenorrhea.
Sexual relations	Not contraindicated during menses (the male should wear a condom to prevent exposure to body fluid). Heightened or decreased sexual arousal may be noticed during menses. Orgasm may increase menstrual flow. It is improbable but not impossible for conception to occur from coitus during menses.
Activities of daily life	Nothing is contraindicated (many people believe incorrectly that things like washing hair are harmful).
Pain relief	Prostaglandin inhibitors such as ibuprofen (Motrin) are specific for menstrual pain. Applying local heat may also be helpful. If a migraine headache occurs, specific drugs for this are now available, such as sumatriptan (Imitrex).
Rest	More rest may be helpful if dysmenorrhea interferes with sleep at night.
Nutrition	Many women need iron supplementation to replace iron lost in menses. Eating pickles or cold food does not cause dysmenorrhea.

BOX 4.3

Nursing Outcomes Classification (NOC) and Nursing Interventions Classification (NIC)

Sex and Sexuality

NOC: Knowledge, Sexual Functioning

Knowledge, sexual functioning is defined as the extent of understanding conveyed about sexual development and responsible sexual practices (Johnson et al., 2000). Some specific indicators that suggest that this outcome has been achieved include the client's ability to describe the following:

- Function of specific reproductive body parts
- Physical and emotional changes associated with puberty
- Reproduction
- Societal influences on sexual behavior
- Safer sex practices
- Effective contraception
- Measures to prevent sexually transmitted infections (STIs)

NIC: Teaching, Safer Sex

Teaching, safer sex is defined as providing instruction about sexual protection during sexual activity (McCloskey and Bulechek, 2000). Some important activities involved when implementing this intervention include the following:

- Discussing client's attitudes about birth control methods and instructing on the use of effective methods as appropriate
- Encouraging client to be selective in choosing sexual partners
- Instructing on low-risk sexual practices and the importance of good hygiene, lubrication, and voiding after intercourse
- Endorsing the use of condoms, including ways for the client to convince partners to use them
- Providing client with condoms and spermicidal products as appropriate
- Encouraging clients at high risk for STIs to seek regular examinations

- Planning sex education classes for groups of clients as appropriate

NIC: Teaching, Sexuality

Teaching, sexuality is defined as assisting individuals to understand physical and psychosocial dimensions of sexual growth and development (McCloskey and Bulechek, 2000). Some important activities involved when implementing this intervention include the following:

- Creating a nonjudgmental, accepting atmosphere
- Explaining human anatomy and physiology of the male and female body and human reproduction
- Discussing signs of fertility, such as ovulation and menstruation
- Supporting parents' role as primary sexuality educators for their children
- Educating parents on sexual growth and development
- Using appropriate questions for client's self-reflection
- Exploring the meaning of sexual roles
- Discussing sexual behavior and appropriate ways to express one's feelings and needs
- Informing children and adolescents of the benefits of postponing sexual activity and on the negative consequences of early childbearing
- Teaching about STIs, including HIV infection and AIDS
- Educating children and adolescents about effective contraception, including assisting adolescents in choosing a method as appropriate
- Facilitating role-playing to aid in resisting peer and social pressures of sexual activity
- Enhancing self-esteem through peer role-modeling and role-playing

---

Biologic gender is the term used to denote a person's chromosomal sex: male (XY) or female (XX). **Gender identity** or sexual identity is the inner sense a person has of being male or female, which may be the same as or different from biologic gender. **Gender role** is the male or female behavior a person exhibits, which, again, may or may not be the same as biologic gender or gender identity.

Development of Gender Identity

Whether gender identity arises from primarily a biologic or a psychosocial focus is controversial. The amount of testosterone secreted in utero (a process termed sex typing) may affect this characteristic. How appealing parents

or other adult role models portray their gender roles may also influence how a child envisions himself or herself. For example, both sons and daughters may relate better to whichever parent is kinder and more caring. This may result in a son's assuming characteristics often regarded as feminine or a daughter's developing interests typically regarded as masculine.

Gender role is also culturally influenced. In Western society, women have in the past been viewed as kind and nurturing, with sole responsibility for childrearing and homemaking. Men were viewed as financial providers for the family. Gender roles today are more interchangeable than they once were: women pursue all kinds of jobs and careers without loss of femininity, and men participate (some as primary homemakers) in childrearing and household duties without loss of masculinity.

An individual's sense of gender identity develops throughout an entire life span, but the stage is set by expectations even before a child is born. Although parents usually respond to the question, "Do you want a boy or a girl?" with the answer, "It doesn't matter as long as it's healthy," many parents actually do have strong preferences for a male or female child. Although some parents may be disappointed if the child is not the gender they hoped for, most adapt quickly and will say later that they always wanted a child of that sex. Children who suspect that their parents wanted a child of the opposite sex are more likely to adopt roles of the opposite sex than if they are confident their parents are pleased with them as they are.

Infancy

Gender identity is established early in life (Fulchiero-Gordon, 2005). From the day of birth, female and male babies are treated differently by their parents. People generally bring girls dainty rattles and dresses with ruffles; on the whole, they are treated more gently by parents and held and rocked more than male babies. People tend to buy boys bigger rattles and sports-related jogging suits. Admonitions given babies can be different. A girl might be told, "Don't cry. You don't look pretty when you cry." A boy might be told, "You've got to learn to be tougher than that if you're going to make it in this world." By the end of the first year, differences in play are usually strongly evident. Boys appear to demonstrate more innate aggression, even at this early stage, than girls do. For more about the infant period, see Chapters 27 and 28.

Preschool Period

Children can distinguish between males and females as early as 2 years of age. By age 3 or 4 years, they can say what sex they are, and they have absorbed cultural expectations of that sex role. Often, boys will play rough-and-tumble games with other boys, and girls will play more quietly with each other, although the two frequently mix at this age.

Sex role modeling is reinforced through behavior toward and expectations of the child, as well as from such things as the color and décor of the child's room and the child's clothing. Social contacts between the child and significant adults contribute to sexual identification and should be encouraged in this developmental period. A positive self-concept grows from parental love, effective relationships with others, success in play activities, and gaining skills and self-control.

Most American parents are not too rigid about what clothing or colors are appropriate for boys and girls. They strive to teach both sons and daughters about expressing feelings, performing household tasks, and engaging in the same play activities. However, some parents have fixed role identifications. Comments such as, "What kind of mommy are you going to be, treating a doll that way?" or "Is that the way a lady sits?" from parents and well-meaning friends help to govern girls' choice of actions. Common sayings such as "all boy" or "boys will be boys"

BOX 4.4 FOCUS ON . . .

FAMILY TEACHING

Gender Identity Concerns

Q. Suzanne Matthews asks you, "Is it all right to call body parts by nicknames, such as 'peter' for penis, when we talk to children? Or should we use the anatomic name?"

A. Although this decision is strictly up to parents, using anatomic names is usually advised. This prevents children from thinking of one part of the body as so different from others (and perhaps dirty or suspect) that it can't be called by its real name.

Q. Kevin Matthews asks you, "Will it be important to give our child unisex toys? Can't girls play with dolls and boys play with trucks anymore?"

A. Developing a sense of gender involves more than the toys that children use for play. If parents are concerned with instituting unisex roles in children, they need to begin by monitoring their own perspective on what they believe are female and male roles. Once they project a feeling that roles are interchangeable, the general home milieu is more important than any one action in teaching this principle to children in their family.

The way people manifest maleness and femaleness is culturally influenced. For example, in certain cultures, a man may be expected to maintain an air of "machismo" or distance while his partner is in labor, rather than move closer to her and be more comforting. Being aware of cultural differences in this way helps you to view people as individuals and better understand their actions in particular situations.

represent the differences expected between the two sexes. The suggestions in Box 4.4 can help parents promote a positive and more unisex gender identity in their child.

Although the development of an Oedipus complex (the strong emotional attachment of a preschool boy for his mother or a preschool girl for her father) may have been overstated by Freud as a result of sexual bias, many children manifest indications that such a phenomenon does occur during this time. The preschool boy shows signs of competing with his father for his mother's love and attention; the preschool girl competes with her mother for her father's attention and love. Parents may need reassurance that this phenomenon of competition and romance in preschoolers is normal and is one step in the development of their child's gender role identity. Preschooler development is discussed further in Chapter 30.

School-Age Child

Early school-age children typically spend play time imitating adult roles as a way of learning gender roles (Fig. 4.18). They form strong impressions of what a female or male role should be. Where once schools promoted differences

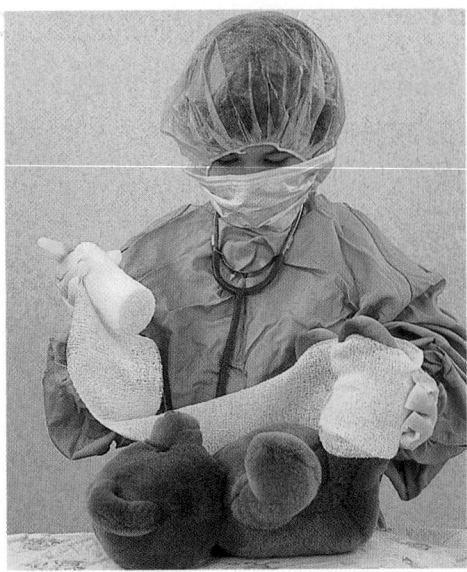

FIGURE 4.18 Early school-age children imitate adult roles to learn more about them. Here a girl "tries on" what being a nurse will feel like. (© Barbara Proud.)

in boys and girls by separating activities and through such beliefs as expecting boys to be poorer readers, to write less neatly, and to act rougher in the school hallways, grade schools have become more attuned to unisex activities. For more information about school-age development, see Chapter 31.

Girls may participate in activities that were once male-dominated, such as Little League and auto repair courses; boys may take cooking courses or ballet lessons, formerly the province of girls.

Adolescent

At puberty, as the adolescent begins the process of establishing a sense of identity, the problem of final gender role identification surfaces again. Most early adolescents maintain strong ties to their gender group, boys with boys and girls with girls. The advent of menstruation may provide a common bond for girls at this stage. Some adolescents choose a child of their own gender a few years older than themselves to use as their model of gender role behavior. This is a way that adolescents can be certain that they understand and feel comfortable with their own sex before they are ready to reach out and interact with members of the opposite sex.

Interviewing adolescents for a sexual history needs to be done tactfully and with confidentiality, because this is a new and sensitive area for them. Although behavior varies in different communities, as many as 50% of adolescents are already sexually active (Centers for Disease Control and Prevention [CDC], 2005). This means that children as young as the early teen years need guidelines for safer sex (Boxes 4.5 and 4.6). Including such instructions as part of sexual counseling should help to reduce the incidence of STIs as well as empower adolescents with better self-care skills. It is important when discussing

safer sex practices to be certain that adolescents not only understand when but how they will incorporate them into their lifestyle. One of the reasons that preventive measures for human immunodeficiency virus (HIV) and other STIs have not been as successful as first predicted may be that adolescents' total lifestyle and interpretation of sexuality were not at first considered (Box 4.7). Chapter 32 discusses adolescence in greater detail.

Adolescence can be a very stressful time for the boy who first realizes that he is gay or the girl who first realizes that she is lesbian. Part of the reason for the high suicide rate in adolescence may be because homosexual teenagers feel so lost in a heterosexual-dominant culture (Rosenberg, 2003).

Young Adult

When young adults move away from home to attend college or establish their own home, they choose the way they will express their sexuality along with other life patterns. Many young adults marry with a commitment to one sexual partner. Others establish relationships (cohabitation) that are less binding by legal definitions but perhaps equally binding in concern and support. Young adults may view cohabitation as a means of learning more about a possible marriage partner on a day-to-day basis, in the hope that a future marriage will then be stronger and more lasting. Homosexuality or bisexuality may be overtly expressed for the first time during this period.

Conflicts in parenting can occur if an individual's gender role does not meet the needs of his or her child and family situation, or if an individual's partner has different expectations regarding gender roles. Parents-to-be need to take time to discuss some of the views they have on parenting and see whether they agree on male and female roles and their relationship with their children. A single parent may be concerned about how both roles can be fulfilled and can benefit from talking with a health care provider about how to discuss this area of concern with a child. Conflicts in the roles parents have chosen often come to light for the first time during pregnancy, as they worry about what type of parents they are going to be or whether they are adequately prepared to be parents. Being able to talk to health care personnel about the gender roles they have adopted in life can be a major step in promoting feelings of adequacy and preparing themselves to raise a child.

Middle-Age Adult

For many women and men in midlife, sexuality has achieved a degree of stability. A sense of masculinity or femininity and comfortable patterns of behavior have been established. This increased security in identity can promote greater intimacy in sexual and social relationships. This may also be a time when adults allow themselves more freedom in exploring and satisfying sexual needs.

Although menopause alters reproductive functioning, it does not physically inhibit sexual functioning. Generally, a woman with a strong self-image, positive sexual and social relationships, and knowledge regarding her body and menopause is likely to progress through this natural biologic stage without problems and remain sexually ac-

BOX 4.9 FOCUS ON . . .

PHARMACOLOGY

Sildenafil Citrate (Viagra)

Classification: Therapy for erectile dysfunction

Action: Causes smooth muscle relaxation and inflow of blood to the corpus cavernosum of the penis, achieving erection (Karch, 2004)

Dosage: 50 mg PO prn 1 hour before sexual activity, up to one dose per day

Possible Adverse Effects: Headache, dizziness, ventricular arrhythmia, impairment of blue/green discrimination

Nursing Implications
- Assess patient for preexisting cardiovascular risk.
- Caution patient that dose should be limited to one time per day; use is contradicted if the patient is taking nitrates.
- Erection lasting more than 4 hours (priapism) can occur. This condition can lead to penile tissue damage.
- Caution patient that this drug does not protect against sexually transmitted infections or pregnancy, so he must use safer sex practices.

in those who are taking medications that contain nitrates), surgical implants to aid erection and the use of vacuum pressure are possible alternatives. Testosterone injections may be helpful in some men. In all instances, frank discussion about the cause of the problem and currently available therapies is helpful. Sildenafil is not FDA-approved for women, but this is a future possibility. Vibration or vacuum devices are also available to increase clitoral enlargement and sexual arousal in women.

Premature Ejaculation

Premature ejaculation is ejaculation before penile-vaginal contact. The term also is often used to mean ejaculation before the sexual partner's satisfaction has been achieved. Premature ejaculation can be unsatisfactory and frustrating for both partners.

The cause of premature ejaculation, like that of ED, can be psychological. Masturbating to orgasm (in which orgasm is achieved quickly owing to lack of time) may play a role. Other reasons suggested are doubt about masculinity and fear of impregnating the woman, which prevents the man from sustaining an erection. Serotonergic antidepressants may be helpful. Sexual counseling for both partners to reduce stress may be helpful in alleviating the problem.

Pain Disorders

Because the reproductive system has a sensitive nerve supply, when pain occurs in response to sexual activities, it can be acute and severe and impair a person's ability to enjoy this segment of life.

Vaginismus

Vaginismus is involuntary contraction of the muscles at the outlet of the vagina when coitus is attempted. This muscle contraction prohibits penile penetration. Vaginismus may occur in women who have been raped. It can also be the result of early learning patterns in which sexual relations were viewed as bad or sinful. As with other sexual problems, sexual or psychological counseling to reduce this response may be necessary.

Dyspareunia/Vestibulitis

Dyspareunia is pain during coitus. Vestibulitis is inflammation of the vestibule (Brotto et al., 2003). These conditions can occur due to endometriosis (abnormal placement of endometrial tissue), vaginal infection, or hormonal changes such as those that occur with menopause and cause vaginal drying. A psychological component may be present. Treatment is aimed at the underlying cause. Encouraging open communication between sexual partners is a nursing intervention that proves useful in all these situations (Shafer, 2005).

Checkpoint Question 5

The Matthews' neighbor Cindy is a woman who has sex with women. Another term for this sexual orientation is

a. Lesbian
b. Celibate
c. Gay
d. Voyeur

Key Points

The reproductive and sexual organs form early in intrauterine life; full functioning becomes possible at puberty.

The female internal organs of reproduction include the ovaries, fallopian tubes, uterus, and vagina.

The female external organs of reproduction include the mons veneris, labia minora and majora, vestibule, clitoris, fourchette, perineal body, hymen, and Skene's and Bartholin's glands.

The male external reproductive structures are the penis, scrotum, and testes. Internal organs are the epididymis, vas deferens, seminal vesicles, ejaculatory ducts, prostate gland, urethra, and bulbourethral glands.

A menstrual cycle is periodic uterine bleeding in response to cyclic hormones. Menarche is the first menstrual period. Menopause is the end of menstruation. Menstrual cycles are possible because of the interplay between the hypothalamus, pituitary, ovaries, and uterus.

Biologic gender is determined by a person's chromosomes (XX or XY) and is set at conception. Gender identity is a person's concept of being male or female. This develops over a lifetime. Gender role is yet a third aspect and is the behavior a person demonstrates based on his or her gender identity as male or female.

Masters and Johnson have identified a sexual response cycle consisting of excitement, plateau, orgasm, and resolution stages. Disorders of sexual dysfunction include failure to achieve orgasm, vaginismus, dyspareunia, inhibited sexual desire, premature ejaculation, and erectile dysfunction.

People present with varying sexual orientations, such as heterosexual, homosexual (women who have sex with women or men who have sex with men), or bisexual. Common sexual expressions are voyeurism, fetishism, and celibacy.

Educating people about reproductive function is an important primary health strategy because it teaches them to better monitor their own health through vulvar or testicular self-examination.

Adolescents should be taught that with sexual maturity comes sexual responsibility. The best protection against either an STI or an unintentional pregnancy is the practice of abstinence or safer sex.

Critical Thinking Exercises

1. At the beginning of the chapter, you met Suzanne and Kevin Matthews, a young adult couple, 12 weeks pregnant, who came to your antepartal clinic for a routine visit. Suzanne, in tears, states, "My husband doesn't seem interested in me anymore. We haven't had sex since I became pregnant." Kevin states, "I'm afraid I'll hurt the baby." How would you counsel them?

2. Kevin's adolescent nephew Mark comes in for an STI. What would you advise Mark regarding safer sex practices?

3. Suzanne tells you that she hopes her new daughter won't be a "tomboy." She asks you what is the best way to convince a girl to be more of a "lady." What advice would you give her? Suppose her daughter was 17 years old? Would your advice be different? Suppose she was concerned because a son was not "boyish" enough? Would your answer be any different?

4. Examine the National Health Goals related to reproductive tract or sexual functioning. Most government-sponsored money for nursing research is allotted based on these goals. What would be a possible research topic to explore pertinent to these goals that would advance evidence-based practice in relation to the Matthews family?

References

Basson, R., et al. (2003). Definitions of women's sexual dysfunction reconsidered: Advocating expansion and revision. *Journal of Psychosomatic Obstetrics and Gynecology, 24*(4), 221–229.

Brotto, L. A., Basson, R., & Gehring, D. (2003). Psychological profiles among women with vulvar vestibulitis syndrome: A chart review. *Journal of Psychosomatic Obstetrics and Gynecology, 24*(3), 195–203.

Cedars, M. I., & Evans, M. (2003). Menopause. In Scott, J. R., et al. (Eds.), *Danforth's obstetrics and gynecology.* Philadelphia: Lippincott Williams & Wilkins.

Centers for Disease Control and Prevention. (2005). *Adolescent pregnancy.* Washington, D.C.: CDC.

Colarusso, C. A. (2005). Midlife transition and crisis. In Sadock, B. J., & Sadock, V. A. (Eds.), *Kaplan and Sadock's comprehensive textbook of psychiatry.* Philadelphia: Lippincott Williams & Wilkins.

De, E., & Wilson, T. (2004). Urinary incontinence. In Siroky, M. B., Oates, R. D., & Babayan, R. K. (Eds.), *Handbook of urology: Diagnosis and therapy* (3rd ed.). Philadelphia: Lippincott Williams & Wilkins.

Department of Health and Human Services. (2000). *Healthy people 2010.* Washington, D.C.: DHHS.

DiGiulio, G. (2003). Sexuality and people living with physical or developmental disabilities: A review of key issues. *Canadian Journal of Human Sexuality, 12*(1), 53–68.

Dimitrakakis, C., et al. (2004). Breast cancer incidence in postmenopausal women using testosterone in addition to usual hormone therapy. *Menopause, 11*(5):531–535.

Drescher, J., Stein, T. S., & Byne, W. M. (2005). Homosexuality, gay and lesbian identities, and homosexual behavior. In Sadock, B. J., & Sadock, V. A. (Eds.), *Kaplan and Sadock's comprehensive textbook of psychiatry.* Philadelphia: Lippincott Williams & Wilkins.

Eisenberg, M. E., et al. (2004). Parents' beliefs about condoms and oral contraceptives: Are they medically accurate? *Perspectives on Sexual and Reproductive Health, 36*(2), 50–57.

Fazio, L., & Brock, G. (2004). Erectile dysfunction: Management update. *Canadian Medical Association Journal, 170*(9), 1429–1437.

Feldman, J., & Bockting, W. (2003). Transgender health. *Minnesota Medicine, 86*(7), 25–32.

Fulchiero-Gordon, M. (2005). Normal child development. In Sadock, B. J., & Sadock, V. A. (Eds.), *Kaplan and Sadock's comprehensive textbook of psychiatry.* Philadelphia: Lippincott Williams & Wilkins.

Green, R. (2005). Gender identity disorders. In Sadock, B. J., & Sadock, V. A. (Eds.), *Kaplan and Sadock's comprehensive textbook of psychiatry.* Philadelphia: Lippincott Williams & Wilkins.

Howard, M., et al. (2004). Young males' sexual education and health services. *American Journal of Public Health, 94*(8), 1332–1335.

Hughes, C., & Evans, A. (2003). Health needs of women who have sex with women. *British Medical Journal, 327*(7421), 939–940.

Johnson, J. (2003). Infertility. In Scott, J. R., et al. (Eds.), *Danforth's obstetrics and gynecology.* Philadelphia: Lippincott Williams & Wilkins.

Johnson, M., Maas, M., & Moorhead, S. (2000). *Nursing outcomes classification* (2nd ed.). St. Louis: Mosby.

Kalman, M. (2003). Taking a different path: Menstrual preparation for adolescent girls living apart from their mothers. *Health Care for Women International, 24*(10), 868–879.

Karch, A. M. (2004). *Lippincott's nursing drug guide.* Philadelphia: Lippincott Williams & Wilkins.

Kosters, J. P., & Gotzsche, P. C. (2004). Regular self-examination or clinical examination for early detection of breast cancer. *Cochrane Database of Systematic Reviews* (2) (CD003373).

Masters, W. H. (1998). *Heterosexuality.* New York: Smithmark.

McCance, K. L., & Huether, S. E. (2004). *Understanding pathophysiology* (3rd ed.). St. Louis: Mosby.

McCloskey, J., & Bulechek, G. (2000). *Nursing interventions classification* (3rd ed.). St. Louis: Mosby.

McEvoy, M., Chang, J., & Coupey, S. M. (2004). Common menstrual disorders in adolescence: Nursing interventions. *MCN: American Journal of Maternal Child Nursing, 29*(1), 41–49.

McKenzie, L. J., & Carson, S. A. (2003). Human sexuality and female sexual dysfunction. In Scott, J. R., et al. (Eds.), *Danforth's obstetrics and gynecology.* Philadelphia: Lippincott Williams & Wilkins.

Nachtigall, L. E., & Nachtigall, M. J. (2004). Menopausal changes, quality of life, and hormone therapy. *Clinical Obstetrics and Gynecology, 47*(2), 485–488.

Person, E. S. (2005): Paraphilias. In Sadock, B. J., & Sadock, V. A. (Eds.), *Kaplan and Sadock's comprehensive textbook of psychiatry.* Philadelphia: Lippincott Williams & Wilkins.

Rosenberg, M. (2003). Recognizing gay, lesbian, and transgender teens in a child and adolescent psychiatry practice. *Journal of the American Academy of Child and Adolescent Psychiatry, 42*(12), 1517–1521.

Sadock, V. A. (2005). Normal human sexuality and sexual dysfunctions. In Sadock, B. J., & Sadock, V. A. (Eds.), *Kaplan and Sadock's comprehensive textbook of psychiatry.* Philadelphia: Lippincott Williams & Wilkins.

Shafer, L. C. (2005). Approach to the patient with sexual dysfunction. In Goroll, A. H., May, L. A., & Mulley, A. G. (Eds.), *Primary care medicine* (5th ed.). Philadelphia: Lippincott Williams & Wilkins.

Speroff, L., & Fritz, M. A. (2005). *Clinical gynecologic endocrinology and infertility* (7th ed.). Philadelphia: Lippincott Williams & Wilkins.

Tanner, J. M. (1990). Fetus into man. In Tanner, J. M. *Physical growth from conception to maturity* (2nd ed.). Cambridge, MA: Harvard University Press.

Tate, F. B., & Longo, D. A. (2004). Homophobia: A challenge for psychosocial nursing. *Journal of Psychosocial Nursing and Mental Health Services, 42*(8), 26–33.

Valente, S. M., & Bullough, V. (2004). Sexual harassment of nurses in the workplace. *Journal of Nursing Care Quality, 19*(3), 234–241.

Wood, W. C., et al. (2005). Malignant tumors of the breast. In DeVita, V. T., Hellman, S., & Rosenberg, S. A. (Eds.), *Cancer: Principles and practice of oncology.* Philadelphia: Lippincott Williams & Wilkins.

Wise, G. J., et al. (2005). Male breast disease. *Journal of the American College of Surgeons, 200*(2), 255–269.

Suggested Readings

Askew, I., & Berer, M. (2003). The contribution of sexual and reproductive health services to the fight against HIV/AIDS: A review. *Reproductive Health Matters, 11*(22), 51–73.

Bakker, L. J., & Cavender, A. (2003). Promoting culturally competent care for gay youth. *Journal of School Nursing, 19*(2), 65–72.

Bustamante-Forest, R., & Giarratano, G. (2004). Changing men's involvement in reproductive health and family planning. *Nursing Clinics of North America, 39*(2), 301–318.

Connell, P., McKevitt, C., & Low, N. (2004). Investigating ethnic differences in sexual health: Focus groups with young people. *Sexually Transmitted Infections, 80*(4), 300–305.

Foy, R., & Crilly, M. (2004). Evidence-based reproductive health care: Getting evidence into practice. *Journal of Family Planning and Reproductive Health Care, 30*(1), 17–20.

Goold, P. C., Ward, M., & Carlin, E. M. (2003). Can the Internet be used to improve sexual health awareness in web-wise young people? *Journal of Family Planning and Reproductive Health Care, 29*(1), 28–30.

Johnson, W. D., Hedges, L. V., & Diaz, R. M. (2005). Interventions to modify sexual risk behaviors for preventing HIV infection in men who have sex with men. *Cochrane Library (Oxford) (1)* (CD001230).

Khalid, A. (2004). Irregular or absent periods: What can an ultrasound scan tell you? *Best Practice and Research in Clinical Obstetrics and Gynaecology, 18*(1), 3–11.

Taleporos, G., & McCabe, M. P. (2003). Relationships, sexuality and adjustment among people with physical disability. *Sexual and Relationship Therapy, 18*(1), 25–43.

Unger, J. (2004). How to assess and treat erectile dysfunction. *Emergency Medicine, 36*(1), 28–30.

CHAPTER 5

Reproductive Life Planning

Key Terms

abstinence
barrier method
cervical cap
coitus interruptus
condom
contraceptive
diaphragm
elective termination of
    pregnancy
fertility awareness
intrauterine device
laparoscopy
natural family planning
reproductive life planning
tubal ligation
vasectomy

Objectives

After mastering the contents of this chapter, you should be able to:

1. Describe common methods of reproductive life planning and the advantages, disadvantages, and risk factors associated with each.
2. Assess clients for reproductive life planning needs.
3. Formulate nursing diagnoses related to reproductive life planning concerns.
4. Identify expected outcomes for couples desiring reproductive life planning.
5. Plan nursing care related to reproductive life planning, such as helping a client select a suitable family planning measure.
6. Implement nursing care related to reproductive life planning, such as educating adolescents about the use of condoms as a safer sex practice as well as to prevent unwanted pregnancy.
7. Evaluate expected outcomes for achievement and effectiveness of care.
8. Identify National Health Goals related to reproductive life planning that nurses can help the nation achieve.
9. Identify areas related to reproductive life planning that could benefit from additional nursing research or application of evidence-based practice.
10. Use critical thinking to analyze ways reproductive health planning can promote reproductive health within a family-centered framework.
11. Integrate reproductive life planning with nursing process to achieve quality maternal and child health nursing care.

Seventeen-year-old Dana Crews has come to a community health clinic for a pelvic examination and Pap smear. During the assessment interview, Dana states that she is sexually active. She and her boyfriend sometimes use a condom. She trusts her boyfriend will "stop in time" when they aren't using one. She doesn't want to take the pill because she can't afford it and she's afraid her parents will find out that she's having sex.

Previous chapters described the anatomy and physiology of the male and female reproductive systems. This chapter adds information about ways to prevent pregnancy or plan and space children. This is important information, because it builds a base for care and health teaching about safer sex practices.

Does Dana need any additional health teaching to be well informed about reproductive life planning?

After you've studied this chapter, access the accompanying website. Read the patient scenario and answer the questions to further sharpen your skills, grow more familiar with RN-CLEX types of questions, and reward yourself with how much you have learned.

Reproductive life planning includes all the decisions an individual or couple make about having children. These decisions usually include whether and when to have children, how many children to have, and how they are spaced. Couples often need counseling about how to avoid conception. Others need information on increasing fertility. Some couples need counseling because contraception has failed.

It is important for the health of children that as many pregnancies as possible be intended, because when a pregnancy is unintended, the mother is less likely to seek prenatal care, less likely to breast-feed, and less careful to protect the fetus from harmful substances. A disproportionate share of the women who bear children whose conception was unintended are unmarried; such women are less apt to complete high school or college and more likely to require public assistance and to live in poverty than their peers who are not mothers. The child of such a pregnancy is at greater risk of low birthweight, dying in the first year, being abused, and not receiving sufficient resources for healthy development (DHHS, 2000).

Until the 1950s, **contraceptive** products (products to prevent pregnancy) were not all that reliable or could not be easily purchased. Today, people have numerous contraceptive choices, which range in reliability and accessibility from fair to good. Reproductive health has become so important that a number of National Health Goals speak directly to this area of care (Box 5.1).

An individual's or a couple's choice of contraceptive method should be made carefully, with complete knowledge about the advantages, disadvantages, and side effects of the various options (Box 5.2). Important things to consider include the following:

- Personal values
- Ability to use a method correctly
- How the method will affect sexual enjoyment
- Financial factors
- Status of a couple's relationship
- Prior experiences
- Future plans

The widespread use of contraceptives in recent years points to both an increased awareness of responsibility for contraception and the options available. Understanding how various methods of contraception work and how they compare in terms of benefits and disadvantages is necessary for successful counseling. Effective use of contraception leads to fewer abortions (Speroff and Fritz, 2005). It is also important to be able to answer questions about elective termination of pregnancy with accurate, up-to-date knowledge and objectivity for couples whose

---

BOX 5.1 FOCUS ON . . .

NATIONAL HEALTH GOALS

A number of National Health Goals speak directly to reproductive life planning:

- Reduce the proportion of females experiencing pregnancy despite use of a reversible contraceptive method from a baseline of 13% to a target of 7%.
- Increase the proportion of pregnancies that are intended from a baseline of 51% to a target of 70%.
- Decrease the proportion of births occurring within 24 months of a previous birth from a baseline of 11% to a target of 6%.
- Increase the proportion of females at risk for unintended pregnancy (and their partners) who use contraception from a baseline of 93% to a target of 100%.
- Increase the number of health care providers who provide emergency contraception (new goal).
- Increase male involvement in pregnancy prevention and family planning efforts (new goal; baseline to be determined) (DHHS, 2000).

Nurses can help the nation achieve these objectives by teaching people, especially adolescents, about contraceptive options. This instruction must be done carefully to avoid indirectly encouraging sexual activity among teens. Investigation into which contraceptives adolescents prefer and why they make the choices they do could be an important area of nursing research.

BOX 5.2 FOCUS ON . . .

COMMUNICATION

You notice that Dana, 17 years old, is reading a pamphlet on oral contraceptives while she waits to be seen by the nurse practitioner.

Less Effective Communication

Nurse: Is that pamphlet helpful? Tell you everything you need to know?

Dana: Not really. Does this come with some way to remind me to take a pill every day?

Nurse: If you're old enough to be sexually active, you should be responsible enough to do that without a separate reminder.

More Effective Communication

Nurse: Is that pamphlet helpful? Tell you everything you need to know?

Dana: Not really. Does this come with some way to remind me to take a pill every day?

Nurse: Will that be a problem?

Dana: I think so.

Nurse: It's good to see you considering your individual lifestyle before making a choice. If you'd like, I could show you how to make out a reminder chart. There are other methods that don't require reminders. Be sure to discuss all options with your nurse practitioner.

Reproductive life planning measures must be individualized to fit a person's lifestyle; otherwise, they will be quickly discontinued. Taking the time to help a woman assess how particular measures fit her lifestyle is better than just giving advice with a "one size fits all" philosophy.

contraceptive method has failed. Legal and ethical issues (e.g., enforced use of contraception for the physically or cognitively challenged) must also be considered when counseling clients on the use of contraceptives. With information and the ability to discuss specific concerns, clients are better prepared to make the decisions that are right for them.

Nursing Process Overview

For Reproductive Health

● *Assessment*

As a result of changing social values and lifestyles, many people are able to talk easily about reproductive life planning. However, others are uncomfortable with this topic and may not voice their interest in the subject independently (Box 5.3). For this reason, at health assessments, clients should be asked if they want more information or need any help with reproductive life planning. Important assessments before the initiation of a contraceptive method include the following:

• A Pap smear, pregnancy test, gonococcal and chlamydial screening, and perhaps hemoglobin for detection of anemia
• Obstetric history, including sexually transmitted infections (STIs), past pregnancies, previous elective abortions, failure of previously used methods, and compliance record
• Subjective assessment of the client's desires, needs, feelings, and understanding of conception (e.g., teens may believe that nothing can happen to them; many women in the immediate postpartum period may believe that they cannot conceive immediately, especially if they are breast-feeding)
• Sexual practices, such as frequency, number of partners, feelings about sex and body image (Box 5.4).

● *Nursing Diagnosis*

Because reproductive life planning touches on so many facets of life, nursing diagnoses can differ greatly depending on the circumstances. Examples

BOX 5.3 FOCUS ON . . .

DIVERSITY OF CARE

People differ greatly in the ways that they desire or accept information on reproductive planning, depending on individual preferences and sociocultural influences. Be certain while counseling people about reproductive planning that you do not impose your own values but, rather, respect the patient's, and that you work together to identify a system that the patient will be able to follow consistently.

BOX 5.4 ASSESSMENT

Assessing the Client for Possible Contraindications to Contraceptive Use

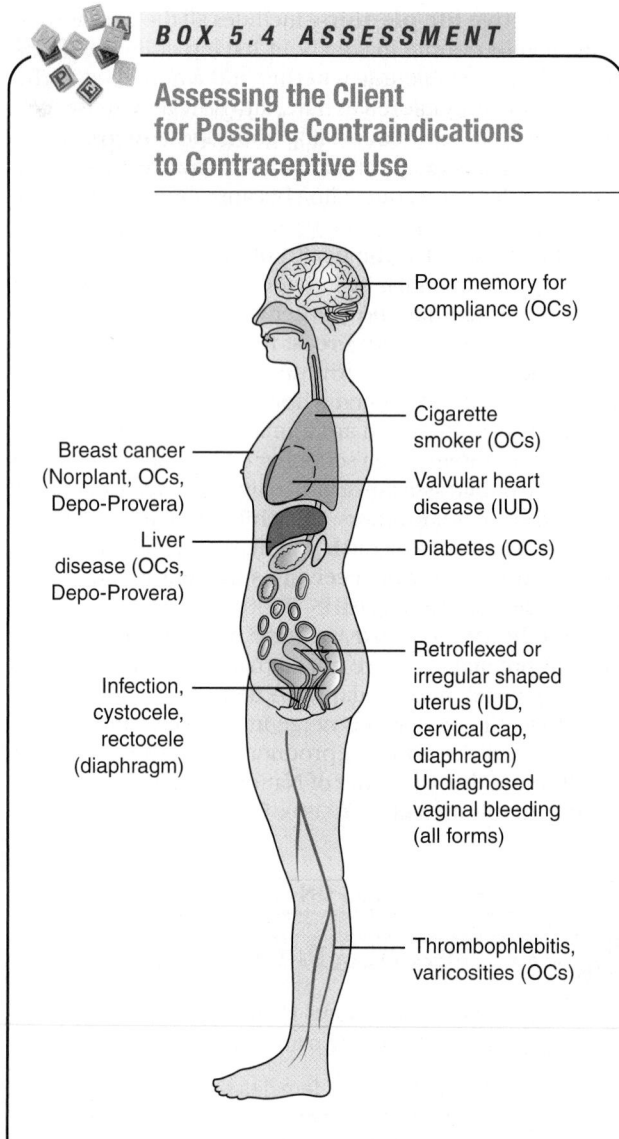

- Poor memory for compliance (OCs)
- Cigarette smoker (OCs)
- Breast cancer (Norplant, OCs, Depo-Provera)
- Valvular heart disease (IUD)
- Liver disease (OCs, Depo-Provera)
- Diabetes (OCs)
- Infection, cystocele, rectocele (diaphragm)
- Retroflexed or irregular shaped uterus (IUD, cervical cap, diaphragm) Undiagnosed vaginal bleeding (all forms)
- Thrombophlebitis, varicosities (OCs)

of nursing diagnoses applicable to reproductive life planning include the following:

• Health-seeking behaviors regarding contraception options related to desire to prevent pregnancy
• Deficient knowledge related to use of diaphragm
• Decisional conflict regarding choice of birth control because of health concern
• Decisional conflict related to unwanted pregnancy
• Powerlessness related to failure of chosen contraceptive
• Altered sexuality patterns related to fear of pregnancy

● *Planning and Implementation*

When establishing expected outcomes for care in this area, be certain that they are realistic for the individual. If a woman has a history of poor compliance with medication, for instance, it might not be realistic for her to plan to take an oral contraceptive every day. Be certain to be sensitive to a couple's religious, cultural, and moral beliefs before suggesting possible methods. It is equally important to explore your own beliefs and values. This not only helps develop self-awareness of how these beliefs affect nursing care, but it allows you to become more sensitive to the beliefs of others.

Education is an important nursing role in this area. Some couples cannot make realistic plans about contraception because they are uninformed or misinformed about the options. An organization that is helpful for referral for reproductive life planning is Planned Parenthood (*www.plannedparenthood.org*). When counseling, be certain to emphasize safer sex measures as well as contraceptive ones (see Box 4.5). For example, although many contraceptive options offer reliable pregnancy prevention, only condoms provide protection against STIs, an important concern if the relationship is not a monogamous one.

Many postpartum services print information on contraception, which they distribute to women to read before discharge. Women are then invited to ask questions as necessary about the material. Read these materials to see that they are accurate, and if suggestions are needed, make them to the correct health care committee. Be certain that unlicensed assistive personnel understand that if a woman has a question about the written material, their job is not to answer it but to refer the woman to someone (such as a nurse) who is more knowledgeable about the subject. Otherwise, they may suggest what method works for them rather than offering unbiased advice. This can result in a woman's choosing a contraceptive method that is not appropriate for her lifestyle and that may then be ineffective for her.

Clients are required to provide informed consent for surgical contraceptive methods or procedures. The risks, benefits, alternatives, and proper use of the method and the client's understanding of his or her rights and responsibilities should be included in the consent form. If you are helping to obtain a signature for consent, always do so in the presence of a witness. Informed consent helps ensure that clients have weighed their options and chosen a method that best meets their needs.

● *Outcome Evaluation*

Evaluation is important in reproductive life planning, because anything that causes clients to discontinue or misuse a particular method will leave them at risk of pregnancy. It is important to reassess early (within 1 to 3 weeks) after a couple begins a new method of contraception, to prevent such an occurrence. Evaluation is much broader than simply ensuring that no unwanted conception occurs, however. The satisfaction of a woman and her sexual partner with the method chosen is also important. Examples of expected outcomes include the following:

- Client voices confidence in chosen method by next visit.
- Client expresses satisfaction with chosen method at follow-up visit.
- Client consistently uses chosen method without pregnancy for next year.

CONTRACEPTIVES

Although as many as 49% of pregnancies in the United States are unintended, as many as 40 million women in the United States use some form of contraception, a figure that represents 65% of women of childbearing age (Centers for Disease Control and Prevention, 2005). To be ideal, a contraceptive should have the following characteristics:

- Safe
- 100% effective
- Free of side effects
- Easily obtainable
- Affordable
- Easy to use and acceptable to both user and sexual partner
- Free of effects on future pregnancies

The most frequently used contraceptive methods and their effectiveness are shown in Table 5.1. This table gives the predicted number of pregnancies that will occur for each method in the first year of use for couples who use the method consistently and correctly and also the expected failure rate for routine use (less than perfect). A method that shows a large difference in these rates is a method that may not be easy and convenient to use.

Box 5.5 provides details on how to implement a plan of care for an adolescent seeking contraceptive information. Box 5.6 highlights appropriate outcomes and interventions using the terminology identified by the Nursing Outcomes Classification and Nursing Interventions Classification (NOC and NIC).

Abstinence

Obviously, the most effective way to protect against conception is to abstain from sexual intercourse (**abstinence**). Abstinence has a theoretical 0% failure rate and is also the most effective way to prevent STIs. However, clients, particularly adolescents, may find it difficult to adhere to abstinence, or they may completely overlook it as an option. Because it fails as an effective birth prevention measure for so many people, use of no contraceptive has a failure rate of 85% (Trussell, 2003). In a moment of passion, many otherwise responsible people may fail to consider abstinence as an option. It is important to present it as a contraceptive option and provide information on ways to comply with this method (Box 5.7). Education about abstinence has resulted in less unprotected sexual activity among adolescents (Santelli et al., 2004).

Natural Family Planning

Natural family planning methods, as the name implies, are those that involve no introduction of chemical or foreign material into the body.

Many people hold religious beliefs that rule out the use of birth control pills or devices; others simply prefer natural methods because no expense or foreign substance is involved; still others believe that a "natural" way of planning pregnancies is best for them. These people are the candidates for natural family planning methods. The effectiveness of these methods varies greatly, depending mainly

TABLE 5.1

Contraceptive Failure Rates

Type of Contraceptive	Ideal Failure Rate* (%)	Typical Use Failure Rate* (%)	% of Women Still Using at 1 Year	Advantages	Disadvantages
No method	85	85	—	No cost	High motivation needed; highly unreliable
Lactation, amenorrhea	—	—	0	Effective for short term	Temporary measure; not reliable if infant takes supplemental feedings
Spermicides	15	29	42	No major health risk; no prescription necessary	Unaesthetic to some; must be properly inserted
Withdrawal	4	27	43	No cost	Not recommended for adolescents
Periodic abstinence	—	25	—	No cost; acceptable to Roman Catholic church	Requires high motivation and periods of abstinence
Calendar	9	—	—	No cost	Requires motivation, cooperation
Ovulation method	3	—	—	No cost	Requires motivation, cooperation
Sympto-thermal	2	—	—	No cost	Requires motivation, cooperation
Postovulation	1	—	—	—	Needs funds for monthly kit
Cervical cap (parous woman)	26	32	46	Can use for several days if desired	May be difficult to insert; can irritate cervix
Cervical cap (nulliparous woman)	9	16	57	Can use for several days if desired	May be difficult to insert; can irritate cervix
Sponge (parous woman)	20	32	46	Easy to insert; no prescription	May cause leakage
Sponge (nulliparous woman)	9	16	57	Easy to insert; no prescription	May cause leakage
Diaphragm	6	16	57	Easy to insert	Prescription needed
Female condom	5	21	49	Protection against STIs	Insertion may be difficult
Male condom	2	15	53	Protects against STIs; male responsibility; no prescription necessary	Requires interruption of sexual activity
Transdermal patch	0.3	8	68	Easy to apply	Irritation at local site
Vaginal ring	0.3	8	68	Easy to insert	May need reminder to insert
IUD (Progesterone T)	1.5	2	81	No memory or motivation needed	Cramping, bleeding; expulsion possible; not recommended if risk of STIs
IUD (copper T)	0.6	0.8	78	No memory or motivation needed	Cramping, bleeding; expulsion possible; not recommended if risk of STIs
IUD (Levonorgestrel 20 Mirena)	0.1	0.1	81	No memory or motivation needed	Cramping, bleeding; expulsion possible; not recommended if risk of STIs
Combination oral contraceptives (COCs)	0.3	8	68	Coitus independent	Continual cost; possible side effects
Injectable progesterone (Depo-Provera)	0.3	3	56	Coitus independent; dependable for 4 to 12 weeks	Continual cost; continual injections
Implanted progesterone (Norplant)	0.05	0.05	84	Coitus independent; dependable for 5 years	Initial cost; appearance on arm
Female sterilization	0.5	0.5	100	Permanent and highly reliable	Initial cost; irreversible
Male sterilization	0.1	0.15	100	Permanent and highly reliable	Initial cost; irreversible

*Among couples who use the method consistently and correctly during a year's time.
Modified from Trussell, J. (2003). In Hatcher, R. A., Trussell, J., Stewart, F., et al. (Eds.). *Contraceptive technology* (18th ed.). New York: Ardent Media.

BOX 5.5: Focus on Nursing Care Planning

A Multidisciplinary Care Map for An Adolescent Seeking Contraceptive Information

•

Seventeen-year-old Dana Crews has come to a community health clinic for a pelvic examination and a Pap smear. During the assessment interview, Dana states that she is sexually active. She and her boyfriend sometimes use a condom. She trusts that her boyfriend will "stop in time" when they aren't using one. She doesn't want to take the pill because she can't afford it, and she's afraid that her parents will find out that she's having sex.

Family Assessment
Client lives at home with parents and younger sister, 12 years old. Father works as Boy Scout Administrator. Mother is stay-at-home Mom. Client states family finances are "good; no problem."

Client Assessment
Past medical history is negative for major health problems. Menarche was at age 12. Menstrual cycles range from 28 to 35 days, with a moderately heavy flow lasting 5 to 7 days. She has enough cramping monthly that she "usually has to stay home from school for one day." Last menstrual flow was 1 week ago. Uses contraception inconsistently. Denies any history of sexually transmitted infections or other reproductive problems. Her weight is appropriate for her height. Secondary sex characteristics are present. You notice her smoking a cigarette in the hallway. Following her health care visit, she is prescribed Ortho-ovum 7/7/7, a 28-day-cycle triphasic oral contraceptive.

Nursing Diagnosis
Health-seeking behaviors related to knowledge deficit concerning contraception

Outcome Criteria
Client identifies options available to her; states valid reasons for method chosen; demonstrates correct use of and appropriate follow-up care for chosen method; voices satisfaction with method chosen by 1 month's time.

Team Member Responsible	Assessment	Intervention	Rationale	Expected Outcome
Activities of Daily Living				
Nurse	Assess client's lifestyle.	Discuss when she will take pill and where she will store them. Caution against smoking while taking an estrogen-based pill.	Reviewing lifestyle may provide clues to possible reasons why the method will be ineffective or not continued.	Client describes lifestyle to health care provider and actively participates in devising lifestyle changes that will add to contraceptive's effectiveness.
Consultations				
Nurse	Consult with M.D., N.P., or nurse-midwife to determine whether method client chooses will be optimal, safe, and effective.	Secure prescription for medication.	Effective health care is a collaborative effort drawing on interdisciplinary expertise.	Consultation reveals that the contraceptive method chosen will be optimal, safe, and effective; client receives prescription.

(continued)

Team Member Responsible	Assessment	Intervention	Rationale	Expected Outcome
Procedures/Medications				
Physician/ Nurse Practitioner	Assess what form of contraceptive client thinks she could use most effectively.	Complete preprescription procedures such as a Pap test and pelvic examination. Review method of administration with client and steps to take if she forgets to take a pill.	Medication administration invariably requires discussion to help clients comply.	Any procedure necessary for prescription of a contraceptive is carried out safely with optimal respect for client privacy and concern.
Nurse	Determine whether client has any questions regarding pelvic examination or other procedures scheduled.	Assist with procedures such as Pap test; meet with client to answer any questions regarding contraceptive chosen.	Nurses can be instrumental in lending psychological and physical support during procedures.	Client states that she understands the importance of prescription procedures to ensure her safety.
Nutrition				
Nurse/ Nutritionist	Determine whether client commonly eats a dietary source of folic acid.	Discuss with client that oral contraceptive use can lead to folic acid deficiency.	Knowledge of side effects is important to create informed consumers.	Client acknowledges that she needs to be conscious of the need for folic acid; names two good sources of folic acid in food.
Patient/Family Education				
Nurse	Determine whether client has any further questions regarding chosen contraceptive measure.	Instruct the client about the method selected, including any specific measures needed to ensure success of the method. Have client repeat information for return demonstration.	Instruction provides an opportunity for learning to improve compliance.	Client describes the action of oral contraceptives and the need to take them conscientiously.
Psychosocial/Spiritual/Emotional Needs				
Nurse	Assess if client has discussed with boyfriend that contraception is different than safer sex practices.	Review and discuss the need for safer sex practices in addition to contraception.	Safer sex practices promote health, empower the client, and minimize the risk of sexually transmitted infections. Discussion provides additional feedback and support and permits a safe outlet for expression of concerns and feelings.	The client acknowledges the need for safer sex practices to prevent sexually transmitted infections.
Discharge Planning				
Nurse	Assess if client understands she will need continued health supervision while on an oral contraceptive.	Explain the need for routine follow-up in 1 month and yearly pelvic examinations.	Follow-up is essential for evaluating adherence and satisfaction and for reducing the risk of possible complications.	Client states that she will return for a follow-up visit in 1 month and every year after that.

BOX 5.6

Nursing Outcomes Classification (NOC) and Nursing Interventions Classification (NIC)

Contraception

NOC: Knowledge, Conception Prevention

Knowledge, conception prevention, is defined as the extent of understanding conveyed about pregnancy prevention (Johnson et al., 2000). Some specific indicators suggesting that this outcome has been achieved include the client's ability to describe the following:

- Various methods such as periodic abstinence, chemical and mechanical barriers, hormonal therapy, and surgical intervention
- Method for how chosen contraceptive works
- Correct use of chosen method (including a demonstration of its use)
- Effectiveness on STI transmission
- How conception occurs
- Advantages and disadvantages of having a child
- Influence of personal and religious values on contraception

NIC: Family Planning, Contraception

Family planning, contraception, is defined as the facilitation of pregnancy prevention by providing information about the physiology of reproduction and methods to control conception (McCloskey & Bulechek, 2000). Some important activities involved when implementing this intervention include the following:

- Determining the need for family planning
- Explaining reasons for most unplanned pregnancies
- Determining ability and motivation of client and partner to use contraception correctly and regularly
- Appraising client's knowledge of contraception and plans for selecting a method
- Explaining female reproductive cycle and advantages and disadvantages of methods
- Assisting female client to determine ovulation through basal body temperature, changes in vaginal secretions, and other physiologic indicators
- Instructing client in use of chemical, hormonal, or mechanical contraceptives
- Referring client to community resources for family planning

---

BOX 5.7 FOCUS ON . . .

FAMILY TEACHING

Suggestions for Promoting Abstinence

Q. Suppose Dana, the 17-year-old you met at the beginning of the chapter, asks you how she can avoid being pressured into unwanted sex?

A. Here are a few suggestions:

- Discuss with your partner in advance what sexual activities you will permit and what you will not.
- Try to avoid high-pressure situations (e.g., a party with known drug use, excessive alcohol consumption, and no adult supervision).
- If pressured, say "no," and be sure that your partner understands that you mean it.
- Be certain your partner understands that you consider being forced into relations against your wishes the same as rape, not simply irresponsible conduct.
- Don't accept any drugs to "help you relax" or "be cool," as such a drug would impair your judgment. The drug could also be the "date rape" drug, flunitrazepam (Rohypnol).

on the couple's ability to refrain from having sex on fertile days. Failure rates are usually about 25% (Trussell, 2003), although the theoretical failure rate is as low as 1% to 9%. If pregnancy should occur, the continued use of these methods poses no risk to the fetus.

Fertility Awareness Methods

Fertility awareness methods rely on detecting when a woman is capable of impregnation (fertile) and using periods of abstinence or contraceptive use during that time (VandeVusse et al., 2003). Couples are then free to go without contraception during the rest of the month. As described later, there are a variety of ways to determine a fertile period. Couples may calculate the period based on a set formula, measure the woman's body temperature, observe the consistency of cervical mucus, use an over-the-counter (OTC) ovulation test kit, or employ a combination of these methods.

Calendar (Rhythm) Method. The calendar method requires a couple to abstain from coitus on the days of a menstrual cycle when the woman is most likely to conceive (3 or 4 days before until 3 or 4 days after ovulation). To plan for this, the woman keeps a diary of six menstrual cycles. To calculate "safe" days, she subtracts 18 from the shortest cycle documented. This number represents her first fertile day. She subtracts 11 from her longest cycle.

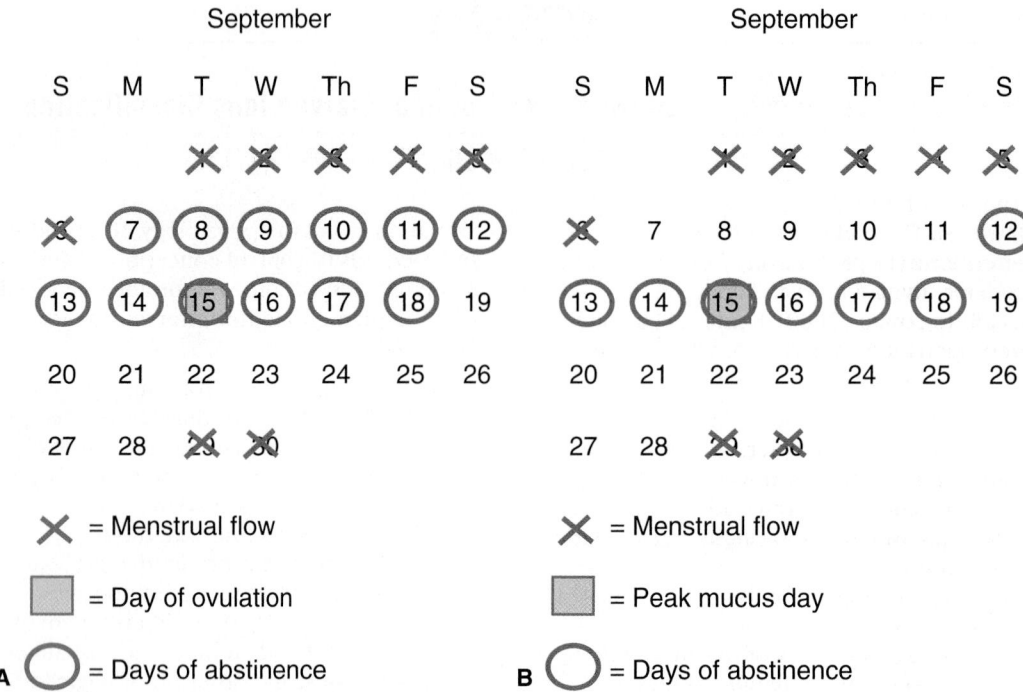

FIGURE 5.1 (A) A typical month using the calendar method as a natural family planning method. **(B)** A typical month using the cervical mucus method of natural family planning. Unmarked days are those safe for sexual relations.

This represents her last fertile day. If she had six menstrual cycles ranging from 25 to 29 days, her fertile period would be from the 7th day (25 minus 18) to the 18th day (29 minus 11). To avoid pregnancy, she would avoid coitus or use a contraceptive such as vaginal foam during those days (Fig. 5.1A).

Basal Body Temperature Method. Just before the day of ovulation, a woman's basal body temperature (BBT) falls about 0.5°F. At the time of ovulation, her BBT rises a full degree because of the influence of progesterone. This higher level is then maintained for the rest of her menstrual cycle. This pattern is the basis of the BBT method of contraception.

To use this method, the woman takes her temperature each morning immediately after waking, before she undertakes any activity; this is her BBT. As soon as she notices a slight dip in temperature followed by an increase, she knows that she has ovulated. She refrains from having sex for the next 3 days (the life of the discharged ovum). Because sperm can survive for at least 4 days in the female reproductive tract, it is usually recommended that the couple combine this method with a calendar method, so that they abstain for a few days before ovulation as well. The calendar method has an ideal failure rate of 9% (Trussell, 2003). For more information on BBT and its use in aiding fertility, see Chapter 6 and Figure 6.2.

A problem with this method is that many factors can affect the BBT. For example, a temperature rise caused by illness could be mistaken as the signal of ovulation. If this happens, a woman could mistake a fertile day for a safe one. Changes in the woman's daily schedule, such as starting an aerobic program, can also influence the BBT.

A woman who works nights should take her temperature after awakening from her longer sleep period, no matter what the time of day.

Cervical Mucus (Billings) Method. Another method to predict ovulation is to use the changes in cervical mucus that occur naturally with ovulation. Before ovulation each month, the cervical mucus is thick and does not stretch when pulled between the thumb and finger. Just before ovulation, mucus secretion increases. With ovulation (the peak day), cervical mucus becomes copious, thin, watery, and transparent. It feels slippery and stretches at least 1 inch before the strand breaks, a property known as *spinnbarkeit.* In addition, breast tenderness and an anterior tilt to the cervix occur. All the days on which the mucus is copious, or at least 3 days after the peak day, are considered to be fertile days, or days on which the woman should abstain from sex to avoid conception.

A woman using this method must be conscientious about assessing her vaginal secretions daily, or she will miss the change in cervical secretions. The feel of vaginal secretions after sexual relations is unreliable, because seminal fluid (the fluid containing sperm from the male) has a watery, postovulatory consistency and can be confused with ovulatory mucus. Figure 5.1B shows a hypothetical month using this method. The ideal failure rate is 3% (Trussell, 2003).

Symptothermal Method. The symptothermal method of birth control combines the cervical mucus and BBT methods. The woman takes her temperature daily, watching for the rise in temperature that marks ovulation. She also analyzes her cervical mucus daily. The couple must abstain from intercourse until 3 days after the rise in temperature or the fourth day after the peak of mucus change, because these are the woman's fertile days. The symptothermal method is more effective than either the BBT or the cervical mucus method alone (ideal failure rate, 2%).

Ovulation Awareness. Yet another method to predict ovulation is the use of an OTC ovulation detection kit (Freundl et al., 2003). These kits detect the midcycle surge of luteinizing hormone (LH) that can be detected in urine 12 to 24 hours before ovulation. Such kits are 98% to 100% accurate in predicting ovulation. Although they are fairly expensive, use of such a kit in place of cervical mucus testing makes this form of natural family planning more attractive to many women.

Lactation Amenorrhea Method. As long as a woman is breast-feeding an infant, there is some natural suppression of ovulation. However, if the infant is receiving a supplemental feeding, the use of lactation as an effective birth control method is questionable. Because women may ovulate but not menstruate while breast-feeding, the woman may still be fertile even if she has not had a period since childbirth (Van der Wijden et al., 2005). As a rule of thumb, after 6 months of breast-feeding, the woman should be advised to choose another method of contraception (Peterson, 2003).

Coitus Interruptus. **Coitus interruptus** is one of the oldest known methods of contraception. The couple proceeds with coitus until the moment of ejaculation. Then the man withdraws and spermatozoa are emitted outside the vagina. Unfortunately, ejaculation may occur before withdrawal is complete and, despite the care used, some spermatozoa may be deposited in the vagina. Furthermore, because there may be a few spermatozoa present in preejaculation fluid, fertilization may occur even if withdrawal seems controlled. For these reasons, coitus interruptus offers little protection against conception. Adolescent boys, especially, may lack the control or experience to use the method effectively (De Visser, 2004).

Effect on Sexual Enjoyment

Once a couple is certain of a woman's nonfertile days using one of the natural planning methods, more spontaneity in sexual relations is possible than with methods that involve vaginal insertion products (VandeVusse, 2003). On the other hand, the required days of abstinence may make a natural planning method unsatisfactory and unenjoyable for a couple. Coitus interruptus may be unenjoyable because of the need to withdraw before ejaculation.

Use by the Adolescent

Natural methods of family planning (with the exception of abstinence) are usually not the contraceptive method of choice for adolescents. Girls tend to have occasional anovulatory menstrual cycles for several years after menarche, and they do not always experience definite cervical changes or an elevated body temperature. Also, these methods require adolescents to say "no" to sexual intercourse on fertile days, a task that may be difficult to complete under peer pressure.

Checkpoint Question 1

Suppose Dana, 17 years old, tells you she wants to use a fertility awareness method of contraception. How will she determine her fertile days?

a. She will notice that she feels hot, as if she has an elevated temperature.
b. She should assess whether her cervical mucus is thin and watery.
c. She should monitor her emotions for sudden anger or crying.
d. She should assess whether her breasts feel sensitive to cool air.

Oral Contraception

Oral contraceptives, commonly known as the pill or COCs (for **c**ombination **o**ral **c**ontraceptives), are composed of varying amounts of synthetic estrogen combined with a small amount of synthetic progesterone (progestin) (Peterson, 2003). The estrogen acts to suppress follicle-stimulating hormone (FSH) and LH, thereby suppressing ovulation. The progesterone action complements that of estrogen by causing a decrease in the permeability of cervical mucus, thereby limiting sperm motility and access to ova. Progesterone also interferes with tubal transport and endometrial proliferation to such degrees that the possibility of implantation is significantly decreased.

Popular COCs prescribed in the United States are monophasic (i.e., they provide fixed doses of both estrogen and progestin throughout the 21-day cycle). Biphasic preparations deliver a constant amount of estrogen throughout the cycle but an increased amount of progestin during the last 11 days. Triphasic preparations vary in both estrogen and progestin content throughout the cycle. Triphasic types more closely mimic a natural cycle, thereby reducing breakthrough bleeding (bleeding outside the normal menstrual flow).

COCs must be prescribed by a physician, nurse practitioner, or nurse-midwife after a pelvic examination and a Papanicolaou (Pap) smear (Fig. 5.2). When used correctly, they are 99.7% effective in preventing conception. Because women occasionally forget to take them, and because of individual physiologic differences, the typical failure rate is about 8% (Trussell, 2003).

Noncontraceptive benefits to women who take COCs include decreased incidences of the following conditions:

- Dysmenorrhea, due to lack of ovulation
- Premenstrual dysphoric syndrome, because of the increased progesterone levels
- Iron deficiency anemia, due to the reduced amount of menstrual flow
- Acute pelvic inflammatory disease (PID) and the resulting tubal scarring
- Endometrial and ovarian cancer and ovarian cysts
- Fibrocystic breast disease
- Possibly osteoporosis and uterine myomata (fibroid uterine tumors)
- Colon cancer

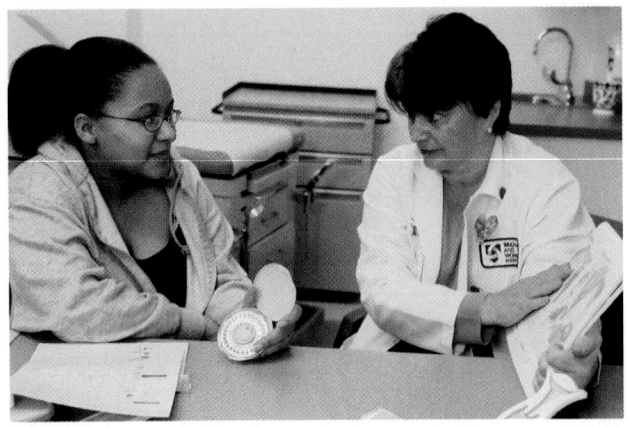

FIGURE 5.2 Counseling women on how to follow an oral contraceptive schedule and what to do if they miss a day or more is an important nursing responsibility. (© Caroline Brown, RNC, MS, DEd.)

In addition, COCs may have some metabolic effects over and above their contraceptive action, because estrogen interferes with lipid metabolism, lowering the concentration of low-density lipoproteins (LDL) and increasing the high-density lipoprotein (HDL) level.

COCs are packaged in convenient dispensers. The instructions for taking them are roughly similar for all brands. They are packaged 21 or 28 pills to a container. It is generally recommended that the first pill be taken on a Sunday (the first Sunday after the beginning of a menstrual flow), although a woman may choose to begin on any day. After childbirth, a woman should start the contraceptive on the Sunday closest to 2 weeks after delivery; after an abortion, then on the first Sunday after the procedure. Because pills are not effective for the first 7 days, she should be advised to use a second form of contraception during the initial 7 days on which she takes pills. A woman prescribed a 21-day cycle brand takes a pill at the same time every day for 21 days. Pill taking by this regimen will end on a Saturday. The woman would then not take any pills for 1 week. She would restart a new month's supply of pills on the Sunday 1 week after she stopped. A menstrual flow begins about 4 days after the woman finishes a cycle of pills.

To eliminate having to count days between pill cycles, certain brands of oral contraceptives are packaged with 28 pills—21 active pills and 7 placebo pills. With these brands, a woman starts a second dispenser of pills the day after finishing the first dispenser. There is no need to skip days because of the placebo tablets. Menstrual flow begins during the 7 days on which she is taking the placebo tablets.

A woman who does not want to have menstrual flows can eliminate them by beginning a new 21-day cycle of pills immediately after finishing a first one rather than waiting the usual 7 days to begin a new cycle (with the 28-day cycle regimens, she can omit taking the placebo pills and immediately begin a new dispenser). It is not advised that women do this on a continual basis, but the advice can be helpful to cover certain special occasions.

For ovulation suppressants to be effective, they must be taken consistently and conscientiously. Some women leave them in plain sight on the bathroom or kitchen counter so that they are easily reminded to take them. Women with young children in the house need to be cautioned that this is a dangerous practice. Poisoning with increased blood clotting from the high estrogen content could result if a small child ingested the pills accidentally. Women who have difficulty remembering to take a contraceptive in the morning may find it easier to take a daily pill at bedtime or with a meal (the time of day makes no difference; it is the consistency that is important). Also, some women find that taking pills at bedtime rather than in the morning eliminates any nausea they otherwise experience (Box 5.8).

Side Effects and Contraindications

For a listing of risk factors and contraindications associated with COCs, see Box 5.9. The main side effects that women may experience are the following:

- Nausea
- Weight gain
- Headache
- Breast tenderness
- Breakthrough bleeding (spotting outside the menstrual period)

BOX 5.8 FOCUS ON . . .

FAMILY TEACHING

Suggestions on Oral Contraceptive Management

Q. Suppose that Dana, the 17-year-old you met at the beginning of the chapter, asks what to do if she forgets to take an oral contraceptive pill. What do you tell her?

A. The answer differs, depending on your situation:

1. If you forget to take one pill, take it as soon as you remember. Continue the following day with your usual schedule. Doing so might mean taking two pills on one day, if you don't remember until the second day. *Missing one pill this way should not initiate ovulation.*

2. If you miss two consecutive pills, take two pills as soon as you remember and two pills again the following day. Then continue the following day with your usual schedule. You may experience some breakthrough bleeding (vaginal spotting) with two forgotten pills. Do not mistake this bleeding for your menstrual flow. *Missing two pills may allow ovulation to occur, so an added contraceptive should be used for the remainder of the month.*

3. If you miss three or more pills in a row, throw out the rest of the pack and start a new pack of pills the following Sunday. *You might not have a period because of this routine and should use extra protection until 7 days after starting a new pack of pills.*

BOX 5.9

Contraindications to Oral Contraceptive Use

- Breast-feeding and less than 6 weeks postpartum
- Age 35 years or older and smoking 15 or more cigarettes per day
- Multiple risk factors for arterial cardiovascular disease, such as older age, smoking, diabetes, hypertension
- Elevated blood pressure of 160 mm Hg systolic or above or 100 mm Hg diastolic or above
- Current or history of deep vein thrombosis or pulmonary embolism
- Major surgery that requires prolonged immobilization
- Current or history of ischemic heart disease
- Stroke
- Complicated valvular heart disease
- Migraine with focal neurologic symptoms (migraine with aura)
- Migraine without focal neurologic symptoms and age 35 years or older
- Current breast cancer
- Diabetes with nephropathy, retinopathy, neuropathy, vascular disease, or diabetes of more than 20 years' duration
- Severe cirrhosis
- Liver tumors

Peterson, H. B., et al. (2003). Contraception. In Scott, J. R., et al. (eds.). *Danforth's obstetrics and gynecology.* Philadelphia: Lippincott Williams & Wilkins, pp. 541–559.

- Monilial vaginal infections
- Mild hypertension
- Depression

These side effects usually subside after a few months of use, or they may be managed by using a different routine or brand of contraceptive.

It is no longer believed that the use of COCs leads to an increased risk of myocardial infarction, and the risk of increased clotting or blood pressure elevation is low. Nevertheless, COCs are not routinely prescribed for women with a history of thromboembolic disease or a family history of cerebral or cardiovascular accident, because of the increased tendency toward clotting as an effect of increased estrogen. The risk of abnormal clotting is 5/100,000 for the average woman, 15–30/100,000 for pill users, and 60/100,000 for pregnant women (Peterson, 2003).

All women taking COCs are advised to notify their health care provider if the following symptoms, which are indicative of myocardial or thromboembolic complications, occur:

- Chest pain (pulmonary embolus or myocardial infarction)
- Shortness of breath (pulmonary embolus)
- Severe headaches (cerebrovascular accident)
- Severe leg pain (thrombophlebitis)
- Eye problems such as blurred vision (hypertension, cerebrovascular accident)

Early studies found that breast-fed infants had lower weight gains when the mother was taking an oral contraceptive containing a high level of estrogen during breast-feeding, because the estrogen content decreased the woman's milk supply. Although there is less estrogen in today's preparations, it is still not recommended that breast-feeding women take estrogen-based COCs until their milk supply is well established. Women may take progesterone-only pills (mini-pills) during breast-feeding (see later discussion).

COCs have been known to interfere with glucose metabolism. For this reason, women with diabetes mellitus or a history of liver disease, including hepatitis, should be evaluated individually before COCs are prescribed. COCs may increase the risk of breast cancer in women who have other risks such as increased blood pressure, hyperlipidemia, or a history of smoking, so these women also are not acceptable candidates for COCs (Peterson, 2003).

A number of drugs, such as barbiturates, griseofulvin, isoniazid, penicillin, and tetracycline, decrease the effectiveness of COCs, so women might want to change their contraceptive method temporarily while taking these drugs (Karch, 2004). COCs may interact with a number of drugs such as acetaminophen, anticoagulants, and some anticonvulsants, reducing their therapeutic effect. Typically, COCs increase or strengthen the action of caffeine and corticosteroids.

The cost of oral contraceptives and the woman's ability to follow instructions faithfully must both be considered before COCs are prescribed. The woman using COCs should return for a follow-up visit yearly (for a pelvic examination, Pap smear, and breast examination), as long as she continues to use this form of birth control. Women without risk factors may continue to take low-dose oral contraceptives until they reach menopause.

Effect on Sexual Enjoyment

For the most part, not having to worry about pregnancy because the contraceptive being used is so reliable makes sexual relations more enjoyable for couples. Some women appear to lose interest in coitus after taking the pill for about 18 months, possibly because of the long-term effect of altered hormones in their body. Sexual interest increases again after they change to another form of contraception. Some women experience nausea with the pill and find that this interferes with sexual enjoyment as well as with other activities. If they are having side effects with one brand, they might be able to take another brand that has a different strength of estrogen without problems.

Effect on Pregnancy

If a woman taking a COC suspects that she is pregnant, she should discontinue taking the pill if she intends to continue the pregnancy. High levels of estrogen or progesterone might be teratogenic to a growing fetus, although the actual risk is now thought to be no higher than normally occurs (23.3%) (Speroff & Fritz, 2005).

Use by the Adolescent

It is usually recommended that adolescent girls have well-established menstrual cycles for at least 2 years before beginning COCs. This reduces the chance that the COC will cause permanent suppression of pituitary-regulating activity. Estrogen has the side effect of causing the epiphyses of long bones to close and growth to halt; therefore, waiting at least 2 years also ensures that the preadolescent growth spurt will not be halted. Because adolescents' compliance with most medications is low, adolescent girls may not take pills reliably enough to make them effective. In addition, the cost of a continuing supply of pills may be prohibitive for teens. COCs have side benefits of improving facial acne in some girls because of the increased estrogen/androgen ratio created, and of decreasing dysmenorrhea, a problem for many adolescents. The pill may be prescribed to some adolescents specifically to decrease dysmenorrhea, especially if endometriosis is present (see Chapter 47).

Discontinuing Use

After a woman stops taking a COC, she may not be able to become pregnant for 1 or 2 months, and possibly 6 to 8 months, because the pituitary gland requires a recovery period to begin cyclic gonadotropin stimulation again. If ovulation does not return spontaneously after this time, it can be stimulated by clomiphene citrate (Clomid) therapy.

Continuous or Extended Regimen Pills

Women may be prescribed extended programs for pills (91-day regimens, or 84 days of pills followed by 7 days of placebo). Although some women experience breakthrough bleeding, such regimens limit menstrual periods to only four times a year and provide effective birth control (Anderson & Hait, 2003).

Mini-pills

Oral contraceptives containing only progesterone are popularly called mini-pills. Without estrogen content, ovulation may occur but, because the progestins have not allowed the endometrium to develop fully, implantation will not take place. Such a pill has advantages for the woman who cannot take an estrogen-based pill because of the danger of thrombophlebitis but who wants high-level contraception assurance. This type of pill is taken every day, even through the menstrual flow. Because it does not interfere with milk production, it may be taken during breast-feeding.

Estrogen/Progesterone Patch

Transdermal patches that slowly but continuously release a combination of estrogen and progesterone were approved by the U.S. Food and Drug Administration (FDA) in 2001 and reached the market in 2002 (Fig. 5.3). Patches are applied once a week for 3 weeks. During the week on which the woman is patch free, a menstrual flow will occur. The efficiency of transdermal patches is equal to that of COCs, although they may be less effective in women who weigh more than 90 kg. Transdermal patches have the potential to increase adherence, because the woman does not need to remember to take a daily pill. A second advantage is easy concealment. Mild breast discomfort and irritation at the application site may occur (Rubinstein et al., 2004).

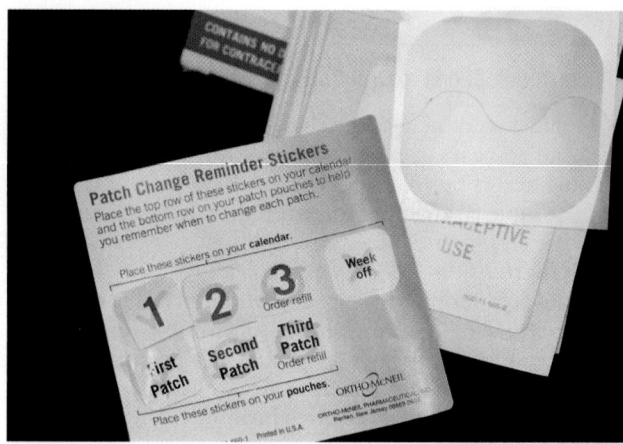

FIGURE 5.3 Estrogen/progesterone based patches help adherence because they need attention only once a week. They may be applied on arms, the trunk, or buttocks.

Patches may be applied to one of four areas: upper outer arm, upper torso (front or back, excluding the breasts), abdomen, or buttocks. It should not be placed on any area where makeup, lotions, or creams will be applied or where the skin is red, irritated, or has an open lesion.

Patches can be worn in the shower, while bathing, or while swimming. If a patch comes loose, the woman should remove it and immediately replace it with a new patch. No additional contraception is needed if the woman is sure the patch has been loose for less than 24 hours. If the woman is not sure how long the patch has been loose, she should remove it and apply a new patch, but this will start a new 4-week cycle, with a new day 1 and a new day to change the patch. She also should use a backup contraception method, such as a condom or spermicide, for the first week of this new cycle (Box 5.10).

Vaginal Rings

A vaginal ring (a silicone ring that surrounds the cervix and continually releases a combination of estrogen and progesterone) was also FDA approved in 2001 (Fig. 5.4). The ring is inserted by the woman and left in place for 3 weeks, then removed for 1 week (Johansson & Sitruk-Ware, 2004). Menstrual bleeding occurs during the ring-free week. The hormones released are absorbed directly by the mucous membrane of the vagina, thereby avoiding a "first pass" through the liver, as happens with COCs; this is an advantage for women with liver disease. The efficiency is 99.7%, equal to that of COCs. Fertility returns immediately after removal of the ring (Peterson, 2003). Women may need to make out a calendar that they post conspicuously to remind themselves to remove and replace the ring.

Emergency Postcoital Contraception

A number of regimens are available for emergency postcoital contraception. These are often referred to as "morning-after pills." The high level of estrogen they contain apparently interferes with the production of proges-

BOX 5.10 FOCUS ON . . .

EVIDENCE-BASED PRACTICE

Can adolescents use transdermal contraceptive patches effectively?

To answer this question, researchers followed 50 adolescent girls, ages 15 to 18 years, who were prescribed transdermal contraceptive patches as their method of birth control for 1 and 3 months. Forty girls (80%) completed 1 month of treatment, and 31 (62%) completed all 3 months. No pregnancies occurred during the time the patches were in place. At the 3-month follow-up, 87% of participants reported conscientious use. They mentioned ease of use, no need for daily attention, and ease of concealment as the patch's main advantages. About 77% of participants who completed the study planned to continue with patch use. Disadvantages reported were irritation at the application site, breast discomfort, and detachment of the patch.

This is an important study for nurses, because nurses are the people who perform a high percentage of reproductive life planning counseling. Knowing that adolescents found patches easy to use, but that patches also can detach during active lifestyles, can open up teaching opportunities.

Rubinstein, M. L., Halpern-Felsher, B. L., & Irwin, C. E. (2004). An evaluation of the use of the transdermal contraceptive patch in adolescents. *Journal of Adolescent Health, 34*(5), 395–401.

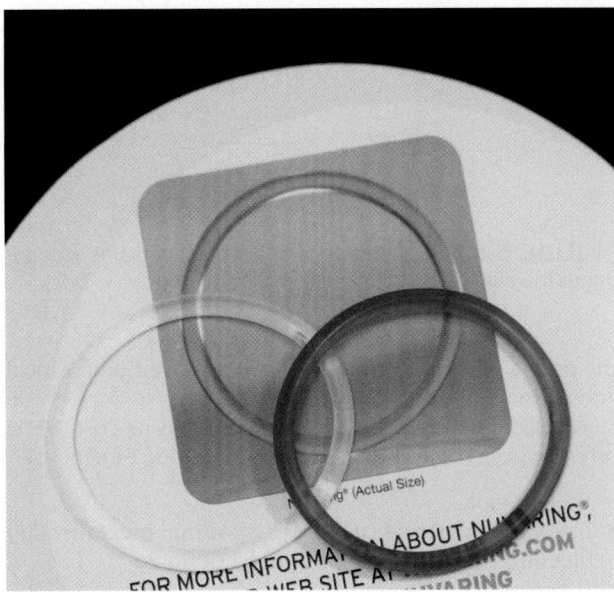

FIGURE 5.4 A vaginal ring. Progesterone is gradually released to be absorbed by the vaginal walls.

terone, thereby prohibiting good implantation. The Yuzpe regimen consists of the administration of two fixed-dose combination pills (usually Ovral), taken within 72 hours after unprotected intercourse (Croxatto et al., 2003). This is followed by two additional pills 12 hours later. This high dose of estrogen (200 mcg) almost always causes nausea and vomiting. Pretreatment with an antiemetic, such as 50 mg meclizine (Bonine), is usually recommended to decrease the possibility of vomiting. If vomiting should occur within 2 hours after administration, the pills should be repeated.

A specially designed emergency contraceptive kit (Preven) is available for use after unprotected sexual intercourse, particularly after a sexual assault has occurred (Weismiller, 2004). The kit consists of a urine pregnancy test to determine whether pregnancy has occurred and four pills that contain concentrations of estrogen/progestin (the first two taken within 72 hours after intercourse and the next two 12 hours later).

A progestin-only method termed "Plan B" is also available. With this plan, two pills containing high doses of levonorgestrel are taken (one pill immediately and one 12 hours later). This plan results in less nausea and may actually prevent more pregnancies than the estrogen-based regimen (Steinbrook, 2004). Legislation is being planned in a few states to allow pharmacists to distribute Plan B tablets without a prescription (Raine et al., 2005).

Overall, the rate of effectiveness for emergency postcoital methods of contraception is between 75% and 85% (Trussell, 2003). The method should always be used cautiously, because high levels of estrogen have been associated with congenital anomalies if the pregnancy is not prevented. Mifepristone, discussed later as an abortifacient, or an intrauterine device may also be prescribed for emergency postcoital contraception.

Checkpoint Question 2

Suppose Dana, 17 years old, chooses to use a combination oral contraceptive (COC) as her family planning method? What is a danger sign of COCs you would ask her to report?

a. A stuffy or runny nose
b. Arthritis-like symptoms
c. Slight weight gain
d. Migraine headache

Subcutaneous Implants

Norplant consists of six nonbiodegradable Silastic implants, about the width of a pencil lead, that are filled with levonorgestrel (a synthetic progesterone) and embedded just under the skin on the inside of the upper arm (Fig. 5.5). Once embedded, the implants appear as irregular lines on the skin, simulating small veins (Alvarez et al., 2003). Over the next 5 years, the implants slowly release the hormone, suppressing ovulation, stimulating thick cervical mucus, and changing the endometrium so that implantation is difficult.

The implants are inserted with the use of a local anesthetic, during the menses or no later than day 7 of the menstrual cycle, to be certain that the woman is not pregnant at the time of insertion. They can be inserted immediately after an abortion or 6 weeks after the birth of a baby. The failure rate is less than 1% (Trussell, 2003). At

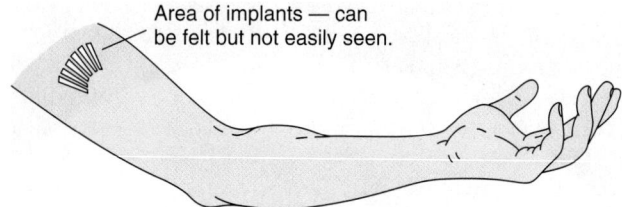

Area of implants — can be felt but not easily seen.

FIGURE 5.5 The appearance of Norplant implants placed under the skin.

the end of 5 years, the implants are removed under local anesthesia.

A disadvantage of the implant method is its cost ($500 on average). The following are possible side effects:

- Weight gain
- Irregular menstrual cycle (e.g., spotting, breakthrough bleeding, amenorrhea, prolonged periods)
- Hair loss
- Depression
- Scarring at the insertion site
- Need for removal

A major advantage of this long-term reversible contraceptive is that it offers an effective and reliable alternative to COCs and their estrogen-related side effects. Compliance issues associated with COCs are eliminated. Sexual enjoyment is not inhibited, as may be the case with condoms, spermicides, diaphragms, and natural family planning methods. Implants can be used during breast-feeding without an effect on milk production. Also, implants can be used safely in adolescents. The rapid return to fertility (about 3 months after removal) is an advantage for women who wish to have children (Speroff & Fritz, 2005).

Contraindications to Norplant are pregnancy, desire to be pregnant within 1 to 2 years, and undiagnosed uterine bleeding. A complication (rare) that can occur is an infection at the insertion site. If pregnancy does occur with the rods in place, they can be removed to reduce the small possibility of birth defects in the fetus.

Intramuscular Injections

A single injection of medroxyprogesterone acetate (Depo-Provera) given every 12 weeks or injections of Lunelle (a synthetic estrogen and progesterone) given every 30 days inhibit ovulation, alter the endometrium, and change the cervical mucus (Box 5.11). The effectiveness rate of these methods is almost 100%, making them an increasingly popular contraceptive method (Trussell, 2003). Depo-Provera, because it contains only progesterone, can be used during breast-feeding. Potential side effects are similar to those of subcutaneous implants: irregular menstrual cycle, headache, weight gain, and depression. Depo-Provera may impair glucose tolerance in women at risk for diabetes. Because there also may be a slight increase in the risk for osteoporosis, women should be advised to include an adequate amount of calcium in their diet (up to 1,200 mg/day) and to engage in weight-bearing exercise daily to minimize this risk.

BOX 5.11 FOCUS ON . . .

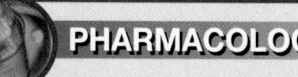

PHARMACOLOGY

Medroxyprogesterone Acetate (Depo-Provera)

Classification: Contraceptive

Action: Medroxyprogesterone acetate (Depo-Provera) is a progesterone derivative that inhibits the secretion of pituitary gonadotropins, thereby altering the endometrium and preventing follicular maturation and ovulation (Karch, 2004).

Pregnancy Category: X

Dosage: 150 mg intramuscular injection every 3 months

Possible Adverse Effects: Spotting, breakthrough bleeding, amenorrhea, irregular menstrual flow, headaches, weight fluctuations, fluid retention, edema, rash or acne, abdominal discomfort, glucose intolerance, pain at injection site

Nursing Implications
- Advise client to have an annual physical examination that includes breast examination, pelvic examination, and Pap smear.
- Caution the client about potential side effects.
- Advise the client to report pain or swelling of the legs, acute chest pain or shortness of breath, tingling or numbness in the extremities, loss of vision, sudden severe headaches, dizziness, or fainting; these are signs of cardiovascular complications.

Like subcutaneous implants, intramuscular injections have the advantage of longer-term reliability without many of the side effects and contraindications associated with COCs. An advantage of intramuscular injections over implants is that there is no visible sign that a birth control measure is being used. Two disadvantages are that the woman must return to a health care provider for a new injection every 4 to 12 weeks for the method to remain reliable, and the return to fertility is often delayed by about 6 to 12 months. A reminder system, such as a postcard mailed by the prescribing agency, may be necessary to be certain that women return on time for their next injection. Alternative methods of administration, such as allowing pharmacists to give the injections or selling them OTC so that women can inject themselves, are being studied (Plourd & Rayburn, 2003).

Intrauterine Devices

The **intrauterine device** (IUD) is a small plastic object that is inserted into the uterus through the vagina. IUDs became popular as a method of birth control in the 1980s, but they are used by only a small number of U.S. women today; few manufacturers continue to provide them since a number of lawsuits were filed in association with the increased incidence of PID (infection of the pelvic organs) in women using one particular brand, now no longer

> ## Checkpoint Question 3
>
> Suppose Dana, 17 years old, chooses subcutaneous implants (Norplant) as her method of reproductive life planning. How long will these implants be effective?
>
> a. One month
> b. Twelve months
> c. Five years
> d. Ten years

available (Hubacher & Cheng, 2004). The rate of IUD use is only 1% in the United States; worldwide, the rate is 20% (Peterson, 2003).

Although the insertion of foreign objects into the uterus for contraceptive purposes dates back thousands of years (ancient camel drivers used the technique on their animals), the mechanism of action for the method is still not fully understood. Originally, it was thought that the presence of a foreign substance in the uterus interfered with the ability of an ovum to develop as it traversed the fallopian tube. Today, the IUD is thought to be preventing fertilization as well as creating a local sterile inflammatory condition that prevents implantation. When copper is added to the device, sperm mobility appears to be affected. This decreases the possibility that sperm will successfully cross the uterine space and reach the ovum.

An IUD must be fitted by a physician, nurse practitioner, or nurse-midwife, who first performs a Pap test and pelvic examination. The device is inserted before the client has had coitus after a menstrual flow, so the health care provider can be assured that the woman is not pregnant at the time of insertion. Insertion may be done immediately after childbirth: an IUD inserted soon after childbirth does not affect uterine involution or its return to a prepregnant uterine size.

The insertion procedure is performed in an ambulatory setting such as a physician's office or a reproductive planning clinic. The device is inserted in a collapsed position, then enlarged to its final shape in the uterus when the inserter is withdrawn. The woman may feel a sharp cramp as the device is passed through the internal cervical os, but she will not feel the IUD after it is in place. Properly fitted, such devices are contained wholly within the uterus, although the attached string protrudes through the cervix into the vagina (Johnson, 2005).

Three common types of IUDs used in the United States are the Copper T380 (ParaGard), a T-shaped plastic device wound with copper, and Progestasert and Mirena, which hold a drug reservoir of progesterone in the stem (Fig. 5.6). The progesterone in the drug reservoir gradually diffuses into the uterus through the plastic; it both prevents endometrium proliferation and thickens cervical mucus. The Progestasert must be changed yearly, because the progesterone supply becomes depleted. The newer Mirena type is effective for 5 years (possibly as long as 7 years). Both

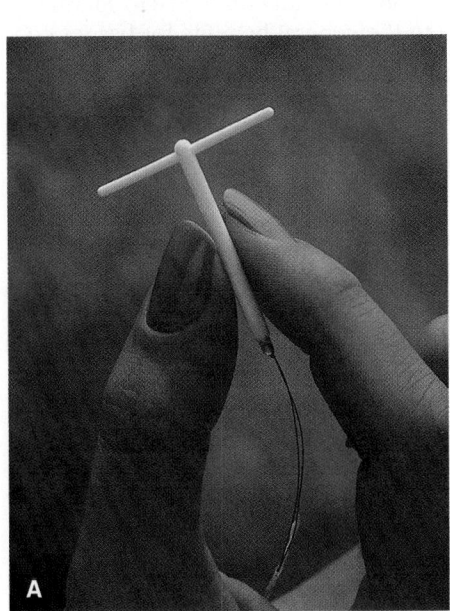

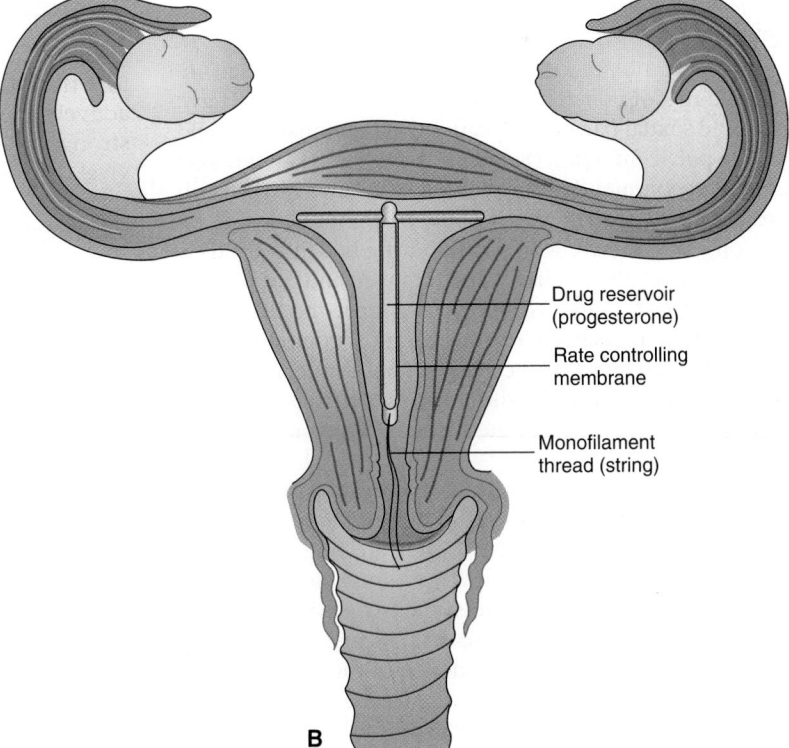

Drug reservoir
(progesterone)

Rate controlling
membrane

Monofilament
thread (string)

FIGURE 5.6 (A) Intrauterine device; **(B)** an IUD in place in the uterus. (Courtesy of ALZA Pharmaceuticals, Palo Alto, CA.)

have a failure rate as low as 0.1% to 1.5%. The Copper T380, because of the added copper, has a comparable failure rate (Trussell, 2003). It is effective for 10 years, after which time it should be removed and replaced with a new IUD.

IUDs have several advantages over other contraceptives. Only one insertion is necessary, so there is no continuing expense. The device does not require daily attention or interfere with sexual enjoyment. It is appropriate for women who are at risk for complications associated with COCs or who wish to avoid some of the systemic hormonal side effects. The woman should regularly check after each menstrual flow, to make sure the IUD string is in place, and obtain a yearly pelvic examination.

Side Effects and Contraindications

A woman may notice some spotting or uterine cramping the first 2 or 3 weeks after IUD insertion; as long as this is present, she should use an additional form of contraception, such as vaginal foam. A woman with an IUD in place may have a higher than usual risk for PID, although the copper-wound devices may actually carry a lower risk. Some women have a heavier than usual menstrual flow for 2 or 3 months and experience more dysmenorrhea than other women do. Ibuprofen, a prostaglandin inhibitor, is helpful in relieving the pain. Occasionally, a woman continues to have cramping and spotting after insertion; in such cases, she is likely to expel the device spontaneously. Women with IUDs in place should take active steps to avoid toxic shock syndrome (TSS; a staphylococcal infection from the use of tampons), because infection might travel by the IUD string into the uterus to cause uterine infection. TSS is discussed in Chapter 47.

IUDs are not recommended for women with an increased risk of contracting STIs, such as those who have multiple sexual partners, because this combination could lead to pelvic infection (Steen & Shapiro, 2004). They also are not recommended for women who have never been pregnant (their small uterus could be punctured with insertion) or who have a history of having had PID. If PID is suspected, the device should be removed and the woman should receive antibiotic therapy to treat the infection. Women with IUDs need to know the most common symptoms of PID (fever, lower abdominal tenderness, and pain on intercourse) so they can report these to their health care provider immediately if they occur (see Chapter 47).

IUDs are also contraindicated in the woman whose uterus is distorted in shape (the device might perforate an abnormally shaped uterus). They are not advised for women with severe dysmenorrhea (painful menstruation), menorrhagia (bleeding between menstrual periods), or a history of ectopic (tubal) pregnancy, because their use may increase the symptoms or incidence of these conditions. Women with valvular heart disease may be advised against the use of an IUD because the increased risk of PID could lead to accompanying valvular involvement from bacterial endocarditis. Because IUDs can cause a heavier than usual

menstrual flow, women with anemia are also not usually considered to be good candidates for IUD use.

Effect on Pregnancy

If a woman with an IUD in place suspects that she is pregnant, she should alert her primary health care provider. Although the IUD may be left in place during the pregnancy, it is usually removed vaginally to prevent the possibility of infection or spontaneous abortion during the pregnancy. The woman should receive an early sonogram to document placement of the IUD (Schiesser et al., 2004). This can also rule out ectopic pregnancy, which has an increased incidence among IUD users who become pregnant with the IUD in place.

Use by the Adolescent

IUDs are rarely prescribed for adolescents, because teens tend to have variable sexual partners and no prior pregnancies, both contraindications to IUD use.

Barrier Methods

Barrier methods are forms of birth control that work by the placement of a chemical or other barrier between the cervix and advancing sperm so that sperm cannot enter the uterus or fallopian tubes and fertilize the ovum. A major advantage of barrier methods is that they lack the hormonal side effects associated with COCs. However, compared with COCs, their failure rates are higher and sexual enjoyment may be lessened.

Vaginally Inserted Spermicidal Products

Spermicidal agents cause the death of spermatozoa before they can enter the cervix. These agents are not only actively spermicidal but also change the vaginal pH to a strong acid level, a condition not conducive to sperm survival. In addition to the general benefits for barrier contraceptives, the advantages of spermicides include the following:

- They may be purchased without a prescription or an appointment with a health care provider, so they allow for greater independence and lower costs.
- When used in conjunction with another contraceptive, they increase the other method's effectiveness.
- Various preparations are available, including gels, creams, sponges, films, foams, and suppositories. Gels or creams are inserted into the vagina before coitus with an applicator (Fig. 5.7). The woman should do this no more than 1 hour before coitus for the most effective results. She should not douche for 6 hours after coitus, to ensure that the agent has completed its spermicidal action.

Another form of spermicidal protection is a film of glycerin impregnated with a spermicidal agent that is folded and inserted vaginally. On contact with vaginal secretions or precoital penile emissions, the film dissolves and a carbon dioxide foam forms to protect the cervix against invading spermatozoa. The use of this method is not rec-

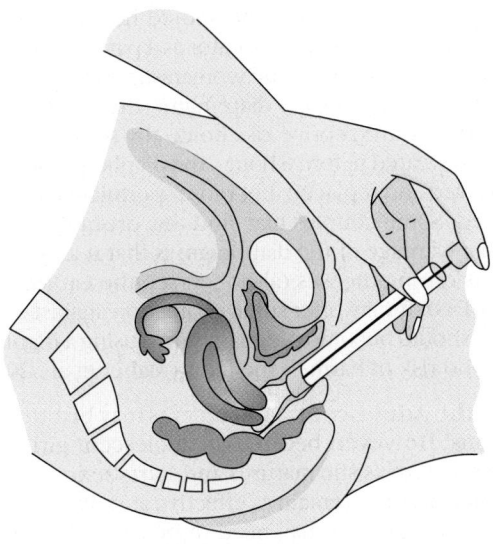

FIGURE 5.7 Vaginal insertion of a spermicidal agent.

ommended for women near menopause, a time in life when vaginal secretions are lessening.

Still other vaginal products are cocoa butter- and glycerin-based vaginal suppositories filled with a spermicide. Inserted vaginally, these dissolve and release the spermicidal ingredients. Because it takes about 15 minutes for a suppository to dissolve, it must be inserted 15 minutes before coitus.

Sponges are foam-impregnated synthetic sponges that are inserted vaginally to block sperm access to the cervix (Kuyoh et al., 2003). Well liked by most users, they are easy to insert and have an efficiency rate of 80% (ideal) and a typical use failure rate of 68% (Trussell, 2003). They should remain in place for 6 hours after intercourse to ensure sperm destruction.

Side Effects and Contraindications. Vaginally inserted spermicidal products are contraindicated in women with acute cervicitis, because they might further irritate the cervix. They are generally inappropriate for couples who must prevent conception (perhaps because the woman is taking a drug that is teratogenic, or the couple absolutely does not want the responsibility of children), because the overall failure rate of all forms of these products is about 20%. Some women find the vaginal leakage after use of these products bothersome. Vaginal suppositories, because of the cocoa butter or glycerin base, are the most bothersome in this regard.

Effect on Sexual Enjoyment. Although spermicidal products must be inserted fairly close to the time of coitus, they also are so easily purchased OTC that many couples find the inconvenience of insertion only a minor problem. If a couple is concerned that the method does not offer enough protection, worry about becoming pregnant may interfere with sexual enjoyment. Some couples find the foam or moisture irritating to vaginal and penile tissue during coitus and therefore are unable to use them.

Effect on Pregnancy. If conception should occur, there is no reason to think that the fetus will be affected by the spermicide. Some women worry that a sperm that survived the spermicide must have been weakened by migrating through it and therefore will produce a defective child. They can be assured that conception occurred most likely because the product did not completely cover the cervical os, so the sperm that reached the uterus is free of the product and unharmed.

Use by the Adolescent. Many adolescents use vaginal products as their chief method of birth control because no parental permission or extensive expense is involved. Adolescents should be cautioned that this method has a high failure rate (20%). All women need to be cautioned that preparations labeled "feminine hygiene" products are for vaginal cleanliness and are not spermicidal; therefore, they are not effective contraceptives.

Because of the nontraditional settings in which adolescents may engage in coitus (e.g., in cars, on couches), some young women find inserting the product awkward and consequently do not use it, even though they have purchased it and intended to be more cautious.

Diaphragms

A **diaphragm** is a circular rubber disk that is placed over the cervix before intercourse; it forms a barricade against the entrance of spermatozoa (Fig. 5.8) (Kuyoh et al., 2003). Although use of a spermicide is not required, use of a spermicidal gel with a diaphragm combines a barrier and a chemical method of contraception. The failure rate of the diaphragm may be as low as 6% (ideal) to 16% (typical use) (Trussell, 2003).

A diaphragm is prescribed and fitted initially by a physician, nurse practitioner, or nurse-midwife to ensure a correct fit. Because the shape of the cervix changes with

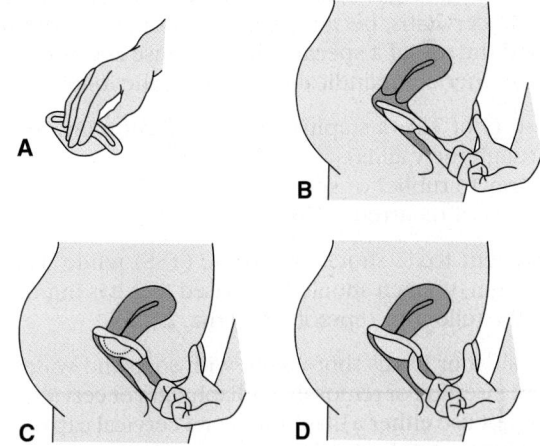

FIGURE 5.8 Proper insertion of a diaphragm. (**A**) After spermicidal jelly or cream is applied to the rim, the diaphragm is pinched between the fingers and thumb. (**B**) The folded diaphragm is then gently inserted into the vagina and pushed backward as far as it will go. (**C**) To check for proper positioning, the woman should feel the cervix to be certain it is completely covered by the soft rubber dome of the diaphragm. (**D**) To remove the diaphragm, a finger is hooked under the forward rim and the diaphragm is pulled down and out.

pregnancy, miscarriage, cervical surgery (dilatation and curettage [D&C]), or therapeutic abortion, a woman must return for a second fitting if any of these occur. The woman should also have the fit of the diaphragm checked if she gains or loses more than 15 lb, because this could change her pelvic and vaginal contours. A diaphragm is inserted into the vagina, after first coating the rim with a spermicide gel, by sliding it along the posterior wall and pressing it up against the cervix so that it is held in place by the vaginal fornices. A woman needs to check her diaphragm with a finger after insertion to be certain that it is fitted well up over the cervix; this is determined by palpating the cervical os through the diaphragm.

A diaphragm should be kept in place for at least 6 hours after coitus, because spermatozoa remain viable in the vagina for that duration. It may be left in place for as long as 24 hours. If it is left in the vagina longer than this, the stasis of fluid may cause cervical inflammation (erosion) or urethral irritation. The woman removes the diaphragm by inserting a finger into the vagina and loosening the diaphragm by pressing against the anterior rim and then withdrawing it vaginally. After use, she washes the diaphragm in mild soap and water, dries it gently, and stores it in its protective case. With this care, a diaphragm will last for 2 to 3 years.

Side Effects and Contraindications. Users of diaphragms may experience a higher number of urinary tract infections (UTIs) than nonusers, probably because of pressure on the urethra. Diaphragms may not be effective if the uterus is prolapsed, retroflexed, or anteflexed to such a degree that the cervix is also displaced in relation to the vagina. Intrusion on the vagina by a cystocele or rectocele, in which the walls of the vagina are displaced by bladder or bowel, may make insertion of a diaphragm difficult. Diaphragms should not be used in the presence of acute cervicitis, because the close contact of the rubber and the use of a spermicide can cause additional irritation. Other contraindications include the following:

- History of TSS (a staphylococcal infection introduced through the vagina)
- Allergy to rubber or spermicides
- History of recurrent UTIs

To prevent toxic shock syndrome (TSS) while using a diaphragm, women should be advised that it is important to do the following (Speroff and Fritz, 2005):

1. Wash your hands thoroughly with soap and water before insertion or removal of a diaphragm or cervical cap.
2. Do not use either a diaphragm or a cervical cap during your menstrual period.
3. Do not leave the diaphragm in place longer than 24 hours.
4. Be aware of the symptoms of TSS, such as elevated temperature, diarrhea, vomiting, muscle aches, and a sunburn-like rash.
5. If symptoms of TSS should occur, immediately remove the diaphragm and telephone your health care provider.

Effect on Sexual Enjoyment. Some women dislike using diaphragms because they must be inserted before coitus (although they may be inserted up to 2 hours beforehand,

minimizing this problem) and should be left in place for 6 hours afterward. Use of a vibrator as a part of foreplay, frequent penile insertion, or the woman-superior position during coitus may dislodge a diaphragm; therefore, this may not be the contraceptive of choice for some couples. If coitus is repeated before 6 hours, the diaphragm should not be removed and replaced, but more spermicidal gel should be added. Some couples may find this precaution restricting. An advantage of the diaphragm is that it allows sexual relations during menses (although see the earlier precaution on TSS). It may offer some protection against STIs. If a woman should become pregnant while using a diaphragm, there is no risk of harm to the fetus (Maher et al., 2004).

Use by the Adolescent. Adolescents may be fitted for diaphragms. However, because an adolescent girl's vagina will vary in size as she matures and starts sexual relations, the device may not remain as effective as it does with older women. Adolescents may need to be reminded that continuing pelvic examinations are necessary to ensure that it continues to fit properly. Some adolescents may not know where their cervix is or how to feel for it when checking the placement of the diaphragm; an anatomic diagram can be used for education, or they can be shown their cervix during a pelvic examination by the use of a mirror.

What if... Dana, 17 years old, tells you that she and a friend intend to share a diaphragm because they don't have enough money for each to buy one? What would you recommend? Why?

Cervical Caps

A **cervical cap** is yet another barrier method of contraception. Caps are made of soft rubber, are shaped like a thimble, and fit snugly over the uterine cervix (Fig. 5.9). The failure rate is estimated to be as high as 26% (ideal) to 32% (typical use) (Trussell, 2003).

Many women cannot use cervical caps because their cervix is too short for the cap to fit properly. Also, caps tend to dislodge more readily than diaphragms during coitus. An advantage is that cervical caps can remain in place longer than diaphragms, because they do not put pressure on the vaginal walls or urethra; however, this period should not exceed 48 hours, to prevent cervical irritation (Peterson, 2003). Cervical caps, like diaphragms, must be fitted individually by a health care provider. They are contraindicated in women with any of the following conditions:

- An abnormally short or long cervix
- A previous abnormal Pap smear
- A history of TSS
- An allergy to latex or spermicide
- A history of PID, cervicitis, or papillomavirus infection
- A history of cervical cancer
- Undiagnosed vaginal bleeding

Male Condoms

A **condom** is a latex rubber or synthetic sheath that is placed over the erect penis before coitus begins (Fig. 5.10).

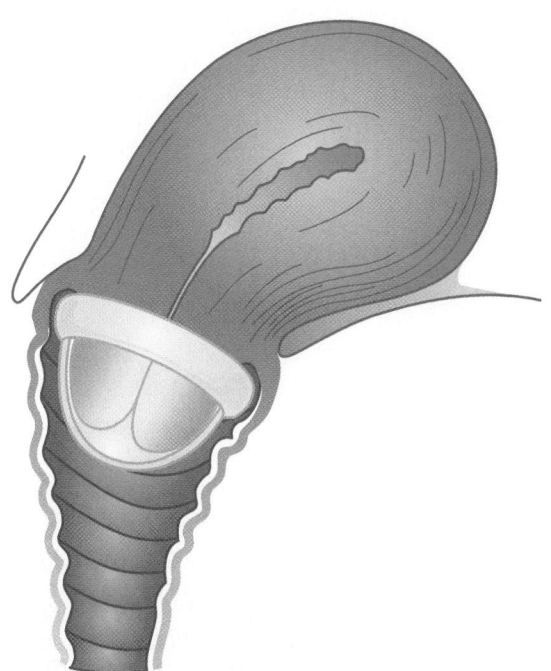

FIGURE 5.9 A cervical cap is placed over the cervix and used with a spermicidal jelly the same as a diaphragm.

It prevents pregnancy, because spermatozoa are deposited not in the vagina but in the tip of the condom. The use of condoms has an ideal failure rate of 2% and a typical failure rate of about 15%, because breakage or spillage occurs in up to 15% of uses (Trussell, 2003). A big advantage of con-

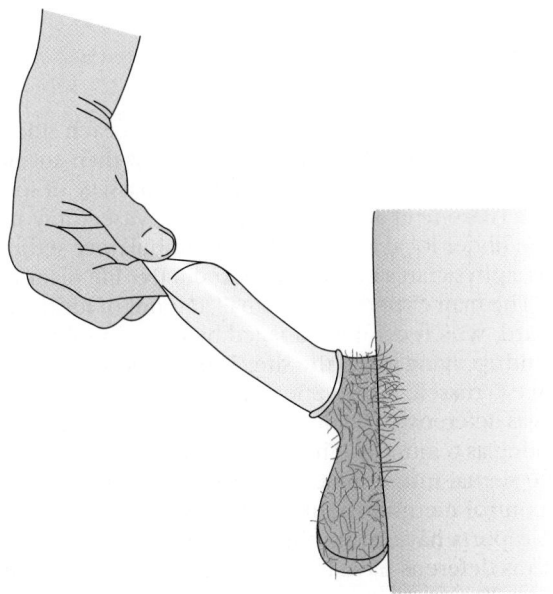

FIGURE 5.10 Male condom. Being certain that space is left at the tip helps to ensure the condom will not break with ejaculation.

doms is that they are one of the few "male-responsibility" birth control measures available, and no health care visit or prescription is needed. Latex condoms have the additional potential of preventing the spread of STIs, and their use has become a major part of the fight to prevent infection with human immunodeficiency virus (HIV). It is recommended that they always be worn during coitus between partners who do not maintain a monogamous relationship (Eisenberg et al., 2004).

Side Effects and Contraindications. There are no contraindications to the use of condoms except for a sensitivity to latex.

Effect on Sexual Enjoyment. To be effective, condoms must be applied before any penile-vulvar contact, because even pre-ejaculation fluid may contain some sperm. The condom should be positioned so that it is loose enough at the penis tip to collect the ejaculate without placing undue pressure on the condom. The penis (with the condom held carefully in place) must be withdrawn before it begins to become flaccid after ejaculation. If it is not withdrawn at this time, sperm may leak from the now loosely fitting sheath into the vagina. Some men find that condoms dull their enjoyment of coitus; some couples do not like the fact that the male must withdraw promptly after ejaculation. Concern that the condom may break or slip also may inhibit sexual pleasure.

Use by the Adolescent. Male adolescents are showing an increase in their ability to use condoms responsibly. Adolescent boys who have infrequent coitus may use condoms that they have owned and stored for a long time. The effectiveness of these old condoms, especially if they are carried in a warm pocket, is questionable. Adolescents may need to be cautioned that condoms should never be reused, because even a pinpoint hole can allow thousands of sperm to escape. For many adolescent couples, use of a dual method, such as a vaginally inserted spermicide by the girl and a condom by her partner, is the preferred method of birth control (Anderson et al., 2003). The effectiveness of these two methods used in conjunction becomes about 95%.

Female Condoms

Condoms for females are latex sheaths made of polyurethane and prelubricated with a spermicide. The inner ring (closed end) covers the cervix, and the outer ring (open end) rests against the vaginal opening. The sheath may be inserted any time before sexual activity begins and then removed after ejaculation occurs. Like male condoms, they are intended for one-time use and offer protection against both conception and STIs (Fig. 5.11). Female condoms can be purchased OTC but are more expensive than male condoms. Male and female condoms should not be used together. The failure rate in preliminary studies was somewhat greater than the failure rate for male condoms, 5% to 21% (Trussell, 2003). Most of these pregnancies occurred because of incorrect or inconsistent use. They have not gained great popularity, because women have found them difficult to use.

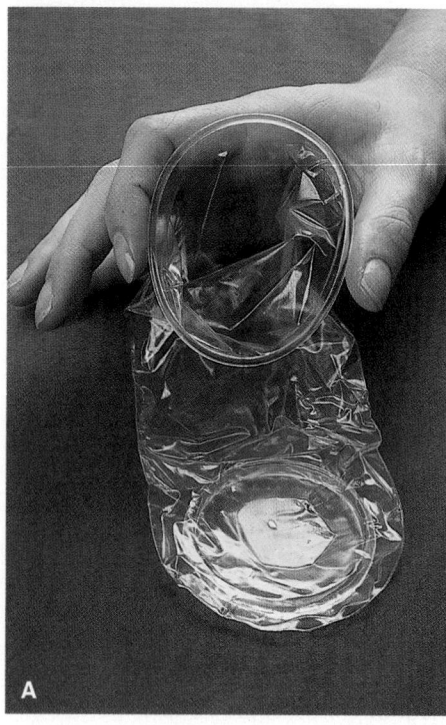

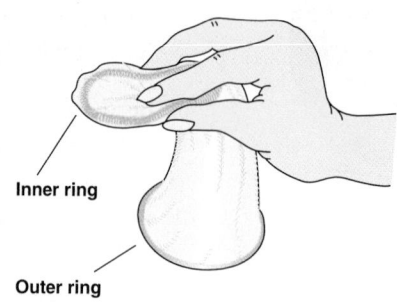

Inner ring

Outer ring

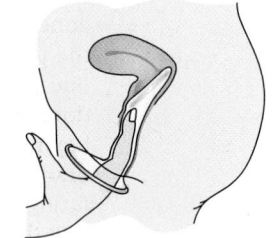

A

B

FIGURE 5.11 A female condom. Such a device is effective protection against both STIs and pregnancy. (**A**) The REALITY (WP-333) female condom. (© Barbara Proud.) (**B**) Insertion technique. (Courtesy of Wisconsin Pharmaceutical Company, Inc.)

Checkpoint Question 4

Dana, 17 years old, wants to try female condoms as her reproductive planning method. Which instruction would you give her?

a. The hormone the condom releases may cause mild weight gain.

b. She should insert the condom before any penile penetration.

c. She should coat the condom with a spermicide before use.

d. Female condoms, unlike male condoms, can be reused.

Surgical Methods of Reproductive Life Planning

Surgical methods of reproductive life planning include sterilization (tubal ligation for women and vasectomy for men). About 28% of all women in the United States of childbearing age choose a sterilization procedure to prevent unwanted pregnancy. Vasectomy is the contraceptive method of choice for about 11% of men, making these two procedures the most frequently used methods of contraception in the United States for couples older than 30 years of age (Peterson, 2003). Many people choose these surgical methods because they are the most effective methods of contraception besides abstinence and because they have no effect on sexuality.

Although procedures for the reversal of both male and female sterilization do exist, such techniques are much more complicated and expensive than the sterilization itself, and success rates vary greatly (Ribeiro et al., 2004). For this reason, surgical methods should be chosen with great thought and care and should be considered permanent. Counseling should be especially intensive for men and women younger than 25 years of age, because the possibility of divorce, death of a sexual partner, loss of a child, or remarriage could change their philosophy toward childbearing in the future. In addition, sterilization is not recommended for individuals whose fertility is important to their self-esteem.

Vasectomy

In a **vasectomy,** a small incision is made on each side of the scrotum. The vas deferens at that point is then cut and tied, cauterized, or plugged, blocking the passage of spermatozoa (Barone et al., 2004) (Fig. 5.12). Vasectomy can be done under local anesthesia in an ambulatory setting, such as a physician's office or a reproductive life planning clinic. The man experiences a small amount of local pain afterward, which can be managed by taking a mild analgesic and applying ice to the site. The procedure is 99.5% effective (Trussell, 2003). Spermatozoa that were present in the vas deferens at the time of surgery can remain viable for as long as 6 months. Therefore, although the man can resume sexual intercourse within 1 week, an additional birth control method should be used until two negative sperm reports have been obtained (proof that all sperm in the vas deferens have been eliminated, usually requiring 10 to 20 ejaculations).

Some men resist the concept of vasectomy because they are not sufficiently aware of their anatomy to know exactly what the procedure involves. They can be assured

Some evidence of endometriosis occurs in as many as 50% of women, most probably from regurgitation through the fallopian tubes at the time of menstruation. Viable particles of endometrium that have been regurgitated in this way begin to proliferate and grow at the new sites, impeding fertility in a variety of ways. If growths occur in the fallopian tube, tubal obstruction may result or adhesions forming from these growths may displace fallopian tubes away from the ovaries, preventing the entrance of ova into the tubes. Peritoneal macrophages that are drawn to these distant sites when the abnormal tissue is recognized can destroy sperm. The occurrence of endometriosis may indicate that the endometrial tissue has different or more friable qualities than normal endometrium (perhaps due to a luteal phase defect) and therefore is a type of endometrium that does not support embryo implantation as well as usual. Endometriosis can be treated both medically and surgically (see Chapter 47).

Cervical Problems

At the time of ovulation, the cervical mucus is thin and watery and can be easily penetrated by spermatozoa for a period of 12 to 72 hours. If coitus is not synchronized with this time period, the cervical mucus may be too thick to allow spermatozoa to penetrate the cervix. Infection or inflammation of the cervix (erosion) may cause so much thickening in cervical mucus that spermatozoa cannot penetrate it easily or survive in it. A stenotic cervical os or obstruction of the os by a polyp may further compromise penetration. However, this is rarely enough of a problem to be the sole cause of infertility. A woman who has undergone dilatation and curettage (D&C) procedures several times or cervical conization (cervical surgery) should be evaluated in light of the possibility that scar tissue and tightening of the cervical os has occurred.

Vaginal Problems

Infection of the vagina can cause the pH of the vaginal secretions to become acidotic, limiting or destroying the motility of spermatozoa. Some women appear to have sperm-immobilizing or sperm-agglutinating antibodies in their blood plasma that act to destroy sperm cells in the vagina or cervix. Either of these problems can limit the ability of sperm to enter the uterus (Speroff & Fritz, 2005).

Unexplained Infertility

In a small proportion of couples, no known cause for infertility can be discovered. Possibly the problems of either partner alone are not significant, but when combined they become sufficient to create infertility. It is obviously discouraging for couples to complete a fertility evaluation and be told that their inability to conceive cannot be explained. Such couples need support from health care providers to find alternative solutions, such as continuing to try to conceive, using an assistive reproductive technique, choosing to adopt, or agreeing to a child-free life.

Checkpoint Question 2

Cheryl Carl is diagnosed as having endometriosis. This condition interferes with fertility because:

a. The ovaries stop producing adequate estrogen.
b. The uterine cervix becomes inflamed and swollen.
c. Pressure on the pituitary leads to decreased FSH levels.
d. Endometrial implants can block the fallopian tubes.

FERTILITY ASSESSMENT

Not all couples who desire fertility testing want to have children immediately. Some just want to know for their own peace of mind that they are fertile. Others want to know that they are indeed infertile, so that they can discontinue contraceptive measures (although they need to be cautioned to maintain safer sex practices).

The age of the couple and the degree of apprehension they feel about possible infertility make a difference in determining when they should be referred for fertility evaluation. Although some health care plans or specific settings set limits on the age range in which fertility testing can be scheduled (e.g., not before age 18 years and not after age 45 years), other settings do not establish such limits, allowing couples of any age to benefit from assessment. Both maternal and paternal aging reduce fertility (de La Rochebrochard & Thonneau, 2003). As a rule of thumb, if the woman is younger than 35 years of age, she should be referred for evaluation after 1 year of infertility; if older than 35 years, after 6 months of infertility. Referral is recommended sooner for older women because of possible age limitations associated with adoption, IVF, and embryo transfer, common alternatives to natural childbearing. It would be doubly unfortunate if a couple delayed fertility testing so long that they not only learned they could not conceive but also were considered by an adoption agency to be "too old" to be prospective parents. If the couple is extremely apprehensive or know of a specific problem, studies should never be delayed, regardless of the couple's age.

Basic fertility assessment begins with a health history and physical examination of both sexual partners.

Health History

Nurses often assume the responsibility for initial history taking with an infertile couple. Because of the wide variety of factors that may be responsible for infertility, it is important that a history be thorough. A minimum history for the man should include the following:

- General health
- Nutrition
- Alcohol, drug, or tobacco use
- Congenital health problems such as hypospadias or cryptorchidism
- Illnesses such as mumps orchitis, urinary tract infection, or sexually transmitted diseases
- Operations such as surgical repair of a hernia, which could have resulted in a blood compromise to the testes

- Current illnesses, particularly endocrine illnesses or low-grade infections
- Past and current occupation and work habits (e.g., does his job involve sitting at a desk all day or exposure to x-rays or other forms of radiation?)

It is important to document sexual practices such as the frequency of coitus and masturbation, failure to achieve ejaculation, premature ejaculation, coital positions used, use of lubricants and past contraceptive measures, and existence of any children produced from a previous relationship (Box 6.3).

Most couples assume that infertility is the woman's problem. Many women, even after careful explanation that the problem is their male partner's and not theirs, continue to show low self-esteem, as if the fault rested with them. A woman should be asked about current or past reproductive tract problems, such as infections; her overall health, emphasizing endocrine problems such as galactorrhea (breast nipple secretions) or symptoms of thyroid dysfunction; and any abdominal or pelvic operations she has had that could have compromised blood flow to pelvic organs. Additional questions focus on the frequency of using douches or intravaginal medications or sprays (which may interfere with vaginal pH); exposure to occupational hazards such as x-rays or toxic substances; and nutrition, especially folic acid intake.

Also obtain information from the woman about whether she can detect ovulation. Pay particular attention to the typical symptoms, such as breast tenderness and midcycle "wetness," that indicate ovulation.

In addition to the above items, a menstrual history should be obtained, including the following:

- Age of menarche
- Length, regularity, and frequency of menstrual periods
- Amount of flow
- Any difficulties experienced, such as dysmenorrhea or premenstrual dysphoric disorder

BOX 6.3 FOCUS ON . . .

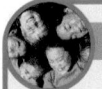

DIVERSITY OF CARE

Do Cultural Traditions Ever Interfere With Fertility?

Obtaining a sexual history, which is necessary for a fertility evaluation, is often difficult because cultural taboos can make couples feel uncomfortable discussing this part of their life. Simple factors, such as how often couples engage in sexual relations, are influenced by culture and religion. According to Orthodox Jewish law, for example, a couple may not engage in sexual relations for 7 days following menstruation (the *nida* period). This practice can result in fertility problems if the woman ovulates within the 7-day period. Being aware that cultural differences can influence how a couple reacts to a diagnosis of infertility can help you appreciate the meaning of this diagnosis to an individual couple.

- History of contraceptive use
- History of any previous pregnancies or abortions

While obtaining the history, take time with each partner individually and as a couple to encourage questions and to discuss overall attitudes toward sexual relations, pregnancy, and parenting. A frank discussion centered on resolving the couple's fears and clearing up any long-standing confusion or misinformation will help to set a positive tone for future interactions, establish a feeling of trust with health care personnel, and increase self-esteem. Talking with both partners can also help them clarify their feelings about infertility and why they are seeking help in this area (Box 6.4).

Physical Assessment

After a thorough history, both men and women need a complete physical examination. For the man, inspect in particular for secondary sexual characteristics and genital abnormalities, such as the absence of a vas deferens or the presence of undescended testes or a varicocele (enlargement of a testicular vein). The presence of a hydrocele (collection of fluid in the tunica vaginalis of the scrotum) is rarely associated with infertility but should be documented if present.

For the woman, a thorough physical assessment including breast and thyroid examination is necessary to rule out current illness. Of particular importance are secondary sex characteristics, which indicate maturity and good pituitary function (see Chapter 32 for a discussion of Tanner stages). A complete pelvic examination including a Pap test (see Chapter 10) is needed to rule out anatomic disorders and infection.

Fertility Testing

Basic fertility testing involves only three tests: semen analysis in the male and ovulation monitoring and tubal patency assessment in the female.

Nurses play key roles in preparing couples for these tests, helping them schedule the studies appropriately, and supporting them while they wait for results. It is important that all personnel involved work cooperatively so that couples do not receive conflicting reports to add to their stress level (Box 6.5).

Additional testing for men, if warranted, can include urinalysis; a complete blood count; blood typing, including Rh factor; a serologic test for syphilis; a test for the presence of human immunodeficiency virus (HIV); erythrocyte sedimentation rate (an increased rate indicates inflammation); protein-bound iodine (a test for thyroid function); cholesterol level (arterial plaques could interfere with pelvic blood flow); and gonadotropin, prolactin, and testosterone levels.

Advanced testing for the woman may include a rubella titer, a serologic test for syphilis, and an HIV evaluation. If a woman has symptoms of thyroid dysfunction, a thyroid uptake determination and thyroid-stimulating hormone level may be ordered. If a woman has a history of menstrual irregularities, blood may be assayed for FSH, estrogen, LH, and progesterone levels. If a woman has a history

BOX 6.4: Focus on Nursing Care Planning

A Multidisciplinary Care Map for A Family Seeking a Fertility Evaluation

•

Cheryl and Bob Carl, married when they were both 25 years old, planned to wait 5 years before beginning their family, so that they would have time to save money for a house. At the end of 5 years, they bought the house. On the day they moved in, Mrs. Carl stopped taking her birth control pills. At the end of a year, however, she still was not pregnant. Three years later, the Carls began fertility testing. They are now undergoing their second cycle of in vitro fertilization and embryo transfer. The Carls have applied for a second mortgage on their house to finance the fertility testing and fertilization procedures. At her last visit, Mrs. Carl stated, "This is my fault because I'm so rigid. I can't relax enough to get pregnant. Look at the way I had to buy the house before I could even consider getting pregnant, and now we'll probably lose it. Besides that, it feels like our whole life revolves around trying to get pregnant."

Family Assessment
Couple live in three bedroom middle-income home; husband works as a bank manager; wife works as a receptionist in a medical office. Husband reports finances as "not good." Couple both appear discouraged about their apparent inability to have children.

Client Assessment
Past medical history negative for any major health problems; reports a menstrual cycle of 5 days' duration with moderate flow every 30 to 32 days; moderate dysmenorrhea for the first 2 days of her menses. Oral contraceptive use for 6 years; discontinued 3 years ago. Baseline laboratory studies and vital signs within normal limits.

Nursing Diagnosis
Situational low self-esteem related to seeming inability to conceive

Outcome Criteria
Couple verbalizes feelings about possible infertility and effect on self-esteem; participates actively in care and treatment decisions; states they feel some control over situation and required treatment.

Team Member Responsible	Assessment	Intervention	Rationale	Expected Outcome
Activities of Daily Living				
Nurse	Assess couple's lifestyle to identify areas in which they are successful.	Review and reinforce with client couple activities they have achieved successfully.	Identifying positive attributes can provide a foundation for rebuilding self-esteem.	Couple names at least three positive achievements, such as organizing at work or planting garden.
Nurse	Assess if there is a common interest they could draw upon.	Ask couple to propose a new activity that would interest both of them.	Beginning a new activity can eliminate total concentration on fertility management.	Couple names and begins to participate in a new activity by 2 weeks' time.

(continued)

Team Member Responsible	Assessment	Intervention	Rationale	Expected Outcome
Consultations				
Nurse/Social Worker	Assess the couple's community for available community resources.	Ask couple if they would like a referral to a support group such as Resolve.	A national organization can help supply effective support during a family crisis.	Couple confirms that they have contacted an outside support group and have attended at least one meeting or on-line chat group.
Procedures/Medications				
Nurse/Physician/Nurse Practitioner	Assess whether couple understands what procedures will be scheduled for a basic fertility series.	Encourage clients to ask questions about procedures; if prescribed an ovulation stimulant, review dosage and administration schedule.	Fully informed clients are better able to participate in their own care.	Clients show interest in procedures and medication by asking questions and demonstrating successful medication adherence.
Nutrition				
Nurse/Nutritionist	Assess whether couple ingests a healthy diet in light of busy lifestyle.	Remind client to continue to take prenatal vitamin (because of folic acid content) during fertility studies to be well prepared when pregnancy is achieved.	Folic acid is necessary in early pregnancy to help prevent spinal cord anomalies. Overall health may contribute to fertility.	Client demonstrates that she has renewed her prenatal vitamin prescription and confirms that she takes them. Client lists a healthy diet and states that she does not smoke or take recreational drugs.
Patient/Family Education				
Nurse	Assess whether couple understands why ovulation and conception occur.	Discuss new fertility measures being instituted; include both members of couple in discussion as appropriate.	Discussing conception-related factors helps to provide a baseline for understanding possible procedures and treatments. Including the partners as a couple helps promote family-centered care.	Couple discusses options they need to follow for fertility testing.
Spiritual/Psychosocial/Emotional Needs				
Nurse	Attempt to identify the meaning of fertility to each client individually and to the couple.	Clarify any misconceptions clients may have about fertility and infertility.	Misconceptions can negatively affect self-esteem.	Clients accurately describe situation and manifest adequate self-esteem.
Discharge Planning				
Nurse	Assess whether couple has any further questions about fertility testing and how they are active partners in it.	Stress that waiting for a much-desired pregnancy to come to term can be just as stressful as waiting for fertility measures to be effective.	Identifying stressful situations can help the couple prepare for them.	Couple states they feel well equipped to manage stress following fertility assessment.
Nurse	Determine who the couple has to turn to for support outside of health care providers.	Discuss possible support persons and groups.	Additional support can assist in reinforcing positive attributes, thus enhancing self-esteem.	Clients list appropriate persons or groups to use as support people.

BOX 6.5 FOCUS ON . . .

EVIDENCE-BASED PRACTICE

Can psychosocial counseling increase the conception rate in infertile couples?

Many infertility services offer some form of counseling to couples undergoing fertility assessment and treatment. To discover whether these services make a difference in the final fertility outcome, a researcher reviewed the literature for studies that provided some time of psychosocial intervention for infertile couples. A total of 380 studies were identified and analyzed. Results of this systematic review showed that pregnancy rates were unlikely to be affected by psychosocial interventions. Interestingly, though, group interventions that emphasized education and skills training such as relaxation training were significantly more effective in producing attitude changes than counseling interventions that emphasized emotional expression and support.

This is an important study for nurses, because nurses are often the people responsible for designing and offering counseling at health care centers. The study suggests that planning a program that emphasizes learning a new skill will be better received than one that just discusses thoughts and feelings.

Source: Boivin, J. (2003). A review of psychosocial interventions in infertility. *Social Science & Medicine, 57*(12), 2325–2341.

BOX 6.6 FOCUS ON . . .

FAMILY TEACHING

Tips for Ensuring an Accurate Semen Analysis

Q. Bob Carl asks you, "What can I do to make sure that the analysis of my semen sample is as accurate as possible?"

A. To ensure accurate results, use the following guidelines when obtaining a semen sample for analysis:

- Use a clean, dry plastic or glass container with a secure lid to collect the sample.
- Collect the specimen as close as possible to your usual schedule of sexual activity.
- Avoid using any lubricants when you collect the specimen.
- After you've collected the specimen in the container, close it securely and write down the time you collected it.
- Keep the specimen at body temperature while transporting it. Carrying it next to your chest is one way to do this.
- Take the specimen to the laboratory or health care provider's office immediately so it can be analyzed within 1 hour of collection.

of galactorrhea, a serum prolactin level will be obtained. A pelvic sonogram may be performed to rule out ovarian, tubal, or uterine structural disorders.

Semen Analysis

For a semen analysis, after 2 to 4 days of sexual abstinence, the man ejaculates by masturbation into a clean, dry specimen jar, and the spermatozoa are examined under a microscope within 1 hour (Box 6.6). The number of sperm in the specimen are counted, and their appearance and motility are noted. An average ejaculation should produce 2.5 to 5.0 mL of semen and should contain a minimum of 20 million spermatozoa per milliliter of fluid (the average normal sperm count is 50 to 200 million per milliliter). The analysis may need to be repeated after 2 or 3 months, because spermatogenesis is an ongoing process, and 30 to 90 days is needed for new sperm to reach maturity (Speroff & Fritz, 2005).

Sperm Penetration Assay and Antisperm Antibody Testing

For impregnation to take place, sperm must be mobile enough to reach the ova. Although sperm penetration studies are rarely necessary, they may be carried out to determine whether a man's sperm, once they reach an ovum, can penetrate it effectively. With the use of an artificial reproductive technique such as IVF, poorly mobile sperm or those with poor penetration can be injected into the woman's ovum under laboratory conditions (intracyto-

plasmic sperm injection), bypassing the need for sperm to be fully mobile.

Ovulation Monitoring

The least costly way to determine a woman's ovulation pattern is to ask her to record her basal body temperature (BBT) for at least 1 month. To determine this, the woman takes her temperature each morning, before getting out of bed or engaging in any activity, eating, or drinking, using a special BBT or tympanic thermometer. She plots this daily temperature on a monthly graph, noticing conditions that might affect her temperature (e.g., colds, other infections, sleeplessness). At the time of ovulation, the basal temperature can be seen to dip slightly (about 0.5°F); it then rises to a level no higher than normal body temperature and stays at that level until 3 or 4 days before the next menstrual flow. This increase in BBT marks the time of ovulation, because it occurs immediately after ovulation (actually at the beginning of the luteal phase of the menstrual cycle, which can occur only if ovulation occurred). A temperature rise should last approximately 10 days. If it does not, a luteal phase defect is suggested (i.e., progesterone production begins but is not sustained). Typical graphs of BBT are shown in Figure 6.2.

Ovulation Determination by Test Strip

Various brands of commercial kits are available for assessing the upsurge of LH that occurs just before ovulation

Basal body temperature

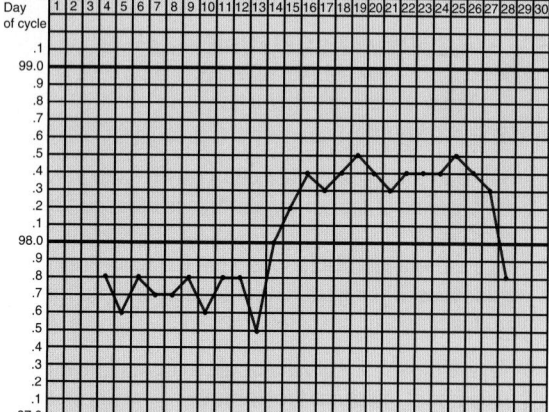

A Ovulation without conception

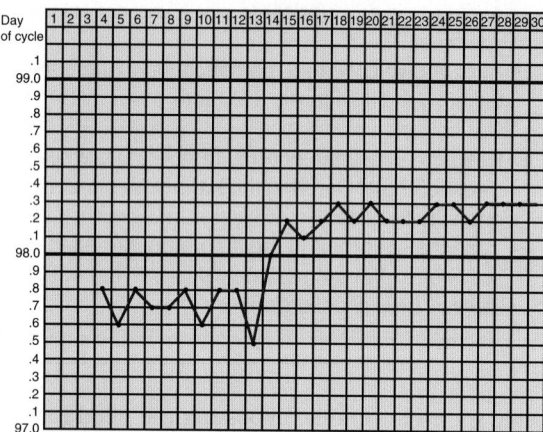

B Ovulation with conception

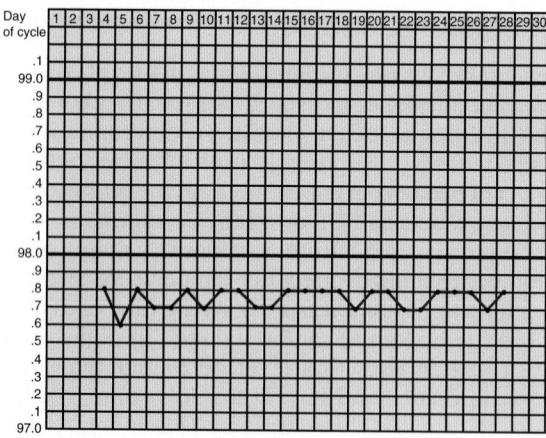

C Anovulatory cycle

FIGURE 6.2 Basal body temperature graph. (**A**) The woman's temperature dips slightly at midpoint in the menstrual cycle, then rises sharply, an indication of ovulation. Toward the end of the cycle (the 24th day), her temperature begins to decline, indicating that progesterone levels are falling and that she did not conceive. (**B**) The woman's temperature rises at the midpoint in the cycle and remains at that elevated level past the time of her normal menstrual flow, suggesting that pregnancy has occurred. (**C**) There is no preovulatory dip, and no rise of temperature anywhere during the cycle. This is the typical pattern of a woman who does not ovulate.

(Smith et al., 2003). These can be used in place of BBT monitoring. The woman dips a test strip into a midmorning urine specimen and then compares it with the kit instructions for a color change. Such kits are purchased over the counter, are easy to use, and have the advantage of marking the point just before ovulation occurs rather than after ovulation, as is the case with BBT. They are not as economical as simple temperature recording, but they are advantageous for women with irregular work or daily activity schedules (e.g., working the night shift, arising at varying times in the morning), which can make BBT measurements inaccurate.

What if... Cheryl Carl has been asked to record her daily basal body temperature. What if she tells you she works nights as a cocktail waitress, goes to bed at 4 AM, then wakes at 6 AM to drive her husband to work? Starting at noon, she sleeps for 4 or 5 hours before getting up to go to work. When during the day should she record her basal body temperature?

Tubal Patency

Tubal patency can be assessed in a number of ways. Both ultrasound and x-ray imaging can be used, not only to determine the patency of fallopian tubes but also to assess the depth and consistency of the endometrial lining.

Sonohysterography. Sonohysterography is an ultrasound technique designed for inspecting the uterus. The uterus is filled with sterile saline, introduced through a narrow catheter inserted into the uterine cervix. A transvaginal ultrasound transducer is then inserted into the vagina to inspect the uterus for abnormalities such as septal deviation or the presence of a myoma. Because this is a minimally invasive technique, it can be done at any time during the menstrual cycle.

Hysterosalpingography. Hysterosalpingography (uterosalpingography), a radiologic examination of the fallopian tubes using a radiopaque medium, is the most frequently used method of assessing tubal patency. This is scheduled immediately after the menstrual flow to avoid reflux of menstrual debris up the tubes and unintentional irradiation of a growing zygote. It is contraindicated if infection of the vagina, cervix, or uterus is present (infectious organisms might be forced into the pelvic cavity). For the procedure, iodine-based radiopaque material is introduced into the cervix under pressure (Fig. 6.3). The radiopaque material outlines the uterus and both tubes, provided that the tubes are patent. Because the medium is thick, it distends the uterus and tubes slightly, causing momentary painful uterine cramping. After the study, the contrast medium drains out through the vagina. The instillation of radiopaque material may be therapeutic as well as diagnostic: the pressure of the solution may actually break up adhesions as it passes through the fallopian tubes, thereby increasing their patency. Although extremely rare, the procedure carries a small risk of infection, allergic reaction to the contrast medium, or embolism

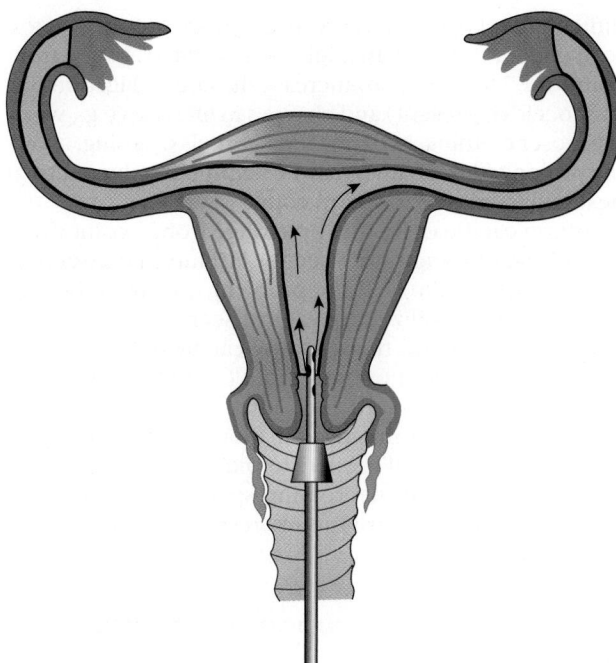

FIGURE 6.3 Insertion of a dye for a hysterosalpingogram. The contrast dye outlines the uterus and fallopian tubes on x-ray to demonstrate patency.

from dye entering a uterine blood vessel (Papaioannou et al., 2004).

Advanced Surgical Procedures

If the assessments already listed do not reveal the cause of infertility, a number of surgical procedures may be scheduled.

Uterine Endometrial Biopsy

Uterine endometrial biopsy may be used as a test for ovulation or to reveal an endometrial problem such as a luteal phase defect. If the endometrium resembles a corkscrew (a typical progesterone-dominated endometrium), this suggests that ovulation has occurred. Endometrial biopsies are being performed less commonly, having been replaced with serum progesterone level evaluations (Smith et al., 2003).

The biopsy is usually done 2 or 3 days before the expected menstrual flow (day 25 or 26 of a typical 28-day menstrual cycle). After a paracervical block, a thin probe and biopsy forceps are introduced through the cervix. The woman may experience mild to moderate discomfort from the maneuvering of the instruments. There may be a moment of sharp pain as the biopsy specimen is taken from the anterior or posterior uterine wall. Possible complications include pain, excessive bleeding, infection, and uterine perforation. This procedure is contraindicated if pregnancy is suspected (although the chance that it would interfere with a pregnancy is probably less than 10%) or if an infection such as acute PID or cervicitis is present. The woman should be cautioned to expect a small amount of vaginal spotting after the procedure. She should be in-

structed to call her primary care provider if she develops a temperature greater than 101°F, has a large amount of bleeding, or passes clots. It is important to advise the woman to telephone the health care agency when she has her next menstrual flow. This helps "date" the endometrium and the accuracy of the analysis.

Hysteroscopy

Hysteroscopy is visual inspection of the uterus through the insertion of a hysteroscope, a thin hollow tube, through the cervix. This is helpful if uterine adhesions or other abnormalities were discovered on the hysterosalpingogram.

Laparoscopy

Laparoscopy is the introduction of a thin, hollow, lighted tube (a fiberoptic telescope or laparoscope) through a small incision in the abdomen, just under the umbilicus, to examine the position and state of the fallopian tubes and ovaries. It is rarely done unless the results of uterosalpingography are abnormal. It is scheduled during the follicular phase of a menstrual period and is done under general anesthesia because of the pain caused by extensive maneuvering. This also allows for good relaxation and a steep Trendelenburg position (which brings the reproductive organs down out of the pelvis). Carbon dioxide is introduced into the abdomen to move the abdominal wall outward and offer better visualization. Women may feel bloating of the abdomen after such a procedure. If some carbon dioxide escapes under the diaphragm, they may feel extremely sharp shoulder pain from pressure.

Laparoscopy technique (see Fig. 5.13) may be used to view the proximity of the ovaries to the fallopian tubes. If this distance is too great, the discharged ovum cannot enter the tube. During the procedure, dye can be injected into the uterus through a polyethylene cannula placed in the cervix to assess tubal patency. Tubes are patent if the dye appears in the abdominal cavity. A scope may be passed directly into a fallopian tube to reveal information about the presence and condition of the fimbria and endometrium lining the tube. If the fimbria have been destroyed by PID, the chance for a normal conception is in doubt, because ova seem to be unable to enter a tube if fimbrial currents are absent.

 Checkpoint Question 3

Cheryl Carl is scheduled to have a hysterosalpingogram. Which of the following instructions would you give her regarding this procedure?

a. She may feel some mild cramping when the dye is inserted.
b. The sonogram of the uterus will reveal any tumors present.
c. She will not be able to conceive for 3 months after the procedure.
d. Many women experience mild bleeding as an aftereffect.

INFERTILITY MANAGEMENT

Management of infertility focuses on correction of any underlying problem that was discovered on assessment. In the meantime, all couples can benefit from some practical information on how to increase the chances of achieving conception on their own. Some suggestions to discuss with a couple are included in Box 6.7.

Correction of the Underlying Problem

The overall management of infertility involves treating such underlying causes as chronic disease, inadequate hormone production, endometriosis, or infection. If correction of these problems does not yield success, infertility management focuses on achieving conception through an assisted reproductive technology such as IVF or sperm donation.

Increasing Sperm Count and Motility

If sperm are not motile because the vas deferens is obstructed, the obstruction is most likely to be extensive and difficult to relieve by surgery. If sperm are present but the total count is low, a man might be advised to abstain from coitus for 7 to 10 days to increase the count. Ligation of a varicocele (if present) and changes in lifestyle (e.g., wearing looser clothing, avoiding long periods of sitting, avoiding prolonged hot baths) may be helpful to reduce scrotal heat and increase the sperm count.

Sperm can be extracted by syringe from a point proximal to the blockage and used for intrauterine insemination (Johnson, 2003). If the problem appears to be that sperm are immobilized by vaginal secretions due to an immunologic factor, the response can be reduced by abstinence or condom use for about 6 months. However, to avoid this prolonged time interval, washing of the sperm and intrauterine insemination may be preferred. The administration of corticosteroids to the woman may have some effect in decreasing sperm immobilization because it reduces her immune response and antibody production.

Reducing the Presence of Infection

If a vaginal infection is present, the infection will be treated according to the causative organism based on culture reports (see Chapter 14). Vaginal infections such as trichomoniasis and moniliasis tend to recur, requiring close supervision and follow-up. The possibility that the sexual partner is reinfecting the woman needs to be considered. Women who are prescribed metronidazole (Flagyl) for a trichomonal infection should be cautioned that it can be teratogenic early in pregnancy and therefore should not be continued if a pregnancy is suspected.

Hormone Therapy

If the problem appears to be a disturbance of ovulation, administration of GnRH is a possibility. Therapy with clomiphene citrate (Clomid, Serophene) may also be used to stimulate ovulation (Box 6.8). In other women, ovarian follicular growth can be stimulated by the administration of human menopausal gonadotropins (Pergonal) in conjunction with administration of human chorionic gonadotropin (hCG) to produce ovulation (Box 6.9). Human menopausal gonadotropins (derived from postmenopausal urine) are combinations of FSH and LH. If increased prolactin levels are identified, bromocriptine (Parlodel) is added to the medication regimen to reduce prolactin levels and allow for the rise of gonadotropins (Karch, 2004).

Administration of either clomiphene citrate or human menopausal gonadotropins may overstimulate an ovary, causing multiple ova to come to maturity and possibly resulting in multiple births (Jain et al., 2004). Women who receive these agents should be counseled that this is a possibility, although it is less of a problem when follicular growth is monitored by ultrasound. If sperm do not appear to survive in the vaginal secretions because secretions are too scant or tenacious, the woman may be prescribed low-dose estrogen therapy to increase mucus production during days 5 to 10 of her cycle. Conjugated estrogen (Premarin) is a type of estrogen used for this purpose.

If the problem appears to be a luteal phase defect, this may be corrected by progesterone vaginal suppositories

---

BOX 6.7 FOCUS ON . . .

FAMILY TEACHING

Suggestions to Aid Conception

Q. Cheryl Carl asks, "Is there anything that we can do to help increase our chances for conception?"

A. Use the following suggestions to help aid conception:

- Couples can determine the woman's time of ovulation through the use of basal body temperature, analysis of cervical secretions, or a commercial ovulation determination kit. Planning sexual relations for every other day around the time of ovulation is ideal.
- Although frequent intercourse may stimulate sperm production, men need sperm recovery time after ejaculation to maintain an adequate sperm count. This is why coitus every other day, rather than every day, during the fertile period will probably yield faster results.
- The male-superior position is the best position for intercourse to achieve conception because it places sperm closest to the cervical opening.
- The male should try for deep penetration so ejaculation places sperm as close as possible to the cervix. Elevating the woman's hips on a small pillow is another way to facilitate sperm collection near the opening to the cervix.
- The woman should remain on her back with knees drawn up for at least 20 minutes after ejaculation to help sperm remain near the cervix.
- No artificial lubricants should be used because they may interfere with sperm motility.
- No douching or lubricants should be used before or after intercourse so vaginal pH is unaltered.

BOX 6.8 FOCUS ON . . .

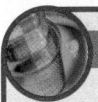

PHARMACOLOGY

Clomiphene Citrate (Clomid)

Action: Clomiphene citrate (Clomid) is an estrogen agonist used to stimulate the ovary. The drug binds to estrogen receptors, decreasing the number of available estrogen receptors and falsely signaling the hypothalamus to increase FSH and LH secretion (Karch, 2004).

Pregnancy category: X

Dosage: Initially, 50 mg/day orally for 5 days (started anytime if no uterine bleeding has occurred recently or about the fifth day of the cycle if uterine bleeding occurs) followed by 100 mg/day for 5 days, started as early as 30 days after the initial course of therapy. This second course may be repeated one more time.

Possible adverse effects: Abdominal discomfort, distention, bloating, nausea, vomiting, breast tenderness, vasomotor flushing, ovarian enlargement, ovarian overstimulation, multiple births, visual disturbances.

Nursing Implications
• Ensure that the woman has had a pelvic examination and baseline hormonal studies before therapy.
• Instruct the client in medication scheduling. Use a calendar to mark treatment schedule and plot ovulation. Remind client that timing intercourse with ovulation is important for achieving pregnancy.
• Explain about the signs of estrogen and progesterone activity.
• Advise the client that 24-hour urine samples may be necessary periodically.
• Caution client to report any bloating, stomach pain, blurred vision, unusual bleeding, bruising, or visual changes.
• Inform the client that therapy can be repeated for a total of three courses; if no results are obtained, therapy will be discontinued at that point.

BOX 6.9 FOCUS ON . . .

PHARMACOLOGY

Menotropins (Pergonal, Humegon)

Action: Menotropins are purified preparations of human gonadotropins that produce ovarian follicular development and growth. When followed by administration of human chorionic gonadotropin (hCG), they produce ovulation.

Pregnancy category: C

Dosage: To achieve ovulation, 5 IU FSH/7.5 IU LH intramuscularly daily for 9 to 12 days, followed by administration of 10,000 IU hCG 1 day later.

Possible adverse effects: Ovarian enlargement, hyperstimulation syndrome, febrile reactions, multiple pregnancies.

Nursing Implications
• Explain the drug's action so that the client understands the importance of coordinating sexual relations with ovulation.
• Instruct the client and partner in the procedure for intramuscular injection, if appropriate.
• Monitor the client at least every other day during treatment and for 2 weeks afterward for signs of possible ovarian enlargement. If it occurs, discontinue the drug and notify the primary health care provider. Prepare the client for possible admission to the health care facility.
• Assist client in preparing a calendar to show treatment schedule to assist with compliance.
• Provide explanations about the signs of estrogen and progesterone activity to watch for.
• Advise the client to have intercourse daily beginning on the day before hCG therapy to achieve the desired effects.
• Counsel the client and partner about possible breast enlargement and also about the possibility of multiple births.

begun on the third day of the temperature rise and continued for the next 6 weeks (if pregnancy occurs) or until the menstrual flow resumes.

Surgery

If a myoma (fibroid tumor) is interfering with fertility, a myomectomy, or surgical removal of the tumor, may be necessary. Myomectomy may be done by a hysteroscopic ambulatory procedure if the growth is small. Uterine adhesions may also be lysed by hysteroscopy. After this procedure, the woman is prescribed estrogen for 3 months to prevent adhesions from reforming, and an IUD is inserted to help prevent the uterine sides from touching. This treatment can be difficult for a woman to accept, because preventing pregnancy (using an IUD) is exactly what she does not want to do.

For problems of abnormal uterine formation, such as a septate uterus, surgery is also available. However, these defects are usually related to early pregnancy loss, not infertility.

If the problem is tubal insufficiency from inflammation, diathermy or steroid administration may be helpful in reducing adhesions. Hysterosalpingography can be repeated to determine whether it produces a therapeutic effect. Canalization of the fallopian tubes and plastic surgical repair (microsurgery) are possible treatments. If peritoneal adhesions or nodules of endometriosis are holding the tubes fixed and away from the ovaries, they can be removed by laparoscopy or laser surgery. Additional therapy for endometriosis is discussed in Chapter 47.

Assisted Reproductive Techniques

If ovulation, sperm production, or sperm mobility problems cannot be corrected, assisted reproductive strategies are available (Richlin et al., 2003). Box 6.10 highlights outcomes and interventions for these problems using the terminology identified by the Nursing Outcomes Classification (NOC) and Nursing Interventions Classification (NIC).

Artificial Insemination

Artificial insemination is the instillation of sperm into the female reproductive tract to aid conception (O'Brien & Vandekerckhove, 2005). The sperm can be instilled into the cervix (intracervical insemination) or into the uterus (intrauterine insemination). Either the husband's sperm (artificial insemination by husband) or donor sperm (artificial insemination by donor or therapeutic donor insemination) can be used. These techniques can be used if the man has an inadequate sperm count or the woman has a vaginal or cervical factor that interferes with sperm motility. They can also be used if the man has a known genetic disorder that he does not want transmitted to offspring or if the woman has no male partner. It is useful for men who, feeling their family was complete, underwent a vasectomy that cannot now be reversed but who now wish to have children. In the past, men who underwent chemotherapy or radiation for testicular cancer had to accept being child-free afterward if they were no longer able to produce sperm. Today, sperm can be cryopreserved (frozen) in a sperm bank before radiation or chemotherapy, and then used for insemination afterward (Meistrich et al., 2005).

One disadvantage of using frozen sperm is that it tends to have slower motility than unfrozen specimens. However, although the rate of conception may be lower from this source, there appears to be no increase in the incidence of congenital anomalies in children conceived by this method. An advantage of cryopreserved sperm is that it can be used even after years of storage. However, this has resulted in ethical, legal, and religious dilemmas.

> *What if...* Bob Carl had some sperm cryopreserved so that Cheryl could become pregnant, but he and Cheryl divorce before it was used? To whom would the cryopreserved sperm belong at that point?

To prepare for artificial insemination, a woman must record her BBT, assess her cervical mucus, or use an ovulation predictor kit to predict her likely day of ovulation. On the day after ovulation, the selected sperm are delivered to her cervix using a device similar to a cervical cap or diaphragm, or they are injected directly into the uterus using a flexible catheter (Fig. 6.4).

If therapeutic donor insemination is selected, the donors are usually volunteers who have no history of disease and no family history of possible inheritable disorders. The blood type, or at least the Rh factor, can be matched with the woman's to prevent incompatibility. If a woman desires, frozen sperm from sperm banks can be selected according to desired physical or mental characteristics.

With artificial insemination, especially therapeutic donor insemination, legal issues must be considered. Some states have specific laws regarding inheritance, child support, and responsibility concerning children conceived by this method. Some couples have religious or ethical beliefs

---

BOX 6.10

Nursing Outcomes Classification (NOC) and Nursing Interventions Classification (NIC)

Reproductive Technologies

NOC: Knowledge, Treatment Procedures
Knowledge, treatment procedures is defined as the extent of understanding conveyed about procedures required as part of a treatment regimen (Johnson et al., 2000). Some specific indicators that suggest that this outcome has been achieved include the client's ability to describe the following:

- Treatment procedure and purpose
- Steps of the procedure, including how the procedure works
- Any restrictions or precautions for or care associated with the procedure
- Possible complications, including any actions to take should complications arise

NIC: Reproductive Technology Management
Reproductive technology management is defined as assisting a client through the steps of complex infertility treatment (McCloskey and Bulechek, 2000).

Some important activities involved when implementing this intervention include the following:

- Providing education about the various treatment methods
- Discussing ethical dilemmas before initiating a particular method
- Teaching ovulation prediction and detection techniques and administration of ovulatory stimulants
- Assisting with fertilization procedures
- Providing anticipatory guidance for client about typical emotional reactions associated with fertilization procedures
- Discussing the risks associated with a planned procedure
- Performing pregnancy tests, including providing support when implantation fails
- Scheduling follow-up medications, tests, and examinations
- Referring to an infertility support group as needed

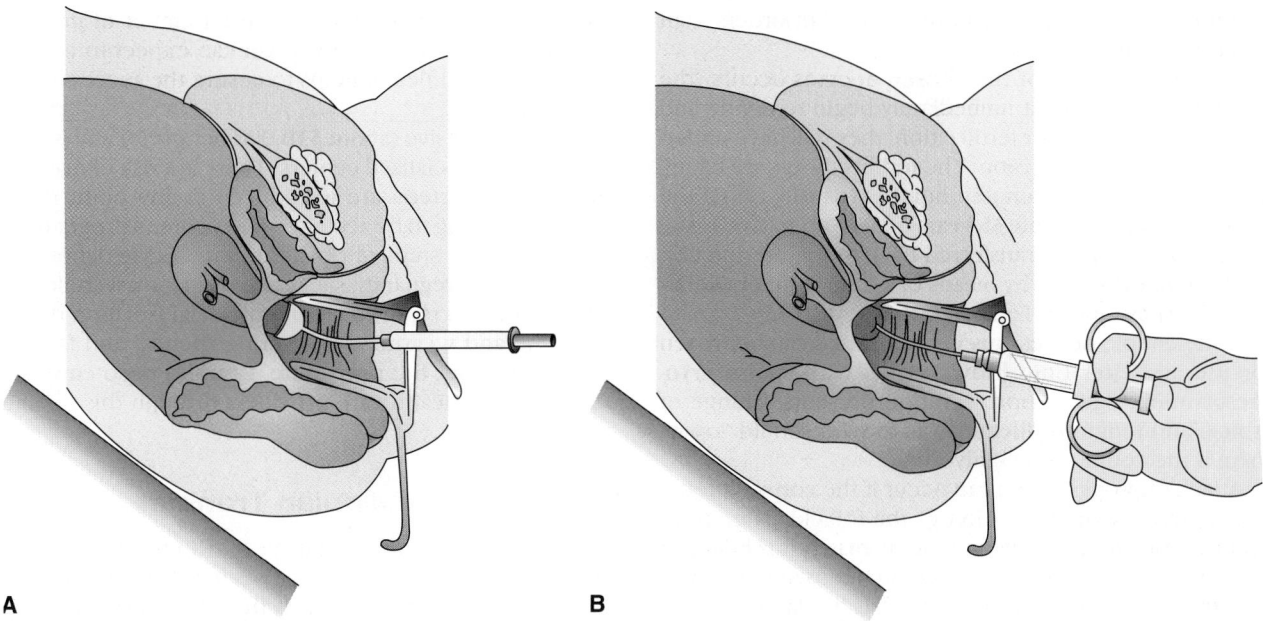

A   **B**

FIGURE 6.4 Artificial insemination. Sperm are deposited next to the cervix (**A**) or injected directly into the uterine cavity (**B**).

that prohibit them from using artificial insemination. In addition, because artificial insemination takes an average of 6 months to achieve conception, it may be a discouraging process for couples.

Checkpoint Question 4

Bob Carl asks you what artificial insemination by donor entails. Which would be your best answer?

a. Artificial sperm are injected vaginally to test tubal patency.
b. Donor sperm are introduced vaginally into the uterus or cervix.
c. The husband's sperm is administered intravenously weekly.
d. Donor sperm are injected intraabdominally into each ovary.

In Vitro Fertilization

In IVF, one or more mature oocytes are removed from a woman's ovary by laparoscopy and fertilized by exposure to sperm under laboratory conditions outside the woman's body. About 40 hours after fertilization, the laboratory-grown fertilized ova are inserted into the woman's uterus, where ideally one or more of them will implant and grow (Smith et al., 2003).

IVF is most often used for couples who have not been able to conceive because the woman has blocked or damaged fallopian tubes. It is also used when the man has oligospermia or a low sperm count, because the controlled, concentrated conditions in the laboratory require only 1 sperm. IVF may be helpful to couples when an absence of cervical mucus prevents sperm from traveling to or entering the cervix, or antisperm antibodies cause immobilization of sperm. In addition, couples with unexplained infertility of long duration may be helped by IVF.

A donor ovum, rather than the woman's own ovum, also can be used for the woman who does not ovulate or who carries a sex-linked disease that she does not want to pass on to her children.

Before the procedure, the woman is given an ovulation-stimulating agent such as GnRH, clomiphene citrate (Clomid), or human menopausal gonadotropin (Pergonal). Beginning about the 10th day of the menstrual cycle, the ovaries are examined daily by sonography to assess the number and size of developing ovarian follicles. When a follicle appears to be mature, the woman is given an injection of hCG, which causes ovulation in 38 to 42 hours.

A needle is then introduced intravaginally, guided by ultrasound, and the oocyte is aspirated from its follicle. Often, many oocytes ripen at once, and perhaps as many as 3 to 12 can be removed. The oocytes are incubated for at least 8 hours to ensure viability. In the meantime, the husband or donor supplies a fresh semen specimen. The sperm cells and oocytes are mixed and allowed to incubate in a growth medium.

In the past, many sperm were necessary, to allow sperm to make their way through the resistant zona pellucida surrounding the ovum. A number of techniques, such as creating passages through the resistant cells (zona drilling), have been discovered to help sperm cross the zona. In some instances, it has been possible to inject sperm directly under the zona pellucida (intracytoplasmic sperm injection). This is the technique that makes it possible for fertilization to take place with only one sperm. Worry that this technique could lead to an increased number of birth defects is unproven but may be related to a tendency for infertile men to have more chromosomal disorders than other men (Foresta, 2005).

After fertilization of the chosen oocytes occurs, the zygotes formed almost immediately begin to divide and grow. By 40 hours after fertilization, they will have undergone their first cell division. The fertilized eggs are examined and, if normal, a chosen number (usually two if the woman is younger than 35 years of age; up to five if she is older than 40) are transferred back to the uterine cavity through the cervix by means of a thin catheter (Rebar & DeCherney, 2004) (Fig. 6.5).

If the couple desires, any eggs not used can be frozen for use at a later time. However, as with sperm cryopreservation, egg cryopreservation presents a range of ethical and religious dilemmas as to who should "own" them if the couple should divorce.

A lack of progesterone can occur if the corpus luteum was injured by the aspiration of the follicle. Therefore, progesterone may be given to the woman if it is believed that she will not produce enough on her own to support implantation. Proof that the zygote has implanted can be demonstrated by a routine serum pregnancy test as early as 11 days after transfer.

In some centers, nurse practitioners are the health care providers who complete oocyte removal and transfer. In all centers, nurses need to supply support and counseling to sustain the couple through the process. The recovery rate for harvesting ripened eggs is high (about 90%), as is the ability to fertilize eggs by sperm in vitro. However, the overall pregnancy rate by IVF is as low as 20% to 30% per treatment cycle (Richlin et al., 2003). Although IVF programs do not result in an increase in birth defects, about 25% of pregnancies end in spontaneous abortion (the same rate as for natural pregnancies). Once a pregnancy has been successfully established, the woman's prenatal care is the same as that for any pregnancy. Research has shown that, because the couple was so committed to the procedure, they adjust to pregnancy and parenthood well.

If a sonogram reveals that a multiple pregnancy of more than two or three zygotes has been achieved, selective termination of gestational sacs until only two are remaining may be recommended. This is done by intraabdominal injection of potassium chloride into the gestational sacs chosen to be eliminated. Reducing the number of growing embryos to a number the woman can expect to carry to term without difficulty helps to ensure the success of the pregnancy.

IVF is expensive (about $10,000 per cycle) and is available only at specialized centers. There is a risk of maternal infection if bacteria are introduced at any point in the transfer. Waiting to be accepted by a center's program and waiting for the steps of obtaining the oocyte, laboratory growth, and pregnancy success is a major psychological strain. Couples report a feeling of social isolation during this time and weariness answering friends' and family's questions about the procedure. Couples need empathic support from health care providers through this difficult time (Box 6.11).

Gamete Intrafallopian Transfer

In gamete intrafallopian transfer (GIFT) procedures, ova are obtained from ovaries exactly as in IVF. Instead of waiting for fertilization to occur in the laboratory, however, both ova and sperm are instilled within a matter of hours, using a laparoscopic technique, into the open end of a patent fallopian tube. Fertilization then occurs in the tube, and the zygote moves to the uterus for implantation. This procedure has a pregnancy rate equal to that of IVF. The procedure is contraindicated if the woman's fallopian tubes are blocked, because this could lead to ectopic (tubal) pregnancy (Lodhi et al., 2004).

Zygote Intrafallopian Transfer

Zygote intrafallopian transfer (ZIFT) involves oocyte retrieval by transvaginal, ultrasound-guided aspiration, followed by culture and insemination of the oocytes in the laboratory (Duckitt, 2005). Within 24 hours, the fertilized eggs are transferred by laparoscopic technique into the end of a waiting fallopian tube. ZIFT differs from GIFT in that fertilization takes place outside the body, allowing health care providers to be certain that fertilization has occurred before the growing structure is reintroduced. As in GIFT, a woman must have one functioning fallopian tube for the technique to be successful, because the zygotes are

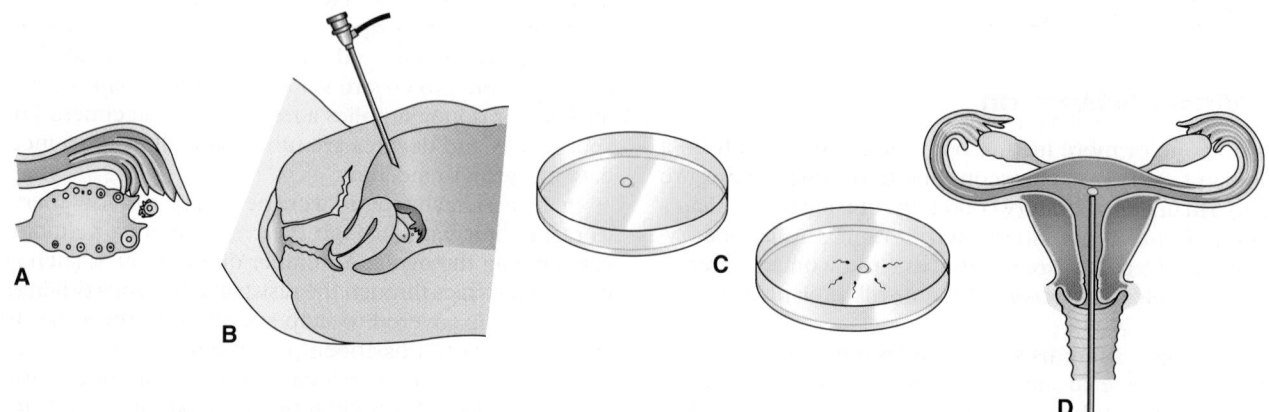

FIGURE 6.5 Steps involved in in vitro fertilization. (**A**) Ovulation. (**B**) Capture of ova (done here intra-abdominally). (**C**) Fertilization of ova and growth in culture medium. (**D**) Insertion of fertilized ova into uterus.

BOX 6.11 FOCUS ON . . .

COMMUNICATION

Cheryl Carl has been trying to get pregnant for 4 years. She and her husband agreed to in vitro fertilization at a cost of approximately $10,000 per month, even though her religion does not approve of this technique. Every time you see her at the fertility clinic, she seems sadder than the previous time.

Less Effective Communication

Nurse: How is everything going, Mrs. Carl?
Mrs. Carl: Fine. I'm just tired of no results.
Nurse: That's partly your fault, Mrs. Carl. You waited a long time before you came for an evaluation.
Mrs. Carl: Making wise choices is difficult for me. I'll probably make a lousy parent if I ever do get pregnant.

More Effective Communication

Nurse: How is everything going, Mrs. Carl?
Mrs. Carl: Fine. I'm just tired of no results.
Nurse: Considering that you have been trying for such a long time, I think you've done very well. Infertility management is always difficult.
Mrs. Carl: I've learned to be patient. I figure that will stand me in good stead the day I do have a child.

Clients often may not make the same choices about fertility testing or management that a health care provider might make; such decisions are based on individual circumstances and situations. Be careful not to criticize clients for making choices that you think are poor ones. A more effective technique is to support them at that point and help them find ways to continue to feel good about themselves and maintain self-esteem.

implanted into the fimbriated end of a tube rather than into the uterus.

Surrogate Embryo Transfer

Surrogate embryo transfer is an assisted reproductive technique for a woman who does not ovulate. The process involves use of an oocyte that has been donated by a friend or relative or provided by an anonymous donor (Brinsden, 2003). The menstrual cycles of the donor and recipient are synchronized by administration of gonadotropic hormones. At the time of ovulation, the donor's ovum is removed by a transvaginal, ultrasound-guided procedure. The oocyte is then fertilized by the recipient woman's male partner's sperm (or donor sperm) and placed in the recipient woman's uterus by embryonic transfer. Once pregnancy occurs, it progresses the same as an unassisted pregnancy.

Preimplantation Genetic Diagnosis

The individual retrieval of oocytes and their fertilization under laboratory conditions has led to close inspection and recognition of differences in sperm and oocytes. Before the oocyte is fertilized, the DNA of both sperm and oocytes can be examined for specific genetic characteristics or other abnormalities (Pickering & Braude, 2003).

Couples participating in intrauterine transfer and artificial insemination can have the sex of their offspring predetermined using these methods. Such techniques can be useful, because popular methods to influence the sex of a child (such as douching with a baking soda mixture before coitus to have a boy or with a vinegar solution to have a girl) have proved to be more folklore than scientific fact.

ALTERNATIVES TO CHILDBIRTH

For some couples, even treatment for infertility with procedures such as IVF are not successful. These couples need to consider still other options.

Surrogate Mothers

A surrogate mother is a woman who agrees to carry a pregnancy to term for an infertile couple (Jadva et al., 2003). The surrogate may provide the ova and be impregnated by the man's sperm. In other instances, the ova and sperm both may be donated by the infertile couple, or donor ova and sperm may be used. Surrogate mothers are often friends or family members who assume the role out of friendship or compassion, or they can be referred to the couple through an agency or attorney and receive monetary reimbursement for their service. The infertile couple can enjoy the pregnancy as they watch it progress in the surrogate.

A number of ethical and legal problems can arise if the surrogate mother decides at the end of pregnancy that she has formed an attachment to the fetus and wants to keep the baby despite the prepregnancy agreement she signed. Court decisions have been split on whether the surrogate or the infertile couple has the right to the child. Another potential problem occurs if the child is born imperfect and the infertile couple then no longer wants the child. Who should have responsibility in this instance? For these reasons, the couple and the surrogate mother must be certain they have given adequate thought to the process, and to what will be the outcome should these problems occur, before they attempt it.

Adoption

Adoption, once a ready alternative for infertile couples, is still a viable alternative, although today there are fewer children available for adoption from official agencies than formerly. Often it takes longer to find a child for adoption than it once did, unless the couple considers foreign-born or physically or cognitively challenged children or children of other races. Also, like other alternatives, adoption may not be right for every couple. Issues of adoptive families are discussed in Chapter 2.

Child-Free Living

Child-free living is an alternative lifestyle available to both fertile and infertile couples. For many infertile couples who have been through the rigors and frustrations of infertility testing and unsuccessful treatment regimens, child-free living may emerge as the option they finally wish to pursue. A couple in the midst of fertility testing may begin to re-examine their motives for pursuing pregnancy and may decide that pregnancy and parenting are not worth the emotional or financial cost of future treatments. They may decide that the additional stress of going through an adoption is not for them, or they may simply decide that children are not necessary for them to complete their family unit. For these couples, child-free living is a positive choice.

Child-free living has advantages for a couple in that it allows time for both to pursue careers. They can travel more or have more time to pursue hobbies or continue their education. If a couple still wishes to include children in their lives in some way, many opportunities are available to do this: through family connections (most parents welcome offers from siblings or other family members to share in childrearing), through volunteer organizations (such as Big Brother or Big Sister programs), or through local schools and town recreational programs.

Child-free living can be as fulfilling as having children, because it allows a couple more time to help other people and to contribute to society through personal accomplishments. Many couples who believe that overpopulation is a major concern choose child-free living even if infertility is not present.

Checkpoint Question 5

Cheryl Carl is having a GIFT procedure. What makes her a good candidate for this procedure?

a. She has patent fallopian tubes, so fertilized ova can be implanted into them.

b. She is Rh negative, a necessary stipulation to rule out Rh incompatibility.

c. She has a normal uterus, so sperm can be injected through the cervix into it.

d. Her husband is taking sildenafil (Viagra), so all his sperm will be motile.

Key Points

Infertility is said to exist when a pregnancy has not occurred after 1 year of unprotected coitus. Sterility refers to the inability to conceive due to a known condition.

About 14% of couples today experience infertility. The incidence increases with the age of the couple.

Infertility testing can be an intense psychological stressor for couples. Support from health care personnel is necessary during this time, not only to help couples through the experience on an individual basis but also to help them maintain their relationship as a couple.

Couples who are told that an infertility problem has been discovered are apt to suffer a loss of self-esteem. The nursing role includes offering support to help them look at other aspects of their lives in which they do achieve and to recognize that they are productive, healthy people in many ways.

Male factors that contribute to infertility are inadequate sperm count, obstruction or impaired sperm motility, and problems with ejaculation. Female factors that cause infertility are problems with ovulation, tubal transport, or impaired implantation.

Basic infertility assessment procedures consist of a health history, physical examination, laboratory tests to document general health, and specific tests for semen, ovulation, and tubal patency.

Measures to induce fertility are aimed at improving sperm number and transport, decreasing infections, stimulating ovulation, and regulating hormones.

Artificial insemination, donor egg transfer, IVF, adoption, surrogate motherhood, and child-free living are all possible solutions for infertility.

Critical Thinking Exercises

1. Cheryl Carl, whom you met at the beginning of the chapter, stated that she believed her infertility problem was her fault because she was too rigid. She said, "It feels like our whole life revolves around trying to get pregnant." Does a rigid personality affect infertility? Does relaxation aid conception?

2. The Carls want to have a child as soon as possible. In addition to their infertility assessment, what advice would you give them to help increase their chances of conceiving quickly?

3. Cheryl Carl is scheduled for a hysterosalpingogram. How would you prepare her for this procedure? What should she expect when the procedure is over?

4. Examine the National Health Goals related to infertility. Most government-sponsored money for nursing research is allotted based on these goals. What would be a possible research topic to explore pertinent to these goals that would be applicable to the Carl family and also advance evidence-based practice?

References

Boivin, J. (2003). A review of psychosocial interventions in infertility. *Social Science and Medicine, 57*(12), 2325–2341.

Brinsden, P. R. (2003). Gestational surrogacy. *Human Reproduction Update, 9*(5), 483–491.

De La Rochebrochard, E., & Thonneau, P. (2003). Paternal age over or equal to 40 years: An important risk factor for infertility. *American Journal of Obstetrics and Gynecology, 189*(4), 901–905.

Department of Health and Human Services. (2000). *Healthy people 2010*. Washington, D.C.: DHHS.

Duckitt, K (2005). Infertility and subfertility. In Godlee, F. (Ed.), *Clinical evidence.* London: BMJ Publishing Group Ltd.

Eschenbach, D. A. (2003). Pelvic infections and sexually transmitted diseases. In Scott, J. R., et al. (Eds.), *Danforth's obstetrics and gynecology* (9th ed.). Philadelphia: Lippincott Williams & Wilkins.

Foresta, C., et al. (2005). Genetic abnormalities among severely oligospermic men who are candidates for intracytoplasmic sperm injection. *Journal of Clinical Endocrinology and Metabolism, 90*(1), 152-156.

Hamilton-Fairley, D., & Taylor, A. (2003). Anovulation. *BMJ, 327*(7414), 546-549.

Hirsh, A. (2003). ABC of subfertility: Male subfertility. *BMJ, 327*(7416), 669-672.

Jadva, V., et al. (2003). Surrogacy: The experiences of surrogate mothers. *Human Reproduction, 18*(10), 2196-2204.

Jain, T., Missmer, S. A., & Hornstein, M. D. (2004). Trends in embryo-transfer practice and in outcomes of the use of assisted reproductive technology in the United States. *New England Journal of Medicine, 350*(16), 1639-1645.

Johnson, J. (2003). Infertility. In Scott, J. R., et al. (Eds.), *Danforth's obstetrics and gynecology* (9th ed.). Philadelphia: Lippincott Williams & Wilkins.

Johnson, M., Maas, M., & Moorhead, S. (2000). *Nursing outcomes classification* (2nd ed.). St. Louis: Mosby.

Karch, A. M. (2004). *Lippincott's nursing drug guide.* Philadelphia: Lippincott Williams & Wilkins.

Khalaf, Y. (2003). Tubal subfertility. *BMJ, 327*(7415), 610-613.

Lodhi, S., et al. (2004). Gamete intra-fallopian transfer or intrauterine insemination after controlled ovarian hyperstimulation for treatment of infertility due to endometriosis. *Gynecological Endocrinology, 19*(3), 152-159.

McCloskey, J., & Bulechek, G. (2000). *Nursing interventions classification* (3rd ed.). St. Louis: Mosby.

Meistrich, M. L., et al. (2005). Gonadal dysfunction. In DeVita, V. T., Hellman, S., & Rosenberg, S. A. (Eds.), *Cancer: Principles and practice of oncology* (7th ed.). Philadelphia: Lippincott Williams & Wilkins.

O'Brien, P., & Vandekerckhove, P. (2005). Intra-uterine versus cervical insemination of donor sperm for subfertility. *Cochrane Library (Oxford) (2)* (CD000317).

Papaioannou, S., et al. (2004). Tubal evaluation in the investigation of subfertility: A structured comparison of tests. *BJOG: An International Journal of Obstetrics and Gynecology, 111*(12), 1313-1321.

Pasqualotto, F. F., et al. (2005). Semen profile, testicular volume, and hormonal levels in infertile patients with varicoceles compared with fertile men with and without varicoceles. *Fertility and Sterility, 83*(1), 74-77.

Pickering, S., & Braude, P. (2003). Further advances and uses of assisted conception technology. *BMJ, 327*(7424), 1156-1158.

Rebar, R. W., & DeCherney, A. H. (2004). Assisted reproductive technology in the United States. *New England Journal of Medicine, 350*(16), 1603-1604.

Richlin, S. S., Shanti, A., & Murphy, A. A. (2003). Assisted reproductive technology. In Scott, J. R., et al. (Eds.), *Danforth's obstetrics and gynecology* (9th ed.). Philadelphia: Lippincott Williams & Wilkins.

Schenken, R. S. (2003). Endometriosis. In Scott, J. R., et al. (Eds.) *Danforth's obstetrics and gynecology* (9th ed.). Philadelphia: Lippincott Williams & Wilkins.

Smith, S., et al. (2003). Diagnosis and management of female infertility. *Journal of the American Medical Association, 290*(13), 1767-1770.

Speroff, L., & Fritz, M. A. (2005). *Clinical gynecologic endocrinology and infertility* (7th ed.). Philadelphia: Lippincott Williams & Wilkins.

Steen, R., & Shapiro, K. (2004). Intrauterine contraceptive devices and risk of pelvic inflammatory disease. *Reproductive Health Matters, 12*(23), 136-143.

Suggested Readings

Barber, D. (2004). Endometriosis: Diagnosis and management of symptoms. *Community Practitioner, 77*(6), 227-228.

Chervenak, F. A., McCullough, L. B., & Rosenwaks, Z. (2003). Ethical considerations in newer reproductive technologies. *Seminars in Perinatology, 27*(6), 427-434.

Collopy, K. S. (2004). "I couldn't think that far": Infertile women's decision making about multifetal reduction. *Research in Nursing and Health, 27*(2), 75-86.

Klonoff-Cohen, H. S., & Natarajan, L. (2004). The effect of advancing paternal age on pregnancy and live birth rates in couples undergoing in vitro fertilization or gamete intrafallopian transfer. *American Journal of Obstetrics and Gynecology, 191*(2), 507-514.

Lee, S. (2003). Effects of using a nursing crisis intervention program on psychosocial responses and coping strategies of infertile women during in vitro fertilization. *Journal of Nursing Research, 11*(3), 197-207.

Peters, K. (2003). In pursuit of motherhood: The IVF experience. *Contemporary Nurse, 14*(3), 258-270.

Pickering, S., & Braude, P. (2003). Further advances and uses of assisted conception technology. *BMJ, 327*(7424), 1156-1158.

Pook, M., & Krause, W. (2005). Stress reduction in male infertility patients: A randomized, controlled trial. *Fertility and Sterility, 83*(1), 68-73.

Rapport, F. (2003). Exploring the beliefs and experiences of potential egg share donors. *Journal of Advanced Nursing, 43*(1), 28-42.

Rowell, P., & Braude, P. (2003). Assisted conception: General principles. *BMJ, 327*(7418), 799-801.

Stern, J. E., et al. (2003). Determining access to assisted reproductive technology: Reactions of clinic directors to ethically complex case scenarios. *Human Reproduction, 18*(6), 1343-1352.

Taylor, A. (2003). ABC of subfertility: Extent of the problem. *BMJ, 327*(7412), 434-436.

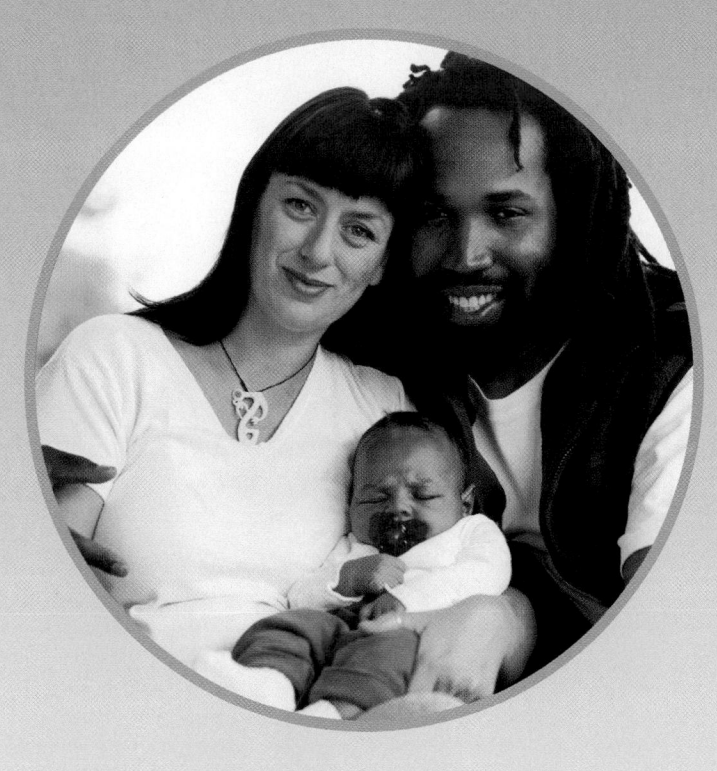

UNIT THREE

The Nursing Role in Caring for the Pregnant Family

•

CHAPTER 7

Genetic Assessment and Counseling

Key Terms

alleles
chromosomes
dermatoglyphics
dominant gene
genes
genetics
genome
genotype
heterozygous
homozygous
imprinting
karyotype
meiosis
nondisjunction
phenotype
recessive gene

Objectives

After mastering the contents of this chapter, you should be able to:

1. Describe the nature of inheritance, patterns of recessive and dominant mendelian inheritance, and common chromosomal aberrations such as nondisjunction syndromes.
2. Assess a family for the probability of inheriting a genetic disorder.
3. Formulate nursing diagnoses related to genetic disorders.
4. Establish expected outcomes that meet the needs of the pregnant family undergoing genetic assessment and counseling.
5. Plan nursing care related to an alteration in genetic health, such as assisting with an amniocentesis.
6. Implement nursing care related to identification of or counseling for a genetic disorder.
7. Evaluate expected outcomes for achievement and effectiveness of nursing care.
8. Identify National Health Goals and specific measures related to genetic disorders that nurses can help the nation achieve.
9. Identify areas related to genetic assessment that could benefit from additional nursing research or application of evidence-based practice.
10. Use critical thinking to analyze ways that nurses can contribute to health education and family-centered counseling for genetic issues.
11. Integrate knowledge of genetic inheritance with nursing process to achieve quality maternal and child health nursing care.

*A*my Alvarez is a woman you meet at a genetic counseling center. She was adopted as a newborn and never felt a need to locate her birth parents because her adoptive parents provided a "close to perfect" childhood for her. After college, she married the most eligible bachelor in her hometown. She is now pregnant with her first child. At 15 weeks into the pregnancy, she has been advised her child may have translocation Down syndrome. She asks you, "Why is this happening? There's no disease like this in either of our families."

Previous chapters described techniques for caring for women and their families preparing for childbearing and childrearing. This chapter discusses the basic principles by which disorders are inherited and information about the necessary assessments, care, and guidelines for counseling of the woman and her family if it is discovered that there is a possibility of a genetic disorder in a child. This is important information, because it can influence the health of a family for generations to come.

How would you answer Amy?

After you've studied this chapter, access the accompanying website. Read the patient scenario and answer the questions to further sharpen your skills, grow more familiar with RN-CLEX types of questions, and reward yourself with how much you have learned.

As many as 1 in 20 newborns inherits a genetic disorder. More than 30% of pediatric hospital admissions are for genetic-influenced disorders (Ward, 2003). The possibility that a child could have a genetic disorder crosses the minds of most pregnant women and their partners at some point in a pregnancy, whether or not there is any family history of genetic disorders. Many pregnant couples ask health care providers about their chances of having a child with a genetic disorder and about genetic testing, because advances in screening techniques have made genetic testing a common feature of prenatal care. The importance of the Human Genome Project and the necessity to improve techniques of screening for genetic disorders have become a national priority (Box 7.1). Nurses can be instrumental in fostering the achievement of these goals (Siegel & Milunsky, 2004).

Women are offered routine screening of maternal serum levels of alpha-fetoprotein (MSAFP) early in pregnancy to evaluate for neural tube or chromosomal disorders in the fetus. Chorionic villi sampling (CVS) and amniocentesis are follow-up techniques that may be offered to women who are older than 35 years of age, and to those whose MSAFP level is abnormal, to further screen for genetic disorders. Couples who already know of the existence of a genetic disorder in their family and those who have had a previous child born with a congenital anomaly require still additional, more extensive testing. After a positive test for a genetic disorder, they will almost certainly undergo an emotional period of decision making as they decide how to prepare for an ill child or make a decision to end the pregnancy. Informative and sensitive genetic counseling by health care providers educated in the specialty of genetics is essential for these couples. Because most screening takes place in an ambulatory setting, a nurse can play a vital role as educator, supporter, and communicator for the family (Pelchat et al., 2004).

Nursing Process Overview

For Genetic Assessment and Counseling

● *Assessment*

Assessment is a crucial step in any nursing intervention, but it plays an especially vital role in genetic screening and counseling. Assessment measures include a detailed family history, physical examination of both the parents and the affected child, and an ever-growing series of laboratory assays of blood, amniotic fluid, and maternal and fetal cells. Nurses serve as members of genetic assessment and counseling teams in many roles, especially when helping to obtain the initial family history, assisting with the preliminary physical examination, obtaining blood serum for analysis, or assisting with procedures such as amniocentesis.

● *Nursing Diagnosis*

Typical nursing diagnoses related to the area of genetic disorders are the following:

- Decisional conflict related to testing for an untreatable genetic disorder
- Fear related to outcome of genetic screening tests
- Situational low self-esteem related to identified chromosomal abnormality
- Deficient knowledge related to inheritance pattern of the family's inherited disorder
- Health-seeking behaviors related to potential for genetic transmission of disease
- Altered sexuality pattern related to fear of conceiving a child with a genetic disorder

● *Outcome Identification and Planning*

Outcome identification and planning for families involved with genetic assessment differ according to the types of assessments performed and the results obtained. They may include determining what information the couple needs to know before testing can proceed or helping couples to arrange for further assessment measures during a pregnancy. Goals must be realistic and consistent with the individual's or couple's lifestyle (not all people want to be totally informed about family illnesses).

● *Implementation*

Parental reaction to the knowledge that their child has a possible genetic disorder or to the birth of a child with a genetically inherited disorder usually involves a grief reaction, similar to that experienced by parents whose child has died at birth. Both parents must work through the stages of shock and denial ("This cannot be true"), anger ("It's not fair that this happened to us"), and bargaining ("If only this would go away") to reorganization and acceptance ("It has happened to us and it is all right"). For some couples, a genetic disorder is diagnosed during the pregnancy; it may not be discovered until birth, or possibly not even until the child is of

---

BOX 7.1 FOCUS ON . . .

NATIONAL HEALTH GOALS

Two National Health Goals speak directly to genetic disease and screening:

- Increase to at least 90% the proportion of women enrolled in prenatal care who are offered screening and counseling for prenatal detection of fetal abnormalities.
- Increase to at least 95% the proportion of newborns screened by state-sponsored programs for genetic disorders and other disabling conditions and to 90% the proportion of newborns testing positive for disease who receive appropriate treatment (DHHS, 2000).

Nurses can help the nation achieve these goals by being sensitive to the need for genetic screening and counseling in prenatal and birth settings. Answers to questions provided by nursing research, such as when people are most responsive to genetic counseling or what effect on bonding occurs, if any, when the parents learn about an abnormal alpha-fetoprotein level during pregnancy, can also help meet these goals.

school age. For these parents, the reaction will occur at that later point of diagnosis.

As a rule, when parents are under stress, it is most helpful to guide them to concentrate on short-term goals and actions. Help them look first at the immediate needs of their family, the fetus, and the newborn, and later on at what type of continued follow-up will be necessary. For instance, after the birth, will the baby need to be hospitalized for immediate surgical correction of accompanying congenital anomalies, or will the parents be able to take the baby home? These decisions must be made immediately. What kind of special schooling the child will need is a decision that can wait until a later date.

Identifying support people who can be helpful to the parents during their time of disorganization and shock is also important. These people may be the usual family resources, such as grandparents or other family members. In some families, these people are as disturbed by the diagnosis as the parents and therefore cannot offer their usual support. Secondary support sources may be necessary, including organizations such as the March of Dimes Birth Defects Foundation (*www.marchofdimes.com*), the American Association of Klinefelter Syndrome Information and Support (*www.AAKSIS.org*), the National Fragile X Foundation (*www.NFXF.org*), the National Down Syndrome Society (*www.ndss.org*), and the Turner Syndrome Society (*www.Turner-syndrome-us.org*). Not all parents are ready to talk to members of such organizations at the time of diagnosis. To join such an organization may make the diagnosis seem "real" or move them out of denial before they are ready.

Identifying health care personnel and ensuring clear communication among health care providers with whom the parents will need to maintain contact during the next few months can offer additional support. Ensuring that the parents have health care providers they know they can turn to, especially when they are moving out of denial, helps them move forward.

● *Outcome Evaluation*

Examples of expected outcomes for a family with a known genetic disorder include the following:

• Couple states they feel capable of coping no matter what the outcome of genetic testing.
• Client accurately states the chances of a genetic disorder occurring in her next child.
• Couple states they have resolved their feelings of low self-esteem related to birth of a child with a genetic disorder.

A couple's decisions about genetic testing and childbearing may change over time. For example, a decision made at age 25 not to have children because of a potential genetic disorder may be difficult to maintain at age 30, as the couple sees many of their friends with growing families. Individuals and couples who have asked for genetic counseling should be given the phone number of a genetic counselor and urged to call periodically for news of recent advances in genetic screening techniques or disease treatments, so they can remain current.

GENETIC DISORDERS

Inherited or genetic disorders are disorders that can be passed from one generation to the next. They result from some disorder in gene or chromosome structure. **Genetics** is the study of the ways such disorders occur.

Genetic disorders can occur at the moment an ovum and sperm fuse or even earlier, in the meiotic division phase of the gametes (ovum and sperm). Some genetic abnormalities are so severe that normal fetal growth cannot continue. This results in early spontaneous abortion. Genetic disorders are so common that as many as 50% of first-trimester spontaneous miscarriages may be the result of chromosomal abnormalities (Ward, 2003). Other genetic disorders do not affect life in utero, so the result of the disorder becomes apparent only at the time of fetal testing or after birth. In the near future, it may be possible not only to identify aberrant genes for disorders but also to insert healthy genes in their place using stem cells. Gene replacement therapy is encouraging in the treatment of blood, spinal cord, and immunodeficiency syndromes (Jones et al., 2003).

Nature of Inheritance

Genes are the basic units of heredity that determine both the physical and cognitive characteristics of people. Composed of segments of DNA (deoxyribonucleic acid), they are woven into strands in the nucleus of all body cells to form **chromosomes.**

In humans, each cell, with the exception of the sperm and ovum, contains 46 chromosomes (44 autosomes and 2 sex chromosomes). Spermatozoa and ova each carry only half of the chromosome number, or 23 chromosomes. For each chromosome in the sperm cell, there is a like chromosome of similar size and shape and function (autosome, or homologous chromosome) in the ovum. Because genes are always located at fixed positions on chromosomes, two like genes (**alleles**) for every trait are represented in the ovum and sperm on autosomes. The one chromosome in which this does not occur is the chromosome for determining sex. If the sex chromosomes are both type X (large symmetric) in the zygote formed from the union of a sperm and ovum, the individual is female (Fig. 7.1*A*). If one sex chromosome is an X and one a Y (a smaller type), the individual is a male (Fig. 7.1*B*).

A person's **phenotype** refers to his or her outward appearance or the expression of the genes. A person's **genotype** refers to his or her actual gene composition. A person's **genome** is the complete set of genes present (about 50,000 to 100,000). A normal genome is abbreviated as 46XX or 46XY (designation of the total number of chromosomes plus a graphic description of the sex chromosomes present). If a chromosomal aberration exists, it is listed after the sex chromosome pattern. In such abbreviations, the letter *p* stands for short arm defects and *q* stands for defects on the long arm of the chromosome. The abbreviation 46XX5p–, for example, is the abbreviation for a female with 46 total chromosomes but with the short arm of chromosome 5 missing (cri-du-chat syndrome). In Down syndrome, the person has an extra

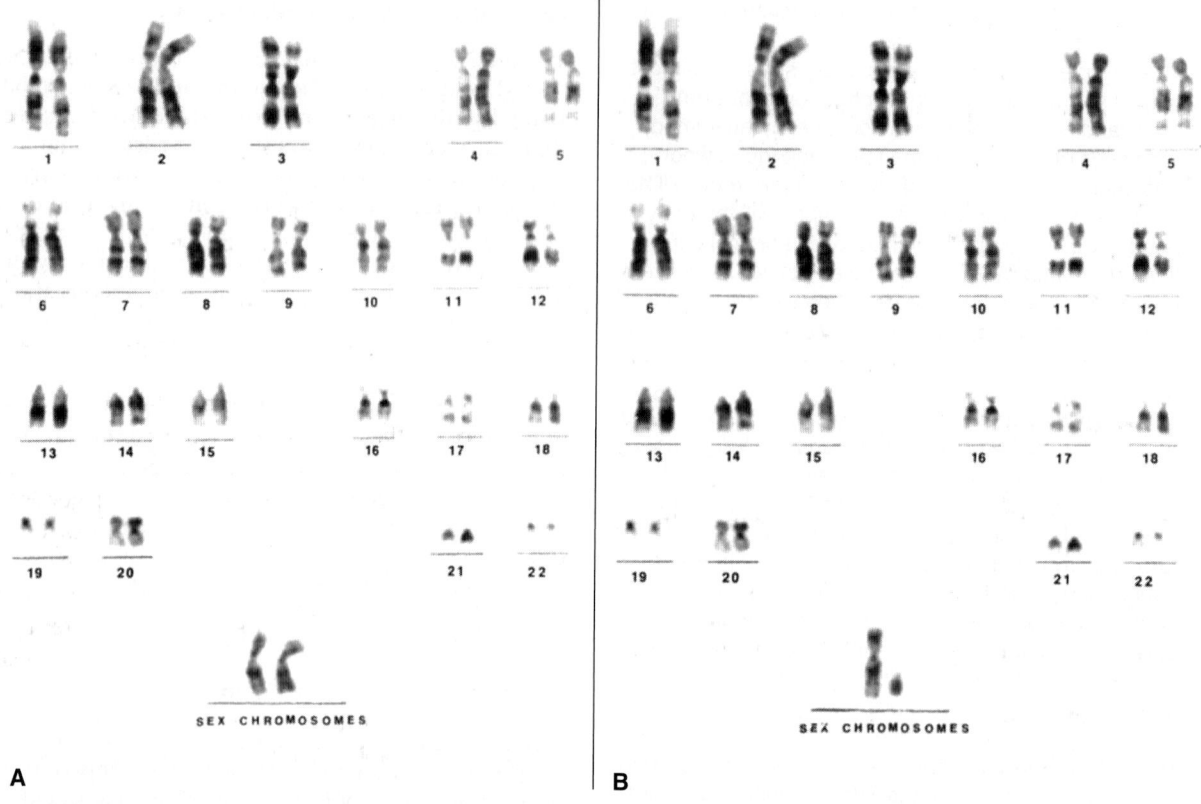

A   B

FIGURE 7.1 Photomicrographs of human chromosomes (karyotypes [photograph of chromosomes arranged in a standard classification]). If a blood sample is taken from a child or adult and the white blood cells are examined at the mitotic division phase of reproduction, transferred to slides, and photographed under high-power magnification, the individual chromosomes can be cut from the photograph and arranged according to size and shape. (**A**) Normal female karyotype. (**B**) Normal male karyotype.

chromosome 21, which is abbreviated as 47XX21+ or 47XY21+.

Mendelian Inheritance: Dominant and Recessive Patterns

The principles of genetic inheritance of disease are the same as those that govern genetic inheritance of other physical characteristics, such as eye or hair color. These principles were discovered and described by Gregor Mendel, an Austrian naturalist, in the 1800s, and they are known as mendelian laws.

A person who has two like genes for a trait—for blue eyes, for example (one from the mother and one from the father)—on two like chromosomes is said to be **homozygous** for that trait. If the genes differ (a gene for blue eyes from the mother and a gene for brown eyes from the father, or vice versa), the person is said to be **heterozygous** for that trait. Many genes are dominant in their action over others; that is, when paired with other genes, **dominant genes** are always expressed in preference to the other genes. A gene that is not dominant is **recessive.** For example, brown eye color is dominant over blue, so a person with a heterozygous pattern would appear to have brown eyes. An individual with two homozygous

genes for a dominant trait is said to be homozygous dominant; an individual with two genes for a recessive trait is homozygous recessive.

Mendelian laws permit the prediction of inheritance of traits, such as eye color, or the chance that a child born to parents with a certain genotype will be born with a disorder. Inheritance patterns for eye color or hair color provide a useful example of these principles. If the father is homozygous dominant (has two dominant genes for brown eye color) and the mother is homozygous recessive (has two genes for blue eye color), it can be predicted that their children have a 100% chance of being heterozygous for the trait (Fig. 7.2*A*); they will appear brown-eyed (the phenotype) but will carry a recessive gene for blue eyes (the genotype). If the father, however, is heterozygous (has one dominant gene and one recessive gene), a child born to this couple will have an equal chance of being brown-eyed or blue-eyed (Fig. 7.2*B*).

Suppose the mother is heterozygous instead of homozygous recessive and the father is homozygous dominant. When this pairing occurs, the chances are equal that their child will be homozygous dominant like the father or heterozygous like the mother. All the children's phenotypes will be brown eyes (Fig. 7.2*C*).

Suppose both parents are heterozygous. There is a 25% chance of their child's being homozygous recessive

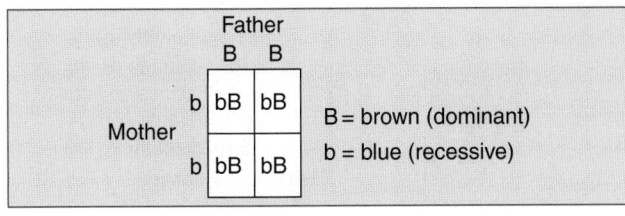

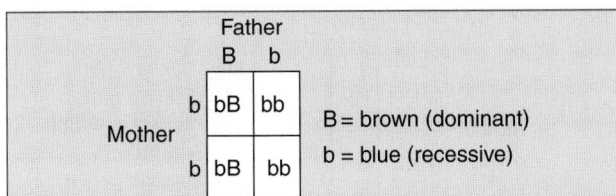

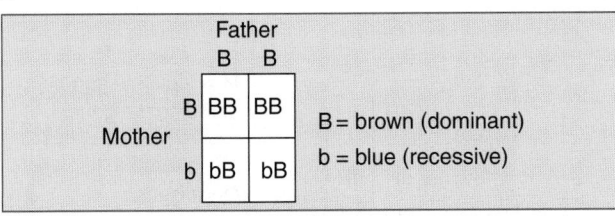

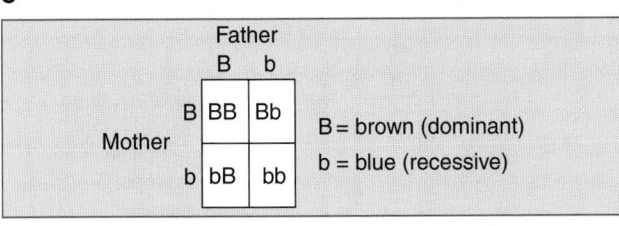

FIGURE 7.2 Possible inheritance of eye color.

(appearing blue-eyed), a 50% chance of being heterozygous (appearing brown-eyed), and a 25% chance of being homozygous dominant (appearing brown-eyed). This is how two brown-eyed parents can produce a blue-eyed child (Fig. 7.2D), and it confirms that it is impossible to predict a person's genotype from the phenotype, or outward appearance.

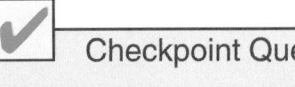 **Checkpoint Question 1**

Amy Alvarez is pregnant with her first child. Her phenotype refers to:

a. Her concept of herself as male or female.
b. Whether she has forty-six chromosomes or not.
c. Her actual genetic composition.
d. Her outward appearance.

Inheritance of Disease

Since the entire human genome has been mapped, an increasing number of types of disease inheritance have been identified.

Autosomal Dominant Disorders

Although more than 3,000 autosomal dominant disorders are known, only a few are commonly seen. Most of them cause structural defects. With an autosomal dominant condition, either a person has two unhealthy genes (homozygous dominant) or is heterozygous, with the gene causing the disease stronger than the corresponding healthy recessive gene for the same trait. Huntington disease is a progressive neurologic disorder that usually manifests symptoms between 35 and 45 years of age and is characterized by loss of motor control and intellectual deterioration. It an example of a heterozygous inherited autosomal dominant disorder. It is now possible to detect people who will develop this disorder by analyzing for a specific gene on chromosome 4. Unfortunately, there is no cure for Huntington disease, so potentially affected individuals must make a difficult choice in deciding to undergo the analysis when there is nothing but palliative care for this ultimately fatal disorder (Dawson et al., 2004).

Other examples of autosomal dominantly inherited disorders include facioscapulohumeral muscular dystrophy (a disorder that results in muscle weakness), a form of osteogenesis imperfecta (a disorder in which bones are exceedingly brittle), and Marfan syndrome (a disorder of connective tissue in which the child is thinner and taller than normal and may have associated heart defects). If a person who is heterozygous for an autosomal dominant trait such as facioscapulohumeral muscular dystrophy mates with a person who is free of the trait, as shown in Figure 7.3A, the chances are even (50%) that a child born to the couple would have the disorder or would be disease- and carrier-free (i.e., carrying no affected gene for the disorder).

Two heterozygous people with a dominantly inherited disorder are unlikely to choose each other as reproductive partners. If they do, however, their chances of having children free from the disorder decline (Fig. 7.3B): there would be only a 25% chance of a child's being disease- and carrier-free, a 50% chance that the child would have

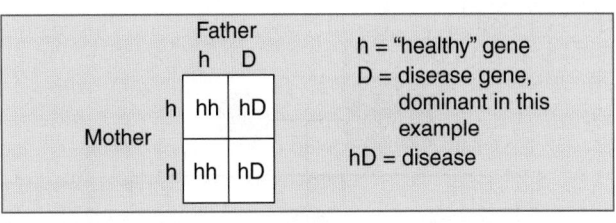

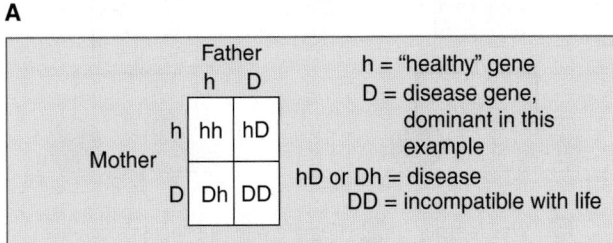

FIGURE 7.3 Autosomal dominant inheritance.

the disorder as both parents do, and a 25% chance that a child would be homozygous dominant (i.e., have two dominant disorder genes), a condition that probably would be incompatible with life.

In assessing family genograms (maps of family relationships) for the incidence of inherited disorders, a number of common findings are usually discovered when a dominantly inherited pattern is present in the family:

1. One of the parents of a child with the disorder also will have the disorder (a vertical transmission picture).
2. The sex of the affected individual is unimportant in terms of inheritance.
3. There is usually a history of the disorder in other family members.

Figure 7.4 shows a typical genogram of a family with an autosomal dominantly inherited disorder.

Autosomal Recessive Inheritance

More than 1,500 autosomal recessive disorders have been identified. In contrast to structural disorders, these tend to be biochemical or enzymatic. Such diseases do not occur unless two genes for the disease are present (i.e., a homozygous recessive pattern). Many inborn errors of metabolism are recessively inherited in this way. Examples include cystic fibrosis, adrenogenital syndrome, albinism, Tay-Sachs disease, galactosemia, phenylketonuria, limb-girdle muscular dystrophy, and Rh-factor incompatibility.

An example of autosomal recessive inheritance is shown in Figure 7.5A. Both parents are disease-free of cystic fibrosis, but both are heterozygous in genotype, so they carry a recessive gene for cystic fibrosis. When this occurs, there is a 25% chance that a child born to them will be disease- and carrier-free (homozygous dominant for the healthy gene); a 50% chance that the child will be, like the parents, free of disease but carrying the unexpressed disease gene (heterozygous); and a 25% chance that the child will have the disease (homozygous recessive).

Suppose a woman with the heterozygous genotype shown in Figure 7.5A mates with a man who has no trait for cystic fibrosis. There is a 50% chance that a child born

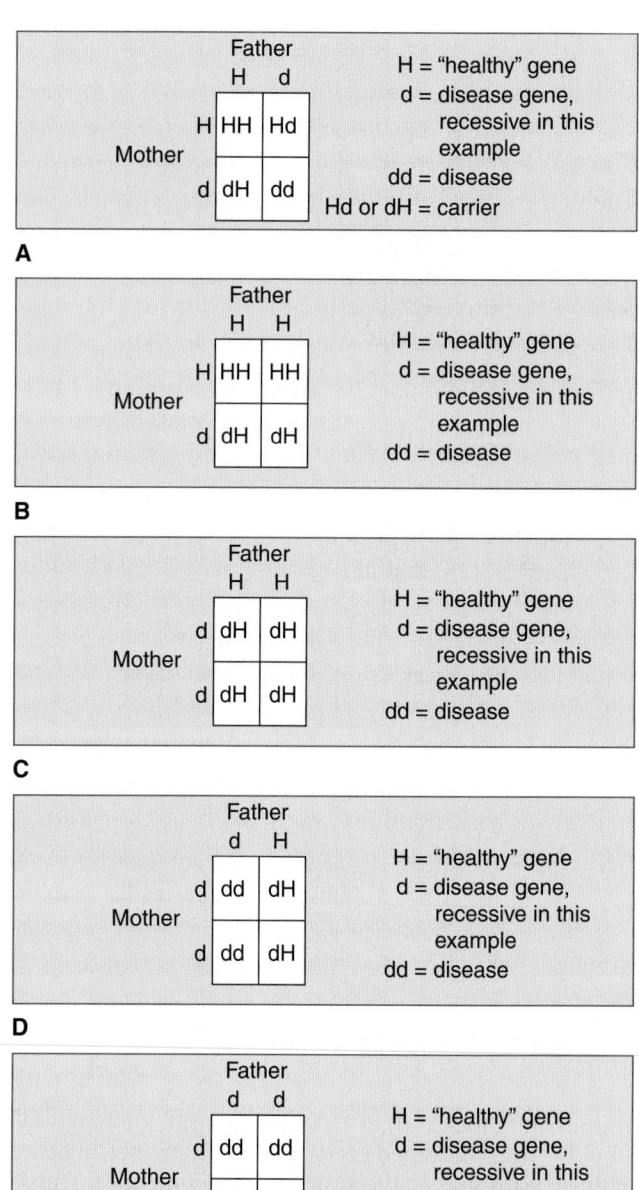

A

B

C

D

E

FIGURE 7.5 Autosomal recessive inheritance.

to them will be completely disorder- and carrier-free, like the father. Likewise, there is a 50% chance that their child will be heterozygous (i.e., a carrier), like the mother (see Fig. 7.5B). There is no chance in this case that any of their children will have the disorder. However, they should be aware that if a child of theirs who carries the trait eventually has children with a sexual partner who also has a recessive gene for the trait, the grandchildren may manifest the disease. Cystic fibrosis is caused by an errant gene on the seventh chromosome. As many as 1 in every 29 Caucasian people carries the trait. People who are concerned as to whether they have a recessive gene for the disorder can have a DNA analysis to reveal their status (Farrell & Farrell, 2003).

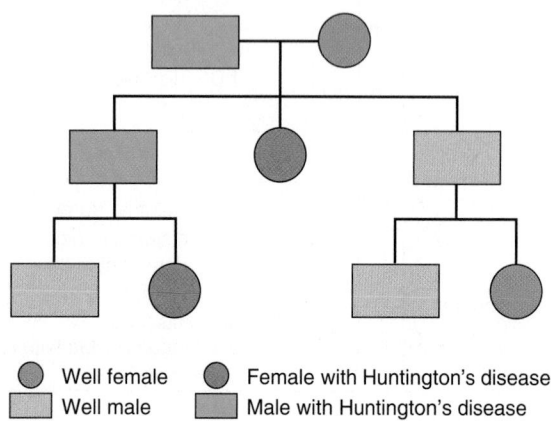

FIGURE 7.4 Family genogram: autosomal dominant inheritance.

Twenty years ago, most children with cystic fibrosis died in early childhood and therefore never reached child-bearing age. Today, with good management, such children can live to adulthood and have children of their own. If a person with cystic fibrosis (homozygous recessive) should choose a sexual partner without the trait, none of their children would have the disorder, but all would be carriers of a recessive gene for the disorder (see Fig. 7.5C).

If a person with cystic fibrosis mated with a person with an unexpressed gene for the disease, there would be a 50% chance that a child would have the disorder (homozygous) and a 50% chance that he or she would be heterozygous for the disorder (see Fig. 7.5D). If a person with the disorder mated with a person who also had the disorder, as shown in Figure 7.5E, there is a 100% chance that their child would have the disorder.

When family genograms are assessed for the incidence of inherited disease, situations commonly discovered when a recessively inherited disease is present in the family include the following:

1. Both parents of a child with the disorder are clinically free of the disorder.
2. The sex of the affected individual is unimportant in terms of inheritance.
3. The family history for the disorder is negative—that is, no one can identify anyone else who had it (a horizontal transmission pattern).
4. A known common ancestor between the parents sometimes exists. This explains how both male and female came to possess a like gene for the disorder.

Figure 7.6 shows a typical genogram of a family with an autosomal recessive inherited disorder.

X-Linked Dominant Inheritance

Some genes for disorders are located on, and therefore transmitted only by, the female sex chromosome (the X chromosome). There are about 300 known X-linked disorders, and their transmission is called X-linked inheritance. If the gene is dominant, only one X chromosome

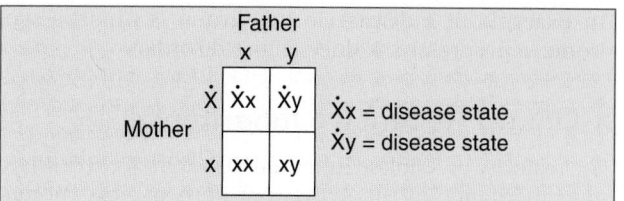

A

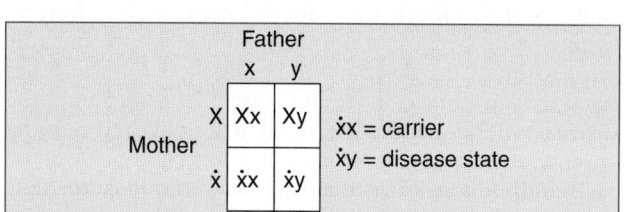

B

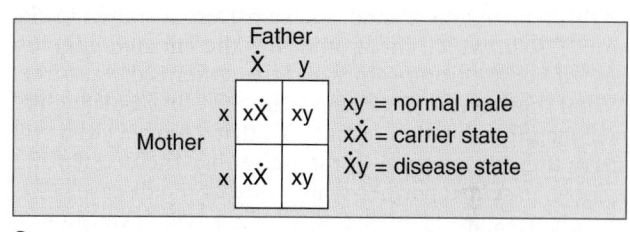

C

FIGURE 7.7 Sex-linked inheritance: (**A**) sex-linked dominant; (**B, C**) sex-linked recessive.

with the trait need be present for symptoms of the disorder to be manifested (Fig. 7.7A). Family characteristics seen with this type of inheritance include the following:

1. All individuals with the gene are affected.
2. All female children of affected men are affected; all male children of affected men are unaffected.
3. It appears in every generation.
4. All children of homozygous affected women are affected. Fifty percent of the children of heterozygous affected women are affected (Fig. 7.8).

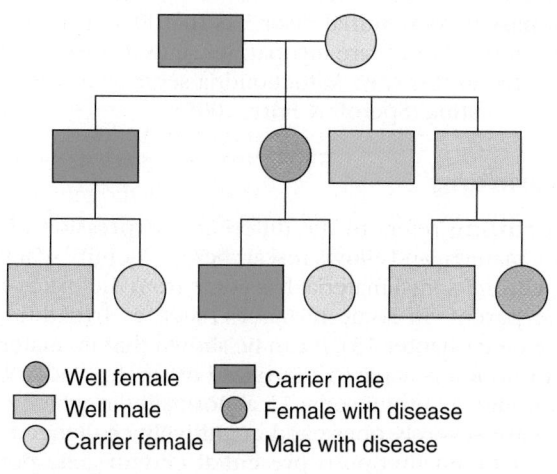

Legend:
- ○ Well female
- □ Well male
- ○ Carrier female
- ■ Carrier male
- ● Female with disease
- ▨ Male with disease

FIGURE 7.6 Family genogram: autosomal recessive inheritance.

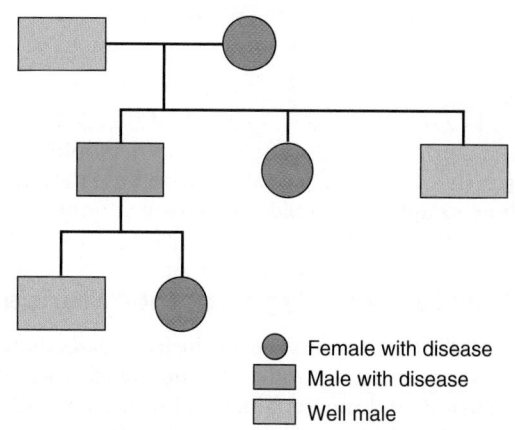

Legend:
- ● Female with disease
- ■ Male with disease
- ▨ Well male

FIGURE 7.8 Family genogram: X-linked dominant inheritance.

An example of a disease in this group is Alport's syndrome, a progressive kidney failure disorder.

X-Linked Recessive Inheritance

The majority of X-linked inherited disorders are recessive, and inheritance of the gene from both parents (homozygous recessive) is incompatible with life. Therefore, females who inherit the affected gene will be heterozygous, and, because a normal gene is also present, the expression of the disease will be blocked. On the other hand, because males have only one X chromosome, the disease will be manifested in any male children who receive the affected gene from their mother.

Hemophilia A, Christmas disease (a blood-factor deficiency), color blindness, Duchenne (pseudohypertrophic) muscular dystrophy, and fragile X syndrome are examples of this type of inheritance. Such a pattern is shown in Figure 7.7B, in which the mother has the affected gene on one of her X chromosomes and the father is disease-free. When this occurs, the chances are 50% that a male child will manifest the disease and 50% that a female child will carry the disease gene. If the father has the disease and chooses a sexual partner who is free of the disease gene, the chances are 100% that a daughter will have the sex-linked recessive gene, but there is no chance that a son will have the disease (see Fig. 7.7C).

When family genograms are assessed for inherited disorders, the following findings usually are apparent if an X-linked recessive inheritance disorder is present in the family:

1. Only males in the family will have the disorder.
2. A history of girls dying at birth for unknown reasons often exists (females who had the affected gene on both X chromosomes).
3. Sons of an affected man are unaffected.
4. The parents of affected children do not have the disorder.

Figure 7.9 shows a typical family genogram in which there is an X-linked recessive inheritance pattern.

Y-Linked Inheritance. Although genes responsible for features such as height and tooth size are found on the Y chromosome, no known disease genes are inherited by Y-chromosome transmission (Ward, 2003).

? *What if...* Amy Alvarez had a recessive X-linked chromosome disorder, such as hemophilia, and said that she wanted to have all boys because they would not show symptoms? Would she be well informed?

Multifactorial (Polygenic) Inheritance

Many childhood disorders such as heart disease, diabetes, pyloric stenosis, cleft lip and palate, neural tube disorders, hypertension, and mental illness tend to have a higher-than-usual incidence in some families. Diabetes is one example that has been studied closely. Certain human

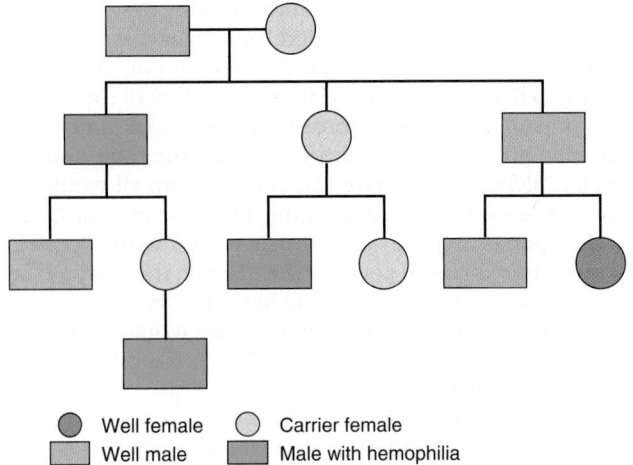

Well female   Carrier female
Well male   Male with hemophilia

FIGURE 7.9 Family genogram: X-linked recessive inheritance.

lymphocyte antigens (HLAs) inherited from both parents appear to play a role in genetic susceptibility to diabetes mellitus. Children who will develop diabetes mellitus can be shown to have an increased frequency of HLA B8, B15, DR3, and DR4 on chromosome 6. They lack DR2, an HLA that appears to be protective against diabetes mellitus.

Diseases caused by multiple factors do not follow the mendelian laws of inheritance, probably because more than a single gene or HLA is involved. Environmental influences may be instrumental in determining whether the disorder is expressed. It may be difficult for parents to understand these disorders because their occurrence is so unpredictable. A family history, for instance, may reveal no set pattern. Some of these conditions have a predisposition to occur more frequently in one sex (e.g., cleft palate occurs more often in girls), but they can occur in either sex.

Mitochondrial Inheritance. Mitochondria are cell organelles that are found outside the cell nucleus. They are inherited solely from the cytoplasm of the ovum. Male carriers cannot pass a disorder carried in the mitochondria to any of their children. Females, on the other hand, will pass mitochondrial disorders to 100% of their children. A number of rare myopathies (muscle diseases) are inherited in this way. Mitochondria serve as markers for genetic testing (Speroff & Fritz, 2005).

Imprinting

Imprinting refers to the differential expression of genetic material and allows researchers to identify whether the chromosomal material has come from the male or female parent. In some instances, such as hydatidiform mole (see Chapter 15), it can be shown that no maternal contribution is made to a fertilized ovum. In Prader-Willi syndrome, a chromosome 15 abnormality in which children are severely obese and cognitively challenged, no paternal contribution is present at certain gene points (Goldstone, 2004).

Chromosomal Abnormalities (Cytogenic Disorders)

In some instances of genetic disease, the abnormality occurs not because of dominant or recessive gene patterns but through a fault in the number or structure of chromosomes. When chromosomes are photographed and displayed, the result is termed a **karyotype.** Specific parts of chromosomes can be identified by karyotyping or by a process termed fluorescent in situ hybridization (FISH).

Nondisjunction Abnormalities

Meiosis is the type of cell division in which the number of chromosomes in the cell is reduced to the haploid (half) number for reproduction (i.e., 23 rather than 46 chromosomes). All sperm and ova undergo a meiosis cell division early in formation. During this division, half of the chromosomes are attracted to one pole of the cell and half to the other pole. The cell then divides cleanly, with 23 chromosomes in the first new cell and 23 chromosomes in the second new cell. Chromosomal abnormalities occur if the division is uneven (**nondisjunction**). The result may be that one new sperm cell or ovum has 24 chromosomes and the other has only 22 (Fig. 7.10). If a defective spermatozoon or ovum with 24 or 22 chromosomes fuses with a normal spermatozoon or ovum, the zygote (sperm and ovum combined) will have either 47 or 45 chromosomes, not the normal 46. The presence of 45 chromosomes does not appear to be compatible with life, and the

embryo or fetus probably will be aborted. Down syndrome (trisomy 21) (47XX21+ or 47XY21+) is an example of a disease in which the individual has 47 chromosomes. There are three rather than two copies of chromosome 21 (Fig. 7.11).

The incidence of Down syndrome increases with increasing maternal age and is highest if the mother is older than 35 years of age and the father is older than 55. Thus, aging seems to present an obstacle to clean cell division. The incidence is 1:100 in women older than 40 years of age, compared with 1:1,500 in women younger than 20 years (Ward, 2003). Other examples of cell nondisjunction include trisomy 13 (Fig. 7.12) and trisomy 18 (cognitive challenged syndromes).

If nondisjunction occurs in the sex chromosomes, other types of abnormalities occur. Turner and Klinefelter syndromes are the most common types. In Turner syndrome (45XO), which is marked by webbed neck, short stature, sterility, and possibly cognitive challenge, the individual, although female, has only one X chromosome (or has two X chromosomes but one is defective). She appears to be female (female phenotype) because of the one X chromosome. In Klinefelter syndrome (marked by sterility and possibly cognitive challenge), the individual has male genitals but the sex chromosomal pattern is 47XXY.

Deletion Abnormalities

Deletion abnormalities are a form of chromosome disorder in which part of a chromosome breaks during cell division,

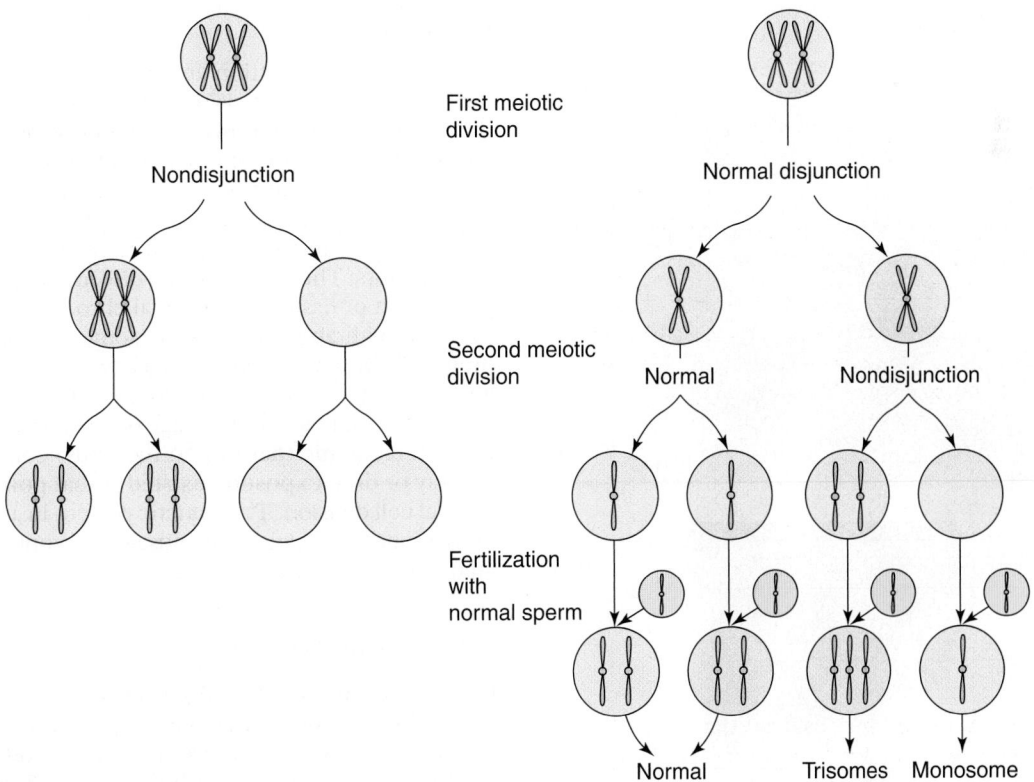

FIGURE 7.10 Process of nondisjunction at the first and second meiotic divisions of the ovum and fertilization with normal sperm.

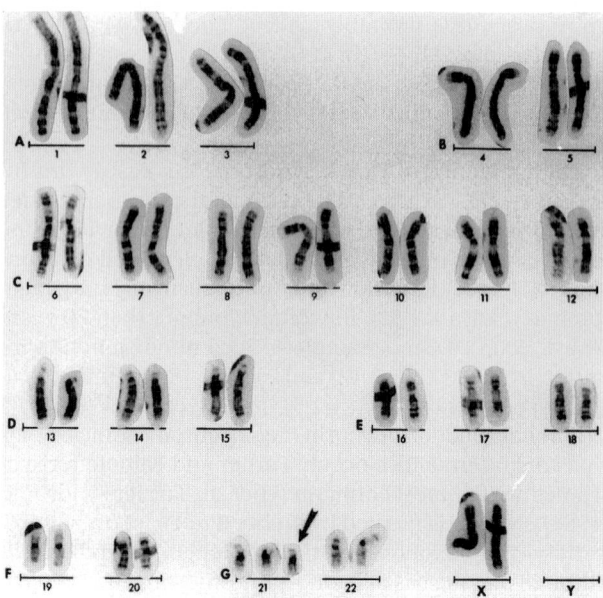

FIGURE 7.11 Karyotype of trisomy 21. (Courtesy of Dr. Kathleen Rao, Dept. of Ped., UNC.)

causing the affected person to have the normal number of chromosomes plus or minus an extra portion of a chromosome, such as 45.75 chromosomes or 47.5. For example, in cri-du-chat syndrome (46XY5q–), one portion of chromosome 5 is missing (see discussion later in this chapter).

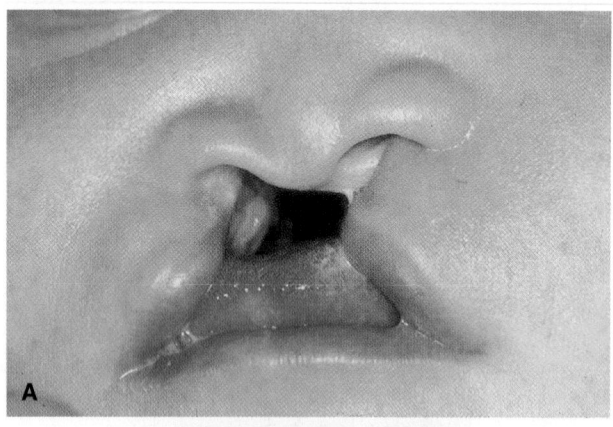

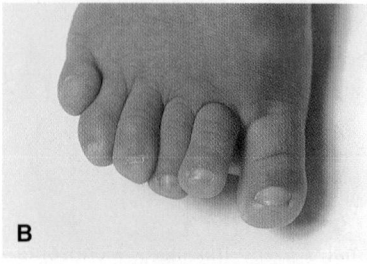

FIGURE 7.12 An infant with trisomy 13 has (**A**) a cleft palate and (**B**) supernumerary digits (polydactyly). (© NMSB/Custom Medical Stock Photo.)

Translocation Abnormalities

Translocation abnormalities are perplexing situations in which a child gains an additional chromosome through another route. A form of Down syndrome occurs as a translocation abnormality. In this instance, one parent of the child has the correct number of chromosomes (46), but chromosome 21 is misplaced; it is abnormally attached to another chromosome, such as chromosome 14. The parent's appearance and functioning are normal because the total chromosome count is a normal 46. He or she is termed a balanced translocation carrier (Pastva et al., 2004).

If, during meiosis, this abnormal chromosome 14 (carrying the extra 21 chromosome) and a normal chromosome 21 from the other parent are both included in one sperm or ovum, the resulting child will have a total of 47 chromosomes because of the extra number 21. Such a child is said to have an unbalanced translocation syndrome. The phenotype (appearance) of the child will be indistinguishable from that of a child with the form of Down syndrome that occurs from nondisjunction.

About 2% to 5% of children with Down syndrome have this type of chromosome pattern. It is important to identify parents who are translocation carriers, because their chance of having a child born with Down syndrome is higher than normal. If the father is the carrier, this risk is about 5%; if the mother is the carrier, the risk is about 15%. As many as 15% of couples who have frequent early spontaneous miscarriages may have this type of chromosomal aberration (Ward, 2003).

Mosaicism

Usually, a nondisjunction abnormality occurs during the meiosis stage of cell division, when sperm and ova halve their number of chromosomes. Mosaicism is an abnormal condition that is present when the nondisjunction disorder occurs after fertilization of the ovum, as the structure begins mitotic (daughter-cell) division. If this occurs, different cells in the body will have different chromosome counts. The extent of the disorder depends on the proportion of tissue with normal chromosome structure to tissue with abnormal chromosome constitution. Children with Down syndrome who have near-normal intelligence may have this type of pattern. The occurrence of such a phenomenon at this stage of development suggests that a teratogenic (harmful to the fetus) condition, such as x-ray or drug exposure, existed at that point to disturb normal cell division. This genetic pattern in a female with Down syndrome caused by mosaicism would be abbreviated as 46XX/47XX21+.

Isochromosomes

If a chromosome accidentally divides not by a vertical separation but by a horizontal one, a new chromosome with mismatched long and short arms can result. This is an isochromosome. It has much the same effect as a translocation abnormality when an entire extra chromosome exists. Some instances of Turner syndrome (45XO) may occur because of isochromosome formation.

Checkpoint Question 2

Amy Alvarez is a balanced translocation carrier for Down syndrome. This term means that:

a. All of her children will be born with some aspects of Down syndrome.

b. All of her female and none of her male children will have Down syndrome.

c. She has a greater than average chance a child will have Down syndrome.

d. It's impossible for any of her children to be born with Down syndrome.

GENETIC COUNSELING

Anyone concerned about the possibility of transmitting a disease to his or her children should have access to genetic counseling for advice on the inheritance of disease. Such counseling can serve the following purposes:

- Provide concrete, accurate information about inherited disorders
- Reassure people who are concerned that their child may inherit a particular disorder that the disorder will not occur
- Allow people who are affected by inherited disorders to make informed choices about future reproduction
- Educate people about inherited disorders and the process of inheritance
- Offer support by skilled health care professionals to people who are affected by genetic disorders

Genetic counseling may result in making individuals feel "well" or free of guilt for the first time in their lives. They may discover that the disorder they were worried about was not an inherited one but was rather a chance occurrence.

In other instances, counseling results in informing individuals that they are carriers of a trait that is responsible for a child's condition. Even when people understand that they have no control over this, knowledge about passing along a genetic disorder can cause guilt and self-blame. Marriages and relationships can suffer unless both partners are given adequate support.

It is essential that information revealed in genetic screening be kept confidential, because such information could be used to damage a person's reputation or harm a future career or relationship. This necessity to maintain confidentiality prevents health care providers from alerting other family members about the inherited characteristic unless the member requesting genetic assessment has given consent. In some instances, a genetic history reveals new information, such as that a child has been adopted or is the result of artificial insemination, or that a current husband is not the child's father. The member of the family seeking counseling has the right to decide whether this information may be shared with other family members.

The timing of genetic counseling is also important. The ideal time is before the first pregnancy. Some couples take this step before committing themselves to marriage, offering out of compassion for the partner not to involve him or her in a marriage commitment if children of the marriage would be subject to a serious inherited disorder. Other couples first become aware of a need for genetic counseling after the birth of a first child with a disorder. Couples who seek counseling after a first affected child is born need counseling before a second pregnancy occurs. They may not be ready for this, however, until the initial shock of their first child's condition and the grief reaction that may accompany it have run their course. Only then are they ready for information and decision making (Wallerstedt et al., 2003) (Box 7.2).

Even if a couple decides not to have any more children, it is important that they know that genetic counseling is available should their decision change. They also

BOX 7.2 FOCUS ON . . .

 FAMILY TEACHING

Genetic Screening

Q. Amy Alvarez is anxious to have her fetus' health confirmed. She asks you, "Why do I have to wait so late in pregnancy for genetic studies by amniocentesis?"

A. Genetic analysis is done on skin cells obtained from amniotic fluid. The test cannot be scheduled until enough amniotic fluid is present for analysis. Fortunately, this analysis now can be done as early as the 12th week of pregnancy.

Q. Why do laboratories take so long to return karyotyping results?

A. Karyotyping has traditionally (and by necessity) been done on cells at the metaphase (center phase) of division, so the laboratory has had to delay testing until the cells grow to reach this phase. New techniques

now allow analysis to be done immediately so that results are available much sooner.

Q. There are no inherited diseases that we know of in our family, but should my husband and I have a karyotype done "just to be sure" before we have our first baby?

A. A genetic analysis is not routinely recommended unless there is evidence or suspicion of genetic disease in the family. Remember that karyotyping reveals only diseases that are present on chromosomes. A "perfect" karyotype doesn't guarantee that a newborn will not be ill in a noninherited way.

Q. If chorionic villi are part of the placenta, how does testing them reveal the chromosome picture of the fetus?

A. Because the fetus and all accessory structures arise from the same single ovum and sperm, the placenta contains the same cells as the fetus.

should be aware that as their children reach reproductive age, they too may benefit from genetic counseling. Couples who are most apt to benefit from a referral for genetic testing or counseling include the following:

• *A couple who has a child with a congenital disorder or an inborn error of metabolism.* Many congenital disorders occur because of teratogenic invasion during pregnancy that has gone unrecognized. Learning that the abnormality occurred by chance rather than inheritance is important, because the couple will not have to spend the remainder of their childbearing years in fear that another child may be born with the disorder (although a chance circumstance could occur again). If a definite teratogenic agent, such as a drug the woman took during pregnancy, can be identified, the couple can be advised about preventing this occurrence in a future pregnancy.

• *A couple whose close relatives have a child with a genetic disorder, including a congenital disorder or inborn error of metabolism.* It is difficult to predict the expected occurrence of "familial" or multifactorial disorders. Therefore, counseling should be aimed at educating the couple about the disorder, available treatment, and the prognosis or outcome. Based on this information, the couple can make an informed reproductive choice.

• *Any individual who is a known balanced translocation carrier.* Understanding of his or her own chromosome structure and the process by which future children could be affected can help the individual make an informed choice about reproduction or can alert him or her to the importance of fetal karyotyping during any future pregnancy (Box 7.3).

• *Any individual who has an inborn error of metabolism or chromosomal disorder.* Any person with a

BOX 7.3 :   Focus on Nursing Care Planning

A Multidisciplinary Care Map for A Couple Concerned About Genetic Disorders in Future Offspring

•

Amy Alvarez is a woman you meet at a genetic counseling center. She was adopted as a newborn and never felt a need to locate her birth parents because her adoptive parents provided a "close to perfect" childhood for her. After college, she married the most eligible bachelor in her hometown. She is now pregnant with her first child. At 15 weeks into the pregnancy, she has been advised her child may have translocation Down syndrome. She asks you, "Why is this happening? There's no disease like this in either of our families."

Family Assessment
Client's family history is unknown because of adoption. Husband's family has no history of Down syndrome. Client is presently attending law school. Husband works as a county public defender. Family lives in condo by lake front. Finances rated as "good."

Client Assessment
Client's and husband's past medical histories show no evidence of major health problems. Pregnancy is at 15 weeks. Maternal serum alpha-fetoprotein showed decreased level; amniocentesis with karyotyping revealed fetal translocation.

Nursing Diagnosis
Health-seeking behaviors related to knowledge of possible genetic disorder inheritance

Outcome Criteria
Couple accurately states the cause of this genetic disorder; describes range of options open to them so any decision they make regarding the pregnancy is an informed one.

(continued)

Team Member Responsible	Assessment	Intervention	Rationale	Expected Outcome
History				
Nurse Practitioner/ Nurse	Obtain a detailed history and physical examination of the client and spouse, including information about each family member and other relatives.	Perform a physical examination to document current health.	A thorough history and physical examination provide baseline information to direct need for follow-up testing.	Couple participates fully in health examination, so family history obtained is as complete as possible.
Activities of Daily Living				
Nurse	Explore the meaning of genetic testing with the couple and ask how this will affect their everyday life.	Encourage couple to verbalize feelings and concerns. Allow time for questions and answers.	Exploration, verbalization, and active questioning provide a safe outlet for feelings, help to increase the other partner's awareness of needs, and open lines of communication.	Couple describes the effect on their life of needing genetic screening; asks questions as needed.
Consultations				
Physician/ Nurse	Assess whether couple would like to speak to an expert in the field of genetics to clarify their understanding.	Refer client to genetic counselor so she can be made aware of exact inheritance pattern and options available.	Couples cannot make informed choices without being aware of extent of problem.	Couple meets with genetic counselor within 1 week's time
Procedures/Medications				
Physician/ Nurse	Develop a family genogram for client and spouse.	Be certain couple receives written documentation of chromosome disorder to take to genetic counselor.	Good communication between health care providers helps to ensure a positive outcome. A family genogram may provide additional information about the client's and spouse's family histories.	Couple receives results of tests in a timely and appropriate manner. A family genogram is developed and maintained with health documentation.
Nutrition				
Dietitian/ Nurse	Assess the couple's nutrition patterns.	Analyze whether couple maintains healthy diet during testing and consultation period	A healthy diet during pregnancy is important if pregnancy will be continued.	Client confirms that she continues to take prenatal vitamins and adequate protein intake.
Patient/Family Education				
Nurse Practitioner/ Nurse	Ask couple if they have further questions about their particular inheritance pattern.	Review with the couple the mode of transmission and chances for manifesting Down syndrome in offspring.	Down syndrome may be inherited at a higher incidence in a balanced translocation carrier than in others.	Couple describes accurately the mode of transmission of Down syndrome.

(continued)

Team Member Responsible	Assessment	Intervention	Rationale	Expected Outcome
Spiritual/Psychosocial/Emotional Needs				
Nurse	Assess whether couple would be interested in learning some activities to reduce stress.	Instruct the couple in positive coping mechanisms. Include activities such as information sharing, relaxation and breathing exercises, and physical activity. Provide emotional support and guidance to the couple throughout testing.	Positive coping mechanisms assist in controlling fear and minimizing its intensity, thus promoting effective problem solving. Emotional support from a variety of sources helps to alleviate some of the stress and anxiety associated with genetic testing.	Couple demonstrates positive coping mechanisms. Couple states that the emotional support they received throughout their period of genetic screening and counseling was adequate.
Discharge Planning				
Social worker/ Nurse	Assess community for support organizations available.	Because the couple has chosen to continue pregnancy, refer them to national support group (Down Syndrome Foundation) and local parents support group.	Additional counseling and support may be necessary as pregnancy progresses or at birth of child. Use of community resources can provide additional support and help reduce feelings of isolation and loneliness.	Couple records the names and telephone numbers of support groups as well as the genetic counseling team and states they will keep numbers available if they should need further future information.

disease should know the inheritance pattern of the disease and, like those who are balanced translocation carriers, should be aware of prenatal diagnosis, if possible, for his or her particular disorder.

- *A consanguineous (closely related) couple.* The more closely related two people are, the more genes they have in common, so the more likely it is that a recessively inherited disease will be expressed. A brother and sister, for example, have about 50% of their genes in common; first cousins have about 12% of their genes in common.
- *Any woman older than 35 years of age and any man older than 45 years of age.* This is directly related to the association between advanced parental age and the occurrence of Down syndrome.
- *Couples of ethnic backgrounds in which specific illnesses are known to occur.* Mediterranean people, for example, have a high incidence of thalassemia, a blood disorder; those with a Chinese ancestry have a high incidence of another blood disorder, glucose-6-phosphate dehydrogenase (G6PD) deficiency (Box 7.4).

Nursing Responsibilities

Nurses play important roles in assessing for signs and symptoms of genetic disorders, in offering support to individuals who seek genetic counseling, and in helping with reproductive genetic testing procedures. Nurses can be instrumental in the following ways:

- Alerting a couple to what procedures they can expect to undergo

- Explaining how different genetic screening tests are done and when they are usually offered
- Supporting a couple during the wait for test results
- Assisting couples in values clarification, planning, and decision making based on test results

A great deal of time may need to be spent offering support for a grieving couple confronted with the reality of how tragically the laws of inheritance have affected their lives.

BOX 7.4 FOCUS ON . . .

DIVERSITY OF CARE

Certain genetic disorders are more commonly found in some ethnic groups than in others, because people often marry within their own racial or ethnic group. β-Thalassemia, for example, occurs most frequently in families of Greek or Italian heritage, whereas α-thalassemia occurs most often in persons from the Philippines or Southeast Asia. Sickle cell anemia occurs most often in African Americans. Tay-Sachs disease occurs most often in people of Jewish ancestry.

It is important that families who are at high risk for particular genetic disorders because of their ethnic heritage be informed of the incidence of these disorders and offered genetic screening as appropriate.

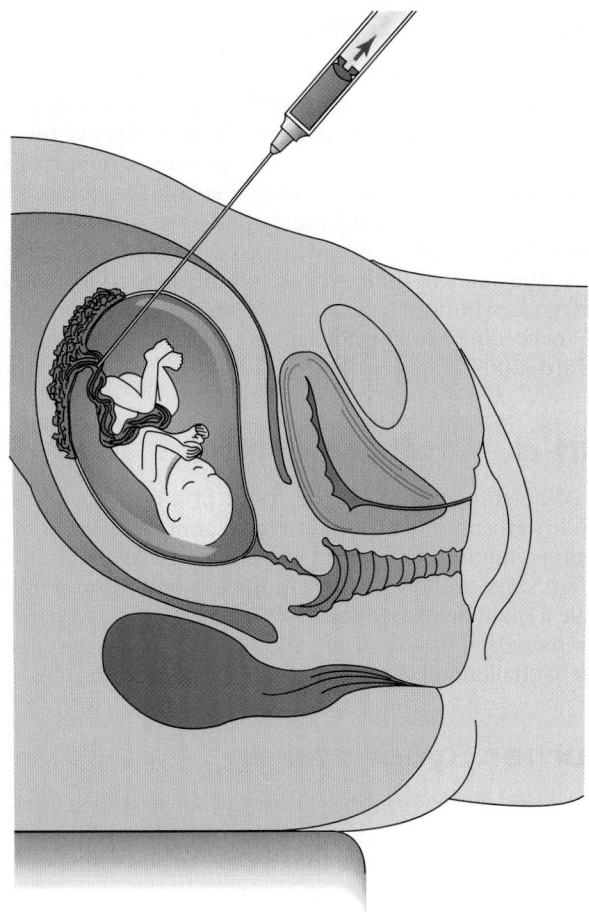

FIGURE 7.14 Percutaneous umbilical blood sampling. Blood is withdrawn from the cord using amniocentesis technique.

into the uterus and membranes to visually inspect the fetus for gross abnormalities. It can be used to confirm a sonography finding, to remove skin cells for DNA analysis, or to perform surgery for a congenital disorder such as a stenosed urethra.

Preimplantation Diagnosis. It may be possible in the future for a fertilized ovum to be removed from the uterus by lavage before implantation and biopsied for DNA analysis. The ovum would then be reinserted or not, depending on the findings and the parents' wishes. This would provide genetic information extremely early in a pregnancy. The technique is currently possible with in vitro fertilization procedures used in fertility treatment. This technique may also allow healthy genes to be inserted to correct underlying disorders very early in pregnancy (therapeutic cloning or stem cell transfer) (Hochedlinger & Jaenisch, 2003).

Reproductive Alternatives

Some couples are reluctant to seek genetic counseling because they are afraid they will be told it would be unwise to have children. Helping them to realize that viable alternatives for having a family exist for them allows them to seek the help they need.

Artificial insemination by donor (AID) is an option for couples if the genetic disorder is one inherited by the male partner or is a recessively inherited disorder carried by both partners. AID is available in all major communities and can permit the couple to experience the satisfaction and enjoyment of a normal pregnancy.

If the inherited problem is one arising from the female partner, surrogate embryo transfer is an assisted reproductive technique that is a possibility. An oocyte donated by a friend or relative or provided by an anonymous donor is fertilized by the husband's sperm in the laboratory and then implanted into the woman's uterus (Brinsden, 2003). Like AID, donor embryo transfer offers the couple a chance to experience a normal pregnancy.

Use of a surrogate mother (a woman who agrees to be artificially inseminated, typically by the male partner's sperm, and bear a child for the couple) is still another possibility (Jadva et al., 2003). All of these procedures are expensive and, depending on individual circumstances, may have disappointing success rates. Assisted reproductive techniques are discussed in more detail in Chapter 6.

Adoption is an alternative many couples find rewarding (see Chapters 2 and 6). Also, choosing to remain child-free should not be discounted as a viable option. Many couples who have every reason to think they would have normal children choose this alternative because they believe their existence is full and rewarding without the presence of children.

Diagnosis of a disorder during pregnancy with prompt treatment at birth to minimize the prognosis and outcome of the disorder is another route to explore. Termination of a pregnancy that reveals a chromosomal or metabolic abnormality is a final option.

Couples need support from health care personnel to decide on an alternative that is correct for them, not one that they sense a counselor feels would be best. They may need to consider the ethical philosophy or beliefs of other family members when making their decision, although ultimately they must do what they believe is best for them as a couple. A useful place to start counseling might be with values clarification, to be certain the couple understands what is most important to them.

Future Possibilities

Stem cell research is looking at the possibility that immature cells from a healthy embryo (stem cells) could be implanted into an embryo with a known abnormal genetic makeup, replacing the abnormal cells or righting the affected child's genetic composition (Hochedlinger & Jaenisch, 2003). Stem cell research is costly, however, and produces some ethical questions (e.g., what will be the source of donor oocytes for the new technology?).

Legal and Ethical Aspects of Genetic Screening and Counseling

Nurses can be instrumental in seeing that couples who seek genetic counseling receive results in a timely manner and with compassion about what their results may mean to future childbearing. It is important to keep in mind several legal responsibilities of genetic testing, counseling, and therapy, including the following:

- Participation by couples or individuals in genetic screening must be elective.
- People desiring genetic screening must sign an informed consent for the procedure.
- Results must be interpreted correctly yet provided to the individuals as quickly as possible.
- The results must not be withheld from the individuals and must be given only to those persons directly involved.
- After genetic counseling, persons must not be coerced to undergo procedures such as abortion or sterilization. Any procedure must be a free and individual decision.

Failure to heed these guidelines could result in charges of invasion of privacy, breach of confidentiality, or psychological injury caused by "labeling" someone or imparting unwarranted fear and worry about the significance of a disease or carrier state. All couples who seek counseling and are identified as being at risk for having a child with a genetic disorder must be informed of the risk and offered appropriate diagnostic procedures (e.g., amniocentesis). "Wrongful birth" lawsuits have been initiated against health care providers for not making this information available.

? *What if...* Amy Alvarez were pregnant with twins? One twin fetus is diagnosed as having Down syndrome, and the other is not. How would you counsel her if she wanted to abort the affected child, when the procedure also might endanger the child without the disorder?

COMMON CHROMOSOMAL DISORDERS RESULTING IN PHYSICAL OR COGNITIVE DEVELOPMENTAL DISORDERS

A number of chromosomal disorders, particularly nondisjunction disorders, are easily detected at birth on physical examination. Many of these disorders leave children cognitively challenged. Care of the child who is cognitively challenged is discussed in Chapter 54.

Trisomy 13 Syndrome

In trisomy 13 syndrome (Patau syndrome), the child has an extra chromosome 13 and is severely cognitively challenged. The incidence of the syndrome is low, approximately 0.45 per 1,000 live births. Midline body disorders such as cleft lip and palate, heart defects, particularly ventricular septal defects, and abnormal genitalia are present. Other common findings include microcephaly with abnormalities of the forebrain and forehead; eyes that are smaller than normal (microphthalmos) or absent; and low-set ears. Most of these children do not survive beyond early childhood (see Fig. 7.12).

Trisomy 18 Syndrome

Children with trisomy 18 syndrome have three copies of chromosome 18. They are severely cognitively challenged. The incidence is approximately 0.23 per 1,000 live births. These children tend to be small for gestational age at birth and have markedly low-set ears, a small jaw, congenital heart defects, and usually misshapen fingers and toes (the index finger tends to deviate or cross over other fingers). Also, the soles of their feet are often rounded instead of flat (rocker-bottom feet). As in trisomy 13 syndrome, most of these children do not survive beyond early infancy (Ward, 2003).

Cri-du-Chat Syndrome

Cri-du-chat syndrome is the result of a missing portion of chromosome 5. In addition to an abnormal cry, which sounds much more like the sound of a cat than a human infant's cry, children with cri-du-chat syndrome tend to have a small head, wide-set eyes, and a downward slant to the palpebral fissure of the eye. They are severely cognitively challenged (Sarimski, 2003).

Turner Syndrome

The child with Turner syndrome (gonadal dysgenesis; 45XO) has only one functional X chromosome. The child is short in stature. The hairline at the nape of the neck is low-set, and the neck may appear to be webbed and short. A newborn may have appreciable edema of the hands and feet and a number of congenital anomalies, most frequently coarctation (stricture) of the aorta and kidney disorders. The child has only streak (small and nonfunctional) gonads, so that, with the exception of pubic hair, secondary sex characteristics do not develop at puberty. Lack of ovarian function results in sterility. The incidence is approximately 1 per 10,000 live births (Parker et al., 2003).

Although children with Turner syndrome may be severely cognitively challenged, difficulties in this area are more commonly limited to learning disabilities. Socioemotional adjustment problems may accompany the syndrome as well because of the lack of fertility and if the nuchal folds are prominent.

Human growth hormone administration may help children with Turner syndrome to achieve additional height (Cave et al., 2005). If treatment with estrogen is begun at approximately 13 years of age, secondary sex characteristics will appear, and osteoporosis may be prevented (Box 7.6). If females continue taking estrogen for three out of every four weeks, they will have withdrawal bleeding that results in a menstrual flow. This flow, however, does not correct the problem of sterility. Gonadal tissue is scant and inadequate for ovulation because of the basic chromosomal aberration.

Klinefelter Syndrome

Infants with Klinefelter syndrome are males with an XXY chromosome pattern (47XXY). Characteristics of the syn-

BOX 7.6 FOCUS ON . . .

EVIDENCE-BASED PRACTICE

Should adolescents with Turner syndrome be prescribed estrogen replacement therapy?

This is an interesting question, because estrogen replacement therapy (ERT) is no longer recommended routinely for the average woman. To investigate whether the usual guidelines applied to women with Turner syndrome, researchers interviewed 50 women with Turner syndrome, 30 to 59 years of age. The findings revealed that 70% of these women were taking ERT. Others had never had it prescribed or didn't follow a routine conscientiously. Bone density scans revealed that women who took estrogen had significantly greater bone density than those women not taking the replacement estrogen. The main reason revealed for good adherence was education by a health care provider about the importance of adherence to help prevent osteoporosis.

This is an important study for nurses, because nurses are often the health care provider who is asked about the benefits or nonbenefits of ERT. It's important for the health of women with Turner syndrome to know they are an exception to usual guidelines.

Source: Hanton, L., et al. (2003). The importance of estrogen replacement in young women with Turner syndrome. *Journal of Women's Health, 12*(10), 971–977.

drome may not be noticeable at birth. At puberty, secondary sex characteristics do not develop; the child has small testes that produce ineffective sperm. Affected individuals tend to develop gynecomastia (increased breast size). The incidence is about 1 per 1,000 live births. Karyotyping can be used to reveal the additional X chromosome (Hall et al., 2003).

Fragile X Syndrome

Fragile X syndrome is an X-linked disorder in which one long arm of an X chromosome is defective. The incidence is about 1 in 1,000 live births. It is the most common cause of cognitive challenge in boys.

Before puberty, boys with fragile X syndrome typically may have maladaptive behaviors such as hyperactivity and autism. They are apt to have reduced intellectual functioning, with marked deficits in speech and arithmetic. They may be identified by the presence of a large head, a long face with a high forehead, a prominent lower jaw, and large protruding ears. Hyperextensive joints and cardiac disorders may also be present. After puberty, enlarged testicles may become evident. Affected individuals are fertile and can reproduce (Medved & Brockmeier, 2004).

Carrier females may show some evidence of the physical and cognitive characteristics. Although intellectual function from the syndrome cannot be improved, both folic acid and phenothiazine administration may improve symptoms of poor concentration and impulsivity.

Down Syndrome (Trisomy 21)

Trisomy 21, the most frequently occurring chromosomal abnormality, occurs in about 1 in 800 live births. It occurs most frequently in the pregnancies of women who are older than 35 years of age (the incidence is as high as 1 in 100 live births for these women). Paternal age (older than 55 years) may also contribute to the increased incidence in this age group.

The physical features of children with Down syndrome are so marked that fetal diagnosis is possible by sonography in utero. The nose is broad and flat. The eyelids have an extra fold of tissue at the inner canthus (an epicanthal fold), and the palpebral fissure (opening between the eyelids) tends to slant laterally upward. The iris of the eye may have white specks in it, called Brushfield spots. Even in the newborn, the tongue may protrude from the mouth because the oral cavity is smaller than normal. The back of the head is flat, the neck is short, and an extra pad of fat at the base of the head causes the skin to be so loose it can be lifted up (like a puppy's skin). The ears may be low-set. Muscle tone is poor, giving the baby a rag-doll appearance. This can be so lax that the child's toe can be touched against the nose (not possible in the average mature newborn). The fingers of many children with Down syndrome are short and thick, and the little finger is often curved inward. There may be a wide space between the first and second toes and between the first and second fingers. The palm of the hand shows a peculiar crease (a simian line), which is a single horizontal palm crease rather than the normal three creases in the palm (Fig. 7.15).

Children with Down syndrome usually are cognitively challenged to some degree. The challenge can range from that of an educable child (intelligence quotient [IQ] of 50 to 70) to one who is profoundly affected (IQ less than 20). The extent of the cognitive challenge is not evident at birth. Educable children may represent mosaic chromosomal patterns. The fact that the brain is not developing well is evidenced by a head size that is usually smaller than the 10th or 20th percentile at well-child visits.

These children also appear to have altered immune function and are prone to upper respiratory tract infections. Congenital heart disease, especially atrioventricular defects, is common. Stenosis or atresia of the duodenum, strabismus, and cataract disorders are also common. For unknown reasons, acute lymphocytic leukemia occurs approximately 20 times more frequently in children with Down syndrome than in the general population. Even if children are born without an accompanying disorder such as heart disease, their lifespan usually is only 50 to 60 years, because aging seems to occur faster than normal (Benke, 2004).

Children with Down syndrome need to be exposed to early educational and play opportunities (see Chapter 54).

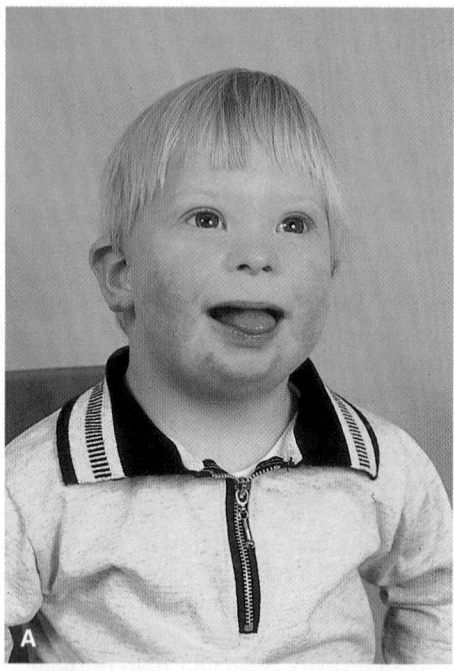

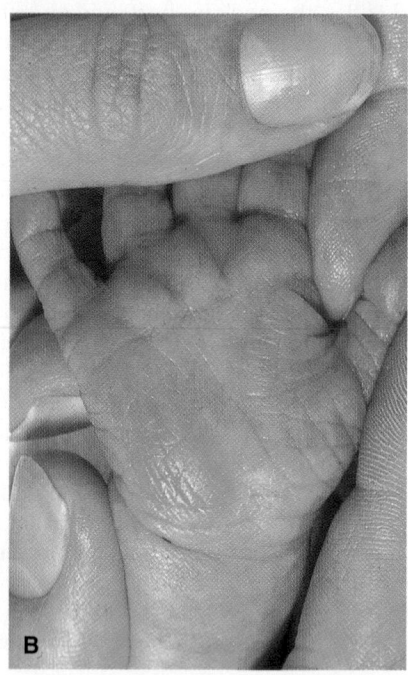

FIGURE 7.15 **(A)** Typical facial features of the child with Down syndrome. (© Barbara Proud.) **(B)** A simian line, a horizontal crease seen in children with Down syndrome. (SPL/Custom Medical Stock Photo.)

Checkpoint Question 4

Amy Alvarez's child is born with Down syndrome. What is a common physical feature of newborns with this disorder?

a. Spastic and stiff muscles
b. Loose skin at back of neck
c. A white lock of forehead hair
d. Wrinkles on the soles of the feet

Key Points

Genetic disorders are disorders resulting from a defect in the structure or number of genes or chromosomes. Genetics is the study of how and why such disorders occur.

A phenotype is a person's outward appearance. Genotype refers to the actual gene composition. A person's genome is the complete set of genes present. A karyotype is a graphic representation of the chromosomes that are present.

A person is homozygous if he or she has two like genes for a trait and heterozygous if he or she has two unlike genes for a trait.

Mendelian laws can predict the likely incidence of recessive or dominant diseases in offspring. Division disorders, including nondisjunction abnormalities, deletion, translocation, and mosaicism, also create genetic disorders.

Genetic counseling can be a role for nurses if they receive proper preparation and education. Assessment of genetic disorders consists of a health history, physical examination, and diagnostic studies such as CVS, amniocentesis, and MSAFP analysis.

Some karyotyping tests, such as CVS and amniocentesis, introduce a risk of spontaneous or threatened miscarriage. Be certain that women undergoing these tests remain in the health care facility for at least 30 minutes after the procedure to be sure that a complication such as vaginal bleeding, uterine cramping, or abnormal fetal heart rate is not present. Women with an Rh-negative blood type need Rh immune globulin administration after these procedures.

An important aspect of genetic counseling is respecting a couple's right to privacy. Be certain that information remains confidential and is not given indiscriminately to others, including other family members.

People who are told that a genetic abnormality does exist in their family may suffer a loss of self-esteem. Offering support to help them deal with

Because they are prone to infections, sensible precautions such as using good handwashing technique are important when caring for them. The enlarged tongue may interfere with swallowing and cause choking unless the child is fed slowly. As with all newborns, these infants need physical examination at birth to enable detection of the genetic disorder and initiation of parental counseling and support.

TABLE 8.1

Terms Used to Denote Fetal Growth

Name	Time Period
Ovum	From ovulation to fertilization
Zygote	From fertilization to implantation
Embryo	From implantation to 5–8 weeks
Fetus	From 5–8 weeks until term
Conceptus	Developing embryo or fetus and placental structures throughout pregnancy

fully developed fetus ready to be born. Table 8.1 lists common terms used to describe the fetus at various stages in this growth.

Fetal growth and development is typically divided into three periods: pre-embryonic (first 2 weeks, beginning with fertilization), embryonic (weeks 3 through 8), and fetal (from week 8 through birth).

Fertilization: The Beginning of Pregnancy

Fertilization (also referred to as conception, impregnation, or fecundation) is the union of an ovum and a spermatozoon. This usually occurs in the outer third of a fallopian tube, the ampullar portion (Speroff & Fritz, 2005).

Usually only one ovum reaches maturity each month. Once it is released, fertilization must occur fairly quickly because an ovum is capable of fertilization for only 24 hours (48 hours at the most). After that time, it atrophies and becomes nonfunctional. Because the functional life of a spermatozoon is about 48 hours, possibly as long as 72 hours, the total critical time span during which sexual relations must occur for fertilization to be successful is about 72 hours (48 hours before ovulation plus 24 hours afterward).

As the ovum is extruded from the graafian follicle of an ovary with ovulation, it is surrounded by a ring of mucopolysaccharide fluid (the zona pellucida) and a circle of cells (the corona radiata). The ovum and these surrounding cells (which increase the bulk of the ovum and serve as protective buffers against injury) are propelled into a nearby fallopian tube by currents initiated by the fimbriae—the fine, hairlike structures that line the openings of the fallopian tubes. A combination of peristaltic action of the tube and movements of the tube cilia help propel the ovum along the length of the tube.

Normally, an ejaculation of semen averages 2.5 mL of fluid containing 50 to 200 million spermatozoa per milliliter, or an average of 400 million sperm per ejaculation. At the time of ovulation, there is a reduction in the viscosity (thickness) of the cervical mucus, which makes it easier for spermatozoa to penetrate it. Sperm transport is so efficient close to ovulation that spermatozoa deposited in the vagina during intercourse generally reach the cervix within 80 seconds and the outer end of a fallopian tube within 5 minutes after deposition. This is one reason why douching is not an effective contraceptive measure.

Spermatozoa move by means of their flagella (tails) and uterine contractions through the cervix and the body of the uterus and into the fallopian tubes, toward the waiting ovum. The mechanism whereby spermatozoa are drawn toward an ovum is probably a species-specific reaction, similar to an antibody–antigen reaction. Capacitation is a final process that sperm must undergo to be ready for fertilization. This process, which happens as the sperm move toward the ovum, consists of changes in the plasma membrane of the sperm head, which reveal the sperm-binding receptor sites.

All of the spermatozoa that achieve capacitation reach the ovum and cluster around the protective layer of corona cells. Hyaluronidase (a proteolytic enzyme) is apparently released by the spermatozoa and acts to dissolve the layer of cells protecting the ovum. It is believed that one reason an ejaculation contains large numbers of sperm is to provide enough enzymes to dissolve the corona cells. Under ordinary circumstances, only one spermatozoon is able to penetrate the cell membrane of the ovum. Once it penetrates the cell, the cell membrane changes composition to become impervious to other spermatozoa. An exception to this is the formation of hydatidiform mole, in which multiple sperm enter; this leads to abnormal growth (see Chapter 15).

Immediately after penetration of the ovum, the chromosomal material of the ovum and spermatozoon fuse. The resulting structure is called a **zygote.** Because the spermatozoon and ovum each carried 23 chromosomes (22 autosomes and 1 sex chromosome), the fertilized ovum has 46 chromosomes. If an X-carrying spermatozoon entered the ovum, the resulting child will have two X chromosomes and will be female (XX). If a Y-carrying spermatozoon fertilized the ovum, the resulting child will have an X and a Y chromosome and will be male (XY).

Fertilization is never a certain occurrence, because it depends on at least three separate factors: equal maturation of both sperm and ovum, the ability of the sperm to reach the ovum, and the ability of the sperm to penetrate the zona pellucida and cell membrane and achieve fertilization.

From the fertilized ovum (zygote), the future child and also the accessory structures needed for support during intrauterine life (e.g., placenta, fetal membranes, amniotic fluid, umbilical cord) are all formed.

 Checkpoint Question 1

Liz Calhorn asks how much longer her doctor will refer to the baby inside her as an embryo. What would be your best explanation?

a. This term is used during the time before fertilization.
b. Her baby will be a fetus as soon as the placenta forms.
c. After the 20th week of pregnancy, the baby is called a zygote.
d. From the time of implantation until 5 to 8 weeks, the baby is an embryo.

Implantation

Once fertilization is complete, the zygote migrates over the next 3 to 4 days toward the body of the uterus, aided by the currents initiated by the muscular contractions of the fallopian tubes. During this time, mitotic cell division, or cleavage, begins. The first cleavage occurs at about 24 hours; cleavage divisions continue to occur at a rate of one about every 22 hours. By the time the zygote reaches the body of the uterus, it consists of 16 to 50 cells. At this stage, because of its bumpy outward appearance, it is termed a **morula** (from the Latin word *morus,* meaning mulberry).

The morula continues to multiply as it floats free in the uterine cavity for 3 or 4 more days. Large cells tend to collect at the periphery of the ball, leaving a fluid space surrounding an inner cell mass. At this stage, the structure is termed a **blastocyst.** It is this structure that attaches to the uterine endometrium. The cells in the outer ring are known as **trophoblast** cells. They are the part of the structure that will later form the placenta and membranes. The inner cell mass (embryoblast cells) is the portion of the structure that will form the embryo.

Implantation, or contact between the growing structure and the uterine endometrium, occurs approximately 8 to 10 days after fertilization. After the 3rd or 4th day of free floating (about 8 days since ovulation), the last residues of the corona and zona pellucida are shed by the growing structure. The blastocyst brushes against the rich uterine endometrium (in the second [secretory] phase of the menstrual cycle), a process termed apposition. It attaches to the surface of the endometrium (adhesion) and settles down into its soft folds (invasion). Stages to this point are depicted in Figure 8.1.

The blastocyst is able to invade the endometrium because, as the trophoblast cells on the outside of the structure touch the endometrium, they produce proteolytic enzymes that dissolve the tissue they touch. This action allows the blastocyst to burrow deeply into the endometrium and receive some basic nourishment of glycogen and mucoprotein from the endometrial glands. As invasion continues, the structure establishes an effective communication network with the blood system of the endometrium. The touching or implantation point is usually high in the uterus, on the posterior surface. If the point of implantation is low in the uterus, the growing placenta may occlude the cervix and make birth of the child difficult (placenta previa).

Implantation is an important step in pregnancy, because as many as 50% of zygotes never achieve it. In these instances, the pregnancy ends as early as 8 to 10 days after conception, often before the woman is even aware it had begun. Occasionally, a small amount of vaginal spotting appears with implantation, because capillaries are ruptured by the implanting trophoblast cells. A woman who normally has a particularly scant menstrual flow may mistake implantation bleeding for her menstrual period. If this happens, the predicted date of birth of her baby (based on the time of her last menstrual period) will be calculated 4 weeks late. Once implanted, the zygote is an **embryo.**

EMBRYONIC AND FETAL STRUCTURES

The Decidua

After fertilization, the corpus luteum in the ovary continues to function rather than atrophying, because of the influence

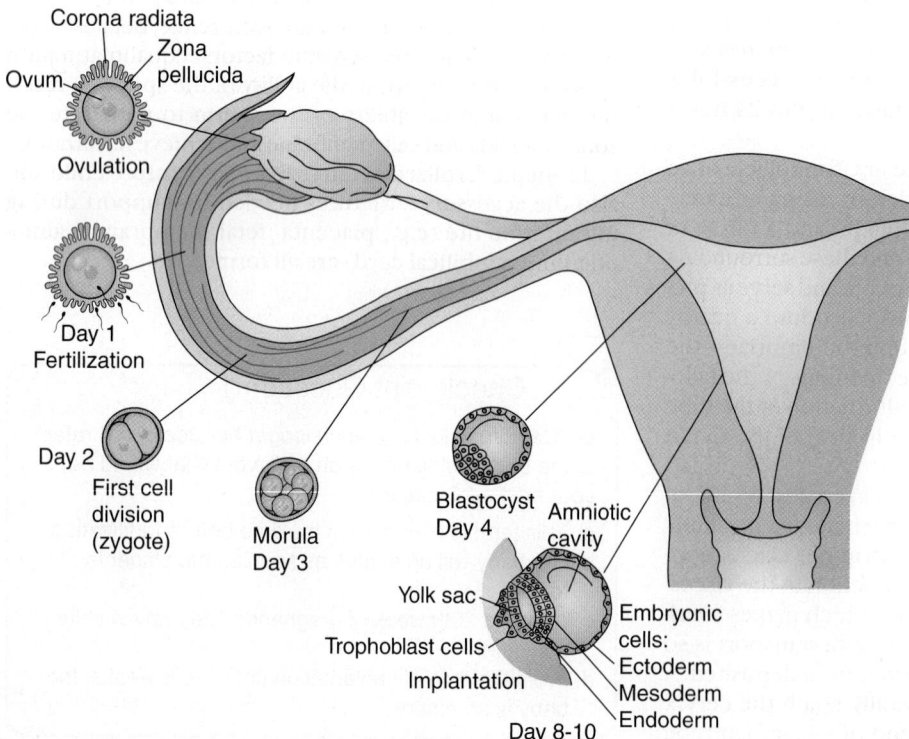

FIGURE 8.1 Schema of ovulation, fertilization, and implantation. At the time of implantation, the blastocyst is already differentiated into germ layers (ectoderm, mesoderm, and endoderm). Cells at the periphery of the structure are trophoblast cells that mature into the placenta.

of human chorionic gonadotropin (hCG), a hormone secreted by the trophoblast cells. The uterine endometrium, instead of sloughing off as in a normal menstrual cycle, continues to grow in thickness and vascularity. The endometrium is now termed the **decidua** (the Latin word for falling off), because it will be discarded after the birth of the child. The decidua has three separate areas (Fig. 8.2):

1. Decidua basalis, the part of the endometrium that lies directly under the embryo (or the portion where the trophoblast cells are establishing communication with maternal blood vessels)
2. Decidua capsularis, the portion of the endometrium that stretches or encapsulates the surface of the trophoblast
3. Decidua vera, the remaining portion of the uterine lining

As the embryo continues to grow, it pushes the decidua capsularis before it like a blanket. Eventually, enlargement brings the structure into contact with the opposite uterine wall. Here, the decidua capsularis fuses with the endometrium of the opposite wall. This is why at birth, the entire inner surface of the uterus is stripped away, leaving the organ highly susceptible to hemorrhage and infection.

Chorionic Villi

Once implantation is achieved, the trophoblastic layer of cells of the blastocyst begins to mature rapidly. As early as the 11th or 12th day, miniature villi, or probing "fingers," termed **chorionic villi,** reach out from the single layer of cells into the uterine endometrium. At term, almost 200 such villi will have formed.

Chorionic villi have a central core of loose connective tissue surrounded by a double layer of trophoblast cells. The central core of connective tissue contains fetal capillaries. The outer of the two covering layers is termed the

syncytiotrophoblast, or the syncytial layer. This layer of cells is instrumental in the production of various placental hormones, such as hCG, somatomammotropin (human placental lactogen [hPL]), estrogen, and progesterone. The inner layer, known as the cytotrophoblast or Langhans' layer, is present as early as 12 days' gestation. It appears to function early in pregnancy to protect the growing embryo and fetus from certain infectious organisms such as the spirochete of syphilis. However, this layer of cells disappears between the 20th and 24th week. This is why syphilis is considered to have a high potential for fetal damage late in pregnancy, when cytotrophoblast cells are no longer present. The layer appears to offer little protection against viral invasion at any point.

The Placenta

The placenta (Latin for pancake, which is descriptive of its size and appearance at term), arises out of trophoblast tissue. It serves as the fetal lungs, kidneys, and gastrointestinal tract and as a separate endocrine organ throughout pregnancy. Its growth parallels that of the fetus, growing from a few identifiable cells at the beginning of pregnancy to an organ 15 to 20 cm in diameter and 2 to 3 cm in depth at term. It covers about half the surface area of the internal uterus.

Circulation

Placental circulation is depicted in Figure 8.3. As early as the 12th day of pregnancy, maternal blood begins to collect in the intervillous spaces of the uterine endometrium surrounding the chorionic villi. By the 3rd week, oxygen and other nutrients, such as glucose, amino acids, fatty acids, minerals, vitamins, and water, diffuse from the maternal blood through the cell layers of the chorionic villi to the villi capillaries. From there, nutrients are transported back to the developing embryo.

For practical purposes, there is no direct exchange of blood between the embryo and the mother during pregnancy. The exchange is carried out only by selective osmosis through the chorionic villi. However, because the chorionic villi layer is only one cell thick, minute breaks do allow occasional fetal cells to cross, as well as enzymes such as alpha-fetoprotein from the fetal liver. Placental osmosis is so effective that all but a few substances are able to cross from the mother into the fetus. Because almost all drugs are able to cross into the fetal circulation, it is important that a woman take no nonessential drugs (including alcohol and nicotine) during pregnancy (Yankowitz, 2003). Alcohol perfuses across the placenta so well that pregnant women are advised to drink no alcohol at all during pregnancy (Galan & Hobbins, 2003). The specific mechanisms that allow nutrients to cross the placenta are shown in Table 8.2. All of these processes are affected by maternal blood pressure and the pH of the fetal and maternal plasma. Specific transport of substances and their effects on the fetus are discussed in Chapter 11.

As the number of chorionic villi increases with pregnancy, the villi form an increasingly complex communication network with the maternal blood. Intervillous spaces grow larger and larger, becoming separated by a series of

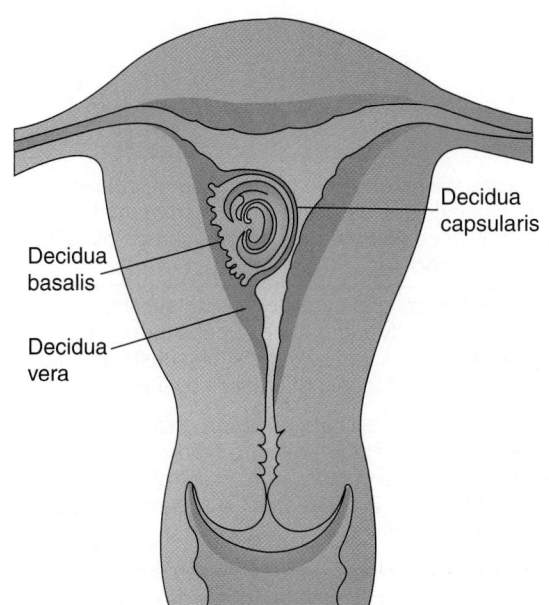

FIGURE 8.2 Division of uterine decidua into three areas.

Decidua capsularis

Decidua basalis

Decidua vera

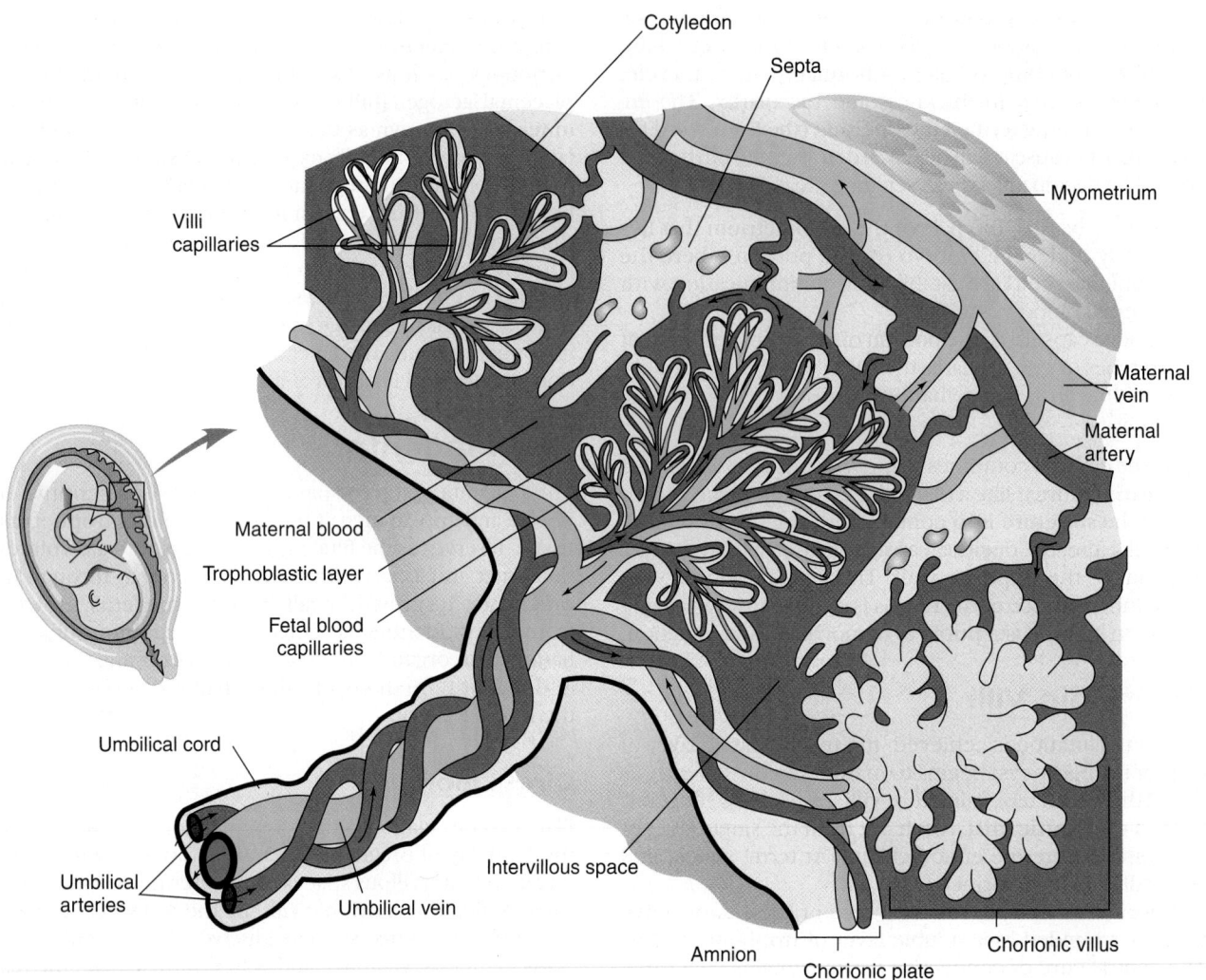

FIGURE 8.3 Placental circulation.

TABLE 8.2

Mechanisms by Which Nutrients Cross the Placenta

Mechanism	Description
Diffusion	When there is a greater concentration of a substance on one side of a semipermeable membrane than on the other, substances of correct molecular weight cross the membrane from the area of higher concentration to the area of lower concentration. Oxygen, carbon dioxide, sodium, and chloride cross the placenta by this method.
Facilitated diffusion	To ensure that the fetus receives enough concentrations of necessary growth substances, some substances cross the placenta more rapidly or more easily without the expenditure of energy than would occur if only simple diffusion were operating. A carrier moves the substance into and through the membrane. Glucose is an example of a substance that crosses by this process.
Active transport	This process requires energy and action of an enzyme to facilitate transport. Essential amino acids and water-soluble vitamins cross the placenta against the pressure gradient or from an area of lower molecular concentration to an area of greater molecular concentration. Amino acid concentrations in the fetal plasma are twice what they are in the mother, a situation that must occur to provide building substances for active fetal growth.
Pinocytosis	Absorption by the cellular membrane of microdroplets of plasma and dissolved substances. Gamma globulin, lipoproteins, phospholipids, and other molecular structures that are too large for diffusion and that cannot participate in active transport cross in this manner. Unfortunately, viruses that then infect the fetus can also cross in this manner.

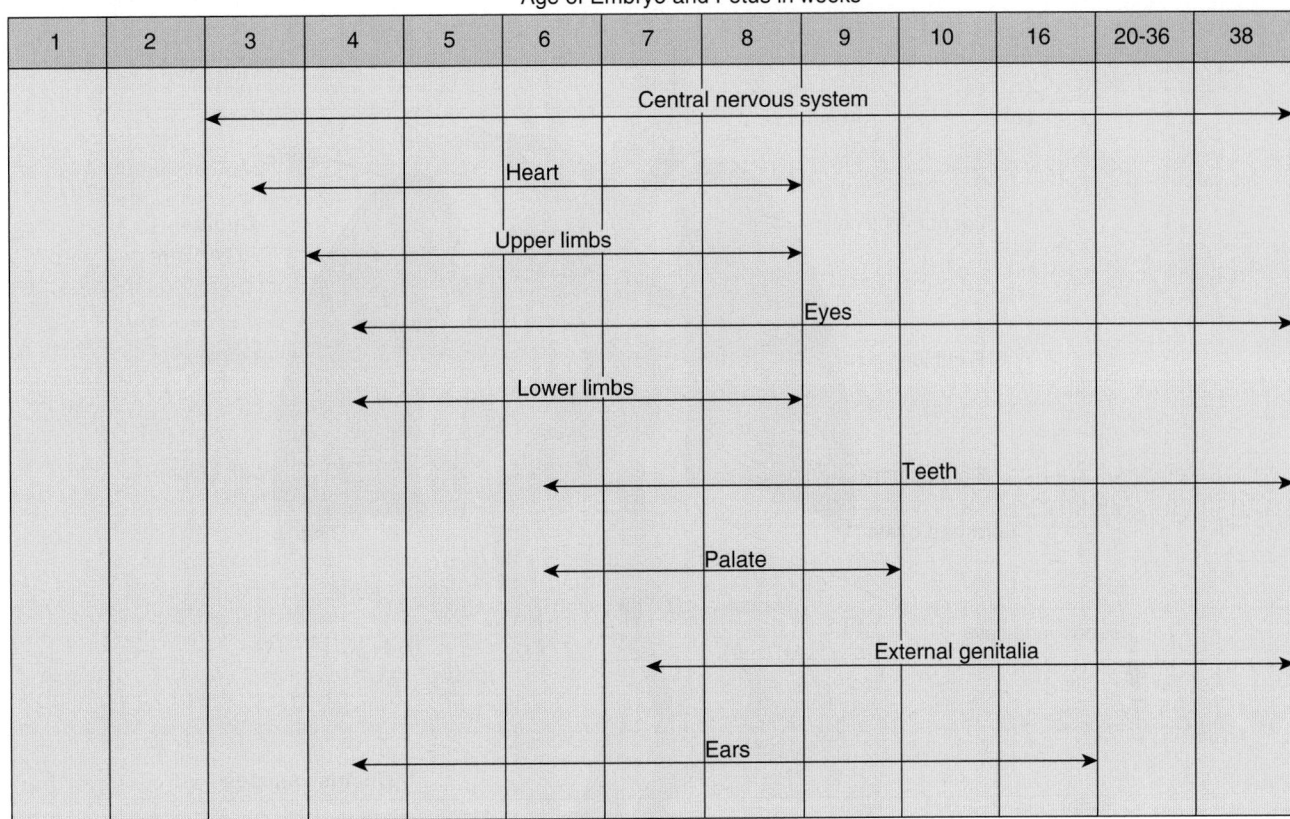

Age of Embryo and Fetus in weeks

FIGURE 8.5 Critical periods of fetal growth.

The blood oxygen saturation level of the fetus is about 80% of a newborn's saturation level. The rapid fetal heart rate during pregnancy (120 to 160 beats per minute) is necessary to supply oxygen to cells, because the red blood cells are never fully saturated. Despite a low blood oxygen saturation level, carbon dioxide does not accumulate in the fetal system because it rapidly diffuses into maternal blood across a favorable placental pressure gradient.

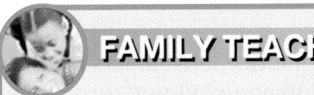

BOX 8.2 FOCUS ON . . .

FAMILY TEACHING

Teratogens at Work

Q. Liz Calhom tells you, "I have to work. How can I guard against fetal teratogens at work?"

A. Here are a number of helpful tips:

• Ask your employer for a statement on hazardous substances at your work site; discuss your need to avoid these substances during pregnancy.
• Avoid rooms, such as coffee rooms, where smokers gather.
• Refrain from drinking alcohol, a frequent accompaniment to work lunches or social functions; make sure that nonalcoholic drinks are available.

Fetal Hemoglobin

Fetal hemoglobin differs from adult hemoglobin in several ways. It has a different composition (two alpha and two gamma chains, compared with two alpha and two beta chains of adult hemoglobin). It is also more concentrated and has greater oxygen affinity, two features that increase its efficiency. So much hemoglobin forms at birth that a newborn's hemoglobin level is about 17.1 g/100 mL, compared with an adult's normal level of 11 g/100 mL; a newborn's hematocrit is about 53%, compared with an adult's normal level of 45%.

The change from fetal to adult hemoglobin levels begins before birth and accelerates after birth. The major blood dyscrasias, such as sickle cell anemia, tend to be defects of the beta hemoglobin chain. That is why clinical symptoms do not become apparent until the bulk of fetal hemoglobin has matured to adult hemoglobin composition, at about 6 months of age (Wilson et al., 2003).

Respiratory System

At the 3rd week of intrauterine life, the respiratory and digestive tracts exist as a single tube. Like all body tubes, initially it is a solid structure, which then canalizes (hollows out). By the end of the 4th week, a septum begins to divide the esophagus from the trachea. At the same time, lung buds appear on the trachea.

Until the 7th week of life, the diaphragm does not completely divide the thoracic cavity from the abdomen. This

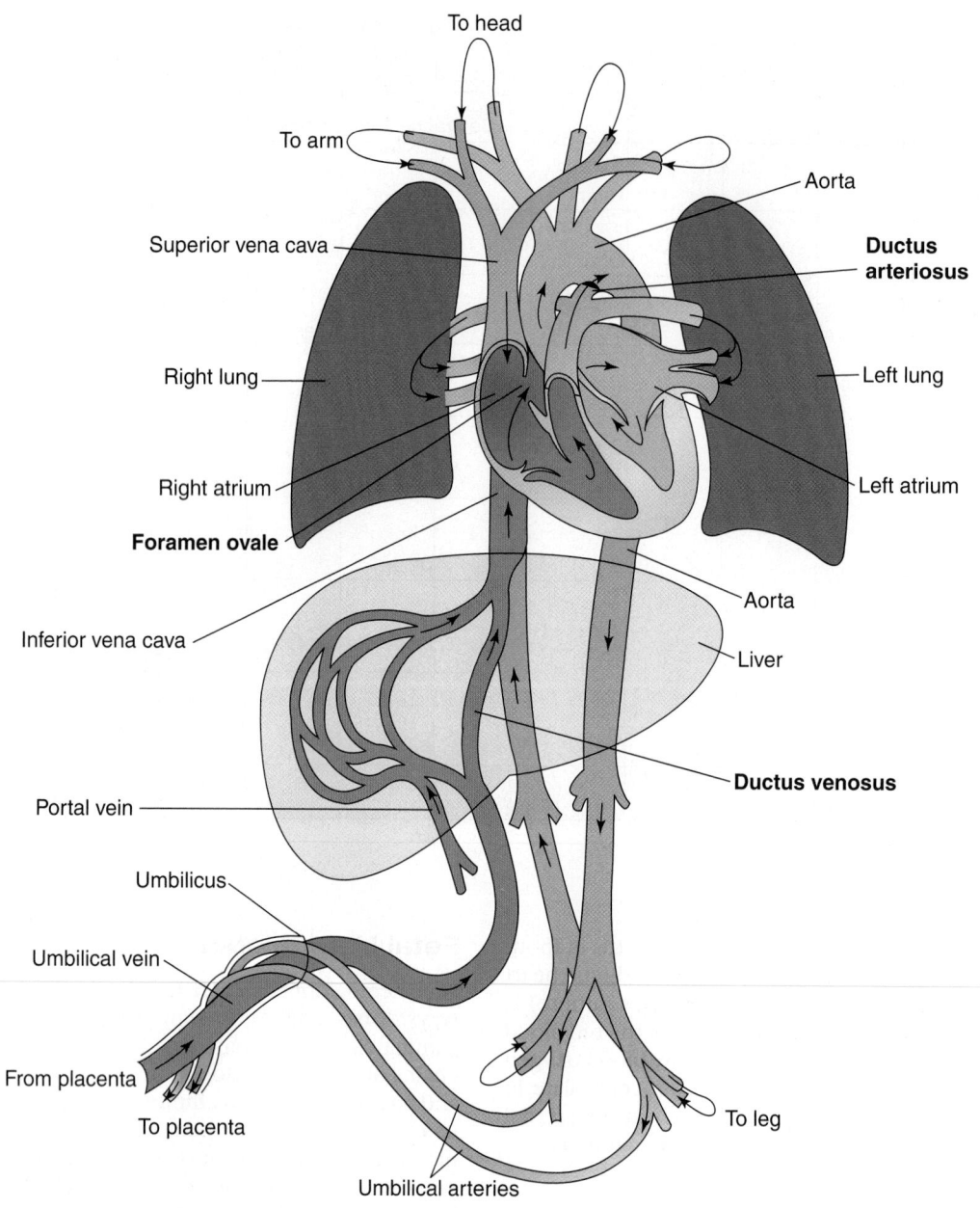

FIGURE 8.6 Fetal circulation.

means that during the 6th week of life lung buds may extend down into the abdomen, re-entering the chest only as the chest's longitudinal dimension increases and the diaphragm becomes complete (at the end of the 7th week). If the diaphragm fails to close completely, the stomach, spleen, liver, or intestines may enter the thoracic cavity. This causes the child to be born with a diaphragmatic hernia or with intestine still present in the chest, compromising the lungs and perhaps displacing the heart (Doughty, 2004).

Important respiratory developmental milestones include the following:

• Alveoli and capillaries begin to form between the 24th and 28th weeks. Both capillary and alveoli development must be complete before gas exchange can occur in the fetal lungs.

• Spontaneous respiratory practice movements begin as early as 3 months' gestation and continue throughout pregnancy.
• Specific lung fluid with a low surface tension and low viscosity forms in alveoli to aid in expansion of the alveoli at birth; it is rapidly absorbed after birth.
• **Surfactant,** a phospholipid substance, is formed and excreted by the alveolar cells at about the 24th week of pregnancy. This decreases alveolar surface tension on expiration, preventing alveolar collapse and improving the infant's ability to maintain respirations in the outside environment (Ainsworth & McCormack, 2004).

The ability to produce surfactant is influenced by a person's genetic makeup (Hallman, 2004). Surfactant has two components: lecithin (L) and sphingomyelin (S). Early in the formation of surfactant, sphingomyelin is the chief component. At about 35 weeks, there is a surge in the production of lecithin, which then becomes the chief component by a ratio of 2:1. With fetal lung movements, surfactant mixes with amniotic fluid. Analysis of the L/S ratio by an amniocentesis technique is one of the primary tests of fetal maturity. Lack of surfactant is a factor associated with the development of respiratory distress syndrome (see Chapter 26). Any interference with the blood supply to the fetus, such as occurs with placental insufficiency from hypertension, appears to enhance surfactant development. This type of stress probably increases steroid levels in the fetus. Although there is little evidence-based information available to document the phenomenon, synthetically increasing steroid levels in the fetus can hurry alveolar maturation (Bloom & Leveno, 2004).

Checkpoint Question 3

Liz Calhorn asks you why her doctor is so concerned about whether her fetus is producing surfactant or not. Your best answer would be:

a. Surfactant keeps lungs from collapsing on expiration, and thus aids newborn breathing.
b. Surfactant is produced by the fetal liver, so its presence reveals liver maturity.
c. Surfactant is the precursor to IGM antibody production, so it prevents infection.
d. Surfactant reveals mature kidney function, as it is produced by kidney glomeruli.

Nervous System

Like the circulatory system, the nervous system begins to develop extremely early in pregnancy. During the 3rd and 4th weeks of life, possibly before the woman even realizes she is pregnant, active formation of the nervous system and sense organs has already begun.

- A neural plate (a thickened portion of the ectoderm) is apparent by the 3rd week of gestation. Its top portion differentiates into the neural tube, which will form the central nervous system (brain and spinal cord), and the neural crest, which will develop into the peripheral nervous system.
- Brain waves can be detected on an electroencephalogram (EEG) by the 8th week.
- All parts of the brain (cerebrum, cerebellum, pons, and medulla oblongata) form in utero, although they are not completely mature at birth. Growth proceeds rapidly during the first year and continues at high levels until 5 or 6 years of age.
- The eye and inner ear develop as projections of the original neural tube.
- By 24 weeks, the ear is capable of responding to sound; the eyes exhibit a pupillary reaction, indicating that sight is present.

The neurologic system seems particularly prone to insult during the early weeks of the embryonic period. Spinal cord disorders such as meningocele may occur because of lack of folic acid (contained in green leafy vegetables and pregnancy vitamins). All during pregnancy and at birth, the system is vulnerable to damage from anoxia.

Endocrine System

As soon as endocrine organs mature in intrauterine life, function begins, including the following processes:

- The fetal adrenal glands supply a precursor for estrogen synthesis by the placenta.
- The fetal pancreas produces the insulin needed by the fetus (insulin does not cross the placenta from the mother to the fetus).
- The thyroid and parathyroid glands play vital roles in metabolic function and calcium balance.

Digestive System

The digestive tract separates from the respiratory tract at about the 4th week and thereafter grows extremely rapidly. Initially solid, the tubes canalize (hollow out) to become patent. Later, the endothelial cells of the gastrointestinal tract proliferate extensively, occluding the lumens once more, and they must canalize again. Atresia or stenosis can develop if either the first or second canalization does not occur. The proliferation of cells shed in the second recanalization forms the basis for meconium (see below).

Because of this rapid intestinal growth, the abdomen, by the 6th week of intrauterine life, becomes too small to contain the intestine. A portion of the intestine, guided by the vitelline membrane (a part of the yolk sac), is pushed into the base of the umbilical cord, where it remains until about the 10th week, when the abdominal cavity has grown large enough to accommodate all of the intestinal mass. As the intestine returns to the abdominal cavity, it must rotate 180 degrees. Failure to do so can result in inadequate mesentery attachments, possibly leading to volvulus of the intestine in the newborn. If any intestinal coils remain outside the abdomen, in the base of the cord, a congenital anomaly develops, termed omphalocele. A similar defect, gastroschisis, occurs when the original midline fusion that occurred at the early cell stage is incomplete (Williams et al., 2003). If the vitelline duct does not atrophy after return of the intestines, a Meckel's diverticulum (a pouch of intestinal tissue) can result (Doughty, 2004).

Meconium, a collection of cellular wastes, bile, fats, mucoproteins, mucopolysaccharides, and portions of the vernix caseosa, the lubricating substance that forms on the fetal skin, forms in the intestines as early as the 16th week. Meconium is sticky in consistency and appears black or dark green (obtaining its color from bile pigment).

The gastrointestinal tract is sterile before birth. Because vitamin K is synthesized by the action of bacteria in the intestines, vitamin K levels are low in the newborn. Sucking and swallowing reflexes are not mature until the fetus is at about 32 weeks' gestation or weighs 1,500 g.

The ability of the gastrointestinal tract to secrete enzymes essential to carbohydrate and protein digestion is mature at 36 weeks. However, amylase, an enzyme found in saliva that is necessary for digestion of complex starches, is not mature until 3 months after birth. Many newborns have not yet developed lipase, an enzyme needed for fat digestion.

The liver is active throughout gestation, functioning as a filter between the incoming blood and the fetal circulation and as a deposit site for fetal stores such as iron and glycogen. However, it is still immature at birth, possibly leading to hypoglycemia and hyperbilirubinemia, two serious problems, in the first 24 hours after birth. It does not prevent recreational drugs or alcohol ingested by the mother from entering the fetal circulation.

Musculoskeletal System

The fetus can be seen to move on ultrasonography as early as the 11th week, although the mother usually does not feel this movement (**quickening**) until almost 20 weeks of gestation. During the first 2 weeks of fetal life, cartilage prototypes provide position and support. Ossification of bone tissue begins at about the 12th week. The ossification process continues all through fetal life and actually until adulthood. Carpals, tarsals, and sternal bones generally do not ossify until birth is imminent.

Reproductive System

A child's sex is determined at the moment of conception by a spermatozoon carrying an X or a Y chromosome and can be ascertained as early as 8 weeks by chromosomal analysis. At about the 6th week of life, the gonads (ovaries or testes) form. If testes form, testosterone is secreted, apparently influencing the sexually neutral genital duct to form other male organs (maturity of the wolffian, or mesonephric, duct). In the absence of testosterone secretion, female organs will form (maturation of the müllerian, or paramesonephric, duct). This is an important phenomenon, because if a mother should take an androgen or an androgen-like substance during this stage of pregnancy, a child who is chromosomally female would appear more male than female at birth. If deficient testosterone is secreted by the testes, both the müllerian (female) duct and the male (wolffian) duct could develop (pseudo-hermaphroditism, or intersex).

The testes first form in the abdominal cavity and do not descend into the scrotal sac until the 34th to 38th week. Therefore, many male preterm infants are born with undescended testes. These children should be observed closely to be sure that the testes descend when the child reaches what would have been the 34th to 38th week of gestational age, because testicular descent does not occur as readily in extrauterine life as it would in utero.

Urinary System

Although rudimentary kidneys are present as early as the end of the 4th week, they do not appear to be essential for life before birth, because the placenta clears the fetus of waste products. Urine is formed by the 12th week and is excreted into the amniotic fluid by the 16th week of gestation. At term, fetal urine is being excreted at the rate of 500 mL/day. An amount of amniotic fluid that is less than normal (oligohydramnios) suggests that fetal kidneys are not secreting adequate urine (Hofmeyr, 2005).

The complex structure of the kidneys is gradually developed during intrauterine life and continues for months afterward. The loop of Henle, for example, is not fully differentiated until the child is born. Glomerular filtration and concentration of urine in the newborn are not efficient, because the kidneys are not fully mature even by birth.

Early in the embryonic stage of urinary system development, the bladder extends to the umbilical region. On rare occasions, an open lumen between the urinary bladder and the umbilicus fails to close. Termed a patent urachus, this is discovered at birth by the persistent drainage of a clear, acid-pH fluid (urine) from the umbilicus.

Integumentary System

The skin of a fetus appears thin and almost translucent until subcutaneous fat begins to be deposited at about 36 weeks. Skin is covered by soft downy hairs (lanugo) and a cream cheese–like substance, vernix caseosa, which is important for lubrication and for keeping the skin from macerating in utero.

Immune System

Immunoglobulin G (IgG) maternal antibodies cross the placenta into the fetus primarily during the third trimester of pregnancy, giving a fetus temporary passive immunity against diseases for which the mother has antibodies. These often include poliomyelitis, rubella (German measles), rubeola (regular measles), diphtheria, tetanus, infectious parotitis (mumps), hepatitis B, and pertussis (whooping cough). Little or no immunity to the herpes virus (the virus of cold sores and genital herpes) is transferred to the fetus, and the average newborn is potentially susceptible to these diseases.

The level of these acquired passive IgG immunoglobulins peaks at birth and then decreases over the next 8 months while the infant begins to build up his or her own stores of IgG, as well as IgA and IgM. Because the passive immunity received by the newborn has already declined substantially by about 2 months, immunization against diphtheria, tetanus, pertussis, poliomyelitis, and *Haemophilus influenzae* is typically begun at this time. Passive antibodies to measles have been demonstrated to last for longer than 1 year. Consequently, the immunization for measles is not given until an extrauterine age of 12 months.

It has been shown that a fetus is capable of active antibody production late in a pregnancy. Generally this is not necessary, however, because antibodies are manufactured only after stimulation by an invading antigen, and antigens rarely invade the intrauterine space. However, infants whose mothers have had an infection such as rubella during pregnancy typically have active IgM antibodies to rubella in their blood serum at birth. Because IgA and IgM antibodies cannot cross the placenta, their presence in a newborn is proof that the fetus has been exposed to a disease.

Milestones of Fetal Growth and Development

During pregnancy, couples often ask questions about their baby's appearance and age. To answer these questions effectively and to plan care that safeguards fetal growth, it is helpful to be able to describe the developmental milestones according to the number of weeks of intrauterine life.

Milestones can be confusing, because the life of the fetus is typically measured from the time of ovulation or fertilization (ovulation age), but the length of the pregnancy is usually measured from the first day of the last menstrual period (gestational age). Because ovulation and fertilization take place about 2 weeks after the last menstrual period, the ovulation age of the fetus is always 2 weeks less than the length of the pregnancy or the gestational age.

Both ovulation and gestational age are also sometimes measured in lunar months (4-week periods) or in trimesters (3-month periods) rather than in weeks. In lunar months, a pregnancy is 10 months (40 weeks or 280 days) long; a fetus grows in utero 9.5 lunar months or three full trimesters (38 weeks or 266 days).

The following discussion of fetal developmental milestones is based on gestational weeks, because it is helpful when talking to expectant parents to be able to correlate fetal development with the way they measure pregnancy—from the first day of the last menstrual period. Figure 8.7 illustrates the comparative size and appearance of human embryos and fetuses at different stages.

End of 4th Gestational Week

At the end of the 4th week of gestation, the human embryo is a rapidly growing formation of cells but does not yet resemble a human being.

- Length: 0.75 to 1 cm
- Weight: 400 mg
- The spinal cord is formed and fused at the midpoint.
- Lateral wings that will form the body are folded forward to fuse at the midline.
- Head folds forward and becomes prominent, representing about one third of the entire structure.
- The back is bent so that the head almost touches the tip of the tail.
- The rudimentary heart appears as a prominent bulge on the anterior surface.
- Arms and legs are budlike structures.
- Rudimentary eyes, ears, and nose are discernible.

End of 8th Gestational Week

- Length: 2.5 cm (1 in)
- Weight: 20 g
- Organogenesis is complete.
- The heart, with a septum and valves, is beating rhythmically.
- Facial features are definitely discernible.
- Arms and legs have developed.
- External genitalia are present, but sex is not distinguishable by simple observation.
- The primitive tail is regressing.
- Abdomen appears large because the fetal intestine is growing rapidly.
- Sonogram shows a gestational sac, diagnostic of pregnancy (Fig. 8.8).

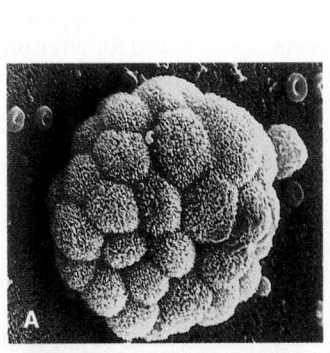
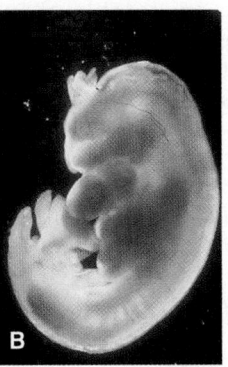
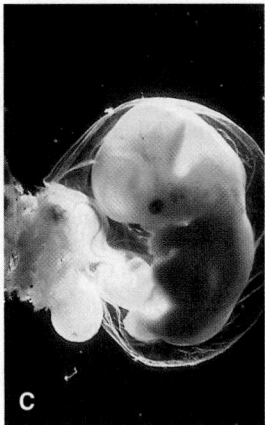
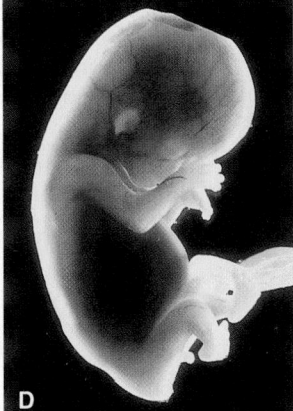
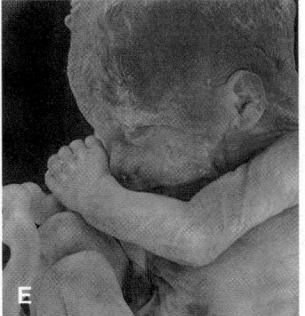

FIGURE 8.7 Human embryos at different stages of life: (**A**) Implantation in uterus 7 to 8 days after conception. (**B**) Embryo at 32 days. (**C**) At 37 days. (**D**) At 41 days. (**E**) Between 12–15 weeks. (Petit Format/Nestle/Science Source/Photo Researchers.)

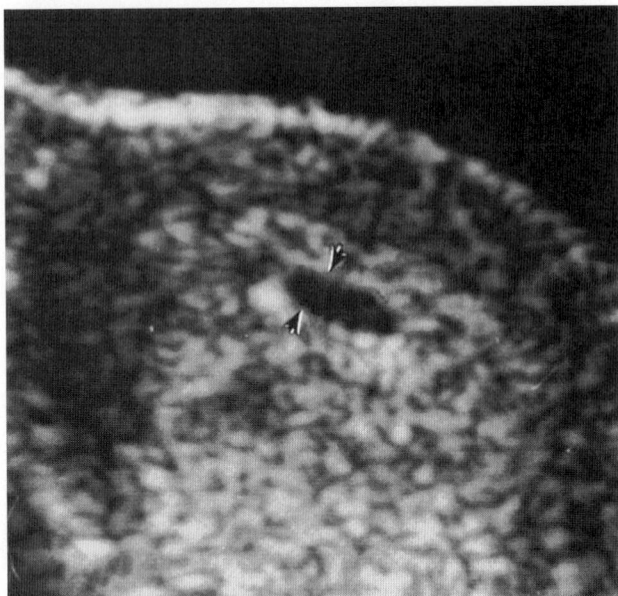

FIGURE 8.8 Sonogram showing the characteristic circle diagnostic of pregnancy (the gestational sac). (Benson, C. B., et al. [1988]. *Atlas of obstetrical ultrasound.* Philadelphia: J. B. Lippincott.)

End of 12th Gestational Week (First Trimester)

- Length: 7 to 8 cm
- Weight: 45 g
- Nail beds are forming on fingers and toes.
- Spontaneous movements are possible, although they are usually too faint to be felt by the mother.
- Some reflexes, such as the Babinski reflex, are present.
- Bone ossification centers are forming.
- Tooth buds are present.
- Sex is distinguishable by outward appearance.
- Kidney secretion has begun, although urine may not yet be evident in amniotic fluid.
- Heartbeat is audible through Doppler technology.

End of 16th Gestational Week

- Length: 10 to 17 cm
- Weight: 55 to 120 g
- Fetal heart sounds are audible with an ordinary stethoscope.
- Lanugo (the fine, downy hair on the back and arms of newborns, which apparently serves as a source of insulation for body heat) is well formed.
- Liver and pancreas are functioning.
- Fetus actively swallows amniotic fluid, demonstrating an intact but uncoordinated swallowing reflex; urine is present in amniotic fluid.
- Sex can be determined by ultrasonography.

End of 20th Gestational Week

- Length: 25 cm
- Weight: 223 g

- Spontaneous fetal movements can be sensed by the mother.
- Antibody production is possible.
- Hair forms, extending to include eyebrows and hair on the head.
- Meconium is present in the upper intestine.
- Brown fat, a special fat that will aid in temperature regulation at birth, begins to be formed behind the kidneys, sternum, and posterior neck.
- Vernix caseosa, which serves as a protective skin covering during intrauterine life, begins to form.
- Definite sleeping and activity patterns are distinguishable (the fetus has developed biorhythms that will guide sleep/wake patterns throughout life).

End of 24th Gestational Week (Second Trimester)

- Length: 28 to 36 cm
- Weight: 550 g
- Passive antibody transfer from mother to fetus probably begins as early as the 20th week of gestation, certainly by the 24th week. Infants born before antibody transfer has taken place have no natural immunity and need more than the usual protection against infectious disease in the newborn period until the infant's own store of immunoglobulins can build up.
- Meconium is present as far as the rectum.
- Active production of lung surfactant begins.
- Eyebrows and eyelashes are well defined.
- Eyelids, previously fused since the 12th week, are now open.
- Pupils are capable of reacting to light.
- When fetuses reach 24 weeks, or 601 g, they have achieved a practical low-end age of viability if they are cared for after birth in a modern intensive care facility.
- Hearing can be demonstrated by response to sudden sound.

End of 28th Gestational Week

- Length: 35 to 38 cm
- Weight: 1,200 g
- Lung alveoli begin to mature, and surfactant can be demonstrated in amniotic fluid.
- Testes begin to descend into the scrotal sac from the lower abdominal cavity.
- The blood vessels of the retina are thin and extremely susceptible to damage from high oxygen concentrations (an important consideration when caring for preterm infants who need oxygen).

End of 32nd Gestational Week

- Length: 38 to 43 cm
- Weight: 1,600 g
- Subcutaneous fat begins to be deposited (the former stringy, "little old man" appearance is lost).
- Fetus responds by movement to sounds outside the mother's body.
- Active Moro reflex is present.
- Birth position (vertex or breech) may be assumed.

- Iron stores, which provide iron for the time during which the neonate ingests only milk after birth, are beginning to be developed.
- Fingernails grow to reach the end of fingertips.

End of 36th Gestational Week

- Length: 42 to 48 cm
- Weight: 1,800 to 2,700 g (5 to 6 lb)
- Body stores of glycogen, iron, carbohydrate, and calcium are deposited.
- Additional amounts of subcutaneous fat are deposited.
- Sole of the foot has only one or two crisscross creases, compared with the full crisscross pattern that will be evident at term.
- Amount of lanugo begins to diminish.
- Most babies turn into a vertex or head-down presentation during this month.

End of 40th Gestational Week (Third Trimester)

- Length: 48 to 52 cm (crown to rump, 35 to 37 cm)
- Weight: 3,000 g (7 to 7.5 lb)
- Fetus kicks actively, hard enough to cause the mother considerable discomfort.
- Fetal hemoglobin begins its conversion to adult hemoglobin. The conversion is so rapid that, at birth, about 20% of hemoglobin is adult in character.
- Vernix caseosa is fully formed.
- Fingernails extend over the fingertips.
- Creases on the soles of the feet cover at least two thirds of the surface.

In primiparas (women having their first baby), the fetus often sinks into the birth canal during the last 2 weeks, giving the mother a feeling that the load she is carrying is less. This event, termed **lightening,** is a fetal announcement that the third trimester of pregnancy has ended and birth is at hand.

Determination of Estimated Birth Date

It is impossible to predict the day an infant will be born with a high degree of accuracy. Traditionally, this date has been referred to as the estimated date of confinement (EDC). Because women are no longer "confined" after childbirth, the abbreviation EDB (**estimated date of birth**) or EDD (estimated date of delivery) is more commonly used today.

Fewer than 5% of pregnancies end exactly 280 days from the last menstrual period; fewer than half end within 1 week of the 280th day.

If fertilization occurred early in a menstrual cycle, the pregnancy will probably end "early"; if ovulation and fertilization occurred later in the cycle, the pregnancy will end "late." Because of these normal variations, a pregnancy ending 2 weeks before or 2 weeks after the calculated EDB is considered well within the normal limit (38 to 42 weeks). Gestational age wheels or birth date calculators, which can be used to predict a birth date, are available. Nagele's rule is the standard method used to predict the length of a pregnancy (Box 8.3).

> **BOX 8.3**
>
> ### Nagele's Rule
>
> To calculate the date of birth by this rule, count backward 3 calendar months from the first day of the last menstrual period and add 7 days. For example, if the last menstrual period began May 15, you would count back 3 months (April 15, March 15, February 15) and add 7 days, to arrive at a date of birth of February 22.

What if... Liz Calhorn, the young woman you met at the beginning of the chapter, first came to your prenatal clinic on August 5. What if she tells you that she had her last menstrual period on March 13 to March 18? What would be her estimated date of birth (EDB)?

ASSESSMENT OF FETAL GROWTH AND DEVELOPMENT

Fetal growth and development can be compromised if a fetus has a metabolic or chromosomal disorder that interferes with normal growth, if the supporting structures such as the placenta or cord do not form normally, or if environmental influences such as cigarette smoking (the nicotine in cigarettes causes fetal growth restriction) or alcohol consumption (alcohol causes a severe cognitive challenge) interfere with fetal growth. Much information about the size and health of the unborn child can be gathered through a variety of assessment techniques. Nursing responsibilities for these assessment procedures include seeing that a signed consent form has been obtained as needed, scheduling the procedure, explaining the procedure to the woman and her support person, preparing the woman physically and psychologically, providing support during the procedure, assessing both fetal and maternal responses to the procedure, providing any necessary follow-up care, and managing equipment and specimens (Box 8.4).

Additional consent to perform a procedure is necessary if the procedure poses any risk to the mother or fetus that would not otherwise be present. Information must be provided about what the procedure entails and what the possible risks are.

Health History

Like all assessments, fetal assessment begins with a health history. Ask specifically about nutritional intake, because, if the mother is not eating a healthy diet, she may not be taking in enough nutrients for fetal growth. Be certain to ask also about personal habits such as cigarette smoking, recreational drug use, and exercise, because all of these also influence fetal growth. Most women actively protect the child growing inside them. Asking if the woman has had any accidents or experienced intimate partner abuse helps reveal whether the fetus could have suffered from

A Multidisciplinary Care Map for A Woman Undergoing Fetal Studies

●

Liz Calborn, an 18-year-old woman, thinks she is 24 weeks pregnant. Today, at a clinic visit, she tells you she felt her fetus move for the first time. She states, "Feeling the baby move made me realize for the first time there's someone inside me, you know what I mean? It made me know it's time I started being more careful with what I do."

Family Assessment

Client lives in one-bedroom apartment; supports self with typing position at insurance agency. States, "My parents would help out if I begged them, but I'm not going to do that." Boyfriend (father of fetus) is supportive, but couple has no plans to marry. Client states, "I'm too young."

Client Assessment

Client smokes a pack of cigarettes a day. Twice during the pregnancy (at the 4th and 10th week), she drank beer at summer picnics. Takes aspirin, 10 g, for almost daily sinus headaches. No spotting or falls since last menstrual period. No recreational drugs.

Nutrition: Skips breakfast to help control her weight. Lunch: A hotdog and salad. One diet cola. Dinner: Macaroni and cheese; applesauce. One cup coffee.

Physical examination: Fundal height is 2.0 cm. Fetal heart tones by Doppler at 160/min. Has been advised to have an ultrasound done to assess for fetal growth and to date pregnancy.

Nursing Diagnosis

Risk for altered fetal growth related to inadequate nutrition, alcohol and nicotine consumption

Outcome Criteria

Client consents to sonogram for fetal growth assessment; reports lessened alcohol and cigarette consumption.

Team Member Responsible	Assessment	Intervention	Rationale	Expected Outcome
Activities of Daily Living				
Nurse	Ask patient to recount a "typical day" to reveal any actions possibly detrimental to fetal growth.	Discuss common actions that are unsafe during pregnancy, such as smoking and drinking alcohol.	Knowing what constitutes unsafe practices during pregnancy is a woman's best safeguard against fetal harm.	Client states that she now knows and will avoid unsafe actions during pregnancy.
Consultations				
Physician/ Nurse	Determine whether sonogram department has appointments free in coming week.	Schedule sonogram 1 week in advance with sonogram department.	Client believes she is 24 weeks pregnant. Fundal height, recent fetal movements correspond more closely to 20 weeks.	Client reports for scheduled ultrasound in 1 week.

(continued)

Team Member Responsible	Assessment	Intervention	Rationale	Expected Outcome
		Procedures/Medications		
Physician	Assess use of over-the-counter and complementary therapies.	Discuss with client in-advisability of taking aspirin during pregnancy; suggest she take acetaminophen (Tylenol) instead.	Acetylsalicylic acid (aspirin) can lead to bleeding or prolong pregnancy.	Client reports at next prenatal visit that she takes acetaminophen for pain during pregnancy.
		Nutrition		
Nurse/ nutritionist	Ask client for a 24-hour recall nutrition history.	Discuss the advisability of eating breakfast while pregnant to help avoid hypoglycemia in fetus.	Knowing what constitutes unsafe practices during pregnancy is a woman's best safeguard against fetal harm.	Client reports at prenatal visits that she eats breakfast of at least toast and orange juice before leaving for work in the morning.
Nutritionist	Assess and analyze the 24-hour recall history.	Discuss advantages of good pregnancy nutrition with client and define healthy pregnancy nutrition.	Client needs to improve total nutrition, especially intake of protein sources, to better support pregnancy.	Client meets with clinic nutritionist to discuss better nutrition pattern.
		Patient/Family Education		
Nurse	Determine whether client understands that ultrasound is not x-ray, so is not harmful to fetus.	Instruct client about preparation for sonogram (drink fluid; avoid emptying bladder).	A well-prepared client is more apt to result in an effective procedure and a satisfied client.	Client will describe accurate preparations for procedure.
		Spiritual/Psychosocial/Emotional Needs		
Nurse/ Physician	Assess the extent of factors, such as alcohol and cigarette use, that could lead to intrauterine growth restriction.	Review the possibility with client that her pregnancy dating may be wrong, because fundal height is below normal. Alternate cause could be fetal growth restriction.	Understanding contributors to fetal health is necessary for women to make informed choices during pregnancy.	Client states that she is aware she needs to improve nutrition and reduce alcohol and cigarette use.
		Discharge Planning		
Nurse	Assess whether client understands where to go and preparation necessary for ultrasound.	Give instructions for ultrasound scheduled for 1 week from today.	Well-prepared clients are more apt to cooperate with procedures and feel satisfaction afterward.	The patient receives printed instructions for ambulatory ultrasound.
Physician	Perform complete assessment to help ensure continuity of care with other services.	Mark chart as high-risk client for intrauterine growth restriction (fundal height below average for weeks gestation).	Documenting risk factors helps to safeguard the fetus.	The patient chart documents high-risk status.

trauma (intimate partner abuse tends to increase during pregnancy because of the stress a pregnancy can create) (Lipsky et al., 2004).

Estimating Fetal Growth

McDonald's rule, a symphysis-fundal height measurement, although not thoroughly documented to be reliable, is a common method of determining, during midpregnancy, that a fetus is growing in utero (McAllion, 2004). Typically, the distance from the uterine fundus to the symphysis pubis in centimeters is equal to the week of gestation between the 20th and 31st weeks of pregnancy. The measurement is made from the notch of the symphysis pubis to over the top of the uterine fundus as the woman lies supine (Fig. 8.9). McDonald's rule becomes inaccurate during the third trimester of pregnancy because the fetus is growing more in weight than in height during this time. Until then, a fundal height much greater than this standard suggests multiple pregnancy, a miscalculated due date, a large-for-gestational-age infant, hydramnios (increased amniotic fluid volume), or possibly even hydatidiform mole (see Chapter 15). A fundal measurement much less than this suggests that either the fetus is failing to thrive (intrauterine growth restriction), the pregnancy length was miscalculated, or an anomaly, such as anencephaly, has developed.

Determining and recording that the fundus has reached typical milestone measurements, such as over the symphysis pubis at 12 weeks, at the umbilicus at 20 weeks, and at the xiphoid process at 36 weeks, is also helpful.

Assessing Fetal Well-Being

A number of actions or procedures are helpful in detecting and documenting that the fetus is healthy.

Fetal Movement

Fetal movement that can be felt by the mother (quickening) begins at approximately 18 to 20 weeks of pregnancy and peaks at 28 to 38 weeks. A healthy fetus moves with

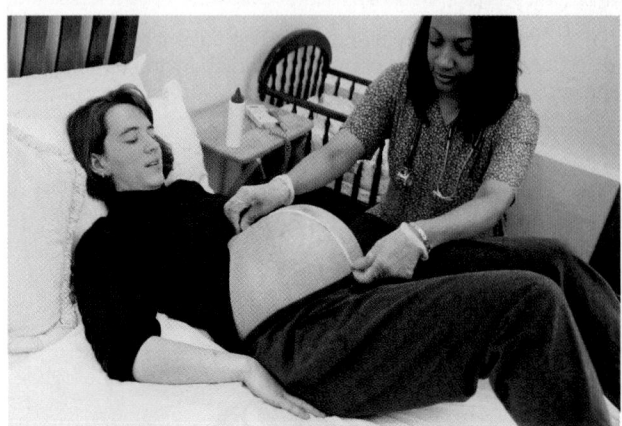

FIGURE 8.9 Measuring fundal height from the superior aspect of the pubis to the fundal crest. The nurse places the tape flat against the abdomen for the measurement.

a degree of consistency, or at least 10 times a day. In contrast, a fetus not receiving enough nutrients because of placental insufficiency has greatly decreased movements. Based on this, asking the mother to observe and record the number of movements the fetus makes daily offers a gross assessment of fetal well-being.

Because of variations in movements among normal, healthy fetuses, as well as variations in different health care providers' level of confidence in the technique, a variety of protocols have been developed by different institutions. One popular way to approach this assessment is to ask the mother to lie in a left recumbent position after a meal and record how many fetal movements she feels over the next hour (the Sandovsky method). In this position, a fetus normally moves a minimum of twice every 10 minutes or an average of 10 to 12 times an hour. If less than 10 movements occur, the mother repeats the test for the next hour. She is instructed to telephone her health care provider if she has felt fewer than 10 movements (half the normal number) during the chosen 2 hours (Spong, 2003). Another protocol is "Count-to-Ten" (the Cardiff method). For this, the mother records the time interval it takes for her to feel 10 fetal movements. Usually, this occurs within 60 minutes. Make sure to instruct the woman that fetal movements do vary, especially in relation to sleep cycles of the fetus and the mother's activity during the observation time. Otherwise, she can become unduly anxious that her fetus may be in jeopardy.

What if... You give instructions to Liz Calhorn, the mother described at the beginning of the chapter, to count fetal movements for 1 hour three times a day after meals. What if she tells you that she snacks all day long rather than eating at regular times? How would you modify your instructions? Which is more important, that she count movements after meals, or that she does it three times a day?

Fetal Heart Rate

Fetal hearts beat at 120 to 160 beats per minute throughout pregnancy. Fetal heart sounds can be heard and counted as early as the 10th to 11th week of pregnancy by the use of an ultrasonic Doppler technique (Neilson & Alfirevic, 2005) (Fig. 8.10). Box 8.5 highlights appropriate outcomes and interventions using terminology identified by the Nursing Outcomes Classification (NOC) and Nursing Interventions Classification (NIC) in relation to assessing fetal heart rates.

Rhythm Strip Testing. The term "rhythm strip testing" has come to mean assessment of the fetal heart rate for whether a good baseline rate and long- and short-term variability are present. For the test, the woman is placed in a semi-Fowler's position (either in a comfortable lounge chair or on an examining table or bed with an elevated backrest) to prevent the uterus from compressing the vena cava and causing supine hypotension syndrome during the test. External fetal heart rate and uterine contraction monitors are attached abdominally (Fig. 8.11*A*). The fetal heart rate is then recorded for 20 minutes.

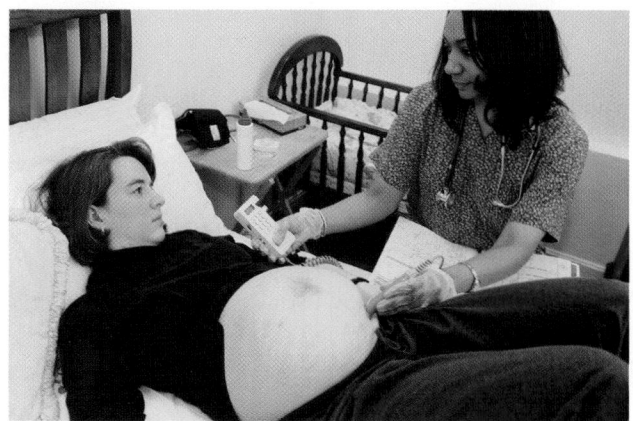

FIGURE 8.10 Measuring fetal heart rate with a Doppler transducer, which detects and broadcasts the fetal heart rate so the parents-to-be as well as you can hear it. (© Barbara Proud.)

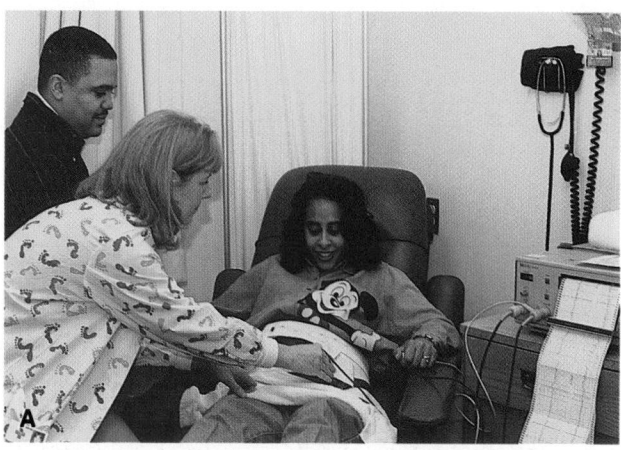

FIGURE 8.11 Rhythm strip and nonstress testing of fetal heart rate. (**A**) The woman sits in a comfortable chair to avoid supine hypotension. Both a uterine contraction monitor and fetal heart rate monitor are in place on her abdomen. (Photo by Melissa Olson, with permission of Chestnut Hill Hospital, Philadelphia, PA.) (*continued on next page*)

BOX 8.5

Nursing Outcomes Classification (NOC) and Nursing Interventions Classification (NIC)

Assessing Fetal Well-Being

NOC: Fetal Status, Antepartum

Fetal status, antepartum, is defined as the conditions indicative of fetal physical well-being from conception to the onset of labor (Johnson et al, 2000). Some specific indicators that this outcome has been achieved include the following parameters demonstrated within the expected range:

- Fetal heart rate
- Deceleration patterns
- Variability
- Fetal ultrasound growth measurements
- Fetal movement frequency and pattern
- Nonstress test
- Contraction stress test
- Biophysical profile score
- Amniotic fluid sample findings
- Umbilical artery blood flow velocity

NIC: Electronic Fetal Monitoring, Antepartum

Electronic fetal monitoring, antepartum, is defined as the electronic evaluation of fetal heart rate response to movement, external stimuli, or uterine contractions during antepartal testing (McCloskey and Bulechek, 2000). Some important activities involved when implementing this intervention include the following:

- Reviewing obstetric history for risk factors requiring antepartal testing

- Determining client's knowledge about reasons for testing
- Assessing maternal vital signs and inquiring about oral intake
- Verifying maternal and fetal heart rates before initiating electronic fetal monitoring
- Instructing client about reasons for monitoring
- Performing Leopold maneuver to determine fetal position
- Applying transducer as appropriate
- Distinguishing and differentiating among multiple fetuses
- Reassuring mother about normal fetal heart rate signs; adjusting monitors to achieve and maintain tracing clarity
- Obtaining baseline fetal heart rate tracing per protocol
- Interpreting electronic monitor strip for baseline heart rate, long-term variability, and presence of spontaneous accelerations, decelerations, or contractions
- Initiating intravenous infusion, ultrasound, or vibroacoustic stimulation per protocol
- Interpreting tracing based on test
- Providing anticipatory guidance for abnormal test results
- Providing written discharge instructions for future testing and return for follow-up as indicated

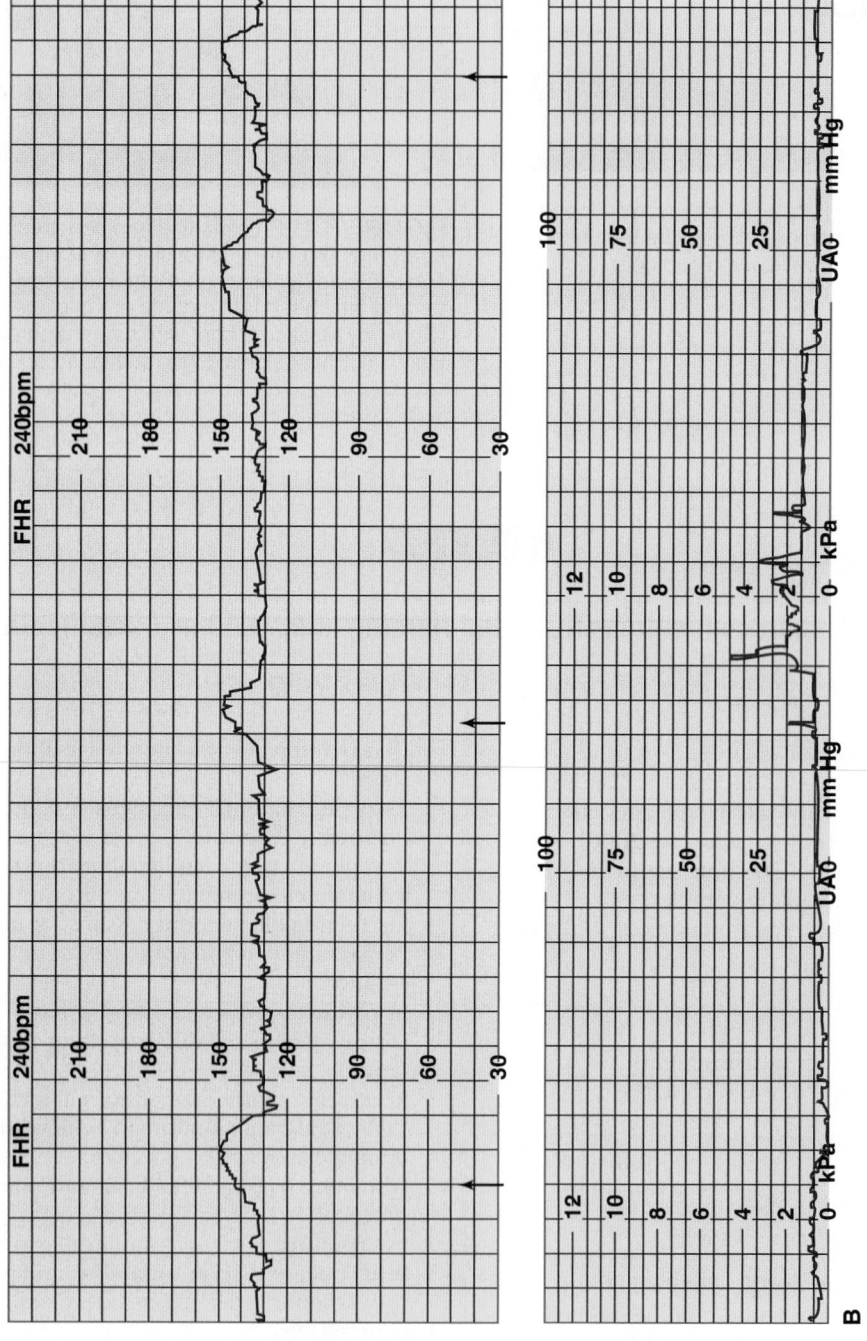

FIGURE 8.11 **(continued)** **(B)** A rhythm strip. The upper strip signifies heart rate; the lower strip indicates uterine activity. *Arrows* signal fetal movement. (*continued*)

long-term testing is not yet available), MRI has the potential to replace or complement ultrasonography as a fetal assessment technique. It may be most helpful in diagnosing complications such as ectopic pregnancy or trophoblastic disease (see Chapter 15), because later in a pregnancy fetal movement (unless the fetus is sedated) can obscure the findings.

Maternal Serum Alpha-Fetoprotein

Alpha-fetoprotein (AFP) is a substance produced by the fetal liver that is present in amniotic fluid and maternal serum. The level is abnormally high in the maternal serum (MSAFP) if the fetus has an open spinal or abdominal defect, because the open defect allows more AFP to appear. Although the reason is unclear, the level is low if the fetus has a chromosomal defect such as Down syndrome. MSAFP levels begin to rise at 11 weeks' gestation and then steadily increase until term. Traditionally assessed at the 15th week of pregnancy, between 85% and 90% of neural tube defects and 80% of Down syndrome babies can be detected by this method (Spong, 2003).

Triple Screening

Triple screening, or analysis of three indicators (MSAFP, unconjugated estriol, and hCG), may be performed in place of AFP testing alone to yield even more reliable results. As with the measurement of MSAFP, it requires only a simple venipuncture of the mother.

Chorionic Villi Sampling

Chorionic villi sampling (CVS) is a biopsy and chromosomal analysis of chorionic villi that is done at 10 to 12 weeks of pregnancy. This procedure is discussed in Chapter 7. Coelocentesis (transvaginal aspiration of fluid from the extraembryonic cavity) is an alternative method to remove cells for fetal analysis.

Amniocentesis

Amniocentesis (from the Greek *amnion* for sac and *kentesis* for puncture) is the aspiration of amniotic fluid from the pregnant uterus for examination. The procedure can be done in a physician's office or in an ambulatory clinic. It is typically scheduled between the 14th and 16th weeks of pregnancy to allow for a generous amount of amniotic fluid to be present. The technique can be used again near term to test for fetal maturity.

Amniocentesis is a technically easy procedure, but it can be frightening to a woman. Because it involves penetration of the integrity of the amniotic sac, there also is a risk to the fetus, although this risk is low (less than 0.5%) (Fischbach, 2004). It can lead to complications such as hemorrhage from penetration of the placenta, infection of the amniotic fluid, and puncture of the fetus. It can lead to irritation of the uterus, causing premature labor.

In preparation for amniocentesis, ask the woman to void (to reduce the size of the bladder, thus preventing inadvertent puncture). Place her in a supine position on the examining table and drape her appropriately, exposing only her abdomen. Place a folded towel under her right buttock to tip her body slightly to the left and move the uterus off the vena cava, to prevent supine hypotension syndrome. Attach fetal heart rate and uterine contraction monitors. Take the maternal blood pressure and measure the fetal heart rate for baseline levels.

Explain that a sonogram will be done to determine the position of the fetus, a pocket of amniotic fluid, and the placenta. Then the abdomen will be washed with an antiseptic solution, and a local anesthetic will be given. Caution the woman that she may feel a sensation of pressure as the needle used for aspiration, a 3- or 4-in, 20- to 22-gauge spinal needle, is introduced. Do not suggest that she take a deep breath and hold it as a distraction against discomfort: this lowers the diaphragm against the uterus and shifts intrauterine contents.

The needle is inserted into the amniotic cavity over a pool of amniotic fluid, carefully avoiding the fetus and placenta (Fig. 8.14). A syringe is attached, and about 15 mL of amniotic fluid is withdrawn. The needle is then removed, and the woman rests quietly for about 30 minutes. During the procedure and for the 30 minutes afterward, observe the fetal heart rate monitor to be certain the rate remains normal, and observe the uterine contraction monitor to be sure than no contractions are occurring.

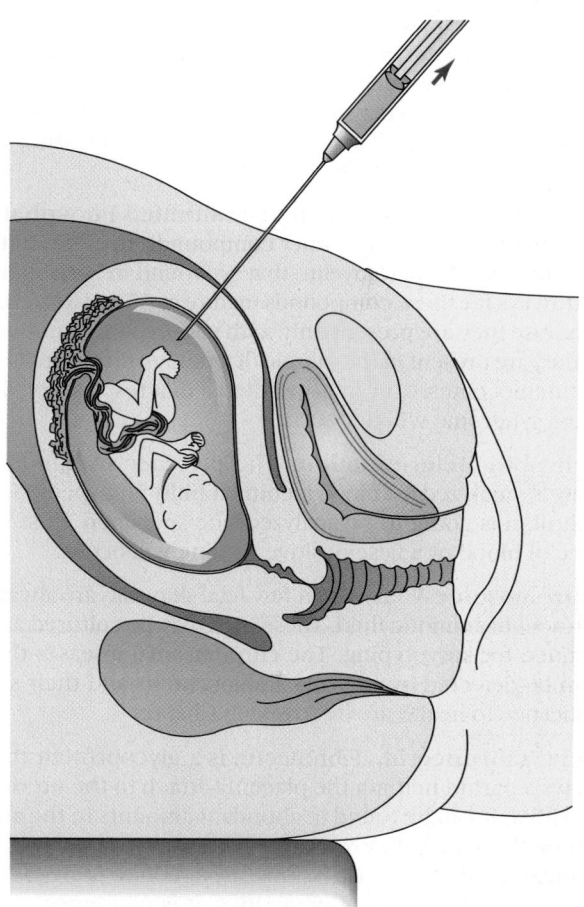

FIGURE 8.14 Amniocentesis. A pocket of amniotic fluid is located by sonogram. A small amount of fluid is removed by aspiration.

If the woman has Rh-negative blood, Rho(D) immune globulin (RhIG; RhoGAM) may be administered after the procedure to prevent fetal isoimmunization. This is to ensure that maternal antibodies will not form against any placental red blood cells that might have accidentally been released during the procedure.

Amniocentesis can provide information in a number of areas.

Color. Normal amniotic fluid is the color of water; late in pregnancy, it may have a slightly yellow tinge. A strong yellow color suggests a blood incompatibility (the yellow results from the presence of bilirubin released with the hemolysis of red blood cells). A green color suggests meconium staining, a phenomenon associated with fetal distress.

Lecithin/Sphingomyelin Ratio. Lecithin and sphingomyelin are the protein components of the lung enzyme surfactant that the alveoli begin to form at about the 22nd to 24th weeks of pregnancy. After amniocentesis, the L/S ratio may be determined quickly by a shake test (if bubbles appear in the amniotic fluid after shaking, the ratio is mature) or sent for laboratory analysis. An L/S ratio of 2:1 is traditionally accepted as lung maturity.

Infants of mothers with severe diabetes may have false-mature readings of lecithin because the stress to the infant in utero tends to mature lecithin pathways early. This means that fetal values must be considered in light of the presence of maternal diabetes, or the infant may be born with mature lung function but be immature overall (fragile giants) and thus may not do well in postnatal life. Some laboratories interpret a ratio of 2.5:1 or 3:1 as a mature indicator in infants of diabetic mothers.

Phosphatidyl Glycerol and Desaturated Phosphatidylcholine. These are other compounds, in addition to lecithin and sphingomyelin, that are found in surfactant. Pathways for these compounds mature at 35 to 36 weeks. Because they are present only with mature lung function, if they are present in the sample of amniotic fluid obtained by amniocentesis, it can be predicted that respiratory distress syndrome will not occur.

Bilirubin Determination. The presence of bilirubin may be analyzed if a blood incompatibility is suspected. If bilirubin is going to be analyzed, the specimen must be free of blood or a false-positive reading will occur.

Chromosome Analysis. A few fetal skin cells are always present in amniotic fluid. These cells may be cultured and stained for karyotyping. The chromosomal diseases that can be detected by prenatal amniocentesis and their significance to health are discussed in Chapter 7.

Fetal Fibronectin. Fibronectin is a glycoprotein that plays a part in helping the placenta attach to the uterine decidua. It can be found in abundant amounts in the amniotic fluid. Early in pregnancy, it can be assessed in the woman's cervical mucus, but the amount then fades until, after 20 weeks of pregnancy, it is no longer present. As labor approaches and cervical dilation begins, it can be assessed again in cervical or vaginal fluid. Damage to fetal membranes releases a great deal of the substance, so detection of fibronectin in the amniotic fluid

or in the mother's vagina can serve as an announcement that preterm labor may be beginning.

Inborn Errors of Metabolism. Some inherited diseases that are caused by inborn errors of metabolism can be detected by amniocentesis. For a condition to be identified, the enzyme defect must be present in the amniotic fluid as early as the time of the procedure. Examples of illnesses that can be detected in this way are cystinosis and maple syrup urine disease (amino acid disorders).

Alpha-Fetoprotein. If the fetus has an open body defect, such as anencephaly, myelomeningocele, or omphalocele, increased levels of AFP will be present in the amniotic fluid because of leakage of AFP into the fluid. The level will be decreased in the amniotic fluid of fetuses with chromosomal defects such as Down syndrome. Acetylcholinesterase is another compound that is obtained from amniotic fluid in high levels if a neural tube defect is present.

Percutaneous Umbilical Blood Sampling

PUBS (also called cordocentesis or funicentesis) is the aspiration of blood from the umbilical vein for analysis. After the umbilical cord is located by sonography, a thin needle is inserted by amniocentesis technique into the uterus and is guided by ultrasound until it pierces the umbilical vein. A sample of blood is then removed for blood studies, such as a complete blood count, direct Coombs' test, blood gases, and karyotyping. To ensure that the blood obtained is fetal blood, it is submitted to a Kleihauer-Betke test. If a fetus is found to be anemic, blood may be transfused using this same technique. Because the umbilical vein continues to ooze for a moment after the procedure, fetal blood could enter the maternal circulation, so RhIG is given to Rh-negative women to prevent sensitization. The fetus is monitored by a nonstress test before and after the procedure to be certain that uterine contractions are not present and by ultrasound to see that no bleeding is evident. This procedure carries little additional risk to the fetus or mother over amniocentesis and can yield information not available by any other means, especially about blood dyscrasias (Speroff & Fritz, 2005).

Amnioscopy

Amnioscopy is the visual inspection of the amniotic fluid through the cervix and membranes with an amnioscope (a small fetoscope). The main use of the technique is to detect meconium staining. It carries some risk of membrane rupture.

Fetoscopy

Fetoscopy, in which the fetus is visualized by inspection through a fetoscope (an extremely narrow, hollow tube inserted by amniocentesis technique), is sometimes helpful in assessing fetal well-being. A photograph can be taken through the fetoscope to reassure parents that their infant is well and perfectly formed. The procedure may be used for the following purposes:

- To confirm the intactness of the spinal column
- To obtain biopsy samples of fetal tissue and fetal blood samples

- To perform elemental surgery, such as inserting a polyethylene shunt into the fetal ventricles to relieve hydrocephalus or anteriorly into the fetal bladder to relieve a stenosed urethra (Cortes & Farmer, 2004).

The earliest time in pregnancy that fetoscopy can be performed is about the 16th or 17th week. For the procedure, the mother is prepared and draped as for amniocentesis. A local anesthetic is injected into the abdominal skin. The fetoscope is then inserted through a minor abdominal incision. If the fetus is very active, meperidine (Demerol) may be administered to the mother. This drug crosses the placenta and sedates the fetus, to avoid fetal injury by the scope and to allow better observation.

Fetoscopy carries a small risk of premature labor. Amnionitis (infection of the amniotic fluid) may occur. To avoid this, the mother may be prescribed 10 days of antibiotic therapy after the procedure. The number of procedures performed by fetoscopy is limited because of the manipulation involved and the ethical quandary of the mother's autonomy being compromised by fetal needs if further procedures are necessary (e.g., asking the mother to undergo general anesthesia so that the fetus can have surgery).

Biophysical Profile

A biophysical profile combines five parameters (fetal reactivity, fetal breathing movements, fetal body movement, fetal tone, and amniotic fluid volume) into one assessment. The fetal heart and breathing record measures short-term central nervous system function; the amniotic fluid volume helps measure long-term adequacy of placental function. The scoring for a complete profile is shown in Table 8.5. By this system, each item has the potential for scoring a 2, so 10 would be the highest score possible. A biophysical profile is more accurate in predicting fetal well-being than any single assessment (Alfirevic & Nielson, 2005). Because the scoring system is similar to that of the Apgar score determined at birth on infants, it is popularly called a fetal Apgar.

Biophysical profiles may be done as often as daily during a high-risk pregnancy. If the fetus score on a complete profile is 8 to 10, the fetus is considered to be doing well. A score of 6 is considered suspicious; a score of 4 denotes a fetus in jeopardy. More recently, some centers use only two assessments (amniotic fluid index and nonstress test) for assessment. Referred to as a modified biophysical profile, it predicts short-term viability by the nonstress test and long-term viability by the amniotic fluid index. Nurses play a large role in obtaining the information for both the modified and the full biophysical profile by obtaining either the nonstress test or the sonogram reading.

Checkpoint Question 5

Liz Calhorn is scheduled to have an amniocentesis to test for fetal maturity. What instruction would you give her before this procedure?

a. Void immediately before the procedure to reduce your bladder size.

b. The x-ray used to reveal your fetus' position has no long-term effects.

c. The intravenous fluid infused to dilate your uterus does not hurt the fetus.

d. No more amniotic fluid forms afterward, which is why only a small amount is removed.

Key Points

The union of a single sperm and egg (fertilization) signals the beginning of pregnancy.

The fertilized ovum (zygote) travels by way of a fallopian tube to the uterus, where implantation takes place in about 8 days. From implantation to 5 to 8 weeks, the growing structure is called an embryo.

TABLE 8.5

Biophysical Profile Scoring

Assessment	Instrument	Criteria for a Score of 2
Fetal breathing	Sonogram	At least one episode of 30 sec of sustained fetal breathing movements within 30 min of observation
Fetal movement	Sonogram	At least three separate episodes of fetal limb or trunk movement within a 30-min observation
Fetal tone	Sonogram	The fetus must extend and then flex the extremities or spine at least once in 30 min
Amniotic fluid volume	Sonogram	A pocket of amniotic fluid measuring more than 1 cm in vertical diameter must be present
Fetal heart reactivity	Nonstress test	Two or more fetal heart rate accelerations of at least 15 beats/min above baseline and of 15 sec duration occur with fetal movement over a 20-min time period

The period after 8 weeks until birth is the fetal period.

Growth of the umbilical cord, amniotic fluid, and amniotic membranes proceeds in concert with fetal growth. The placenta produces a number of important hormones: estrogen, progesterone, hPL, and hCG.

Various methods to assess fetal growth and development include fundal height, fetal movement, fetal heart tones, ultrasonography, MRI, MSAFP, amniocentesis, PUBS, amnioscopy, and fetoscopy.

A biophysical profile is a combination of fetal assessments that predicts fetal well-being better than single parameters do.

Critical Thinking Exercises

1. Liz Calhorn, whom you met at the beginning of the chapter, has stated that her feelings have changed since she felt her baby move inside her. How would you modify your health teaching with her because of this statement?

2. When Liz is scheduled for an ultrasound examination at 20 weeks' gestation, she tells you she doesn't want to know the sex of her fetus. Why do some women want to know this, whereas some do not? Is there an advantage to knowing or not knowing?

3. Late in pregnancy, Liz is scheduled for weekly non-stress tests. She invariably comes late for these tests because they are "time-consuming and boring." How could you make such tests more appealing to help increase her cooperation?

4. Examine the National Health Goals related to fetal growth and assessment. Most government-sponsored money for nursing research is allotted based on these goals. What would be a possible research topic to explore pertinent to these goals that would advance evidence-based practice in relation to Liz Calhorn or her family?

References

Ainsworth, S. B., & McCormack, K. (2004). Exogenous surfactant and neonatal lung disease: An update on the current situation. *Journal of Neonatal Nursing, 10*(1), 6–11.

Alfirevic, Z., & Neilson, J. P. (2005). Biophysical profile for fetal assessment in high risk pregnancies. *Cochrane Library (Oxford) (2)* (CD000038).

Bloom, S. L., & Leveno, K. J. (2004). Corticosteroid use in special circumstances: Preterm ruptured membranes, hypertension, fetal growth restriction, multiple fetuses. *Clinical Obstetrics and Gynecology, 46*(1), 150–160.

Bricker, L., & Neilson, J. P. (2005). Routine Doppler ultrasound in pregnancy. *Cochrane Library (Oxford) (2)* (CD001450).

Chen, W. A., et al. (2003). Alcohol and the developing brain: Neuroanatomical studies. *Alcohol Research and Health, 27*(2), 174–180.

Cortes, R. A., & Farmer, D. L. (2004). Recent advances in fetal surgery. *Seminars in Perinatology, 28*(3), 199–211.

Department of Health and Human Services. (2000). *Healthy people 2010.* Washington, D.C.: DHHS.

Doughty, D. (2004). Structure and function of the gastrointestinal tract in infants and children. *Journal of the Wound, Ostomy and Continence Nurses Society, 31*(4), 207–214.

Fischbach, F. T. (Ed.). (2004). *Manual of laboratory and diagnostic tests* (7th ed.). Philadelphia: Lippincott Williams & Wilkins.

Galan, H. L., & Hobbins, J. C. (2003). Intrauterine growth restriction. In Scott, J. R., et al. (Eds.), *Danforth's obstetrics and gynecology.* Philadelphia: Lippincott Williams & Wilkins.

Hallman, M. (2004). Lung surfactant, respiratory failure, and genes. *New England Journal of Medicine, 350*(13), 1278–1280.

Hochedlinger, K., & Jaenisch, R. (2003). Mechanisms of disease: Nuclear transplantation, embryonic stem cells, and the potential for cell therapy. *New England Journal of Medicine, 349*(3), 275–286.

Hofmeyr, G. J. (2005). Prophylactic versus therapeutic amnioinfusion for oligohydramnios in labour. *Cochrane Library (Oxford) (2)* (CD000176).

Johnson, M., Mass, M., & Moorhead, S. (2000). *Nursing outcomes classification* (2nd ed.). St. Louis: Mosby.

LaMar, K., & Hamernik, C. (2003). Life inside the womb: Implications for newborn and infant nurses. *Newborn and Infant Nursing Reviews, 3*(4), 136–142.

Lanza, R., & Rosenthal, N. (2004). The stem cell challenge. *Scientific American, 290*(6), 92–99.

Lipsky, S., et al. (2004). Police-reported intimate partner violence during pregnancy and the risk of antenatal hospitalization. *Maternal and Child Health Journal, 8*(2), 55–63.

Mazurek, P. (2004). Congenital heart defects in children. *Journal of Emergency Medical Service, 29*(2), 90–100.

McAllion, D. (2004). Fundal height measurement and low birth weight. *British Journal of Midwifery, 12*(2), 101–104.

McCloskey, J., & Bulechek, G. (2000). *Nursing interventions classification* (3rd ed.). St. Louis: Mosby.

Mitchell, L. M. (2004). Women's experiences of unexpected ultrasound findings. *Journal of Midwifery and Women's Health, 49*(3), 228–234.

Neilson, J. P., & Alfirevic, Z. (2005). Doppler ultrasound for fetal assessment in high risk pregnancies. *Cochrane Library (Oxford) (2)* (CD000073).

Nelson, K. H., & Nelson, L. H. (2003). Ultrasound in obstetrics. In Scott, J. R., et al. (Eds.), *Danforth's obstetrics and gynecology.* Philadelphia: Lippincott Williams & Wilkins.

Rados, C. (2004). FDA cautions against ultrasound "keepsake" images. *FDA Consumer, 38*(1), 12–16.

Spar, D. (2004). The business of stem cells. *New England Journal of Medicine, 351*(3), 211–213.

Speroff, L., & Fritz, M. A. (2005). *Clinical gynecologic endocrinology and infertility* (7th ed.). Philadelphia: Lippincott Williams & Wilkins.

Spong, C. Y. (2003). Fetal monitoring. In Scott, J. R., et al. (Eds.), *Danforth's obstetrics and gynecology.* Philadelphia: Lippincott Williams & Wilkins.

Stallard, T. C., & Burns, B. (2003). Emergency delivery and perimortem C-section. *Emergency Medicine Clinics of North America, 21*(3), 679–693.

Tan, K. H., & Smyth, R. (2005). Fetal vibroacoustic stimulation for facilitation of tests of fetal well-being. *Cochrane Library (Oxford) (2)* (CD002963).

Williams, T., Butler, R., & Sundem, T. (2003). Management of the infant with gastroschisis: A comprehensive review of the literature. *Newborn and Infant Nursing Reviews, 3*(2), 55–56.

Wilson, R. E., Krishnamurti, L., & Kamat, D. (2003). Management of sickle cell disease in primary care. *Clinical Pediatrics, 42*(9), 753–761.

Yankowitz, J. (2003). Drugs in pregnancy. In Scott, J. R., et al. (Eds.), *Danforth's obstetrics and gynecology*. Philadelphia: Lippincott Williams & Wilkins.

Suggested Readings

Alfirevic, Z., & Neilson, J. P. (2005). Biophysical profile for fetal assessment in high risk pregnancies. *Cochrane Library (Oxford) (2)* (CD000038).

Baston, H. (2003). Monitoring fetal well-being during routine antenatal care. *Practising Midwife, 6*(4), 29–33.

Bloom, K. C., et al. (2004). Barriers to prenatal care for homeless pregnant women. *JOGNN: Journal of Obstetric, Gynecologic, and Neonatal Nursing, 33*(4), 428–435.

Cortes, R. A., & Farmer, D. L. (2004). Recent advances in fetal surgery. *Seminars in Perinatology, 28*(3), 199–211.

Farmer, D. L., et al. (2003). In utero repair of myelomeningocele: Experimental pathophysiology, initial clinical experience, and outcomes. *Archives of Surgery, 138*(8), 872–878.

Kirschbaum, M. J. (2004). Gestational age/developmental guidelines tool. *Neonatal Network: Journal of Neonatal Nursing, 23*(2), 71–73.

Leviton, A., et al. (2005). The wealth of information conveyed by gestational age. *Journal of Pediatrics, 146*(1), 123–127.

Little, B. B., et al. (2003). Treatment of substance abuse during pregnancy and infant outcome. *American Journal of Perinatology, 20*(5), 255–262.

Lockwood, C. J. (2003). Testing for risk of preterm delivery. *Clinics in Laboratory Medicine, 23*(2), 345–360.

Porreco, R. P., et al. (2005). Expectation of pregnancy outcome among mature women. *American Journal of Obstetrics and Gynecology, 192*(1), 38–41.

Schwarz, U., & Galinkin, J. L. (2003). Anesthesia for fetal surgery. *Seminars in Pediatric Surgery, 12*(3), 196–201.

Smith, G. C. (2005). Estimating risks of perinatal death. *American Journal of Obstetrics and Gynecology, 192*(1), 17–22.

Stenhouse, E., et al. (2003). How well do midwives estimate the date of delivery? *Midwifery, 19*(2), 125–131.

Sydorak, R. M., & Harrison, M. R. (2003). Congenital diaphragmatic hernia: Advances in prenatal therapy. *Clinics in Perinatology, 30*(3), 465–479.

CHAPTER 9

Psychological and Physiologic Changes of Pregnancy

Key Terms

ballottement
Braxton Hicks contractions
Chadwick's sign
couvade syndrome
diastasis
Goodell's sign
Hegar's sign
hyperptyalism
melasma
Montgomery's tubercles
multipara
operculum
polyuria
positive signs of pregnancy
presumptive signs of
   pregnancy
primigravida
probable signs of pregnancy
pseudoanemia
striae gravidarum

Objectives

After mastering the contents of this chapter, you should be able to:

1. Describe common psychological and physiologic changes that occur with pregnancy, the underlying principles for these changes, and the relationship of the changes to pregnancy diagnosis.
2. Assess a woman for the psychological and physical changes that occur with pregnancy through health history and physical examination.
3. Formulate nursing diagnoses related to the psychological and physical changes of pregnancy.
4. Identify expected outcomes for a family's psychological and physical adaptation to pregnancy.
5. Plan nursing care related to the changes and diagnosis of pregnancy, such as helping a woman plan to get adequate rest.
6. Implement nursing care, such as health teaching related to the expected changes of pregnancy.
7. Evaluate outcome criteria for the achievement and effectiveness of care.
8. Identify National Health Goals that nurses can help the nation achieve.
9. Identify areas of nursing care related to the psychological and physiologic changes of pregnancy that could benefit from additional nursing research or application of evidence-based practice.
10. Use critical thinking to analyze how the physical and psychological changes of pregnancy affect family functioning, and develop ways to make nursing care more family-centered.
11. Integrate knowledge of the psychological and physiologic changes of pregnancy with nursing process to achieve quality maternal and child health nursing care.

Lauren Maxwell is a part-time model who has come to your clinic for her first prenatal visit. She tells you she missed her period 4 weeks ago and immediately took a home pregnancy test. She's excited that it was positive, because she and her husband have been trying for several months to get pregnant. She is also anxious: "I know there's no turning back now, but I wonder what this will do to my career," she tells you. She says that her husband, John, doesn't seem a bit scared: "I don't know if that's a good thing or not," she confides. She's also worried about being a good parent: "I'd die," she says, "if I turned into the same kind of parent my parents were."

In addition to the positive home pregnancy test, Lauren presents with amenorrhea, breast tenderness, fatigue, and morning sickness. Lauren is interested in knowing when she will begin to look pregnant and what she can do for the morning sickness.

Previous chapters discussed normal anatomy and physiology before pregnancy. This chapter adds information to your knowledge base about the physical and psychological changes that occur in both a woman and her partner during pregnancy. This is important information because it can help protect the health of both a woman and her fetus for the next 9 months.

What psychological development tasks of pregnancy will Lauren need to complete? What suggestions could you make to ease her worry about being a good parent?

After you've studied this chapter, access the accompanying website. Read the patient scenario and answer the questions to further sharpen your skills, grow more familiar with RN-CLEX types of questions, and reward yourself with how much you have learned.

Pregnancy brings both psychological and physical changes to a woman and her partner. Clients are often interested in learning more about the changes pregnancy brings, because these changes verify the reality and mark the progress of a pregnancy.

The physiologic changes of pregnancy occur gradually but eventually affect all organ systems of a woman's body. Changes are necessary to allow a woman to be able to provide oxygen and nutrients for her growing fetus, as well as extra nutrients for her own increased metabolism during the pregnancy. They also ready her body for labor and birth and for lactation once the baby is born. Although the physiologic changes that occur with pregnancy are extensive, women are usually happy to learn that they are also temporary: when pregnancy ends, the woman's body will return virtually to its prepregnant state. Psychological changes occur in response not only to the physiologic alterations that are occurring but also to the increased responsibility associated with welcoming a new and completely dependent person to the family.

Despite the magnitude of some of these changes, they are all extensions of normal physiology. This makes pregnancy represent a time of wellness, not illness. Because of this, the major responsibility of a nurse caring for a pregnant woman and family is to help the family maintain a state of wellness throughout the pregnancy and into early parenthood. A National Health Goal relevant to this issue is shown in Box 9.1.

Nursing Process Overview

For Healthy Adaptation to Pregnancy

● Assessment

Ideally, assessment for pregnancy begins before the pregnancy. During a preconception assessment, it is important to evaluate the woman's health status, nutritional intake (e.g., sufficient intake of folic acid), and lifestyle (e.g., drinking and smoking habits); identify any potential problems (e.g., potential for ectopic pregnancy resulting from tubal scarring); and identify the woman's understanding and expectations of conception, pregnancy, and parenthood.

In early pregnancy, be certain that you establish a trusting relationship with a woman so she will see you as a person who is capable of counseling her and helping her solve problems and in whom she is willing to confide. It is important to assess the woman's health and nutritional status, as well as the well-being of the fetus, throughout pregnancy. Document the woman's physiologic adaptations and the family's psychological adaptations to pregnancy, noting any abnormal findings. Physical findings are gained through the health history, physical assessment, and laboratory tests. Assessment in psychological areas is obtained primarily through interviewing and should include societal, cultural, family, and personal influences on the client's adaptation to pregnancy.

BOX 9.1 FOCUS ON . . .

NATIONAL HEALTH GOALS

At least one National Health Goal speaks directly to the physiologic and psychological changes of pregnancy:

- Increase to at least 60% the proportion of primary care providers who provide age-appropriate preconception care and counseling (DHHS, 2000).

Nurses can help the nation achieve this objective by being certain that adolescents receive counseling in nutrition and safer sex practices so they can enter intended pregnancies in good health. Nursing research to identify the best way to reach mature women with preconception counseling is also important.

● Nursing Diagnosis

Examples of nursing diagnoses involving the changes that occur with pregnancy include:

- Anxiety related to unexpected pregnancy
- Altered breathing pattern related to respiratory system changes of pregnancy
- Disturbed body image related to weight gain with pregnancy
- Deficient knowledge related to normal changes of pregnancy
- Imbalanced nutrition, less than body requirements, related to morning sickness

● Outcome Identification and Planning

Although a woman may have read pamphlets or talked to her friends about the physiologic changes of pregnancy, she is often surprised to see these changes occurring in herself. She may say, "I knew I'd be tired, but I never guessed it would be this bad," or "I've read about dark pigment forming on my abdomen, but is it normal for it to be this dark? Will this go away?"

Planning nursing care in connection with the physiologic and psychological changes of pregnancy should involve a plan to review these types of concerns with the woman as well as a plan to ask about the individual responses she is experiencing.

● Implementation

The changes of pregnancy may appear insignificant if taken one by one, but together they add up to major changes.

Most women of childbearing age have a mental picture of themselves or a good idea of how they will look in a dress before they try it on in a store. They participate in sports or other activities that conform to that self-image. Then, in 9 months, a woman gains 25 to 30 lb and her figure changes so drastically that none of her prepregnancy clothes any longer fit. At the beginning of pregnancy, she may feel constantly nauseated. Toward the end, the extra weight and the strain of waiting may make her feel tired and short of breath. Endocrine changes can make her feel moody and quick to cry.

She may never have been concerned with her health before; now, every month (and toward the end of pregnancy, every week), she reports to a health care provider for a prenatal checkup. She may worry that she will never lose all the weight she has gained, that the stretch marks on her abdomen will remain forever, and that she will always be as tired or as nauseated as she feels during various stages of her pregnancy.

Help women at prenatal visits to voice their concerns about either physiologic or psychological changes of pregnancy, so the worry brought on by these changes doesn't compound an already potentially stressful situation for her. She may need suggestions on exercise and nutrition to prepare for pregnancy and to follow during pregnancy. For many women, pregnancy is the first time they have seen a health care provider since childhood. Nursing interventions can be instrumental in not only guiding a woman safely through a pregnancy but also connecting her back with ongoing health care.

● *Outcome Evaluation*

Evaluation should determine whether the woman has really "heard" your teaching despite the stress of her pregnancy. People under stress do not always comprehend well, so it is not unusual for a woman to pocket away information, thinking, "I'll concentrate on what that means when it happens to me, not now." Then, when a particular change has happened, she realizes she has forgotten what you said. Evaluation that reveals learning did not take place confirms that pregnancy is a period of stress more often than it reflects the quality of teaching. Examples of outcome criteria you might strive for include:

- Client states she is able to continue her usual lifestyle throughout pregnancy.
- Family members describe ways they have adjusted their lifestyles to accommodate the mother's fatigue.
- Couple states they accept the physiologic changes of pregnancy as normal.

PSYCHOLOGICAL CHANGES OF PREGNANCY

Pregnancy is such a huge change in a woman's life that it brings about more psychological changes than any other life event besides puberty (Katz, 2003). A woman's attitude toward a pregnancy depends a great deal on psychological aspects such as the environment in which she was raised, the messages about pregnancy her family communicated to her as a child, the society and culture in which she lives as an adult, and whether the pregnancy has come at a good time in her life.

Social Influences

Until recently, the heavy emphasis on medical management for women during pregnancy conveyed the idea that pregnancy was a 9-month-long illness. The pregnant woman went alone to a physician's office for care; at the time of birth, she was separated from her family and admitted to a hospital. She was hospitalized in seclusion from visitors and even from the new baby for a week afterward.

Today, our society has come to view pregnancy as a time of health. Nurses have played an important role in helping to convince other health care providers that certain long-standing protocols that separated women from their families are no longer appropriate. As a result, instead of coming alone for prenatal care, women now bring their families. Instead of being given general anesthetics so they can "sleep through" labor and birth, they are urged to participate actively in the experience. The addition of birthing rooms and an emphasis on family-centered care have helped involve families, not just the woman, in childbirth.

The way a pregnant woman and her partner feel about pregnancy and childbirth may be affected by their cultural background, their personal experiences, and the experiences of friends and relatives, as well as by the current public philosophy of childbirth. People's opinions about adolescent pregnancies, "late in life" pregnancies, or lesbian pregnancies have changed markedly. By informing women about their new health care options and continuing to work with other health care providers to "demedicalize" childbirth, nurses can help make pregnancy and childbirth even more enjoyable for clients and their families.

Cultural Influences

A woman's cultural background may strongly influence how active a role she wants to take in her pregnancy, because certain beliefs and taboos may place restrictions on her behavior and activities (Andrews & Boyle, 2002). To learn about the beliefs of a particular woman and her partner, ask at prenatal visits if there is anything they believe should or should not be done to make the pregnancy successful and keep the baby healthy. Supporting these beliefs shows respect for the individuality of the woman and her knowledge of good health (Box 9.2).

BOX 9.2 FOCUS ON . . .

DIVERSITY OF CARE

Superstitions and Pregnancy

Before evidence-based practice was available to scientifically disprove or prove happenings in pregnancy, every culture circulated explanations about what people thought causes complications of pregnancy. Because these myths are well engrained in cultures, they persist. For example, beliefs that lifting your arms over your head during pregnancy will cause the cord to twist, or that watching a lunar eclipse will cause birth deformities, are typical of this type of myth. Listen to such "tall tales" to show respect for the person's beliefs, but encourage a woman to ask her health care provider to find out if there is any substance to them.

Family Influences

The family in which a woman was raised can be as influential to her beliefs about pregnancy as her cultural environment. If she and her siblings were loved and seen as the pleasant outcome of a happy marriage, she is more likely to have a positive attitude toward her pregnancy than if she and her siblings were seen as intruders or were blamed for the breakup of a marriage. No matter how often a woman is told that pregnancy is natural and simple, she will not be overjoyed to find herself pregnant if all she has heard are stories about excruciating pain and endless suffering in labor. If her mother constantly reminded her, "If you hadn't come along, I could have gone to college" or "I could have had a career," the daughter may view pregnancy as a disaster.

"People love as they have been loved" is said so often it has become a cliché. It is highly relevant, however, to whether pregnancy and childbirth will be viewed in a positive or a negative light. If a woman has had difficulty loving others because she has not received love, she may worry that she will have difficulty loving and accepting the fetus growing within her. To mother her baby well, she should be able to feel a pleasurable anticipation at the prospect of rearing a child; becoming a mother is a second adjustment above and beyond being pregnant. The woman who views mothering as a positive activity is more likely to be pleased when she becomes pregnant than one who devalues mothering (Jaccard et al., 2003).

Individual Influences

A woman's ability to cope with or adapt to stress plays a major role in how she will resolve conflict and adapt to the new life contingencies that are coming. This ability to adapt—to being a mother without needing mothering, to loving a child as well as a husband, to becoming a mother of each new child—depends, in part, on her basic temperament, on whether she adapts to new situations quickly or slowly, whether she faces them with intensity or maintains a low-key approach, and whether she has had experiences coping with change and stress.

The extent to which a woman feels secure in her relationship with the people around her, especially the father of her child, is usually also important to her acceptance of a pregnancy. Acceptance is usually easier if she has confidence in the stability of her relationship with the child's father and knows that he will be there to give her emotional support. Worrying whether her partner may soon disappear, leaving her alone to raise the child, may make her reexamine whether the pregnancy is a wise life step.

A woman who thinks of brides as young but mothers as old may believe pregnancy will rob her of her youth. If she thinks children are sticky-fingered and time-consuming, she may view the pregnancy as taking away her freedom. If she has heard that pregnancy will permanently stretch her abdomen and breasts, her concern may be that she will lose her looks. She may feel that pregnancy will rob her financially and ruin her chances of job promotion. These are real feelings and must be taken seriously when counseling pregnant women. Such concerns cannot be shrugged off with simple clichés ("One door closes, another one opens") or with repression ("You shouldn't think that way; you'll love having a baby in the house"). The woman needs an opportunity to express these feelings and become aware of their intensity to resolve them. Women who do not have a supportive partner need to locate a support person during pregnancy. Often this is another woman who relates to the wonder and excitement of pregnancy and birth. In many instances, it is a health care provider.

Whether the father of the child is able to accept the pregnancy and the coming child depends on the same factors that affect the woman: cultural background, past experience, and relationship with family members. If he was raised to believe that men should not show their emotions, he may not be able to say easily, "I want this baby" or "I'm glad" when his partner tells him of the positive diagnosis. He may not be able to say such things as, "It's great to feel it kick."

Although men may be inarticulate in these ways, they may be able to convey such emotions by a touch or a caress, one reason men's presence is always desirable at a prenatal visit and certainly in the birthing room. Their partner will know that a hand on hers is as meaningful an expression of emotion as a spoken word.

THE PSYCHOLOGICAL TASKS OF PREGNANCY

During the 9 months of pregnancy, a woman and her partner run a gamut of emotions ranging from surprise at finding out the woman is pregnant (or wishing she were not) to pleasure and acceptance of the fact as they begin to identify with the coming child, to worry for themselves and the child, to impatience near the end of pregnancy (Table 9.1). Once the child is born, the woman and her partner may feel surprised again that the pregnancy is over and that the mother has really given birth.

From a physiologic standpoint, it is fortunate that a pregnancy is 9 months long, because this gives the fetus time to mature and be prepared for life outside the protective uterine environment. From a psychological standpoint, the 9-month period is fortunate for the family as well, because it gives them time to prepare emotionally as well. These psychological changes are frequently termed "guaranteeing safe passage" for the fetus. How well a woman adjusts to the potential stress of pregnancy can affect her relationship with the child and may even influence whether she is able to carry the pregnancy to term (Box 9.3).

First Trimester: Accepting the Pregnancy

The Woman

The task of women during the first trimester is to accept the reality of the pregnancy. Most cultures structure their celebrations around important life events. Coming of age, marriages, birthdays, and deaths all have rituals to help individuals take a step forward or accept the coming change in their lives. A diagnosis of pregnancy is a similar rite of passage. This aura of initiation into one of the large

TABLE 9.1

Common Psychosocial Changes That Occur With Pregnancy

Psychosocial Change	Description
First Trimester	
Task: Accepting the pregnancy	Woman and partner both spend time recovering from shock of learning they are pregnant and concentrate on what it feels like to be pregnant. A common reaction is ambivalence, or feeling both pleased and not pleased about the pregnancy.
Second Trimester	
Task: Accepting the baby	Woman and partner move through emotions such as narcissism and introversion as they concentrate on what it will feel like to be a parent. Role-playing and increased dreaming are common.
Third Trimester	
Task: Preparing for the baby and end of pregnancy	Woman and partner grow impatient with pregnancy as they ready themselves for birth.

mysteries of life gives special meaning to the health care visit in which the diagnosis of pregnancy is confirmed, making it more than an ordinary visit to a health care facility. Receiving confirmation of pregnancy at a health care provider's office makes a woman feel "more pregnant."

BOX 9.3 FOCUS ON . . .

EVIDENCE-BASED PRACTICE

Can psychological factors affect pregnancy outcome?

To answer this question, nurse researchers followed 120 pregnant women from three clinic populations in rural Appalachia during their 16th to 28th weeks of pregnancy. They found that women with symptoms of depression, low levels of self-esteem, or a negative perception of pregnancy had significantly higher odds of delivering a preterm baby. Further investigation is necessary to reveal the mechanism by which these psychological factors cause early birth, but the findings suggest that women who respond this way to pregnancy may not eat as well or in other ways "protect" their pregnancies.

This is an important study for nurses, because nurses are often the health care providers who take initial health histories, so they are the first people who can detect if a woman is depressed or not feeling good about her pregnancy.

Source: Jesse, D. E., Seaver, W., & Wallace, D. C. (2003). Maternal psychosocial risks predict preterm birth in a group of women from Appalachia. *Midwifery, 19*(3), 191–202.

The availability of family planning measures today, in theory, would seem to prevent the diagnosis of pregnancy from being a surprise. In reality, as many as 50% of pregnancies are still unintended, unwanted, or mistimed (DHHS, 2000). Because no woman can be absolutely confident in advance that she will be able to conceive until it happens, every pregnancy is a surprise to some extent, either because the woman had not planned on becoming pregnant, or because she had been looking forward to being pregnant but cannot believe it has happened so quickly. If pregnancy announced itself with more reliable signs than a missed period, slight breast tenderness, or vague nausea and tiredness, women could become more certain how they feel about being pregnant sooner. Home pregnancy test kits have helped women in this regard by confirming pregnancy early on. Until it is verified by a home test or a health care visit, however, the uncertainty of the symptoms makes pregnancy a vague theoretical possibility and leaves room for denial.

Often women immediately experience something less than pleasure and closer to disappointment or anxiety at the news that they are pregnant. This emotional response of ambivalence is further discussed later in this chapter. Fortunately, most women are able to change their attitude toward the pregnancy by the time they feel the child move inside them. Some health care plans provide for a routine sonogram at 4 months of pregnancy. Seeing a fetal outline on the monitor screen during a sonogram can be a major step in promoting acceptance (Chervenak & McCullough, 2005).

The Partner

Once partners were forgotten in the childbearing process (Daniel, 2004). Unwed fathers, in particular, were often dismissed as not interested in the pregnancy or the woman's health. A lesbian partner was completely ignored. It is recognized today that all partners have an important role and should be encouraged to have an emotional interest in the pregnancy. This means that, as a woman adapts to pregnancy, her partner may go through some of the same psychological changes.

For partners, accepting the pregnancy means not only accepting the certainty of the pregnancy and the reality of the child to come but also accepting the woman in her changed state. A partner should try to give the woman emotional support while she is learning to accept the reality of pregnancy, and she should reciprocate when the partner begins to go through the process.

Like women, partners' feelings regarding the pregnancy vary. Often partners are proud and happy about the pregnancy, facilitating acceptance of it. However, partners may experience some feelings that make this task more difficult. It is not unusual for a partner to feel both overwhelmed with what the loss of the woman's salary will mean to the family, if she means to quit work, and somewhat jealous of the growing baby, who, although not yet physically apparent, seems to be taking up a great deal of the woman's time and thought.

An unwed father may have a great deal of difficulty accepting a pregnancy unless he is actively involved in prenatal care. He tries to picture himself as a father but

reason for these changes to allow a woman to accept them without worrying.

Cardiovascular System

Changes in the circulatory system are extremely significant to the health of the fetus, because they are necessary for adequate placental and fetal circulation. Table 9.5 summarizes these changes.

Blood Volume. To provide for an adequate exchange of nutrients in the placenta and to provide adequate blood to compensate for blood loss at birth, the total circulatory blood volume of the woman's body increases by at least 30% (and possibly as much as 50%) during pregnancy. Blood loss at a normal vaginal birth is about 300 to 400 mL; blood loss from a cesarean birth can be as high as 800 to 1,000 mL. The increase in blood volume occurs gradually, beginning at the end of the first trimester. It peaks at about the 28th to the 32nd week and then continues at this high level throughout the third trimester. Because the plasma volume increases faster than red blood cell production does, the concentration of hemoglobin and erythrocytes may decline, giving the woman a **pseudoanemia** early in pregnancy. The woman's body compensates for this change by producing more red blood cells, creating near-normal levels of red blood cells again by the second trimester.

Iron Needs. Almost all women need some iron supplementation during pregnancy because of a variety of factors. The fetus requires a total of about 350 to 400 mg of iron to grow. The increases in the mother's circulatory red blood cell mass require an additional 400 mg of iron. This is a total increased need of about 800 mg. Because the average woman's store of iron is less than this amount (about 500 mg), and because iron absorption may be impaired during pregnancy as a result of decreased gastric acidity (iron is absorbed best from an acid medium), additional iron is often prescribed during pregnancy to prevent a true anemia.

Either a hemoglobin concentration of less than 11.5 g/100 mL or a hematocrit value below 30% is considered true anemia, for which iron therapy above normal supplementation is advocated. (See Chapter 14 for additional information on anemia in pregnancy.) The need for folic acid increases even more during pregnancy; if the intake of folic acid is not great enough, megalohemoglobinemia (large, nonfunctioning red blood cells) will result. Inadequate folic acid levels have also been linked to an increased risk for neural tube disorders in fetuses. Women should be certain to eat foods that are high in folic acid (e.g., spinach, asparagus, legumes), both during the prepregnancy period and during pregnancy. Prenatal vitamins that contain folic acid are routinely prescribed (de Jong-Van den Berg et al., 2005).

Heart. To handle the increase in blood volume in the circulatory system, a woman's cardiac output increases significantly, by 25% to 50%; the heart rate increases by 10 beats per minute. Like the circulating volume increase, the bulk of the cardiac work increase occurs during the second trimester, with a small increase in the third trimester. The average woman is unaware of the significant circulatory system changes that are occurring inside her to supply adequate blood to the placenta. However, this rise in circulating load has implications for the woman with cardiac disease. Although the average woman's heart is able to adjust to these changes readily, a woman whose heart has difficulty handling her normal circulating load can be overwhelmed by the requirements placed on it when she is pregnant.

Because the diaphragm is pushed upward by the growing uterus late in pregnancy, the heart is shifted to a more transverse position in the chest cavity, a position that may make it appear enlarged on x-ray examination. Some women have audible functional (innocent) heart murmurs during pregnancy, probably because of the altered heart position.

Palpitations of the heart are not uncommon during pregnancy, particularly on quick motion. You can caution women not to feel frightened if palpitations do occur. Palpitations in the early months of pregnancy are probably caused by sympathetic nervous system stimulation; in later months, they may result from increased thoracic pressure caused by the pressure of the uterus against the diaphragm.

Blood Pressure. Despite the hypervolemia of pregnancy, the blood pressure does not normally rise because the increased heart action takes care of the greater amount of circulating blood. Average blood pressures for adult women are shown in Appendix G.

TABLE 9.5

Changes in the Cardiovascular System During Pregnancy

Assessment Factor	Prepregnancy	Pregnancy
Cardiac output		25%–50% increase
Heart rate (bpm)	70–80	80–90
Plasma volume (mL)	2,600	3,600
Blood volume (mL)	4,000	5,250
Red blood cell mass (mm^3)	4,200,000	4,650,000
Leukocytes (mm^3)	7,000	20,500
Total protein (g/dL)	7.0	5.5–6.0
Fibrinogen (mg/dL)	300	450
Blood pressure		Decreases in 2nd trimester, at prepregnancy level in 3rd trimester

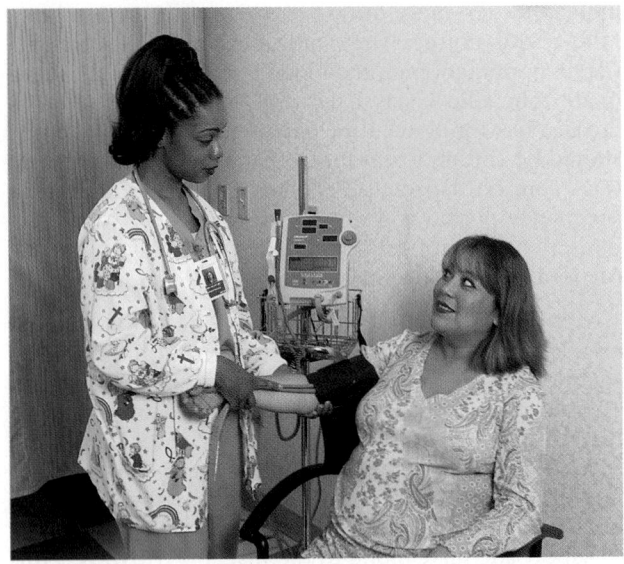

FIGURE 9.7 Blood pressure determination is an important assessment during pregnancy; normally, blood pressure does not elevate during pregnancy.

In most women, blood pressure actually decreases slightly during the second trimester because the peripheral resistance to circulation is lowered as the placenta expands rapidly. During the third trimester, the blood pressure rises again to first-trimester levels (Fig. 9.7).

Peripheral Blood Flow. During the third trimester of pregnancy, blood flow to the lower extremities is impaired by the pressure of the expanding uterus on veins and arteries. This decrease in blood flow in the venous system can lead to edema and varicosities of the vulva, rectum, and legs.

Supine Hypotension Syndrome. When a pregnant woman lies supine, the weight of the growing uterus presses the vena cava against the vertebrae, obstructing blood flow from the lower extremities. This causes a decrease in blood return to the heart and, consequently, decreased cardiac output and hypotension (Fig. 9.8). This maternal hypotension is potentially dangerous because it can cause fetal hypoxia. A woman experiences this hypotension as lightheadedness, faintness, and palpitations (Katz, 2003).

Supine hypotension syndrome can easily be corrected by having the woman turn onto her side (preferably the left side), so that blood flow through the vena cava increases again. To lessen the possibility of occurrence of this phenomenon, women develop an increase in collateral blood circulation during pregnancy. Teach women always to rest on the left side rather than the back, because even with additional collateral circulation, a supine position tends to lead to hypotension.

Blood Constitution. The level of circulating fibrinogen, a constituent of the blood that is necessary for clotting, increases as much as 50% during pregnancy, probably because of the increased level of estrogen. Other clotting factors, such as factors VII, VIII, IX, and X, and the platelet count also increase. These increases are a safeguard against major bleeding should the placenta be dislodged and the uterine arteries or veins be opened. Total white blood cell count rises slightly, both as a protective mechanism and as a reflection of the woman's total blood volume (up to about 20,000 cells/mm^3). The total protein level of blood decreases, perhaps indicating the amount of protein being used by the fetus. Because the circulating system has a lower total protein load and hypervolemia, fluid readily leaves the blood vessels to equalize osmotic and hydrostatic pressure. This causes the common ankle and foot edema of pregnancy (not to be confused with nondependent or generalized edema, which is a symptom of pregnancy-induced hypertension).

Blood lipids increase by one third, and the cholesterol serum level increases by 90% to 100%. These increases provide a ready supply of available energy for the fetus.

What if... Lauren Maxwell, the woman you met at the beginning of this chapter, stated that some of her concerns were morning sickness and fatigue. What if you discovered she was homeless? Would your advice for her be any different?

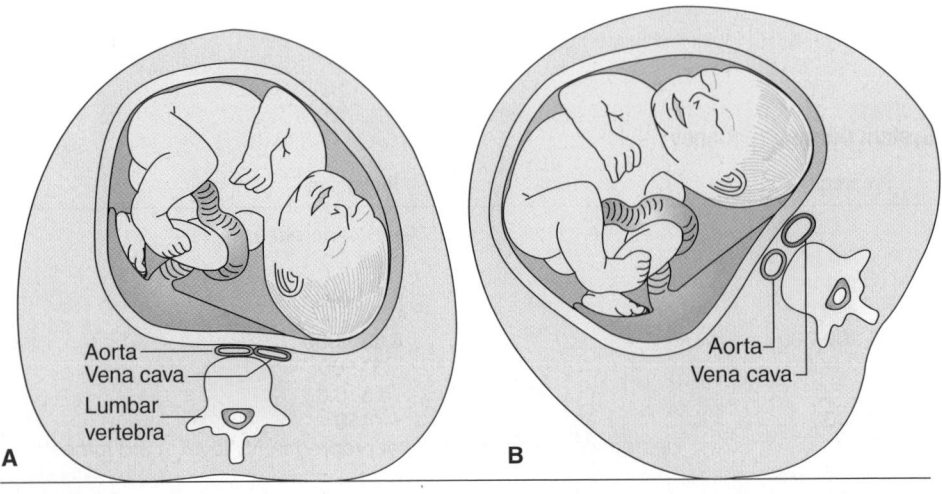

FIGURE 9.8 Supine hypotension can occur if a pregnant woman lies on her back. (**A**) The weight of the uterus compresses the vena cava, trapping blood in the lower extremities. (**B**) If a woman turns on her side, pressure is lifted off of the vena cava.

Gastrointestinal System

As the uterus increases in size, it tends to push the stomach and intestines toward the back and sides of the abdomen. At about the midpoint of pregnancy, this pressure may be sufficient to slow intestinal peristalsis and the emptying time of the stomach, leading to heartburn, constipation, and flatulence. Pressure from the uterus on veins returning from the lower extremities can lead to hemorrhoids (Tiran, 2003). Relaxin, a hormone produced by the ovary, may contribute to decreased gastric motility; this natural slowing is helpful, because the blood supply may be reduced to the gastrointestinal tract (i.e., blood is drawn to the uterus). Progesterone also has an effect on smooth muscle, such as that in the intestine, making it less active.

At least 50% of women experience some nausea and vomiting early in pregnancy. This is one of the first sensations a woman may experience with pregnancy (sometimes it is noticed even before the first missed menstrual period). It is most apparent early in the morning, on rising, or if the woman becomes fatigued during the day. It is more frequent in women who smoke cigarettes. Known as morning sickness, nausea and vomiting begin to be noticed at the same time levels of hCG and progesterone begin to rise. Sickness may occur as a systemic reaction to increased estrogen levels or decreased glucose levels, because glucose is being used in such great quantities by the growing fetus (Box 9.9). Many alternate or complementary methods to help reduce nausea with pregnancy are available (Cummings, 2004). These are discussed in Chapter 12.

This common feeling of nausea usually subsides after the first 3 months, after which time the woman may have a voracious appetite. Although the acidity of stomach

---

BOX 9.9: Focus on Nursing Care Planning

A Multidisciplinary Care Map for A Woman Experiencing a First Pregnancy

●

Lauren Maxwell is a part-time model who has come to your clinic for her first prenatal visit. She tells you she missed her period 4 weeks ago and immediately took a home pregnancy test. She's excited that it was positive, because she and her husband have been trying for several months to get pregnant. She tells you she is also anxious. She says that her husband, John, doesn't seem a bit scared: "I don't know if that's a good thing or not," she confides. She's also worried about being a good parent: "I'd die," she says, "if I turned into the same kind of parent my parents were."

Family Assessment

The Maxwells have been married for 3½ years. They live in student housing next to the university campus. Husband, John, works as a chef in nearby Italian restaurant. Client, Lauren, works part time as a model while she attends cooking school. Finances are listed as "tight" but "okay."

Client Assessment

Lauren presents with amenorrhea, breast tenderness, fatigue, and morning sickness. She is interested in when she will begin to look pregnant and what she can do for the morning sickness (she has eaten almost nothing for 2 days).

Nursing Diagnoses

Altered nutrition pattern related to nausea of early pregnancy
Anxiety related to pregnancy and becoming a parent

Outcome Criteria

Client states that she is able to eat at least one full meal a day even in light of nausea; names two complementary therapies she is using to decrease nausea; states that she is managing anxiety by self-help measures, with support from significant others.

(continued)

Team Member Responsible	Assessment	Intervention	Rationale	Expected Outcome
Activities of Daily Living				
Nurse	Determine whether client is able to carry out usual activities (attending work, school, keeping house) by obtaining a health history.	Work with client to see if modifications (going to work later, giving more home responsibility to husband) will help alleviate symptoms.	Documenting whether client can complete normal activities helps to document extent of concerns.	Client reports that she is able to attend school and work part time as long into pregnancy as she desires.
Consultations				
Nurse	Assess if client needs additional suggestions from team expert for dealing with nausea.	Consult with nutritionist if nausea still interferes with eating by 1 week's time.	Nausea in early pregnancy can become extreme if not recognized as potentially serious in early pregnancy.	Client meets with nutritionist if she still describes incapacitating nausea at 1 week telephone follow-up.
Procedures/Medications				
Physician/ Nurse midwife	Assess whether client would like to try a complementary therapy, such as ginger before meals.	Review pros and cons of any alternative therapy chosen by client.	Many alternative therapies are effective at reducing symptoms of nausea during pregnancy.	Client states she is using at least one alternative therapy by 1 week follow-up telephone call.
Nutrition				
Nurse/Team nutritionist	Ask client to list 24-hour recall nutrition history.	Examine 24-hour recall history and analyze for nutrition deficits. Make suggestions for better intake.	Documenting the problem best identifies its extent.	Client gives 24-hour recall history and helps determine any nutritional deficits and possible solutions.
Nurse	Assess whether client feels that anxiety or worry over gaining weight is adding to her nausea.	Discuss with client that anxiety can add to nausea; weight gained during pregnancy can be lost after pregnancy.	Identifying the cause of anxiety is the first step in determining how to best relieve it.	Client states that she recognizes anxiety is normal for her situation. No longer anxious about pregnancy weight gain.
Patient/Family Education				
Nurse	Determine whether client is aware that nausea is a common, normal sign of pregnancy.	Provide clinic pamphlet, *So You're Pregnant,* to client and discuss early symptoms of pregnancy.	Recognizing that a symptom is normal helps client to accept discomfort.	Client reports at 1 week follow-up phone call that she recognizes nausea as part of early pregnancy.
Nurse	Ask if client is aware that anxiety is a common response to pregnancy diagnosis.	Discuss with client how she normally manages anxiety. Offer suggestions as necessary.	Mild anxiety responds to many self-help measures, such as meditation or quiet reflection.	Client reports that she is managing anxiety by suggested self-help measures.
Psychosocial/Spiritual/Emotional Needs				
Nurse	Determine whether client feels it would be helpful for nurse to meet with husband.	If desired, schedule a time to meet with husband to explain early pregnancy symptoms.	Significant others may be unable to give support if they are not well informed.	Client asks for help as needed by 1 week follow-up phone call.

(continued)

Team Member Responsible	Assessment	Intervention	Rationale	Expected Outcome
Psychosocial/Spiritual/Emotional Needs				
Nurse	Assess if client is concerned that differences in husband's and her feelings toward pregnancy will interfere with their relationship.	Urge client to discuss pregnancy fears with husband.	Differences in reactions to pregnancy can potentially interfere with degree of support from significant other.	Client says she has discussed her fears with her husband and will continue to do so as pregnancy progresses.
Discharge Planning				
Nurse	Assess if client has any further questions before she leaves the clinic.	Meet with client after physical examination to be certain all her questions have been answered.	Unanswered questions can lead to increased anxiety over coming weeks.	Client confirms that her questions have been answered; has telephone number for clinic if further concerns arise.

secretions decreases during pregnancy, heartburn may result from reflux of stomach contents into the esophagus, caused by upward displacement of the stomach by the uterus, and a relaxed cardioesophageal sphincter, caused by the action of relaxin. Interventions for heartburn are also discussed in Chapter 12.

Women with chronic gastric reflux usually find their condition improved during pregnancy because the acidity of the stomach is decreased. Due to the gradual slowing of the gastrointestinal tract, decreased emptying of bile from the gallbladder may result. This can lead to reabsorption of bilirubin into the maternal bloodstream, giving rise to a symptom of generalized itching (subclinical jaundice). A woman who has had gallstones may have an increased tendency to stone formation during pregnancy as a result of the increased plasma cholesterol level and additional cholesterol incorporated in bile.

Some pregnant women notice hypertrophy at their gumlines and bleeding of gingival tissue when they brush their teeth. There may be increased saliva formation (**hyperptyalism**), probably as a local response to increased levels of estrogen. This is an annoying but not serious problem. A lower than normal pH of saliva may lead to increased tooth decay if tooth brushing is not done conscientiously. This can be a problem for homeless women or any other women who do not have frequent access to a place to brush their teeth.

Urinary System

Like other systems, the urinary system undergoes many physiologic changes during pregnancy. These include alterations in fluid retention and renal, ureter, and bladder function. Changes in the urinary system are summarized in Table 9.6. These changes result from the following:

- Effects of high estrogen and progesterone levels
- Compression of the bladder and ureters by the growing uterus
- Increased blood volume
- Postural influences

Fluid Retention. To provide sufficient fluid volume for effective placental exchange, total body water increases to 7.5 L; this requires the body to increase its sodium reabsorption in the tubules to maintain osmolarity. Under the influence of progesterone, there is an increased response of the angiotensin-renin system in the kidney, which leads to an increase in aldosterone production. Aldosterone aids sodium reabsorption. Progesterone appears to be potassium-sparing, so that even with an increased urine output, potassium levels remain adequate.

Water is retained during pregnancy to aid the increase in blood volume and to serve as a ready source of nutrients to the fetus. Because nutrients can pass to the fetus only when dissolved in or carried by fluid, this ready fluid supply is a fetal safeguard.

At one time, pregnant women were administered diuretics to help clear this excess fluid from their system.

TABLE 9.6

Urinary Tract Changes During Pregnancy

Variable	Change
Glomerular filtration rate	Increased by 50%
Renal plasma flow	Increased by 25%–80%
Blood urea nitrogen	Decreased by 25%
Plasma creatinine level	Decreased by 25%
Renal threshold for sugar	Decreased to allow slight spillage
Bladder capacity	Increased by 1,000 mL
Diameter of ureters	Increased by 25%
Frequency of urination	Increased 1st trimester, last 2 weeks of pregnancy to 10–12 times/day

A sodium-restricted diet was also recommended. Today, it is recognized that these practices are actually harmful, because the increased fluid volume provides physiologic benefits for the fetus. In addition, the excess fluid can serve to replenish the mother's own blood volume, should hemorrhage occur.

Renal Function. During pregnancy, a woman's kidneys must excrete not only the waste products of her body but also those of the growing fetus. Also, her kidneys must be able to excrete additional fluid and manage the demands of increased renal blood flow. The kidneys may increase in size, changing their structure and ultimately affecting their function.

During pregnancy, urinary output gradually increases (by about 60% to 80%). The specific gravity decreases. The glomerular filtration rate (GFR) and renal plasma flow begin to increase in early pregnancy to meet the increased needs of the circulatory system. By the second trimester, both the GFR and the renal plasma flow have increased by 30% to 50%, and they remain at these levels for the duration of the pregnancy. This rise is consistent with that of the circulatory system increase, peaking at about 24 weeks. This efficient GFR level leads to a lowered blood urea nitrogen (BUN) and low creatinine levels in maternal plasma. A BUN of 15 mg/100 mL or higher or a serum creatinine concentration greater than 1 mg/100 mL are considered abnormal and reflect the kidney's difficulty in handling the increased blood load. The higher GFR leads to increased filtration of glucose into the renal tubules. Because reabsorption of glucose by the tubule cells occurs at a fixed rate, there will be some accidental spilling of glucose into the urine during pregnancy. Lactose, which is being produced by the mammary glands but is not used during pregnancy, will also be spilled into the urine. Although minimal spilling of glucose into the urine may occur, the finding of more than a trace of glucose in a routine sample of urine from a pregnant woman is considered abnormal until proven otherwise, because this can be a sign of gestational diabetes (see Chapter 14).

Creatinine clearance has become the standard test for renal function during pregnancy, because creatinine is cleared from the body at a steady rate in relation to GFR. A normal pregnancy value is 90 to 180 mL/min. This is analyzed from a 24-hour urine sample.

Ureter and Bladder Function. A pregnant woman may notice an increase in urinary frequency during the first 3 months of pregnancy, until the uterus rises out of the pelvis and relieves pressure on the bladder. Frequency of urination may return at the end of pregnancy, as lightening occurs and the fetal head exerts renewed pressure on the bladder.

Because of the increased level of progesterone during pregnancy, the ureters increase in diameter and the bladder capacity increases to about 1,500 mL. The uterus tends to rise on the right side of the abdomen because it is pushed slightly in that direction by the greater bulk of the sigmoid colon. As a result, pressure on the right ureter may lead to urinary stasis and pyelonephritis if not relieved (August & Lindheimer, 2005). Pressure on the urethra may lead to poor bladder emptying and bladder infection. Such infections are potentially dangerous to the

pregnant woman, because they can ascend to become kidney infections. They are potentially dangerous to the fetus, because urinary tract infections are associated with preterm labor.

Skeletal System

Calcium and phosphorus needs are increased during pregnancy, because the fetal skeleton must be built. As pregnancy advances, there is a gradual softening of the woman's pelvic ligaments and joints to create pliability and to facilitate passage of the baby through the pelvis at birth. This softening is probably caused by the influence of both the ovarian hormone relaxin and placental progesterone. Excessive mobility of the joints can cause discomfort. A wide separation of the symphysis pubis, as much as 3 to 4 mm by 32 weeks of pregnancy, may occur. This makes women walk with difficulty because of pain.

To change her center of gravity and make ambulation easier, a pregnant woman tends to stand straighter and taller than usual. This stance is sometimes referred to as the "pride of pregnancy." Standing this way, with the shoulders back and the abdomen forward, creates a lordosis (forward curve of the lumbar spine), which may lead to backache (Box 9.10).

Endocrine System

Almost all aspects of the endocrine system increase during pregnancy (Table 9.7).

Placenta. The most striking change in the endocrine system during pregnancy is the addition of the placenta as an

---

BOX 9.10 FOCUS ON . . .

FAMILY TEACHING

Backache During Pregnancy

Q. You notice Lauren Maxwell rubbing her back at a prenatal visit. She asks you how she can keep her backache from becoming worse.

A. Backache is a common symptom of pregnancy because of the strain the extra uterine weight puts on lower vertebrae. It may be serious if
- It is experienced as waves of pain (could be preterm labor).
- There are accompanying urinary symptoms, such as frequency and pain on urination (could be a urinary tract infection).
- The back is tender at the point of backache (could be pyelonephritis or a kidney infection).
- Rest doesn't relieve it (could be a muscle strain).

Measures to relieve backache in pregnancy are
- Limit the use of high heels, because they add to the natural lordosis of pregnancy.
- Try to rest daily with feet elevated.
- Walk with head high, pelvis straight.
- Pelvic rocking at the end of the day may relieve pain for the night.

Prenatal care, essential for ensuring the overall health of newborns and their mothers, is a major strategy for helping to reduce the number of low-birthweight babies born yearly (Wessel, Endrikat, & Buscher, 2003). It is seen as so important that a number of National Health Goals speak directly to it (Box 10.1). Ideally, prenatal care begins during the mother's childhood. It includes balanced nutrition with adequate intake of calcium and vitamin D during infancy and childhood to prevent rickets (which can distort pelvic size); adequate immunizations against contagious diseases for protection against viral diseases such as rubella during pregnancy; and a healthy daily diet to ensure the best state of health possible for a woman and her partner when entering pregnancy.

Promoting prenatal health also includes developing positive attitudes about sexuality, womanhood, and childbearing. Once a woman becomes sexually active, preparation for a successful pregnancy includes practicing safer sex, regular pelvic examinations, and prompt treatment of any sexually transmitted infection to prevent complications that could lead to infertility. Acquisition and use of reproductive life planning information may help to ensure that each pregnancy is planned.

Women who maintain a healthy lifestyle come to a first prenatal visit prepared to follow health-promotion strategies. For many women, this visit may be the first time they have been to a health care facility since the routine health maintenance visits of childhood. It also may be the first time they have had an appointment that focuses more on health promotion than on the diagnosis of disease. A woman may have a specific reason (her agenda) for coming to the first prenatal visit (e.g., to confirm the diagnosis of pregnancy). A prenatal visit is also a time for additional health promotion, pregnancy education, and development of a positive pattern of healthy behaviors for the family to use in the future (your agenda). What and how much is needed varies depending on the age and parity of the woman and her degree of family support.

BOX 10.1 FOCUS ON . . .

NATIONAL HEALTH GOALS

A number of National Health Goals speak directly to the importance of prenatal care:

- Increase to at least 80% the proportion of primary care providers who provide age-appropriate preconception care and counseling.
- Increase to at least 90% the proportion of all pregnant women who receive prenatal care in the first trimester of pregnancy from a baseline of 76% (DHHS, 2000).

Nurses can help the nation to achieve these goals by educating women and their families about the importance of prenatal care and by making sites of prenatal care receptive to women and families. Additional nursing research to investigate ways to promote prenatal care or to enlarge the scope of nursing involvement in prenatal care would be important to help the nation meet these goals.

Nursing Process Overview

For Prenatal Care

● Assessment

The first prenatal visit is a time to establish baseline data relevant to health assessment and planning health-promotion strategies now and with every subsequent visit. Explaining why specific assessment data are relevant to the pregnancy may be the first step in this process. For instance, when weighing a woman, discussing what routine weight gain is to be expected in the next few months supplies important information while showing that weight measurement is an important routine procedure. Relating assessment information and health-promotion activities throughout the pregnancy helps keep the woman and her family well informed and eager to comply with further health care recommendations. Obtaining a health history, including screening for the presence of teratogens (any factor that may adversely affect the fetus) and any problems the woman may be experiencing, is important initially and at subsequent visits.

● Nursing Diagnosis

Although most women probably have used a home pregnancy detection kit to find out if they are pregnant, the first prenatal visit officially serves to confirm this, so nursing diagnoses may focus on the response of the woman and her family to that information. For example:

- Decisional conflict related to desire to be pregnant
- Risk for ineffective coping related to confirmation of unplanned pregnancy

Nursing diagnoses appropriate to prenatal care in general include:

- Health-seeking behaviors related to guidelines for nutrition and activity during pregnancy
- Deficient knowledge regarding exposure to teratogens during pregnancy
- Risk for injury to fetus related to current lifestyle behaviors

● Outcome Identification and Planning

Sufficient time should be reserved at prenatal visits so they can be thorough, allowing enough time to set realistic goals and expected outcomes with both the woman and her partner, if desired. Make sure that a woman leaving an initial prenatal visit schedules an appointment for a following visit, as this may not occur to a woman who may be excited or overwhelmed by all the new things that are happening to her and her family. Establishing a pattern of regular appointments is crucial to providing effective prenatal care. Although many settings are looking at whether the number of prenatal visits traditionally scheduled is needed during a normal pregnancy, return appointments are usually scheduled every 4 weeks through the 28th week of pregnancy, every 2 weeks through the 36th week, and then every week until birth. Women categorized as high risk are followed more closely.

● *Implementation*

The purposes of prenatal care are to:

• Establish a baseline of present health
• Determine the gestational age of the fetus
• Monitor fetal development
• Identify women at risk for complications
• Minimize the risk of possible complications by antici-pating and preventing problems before they occur
• Provide time for education about pregnancy, lactation and newborn care

During prenatal visits, much time is spent on teaching about prenatal care. In addition, it may be helpful to give a woman and her partner pamphlets or books that cover the same topics. Be sure you have read all the printed material you give families. This prepara-tion helps to ensure that a pamphlet's advice is con-sistent with what you have already said and with the views of the woman's primary care physician or nurse-midwife. A beautiful picture on the cover of a pamphlet does not ensure the quality of the advice in-side. In addition, reinforce instructions that the woman may call the health care setting if she has any problems or questions between visits. Some women may feel reluctant to "bother" a health care provider outside of scheduled visits unless you give them permission to do this.

● *Outcome Evaluation*

Evaluation during prenatal visits should concentrate on the woman's initial progress toward understanding goals of care for pregnancy and assessing outcomes established for specific diagnoses. Examples of expected outcomes might include:

• Couple states they have reached a decision about maintaining or discontinuing the pregnancy.
• Client states she feels well informed about the com-mon discomforts of pregnancy and actions to take to relieve them.
• Client lists ways to avoid exposure to teratogens during pregnancy.

HEALTH PROMOTION DURING PREGNANCY

The Preconceptual Visit

Ideally, women schedule appointments with a physician or nurse-midwife before becoming pregnant to obtain ac-curate reproductive life planning information, receive re-assurance about fertility (as much as can be given based on a health history and a routine physical examination), and detect any problems that may need correction through a health history, pelvic examination, and Papanicolaou (Pap) test. At this visit, hemoglobin level and blood type (including Rh factor) can be determined; minor vaginal in-fections such as those arising from *Candida* or chlamydia can be corrected to help ensure fertility; and the woman

can be counseled on the importance of a good protein diet, adequate intake of folic acid, and early prenatal care if she does become pregnant (Moos, 2004). More often, however, women arriving for their first prenatal visit will not have had a recent health care appointment oriented toward reproduction. Thus, the first prenatal visit usually covers a wide range of assessment criteria. Box 10.2 high-lights appropriate outcomes and interventions for pre-conception care using the terminology identified by the Nursing Outcomes Classification (NOC) and Nursing In-terventions Classification (NIC).

Choosing a Health Care Provider for Pregnancy and Childbirth

Once a woman is or suspects that she may be pregnant, she chooses a primary health care provider to care for her throughout the pregnancy and birth. Various options are available, including a prenatal clinic, her HMO health care provider, a nurse-midwife, an obstetrician, or a family prac-titioner. Regardless of the type of health care provider cho-sen, prenatal care needs to be initiated early and continued throughout pregnancy (Box 10.3).

Nurses can contribute to the success of prenatal care by listening, counseling, and teaching, three areas of nurs-ing expertise. Many clinics and group practices provide an initial educational seminar for women in the early stages of their pregnancy, often led by a nurse or nurse practitioner. Some practices form cohorts of women to meet monthly and discuss their concerns, termed "cen-tered pregnancy care" (McCartney, 2004). Box 10.4 summarizes ways that prenatal care can be improved and individualized so that all women are interested in obtain-ing it.

HEALTH ASSESSMENT DURING THE FIRST PRENATAL VISIT

Prenatal care is important because lack of it is associated with the birth of preterm infants and various complica-tions for the woman (Villar et al., 2005). The major causes of death during pregnancy today for women are ectopic pregnancy, hypertension, hemorrhage, embolism, infec-tion, and anesthesia-related complications such as intra-partum cardiac arrest (DHHS, 2000). An important focus of all prenatal visits, therefore, is to screen for danger signs that might reveal any of these conditions (see Chapter 11).

Box 10.5 highlights appropriate outcomes and inter-ventions for prenatal care using the terminology identi-fied by the Nursing Outcomes Classification and Nursing Interventions Classification.

The first visit includes an extensive health history, a complete physical examination, including a pelvic ex-amination, and blood and urine specimens for labora-tory work. Manual pelvic measurements can be taken to determine pelvic adequacy. Following this, time should be set aside to begin health education about pregnancy (Box 10.6).

BOX 10.2

Nursing Outcomes Classification (NOC) and Nursing Interventions Classification (NIC)

Preconception

NOC: Knowledge, Preconception

Knowledge, preconception is defined as the extent of understanding conveyed about maternal health prior to conception to ensure a healthy pregnancy (Johnson, Maas, & Moorhead, 2000). Some specific indicators that suggest that this outcome has been achieved include the client's ability to:

- Describe factors to consider when deciding about pregnancy
- Describe components of a healthy pregnancy, including healthy diet, appropriate rest and exercise, and potential adverse effects of alcohol, tobacco, and drug use
- Identify maternal risk factors associated with pregnancy and fetal development, environmental hazards, and risk for hereditary diseases
- Describe potential personal and family adjustments to pregnancy and addition of new family member

NIC: Preconception Counseling

Preconception counseling is defined as screening and providing information and support to individuals of childbearing age before pregnancy to promote health and reduce risks (McCloskey & Bulechek, 2000). Some important activities involved when implementing this intervention include:

- Obtaining client history, including thorough sexual history, and determining readiness for pregnancy with both partners
- Providing information about risk factors
- Referring for genetic counseling or prenatal diagnostic testing as needed
- Encouraging dental examination to minimize exposure to x-ray examinations and anesthetics
- Instructing about the relationships among early fetal development and personal habits, medication use, teratogens, and self-care needs
- Recommending self-care measures needed during the preconception period
- Educating about ways to avoid teratogens
- Discussing ways to prepare for pregnancy socially, financially, and psychologically
- Identifying real and perceived barriers to obtaining family planning services
- Encouraging contraception until prepared for pregnancy
- Discussing methods of identifying fertility, signs of pregnancy, and ways to confirm pregnancy
- Emphasizing the need for early and continued prenatal care once pregnant

---

 Checkpoint Question 1

Sandra Czerinski feels well. She asks you why she needs to come for prenatal care. The best reason for her to receive regular care is:

a. Discovering allergies can help eliminate early birth.

b. It helps document how many pregnancies occur each year.

c. It provides time for education about pregnancy and birth.

d. It determines whether pregnancies today are planned or not.

The Initial Interview

Interviewing expectant women often elicits contradictory information. Women are likely to want to talk about their past health and current pregnancy, so interviewing them should go smoothly and be productive. On the other hand, pregnancy symptoms are subtle, so a woman may not regard certain information as important, providing vague

answers to questions about these areas. Perhaps she is unaware that she is the only person who knows the answers to a number of vital questions ("How do you feel about being pregnant?" or "Have you been taking anything for your morning nausea?"). Outside pressures, such as having to report for work or older children coming home from school, may interfere with the effectiveness of the interview. Late in pregnancy, a woman may feel uncomfortable sitting for a long time.

Interviewing is best accomplished in a private, quiet setting. Trying to talk to a woman in a crowded hallway or a full waiting room is rarely effective. Pregnancy is too private an affair to be discussed under these circumstances.

It is helpful if the person scheduling the appointment cautions a woman that the first visit may be long. This prevents her from trying to fit the visit in between other errands or from having to terminate the interview because of another appointment.

Be certain to ask what name a woman wants you to use when addressing her in a prenatal setting, and make certain that she knows your name and understands your role correctly. If she views you as someone only gathering preliminary data, she will be willing to discuss superficial facts (name, address, phone number, and the like) but will resist

BOX 10.3 FOCUS ON . . .

EVIDENCE-BASED PRACTICE

Is continuity of care important in prenatal settings?

To answer this question, researchers completed a meta-analysis of two studies involving 1,815 women who were cared for at prenatal visits by midwives who offered continuity of care or cared for by a system of inconsistent caregivers (either a physician or a midwife). Results showed that women who had continuity of care from a team of midwives were less likely to be admitted to the hospital during pregnancy and more likely to attend antenatal education programs. They were also less likely to use drugs for pain relief during labor, and their newborns were less likely to require resuscitation. They were more likely to be pleased with their antenatal, intrapartum, and postnatal care. There were no differences between the two groups in Apgar scores or in rates of low birthweight and stillbirths or neonatal deaths. The researchers concluded that continuity of care at prenatal visits has noticeable advantages for women.

This is an important study for nurses because nurses are the people who typically make or assist women to make return visits to the health care facility. Knowing that continuity of care is important can serve as a guide for scheduling visits.

Source: Hodnett, E. D. (2005). Continuity of caregivers for care during pregnancy and childbirth. *The Cochrane Library, (Oxford) (3).* (ID #CD000062).

discussing more intimate things (her feelings toward this pregnancy, the difficulty she has reworking old fears, how scared she is about birth).

Because initial health history taking is often time-consuming, a woman may be asked to complete some of the forms. Good interviewing technique, however, is important to obtain thorough and meaningful health histories. The rapport established by face-to-face interviewing gives a woman the feeling that she is more than just a client number or chart. It may be as much a reason she returns for follow-up care as her desire to be assured that her pregnancy is progressing normally.

Components of the Health History

An initial interview serves several purposes:

- Establishing rapport
- Gaining information about the woman's physical and psychosocial health
- Obtaining a basis for anticipatory guidance for the pregnancy

Establishing a baseline health picture at the initial pregnancy visit is important. If on subsequent visits a symptom is mentioned, you can then check your records to verify that it is truly a new symptom. It may be that the woman is just becoming more aware of it. General interviewing techniques are discussed in Chapter 33. Included in the following section are the elements pertinent to a pregnancy history.

Demographic Data

Demographic data usually obtained include name, age, address, telephone number, religion, and health insurance information.

Chief Concern

The chief concern is the reason the woman has come to the health care setting—in this instance, the fact that she is or thinks she is pregnant.

To help confirm pregnancy, inquire about the date of her last menstrual period and whether she has had a preg-

BOX 10.4

Suggestions for Improving Prenatal Care Services

- Schedule appointments for women within a week after they first call the health care setting. This initial contact can be done through a group orientation session, individually by a health team member, or, if risk status warrants, by a physician. Try to schedule further appointments at times convenient for the client and her support people to encourage attendance.
- Make waiting time educational by providing materials such as pamphlets or videotapes in the waiting room.
- Provide privacy for assessments such as blood pressure, weight, and urine checks.
- Encourage women to feel responsible for their health record. If a woman's first language is not English, make sure to record pregnancy information so she can read it.

- Be certain that pregnant women meet health care providers while fully clothed and upright, not naked and in a lithotomy position on an examining table.
- Encourage family members and friends to accompany the woman for prenatal care. Allow them to enter the examination room and participate in all aspects of care to the extent they and the client desire.
- Schedule appointments to provide continuity of care. Be certain that women have a specific person's name as a phone or e-mail contact for pregnancy-related questions. Without this information, they tend not to call.
- Educate pregnant women about care options and encourage them to participate in making decisions about their care.

BOX 10.5

Nursing Outcomes Classification (NOC) and Nursing Interventions Classification (NIC)

Prenatal Care

NOC: Knowledge, Pregnancy

Knowledge, pregnancy is defined as the extent of understanding conveyed about maintenance of a healthy pregnancy and prevention of complications (Johnson, Maas, & Moorhead, 2000). Some specific indicators that suggest that this outcome has been achieved include evidence of the following:

- Acknowledgment of the importance of prenatal care and prenatal education along with discussion of options for providing prenatal health care and childbirth
- Identification of the danger signs of pregnancy and possible complications
- Description of the following: major fetal developmental milestones; physical and psychological changes of pregnancy; appropriate health-promotion behaviors such as proper body mechanics, adequate rest and sleep, and exercise; measures to promote self-care for discomforts of pregnancy; healthy weight gain patterns and correct use of dietary supplements; importance of dental care; safer sex practices; and proper use of safety devices in an automobile
- Description of the signs of labor and techniques to facilitate effective labor
- Identification of possible fetal teratogens and environmental hazards
- Discussion of ways to prepare family members

NIC: Prenatal Care

Prenatal care is defined as the monitoring and managing of a patient during pregnancy to prevent complications and promote a healthy outcome for both the mother and infant (McCloskey & Bulechek, 2000).

Some important activities involved when implementing this intervention include:

- Instructing client on importance of regular prenatal care throughout pregnancy, necessary nutrition, exercise, rest, desired weight gain, danger signs, fetal growth and development, self-care strategies for common discomforts, and harmful effects of teratogens
- Encouraging client's partner to participate in prenatal care, including attending prenatal classes
- Monitoring physiologic parameters including nutritional status, blood pressure, laboratory studies such as urine glucose and protein and hemoglobin, edema of ankles, hands and face, deep tendon reflexes
- Measuring fundal height with comparison to gestational age
- Assessing fetal heart rate and fetal growth and development
- Providing anticipatory guidance about physical and psychological changes during pregnancy
- Monitoring psychological adjustment of client and family, along with counseling client about changes in sexuality and body image during pregnancy
- Assessing social support system and assisting client to develop and use social support
- Instructing client on how to monitor fetal activity
- Guiding client in imaging her unborn child as appropriate
- Providing parents with opportunity to hear fetal heart tones and see ultrasound image of the fetus
- Referring client to childbirth preparation and child care and parenting classes as appropriate

nancy test or used a home test kit. Elicit information about the signs of early pregnancy, such as nausea, vomiting, breast changes, or fatigue. Question her about any discomforts of pregnancy, such as constipation, backache, or frequent urination. Also, ask about any danger signs of pregnancy, such as bleeding, continuous headache, visual disturbances, or swelling of the hands and face.

Ask if the pregnancy was planned. If you feel uncomfortable asking directly, using a statement such as, "All pregnancies are a bit of a surprise. Is that how it was with this one?" may help provide you with this information. Another way to word such a question would be, "Some couples plan on having children right away; some plan on waiting. How was it with you?" If the woman says the pregnancy was not planned, explore to learn if she has reached a decision about whether to continue with the pregnancy. A question such as, "Some women change their mind about wanting a baby once they realize they are pregnant; some don't. How

has it been for you?" may be effective for obtaining this type of information because it says either option is possible. You just want her to tell you which is happening.

Family Profile

In the past, the social history or family setting history (family profile) was left until the end of a health interview. More often, it is now obtained at the beginning of the interview, following the chief concern. Doing so can help you get to know a woman earlier, identify support persons, shape the nature and kind of questions asked, and evaluate the possible impact of the client's culture on care. Ask about marital status. As a rule, both married and unmarried women want you to know this as they want to alert you if they do not have support people readily available.

It is important to know the size of the apartment or house in which a woman lives because you will be talking

BOX 10.6: Focus on Nursing Care Planning

A Multidisciplinary Care Map for
A First Prenatal Visit
●

Sandra Czerinski is a 29-year-old woman, 16 weeks pregnant, who comes for a first prenatal visit. She is concerned because she didn't realize she was pregnant until a week ago. Because of this, she has been actively dieting (two diet drinks plus one meal of mainly vegetables daily) plus lifting weights at a health club. She wants her urine tested because "I have to go all the time." She does not want any blood work done because she doesn't have health insurance. She hasn't had a pelvic examination since she was in high school, when she had a vaginal infection. She remembers that as being very painful.

Family Assessment

Single woman; lives by self in one-bedroom apartment. Works at a laundry. Boyfriend is a roofing salesman; out of town 4 days a week.

Client Assessment

Gravida 1, para 0. Last menstrual period 4 months ago. Had nausea last month but thought this was "flu."

Menarche at age 11; menstrual cycle every 29 days, 6 days' duration with moderate flow and mild cramps. Past history positive for sinusitis and appendectomy at age 12 years. Smokes about ½ pack per day, "more when I'm stressed at work"; denies alcohol use. "I drink club soda with lime or mineral water."

ROS: Height 5 feet 5 inches; weight 195 pounds. Slight gingival hyperplasia; breasts full and slightly tender.

Pelvic examination by nurse-midwife: cervical os round, clean, and slightly soft; uterus enlarged and soft; + Chadwick's sign, + Hegar's sign, + Goodell's sign. Uterine height palpable at three fingers over symphysis pubis. Fetal heart rate via Doppler at 152 beats per minute.

Remainder of physical examination within normal limits. Serum hCG and ultrasound positive for pregnancy.

Nursing Diagnosis

Health-seeking behaviors related to guidelines for pregnancy

Outcome Criteria

Client states the need to stop smoking; identifies measures she will take to reduce number of cigarettes smoked, and states she will no longer try to lose weight. Makes appointment for follow-up visits.

Nursing Interventions and Care Mapping

Team Member Responsible	Assessment	Intervention	Rationale	Expected Outcome
Activities of Daily Living				
Nurse/ nurse-midwife	Assess client's expectations about this pregnancy, including whether she expects to continue to work, continue present lifestyle.	Discuss the effect of pregnancy on her partner and any religious or cultural beliefs that would interfere with her ability to adapt to pregnancy changes.	Assessing expectations is important to assist the client in identifying areas of need and adapting to the pregnancy to ensure the optimal outcome for the mother, fetus, and partner.	Client describes the likely effect of the pregnancy on herself and partner; identifies areas where she anticipates life changes.

(continued)

Team Member Responsible	Assessment	Intervention	Rationale	Expected Outcome
Consultations				
Nurse-midwife	Fully assess symptoms of urinary frequency to rule out urinary tract infection	Consult with primary care provider about further investigation of urinary tract infection if indicated.	Urinary tract infections are associated with preterm birth.	Primary care physician will document urinary tract infection if signs/symptoms warrant and will prescribe appropriate antibiotic.
Procedures/Medications				
Nurse-midwife/nurse	Obtain a gynecologic and obstetrics health history.	Perform initial assessment, including vital signs, height and weight measurement, and history and physical examination.	Initial assessment provides a baseline for future comparison and identification of factors that may place the client at risk for pregnancy concerns.	Client receives a thorough initial assessment, to lay a psychological and physiologic foundation of health care information for pregnancy care.
Nurse	Obtain usual weight before pregnancy and weight at each visit. Obtain urine and blood specimens.	Establish client BMI. Monitor weight at every visit. Explain that blood assessment is not done at every visit.	A baseline weight is necessary for future comparison. Adequate weight gain during pregnancy (typically 25 to 30 pounds) is necessary for optimal fetal growth and development. Present BMI is 32.4.	Client's weight is monitored and compared with previous weights at each prenatal visit. Client states she understands importance of initial bloodwork, urinalysis.
Nutrition				
Nurse/nutritionist	Obtain a 24-hour nutrition recall.	Discuss with the client her increased nutritional needs during pregnancy. Provide information about a well-balanced diet, including food selections, such as fresh fruits and vegetables, milk products, and high-protein foods, fluid intake, and prenatal vitamin supplementation.	A well-balanced diet with adequate fluid intake and use of prenatal vitamins helps to ensure an optimal environment for fetal growth and development. Dieting is contraindicated during pregnancy.	Client voices an understanding of the increased nutritional needs during pregnancy and describes her plan to provide for these needs. Voices understanding of why she should discontinue dieting.
Patient/Family Education				
Nurse	Assess if client is interested in decreasing smoking during pregnancy.	Instruct the client in the effects of smoking on the fetus. Assist client with methods to reduce and stop, if possible.	Nicotine in cigarettes has been shown to be teratogenic to the fetus.	Client describes the effect on a fetus of smoking during pregnancy and her plan to stop smoking at least until after the birth and, ideally, long term.
Nurse	Assess if client is aware of the danger signs of pregnancy that she will need to report immediately should they occur.	Instruct the client about possible danger signs to report immediately. Emphasize that although these signs are important, they do not necessarily mean that something is wrong.	Knowledge of possible danger signs allows for early detection and prompt intervention should it be necessary.	Client and intimate partner list danger signs of pregnancy to report immediately. They acknowledge that these signs suggest, but do not necessarily mean, that the pregnancy is at risk.

(continued)

Team Member Responsible	Assessment	Intervention	Rationale	Expected Outcome
Psychosocial/Spiritual/Emotional Needs				
Nurse	Assess if client has concerns about success of pregnancy.	Assure client that concern during pregnancy is a normal response. Include information about physiologic and psychological changes of pregnancy.	Anxiety can interfere with client's ability to adjust to pregnancy. Reviewing information reinforces understanding of what is to come and helps to alleviate fears and anxieties related to pregnancy.	Client describes any concerns about pregnancy and receives appropriate assurance.
Discharge Planning				
Nurse	Assess whether client will have any difficulty continuing with prenatal care.	Assist client with setting up appointments for visits and tests to evaluate fetal well-being as necessary, despite lack of health insurance.	Assisting with appointment setting helps to ensure adherence.	Client states plan for expected antepartal care visits and affirms her willingness to adhere to the plan.

with her in the coming months about a bedroom or space for a baby's bed. It also is important to know whether the essential rooms are on the ground floor or upstairs in case she is restricted from climbing stairs more than once or twice a day during the last part of pregnancy or after birth.

Before you can begin to offer a woman any more than stereotyped health care instruction, get to know her and her sexual partner's age (additional testing such as genetic screening may be necessary if she is over 35), their educational levels (offers an estimation of the level of teaching you will plan), and occupation (does the woman's work involve heavy lifting, long hours of standing in one position, handling of a toxic substance?).

Adaptation to pregnancy is highly individualized. A change in status from independence to dependence because of stopping work, chronic illness at home, the death or loss of a significant person during pregnancy, geographic moves, financial hardship, and lack of support people are examples of situations that can hinder a woman's ability to accept her pregnancy and child. No one in the health care setting will be aware of these potentially harmful situations unless questions about family profile are asked.

History of Past Illnesses

Questions about a woman's past medical history are an important part of an interview because a past condition may become active during or immediately following pregnancy. Representative diseases that can pose a potential difficulty during pregnancy include kidney disease, heart disease (coarctation of the aorta and rheumatic fever cause problems most often), hypertension, sexually transmitted infection (including hepatitis B and human immunodeficiency virus [HIV]), diabetes, thyroid disease, recurrent seizures, gallbladder disease, urinary tract infections, varicosities, phenylketonuria, tuberculosis, and asthma. It is important

to find out whether a woman had childhood diseases such as chickenpox (varicella), mumps (epidemic parotitis), measles (rubeola), German measles (rubella), or poliomyelitis. From this information, you can estimate the degree of antibody protection the client has against these diseases if she is exposed to them during her pregnancy. While pregnant, she can be immunized against poliomyelitis by the Salk (killed virus) vaccine. However, she cannot be immunized against the other diseases because the vaccines against these contain live viruses, as does the oral Sabin poliomyelitis vaccine. Live virus vaccines could be harmful to the fetus if the virus crossed the placenta.

Also ask about any allergies, including any drug sensitivities. As a rule, women with allergies of any magnitude should be urged to breast-feed rather than bottle-feed their infants to avoid possible milk allergy in the infant (Hanson, Korotkova, & Telemo, 2003). Any past surgical procedures are also important because adhesions resulting from past abdominal surgery may interfere with uterine growth.

What if... Sandra Czerinski tells you she has no idea what childhood diseases or immunizations she had? How would you suggest that she obtain this information?

History of Family Illnesses

A family history documents illnesses that occur frequently in the family and helps to identify potential problems in the mother during pregnancy or in the infant at birth. Ask specifically about cardiovascular and renal disease, cognitive impairment, blood disorders, or any known genetically inherited diseases or congenital anomalies (McGregor & Parker, 2003).

Day History/Social Profile

Information about a woman's current nutrition, elimination, sleep, recreation, and interpersonal interactions can be elicited best by asking the woman to describe a typical day of her life. If any of this information is not reported spontaneously as she describes her day, ask for additional details.

Nutrition is an important part of a day history to obtain, particularly in light of the number of young adults with eating disorders today. A "24-hour recall" is helpful to obtain accurate nutrition information because by doing this, the woman tells you what she actually ate, not what she should have eaten (Box 10.7).

Ask about the type, amount, and frequency of exercise to determine her routine pattern and whether it will be consistent with a recommended level for pregnancy. If she hikes or camps, she is at risk for exposure to Lyme disease. Ask about hobbies. Certain hobbies, such as working with lead-based glazes and ceramics, might not be wise to continue during pregnancy because lead is teratogenic.

Because smoke, whether first-hand or second-hand, has been shown to be harmful to fetal growth (Albrecht et al., 2004), obtain information about the client's smoking habits. Excessive alcohol intake can lead to poor nutrition, can be directly responsible for fetal alcohol syndrome, and may cause preterm birth (Albertsen et al., 2004). If a woman answers vaguely about how much she smokes or drinks alcohol ("I drink socially" or "I only smoke occasionally"), attempt to determine exactly what she means so you can more accurately evaluate the frequency of these events.

Pregnant women, especially adolescents, are at an increased risk for intimate partner abuse. Ask enough questions to be certain the woman is not involved in an abusive partnership (Katz, 2003).

A medication history is also important. Ask whether the woman takes any medications, prescribed or over-the-counter, because their effect on a growing fetus will have to be evaluated. This also includes any herbal preparations that a woman might be using. Even seemingly innocent medications for simple conditions can be detrimental during pregnancy. For example, isotretinoin (Accutane), a vitamin A preparation taken for acne, is associated with spontaneous miscarriage and congenital anomalies. Herbal supplements should be evaluated carefully before being taken by pregnant women to be certain they don't stimulate uterine contractions (Buehler, 2003).

Ask about the use of any recreational drugs, such as marijuana or cocaine, as these also can be deleterious to fetal growth. Include intravenous drug use because of the increased risk for exposure to HIV or hepatitis B. Although this type of information is not usually readily revealed, most women will answer these questions honestly during pregnancy because they are concerned about protecting the health of their fetus.

Gynecologic History

In the past, most women had children early in their childbearing years, so the number of reproductive tract or women's health problems, such as breast disease, they had experienced before pregnancy were few. Today, however, women often delay conception of their first child past 30 years of age. Therefore, it is not unusual to discover a woman who has had a reproductive tract or breast problem. Table 10.1 lists common gynecologic illnesses and their possible significance in pregnancy.

BOX 10.7 FOCUS ON . . .

COMMUNICATION

Sandra Czerinski has come to her obstetrician's office for a first prenatal visit.

Less Effective Communication

Nurse: The next thing I need, Ms. Czerinski, is for you to tell me what a typical day is like for you.

Ms. Czerinski: I don't usually have typical ones. Or very interesting ones.

Nurse: What about yesterday? Could you describe that to me?

Ms. Czerinski: Okay. I was up at 7:00, was at work by 9:00. A friend picked me up after work and we celebrated his birthday. I was back home and in bed by 10:00. That's pretty much the day.

Nurse: You're right. It doesn't sound very interesting. Next, let me ask you about your family medical history.

More Effective Communication

Nurse: The next thing I need, Ms. Czerinski, is for you to tell me what a typical day is like for you.

Ms. Czerinski: I don't usually have typical ones. Or very interesting ones.

Nurse: What about yesterday? Could you describe that to me?

Ms. Czerinski: Okay. I was up at 7:00, was at work by 9:00. A friend picked me up after work and we celebrated his birthday. I was back home and in bed by 10:00. That's pretty much the day.

Nurse: What did you have for breakfast?

Ms. Czerinski: Nothing. I was too rushed to eat.

Nurse: Dinner?

Ms. Czerinski: We were celebrating at a bar. Cheese blintzes, I think. And beer. A lot of beer.

Most people are not aware how much information can be revealed by a day history, so they give only a scant description of their day. Asking additional questions to make them elaborate on various parts often reveals poor nutrition, poor exercise, or risky behavior patterns.

TABLE 10.1

Gynecologic Disorders

Disorder	Possible Symptoms	Significance and Suggested Therapy
Vulva		
Cysts of Skene's or Bartholin's glands	Asymptomatic swelling at the sides of the urinary meatus or vestibule	Such cysts are surgically incised to prevent blockage of gland duct.
Condylomata acuminata	Cauliflower-like lesion on vulva	This lesion tends to occur in women with chronic vaginitis. Caused by the epidermatrophic virus that causes common warts. Removed by cryocautery or knife excision.
Lichen sclerosus	Whitish papules on the vulva; asymptomatic	There is no need for removal; the area is biopsied because leukoplakia, a potentially cancerous condition, has an almost identical appearance.
Leukoplakia	Thick, gray, patchy epithelium that cracks; possibly a pre-malignant state and infects easily, accompanied by itching and pain	Therapy involves hydrocortisone and frequent return visits to health care personnel (every 6 months) for observation to detect any changes suggestive of carcinoma.
Carcinoma of the vulva	A shallow vulvar ulcer that does not heal	Vulvar cancer occurs most often in postmenopausal women; represents only 3% to 4% of all reproductive tract cancers in women. Therapy is vulvectomy—vagina is left intact, and sexual relations and pregnancy, with cesarean birth to prevent tearing of fibrotic vulvar tissue, may be possible.
Vagina and Cervix		
Adenosis	Asymptomatic vaginal cysts with columnar rather than squamous epithelium present on vaginal walls	This condition is caused by diethylstilbestrol (DES) administration while in utero. Has the potential for becoming malignant (clear cell adenocarcinoma). If adenosis is present, an examination two or three times a year with a Pap test and Lugol's staining is necessary, and the woman should not use estrogen sources such as oral contraceptives. If adenocarcinoma occurs, local destruction of atypical cells can be achieved by excision, cautery, or cryosurgery. This condition is rarely seen today because DES is no longer prescribed during pregnancy.
Cervical polyp	Red, vascular, protruding pedunculated tissue that bleeds readily with trauma	A polyp may be discovered because of vaginal spotting on coitus, tampon insertion, or vaginal examination. Removed vaginally by excision. Often associated with chronic cervical inflammation.
Cervicitis (erosion)	Reddened cervical tissue with a whitish exudate	Douching with a vinegar solution aids healing. May be treated with cryosurgery if extensive.
Nabothian cyst	Clear shining circles on cervix from blocked gland ducts	No therapy is necessary.
Cervical carcinoma	Postcoital spotting, unexplained vaginal discharge or spotting between menstrual periods	Cervical cancer is the most frequent type of reproductive tract malignancy; risk factors include coitus with multiple partners or uncircumcised males, herpes type II infections, or DES use during pregnancy. Diagnosed by Pap test or colposcopy. Therapy is conization, radiation, or surgical excision. Pregnancy is possible following cervical carcinoma; cesarean birth may be necessary because of fibrotic cervical tissue.
Ovaries		
Endometrial cyst	Chocolate-brown cyst on tender enlarged ovary; may cause acute pain if rupture occurs	Endometriosis is the cause; occurs in women aged 20 to 40 years. Therapy is surgical excision; ovary may or may not be removed depending on extent of cyst.
Follicular cyst	Amenorrhea and possibly dyspareunia; ovary tender and enlarged	Cysts typically regress after 1 or 2 months; low-dose oral contraceptive may be prescribed for 6 to 12 weeks to suppress ovarian activity; estrogen may be continued for 6 months.
Polycystic disease	Multiple follicular cysts of both ovaries	Excess adrenal supply of estrogen leads to inhibition of follicle-stimulating hormone and anovulation. Clomiphene citrate therapy to induce ovulation or wedge resection of the ovaries is used as therapy.

TABLE 10.1

Gynecologic Disorders (continued)

Disorder	Possible Symptoms	Significance and Suggested Therapy
Corpus luteum cyst	Delayed menstrual flow followed by prolonged bleeding; ovary enlarged and tender	A corpus luteum has persisted rather than atrophied. Most regress in about 2 months; a low-dose oral contraceptive may be prescribed for 6 weeks to suppress ovarian activity.
Dermoid cyst	Asymptomatic; ovary enlarged on examination	Cyst originates from embryonic tissue; may contain hair, cartilage, and fat. Most common ovarian tumor of childhood; also occurs at 30 to 50 years. Therapy is surgical resection.
Serous cystadenoma	Bilateral; asymptomatic except for signs of pelvic pressure	This is the most common type of benign ovarian cyst; high malignancy rate of 20% to 30%. Therapy is surgical resection.
Carcinoma	Asymptomatic; intermenstrual bleeding	Ovarian cancer originates in epithelial tissue most often in women over 50 years of age. Tendency may be inherited; environmental contamination may play a role in development. Therapy is hysterectomy and salpingo-oophorectomy.
Uterus Endometrial polyp	Intermenstrual bleeding	Polyp is removed by dilatation and curettage.
Leiomyomas (fibroids)	Asymptomatic or with increased menstrual flow	Muscle and fibrous connective tissue form in response to estrogen stimulation. May increase in size during pregnancy; may cause interference with cervical dilatation and result in postpartal hemorrhage. Stress to the myometrium by uterine contractions may be the original cause of formation. Therapy is surgical resection (myomectomy) or hysterectomy if child-bearing is complete.
Endometrial carcinoma	Vaginal bleeding between menstrual periods	Diagnosis is by endometrial washing, not Pap test. Therapy is hysterectomy.
Uterine prolapse	Vaginal pressure and low back pain	The uterus has descended in the vagina due to overstretching of uterine supports and trauma to the levator ani muscle. Occurs most often in women who had insufficient prenatal care, birth of a large infant, a prolonged second stage of labor, bearing-down efforts or extraction of a baby before full dilatation, instrument birth, and poor healing of perineal tissue postpartally. Therapy is surgery to repair uterine supports or placement of a pessary, a plastic uterine support. Women with pessaries in place need to return for a pelvic examination every 3 months to have the pessary removed, cleaned, and replaced and the vagina inspected; otherwise, vaginal infection or erosion of the vaginal walls can result.

A woman's past experience with her reproductive system may have some influence on how well she accepts a pregnancy. Obtain information about her age of menarche (first menstrual period) and how well she was prepared for it as a normal part of life. Ask about her usual cycle, including the interval, duration, amount of menstrual flow, and any discomfort she feels. Ascertain her degree of discomfort, including when it occurs, how long it lasts, and what she does to relieve it. If she describes menstrual cramps as "horrible" and wonders "how I live through them some months," anticipate the need for additional counseling to help her prepare for labor. Some women with severe dysmenorrhea look forward to pregnancy as it will mean 9 months without discomfort. Anticipate their need for counseling in the postpartum period about active ways to relieve their menstrual discomfort when their periods resume (see Chapter 47).

Also ask if a woman does a monthly perineum self-examination (see Chapter 33 for this technique) to evaluate her interest in self-care. Breast self-examination is no longer thought to yield enough reliable information to be continued as a self-care routine (Kosters & Gotzsche, 2005).

Ask about past surgery on the reproductive tract. For example, if a woman has had tubal surgery, such as for an ectopic pregnancy, the statistical risk of another tubal pregnancy increases. If she has had uterine surgery, a cesarean birth may be necessary because her uterus may not be able to expand and contract as efficiently as usual because of the surgical scar. If she has undergone frequent dilatation and curettage of the uterus, her cervix may be weakened or unable to remain closed for 9 months. This could lead to premature birth unless she has a surgical procedure (cerclage) for this (see Chapter 15).

Ask also about what reproductive planning methods, if any, have been used. Occasionally, a woman may become pregnant with an intrauterine device (IUD) in place. If this occurs, it will be removed to prevent infection during pregnancy. Another woman, not realizing she is pregnant, may continue to take an oral contraceptive for some time into the pregnancy. Document whether such use occurred, because some evidence suggests that estrogen can harm fetal growth. Be certain to include a sexual history, including the number of sexual partners and use of safer sex practices, to establish the woman's risk for contracting a sexually transmitted infection.

As part of any woman's gynecologic history, assess for the possibility of stress incontinence (incontinence of urine on laughing, coughing, deep inspiration, jogging, or running). With these actions, the diaphragm descends, increasing abdominal pressure, which increases bladder tension and causes emptying. Stress incontinence occurs from lack of strength in the perineal muscles and bladder supports. Commonly, weakness occurs from difficult births, the birth of large infants, grand multiparity, and instrumented births. During pregnancy, stress incontinence can become intensified from the increasing abdominal pressure. Some women accept this incontinence as a normal consequence of childbearing and may not report it unless asked.

Women can relieve stress incontinence to some degree by strengthening the perineal muscles with the use of Kegel exercises (periodic tightening of the perineal muscles; see Chapter 11). Surgical correction to increase support to the bladder neck also could be performed following the pregnancy.

Obstetric History

Do not assume that the current pregnancy is a woman's first pregnancy simply because she is very young or says she has only recently been married. For each previous pregnancy, document the child's sex and the place and date of birth. Review the pregnancy briefly:

- Was it planned?
- Did she have any complications, such as spotting, swelling of her hands or feet, falls, or surgery?
- Did she take any medication? If so, what and why?
- Did she receive prenatal care? If so, when did she start?
- What was the duration of the pregnancy?
- What was the duration of labor?
- Was labor what she expected? Worse? Better?
- What was the type of birth?
- What type of anesthesia, if any, was used?
- Did she have stitches following birth?
- Did she have any complications, such as excessive bleeding or infection following the birth?
- What was the infant's birthweight and sex?
- What was the condition of the infant at birth? Did the infant cry right away?
- What was the infant's Apgar score? (Most mothers know this.)
- Was any special care needed for the baby, such as suctioning, oxygen, or an incubator?
- Was the baby discharged from the health care setting with her?

- What is the child's present state of health?
- How was the pregnancy overall for her?

Ask about any previous miscarriages or abortions and whether she had any complications during or following them. **Abortion** is the medical term for any pregnancy terminated before the age of viability, commonly called a miscarriage. The **age of viability** is the earliest age at which fetuses could survive if they were born at that time, generally accepted as 24 weeks, or fetuses weighing more than 400 g. If the woman's blood type is Rh negative, ask if she received Rh immune globulin (RhIG [RhoGAM]) after miscarriages or abortions or previous births so you will know whether Rh sensitization could have occurred. Ask if she has ever had a blood transfusion to establish possible risk of hepatitis B or HIV exposure or Rh sensitization.

After a history of previous pregnancies is obtained, determine the woman's status with respect to the number of times she has been pregnant, including the present pregnancy (**gravida**), and the number of children above the age of viability she has previously borne (**para**). Table 10.2 explains these terms. For example, a woman who has had two previous pregnancies, has given birth to two term children, and is again pregnant is gravida 3, para 2. A woman who has had two miscarriages at 12 weeks (under the age of viability) and is again pregnant is a gravida 3, para 0.

A more comprehensive system for classifying pregnancy status (GTPAL or GTPALM) provides greater detail on a woman's pregnancy history. By this system, the gravida classification remains the same, but para is broken down into:

T: The number of full-term infants born (infants born at 37 weeks or after)
P: The number of preterm infants born (infants born before 37 weeks)

TABLE 10.2

Terms Related to Pregnancy Status

Term	Definition
Para	The number of pregnancies that reached viability, regardless of whether the infants were born alive or not
Gravida	A woman who is or has been pregnant
Primigravida	A woman who is pregnant for the first time
Primipara	A woman who has given birth to one child past age of viability
Multigravida	A woman who has been pregnant previously
Multipara	A woman who has carried two or more pregnancies to viability
Nulligravida	A woman who has never been and is not currently pregnant

A: The number of spontaneous or induced abortions
L: The number of living children
M: Multiple pregnancies

Using this system, the woman in the first example above would be gravida 3, para 2002 (GTPAL) or 320020 (GT-PALM). A multigestation pregnancy is considered as one para. For example, a woman who had term twins, then one preterm infant, and is now pregnant again would be a gravida 3, para 21031 (GTPALM).

A pregnant woman who had the following past history—a boy born at 39 weeks' gestation, now alive and well; a girl born at 40 weeks' gestation, now alive and well; a girl born at 33 weeks' gestation, now alive and well—would have her pregnancy information summarized as follows: gravida 4; para 21030 (GTPALM).

Review of Systems

A review of systems completes the subjective information. Use a systematic approach, such as head to toe, and explain what you'll be doing. For example, "I'm going to start at the top of your head and go through to your toes, asking about body parts or systems and any diseases that you may have had." A review of systems helps women recall diseases they forgot to mention earlier, such as a urinary tract infection, a disease that can influence the outcome of pregnancy and so would be important to your history taking.

The following body systems and questions about conditions constitute the minimum information to be addressed in a review of systems for a first prenatal visit:

- *Head:* Headache? Head injury? Seizures? Dizziness? Fainting?
- *Eyes:* Vision? Glasses needed? Diplopia? Infection? Glaucoma? Cataract? Pain? Recent changes?
- *Ears:* Infection? Discharge? Earache? Hearing loss? Tinnitus? Vertigo?
- *Nose:* Epistaxis (nose bleeds)? Discharge? How many colds a year? Allergy? Postnasal drainage? Sinus pain?
- *Mouth and pharynx:* Dentures? Condition of teeth? Toothaches? Any bleeding of gums? Hoarseness? Difficulty in swallowing? Tonsillectomy?
- *Neck:* Stiffness? Masses?
- *Breasts:* Lumps? Secretion? Pain? Tenderness?
- *Respiratory system:* Cough? Wheezing? Asthma? Shortness of breath? Pain? Serious chest illness, such as tuberculosis or pneumonia?
- *Cardiovascular system:* History of heart murmur? History of heart disease such as rheumatic fever or Kawasaki disease? Hypertension? Any pain? Palpitations? Anemia? Does she know her blood pressure? Has she ever had a blood transfusion?
- *Gastrointestinal system:* What was her prepregnancy weight? Vomiting? Diarrhea? Constipation? Change in bowel habits? Rectal pruritus? Hemorrhoids? Pain? Ulcer? Gallbladder disease? Hepatitis? Appendicitis?
- *Genitourinary system:* Urinary tract infection? Hematuria? Frequent urination? Sexually transmitted infection? Pelvic inflammatory disease? Hepatitis B? HIV?
- *Extremities:* Varicose veins? Pain or stiffness of joints? Any fractures or dislocations?
- *Skin:* Any rashes? Acne? Psoriasis?

Conclusion

End an interview by asking if there is something you have not covered that the woman wants to discuss. This gives her one more chance to ask any questions she has about this new life experience.

Support Person's Role

More and more partners accompany women for prenatal care today. Young children may also accompany their mothers on these visits. Some women bring a female friend as their best support person. If family members are present, should they be included in an initial interview? As a whole, interviewing is most effective if it is a one-to-one interaction. A woman may be unwilling to mention certain concerns when her family is present for fear of worrying them. A husband may not be the father of her child, and she may be unable to voice her concern over this fact or alert you to the possibility she is worried about blood incompatibility because another man is the father.

If childbearing is to be a family affair, however, it is important to determine the partner's degree of acceptance of the pregnancy and of assuming a new parenting role. Including siblings in a prenatal visit provides them with an opportunity to involve them with the pregnancy planning and coming baby. Interviewing the woman alone and then inviting the support person and family to join her while you talk about pregnancy symptoms with them as a family is an effective solution (Fig. 10.1). Providing some private interview time with a partner allows the partner to express any concerns or worries. The main areas you should investigate with the partner include his current health, his feelings and concerns about the pregnancy, and his knowledge of pregnancy and childbirth. If the woman wishes, the partner can accompany her during the physical examination. After the confirmation of pregnancy, the partner should be included when health care information is given (Box 10.8).

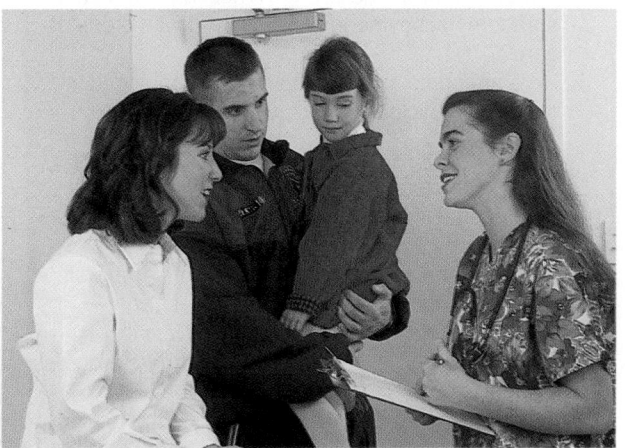

FIGURE 10.1 Include support people in a prenatal visit so that visits are family centered. Here a husband, wife, and child are included in the initial prenatal interview, making all feel a part of the pregnancy. (© Barbara Proud.)

Checkpoint Question 2

Why is it important to ask Sandra about past surgery on a pregnancy health history?

a. To test her recent and long term memory.
b. Adhesions from surgery could limit uterine growth.
c. To assess whether she could be allergic to any medication.
d. To determine if she has effective health insurance.

Physical Examination

After a health history is obtained, women have a physical examination. If a woman voids for a clean-catch urine before the exam, this can reduce bladder size and make the pelvic examination more comfortable, allow easier identification of pelvic organs, as well as providing a urine specimen for laboratory testing. The urine specimen is sent to the laboratory for evaluation of bacteria, protein, glucose, and ketones, or these can be immediately tested by dipstick analysis. Box 10.9 provides instructions on how to obtain a clean-catch urine sample.

A physical examination at a first prenatal visit typically includes inspection of body systems, with emphasis on the changes that occur with pregnancy or that could signal a developing problem. General techniques of physical examination are discussed in Chapter 33.

BOX 10.8 FOCUS ON . . .

FAMILY TEACHING

Suggestions for Encouraging Partner Participation in Prenatal Visits

Q. Sandra Czerinski asks you, "What can I do to make sure that my boyfriend feels involved with prenatal care?"

A. Here are some suggestions for encouraging your partner's participation:

- Ask for appointments to be scheduled at a time that is convenient for both of you.
- Be certain that your partner reserves enough time so the visit doesn't become more of an inconvenience than an enjoyable event. A prenatal visit can be lengthy.
- Ask your partner to accompany you into the examining room at visits so you both can share progress or decisions.
- Be certain that your partner listens to the fetal heart at visits as soon as it can be heard.
- If a sonogram is scheduled, ask your partner to view it with you (it's an exciting moment for both of you to see your fetus moving).

Baseline Height/Weight and Vital Sign Measurement

A woman's weight and height are obtained at a first prenatal visit to establish a baseline for future comparison. Record this assessment with her prepregnancy weight, if available, to determine how much weight she has already gained or lost (Fig. 10.2). When weighing, be certain to convey an air of "accuracy is what counts" instead of censoring weight gain so the woman feels comfortable gaining 30 to 35 lb during pregnancy (many adolescents need to gain 40 lb to ensure a healthy fetus).

Vital signs, including blood pressure, respiratory rate, and pulse rate, are measured for baseline information. A sudden increase in blood pressure, like a sudden weight gain, is a danger sign of hypertension of pregnancy. A sudden increase in pulse or respirations may suggest bleeding. If close monitoring will be necessary during pregnancy, a support person or the woman herself can be taught the technique of blood pressure recording.

Assessment of Systems

General Appearance and Mental Status. Physical examination always begins with an inspection of general appearance to form an overall impression of the woman's health and well-being. General appearance is important because it reveals how people feel about themselves by the manner in which they dress, the way they speak, and the body posture they assume. Not all women are happy about being pregnant. Closely inspect for signs such as careless hygiene, unwashed hair, inappropriate or soiled clothing, and sad facial expression that may suggest fatigue or depression (Marcus et al., 2003).

If the woman has any bandages and other dressings in place, be sure to remove and replace them because they could hide an important finding such as a malignant melanoma or skin cancer, which are increasing problems in young adults (Freak, 2004).

A second increasing problem, or perhaps one receiving increased recognition, is intimate partner abuse, a condition that not only is dangerous to the woman but also may lead to early pregnancy loss (Janssen et al, 2003). Ask when and how any skin abnormality, such as an ecchymotic area, occurred. Most marks from battering occur on the face, the ulnar surfaces of the forearms (from a woman raising her arms to defend herself), the abdomen or buttocks (from being kicked), or the upper arms (from being grabbed and held forcefully). Noting the color of ecchymotic spots helps to date when they occurred. Such marks typically progress through purple to yellow changes.

Head and Scalp. Examine the woman's head for symmetry, normal contour, and tenderness and the hair for presence, distribution, thickness, excessive dryness or oiliness, cleanliness, or the use of hair dye (hair dye may be carcinogenic over an extended period of time). Look for **chloasma** (extra pigment on the face that occurs from melanocyte-stimulating hormone), which may accompany pregnancy. Hair growth speeds up during pregnancy as a result of the overall increased metabolic rate, and women may comment they have noticed this. Dryness

BOX 10.9 NURSING PROCEDURE

Obtaining a clean-catch urine specimen

Purpose
Helping a woman obtain a clean-catch urine specimen

PROCEDURE	PRINCIPLE
1. Ask the client to wash her hands.	1. Handwashing helps prevent the spread of micro-organisms.
2. Have the client open the commercial clean-catch urine specimen kit and moisten the cotton balls with the antiseptic solution or open the prepared antiseptic wipes.	2. Preparation enhances efficiency and decreases the possibility of contamination during the procedure.

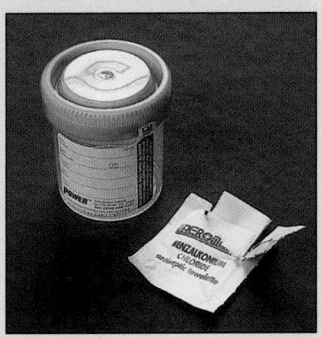

3. a. Have the client sit on the commode and separate her labia with her nondominant hand.

3. Cleansing helps prevent microorganisms from entering the urine specimen. Cleansing from front to back prevents bringing rectal contamination forward and prevents transmission of microorganisms.

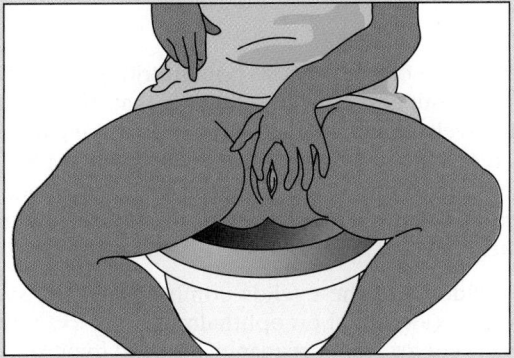

b. Tell her to cleanse her perineum, washing from front to back, using a cotton ball or wipe for only one stroke, then discarding it.

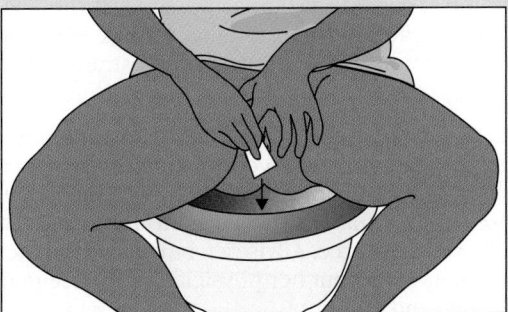

(continued)

PROCEDURE	PRINCIPLE
4. Advise the client to avoid touching the inside of the container or cap.	**4.** Careful handling of equipment prevents contamination.
5. Ask her to begin urinating, allowing the first urine to flow into the toilet. Then tell her to hold the container under the urine stream to obtain the specimen, removing the container after approximately 10 to 20 mL has been obtained. Once obtained, advise the client to remove the container, release her hand from her labia, and finish voiding in the toilet.	**5.** The first flow of urine washes microorganisms and debris from the urinary meatus. Collecting the specimen midstream ensures a sterile specimen is obtained.

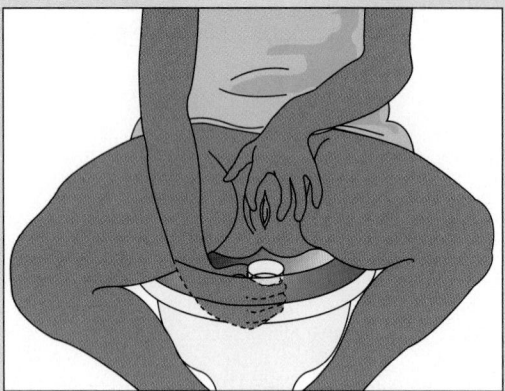

PROCEDURE	PRINCIPLE
6. Tell the woman to cap the specimen container, wash her hands, and bring it to you. Encourage her to report any pain on urination.	**6.** Capping the container prevents inadvertent spilling and possible contamination of the specimen. Pain on urination is a symptom of urinary tract infection.

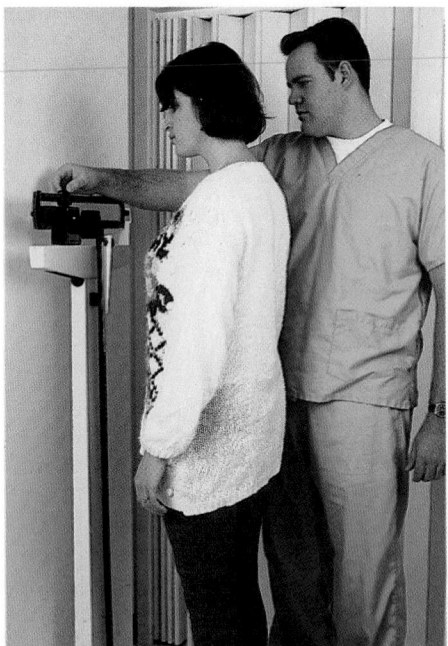

FIGURE 10.2 A woman weighs in at a prenatal visit. Pregnant women may need reassurance that gaining weight aids fetal growth. (© Barbara Proud.)

or sparseness of hair suggests poor nutrition. Lack of cleanliness may suggest fatigue, reflecting that the woman has not felt well enough to wash it recently. Urge women during pregnancy to let some other task go and save energy for self-care so they can continue to feel good about themselves. Dandruff shampoos may be used during pregnancy because they are not absorbed.

Eyes. Edema of the eyelids combined with a swollen optic disk (identified on ophthalmoscopic examination) suggests edema from pregnancy-induced hypertension, a potentially dangerous condition in pregnancy. On interview, women with pregnancy-induced hypertension also usually report spots before their eyes or diplopia (double vision). Teach pregnant women to recognize symptoms of poor vision as a potential danger sign of pregnancy that should be reported as soon as possible. If they do close desk work, caution them to take a break every hour so they do not confuse sensations of eyestrain with actual danger signs.

Nose. The increased level of estrogen associated with pregnancy may cause nasal congestion or the appearance of swollen nasal membranes. Even topical medicines such as nose drops or nasal sprays used to reduce this are absorbed to some degree. Advise a woman to avoid these during pregnancy without her physician's or nurse-midwife's knowledge and consent.

Ears. The nasal stuffiness that accompanies pregnancy may lead to blocked eustachian tubes and therefore a feeling of "fullness" in the ears or dampening of sound during early pregnancy. Usually this disappears as the body adjusts to the new estrogen level. Normal hearing level and normal tympanic landmarks should be present.

Sinuses. Sinuses should feel nontender. Establishing that tenderness over sinuses does not exist helps to evaluate that a client's reports of headache during pregnancy (a danger sign until ruled otherwise) is probably not sinus-related.

Mouth, Teeth, and Throat. Gingival (gum) hypertrophy may result from estrogen stimulation during pregnancy. The gums may be slightly swollen and tender to the touch, but not reddened. The pregnant woman is prone to vitamin deficiency because of the rapid growth of the fetus. Assess carefully for cracked corners of the mouth, which would reveal vitamin A deficiency. Assess carefully for pinpoint lesions with an erythematous base on the lips; these suggest a herpes infection (a herpes lesion on the gumline is more often a shallow ulcer). Because newborns are susceptible to herpes infection, lesions present at birth may necessitate limiting the woman's contact with her newborn.

Teach all women not to neglect good dental hygiene or yearly dental visits while pregnant. They should maintain thorough toothbrushing (some stop thorough brushing because they notice slightly blood-tinged saliva due to gingival hypertrophy).

If many dental caries are obvious, the woman should be referred to a dentist or dental clinic. Carious teeth are a source of infection and should be treated before abscesses develop and cause more serious problems. Contrary to what many women believe, dental x-rays can be taken during pregnancy as long as the woman reminds her dentist she is pregnant and is given a lead apron to shield her abdomen. Urge her to obtain permission from her primary care provider before consenting to extensive dental work requiring anesthesia.

Neck. Slight thyroid hypertrophy may occur with pregnancy because the overall metabolic rate is increased. All women should eat seafood once weekly to supply enough iodine for the accompanying increased thyroxine production (eating tuna more often than that is contraindicated, however, because of potentially high mercury content) (Stephenson, 2004). Encourage a woman who uses iodized salt to continue using this during pregnancy. Without this precaution, some women will view iodine as an unnecessary additive and discontinue using it during pregnancy.

Lymph Nodes. No palpable lymph nodes should be present; however, because pregnant women may develop an increased number of upper respiratory infections due to reduced immunologic resistance, one or two pea-sized cervical lymph nodes may be palpable. If a woman has a tooth abscess from bacterial growth under hypertrophied gingival tissue (periodontal disease), submaxillary lymph nodes may be palpable.

Breasts. Breast changes may be one of the first things women notice in pregnancy:

- Areolae darken.
- Secondary areolae may develop surrounding the natural ones.
- Montgomery tubercles (sebaceous glands in the areolae) become prominent.
- Overall breast size increases.
- Breast consistency firms.
- Blue streaking of veins becomes prominent.
- Colostrum may be expelled as early as the 16th week of pregnancy.
- Any supernumerary nipple also may become darker and enlarge in size.

Benign breast lesions that might be discovered on physical examination are discussed in Chapter 47.

Heart. Heart rate typically ranges from 70 to 80 beats per minute, and no accessory sounds or murmurs should be present. Occasionally, a woman may develop an innocent (functional) heart murmur during pregnancy because of the increased vascular volume. If this occurs, she needs further evaluation to ensure that it is only a physiologic change of pregnancy and not a previously undetected heart condition. Many women notice occasional palpitations (heart skipping a beat) during pregnancy, especially when lying supine. Teach pregnant women always to rest or sleep on their side (left side is best) to help avoid this problem.

Lungs. Assess respiratory rate and rhythm. Although lung tissue assumes a more horizontal position during pregnancy, vital capacity is not reduced. Late in pregnancy, diaphragmatic excursion (diaphragm movement) is lessened because the diaphragm cannot descend as fully as usual because of the distended uterus.

Back. The lumbar curve in many pregnant women is accentuated on standing so that they can maintain body posture in the face of increasing abdominal size. This response may cause considerable back pain during pregnancy. Assess the spine for any abnormal curve that would suggest scoliosis. Young women with scoliosis may need a referral to their orthopedist during pregnancy to be certain that their condition is not worsening.

Rectum. Assess the rectum closely for hemorrhoidal tissue, which commonly occurs from uterine pressure on pelvic veins preventing venous return. Hemorrhoids can be very uncomfortable for women and worrisome if they are not assured that hemorrhoids are a normal discomfort of pregnancy.

Extremities and Skin. Many women develop palmar erythema and itching early in pregnancy from a high estrogen level and perhaps subclinical jaundice (jaundice that is not yet apparent by a color change) from reabsorbed bilirubin due to slowed intestinal peristalsis. Assess the lower extremities carefully for varicosities, filling time of the toenails (which should be under 5 seconds), and the presence of edema caused by impaired venous return from the lower extremities. Any edema more than ankle swelling may be a danger sign of pregnancy.

Assess the gait of pregnant women to see that they are keeping their pelvis tucked under the weight of their abdomen. This position prevents them from developing muscle strains from abnormal abdominal muscle tension. Many pregnant women develop a "waddling" gait late in pregnancy from relaxation of the symphysis pubis. This relaxation may cause pain if the cartilage is actually so unstable that it moves on walking.

Measurement of Fundal Height and Fetal Heart Sounds

At about 12 to 14 weeks of pregnancy, the uterus is palpable over the symphysis pubis as a firm globular sphere. It reaches the umbilicus at 20 to 22 weeks and the xiphoid process at 36 weeks, and then often returns to about 4 cm below the xiphoid due to "lightening" at 40 weeks. If the woman is past 12 weeks of a pregnancy, palpate the fundus location, measure the fundal height (from the notch above the symphysis pubis to the superior aspect of the uterine fundus), and plot the height on a graph such as the one shown in Figure 10.3. Plotting uterine growth at each visit can help detect any unusual variation in fetal growth. If an abnormality is detected, further investigation with ultrasound can be done to determine the cause of the unusual increase or decrease in growth.

Auscultate for fetal heart sounds (120 to 160 beats per minute). These can be heard at 10 to 12 weeks if a Doppler technique is used but not until 18 to 20 weeks if a regular stethoscope is used. Palpate for fetal outline and position after the 28th week.

Checkpoint Question 3

Sandra reports that the palms of her hands are always itchy. You notice scratches on them when you do a physical exam. What is the most likely cause of this finding during pregnancy?

a. She must have become allergic to dishwashing soap.
b. She has an allergy to her fetus and will probably abort.
c. Her weight gain has stretched the skin over her hands.
d. This is a common reaction to increasing estrogen levels.

Pelvic Examination

A pelvic examination reveals information on the health of both internal and external reproductive organs. It requires the following equipment: a **speculum** (a metal or plastic instrument with movable flat blades; Fig. 10.4), a spatula for cervical scraping, a clean examining glove, lubricant, a glass slide or liquid collection device for the Pap smear, a culture tube, two or three sterile cotton-tipped applicators or cytobrushes for obtaining cervical cultures, a good examining light, and a stool at correct sitting height (Keye & Damewood, 2003).

Be aware that pelvic examinations have the reputation of being painful and, of course, cause a loss of modesty. If this is a first pregnancy, it may be the first time a woman has ever had this type of exam. Having heard stories about how painful these examinations are may cause her to tense just thinking about it. When the pelvic muscles are tight and tense, not only does the examination become painful, but also the examiner has difficulty assessing the status of the pelvic organs.

Allow the woman the opportunity to talk with the person performing the examination while sitting up, before being placed in a lithotomy position (Fig. 10.5): it may enhance her sense of self-esteem and control to meet her examiner first while in this position. Many women want their support person to remain with them at the head of the table during the examination. In addition, it is customary, especially on an initial visit, for a nurse or a nursing assistant to be in the room with a woman for the pelvic examination to offer additional support. This is true whether the examiner is male or female.

When serving as a support person, remain at the head of the table; do not stand at the foot of the table. Being at the head of the table enables you to hold the woman's hand or put a hand on her shoulder if she needs the support of physical contact. Explanations of what is happening or what the examiner is doing are helpful. Conversation with the examiner over her head is not. Suggesting that a woman breathe in and out (not hold her breath as she is likely to do) is another technique to help her relax (holding her breath pushes the diaphragm down and makes the pelvic organs tense and unyielding).

Before a pelvic examination, a woman should void to reduce her bladder size and then lie in a **lithotomy posi-**

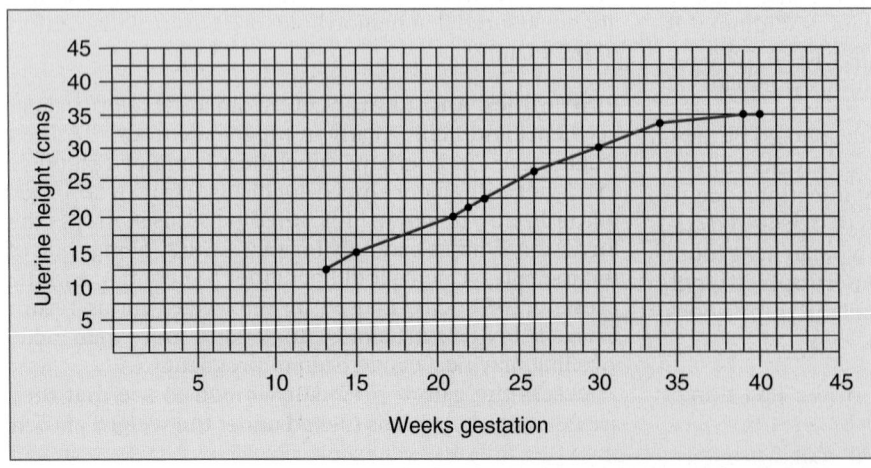

FIGURE 10.3 Plotting uterine height on a uterine height graph at prenatal visits (typically after 12 weeks gestation) helps to monitor whether fundal height is adequate.

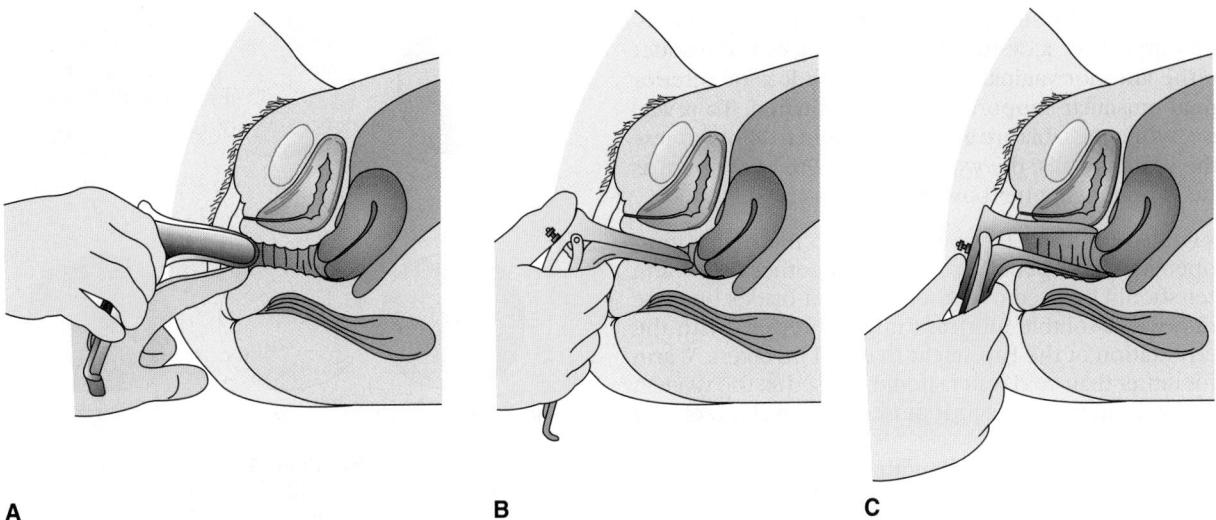

FIGURE 10.4 Insertion of a vaginal speculum. (**A**) Blades held obliquely on entering the vagina. (**B**) Blades rotated to horizontal position as they pass the introitus. (**C**) Blades separated by depressing thumbpiece and elevating handle. The position of the blades is maintained by adjusting a thumbscrew.

tion (on her back with her thighs flexed and her feet resting in the examining table stirrups (see Fig. 10.5). Make sure her buttocks extend slightly beyond the end of the examining table. Place a pillow under her head to help her relax her abdominal muscles.

Properly drape her with a draw sheet over her abdomen that extends over her legs. Be sure pregnant women remain in a lithotomy position for as short a time as possible to help prevent thromboembolism and supine hypotension syndrome.

If desired, a woman may watch the pelvic examination with an overhead mirror or a mirror held by herself or the examiner. Seeing vaginal cervical pathology can help her to understand any kind of problem present and the interventions necessary to improve it. If not already doing so, sexually active women should be taught how to do a monthly perineal examination (holding a mirror) so they can detect perineal lesions such as herpes simplex 2 viral infections.

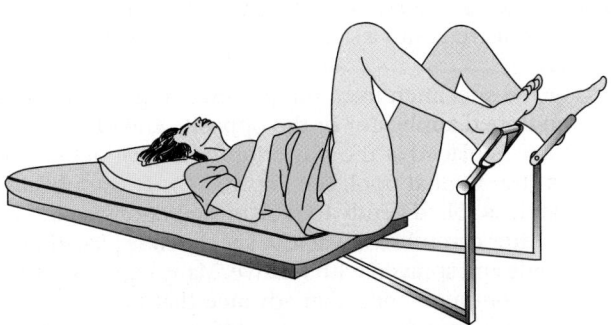

FIGURE 10.5 A lithotomy position used for a pelvic examination. Help position the woman with her buttocks just over the edge of the table. Drape appropriately for modesty.

? What if... the foot of an examining table in a clinic faces the room door, leaving women to feel exposed if someone should walk in unexpectedly? Is this the best position for the table? What could you do about this?

External Genitalia. A pelvic examination begins with inspection of the external genitalia. Any signs of inflammation, irritation, or infection, such as redness, ulcerations, or vaginal discharge, are noted.

A herpes simplex 2 virus infection appears as clustered, pinpoint vesicles on an erythematous (reddened) base on the vulva. These feel painful when touched or irritated. It is important to detect these during pregnancy as the presence of herpes lesions on the vulva or vagina at the time of birth may necessitate cesarean birth to prevent exposing the fetus to the virus during passage through the birth canal. There may be an association between cervical cancer and herpes simplex 2 infections. Note in the record the presence of a herpes infection for future follow-up with cytologic (Pap) smears for cervical cancer.

The Skene glands that empty into the urethra are checked for infection. To do this, a sterile gloved finger is inserted into the vagina and pressed against the anterior vaginal wall to see if any pus can be extruded from the openings to the glands at the urethral opening. The woman is also evaluated for possible infection of the Bartholin glands that enter into the distal vagina. The sites of the Bartholin glands (5 and 7 o'clock positions) are palpated between the vaginal finger and the thumb of the same hand. If a discharge is produced from any of these gland ducts (Skene or Bartholin), a culture is obtained. Infection here could be caused by something as simple as streptococci; often it is gonorrhea.

Problems with vascular muscle wall support, such as a rectocele (a forward pouching of the rectum into the posterior vaginal wall due to loss of posterior vaginal muscular support) or a cystocele (a pouching of the bladder into the anterior vaginal wall, caused by loss of anterior vaginal muscular support), are also evaluated. To reveal these, while the labia are gently separated to allow a view of the vaginal walls, the woman is asked to bear down as if she were moving her bowels.

Internal Genitalia. To view the cervix, the vagina must be opened with a speculum. No lubricant other than warm water should be used over the speculum blades because even a water-soluble lubricant might interfere with the interpretation of the Pap smear that will be taken. Warm water rather than cold water should be used so the woman does not contract her vaginal muscles when she feels the cold instrument.

A speculum is introduced with the blades in a closed position and directed toward the posterior rather than the anterior vaginal wall because the posterior wall is less sensitive (see Fig. 10.4A). A speculum enters most readily if it is inserted at an oblique angle (the crease of the blades directed to 4 or 8 o'clock), then rotated to a horizontal position when fully inserted (the crease of the blades pointing to a 3 or 9 o'clock position) (see Fig. 10.4B). When fully inserted and rotated to a horizontal position, the blades are opened so the cervix is visible and are secured in the open position by tightening the thumb screw at the side (see Fig. 10.4C).

With the speculum in place, the cervix can be inspected for its position. Normally it is centered on the vagina; a retroverted uterus has a cervix positioned anteriorly, and an anteverted uterus has its cervix positioned posteriorly. The cervix color (a nonpregnant cervix is light pink; in pregnancy it changes to almost purple) and any lesions, ulcerations, discharge, or otherwise abnormal appearance are documented.

In a **nulligravida** (a woman who is not or never has been pregnant), the cervical os is round and small. In a woman who has had a previous pregnancy with a vaginal birth, the cervical os has much more of a slitlike appearance (Fig. 10.6A). If the woman had a cervical tear during a previous birth, the cervical os may appear as a transverse crease the width of the cervix or a typical starlike (stellate) formation. If a cervical infection is present, a mucus discharge may be present. With infection, the epithelium of the cervical canal often enlarges and spreads onto the area surrounding the os, giving the cervix a reddened appearance (**erosion;** see Fig. 10.6C). This area bleeds readily if it is touched.

Trichomoniasis, a protozoal infection, generally gives signs of redness; a profuse, whitish, bubbly discharge; and petechial spots on the vaginal walls. Candidal (*Monilia*) infection typically presents with thick, white vaginal patches that may bleed if scraped away. A gonorrhea infection typically presents with a thick, greenish-yellow discharge and extreme inflammation. Chlamydia infection, in contrast, shows few symptoms except slight cervical redness.

Carcinoma of the cervix appears as an irregular, granular growth at the os. Cervical polyps (red, soft, pedunculated protrusions) also are occasionally seen at the os.

Pap Smear. A Pap smear is taken for early detection of cervical cancer and diagnosis of precancerous and can-

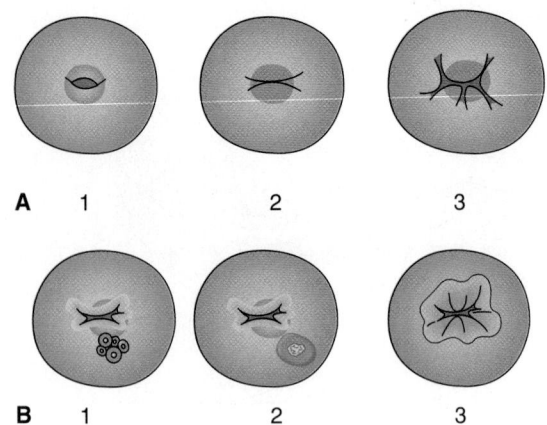

FIGURE 10.6 (A) Appearances of the cervix. (1) Nulligravida cervix. (2) Cervix after childbirth. (3) "Stellate" cervix seen after mild cervical tearing. **(B)** Possible cervical lesions. (1) Herpes II. (2) Chancre of syphilis. (3) Erosion or infection.

cerous conditions of the vulva and vagina; it also reveals inflammatory and infectious diseases. Although only an endocervical smear (one from inside the cervix) may be taken to be plated for a Pap test in some centers, in others three separate specimens—one from the endocervix, one from the cervical os, and one from the posterior vaginal fornix—are obtained (Fig. 10.7). In addition, a cervicogram (a photograph of the cervix) may be taken. Cervicograms serve as complements to Pap smears as a weapon for detecting cervical cancer and documenting that lesions from infections are healing.

To obtain an endocervical specimen for a Pap smear, a sterile cotton applicator, wet with saline, is inserted through the speculum into the os of the cervix and gently rotated, first clockwise, then counterclockwise (see Fig. 10.7A). It is then removed without touching the sides of the vagina. The specimen is then gently painted on a glass slide. The slide is sprayed with a fixative to preserve the cells. Use of cytobrushes for pregnant women is not recommended, because they can cause cervical bleeding due to increased cervical softening (Fischbach, 2004).

To take a cervical os specimen, the uneven end of a spatula is inserted through the speculum and pressed on the os of the cervix and rotated to scrape cells in a circle around the os (see Fig. 10.7B). After removal, the spatula is then smeared onto a slide and the slide is sprayed with fixative.

For the specimen from the posterior vaginal fornix, a cotton-tipped applicator or the opposite end of the spatula blade is placed at the posterior fornix just below the cervix (the vaginal pool; see Fig. 10.7C). The applicator or spatula is rolled gently to pick up secretions collected there. After careful removal, the specimen is placed on a third slide and sprayed with fixative. Many Pap smears are read by computer today, an advance that has made the collection of specimens slightly different. If a ThinPrep Pap smear is being taken, a small broomlike collection device is inserted into the endocervical canal deep enough

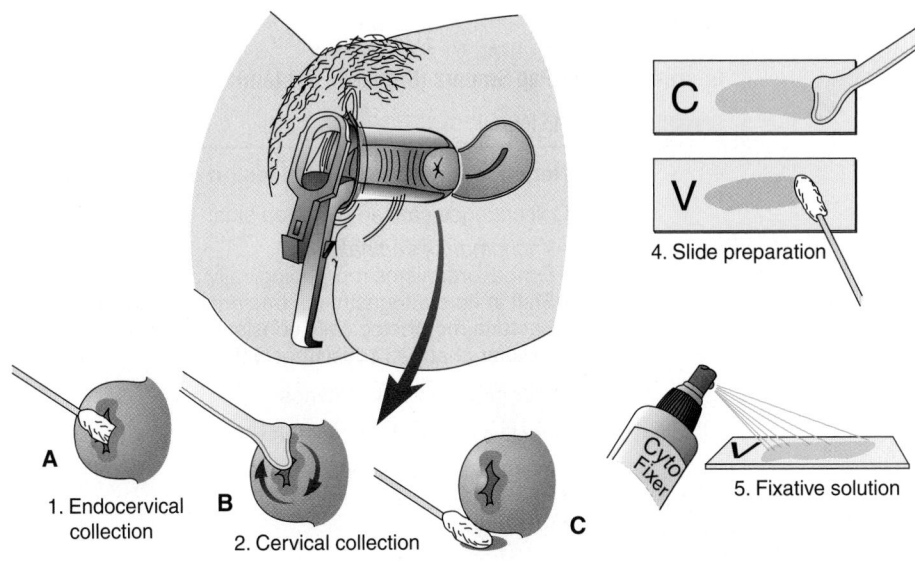

FIGURE 10.7 Obtaining a traditional Pap smear. (**A**) Specimen taken from endocervix. (**B**) Specimen taken from cervix. (**C**) Specimen taken from vaginal pool.

1. Endocervical collection

2. Cervical collection

3. Vaginal pool collection

4. Slide preparation

5. Fixative solution

to allow the short bristles to contact the endocervix, and it is rotated in a clockwise direction five times. The device is then rinsed off in a special solution-filled collection vial; the vial is then capped, labeled, and sent to the laboratory (Fischbach, 2004; Fig. 10.8).

The classification of Pap smears is constantly being revised as the meaning of abnormal cells is further defined (Davey, 2003). The Bethesda classification of Pap smears is shown in Table 10.3. Be certain when discussing these reports with women that they do not overinterpret the results. The first category means only normal cells were found. The second category means cells are inflamed because infection is present (the woman needs to be treated and reexamined in about 3 months). At the next level (LSIL), cells are moderately suspicious for malignancy. The HSIL category identifies that precancerous cells are present.

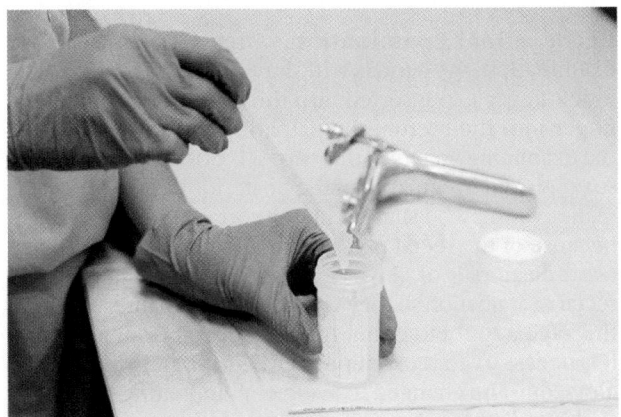

FIGURE 10.8 For liquid Pap tests, the collecting instrument is placed in a commercial vial and capped rather than being smeared onto a slide.

This level requires a colposcopy examination for further evaluation. Only the last category is indicative that squamous cell carcinoma is present. Therapy at this level will include colposcopy, biopsy, and removal of the affected cells, usually by conization.

Many women ask how often repeat Pap smears are necessary because the recommendations have changed. The American Cancer Society recommends women begin to have Pap smears when they turn 18 or become sexually active (whichever is first). They may be necessary as infrequently as every 3 years in women who have had two consecutive negative tests a year apart. Women who should have them more frequently are those who have multiple sexual partners, who have a history of human papillomavirus (HPV) infection, who smoke cigarettes, or who were active sexually before age 21. Screening as infrequently as every 3 years could miss pathology in these women.

Women who engage in anal intercourse may have an anal swab taken as well as vaginal swabs to detect anal squamous neoplasms. The technique for obtaining anal Pap smears is the same as that for vaginal specimens (a cytobrush is used). Caution the patient that she may have slight rectal bleeding following the procedure.

Vaginal Inspection. Before the speculum is removed, a culture for gonorrhea, chlamydia, or group B streptococcus may be taken. After gently swabbing the cervix using cotton-tipped applicators, the specimens obtained are then plated onto a medium to allow for their growth. All these organisms can cause disease in the newborn, so it is best if they can be eradicated during pregnancy.

A speculum must be unlocked and partially closed before removal; otherwise, pain from excessive stretching could occur. If the speculum is kept partially open as it is removed, it should not cause any pain, and the sides of the vagina can be inspected as it is withdrawn. In a nonpregnant woman, vaginal walls are light pink; pregnancy

TABLE 10.3

Interpretation of Pap Smears (Bethesda System)

Classification	Findings
1	**Negative for intraepithelial lesion or malignancy** Cell changes caused by organisms: • *Trichomonas vaginalis* • Fungal organisms morphologically consistent with *Candida* species • Shift in flora suggestive of bacterial vaginosis (coccobacillus) • Bacteria morphologically consistent with *Actinomyces* species • Cellular changes consistent with herpes simplex virus Other nonneoplastic findings Reactive changes associated with: • Inflammation (includes repair) • Radiation • IUD use Atrophy Glandular cells status after hysterectomy Endometrial cells (in women >40 years of age)
2	**Atypical squamous cells of undetermined significance (ASCUS)**
3	**Low-grade squamous intraepithelial lesion (LSIL)** Changes include those caused by: • Human papillomavirus (HPV) • Mild dysplasia • Cervical intraepithelial neoplasm (CIN) grade 1 (low-grade precursor)
4	**High-grade squamous intraepithelial lesion (HSIL)** Changes include those caused by: • Moderate to severe dysplasia • CIN grades 2 and 3 (high-grade precursors)—formerly carcinoma in situ (CIS) Has features suspicious for invasion
5	**Squamous cell carcinoma**

turns them dark blue to purple. Any areas of inflammation, ulceration, lesions, or discharge should be noted.

Examination of Pelvic Organs. Following the speculum examination, a bimanual (two-handed) examination is performed to assess the position, contour, consistency, and tenderness of pelvic organs (Fig. 10.9). The index and middle fingers of one gloved hand are lubricated and inserted into the vagina so the walls of the vagina can be palpated for abnormalities. The other hand is then placed on the woman's abdomen and pressed downward toward the hand still in the vagina until the uterus can be felt between them. If a uterus is extremely retroverted, it may not be palpable abdominally. Next, the right and left ovaries are identified by the same method. Ovaries are normally slightly tender, so the pressure caused by palpation may cause the woman some discomfort.

Abnormalities that can be noted by bimanual examination include ovarian cysts, enlarged fallopian tubes (perhaps from pelvic inflammatory disease), and an enlarged uterus (see Table 10.1). An early sign of pregnancy (Hegar's

sign) is elicited on bimanual examination as well (see Fig. 9.4).

Rectovaginal Examination. After a bimanual pelvic examination, the hand is withdrawn from the vagina. The index finger is reinserted into the vagina and the middle finger into the rectum. By palpating the tissue between the examining fingers in this way, it is possible to assess the strength and irregularity of the posterior vaginal wall. This maneuver may be slightly uncomfortable for the woman because of the rectal pressure involved. Some examiners use a clean pair of gloves before they perform a vaginal-rectal examination so they will not spread an infection from the vagina to the rectum. After the rectal examination, if it is necessary to reexamine the vagina for any reason, the glove must be changed to avoid contaminating the vagina with fecal material.

After completing the examination, any excess lubricant is wiped away from the vaginal and rectal openings. It is important to wipe front to back to prevent bringing rectal contamination forward to the vaginal introitus.

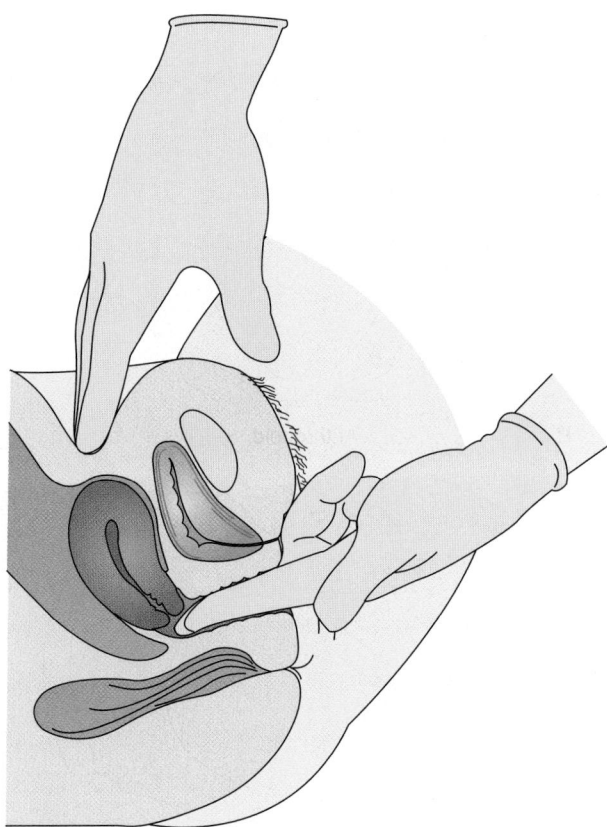

FIGURE 10.9 A bimanual examination to determine uterine size.

 Checkpoint Question 4

Sandra has not had a pelvic exam since she was in high school. What advice would you give her to help her relax during her first prenatal pelvic exam?

a. Have her take a deep breath and hold it during the exam.
b. Tell her to bear down slightly as the speculum is inserted.
c. Singing out loud helps, because it pushes down the diaphragm.
d. She should breathe slowly and evenly during the exam.

Estimating Pelvic Size

It is impossible to predict from the outward appearance of a woman whether her pelvic ring will be adequate for a fetus to pass through its center. Some women look as if they have a wide pelvis but, in reality, have only wide iliac crests and a normal or even smaller-than-normal internal ring. Other women appear as if their pelvis will be small because the iliac crests are nonflaring, but the internal pelvis, the part that must be sufficiently large for childbirth, is of average size, allowing them to give birth vaginally without difficulty. Differences in pelvic contour and development occur mainly because of hereditary factors, but disease

(e.g., rickets, now rarely seen in the United States, which may cause contraction of the pelvis) or injury (inadequate repair following an accident) also may play a role.

If on this initial visit the primary care provider establishes that the woman is pregnant, and if she has never given birth vaginally before, pelvic measurements may be taken. Some care providers prefer to take these measurements later in pregnancy, when the woman's pelvic muscles are more relaxed, making measurement easier. If a routine sonogram is scheduled, estimations may be made by a combination of pelvic pelvimetry and fetal sonography. Estimation of pelvic adequacy must be done at least by the 24th week of pregnancy, because by this time there is danger that the fetal head will reach a size that will interfere with safe passage and birth if the pelvic measurements are small.

Once a woman has given birth vaginally, her pelvis has been proven adequate. Thus, it is not necessary to take her pelvic measurements again unless she has had an intervening history of trauma to the pelvis.

The types of pelves found in women can be categorized into four groups (Fig. 10.10): android, anthropoid, gynecoid, and platypelloid.

Internal pelvic measurements give the actual diameters of the inlet and outlet through which the fetus must pass. The following measurements are made most commonly:

1. The **diagonal conjugate.** This is the distance between the anterior surface of the sacral prominence and the anterior surface of the inferior margin of the symphysis pubis (Fig. 10.11*A*). The most useful measurement for estimation of pelvic size, it suggests the anteroposterior diameter of the pelvic inlet (the narrower diameter at that level, or the one that is most apt to cause a misfit with the fetal head). The diagonal conjugate is measured while the woman is in a lithotomy position. To measure it, two fingers are introduced vaginally and pressed inward and upward until the middle finger touches the sacral prominence. With the other hand, the part of the examining hand where it touches the symphysis pubis is marked (see Fig. 10.11*A*). After withdrawing the examining hand, the distance between the tip of the middle finger and the marked point on the glove on that hand is measured by comparing it with a ruler or, for greater accuracy, a pelvimeter. Caution the client that the measurement may be slightly painful, because she may feel the pressure of the examining finger as it stretches to touch the sacral prominence. If the examiner's hand is small with short fingers, manual pelvic measurements may not be possible, because the fingers may not reach the sacral prominence. If the measurement obtained is more than 12.5 cm, the pelvic inlet is rated as adequate for childbirth (the diameter of the fetal head that must pass that point averages 9 cm in diameter).

2. The **true conjugate** or **conjugate vera** is the measurement between the anterior surface of the sacral prominence and the posterior surface of the inferior margin of the symphysis pubis. This measurement cannot be made directly, but it can be estimated from the measurement made of the diagonal conjugate. To do this, the usual depth of the symphysis pubis (assumed to be 1.5 to 2 cm) is subtracted from the diagonal conjugate measurement. The distance remaining will be the

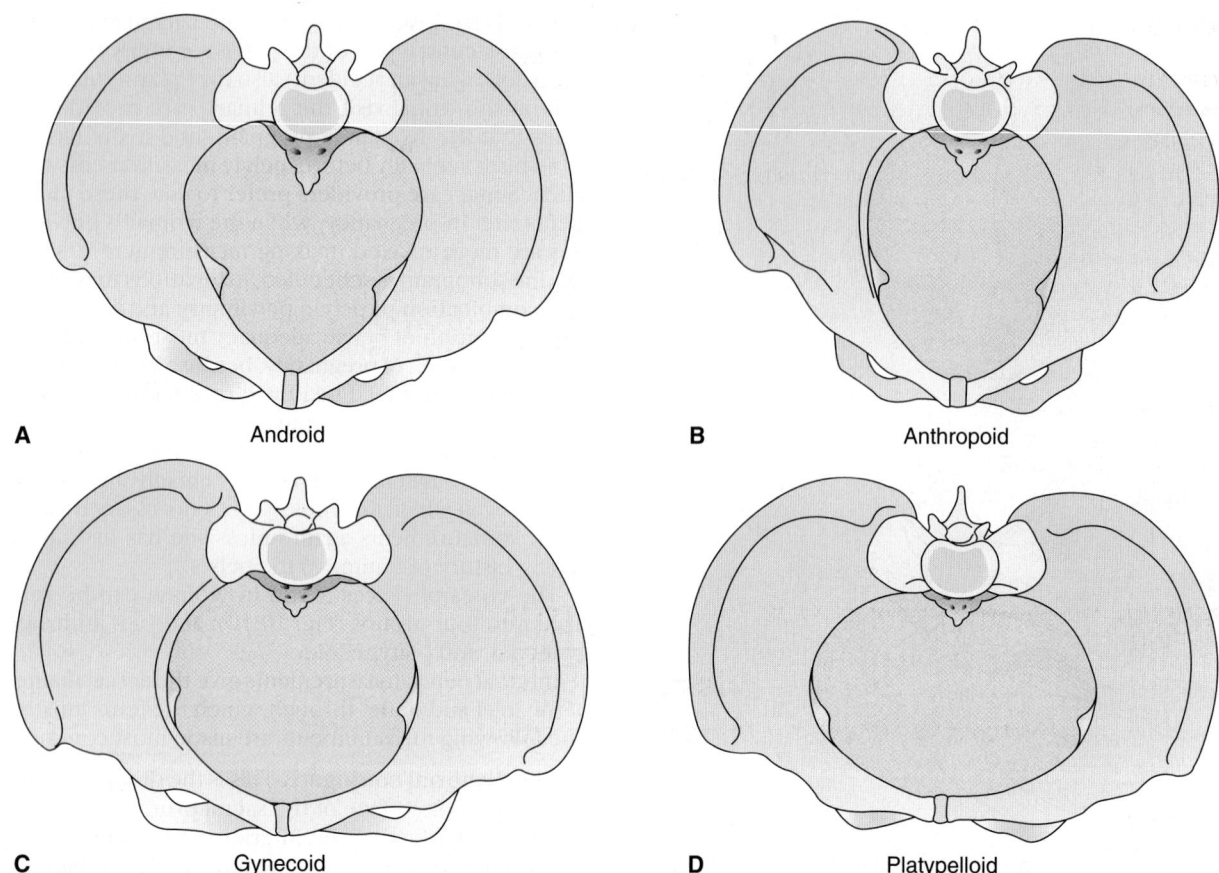

A   Android

B   Anthropoid

C   Gynecoid

D   Platypelloid

FIGURE 10.10 Types of pelves. (**A**) *Android* pelvis—"male" pelvis. The pubic arch in this pelvis type forms an acute angle, making the lower dimensions of the pelvis extremely narrow. A fetus may have difficulty exiting from this type of pelvis. (**B**) *Anthropoid* pelvis— "ape-like" pelvis. The transverse diameter is narrow, and the anteroposterior diameter of the inlet is larger than normal. This structure does not accommodate a fetal head as well as a gynecoid pelvis. (**C**) *Gynecoid* pelvis—"normal" female pelvis. The inlet is well rounded forward and backward; the pubic arch is wide. This pelvic type is ideal for childbirth. (**D**) *Platypelloid* pelvis—"flattened" pelvis. The inlet is an oval, smoothly curved, but the anteroposterior diameter is shallow. A fetal head might not be able to rotate to match the curves of the pelvic cavity in this type of pelvis.

true conjugate, or the actual diameter of the pelvic inlet through which the fetal head must pass. The average true conjugate diameter is, therefore, 12.5 cm minus 1.5 or 2 cm, or 10.5 to 11 cm.

3. The **ischial tuberosity** diameter. This measurement is the distance between the ischial tuberosities, or the transverse diameter of the outlet (the narrowest diameter at that level, or the one most apt to cause a misfit). It is made at the medial and lowermost aspect of the ischial tuberosities at the level of the anus (see Fig. 10.11*B*). A pelvimeter is generally used, although the diameter can be measured by a ruler or by comparing it with a known hand span or clenched fist measurement. A diameter of 11 cm is considered adequate because it will allow the widest diameter of the fetal head, or 9 cm, to pass freely through the outlet.

Laboratory Assessment

A number of laboratory studies are included in assessment measures at a first prenatal visit to confirm general health

and rule out sexually transmitted infection that could injure the growing fetus. Normal levels for these studies are shown in Appendix F.

Blood Studies

The following blood studies are usually done at a first prenatal visit:

1. A complete blood count, including hemoglobin or hematocrit and red cell index to determine the presence of anemia, a white blood cell count to determine infection, and a platelet count to estimate clotting ability.
2. Women are advised to have a blood sample taken for a genetic screen for commonly ethnically inherited diseases. African-American women may have a blood sample taken to screen for sickle cell trait or disease and possibly glucose-6-phosphate dehydrogenase. Asian and Mediterranean women may have this done for beta-thalassemia; those with Jewish ancestry may have this done for Tay-Sachs disease, and Caucasian women may

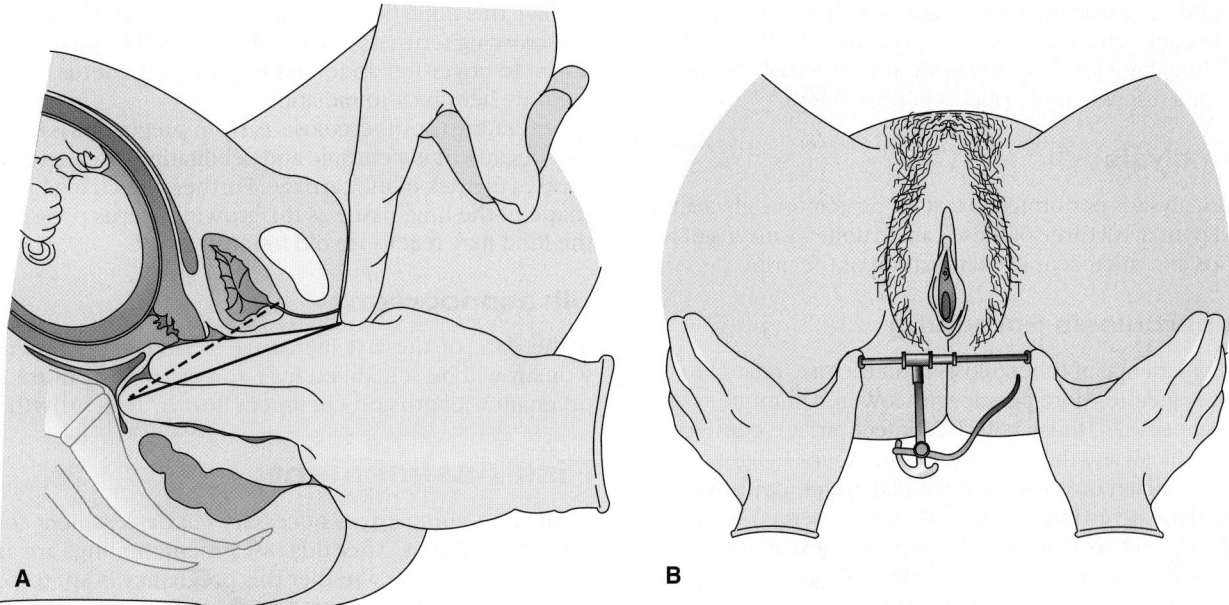

FIGURE 10.11 (A) Measurement of diagonal conjugate diameter. *Solid line* = diagonal conjugate; *dotted line* = true conjugate. **(B)** Measurement of ischial tuberosity diameter.

be tested for cystic fibrosis (see Chapter 7 for a discussion of these disorders).

3. A serologic test for syphilis (VDRL or rapid plasma reagin test). If syphilis is present, it must be treated early in pregnancy before fetal damage occurs. A blood sample for a serologic test for gonorrhea may be drawn on women suspected of having this disease.

4. Blood typing (including Rh factor). Blood type is documented because blood may have to be made available if the woman has bleeding early in her pregnancy.

5. Maternal serum for AFP (MSAFP). This level will be elevated if a neural tube or abdominal defect is present in the fetus; it may be decreased if a chromosomal anomaly is present. This test is done at 16 to 18 weeks of pregnancy. The level in serum is expressed as "multiples of the mean" (MOM). A normal value is 2.5 MOM. If this is elevated or decreased, a sonogram or amniocentesis will be ordered to assess for a fetal disorder.

6. An indirect Coombs' test (determination if Rh antibodies are present in an Rh-negative woman). This test is generally repeated at 28 weeks of pregnancy. If the titers are not elevated, an Rh-negative woman will receive RhIG (RhoGAM) at 28 weeks of pregnancy and after any procedure that might cause placental bleeding, such as amniocentesis or external version.

7. Antibody titers for rubella and hepatitis B (HBsAg). These tests determine whether the woman is protected against rubella if exposure should occur during pregnancy and whether a newborn will have a chance of developing hepatitis B. HBsAg testing may be repeated at about 36 weeks. Antibodies for varicella (chickenpox) may also be assessed. Vaccine against these diseases can be offered in the postpartum period.

8. HIV screening. All women can be asked, and those at high risk for contracting HIV infection should be asked, whether they want to be screened for this disease early in pregnancy. High-risk criteria include women who

have used or are using intravenous drugs; have engaged in sex with multiple partners; have had sexual partners who are infected or are at risk because they are bisexual, intravenous drug abusers, or hemophiliacs; or received a blood transfusion between 1977 and 1985 (Minkoff & Gibbs, 2003).

Screening is done by an enzyme-linked immunosorbent assay (ELISA) on a blood sample. If this is positive, the finding is confirmed by a second test (a Western blot). Testing for HIV early in pregnancy allows a woman who is found to be HIV antibody positive the opportunity to begin therapy with zidovudine (AZT), which can decrease the risk of her infant acquiring the virus. It also allows the woman the option of choosing to terminate a pregnancy to avoid giving birth to an infant who has a high risk of HIV infection.

As there is still no cure for HIV infection, some women may choose not to have a blood titer taken because they would rather not know that they have the illness. This is their option. Screening cannot be mandatory in prenatal settings. Health care providers need to be certain that test results given to clients are accurate (a high blood antibody titer means the person has been exposed to the virus, not that he or she necessarily is infected) and are presented with tact and compassion, with respect for the meaning of the results to the client. Results of HIV testing are kept confidential; be certain not to report this information to anyone other than the client.

9. If the woman has a history of previously unexplained fetal loss, has a family history of diabetes, has had babies who were large for gestational age (9 lb or more at term), is obese, or has glycosuria, she will need to be scheduled for a 50-g oral 1-hour glucose loading or tolerance test toward the end of the first trimester to rule out gestational diabetes. If not, she will have this done routinely at the 24th to 28th week to evaluate insulin-antagonistic

effects of placental hormones, which can register a noticeable effect at this time. The plasma glucose level should not exceed 140 mg/dL at 1 hour (see Chapter 14 for a discussion of diabetes in pregnancy).

Urinalysis

A urinalysis is performed to test for proteinuria, glycosuria, and pyuria. All three of these can be done by means of test strips and microscopic examination of the urine.

Tuberculosis Screening

The incidence of tuberculosis is on the rise, related to the HIV epidemic. More people with lowered immune system resistance (i.e., those with HIV infection) are contracting tuberculosis and then spreading it to others. In light of this, the physician or nurse-midwife may order a purified protein derivative (PPD) tuberculin test to screen for tuberculosis. Any woman who has a positive reaction would then require a chest x-ray for further diagnosis.

If a woman has a history of tuberculosis or has received a BCG vaccine for tuberculosis, a tuberculin skin test should not be given because the reaction would be extreme. Although BCG vaccine is not administered in the United States, immigrants from other countries may have received this. To assess a woman's current disease status, a chest x-ray may be ordered. A woman is often reluctant to have this done because she knows radiation is harmful to a growing fetus. Assure her that she will be given a lead apron to cover her abdomen to protect the fetus, exposing only her chest to radiation.

Screening for tuberculosis early in pregnancy is important because it is a chronic and debilitating disease that increases the risk of miscarriage. Further, the change in the shape of the lung tissue as the growing uterus presses on the lung may reactivate old lesions.

Ultrasonography

If the date of the last menstrual period is unknown, a woman will be scheduled for a sonogram to confirm the pregnancy length and document healthy fetal growth.

Risk Assessment

Table 10.4 summarizes necessary data assessment for a first prenatal visit. After this assessment, findings are analyzed to determine whether this pregnancy is apt to continue with a good outcome or there is some risk that it will end before term or with an unfavorable fetal or maternal outcome (a high-risk pregnancy).

Many factors enter into the categorization of high risk. Most health care agencies use some tool to determine high risk, but no tool is perfect because the concept of high risk is a very individualized one. Table 10.5 lists factors

TABLE 10.4

Assessments for a First Pregnancy Visit

Health History

Demographic data	Name, address, age, telephone number, health insurance
Chief concern	Was pregnancy planned? When was last menstrual period? Any exposure to infectious diseases or ingestion of drugs since she thinks she has been pregnant?
Family and social profile	What is family composition? Who is her chief support person? What is her occupation? Source of income? Level of exercise? Hobbies? Recreational drug use? Living conditions? Nutrition? Sleep pattern?
Past medical history	Any abdominal surgery, kidney, heart, hypertension, sexually transmitted infections, diabetes, allergies?
Gynecologic history	When was menarche? What is length and duration of menstrual cycle?
Obstetric history	Any previous pregnancies? When? Type and outcome of birth? Any history of previous miscarriages?
Review of systems	Brief review of all body systems

Physical Examination

Baseline data	Height, weight, vital signs, fundal height measurements (after 12 weeks), fetal heart sounds
System assessment	Full physical examination to confirm general health
Pelvic examination	General assessment, Pap smear, cultures for chlamydia, gonorrhea, group B streptococcus, pelvic measurements

Laboratory Assessment

Blood assessment	Complete blood count, serologic test for syphilis, blood type and Rh, alpha-fetoprotein, antibody titer against Rh, hepatitis B, rubella, and possibly varicella and HIV.
Urinalysis	Clean catch for glucose, protein, ketones, and culture
Tuberculosis	PPD test
Ultrasound	To date pregnancy or confirm fetal health (if date of last menstrual period is unknown)

TABLE 10.5

Assessments That Might Categorize a Pregnancy as At Risk

Obstetric History	History of infertility or grand multiparity
	Premature cervical dilatation
	Uterine or cervical anomaly
	Previous preterm labor or preterm birth or cesarean birth
	Previous macrosomic infant
	Two or more spontaneous or elective abortions
	Previous hydatidiform mole/choriocarcinoma
	Previous ectopic pregnancy or stillborn/neonatal death
	Previous multiple gestation
	Previous prolonged labor
	Previous low-birthweight infant
	Previous midforceps delivery
	Last pregnancy less than 1 year previous
	Previous infant with neurologic deficit, birth injury, or congenital anomaly
Medical History	Cardiac or pulmonary disease, chronic hypertension
	Metabolic disease
	Renal disease, recent urinary tract infection, or bacteriuria
	Gastrointestinal disorders
	Seizure disorders
	Family history of severe inherited disorders
	Surgery during pregnancy
	Emotional disorders or cognitive challenge
	Previous surgeries, particularly involving reproductive organs
	Endocrine disorders
	Hemoglobinopathies
	Sexually transmitted infections
	Reproductive tract anomalies, history of abnormal Pap smear, malignancy
Current Obstetric Status	Inadequate prenatal care
	Intrauterine growth-restricted fetus
	Large-for-gestational-age fetus
	Pregnancy-induced hypertension or preeclampsia
	Abnormal fetal surveillance tests
	Polyhydramnios
	Placenta previa
	Abnormal presentation
	Maternal anemia
	Weight gain under 10 lb or weight loss over 5 lb
	Over/underweight
	Fetal or placental malformation
	Rh sensitization
	Preterm labor
	Multiple gestation
	Premature rupture of membranes
	Abruptio placentae
	Postdate pregnancy
	Fibroid tumors
	Fetal version
	Cervical cerclage
	Sexually transmitted infection
	Other maternal infection
	Poor immunization status
Psychosocial Factors	Inadequate finances
	Lack of support person
	Adolescent
	Poor nutrition
	More than two children at home; no help
	Lack of acceptance of pregnancy
	Attempt or ideation of suicide
	Inadequate or poor housing
	Father of baby uninvolved
	Minority status
	Dangerous occupation

(continued)

TABLE 10.5

Assessments That Might Categorize a Pregnancy as At Risk (continued)

Psychosocial Factors	Dysfunctional grieving Psychiatric history
Demographic Factors	Maternal age under 16 or over 35 Education under 11 years
Lifestyle	Cigarette smoking greater than 10 cigarettes a day Substance abuse Long amounts of time spent commuting Nonuse of seatbelts Alcohol intake Heavy lifting or long periods of standing Unusual stress No in-home smoke detectors

that would identify a pregnancy as being at high risk. The woman identified this way needs close observation during pregnancy to see that the pregnancy is progressing well; the infant born of a woman identified this way needs close observation in the neonatal period until it is confirmed that no anomalies exist.

Risk assessment should be updated at each pregnancy visit, as the failure to identify risk potential in pregnancy leads to increased perinatal mortality. See Chapters 14 through 17 for a more detailed discussion of high-risk pregnancy and its management.

Important aspects of ongoing prenatal care are discussed in Chapter 11. Box 10.10 lists components of assessments and care done during continuing prenatal visits.

Checkpoint Question 5

Sandra has pelvic measurements taken. What size should the ischial tuberosity diameter be to be considered adequate?

a. 6 cm
b. Twice the width of the conjugate diameter
c. 11 cm
d. Half the width of the symphysis pubis

BOX 10.10

Assessments and Care for Continuing Prenatal Visits

Mother's Health
Health Interview
  Interim history or new personal or family
    developments since last visit
    Review danger signs of pregnancy
    Review symptoms of beginning labor
Physical exam
  Blood pressure (every visit)
  Clean-catch urine for glucose, protein, and
    leukocytes (every visit)
  Blood serum level for alpha-fetoprotein (MSAFP)
    (16 weeks)
  VDRL test for syphilis if possibility of new
    exposure
  Glucose screen (28 weeks)
  Glucose challenge (24 to 28 weeks) if warranted
  Anti-Rh titer (28 weeks)
  Group B streptococcus (GBS) (35 to 37 weeks)

Fetal Health
Fetal heart rate
Fundal height
Quickening or fetal movement
Ultrasound dating of pregnancy

Key Points

Prenatal care has the potential to reduce the incidence of preterm birth and congenital anomalies and the infant mortality rate. Its purposes include establishing a baseline of present health, determining the gestational age of the fetus, monitoring fetal development, identifying the woman at risk for complications, minimizing the risk of possible complications by anticipating and preventing problems before they occur, and providing time for education about pregnancy and possible dangers.

A first prenatal visit confirms a pregnancy, but it is also a time for important assessments such as a health history, physical examination, and laboratory tests. The physical examination could include measurement of fundal height and assessment of fetal heart sounds if the pregnancy is beyond 12 weeks, a pelvic examination (including a Pap test), and possibly an estimation of pelvic size.

A first prenatal visit sets the tone for visits to follow. Maintaining a supportive manner is helpful in establishing rapport and allowing a woman to feel comfortable to return for future care. Remember that a family, not a woman alone, is having a baby, and include family members in procedures and health teaching as desired.

For a pelvic exam, pregnant women should remain in a lithotomy position for as short a time as possible to help prevent thromboembolism and supine hypotension syndrome.

Common pelvic types include gynecoid (well-rounded with a wide pubic arch), anthropoid (narrow), platypelloid (flattened), and android (male or with a sharp pubic arch). A gynecoid pelvis is ideal for childbearing.

The true conjugate (conjugate vera) is the measurement between the anterior surface of the sacral prominence and the posterior surface of the inferior margin of the symphysis pubis (the anterior-posterior diameter of the pelvic inlet). The average is 10.5 to 11 cm. The ischial tuberosity diameter is the distance between the ischial tuberosities or the transverse diameter of the outlet. The average is 11 cm.

Critical Thinking Exercises

1. Sandra Czerinski, whom you met at the beginning of the chapter, was worried about having a pelvic examination. How could you help relieve her concern?
2. Sandra works at a commercial laundry ironing sheets. Is there any type of pregnancy risk for her at this job? Is this a job that probably keeps her on her feet for long periods? Is she apt to be exposed to toxic substances at work? Is there a greater opportunity than usual for her to develop upper respiratory infections?
3. Sandra's boyfriend rarely comes with her to prenatal visits. Another woman has a supportive husband who always comes. Would your role be different in these two situations?
4. Examine the National Health Goals related to prenatal care. Most government-sponsored money for nursing research is allotted based on these goals. What would be a possible research topic to explore pertinent to these goals that would be applicable to the Czerinski family and also advance evidence-based practice?

References

Albertson, K., et al. (2004). Alcohol consumption during pregnancy and the risk of preterm delivery. *American Journal of Epidemiology, 159*(2), 155-161.

Albrecht, S. A., et al. (2004). Smoking cessation counseling for pregnant women who smoke. *JOGNN: Journal of Obstetric, Gynecologic, and Neonatal Nursing, 33*(3), 298-305.

Buehler, B. A. (2003). Interactions of herbal products with conventional medicines and potential impact on pregnancy. *Birth Defects Research: Developmental and Reproductive Toxicology, 68*(6), 494-495.

Davey, D. D. (2003). Cervical cytology classification and the Bethesda System. *Cancer Journal, 9*(5), 327-334.

Department of Health and Human Services. (2000). *Healthy people 2010.* Washington, DC: DHHS.

Fischbach, F. T. (Ed.) (2004). *Manual of laboratory & diagnostic tests.* Philadelphia: Lippincott Williams & Wilkins.

Freak, J. (2004). Promoting knowledge and awareness of skin cancer. *Nursing Standard, 18*(35), 45-54.

Hanson, L. A., Korotkova, M., & Telemo, E. (2003). Breastfeeding, infant formulas, and the immune system. *Annals of Allergy, Asthma, & Immunology, 90*(6), Suppl. 3, 59-63.

Hodnett, E. D. (2004). Continuity of caregivers for care during pregnancy and childbirth. *The Cochrane Library (Oxford) (3)* (CD000062).

Janssen, P. A., et al. (2003). Intimate partner violence and adverse pregnancy outcomes: a population-based study. *American Journal of Obstetrics and Gynecology, 188*(5), 1341-1347.

Johnson, M., Maas, M., & Moorhead, S. (2000). *Nursing outcomes classification* (2nd ed.). St. Louis: Mosby.

Katz, V. (2003). Prenatal care. In J. R. Scott et al., *Danforth's obstetrics and gynecology* (9th ed.). Philadelphia: Lippincott Williams & Wilkins.

Keye, W. R., & Damewood, M. D. (2003). Office gynecology. In J. R. Scott et al., *Danforth's obstetrics and gynecology* (9th ed.) Philadelphia: Lippincott Williams & Wilkins.

Kosters, J. P., & Gotzsche, P. C. (2004). Regular self-examination or clinical examination for early detection of breast cancer. *The Cochrane Library (Oxford) (3)* (CD003373).

Marcus, S. M., et al. (2003). Depressive symptoms among pregnant women screened in obstetrics settings. *Journal of Women's Health, 12*(4), 373-380.

McCartney, P. R. (2004). Centering pregnancy: a renaissance in prenatal care? *MCN: The American Journal of Maternal/Child Nursing, 29*(4), 261-262.

McCloskey, J., & Bulechek, G. (2000). *Nursing interventions classification* (3rd ed.). St. Louis: Mosby.

McGregor, S., & Parker, E. (2003). Family matters: taking a genetic history. *Practising Midwife, 6*(10), 26-28.

Minkoff, H. L., & Gibbs, R. S. (2003). Obstetric and perinatal infections. In J. R. Scott et al., *Danforth's obstetrics and gynecology* (9th ed.). Philadelphia: Lippincott Williams & Wilkins.

Moos, M. (2004). Preconceptional health promotion: progress in changing a prevention paradigm. *Journal of Perinatal and Neonatal Nursing, 18*(1), 2-13.

Stephenson, J. (2004). FDA warns on mercury in tuna. *JAMA, 291*(2), 171.

Villar, J., et al. (2005). Patterns of routine antenatal care for low-risk pregnancy. *The Cochrane Library (Oxford) (3)* (CD000934).

Wessel, J., Endrikat, J., & Buscher, U. (2003). Elevated risk of neonatal outcome following denial of pregnancy: results of a one-year prospective study compared with control groups. *Journal of Perinatal Medicine, 31*(1), 29-35.

Suggested Readings

Browne-Krimsley, V. (2004). Lessons learned: providing culturally competent care in a nurse-managed center. *ABNF Journal, 15*(4), 71-73.

Dillard, R. G. (2004). Improving pre-pregnancy health is key to reducing infant mortality. *North Carolina Medical Journal, 65*(3), 147-148.

Gramling, L., Hickman, K., & Bennett, S. (2004). What makes a good family-centered partnership between women and their practitioners? *Birth, 31*(1), 43-48.

Higgins, L. P. & Hawkins, J. W. (2005). Screening for abuse during pregnancy. *MCN: The American Journal of Maternal/Child Nursing, 30*(2), 109-114.

Jesse, D. E., & Graham, M. (2005). Are you often sad and depressed? Brief measures to identify women at risk for depression in pregnancy. *MCN: The American Journal of Maternal/Child Nursing, 30*(1), 40-45.

Jesse, D. E., Seaver, W., & Wallace, D. C. (2003). Maternal psychosocial risks predict preterm birth in a group of women from Appalachia. *Midwifery, 19*(3), 191-202.

Lazarus, E. (2003). What's new in first trimester ultrasound. *Radiologic Clinics of North America, 41*(4), 663-679.

Lewallen, L. P. (2004). Healthy behaviors and sources of health information among low-income pregnant women. *Public Health Nursing, 21*(3), 200-206.

Sackett, K., Pope, R. K., & Erdley, W. S. (2004). Demonstrating a positive return on investment for a prenatal program at a managed care organization: an economic analysis. *Journal of Perinatal and Neonatal Nursing, 18*(2), 117-127.

Schrag, S. J., et al. (2003). Prenatal screening for infectious diseases and opportunities for prevention. *Obstetrics and Gynecology, 102*(4), 753-760.

Singer, L. T., et al. (2004). Cognitive outcomes of preschool children with prenatal cocaine exposure. *JAMA, 292*(2), 171.

Vidaeff, A. C., Franzini, L., & Low, M. D. (2003). The unrealized potential of prenatal care: a population health approach. *Journal of Reproductive Medicine, 48*(11), 837-842.

CHAPTER 11

Promoting Fetal and Maternal Health

Key Terms

cytomegalovirus
fetal alcohol syndrome
leukorrhea
Sims' position
teratogen
toxoplasmosis

Objectives

After mastering the contents of this chapter, you should be able to:

1. Describe health practices important for a healthy pregnancy outcome.
2. Assess a woman for health practices and concerns during pregnancy.
3. Formulate nursing diagnoses concerned with healthy pregnancy.
4. Identify expected outcomes to promote a healthy pregnancy.
5. Plan health-promotion strategies to limit exposure to teratogens or reduce the minor discomforts of pregnancy.
6. Implement care to promote positive health practices during pregnancy.
7. Evaluate outcomes for achievement and effectiveness of care.
8. Identify National Health Goals related to pregnancy care that nurses can help the nation achieve.
9. Identify areas of prenatal care that could benefit from additional nursing research or the application of evidence-based practice.
10. Use critical thinking to analyze ways to promote individualized and family-centered prenatal care.
11. Integrate knowledge of health-promotion strategies with the nursing process to achieve quality maternal and child health nursing care.

*J*ulberry Adams, a single woman, is 4 months pregnant when you see her in a prenatal clinic. She works as a curator for an art gallery but has missed work this last week because of nausea. She is worried she will not be able to work past 6 months of her pregnancy because her job involves a great deal of walking. She has already stopped volunteer work teaching children's swimming at the YMCA. She wonders how she will be able to afford her apartment if she has to quit work. She wants to travel to see her sister in St. Louis because her sister is very ill but has heard that pregnant women shouldn't drive over 100 miles. She asks you if marijuana reduces early pregnancy nausea.

Previous chapters discussed normal anatomy and physiology and the changes of pregnancy. This chapter adds information about the health teaching that women need during pregnancy to ensure a healthy outcome for themselves and their child. This is important information because it can help protect the health of both women and newborns.

What additional health teaching does Ms. Adams need?

After you've studied this chapter, access the accompanying website. Read the patient scenario and answer the questions to further sharpen your skills, grow more familiar with RN-CLEX types of questions, and reward yourself with how much you have learned.

The health of a fetus and the health of the mother are inextricably linked. Generally, a woman who eats well and takes care of her own health during pregnancy provides a healthy environment for fetal growth and development. However, she may need instructions on exactly what constitutes a healthy lifestyle for herself and her baby. Most women have questions regarding how much extra rest they need, what type of exercise they can continue, and whether all the changes going on in their bodies, some of which bring them daily discomfort, are normal. Therefore, a major role in promoting maternal and fetal health is education. Providing empathetic advice about ways to alleviate the minor discomforts of pregnancy, alerting a woman to the danger signs of pregnancy, and keeping abreast of the latest evidence-based practice studies done on maternal exposure to **teratogens** (factors detrimental to fetal health) are all part of this role. National Health Goals have been established to increase the number of women receiving prenatal care (Box 11.1).

Encourage a pregnant woman to discuss whatever concerns she has during visits. Although some of these concerns may represent minor common discomforts associated with normal pregnancy, others may be early indicators of potential problems (Box 11.2). You need to know what is going on as soon as possible—first, so you can provide information and guidance on ways to alleviate the discomforts of pregnancy and, second, so you can alert the woman's physician or nurse-midwife of your findings early in the pregnancy. Early detection and continued monitoring of conditions such as pregnancy-induced hypertension (PIH) and diabetes reduce the risks of their danger.

Unless women bring problems to their health care provider's attention early in pregnancy, they may not learn to take the necessary measures to prevent further discomfort during or after the pregnancy. Many women do not mention any concerns or discomforts unless specifically asked because they may not be aware of

Nursing Process Overview

For Health Promotion of a Fetus and Mother

● *Assessment*

A thorough health history, physical evaluation, and initial laboratory data are obtained at the first prenatal visit. Continuing assessment concentrates on screening for any abnormalities in physical or emotional health that might be occurring and for the possibility of teratogens in the pregnant woman's environment.

BOX 11.1 FOCUS ON . . .

NATIONAL HEALTH GOALS

A number of National Health goals speak to the importance of prenatal care. These goals are:

- Increase to 94% the proportion of pregnant women who abstain from alcohol, cigarettes, and illicit drugs.
- Increase the proportion of pregnant females screened for sexually transmitted infections during prenatal health care visits.
- Increase to at least 90% the proportion of all pregnant women who receive early and adequate prenatal care, from a baseline of 74% (DHHS, 2000).

Because nurses are important members of prenatal health care teams, they play an important role in seeing that services include preconceptual care and that women are aware that early pregnancy care is important. Evidence-based practice and nursing research to answer such questions as what aspects of preconceptual care are most important in reducing pregnancy complications, and what are effective incentives to make women come early for prenatal care, are important to help the nation meet these goals.

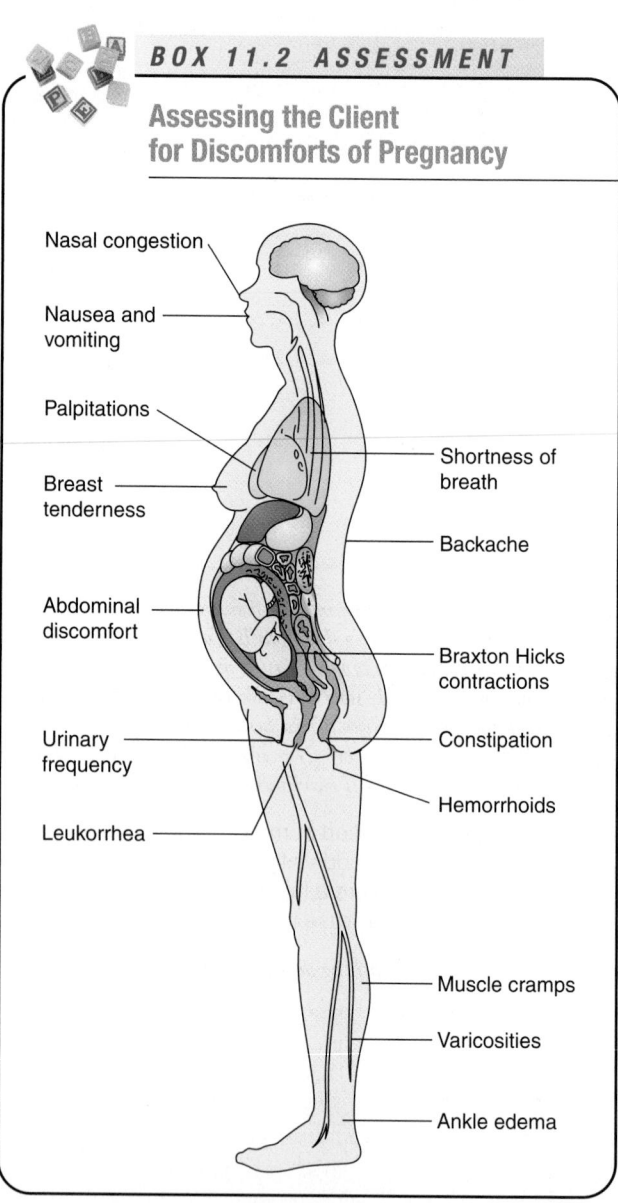

BOX 11.2 ASSESSMENT

Assessing the Client for Discomforts of Pregnancy

- Nasal congestion
- Nausea and vomiting
- Palpitations
- Breast tenderness
- Abdominal discomfort
- Urinary frequency
- Leukorrhea
- Shortness of breath
- Backache
- Braxton Hicks contractions
- Constipation
- Hemorrhoids
- Muscle cramps
- Varicosities
- Ankle edema

their significance or are reluctant to take up a busy health care provider's time for these things (Corbett, Ryan, & Weinrich, 2003). For example, women experiencing constipation may not take care of the problem early or well enough to prevent the occurrence of hemorrhoids, which can then become a long-term problem not only throughout the pregnancy but afterward as well.

● Nursing Diagnosis

Examples of nursing diagnoses related to health promotion of the pregnant woman and fetus are:

- Health-seeking behaviors related to interest in maintaining optimal health during pregnancy
- Anxiety related to minor symptoms of pregnancy
- Risk for deficient fluid volume related to nausea and vomiting of pregnancy
- Constipation related to reduced peristalsis during pregnancy
- Disturbed body image related to change of appearance with pregnancy
- Risk for altered sexuality patterns related to fear of harming fetus during pregnancy
- Disturbed sleep pattern related to frequent need to empty bladder during night
- Fatigue related to increased metabolic needs of pregnancy
- Risk for fetal injury related to maternal cigarette smoking

● Outcome Identification and Planning

When establishing goals and outcomes, be certain that plans are realistic for a woman's situation and family lifestyle (Box 11.3). Try to turn long-term goals into more manageable, short-term ones if possible. For example, a goal of reducing smoking during the pregnancy may be more realistic than a goal of stopping smoking forever. Eliminating the pressure of making a major permanent lifestyle change can help a woman concentrate her efforts on herself and a fetus over the next several months. Continued reinforcement of her progress may help her to continue reducing the number of cigarettes smoked or to quit smoking altogether after the baby is born, providing a smoke-free environment for her child. Similarly, you cannot set a goal for a woman to be free of the nausea of early pregnancy. The best you can expect to accomplish is to maintain good nutrition and adequate weight gain in the face of it. Nor can you do much about the frequency of urination, backache, or fatigue that occur with pregnancy except to help a woman adapt her lifestyle to these symptoms (e.g., encourage her to drink more liquids during the day and less in the early evening; schedule regular rest periods if possible; see Box 11.3).

Often, helping a woman plan to avoid teratogens is difficult because a total change in lifestyle, such as not smoking, not drinking alcohol, or changing a work environment, may be involved. Fortunately, most women are highly motivated to complete a pregnancy satisfactorily. With this level of motivation, planning becomes the task of determining the best route to achieve a goal rather than educating about the need for goal achievement.

When planning teaching strategies, a woman's receptiveness to instruction is key. Regardless of how excited and pleased a woman is about being pregnant, she can assimilate only so much information at one particular time. Therefore, be selective about the health information you provide and include those points most relevant to the individual woman. For example, you'd want to discuss varicosity prevention more for a woman with a history of varicosities in a former pregnancy than for one who is pregnant for the first time and is very athletic. Keep in mind that the health measures being taught must be maintained for an extended time—40 weeks. To help a woman follow changes this long, choose priorities and make health advice meaningful and individualized.

Remember that a basic tenet of teaching and learning is that learning is enhanced when the information has direct application to that person. This principle means that devising a plan that spaces out health-promotion and health-maintenance information based on the changes associated with early and late pregnancy is most helpful. Teach those measures that are immediately applicable first; those that have relevance only toward the end of pregnancy can be taught then.

● Implementation

The major intervention associated with health promotion during pregnancy is education. Although the average woman is aware that some discomforts may occur, these discomforts may seem extreme when they are happening to her. Often, adolescent girls are uninformed about the common discomforts of pregnancy because they lack a set of peers with pregnancy

---

BOX 11.3 FOCUS ON . . .

DIVERSITY OF CARE

Recent immigrants may have limited English proficiency, so providing meaningful preconceptual or prenatal education can be challenging. Women from cultures that view pregnancy as a wellness state may not seek care because they do not view pregnancy as a time when medical intervention is necessary. Other women may be extremely modest and avoid health visits because they find pelvic examinations difficult, intrusive, and embarrassing. Some women may rely on herbs and folk remedies to manage the common discomforts of pregnancy, so they don't feel a need for medical management. This variety of cultural backgrounds makes individualized assessment mandatory.

Planning prenatal care to meet the needs of all of the different cultures represented in the United States may include furnishing interpreters to aid in communication, providing classes in prenatal health, explaining how health-promotion regimens fit with women's cultural belief systems, and maintaining an attitude of advocacy to help women adjust to a formal health care system.

experience. One who knows that it is normal for breast tenderness to occur during pregnancy may not be sure that the amount of breast tenderness she is having is normal. A woman who had a mental image of herself as someone who would not gain much weight during pregnancy may be very concerned that she is, in fact, gaining a great deal of weight. It is crucial to any teaching to be certain all women understand that they should double-check with their primary care provider before taking any nonessential medication during pregnancy.

Other important interventions include good role modeling, such as not smoking in prenatal settings, and exhibiting a healthy lifestyle through adequate nutrition and exercise.

● *Outcome Evaluation*

Evaluation is an ongoing process at regular prenatal health care visits. Expected outcomes developed with a woman at one prenatal visit need to be assessed at the next. Examples of appropriate outcomes may include:

- The client states measures she will use to manage the common discomforts of pregnancy.
- The client reports resting for a half-hour twice a day.
- The client verbalizes positive statements about her appearance.
- The client states she has stopped smoking.
- The client documents that she walks the length of a city block daily.

HEALTH PROMOTION DURING PREGNANCY

Health promotion during pregnancy begins with reviewing self-care.

Self-Care Needs

Because pregnancy is not an illness, few special care measures other than common sense about self-care are required. Many women, however, have heard different warnings about what they should or should not do during pregnancy, so the average woman needs some help separating fact from fiction so that she can enjoy her pregnancy unhampered by unnecessary restrictions. Be alert to the common misunderstandings of pregnancy. In no other area of nursing, except possibly for infant feeding, does there seem to be as many misconceptions or inappropriate information available to women.

Bathing

At one time, tub baths were restricted during pregnancy because it was feared that bath water would enter the vagina and cervix and contaminate the uterine contents. Further, it was believed that hot water touching the abdomen might initiate labor. Because the vagina normally is in a closed position, however, the danger of tub bath water entering the cervix is minimal. In addition, water

temperature has no documented effect on initiating labor. During pregnancy, sweating tends to increase because a woman excretes waste products for herself and a fetus. She also has an increase in vaginal discharge. For these reasons, daily tub baths or showers are now recommended.

As pregnancy advances, a woman may have difficulty maintaining her balance when getting in and out of a bathtub. If so, she should change to showering or sponge bathing for her own safety. If membranes rupture or vaginal bleeding is present, tub baths are contraindicated because then there might be a danger of contamination of uterine contents. During the last month of pregnancy, when the cervix may begin to dilate, some health care providers restrict tub bathing for the same reason.

Breast Care

A few precautions during pregnancy are helpful to prevent breast discomfort. A general rule is for a woman to wear a firm, supportive bra with wide straps to spread weight across the shoulders. A woman may need to buy a larger bra halfway through pregnancy to accommodate increased breast size. If she plans on breast-feeding her newborn, she might choose to buy bras suitable for breast-feeding so she can continue to use them after the baby's birth.

At about the 16th week of pregnancy, colostrum secretion begins in the breasts. The sensation of a fluid discharge from the breasts can be frightening unless a woman is warned that this is a possibility. Instruct her to wash her breasts with clear tap water (no soap, because that could be drying) daily to remove the colostrum and reduce the risk of infection. Afterward, she should dry her nipples well by patting them.

If colostrum secretion is profuse, a woman may need to place gauze squares or breast pads inside her bra, changing them frequently to maintain dryness. Otherwise, constant moisture next to the breast nipple can cause nipple excoriation, pain, and fissuring.

Dental Care

Gingival tissue tends to hypertrophy during pregnancy. Unless a pregnant woman brushes well, pockets of plaque form readily between the enlarged gumline and teeth. In addition, encourage pregnant women to see their dentists regularly for routine examination and cleaning. Nine months is a fairly long time to be without preventive dental care. Although a pregnant woman should question the need for x-rays during pregnancy, if these are necessary for dental health, they can be done safely as long as a woman's abdomen is shielded with a lead apron.

Tooth decay occurs from the action of bacteria on sugar. This action lowers the pH of the mouth, creating an acid medium that leads to etching or destruction of the enamel of teeth. Encourage the woman to snack on nutritious foods, such as fresh fruits and vegetables like apples and carrots to avoid sugar coming in contact with the teeth. If a client has trouble avoiding sweet snacks such as candy, suggest eating sweet snacks that dissolve easily (like a chocolate bar) rather than those that remain in the mouth a long time (like chewy candy). This helps to minimize the level of sugar in the mouth.

Perineal Hygiene

Although women have increased vaginal discharge during pregnancy, douching is contraindicated because the force of the irrigating fluid could cause it to enter the cervix and lead to infection. In addition, douching alters the pH of the vagina, leading to an increased risk of bacterial growth.

Dressing

The days when a woman had to purchase a completely new maternity wardrobe have disappeared. Although economically advantageous, this may be disappointing to a woman who wants to announce her pregnancy early by wearing maternity clothing.

A woman should avoid garters, extremely firm girdles with panty legs, and knee-high stockings because these may impede lower-extremity circulation. Suggest wearing shoes with a moderate to low heel to minimize pelvic tilt and possible backache. Otherwise, the rules are common sense and comfort.

Sexual Activity

Some women are embarrassed to ask questions about sexual relations during pregnancy. However, most women are concerned about whether sexual intercourse should be restricted. Many need information to refute some of the myths about sexual relations in pregnancy that still exist, such as:

- Coitus on the expected date of her period will initiate labor.
- Orgasm will initiate labor, but participating in sexual relations without orgasm will not.
- Coitus during the fertile days of a cycle will cause a second pregnancy or twins.
- Coitus might cause rupture of the membranes.

None of these is true. Asking a woman at a prenatal visit if she has any questions about sexual activity allows her to voice such concerns (Box 11.4). Then you can help dispel these myths, allowing a woman to feel more comfortable and secure that coitus is not harming her child.

Women with a history of spontaneous miscarriage may be advised to avoid coitus during the time of the pregnancy when a previous miscarriage occurred. Women whose membranes have ruptured or who have vaginal spotting should be advised against coitus until examined to prevent possible infection (Read, 2004). Advise caution about male oral–female genital contact, because accidental air embolism has been reported from this act during pregnancy (Katz, 2003). Otherwise, there are no sexual restrictions during pregnancy.

Early in pregnancy, a woman may experience a decreased desire for coitus resulting from the increased estrogen level in her body. Breast tenderness may limit a usual pattern of sexual arousal. As pelvic congestion increases from the additional uterine blood supply, most women notice increased clitoral sensation. Some women may experience orgasm for the first time during pregnancy because of the increased pelvic congestion. As pregnancy advances and a woman's abdomen increases in size, she and her sexual partner may need to use new positions for intercourse. A side-by-side position or a woman in a superior position may be more comfortable. As vaginal secretions

change, a woman may find a water-soluble lubricant helpful. If she begins to experience discomfort from penile penetration, mutual masturbation or female oral–male genital relations might be satisfying to both partners. Caution women with a non-monogamous sexual partner that the partner needs to use a condom to prevent transmission of a sexually transmitted infection during pregnancy. Women may use female condoms throughout pregnancy.

BOX 11.4 FOCUS ON . . .

COMMUNICATION

Julberry Adams is 4 months pregnant and no longer lives with the father of her baby.

Less Effective Communication

Nurse: Do you have any questions, Mrs. Adams?
Julberry: I'm not Mrs. Adams.
Nurse: I'm sorry, Ms. Adams. Do you have any questions?
Julberry: How long into pregnancy can I have sex?
Nurse: Well, since you're single, you don't really need that kind of advice. Let's talk about exercise and nutrition instead.

More Effective Communication

Nurse: Do you have any questions, Mrs. Adams?
Julberry: I'm not Mrs. Adams.
Nurse: I'm sorry, Ms. Adams. Do you have any questions?
Julberry: How long into pregnancy can I have sex?
Nurse: Basically, as long as you're comfortable and you don't have any complications.
Julberry: Good. My new boyfriend made me promise to ask today.

Health teaching is an art separate from teaching morality. In the first scenario, the nurse cuts off communication by making a judgment and thus supplying the information that the nurse thinks the client needs. In the second scenario, the nurse actively listens to the client, focuses on her needs and concerns, and supplies the information the client has requested.

✔ Checkpoint Question 1

Which statement by Julberry Adams would alert you that she needs more teaching about safe practices during pregnancy?

a. "I take either a shower or tub bath, because I know both are safe."
b. "I wash my breasts with clear water, not with soap, daily."
c. "I'm glad I don't have to ask my boyfriend to use condoms anymore."
d. "I'm wearing low-heeled shoes to try and avoid backache."

Exercise

Exercise during pregnancy is important to prevent circulatory stasis in the lower extremities. It also can offer a general feeling of well-being (Kramer, 2005). For some women, teaching about exercise focuses on helping them realize the need for exercise and urging them to get enough. Others may need to be cautioned to restrict exercise or participation in contact sports.

Extreme exercise has been associated with a lower birth rate. The American College of Obstetricians and Gynecologists (ACOG) recommends that the average, well-nourished women should exercise during pregnancy every day for 30 consecutive minutes (ACOG, 2002). An exercise program should consist of 5 minutes of warm-up exercises, an active "stimulus" phase of 20 minutes, and then 5 minutes of cool-down exercises. The type of activity chosen depends on a woman's interests. Exercises that exercise large muscle groups rhythmically, such as walking, are best. The intensity of the exercise program depends on a woman's cardiopulmonary fitness. Before she begins any exercise program, make sure a woman has consulted her physician or nurse-midwife. If any complication of pregnancy should occur, such as bleeding or pregnancy-induced hypertension (PIH), a woman should discontinue her exercise program until she rechecks with her primary health care provider about continuing the program.

Both pregnant and nonpregnant women should exercise at 70% to 85% of their maximum heart rate. The easiest way to calculate this is to subtract a woman's age from 220, then multiply this by 70% or 85%. For example, after exercise a 23-year-old woman should have a pulse range of 137 to 167 (220 minus 23 times 70% and 85%). For a woman of 35, this target range would be 129 to 157.

Teach the client how to assess quickly if she is exercising too strenuously by evaluating her ability to continue talking while exercising. If she is too short of breath to do this, she is exercising beyond her target heart rate.

A planned exercise program may have long-term benefits such as:

- Lowered cholesterol level
- Reduced risk of osteoporosis
- Increased energy level
- Maintenance of healthy body weight
- Decreased risk of heart disease
- Increased self-esteem and well-being

As a rule, a woman can continue any sport she participated in before pregnancy unless it was one that involved body contact, such as soccer. If a woman is a competent horsewoman, for example, there is little reason for her to discontinue riding until it becomes uncomfortable. Pregnancy is not the time to learn to ride, however, because a beginning rider is at greater risk for being thrown than an experienced one. The same principles apply to skiing and bicycling. An accomplished skier or bicyclist may continue the activity in moderation until balance becomes a problem. Pregnancy is not the time to learn to ski or ride a bicycle, however, because the lack of skill may result in many falls.

Swimming is a good activity for pregnant women and, like bathing, is not contraindicated as long as the membranes are intact. It may help relieve backache during pregnancy (Young & Jewell, 2005). Long-distance swimming or any other activity carried out to a point of extreme fatigue should be avoided. A high-impact aerobics program is contraindicated because this can be strenuous to both pelvic and knee joints. In addition, it may lead to hyperthermia for the mother and fetus. Epidemiologic studies suggest that an elevation of maternal body temperature by 2 degrees C for at least 24 hours can cause a range of developmental defects, but there is little information on thresholds for shorter exposures (Edwards, Saunders, & Shiota, 2003). Use of hot tubs and saunas after workouts longer than 15 minutes is contraindicated, however, on the chance these could raise the internal fetal temperature.

Walking is the best exercise during pregnancy, and women should be encouraged to take a walk daily unless inclement weather, many levels of stairs, or an unsafe neighborhood are contraindications. Jogging, in contrast, is questioned because of the strain that the extra weight of pregnancy places on the knees. Late in pregnancy, jogging can cause pelvic pain from relaxed symphysis pubis movement. Guidelines for exercise during pregnancy are highlighted in Box 11.5.

Sleep

The optimal condition for body growth occurs when growth hormone secretion is at its highest level—that is, during sleep. This, plus the overall increased metabolic demand of pregnancy, appears to be the physiologic reason pregnant women need an increased amount of sleep or at least rest to build new body cells during pregnancy.

Pregnant women rarely have difficulty falling asleep at night because of this increased physiologic need for sleep. If a woman has trouble falling asleep, drinking a glass of warm milk may help. Relaxation exercises (lying quietly, systematically relaxing neck muscles, shoulder muscles, arm muscles, and so on) also may be effective.

Late in pregnancy, a woman often finds herself awakened from sleep at short, frequent intervals by the activity of her fetus. Frequent waking this way leads to loss of REM (rapid eye movement) sleep. On arising, a woman may feel anxious or not well rested, although she has slept her usual number of hours. She also may awaken with pyrosis or dyspnea if she has been lying flat. In this instance, sleeping on two pillows or on a couch with an armrest may be helpful.

To obtain enough sleep and rest during pregnancy, most pregnant women need a rest period during the afternoon as well as a full night of sleep. A good resting or sleeping position is a modified **Sims' position,** with the top leg forward (Fig. 11.1). This puts the weight of the fetus on the bed, not on the woman, and allows good circulation in the lower extremities.

Be certain the client knows to avoid resting in a supine position, as supine hypotension syndrome (faintness, diaphoresis, and hypotension from the pressure of the expanding uterus on the inferior vena cava) can develop in this position. Also be certain she knows not to rest with her knees sharply bent either when sitting or lying down, because of the increased risk of venous stasis this causes below the knee.

BOX 11.5 FOCUS ON . . .

FAMILY TEACHING

Guidelines for Exercise in Pregnancy

Q. Julberry Adams asks you, "Now that I'm pregnant, what kinds of exercise should I do?"

A. Use the following recommendations as guidelines for exercising while you are pregnant:

1. Perform regular exercise (about three times per week) rather than engaging in intermittent activity.
2. Do not perform vigorous exercise in hot, humid weather or if you have a fever to avoid over-exerting yourself or developing hyperthermia.
3. Avoid activities that require jumping, jarring motions, or rapid changes in direction, because your joints may be unstable.
4. Exercise on a wooden floor or a tightly carpeted surface to reduce shock to the abdomen or knees and provide a sure footing.
5. To avoid muscle cramping, avoid exercises and motions that involve deep flexion or joint extension, such as stretching with the toes extended.
6. Always start your exercise program by warming up for approximately 5 minutes with activities such as slow walking or stationary cycling with low resistance.
7. End your exercise program with a period of gradually declining activity that includes gentle, stationary stretching. Because of the increased risk of joint injury, do not stretch to the point of maximum resistance.
8. Measure your heart rate at times of peak activity. Talk with your primary care provider about target heart rate and limits, and don't exceed them.
9. When getting up from lying on the floor, do so gradually to prevent dramatic blood pressure changes or stretching of the round ligament.
10. Drink liquids liberally before and after exercise to prevent dehydration. If necessary, interrupt your activity to replenish fluids.
11. If you were sedentary before pregnancy, begin your exercise program with physical activity of very low intensity and advance your activity level gradually.
12. Stop any activity and contact your primary care provider if any unusual symptoms appear.
13. Perform strenuous activities for no longer than 20 minutes.
14. To prevent supine hypotension do not exercise in the supine position (lying down flat) after the 4th month of pregnancy.
15. Avoid exercises that employ the Valsalva maneuver (holding your breath, bearing down) because these actions decrease blood supply to the fetus.
16. Make sure your caloric intake is adequate to meet not only the extra energy needs of pregnancy but also those of the exercise performed.

Employment

Unless a woman's job involves exposure to toxic substances, lifting heavy objects, other kinds of excessive physical strain, long periods of standing, or having to maintain body balance, there are few reasons a woman cannot continue to work throughout pregnancy (Saurel-Cubizolles et al., 2004). Changes in public assistance laws that encourage women to seek employment have led to more women working during pregnancy than ever before. To protect women from loss of employment benefits during pregnancy, Congress passed an employment rights law in 1978 (Public Law 95-555). However, this law does not cover women who work for companies with fewer than 15 employees.

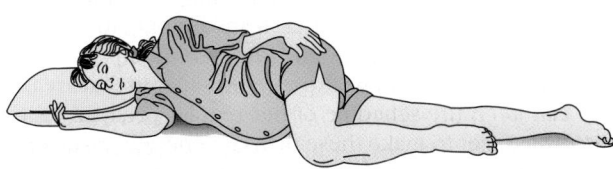

FIGURE 11.1 A modified Sims' position is a good rest position during pregnancy. Notice that the weight of the fetus rests on the bed.

According to this law, an employer cannot:

- Deprive women of seniority rights, in pay or promotion, because they take a maternity leave
- Treat women returning from maternity leave as new hires, starting over on the eligibility period for pension and other benefits
- Force pregnant women to leave if they are able to and want to continue working
- Refuse to hire women just because they are pregnant or fire them for the same reason
- Refuse to cover employees' normal pregnancy and delivery expenses in the company health plan or pay less for pregnancy than for other medical conditions
- Refuse to pay sick leave or disability benefits to women whose difficult pregnancies keep them off the job

Passed in 1993, the Family Leave Act, another federal law, guarantees women the right to 12 weeks of unpaid, job-protected leave on the birth of a child, the adoption or foster placement of a child, when a woman is needed to care for a parent, spouse, or child with a serious health condition, or because of a serious health condition in herself (29 CFR 825.11). Specifically mentioned in the law is any period of incapacity due to pregnancy or for prenatal care (American Public Health Association, 2001). Families need to be educated about this important law because many women are still not aware that they can take time off from work during pregnancy or spend time with a new baby. Additional women may be able to qualify for provisions under the Americans With Disabilities Act.

Some occupations are hazardous during pregnancy because they bring women into contact with harmful substances. For example, nurses working with anesthetic gases in operating rooms or dental offices are reported to have a higher incidence of spontaneous miscarriage and, possibly, congenital anomalies in children than nurses working in other locales, probably due to exposure to nitrous oxide (National Institute of Occupational Safety and Health, 2000). This finding suggests that breathing even a low dose of anesthetic gases such as nitrous oxide can be a serious occupational hazard for nurses. Nurses working with chemotherapy agents should wear gloves to protect themselves from exposure to these drugs, which are possibly teratogenic. Ribavirin (Virazole), an antibiotic used to treat respiratory syncytial infections, is also apparently teratogenic if inhaled by health care providers (Karch, 2004).

A number of studies suggest that preterm birth may occur more frequently in women who work at strenuous jobs or those that require long periods of standing (Saurel-Cubizolles et al., 2004). Other problems that can occur with employment include interference with adequate rest and nutrition. Urge a woman who works outside her home to put her feet up to rest when performing tasks that can be done in that position. Review what she eats at fast-food restaurants or packs for herself to be certain she plans ways to make this type of lunch as nutritious as if she were eating at home.

Remember, most women work to augment or supply the family income, not for fun. Even those who could afford to leave their jobs may not be willing to sacrifice the collegial relationships and sense of fulfillment derived from work, or the lifestyle their income has allowed them to enjoy. Counseling them to reserve periods during the day for rest and to eat a healthy diet is more effective than suggesting they resign from their jobs during pregnancy to get more rest (Box 11.6).

BOX 11.6 FOCUS ON . . .

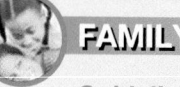

FAMILY TEACHING

Guidelines for Pregnant Working Women

Q. Julberry Adams asks you, "Now that I'm pregnant, can I continue to work outside of the home?"

A. Use the following suggestions as guidelines for safe pregnancy practices:

- Plan to rest during your break periods rather than running errands, etc.
- Try to use at least part of your lunch hour to rest. Lie on your left side in a break room if possible. If this is not possible, then rest sitting with your legs elevated.
- If your job involves long periods of standing, think of times you could stop and elevate your legs (working in a low file drawer, reading time in a classroom, etc.).
- Walk around periodically to avoid prolonged standing in one position if possible; stretch your back periodically to avoid backache.
- Wear support hose to improve venous return to your lower extremities.
- Avoid excessive overtime or working longer than 8-hour shifts.
- Empty your bladder every 2 hours to help prevent bladder infection.
- Get extra rest on weekends or days off.
- Take great caution when working around equipment that requires good balance. Avoid ladders or climbing late in pregnancy, when balance can be a problem.
- Learn your target heart rate for exercise. If your job involves strenuous exercise, stop and rest at the point your target heart rate is exceeded.
- Be sure you are not relying on fast foods for meals. Take time to pack or purchase nutritious foods.

 Checkpoint Question 2

Julberry Adams describes her typical day to you. What would alert you that she may need further pregnancy advice?

a. "I jog rather than walk every time I can for exercise."
b. "I always go to sleep on my side, not on my back."
c. "I pack my lunch in the morning when I'm not so tired."
d. "I walk around my desk every hour to prevent varicosities."

Travel

Many women have questions about travel during pregnancy (Kingman & Economides, 2003). Early in a normal pregnancy, there are no restrictions. If a woman is susceptible to motion sickness, she should not take any medica-

tion for this unless it is specifically prescribed or approved by her physician or nurse-midwife. Late in pregnancy, travel plans should take into consideration the possibility of early labor, requiring birth at a strange setting where a woman's obstetric history will be unknown.

Regardless of the month of her pregnancy, if a woman plans to spend time at a remote location, such as a campsite, be certain she knows the location of a nearby health care facility should an unexpected complication occur. Caution her not to eat uncooked fruits, vegetables, and meat or drink unpurified water. If she is going to be away from home for an extended time, she needs to make arrangements to visit a health care provider in that area so she can keep the schedule of her regular prenatal visits. Encourage her to make these plans far enough in advance so that her records can be copied and sent with her or be forwarded to the interim health care provider. Be aware that you need her written permission to send records. Also, make sure she has enough of her prescribed vitamin supplement plus adequate prescriptions for refills as necessary.

Advise a woman who is taking a long trip by automobile to plan for frequent rest or stretch periods. Preferably every hour, but at least every 2 hours, she should get out of the car and walk a short distance. This break will relieve stiffness and muscle ache and improve lower extremity circulation, helping to prevent varicosities, hemorrhoids, and thrombophlebitis.

Pregnant women may drive as long as they fit comfortably behind the steering wheel. They should use seat belts like everyone else (Box 11.7). Occasionally, uterine rupture has been reported from seat belt use, but overall evidence suggests that seat belts reduce mortality among pregnant women in car accidents, as they do for everyone. Both shoulder harnesses and lap belts should be used. The lap belt should be worn as snugly as comfortable so that it fits under the abdominal bulge and across the pelvic bones. The shoulder harness should be snug but comfortable, worn across the shoulder, chest, and upper abdomen. A pad may be placed under the shoulder harness at the neck to avoid chafing (Fig. 11.2).

Pregnancy is also a time for a family to think about transportation safety for the newborn. Purchasing a car seat is an investment that not only is legally required for transporting infants but also helps guarantee their safety. Families who cannot afford to purchase an infant car seat may

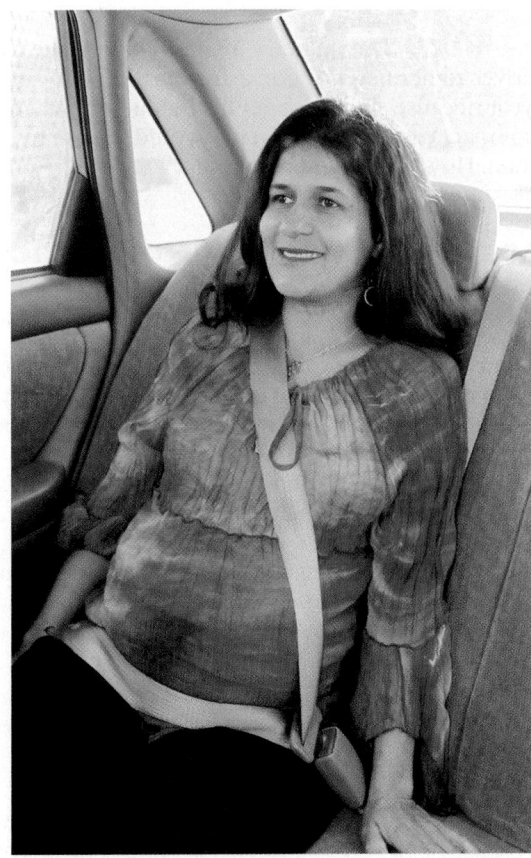

FIGURE 11.2 Encourage women to wear seatbelts during pregnancy. The bottom strap should cross beneath the abdomen.

BOX 11.7 FOCUS ON . . .

EVIDENCE-BASED PRACTICE

Do pregnant women use seat belts?

To answer this question, researchers asked 450 women attending a prenatal clinic about their seat belt use. Results showed that nearly all subjects (95%) were either maintaining or increasing their pre-pregnancy frequency of using seat belts. Seventy-two percent of subjects were able to demonstrate correct placement of a seat belt. Sixty percent said they were aware that a restraint would protect their baby if they were in an accident. In contrast, 48% thought the restraint would cause injury to their baby. As expected, those women who said they believed a restraint would protect them wore their seat belts significantly more than those who didn't believe that seat belts protected them. The most common reasons given for not wearing seat belts were lack of comfort and forgetfulness. Disappointingly, only 36% of the sample said they had received information about seat belt use during their current pregnancy.

This is an important study for nurses because nurses in prenatal sites are often the people who give women prenatal instructions about such everyday actions as seat belt use. Being certain that pregnant women receive information about the importance of seat belts could increase seat belt use and the safety of pregnant women.

Source: McGwin, G., et al. (2004). Knowledge, beliefs, and practices concerning seat belt use during pregnancy. *Journal of Trauma-Injury Infection & Critical Care, 56*(3), 670–675.

want to ask friends or relatives about the possibility of borrowing one no longer needed. Many hospitals and local Red Cross chapters provide infant seats on a rental or loan basis for families who may find it difficult to obtain one in other ways.

Traveling by plane is not contraindicated as long as the plane has a well-pressurized cabin (true of commercial airlines but not of all small private planes). Some airlines do not permit women who are more than 7 months pregnant on board; others require written permission from a woman's primary care provider. Advise a woman to investigate these restrictions by calling the airline or a travel agency before making travel plans.

With businesses becoming global, more women than ever before are asked to travel internationally. Women who travel abroad may need additional immunizations, such as cholera vaccine, for entry into certain countries (Schmidt, Kroger, & Roy, 2004). All live virus vaccines (measles, mumps, rubella, and yellow fever) are contraindicated during pregnancy and should not be administered unless the risk of the disease outweighs the risk to the pregnancy. Before any immunization during pregnancy, the woman should ask her primary care provider to verify it will be safe. Pregnancy does not alter indications for rabies vaccine because without the vaccine, a fatal disease could occur. Tetanus is also treated the same in pregnant women as in others (Sheffield & Ramin, 2004).

What if... Julberry Adams tells you she usually drives to her parents' house for vacation but can't this year because she no longer fits behind the wheel of her compact car. She asks you if it would be safe to take the train. How would you respond?

Discomforts of Early Pregnancy: The First Trimester

Although most women are pleased to be pregnant, the symptoms of early pregnancy tend to cause discomfort to a woman rather than provide evidence that she is carrying a child. As such, a woman may become frustrated, expecting pregnancy to be a time of glowing good health. Providing empathetic and sound advice about measures to relieve these discomforts helps promote overall health and well-being. Although the symptoms discussed below are classified as minor, they may not seem minor to a woman who wakes up each morning feeling nauseated, wondering if she will ever feel like herself again. Also, each of these symptoms has the potential to lead to problems that are more serious.

Nursing Diagnoses

Listening, observing carefully, and developing nursing diagnoses based on assessment data are important steps in prenatal care. Keep in mind that although many women will experience one or several of these symptoms, each woman's experience is unique and nursing diagnoses must be developed according to each woman's individual needs. Examples of nursing diagnoses that might be developed for women experiencing the discomforts of early pregnancy are:

- Health-seeking behaviors related to interest in using herbal remedies to relieve discomforts of pregnancy
- Disturbed body image related to breast and abdominal enlargement in pregnancy
- Constipation related to reduced peristalsis in pregnancy
- Fatigue related to increased physiologic need for sleep and rest during pregnancy
- Acute pain related to frequent muscle cramps secondary to physiologic changes of pregnancy
- Disturbed sleep pattern related to frequent need to empty bladder during night

Breast Tenderness

Breast tenderness is often one of the first symptoms noticed in early pregnancy; it may be most noticeable on exposure to cold air. For most women, the tenderness is minimal and transient, something they are aware of but not something that overly concerns them. If the tenderness is enough to cause discomfort, encourage a woman to wear a bra with a wide shoulder strap for support and to dress warmly to avoid cold drafts if cold increases symptoms. If actual pain exists, the presence of conditions such as nipple fissure or other explanations for the pain, such as breast abscess, should be ruled out.

Palmar Erythema

Palmar erythema, or palmar pruritus, occurs in early pregnancy and is probably caused by increased estrogen levels. Constant redness or itching of the palms may make a woman believe she has developed an allergy. Explain that this type of itching in early pregnancy is normal before she spends time and effort trying different soaps or detergents or attempting to implicate certain foods she has eaten. For some women, calamine lotion is soothing. As soon as her body adjusts to the increased level of estrogen, the erythema and pruritus disappear.

Constipation

As the weight of the growing uterus presses against the bowel and peristalsis slows, constipation may occur (Wald, 2003). Discuss preventive measures with a woman early in pregnancy to help her avoid this problem. Encourage her to evacuate her bowels regularly (many women neglect this first simple rule); to increase the amount of roughage in her diet by eating raw fruits, bran, and vegetables; and to drink at least eight 8-oz glasses of water daily.

Some women find their prescribed oral iron supplement contributes to constipation. Reinforce the need for this supplement to build fetal iron stores. Help a woman find a method to relieve or prevent constipation other than not taking the supplement.

Advise a woman not to use mineral oil to relieve constipation, because it can absorb fat-soluble vitamins (A, D, K, and E), which are necessary for both good fetal and maternal health, and flush them out of the body.

Enemas also should be avoided because their action might initiate labor. Over-the-counter laxatives are contraindicated, as are all nonessential drugs during pregnancy unless specifically prescribed or sanctioned by a woman's physician or nurse-midwife (Yankowitz, 2003). If dietary measures and attempts at regular bowel evacuation fail, a stool softener, such as docusate sodium (Colace), or evacuation suppositories, such as glycerin, may be prescribed. Some women have extensive flatulence accompanying constipation. Recommend avoiding gas-forming foods, such as cabbage or beans, to help control this problem.

Nausea, Vomiting, and Pyrosis

At least half of pregnant women experience other gastrointestinal symptoms such as nausea, vomiting, and pyrosis. Because these symptoms also interfere with nutrition, they are discussed in Chapter 12.

Fatigue

Fatigue is extremely common in early pregnancy, probably due to increased metabolic requirements. Much of it can be relieved by increasing the amount of rest and sleep. Some women are reluctant to take time out of their day for rest. They know that pregnancy is not an illness, and so they proceed as if nothing is happening to them. Rarely is there justification during a normal pregnancy for women to take extra days off from work because of their condition, but it is also unrealistic to proceed as if nothing is happening. Fatigue can increase the amount of morning sickness a woman experiences. If she becomes too tired, she may not eat properly and nutrition can suffer. If she remains on her feet without at least one break during the day, the risk for varicosities and the danger of thromboembolic complications increase.

For all these reasons, ask women at prenatal visits whether they manage to have at least one short rest period every day. A good resting position is a modified Sims' position, with the top leg forward (see Fig. 11.1). This position puts the weight of the fetus on the bed, not on the woman, and allows good circulation in the lower extremities.

A woman who works outside her home at a job that requires her to be on her feet most of the day might use part of her lunch hour to sit with her feet elevated, such as on an adjoining chair (Fig. 11.3). After she returns home from work in the evening, she may need to modify her customary routine from typical activities such as cooking dinner or watching a child's soccer game to resting, then cooking dinner or going to the soccer game, or resting while her partner cooks dinner (part of "we are having a baby at our house" for a partner who does not usually share in household chores). Women who work at sedentary jobs, inside or outside their home, may, in contrast, need to use this time to increase their activity, such as taking a walk or using a treadmill.

Muscle Cramps

Decreased serum calcium levels, increased serum phosphorus levels, and, possibly, interference with circulation commonly cause muscle cramps of the lower extremities during pregnancy. These problems are best relieved if a woman lies on her back momentarily and extends her involved leg while keeping her knee straight and dorsiflexing the foot until the pain disappears (Fig. 11.4).

If a woman is experiencing frequent leg cramps, she may need a prescription for aluminum hydroxide gel (Amphojel), which binds phosphorus in the intestinal tract and thereby lowers its circulating level. Lowering milk intake to only a pint daily and supplementing this with calcium lactate may also help to reduce the phosphorus level. Elevating lower extremities frequently during the day to

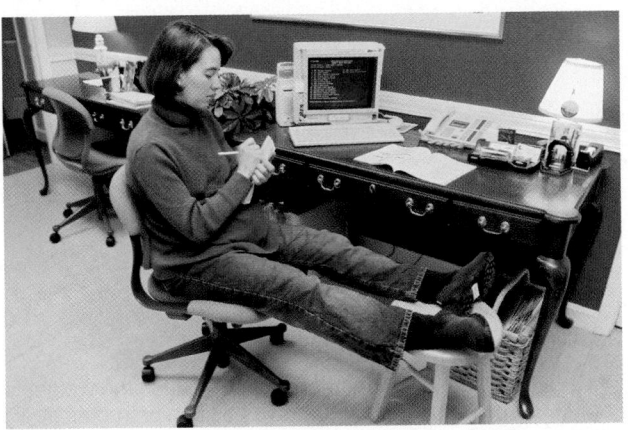

FIGURE 11.3 A "feet-up" break during a workday helps prevent ankle edema. (© Caroline Brown, RNC, MS, DEd.)

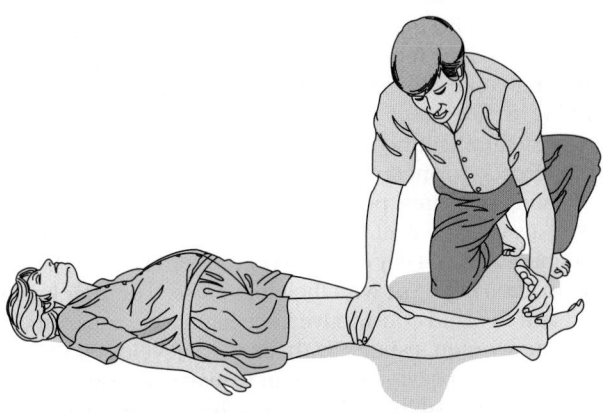

FIGURE 11.4 Relieving a leg cramp in pregnancy. Pressing down on the knee and pressing the toes backward (dorsiflexion) relieves most cramps. Here, a woman's partner helps.

improve circulation and avoiding full leg extension, such as stretching with the toes pointed, may be helpful prevention. Typically, muscle cramps are a minor symptom of pregnancy, but the pain is extreme and the intensity of the contraction can be frightening. Always ask at prenatal visits if this is a problem. Otherwise, women may not realize that cramping is pregnancy-related and so fail to report it.

Pregnant women also have a higher incidence of "restless leg syndrome" (waking at night because of spontaneous leg movement) than nonpregnant women (Manconi et al., 2004). This movement can be so annoying and frequent that women have difficulty sleeping.

Hypotension

Supine hypotension is a symptom that occurs when a woman lies on her back and the uterus presses on the vena cava, impairing blood return to her heart. A woman experiences an irregular heart rate and a feeling of apprehension. To relieve the problem is simple: if a woman turns or is turned onto her side, pressure will be removed from the vena cava, blood flow will be restored, and the symptoms will quickly fade.

If a woman rises suddenly from a lying or sitting position or stands for an extended time in a warm or crowded area, she may faint from the same phenomenon (blood pooling in the pelvic area or lower extremities). Rising slowly and avoiding extended periods of standing prevent this problem. If a woman should feel faint, sitting with her head lowered—the same action as for any person who feels faint—will alleviate the problem.

Varicosities

Varicosities, or the development of tortuous leg veins, are common in pregnancy because the weight of the distended uterus puts pressure on the veins returning blood from the lower extremities (Katz, 2003). This causes pooling of blood and distention of the vessels. The veins become engorged, inflamed, and painful. Although usually confined to the lower extremities, varicosities can extend up to and include the vulva. They occur most frequently in women with a family history of varicose veins and those who have a large fetus or a multiple pregnancy. Urge such women to take active measures to prevent varicosities beginning in early pregnancy; if left until the second trimester, the best they will be able to accomplish is relief of pain from already formed varicosities.

Resting in a Sims' position or on the back with the legs raised against the wall or elevated on a footstool for 15 to 20 minutes twice a day is a good precaution (Fig. 11.5). Caution women not to sit with their legs crossed or their knees bent and to avoid constrictive knee-high hose or garters.

Some women, especially those who developed varicosities during a previous pregnancy, may need elastic support stockings such as TEDS for relief of varicosities. A woman should don the support stockings before she arises in the morning. Once she is on her feet, the pooling of blood has already begun, and the stockings will be less effective. When applied properly, the stockings should reach an area above the point of distention. Before a woman buys stockings, be certain she understands that the stockings should be labeled "medical support hose." Many pantyhose manufacturers advertise their stockings as giving "firm support," and a woman may assume erroneously this is sufficient for her.

Because it stimulates venous return, exercise is as effective as rest periods at alleviating varicosities. Most women assume they do not need set exercise periods during pregnancy because they work hard at other activities. If they analyze the type of work they do, however, they may realize that a great deal of their work leads to venous stasis of the lower extremities. Women stand in one position to wash dishes, cook dinner, run a copying machine, defend a client in court, process a part on an assembly line, or teach a class. Sitting at a desk for prolonged periods of time with legs dependent also encourages venous stasis. Advise women to break up these long periods of sitting or standing with a "walk break" at least twice a day. As a rule, their families will benefit by accompanying them. Partners may discover that they, too, walk very little during their workday.

Vitamin C may be helpful in reducing the size of varicosities because it is necessary for the formation of blood vessel collagen and endothelium. Ask at prenatal visits if women include fresh fruit in their diet every day.

Hemorrhoids

Hemorrhoids (varicosities of the rectal veins) occur commonly in pregnancy because of pressure on these veins from the bulk of the growing uterus. Daily bowel evacuation to relieve constipation and resting in a modified Sims' position daily are both helpful. At day's end, assuming a knee–chest position (Fig. 11.6) for 10 to 15 minutes is an excellent way to reduce the pressure on rectal veins. Keep in mind that a knee–chest position may make a woman feel lightheaded initially. Therefore, instruct her to remain in this position for only a few minutes at first, and then gradually increase the time until she can maintain the position comfortably for about 15 minutes. Stool softeners may be recommended for a woman who already has hemorrhoids. Applying witch hazel or cold compresses to external hemorrhoids may help to relieve pain. Replacing hemorrhoids with gentle finger pressure can be helpful. As with varicosities, think prevention, not just providing help for already established hemorrhoids.

Checkpoint Question 3

Julberry Adams tells you she is developing painful hemorrhoids. Advice you would give her would be:

a. Take a tablespoon of mineral oil with each of your meals.
b. Omit fiber from your diet. This will prevent constipation.
c. Lie on your stomach daily to drain blood from rectal veins.
d. Witch hazel pads feel cool against swollen hemorrhoids.

Heart Palpitations

On sudden movement, such as turning over in bed, a pregnant woman may experience a bounding palpitation of the heart. This is probably due to the circulatory adjustments necessary to accommodate her increased blood supply dur-

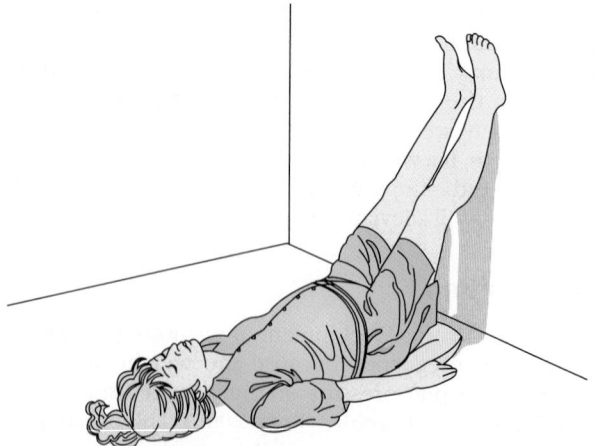

FIGURE 11.5 Position to relieve varicosities. The mother keeps a pad under her right hip to prevent supine hypotensive syndrome.

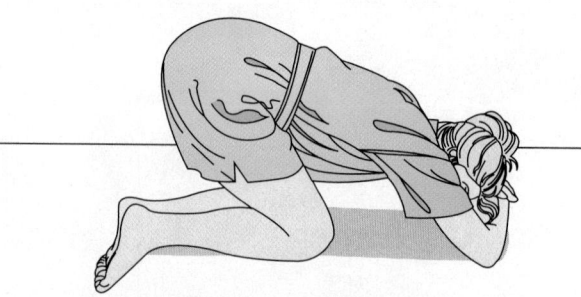

FIGURE 11.6 Knee–chest position. Because the weight of the uterus is shifted forward, this position promotes free flow of urine from the kidneys (preventing urinary tract stasis and infection) and better circulation in the rectal area (preventing hemorrhoids).

ing pregnancy. Although only momentary, the sensation can be frightening because the heart seems to have skipped a beat. It is reassuring for women to know that palpitations are normal and to be expected on occasion. Only if they occur very frequently or continuously or are accompanied by pain are they a concern. Gradual, slow movements will help prevent this from happening so frequently.

Frequent Urination

Frequent urination occurs in early pregnancy due to the pressure of the growing uterus on the anterior bladder. The sensation may last for about 3 months, sometimes beginning as early as the first or second missed menstrual period, disappear in midpregnancy when the uterus rises above the bladder, and return again in late pregnancy as the fetal head presses against the bladder (Fig. 11.7).

When a woman describes frequency of urination, be certain this is the only urinary symptom she is experiencing. Ask her about any burning or pain on urination or whether she has noticed any blood in her urine, signs of urinary tract infection.

There are no solutions for decreasing the frequency of urination. Women should not restrict their fluid intake, as fluids are necessary to allow their blood volume to double. Suggesting that a woman reduce the amount of caffeine she is drinking may be helpful. Most importantly, a woman needs to understand that voiding more frequently is a normal phenomenon. Unless a woman is cautioned that the sensation of frequency returns after lightening (the settling of the fetal head into the inlet of the pelvis at pregnancy's end), she may worry at that time that she has a urinary tract infection. Again, unless other symptoms are present, she can be assured this a normal finding.

Occasionally, a woman notices stress incontinence (involuntary loss of urine on coughing or sneezing) during pregnancy. Although this is largely unpreventable, doing Kegel exercises (alternately contracting and relaxing perineal muscles; Box 11.8) helps strengthen uri-

---

> ### BOX 11.8
>
> ### Kegel Exercises
>
> Kegel exercises are exercises designed to strengthen the pubococcygeal muscles. Each is a separate exercise and should be done about three times a day. Exercises are as follows:
>
> 1. Squeeze the muscles surrounding the vagina as if stopping the flow of urine. Hold for 3 seconds. Relax. Repeat this sequence 10 times.
> 2. Contract and relax the muscles surrounding the vagina as rapidly as possible 10 to 25 times.
> 3. Imagine that you are sitting in a bathtub of water and squeeze muscles as if sucking water into the vagina. Hold for 3 seconds. Relax. Repeat this action 10 times.
>
> It may take as long as 6 weeks of exercise before pubococcygeal muscles are strengthened. In addition to strengthening urinary control and preventing stress incontinence, Kegel exercises can lead to increased sexual enjoyment because of the tightened vaginal muscles.

nary control, directly strengthens perineal muscles for birth, and decreases the possibility of stress incontinence (Harvey, 2003).

Abdominal Discomfort

Some women experience uncomfortable feelings of abdominal pressure early in pregnancy. Women with a multiple pregnancy may notice this throughout pregnancy. Typically, pregnant women stand with their arms crossed in front of them because the weight of their arms resting on their abdomen relieves this discomfort.

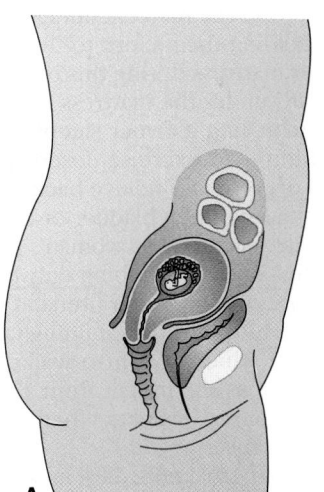 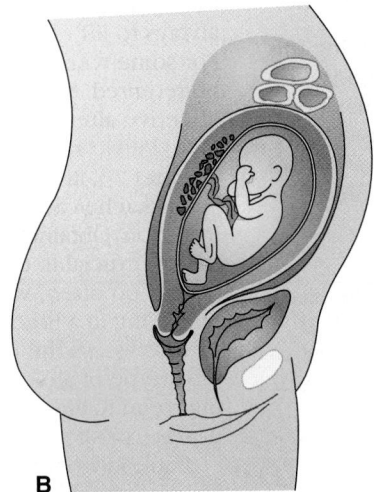 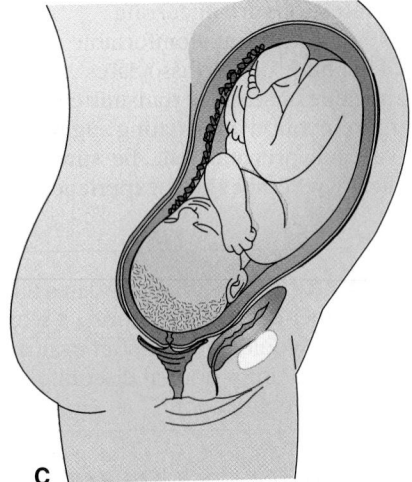

A **B** **C**

FIGURE 11.7 Bladder changes during pregnancy. **(A)** Early pregnancy: the uterus presses against the bladder, causing frequent urination. **(B)** Middle pregnancy: urinary frequency is relieved. **(C)** Late pregnancy: the uterus is again pressing on the bladder, leading to the recurrence of urinary frequency.

When women stand up quickly, they may experience a pulling, sometimes sharp and frightening, pain in the right or left lower abdomen from tension on a round ligament. They can prevent this by always rising slowly from a lying to a sitting, or from a sitting to a standing position. Because round ligament pain may simulate the abrupt pain that occurs with ruptured ectopic pregnancy, the client's description of the pain must be evaluated carefully (Katz, 2003).

Leukorrhea

Leukorrhea, a whitish, viscous vaginal discharge or an increase in the amount of normal vaginal secretions, occurs in response to the high estrogen levels and the increased blood supply to the vaginal epithelium and cervix in pregnancy. A daily bath or shower to wash away accumulated secretions and prevent vulvar excoriation usually controls this problem. Wearing cotton underpants and sleeping at night without underwear can be helpful to reduce moisture and possible vulvar excoriation. Some women may need to wear a perineal pad to control the discharge. Caution women not to use tampons because this could lead to stasis of secretions and subsequent infection. Advise women to contact their physician or nurse-midwife if there is a change in the color, odor, or character of this discharge, which might suggest infection. Caution women not to douche; douching is contraindicated throughout pregnancy because fluid could be forced into the uterine cervix.

A woman with vulvar pruritus needs evaluation because this strongly indicates infection. Be certain she is describing pruritus-like symptoms and is not describing burning on urination, a sign of an early bladder infection (which also needs therapy, but of a different type). Common vaginal infections such as Candida that present with pruritus are discussed in Chapter 47.

Avoiding tight underpants and pantyhose may help prevent vulvar and vaginal infections, particularly yeast infections. Although over-the-counter medications for yeast infections are available, caution women to contact their health care provider rather than self-treat vaginal infections during pregnancy so their health care provider knows infections are occurring.

A woman who is uncomfortable about discussing this part of her body or who associates vaginal infections with poor hygiene or sexually transmitted infection may be reluctant to mention an irritating vaginal discharge. Therefore, at each prenatal visit, be sure to ask the woman specifically whether she is experiencing this problem.

What if... Julberry Adams tells you she has urinary frequency. She also reports a white vaginal discharge. How would you go about evaluating whether she is experiencing a normal discomfort of pregnancy or a urinary tract infection?

Discomforts of Middle to Late Pregnancy

At approximately the 20th to 24th weeks, the midpoint of pregnancy, a woman is usually ready for further health teaching that relates to the new developments that will occur in the latter half of pregnancy. As she starts to view the child within her as a separate person, she becomes interested in discussing and making plans for the signs and symptoms of beginning labor, birth, and the infant's care. The midpoint of a pregnancy also is a good time to describe the new minor symptoms that may occur and to review the precautionary measures to prevent constipation, varicosities, and hemorrhoids, as these increase in intensity late in pregnancy.

Nursing Diagnoses

Examples of possible nursing diagnoses associated with the discomforts of middle to late pregnancy are:

- Health-seeking behaviors related to discomforts of middle to late pregnancy
- Acute pain related to sudden postural change in pregnancy
- Anxiety related to shortness of breath resulting from expanding uterine pressure on diaphragm
- Deficient knowledge related to occurrence of Braxton Hicks contractions in late pregnancy

Box 11.9 highlights appropriate outcomes and interventions related to monitoring the mother in the later part of pregnancy, using the terminology identified by the Nursing Outcomes Classification (NOC) and Nursing Interventions Classification (NIC).

Backache

As pregnancy advances, a lumbar lordosis occurs and postural changes necessary to maintain balance may lead to backache. Wearing shoes with low to moderate heels reduces the amount of spinal curvature necessary to maintain an upright posture. Encouraging a woman to walk with her pelvis tilted forward (putting pelvic support under the weight of the fetus) is also helpful. In addition, applying local heat may aid in relieving backache.

To avoid back strain, advise women to squat rather than bend over to pick up objects. Also encourage them always to lift objects by holding them close to the body. For some women, a firmer mattress during this time may be required. Sliding a board under the mattress is a cost-effective alternative for achieving a firmer sleeping surface. Pelvic rocking or tilting, an exercise described in Chapter 13, also helps to prevent and relieve backache.

Backache can be an initial sign of a bladder or kidney infection. Obtaining a detailed account of a woman's symptoms is crucial to ensure that she is describing only backache. Too often, women are observed at a prenatal visit only lying in a lithotomy position on an examining table. Always assess the manner in which a woman walks and what type of shoes she wears as she moves from a waiting room to an examining room to evaluate whether her posture or shoes could be a cause.

Caution women not to take herbal remedies, muscle relaxants, or analgesics (or any other medication) for back pain without first consulting their physician or nurse-midwife. Generally, acetaminophen (Tylenol) is considered to be safe and effective for relieving this type of pain during pregnancy.

BOX 11.9

Nursing Outcomes Classification (NOC) and Nursing Interventions Classification (NIC)

Monitoring in Late Pregnancy

NOC: Maternal Status, Antepartum

Maternal status, antepartum is defined as the conditions and behaviors indicating maternal well-being from conception to the onset of labor (Johnson, Maas, & Moorhead, 2000). Some specific indicators that suggest that this outcome has been achieved include:

- Evidence of emotional attachment to the fetus
- Ability to cope with discomforts of pregnancy
- Weight change within expected range
- Vital signs within expected parameters
- Laboratory test results such as urine protein and glucose, blood glucose, hemoglobin, and liver enzymes within expected range

NOC: Fetal Status, Antepartum

Fetal status, antepartum is defined as the conditions indicating fetal physical well-being from conception to the onset of labor (Johnson, Maas, & Moorhead, 2000). Some specific indicators that suggest that this outcome has been achieved include:

- Fetal heart rate between 120 and 160 beats per minute
- Fetal ultrasound growth and movement frequency and pattern within expected range

NIC: Surveillance, Late Pregnancy

Surveillance, late pregnancy is defined as the purposeful and ongoing acquisition, interpretation, and synthesis of maternal-fetal data for treatment, observation, or admission (McCloskey & Bulechek, 2000). Some important activities to include when implementing this intervention include:

- Determining maternal-fetal health risks through client interview
- Monitoring maternal vital signs
- Inquiring about presence and quality of fetal movements
- Monitoring for signs of PIH, urinary tract infection, and preterm labor
- Assessing elimination patterns
- Interpreting results of diagnostic tests
- Monitoring comfort level, nutritional status, changes in sleep patterns, and uterine activity
- Obtaining history of sexually transmitted diseases and frequency of intercourse as appropriate
- Instituting appropriate treatment according to standard protocols

Headache

Many women experience headache during pregnancy, apparently from their expanding blood volume, which puts pressure on cerebral arteries. Trying to reduce any possible causative situations, such as eye strain or tension, may lessen the number of headaches they experience. Resting with cold towels on their forehead and taking usual adult doses of acetaminophen usually furnish adequate relief. Although a few women who have migraine headaches find these worsen during pregnancy, most women notice considerable improvement with this type of headache (Gladstone, Eross, & Dodick, 2004) (see Chapter 49). Caution women that if a headache is unusually intense or continuous, they should report it to their primary care provider. This type of headache may be a danger sign of pregnancy caused by high blood pressure.

Dyspnea

As the expanding uterus puts pressure on the diaphragm, it causes lung compression and shortness of breath. A woman will notice this primarily at night when her body is flat. She also will definitely notice it on exertion. To relieve nighttime dyspnea, advise her to sleep upright, allowing the weight of the uterus to fall away from her diaphragm. As pregnancy progresses, she may require two or more pillows to sleep on at night to avoid the problem. Caution her to limit her activities during the day to prevent exertional dyspnea. Always question women about this important symptom at prenatal visits to be certain the sensation is not continuous, which describes more than usual involvement.

Ankle Edema

Most women experience some swelling of the ankles and feet during late pregnancy, most noticeably at the end of the day. Women are often conscious of this first when they kick off their shoes and then cannot put them on again comfortably.

As long as proteinuria and hypertension are absent, ankle edema of this nature is a normal occurrence of pregnancy. It is probably caused by reduced blood circulation in the lower extremities due to uterine pressure and general fluid retention. This simple edema can be relieved best by resting in a left side-lying position because this increases the kidney's glomerular filtration rate and allows good venous return. Sitting for half an hour in the afternoon and again in the evening with the legs elevated is also helpful. Women should avoid wearing constricting clothing such as panty girdles or knee-high stockings because these impede lower extremity circulation and venous return.

Some women need reassurance that ankle edema is normal during pregnancy. Otherwise, they worry that it is a beginning sign of pregnancy-induced hypertension (PIH). On the other hand, do not dismiss a report of lower extremity edema lightly until you are certain a woman does not exhibit any signs of proteinuria or edema of other, non-dependent parts, or has had a sudden increase in weight indicative of PIH.

Braxton Hicks Contractions

Beginning as early as the 8th to 12th week of pregnancy, the uterus periodically contracts and then relaxes again. Early in pregnancy, these contractions, termed Braxton Hicks contractions, are not noticeable. By middle or late pregnancy, the contractions become stronger, and a woman who tenses at the sensation may even experience some minimal pain, similar to a hard menstrual cramp. Although these contractions are not a sign of beginning labor, women should telephone or e-mail their primary care provider to report them so that they can be evaluated. A rhythmic pattern of even very light contractions can be a beginning sign of labor.

> ### Checkpoint Question 4
>
> Julberry Adams has ankle edema by the end of each day. Which statement by her would reveal that she understands what causes this?
>
> a. "I know this is a beginning complication; I'll call my doctor tonight."
> b. "I understand this is from eating too much salt; I'll restrict that more."
> c. "I'll rest in a Sims' position to take pressure off lower extremity veins."
> d. "I walk for half an hour every day to relieve this; I'll try walking more."

DANGER SIGNS OF PREGNANCY

Although most danger signs of pregnancy occur toward the end of pregnancy, women need to know about them from the beginning. To introduce these, assure a pregnant woman you have every reason to believe she is going to have a normal, uncomplicated pregnancy (assuming that is true) as well as no reason to think she is going to experience any serious problems, but if any of the things described below do occur, she should inform her health care provider by telephone or e-mail immediately. Be certain you give her an alternate contact number to call if the health care facility is closed. Emphasize that if one of these danger signs should occur, it serves merely as a signal of the possibility that something may happen, not that something serious has happened. It is important for her to report it immediately, though, so it can be dealt with before something harmful does occur.

Vaginal Bleeding

A woman should report vaginal bleeding, no matter how slight, because some of the serious bleeding complica-

tions of pregnancy begin with only slight spotting. When talking with a woman, ask her how she discovered the spotting. If she discovered it on toilet paper following a bowel movement, she's probably reporting spotting from hemorrhoids. Until the bleeding is found to be innocent, however, all women with spotting need further evaluation.

Persistent Vomiting

Once- or twice-daily vomiting is not uncommon during the first trimester of pregnancy. However, persistent, frequent vomiting is not normal. Vomiting that continues past the 12th week of pregnancy is also extended vomiting. Persistent or extended vomiting depletes the nutritional supply available to a fetus and is a danger to the pregnancy. (See Chapter 12 for a discussion of persistent vomiting [hyperemesis gravidarum].)

Chills and Fever

Chills and fever may indicate an intrauterine infection, a serious complication for both a woman and a fetus. These also may be symptoms of a relatively benign gastroenteritis. However, because a woman cannot make a definite determination about the cause, further evaluation by a health care provider is necessary.

Sudden Escape of Clear Fluid From the Vagina

When a gush of clear fluid is discharged suddenly from the vagina, it means the membranes have ruptured and mother and fetus are now both threatened, because the uterine cavity is no longer sealed against infection. If a fetus is small and the head does not fit snugly into the cervix, the umbilical cord may prolapse following membrane rupture. If the cord is then compressed by the fetal head, oxygenation is compromised and a fetus will be in immediate and grave danger. Alerting a health care provider to any sudden escape of fluid is crucial so a safe and controlled birth can be planned. Occasionally, a woman confuses stress incontinence (involuntary loss of urine on coughing or sneezing or lifting a heavy object) for this. In this situation, vaginal examination typically reveals that the membranes are still intact.

Abdominal or Chest Pain

Abdominal pain at any time is a signal that something is abnormal, so the woman should report it immediately. Some women may think that it is normal because the growing uterus is deflecting their other organs from their usual alignment, but actually the uterus expands painlessly. Abdominal pain is a sign of some other problem, such as a tubal (ectopic) pregnancy, separation of the placenta, preterm labor, or something unrelated to the pregnancy but perhaps equally as serious, such as appendicitis, ulcer, or pancreatitis. Chest pain may indicate a pulmonary embolus, a complication that can follow thrombophlebitis.

Pregnancy-Induced Hypertension (PIH)

PIH refers to a potentially severe and even fatal elevation of blood pressure that occurs during pregnancy. A number of symptoms signal that PIH is developing:

- Rapid weight gain (over 2 lb per week in the second trimester, 1 lb per week in the third trimester)
- Swelling of the face or fingers
- Flashes of light or dots before the eyes
- Dimness or blurring of vision
- Severe, continuous headache
- Decreased urine output

Some edema of the ankles during pregnancy is normal, particularly if it occurs after a woman has been on her feet for a long period of time. Swelling of the hands (ask if she has noticed that her rings are tight) or face (difficulty opening eyes in the morning due to edema of the eyelids) indicates edema too extensive to be normal. Visual disturbances or a continuous headache may signal cerebral edema or acute hypertension. Be certain a woman is not reporting symptoms she had before she became pregnant. If she had the same visual difficulties and headaches before pregnancy as she is reporting now, she may need to see an ophthalmologist rather than her obstetrician for help with the problem. (See Chapter 15 for more on PIH.)

Increase or Decrease in Fetal Movement

Because a fetus normally moves more or less the same amount every day, an unusual increase or decrease in movement suggests that a fetus is responding to the need for oxygen. Be sure to ask the woman about typical fetal movements and whether she has noticed any increase or decrease in this rate recently. Also emphasize the need for a woman to report any changes she notices so that further testing and follow-up can be done. Tests of fetal movement are discussed in Chapter 8.

PREVENTING FETAL EXPOSURE TO TERATOGENS

A **teratogen** is any factor, chemical or physical, that adversely affects the fertilized ovum, embryo, or fetus. To reach maturity in optimal health, a fetus needs sound genes (see Chapter 7) and a healthy intrauterine environment that protects it from the influence of teratogens.

At one time, it was assumed that a fetus in utero was protected from chemical or physical injury by the presence of the amniotic fluid and by the absence of any direct placental exchange between mother and fetus. When infants were born with disorders, it was attributed to the influence of fate, bad luck, or, in some cultures, evil spirits. Today, it is acknowledged that a fetus is extremely vulnerable to environmental injury. Although the causes of many anomalies occurring in utero are still unknown, many teratogenic factors have been isolated.

Effects of Teratogens on a Fetus

Several factors influence the amount of damage a teratogen can cause. The strength of the teratogen is one factor. For example, radiation is a known teratogen. In small amounts (everyone is exposed to some radiation every day, such as from sun rays), it causes no damage. However, in large doses (e.g., the amount of radiation necessary to treat cancer of the cervix), serious fetal defects or death can occur.

The timing of the teratogenic insult is another factor that makes a significant difference. If a teratogen is introduced before implantation, either the zygote is destroyed or it appears unaffected. If the insult occurs when the main body systems are being formed (in the 2nd to 8th weeks of embryonic life), a fetus is very vulnerable to injury. During the last trimester, the potential for harm again decreases because all the organs of a fetus are formed and are merely maturing. The times when different anatomic areas of a fetus are most likely to be affected by teratogens are shown in Figure 8.5.

Two exceptions to the rule that deformities usually occur in early embryonic life are the effects caused by the organisms of syphilis and toxoplasmosis. These two infections can cause abnormalities in organs that were originally formed normally.

A third factor determining the effects of a teratogen is the teratogen's affinity for specific tissue. Lead, for instance, attacks and disables nervous tissue. Thalidomide causes limb defects. Tetracycline causes tooth enamel deficiencies and, possibly, long bone deformities. The rubella virus, on the other hand, can affect many organs: the eyes, ears, heart, and brain are the four most commonly attacked.

Nursing Diagnoses

Much of the health history information obtained at prenatal visits helps to determine whether a woman has been exposed to a teratogen since the last visit.

Examples of nursing diagnoses associated with maternal exposure to teratogens are:

- Health-seeking behavior related to mother's interest in avoiding exposure to substances harmful to a fetus during pregnancy
- Risk for fetal injury related to lack of knowledge about teratogenicity of alcohol, drugs, and cigarettes
- Risk for infection related to fetal transmission from maternal exposure to genital herpes

Teratogenic Maternal Infections

Teratogenic maternal infections can involve either sexually transmitted or systemic infections. Organisms that cross the placenta can be viral, bacterial, or protozoan. Most cause relatively mild, flulike symptoms in a woman but can have much more serious effects on a fetus or newborn. Preventing and predicting fetal injury from infection is complicated because a disease may be subclinical (without any symptoms in the mother) and yet may injure a fetus.

When diseases that are known to cross the placenta and cause fetal harm are tested for, they are described collectively under the umbrella term TORCH, an abbreviation for toxoplasmosis, rubella, cytomegalovirus, and herpes simplex virus. (Some sources identify the O with "other infections," which could include syphilis, hepatitis B virus [HBV], and human immunodeficiency virus [HIV].) The TORCH screen is an immunologic survey to determine whether these infections exist in either the pregnant woman (to identify fetal risk factors) or the newborn (to detect if antibodies against the common infectious teratogens are present). Although it is now known that many more than the original four or five maternal infections can cause harm to a fetus or newborn (a chlamydia or streptococcal B infection, for example, can cause pneumonia in the newborn [see Chapter 26]), the TORCH screen still provides a quick way to assess the potential risk of teratogenic infection in pregnant women or newborns. Both hepatitis B and HIV infections are discussed in Chapter 14. TORCH screen infections are described in more detail below.

Toxoplasmosis

Toxoplasmosis, a protozoan infection, is spread most commonly through contact with uncooked meat, although it may also be contracted through handling cat stool in soil or cat litter (Ricci et al., 2003). A woman experiences almost no symptoms of the disease except a few days of malaise and posterior cervical lymphadenopathy. Even in light of these mild symptoms, if the infection crosses the placenta, the infant may be born with central nervous system damage, hydrocephalus, microcephaly, intracerebral calcification, and retinal deformities. If the diagnosis is established by serum analysis during pregnancy, therapy with sulfonamides may be prescribed. However, the prevention of fetal deformities is uncertain, and sulfa may lead to increased bilirubin levels in the newborn. Pyrimethamine, an antiprotozoal agent, may also be used. This drug is an antifolic acid drug, so it is administered with caution early in pregnancy to prevent reducing folic acid levels.

As many as 1 in 900 pregnancies may be affected by toxoplasmosis (Minkoff & Gibbs, 2003). Prepregnancy serum analysis can be done to identify women who have never had the disease and so are susceptible (about 50% of women). Removing a cat from the home during pregnancy as a means of prevention is not necessary as long as the cat is healthy. On the other hand, taking in a new cat is unwise. Instruct pregnant women to avoid undercooked meat and also not to change a cat litter box or work in soil in an area where cats may defecate.

Rubella

The rubella virus usually causes only a mild rash and mild systemic illness in the mother, but the teratogenic effects on a fetus can be devastating (Gerber & Hohlfeld, 2003). Fetal damage from maternal infection with rubella (German measles) includes deafness, mental and motor challenges, cataracts, cardiac defects (most commonly patent ductus arteriosus and pulmonary stenosis), restricted intrauterine growth (small for gestational age), thrombo-

cytopenic purpura, and dental and facial clefts, such as cleft lip and palate.

Typically, a rubella titer is obtained on the first prenatal visit. A titer greater than 1:8 suggests immunity to rubella. A titer of less than 1:8 suggests that a woman is susceptible to viral invasion. A titer that is greatly increased over a previous reading or is initially extremely high suggests that a recent infection has occurred.

A woman who is not immunized before pregnancy cannot be immunized during pregnancy because the vaccine uses a live virus that would have effects similar to those occurring with a subclinical case of rubella. After a rubella immunization, a woman is advised not to become pregnant for 3 months, until the rubella virus is no longer active. Immediately after a pregnancy, assess whether a woman with low rubella titers would like to be immunized to provide protection against rubella in future pregnancies (Speroff & Fritz, 2005).

An increasing concern is women who demonstrate antibodies against rubella yet still become reinfected during pregnancy. Because of this, all pregnant women should avoid contact with children with rashes. Infants who are born to mothers who had rubella during pregnancy may be capable of transmitting the disease after birth. The infant needs to be isolated from other newborns during the newborn period. The mother should be made aware of the possibility that her infant might infect others, including pregnant women. Nurses who care for pregnant women or newborns should receive immunization against rubella to ensure that they neither spread nor contract the disease.

Cytomegalovirus

Cytomegalovirus (CMV), a member of the herpes virus family, is another teratogen that can cause extensive damage to a fetus while causing few symptoms in a woman (Minkoff & Gibbs, 2003). It is transmitted by droplet infection from person to person. If a woman acquires a primary CMV infection during pregnancy and the virus crosses the placenta, the infant may be born severely neurologically challenged (hydrocephalus, microcephaly, spasticity) or with eye damage (optic atrophy, chorioretinitis), deafness, or chronic liver disease. The child's skin may be covered with large petechiae ("blueberry-muffin" lesions). Because a woman has almost no symptoms, she may not be aware that she has contracted an infection. However, diagnosis in the mother or infant can be established by the isolation of CMV antibodies in blood serum. Unfortunately, no treatment for the infection exists even if it presents in the mother with enough symptoms to allow detection. Because there is no treatment or vaccine for the disease, routine screening for CMV during pregnancy is not recommended. Women can help prevent exposure by thorough handwashing before eating and avoiding crowds of young children at daycare or nursery settings.

Like herpes simplex, a primary CMV infection may become latent and then reactivate periodically. These recurrences are not thought to have a teratogenic effect on a fetus, but they can cause infection of the newborn during birth from genital secretions, or postpartum from exposure to CMV-infected breast milk. CMV infection contracted at or shortly after birth is not associated with serious adverse effects except in babies of very low birth-weight (1,200 g).

Herpes Simplex Virus (Genital Herpes Infection)

A primary, first-episode genital herpes infection in a pregnant woman poses a substantial risk to a fetus (Sheffield et al., 2004). The first time a woman contracts a genital herpes infection, systemic involvement occurs. The virus spreads into the bloodstream (viremia) and crosses the placenta to a fetus.

If the infection takes place in the first trimester, severe congenital anomalies or spontaneous miscarriage may occur. If the infection occurs during the second or third trimester, there is a high incidence of premature birth, intrauterine growth restriction, and continuing infection of the newborn at birth. Unless recognized and treated, the fetal mortality and morbidity rates are as high as 80% (Brown, 2004).

If a woman has had herpes simplex virus type 1 infections before the genital herpes invasion or if the genital herpes (type 2) infection is a recurrence, antibodies to the virus in her system prevent spread of the virus to a fetus across the placenta. If genital lesions are present at the time of birth, however, a fetus may contract the virus from direct exposure during birth. For women with a history of genital herpes and existing genital lesions, cesarean birth is often advised to reduce the risk of this route of infection. This awareness of the placental spread of herpes simplex virus has increased the importance of obtaining information about exposure to genital herpes or any painful perineal or vaginal lesions that might indicate this infection at prenatal visits.

Intravenous or oral acyclovir (Zovirax) can be administered to women during pregnancy (Karch, 2004). The primary mechanism for protecting a fetus, however, focuses on disease prevention. Urging women to practice safer sex is important to lessen their exposure to this and other sexually transmitted infections.

Other Viral Diseases

It has been difficult to demonstrate other viral teratogens, but rubeola (measles), coxsackievirus, mumps, varicella (chickenpox), poliomyelitis, influenza, and viral hepatitis all may be teratogenic. Parvovirus B19, the causative agent of erythema infectiosum (also called fifth disease), if contracted during pregnancy, can cross the placenta and attack the red blood cells of a fetus. Infection during early pregnancy is associated with fetal death. If the infection occurs late in pregnancy, the infant may be born with severe anemia and congenital heart disease (Al-Khan, Caligiuri, & Apuzzio, 2003).

Syphilis. Syphilis, a sexually transmitted infection, is of great concern for the maternal–fetal population despite the availability of accurate screening tests and proven medical treatment, as it places a fetus at risk for intrauterine or congenital syphilis (Dobson, 2004). Early in pregnancy, when the cytotrophoblast layer of the chorionic villi is still intact, the causative spirochete of syphilis, *Treponema pallidum,* cannot cross the placenta and damage the fetus. When the cytotrophoblastic layer atrophies at about the 16th to 18th week of pregnancy, the spirochete then can cross and cause extensive damage. If syphilis is detected and treated with an antibiotic such as benzathine penicillin in the first trimester, therefore, a fetus is rarely affected. If left untreated beyond the 18th week of gestation, deafness, cognitive challenge, osteochondritis, and fetal death are possible.

For this reason, serologic screening (either a VDRL or a rapid plasma reagin) should be done at the first prenatal visit; the test may then be repeated again close to term (the 8th month) if exposure is a concern. Even when a woman has been treated with appropriate antibiotics, the serum titer remains high for more than 200 days; an increasing titer, however, suggests that reinfection has occurred. In an infant born to a woman with syphilis, the serologic test for syphilis may remain positive for up to 3 months even though the disease was treated during pregnancy.

The newborn with congenital syphilis may have congenital anomalies, extreme rhinitis (sniffles), and a characteristic syphilitic rash, all of which identify the baby as high risk at birth. When the baby's primary teeth come in, they are oddly shaped (Hutchinson teeth). Medical and nursing care of the newborn with congenital syphilis is discussed in Chapter 26.

Lyme Disease. Lyme disease, a multisystem disease caused by the spirochete *Borrelia burgdorferi,* is spread by the bite of a deer tick. The highest incidence occurs in the summer and early fall. The largest outbreaks of the disease are found on the east coast of the United States (Eppes, 2003). After the tick bite, a typical skin rash, *erythema chronicum migrans* (large, macular lesions with a clear center), develops. Pain in large joints such as the knee may be present. Infection in pregnancy can result in spontaneous miscarriage or severe congenital anomalies.

Women anticipating becoming pregnant or who are pregnant should avoid areas such as wooded or tall grassy areas where they are apt to be bitten by ticks. If hiking in these areas, a woman should avoid the use of tick repellents containing diethyltoluamide because this ingredient is teratogenic. Instead, she should wear long, light-colored slacks tucked into her socks to prevent her legs from being exposed. To spread the spirochete, the tick must be present on the body possibly as long as 24 hours. After returning home from an outing, therefore, a woman should inspect her body carefully and immediately remove any ticks found. If she has any symptoms that suggest Lyme disease or knows she has been bitten, she should contact her primary health care provider immediately. Treatment of Lyme disease for pregnant women differs from that for nonpregnant women. The drugs used for nonpregnant adults, tetracycline and doxycycline, cannot be used during pregnancy because they cause tooth discoloration and, possibly, long-bone malformation in a fetus. A course of penicillin will be prescribed to reduce symptoms in the pregnant woman.

Because the symptoms of Lyme disease are chronic but not dramatic (a migratory rash and joint pain), women may not report them at a prenatal visit unless they are educated about their importance and are asked at prenatal visits if such symptoms are present.

Infections That Cause Illness at Birth. A number of infections are not teratogenic to a fetus during pregnancy but are harmful if they are present at the time of birth. Gonorrhea, candidiasis, chlamydia, streptococcus B, and hepatitis B infections are examples of these. Chapters 26 and 47 discuss the effects of these infections on maternal, fetal, and neonatal health.

Potentially Teratogenic Vaccines

Live virus vaccines, such as measles, mumps, rubella, and poliomyelitis (Sabin type), are contraindicated during pregnancy because they may transmit the viral infection to a fetus (Katz, 2003). Care must be taken in routine immunization programs to make sure that adolescents about to be vaccinated are not pregnant. Women who work in biologic laboratories where vaccines are manufactured are well advised not to work with live virus products during pregnancy.

Teratogenic Drugs

Many women, assuming that the rule of being cautious with drugs during pregnancy applies only to prescription drugs, take over-the-counter drugs or herbal supplements freely. Although not all drugs cross the placenta (e.g., heparin does not because of its large molecular size), most do. Also, even though most herbs are safe, ginseng, for example, used to improve general well-being, or senna, used to relieve constipation, may not be safe (Rousseaux & Schachter, 2003).

To identify drugs that are unsafe for ingestion during pregnancy, the U.S. Food and Drug Administration (FDA) has established five categories of safety (Table 11.1). Two principles govern drug intake during pregnancy:

- Any drug or herbal supplement, under certain circumstances, may be detrimental to fetal welfare. Therefore, during pregnancy, women should not take any drug or supplement not specifically prescribed or approved by their physician or nurse-midwife.
- A woman of childbearing age and ability should take no drugs other than those prescribed by a physician or nurse-midwife to avoid exposure to a drug should she become pregnant.

The classic teratogenic drug is thalidomide, once liberally prescribed for morning sickness in Europe. Never approved for use in the United States, thalidomide caused amelia or phocomelia (total or partial absence of extremities) in 100% of instances when taken between the 34th and 45th day of pregnancy. Thalidomide is again available as an anti-cancer drug for use particularly with patients with multiple myeloma (Rajkumar, 2004). Patients taking this must be conscientious not to do so if they are pregnant. Other examples of drugs capable of being teratogenic are shown in Table 11.2.

The use of recreational drugs during pregnancy puts a fetus at risk in two ways: the drug may have a direct teratogenic effect, and intravenous drug use also risks exposure to diseases such as HIV and hepatitis B.

Narcotics such as meperidine (Demerol) and heroin have long been implicated as causing intrauterine growth restriction. The use of marijuana alone apparently does not, although the long-term effects of marijuana during pregnancy are still unstudied. Cocaine, particularly its crack form, is potentially harmful to a fetus because it causes severe vasoconstriction in the mother, compromising placental blood flow and so interfering with the fetal nutrient supply. Its use is associated with spontaneous miscarriage, preterm labor, meconium staining, and intrauterine growth restriction (Ogunyemi & Hernandez-Loera, 2004). Whether cocaine causes long-term effects remains controversial (Rayburn & Bogenschutz, 2004). See Chapter 17 for more information on the potential hazards of cocaine or heroin use during pregnancy.

TABLE 11.1

Pregnancy Risk Categories of Drugs

Category	Description	Example
A	Adequate studies in pregnant women have failed to show a risk to the fetus in the first trimester of pregnancy; there is no evidence of risk in later trimesters.	Thyroid hormone
B	Animal studies have not shown an adverse effect on the fetus, but there are no adequate clinical studies in pregnant women.	Insulin
C	Animal studies have shown an adverse effect on the fetus, but there are no adequate studies on humans, or there are no adequate studies in animals or humans. Pregnancy risk is unknown.	Docusate sodium (Colace)
D	There is evidence of risk to the human fetus, but the potential benefits of use in pregnant women may be acceptable despite potential risks.	Lithium citrate
X	Studies in animals or humans show fetal abnormalities, or adverse reaction reports indicate evidence of fetal risk. The risks involved clearly outweigh potential benefits.	Isotretinoin (Accutane)

Karch, A.M. (2004). *Lippincott's nursing drug guide.* Philadelphia: Lippincott Williams & Wilkins.

TABLE 11.2

Some Potentially or Positively Teratogenic Drugs

Category	Drug	Drug Use	Teratogenic Effect
Vitamin A derivatives	Isotretinoin (Accutane) Etretinate (Tegison)	Acne Psoriasis	Craniofacial, cardiac, CNS anomalies Craniofacial, cardiac, CNS anomalies
Alcohol	Wine, whiskey	Social use	Fetal alcohol syndrome
Analgesics	Acetylsalicylic acid (aspirin) NSAIDs	Minor pain relief	Prolonged pregnancy; maternal bleeding Patent ductus arteriosus
Antineoplastics	Methotrexate Cyclophosphamide (Cytoxan)	Chemotherapy Chemotherapy	Multiple anomalies Multiple anomalies
Androgens	Danazol	Endometriosis	Masculinization of female fetus
Anticonvulsants	Phenytoin (Dilantin) Valproic acid Carbamazepine Lamotrigine	Seizures	Fetal hydantoin syndrome Neural tube defects Neural tube defects Possibly fetal anomalies
Anticoagulants	Warfarin (Coumarin)	Anticoagulation	Fetal bleeding or anomalies
Antidepressants	Imipramine (Tofranil)	Elevate mood	Cardiovascular anomalies
Antischizophrenic	Lithium	Schizophrenia	Hydramnios
Antithyroid	Methimazole	Hypothyroidism	Hypothyroidism in fetus
Antibiotics	Ribavirin Sulfonamides Tetracycline	Respiratory infection Infection Infection	Multiple anomalies Hyperbilirubinemia in newborn Teeth and bone deformities
Antihelmintics	Lindane	Eradication of lice	Manufacturer recommendation of limiting exposure to 2 doses
Angiotensin-converting enzyme inhibitors	Enalapril (Vasotec) Captopril (Capoten)	Reduce hypertension	Oligohydramnios
Caffeine	Caffeine	Coffee, soft drinks, chocolate	Low birthweight
Hypoglycemics	Tolbutamide (Orinase)	Type II diabetes	Profound hypoglycemia in newborn
Nicotine		Cigarette smoke	Growth retardation
Radiopharmaceuticals	Iodide-131	Diagnostic studies	May destroy thyroid of fetus
Narcotics	Cocaine Heroin	Social pleasure	Dysmorphic and CNS anomalies Growth retardation; narcotic withdrawal in newborn
Tranquilizers	Benzodiazepine (diazepam)	Reduce anxiety	Growth retardation; CNS dysfunction Hypotonia, respiratory depression
Vaccines (live)	Rubella	Provide immunity	Possible infection in fetus

Yankowitz, J. (2003). Drugs in pregnancy. In J.R. Scott, et al. *Danforth's obstetrics and gynecology* (9th ed.). Philadelphia: Lippincott Williams & Wilkins.

An area of recreational drug use that needs to be examined is that of inhalant abuse ("huffing"). Substances frequently used as inhalants include gasoline, butane lighter fluid, Freon, glue, and nitrous oxide (NIOSH, 2000). Although the teratogenic properties of inhalants are not well studied, they all carry the possibility of respiratory distress, which could limit the oxygen supply to a fetus.

Teratogenicity of Alcohol

Evidence over the years has shown that when women consume a large quantity of alcohol during pregnancy, their babies show a high incidence of congenital deformities and cognitive impairment. It was assumed that these defects were the result of the mother's poor nutritional status (drinking alcohol rather than eating food), not necessarily the direct result of the alcohol. However, alcohol has now been firmly isolated as a teratogen. Fetuses cannot remove the breakdown products of alcohol from their body. The large buildup of these leads to vitamin B deficiency and accompanying neurologic damage.

Women during pregnancy should be screened for alcohol use because an infant born with **fetal alcohol syndrome** is not only small for gestational age but can be cognitively challenged (Mukherjee et al., 2005). The infant typically has a characteristic craniofacial deformity including short palpebral fissures, a thin upper lip, and an upturned nose (Yankowitz, 2003). Because of individual variations in metabolism, it is impossible to define a safe level of alcohol consumption. Women are best advised, therefore, to abstain from alcohol completely. Women with alcohol addiction should be referred to an alcohol treatment program as early in pregnancy as possible to help them reduce their alcohol intake (Box 11.10).

Teratogenicity of Cigarettes

Cigarette smoking is associated with infertility in women. Cigarette smoking by a pregnant woman has been shown to have teratogenic effects on a fetus, especially growth restriction (Katz, 2003). In addition, these children may be at greater risk than others for sudden infant death syndrome. Low birthweight in infants of smoking mothers results from vasoconstriction of the uterine vessels, an effect of nicotine that limits the blood supply to a fetus. Another contributory effect may be related to inhaled carbon monoxide. Secondary smoke, or inhaling the smoke of another person's cigarettes, may be as harmful as actually smoking

---

BOX 11.10 : Focus on Nursing Care Planning

A Multidisciplinary Care Map for a Pregnant Woman With Threats to Fetal Health

●

Julberry Adams, a single woman, is 4 months pregnant when you see her in a prenatal clinic. She works as a curator for an art gallery but has missed work this last week because of nausea. She has stopped volunteer work teaching children's swimming at the YMCA. She wonders how she will be able to afford her apartment if she has to quit work. She wants to travel to see her sister in St. Louis because her sister is very ill but has heard that pregnant women shouldn't drive over 100 miles. She asks you if marijuana reduces early pregnancy nausea.

Family Assessment
Client lives by herself in one-family loft in downtown city. Rates finances as "good, unless I have to quit work because of pregnancy." She asks you, "Will I have to have an ultrasound? I'm worried about that."

Client Assessment
Gravida 1, para 0. Unsure of date of last menstrual period, but it was about 11 weeks ago. Uterine height barely above symphysis. Fetal heart rate at 148 beats per minute by Doppler. History of frequent sinus headaches. "I use Sudafed (pseudoephedrine) at least 3 to 4 times a week; sometimes other things." Smokes one half pack of cigarettes "some days." Drinks 2 to 3 glasses of wine per week at art gallery functions. Denies history of marijuana or other recreational drug use.

Nursing Diagnosis
Risk for fetal injury related to knowledge deficit concerning possible fetal exposure to teratogens

Outcome Criteria
Client reports a decrease in smoking to at least 10 cigarettes per day or less and no alcohol consumption
Verbalizes no use of recreational drugs including marijuana
States she has contacted health care provider about use of sinus medications

(continued)

Team Member Responsible	Assessment	Intervention	Rationale	Expected Outcome
Activities of Daily Living				
Nurse	Assess what activities client wants to participate in during pregnancy.	Discuss desired activities and any modification necessary for pregnancy with client.	Finding a match between desired activities and preferred activities will help with adherence.	Client discusses what activities she intends to continue during pregnancy and ways to modify them as necessary.
Physician	Assess what work or travel plans entail.	Assure client she can continue work, travel to sister's home.	Reassurance helps clients maintain normal lifestyle.	Client states she will continue work, maintain contact with sister.
Consultations				
Nurse	Assess what medications client is currently taking.	Consult with client's primary and maternal health care providers about safety of over-the-counter (OTC) medications.	Not all OTC medications are safe during pregnancy.	Client states she will follow recommendations of primary health care provider regarding medications.
Procedures/Medications				
Physician/ nurse-midwife	Anticipate the need for follow-up ultrasound examination for fetal growth evaluation.	Explain the need for ultrasound exam to assess for fetal growth restriction because of alcohol and cigarette smoking habits.	Teratogen exposure may have slowed fetal growth, which will be revealed by ultrasound exam.	Client states that she is aware of purpose of ultrasound exam and will allow exam to be scheduled.
Nutrition				
Nurse	Assess client's lifestyle to see what foods she could substitute for alcohol, what measures she could use best for nausea.	Suggest client replace alcohol consumption with caffeine-free beverages.	Alcohol consumption during pregnancy is associated with fetal alcohol syndrome.	Client voices intent to replace alcohol consumption with caffeine-free beverages.
		Suggest measures to combat nausea and vomiting, such as dry crackers, acupuncture band.	Decreasing nausea to increase food intake aids fetal growth and development.	Client suggests measures that appeal to her to reduce nausea and vomiting.
			Client participation helps to individualize care, increase feelings of control, and promote adherence.	
Patient/Family Education				
Nurse/ nurse-midwife	Assess whether client has tried any non-medicinal measures to relieve sinus headaches.	Discuss with client possible non-medicinal measures to assist with sinus headache relief, including saline nasal sprays, humidification, and warm compresses to nasal area.	Complementary comfort measures may provide symptomatic relief without danger to a fetus.	Client describes two complementary therapies she will use to relieve sinus congestion.

(continued)

Team Member Responsible	Assessment	Intervention	Rationale	Expected Outcome
Psychosocial/Spiritual/Emotional Needs				
Nurse/social worker	Discuss with client whether her current support system is reliable.	Help client locate at least one person she can depend on if a pregnancy emergency should arise.	Pregnancy can be a very stressful time for a woman who has an insecure support system.	Client telephones or e-mails the health care facility with questions rather than relying on non-experienced friends for information; names one support person.
Discharge Planning				
Nurse	Assess extent of cigarette smoking.	Encourage the client to decrease smoking and quit if possible. Offer suggestions to accomplish this goal, including use of sugar-free gums or candies, distraction, and activity. Refer to a smoking-cessation group if appropriate.	Cigarette use during pregnancy can lead to fetal growth restriction. Support and suggestions provide concrete measures to assist client with cutting down and quitting.	Client voices intention to decrease smoking and if possible quit smoking during pregnancy.

the cigarettes. All prenatal health care settings should be smoke-free environments for this reason.

If a woman cannot stop smoking during pregnancy (and, realistically, many women cannot), reducing the number of cigarettes smoked per day should help diminish adverse effects on a fetus as well as also protect a woman's own health from long-term illnesses such as chronic respiratory diseases.

The best way to urge women to discontinue smoking is to educate them about the risks to themselves and their fetus at the first prenatal visit. It may be effective to encourage women to sign a contract with a health care provider to try to stop or to join a smoking-cessation program. Be certain pregnant women know that they should not enter a stop-smoking program that uses drug therapy such as nicotine patches, because the substitute drug may be as harmful to a fetus as smoking.

Environmental Teratogens

Teratogens from environmental sources can be as damaging to a fetus as those that are directly or deliberately ingested. Women can be exposed to these through contact at home or at work sites. For example, washing children's hair with a shampoo such as lindane (Kwell) to remove lice should be limited to two exposures because of potential toxicity (Karch, 2004).

Metal and Chemical Hazards

Pesticides and carbon monoxide such as from automobile exhaust are examples of chemical teratogens that are harmful and so should be avoided. Arsenic, a byproduct of copper and lead smelting, used in pesticides, paints, and leather processing; formaldehyde, used in paper ma-

nufacturing; and mercury, used in the manufacture of electrical apparatuses, are all teratogens that can be contacted at work sites. Additional information on specific chemicals can be obtained from the National Institute for Occupational Safety and Health (NIOSH) at their web site (*www.cdc.gov/NIOSH*).

Lead poisoning generally is considered a problem of young children eating lead-based paint chips, but it also can be a fetal hazard. Women may ingest lead by drinking water that travels through old pipes that are leaching lead or by "sniffing" gasoline. Lead ingestion during pregnancy may lead to a newborn who is cognitively or neurologically challenged (Hackley & Katz-Jacobson, 2003).

Radiation

Rapidly growing cells are extremely vulnerable to destruction by radiation. Radiation has been proven to be a potent teratogen to unborn children because of the high proportion of rapidly growing cells present. It produces a range of malformations depending on the stage of development of the embryo or fetus and the strength and length of exposure. If the exposure occurs before implantation, the growing zygote apparently is killed. If the zygote is not killed, it survives apparently unharmed. The most damaging time for exposure and subsequent damage is from implantation to 6 weeks after conception (when many women are not yet aware that they are pregnant). The nervous system, brain, and the retinal innervation are most affected.

As a rule, therefore, all women of childbearing age should be exposed to pelvic x-rays only in the first 10 days of a menstrual cycle (when pregnancy is unlikely because ovulation has not yet occurred), except in emergency situations. A serum pregnancy test can be done on all women who have reason to believe they might be pregnant before diagnostic tests involving x-rays are performed.

Radiation of the pelvis should be avoided all during pregnancy if possible. It should be undertaken only at term if the data obtained are important for birth and cannot be obtained by any other means. Sonography and magnetic resonance imaging have replaced x-ray examination for confirmation of situations such as multiple pregnancy because these do not appear to be teratogenic.

In addition to immediate fetal damage, evidence exists that radiation can have long-lasting effects on the health of the child. There appears to be an increased risk of cancer in children exposed to radiation in utero. Exposure of the fetal gonads could lead to a genetic mutation that will not be evident until the next generation (Katz, 2003).

If a woman needs non-pelvic radiation during pregnancy (e.g., dental x-rays, arm or leg x-ray after a fall), she should be given a lead apron to shield her pelvis during the procedure. Even fluoroscopy, which uses lower radiation doses than regular x-ray photography, can cause fetal deformities and should be avoided during pregnancy—again, except in an emergency. Although still being investigated, long-term use of slight radiation sources, such as a word processor, computer, or cellular phone, does not appear to be teratogenic.

Hyperthermia and Hypothermia

Hyperthermia to a fetus may be detrimental to growth because it interferes with cell metabolism. Hyperthermia can occur from the use of saunas, hot tubs, or tanning beds, or from a work environment next to a furnace, such as in welding or steel making. For this reason, pregnant women should avoid hot tubs or saunas. Women who use a hot tub at 40°C should not stay in it for longer than about 10 minutes at one time. Maternal fever early in pregnancy (4 to 6 weeks) may cause abnormal fetal brain development and possibly seizure disorders, hypotonia, and skeletal deformities (Edwards, Saunders, & Shiota, 2003).

The effect of hypothermia on pregnancy is not well known. Because the uterus is an internal organ, a woman's body temperature would have to be lowered significantly before a great deal of fetal change would result.

Teratogenic Maternal Stress

Many myths exist about the effect of being frightened or surprised while pregnant. For example:

- If a woman sees a mouse during pregnancy, her child will be born with a furry or molelike birthmark.
- Eating strawberries causes strawberry birthmarks.
- Looking at a handicapped child while pregnant will cause a child in utero to be handicapped the same way.

Common sense and awareness of fetal–maternal physiology have dispelled these superstitions. There is some evidence, however, that an emotionally disturbed pregnancy, one filled with anxiety and worry beyond the usual amount, could produce physiologic changes through its effect on the sympathetic division of the autonomic nervous system. The primary changes this could cause include

constriction of the peripheral blood vessels (a fight-or-flight syndrome). If the anxiety is prolonged, the constriction of uterine vessels (the uterus is a peripheral organ) could interfere with the blood and nutrient supply to a fetus.

These phenomena are characteristic only of long-term, extreme stress, not of the normal anxiety of pregnancy. Illness or death of one's partner, difficulty with relatives, marital discord, and illness or death of another child are examples of stressful situations that might provoke excessive anxiety.

Helping a woman resolve these complex problems during pregnancy is not easy. If maternal stress is severe, however, securing counseling is as important as ensuring good physical care.

PREPARING FOR LABOR

At about the midpoint of pregnancy, along with cautioning women about discomforts of pregnancy and possible teratogen situations, it is time to review the events that signal the beginning of labor so that women will not be surprised by these happenings or dismiss them as something other than what they are.

Lightening

Lightening is the settling of the fetal head into the inlet of the true pelvis. It occurs approximately 2 weeks before labor in primiparas but at unpredictable times in multiparas. A woman notices she is not as short of breath as she was. Her abdominal contour is definitely changed, and on standing she may experience frequency of urination or sciatic pain (pain across her buttock radiating down her leg) from the lowered fetal position.

Show

Show is the common term used to describe the release of the cervical plug (operculum) that formed during pregnancy. It consists of a mucous, often blood-streaked vaginal discharge and indicates the beginning of cervical dilatation.

Rupture of the Membranes

A sudden gush of clear fluid (amniotic fluid) from the vagina indicates rupture of the membranes. A woman should telephone her primary care provider immediately when this occurs. After rupture of the membranes, there is a danger of cord prolapse and uterine infection.

Excess Energy

Feeling extremely energetic is a sign of labor important for women to recognize. It occurs as part of the body's physiologic preparation for labor. If a woman does not recognize the sensation for what it is, she may use this burst of energy to clean her house or finish paperwork at the office and exhaust herself before labor begins. If she can recognize this symptom as an initial sign of labor, she can conserve her energy in preparation for labor.

Uterine Contractions

For most women, labor begins with contractions. True labor contractions usually start in the back and sweep forward across the abdomen like the tightening of a band. They gradually increase in frequency and intensity. Advise a woman to telephone her primary care provider when contractions begin to alert health care personnel that she is in labor. Inform her at what point in labor her physician or nurse-midwife wants her to come to the health care facility (such as when contractions are 5 minutes apart). Be certain she knows this is not a hard-and-fast rule, however. If she should become exceptionally anxious, be home alone, or have a long drive, she should be given the option of using common sense to determine when to leave home.

Checkpoint Question 5

Julberry Adams makes the following statements. Which one is the safest practice?

a. "My brother takes medicine for heartburn; if I get that, I'll just borrow his."
b. "I'm going to get a measles shot; I don't want measles while I'm pregnant."
c. "There are so many medicines for headache, I have to ask my doctor what to take."
d. "I know all over-the-counter medicine is safe; it's why it's over the counter."

Key Points

Prenatal education is an important part of prenatal care. The more women know about measures they should take during pregnancy to safeguard their health, the more likely they will avoid substances or activities harmful to fetal growth.

Urge women to find the best way for them to modify their lifestyle for pregnancy. Pregnancy is 9 months long, so modifications must be agreeable to a woman or she will not maintain them over such a long time span.

Discussion and health-teaching periods during pregnancy should cover self-care topics such as bathing, sexual activity, sleep, and exercise.

Women need to make provisions for rest periods during their day and to be aware of any potential teratogens at a work site, such as exposure to radiation or heavy metals.

Women who travel should plan for break periods to avoid congestion in the lower extremities. Seat belts should be used when traveling by car.

Common discomforts of early pregnancy include breast tenderness, constipation, palmar erythema, nausea and vomiting, fatigue, muscle cramps, pain from varicosities or hemorrhoids, heart palpitations, frequency of urination, and leukorrhea. If women know that these symptoms may occur, they will not interpret them as complications.

Minor discomforts of middle or late pregnancy include backache, dyspnea, ankle edema, and Braxton Hicks contractions. Caution women that contractions could be a sign of labor.

Danger signs for women to report during pregnancy are vaginal bleeding, persistent vomiting, chills and fever, escape of fluid from the vagina, abdominal or chest pain, swelling of the face and fingers, vision changes or continuous headache, rhythmic cramping, burning with urination, or a pronounced decrease in fetal movement.

Women should take active measures to avoid exposure to infectious diseases such as rubella, HIV, cytomegalovirus, herpes simplex virus, syphilis, Lyme disease, and toxoplasmosis during pregnancy.

Counsel women about the necessity to avoid the use of any drugs or herbal supplements not specifically approved by their physician or nurse-midwife during pregnancy, as well as alcohol and cigarettes.

It is almost impossible for a woman to modify a behavior, such as smoking, if her support person does not agree to change also. Including the family in care is an important way of helping support persons understand the need for the modification and increasing cooperation.

Beginning signs of labor for which the pregnant woman should be alert include lightening, show, excess energy, rupture of membranes, and uterine contractions.

Critical Thinking Exercises

1. Julberry Adams, the woman you met at the beginning of the chapter, voiced a number of concerns, including whether she should stop work and whether it would be safe to take a long trip. What advice would you give her regarding these questions?
2. Although Julberry describes a day she says involves a lot of walking, she also has long periods of sitting with almost no exercise. What would be some recommendations you could make to help her prevent blood clots from the sharp bend in her knee while sitting?
3. Julberry is having trouble remembering to take her prenatal vitamin. What are some suggestions you could make to help her remember to take this daily?
4. Examine the National Health Goals related to prenatal care. Most government-sponsored money for nursing research is allotted based on these goals. What would be a possible research topic to explore pertinent to these goals that would be applicable to Julberry and her family and also advance evidence-based practice?

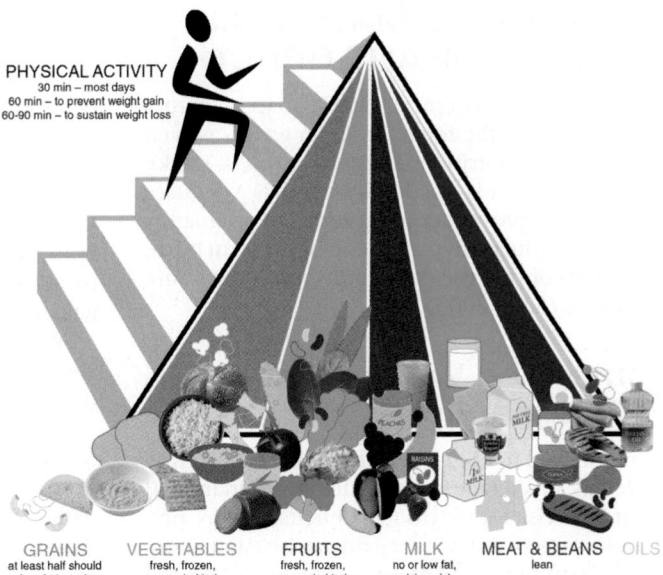

FIGURE 12.1 The food pyramid. (Department of Agriculture. [2005]. *Food guide pyramid: A guide to daily food choices*. Washington, D.C.: DOA.)

PHYSICAL ACTIVITY
30 min – most days
60 min – to prevent weight gain
60-90 min – to sustain weight loss

| GRAINS | VEGETABLES | FRUITS | MILK | MEAT & BEANS | OILS |
| at least half should be whole grain | fresh, frozen, canned, dried | fresh, frozen, canned, dried | no or low fat, calcium rich | lean | |

unrewarding endeavor as results can occur slowly. Begin by emphasizing the physiologic basis for nutritional needs in pregnancy (a woman is building a whole new person). Based on this, explain what nutritional deficits you have found, and then show the pregnant woman how to change her nutritional patterns to improve this situation. Pregnant women are usually highly motivated to adopt healthy behaviors for the sake of their baby's health, although they still need support and encouragement because this can involve a major life change, such as eating a different lunch than everyone around them is eating; getting up 15 minutes earlier in the morning to prepare breakfast rather than just dashing to work with only coffee; or resisting having a soft drink with dinner and drinking orange juice or milk instead. Asking women to list what foods they eat daily and to bring in the chart to show you at a health maintenance visit is an effective motivating technique for many people. In research studies, this is called a **Hawthorne effect,** in which people who are being watched do better than those who are not. With this system, the average woman will eat better than she usually does so her list looks better when she presents it. As soon as she realizes that these better eating patterns are making her feel better, it is hoped she will continue them indefinitely.

Be careful with issuing general statements such as, "Eat high-protein foods." Food in the supermarket is not labeled "high-protein." Instead, provide advice in more specific terms: "Eat three servings of some type of meat or fish every day."

The word "diet" has come to mean a form of unpleasant food denial. Rather than a "pregnancy diet," therefore, it is better to talk about "foods that are best for you during pregnancy" or "pregnancy nutrition." These statements are more positive and refer more closely to what you are encouraging a woman to do. Giving a woman a clearly written list of suggested foods may help. Be sure the list is short, clear, and specific. Complicated lists of foods or a list of don'ts can be overwhelming and, therefore, will be ignored.

● **Outcome Evaluation**

When evaluating whether your client's nutritional pattern has been improved, rely on the most important assessments: weight, energy level, general appearance, bowel function, and, when available, hemoglobin and urinalysis findings. Urge women to be honest about whether they are actually following the nutrition plan. If they are not, it probably means that more planning is needed, because the plan did not fit their lifestyle or degree of motivation. Examples of outcomes that would demonstrate improved nutrition are:

- Client plans weekly menus that include three main meals and two snacks per day.
- By next prenatal visit, client demonstrates knowledge of meat and non-meat sources of protein by providing menus of meals eaten in the last week that include fish, eggs, beans, or peanut butter.
- Client verbalizes correct information about calcium needs during pregnancy.
- Client states she is able to make up later in each day meals missed because of nausea.
- Client's food lists for 1 week include three sources of calcium per day.
- Client describes pattern she is using to increase fluid intake to six glasses daily.

Remember that people have some degree of "backsliding," especially at holidays and special events. To prevent this, help a woman make definite, concrete plans for an upcoming holiday or event. Also, be certain to comment on the things a woman is doing correctly. Positive reinforcement, a basic rule of teaching, enhances learning, self-esteem, and compliance.

RELATIONSHIP OF MATERNAL NUTRITION TO INFANT HEALTH

During pregnancy, a woman must eat adequately to supply enough nutrients to the fetus, so it can grow, as well as to support her own nutrition. Adequate protein intake is vital because so much is needed by a fetus. Adequate protein may also help prevent complications of pregnancy such as pregnancy-induced hypertension or preterm birth. Either deficiencies or overuse of vitamins may contribute to birth anomalies (Katz, 2003).

Recommended Weight Gain During Pregnancy

A weight gain of 11.2 to 15.9 kg (25 to 35 lb) is currently recommended as an average weight gain in pregnancy. If a woman is at high risk for nutritional deficits, a more precise estimation of adequate weight gain can be calculated. This is done by computing **body mass index** (BMI), the ratio of weight to height (Box 12.2; see also Appendix E). Women who are high or low in weight for their height (BMI below 18.5 or above 25) need to have expected outcomes for weight gain adjusted.

Weight gain in pregnancy occurs from both fetal growth and accumulation of maternal stores (Box 12.3) and occurs at approximately 0.4 kg (1 lb) per month during the first trimester and then 0.4 kg (1 lb) per week during the last two trimesters (a trimester pattern of 3-12-12). As a general rule, in the average woman, weight gain is considered excessive if it is more than 3 kg (6.6 lb) a month during the second and third trimesters; it is less than usual if it is under 1 kg (2.2 lb) per month during the second and third trimesters. Women can be assured that most of the weight gained with pregnancy will be lost afterward (Katz, 2003).

Women who are underweight coming into pregnancy should gain slightly more weight than the average woman (0.5 kg per month or week rather than 0.4, or 30 to 40 lb). An obese woman might be advised to gain less than average (0.3 kg or 15 lb). However, to ensure adequate fetal nutrition, advise women not to diet to lose weight during pregnancy. Weight gain will be higher for a multiple pregnancy than for a single pregnancy. You can encourage women pregnant with multiple fetuses to gain at least 1 lb per week

---

BOX 12.2

Calculating Body Mass Index

To calculate body mass index (BMI):

1. Convert weight into kilograms (divide weight in pounds by 2.2).
2. Convert height into centimeters (multiply height in inches by 2.5).
3. Convert centimeters into meters (divide result by 100).
4. Square height in meters.
5. Divide weight in kilograms by height in meters squared.

For example: Mrs. Alarino is 5′6″ tall and weighs 150 lbs. To determine her BMI:

1. Convert weight into kilograms: 150 lb ÷ 2.2 = 68 kg.
2. Convert height into centimeters: 5′6″ = 66″
   ($5 \times 12 = 60 + 6 = 66$ inches)
   $66 \times 2.5 = 165$ cm
   $165 \div 100 = 1.65$ m
3. Square height in meters ($1.65 \times 1.65 = 2.72$).
4. Divide weight (kg) by m^2 ($68 \div 2.72 = 25$ BMI).

Normal Prepregnancy BMI

Underweight	Under 18.5
Normal weight	18.5–24.9
Overweight	25.0–29.9
Obese	Above 30.0

With a BMI of 25, Mrs. Alarino enters pregnancy slightly overweight.

Department of Health & Human Resources. (2005). *BMI: body mass index.* Hyattsville, MD: DHHS.

BOX 12.3 ASSESSMENT

Assessing Maternal Weight Gain

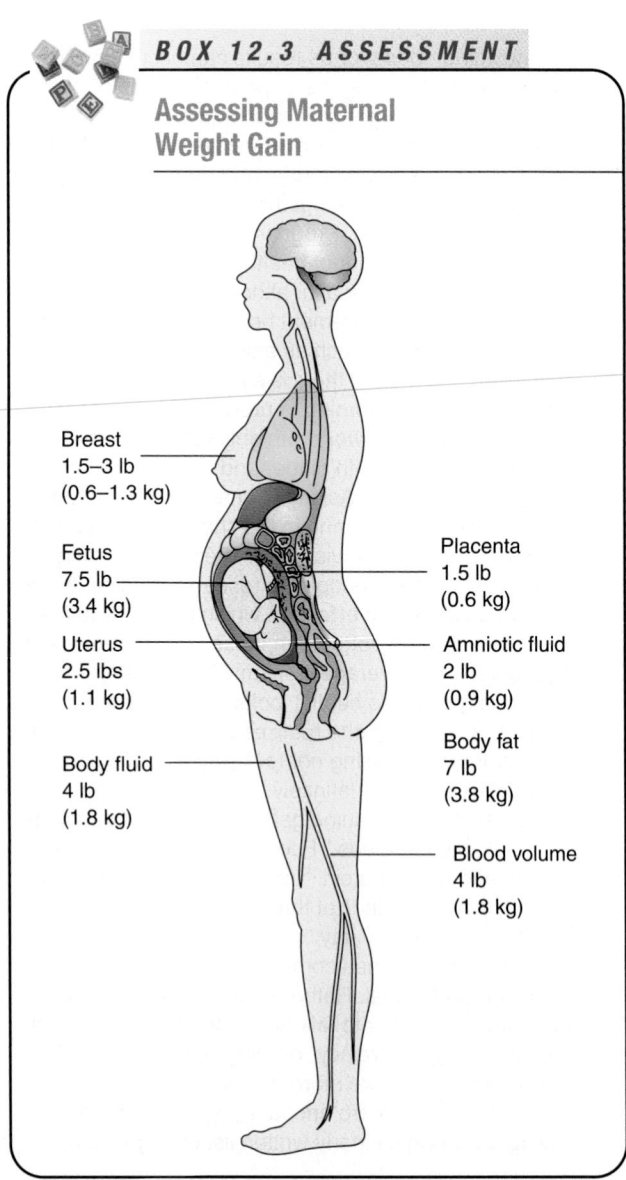

Breast
1.5–3 lb
(0.6–1.3 kg)

Fetus
7.5 lb
(3.4 kg)

Uterus
2.5 lbs
(1.1 kg)

Body fluid
4 lb
(1.8 kg)

Placenta
1.5 lb
(0.6 kg)

Amniotic fluid
2 lb
(0.9 kg)

Body fat
7 lb
(3.8 kg)

Blood volume
4 lb
(1.8 kg)

for a total of 40 to 45 lb (Dudek, 2004). Sudden increases in weight that suggest fluid retention or polyhydramnios (excessive amniotic fluid) or a loss of weight that suggests illness should be carefully evaluated at prenatal visits.

Components of Healthy Nutrition for the Pregnant Woman

The old saying that a pregnant woman must "eat for two" is not a myth; it is a scientific fact. However, this does not mean that a woman needs to eat enough for two adults, just enough to provide nutrients for the growing fetus. To do this, many women will not have to increase by much the quantity of food eaten, but they will have to increase the quality of their intake.

The dietary reference intake (DRI) values for girls and women and the requirements during pregnancy are shown in Table 12.1. Foods eaten should also represent the food groups in a food pyramid (see Fig. 12.1). When discussing nutrition, refer to servings of food rather than milligrams or percentages, because this is how women measure amounts.

Calorie Needs

The DRI of calories for women of childbearing age is 2,200. An additional 300 calories, or a total caloric intake of 2,500 calories, is recommended to meet the increased needs of pregnancy. In addition to supplying energy for a fetus and placenta, this increase provides calories to sustain an elevated metabolic rate from increased thyroid function and an increased workload from the extra weight a woman must carry. An inadequate intake of carbohydrates may lead to protein breakdown for energy, depriving a fetus of essential protein, and possibly resulting in ketoacidosis, a possible cause of fetal and neurologic disorders. Don't recommend sugar substitutes, because a woman needs sugar to maintain glucose levels. Even obese women should never consume fewer than 1,500 calories per day.

When helping a woman plan an increased caloric intake, consider her lifestyle. For example, many women commonly skip meals, have erratic eating patterns, or rely on fast and convenience foods. For pregnancy, help a woman plan to add calories by eating foods rich in protein, iron, and other essential nutrients rather than eating more fast-food, empty-calorie foods such as pretzels and doughnuts. Suggest preparing snacks such as carrot sticks or cheese and crackers early in the day when fatigue is usually less, keeping them readily available in the refrigerator. Otherwise, later in the day when she is tired, a woman may snack on empty-calorie foods simply because they require no preparation.

The easiest method for determining if a woman's caloric intake is adequate is assessing the weight she is gaining. Keep in mind that the weight gain pattern is as important as the total weight gain. Even if a woman has surpassed her target weight before the end of the third trimester,

TABLE 12.1

Dietary Reference Intakes for Pregnant and Nonpregnant Women

	Nonpregnant Women			
	Age 11–14	*Age 15–18*	*Age 19–30*	**Pregnant Women**
Calories (kcal)	2,200	2,200	2,200	2,500
Protein (g)	46	44	50	60
Fat-Soluble Vitamins				
Vitamin A (µg)	800	800	800	800
Vitamin D (µg)	10	10	5	5
Vitamin E (mg)	8	8	15	15
Water-Soluble Vitamins				
Ascorbic acid (mg) Vitamin C	50	60	75	85
Folic acid (µg)	150	180	400	600
Niacin (mg)	15	15	14	17
Riboflavin (mg)	1.3	1.3	1.3	1.6
Thiamine (mg) (B_1)	1.1	1.1	1.1	1.4
Vitamin B_{12} (µg)	2.0	2.0	2.4	2.6
Vitamin B_6 (mg)	1.4	1.5	1.3	2.0
Vitamin D (µg)	5	5	5	5
Minerals				
Calcium (mg)	1,200	1,200	1,200	1,200
Phosphorus (mg)	1,200	1,200	700	700
Iodine (µg)	150	150	150	175
Iron (mg)	15	15	15	30
Magnesium (mg)	280	300	310	350
Zinc (mg)	12	12	12	15
Fluoride (mg)	2	3	3	3

Institute of Medicine (2004). *Summary tables: dietary reference intakes.* Washington, DC: IOM.

encourage her not to restrict her caloric intake. She should continue to gain weight because a fetus is growing rapidly during these final weeks.

Protein Needs

The DRI for protein in women is 44 to 50 g. During pregnancy, the need for protein increases to 60 g daily. If protein needs are met, overall nutritional needs are likely to be met as well (with the possible exceptions of vitamin C, A, and D) because of the high incorporation of other nutrients with protein foods. If protein intake is inadequate, iron, B vitamins, calcium, and phosphorus also will probably be inadequate. Vitamin B_{12} is found almost exclusively in animal protein, so if animal protein is excluded from the diet, a vitamin B_{12} deficiency can occur unless this is supplemented.

Extra protein is best supplied by meat, poultry, fish, yogurt, eggs, and milk, because the protein in these forms contains all nine essential amino acids, or is **complete protein.** The protein in non-animal sources does not contain all essential amino acids (and so is **incomplete protein**). It is possible to provide all amino acids by combining non-animal proteins. Proteins that when cooked together provide all essential amino acids are termed complementary proteins. Examples are beans and rice, legumes and rice, or beans and wheat.

A woman with a family history of high cholesterol levels (**hypercholesterolemia**) probably should not eat more than two or three eggs per week because of the high cholesterol content of eggs. Encourage such women to eat lean meat, to cook with olive oil instead of lard or butter, and to remove the skin from poultry to reduce its fat content. She also should not eat lunch meats such as bologna or salami as food staples, because their protein content may not be high and their fat content is invariably exceptionally high.

Milk is a rich source of protein. Unfortunately, some women resist drinking it because it can be high in calories as well as fat. Others cannot drink it because of lactose intolerance. Some women find it difficult to drink a quart of milk a day because they simply do not like its taste. Nonfat milk supplies the same protein and half the calories as regular milk and is very low in fat. Buttermilk can be substituted, although it contains a large amount of sodium, or chocolate or another flavoring can be added to make milk palatable. Yogurt or cheese may also be substituted for milk, or milk may be incorporated into custards, eggnogs, or cream soups. Women who are lactose intolerant can add a lactase supplement purchased over the counter, which predigests milk and makes it palatable, or take a calcium supplement.

Checkpoint Question 1

Suppose Tori Alarino has a normal BMI. What would be the recommended weight gain for her during pregnancy?

a. 10 lbs.
b. 20 lbs.
c. 30 lbs.
d. 60 lbs.

Fat Needs

Only linoleic acid, an essential fatty acid necessary for new cell growth, cannot be manufactured in the body from other sources. Because linoleic acid must be obtained from food, women must be sure to consume a source of this nutrient during pregnancy. Vegetable oils are a good source. In addition, using vegetable oils (e.g., safflower, corn, olive, peanut, and cottonseed) that have a low cholesterol content rather than animal oils (butter) is recommended for all adults as a means of preventing hypercholesterolemia and coronary heart disease.

Vitamin Needs

The intake of vitamins as a daily dietary supplement has become so common that their importance may be underestimated by some women. Requirements for both fat-soluble and water-soluble vitamins increase during pregnancy to support the growth of new fetal cells (see Table 12.1). Vitamin deficiency can result in several problems. For example, vitamin D, essential for calcium absorption, when lacking can begin to diminish both fetal and maternal mineral bone density.

Although vitamin needs do increase during pregnancy, most of the vitamin intake requirements (with the exception of folic acid) can be met by eating a healthy, varied diet with plenty of fruits and vegetables. Women who were taking oral contraceptives before they became pregnant should be certain to include good sources of vitamins A and B and folic acid in early pregnancy because oral contraceptives may deplete stores of these vitamins. Counsel women not to use mineral oil as a laxative because it can prevent absorption of fat-soluble vitamins from the gastrointestinal tract, limiting their availability to the body.

Commonly, a specially designed multivitamin supplement is prescribed during pregnancy (Box 12.4). Caution women to avoid taking megadoses of vitamins. The mechanism of placental transfer of water-soluble vitamins makes fetal blood levels regularly higher than maternal blood levels, so a maternal overdosage can cause fetal toxicity. Megadoses of vitamin C may cause withdrawal scurvy in the infant at birth. The fat-soluble vitamins are stored in the body rather than excreted and so can reach toxic levels. There may be an association between excessive vitamin A intake and fetal malformation. It is well documented that the intake of excessive vitamin A in the form of isotretinoin (Accutane), a medication prescribed for acne, causes congenital anomalies (Karch, 2004).

When cautioning women about vitamin use, advise them not to leave prenatal vitamins within reach of small children. The excessive folic acid and iron in them can cause poisoning in small children.

Although folic acid (folacin) belongs to the B-vitamin group, its importance during pregnancy warrants a separate discussion. Found predominately in fresh fruits and vegetables, folic acid is necessary for red blood cell formation. As a woman's blood volume doubles during pregnancy, this makes her folic acid needs increase substantially. Without adequate folic acid, a megaloblastic anemia (large but ineffective red blood cells) may develop. If a woman

BOX 12.4 FOCUS ON . . .

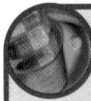

PHARMACOLOGY

Prenatal Vitamins (Natalins)

Action: Supplements nutrition to ensure adequate intake of vitamins and minerals during pregnancy. The folic acid content helps prevent megaloblastic anemia in the mother and neural tube defects in the fetus (Karch, 2004).

Ingredients: Vitamin A (4,000 U), vitamin D (400 U), vitamin E (15 U), vitamin C (80 mg), vitamin B_1 (1.5 mg), vitamin B_2 (2.0 mg), vitamin B_6 (4 mg), vitamin B_{12} (2.5 μg), niacin (17 mg), folic acid (1.0 mg), pantothenic acid (7 mg), calcium (200 mg), iron (54 mg), copper (3 mg), zinc (25 mg), and magnesium (100 mg)

Dosage: One tablet daily

Possible Adverse Effects: None known. Folic acid may mask the signs of pernicious anemia.

Nursing Implications

- Encourage women to take the medication exactly as prescribed; caution women not to exceed the recommended dosage.
- Assist with ways to remind women to take the medication, such as a note on the refrigerator.
- Advise women to keep vitamins, like all medications, out of the reach of small children to prevent accidental poisoning.

has this blood pattern at the time of birth, the infant may be affected as well.

For these reasons, as well as its importance in preventing neural tube defects, women should eat foods high in folic acid such as vegetables and fruit and should take a prenatal vitamin that contains a folic acid supplement of 0.4 to 1.0 mg (Dudek, 2004).

Mineral Needs

Minerals are necessary for new cell building in a fetus. Because they are found in so many foods and because mineral absorption improves during pregnancy, mineral deficiency, with the exceptions of calcium, iodine, and iron, is rare.

Calcium and Phosphorus. The skeleton and teeth constitute a major portion of a fetus. Tooth formation begins as early as 8 weeks in utero. Bones begin to calcify at 12 weeks. To supply adequate calcium and phosphorus for bone formation, pregnant women need to eat foods high in calcium and vitamin D (necessary for calcium to be absorbed from the gastrointestinal tract and to enter bones). The recommended amount of calcium during pregnancy is 1,200 to 1,500 mg. If a woman cannot drink milk or eat milk products such as cheese, she can be prescribed a daily calcium supplement. Most foods high in protein are also high in phosphorus, so by eating high-protein foods,

women receive enough phosphorus, also important for bone growth.

Before nutrition counseling in pregnancy became common, women expected to lose "a tooth a child"—that is, they believed a fetus, as he or she grew, would drain calcium from their teeth. Although it is unlikely that a woman will lose a tooth with pregnancy today, the concern reflected in this myth about a fetus taking calcium from the mother is well founded. However, the calcium in teeth is not as readily absorbed as that of bone. It is more likely that inadequate calcium intake will result in diminished maternal bone density rather than weakened teeth. With an adequate calcium intake during pregnancy, a fetus will receive the needed calcium for growth and mineralization of the fetal skeleton without taking any away from the maternal bones or teeth.

Iodine. Iodine is essential for the formation of thyroxine and, therefore, for the proper functioning of the thyroid gland. As thyroid function increases during pregnancy, a woman needs to ingest enough iodine during pregnancy to supply this increased need. If iodine deficiency occurs, it can cause thyroid enlargement (goiter) in a woman. In extreme instances, it may cause hypothyroidism in a fetus. Thyroid enlargement in a fetus at birth is serious because the increased pressure of the enlarged gland on the airway could lead to early respiratory distress. If not discovered at birth, hypothyroidism may lead to the infant's being cognitively challenged. The DRI for iodine is 175 μg daily during pregnancy. Seafood is the best source.

In areas where the water and soil are known to be deficient in iodine, it is suggested that women use iodized salt and include a serving of seafood in their diet at least once a week.

Iron. A fetus at term has a hemoglobin level of 17 to 21 g per 100 mL of blood, a level that is necessary to oxygenate the blood during intrauterine life. Iron is needed to build this high level of hemoglobin. In addition, after week 20 of pregnancy, a fetus begins to store iron in the liver to last through the first 3 months of life, when intake will consist mainly of milk, typically low in iron. In addition to supplying these high fetal needs, a woman needs iron to build an increased red cell volume for herself and to protect against iron lost in blood at delivery (Cogswell et al., 2003).

The DRI for iron for pregnant women is 30 mg. An average diet supplies about 6 mg iron per 1,000 calories. If a woman eats a 2,500-calorie diet daily, her daily intake, therefore, is about 15 mg iron. Because only 10% to 20% of dietary iron is absorbed, she is actually taking in less than this amount (closer to 1.5 mg to 3 mg). Therefore, dietary supplementation with 15 mg iron per day helps ensure that adequate iron is ingested and absorbed. Stress to women that iron supplementation is intended as a supplement to, not a replacement for, iron-rich foods.

Women with low incomes may find it difficult to eat adequate iron-rich foods, because the foods richest in iron (e.g., organ meats; eggs; green, leafy vegetables; whole grain; enriched breads; dried fruits) are also expensive. Iron absorption increases in an acid environment, so eating iron-rich foods or swallowing iron pills with orange juice may increase absorption. Oral iron compounds can be irritating to the stomach, turn stools black, and cause constipation in some women. If this happens, urge women not to stop taking the iron compound but always take the iron pills with food and increase fluid intake or fiber to relieve the constipation. Some women may need a prescribed stool softener such as docusate sodium (Colace); this stool softener is not associated with teratogenic action, so it can be taken safely during pregnancy.

Fluoride. Because fluoride aids in the formation of sound teeth, a pregnant woman should drink fluoridated water. In an area where the water is not fluoridated either naturally or artificially, supplemental fluoride may be recommended. Fluoride in large amounts causes brown-stained teeth, so a woman should not take the supplement more often than prescribed or if tap water in her area is already fluoridated. Many women, worried about added chemicals in their city water supply, switch to bottled water during pregnancy. If they do this, advise them to buy a fluoridated type or alert their health care providers that they may need supplements.

Sodium. Sodium is the major electrolyte that acts to maintain fluid in the body: when sodium is retained rather than excreted by the kidneys, an equal or balancing amount of fluid is also retained. Retaining enough fluid during pregnancy in the maternal circulation is important to ensure a pressure gradient to allow optimal exchange of nutrients across the placenta.

Unless a woman is hypertensive or has heart disease with required sodium restriction when she enters pregnancy, she should continue to salt foods as usual during pregnancy. However, she should use moderation with foods that are extremely salty, such as lunch meats or potato chips, or with the additive monosodium glutamate. Too much salt could result in retention of excessive amounts of fluid, putting a strain on her heart as blood volume doubles.

Zinc. Zinc is necessary for the synthesis of DNA and RNA. Although not proven, zinc deficiency may be associated with preterm birth. The DRI for zinc during pregnancy is 15 mg, or an increase of 3 mg over prepregnancy needs. Most people who take in adequate protein also take in adequate zinc because zinc is contained in foods such as meat, liver, eggs, and seafood. It is also a component of prenatal vitamins to help ensure an adequate intake (Dudek, 2004).

Fluid Needs

Extra amounts of water are needed during pregnancy to promote kidney function because a woman must excrete waste products for two. Two glasses of fluid daily over and above a daily quart of milk is a common recommendation (a total of six glasses).

Fiber Needs

Constipation can occur during pregnancy from slowed peristalsis due to the pressure of the uterus on the intestine. Eating fiber-rich foods, foods consisting of parts of the plant cell wall resistant to normal digestive enzymes of the small intestine, such as broccoli and asparagus, are a natural way of preventing constipation, because the bulk of the fiber left in the intestine aids evacuation. Fiber also has the advantage of lowering cholesterol levels and may remove carcinogenic contaminants from the intestine. Encourage women to eat plenty of fresh fruits and vegetables, especially green, leafy vegetables, to provide fiber. Eating fiber-rich foods this way is a better choice for preventing constipation than taking a fiber laxative. Doing so allows a woman to receive nutrients from the food as well as preventing constipation.

Foods to Avoid in Pregnancy

As discussed in Chapter 11, alcoholic beverages should not be ingested by a pregnant woman because of their potentially teratogenic effects on a fetus. Other foods to be avoided are those that contain food additives, because the effect of many of these is unknown.

Foods With Caffeine

Caffeine is thought of by many women as just an incidental ingredient in beverages. Actually, it is a central nervous system stimulant capable of increasing heart rate, urine production in the kidney, and secretion of acid in the stomach (Dudek, 2004).

A daily intake of caffeine of two or three cups of coffee has not been associated with low birthweight, but drinking over eight cups is associated with an increased rate of stillbirth (Wisborg et al., 2003). To limit their caffeine intake, women may need to limit not only the amount of coffee they drink but also other sources of caffeine such as chocolate, soft drinks, and tea. If a woman has difficulty omitting these common foods from her diet, she can still reduce the amount of caffeine she ingests by modifying their preparation. For example, instant coffee has less caffeine than brewed coffee; percolated coffee has less caffeine than dripped coffee. Decaffeinated coffee, as the name implies, contains almost no caffeine.

Tea, like coffee, varies in caffeine content depending on the type and time of brewing. The longer tea brews, the greater the caffeine content. Green tea has less caffeine than black tea. Both herbal teas and decaffeinated tea are available.

The cocoa bean that is used to make chocolate and cocoa is yet another natural source of caffeine. Chocolate sources tend to be low in caffeine, however, when compared with coffee. A cup of coffee contains approximately 120 mg of caffeine, whereas a cup of hot chocolate contains only 10 mg. Baking chocolate, used for cake frostings and glazes, is proportionately higher, containing about 35 mg of caffeine per ounce.

Soft drinks do not naturally contain caffeine; it is added to improve their appeal. To limit the amount of caffeine consumed, encourage pregnant women to choose caffeine-free types.

Artificial Sweeteners

Artificial sweeteners are used to improve the taste and limit the caloric content of foods. Federal regulations control the addition of these ingredients, but it is probably safest for pregnant women to reduce their intake. For instance, although the sweetener aspartame has been approved by the FDA for consumption and is apparently safe during pregnancy, large amounts of the compound should be avoided by pregnant women until its safety is thoroughly confirmed. The use of saccharine is not recommended during pregnancy because it is eliminated slowly from the fetal bloodstream. In any event, pregnant women need carbohydrates furnished by sugar rather than artificial substances (Dudek, 2004).

 What if... Tori Alarino states, "I love coffee. There's always a pot brewing at my office. And I love a cup of cappuccino for lunch." What suggestions could you make to help her reduce her caffeine intake?

Weight Loss Diets

As a rule, reducing diets and calorie restrictions are contraindicated during pregnancy because they may lead to fetal ketoacidosis and poor growth. If women have been following such diets before becoming pregnant, they may have few nutritional stores, and additional vitamin supplementation may be necessary.

✔ **Checkpoint Question 2**

Which statement by Tori lets you know she understands how iron is best absorbed?

a. I always take my iron pills with milk.
b. I take iron pills mixed with mashed potatoes.
c. I take the pills with ice cream to disguise their taste.
d. I swallow my iron pills with orange juice.

ASSESSMENT OF NUTRITIONAL HEALTH

The best method for assessing nutritional intake is to ask for a "typical day" history or a 24-hour nutrition recall to isolate usual patterns and possible nutritional risk factors (Table 12.2). First, ask if yesterday was a typical day. If it was, then ask a woman to list all the food she ate within the past 24 hours, starting with when she awakened until she went to sleep. Be certain she includes all the snack foods she ate, as well as sit-down meals. This method of history taking yields much more accurate information about actual intake than if a woman is asked how often during the week she eats citrus fruit, or how much milk she drinks every day. A woman who knows how much milk she ought to drink a day will probably say she drinks a quart a day during pregnancy. However, if asked to list the foods she ate the day before, she may report that she drank only one glass of milk all day.

After obtaining the day's list of food, compare the types and amounts on the list with those shown in Figure 12.1 to see if all food groups and adequate amounts are included. Comparing foods from the person's 24-hour recall with a guide is a helpful way to show clients that what they thought was a "perfect" intake is imperfect, or what they thought was a "little" problem actually involves the loss of an entire food group. Once a woman sees that a deficit exists, she may be more motivated to improve her nutrition. Such a picture also offers an instant reward for a woman who is ingesting adequate foods.

In addition to actual food intake, ask a woman if she thinks she has any problem with nutrition (such as cravings). Also, assess the circumstances of eating, such as cultural preferences, who prepares food in the family, and how many meals are eaten outside the home weekly (Table 12.3).

To strengthen history findings, assess a woman's prepregnancy weight and calculate her BMI. People with

---

TABLE 12.2

Nutritional Risk Factors During Pregnancy

Risk	Rationale
Adolescent (less than 18 years old at LMP)	An adolescent has increased nutritional needs.
Short intervals between pregnancies	The woman's body has not had time to replace nutritional stores depleted during previous pregnancy(ies).
Low income	Family may not have resources to purchase adequate foods to meet pregnancy nutritional needs.
Follows food fads	Foods eaten may not be those adequate for pregnancy.
Drug use (including cigarettes and alcohol)	Drugs may be ingested in preference to healthy foods.
Existence of a chronic illness requiring a special diet	Intake may be low in an essential substance such as carbohydrate or protein.
Underweight or overweight	Underweight and overweight status may indicate chronic inadequate dietary patterns.
Multiple pregnancy	The woman must supply enough nutrition for multiple fetal development.
Anemic at conception	The woman has no iron stores for fetal growth.
Lactose intolerance	The woman may not be ingesting adequate calcium for fetal skeletal growth.

TABLE 12.3

Areas to Be Assessed for a Total Nutrition History

Area of Assessment	Pertinent Questions
Food preparation	Who does the cooking? How many people does the woman cook for? How are foods usually prepared (fried or baked)? What spices or condiments are commonly used? What type oil is used for frying (saturated or unsaturated)?
Food pattern	How many meals are eaten a day? Which is the biggest meal? What types of food are eaten? How many snacks are eaten a day? What are they? How many meals are eaten outside the home? Where are they eaten? Cafeteria? Fast-food store? Restaurant? Bagged lunch? Any foods that she cannot or will not eat? Why?
Financial concerns	Is there enough money for food? Who does the shopping? Would the woman eat differently if more money were available? Is any supplementary financial program used?
Activity level	Is she normally active or sedentary? (Could increase calorie need.)
Health	Does she know of any allergies to food? Does she have any trouble with chewing or digestion? What is bowel movement frequency? Was she taking oral contraceptives before pregnancy? Does she take supplemental vitamins? What type? How many? Does she drink alcohol? What type? How much? Does she smoke cigarettes? What is her stress level? Does stress affect her appetite?
Personal food preferences	Are there any foods she particularly enjoys or dislikes? Are there any foods she feels are harmful or particularly beneficial to her? Are there any cultural or religious preferences?
Family dietary patterns	Does anyone in the family eat a special diet? Is anyone obviously overweight or underweight? Does the family eat meals together? Is mealtime a social time?

poor nutrition are typically over- or underweight and show typical physical signs. Table 12.4 lists important physical examination assessments that suggest a good nutritional intake or evidence of poor nutrition.

Hemoglobin or hematocrit determinations (see Appendix F) are also important assessments of good nutrition. These may reveal smoking habits, as cigarette smokers have higher HgB levels than nonsmokers. These values are measured early in pregnancy and then usually repeated close to term and again at birth. A urinalysis can also be important because a finding such as elevated urine specific gravity could suggest a less-than-adequate fluid intake, and elevated urine glucose levels suggest gestational diabetes (see Chapter 14).

PROMOTING NUTRITIONAL HEALTH DURING PREGNANCY

Setting Nutritional Outcomes

Be certain that plans for improving nutritional patterns take into account a woman's lifestyle, family preferences, finan-

cial resources, customs, and cultural desires, because she and her family must follow them for 9 months (Fig. 12.2; Box 12.5).

Family Considerations

Meal planning is best if it involves the entire family because even if a woman is receptive to changing her eating habits, she may have difficulty carrying out recommendations if her family resists the change. In families where a member has a special nutritional need, such as restricted sodium, change may be even more difficult. You may need to speak with the person who prepares meals for an adolescent as well as the adolescent to be sure recommended changes will be carried out.

Financial Considerations

Food is costly, so to provide the extra servings required during pregnancy, a woman must spend more on food for herself per week than she is used to spending. Women generally view this increased expense as an investment in

TABLE 12.4

Physical Signs and Symptoms of Adequate Pregnancy Nutrition

Assessment Area	Signs of Good Nutrition	Signs of Poor Nutrition
Hair	Shiny; strong with good body	Hair dull and lifeless (possible protein deficit)
Eyes	Good eyesight, particularly at night; conjunctiva moist and pink	Pale and dry conjunctiva (iron & fluid deficit); difficulty with night vision (vitamin A deficit)
Mouth	No cavities in teeth; no swollen or inflamed gingiva; no cracks or fissures at corners of mouth; mucous membrane moist and pink; tongue smooth and nontender	Fissures at corners of mouth; tongue rough and tender (vitamin A deficit); mucous membrane pale (iron deficit)
Neck	Normal contour of thyroid gland	Thyroid gland enlarged (iodine deficit)
Skin	Smooth, with normal color and turgor; no ecchymotic or petechial areas present	Rough texture; poor turgor (fluid deficit)
Extremities	Normal muscle mass and circumference; normal strength and mobility; edema limited to slight ankle involvement; normal reflexes	Poor muscle tone; diminished reflexes (protein deficit)
Finger- and toenails	Smooth; pink; normal contour	Pale; break easily; little growth (protein deficit)
Weight	Within normal limits of ideal weight before pregnancy; following normal pattern of pregnancy weight gain	Over- or underweight; unusually slow or rapid weight gain (inadequate or excessive carbohydrate).
Blood pressure	Within normal limits for length of pregnancy	Decreased from anemia (iron deficit); increased from hypertension

their child's health and do not regard it as a burden. However, a woman on a marginal income, although she may be willing to shoulder the additional cost, may have trouble actually doing so. If this occurs, review what foods the woman is eating to be certain she is not buying only starchy foods because they are more filling and less expensive than protein foods. Help her secure available financial assistance such as food stamps, or inform her about nutritional aid

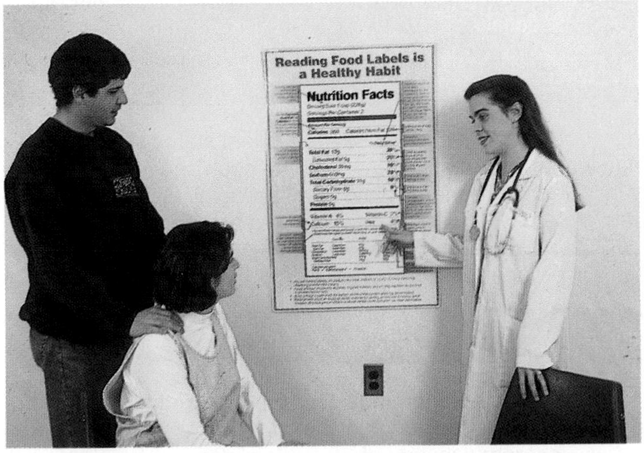

FIGURE 12.2 Encourage pregnant women and their partners to eat a varied diet with a high iron and protein content. This may be difficult for a woman early in pregnancy because of nausea, late in pregnancy because of fatigue. (© Barbara Proud.)

programs such as the Women, Infants and Children Special Supplemental Food Program (WIC).

Under the food stamp program, a family with a low income can buy stamps that can be redeemed at grocery stores for any food items except alcohol or pet food. The cost of stamps varies, but the use of food stamps can increase a family's buying power as much as $150 a month.

The advantage of this type of program is that it helps to supplement the cost of food but places almost no restrictions on what foods can be selected and purchased. It can make the difference for a low-income family between being able to eat meat or living on a starchy diet. Rules concerning eligibility for these programs are changing because of new government restrictions that allow persons to remain on this type of assistance for a limited time only.

WIC is a federal program that provides nutritional support for low-income women and children to reduce not only the risk of low birthweight but also medical costs by preventing costly newborn care. Established in 1972, WIC is funded by the Food and Nutrition Service of the U.S. Department of Agriculture (*www.fns.usda.gov/wic*). The program supplies supplemental foods and nutrition education for:

- Pregnant women
- Postpartum women up to 6 months
- Nursing mothers up to 1 year
- Children from birth to age 5

Each state defines the income eligibility level for its citizens, but the eligibility for all programs is based on income level, geographic area, and nutritional risk. To receive food,

BOX 12.5: Focus on Nursing Care Planning

Multidisciplinary Care Map for a Pregnant Client with Inadequate Nutritional Pattern

●

Tori Alarino, 28, is 4 months pregnant and works at a fast-food restaurant during the day. She eats her breakfast and lunch at work. Her husband works four evenings a week, so she cooks for herself on those evenings. She dislikes milk, so she drinks milkshakes as a source of calcium. She is concerned because she has already gained 23 lb. She craves oranges, eating six to eight of them a day. She tells you, "I thought pregnant women always craved pickles and ice cream. What's wrong with me?"

Family Assessment

Client lives with husband in four-bedroom home; husband works as an electrician. Client's father (aged 58) lives with them since recent divorce.

Client Assessment

Primigravida; LMP 16 weeks ago. Height 5′6″. Prepregnancy weight: 110 lb (10 lb under desirable weight for height); BMI 17.8.

Weight today: 133 lb. History of weight problem during adolescence; currently controls weight by eating only one main meal per day. 24-hour dietary recall: Breakfast—1 cup coffee with 2 Danish pastries; lunch—1 milkshake; dinner—1 hamburger with French fries, 1 milkshake; snacks—8-ounce soft drink, 1 serving fried chicken pieces.

Nursing Diagnosis

Imbalanced nutrition, less than body requirements, related to desire to control weight

Outcome Criteria

Client reports increased intake of foods adequate in calories, high in iron, calcium, and protein by next prenatal visit.

Demonstrates weight gain appropriate for stage of pregnancy and prepregnancy weight.

Team Member Responsible	Assessment	Intervention	Rationale	Expected Outcome
Activities of Daily Living				
Nurse	Assess if the fatigue client reports is interfering with adequate food preparation.	If fatigue is a problem, recommend preparing nutritious lunch early in day when less fatigued.	Fatigue can increase nausea/vomiting in early pregnancy; interfere with food preparation all through pregnancy.	Client states she is able to cook and realizes eating all fast foods may not be her best action.
Consultations				
Nurse/ physician/ women's health practitioner	Assess nutrition requirements based on client's BMI and individual preferences.	Consult with nutritionist about recommended caloric and mineral requirements.	Caloric recommendations may need to be increased in light of client's BMI and prepregnancy and current weight.	An ideal nutrition plan is created and presented to client.

(continued)

Team Member Responsible	Assessment	Intervention	Rationale	Expected Outcome
Procedures/Medications				
Nurse	Assess if client has experience with keeping a journal.	Instruct client to keep a journal recording all food and fluid intake for 1 week, and review with client on next visit.	Keeping a journal provides concrete evidence of client's adherence to nutritional plan.	Client brings log to next prenatal visit and reviews it with prenatal staff.
Nutrition				
Nutritionist	Assess the nutritional requirements based on client's BMI and individual choices.	Provide client with food suggestions. Provide written information as needed.	Assistance from a dietitian ensures a nutritionally sound diet with culturally acceptable food choices. Printed information enhances learning.	Client lists an "ideal" nutrition plan for healthy pregnancy nutrition.
Patient/Family Education				
Nurse/ nutritionist	Assess if client is aware of the importance of healthy nutrition for pregnancy.	Review healthy pregnancy nutrition with client.	Knowledgeable clients can best follow a nutritious meal plan.	Client lists foods she will include for healthy pregnancy nutrition.
Psychosocial/Spiritual/Emotional Needs				
Nurse	Question client about food likes and dislikes. Investigate any cultural influences on food choices.	Ask client to list foods in each food group that are her favorites and she enjoys cooking.	Ascertaining food preferences and cultural influences provides a baseline for future food selections and suggestions.	Client lists foods she prefers and knows she can eat consistently.
Discharge Planning				
Nurse	Assess best times for client to return for prenatal appointments based on work/family obligations.	Schedule a follow-up appointment in 1 week.	Changing nutritional habits and behaviors can be difficult. Scheduling close follow-up provides an opportunity for evaluation and instruction.	Client states she will return for follow-up nutritional counseling.

clients must live in an area that has been designated as a funding area. The nurse or nutritionist in the health care facility determines possible risk and nutritional need. Factors considered that put pregnant women at nutritional risk include age (adolescent or woman over 40); poor obstetric history such as previous spontaneous miscarriage, a short period between pregnancies, previous low-birthweight infant, or gestational diabetes; anemia; poor weight gain; or inadequate consumption of food by nutrition history.

For the pregnant woman, foods typically offered by the program include those with high-quality protein, iron, calcium, and vitamins A and C, such as fruit juice, eggs, milk, and cheese. At predetermined intervals, WIC clients are reevaluated to see if the program supplements are still necessary. WIC has been successful in improving nutrition

during pregnancy because it supplies additional food to recipients and also the periodic evaluations provide time for nutritional counseling (Bitler & Currie, 2005).

School lunch programs are yet another way that some pregnant adolescents can receive help with nutrition. Millions of schoolchildren qualify for free or reduced-price school lunches. A school lunch (type A) is designed to provide one third of a child's DRI. For many adolescents, these school lunches may be the most nutritious meal they eat in a day.

Cultural Considerations

When helping plan nutrition during pregnancy, try to suggest foods that are individually or culturally favored, as these are the foods women tend to enjoy and will eat most consistently. Common cultural differences to be aware of in nutritional counseling are shown in Box 12.6.

 Checkpoint Question 3

You need to obtain a nutrition history from Tori. What is the best way to do this?

a. Ask her to tell you how much protein she eats daily.
b. Assess if Tori feels satisfied or not with her nutrition.
c. Ask Tori to describe what she ate in the last 24 hours.
d. Tell Tori to describe her concept of ideal nutrition.

Managing Common Problems Affecting Nutritional Health

Specific nutrition problems may result during pregnancy from a number of factors or circumstances. Discomforts such as constipation and flatulence that can result from food choices, and possible solutions to these concerns, have already been discussed (see Chapter 11).

Nausea and Vomiting

As many as 50% of pregnant women report nausea and vomiting (Katz, 2003). No definite cause has been established for this symptom of early pregnancy, but it may be related to:

- Sensitivity to the high level of chorionic gonadotropin hormone produced by the trophoblast cells
- High estrogen or progesterone levels
- Lowered maternal blood sugar levels caused by the needs of the developing embryo
- Lack of pyridoxine (vitamin B$_6$)
- Diminished gastric motility

Nausea is aggravated by fatigue and may be aggravated by emotional disturbance.

Most women notice the sensation of nausea as early as the first missed menstrual period and experience it through the first 3 months of pregnancy. The sensation is usually most intense on arising but may occur while a woman is preparing meals or smelling food. Vomiting at least once a day is common. Women who work nights and sleep days often experience "evening sickness," because that is when they arise.

Methods such as acupressure, anti-motion sickness wrist bands, or avoiding fluid with meals are effective for some women. Increasing carbohydrate intake seems to relieve nausea better than any other nutrition remedy. The traditional solution is for women to keep dry crackers, such as saltines, by their bedside and eat a few before rising; sourball candies may serve the same purpose. A woman can then eat a light breakfast or delay breakfast until 10 or 11 AM, past the time her nausea seems to persist. To be certain she maintains a good food intake during pregnancy even in the face of nausea, she should compen-

sate for any missed meals later in the day. If preparing food for others makes her feel queasy, she might try to give these responsibilities to another family member, at least through the worst phase of this symptom. Preparing and freezing meals ahead of time, perhaps at night when the nausea is less bothersome, may also help.

It is a good rule for women not to go longer than 12 hours between meals during pregnancy to prevent hypoglycemia. A woman may need to eat a late-evening snack to compensate for a late breakfast. She may be able to tolerate fruit and raw vegetables during the morning before other food. Urge her to experiment with soups or vegetable drinks that she may not usually think of as breakfast foods but that will give her early-morning calories.

Caution women against self-medicating for nausea by taking antacids. Excessive use of antacids containing sodium bicarbonate may cause fluid retention because of the sodium content. Remember that a woman should not take any medication during pregnancy unless prescribed by her physician or nurse-midwife (Box 12.7).

Fortunately, nausea usually disappears spontaneously as a woman enters her fourth month of pregnancy. If it persists beyond this month or is so extreme in early pregnancy that it interferes with nutrition, it may indicate the development of hyperemesis gravidarum, a complication of pregnancy (see discussion later in this chapter).

Cravings

Cravings for food or aversions to certain foods during pregnancy are so common that they are considered a normal part of adaptation to pregnancy. It was formerly considered that these strange desires for food reflected a woman's need to call attention to the pregnancy or were a reaction to her imposed dependent state. However, cravings are actually more likely the result of a physiologic need for more carbohydrates or particular vitamins and minerals.

Now that recommended pregnancy nutrition allows for more calories and a greater pregnancy weight gain is encouraged, cravings are seen less often than before. When taking a nutritional history, ask if a woman notices any particular cravings. As long as this is a healthy type of food, help her plan a nutrition intake that includes the food, at least in moderation. This is a positive approach to nutrition counseling: it allows her to enjoy her pregnancy without feeling guilty because she is eating foods she craves.

During pregnancy, some women report an abnormal craving for nonfood substances (termed **pica** from the Latin for magpie, a bird that is an indiscriminate eater). The most common form of pica in the past was a craving for laundry starch. Today, women are more apt to report cravings for clay, dirt, cornstarch, or ice cubes (Kettaneh et al., 2005). Although some of these items can do no harm in themselves, the ingestion of large quantities can leave a woman deficient in protein, iron, and calcium, nutrients essential for a healthy pregnancy outcome (Box 12.8).

Always ask women at prenatal visits if they crave any nonfood items, as most women do not supply this information unless asked directly. They worry that you will find their behavior odd, or they may not realize their habit is pregnancy-related as much as being a nervous habit.

BOX 12.6 FOCUS ON . . .

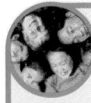

DIVERSITY OF CARE

Characteristics of Certain Ethnic Diets

Group and Place of Origin	Staple Foods	Comments
Hispanic Americans from Puerto Rico	Steamed white rice; many varieties of beans; wheat breads; starchy vegetables such as cassavas, yams, breadfruit, plantains, and green bananas; green peppers; tomatoes; garlic; dried, salted fish; salt pork, bacon; lard; olive oil; sugar; jams and jellies, sweet pastries; sugared fruit juices; cafe con leche (coffee and hot milk)	Milk is rarely consumed as a beverage. Most food is cooked for long periods of time or fried. Malt beer is believed to be nutritious and may be given to children and breast-feeding mothers.
Hispanic Americans from Mexico, Central America	Many varieties of beans; steamed rice; corn products such as tortillas made from lime-soaked cornmeal; chili peppers, tomatoes; mangoes; prickly pear fruit; potatoes; meat and sausages; fish; poultry; eggs; milk cheeses; milk custards and bread puddings; lard; sweet chocolate and coffee drinks; cakes, pastries	Most vegetables are cooked so long that they lose most of their nutritional value. Diet is high in fiber and starch. Animal fat is frequently added during food preparation. Because milk, green leafy vegetables, and fruit intakes are low, diet may be inadequate in calcium, iron, vitamin A, and vitamin C. Obesity is common.
Hispanic Americans from Cuba	Stews and casseroles flavored with sage, parsley, bay leaf, thyme, cinnamon, curry, capers, onion, cloves, garlic, saffron. Soup is served daily. Fried foods, especially fish, poultry, eggs; rice; many varieties of beans	Fruits and vegetables are not eaten on a regular basis. Main meal is usually served at lunch.
Southern African-Americans from West Africa (many generations in United States)	Hominy grits; biscuits; cornmeal and corn bread; rice; legumes; potatoes; onions; tomatoes; hot peppers; green leafy vegetables cooked in fatback or salt pork; okra; sweet potatoes; squashes; corn; cabbage; melons; peaches; pecans; all parts of a pig; fresh meats and poultry; fish; thick stews; butter, shortening, and lard; sugar; bread puddings; pies and sweets	African-American food patterns are similar to whites in same region. Northern African-Americans may be unfamiliar with "soul food." Frying is common; diet tends to be high in fat and salt, low in calcium. High rate of obesity.
Chinese Americans (diets vary sometimes with region)	Rice and rice gruel; wheat noodles; corn; green vegetables, especially from the cabbage family; squashes; cucumbers; eggplant; leafy vegetables; various shoots, including bamboo, mung, and soy; sweet potatoes; radishes; onions; peas and pods; mushrooms; roots; many local, seasonal vegetables; pickled vegetables; sea vegetables; plums; peaches; tangerines; kumquats and other citrus fruits; litchis; longans; mangoes; papayas; pomegranates; soybean products such as tofu (soybean curd), soy sauces, bean noodles, and soy milk; tiny portions of meat, fish with bones, or poultry; seafood; soup or tea as beverage; sugar as seasoning	Yin (feminine)–yang (masculine) concept of balancing intake; moderation is valued. Obesity is rare. Regional differences in food choices exist. Rice symbolizes life and fertility. Raw vegetables are rarely served. Diet is high in fiber and many nutrients, is low in fat, and may be low in protein.
Japanese Americans	Rice; vegetables; pickled vegetables; soy as miso (soup), tofu, bean paste, and soy sauce; fruits; salads; fish with bones; sugar as seasoning; sea vegetables; seafood; ginseng; green tea	Common preparation methods include broiling, steaming, boiling, and stir-frying. Meat portions are small. Milk is rarely used by adults. Diet is low in fat, rich in nutrients, high in sodium.

(continued)

BOX 12.6 FOCUS ON . . . (continued)

DIVERSITY OF CARE

Vietnamese Americans	Rice, rice noodles; French bread and croissants with butter; hot peppers; curries of asparagus and potatoes; salads; tropical fruits and vegetables; lemons and limes; small portions of poultry; eggs; fish pats; nuoc mam (a strong, fermented fish sauce added to almost every cooked dish); sweets, candies, sweetened drinks; coffee; tea	Rice may be eaten at every meal. Fresh milk is not readily available; lactose intolerance is common. Little fat is used in preparation. Diet may be low in iron and calcium.
Native Americans	Southeast: corn; cornmeal; coontie (flour from a palmlike plant); fried breads; swamp cabbage (now illegal to harvest); pumpkins; squashes; papayas; alligator, snake, wild hog, duck, fish, and shellfish. Northeast: blueberries; cranberries; beans; corn; pumpkins; fish; lobster; wild game; maple syrup. Midwest: bison; beans; corn; melons; squashes; tomatoes. Southwest: corn (many colors and varieties); beans; squash; pumpkins; chili peppers; melons; pinenuts; cactus. Northwest: salmon; caviar; other fish; otter; seal; whale; bear; elk; other game; wild fruits; acorns (and other wild nuts); wild greens	Food has great religious and social significance. Corn is a status food for most tribes. Milk is seldom used; calcium intake is usually low. Diets on some reservations are considered poor. High rate of obesity.

Dudek, S. (2004). *Nutrition handbook for nursing practice* (4th ed.). Philadelphia: Lippincott Williams & Wilkins.

BOX 12.7 FOCUS ON . . .

FAMILY TEACHING

Measures to Reduce and Evaluate Nausea During Pregnancy

Q. Tori Alarino tells you, "I've been nauseated ever since I became pregnant. What can I take to make this better?"

A. If nausea and vomiting are causing a fluid imbalance, medications can be prescribed. Common nonpharmacologic measures you can take to reduce nausea are:

- Be aware that at least 50% of women experience nausea during pregnancy, so what you are experiencing is normal.
- Eat a few dry crackers, toast, or a sourball before you get out of bed in the morning to increase your carbohydrate intake.
- Eat small but frequent meals rather than large infrequent ones.
- Avoid greasy or highly seasoned food.
- Delay breakfast until nausea passes (dinner if it is evening nausea).
- Make up missed meals at some other time of the day to maintain nutrition.
- Avoid sudden movements and fatigue because these may increase or cause nausea.

- Eat a snack before bedtime so delaying breakfast won't cause you to go a long time between meals.
- Purchase a wrist acupressure band (purchased in travel stores for motion sickness).

If nausea is present:
- Try sipping a carbonated beverage, water, or an herbal noncaffeinated tea.
- Try a walk outside in the fresh air or take deep breaths through an open window.

Notify your health care provider if:
- You are losing weight rather than gaining it.
- You have not gained the projected amount of weight for your week of pregnancy.
- You are unable to make up for lost meals some other time of the day.
- You have signs of dehydration such as little urine output.
- Nausea has lasted past 12 weeks of pregnancy.
- You vomit more than once daily.

BOX 12.8 FOCUS ON . . .

EVIDENCE-BASED PRACTICE

Does the practice of pica influence fetal health?

To answer this question, nurse researchers interviewed 128 women attending a prenatal clinic in a southern state as to whether they ate nonfood substances during pregnancy. The majority of the participants were African-American, single, in their early 20s, with a high school education, unemployed, and without a religious preference. This was the first pregnancy for 41% of the women. Of the sample, 75% were participants in the Special Supplemental Nutrition Program for Women, Infants, and Children program (WIC). Seventy-six percent of women reported they took daily prenatal vitamin and iron supplementation. Results of the study showed that 48 women (38%) craved a nonfood substance such as ice, laundry starch, cornstarch, or clay dirt. Interestingly, of the 48 women identified as experiencing pica, only 36 (75%) had this noted in their medical chart. Results showed that women who experience pica daily had lower hematocrit levels than women who did not experience pica or experience pica only intermittently, although these levels were not low enough for a diagnosis of anemia. The researchers recommend that nurses ask women during pregnancy if they are experiencing pica, because women may not reveal this to health care personnel unless asked directly.

This is an important study because it reveals that the incidence of pica in this sample of pregnant women was higher (38%) than is usually reported. It stresses how important it is for nurses to be aware that a proportion of women in any prenatal setting may be eating nonfood substances in preference to healthy prenatal foods.

Source: Corbett, R. W., Ryan, C. & Weinrich, S. P. (2003). Pica in pregnancy: does it affect pregnancy outcomes? *MCN, American Journal of Maternal Child Nursing, 28*(3), 183–189.

Encouraging a woman to stop eating the nonfood substance may not be effective because the habit may be deeply ingrained. Because pica is a symptom that often accompanies iron-deficiency anemia, correcting this underlying problem with an iron supplement may correct the pica. At subsequent visits, be certain to assess if a woman's hemoglobin is increasing and ask if she notices any difference in her cravings.

Pyrosis

Pyrosis (heartburn) is a burning sensation along the esophagus caused by regurgitation of gastric contents into the lower esophagus. In pregnancy, it may accompany early nausea, but it may persist beyond the resolution of nausea and even increase in severity as pregnancy advances.

Pyrosis is probably caused by decreased gastric motility, which slows gastric emptying, and pressure of the expanding uterus against the stomach. Common suggestions to help prevent reflux into the esophagus are to eat small meals frequently, sleep with two pillows, and don't lie down immediately after eating. Aluminum hydroxide (Amphojel) or a combination of aluminum and magnesium hydroxide (Maalox) may be prescribed for relief. If those do not relieve the discomfort, a histamine antagonist such as cimetidine (Tagamet) or ranitidine (Zantac) may be prescribed (Yankowitz, 2003). Be certain a woman understands that this "chest" pain is from her gastrointestinal tract and that, although it is called heartburn, it has nothing to do with her heart.

Hypercholesterolemia

Women with a family history of hypercholesterolemia may enter pregnancy with an elevated cholesterol level. During pregnancy, increasing progesterone levels cause a further elevation of cholesterol. Combined with intrahepatic cholestasis, this can lead to an increased risk for gallstone formation (cholelithiasis) and cardiovascular disease. Preventing cholelithiasis during pregnancy is important because gallstones can cause extremely sharp pain. Fortunately, surgery to remove gallstones during pregnancy is possible with new ambulatory laparotomy techniques (Rollins, Chan, & Price, 2004).

A woman who has had difficulty with hypercholesterolemia before pregnancy may need to continue to eat only moderate amounts of fat during pregnancy to prevent any increase in cholesterol. Helpful ways to reduce cholesterol may include:

- Exercising daily
- Eating oat cereal
- Broiling meat rather than frying it
- Using a minimum of salad oils
- Substituting new omega-3 products for butter
- Eating fish high in omega-3 oil, such as salmon or trout

Although tuna is also high in omega-3 oil, currently recommendations are that pregnant women should limit their intake of tuna to no more than one serving a week, because it may have a high mercury content (Jarup, 2003).

Urge women to check with their health care provider about the wisdom of continuing to take cholesterol-lowering drugs during pregnancy, because these drugs may be teratogenic (Karch, 2004). A low-cholesterol diet will automatically be lower in calories than the average diet, because oils and fats add many calories. Therefore, assess these women carefully for adequate weight gain during pregnancy. Make sure that a woman does include some oil daily (perhaps as olive oil on a salad) so she has included a source of linoleic acid in her daily intake.

 Checkpoint Question 4

Which statement by Tori would best suggest she has pica?

a. I love snacking on ice cubes; no food, just ice cubes.
b. I can't eat a thing before 11 every morning.
c. I notice I've been eating more sweet stuff than usual.
d. I crave oranges; can't get enough of them every day.

Promoting Nutritional Health in Women With Special Needs

The Adolescent

The pregnant adolescent needs a higher caloric intake (2,500 calories per day) to supply energy for her high level of activity and growth than mature women. The nutrients most often lacking from a typical adolescent diet tend to be calcium, iron, folic acid, and total calories. Look for sources of these when analyzing a teenager's pregnancy intake.

Good nutrition can be a problem with pregnant teenagers because of the dual demands of consuming enough food to provide for fetal growth and their own continuing growth. Often adolescents, in their search for identity, avoid foods that their parents see as important for them (e.g., milk, warm cereal, vegetables, or fruit), and indulge instead in foods such as soft drinks, potato chips, and French fries. To help an adolescent plan nutritional intake for pregnancy, respect her right to reject traditional foods as long as what she does eat includes sufficient nutrients. A cheese and sausage pizza, a glass of milk, and an apple is a lunch that provides all basic food groups (meat: sausage; bread: pizza crust; vegetable: tomato sauce; dairy: cheese and milk; fruit: apple). A hamburger "with everything" plus a tangerine and milk provides the same (Box 12.9).

Most adolescents snack frequently during the day. Toward the end of pregnancy, when fatigue may be a problem, they may begin to eat more and more "junk food" because preparing nutritious snacks takes more effort. Advise them to prepare some nutritious snacks such as carrot sticks or cheese bites early each day when they have more energy so that later in the day, when they are tired, eating a nutritious snack will not involve much effort.

Counseling adolescents about pregnancy nutrition may not be effective, because they often are not responsible for cooking the food they eat. You may need to speak to their parents or support persons (with permission) about certain foods to prepare before you can alter their nutrition pattern. If possible, suggest a number of foods that would fill a deficit and let the adolescent choose from them to provide a sense of control (Symon & Wrieden, 2003).

A Woman Over Age 40

Today, many women are older than 40 by the time they have their first child, and many more are older than 40 when they have their second or third child (Bastian et al., 2005). The nutritional needs of women in this age group are poorly studied, but it is obvious these women should maintain the same careful pregnancy nutrition as younger women. Because women in this age group may have slightly decreased kidney function, they should be sure to maintain a high fluid intake to remove waste products for themselves and for a fetus. Many women at this point in life are caring for elderly parents, and many have delayed childbearing to establish a career; this means they may eat whatever they are preparing for elderly parents or depend on packed or fast-food lunches for at least part of their nutrition each week. Focus your nutrition counseling on maintaining adequate nutrition during pregnancy, based on these changing lifestyles.

FOCUS ON 12.9 . . .

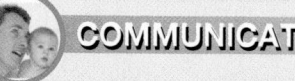

COMMUNICATION

Tori comes to your prenatal clinic for her first visit. You want to obtain a nutrition history from her.

Less Effective Communication

Nurse: Hi, Tori. Are you eating a nutritious diet?
Tori: I can't get enough food since I've been pregnant. No problem.
Nurse: Have you ever compared what you eat to a food pyramid to see if you're eating all the different types of food it shows?
Tori: Sure. Grain is on one side; meat is on the other. I eat both of those.
Nurse: It's important to drink at least a quart of milk a day during pregnancy. Are you doing that?
Tori: I'm drinking milkshakes so I not only get calcium but extra calories.
Nurse: That's great. Good nutrition is so important during pregnancy. I'm glad you're so aware of it.

More Effective Communication

Nurse: Hi, Tori. Are you eating a nutritious diet?
Tori: I can't get enough food since I've been pregnant. No problem.
Nurse: Tell me what you ate yesterday.
Tori: A muffin for breakfast, French fries for lunch, a hamburger for supper. A milkshake before bed.
Nurse: That's sounds good, but let's talk about ways you might get some fruit and vegetables into your day.

Most people believe they eat well, so if just asked general questions about nutrition, they respond that their nutrition is adequate. Only when they are asked to actually describe what they ate during one day is the truth revealed.

A Woman With Decreased Nutritional Stores

A woman with high parity or a short interval between pregnancies or one who has been dieting rigorously to lose weight before pregnancy may enter pregnancy with such depleted nutritional reserves that she has little to draw on during the first part of pregnancy. If her folic acid intake has been inadequate, her fetus may also be susceptible to neural tube defects (Carmichael et al., 2003). This shortage of nutrients may become critical during the time she is unable to eat well because of the normal nausea and vomiting of pregnancy. In addition, nutritional stores may be affected by other variables. Be alert to the following:

- Women from low-income families may enter pregnancy with anemia.
- Women who used diuretics for a dieting program may be deficient in potassium.

- Women who have been taking oral contraceptives may have decreased folate stores.
- Women who were using intrauterine devices or who have menorrhagia may be deficient in iron from excessive blood loss with menstrual flows.
- Women who drink alcohol excessively may be deficient in thiamine.

Women with these decreased nutritional stores need to be identified early in pregnancy through history taking so they can be referred to a nutritionist for specific nutritional counseling. They may need additional supplements during pregnancy to restore a particular nutrient.

A Woman Who Is Underweight

Today's emphasis on slim, model-like female figures makes it easy to overlook the health problem of a woman who is underweight. A woman who enters a pregnancy underweight, however, needs nutritional counseling just as much as any pregnant client.

Underweight is defined as a state in which a woman's weight is 10% to 15% less than the ideal weight for her height, or a BMI of less than 18.5. Most women who are underweight tire easily because they have an accompanying iron-deficiency anemia. Even when underweight women gain excessive weight during pregnancy, they still tend to have a higher-than-usual incidence of low-birthweight infants, probably because of depleted nutrient stores at the pregnancy's beginning. This is one reason why preconceptual health care visits and assessments are so important (Katz, 2003).

Being underweight may occur for a variety of reasons:

- Dieting for weight loss
- Poverty and the inability to buy adequate food (however, many poor women are obese, not underweight, because starchy foods are less expensive than those that have a higher protein content, such as meat and eggs)
- Excessive worry or stress, emotions that can lead to a loss of appetite
- Depression, which causes a chronic loss of appetite
- An eating disorder, such as anorexia nervosa or bulimia, conditions in which a woman has developed a revulsion to food (see Chapter 54)

However, the major reason for being underweight is insufficient intake of food due to chronic poor nutritional habits.

Convincing women who are underweight to eat more may be difficult because you are asking a woman to change lifelong eating habits. Counseling also can be challenging because during the first trimester of pregnancy, when fetal need is greatest and at a time when she has nausea and vomiting, possibly losing all desire to eat, you are asking her to take in additional food.

Begin counseling by asking a woman for a 24-hour nutrition recall. If she is just asked if she eats well, she will usually say she does (it seems adequate to her because it is her usual pattern).

Total daily caloric intake for the underweight woman may need to be 3,500 calories (500 to 1,000 calories more than the usual specified daily amount). Work with women to develop menus based on well-planned meals rather than on quick take-out foods. Suggest additional calories in the form of a concentrated formula such as an instant liquid breakfast drink. Be certain a woman understands this should not be a high-protein drink used for high-protein dieting regimens. Such diet drinks deliver a concentrated solute load (breakdown products of protein) to the kidney (already working to capacity because of the pregnancy) and provide so little carbohydrate in proportion to protein that they encourage the breakdown of protein for body energy, a process that results in acidosis. High-protein diets of this nature are not recommended for long-term use by anyone, but they should be totally avoided by women during pregnancy.

A 500-calorie increase over normal requirements should result in a weight gain of an additional pound per week. Be certain to plan for this additional gain when the total weight gain during pregnancy is calculated at each office visit. Otherwise, the total weight gain of a woman may seem excessive when it is actually healthy.

If a lack of nutritional stores makes a woman feel tired, urge her to schedule adequate rest periods daily so she can feel sufficiently energetic to prepare nutritious meals. Be certain she is taking her prescribed vitamin and iron supplements. Additional nutritional counseling in the postpartum period may be necessary so she can maintain better nutrition throughout her life and can enter a subsequent pregnancy (if she desires one) in a state of nutritional health.

A Woman Who Is Overweight

A woman is considered **overweight** if she is 20% above ideal weight or has a BMI over 25. She is considered **obese** if she weighs more than 200 pounds, she is 50% above ideal body weight for height, or her BMI is above 30. As many as 10% of pregnant women in the United States are overweight. Less-educated women and those living in poverty tend to be more overweight than others. Obesity in pregnancy is serious because it is associated with an increased incidence of gestational diabetes and pregnancy-induced hypertension (Linne, 2004; O'Brien et al., 2004).

Although obesity may occur from hypothyroidism, it most often occurs as a result of excessive caloric intake and decreased energy expenditure. Obesity becomes a problem during pregnancy for a variety of reasons:

- Pregnancy causes circulatory volume to increase 20% to 50% and metabolism to increase to meet the demands of the pregnancy, placing additional stress on a possibly already overworked body.
- It is often difficult to hear fetal heart tones in an obese woman; palpating for position and size of a fetus at birth is also difficult.
- Obese women are at an increased risk for giving birth to infants with macrosomia (excessive fetal growth); this increases the incidence of cesarean births in this population.
- Performing a cesarean birth, if necessary, may be difficult because of the excessive adipose tissue that must be incised to reach the uterus.

- The pregnancies of obese women are more apt to be prolonged, leading to postmature infants.
- Ambulating during pregnancy and immediately afterward is more difficult because of the increased energy expenditure necessary, increasing the risk for complications such as thrombophlebitis and pneumonia.

The habit of overeating has many causes. For some women, this is a coping mechanism for stress; whenever they feel tense or worried, they help themselves to something "comforting" to eat. Because pregnancy is stressful, it may be a particularly difficult time for a woman to change her food intake patterns. Other women overeat because their parents did and they were raised to always "clean their plate." If a woman has been serving her family an excessive intake of calories as well as herself, then the entire family may have to change their eating patterns to bring about a change in a woman's intake.

Dieting to reduce weight is not recommended during pregnancy because if carbohydrates are reduced too much, the body will use protein and fat for energy. This could deprive a fetus of essential nutrients (Carmichael et al., 2003). It could lead to ketoacidosis. Although the long-term effects of mild ketoacidosis on a fetus are not well studied, it can be avoided if the daily caloric intake, even in the most obese woman, does not go below 1,500 to 1,800 per day.

Overweight women tend to exercise less than women of normal weight. Exercising is more awkward and more tiring, and they may feel self-conscious wearing exercise clothing. Try to encourage them to engage in at least a minimum activity program, such as walking around the block once a day, in conjunction with lessened carbohydrate intake.

Helping a woman look at her nutrition in terms of empty-calorie versus nutritious foods may help her to eat more sensibly. Early in pregnancy, when she is eager to appear pregnant, she may resist limiting her intake. Stress that a fetus grows best on nutritious foods, not necessarily those with the most calories. Provide additional nutritional counseling in the postpartum period so she can prepare more nutritious meals in the future for herself and her growing family. If successful, she will not enter another pregnancy severely overweight.

A Woman Who Is a Vegetarian

About 2.5% of the United States population are vegetarians (ADA, 2003). Vegetarian diets are consistent with Dietary Guidelines for Americans. Most women vegetarians are closer to their ideal weight and have lower serum cholesterol levels and lower blood pressure levels than women who eat a more typical American diet. Nurses may find that many pregnant women, therefore, will want to exclude meat from their diets. There are many different types of vegetarians: lacto-ovo-vegetarians (no animal flesh or fish is eaten, but dairy products and eggs are), lacto-vegetarians (no meat, fish, or eggs are eaten, but dairy products are), and vegans (nothing derived from an animal is eaten). Most vegetarians are knowledgeable about their diets and can discuss what foods are high in various nutrients and how they incorporate such foods into their daily intake.

A vegetarian food pyramid is identical to a usual one, except it contains no meat (shows fish and eggs). Women should try to eat three or more servings a day of both fruits and vegetables, six or more servings per day of grains, and two or more servings per day of legumes such as kidney, black, or lima beans.

Special concerns for pregnant vegetarians include lack of vitamin B_{12} (meat is the chief source of this) and an inadequate intake of calcium (recommend dark-green vegetables as sources) and vitamin D (fortified milk and sunlight are the main sources of this). Urge women who are vegetarians to take a daily prenatal supplement, like all women, to ensure adequate iron and folic acid.

A Woman With Phenylketonuria

Phenylketonuria (PKU), named because the breakdown product of phenylalanine, an essential amino acid, is excreted in the urine in this form, is an inherited disorder in which a person cannot convert phenylalanine into tyrosine, the form used for cell growth. Without conversion, phenylalanine accumulates in the person's blood serum, eventually leaving the bloodstream to invade body cells. When brain cells are invaded, severe cognitive challenge and accompanying neurologic damage, such as recurrent seizures, may develop (see Chapter 48). A fetus of a woman with uncontrolled PKU can develop microcephaly, intrauterine growth restriction, and neurologic damage as well (Rouse & Azen, 2004).

Foods high in phenylalanine are those high in protein; examples of foods low in phenylalanine are fruits and vegetables such as orange juice, bananas, squash, spinach, and peas. Children with PKU follow a diet with restricted phenylalanine intake until at least past adolescence. A woman with PKU should consult her internist when she is planning to become pregnant and should plan to return to a low-phenylalanine diet for at least 3 months before she becomes pregnant. A woman typically follows this low-phenylalanine diet during the pregnancy and afterward as long as she is breast-feeding (Waisbren & Azen, 2003).

A woman with PKU needs support during pregnancy to adhere to these nutritional restrictions. It is particularly disappointing if she does not become pregnant immediately after starting the restricted diet, because each month she is "prepregnant" extends the period she must follow the restrictions. A woman with PKU is usually well informed about her particular nutritional needs. She is aware that phenylalanine is destructive to developing brain cells and that not following her restricted plan could leave her future child severely cognitively challenged.

A Woman With a Multiple Pregnancy

A woman with a multiple pregnancy gains more weight overall and with greater speed than a woman carrying a single child because of the increased fetal weight (a total weight gain of 40 to 45 lbs). To sustain her own nutrition stores, she must ingest high levels of protein and carbohydrate. In particular, there is an increased burden on ma-

Cultural and Socioeconomic Factors

Whether women want or are able to take a childbirth and parenting preparation course depends a great deal on cultural and socioeconomic factors and individual choices (Box 13.4). A course may not be helpful if suggestions made regarding infant clothing and supplies, formula or breastfeeding, or maternal nutrition and health are not culturally appropriate. In some cultures, the advice of a friend or family member carries more weight than the advice of a professional health care practitioner. Asking each woman separately whether she is interested in a course and being certain that women are fully informed about the options available to them are two ways to avoid cultural stereotyping and to be certain all women receive as much advice and knowledge as they wish about childbirth. Providing childbirth and parenting information that takes into account the cultural practices and financial needs of individual clients is the best approach to ensure that the information is understood and accepted and that birth experiences are positive.

PRECONCEPTION CLASSES

Preconception classes are held for couples who are planning to get pregnant usually within the next year and who want to know more about what they can expect a pregnancy to be like and what are birth setting/procedure choices. These classes stress that pregnancy brings with it psychological as well as physical changes and include recommended preconception dietary modifications such as a good intake of folic acid (green leafy vegetables) to help prevent neural tube defects.

EXPECTANT PARENTING CLASSES

Expectant parenting classes are designed for couples who are already pregnant. They focus on family health during a pregnancy, covering such topics as the psychological and physical changes of pregnancy, pregnancy nutrition, and newborn care. Many are geared for specific community needs, such as sibling preparation classes, refresher classes for grandparents, classes for expectant adoptive parents, pregnant adolescents, or women with special needs such as those in the military (Schachman, Lee, & Lederman, 2004).

Most preparation for parenthood programs last 4 to 8 hours over a 4- to 8-week period. Both women and their support people are invited, and the curriculum is individualized for the group and its needs. If all the women in the group already have children, for example, they may not need a tour of a maternity unit as part of the program; instead, they may want to learn what is new in baby food or childcare. If all the women in the class work at least part-time, discussion of "brown bag nutrition" and how to include rest periods during work might be most useful. If all the women are teenagers, they may be most interested in what is going to happen to their bodies during pregnancy, or what sports are safe to continue during pregnancy. They may also need more information on how to care for a newborn (Standifird, 2003). They probably will want a tour of the maternity unit (Fig. 13.1). A typical course plan for 8 weeks is shown in Box 13.5 (see also Box 13.6).

Sibling Education Classes

Sibling classes are organized to acquaint older brothers and sisters with what happens during birth and what they can expect a newborn to look like and act like. The classes review how babies grow and things children can do to help their mother during a pregnancy, such as not leaving toys on the floor that need to be picked up and eating healthy foods with her.

If the classes are held at a hospital, a tour of a newborn nursery is included so children can see how small their new sibling will be. A hospital room like the one their mother will occupy may also be visited.

For sibling classes to be successful, age-appropriate information and activities must be provided. See Chapters 28 to 32 for growth and development expectations by age group. Younger children may need reassurance that their

---

BOX 13.4 FOCUS ON . . .

COMMUNICATION

You care for Julia Marco at a prenatal clinic visit. She is in the 16th week of an uncomplicated pregnancy.

Less Effective Communication

Nurse: Have you signed up for childbirth preparation class yet, Julia?

Julia: No.

Nurse: Don't wait too much longer. You're already in your fourth month.

Julia: I'm not sure I'm going to sign up.

Nurse: Everyone can benefit from childbirth preparation. I'll write the telephone number down for you so you don't forget.

More Effective Communication

Nurse: Have you signed up for a childbirth preparation class yet, Julia?

Julia: No.

Nurse: Don't wait too much longer. You're already in your fourth month.

Julia: I'm not sure I'm going to sign up.

Nurse: Why is that?

Julia: Classes are all at the wrong time. And cost too much.

Nurse: Let's work together to find a course that's right for you. We can use the Internet to find out what other options might be available.

It is so important for couples to attend preparation for labor classes that it is easy to ignore the reasons clients present for not wanting to attend them. Careful listening often reveals that time or money concerns are reasons why couples choose not to attend a course. Helping to investigate the many options is the beginning of problem solving.

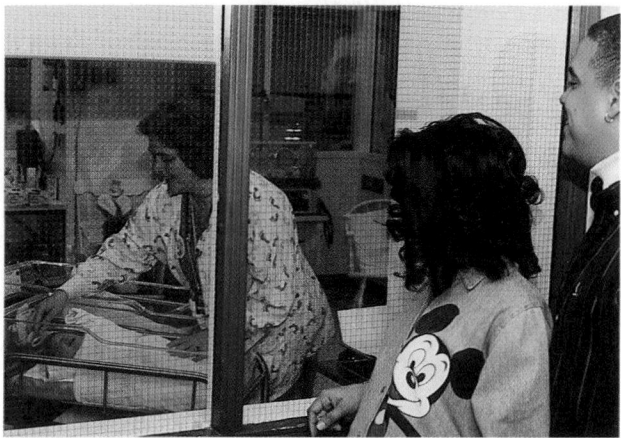

FIGURE 13.1 An enjoyable part of a preparation-for-parenthood class is touring a maternity service. Here, parents-to-be view a newborn nursery. (Photo by Melissa Olson, with permission of Chestnut Hill Hospital, Philadelphia, PA.)

parents will continue to love them after the new baby arrives. Older children may be interested in learning about newborn care and being a part of planning for the newborn.

Breast-Feeding Classes

Breast-feeding classes are designed to help women learn more about breast-feeding so they not only choose breast-feeding over bottle-feeding but also continue with breast-

---

BOX 13.6 FOCUS ON . . .

EVIDENCE-BASED PRACTICE

What is a way to interest more males in preparation-for-childbirth classes?

Emerging evidence suggests that many men want to be more involved in their partner's pregnancy but feel unprepared for parenting and unwelcome in parenting classes. For this study, parenting classes were conducted as they normally were, except that in one class the person conducting the class was male rather than female. When classes ended, participants completed a questionnaire about their satisfaction with the classes. Results showed that men and women who attended sessions where there was a male facilitator reported favorably on this innovation in practice. Satisfaction appeared to have less to do with the information transmitted than with the opportunity for enriched discussion. The researchers concluded that using male class facilitators offers one way of involving men more in prenatal education.

Being certain that childbirth education classes best meet the needs of people in that particular community means that classes should be designed to meet the needs of expectant fathers as well as those of expectant mothers. This is an important study because it suggests a way that classes can be made more "father-friendly."

Source: Symon, A., & Lee, J. (2003). Including men in antenatal education: evaluating innovative practice. *Evidence-Based Midwifery, 1*(1), 12–19.

BOX 13.5

Sample Content for Expectant Parents Class

Lesson 1 Review of Physiologic Changes of
  Pregnancy and Fetal Growth
Lesson 2 Personal Care During Pregnancy
  Nutrition
  Hygiene
  Exercise
  Rest
Lesson 3 Emotional Changes During Pregnancy
Lesson 4 Labor and Birth
  The Process of Birth
  Exercises and Breathing Techniques
  Medication in Labor
Lesson 5 The Postpartum Period
Lesson 6 Infant Care
  Nutrition
  Hygiene
Lesson 7 Plans for Birth
  Birth Settings Available
  Supplies to Take to Birth Settings
  Tour or Film of a Typical Setting
Lesson 8 Reproductive Life Planning

---

feeding for at least 6 months following their child's birth. These classes cover the physiology of breast-feeding as well as psychological aspects. They are often taught by a certified La Leche League instructor.

THE CHILDBIRTH PLAN

Most classes for expectant parents urge couples to make a written childbirth plan or spell out their choice of setting, birth attendant, special needs such as the extent of family participation they wish during labor, birthing positions, medication options, plans for the immediate postpartum period and baby care, and the postpartum stay and family visitation. Some suggestions for a woman and her partner to consider in planning these specific childbirth details are shown in Box 13.7.

Birth planning is usually part of the curriculum for childbirth education classes because a group setting may be the best way for couples to sort out their questions and feelings about how to plan for a healthy and enjoyable birth. Urge couples to make decisions about these issues before the day of birth, or else decisions can be determined by agency policy or the circumstances at the moment without the couple's input. If the expectant family has a strong

BOX 13.7 FOCUS ON . . .

FAMILY TEACHING

Choosing a Birth Setting

Q. Julia and her husband Joe ask you, "There are so many options available for a birth setting. How do we decide which to choose?"

A. Choosing a birth setting is a personal decision. Some questions you might want to ask are:

- What type of caregiver do I want to supervise my prenatal care and labor and birth? Nurse-midwife? Family doctor? Obstetrician?
- Will the same person be present at prenatal visits as for birth? Does the setting offer preparation for childbirth or childrearing classes?
- What settings does a childbirth provider let me choose from? A birthing room? An alternative birthing center? My home?
- Will I be allowed to choose a birth position? Will I have input into the amount of anesthesia used? Can administration of ophthalmic ointment for the baby be delayed? Can I begin breast-feeding immediately? Will nurses who are supportive and informed about breast-feeding be available? Can I use a doula?
- Will the setting allow my partner to participate? Will he or she be allowed to be with me throughout labor and birth? Could he or she cut the cord or help deliver the baby? Can older children participate? Can I record the birth on videotape or by photograph?
- Is early discharge available? Will a follow-up home visit be included in care?
- If I should have a complication during labor or birth, are there adequate supplies and personnel available for emergency care? If the baby should have a complication, is there provision for immediate emergency care or transport to a high-risk facility?

BOX 13.8

Birth Plan: Julia Marco

Birth Attendant
Alexander Coppin, MD, or nurse-midwife Kaitlin Brandywine, whoever is on call for the big day.

Birth Setting
Birthing Room Number 1 at Huntington General

Support Person
Husband Joe (if out of town, my sister Adrienne)

Activities During Labor
I want to walk or rock in the rocking chair or play Monopoly.
I want to wear my own nightgown, and listen to Simon and Garfunkel Central Park Concert tape.
Husband wants to videotape birth.

Birth
Position for birth: squatting
No episiotomy
Husband wants to cut cord.

Postpartum
I want to breast-feed immediately.
I want to use kangaroo care to keep baby warm.
I want to room in.
Husband wants to sleep over on bedside cot.

PREPARATION FOR CHILDBIRTH CLASSES

Preparation for childbirth classes focus on explaining the birth process rather than pregnancy and ways to prevent or reduce the pain of childbirth. Common goals of preparation for childbirth classes are to:

- Prepare the expectant mother and her support person for the childbirth experience
- Create clients who are knowledgeable consumers of obstetric care
- Help clients reduce and manage pain with both pharmacologic and nonpharmacologic methods
- Help increase the couple's overall enjoyment of and satisfaction with the childbirth experience

In addition to teaching about normal labor, they include a number of exercises to ready the body for labor, as well as methods of pain prevention or relief in labor.

Perineal and Abdominal Exercises

Encourage women to maintain an overall active exercise program during pregnancy, as this may help prevent the need for cesarean birth. In childbirth preparation classes, women learn specific exercises to strengthen their pelvic

desire in a certain area, planning ahead will allow them to communicate this so their wish can be accommodated if possible. Be certain all couples understand, however, that the birth plan should be flexible in case a complication or change of plans arises. For example, in the event of a complication of labor or birth that requires an emergency cesarean birth, a preference to have the baby without anesthesia will need to be modified. Box 13.8 illustrates a sample birth plan.

What if... Julia Marco tells you her husband can't be with her during labor. She asks you if it is really important to have someone with her. How would you advise her?

and abdominal muscles and make these both stronger and more supple. Supple perineal muscles allow for ready stretching during birth, reducing discomfort, and help muscles revert more quickly to their normal condition and function more efficiently after childbirth (Holroyd-Leduc & Straus, 2004).

A woman may begin exercises as early in pregnancy as she likes; however, women enrolled in Lamaze preparation programs generally do not begin until the last 8 to 10 weeks of pregnancy. This time frame allows the woman to learn the conditioned responses necessary for prepared labor closer to the time they will be used, but it limits the total amount of time directed to perineal exercises. If labor begins early, a woman may have had little or no practice with perineal exercises.

Women should not participate in a formal exercise program without their physician's or nurse-midwife's approval. They should not attempt to exercise if any of the danger signs of pregnancy appear, and they should never exercise to the point of fatigue. Common safety precautions for preparation for childbirth exercises in pregnancy are summarized in Box 13.9.

Many exercises can be incorporated into daily activities so they will take little time from a woman's day. It is best, however, for a woman to set aside a specific time each day for the task; otherwise, her participation is apt to be sporadic. Initially, women should do each exercise only a few times, gradually increasing the number at each session.

Tailor Sitting

Although many women may be familiar with tailor sitting, they may have to be re-taught the position so it is done in a way that stretches the perineal muscles without occluding blood supply to the lower legs. A woman should not put one ankle on top of the other but should place one leg in front of the other (Fig. 13.2). As she sits in this position, she should gently push on her knees toward the floor until she feels her perineum stretch. This is a good position to use to watch television, read, or talk to friends. It is good to plan on sitting in this position for at least 15 minutes every day. By the end of pregnancy, a woman's perineum should be so supple that when she tailor-sits, her knees will almost touch the floor if pushed.

Squatting

Squatting (Fig. 13.3) also stretches the perineal muscles and can be a useful position for second-stage labor, so a woman should also practice this position for about 15 minutes a day. Most women need a demonstration of effective squatting; otherwise, they tend to squat on their tiptoes. For the pelvic muscles to stretch, a woman must keep her feet flat on the floor. Incorporating squatting into daily activities such as picking up toys from the floor reduces the amount of time a woman must devote to daily exercises.

Pelvic Floor Contractions (Kegel Exercises)

Pelvic floor contractions are another activity that can be done during daily activities. While sitting at her desk or

BOX 13.9 FOCUS ON . . .

FAMILY TEACHING

Exercise Guidelines for Labor Preparation

Q. Julia asks you, "How can I be sure the exercises I'm doing in pregnancy won't hurt me or my baby?"

A. Try following these guidelines:

- Never exercise to the point of fatigue.
- Always rise from the floor slowly, to prevent orthostatic hypotension.
- To rise from the floor, roll over to the side first and then push up to avoid strain on the abdominal muscles or round ligaments.
- To prevent leg cramps when doing leg exercises, never point the toes (extend the heel instead).
- To prevent muscle strain, do not attempt exercises that hyperextend the lower back.
- Do not hold your breath while exercising, because this increases intra-abdominal and intrauterine pressure.
- Do not continue with exercises if any danger signal of pregnancy occurs.
- Do not practice second-stage pushing. Pushing increases intrauterine pressure and could rupture membranes.

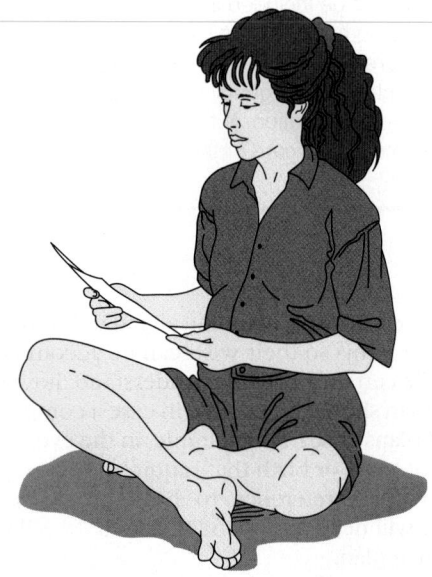

FIGURE 13.2 Tailor sitting strengthens the thighs and stretches perineal muscles to make them more supple. Notice that the legs are parallel so that one does not compress the other. A woman could use this position for television watching, telephone conversations, or playing with an older child.

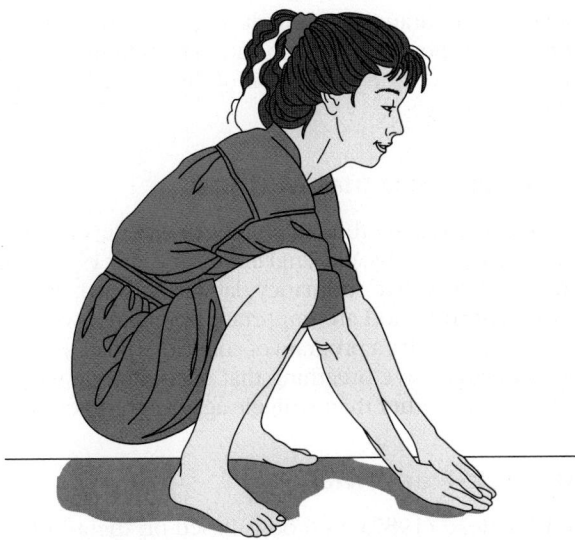

FIGURE 13.3 Squatting helps to stretch the muscles of the pelvic floor. Notice that the feet are flat on the floor for optimum stretching.

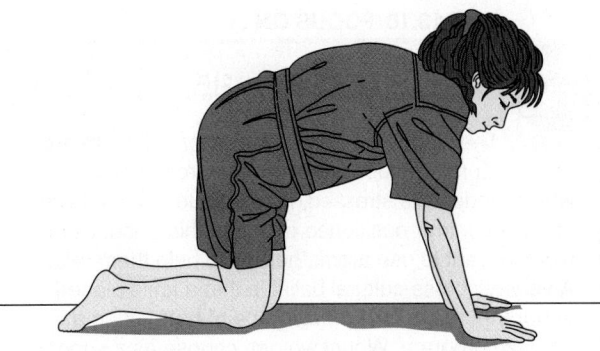

FIGURE 13.4 Pelvic rocking is helpful in relieving backache during pregnancy and labor. The woman hollows her back and then arches it.

working around the house, a woman can tighten the muscles of the perineum by doing Kegel exercises (see Chapter 11, Box 11.8). Such perineal muscle-strengthening exercises will be helpful in the postpartum period to reduce pain and promote perineal healing. They have long-term effects of increasing sexual responsiveness and helping prevent stress incontinence (Holroyd-Leduc & Straus, 2004).

Abdominal Muscle Contractions

Abdominal muscle contractions help strengthen the abdominal muscles during pregnancy and therefore may help prevent constipation as well as help restore abdominal tone after pregnancy. Strong abdominal muscles can also contribute to effective second-stage pushing during labor. Abdominal contractions can be done in a standing or lying position along with pelvic floor contractions. A woman merely tightens her abdominal muscles, then relaxes them. She can repeat the exercise as often as she wishes during the day.

Another way to do the same thing is to practice "blowing out a candle." A woman takes a fairly deep inspiration, then exhales normally. Holding her finger about 6 inches in front of herself, as if it were a candle, she then exhales forcibly, pushing out residual air from her lungs. She can feel her abdominal muscles contract as she reaches the end of her forcible exhalation.

Pelvic Rocking

Pelvic rocking (Fig. 13.4) helps relieve backache during pregnancy and early labor by making the lumbar spine more flexible. It can be done in a variety of positions: on hands and knees, lying down, sitting, or standing. A woman arches her back, trying to lengthen or stretch her spine. She holds the position for 1 minute, then hollows her back. A woman can do this at the end of the day about five times to relieve back pain and make herself more comfortable for the night.

Checkpoint Question 1

Julia Marco asks you which type of exercise is best to strengthen perineal muscles. Your best answer would be:

a. Walk 20 minutes daily at a fairly rapid pace.
b. Alternately tighten and relax perineal muscles as if stopping voiding.
c. Periodically push as if you're moving your bowels.
d. Lift both legs into the air while you lie supine.

Methods for Pain Management

Beginning in the late 1950s, many specific methods for nonpharmacologic pain reduction during labor were developed. These included the Lamaze, Dick-Read, and Bradley methods, all named after the professionals who developed them. More recently, however, childbirth education has been moving away from strict method approaches to more eclectic ones. Much research is being done to verify the effectiveness of each of these many techniques, and in practice many educators are using a variety of approaches in their courses (Box 13.10).

Most of the methods advocated are based on three premises:

1. Discomfort during labor can be minimized if a woman comes into labor informed about what is happening and prepared with breathing exercises to use during contractions. In classes, therefore, a woman learns about her body's response in labor, the mechanisms involved in childbirth, and breathing exercises she can use during labor.
2. Discomfort during labor can be minimized if a woman's abdomen is relaxed and the uterus is allowed to rise freely against the abdominal wall with contractions. Childbirth methods differ only in the manner by which they achieve this relaxation.
3. Pain perception can be altered by **distraction** techniques or by the **gating control theory of pain perception** (Box 13.11).

BOX 13.10 FOCUS ON . . .

DIVERSITY OF CARE

The plans that women make for childbirth are often culturally influenced. A woman from a culture in which modesty is stressed, for example, may not want to have a mirror positioned over a birthing bed. Some women want to use aromatherapy to help them relax. A very old cross-cultural belief is that a knife placed under the mattress will "cut the pain" better than a Lamaze program. Whom women choose as a support person or coach in labor can also differ, depending on their cultural background. Some women would not think of choosing anyone but their male partner; others choose a female relative or friend. Assess each couple individually to be certain that cultural preferences such as these are respected.

The Bradley (Partner-Coached) Method

The Bradley method of childbirth, originated by Robert Bradley (1981), is based on the premise that childbirth is a joyful natural process and stresses the important role of a woman's partner during pregnancy, labor, and the early newborn period. During pregnancy, a woman performs muscle-toning exercises and limits or omits foods that contain preservatives, animal fat, or a high salt content. Pain is reduced in labor by abdominal breathing. In addition, a woman is encouraged to walk during labor and to use an internal focus point as a disassociation technique. The method is used widely in some areas of the United States and at specific centers.

The Psychosexual Method

The psychosexual method of childbirth was developed by Sheila Kitzinger (1990) in England during the 1950s. The method stresses that pregnancy, labor and birth, and the early newborn period are important points in a woman's life cycle. It includes a program of conscious relaxation and levels of progressive breathing that encourages a woman to "flow with" rather than struggle against contractions.

The Dick-Read Method

The Dick-Read (1987) method is based on the approach proposed by Grantly Dick-Read, an English physician. The premise is that fear leads to tension, which leads to pain. If one can prevent this chain of events from occurring, or break the chain between fear and tension or tension and pain, then one can reduce the pain of contractions. A woman achieves relaxation and reduced pain by focusing on abdominal breathing during contractions.

The Lamaze Method

The Lamaze method of prepared childbirth, based on the gating control theory of pain relief, is the one most

---

BOX 13.11

Gate Control Mechanisms

Pain Pathway

1. The endings of small peripheral nerve fibers detect a stimulus.
2. They transmit it to cells in the dorsal horn of the spinal cord.
3. Impulses pass through a dense, interfacing network of cells in the spinal cord (the substantia gelatinosa).
4. Immediately, a synapse occurs that returns the transmission to the peripheral site through a motor nerve. For example, a person touches a candle flame; the impulse travels to the spinal cord and back, and the person jerks his or her hand away from the flame.
5. After this short-circuit synapse, the impulse then continues in the spinal cord to reach the hypothalamus and cortex of the brain.
6. The impulse is interpreted (the candle is hot) and perceived as pain.

Gating Theory of Pain Control

The gating theory of pain refers to gate control mechanisms in the substantia gelatinosa that are capable of halting an impulse at the level of the spinal cord so the impulse is never perceived at the brain level as pain: a process similar to closing a gate.

Techniques to Assist Gating Mechanisms

- *Cutaneous Stimulation.* If large peripheral nerves next to an injury site are stimulated, the ability of the small nerve fibers at the injury site to transmit pain impulses appears to decrease. Therefore, rubbing an injured part or applying transcutaneous electrical nerve stimulation (TENS) or heat or cold to the site (cutaneous stimulation) is an effective maneuver to suppress pain. Effleurage, or light massage used in the Lamaze method, accomplishes this.
- *Distraction.* If the cells of the brain stem that register an impulse as pain are preoccupied with other stimuli, a pain impulse cannot register. Distraction or imagery accomplishes this. Different childbirth classes use different breathing, vocalization, or focusing techniques to accomplish this. (Breathing techniques are most often employed in childbirth classes because they increase oxygenation to the mother and fetus as well as decrease pain.)
- *Reduction of Anxiety.* Pain impulses are perceived more quickly if anxiety is also present. Thus, the third technique of gating is to reduce patient anxiety as much as possible. Teaching a woman what to expect during labor is a means of achieving this.

often taught in the United States. The method is based on the theory that through stimulus-response conditioning, women can learn to use controlled breathing to reduce pain during labor. It was originally termed the **psychoprophylactic** method, as it focuses on preventing pain in labor (prophylaxis) by use of the mind (psyche).

The method was developed in Russia based on Pavlov's conditioning studies but was popularized by a French physician, Ferdinand Lamaze. Formal classes are organized by Lamaze International or the International Childbirth Education Association.

Six major concepts are stressed: (1) labor should begin on its own, not be artificially induced; (2) women should be able to move about freely throughout labor, not be confined to bed; (3) women should receive continuous support during labor; (4) no routine interventions such as intravenous fluid are needed; (5) women should be allowed to assume a non-supine (e.g., upright or side-lying) position for birth; and (6) mother and baby should be housed together following birth, with unlimited opportunity for breast-feeding (Curl et al., 2004).

Three main premises are taught in the prenatal period related to the gating control method of pain relief:

1. Pain occurs to a lesser extent if a woman is relaxed. Much time in class is spent reviewing or teaching reproductive anatomy and physiology and the process of labor and birth with the belief that if women are familiar with what will happen in labor and the nature of contractions, the couple can enter labor with decreased tension.
2. Sensations such as uterine contractions can be blocked from reaching the brain cortex and registering as pain through active interventions. A woman is taught to concentrate on breathing patterns and to use imagery or focusing (concentrating) on a specified object to block incoming pain sensations. The effectiveness of focusing can be observed in athletes who hurt themselves in basketball or football games but do not feel the pain until after the game because they are so focused on winning.
3. Conditioned reflexes can also be used to displace pain during labor. Time in class is spent on learning **conditioned reflexes,** or reflexes that automatically occur in response to a stimulus. Conditioned responses were first noted by Pavlov while conducting studies on salivation in dogs. The same training technique is applied to the birth process in the Lamaze method. A woman is conditioned to relax automatically on hearing a command ("contraction beginning") or on the feel of a contraction beginning. The responses to contractions must be recently conditioned to be effective (because conditioned responses fade if not reinforced). This is the reason it is generally recommended that women attend class in the last trimester of pregnancy.

Classes are kept small so that there is time for individual instruction and attention to each couple (Fig. 13.5). Advise a woman to bring a support person with her to class to practice breathing exercises with her. This person will then act as her coach in labor. Exercises taught in class vary from teacher to teacher, especially in terms of complexity, but have common features shown below. In addition, information to guide a woman and her coach through preg-

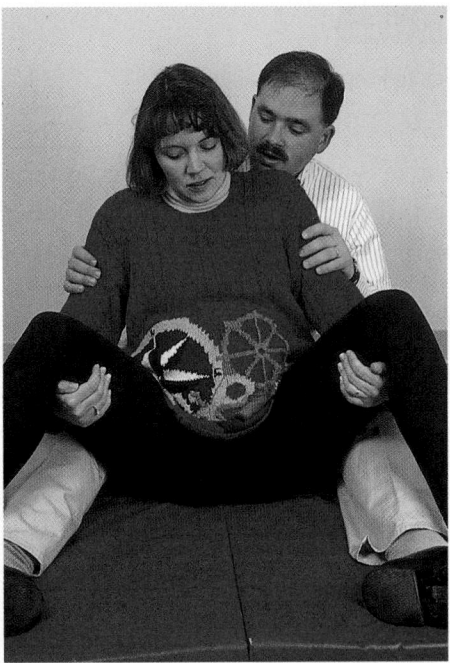

FIGURE 13.5 Every woman needs to be well prepared for birth. Here a couple practices positions for pushing in a childbirth preparation class.

nancy (e.g., prenatal nutrition, exercises, and common discomforts of pregnancy) and prepare them for unexpected circumstances (e.g., malpresentation, cesarean birth, or the need for analgesia or anesthesia) is provided. Supplies that a woman or couple might pack in advance to bring to the hospital may also be discussed (Table 13.1).

Conscious Relaxation. **Conscious relaxation** is learning to relax body portions deliberately so that, unknowingly, a woman does not remain tense and cause unnecessary muscle strain and fatigue during labor. She practices this during pregnancy by deliberately relaxing one set of muscles, then another and another until her body is completely relaxed. Her support person concentrates on noticing symptoms of tension such as a wrinkled brow, clenched fists, or a stiffly held arm. By either placing a comforting hand on the tense body area or telling a woman to relax that area, the support person helps her to achieve complete relaxation (Hotelling, 2004).

The Cleansing Breath. To begin all breathing exercises, a woman breathes in deeply and then exhales deeply (a **cleansing breath**). To end each exercise, she repeats this step. It is an important step to take because it limits the possibility of hyperventilation (blowing off too much carbon dioxide), which can happen with rapid breathing patterns, and so it helps ensure an adequate fetal oxygen supply. If women do become light-headed during labor from hyperventilation (develop respiratory alkalosis), breathing into a paper bag can help, as it causes rebreathing of exhaled carbon dioxide.

Consciously Controlled Breathing. Using **consciously controlled breathing,** or set breathing patterns at specific

TABLE 13.1

Supplies to Prepare for Labor

Item	Purpose
Lip balm	To prevent dry lips
Mouthwash	For rinsing dry mouth
Toothbrush and toothpaste	To prevent dry mouth
Warm socks	Comfort
Small rolling pin covered with soft cloth	Back massage
Focal point	To increase concentration
Busy work (e.g., knitting or magazines)	To pass time
Paper bag	To correct hyperventilation
Extra pillow	For semi-Fowler's position in labor
Watch	For timing contractions
Baby powder	For reducing friction of effleurage
Lollipops	For energy and dry mouth
Snacks (e.g., apples or potato chips)	For coach's comfort
Tapes or compact discs and player	To increase relaxation

rates, provides distraction as well as prevents the diaphragm from descending fully and putting pressure on the expanding uterus. To practice, a woman inhales comfortably but fully, then exhales, with her exhalation a little stronger than her inhalation (to help prevent hypoventilation). She practices breathing in this manner at a controlled pace, depending on the intensity of contractions. Various levels of breathing are:

Level 1. Slow chest breathing at this level consists of comfortable but full respirations at a rate of 6 to 12 breaths per minute. The level is used for early contractions.

Level 2. For this level, breathing is lighter than level 1. The rib cage should expand but be so light the diaphragm barely moves. The rate of respirations is up to 40 per minute. This is a good level of breathing for contractions when cervical dilation is between 4 and 6 cm.

Level 3. Breathing at this level is even more shallow, mostly at the sternum. The rate is 50 to 70 breaths per minute. As the respirations become faster, the exhalation must be a little stronger than the inhalation to allow good air exchange and to prevent hypoventilation. If a woman practices saying "out" with each exhalation, she almost inevitably will make exhalation stronger than inhalation. A woman uses this level for transition contractions. Keeping the tip of her tongue against the roof of her mouth helps pre-

vent the oral mucosa from drying out during such rapid breathing.

Level 4. At this level, a woman uses a "pant-blow" pattern, such as taking three or four quick breaths (in and out), then a forceful exhalation. Because this type of breathing sounds like a train (breath-breath-breath-huff), it is sometimes referred to as "choo-choo" breathing or "hee-hee-hee-hoo" breathing.

Level 5. A woman pants at this level. Chest panting is continuous, very shallow panting at about 60 breaths per minute. It can be used during strong contractions or during the second stage of labor to prevent a woman from pushing before full dilatation.

Some courses stop teaching at the point a woman has mastered the levels of breathing; others have her learn to shift from one level to the other on command or at the point she feels a need for more pain relief. To do this, at the sound of "contraction beginning," she breathes at 12 breaths a minute; at the sound of "contraction getting harder," 40 breaths a minute; "harder still," 70 breaths a minute; and so on, imitating basic shifts she will use in labor.

A woman who can perform the various levels of breathing and maintain relaxation is prepared to handle all labor contractions up to the second stage of labor.

Figure 13.6 illustrates the use of levels of breathing. An early labor contraction is mild. When the contraction begins, the coach says, "Contraction beginning." The woman takes a cleansing breath, then breathes at level 1; she feels no bite from the contraction and so does not need to change to a more involved breathing pattern. Later in labor, the contraction is stronger and longer. Now, at the sound of "Contraction beginning," the woman takes a cleansing breath, then begins level 1 breathing (3 breaths); shifts to level 2 (4 to 6 breaths); then shifts to level 3 (10 breaths). The contraction is lessening. She shifts down to level 2 (4 to 6 breaths), then to level 1 (3 or 4 breaths). The contraction is gone. She takes a final cleansing breath. During actual labor, her coach can tell the strength of contractions by resting a hand on her abdomen or observing a uterine contraction monitor. The coach can tell a woman when to shift breathing levels depending on the coach's estimation of the strength of the contraction with words such as, "contraction beginning, getting stronger, now getting weaker, gone." In the time before transition to the second stage of labor, when contractions are longest and strongest, a woman may need to use her level 4 breathing or continuous light panting as well.

Effleurage. One additional technique to encourage relaxation and displace pain in the Lamaze method is **effleurage,** which is French for light abdominal massage, done with just enough pressure to avoid tickling. To do this, a woman traces a pattern on her abdomen with her fingertips (Fig. 13.7). The rate of effleurage should remain constant even though breathing rates change. Effleurage serves as a distraction technique and decreases sensory stimuli transmission from the abdominal wall, helping limit local discomfort. If an external electronic monitor is in place on the abdomen, effleurage can be done superior or inferior to it or even on the thighs. Effleurage can also be done by the support person.

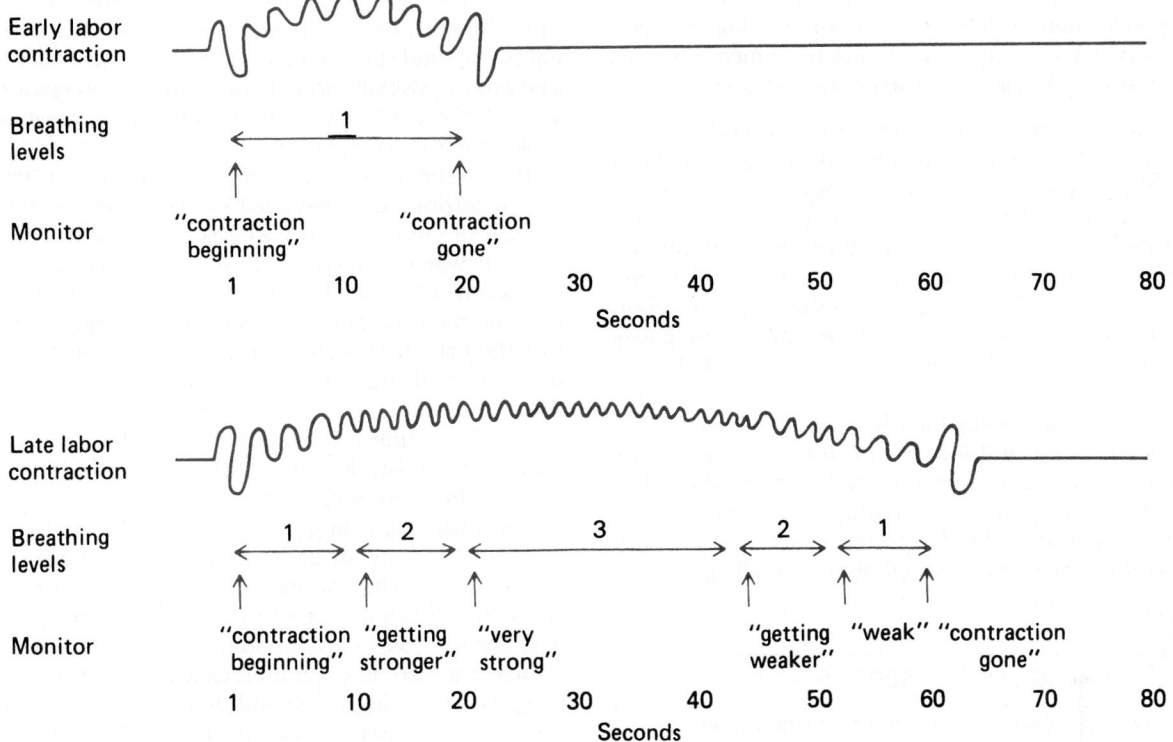

FIGURE 13.6 Example of differing breathing patterns during a single contraction. 1, 2, and 3 are levels of breathing. A cleansing breath is taken at the beginning and end of the contraction.

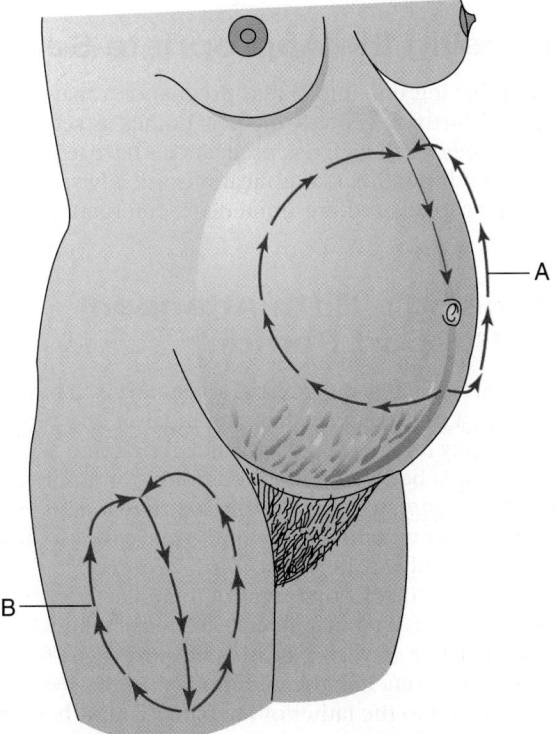

FIGURE 13.7 Effleurage patterns. (**A**) During uterine contractions, a woman traces the pattern on her bare abdomen with her fingers. (**B**) If electronic fetal monitoring is being used, effleurage may be performed on the thigh.

Focusing or Imagery. Focusing intently on an object (sometimes called "sensate focus") is another method of keeping sensory input from reaching the cortex of the brain. A woman brings into labor a photograph of her partner or children, a graphic design, or just something that appeals to her (Fig. 13.8). She concentrates on it during contractions. Be careful not to step into a woman's line of vision during a contraction and break this focused concentration. Other women use imagery by imagining they

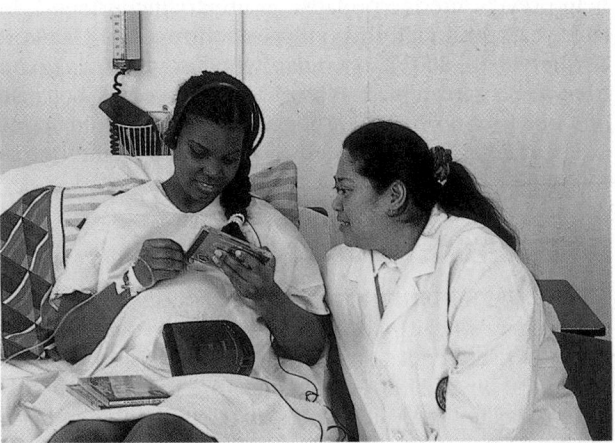

FIGURE 13.8 A woman chooses what object she wishes to focus on during labor. Here, a woman and nurse listen to the taped music the woman will focus on during contractions. (© Barbara Proud.)

are in a calm place such as on a beach watching waves rolling in to them or relaxing on a porch swing (Schardt, 2003). Try not to ask questions or talk to women using this technique or you will break their concentration.

Second-Stage Breathing. During the second stage of labor, when the baby is actually pushed down the birth canal, the type of breathing that is best to use is controversial. In the past, women were told to hold their breath while they pushed. Now it is believed that holding the breath for a prolonged time impairs blood return from the vena cava (a Valsalva maneuver), so this is now discouraged. Teaching women to breathe out while pushing may be helpful. This is called physiologic pushing. Other instructors suggest women breathe any way that is natural for them, except holding their breath.

Women should not practice pushing. The possibility that they would rupture membranes by doing this is too great. They can practice assuming a good position for pushing (squatting, sitting upright, leaning on partner) but should always be cautioned not to actually push.

Checkpoint Question 2

Julia wants to learn Lamaze breathing techniques. What is a principle of Lamaze childbirth?

a. Pain can be interrupted before it registers in the brain as pain.
b. Labor contractions are not pain; they're muscle inflammation.
c. "Brown pain" like labor contractions can be lessened.
d. Labor contractions are intensified by abdominal massage.

Preparation for Cesarean Birth

The fact that cesarean birth may become necessary during labor to ensure a safe birth is covered in most childbirth classes. Cesarean birth is actually offered in some communities to women as an alternative to vaginal birth to help prevent uterine prolapse or urinary incontinence in later years, although this policy is controversial (Minkoff & Chervenak, 2003). A woman who knows she is going to have a cesarean birth as an elective procedure because of a pelvic abnormality or because she is a candidate for a repeat cesarean birth needs additional, specific preparation (see Chapter 20).

THE BIRTH SETTING

The setting for birth that a couple chooses depends on the woman's health and that of her fetus as well as the couple's preferences on how much supervision they desire at the birth. Although hospitals are the usual site for birth today in the United States, that has not always been the case. Up until the late 1800s, childbirth was conducted in the home. Analgesia or anesthesia for childbirth was unpopular until Queen Victoria delivered Prince Leopold under chloroform in 1853. Birth at that point became more complicated and less natural because this extensive level

of anesthesia led to additional interventions. Under anesthesia, women were no longer able to push effectively during the second stage of labor. It became necessary to use a lithotomy position and an episiotomy and forceps for birth as well. Women were asleep for one of the most memorable moments of their life.

Part of the reason for so much anesthesia during birth can be attributed to physicians misinterpreting the type of pain of childbirth. It was assumed that the moment of birth was the major time of discomfort. As a result, women were allowed to labor without any pain medication and then were given anesthesia or analgesia right before the baby was born. In reality, women may not be as uncomfortable during the actual birth as they are during labor. Although the pain felt at birth is intense, it is also over quickly, unlike the hours of labor that precede it. It is also an exhilarating time, directly followed by the reward of the birth of the baby.

Fortunately, birthing practices have changed to better meet women's needs based on their descriptions of the pain of childbirth. If women choose physicians or hospitals who subscribe to more progressive birth practices over the services of more traditional facilities, the overall standard of care in communities leans toward the more progressive settings. The addition of birthing rooms to hospitals in the past 20 years is an example of this. Nurses are in a strong position to advocate for making childbirth a "natural" process in the least restrictive setting possible. At the same time, nurses have a strong responsibility to encourage parents to maintain enough restrictions that birth remains safe.

Choosing the Appropriate Setting

Women having uncomplicated pregnancies may choose hospitals, birthing centers, or their homes as settings for birth. Women with high-risk pregnancies have less choice; women with potential complications are advised to give birth at hospitals, where immediate emergency care is available.

Choosing a Birth Attendant and Support Person

In the United States, most births are supervised by an obstetrician, a physician specializing in labor and birth. As the tendency for specialized physician practice declines, however, it is becoming more common for family medicine practitioners to serve as birth attendants. It is also becoming more common for nurse-midwives to attend births, especially at alternative birth centers.

In addition to selecting who will medically supervise her baby's birth, a woman needs to choose who will support her in labor. In years past, this support was offered by experienced women in the community. In the 1960s, the role was given to the father of the baby. Today, both men and women offer this type of support. In addition to having the father of their baby present, many women choose a doula, or a person specially prepared to assist with birth. Doulas are helpful as fathers may find it hard to provide doula-type support during labor when they are so emotionally involved in the birth. Having such a person present frees the father to enjoy the birth rather than feeling occupied with coaching instructions. Although research in the subject is not extensive, there are suggestions that rates of oxytocin augmentation, epidural anesthesia, and cesarean birth can be reduced by doula support (Bar-Yam, 2003).

Hospital Birth

Advantages and disadvantages of hospital birth are summarized in Box 13.12. The major advantage of a hospital is that supplies and expert personnel are readily available if the mother or fetus or newborn should have a complication.

In evaluating studies that compare the complications of birthing centers or home births to hospitals (women who gave birth in hospitals invariably have more complications than those who give birth in other settings), consider that because high-risk mothers give birth at hospitals, the number of complications in hospital settings is bound to be higher than in other settings.

A woman usually comes to the hospital when her contractions are approximately 5 minutes apart and regular in pattern. If she has preregistered at the hospital, she is admitted to a **birthing room** without any separation time from her support person. Birthing rooms are also called **labor-delivery-recovery rooms** (LDRs) or **labor-delivery-recovery-postpartum rooms** (LDRPs). Such rooms are decorated in a homelike way; couples can bring favorite music or reading materials with them to use during labor; and the bed can be used as a labor bed until birth, when it converts into a **birthing bed** or a lithotomy position bed (Fig. 13.9). Women are expected to use a prepared method of childbirth with a minimum of analgesia and anesthesia (although an advantage of a hospital birth is that anesthesia such as an epidural is readily available if needed). An important aspect of birthing rooms is that the support person and often other family members can stay with a woman throughout labor and birth, allowing the couple and family to feel that they have more control over their birth experience.

At the time of birth, additional cabinets in the room are opened and converted into a space for baby care. Women can choose a birthing position: lithotomy, squatting, supine recumbent, or side-lying. A support person remains with the woman during birth and in some settings can cut the umbilical cord if desired.

Most hospitals screen women in early labor with an external monitor for both fetal heart rate and uterine contractions. If the fetal heart rate is good, such a monitor can usually be removed and used again only for periodic screening as labor progresses. A woman may have intravenous access started as a prophylactic measure. If this is done, the needle should be inserted into a dorsal hand vein so it causes little discomfort and inconvenience for her.

Birthing chairs (Fig. 13.10) are comfortable reclining chairs with a slide-away seat that allows a woman to assume a comfortable position during labor and also furnishes perineal exposure so a birth attendant can assist with the birth. They have the advantage of maintaining a woman in a semi-Fowler's position, a position that acts with gravity and so may speed the second stage of labor.

If a woman chooses to use a supine recumbent position (on her back with knees flexed) rather than a lithotomy position (legs elevated into stirrups) for birth, she uses a birthing bed. Such a position reduces tension on the perineum and may result in fewer perineal tears than with a lithotomy position.

BOX 13.12

Advantages and Disadvantages of Hospital Birth

Advantages
- A woman is encouraged to be prepared to control the discomfort of labor through nonmedication measures such as controlled breathing.
- A woman is encouraged to be knowledgeable about the labor process and make decisions about procedures performed.
- A woman is encouraged to consider breast-feeding to aid uterine contraction and infant bonding.
- Labor, birth, and immediate postpartal care can all be scheduled in a single room.
- A woman is attended by skilled professionals during labor and birth and the postpartal period.
- Emergency care and extended high-risk care are immediately available.

Disadvantages
- Separation of the family for at least one night
- Mother may not feel as much in control of the childbirth experience as she may wish.
- Care may be fragmented, particularly if the woman's physician is not present during the entire labor and birth, or if labor nurses change shifts in the middle of labor. (Many nurse-midwives and physicians make it a point, however, to remain with their client throughout the entire childbirth experience.)

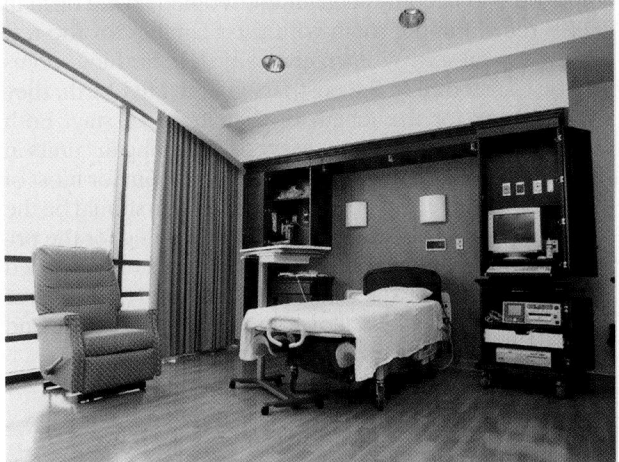

FIGURE 13.9 A birthing (labor-birth-recovery) room designed to maintain a home-like atmosphere in a hospital setting.

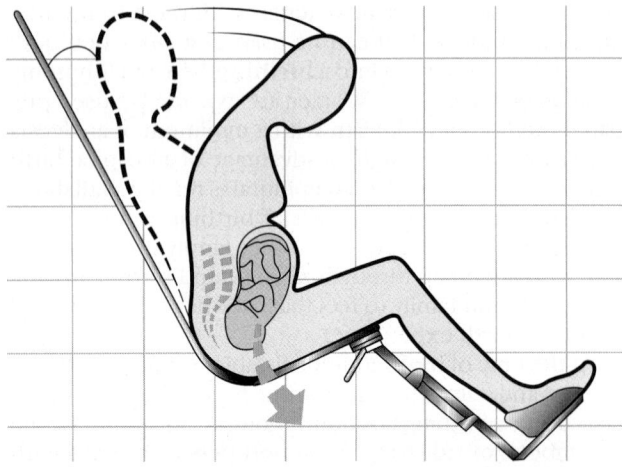

A

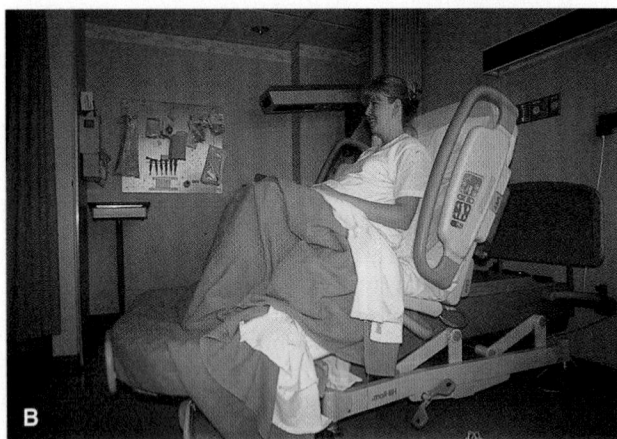

B

FIGURE 13.10 (A) A birthing chair allows the woman to maintain a semi-Fowler's position. **(B)** A birthing chair used during labor. (© Caroline Brown, RNC, MS, DEd.)

Postpartum Care

After birth, encourage mothers to breast-feed immediately. Urge the couple to keep the infant with them so they have ample time to become acquainted. Women giving birth in LDRPs remain in the room with their families for the rest of the hospital stay. Women giving birth in birthing rooms may be transferred to the postpartum unit after birth; they remain there for the length of their hospital stay. Both LDRPs and postpartum units serve as "rooming-in" units in which the infant remains in the mother's room for most of the day. Breast-feeding on demand for infants should be the rule. There should be no restrictions on visiting for the primary support person; in many institutions, a rollaway bed is provided so he or she can remain constantly. Siblings of the newborn should be allowed to visit at least once and touch and become acquainted with the newborn.

Alternative Birthing Centers

Alternative birthing centers (ABCs) are wellness-oriented childbirth facilities designed to remove childbirth from the acute care hospital setting while still providing enough medical resources for emergency care should a

complication of labor and birth arise (Box 13.13). Such a setting is established within or near a hospital, or at least within an easy distance of one. Because it is located outside an acute care setting, where infections abound, the risk of hospital-acquired infection to the mother is thought to be reduced. The birth attendants tend to be nurse-midwives. Women who deliver in ABCs are screened for complications before being admitted. Because women are carefully screened, the mortality rate of mothers and infants is no higher and may be lower in these out-of-hospital settings than in hospital settings.

Like hospitals, ABCs have LDRP rooms where a woman and her support person can invite friends and siblings to participate in the birth. In some centers, a central play area for siblings and cooking facilities are also available. ABCs encourage a woman to express her own needs and wishes during the labor process. A minimum of analgesia and anesthesia is provided, and she can choose a birth position. She can bring her own music or distraction objects, and the partner can perform such tasks as cutting the umbilical cord if he or she chooses. Advantages and disadvantages of ABCs are summarized in Box 13.14.

Women remain in an ABC from 4 to 24 hours after birth. Because a minimum of analgesia or anesthesia is used, a woman recovers quickly after birth and is ready to be discharged this early.

What if... Julia and her husband have a serious disagreement about whether to plan for a home birth or hospital birth? What issues would you suggest they explore? If they cannot agree, how could they compromise?

Home Birth

Home birth is the usual mode of birth in developing countries. Under the supervision of nurse-midwives, it is a popular choice for birth in Europe, but only about 1% of women in the United States choose this method. Home birth may be supervised by a physician, but nurse-midwives are the more likely choice as birth attendants in this setting (Olsen & Jewell, 2005). The Frontier Nursing Service of Kentucky is an example of an organization in the United States that maintains an active and well-accepted program of home birth.

Most women who choose home birth in the United States are well educated and from middle-income families. They choose home birth so they can have the baby close by after birth, can have more control over the childbirth experience, and can give birth in familiar, low-cost surroundings (Hodnett, 2005).

The main advantage of a home birth is that it allows for family integrity: a woman and her family are not separated, so the baby can be immediately integrated into the family (Munday, 2003). On the other hand, it puts the responsibility on a woman to prepare her home for the birth (difficult if she is exhausted toward the end of pregnancy) and to take care of the infant after birth. Some people, however willing, may be unable to take on these roles in a crisis situation such as childbirth. Many women

A Multidisciplinary Care Map for A Family Who Desires Birth at an Alternative Birth Center

●

Julia Marco is pregnant with her second child. During her first pregnancy, she did not attend childbirth classes. She received an epidural for the birth. During a prenatal visit, Julia tells you that she would now like to have a natural birth in a birthing center. She asks you for information on childbirth education courses. Her husband, Joe, wants Julia to go to the hospital and have an epidural like the last time. He insists, "The doctors know what they're doing. We should just let them do their job."

Family Assessment
Family lives with 4-year-old Josh in apartment in central downtown. Julia is a stay-at-home mom; Joe works as a parking garage attendant. Family has limited financial resources, with no medical insurance.

Client Assessment
Pregnancy progressing without evidence of problems or complications. Gravida 2, para 1, 24 weeks' gestation. Client states that she wants to use alternative birth center (ABC); reports concern over previous hospital birth of son. Wants son Josh, now 4 years old, to be a part of new baby's birth. Wants a doula but doesn't know how to contact one. Wants to walk during labor and have a ready supply of "anything chocolate" to eat. No childbirth education classes attended with previous pregnancy; not enrolled in any with this pregnancy at present.

Nursing Diagnosis
Decisional conflict related to choice of birth setting and birth process

Outcome Criteria
Client and partner state advantages and disadvantages of birth setting options; plans for birth and birth setting chosen by 3 weeks.
Client and partner verbalize goal of healthy mother and baby as motivation for choice of birth setting.

Team Member Responsible	Assessment	Intervention	Rationale	Expected Outcome
Activities of Daily Living				
Nurse	Assess the family to see if the couple has a family member to serve as caretaker for son during the birth.	Suggest the couple ask a family member to be caretaker for son during the birth.	A caretaker can enhance the experience for the older child, promoting a positive, family-centered event.	Couple states they have located a suitable caretaker for son.
Consultations				
Nurse midwife	Assess what family expects of a doula for labor.	Give couple list of available doulas in community and help arrange for meeting.	Doulas can offer strong support in labor; pre-arrangements help mutual goals.	Couple confirm they have arranged for a doula to help offer support in labor.

(continued)

Team Member Responsible	Assessment	Intervention	Rationale	Expected Outcome
Consultations				
Nurse/social worker	Investigate the type of birth facilities available in local area in regard to wishes for labor.	Review the requirements, advantages, and disadvantages for birth setting choices available.	Review of options allows the couple to make an informed decision appropriate for their needs.	Client and partner state they understand options available to them.
Procedures/Medications				
Physician/nurse	Determine if there are any contraindications to walking during labor.	Educate client about the few situations, such as placenta previa, that would contradict walking in labor.	Walking during labor has the potential to decrease the time of labor unless contraindicated.	Client states that she will understand the importance of being flexible in regard to wishes in labor based on her and fetal safety.
Nutrition				
Nurse	Assess whether client knows if her chosen food options during labor are approved by local facilities.	Help client modify her goals for nutrition during labor as appropriate based on facility requirements.	As many choices for food exist, coordinating plans with facility should result in least stress during labor.	Client confirms that she has agreed on food type agreeable with chosen agency.
Patient/Family Education				
Nurse	Obtain information about local childbirth education classes available.	Assist couple as necessary with selecting class that fits their resources.	Education can enhance the chances of a positive childbirth experience. Choosing a program that fits the couple's resources helps to promote adherence.	Client attends the chosen preparation for childbirth class before the 38th week of pregnancy.
Nurse	Assess if any classes for sibling preparation for birth are available in community.	Help couple plan for mother and son to attend class on sibling preparation for birth or meet with nurse for instruction.	Adequate preparation for all involved improves the chances of a positive experience.	Couple states that they will either attend a class for sibling preparation or meet with nurse for information.
Psychosocial/Spiritual/Emotional Needs				
Nurse/nurse-midwife	Explore with client and partner past experiences with childbirth and current expectations and beliefs.	Encourage couple to verbalize feelings, concerns, and needs.	Verbalization of feelings permits a safe outlet for emotions and assists in increasing the other person's awareness.	Couple states their overall goal for childbirth is a safe one for mother and new child.
Discharge Planning				
Nurse	Assess if couple has any further questions about birth centers.	Ascertain couple has phone number and directions to chosen birthing center.	Advance planning can help avoid increased stress at time of birth.	Couple states they are happy with birth setting decision and prepared to follow through on plans.
Social worker	Assess the finances the couple will need to complete birth at their chosen setting.	Review financing options with couple.	Advance planning can help avoid increased stress at time of birth.	Couple states they have a plan for financial arrangements.

BOX 13.14

Advantages and Disadvantages of ABCs

Advantages

- A woman is encouraged to be prepared to control the discomfort of labor through non-medication measures such as controlled breathing.
- A woman is encouraged to be knowledgeable about the labor process and to help care providers with decision making.
- A woman is encouraged to breast-feed to aid uterine contraction and infant bonding.
- Family integrity can be maintained because family members may accompany her to the birthing center.
- A woman is attended by skilled professionals during labor and birth.
- Emergency care is immediately available. Extended high-risk care is easily arranged.

Disadvantages

- Extended high-risk care is not immediately available.
- The woman may be fatigued after birth because of early discharge.
- She must independently monitor her postpartal status because of early discharge..

passing through their first postpartum phase, or a "taking-in" phase, may be happier maintaining a dependent passive role than immediately taking responsibility for the infant's care. Advantages and disadvantages of home birth are summarized in Box 13.15.

To be a candidate for a home birth, a woman must be in good health, must be able to adjust to changing circum-

BOX 13.15

Advantages and Disadvantages of Home Birth

Advantages

- A woman is encouraged to become knowledgeable about the birth process and be an active participant in independently reducing the discomfort of labor.
- A woman has the greatest freedom for expressing her individuality.
- There is no separation of the family at birth.

Disadvantages

- Adequate equipment other than first-line emergency equipment is unavailable.
- An abrupt change of goals is necessary if hospitalization is required.
- The woman and support person may become exhausted because of the responsibility placed on them.
- Interference with the "taking-in phase" may occur postpartally because a woman must "take hold."
- A woman must independently monitor her postpartal status.

stances, and must have adequate support people who will sustain her during labor and assist her for the first few days after birth. Women with any complication of pregnancy are not candidates for home birth.

Children Attending the Birth

Most birthing centers and some hospitals allow children to view the birth of a sibling. If older children will be present, a person separate from the main support person needs to be designated to provide entertainment, explanations, food, and a place for them to sleep. Attendance at sibling classes designed to prepare children to witness the birth is often required. The mother must not be expected to provide such supervision during labor, when she becomes introverted and has concern only for herself. A child who is without supervision during this time can remember the experience as a time of rejection rather than an exciting, happy experience.

Help couples consider whether the birth experience will be a positive and enjoyable one for the child. This decision is often based on the child's developmental level. Allowing a child to witness the birth of kittens or puppies might be a more appropriate way to expose a child to birth.

ALTERNATIVE METHODS OF BIRTH

In addition to setting, a number of different methods of childbirth have become popular in the past 15 to 20 years. These include alternative birth methods such as the Leboyer method and birth under water.

Leboyer Method

Frederick Leboyer (1975) is a French obstetrician who postulated that moving from a warm, fluid-filled intrauterine environment to a noisy, air-filled, brightly lit birth room creates a major shock for a newborn. With the **Leboyer method,** the birthing room is darkened so there is no sudden contrast in light; it is kept pleasantly warm, not chilled. Soft music is played, or at least harsh noises are kept to a minimum. The infant is handled gently; the cord is cut late; and the infant is placed immediately after birth into a warm-water bath.

These principles are not drastically different from the usual practice, as infants are always handled gently at birth. Some neonatologists question the wisdom of a warm bath because it could reduce spontaneous respirations and allow a high level of acidosis to occur. Late cutting of a cord can lead to excess blood viscosity in the newborn. Certainly, soft music, gentle handling, and a welcoming atmosphere are important ingredients for all birth attendants to try to incorporate into birth. Providing dim lights (or at least not bright, glaring ones) and providing a warm temperature could be given more consideration in most institutions.

Hydrotherapy and Water Birth

Reclining or sitting in warm water during labor can be soothing; the feeling of weightlessness that occurs under water as well as the relaxation from the warm water both can contribute to reducing discomfort in labor. Using this principle, a number of birthing centers allow women to labor in warm showers or give birth in spa tubs of warm water (McCloghry, 2003). The baby is born underwater and then immediately brought to the surface for a first breath. Some potential difficulties with underwater birth are contamination of the bath water with feces expelled with pushing efforts during the second stage of labor (this could lead to uterine infection in the mother); aspiration of bath water by a fetus, which could lead to pneumonia; and maternal chilling when she leaves the water. Advise women choosing this method that research on the safety and wisdom of the method is ongoing (Cluett et al, 2005).

Checkpoint Question 3

What is a goal of all birth settings?

a. To allow women to eat during labor
b. To keep childbirth pain free
c. To have a safe birth for mother and baby
d. To limit the cost of medical procedures

Key Points

Couples should be encouraged to make a childbirth plan early in pregnancy that includes birth attendant, setting, and any special wishes.

Common exercises taught in pregnancy to strengthen perineal muscles are tailor sitting, squatting, and Kegel exercises. Abdominal muscle-contraction and pelvic rocking exercises strengthen the abdominal muscles and help relieve backache.

Types of childbirth preparation include the Bradley (partner-coached), psychosexual (Kitzinger), Dick-Read, and Lamaze methods. Lamaze is the most common method used in the United States.

Commonly used nonpharmacologic techniques for pain relief in labor are conscious relaxation, consciously controlled breathing, effleurage, focusing, imagery, and hydrotherapy.

Classes for expectant parents provide information on pregnancy, birth, and childcare.

Common sites for childbirth include hospitals, alternative birthing centers, and homes.

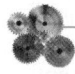

Critical Thinking Exercises

1. Joe Marco, the husband you met at the beginning of the chapter, wants his wife to have their baby at the hospital and have an epidural for pain relief. He insists, "The doctors know what they're doing. We should just let them do their job." After further speaking with Joe, you discover he doesn't want Julia to go through the pain of natural childbirth because he fears he will not be able to help her during labor. How would you convey to Joe that natural childbirth can be a positive experience for him and his wife? How would you assure him that he and Julia can have a safe and active part in the birth of their child?

2. Suppose Julia told you she does not intend to take a preparation for labor class because she wants to have epidural anesthesia as soon as she is admitted to the hospital in labor. Would you advise her to attend a class or not?

3. Suppose Julia wants to have a Leboyer birth. How would you prepare the birthing room?

4. Examine the National Health Goals related to childbirth education. Most government-sponsored money for nursing research is allotted based on these goals. What would be a possible research topic to explore pertinent to these goals that would be applicable to Julia and Joe Marco and also advance evidence-based practice?

References

Bar-Yam, N. B. (2003). Doula care: an age-old practice meets the 21st century. *International Journal of Childbirth Education, 18*(4), 18–21.

Bradley, R. (1981). *Husband-coached childbirth* (3rd ed.). New York: Harper Collins.

Cluett, E. R., et al. (2005). Immersion in water in pregnancy, labour and birth. *The Cochrane Library (Oxford) (2)* (CD000111).

Curl, M., et al. (2004). Overview: childbirth educators, doulas, nurses, and women respond to the six care practices for normal birth. *Journal of Perinatal Education, 13*(2), 42–50.

Department of Health and Human Services. (2000). *Healthy people 2010*. Washington, DC: DHHS.

Dick-Read, G. (1987). *Childbirth without fear: the original approach to natural childbirth* (5th ed.). New York: Harper Collins.

Hodnett, E. D. (2005). Home-like vs. conventional institutional settings for birth. *The Cochrane Library (Oxford) (3)* (CD000012).

Holroyd-Leduc, J. M., & Straus, S. E. (2004). Management of urinary incontinence on women: scientific review. *JAMA: Journal of the American Medical Association, 291*(8), 986–995.

Hotelling, B. A. (2004). Teaching normal birth interactively. *Journal of Perinatal Education, 13*(2), 51–56.

Johnson, M., Maas, M., & Moorhead, S. (2000). *Nursing outcomes classification* (2nd ed.). St. Louis: Mosby.

Kennedy, H. P., & Shannon, M. T. (2004). Keeping birth normal: research findings on midwifery care during childbirth. *JOGNN: Journal of Obstetric, Gynecologic, and Neonatal Nursing, 33*(5), 554–560.

Kitzinger, S. (1990). *The experience of childbirth*. New York: Viking Penguin.

Leboyer, F. (1975). *Birth without violence*. New York: Alfred A. Knopf.

Lu, M. C., et al. (2003). Childbirth education classes: sociodemographic disparities in attendance and the association of attendance with breast-feeding initiation. *Maternal & Child Health Journal, 7*(2), 87–93.

McCloghry, K. (2003). Edgeware Birth Centre: a water birth experience. *British Journal of Midwifery, 11*(5), 314–316.

McCloskey, J., & Bulechek, G. (2000). *Nursing interventions classification* (3rd ed.). St. Louis: Mosby.

Minkoff, H., & Chervenak, F. A. (2003). Elective primary cesarean delivery. *New England Journal of Medicine, 348*(10), 946-950.

Munday, R. (2003). Women's experiences of the postnatal period following planned home birth: a phenomenological study. *MIDIRS Midwifery Digest, 13*(3), 371-375.

Olsen, O., & Jewell, M. D. (2005). Home versus hospital birth. *The Cochrane Library (Oxford) (3)* (CD000352).

Schachman, K. A., Lee, R. K., & Lederman, R. P. (2004). Baby boot camp: facilitating maternal role adaptation among military wives. *Nursing Research, 53*(2), 107-115.

Schardt, D. (2003). Guided imagery: teaching strategies for the childbirth educator. *International Journal of Childbirth Education, 18*(4), 10-12.

Standifird, K. (2003). Teaching teen classes: what works, what doesn't. *International Journal of Childbirth Education, 18*(4), 6-9.

Symon, A., & Lee, J. (2003). Including men in antenatal education: evaluating innovative practice. *Evidence-Based Midwifery, 1*(1), 12-19.

Suggested Readings

Amis, D. (2004). Care practices that promote normal birth #1: Labor begins on it own. *Journal of Perinatal Education, 13*(2), 6-10.

Cooper, T. (2004). Changing the culture: normalising birth. *British Journal of Midwifery, 12*(1), 45-49.

Crenshaw, J. (2004). Care practices that promote normal birth #6: no separation of mother and baby with unlimited opportunity for breast-feeding. *Journal of Perinatal Education, 13*(2), 35-41.

Gagnon, A. J. (2005). Individual or group antenatal education for childbirth/parenthood. *The Cochrane Library (Oxford) (1)* (CD002869).

Hotelling, B., Amis, D., & Green, J. (2004). Care practices that promote normal birth #3: continuous labor support. *Journal of Perinatal Education, 13*(2), 16-22.

Keen, R., DiFranco, J., & Amis, D. (2004). Care practices that promote normal birth #5: non-supine (e.g., upright or side-lying) positions for birth. *Journal of Perinatal Education, 13*(2), 30-34.

Lothian, J., Amis, D., & Crenshaw, J. (2004). Care practices that promote normal birth #4: no routine interventions. *Journal of Perinatal Education, 13*(2), 23-29.

Martell, L. K. (2003). Postpartum women's perceptions of the hospital environment. *JOGNN: Journal of Obstetric, Gynecologic, & Neonatal Nursing, 32*(4), 478-485.

Shilling, T., & DiFranco, J. (2004). Care practices that promote normal birth #2: freedom of movement throughout labor. *Journal of Perinatal Education, 13*(2), 11-15.

van der Hulst, L. A. M., et al. (2004). Does a pregnant woman's intended place of birth influence her attitudes toward and occurrence of obstetric interventions? *Birth, 31*(1), 28-33.

High-Risk Pregnancy: A Woman With a Preexisting or Newly Acquired Illness

Key Terms

deep vein thrombosis
glucose tolerance test
glycosuria
glycosylated hemoglobin
high-risk pregnancy
hyperglycemia
hypoglycemia
megaloblastic anemia
orthopnea
paroxysmal nocturnal dyspnea
peripartal cardiomyopathy
proteinuria
sexually transmitted infections

Objectives

After mastering the contents of this chapter, you should be able to:

1. Define *high-risk pregnancy,* including factors that contribute to its development.
2. Describe common illnesses such as cardiovascular disease, diabetes mellitus, or renal and blood disorders that can result in complications when they exist with pregnancy.
3. Assess a woman with an illness during pregnancy for changes occurring in the illness because of the pregnancy or the pregnancy because of the illness.
4. Formulate nursing diagnoses related to the effect of a preexisting or newly acquired illness on pregnancy.
5. Identify expected outcomes that will contribute to a safe pregnancy outcome when illness occurs with pregnancy.
6. Plan nursing care for a woman with an illness during pregnancy.
7. Implement nursing care for a woman when illness complicates pregnancy.
8. Evaluate expected outcomes to determine achievement and effectiveness of care.
9. Identify National Health Goals related to complications of pregnancy that nurses can help the nation achieve.
10. Identify areas related to illness and pregnancy that could benefit from additional nursing research or application of evidence-based practice.
11. Use critical thinking to analyze ways that nursing care can remain family-centered when a preexisting or newly acquired illness develops.
12. Integrate knowledge of high-risk pregnancy and nursing process to achieve quality maternal and child health nursing care.

*A*ngelina Gomez, a 22-year-old, is pregnant with her first child. She had rheumatic fever with mitral stenosis as a child. She developed gestational diabetes early in this pregnancy. By the 30th week, she has already been hospitalized twice for hyperglycemia. This morning while she was driving to work on the freeway, her compact car was struck by an 18-wheel truck. She has a 3-inch laceration on her right thigh. In the emergency room, her serum glucose level is 207 mg/dL. Her blood pressure is 90/40; her pulse is 130/min; the fetal heart rate is 180/min. An abdominal monitor shows moderate-strength uterine contractions 7 minutes apart. The emergency room physician asks for an ECG to see if her

mitral stenosis is contributing to her low blood pressure. Angelina says to you, "I know everything must be all right. I was wearing my seat belt."

Previous chapters discussed normal pregnancy and the minor discomforts that may occur. This chapter adds information about illnesses and other events that can complicate pregnancy when they occur prior to or during pregnancy.

Does Angelina have a realistic outlook on her condition? Do you think she realizes that pregnancy often becomes high risk not because of any one factor, but an accumulation of them?

After you've studied this chapter, access the accompanying website. Read the patient scenario and answer the questions to further sharpen your skills, grow more familiar with RN-CLEX types of questions, and reward yourself with how much you have learned.

When a woman enters pregnancy with a chronic condition such as cardiovascular or kidney disease, both she and the fetus can be at risk for complications because either the pregnancy can complicate the disease or the disease can complicate the pregnancy, affecting the baby or leaving a woman less equipped to function in the future or undergo a future pregnancy. Nursing care for a woman with a preexisting illness focuses on close observation of maternal health and fetal well-being, education of a woman and her family about danger signs to watch for during pregnancy, and actions to minimize complications whenever possible.

In addition to preexisting illnesses, the pregnant woman, like any other person, may develop non-pregnancy-related illnesses or suffer from trauma during a pregnancy. When this occurs, the illness or injury can adversely affect not only the woman but also the unborn child. Nursing care for the well, pregnant woman focuses on preventing illness and trauma by promoting an especially healthy lifestyle. When accidents and illness occur despite these safeguards, nursing care focuses on:

- Preventing such disorders from affecting the health of the fetus
- Helping the mother regain her health as quickly as possible so she can continue a healthy pregnancy and prepare herself psychologically and physically for labor and birth and the arrival of her newborn

Conditions that cause severe symptoms such as a marked change in fluid and electrolyte balance, altered cardiovascular or respiratory function, or severe blood loss are especially dangerous to a fetus. Some infections, notably toxoplasmosis (see Chapter 11) and some of the sexually transmitted infections, can be just as devastating to the unborn child. National Health Goals related to complications of pregnancy are shown in Box 14.1.

Although pregnancy can be a stressful time, generally women experience overall good health during their pregnancies, perhaps in part because of their extra care and concern in keeping healthy for two. This extra motivation also encourages a woman with a high-risk pregnancy to carefully follow the therapeutic regimen established to keep her and her fetus safe.

BOX 14.1 FOCUS ON . . .

NATIONAL HEALTH GOALS

A number of National Health Goals are aimed at reducing complications of pregnancy that arise from existing or newly acquired disorders. These goals are:

- Reduce the rate of HIV infection in adolescent and young adult females (13 to 24 years of age) to one new case per 100,000 live births, from a baseline of 17 per 100,000.
- Reduce the incidence of gonorrhea to no more than 19 new cases per 100,000 people, from a baseline of 123 per 100,000.
- Reduce the incidence of primary and secondary syphilis to no more than 0.2 cases per 100,000, from a baseline of 3.2 per 100,000.
- Reduce the incidence of genital herpes and genital warts to 14%, from a baseline of 17%.
- Reduce the rate of fetal deaths to 4.1 per 1,000 live births, from a baseline of 6.8 per 1,000.
- Reduce the rate of maternal deaths to 3.3 per 100,000 live births from a baseline of 7.1 per 100,000.
- Reduce the rate of maternal illness during pregnancy to 24 per 100 births, from a baseline of 31.2 per 100 (DHHS, 2000).

Nurses can help the nation reach these goals by educating women about the dangers of and ways to prevent STIs such as syphilis, gonorrhea, and HIV infection. In addition, nurses can help women who have diabetes mellitus understand the importance of prepregnancy care so they enter pregnancy without hyperglycemia, an important effort in reducing congenital anomalies in newborns.

Evidence-based practice and nursing research in areas such as the best way to prevent STIs, how to educate HIV-positive women of the danger of transmitting their infection to a newborn, and specific effects of illnesses on pregnancy or the fetus are needed.

Nursing Process Overview

For Care of a Woman With a Preexisting or Newly Acquired Illness

● *Assessment*

Accurate prenatal assessment of a woman with a preexisting or newly acquired illness requires a thorough understanding of the signs and symptoms of illnesses, such as cardiovascular disease or diabetes mellitus, in addition to an understanding of the course of a normal pregnancy. Assessment techniques include objective measures such as establishing baseline vital signs as well as subjective factors such as the extent of edema or exhaustion (Fig. 14.1). Such assessment is best

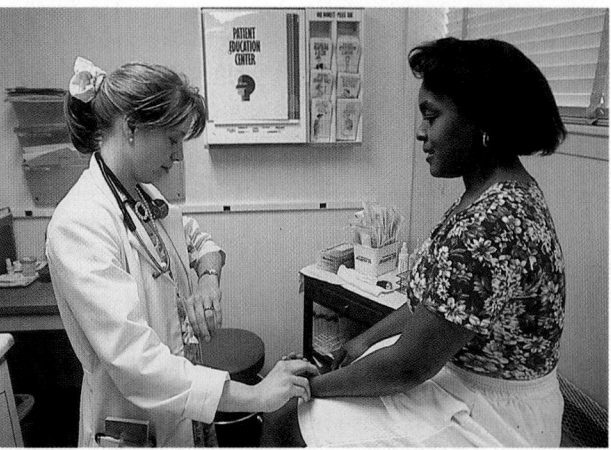

FIGURE 14.1 It is important to establish baseline vital signs in order to later identify a complication related to a preexisting condition. (© Bob Kramer.)

made by the health care personnel who care for a woman consistently throughout the pregnancy so that subtle changes in data can be recognized. In the absence of a consistent care provider, teach a woman to assess her health in relation to objective parameters. She could report exhaustion, for example, in relation to daily activity (e.g., "Two weeks ago I could walk a block without being short of breath. Today I could walk only half a block"; "The last time I was in for a checkup, edema didn't occur until bedtime. Now I notice it every afternoon by the time my son comes home from school").

● *Nursing Diagnosis*

Nursing diagnoses developed for a woman with a high-risk pregnancy address her specific, disease-related condition as well as any therapeutic restrictions her condition might require. Examples of possible nursing diagnoses are:

- Risk for infection transmission related to lack of knowledge of safer sex practices
- Ineffective tissue perfusion (cardiopulmonary) related to poor heart function secondary to mitral valve prolapse during pregnancy
- Pain related to pyelonephritis secondary to pressure on ureters
- Social isolation related to prescribed bed rest during pregnancy secondary to concurrent illness
- Ineffective role performance related to increasing level of daily restrictions secondary to chronic illness and pregnancy
- Knowledge deficit related to normal changes of pregnancy versus illness complications
- Fear regarding pregnancy outcome related to chronic illness
- Health-seeking behaviors related to the effects of illness on pregnancy
- Situational low self-esteem related to diagnosis of HIV infection

● *Outcome Identification and Planning*

Be certain that the expected outcomes established are realistic in light of a woman's pregnancy and the restrictions placed on her by her health. One family member with illness affects all family members; therefore, outcomes should relate to the entire family's health as well.

Try to make plans with a woman who has a pre-existing medical condition based on the pattern of her life before the pregnancy. For example, to ensure that a pregnant woman receives adequate rest during pregnancy, planning for an afternoon rest period a day is usually adequate. However, for a woman with cardiac disease who took two rest periods a day before pregnancy, this could be ineffective because she needs more rest than others. Remember that the additional health supervision needed during pregnancy may involve increased expenses for a family; the family may need to develop new ways to meet these expenses. A primary goal for a woman with a severe chronic condition might be to maintain her health during pregnancy, so she can remain at home as long as

possible, thereby minimizing hospitalization and family disruptions.

Planning after trauma may be difficult for a woman because of the shock of the accident. Be careful, however, not to make plans for her (e.g., "Your best plan would be to allow the doctor to put a cast in place"). Instead, give a woman the available alternatives (e.g., "As the doctor explained, there are two separate therapies for a dislocated knee; let me review with you the advantages and disadvantages of each therapy"). Allowing a woman to choose among alternatives this way helps her to participate in planning care and maintain self-esteem, helping her move a step toward parenthood and assuming care for her family.

● *Implementation*

Nursing interventions for the pregnant woman with a chronic illness may focus on teaching her new or additional measures to maintain health because of the pregnancy. Imaginative solutions to problems may need to be created because the woman may be unable to adjust to the extent of changes she must make.

Provide a pregnant woman who sustains trauma with an opportunity to talk about the event after her emergency care is complete. She may feel guilty that she was not more careful. In some instances, her support person may have been responsible for causing the injury (e.g., by driving carelessly). She may feel both anger at that person's carelessness and yet relief that he or she was not injured and is there to offer support.

A woman and her partner can usually work through these emotions if the pregnancy progresses normally after this point and the fetus was uninjured. If the fetus was injured or the pregnancy disrupted, the event may cause a great deal of stress, and a woman and her partner may need counseling to overcome feelings of guilt and anger about the event.

● *Outcome Evaluation*

If evaluation of outcomes at health care visits reveals that an expected outcome is not being met, new assessment, analysis, and planning need to be done. In some instances, an outcome is not met because a woman did not understand the need for an additional pregnancy measure. In another instance, a woman may need better psychological support to continue to follow a pregnancy routine consistently. Nine months is a long time to adhere to restrictions! Make evaluation ongoing to ensure that you know throughout the pregnancy whether interventions are successful. Some examples of outcomes that might be established are:

- Client states she rests for 2 hours morning and afternoon; dependent edema remains at 1+ or less at next prenatal visit.
- Family members state they are all participating in exercise program since mother developed gestational diabetes.
- Client reports no increase in burning on urination or flank pain at next prenatal visit.

IDENTIFYING THE HIGH-RISK PREGNANCY

A **high-risk pregnancy** is one in which a concurrent disorder, pregnancy-related complication, or external factor jeopardizes the health of the mother, the fetus, or both.

Some women enter pregnancy with a chronic illness that, when superimposed on the pregnancy, makes it high risk. Other women enter pregnancy in good health but then develop a complication of pregnancy that causes it to become high risk. In some instances, a combination of particular circumstances—poverty, lack of support people, poor coping mechanisms, genetic inheritance, or past history of pregnancy complications—can cause a pregnancy to be categorized as high risk (Box 14.2).

In most instances, more than one factor contributes to the classification of a pregnancy as high risk. The pregnancy of a woman who is diabetic, for example, is automatically termed one with greater than normal risk because the fetus is growing in an environment in which **hyperglycemia** (increased serum glucose levels) is the rule. During her pregnancy, the woman, worrying that something will happen to her baby, may fail to begin the "pregnancy work" that she must do so bonding can take place. At birth, her child is in double jeopardy: not only is the baby born with an illness, but he or she also is at high risk for poor maternal–child attachment.

A preterm infant born to a teenage girl, likewise, has a double problem. Not only is the infant immature (and at risk for all the complications that accompany immaturity), but also he or she has a mother who often is immature as well (see Chapter 17 for discussion of the special needs of the pregnant adolescent).

Table 14.1 lists common psychological, social, and physical factors that can cause a pregnancy to be categorized as high risk. Categorizing the risks as minimal, moderate, or extensive differs with each woman because of her individual coping mechanisms and level of support. For example, a woman living in extreme poverty who does not have access to community support would be at high risk for poor nutritional intake during pregnancy, whereas a woman with a similar income who could depend on a nutritional assistance program such as WIC and counseling from a community health nurse might be only at minimal risk.

Remembering that the term "high risk" rarely refers to just one causative factor helps in the planning of holistic and ultimately effective nursing care. Box 14.3 highlights appropriate outcomes and interventions related to high-risk pregnancy care using the terminology identified by the Nursing Outcomes Classification (NOC) and Nursing Interventions Classification (NIC).

Preexisting or newly acquired maternal illnesses that can make a pregnancy high risk are covered in this chapter. Chapter 15 discusses pregnancy-related conditions that can make a pregnancy high risk. Chapter 17 covers populations that are at high risk due to age (younger than 18 years or older than 40 years), the presence of a disability, or drug abuse.

SEXUALLY TRANSMITTED INFECTIONS AND PREGNANCY

Sexually transmitted infections (STIs) are those that are spread through sexual contact with an infected partner. This chapter provides a brief overview of those STIs most important to identify during pregnancy because of their potential effect on the pregnancy, fetus, or newborn. Chapter 26 discusses additional specific care for the newborn.

All STIs can be prevented to some extent by the use of safer sex practices (see Chapter 4), including use of a condom during sexual relations. Little disease immunity is developed against a STI once it has been contracted, so it is possible to become reinfected if preventive measures are not followed. In most instances, an infected partner should also be treated or the disease can recur from cross-infection.

Treatment of most STIs begins with determining the causative organism so that the appropriate antimicrobial or antifungal agent can be prescribed. Women need to be educated about the mode of transmission for these diseases and about measures to reduce the vulvar or vaginal irritation they frequently cause.

BOX 14.2 FOCUS ON . . .

DIVERSITY OF CARE

An illness during pregnancy can complicate not only a pregnancy but also a woman's entire lifestyle and that of her family. Women who think of pregnancy as a time of wellness may have a great deal of difficulty accepting a medical regimen such as daily blood glucose monitoring because this is contradictory to their primary belief about pregnancy. Women in extended families may have an easier time accepting hospitalization during pregnancy than those living in nuclear families, because more people are available to take over their role at home. Conversely, women in extended families may have more difficulty with hospitalization because more people are depending on them to be at home.

Assessing all families individually and asking about the effect on the entire family of an illness during pregnancy helps to identify problems and can lead to timely problem solving.

NURSING DIAGNOSES AND RELATED INTERVENTIONS

Nursing Diagnosis: Pain related to vulvar irritation secondary to existence of STI

Outcome Evaluation: No vaginal discharge or pruritus is present by history or examination. Client reports she is using safer sex practices.

TABLE 14.1

Factors That Categorize a Pregnancy as High Risk

Psychological	Social	Physical
Prepregnancy		
History of drug dependence (including alcohol)	Occupation involving handling of toxic substances (including radiation and anesthesia gases)	Visual or hearing challenges
History of intimate partner abuse		Pelvic inadequacy or misshape
History of mental illness	Environmental contaminants at home	Uterine incompetency, position, or structure
History of poor coping mechanisms	Isolated	Secondary major illness (heart disease, diabetes mellitus, kidney disease, hypertension, chronic infection such as tuberculosis, hemopoietic or blood disorder, malignancy)
Cognitively challenged	Lower economic level	
Survivor of childhood sexual abuse	Poor access to transportation for care	Poor gynecologic or obstetric history
	High altitude	History of previous poor pregnancy outcome (miscarriage, stillbirth, intrauterine fetal death)
	Highly mobile lifestyle	History of child with congenital anomalies
	Poor housing	Obesity
	Lack of support people	Pelvic inflammatory disease
		History of inherited disorder
		Small stature
		Potential of blood incompatibility
		Younger than age 18 years or older than 35 years
		Cigarette smoker
		Substance abuser
Pregnancy		
Loss of support person	Refusal of or neglected prenatal care	Subject to trauma
Illness of a family member	Exposure to environmental teratogens	Fluid or electrolyte imbalance
Decrease in self-esteem		Intake of teratogen such as a drug
Drug abuse (including alcohol and cigarette smoking)	Disruptive family incident	Multiple gestation
Poor acceptance of pregnancy	Decreased economic support	A bleeding disruption
	Conception less than 1 year after last pregnancy or pregnancy within 12 months of the first pregnancy	Poor placental formation or position
		Gestational diabetes
		Nutritional deficiency of iron, folic acid, or protein
		Poor weight gain
		Pregnancy-induced hypertension
		Infection
		Amniotic fluid abnormality
		Postmaturity
Labor and Delivery		
Severely frightened by labor and delivery experience	Lack of support person	Hemorrhage
Inability to participate due to anesthesia	Inadequate home for infant care	Infection
Separation of infant at birth	Unplanned cesarean birth	Fluid and electrolyte imbalance
Lack of preparation for labor	Lack of access to continued health care	Dystocia
Birth of infant who is disappointing in some way (e.g., sex, appearance, or congenital anomalies)	Lack of access to emergency personnel or equipment	Precipitous birth
		Lacerations of cervix or vagina
Illness in newborn		Cephalopelvic disproportion
		Internal fetal monitoring
		Retained placenta

BOX 14.3

Nursing Outcomes Classification (NOC) and Nursing Interventions Classification (NIC)

High-Risk Pregnancy

NOC: Fetal status, Antepartum

Fetal status, antepartum is defined as the conditions indicating fetal physical well-being from conception to the onset of labor (Johnson, Maas, & Moorhead, 2000). Some specific indicators that suggest that this outcome has been achieved include the following:

- Fetal heart rate within range of 120 to 160 beats per minute
- Fetal ultrasound growth measurements, movement frequency, and movement pattern within expected range
- Variability and deceleration patterns in electronic fetal monitor findings within expected parameters

NOC: Maternal status, Antepartum

Maternal status, antepartum is defined as the conditions and behaviors indicating maternal well-being from conception to the onset of labor (Johnson, Maas, & Moorhead, 2000). Some specific indicators that suggest that this outcome has been achieved include the woman's ability to:

- Demonstrate emotional attachment to the fetus
- Cope with discomforts of pregnancy
- Exhibit neurologic reflexes, vital signs, urine protein and glucose, blood glucose, hemoglobin levels,

and other laboratory test results as indicated within expected parameters

NIC: High-risk pregnancy care

High-risk pregnancy care is defined as the identification and management of a high-risk pregnancy to promote healthy outcomes for the mother and baby (McCloskey & Bulechek, 2000). Some important activities involved when implementing this intervention include:

- Determining factors related to poor pregnancy outcomes, including medical risk factors, past pregnancy risk factors, and social and demographic risk factors
- Identifying the woman's knowledge base about potential risk factors
- Providing education to minimize risk factors in conjunction with usual prenatal teaching and self-care activities
- Referring to appropriate support programs as needed
- Instructing on the use of self-monitoring techniques and procedures, including medication therapy
- Providing written guidelines for signs and symptoms that require immediate attention

A Woman With Candidiasis

Candidiasis, a vaginal infection spread by the fungus *Candida,* is so common that as many as 90% of women will have it sometime in their lifetime (Young & Jewell, 2005). It results in a thick vaginal discharge that resembles cream cheese and is extremely pruritic. The vagina appears red and irritated. Candidiasis occurs more frequently during pregnancy than normally because of the increased estrogen level present during pregnancy, which causes the vaginal pH to be less acidic. It also occurs frequently in women being treated with an antibiotic for another infection, in women with gestational diabetes, and in women with HIV infection. Women with repeated infections should have their urine tested for glucose to determine whether gestational diabetes is present.

The disease is diagnosed by microscopic analysis of the vaginal discharge mounted on a wet slide. It is treated by the vaginal application of an over-the-counter antifungal cream such as miconazole (Monistat) for 7 days or a single dose of oral fluconazole (Diflucan) (Scharbo-DeHaan & Anderson, 2003). Treating the infection during pregnancy is important because the profuse vaginal discharge and pruritus can be very uncomfortable. In addition, if infection is present in the vagina at the time of childbirth, it may cause a candidal infection, or thrush, in the newborn (see Chapter 43). Caution pregnant women to telephone their pri-

mary health care provider before using an over-the-counter product to be certain the product is safe to use during pregnancy and also so that her primary care provider can know that a vaginal infection is occurring (Eschenbach, 2003).

A Woman With Trichomoniasis

Trichomoniasis is an infection caused by a single-cell protozoan spread by coitus. A woman notices a yellow-gray, frothy, odorous vaginal discharge. The infection is diagnosed by examination of vaginal secretions on a wet slide that has been treated with potassium hydroxide (KOH) or by a vaginal culture. It is important that trichomoniasis infections be identified and treated because they may be associated with preterm labor, premature rupture of membranes, and post-cesarean infection. The drug of choice is single-dose oral metronidazole (Flagyl) (Scharbo-DeHaan & Anderson, 2003). Metronidazole was once thought to be teratogenic, but the CDC now confirms it is safe in either early or late pregnancy (CDC, 2002).

A Woman With Bacterial Vaginosis

Bacterial vaginosis is local infection of the vagina by the invasion of, most commonly, *Gardnerella vaginalis* organisms. The associated discharge is gray and has a fishy odor. Pruritus may be intense. The treatment is oral metronidazole (Flagyl) or clindamycin for 7 days. Untreated *G. vaginalis* infections are associated with amniotic fluid infections and, perhaps, preterm labor as well as premature rupture of the membranes (Eschenbach, 2003).

A Woman With Chlamydia

Chlamydia is one of the most common types of vaginal infections seen in both pregnant and nonpregnant women. Usually, screening for this infection via a vaginal culture is done during a woman's first prenatal visit. If a woman has multiple sexual partners, screening may be repeated again in the third trimester. The infection, caused by a gram-negative intracellular parasite, causes a heavy, gray-white vaginal discharge. Diagnosis is made by culture of the organism from vaginal secretions using a specific chlamydia culture kit. Therapy for nonpregnant women is usually with doxycycline (Vibramycin), a tetracycline. This is contraindicated during pregnancy because of possible fetal long-bone deformities; azithromycin (Zithromax) or amoxicillin (Amoxil) is used instead (Eschenbach, 2003). A woman's partner also should be treated to prevent her from becoming reinfected. There is a strong association between gonorrhea and chlamydia; therefore, if a chlamydia infection is documented, women are usually tested for gonorrhea as well.

Chlamydia infections must be treated because they are associated with premature rupture of the membranes, preterm labor, and endometritis in the postpartum period. An infant who is born while a chlamydia infection is present in the vagina can suffer conjunctivitis or pneumonia after birth (see Chapters 40 and 50). Long-term effects of chlamydia infections in the mother are pelvic inflammatory disease, possibly leading to infertility (Scharbo-DeHaan & Anderson, 2003).

A Woman With Syphilis

Syphilis is a systemic disease caused by the spirochete *Treponema pallidum.* It is currently increasing in frequency in the United States. The first stage of syphilis results in a painless ulcer (chancre) on the vulva or vagina. Early in pregnancy (before week 18), the placenta appears to provide some protection against the disease. After this time, however, the spirochete crosses the placenta freely and may be responsible for spontaneous miscarriage, preterm labor, stillbirth, or congenital anomalies in the newborn (see Chapter 26). All pregnant women are screened for syphilis at a first prenatal visit by a VDRL, ART, or FTA-ABS antibody reaction test. Those who have multiple sexual partners are tested again at about week 36 of pregnancy. In some institutions, women are screened again at the beginning of labor and newborns are screened for congenital syphilis by a cord blood sample.

One injection of benzathine penicillin G is the drug of choice for the treatment of syphilis during pregnancy (Eschenbach, 2003). After therapy, a woman may experience a sudden episode of hypotension, fever, tachycardia, and muscle aches. This is called a Jarisch-Herxheimer reaction and is caused by the sudden destruction of spirochetes. The reaction lasts about 24 hours and then fades (Pons, 2004).

A Woman With a Herpes Simplex Virus Type 2 Infection

Genital herpes infection is caused by the herpes simplex virus (HSV) type 2. There may be a genetic susceptibility to the herpes virus, as some women appear to be more prone to infection than others. The first time a woman contracts a herpes infection, painful, small, pinpoint vesicles on an erythematous base develop on her vulva or in the vagina, accompanied by a low-grade fever 3 to 7 days after exposure. Although the symptoms fade in a few days, the virus remains in local nerve ganglions, becoming activated again any time she has a break in the skin or also possibly by stress.

If a woman has a primary infection, herpes can be transmitted across the placenta to cause congenital infection in the newborn. If a woman has primary or secondary active lesions in the vagina or on the vulva at the time of birth, herpes infection can be transmitted to the newborn at birth. When infection in the newborn occurs, congenital herpes, a severe systemic infection that is often fatal, can result (see Chapter 26). To help avoid transmission, women with active lesions are scheduled for cesarean birth. If no lesions are present, a vaginal birth is preferable (Minkoff & Gibbs, 2003).

Diagnosis is made by the appearance of the lesions, Pap smear, and enzyme-linked immunosorbent assay (ELISA). The drug of choice for the treatment of herpes infection is oral acyclovir (Zovirax) or valacyclovir (Valtrex) (Karch, 2004). Women can reduce the pain of the lesions by taking sitz baths or applying warm, moist tea bags to the area. Condom use by a woman's partner or by a woman (female condom) is strongly urged to prevent transmission of the virus to a woman's partner.

A Woman With Gonorrhea

Gonorrhea is an STI caused by the gram-negative coccus *Neisseria gonorrhoeae.* A yellow-green vaginal discharge may be present, or a woman may be asymptomatic. Her male partner usually has severe symptoms of pain on urination and a purulent yellow penile discharge. Despite safer sex practices and effective therapy, this disease still spreads at an epidemic rate in young adults.

Gonorrhea is associated with spontaneous miscarriage, preterm birth, and endometritis in the postpartum period. It is also a major cause of pelvic inflammatory disease (PID) and infertility. Diagnosis of gonorrhea is made by culture of the organism from the vagina, rectum, or urethra. Although gonorrhea has traditionally been treated with amoxicillin and probenecid, the incidence of penicillinase-producing strains has made this traditional therapy ineffective. Therefore, oral cefixime (Suprax) or intramuscular ceftriaxone (Rocephin) is the current recommended therapy. Sexual partners also should be treated to prevent reinfection. Because most people who contract gonorrhea also have a chlamydial infection, nonpregnant women should receive doxycycline therapy at the same time. If a woman is pregnant, she should receive amoxicillin or azithromycin. It is

shoveling snow. Make certain a woman's definition of "heavy work" is the same as yours and her physician's or nurse-midwife's.

Many women with heart disease need two rest periods a day (fully resting, not getting up frequently to answer the door or telephone) and a full night's sleep (not tossing and turning because of excess noise or heat in the room) to obtain adequate rest. Rest should be in the left lateral recumbent position to prevent supine hypotension syndrome and increased heart effort.

Promote Healthy Nutrition. A woman with cardiac disease may need closer supervision of nutrition during pregnancy than does the average woman because she must gain enough weight to ensure a healthy pregnancy and a healthy baby, but she must not gain so much weight that she has to supply additional cells with nutrients. This could overburden her heart and circulatory system.

Be certain she is taking her prenatal vitamins. These contain an iron supplement to help prevent anemia. Anemia places an extra burden on the heart because it requires the body to circulate blood more vigorously to distribute oxygen to all body cells. If a woman was following a sodium-restricted diet before pregnancy, this may be continued during pregnancy, although typically a woman's sodium intake is only limited, not severely restricted, during pregnancy. Sodium is necessary for maintaining fluid volume and balance and thus is necessary to allow a woman's body to retain enough blood volume to supply blood to the placenta.

Educate Regarding Medication. Women taking cardiac medication before pregnancy may need to increase their maintenance dose because of their expanded blood volume during pregnancy. A woman who needed digoxin before pregnancy for heart action will continue to require it (and can take it safely) during pregnancy. A woman who was not digoxin-dependent before pregnancy may need such therapy prescribed as pregnancy advances and her cardiac output has to be increased or strengthened. To aid a woman in continuing to think of herself as a fully functioning person, help her to understand that this does not mean her heart function is weakening, but rather that it is being stressed further by the increased circulatory load of pregnancy. Digoxin is sometimes administered to a woman during pregnancy to slow the fetal heart if fetal tachycardia is present. Propranolol (Inderal), a beta-adrenergic blocker frequently used to treat cardiac arrhythmias, is a pregnancy category C drug (unstudied in pregnancy) but apparently does not cause fetal abnormalities. Nitroglycerin, a compound often prescribed for angina, is also a category C drug but is apparently safe (Karch, 2004).

A woman who was taking penicillin prophylactically after rheumatic fever to prevent a recurrence (often taken for 10 years after the occurrence of rheumatic fever, or at least until age 18 years) should continue to take this drug during pregnancy because penicillin is not known to be a fetal teratogen (a category B drug). Close to the anticipated day of birth, some physicians begin a course of an antibiotic such as penicillin for women with heart disease. This is because the postpartum period always involves some mild invasion of bacteria from the denuded placental site on the uterus into the bloodstream. Since this invading bacteria may be streptococci, the bacteria often responsible for subacute bacterial endocarditis, a course of ampicillin, amoxicillin (Amoxil), or clindamycin (Cleocin) at this time offers women needed protection (Reimold & Rutherford, 2003).

It is often difficult to keep healthy women from taking over-the-counter medicines during pregnancy; conversely, it can be just as difficult to encourage them to take the medicine they need during pregnancy. Help women with heart disease to understand that there are valid exceptions to the rule of "no medicine during pregnancy."

Educate Regarding Avoidance of Infection. A systemic infection almost automatically increases body temperature, causing a woman to have to expend more energy and increase her cardiac output, an insult that could be too extreme for a woman with heart disease to withstand. Caution a woman with heart disease to avoid visiting or being visited by people with infections. She should alert health care personnel at the first indication of an upper respiratory tract infection or UTI so that, if warranted, antibiotic therapy can be begun early in the course of the infection. Monthly screening for bacteriuria with a clean-catch urine test may be recommended.

What if... Angelina tells you she has abruptly discontinued the daily penicillin she has been taking for her heart disease since childhood? What would you recommend she do?

Nursing Interventions During Labor and Birth

The anesthetic of choice during labor for women with heart disease is an epidural, because this can make both labor and birth less taxing. Many women with heart disease should not push with contractions; pushing requires more effort than they should expend. If an epidural anesthetic is used, low forceps or a vacuum extractor can be used for birth. A woman may be disappointed that her birth is not more "natural." Stress that these measures can help her achieve her ultimate goals, which are a healthy newborn and a mother able to care for her new baby.

Monitor fetal heart rate and uterine contractions during labor in all women with heart disease. Assess a woman's blood pressure, pulse, and respirations frequently. A rapidly increasing pulse rate (more than 100 bpm) is an indication that a heart is pumping ineffectively and has increased its rate in an effort to compensate. Advise a woman to assume a side-lying position to reduce the possibility of supine hypotension syndrome. If she has some pulmonary edema, it may be necessary for her to have her chest and head elevated (semi-Fowler's position) to ease the work of breathing. Remember, fatigue is a symptom of heart decompensation. If this occurs in labor, evaluate the client carefully to determine whether the fatigue is heart- or labor-related.

Postpartum Nursing Interventions

The period immediately after birth may be a critical time for a woman with heart disease. With delivery of the placenta, the blood that supplied the placenta is now released into the general circulation, subsequently increasing her blood volume 20% to 40%. During pregnancy, the increase in blood volume occurred over a 6-month period, so the heart had time to adjust to this change gradually. After birth, the increase in pressure takes place within 5 minutes, so the heart must make a rapid and major adjustment.

If a woman is in severe congestive heart failure after birth, she needs a program of decreased activity and possibly anticoagulant and digoxin therapy until her circulation stabilizes. Antiembolic stockings and ambulation may be needed to increase venous return from the legs. If prophylactic antibiotics had not been started prior to birth, they will be started immediately after birth to discourage subacute bacterial endocarditis caused by introduction of microorganisms through the placental site.

A woman with heart disease is often interested in close inspection of her baby immediately after birth because she wants to know her infant does not have a heart defect or was not harmed by any medication she took. Be sure to point out that acrocyanosis is normal in newborns, so she does not interpret her baby's severe peripheral cyanosis as cardiac inadequacy.

In the postpartum period, agents to encourage uterine involution such as oxytocin (Pitocin) must be used with caution because they tend to increase blood pressure, and this necessitates increased heart action. As a rule, a woman with heart disease can breast-feed without difficulty. Kegel exercises are acceptable for perineal strengthening immediately, but the woman should not begin postpartum exercises to improve abdominal tone until her physician or nurse-midwife approves them. A stool softener can be prescribed to prevent straining with bowel movements.

Before discharge, be certain a woman has thought through what help she will need at home so she can continue getting periods of rest. Also ensure that she schedules a return appointment for a postpartum checkup for both her gynecologic health and her cardiac status.

What if... Angelina tells you she tries to eat absolutely no salt in an attempt to limit ankle edema and to keep her heart symptoms to a minimum? What would you do?

A Woman With an Artificial Valve Prosthesis

Once, women with heart valve prostheses were advised not to become pregnant. Today, caring for a woman with a valve prosthesis during pregnancy would not be unusual (Elkayam et al., 2004). One potential problem involves the use of oral anticoagulants that a woman takes to prevent the formation of clots at the valve site (Reimold & Ruther-

ford, 2003). Because these medications may increase the risk of congenital anomalies in infants (pregnancy risk category D), women are usually placed on heparin therapy before becoming pregnant to reduce this risk. Heparin does not cross the placenta and so does not interfere with fetal development or fetal coagulation (category C). Subclinical bleeding from the anticoagulant in the mother can cause placental dislodgement. Observe a woman who is taking an anticoagulant for signs of premature separation of the placenta during pregnancy and labor.

A Woman With Chronic Hypertensive Vascular Disease

Women with chronic hypertensive disease come into pregnancy with an elevated blood pressure (140/90 mm Hg or above). Hypertension of this kind is usually associated with arteriosclerosis or renal disease, making it a problem of the older pregnant woman. Chronic hypertension places the mother and fetus at high risk because fetal well-being can be compromised by poor placental perfusion during the pregnancy (Malee, 2003). Management is similar to that of a woman with pregnancy-induced hypertension (see Chapter 15).

A Woman With Venous Thromboembolic Disease

The incidence of venous thromboembolic disease increases during pregnancy due to a combination of stasis of blood in the lower extremities from uterine pressure and hypercoagulability (the effect of increased estrogen; Box 14.7). When the pressure of the fetal head at birth puts additional pressure on lower extremity veins, damage can occur to the walls of vessels. When this triad of effects is in place (stasis, vessel damage, and hypercoagulation), the stage is set for thrombus formation in the lower extremities. The likelihood of **deep vein thrombosis** (DVT) leading to pulmonary emboli increases for women 30 years of age or older because increased age is yet another risk factor for thrombosis formation (Colman-Brochu, 2004).

A woman notices pain and redness usually in the calf of a leg. The risk of thrombus formation can be reduced through common-sense measures such as avoiding the use of constrictive knee-high stockings, not sitting with legs crossed at the knee, and avoiding standing in one position for a long period. If a thrombus does occur during pregnancy, it is diagnosed by a woman's history and Doppler ultrasonography. A woman will be treated with bed rest and intravenous heparin for 24 to 48 hours. After this, she may be prescribed subcutaneous heparin every 12 or 24 hours for the duration of the pregnancy. It is generally recommended that the lower abdomen be used for rotating sites for subcutaneous heparin administration. With pregnancy, however, this site is usually avoided and the injection sites are limited to the arms and thighs. Heparin dosage is regulated by frequent partial thromboplastin time (PTT) determinations. Additional measures of care for a woman with DVT, such as heat, elevation, and bed rest, are discussed in Chapter 25 because 50% of thromboses that occur with pregnancy occur in the postpartum period.

Women taking heparin during pregnancy should not take any additional injections once labor begins to help re-

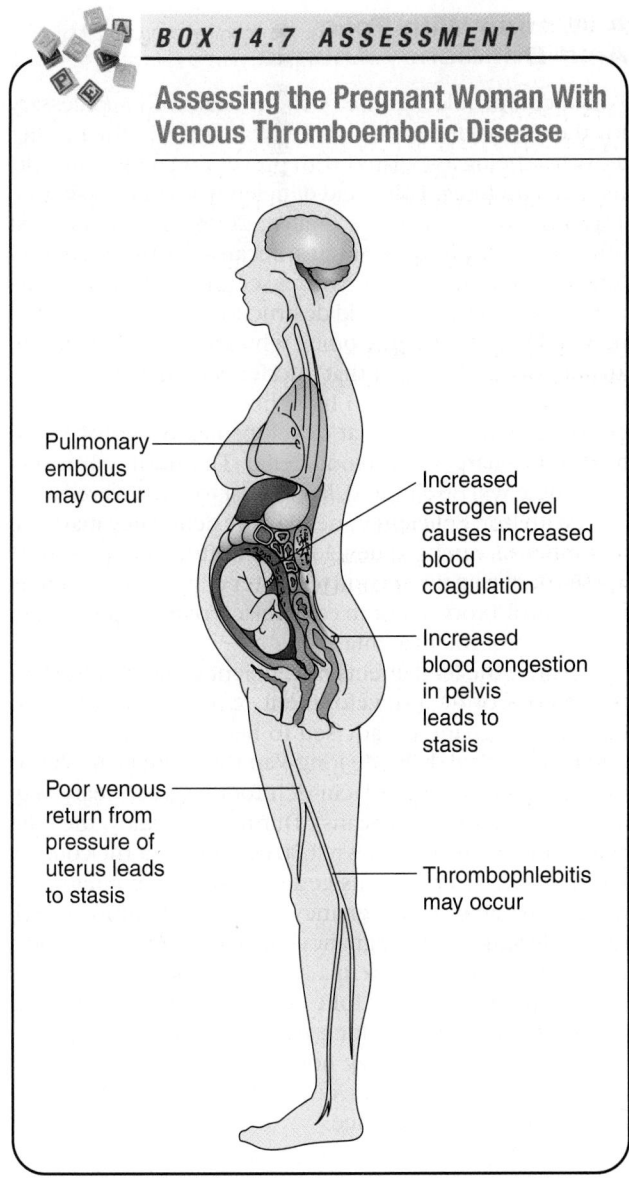

BOX 14.7 ASSESSMENT

Assessing the Pregnant Woman With Venous Thromboembolic Disease

Pulmonary embolus may occur

Increased estrogen level causes increased blood coagulation

Increased blood congestion in pelvis leads to stasis

Poor venous return from pressure of uterus leads to stasis

Thrombophlebitis may occur

A particular group of women has been identified as being more susceptible to thrombi formation, spontaneous miscarriage, fetal death, and hypertension of pregnancy: women with antiphospholipid antibodies (aPLA) (Carp, 2004). It is not known why aPLA occurs in some women and not in others, but these antibodies probably represent an autoimmune process. Women who are identified as aPLA positive may be started on a prophylactic program of aspirin or subcutaneous heparin during pregnancy that is continued postpartum to reduce the possibility of DVT. Administration of a corticosteroid may help to reduce the formation of additional antibodies and so may also be prescribed. After pregnancy, such women should not begin an oral contraceptive because it can increase blood coagulation and the possibility of thrombi formation.

The chief danger of thrombophlebitis is pulmonary embolism or a clot lodging in the pulmonary artery and blocking circulation to the lungs and heart. Symptoms of pulmonary embolism include:

- Chest pain
- Sudden onset of dyspnea
- Cough with hemoptysis
- Tachycardia or missed beats
- Severe dizziness or fainting from lowered blood pressure

Pulmonary embolism needs to be recognized as it is an immediate emergency (McRae & Ginsberg, 2004). Care measures for this are discussed in Chapter 15.

HEMATOLOGIC DISORDERS AND PREGNANCY

Hematologic disorders during pregnancy involve either blood formation or coagulation disorders.

Anemia and Pregnancy

Because the blood volume expands during pregnancy slightly ahead of the red cell count, most women have a pseudoanemia of early pregnancy. This condition is normal and should not be confused with true types of anemia that can occur as complications of pregnancy.

duce the possibility of hemorrhage at birth; they are not candidates for routine episiotomy or epidural anesthesia for this same reason unless at least 4 hours has passed since the last heparin dose was given. PTT determinations should be continued during labor. Either heparin or sodium warfarin (Coumadin) administration can be prescribed after birth.

Checkpoint Question 2

Angelina develops a deep vein thrombosis following an auto accident and is prescribed heparin subq. What should you educate her about in regard to this?

a. Her infant will be born with scattered petechiae on his trunk.
b. Heparin can cause darkened skin in newborns.
c. Heparin does not cross the placenta and so does not affect a fetus.
d. Some infants will be born with allergic symptoms to heparin.

NURSING DIAGNOSES AND RELATED INTERVENTIONS

Nursing Diagnosis: Risk for ineffective tissue perfusion related to maternal anemia during pregnancy.

Outcome Evaluation: Client's hemoglobin is above 12 mg/dL; fetal heart rate is 120 to 160 bpm; client takes prenatal supplement daily.

A Woman With Iron-Deficiency Anemia

Iron-deficiency anemia is the most common anemia of pregnancy, complicating as many as 15% to 25% of all pregnancies (Malee, 2003). Many women enter pregnancy with a deficiency of iron stores resulting from a diet low in iron, heavy menstrual periods, or unwise weight-reducing programs. Iron stores are apt to be low in women who were pregnant less than 2 years before the current pregnancy or those from low socioeconomic levels who have not had iron-rich diets. When the hemoglobin level is below 12 mg/dL (hematocrit under 33%), iron deficiency is suspected. It is confirmed by a corresponding low serum iron level and an increased iron-binding capacity.

Iron is made available to the body by absorption from the duodenum into the bloodstream after it is ingested. In the bloodstream, it is bound to transferrin for transport to the liver, spleen, and bone marrow. At these sites, it is incorporated into hemoglobin or stored as ferritin.

Iron-deficiency anemia is characteristically a microcytic (small red blood cell), hypochromic (less hemoglobin than the average red cell) anemia because when an inadequate supply of iron is ingested, iron is unavailable for incorporation into red blood cells. Both hematocrit and hemoglobin will be reduced (under 33% and 12 mg/dL, respectively). The serum transferrin level will be under 100 mg/dL, the transferrin saturation level will be under 5%, the serum iron level will be under 30 μg/dL, and the mean corpuscular hemoglobin concentration will be under 30; iron-binding capacity, in contrast, will be increased (over 400 μg/dL). Iron-deficiency anemia is mildly associated with low birthweight and preterm birth (Mungen, 2003). Because the body recognizes that it needs increased nutrients, some women develop pica, or the craving and eating of substances such as ice or starch. A woman experiences extreme fatigue and poor exercise tolerance because she can not transport oxygen effectively.

To prevent this common anemia, women should take prenatal vitamins containing an iron supplement of 60 mg elemental iron as prophylactic therapy during pregnancy. In addition, they need to eat a diet high in iron and vitamins (green leafy vegetables, meat, legumes, fruit). Women who develop iron-deficiency anemia will be prescribed therapeutic levels of medication (120 to 180 mg elemental iron/day), usually in the form of ferrous sulfate or ferrous gluconate. Iron is best absorbed from an acid medium. Therefore, advise women to take iron supplements with orange juice or a vitamin C supplement. If they are not already enrolled in a WIC program but are eligible, making a referral could help ensure a better diet. When women begin to take a prescribed iron supplement, new red blood cells should begin to increase, or their reticulocyte counts should rise from a normal range (0.5% to 1.5%) to 3% to 4% by 2 weeks' time. Some women report constipation or gastric irritation when taking oral iron supplements. Increasing roughage in the diet and always taking the pills with food help reduce these symptoms.

If iron-deficiency anemia is severe and a woman has difficulty with oral iron therapy, intramuscular or intravenous iron dextran can be prescribed.

A Woman With Folic Acid-Deficiency Anemia

Folic acid, or folacin, one of the B vitamins, is necessary for the normal formation of red blood cells in the mother as well as being associated with preventing neural tube defects in the fetus. Folic acid-deficiency anemia is seen in 1% to 5% of pregnancies (Malee, 2003). It occurs most often in multiple pregnancies because of the increased fetal demand; in women with a secondary hemolytic illness in which there is rapid destruction and production of new red blood cells; in women who are taking hydantoin, an anticonvulsant agent that interferes with folate absorption; and in women who have been taking oral contraceptives. The anemia that develops is a **megaloblastic anemia** (enlarged red blood cells). The mean corpuscular volume will be elevated, in contrast to the lowered level seen with iron-deficiency anemia. The deficiency may take a number of weeks to develop, so it often becomes most apparent during the second trimester of pregnancy. It may be a contributory factor in early miscarriage or premature separation of the placenta.

Because the fetal effects of deficiency occur in the first few weeks of fetal development, women expecting to become pregnant are advised to begin a supplement of 400 μg folic acid daily (de Jong-Van Den Berg et al., 2005) in addition to eating folacin-rich foods (green leafy vegetables, oranges, dried beans). During pregnancy, the folic acid requirement increases to 600 μg/day. Over-the-counter multivitamin preparations generally do not contain adequate folic acid for pregnancy, whereas vitamins specifically designed for pregnancy do. Women who develop folic acid-deficiency anemia are prescribed even higher or therapeutic levels of folic acid. At prenatal visits, ask whether a woman is taking her prescribed vitamin. To save money, women may not have a prescription filled and may be using over-the-counter, less expensive types, not aware of the difference.

A Woman With Sickle Cell Anemia

Sickle cell anemia is a recessively inherited hemolytic anemia caused by an abnormal amino acid in the beta chain of hemoglobin. If the abnormal amino acid replaces the amino acid valine, sickle hemoglobin (HbS) results; if it is substituted for the amino acid lysine, non-sickling hemoglobin (HbC) results. An individual who is heterozygous (has only one gene in which the abnormal substitution has occurred) has the sickle cell trait (HbAS). If the person is homozygous (has two genes in which the substitution has occurred), sickle cell disease (HbSS) results.

With the disease, the majority of red blood cells are irregular or sickle-shaped so cannot carry as much hemoglobin as normally shaped red blood cells. When oxygen tension becomes reduced, as happens at high altitudes, or blood becomes more viscid than usual (dehydration), the cells tend to clump because of the irregular shape. This clumping can result in vessel blockage with reduced blood flow to organs. The cells then will hemolyze, reducing the number available and causing a severe anemia.

Approximately 1 in every 10 African Americans has the sickle cell trait (i.e., carries a recessive gene for S hemoglobin but is asymptomatic); theoretically, 1 in every 400 African Americans has the disease. Although the sickle cell trait does not appear to influence the course of pregnancy, prematurity, miscarriage, or perinatal mortality rates of these may be higher for women with the homozygous disease (Serjeant et al., 2004). Women with the trait do seem to have an increased incidence of asymptomatic bacteriuria, resulting in an increased incidence of pyelonephritis.

At any time in life, sickle cell anemia is a threat to life if vital blood vessels such as those to the liver, kidneys, heart, lungs, or brain become blocked. In pregnancy, blockage to the placental circulation can directly compromise the fetus, causing low birthweight and possibly fetal death.

Assessment. All African-American women who have not been previously tested should be screened for sickle cell anemia at a first prenatal visit. Hemoglobin levels for all women with sickle cell disease should be obtained throughout pregnancy. A woman with sickle cell disease may normally have a hemoglobin level of 6 to 8 mg/100 mL. Unless she receives active interventions to raise this level, she will maintain it during pregnancy, reducing oxygen to the fetus. Hemolysis in a sickle cell crisis may occur so rapidly that a woman's hemoglobin level can fall to 5 or 6 mg/100 mL in a few hours. There is an accompanying rise in her indirect bilirubin level because she cannot conjugate the bilirubin released from so many red blood cells so quickly destroyed.

Because a pregnant woman with sickle cell anemia is more susceptible to bacteriuria than other women, a clean-catch urine sample is collected periodically during pregnancy to detect developing bacteriuria while a woman is still asymptomatic.

Throughout pregnancy, monitor a woman's diet to be certain she is consuming sufficient amounts of folic acid and possibly an additional folic acid supplement, which may be necessary to build new red blood cells. Her fluid intake should also be carefully monitored. She should consume at least eight glasses of fluids daily. Early in pregnancy, when she may be nauseated, her fluid intake can easily decrease, and dehydration and a subsequent sickle cell crisis may occur.

Assess a woman's lower extremities at prenatal visits for varicosities or pooling of blood in leg veins, which are apt to occur from uterine pressure as pregnancy advances. Such pooling and pressure can lead to red cell destruction. Standing for long periods during the day increases this pressure, whereas sitting on a chair with the legs elevated or lying on the side in a modified Sims' position encourages venous return from the lower extremities. Help a woman plan her day so she has limited long periods of standing and adequate rest periods.

Fetal health is usually monitored during pregnancy by an ultrasound examination at 16 to 24 weeks to assess for intrauterine growth restriction and by weekly nonstress or ultrasound examinations beginning at about 30 weeks. Blood flow through the uterus and placenta may be measured by blood flow velocity. If blood flow velocity is reduced, the chance of intrauterine growth restriction is increased.

Therapeutic Management. Interventions to prevent sickle cell crisis can include periodic exchange transfusions throughout pregnancy to replace sickled cells with normal cells. An exchange transfusion serves a secondary purpose of removing a quantity of the increased bilirubin resulting from the breakdown of red blood cells as well as restoring the hemoglobin level (Malee, 2003). If a crisis occurs, controlling pain, administering oxygen as needed, and increasing the fluid volume of the circulatory system to lower viscosity are important interventions (see Chapter 44 for further discussion of therapy of sickle cell anemia). The fluid administered is often hypotonic (0.45 saline) to keep plasma tension low because of the difficulty a woman has concentrating urine to remove large amounts of fluid. As a rule, women with sickle cell disease are not given an iron supplement during pregnancy. The cells cannot incorporate iron in the usual manner that normal cells can, so excessive iron buildup may result. Women do need a folic acid supplement to keep the new cells produced from being megaloblastic (Katz, 2003).

If a woman develops an infection that raises her temperature and causes her to perspire more than normally (creates dehydration) or contracts a respiratory infection that compromises air exchange so that her PO_2 is lowered, hospitalization for observation may be necessary to rule out the development of a sickle cell crisis and subsequent hemolysis of crowded cells.

When the fetus is mature, the time and method of birth are individualized. Keep a woman well hydrated in labor. If an operative birth is necessary, she generally receives nerve block anesthesia rather than a general anesthetic to avoid the threat of hypoxia.

Women generally are interested in determining at birth whether their child has inherited the disease. Because the disorder is recessively inherited, if one of the parents has the disease and the other is free of the disease and trait, the chances that the child will inherit the disease are zero. If a woman has the disease and her partner has the trait, the chances that the child will be born with the disease are 50% (see Chapter 7). If both parents have the disease, all their children will also have the disease.

Symptoms of sickle cell disease do not become clinically apparent until the child's fetal hemoglobin has converted to a largely adult pattern (in 3 to 6 months). Fetal hemoglobin is composed of two alpha and two gamma chains; adult hemoglobin is composed of two alpha and two beta chains. Because the sickle cell trait is carried on the beta chain, it will not be manifested clinically until this chain appears. Electrophoresis of red blood cells obtained during fetal life by percutaneous umbilical blood sampling or amniocentesis, however, can reveal the presence of the disease on the few beta chains already present in utero. Newborns have approximately 15% adult hemoglobin at birth, so electrophoresis testing at birth can also reveal if the disease is present. Screening is routine in some settings. Nursing care of the child with sickle cell disease is discussed in Chapter 44.

Coagulation Disorders and Pregnancy

Most coagulation disorders are sex-linked or occur only in males and so have little effect on pregnancies. However, von Willebrand disease is a coagulation disorder inherited as an autosomal dominant trait that does occur in women. From the time she was a child, a woman would have noticed menorrhagia or frequent episodes of epistaxis. If these symptoms were not severe, though, the condition may go undiagnosed until pregnancy, when a woman experiences a spontaneous miscarriage or postpartum hemorrhage.

Women with the disorder have normal platelet counts, but bleeding time is prolonged. Levels of factor VIII-related antigen (VIII-R) and factor VIII coagulation activity (VIII-C) are both reduced. Replacement of these factors by infusion of cryoprecipitate or fresh-frozen plasma may be necessary before labor to prevent excessive bleeding.

Hemophilia B (Christmas disease, factor IX deficiency) is a sex-linked disorder, so the actual disease occurs only in males. However, female carriers may have such a reduced level of factor IX (only 33% of normal) that hemorrhage with labor or a spontaneous miscarriage can be a serious complication. Carriers of the disorder need to be identified before pregnancy. Restoration of factor IX levels can be done by infusion of factor IX concentrate or fresh-frozen plasma.

Percutaneous umbilical blood sampling can be used to detect whether a male fetus has hemophilia. If there is a family history of hemophilia, before an internal fetal heart rate monitor is attached or fetal scalp blood sampling is done during labor, the fetal status needs to be determined. If the fetus has a coagulation disorder, these procedures would be contraindicated because they could result in extensive fetal blood loss.

Idiopathic thrombocytopenic purpura (ITP), a decreased number of platelets, can occur at any time of life and occasionally occurs during pregnancy. The cause of the condition is unknown, but it is assumed to be an autoimmune illness (an antiplatelet antibody that destroys platelets is apparently released). Symptoms of the illness usually occur shortly after a viral invasion such as an upper respiratory infection (Malee, 2003).

Without an adequate level of platelets, minute petechiae or large ecchymoses appear on a woman's body. Frequent nosebleeds may occur. Laboratory studies reveal a marked thrombocytopenia (platelet count may be as low as 20,000/mm³ from a normal count of 150,000 mm³).

The illness typically runs a 1- to 3-month limited course, but because the symptoms are similar to pregnancy-induced hypertension with HELLP syndrome, a serious complication of pregnancy (see Chapter 15), they are frightening when they occur during pregnancy. A platelet transfusion or plasmapheresis may be administered to temporarily increase the platelet count. Oral prednisone is also effective. Women with the phenomenon need to be identified during pregnancy because the decreased platelet count can lead to increased bleeding at birth. In addition, the antiplatelet factor can cross the placenta and cause accompanying platelet destruction in the newborn, or allow the newborn to be born with the illness (see Chapter 44 for care of the child with ITP).

Checkpoint Question 3

Which statement by a woman with sickle-cell anemia would alert you she may need further instruction on prenatal care?

a. I understand why folic acid is important for red cell formation.
b. I'm careful to drink at least eight glasses of fluid every day.
c. I take an iron pill every day to help grow new red blood cells.
d. I've stopped jogging so I don't risk becoming dehydrated.

RENAL AND URINARY DISORDERS AND PREGNANCY

Adequate kidney function is important to a successful pregnancy outcome because a woman is excreting waste products not only for herself but also for the fetus. This dual function makes any condition that interferes with kidney or urinary function potentially serious.

A Woman With a Urinary Tract Infection

As many as 4% to 10% of nonpregnant women have asymptomatic bacteriuria (organisms are present in the urine without symptoms of infection). In the pregnant woman, because the ureters dilate from the effect of progesterone, stasis of urine occurs. The minimal glucosuria that occurs with pregnancy allows more than the usual number of organisms to grow. This causes asymptomatic urinary tract infections (UTIs) in as many as 10% to 15% of pregnant women (Morgan, 2004). Asymptomatic infections are dangerous because they can progress to pyelonephritis (infection of the pelvis of the kidney) and are associated with preterm labor and premature rupture of membranes. Women with known vesicoureteral reflux (backflow of urine into the ureters) tend to develop UTIs or pyelonephritis more often than others do. The organism most commonly responsible for UTI is *Escherichia coli* from an ascending infection. A UTI can also occur as a descending infection, or begin in the kidneys from the filtration of organisms present from other body infections. If the infectious organism is determined to be streptococcus B, vaginal cultures should be obtained because streptococcal B infection of the genital tract is associated with pneumonia in newborns.

Assessment

A UTI typically is manifested by frequency and pain on urination. With pyelonephritis, a woman develops pain in the lumbar region (usually on the right side) that radiates downward. The area feels tender to palpation. She may have accompanying nausea and vomiting, malaise, pain, and frequency of urination. Her temperature may be elevated only slightly or may be as high as 103° to 104°F (39° to 40°C). The infection usually occurs on the right side because there is greater compression and urinary stasis on the right ureter from the uterus being pushed that way by the large bulk of the intestine on the left side. A urine culture will reveal over 100,000 organisms per milliliter of urine, a level diagnostic of infection.

Therapeutic Management

Obtain a clean-catch urine sample for culture and sensitivity on women with possible symptoms of UTI (see Chapter 10). Many health care agencies ask women for clean-catch urine specimens at intervals during pregnancy (tested by a rapid dipstick method) to detect infection before it becomes symptomatic. A sensitivity test after a culture will determine which antibiotic needs to be prescribed to combat the infection. Amoxicillin, ampicillin, and cephalosporins are effective against most organisms causing UTIs and are considered safe antibiotics during pregnancy. The sulfonamides can be used early in pregnancy but not near term because they can interfere with protein binding of bilirubin, which then leads to hyperbilirubinemia in the newborn. Tetracyclines are contraindicated in pregnancy; they cause retardation of bone growth and staining of the fetal teeth (Karch, 2004).

NURSING DIAGNOSES AND RELATED INTERVENTIONS

———●———

Nursing Diagnosis: Risk for infection related to stasis of urine with pregnancy

Outcome Evaluation: Oral temperature is below 100.4°F (38°C), and a clean-catch urine specimen has a bacteria count below 100,000 colonies per milliliter.

All women during pregnancy can be reminded of common measures to prevent UTIs, such as:

- Voiding frequently (at least every 2 hours)
- Wiping front to back after bowel movements
- Wearing cotton, not synthetic fiber, underwear
- Voiding immediately after sexual intercourse

The pregnant woman with a UTI needs to take some additional measures, such as drinking an increased amount of fluid to flush out the infection from the urinary tract. Do not merely tell her to "push fluids" or "drink lots of water." Give her a specific amount to drink every day (up to 3 to 4 L per 24 hours) to make certain she does increase her fluid intake sufficiently.

A woman can promote urine drainage by assuming a knee–chest position for 15 minutes morning and evening. In this position, the weight of the uterus is shifted forward, releasing the pressure on the ureters and allowing urine to drain more freely.

If a woman has one UTI during pregnancy, the chances are high that she will develop another late in pregnancy, when urinary stasis tends to be even greater. She may, therefore, be kept on prophylactic antibiotics throughout the remainder of the pregnancy. Ask at prenatal visits whether she is continuing to take this type of prophylactic medicine. When women have pain and symptoms of urinary frequency, they take medication well. When they no longer have any clinical evidence they are sick, their compliance rate, like any other adult's, begins to fall dramatically. A woman may need to post a chart on her refrigerator door or in her bathroom to remind herself to take the medication. Leaving the medicine on a counter to remind herself to take it is not a good habit to develop because soon she will have a new baby in the house; encourage her to keep medicine out of sight and reach to get into the habit of "childproofing" even at this early stage.

Pyelonephritis is an extension of a urinary tract infection or infection that originates or spreads to the kidney (Millar, DeBuque, & Wing, 2003). A woman may be hospitalized for 24 to 48 hours while she is treated with intravenous antibiotics. After this acute episode, she will be maintained on a drug such as oral nitrofurantoin (Macrodantin) for the remainder of the pregnancy. Acidifying urine by the use of ascorbic acid (vitamin C), which is often recommended in nonpregnant women, is not usually recommended during pregnancy because the newborn can develop scurvy in the immediate neonatal period from withdrawal.

After birth, a woman who developed more than one UTI may have an intravenous pyelogram or sonogram scheduled to help detect any urinary tract abnormality that might be present, such as vesicoureteral reflux, to help prevent future infections.

A Woman With Chronic Renal Disease

In the past, females with chronic renal disease did not reach childbearing age or were advised not to have children because of their high risk during pregnancy. Today, women with chronic renal disease are having children because pregnancy does not appear to cause progressive deterioration of kidney lesions. With conscientious prenatal care, even women who have had renal transplants can expect to have healthy pregnancies and healthy children (Basaran et al., 2004).

Women with chronic renal disease may develop severe anemia during pregnancy because their diseased kidneys do not produce erythropoietin, which is necessary for red cell formation. Fortunately, synthetic erythropoietin is now available and is safe to take during pregnancy (Karch, 2004).

Because the glomerular filtration rate normally increases during pregnancy, a woman's serum creatinine level may be actually slightly below normal during pregnancy. The normal serum creatinine level is 0.7 mg/100 mL; during pregnancy, it falls to about 0.5 mg/100 mL. Women with kidney disease who normally have a serum creatinine level of more than 2.0 mg/dL may be advised not to undertake a pregnancy lest the increased strain on already damaged kidneys leads to kidney failure.

Many women with renal disease routinely take a corticosteroid (prednisone) at a maintenance level. This drug therapy typically is continued throughout pregnancy. Although animal studies have shown an increased incidence of cleft palate from corticosteroid use during pregnancy, this does not appear to be true in humans. However, the infant may be hyperglycemic at birth because of the suppression of insulin activity by corticosteroids.

In many women, it is difficult to interpret kidney function during pregnancy based on nonpregnant values (Box 14.8). Trace amounts of glucose and protein in the urine are common during pregnancy because of increased glomerular permeability, so **proteinuria** (protein in urine)

must be compared to a woman's individualized prepregnancy level to be meaningful. If a woman is told proteinuria may occur during pregnancy, she will understand it is an expected change of pregnancy, not a forecast of changing kidney function. Many women with renal disease have elevated blood pressure. To be meaningful, their blood pressure levels during pregnancy must also be compared with prepregnancy levels.

Although successful pregnancy in women with kidney transplants is to be expected, women should be considered individually to determine whether they will be able to carry a pregnancy to term before a pregnancy is initiated. Criteria to be evaluated include:

- A woman's general health and the time since the transplant (preferably more than 2 years)
- Serum creatinine level
- The presence of proteinuria or hypertension or signs of graft rejection
- Medications taken to reduce graft rejection

It is helpful if the drugs a woman is taking are limited to prednisone and azathioprine (an antimetabolite [Imuran], but with no reports of fetal compromise from its use). Women with severe renal disease may require dialysis to aid kidney function during pregnancy (Eroglu et al., 2004). This is associated with a risk of preterm labor, perhaps because progesterone is removed with the dialysis. To prevent this complication, progesterone may be administered intramuscularly before dialysis. If hemodialysis is used, it should be scheduled frequently and for short durations to avoid acute fluid shifts. The heparin administered in connection with hemodialysis is safe during pregnancy because it does not cross the placenta. Even in light of the expanding uterine size, peritoneal dialysis is actually preferred over hemodialysis because it normally causes less drastic fluid shifts. This can be accomplished on an ambulatory basis (continuous ambulatory peritoneal dialysis) throughout pregnancy.

Women with renal disease need a great deal of support during pregnancy. They are aware that kidneys are vital for life and that the stress of pregnancy on damaged kidneys may cause them to fail. They are aware that by being pregnant they are risking not only the life of the child growing inside them but also their own life. They may need extra support and information to know how their fetus is doing. They may need extra time with their infant at birth for bonding because they may have been too concerned during pregnancy to begin this process.

RESPIRATORY DISORDERS AND PREGNANCY

Respiratory diseases range from mild (the common cold) to severe (pneumonia) to chronic (tuberculosis). Any respiratory condition can worsen in pregnancy because the rising uterus compresses the diaphragm, reducing the size of the thoracic cavity and available lung space. Any respiratory disorder can pose serious hazards to the fetus if allowed to progress to the point where the mother's oxygen–carbon dioxide exchange is altered or the mother or fetus cannot receive enough oxygen.

BOX 14.8 ASSESSMENT

Assessing the Pregnant Woman With Renal Disease

Elevated blood pressure from poor kidney function

Flank pain, if pyelonephritis is present

Proteinuria in urine; frequency and burning on urination and bacteriuria if urinary tract infection is present

Elevated serum creatinine from decreased kidney function

Edema from inability of kidneys to evacuate fluid

NURSING DIAGNOSES AND RELATED INTERVENTIONS

Nursing Diagnosis: Risk for ineffective breathing pattern related to respiratory changes during pregnancy

Outcome Evaluation: Respiratory rate is 16 to 20 per minute, PO$_2$ is above 80 mm Hg, PCO$_2$ is below 40 mm Hg, and fetal heart rate is 120 to 160 bpm with good variability.

A Woman With Acute Nasopharyngitis

Acute nasopharyngitis (common cold) tends to be more severe during pregnancy than at other times because during pregnancy, estrogen stimulation normally causes some degree of nasal congestion. This means that even with a minor cold, a woman can find it difficult to breathe. Aspirin should be avoided as a cold remedy during pregnancy because of possible interference with blood clotting in both mother and fetus and the possibility of prolonged pregnancy at term (Karch, 2004). Because common colds are invariably caused by a virus, antibiotic therapy is unnecessary except to prevent a secondary infection. Although most simple cough syrups contain no ingredients that would make them unsafe for use during pregnancy, women should check with their health care provider before taking any over-the-counter medication for a cold (Box 14.9).

A Woman With Influenza

Influenza is caused by a virus, identified as type A, B, or C. The disease spreads in epidemic form and is accompanied by high fever, extreme prostration, aching pains in the back and extremities, and generally a sore, raw throat. Contrary to early reports, influenza infection has not been clearly correlated with congenital anomalies in children or found to be a cause of preterm labor (Malee, 2004). Treatment includes an antipyretic such as acetaminophen (Tylenol) to control fever. Oseltamivir (TamiFlu), a new antiviral drug that is category C, should be used cautiously until its long-term effects are known (Karch, 2004). Because influenza vaccines are made from killed virus, women may be immunized safely against influenza during pregnancy (Harper et al., 2004).

A Woman With Pneumonia

Pneumonia is the bacterial or viral invasion of lung tissue by pathogens such as *S. pneumoniae, Haemophilus influenzae,* and *Mycoplasma pneumoniae.* After the invasion, an acute inflammatory response occurs with exudate of red blood cells, fibrin, and polymorphonuclear leuko-

BOX 14.9 FOCUS ON . . .

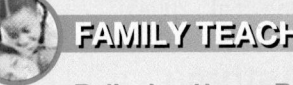

FAMILY TEACHING

Relieving Upper Respiratory Symptoms During Pregnancy

Q. Angelina tells you, "I get a lot of colds. What should I do to keep down symptoms during pregnancy?"

A. Use the following guidelines to help combat common cold symptoms during pregnancy:

- Be sure to get extra rest and sleep and eat a light diet high in vitamin C (orange juice and fruit) to help boost the immune system.
- If you experience any aches and pains, take acetaminophen (Tylenol) every 4 hours.
- Use a room humidifier, especially at night, to moisten nasal secretions and help mucus drain.
- Use only over-the-counter cough drops or syrups that contain natural ingredients such as honey and lemon to help reduce coughing.
- Apply a medicated vapor rub to your chest if you prefer to help relieve nasal congestion.
- Use cool or warm compresses to relieve sinus headaches. Check with your health care provider regarding the use of over-the-counter cough drops, syrups, or decongestants.

cytes into the alveoli. This process confines the bacteria or virus within segments of the lobes of the lungs but also fills alveoli with fluid, blocking off breathing space. If the collection of fluid is extreme, it can limit the oxygen available to the fetus. Therapy usually involves the use of an appropriate antibiotic and perhaps oxygen administration. With severe disease, ventilation support may be necessary. There is a tendency for women with pneumonia late in pregnancy to begin preterm labor (Lim, Macfarlane, & Colthorpe, 2003). If pneumonia is present during labor, oxygen should be administered so the fetus has adequate oxygen resources during contractions.

A Woman With Severe Acute Respiratory Syndrome (SARS)

Severe acute respiratory syndrome (SARS) is a newly emerged infectious disease with the clinical symptoms of persistent fever, chills, muscle aches, malaise, dry cough, headache, and dyspnea. Common laboratory findings are decreased lymphocyte and platelet counts. A coronavirus has been identified as the pathogen responsible for the illness, which appears to have originated in southern China and has spread to become a worldwide pandemic (Hu et al., 2004). SARS spreads by close person-to-person contact via droplet transmission. The incubation period is 2 to 10 days. Therapy is vigorous, with intravenous antibiotics; many people needed respiratory support to survive. SARS during pregnancy creates such an acute illness that it is associated with high incidences of spontaneous miscarriage, preterm delivery, and intrauterine growth restriction. There is no evidence of perinatal SARS infection among infants born to these mothers (Wong et al., 2004).

A Woman With Asthma

Asthma is a disorder marked by reversible airflow obstruction, airway hyperreactivity, and airway inflammation. It complicates about 1% of pregnancies and is associated with an increased risk of perinatal complications (Redding & Stoloff, 2004). Symptoms are often triggered by an irritant (e.g., an inhaled allergen such as pollen or smoke). With inhalation of the allergen, there is an immediate release of bioactive mediators such as histamine and leukotrienes from an IgE/immunoglobulin interaction. This results in constriction of the bronchial smooth muscle, marked mucosal inflammation and swelling, and the production of thick bronchial secretions. These three processes cause a marked reduction in the size of the lumen of air passages. A woman has difficulty pulling in air; on exhalation, she has so much difficulty releasing air that she makes a high-pitched whistling sound (bronchial wheezing) from air being pushed past the bronchial narrowing. Asthma has the potential of reducing the oxygen supply to the fetus if a major attack should occur during pregnancy. Although many women find that their asthma improves during pregnancy due to the high circulating levels of corticosteroids that are present, women with asthma have a higher rate of preterm birth and intrauterine growth restriction than other women. A woman should check with her physician or nurse-midwife about the safety of the medications she routinely takes for this disorder before pregnancy to be certain it will be safe to continue using them during pregnancy and breast-feeding.

The inhaled corticosteroids beclomethasone (Beclovent, Vancenase) and budesonide (Pulmicort, Rhinocort) are commonly used by women with persistent asthma and are the best choice for pregnant women and those who might become pregnant. Women who have been taking a corticosteroid during pregnancy may need parenteral administration of hydrocortisone during labor because of the added stress during this time. Beta-adrenergic agonists such as terbutaline and albuterol may be taken safely during pregnancy, but because they have the potential to reduce labor contractions the dosage is tapered close to term if possible (Karch, 2004).

Women may use cromolyn sodium (Intal), a mast cell stabilizer, to help prevent symptoms. Many adolescents with asthma are prescribed leukotriene receptor antagonists such as montelukast sodium (Singulair) or zafirlukast (Accolate). These are oral medications (pregnancy category B) and so may be continued during pregnancy.

A Woman With Tuberculosis

Tuberculosis is a disease that should have been eradicated in view of the effective treatment available. However, in highly populated areas, the incidence has actually increased and in some areas is at epidemic proportions. Worldwide, it is still one of the leading causes of death (Neralla & Glassroth, 2003).

With tuberculosis, lung tissue is invaded by *Mycobacterium tuberculosis,* an acid-fast bacillus. Macrophages and T lymphocytes surround the bacillus, but rather than actually killing it they merely surround and confine it. Fibrosis, calcification, and a final ring of collagenous scar tissue develop, effectively sealing off the organisms from the body and any further invasion or spread. Antibodies developed will thereafter cause a positive response when tested such as with the Mantoux (purified protein derivative [PPD]) test.

Assessment

In high-risk areas, women should undergo skin testing (a PPD test) at their first prenatal visit. A follow-up chest x-ray can be done for women who show positive reactions. Women need to be cautioned that a positive reaction does not necessarily mean they have the disease; it can mean they have at some time been exposed to tuberculosis and so have antibodies in their system. A chest x-ray to confirm the diagnosis can be done safely during pregnancy if a woman's abdomen is shielded. Symptoms of tuberculosis include:

- Chronic cough
- Weight loss
- Hemoptysis (coughing blood)
- Night sweats
- Low-grade fever
- Chronic fatigue

Therapeutic Management

Women with active tuberculosis need treatment during pregnancy. Isoniazid (INH) and ethambutol hydrochloride (Myambutol), the drugs of choice for tuberculosis, may be given without apparent teratogenic effects. INH may result in a peripheral neuritis if a woman does not take supplemental pyridoxine (vitamin B_6) as well. Ethambutol may cause optic nerve involvement (optic atrophy and loss of green color recognition) in the mother. To detect this, test a woman monthly using the color section of a Snellen (eye test) chart. If symptoms develop, advise her to discontinue the drug.

A woman who had tuberculosis earlier in life and now has a latent form must be especially careful to maintain an adequate level of calcium during pregnancy to ensure that tuberculosis pockets form or are not broken down. With tuberculosis, a woman is usually advised to wait 1 to 2 years after the infection becomes inactive before attempting to conceive. This is because recent inactive tuberculosis is more apt to become active during pregnancy than well-calcified lesions. Pressure on the diaphragm from below changes the shape of the lung, and an incompletely sealed pocket could be broken in this process. Pushing during labor may increase intrapulmonary pressure and cause the same phenomenon. Recent inactive tuberculosis may also become active during the postpartum period as the lung suddenly returns to its more vertical prepregnant position following birth, allowing calcium deposits to break open (Bergeron et al., 2003).

Although tuberculosis can be spread by the placenta to the fetus, it usually is spread to the infant after birth. A woman with a recent history of tuberculosis should have three negative sputum cultures before she holds or cares for her infant. If these are negative, there is no need to isolate the infant from the mother; she can even breast-feed. If active tuberculosis is in the home, the infant is generally discharged on prophylactic INH to prevent infection, with follow-up skin testing at 3-month intervals. If the infant is to be placed on INH, a mother also taking INH should not breast-feed. Otherwise, the combined dosage the infant receives (INH is found in breast milk) could be toxic to the infant.

A Woman With Cystic Fibrosis

Cystic fibrosis is a recessively inherited disease in which there is generalized dysfunction of the exocrine glands. This dysfunction leads to mucous secretions, particularly in the pancreas and lungs, becoming so viscid or thick that normal lung and pancreatic function is compromised.

Many men with cystic fibrosis are sterile because their semen is so thick that sperm cannot be mobile. Fertility may be lessened in women with the disorder because sperm cannot migrate through her viscid cervical mucus. This can make conception a concern. Reproductive technologies such as artificial insemination or in vitro fertilization may be necessary for conception so sperm are not obstructed by cervical mucus or fallopian tubal transport is not impaired.

Persons with the disease typically develop symptoms of chronic respiratory infection and overinflation of their lungs from the thickened mucus as well as an inability to digest fat and protein because the pancreas cannot release amylase. Because of poor pulmonary function that results in inadequate oxygen supply to the fetus, there is an increased risk for preterm labor and perinatal death during pregnancy (Malee, 2004). The presence of cystic fibrosis may be identified by chorionic villi sampling or amniocentesis and identification of the abnormal gene on chromosome 7 during pregnancy or immediately after birth (Richards & Haddow, 2003). It is included in routine neonatal screening programs after birth.

Therapy for the illness consists of pancrelipase (Pancrease) to supplement pancreatic enzymes and a bronchodilator or antibiotic to reduce pulmonary symptoms. Although pancrelipase is a pregnancy risk category C drug (teratogenic effects are unknown), it does not appear to affect the fetus. In addition to pharmacologic measures, women with cystic fibrosis must perform chest physiotherapy daily to reduce the buildup of lung secretions. Although it is a strain on an already stressed respiratory system, pregnancy does not appear to shorten the life span of women with the disorder (Goss et al., 2003).

Modifications for Pregnancy

Because pancrelipase may interfere with iron absorption, a woman is at greater risk for iron-deficiency anemia during pregnancy than other women. Therefore, an iron supplement usually is prescribed. Persons with cystic fibrosis have a higher-than-usual incidence of developing diabetes mellitus due to pancreas involvement; therefore, women need close monitoring of serum glucose levels at

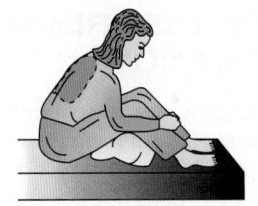

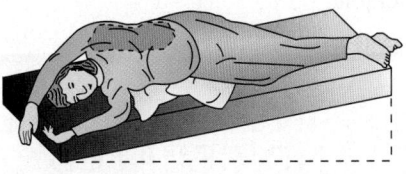

FIGURE 14.2 Modified positions for chest physiotherapy during pregnancy: (**A**) chest physiotherapy for the upper lobes; (**B**) chest physiotherapy for the lower lobes.

prenatal visits to detect the development of gestational diabetes.

Chest physiotherapy becomes difficult late in pregnancy because the process is exhausting. Moving to new positions is difficult, and lying prone, a position used frequently in postural drainage, is contraindicated in late pregnancy. A woman may need to plan more frequent and shorter sessions in modified positions (other than prone) to prevent exhaustion (Fig. 14.2). Fetal health will be monitored by ultrasound and nonstress tests to identify intrauterine growth restriction.

Modifications for the Postpartum Period

Help a woman plan how to conserve her energy for infant care in the immediate postpartum period so she does not become exhausted and can enjoy her newborn. Breast-feeding is usually not recommended because the breast milk of women with cystic fibrosis may contain more fatty acid than usual, and feeding could be tiring for the mother.

 Checkpoint Question 4

Angelina Gomez had tuberculosis as a teenager. What is a danger of this during pregnancy?

a. Calcium deposits that wall off old tuberculosis lesions can break down.
b. Tuberculosis can turn to pneumonia if a woman has a folic acid deficit.
c. PPD tests are negative during pregnancy so TB goes undetected.
d. If tuberculosis spreads to the stomach, it can cause stomach ulcers.

RHEUMATIC DISORDERS AND PREGNANCY

A number of rheumatic disorders occur in young adult women and so are seen during pregnancy. Because most of these illnesses result in discomfort, potential or actual pain related to disease pathology is the primary nursing diagnosis used. Women may not achieve a pain-free outcome because of the nature of these illnesses, but outcomes should center on a woman stating that her pain level is tolerable.

NURSING DIAGNOSES AND RELATED INTERVENTIONS

Nursing Diagnosis: Pain related to rheumatic disorder during pregnancy

Outcome Evaluation: Client states she is moderately comfortable and able to maintain her usual level of daily activity.

A Woman With Juvenile Rheumatoid Arthritis

Juvenile rheumatoid arthritis (sometimes referred to as chronic rheumatoid arthritis), a disease of connective tissue with joint inflammation and contracture, is most likely the result of an autoimmune response. The disease pathology involves synovial membrane destruction. Inflammation with effusion, swelling, erythema, and painful motion of the joints occurs. Over time, formation of granulation tissue can fill the joint space, resulting in permanent disfigurement and loss of joint motion.

Women with juvenile rheumatoid arthritis frequently take corticosteroids and nonsteroidal anti-inflammatory drugs (NSAIDs) to prevent joint pain and loss of mobility. Some women may be taking oral aspirin therapy. Although they should continue to take these medications during pregnancy to prevent joint damage, large amounts of salicylates may lead to increased bleeding at birth or prolonged pregnancy (salicylate interferes with prostaglandin synthesis, so labor contractions are not initiated) (Karch, 2004). The infant may be born with a bleeding defect and may also experience premature closure of the ductus arteriosus due to the drug's effects (Ostensen & Skomsvoll, 2004). For this reason, a woman is asked to decrease her intake of salicylates approximately 2 weeks before term. A few women may be taking low-dose methotrexate, a carcinogen (pregnancy risk category X). They should consult their health care practitioner before becoming pregnant about the advisability of continuing this drug during pregnancy (Chakravarty et al., 2004).

Symptoms of the disease may improve during pregnancy because of the naturally increased circulating level of cor-

ticosteroids in the maternal bloodstream during pregnancy (Malee, 2003). During the postpartum period, when a woman's corticosteroid levels fall to prepregnancy levels again, arthritis symptoms will probably recur.

In the postpartum period, the determination as to the safety of breast-feeding must be individualized based on the medication that each woman is taking. Those taking an NSAID such as ibuprofen can breast-feed. Those taking large doses of aspirin may be advised not to breast-feed because of the danger of increased bleeding in the infant.

Checkpoint Question 5

Angelina Gomez routinely takes acetylsalicylic acid (aspirin) for arthritis. Why should she limit or discontinue this toward the end of pregnancy?

a. Salicylates can lead to increased maternal bleeding at childbirth.
b. Newborns develop withdrawal headaches from salicylates.
c. Aspirin can lead to deep vein thrombosis following birth.
d. Newborns develop a red rash from salicylate toxicity.

A Woman With Systemic Lupus Erythematosus

Systemic lupus erythematosus (SLE) is a multisystem chronic disease of connective tissue that can occur in women of childbearing age: its highest incidence is in women ages 20 to 40 years (Malee, 2003). Widespread degeneration of connective tissue (especially of the heart, kidneys, blood vessels, spleen, skin, and retroperitoneal tissue) occurs with onset of the illness. The most marked skin change is a characteristic erythematous butterfly-shaped rash on the face. In the kidneys, fibrin deposits develop, plugging and blocking the glomeruli and leading to necrosis and scarring. The thickening of collagen tissue in the blood vessels causes vessel obstruction. This can be life-threatening to a woman if blood flow to vital organs becomes compromised and life-threatening to a fetus if blood flow to the placenta is obstructed. Many women with SLE have antiphospholipid antibodies, which increase the tendency for thrombi to form. In contrast, marked thrombocytopenia is present, so clotting may be deficient. A woman may be taking a corticosteroid, NSAIDs, heparin, and salicylates to reduce disease symptoms.

The naturally increased circulation of corticosteroids during pregnancy may lessen symptoms in some women. In others, the chief complication of the disorder—acute nephritis with glomerular destruction—may occur for the first time during pregnancy.

With associated nephritis, a woman's blood pressure will rise. She will develop hematuria and decreased urine output. Proteinuria and edema may begin. It is difficult to differentiate these symptoms from the symptoms of pregnancy-induced hypertension, except that with pregnancy-induced hypertension there is no hematuria.

Frequent monitoring of serum creatinine levels is necessary to assess kidney function. If this value is over 1.5 mg/dL and proteinuria and a decreased creatinine clearance value are also present, the fetus is seriously threatened. Dialysis or plasmapheresis may be necessary to restore platelets to a usual level to guard against hemorrhage at birth.

Women are asked to decrease salicylate use close to birth to reduce the possibility of bleeding in the newborn. Intravenous hydrocortisone may be administered during labor to help a woman adjust to the stress at this time. During the postpartum period, there may be an acute exacerbation of symptoms in a woman as corticosteroid levels again fall to normal. Infants of women with SLE tend to be small for gestational age due to the decreased blood flow to the placenta. There is a greater-than-usual incidence of spontaneous miscarriage and preterm birth. Infants may be born with a lupus-like rash, anemia, thrombocytopenia (low platelet count), and neonatal heart block (Buyon & Clancy, 2003). Newborn symptoms last about 6 months and then fade. Congenital heart block, for which a pacemaker may be necessary, can occur in the newborn. Screening for the exact type of autoantibodies present may be helpful in predicting which newborns are susceptible to this.

GASTROINTESTINAL DISORDERS AND PREGNANCY

Although minor gastrointestinal discomforts (e.g., nausea, heartburn, constipation) are common during pregnancy, acute abdominal pain and protracted vomiting are causes for concern. Pregnancy complications such as premature separation of the placenta or ectopic pregnancy often manifest with acute abdominal pain, so differentiating the cause of abdominal pain is important. In some instances, abdominal pain is associated with a condition completely unrelated to the pregnancy such as ulcerative colitis, hepatitis, hiatal hernia, or cholecystitis. These conditions may be known to a woman before she becomes pregnant, or they may develop or be discovered during her pregnancy. Women who have colostomies can complete pregnancy without difficulty (Aukamp & Sredl, 2004). Even a previous liver transplant is not a contraindication to pregnancy (Armenti, Moritz, & Davidson, 2003).

NURSING DIAGNOSES AND RELATED INTERVENTIONS

Nursing Diagnosis: Imbalanced nutrition, less than body requirements, related to a gastrointestinal disorder during pregnancy

Outcome Evaluation: Client's weight gain is 25 to 30 lb during pregnancy; hemoglobin is above 12 mg/dL; specific gravity of urine is below 1.030.

A Woman With Appendicitis

Appendicitis is inflammation of the appendix. Its incidence is high in young adults, occurring as frequently as approximately 1 in 1,500 to 2,000 pregnancies (Malee, 2003).

Assessment

History taking is important. Appendicitis usually begins with a few hours of nausea, and then an hour or two of generalized abdominal discomfort. A woman may have vomiting during this time. Then comes the typical sharp, peristaltic, lower right quadrant pain of acute appendicitis.

The pain associated with appendicitis is different from the pain that occurs suddenly from an overstretched round ligament during pregnancy. Pain from an overstretched ligament may cause sharp lower quadrant pain if a woman stands up suddenly, but the pain is only transient. Appendicitis pain is also different from that of ectopic pregnancy. With ectopic pregnancy, a woman may have morning sickness; with appendicitis, nausea and vomiting are intense. The pain of ectopic pregnancy may be either diffuse or sharp. In the nonpregnant woman, the pain of appendicitis is sharp and localized at McBurney's point (a point halfway between the umbilicus and the iliac crest on the lower right abdomen). In the pregnant woman, the appendix is often displaced so far up in the abdomen that the localized pain may resemble the pain of gallbladder disease (Fig. 14.3). A complete blood count will reveal leukocytosis. However, because pregnant women have an elevated white blood cell count anyway, this finding is not as helpful in pregnancy as it might be otherwise. Her temperature may be elevated. There are typically ketones in the urine. A sonogram may reveal the inflamed appendix.

Advise a woman not to take food, liquid, or laxatives while she is waiting to be evaluated for possible appendicitis, because increasing peristalsis could cause an inflamed appendix to rupture.

Therapeutic Management

If a woman is near term (past 36 weeks) and the fetus is believed to be mature, a cesarean birth may be performed to deliver the baby and then remove the inflamed appendix at the same time. If appendicitis occurs early in pregnancy, the inflamed appendix is removed by laparoscopy (Bisharah & Tulandi, 2003). As long as the anesthesiologist is aware that a woman is pregnant and carefully controls oxygen levels during anesthesia administration, the outcome of the pregnancy will be good.

If the appendix ruptures before surgery, the risk to both mother and fetus increases dramatically. This is because with rupture, infected fecal material is free in the peritoneum and can spread by the fallopian tubes to the fetus. Also generalized peritonitis is such an overwhelming infection that it is difficult for a woman's body to combat it effectively and also maintain the pregnancy. In addition, peritoneal adhesions may develop after an appendix ruptures, resulting in future infertility due to changes in the placement of fallopian tubes.

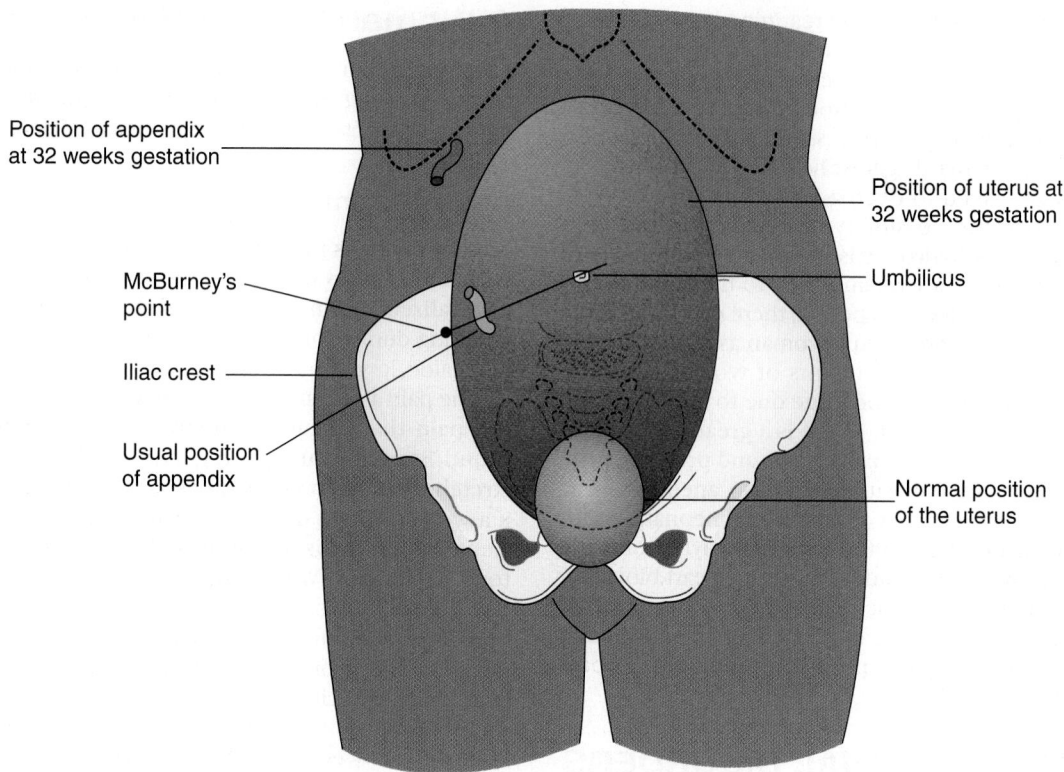

FIGURE 14.3 Change in position of appendix during pregnancy.

A Woman With Gastroesophageal Reflux Disease or Hiatal Hernia

Gastroesophageal reflux disease (GERD) refers to the reflux of acid stomach secretions into the esophagus. Hiatal hernia is a condition in which a portion of the stomach extends and protrudes up through the diaphragm into the chest cavity, trapping stomach acid and causing it to reflux into the esophagus. Although these conditions can be present constantly, symptoms most often occur only sporadically after increased peristaltic action. Both conditions may generate symptoms for the first time during pregnancy as the uterus pushes the stomach up against the esophagus and increases the reflux of acid or the extent of the hernia. Symptoms include:

- Heartburn, which is particularly extreme when lying supine after a full meal
- Gastric regurgitation
- Dysphagia (difficulty swallowing)
- Possible weight loss due to the inability to eat
- Hematemesis (vomiting of blood) if esophageal irritation occurs from the reflux of hydrochloric acid

During pregnancy, these conditions are usually diagnosed by direct endoscopy or ultrasound to avoid exposing a woman to barium x-rays. In most women, antacids will relieve pain. A histamine receptor antagonist, such as ranitidine, can be prescribed to inhibit gastric acid production and help minimize pain. Proton pump inhibitors such as esomeprazole magnesium (Nexium) are also safe

during pregnancy (pregnancy category B) (Richter, 2003). Advise a woman to wear loose clothing and sleep with her head elevated to help confine stomach secretions. After pregnancy, as the uterine pressure is decreased, the symptoms generally become less noticeable or disappear.

A Woman With Cholecystitis and Cholelithiasis

Cholecystitis (gallbladder inflammation) and cholelithiasis (gallstone formation) are most frequently associated with women older than 40 years, obesity, multiparity, and ingestion of a high-fat diet. Symptoms (constant aching and pressure in the right epigastrium, perhaps accompanied by jaundice), therefore, are more apt to occur in the older pregnant woman. Gallstones are formed from cholesterol. It is debated whether the hypercholesterolemia that naturally occurs during pregnancy leads to an increased incidence of cholecystitis or cholelithiasis, but both these conditions are seen with pregnancy.

Medical therapy for both conditions is to lower fat intake. A woman can eat a low-fat but not a fat-free diet during pregnancy because of the importance of linoleic acid for fetal growth. Cholecystitis can be diagnosed by sonogram. If an acute episode occurs during pregnancy, it can generally be managed by administering intravenous fluids to provide fluid and nutrients and analgesics for pain. Surgery for gallbladder removal by laparoscopic technique may be done during pregnancy if a woman's symptoms cannot be controlled by conservative management (Rollins, Chan, & Price, 2004).

A Woman With Pancreatitis

Pancreatitis, inflammation of the pancreas, tends to occur in young adults and so is seen during pregnancy. It is treated the same in pregnancy as in nonpregnant women: nasogastric suction, bowel rest, analgesia (pancreatic pain is sharp), and intravenous hydration. Pancreatic inflammation usually subsides within a week. Pregnancy loss can occur from acidosis, hypovolemia, and fetal hypoxia (Malee, 2003).

A Woman With Hepatitis

Hepatitis is a liver disease that may occur from invasion of the A, B, C, D, or E virus. Hepatitis A is spread mainly by fecal–oral contact (children in day-care settings have a high incidence) or by ingestion of fecally contaminated water or shellfish. It has an incubation period of 2 to 6 weeks. Pregnant women exposed to hepatitis A may be given prophylactic gamma globulin to try to prevent the disease after exposure. This form follows a rather benign course and is not known to be transmitted to the fetus.

Hepatitis B and C are spread by exposure to contaminated blood or blood products. These two types also can be spread by contact with contaminated semen or vaginal secretions and so are considered STIs. Hepatitis D and E are apparently spread by the same methods as hepatitis B but are rarely seen in pregnant women.

Hepatitis B has an incubation period of 6 weeks to 6 months. It occurs in both an acute and chronic form, leading to liver cell necrosis with scarring and inability to convert indirect to direct bilirubin or excrete direct bilirubin. Women exposed to the virus receive immune globulin for prophylaxis; hepatitis B vaccine may be administered to those who are at high risk, such as women who handle blood products. Hepatitis C demonstrates few symptoms, and these may not be present for 12 months after exposure (Hadden, 2004).

Assessment

With all forms of hepatitis, a woman may have nausea and vomiting. Her liver area may feel tender to palpation. Urine will be dark yellow from excretion of bilirubin; stools will be light-colored from lack of bilirubin. Jaundice occurs as a late symptom. On physical examination, hepatomegaly (enlargement of the liver) is noted. The bilirubin level is elevated. Levels of liver enzymes such as transaminase are increased. Specific antibodies against the virus can be detected in the blood serum, so women are routinely screened for this during pregnancy. If a liver biopsy is necessary for diagnosis, this can be performed safely during pregnancy.

Therapeutic Management

A woman is usually prescribed bed rest and encouraged to eat a high-calorie diet because her liver has difficulty converting stored glycogen into glucose in its diseased state. Follow standard precautions to avoid contact with body fluids.

Hepatitis during pregnancy may lead to spontaneous miscarriage or preterm labor. Unlike other diseases, the later in pregnancy the mother contracts hepatitis B infection, the greater the risk the infant will be affected or develop hepatitis B. When this occurs, it is a serious consequence because a proportion of HB Ag-positive infants will develop liver cirrhosis or carcinoma later in life (Malee, 2003). If the mother has anti-HB antibodies present (antibodies toward a virus subgroup), the incidence of this appears to be less. After birth, the infant should be washed well to remove any maternal blood, and hepatitis B immune globulin (HBIG) and immunization against hepatitis B should be administered (see Chapter 23 for additional newborn care). The mother may breast-feed. The infant needs to be observed carefully for symptoms of infection during the first few months of life and chronic liver disease later in life (Boxall et al., 2004).

A Woman With Inflammatory Bowel Disease

Crohn's disease (inflammation of the terminal ileus) and ulcerative colitis (inflammation of the distal colon) occur most often in young adults between ages 12 and 30 years (childbearing years) and so are seen in pregnancy. The cause of these diseases is unknown, but an autoimmune process is thought to be responsible. In both diseases, the bowel develops shallow ulcers. A woman experiences chronic diarrhea, weight loss, occult blood in stool, and nausea and vomiting. If extreme, obstruction and fistula formation with peritonitis can occur. With Crohn's disease, malabsorption, particularly of vitamin B (a substance whose absorption occurs almost entirely in the ileum), occurs.

These diseases obviously have the potential for interfering with fetal growth if extreme malabsorption occurs. Therapy for the disorders is total rest for the gastrointestinal tract by administration of total parenteral nutrition. Although it is possible to sustain a pregnancy by this route, it is obviously not a desirable nutrition pattern. Sulfasalazine (Azulfidine), an anti-inflammatory and a mainstay of therapy, may be continued during pregnancy without fetal injury (Alstead & Nelson-Piercy, 2003). Close to birth, the dosage of sulfasalazine is reduced because it may interfere with bilirubin binding sites and cause neonatal jaundice (Karch, 2004).

NEUROLOGIC DISORDERS AND PREGNANCY

Neurologic illness is not a common problem affecting women of childbearing age. However, any neurologic disease with symptoms of seizures must be carefully managed during pregnancy because the anoxia caused by severe seizures could deprive the fetus of oxygen.

NURSING DIAGNOSES AND RELATED INTERVENTIONS

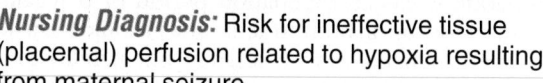

Nursing Diagnosis: Risk for injury (maternal) related to recurrent seizures

Outcome Evaluation: Client states she is seizure-free, with no signs and symptoms of injury; no automobile or other accidents are documented.

A Woman With a Seizure Disorder

Recurrent seizures have a number of causes, such as head trauma or meningitis. The causes of most recurrent seizures, however, are unknown (idiopathic).

Recurrent seizures were at one time so incapacitating and it was believed that seizure control medications caused such a high risk of congenital anomaly that women with seizures were advised not to have children. Today, however, no contraindication to pregnancy exists for women with seizures as long as the medication they take is carefully monitored (Meador & Zupanc, 2004).

Therapeutic Management

Because seizure medications as a group are mildly teratogenic, women with recurrent seizures need to meet with their obstetrician and primary care provider before pregnancy to be certain the medications they are taking are the least teratogenic and the dosage they are taking is the lowest possible to control seizures (Malee, 2003). In the early months of pregnancy, you may need to remind women to continue to take their antiseizure medications despite the nausea or vomiting of early pregnancy. Be certain they understand that the rule "Do not take medication during pregnancy" does not apply to their antiseizure medications. A woman is in the difficult position of having to take drugs to safeguard her own health, but by taking them she may not be safeguarding the health of her fetus. The risk of adverse maternal or fetal outcome from seizures during pregnancy, however, is greater than the risk of teratogenicity from taking anticonvulsant drugs (Karch, 2004).

All women should have evaluations of serum drug levels before pregnancy or early in pregnancy (Penovich, Eck, & Economou, 2004). As the blood volume increases with pregnancy, some women may need their dosage increased. Common drugs prescribed to control seizures are:

- Trimethadione (Tridione) (pregnancy risk category D)
- Valproic acid (sodium valproate and divalproex sodium) (pregnancy risk category D)
- Carbamazepine (Tegretol) (pregnancy risk category C)
- Ethosuximide (Zarontin), a drug often used to control absence seizures (pregnancy risk category C)
- Phenytoin sodium (Dilantin) (pregnancy risk category D). Dilantin can cause a syndrome involving fetal cognitive impairment and a peculiar facial proportion not unlike that of fetal alcohol syndrome. This may occur because of competition for folic acid binding sites. Some infants have an increased danger of neural tube disorders as a result of this folic acid displacement. A sonogram can rule out a neural tube defect.

Women who have been taking phenytoin (Dilantin) may have developed chronic hypertension. For these women, a baseline blood pressure should be established early in pregnancy so that changes can be interpreted correctly. Infants are also prone to hemorrhagic disease of the newborn because of decreased levels of vitamin K coagulation factors at birth from phenytoin. To counteract this, women may be prescribed vitamin K during labor or the last 4 weeks of gestation.

NURSING DIAGNOSES AND RELATED INTERVENTIONS

Nursing Diagnosis: Risk for ineffective tissue (placental) perfusion related to hypoxia resulting from maternal seizure

Outcome Evaluation: Client informs health care personnel about history of seizures; states importance of immediate care and oxygen therapy should she begin a seizure. Apgar score of infant is 7 to 10, with no apparent birth anomalies.

Absence seizures (often just a rapid fluttering of the eyelids or a moment's staring into space) should have no effect on a woman or fetus. Tonic-clonic seizures (sustained, full-body involvement) could affect the fetus because spasm of the chest muscles could lead to hypoxia. If a seizure should occur, a woman must be evaluated to ascertain that the cause of the seizure was the underlying disease, not beginning hypertension of pregnancy. Nonpregnant women experiencing tonic-clonic seizures do not need oxygen during a seizure, but in pregnancy, administering oxygen by mask is good prophylaxis to ensure adequate fetal oxygenation.

Urge a woman to alert hospital personnel at the time of labor that she has recurrent seizures and to report the type of medication she is taking. She should continue to take the medication during labor. If a general anesthetic should be necessary, the anesthesiologist needs to know about her condition before administering anesthesia; otherwise, during the excitement phase of anesthesia induction, a seizure could occur.

Nursing Diagnosis: Risk for impaired parenting related to maternal low self-esteem

Outcome Evaluation: Client accurately states the nature of her disorder (acquired or idiopathic) and the statistical chances of her child inheriting the disorder. After child is born, client identifies sudden jerking movements in her newborn (such as Moro reflex) as healthy newborn characteristics.

A woman who has recurrent seizures may worry that her child will have seizures as the child grows older. If a woman's seizures are the result of an acquired disorder (i.e., infection, such as meningitis or head trauma), a woman can be assured that her child's risk for seizures is no greater than that for any other child. If the etiology of her seizures is unknown, the chance that her child also will have them is slightly higher than in the normal population. This prediction is only theoretical, however, and cannot be made without a thorough review of the onset and nature of a woman's disorder. Be certain a woman has her newborn with her for long periods so she can become acquainted with the sudden jerking motions that occur such as when a newborn is startled (Moro reflex) or quivering of the jaw with prolonged crying. Otherwise she could interpret these normal movements as seizure activity.

A Woman With Myasthenia Gravis

Myasthenia gravis is an autoimmune disorder characterized by the presence of an IgG antibody against acetylcholine receptors in striated muscle. This causes failure of the striated muscles to contract, particularly those of the oropharyngeal, facial, and extraocular groups (Ciafaloni & Massey, 2004).

Myasthenia gravis is treated with anticholinesterase drugs such as pyridostigmine (Mestinon) or neostigmine (Prostigmin) and possibly the corticosteroid prednisone. These medications may be continued during pregnancy, as the fetus will experience no effects from maternal drugs. Plasmapheresis to remove immune complexes from the bloodstream may be prescribed to reduce symptoms further. Plasmapheresis must be carried out gradually during pregnancy to reduce the risk of fluid overload or hypotension. Because smooth muscle is not affected by the disease, labor should occur normally. Magnesium sulfate should be avoided because it can diminish the acetylcholine effect and therefore increase disease symptoms.

An infant born to a woman with myasthenia gravis may demonstrate disease symptoms at birth due to the transfer of antibodies (Jackson, 2003). This is further discussed in Chapter 51.

A Woman With Multiple Sclerosis

Multiple sclerosis (MS) occurs predominantly in women of childbearing age, usually between 20 and 40 years of age (Wingerchuk & Carter, 2003). With MS, nerve fibers become demyelinated and therefore lose function. Women develop symptoms of fatigue, numbness, blurred vision, and loss of coordination. ACTH or a corticosteroid is commonly given to strengthen nerve conduction. These can be administered safely during pregnancy. In contrast, cyclosporine (Sandimmune), azathioprine (Imuran), and cyclophosphamide (Cytoxan), drugs also frequently administered, are not safe for use during pregnancy. The pregnancy safety of interferon has not been tested; as such, it is classified as a pregnancy category C drug. Women may continue with plasmapheresis (withdrawal and replacement of plasma), another treatment regimen, during pregnancy as long as the volume is well controlled. Although women with the disorder may grow increasingly fatigued as pregnancy progresses, pregnancy does not affect the long-term course of MS. MS may actually improve with pregnancy due to the increased circulating corticosteroid levels (Dwosh et al., 2003). UTIs tend to occur as a poorly defined consequence of the illness.

MUSCULOSKELETAL DISORDERS AND PREGNANCY

Women of childbearing age have few musculoskeletal disorders, but one that may be seen is scoliosis.

A Woman With Scoliosis

Scoliosis (lateral curvature of the spine) occurs most often in girls between 12 and 14 years of age. If it is uncorrected at this time, the curvature progresses until it causes deformity, interfering with respiration and heart action because of chest compression. Pelvic distortion can interfere with childbirth, especially at the pelvic inlet. If a woman's spine is extremely curved, spinal or epidural anesthesia may be more difficult to administer.

Girls with scoliosis may wear a body brace during their adolescent years to maintain an erect posture. Although these braces are not as bulky as they once were, unless they are modified, they cannot be worn during the last half of pregnancy. Other girls have stainless-steel rods implanted on both sides of their vertebrae to strengthen and straighten the spine. Such rod implantations do not interfere with pregnancy; a woman will notice some back pain from tension on the back muscles similar to that experienced by the average pregnant woman. If a woman's pelvis is distorted, a cesarean delivery may be necessary to ensure a safe birth. Vaginal birth, if permitted, requires the same management as for any woman. Plot the course of labor on a labor graph so an unusually long first stage, suggesting cephalopelvic disproportion, can be recognized. Chapter 51 discusses in detail the nursing care of adolescents with scoliosis.

ENDOCRINE DISORDERS AND PREGNANCY

Endocrine disorders have the potential to be serious complications of pregnancy because enzymes or hormones control so many specific body functions.

A Woman With a Thyroid Dysfunction

As a normal effect of pregnancy, the thyroid gland enlarges (hypertrophies) slightly due to increased vascularity. A woman with preexisting thyroid problems may have difficulty making this pregnancy transition.

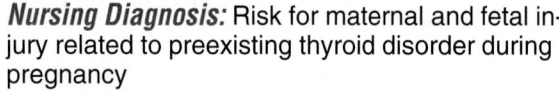

NURSING DIAGNOSES AND RELATED INTERVENTIONS

Nursing Diagnosis: Risk for maternal and fetal injury related to preexisting thyroid disorder during pregnancy

Outcome Evaluation: No congenital anomalies are present in infant at birth; Apgar score is 7 to 10. Mother can continue prepregnancy activities.

A Woman With Hypothyroidism

Hypothyroidism is a rare condition in young adults and especially in pregnancy, because women with symptoms of untreated hypothyroidism may be anovulatory and unable to conceive. A woman who does conceive can have difficulty increasing thyroid functioning to a necessary pregnancy level. This difficulty often causes pregnant women with hypothyroidism to have histories of early spontaneous miscarriage. These women fatigue easily and tend to be obese; their skin is dry (myxedema), and they have little tolerance for cold. During pregnancy, hypothyroidism is associated with extreme nausea and vomiting (hyperemesis gravidarum). It may be associated with breech fetal presentations (Pop et al., 2004).

Most women with hypothyroidism take levothyroxine (Synthroid) to supplement their lack of thyroid hormone. A woman who is taking levothyroxine needs to consult with her obstetrician and internist when she is planning on becoming pregnant. She needs to come for early diagnosis and close follow-up as soon as she suspects she is pregnant (1 week past her missed menstrual period). As a rule, her dose of levothyroxine will be increased as much as 30% for the duration of the pregnancy to simulate the effect that would normally occur in pregnancy (Alexander et al., 2004). Be certain that a woman realizes the importance of taking this increased dose.

After the pregnancy, the dose of levothyroxine prescribed for pregnancy must be gradually tapered back to the prepregnancy level. Be certain a woman does not continue to take her pregnancy dose (trying to be economical and use up her higher-dose pills), or she could pass beyond normal thyroid function and develop hyperthyroidism.

A Woman With Hyperthyroidism

Hyperthyroidism, or overproduction of thyroid hormone, usually causes these symptoms:

- Rapid heart rate
- Exophthalmos (protruding eyeballs)
- Heat intolerance
- Nervousness
- Heart palpitations
- Weight loss

Hyperthyroidism is more apt to be seen in pregnancy than hypothyroidism. If undiagnosed, a woman may develop heart failure during pregnancy because her rapid heart rate cannot adjust to the increasing blood volume occurring with pregnancy. She is more prone to symptoms of hypertension of pregnancy, fetal growth restriction, and preterm labor than the average woman.

Hyperthyroidism is normally diagnosed by a nuclear medicine imaging study involving the radioactive uptake of ^{131}I subtype. This diagnostic procedure should not be used during pregnancy because the fetal thyroid will also incorporate this drug, possibly resulting in destruction of the fetal thyroid.

Treatment for hyperthyroidism is with thioamides (methimazole [Tapazole] or propylthiouracil [PTU]) to reduce thyroid activity (Cooper, 2003). These drugs are, unfortunately, teratogens. They cross the placenta and can lead to congenital hypothyroidism and consequently an enlarged thyroid gland (a goiter) in the fetus. If this abnormal neck growth enlarges enough, it can obstruct the airway and make resuscitation difficult for the infant at birth.

A woman should be regulated on the lowest possible dose of these drugs and cautioned to keep a careful record of doses taken so she does not forget or accidentally duplicate a dose. Surgical treatment to reduce the functioning of the maternal thyroid gland can be accomplished, but this is generally not the treatment of choice during pregnancy due to the need for general anesthesia. After a pregnancy, if a woman desires other children, the procedure might be suggested as an interpregnancy procedure.

If a woman's thyroid function was not regulated during pregnancy, her infant may be born with symptoms of hyperthyroidism because of the excess stimulation he or she received in utero. An assay of fetal cord blood will reveal the level of T4 and thyroid-stimulating hormone and the need for therapy. The infant may appear jittery, and tachypnea and tachycardia may be present. Women receiving smaller or minimal doses of antithyroid drugs may breast-feed, although women receiving large doses of these drugs may be advised not to breast-feed because these drugs are excreted in breast milk (Karch, 2004).

A Woman With Diabetes Mellitus

Diabetes mellitus is an endocrine disorder in which the pancreas cannot produce adequate insulin to regulate body glucose levels. The disorder affects 3% to 5% of all

PLAN	PRINCIPLE
For Unconscious Victim in Supine Position 1. Place the woman in the same position as for external heart compressions (heel of the hand on the lower sternum).	**For Unconscious Victim in Supine Position** 1. Loss of consciousness interferes with the woman's ability to maintain an upright position.
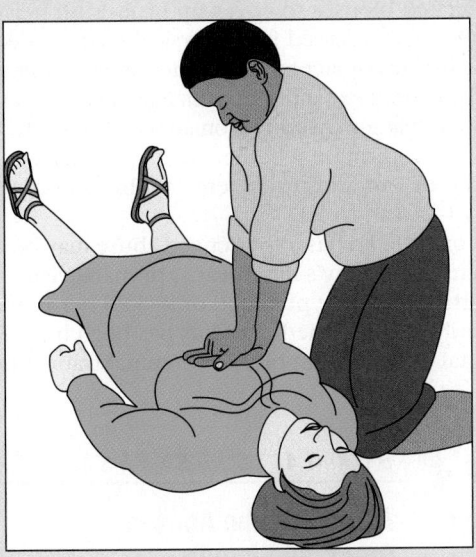 2. Follow Steps 2 and 3 as with standing victim.	2. Compression of the chest forces the object lodged in the airway to move upward. Chest compression can be as effective in the supine position as in the standing position.

landing on her abdomen. Due to her extra weight, this can cause a serious wrist injury. Apply ice to the area to decrease swelling as an immediate first-aid measure. If she has limited motion, an x-ray may be necessary to determine whether a fracture is present. Assure a woman that an x-ray of an extremity is safe during pregnancy as long as her abdomen is shielded during the radiation exposure. Delegate someone to accompany her to the x-ray department and remain with her (outside the actual x-ray room) to ensure that lead protection is offered. Also caution this person to be alert to signs of preterm labor that could suddenly develop as a result of an undetected injury.

Because women of childbearing age are usually healthy, healing of fractures or torn ligaments generally occurs quickly and without complications. Be certain a woman can identify good calcium food sources if she has a fracture so both she and the fetus can have adequate calcium for new bone growth.

Because many more adolescent girls and young adult women participate in sports today than ever before, an increasing number of women of childbearing age have weakened knee cartilage from having dislocated a knee joint during sports (formerly thought of only as a football injury). During pregnancy, when all body cartilage softens, combined with the excessive abdominal weight a woman carries, a woman may dislocate her knee again.

Any woman who has had a previous knee injury should have it reevaluated early in pregnancy. A support device

such as a knee immobilizer may be required for the last 3 months of pregnancy to keep the joint from dislocating again. Discuss with her the advantage of prevention because if the knee cartilage cannot sustain her added weight and dislocates again, she may fall. She can be assured that having a knee immobilizer in place at the time of birth will not interfere with birth; if a lithotomy position and stirrups for birth are necessary, a modified stirrups position can be devised for her.

The laxness of body cartilage may also cause separation of the symphysis pubis if a woman falls with her legs outspread. Many women experience some nagging suprapubic joint pain during pregnancy. A suture separation this way, however, is very painful, especially on walking or turning. To avoid pain and allow the cartilage to heal, a woman needs to remain on bed rest at home for 4 to 6 weeks. If separation of the symphysis pubis is present at the time of birth, this will make labor very painful, especially the pelvic division of labor as the fetus is pushed through the pelvic ring.

Burns

Burns are dangerous in the pregnant woman not only because of the thermal injury that occurs but from the inhalation of carbon monoxide gases from the fire, which can lead to extreme fetal hypoxia as carbon monoxide crosses the placenta in place of oxygen (Malee, 2003).

Smoke is irritating to lung tissue and can result in extensive lung edema; this can cause additional fetal hypoxia due to the lack of oxygen–carbon dioxide exchange space in the mother. Because fluid and electrolyte losses can be great with burns, hypotension from hypovolemia or an electrolyte imbalance can occur. In response to a severe trauma such as a burn, prostaglandins are produced, possibly causing preterm labor. Both maternal and fetal prognoses are poor if burns cover more than 50% of body surface area. Fortunately, few women of childbearing age experience this degree of burn in the United States.

Interestingly, burn tissue heals more quickly than normal during pregnancy. This is probably related to the overall increased metabolism and possibly to the increased corticosteroid serum level that prevents inflammation and damage to tissue from the pressure of edema.

Postmortem Cesarean Birth

If a pregnant woman does not survive serious trauma, it may still be possible for her child to be born safely by a postmortem cesarean birth. This is usually attempted if the fetus is past 24 weeks and less than 20 minutes has passed since the mother died. Infant survival is best in these circumstances if no longer than 5 minutes has passed. By general practice, no consent is necessary for this procedure because the fetus is assumed to want to live but cannot give consent. A classic cesarean incision is used. Personnel should be available to resuscitate the newborn immediately.

Intimate Partner Abuse

As many as 20% to 30% of women seen in emergency departments are there because they have been abused by their intimate partner. Homicide from partner abuse is the number-one cause of death in pregnant women. Abused women may have an unintended pregnancy because they were unable to resist sexual advances from their abusive partner. Another woman may desire the pregnancy very much because she believes having a child will change the partner and make him a better person. She may be grateful for the pregnancy, thinking that by having an infant she will have someone to love her. Intimate partner abuse may increase during pregnancy because stress is often a trigger to abuse, and pregnancy, with all that an expected new child entails (another mouth to feed, body to clothe, or dependent to protect), can increase stress.

Although it is impossible to predict how any individual woman will respond, pregnant abused women may demonstrate behaviors that reveal abuse. A woman may come for care late in pregnancy or not at all, for example, because her partner controls her transportation or money; she may fear that a health care provider will identify and report the abuse; or she may have been pretending the pregnancy did not exist to reduce stress in her home. She may be noticeable in a prenatal setting because she has purchased no maternity clothing (she has no funds for herself and asking for money may incite violence). She may decline laboratory tests if they involve additional transportation or money.

An abused woman may have difficulty following a recommended pregnancy diet (she must cook what her part-

ner wants or she will be beaten). She may grow anxious if her appointment is running late (she must be home to cook dinner or risk a beating). She may call and cancel appointments frequently (or simply not keep appointments) because she has an obvious black eye or a bleeding facial laceration she does not want to reveal. She may dress inappropriately for warm weather, wearing long-sleeved, tight-necked blouses to cover up bruises on her neck or arms. When undressed for a physical examination, there may be bruises or lacerations on her breasts, abdomen, or back she cannot explain. Her neck may reveal linear bruises from strangulation. Ask any woman with bruises to account for them. Determine whether the explanation correlates with the extent and placement of a bruise or laceration (Boxes 14.16 and 14.17).

A woman who has experienced abuse may be anxious to listen to the baby's heartbeat at prenatal visits because her partner recently punched or kicked her in the abdomen and she is worried the fetus has been hurt. Minimal placental infarcts from blunt abdominal trauma may lead

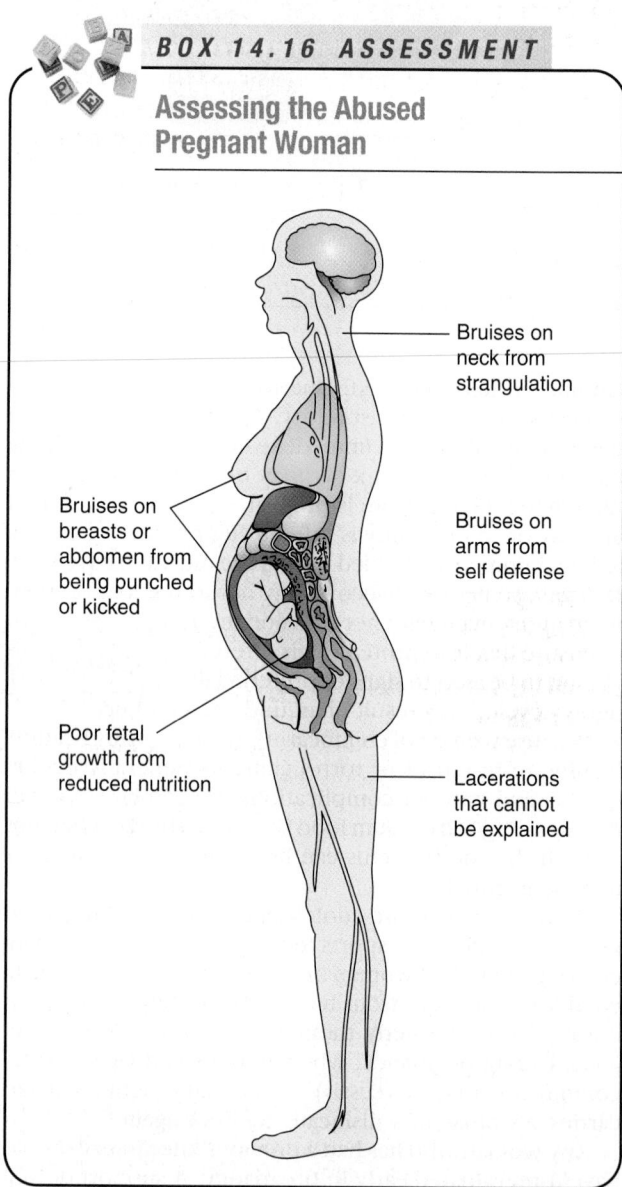

BOX 14.16 ASSESSMENT

Assessing the Abused Pregnant Woman

Bruises on neck from strangulation

Bruises on arms from self defense

Bruises on breasts or abdomen from being punched or kicked

Poor fetal growth from reduced nutrition

Lacerations that cannot be explained

BOX 14.17 FOCUS ON . . .

EVIDENCE-BASED PRACTICE

How big a concern is intimate partner abuse during pregnancy?

To answer this question, researchers investigated the prevalence of abuse among 4,750 women who had recently given birth. Of these women, 1.2% reported they had been exposed to physical violence from an intimate partner during their recent pregnancy, and 1.5% stated they feared their partner might harm them. Researchers then examined pregnancy outcomes among the women who were abused. This analysis revealed that physical violence was associated with an increased risk of hemorrhage, intrauterine growth restriction, and perinatal death. Fear of a partner in the absence of physical abuse was not associated with an elevated risk of adverse pregnancy outcomes. The researchers concluded there is a clear association between physical abuse and poor pregnancy outcomes. Efforts to prevent this could make pregnancy safer.

This is an important study for nurses, because nurses are the health care professionals who often take women's health histories in a health care setting or the people who may have the best opportunity to ask women about the possibility of intimate partner abuse, identify this as a possibility, and help a woman secure help before harm to her pregnancy results.

Source: Janssen, P. A., et al. (2003). Intimate partner violence and adverse pregnancy outcomes: a population-based study. *American Journal of Obstetrics and Gynecology*, 188(5), 1341–1347.

to poor placental perfusion and low birthweight. If abdominal trauma is suspected, a sonogram may be done because this is the most accurate method of assessing fetal health after trauma. Fetal heart tones and fundal height should also be recorded.

NURSING DIAGNOSES AND RELATED INTERVENTIONS

Nursing diagnoses for the abused woman may pertain to physical injuries sustained, but they should also address the emotional manifestations of abuse. Some examples include:

- Powerlessness related to perception that it is impossible to break away from abusing partner
- Fear related to constant threat of violence
- Social isolation related to client's need to hide evidence of her abuse

- Ineffective denial related to inability to face the fact partner is abusive
- Compromised family coping related to dysfunctional relationship between client and abusive partner

Expected outcomes should address specific tasks a woman could accomplish to keep herself safe from further abuse, such as:

- Client carries phone number of home for abused women with her.
- Client and abusive partner continue to attend counseling sessions.
- Client states she has filed restraining order against abusive partner.
- Client states she feels secure living at safe house.

It may be difficult to work with an abused woman who will not leave an abusive relationship because it is so hard to understand why she stays in the situation. A common finding is that a woman cannot leave due to fear of the abusive person (he has threatened that if she leaves, he will find her and kill her) and the guilt and low self-esteem she feels (he has told her so many times this is her fault and she deserves to be treated this way that she believes it). To free herself from this emotional paralysis, she needs outside help. Unfortunately, her low self-esteem and depression lead her to believe that no one would be interested in helping her.

Nursing Diagnosis: Chronic low self-esteem related to continuing physical and mental abuse

Outcome Evaluation: Client identifies positive traits about self; begins to discuss possible reasons why she has remained in an abusive situation; makes concrete, realistic plans for future; states she feels able, with continuing help and outside resources, to protect herself in the future.

Until she can develop better self-esteem, an abused woman may need support to make even simple decisions. Support any ability she has to make constructive decisions. Be familiar with shelters for abused women in your community; discuss with her how she can call the police at any time and they will take her to the shelter. Help her to file charges or obtain a restraining order to keep the abusive person from coming near her again if this is necessary.

After the birth of her child, assuming a woman moved away from the abuser, she may begin to feel a sense of depression from loneliness. This can lead to her having unrealistic expectations of her child, trying to make the infant smile at her and interact with her more than a newborn is capable of in order to have someone to love her. Caution her that her newborn does love her but she has to give the child some time to grow. Demonstrate all the things the child can do, such as attend to the sound of her voice or cuddle against her. Without this awareness, her unrealistic expectations can lead to disappointment and can interfere with mothering.

Do not leave an abused woman without a support system after the birth of her child. If she was depending on prenatal personnel during her pregnancy, the gap must be filled with another support system. This could be a social agency that deals specifically with abused women; it could be a community health nurse who will be visiting her after she returns home. If she is left without a support person, her low self-esteem may not allow her to reach out and seek help. She may decide that suicide or returning to the abuser is her best recourse. If a woman does return to live with an abusive partner, both she and the infant need frequent health care visits scheduled so their health and welfare can be monitored. A child raised in a home where the mother is abused will learn that this is acceptable conduct, and the abuse may extend to yet another generation (see Chapter 55).

Checkpoint Question 7

Angelina received a laceration on her leg from her automobile accident. Why are lacerations of lower extremities potentially more serious in pregnant women than others?

a. A woman is less able to keep the laceration clean because of her fatigue.

b. Increased bleeding can occur from uterine pressure on leg veins.

c. Lacerations can provoke allergic responses because of gonadotropic hormone.

d. Healing is limited during pregnancy, so these will not heal until after birth.

Key Points

A high-risk pregnancy is one in which a concurrent disorder, pregnancy-related complication, or external factor jeopardizes the health of the mother, the fetus, or both.

Pregnancy is a stress to any family because it involves financial expenses plus changes in family roles. If a complication of pregnancy develops, this stress is almost automatically intensified. Families need support during this time to be able to cope with the increased burden.

When women with a preexisting disease become pregnant, a thorough history and physical examination are crucial to obtain at the first prenatal visit to establish a baseline of information on the condition. Documentation of any medication being taken for a secondary condition is also necessary to protect against adverse drug interactions and the possibility of teratogenic action on the fetus.

Teaching is an important nursing intervention because a woman with a preexisting illness must make modifications in her usual therapy to adjust to pregnancy. Pregnancy often stimulates women to learn more about their primary disease as well.

Women who have a complication early in pregnancy may continue to worry about the health of their fetus all during pregnancy. They need to be assured (appropriately) that the episode was temporary and that, with continued monitoring, the fetus should not suffer harm. After giving birth, they may need to spend additional time with their newborns to convince themselves that their infants are healthy so bonding can begin.

Sexually transmitted infections such as candidiasis, trichomoniasis, chlamydia, syphilis, herpes type 2, gonorrhea, papilloma, and HIV may occur during pregnancy. These illnesses need to be treated promptly. Women need to use safer sex practices to help prevent these diseases.

Because blood volume increases by as much as 50% during pregnancy, cardiac function may become inadequate if cardiovascular disease is present. Illnesses that cause difficulty can be either acquired disorders such as Kawasaki disease and rheumatic fever or congenital disorders such as mitral valve stenosis and coarctation of the aorta.

Various forms of anemia can cause complications of pregnancy; iron-deficiency anemia, sickle cell anemia, and folic acid-deficiency anemia are examples. All these anemias can result in fetal distress because of inadequate oxygen transport.

Urinary tract disorders can lead to pregnancy complications because pregnancy increases the workload of the kidneys. UTIs and chronic renal disease are two disorders that may lead to early pregnancy loss.

Acute nasopharyngitis, asthma, pneumonia, influenza, and tuberculosis are respiratory disorders seen in pregnancy. The incidence of tuberculosis is on the increase, and these patients need special assessment and care.

Juvenile rheumatoid arthritis and systemic lupus erythematosus are examples of rheumatic disorders seen in pregnancy. These disorders generally require large doses of NSAIDs for therapy. Women taking salicylates are advised to decrease use 2 weeks before birth to avoid bleeding disorders in the newborn.

Some gastrointestinal illnesses that occur with pregnancy are hiatal hernia, cholecystitis, viral hepatitis, inflammatory bowel disease, and appendicitis. If surgery is necessary for conditions such as chole-cystitis or appendicitis, it can be performed by lap-aroscopic technique during pregnancy, but this may result in preterm labor.

Recurrent seizures are the most frequently seen neu-rologic condition during pregnancy. Many drugs used to control seizures are teratogenic; women need to have their medical regimen evaluated be-fore pregnancy to be certain they are regulated on the fewest medications possible.

The major endocrine disorder seen during pregnancy is diabetes mellitus. Gestational diabetes is diabetes that occurs during pregnancy and fades after it.

Trauma in pregnancy results from sources such as vio-lence, automobile accidents, and falls. Women with traumatic injuries need to be carefully assessed to determine if intimate partner abuse was the cause of the trauma.

Critical Thinking Exercises

1. Angelina Gomez, the woman you met at the begin-ning of the chapter, was seen in an emergency room after an automobile accident. She has a 3-inch lacera-tion on her thigh. Following a severe injury of this kind, what body systems would you assess first?

2. Angelina has developed gestational diabetes. She's re-sistant to learning about her condition, though, be-cause she knows her symptoms are only temporary and will fade at the end of pregnancy. What type of teaching plan would you devise to help her learn in the face of this attitude?

3. One of the most devastating medical diagnoses today is that of HIV infection (infection with the virus that causes AIDS). How is this illness a threat to the new-born as well as the mother? Are there changes a pre-natal clinic would have to make to care for an HIV-positive woman?

4. Examine the National Health Goals related to compli-cations of pregnancy. Most government-sponsored money for nursing research is allotted based on these goals. What would be a possible research topic to ex-plore pertinent to these goals that would be applica-ble to the Gomez family and also advance evidence-based practice?

References

Alexander, A., et al. (2003). Metastatic melanoma in pregnancy: risk of transplacental metastases in the infant. *Journal of Clinical Oncology, 21*(11), 2179–2186.

Alexander, E. K., et al. (2004). Timing and magnitude of in-creases in levothyroxine requirements during pregnancy in women with hypothyroidism. *New England Journal of Medicine, 351*(3), 241–249.

Alstead, E. M., & Nelson-Piercy, C. (2003). Inflammatory bowel disease in pregnancy. *Gut, 52*(2), 159–161.

American Diabetes Association. (2001). *New classifications and recommendations for diabetes mellitus.* New York: ADA.

Armenti, V. T., Moritz, M. J., & Davidson, J. M. (2003). Preg-nancy in female pediatric solid organ transplant recipients. *Pediatric Clinics of North America, 50*(6), 1543–1560.

Aukamp, V., & Sredl, D. (2004). Collaborative care manage-ment for a pregnant woman with an ostomy. *Complemen-tary Therapies in Nursing & Midwifery, 10*(1), 5–12.

Basaran, O., et al. (2004). Pregnancy and renal transplantation. *Transplantation Proceedings, 36*(1), 122–124.

Bergeron, K. G., et al. (2003). Latent tuberculosis in pregnancy: screening and treatment. *Current Women's Health Reports, 3*(4), 303–308.

Bisharah, M., & Tulandi, T. (2003). Laparoscopic surgery in pregnancy. *Clinical Obstetrics & Gynecology, 46*(1), 92–97.

Boxall, E. H., et al. (2004). Natural history of hepatitis B in peri-natally infected carriers. *Archives of Disease in Childhood Fetal & Neonatal Edition, 89*(5), F456–460.

Brocklehurst, P. (2005). Antibiotics for gonorrhea in pregnancy. *The Cochrane Library (Oxford) (4)* (CD000098).

Buyon, J. P., & Clancy, R. M. (2003). Neonatal lupus syndromes. *Current Opinion in Rheumatology, 15*(5), 535–541.

Carp, H. J. (2004). Antiphospholipid syndrome in pregnancy. *Current Opinion in Obstetrics & Gynecology, 16*(2), 129–135.

Centers for Disease Control and Prevention. (2002). Sexually transmitted diseases treatment guidelines, 2002. *MMWR, 51*(1), 1–77.

Chakravarty, E. F., et al. (2004). The use of disease-modifying antirheumatic drugs in women with rheumatoid arthritis of childbearing age: a survey of practice patterns and pregnancy outcomes. *Journal of Rheumatology, 30*(2), 241–246.

Ciafaloni, E., & Massey, J. M. (2004). The management of myas-thenia gravis in pregnancy. *Seminars in Neurology, 24*(1), 95–100.

Colman-Brochu, S. (2004). Deep vein thrombosis in pregnancy. *MCN, American Journal of Maternal Child Nursing, 29*(3), 186–192.

Cooper, D. S. (2003). Hyperthyroidism. *Lancet, 362*(9382), 459–468.

De Jon-Van den Berg, L. T., et al. (2005). Trends and predictors of folic acid awareness and periconceptual use in pregnant women. *American Journal of Obstetrics & Gynecology, 192*(1), 121–128.

Department of Health and Human Services. (2000). *Healthy people 2010.* Washington, DC: DHHS.

Dwosh, E., et al. (2003). The interaction of MS and pregnancy: a critical review. *International MS Journal, 10*(2), 38–42.

Elkayam, U., et al. (2004). Anticoagulation in pregnant women with prosthetic heart valves. *Journal of Cardiovascular Pharmacology & Therapeutics, 9*(2), 107–115.

Eroglu, D., et al. (2004). Pregnancy during hemodialysis: peri-natal outcome in our cases. *Transplantation Proceedings, 36*(1), 53–55.

Eschenbach, D. A. (2003). Pelvic infections and sexually trans-mitted infections. In J. R. Scott et al. (Eds.), *Danforth's ob-stetrics and gynecology* (9th ed.). Philadelphia: Lippincott Williams & Wilkins.

Fey, M. C., & Beal, M. W. (2004). Role of human papilloma virus testing in cervical cancer prevention. *Journal of Midwifery & Women's Health, 49*(1), 4–13.

Gabbe, S. G. (2003). Management of diabetes mellitus complicat-ing pregnancy. *Obstetrics & Gynecology, 102*(4), 857–868.

Geohas, C., & McLaughlin, V. V. (2003). Successful manage-ment of pregnancy in a patient with Eisenmenger syn-drome with epoprostenol. *Chest, 124*(3), 1170–1173.

Goss, C. H., et al. (2003). The effect of pregnancy on survival in women with cystic fibrosis. *Chest, 124*(4), 1460–1468.

Hadden, R. (2004). What nurses need to know. Hepatitis C & pregnancy. *AWHONN Lifelines, 8*(3), 226–231.

Harper, S. A., et al. (2004). Prevention and control of influenza. *MMWR, 53*(RR-6), 1–40.

Hu, D. S. C., et al. (2004). Severe acute respiratory syndrome (SARS): epidemiology and clinical features. *Postgraduate Medical Journal, 80*(2), 279–286.

Hyde, L. K., et al. (2003). Effect of motor vehicle crashes on adverse fetal outcomes. *Obstetrics & Gynecology, 102*(2), 279–286.

Jackson, C. (2003). The effect of myasthenia gravis on pregnancy and the newborn. *Neurology, 61*(10), 1459–1460.

Janssen, P. A., et al. (2003). Intimate partner violence and adverse pregnancy outcomes: a population-based study. *American Journal of Obstetrics & Gynecology, 188*(5), 1341–1347.

Jesse, D. E., & Graham, M. (2005). Are you often sad and depressed? Brief measures to identify women at risk for depression in pregnancy. *MCN: The American Journal of Maternal/Child Nursing, 30*(1), 40–45.

Johnson, M., Maas, M., & Moorhead, S. (2000). *Nursing outcomes classification* (2nd ed.). St. Louis: Mosby.

Karch, A. M. (2004). *Lippincott's nursing drug guide.* Philadelphia: Lippincott Williams & Wilkins.

Katz, V. L. (2003). Prenatal care. In J. R. Scott et al. (Eds.), *Danforth's obstetrics and gynecology.* Philadelphia: Lippincott Williams & Wilkins.

Lallemant, M., et al. (2004). Single-dose perinatal nevirapine plus standard zidovudine to prevent mother-to-child transmission of HIV-1 in Thailand. *New England Journal of Medicine, 351*(3), 217–228.

Langley, R. L. (2004). A review of venomous animal bites and stings in pregnant patients. *Wilderness & Environmental Medicine, 15*(3), 207–215.

Lim, W. S., Macfarlane, J. T., & Colthorpe, C. L. (2003). Treatment of community-acquired lower respiratory tract infections during pregnancy. *American Journal of Respiratory Medicine, 2*(3), 221–233.

Magder, L. S., et al. (2005). Risk factors for in utero and intrapartum transmission of HIV. *JAIDS: Journal of Acquired Immune Deficiency Syndromes, 38*(1), 87–95.

Malee, M. P. (2003). Medical and surgical complications of pregnancy. In J. R. Scott et al. (Eds.), *Danforth's obstetrics and gynecology.* Philadelphia: Lippincott Williams & Wilkins.

Martin, P. S. (2003). CPR: when the patient's pregnant. *RN, 66*(8), 34–40.

McCloskey, J., & Bulechek, G. (2000). *Nursing interventions classification* (3rd ed.). St. Louis: Mosby.

McRae, S. J., & Ginsberg, J. S. (2004). Initial treatment of venous thromboembolism. *Circulation, 110*(9 Suppl 1), I3–9.

Meador, K. J., & Zupanc, M. L. (2004). Neurodevelopmental outcomes of children born to mothers with epilepsy. *Cleveland Clinic Journal of Medicine, 71*(Suppl 2), S38–S41.

Millar, L. K., DeBuque, L., & Wing, D. A. (2003). Uterine contraction frequency during treatment of pyelonephritis in pregnancy and subsequent risk of preterm birth. *Journal of Perinatal Medicine, 31*(1), 41–46.

Minkoff, H. L., & Gibbs, R. S. (2003). Obstetric and perinatal infections. In J. R. Scott et al. (Eds.), *Danforth's obstetrics and gynecology* (9th ed.). Philadelphia: Lippincott Williams & Wilkins.

Morgan, K. L. (2004). Management of UTIs during pregnancy. *MCN, American Journal of Maternal Child Nursing, 29*(4), 254–258.

Mungen, E. (2003). Iron supplementation in pregnancy. *Journal of Perinatal Medicine, 31*(5), 420–426.

Neralla, S., & Glassroth, J. (2003). *Mycobacterium tuberculosis:* the treatment of active disease. *Seminars in Respiratory Infections, 18*(4), 292–306.

Ostensen, M. E., & Skomsvoll, J. F. (2004). Anti-inflammatory pharmacotherapy during pregnancy. *Expert Opinion on Pharmacotherapy, 5*(3), 571–580.

Penovich, P. E., Eck, K. E., & Economou, V. V. (2004). Recommendations for the care of women with epilepsy. *Cleveland Clinic Journal of Medicine, 71*(Suppl 2), S49–57.

Pons, P. T. (2004). Secondary syphilis with Jarisch-Herxheimer reaction. *Annals of Emergency Medicine, 43*(1), 136–138.

Pop, V. J., et al. (2004). Low concentrations of maternal thyroxin during early gestation: a risk factor of breech presentation? *BJOG: International Journal of Obstetrics & Gynaecology, 111*(9), 925–930.

Redding, G., & Stoloff, S. (2004). Changes in recommended treatments for mild and moderate asthma. *Journal of Family Practice, 53*(9), 692–700.

Reece, E. A., & Homko, C. J. (2003). Diabetes mellitus and pregnancy. In J. R. Scott et al. (Eds.), *Danforth's obstetrics and gynecology.* Philadelphia: Lippincott Williams & Wilkins.

Reimold, S. C., & Rutherford, J. D. (2003). Valvular heart disease in pregnancy. *New England Journal of Medicine, 349*(1), 52–59.

Richards, C. S., & Haddow, J. E. (2003). Prenatal screening for cystic fibrosis. *Clinics in Laboratory Medicine, 23*(2), 503–530.

Richter, J. E. (2003). Medical management of patients with esophageal or supraesophageal gastroesophageal reflux disease. *American Journal of Medicine, 115*(Suppl 3A), 179S–187S.

Rollins, M. D., Chan, K. J., & Price, R. R. (2004). Laparoscopy for appendicitis and cholelithiasis during pregnancy: a new standard of care. *Surgical Endoscopy, 18*(2), 237–241.

Scarlatti, G. (2004). Mother-to-child transmission of HIV-1: advances and controversies of the twentieth centuries. *AIDS Reviews, 6*(2), 67–78.

Scharbo-DeHaan, M., & Anderson, D. G. (2003). The CDC 2002 guidelines for the treatment of sexually transmitted diseases: implications for women's health care. *Journal of Midwifery & Women's Health, 48*(2), 96–104.

Serjeant, G. R., et al. (2004). Outcome of pregnancy in homozygous sickle cell disease. *Obstetrics & Gynecology, 103*(6), 1278–1285.

Shah, A. J., & Kilcline, B. A. (2003). Trauma in pregnancy. *Emergency Medicine Clinics of North America, 21*(3), 615–629.

Watts, N. (2004). Screening for domestic violence: a team approach for maternal/newborn nurses. *AWHONN Lifelines, 8*(3), 210–219.

Wingerchuk, D. M., & Carter, J. L. (2003). Practical consultations: multiple sclerosis. *Seminars in Neurology, 23*(3), 253–264.

Wong, S. F., et al. (2004). Pregnancy and perinatal outcomes of women with severe acute respiratory syndrome. *American Journal of Obstetrics & Gynecology, 191*(1), 292–297.

Wren, C., Birrell, G., & Hawthorne, G. (2003). Cardiovascular malformations in infants of diabetic mothers. *Heart, 89*(10), 1217–1220.

Yankowitz, J. (2003). Drugs in pregnancy. In J. R. Scott et al. (Eds.), *Danforth's obstetrics and gynecology.* Philadelphia: Lippincott Williams & Wilkins.

Young, G. L., & Jewell, D. (2005). Topical treatment for vaginal candidiasis (thrush) in pregnancy. *The Cochrane Library (Oxford) (4)* (CD000225).

Suggested Readings

American Diabetes Association. (2003). Evidence-based nutrition principles and recommendations for the treatment and prevention of diabetes and related complications. *Diabetes Care, 26*(Suppl 1), S51–S61.

Andrews, J. I., & Lockwood, C. J. (2004). When does a pregnant patient need antibiotics? *Contemporary OB/GYN, 49*(2), 45–52.

Colwell, C., Murphy, P., & Bryan, T. (2004). Prehospital management of the pregnant patient. *Emergency Medical Services, 33*(3), 59–62.

Duncan, J. (2004). Pregnancy in chronic inflammatory bowel disease. *Gastrointestinal Nursing, 2*(1), 29–34.

Fox, R., et al. (2004). Integrated care pathway for diabetes in pregnancy. *Journal of Integrated Care Pathways, 8*(1), 27–40.

Green, N. S., et al. (2003). Understanding pregnant women's perspectives on preterm birth. *Contemporary OB/GYN, 48*(1), 70–76.

Lange, S. S., & Jenner, M. (2004). Myocardial infarction in the obstetric patient. *Critical Care Nursing Clinics of North America, 16*(2), 211–219.

Murphy, A., Guilar, A., & Donat, D. (2004). Nutrition education for women with newly diagnosed gestational diabetes mellitus: small-group vs. individual counseling. *Canadian Journal of Diabetes, 28*(2), 147–151.

Shehata, H. A., & Okosun, H. (2004). Neurological disorders in pregnancy. *Current Opinion in Obstetrics & Gynecology, 16*(2), 117–122.

Thomas, H. (2004). Women's postnatal experience following a medically complicated pregnancy. *Health Care for Women International, 25*(1), 76–87.

Thompson, J. (2004). Pregnancy: depression and domestic violence. *Community Practitioner, 77*(5), 192–193.

Tuffnell, D. J., West, J., & Walkinshaw, S. A. (2005). Treatments for gestational diabetes and impaired glucose tolerance in pregnancy. *The Cochrane Library (Oxford) (4)* (CD003395).

Walker, G. J. A. (2005). Antibiotics for syphilis diagnosed during pregnancy. *The Cochrane Library (Oxford) (4)* (CD001143).

CHAPTER 15

High-Risk Pregnancy: A Woman Who Develops a Complication of Pregnancy

Key Terms

abortion
ankle clonus
cervical
  cerclage
chorioamnio-
  nitis
Couvelaire
  uterus
early
  pregnancy
  failure
eclampsia
ectopic
  pregnancy
erythroblasto-
  sis fetalis
gestational
  trophoblas-
  tic disease
HELLP
  syndrome
hemolytic
  disease
  of the
  newborn
hydramnios

isoimmuni-
  zation
miscarriage
placenta
  previa
post-term
  pregnancy
preeclampsia
premature
  cervical
  dilatation
premature
  separation
  of the
  placenta
preterm labor
preterm
  rupture of
  membranes
pseudocyesis
recurrent
  pregnancy
  loss
Rh incompa-
  tibility
tocolytic agent

Objectives

After mastering the contents of this chapter, you should be able to:

1. Describe complications of pregnancy that place a pregnant woman and her fetus at high risk.
2. Assess a woman who is experiencing a complication of pregnancy.
3. Formulate nursing diagnoses that address the needs of a woman and her family experiencing a complication of pregnancy.
4. Identify expected outcomes to minimize the risks to a pregnant woman and her fetus when a complication of pregnancy occurs.
5. Plan nursing interventions to meet the needs and promote optimal outcomes for a woman and her family during a complication of pregnancy.
6. Implement nursing actions specific to a woman who has developed a complication of pregnancy.

7. Evaluate outcomes for effectiveness and achievement of nursing care.
8. Identify National Health Goals related to complications of pregnancy and specific measures nurses can take to help the nation achieve these goals.
9. Identify areas of nursing care related to high-risk pregnancy that could benefit from additional nursing research or the application of evidence-based practice.
10. Use critical thinking to analyze ways that nurses can help prevent complications of pregnancy while keeping care family-centered.
11. Integrate knowledge of complications of pregnancy with nursing process to achieve quality maternal and child health nursing care.

---

*B*everly Muzuki is a 20-year-old gravida 2, para 0, 30 weeks pregnant, whom you see in a prenatal clinic. She has had symptoms of a urinary tract infection for the past few days but didn't call the clinic because she knew she had an appointment today and thought getting some help for it could wait until she came in. Yesterday she noticed some mild abdominal pain but thought it was irritation from the bladder infection. During the night, she woke twice because of a nagging backache. This morning, she has intermittent sharp uterine contractions. "Why did this happen?" she asks you. "I didn't do anything wrong."

Previous chapters described normal pregnancy and preexisting and newly acquired conditions that can complicate pregnancy. This chapter adds to your knowledge base information about complications directly related to the pregnancy.

Were Beverly's actions as informed as they could have been?

What additional health teaching might have prevented her from starting labor so early?

After you've studied this chapter, access the accompanying website. Read the patient scenario and answer the questions to further sharpen your skills, grow more familiar with RN-CLEX types of questions, and reward yourself with how much you have learned.

The average woman who enters pregnancy in good health achieves a successful pregnancy and birth without complications. In a few women, however, for reasons that usually are unclear, unexpected deviations or complications from the course of normal pregnancy occur. When this happens, it can place a severe burden on a woman and her family. All families benefit from the support and skill of a professional nurse who helps them work through the tasks of pregnancy and prepare to become new parents. The support and skills of a professional nurse are essential to a family who, in addition to the usual tasks of pregnancy, must take special care to ensure the continuation of the pregnancy and who may be very concerned that the baby cannot be carried to term. Initially, if a pregnant woman develops a complication, hospitalization may be necessary. Once stabilized, a woman may be a candidate for continued follow-up with home care (see Chapter 16).

The leading causes of maternal death during pregnancy are thromboembolism, hemorrhage, infection, pregnancy-induced hypertension, anesthesia complications, ectopic pregnancy, and heart disease (Malee, 2003). These complications have the potential to threaten the life of the mother and the fetus. National Health Goals to reduce complications of pregnancy are shown in Box 15.1.

BOX 15.1 FOCUS ON . . .

NATIONAL HEALTH GOALS

Preventing complications of pregnancy is viewed as so important by most people that this issue is included in the National Health Goals. Four of these goals are:

- Reduce the rate of maternal deaths from pregnancy-related causes to 3.3 per 100,000 live births, from a baseline of 7.1 per 100,000.
- Reduce the rate of maternal illness and complications due to pregnancy to 24 per 100 births, from a baseline of 31 per 100 births.
- Reduce the proportion of preterm births to 7.6%, from a baseline of 11.6%.
- Reduce the incidence of low birthweight to no more than 5% of live births, from a baseline of 7.6%, and of very low birthweight to no more than 0.9% of live births, from a baseline of 1.4% (DHHS, 2000).

Nurses working in prenatal settings can help to ensure that women are well informed about the normal course of pregnancy so they can recognize and alert health care providers when a complication is occurring. They can actively participate in risk assessment at prenatal visits. Nursing research is needed in areas such as what is the best way to determine each woman's individual needs so prenatal instructions can be specifically planned, and whether increasing the number of prenatal visits for high-risk women could reduce complications during pregnancy.

Nursing Process Overview

Caring for a Woman Who Develops a Complication of Pregnancy

● Assessment

Nurses often are the first health care providers to discover that a complication of pregnancy is beginning because they are the people who talk to clients first at prenatal visits. At prenatal visits, always ask women about any symptoms that might indicate a complication. Provide enough time for a thorough health history so problems such as headache, blurred vision, or vaginal spotting can be discovered and investigated thoroughly.

In addition, at the close of a visit, review these symptoms with a woman so she can recognize potential problems and contact the health care center if problems occur. Assure women when giving this information that they are free to call whenever they are concerned. Otherwise, they may wait until their symptoms are acute rather than call when they first notice them.

● Nursing Diagnosis

Many nursing diagnoses pertain to a woman with a pregnancy complication. Some examples are:

- Anxiety related to guarded pregnancy outcome
- Deficient fluid volume related to third-trimester bleeding
- Risk for infection related to incomplete miscarriage
- Risk for ineffective tissue perfusion related to pregnancy-induced hypertension
- Deficient knowledge related to signs and symptoms of possible complications

● Outcome Identification and Planning

Complications of pregnancy produce emergency situations, so outcomes usually focus on a short time frame. Outcomes should address both fetal and maternal welfare and often reflect total family welfare. Treatment protocols, such as those related to bleeding, preterm labor, and pregnancy-induced hypertension, should be regularly updated and maintained so they remain current. Be certain that they reflect a current nursing management level so nurses can act swiftly and independently as needed. Once a woman's condition stabilizes, outcome identification can then focus on long-term objectives.

Many women who develop a pregnancy complication spend a few days in the hospital for therapy and monitoring followed by discharge to their homes, where they may be required to maintain bed rest for a long time. Waiting for a pregnancy to come to term this way can be difficult and anxious. Readmission to the health care facility, especially when a new complication occurs, compounds these feelings. Planning must consider the many feelings this experience can cause.

● *Implementation*

Interventions for a woman experiencing a complication of pregnancy include measures to maintain a number of different areas:

• Continued healthy fetal growth
• A woman's and family's psychological health
• Continuation of the pregnancy as long as possible

Maintaining an optimistic attitude of fetal progress is important so a woman does not begin anticipatory grieving for the fetus and halt the growth of bonding. If the complication can be contained and the pregnancy continues uninterrupted, this will help protect the mental health of the whole family. If the pregnancy cannot be continued, be available to offer support to the family who grieves for the loss of an unborn child and, in rare instances, loss of future childbearing potential or the woman herself.

After a pregnancy with complications, a mother has reason to be especially worried about her infant's health at the time of birth. Be certain she spends enough time with her child to see that although perhaps born before term, her infant is well and healthy. It is helpful to assess the infant for such things as ability to follow a light and respond to a voice while the mother is present. This helps to demonstrate that the infant is well. If an infant is ill at birth, be certain a mother spends time with the child as well, perhaps visiting in an intensive care nursery. This may be difficult because she still may be ill herself.

● *Outcome Evaluation*

Although the success or failure of some nursing interventions cannot be fully evaluated until a child is born or even into the postnatal period, outcomes should be evaluated throughout the pregnancy. Be aware that after a complication of early pregnancy, a woman cannot help but worry during the remainder of the pregnancy that the complication will recur or that the original insult to the fetus was severe enough to cause long-term effects. Evaluate a woman's attitude and physical status at each health care visit to be certain she is coping with the situation and the fear and strain she lives under until the child is born.

Not all fetal outcomes will be optimal. Evaluation will then include the ability of the family to care for an ill infant. Examples of expected outcomes are:

• Client's blood pressure is maintained within acceptable parameters.
• Couple state they feel able to cope with anxiety associated with the pregnancy complication.
• Client remains free of signs and symptoms of pregnancy-induced hypertension.
• Client accurately verbalizes crucial signs and symptoms to report to the health care provider immediately.

BLEEDING DURING PREGNANCY

Vaginal bleeding is a deviation from the normal that may occur at any point during pregnancy. It is never normal, and it is always frightening. It must always be carefully investigated because if it occurs in sufficient amount or for sufficient cause, it can impair both the outcome of the pregnancy and a woman's life or health. The primary causes of bleeding during pregnancy are summarized in Table 15.1.

Bleeding and the Development of Shock

Although vaginal bleeding may be innocent, any degree of vaginal bleeding during pregnancy is potentially serious because the amount visualized may be only a fraction of the blood actually lost. This happens because an undilated cervix and intact membranes can contain blood within the uterus. A woman with any degree of bleeding, therefore, needs to be evaluated for the possibility that she is experiencing a significant blood loss and for hypovolemic shock.

The process of shock due to blood loss is shown in Figure 15.1. Note that because the uterus is a nonessential body organ, danger to the fetal blood supply occurs when a woman's body begins to decrease blood flow to peripheral organs (although the increased blood volume of pregnancy allows more than normal blood loss before hypovolemic shock occurs). Signs of hypovolemic shock (Table 15.2) occur when 10% of blood volume, or approximately two units of blood, have been lost; fetal distress occurs when 25% of blood volume is lost (Box 15.2). Because "normal" blood pressure varies from woman to woman, it is important to know the baseline blood pressure for a pregnant woman. Inform women of their blood pressure at prenatal visits; for example, "Your blood pressure is 110 over 70—that's normal," not just "Your pressure is normal." Then if blood loss should occur, a woman may remember her baseline pressure.

NURSING DIAGNOSES AND RELATED INTERVENTIONS

———●———

Nursing Diagnosis: Risk for deficient fluid volume related to bleeding during pregnancy

Outcome Evaluation: Client's blood pressure is maintained at above 100/60 mm Hg; pulse rate is below 100 beats per minute; only minimal bleeding is apparent; fetal heart rate is maintained at 120 to 160 bpm, with adequate short-term and long-term variability; urine output is greater than 30 mL/hour.

Therapy for hypovolemic shock is aimed at restoring blood volume and halting the source of hemorrhage (Table 15.3). Monitoring urine output is a good gauge of blood loss because kidneys need sufficient arterial blood flow and pressure to function. Obtaining hemoglobin and hematocrit levels and securing a blood sample for typing or cross-matching are essential, as hypovolemic shock can

TABLE 15.1

Summary of Causes of Bleeding During Pregnancy

Time	Type	Cause	Assessment	Cautions
First trimester	Threatened miscarriage (early—under 16 weeks; late—16 to 24 weeks)	Unknown; possibly chromosomal, uterine abnormalities	Vaginal spotting, perhaps slight cramping	
	Imminent (inevitable) miscarriage		Vaginal spotting, cramping, cervical dilatation	
	Missed miscarriage		Vaginal spotting, perhaps slight cramping; no apparent loss of pregnancy	Disseminated intravascular coagulation associated with missed miscarriage
	Incomplete miscarriage		Vaginal spotting, cramping, cervical dilatation, but incomplete expulsion of uterine contents	
	Complete miscarriage		Vaginal spotting, cramping, cervical dilatation, and complete expulsion of uterine contents	
	Ectopic (tubal) pregnancy	Implantation of zygote at site other than in uterus; tubal constricture, adhesions associated	Sudden unilateral lower abdominal quadrant pain; minimal vaginal bleeding, possible signs of shock or hemorrhage	May have repeat ectopic pregnancy in future if tubal scarring is bilateral
Second trimester	Hydatidiform mole (gestational trophoblastic disease)	Abnormal proliferation of trophoblast tissue; fertilization or division defect	Overgrowth of uterus; highly positive human chorionic gonadotropin (hCG) test; no fetus present on sonogram; bleeding from vagina of old or fresh blood accompanied by cyst formation	Retained trophoblast tissue may become malignant (choriocarcinoma); follow for 6 months to 1 year with hCG testing
	Premature cervical dilatation	Cervix begins to dilate and pregnancy is lost at about 20 weeks; unknown cause, but cervical trauma from dilatation and curettage (D&C) may be associated	Painless bleeding leading to expulsion of fetus	Can have cervical sutures placed to ensure a second pregnancy
Third trimester	Placenta previa	Low implantation of placenta possibly due to uterine abnormality	Painless bleeding at beginning of cervical dilatation	No vaginal examinations to minimize placental trauma
	Premature separation of the placenta (abruptio placentae)	Unknown cause; associated with hypertension; placenta separates from uterus	Sharp abdominal pain followed by uterine tenderness; vaginal bleeding; signs of maternal shock, fetal distress	Disseminated intravascular coagulation associated with condition
	Preterm labor	Many possible etiologic factors such as trauma, substance abuse, pregnancy-induced hypertension or cervicitis; increased chance in multiple gestation, maternal illness	Show (pink-stained vaginal discharge) accompanied by uterine contractions becoming regular and effective	Preterm labor may be halted if the cervix is less than 4 cm dilated and the membranes are intact

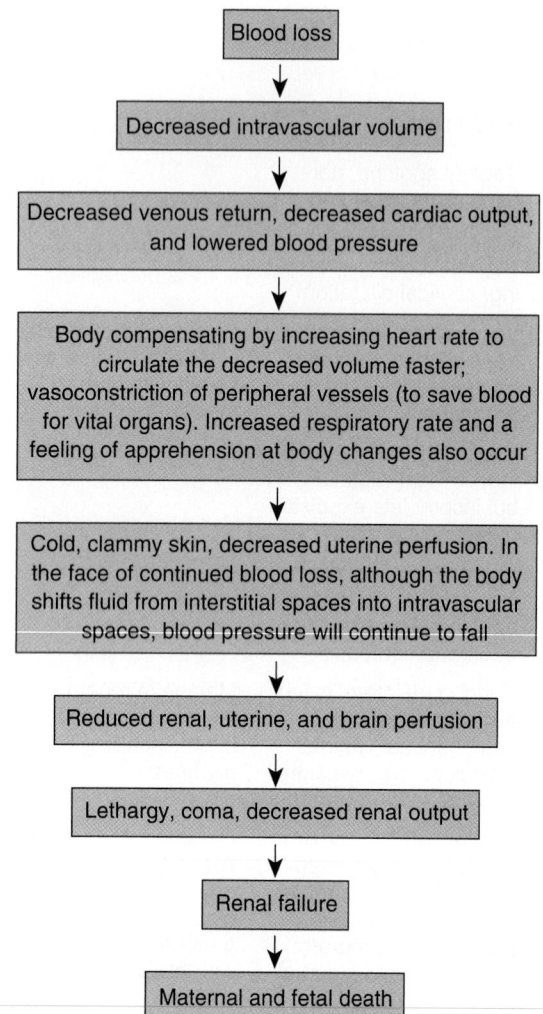

FIGURE 15.1 The process of shock due to blood loss (*hypovolemia*).

TABLE 15.2

Signs and Symptoms of Hypovolemic Shock

Assessment	Significance
Increased pulse rate	Heart is attempting to circulate decreased blood volume
Decreased blood pressure	Less peripheral resistance because of decreased blood volume
Increased respiratory rate	Increases gas exchange to better oxygenate decreased red blood cell volume
Cold, clammy skin	Vasoconstriction occurs to maintain blood volume in central body core
Decreased urine output	Inadequate blood is entering kidney due to decreased blood volume
Dizziness or decreased level of consciousness	Inadequate blood is reaching cerebrum due to decreased blood volume
Decreased central venous pressure	Decreased blood is returning to heart due to reduced blood volume

a wedge under one hip to minimize uterine pressure on the vena cava and to prevent blood from being trapped in the lower extremities (supine hypotension syndrome).

CONDITIONS ASSOCIATED WITH FIRST-TRIMESTER BLEEDING

The time during pregnancy at which bleeding occurs helps to identify its cause. The two most common causes of bleeding during the first trimester are spontaneous miscarriage and ectopic pregnancy.

Spontaneous Miscarriage

An **abortion** is the medical term for any interruption of a pregnancy before a fetus is viable (able to survive outside the uterus if born at that time). A viable fetus is usually defined as a fetus of more than 20 to 24 weeks of gestation or one that weighs at least 500 g. A fetus born before this point is considered a premature or immature birth.

Elective abortion, discussed in Chapter 5, is the planned medical termination of a pregnancy. When the interruption occurs spontaneously, it is clearer to refer to it as a **miscarriage.**

Spontaneous miscarriage occurs in 15% to 30% of all pregnancies and occurs from natural causes (Branch & Scott, 2003). A spontaneous miscarriage is an early miscarriage if it occurs before week 16 of pregnancy and a late miscarriage if it occurs between weeks 16 and 24. For the first 6 weeks of pregnancy, the developing placenta is tentatively attached to the decidua of the uterus; during weeks 6 to 12, a moderate degree of attachment to the myometrium is accomplished. After week 12, the attachment is

lead to multiorgan failure (Poole, 2004). A woman may have a central venous pressure or a pulmonary artery catheter (to measure pulmonary capillary wedge pressure) inserted (see Chapter 41). During pregnancy, these values differ from the average, so they should be evaluated in light of the pregnancy. Central venous pressure during pregnancy is 2 to 7 mm Hg; pulmonary capillary wedge pressure is 6 to 10 mm Hg.

A woman suspected of having serious bleeding needs intravenous fluid replacement as an early intervention. Use a large-gauge Angiocath (16 or 18) for rapid fluid expansion with a solution such as Ringer's lactate. This allows a blood transfusion to be administered through the same site as soon as blood is available. If respirations are rapid, administer oxygen by mask and monitor oxygen saturation levels by pulse oximetry. Obtain arterial blood gases as ordered. Frequent assessments of vital signs should be done, and continuous fetal monitoring by an external monitoring device should be started. Urge the woman to lie in a lateral position. If this is not possible, position her on her back, with

a possibility. Monitor vital signs for changes to detect possible hypovolemic shock. If excessive vaginal bleeding is occurring, immediately position a woman flat and massage the uterine fundus to aid contraction (see Chapter 22). This may be impossible with an early pregnancy because the small uterus isn't palpable above the symphysis pubis. A woman may need a D&C or suction curettage to empty the uterus of the material that is preventing it from contracting and achieving hemostasis. A transfusion may be necessary to replace blood loss. Direct replacement of fibrinogen or another clotting factor may be used to aid coagulation.

After a self-limiting complete miscarriage, a woman needs clear instructions on how much bleeding is abnormal (a rule of thumb is that more than one sanitary pad per hour is excessive) and what color changes she should expect in bleeding (gradually changing to a dark color and then to the color of serous fluid as it does with the postpartum woman). She should know that any unusual odor or passing of large clots is also abnormal. If her physician has prescribed an oral medication such as oral methylergonovine maleate (Methergine) to aid with contraction, be sure she understands why it is being prescribed and the importance of taking it. Some women repress their feelings, anxious to forget the experience as quickly as possible. Repression helps them to handle their anger or grief at the loss of the pregnancy. Be careful that in repressing the experience, however, the woman does not also repress the memory of her medication and leave herself open to hemorrhage.

Infection. The possibility of infection is minimal when pregnancy loss occurs over a short time, bleeding is self-limiting, and instrumentation is limited. However, there's always a possibility it may occur.

Infection tends to occur in women who have lost appreciable amounts of blood, most likely from the debilitating effect of blood loss. Such women need especially close observation to rule out this second and possibly fatal complication.

After a miscarriage, be certain a woman knows the danger signs of infection, such as fever, abdominal pain or tenderness, and a foul vaginal discharge. Fever can be a transient reaction to a period of decreased fluid intake that preceded the miscarriage. In other instances, the fever may be a systemic reaction to the miscarriage process. All fevers of more than 100.4°F (38.0°C) require careful evaluation to avoid overlooking the possibility of infection.

The organism responsible for infection after miscarriage is usually *Escherichia coli* (spread from the rectum forward into the vagina). Caution a woman to wipe her perineal area from front to back after voiding and particularly after defecation to prevent the spread of bacteria from the rectal area. Caution her not to use tampons to control vaginal discharge, because stasis of any body fluid increases the risk of infection. Be careful about using statements such as, "You'll have some vaginal flow now, almost exactly like a menstrual flow." Otherwise, a woman might treat it as a menstrual period and use tampons.

If infection occurs, endometritis (infection of the uterine lining) is the type that usually occurs. It may be more extensive, however, and parametritis, peritonitis, thrombophlebitis, and septicemia can develop. The management of these infections is the same as if they were occurring after the safe delivery of a child (see Chapter 23).

Septic Abortion. A septic abortion is an abortion that is complicated by infection (Rana et al., 2004). Infection can happen after a spontaneous miscarriage, but more frequently it occurs in women who have tried to self-abort or were aborted illegally using a nonsterile instrument such as a knitting needle. Because the uterus is a warm, moist, dark cavity, infectious organisms, once introduced, grow rapidly in this environment, particularly if products of conception such as necrotic membranes are still present.

A woman has symptoms of fever and crampy abdominal pain, and her uterus feels tender to palpation. Left untreated, such an infection can lead to toxic shock syndrome, septicemia, kidney failure, and death.

Women with septic abortion need immediate, intensive assessment and treatment. Typically, complete blood count, serum electrolytes, serum creatinine, blood type and cross-match, and cervical, vaginal, and urine cultures are obtained. An indwelling urinary (Foley) catheter may be inserted to monitor urine output hourly to assess kidney function. Intravenous fluid to restore fluid volume and to provide a route for high-dose, broad-spectrum antibiotic therapy is started. A combination of penicillin (gram-positive coverage), gentamicin (gram-negative aerobic coverage), and clindamycin (gram-negative anaerobic coverage) is commonly used.

A central venous pressure or pulmonary artery catheter may be inserted to monitor left atrial filling pressure and hemodynamic status. The removal of all infected or necrotic tissue from the uterus is important, so a D&C or D&E will be performed. Tetanus toxoid given subcutaneously or tetanus immune globulin given intramuscularly will be ordered for prophylaxis against tetanus.

Infection can be so severe that a woman is admitted to an intensive care setting for continuing care. Dopamine and digitalis may be necessary to maintain sufficient cardiac output. Oxygen and perhaps ventilatory support may be necessary to maintain respiratory function.

Assuming a woman recovers from the intense episode, septic abortion may lead to infertility due to uterine scarring or fibrotic scarring of the fallopian tubes. If a woman caused the infection by trying to self-abort, she needs follow-up counseling to assist her to learn better problem-solving methods for the future.

Isoimmunization. Whenever a placenta is dislodged, either by spontaneous birth or by a D&C at any point in pregnancy, some blood from the placental villi (the fetal blood) may enter the maternal circulation. If the fetus was Rh positive and the woman is Rh negative, enough Rh-positive fetal blood may enter her circulation to cause **isoimmunization**—the production of antibodies against Rh-positive blood by her immunologic system. If her next child should have Rh-positive blood, these antibodies would attempt to destroy the red blood cells of the next infant during the months that infant is in utero.

After a miscarriage, because the blood type of the conceptus is unknown, all women with Rh-negative blood should receive Rh (D antigen) immune globulin (RhIG) to prevent the buildup of antibodies in the event the conceptus was Rh positive.

Powerlessness or Anxiety. As with pregnancy loss for any reason, assess a woman's adjustment to a spontaneous miscarriage (Brier, 2004). Sadness and grief over the loss or a feeling that a woman has lost control of her life is to be expected. Don't forget to assess a partner's feelings as well, or that person's grief over the pregnancy loss can be missed (Box 15.5).

Spontaneous miscarriage can be particularly heartbreaking for an older woman, because she realizes that her window of childbearing is limited.

Checkpoint Question 1

Beverly Muzuki, the woman you met at the beginning of the chapter, had a miscarriage when she was younger. What would be the best advice to give a woman who tells you she is miscarrying?

a. Lie down and don't move for 24 hours to stop the bleeding.
b. Don't do anything special; early miscarriages happen all the time.
c. Save any clots or material passed for your health care provider.
d. Use a tight tampon to put pressure on your cervix and stop the bleeding.

BOX 15.5 FOCUS ON . . .

EVIDENCE-BASED PRACTICE

Do women's partners grieve at the same level as women after a pregnancy loss?

To answer this question, a sociologist interviewed 32 midwives or nurses and 14 men who attended a pregnancy loss self-help group in Northern Ireland. The study uncovered several recurring themes of how men feel after a pregnancy loss, including self-blame, loss of identity, and the need to appear strong and hide feelings of grief and anger. The researcher concluded that when a baby dies before birth, the loss can be extremely devastating for fathers. At the same time, friends and health care personnel tend to discount the loss, omitting the emotional support and cultural rituals that are normally available to bereaved individuals. Asking men to be emotionally strong and support their grieving wives may be asking too much when this situation has created a very personal emotional tragedy for the man as well as the woman. Acknowledging the male partner's grief could lead to better communication about his feelings and better resolution of his grief.

This is an important study for nurses because in the emergency atmosphere of an impending pregnancy loss, it is easy to concentrate on the woman, forgetting that her partner is also suffering from the pregnancy loss.

Source: McCreight, B. S. (2004). A grief ignored: narratives of pregnancy loss from a male perspective. *Sociology of Health and Illness, 26*(3), 326–350.

Ectopic Pregnancy

An **ectopic pregnancy** is one in which implantation occurs outside the uterine cavity. The implantation may occur on the surface of the ovary or in the cervix. The most common site (in approximately 95% of such pregnancies) is in a fallopian tube (Fig. 15.2). Of these fallopian tube sites, approximately 80% occur in the ampullar portion, 12% occur in the isthmus, and 8% are interstitial or fimbrial (Heard & Buster, 2003).

With ectopic pregnancy, fertilization occurs as usual in the distal third of the fallopian tube. Immediately after the union of ovum and spermatozoon, the zygote begins to divide and grow normally. Unfortunately, because an obstruction is present, such as an adhesion of the fallopian tube from a previous infection (chronic salpingitis or pelvic inflammatory disease), congenital malformations, scars from tubal surgery, or a uterine tumor pressing on the proximal end of the tube, the zygote cannot travel the length of the tube. It lodges at the strictured site along the tube and implants there instead of in the uterus.

Approximately 2% of pregnancies are ectopic; ectopic pregnancy is the second most frequent cause of bleeding early in pregnancy. The incidence is increasing because of the increasing rate of pelvic inflammatory disease, which leads to tubal scarring. Ectopic pregnancy occurs more frequently in women who smoke compared to those who do not. There is some evidence that intrauterine devices (IUDs) used for contraception may slow the transport of the zygote and lead to an increased incidence of tubal or ovarian implantation. The incidence also increases following in vitro fertilization. Women who have one ectopic pregnancy have a 10% to 20% chance that a subsequent pregnancy will also be ectopic. This is because salpingitis

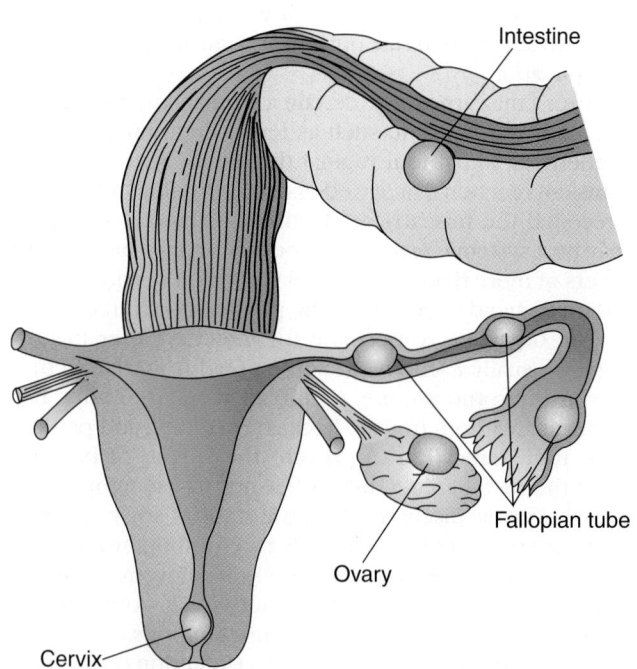

FIGURE 15.2 Sites at which an ectopic pregnancy may occur.

that leaves scarring is usually bilateral. Congenital anomalies such as webbing (fibrous bands) may also be bilateral. Surprisingly, oral contraceptives may reduce the possibility of ectopic pregnancy (Speroff & Fritz, 2005).

Assessment

With ectopic pregnancy, there are no unusual symptoms at the time of implantation. The corpus luteum of the ovary continues to function as if the implantation were in the uterus. No menstrual flow occurs. A woman may experience the nausea and vomiting of early pregnancy, and a pregnancy test for hCG will be positive.

At weeks 6 to 12 of pregnancy (2 to 8 weeks after a missed menstrual period), the zygote grows large enough to rupture the slender fallopian tube or the trophoblast cells break through the narrow base. Tearing and destruction of the blood vessels in the tube result. The extent of the bleeding that occurs depends on the number and size of the ruptured vessels. If implantation is in the interstitial portion of the tube (where the tube joins the uterus), rupture can cause severe intraperitoneal bleeding. Fortunately, the incidence of tubal pregnancies is highest in the ampullar area (the distal third), where the blood vessels are smaller and profuse hemorrhage is less likely. However, continued bleeding from this area may in time result in a large amount of blood loss. Therefore, a ruptured ectopic pregnancy is serious regardless of the site of implantation.

A woman usually experiences a sharp, stabbing pain in one of her lower abdominal quadrants at the time of rupture, followed by scant vaginal spotting. With placental dislodgment, progesterone secretion stops and the uterine decidua begins to slough, causing additional bleeding. The amount of bleeding evident with a ruptured ectopic pregnancy often does not reveal the actual amount present, however, because the products of conception from the ruptured tube and the accompanying blood may be expelled into the pelvic cavity rather than into the uterus. Therefore, this blood does not reach the vagina to become evident. If internal bleeding progresses to acute hemorrhage, a woman may experience lightheadedness and rapid pulse, signs of shock.

When helping determine the possibility of an ectopic pregnancy, ask a woman whether she has pain or vaginal bleeding. Any woman with sharp abdominal pain and vaginal spotting needs to be evaluated by her health care provider to rule out the possibility of ectopic pregnancy. Occasionally, a woman will move suddenly and pull one of her round ligaments, the anterior uterine supports. This can cause a sharp, but momentary and innocent, lower quadrant pain. However, it would be rare for this phenomenon to be reported in connection with vaginal spotting.

By the time a woman with a ruptured ectopic pregnancy arrives at the hospital or physician's office, she may already be in severe shock, as evidenced by a rapid, thready pulse, rapid respirations, and falling blood pressure. Leukocytosis may be present, not from infection but from the trauma. Temperature is usually normal. A transvaginal sonogram will demonstrate the ruptured tube and blood collecting in the peritoneum. Either a falling hCG or serum progesterone level suggests that the pregnancy has ended. If the diagnosis of ectopic pregnancy is in doubt,

a physician may insert a needle through the postvaginal fornix into the cul-de-sac under sterile conditions to see whether blood can be aspirated. A laparoscopy or culdoscopy can be used to visualize the fallopian tube if the symptoms alone do not reveal a clear picture of what has happened. However, sonography alone usually reveals a clear-cut diagnostic picture (Heard & Buster, 2003).

If a woman waits before seeking help, gradually her abdomen becomes rigid from peritoneal irritation. Her umbilicus may develop a bluish tinge (Cullen's sign). A woman may have continuing extensive or dull vaginal and abdominal pain; movement of the cervix on pelvic examination may cause excruciating pain. There may be pain in her shoulders from blood in the peritoneal cavity causing irritation to the phrenic nerve. A tender mass is usually palpable in Douglas' cul-de-sac on vaginal examination.

Therapeutic Management

Although some ectopic pregnancies spontaneously end and then are reabsorbed, requiring no treatment, it is difficult to predict when this will happen, so when an ectopic pregnancy is revealed by an early sonogram, some action is taken. If an ectopic pregnancy can be diagnosed by a sonogram before the tube has ruptured, it can be treated medically by the oral administration of methotrexate followed by leucovorin. Methotrexate, a folic acid antagonist chemotherapeutic agent, attacks and destroys fast-growing cells (Periti et al., 2004). Because trophoblast and zygote growth is rapid, the drug is drawn to the site of the ectopic pregnancy (see Chapter 53 for a general discussion of chemotherapy agents). Women are treated until a negative hCG titer is achieved. A hysterosalpingogram or sonogram is usually performed after the chemotherapy to assess whether the tube is fully patent. Mifepristone, an abortifacient, is also effective at causing sloughing of the tubal implantation site. The advantage of these therapies is that the tube is left intact, with no surgical scarring that could cause a second ectopic implantation (Heard & Buster, 2003).

If an ectopic pregnancy ruptures, it is an emergency situation. Keep in mind the amount of blood evident is a poor estimate of the actual blood loss. A blood sample needs to be drawn immediately for hemoglobin level, typing and cross-matching, and possibly hCG level for immediate pregnancy testing, if pregnancy has not yet been confirmed. Intravenous fluid using a large-gauge catheter to restore intravascular volume is begun. Blood then can be administered through this same line when matched.

The therapy for a ruptured ectopic pregnancy is laparoscopy to ligate the bleeding vessels and to remove or repair the damaged fallopian tube. A rough suture line on a fallopian tube may lead to another tubal pregnancy, so either the tube will be removed or suturing on the tube is done with microsurgical technique.

If a tube is removed, a woman is theoretically only 50% fertile, because every other month, when she ovulates from the ovary next to the removed tube, sperm cannot reach the ovum on that side. However, this is not a reliable contraceptive measure. Research in rabbits has shown that translocation of ova can occur—that is, an ovum released from the right ovary can pass through the pelvic cavity to the opposite (left) fallopian tube and become fertilized, and vice versa.

As with miscarriage, women with Rh-negative blood should receive Rh (D) immune globulin (RhIG) after an ectopic pregnancy for isoimmunization protection in future childbearing.

NURSING DIAGNOSES AND RELATED INTERVENTIONS

Nursing Diagnosis: Powerlessness related to early loss of pregnancy secondary to ectopic pregnancy

Outcome Evaluation: Client states she feels sad at pregnancy loss but is able to deal with situation; has returned to work and has forward-thinking plans.

A woman who has had an ectopic pregnancy not only has grief stages to work through (she has lost a child) but also may have problems of diminished self-image and a sense of powerlessness to resolve if surgery included removal of a fallopian tube. She may believe that she is now "half a woman" if she equated reproductive structures and childbearing with being a woman. Encourage her to verbalize her concerns about this and future childbearing. The process of working through grief and role images takes weeks to months. It should begin in the hospital, however, where a woman has professional people to help her through the first days and to determine whether she will need counseling.

Abdominal Pregnancy

Very rarely after an ectopic pregnancy rupture—so rarely that the instances are difficult to document—the products of conception are expelled into the pelvic cavity with a minimum of bleeding. The placenta continues to grow in the fallopian tube, spreading perhaps into the uterus for a better blood supply; or it may escape into the pelvic cavity and implant on an organ such as an intestine. The fetus will grow in the pelvic cavity (an abdominal pregnancy).

In an abdominal pregnancy, the fetal outline is easily palpable because it is directly below the abdominal wall, not inside the uterus. A woman may not be as aware of movements as she would be normally, or she may experience painful fetal movements and abdominal cramping with fetal movements.

A woman may report she noticed sudden lower quadrant pain earlier in the pregnancy. A sonogram or magnetic resonance imaging will reveal the fetus outside the uterus.

The danger of abdominal pregnancy is that the placenta will infiltrate and erode a major blood vessel in the abdomen, leading to hemorrhage. If implanted on the intestine, it may erode so deeply that it causes bowel perforation and peritonitis. The fetus is also at high risk because without

a good uterine blood supply, nutrients may not reach the fetus in adequate amounts. The survival rate in an abdominal pregnancy is only approximately 60% because of poor nutrient supply. In infants who do survive, there is an increased threat of fetal deformity or growth restriction from an inadequate nutrient supply.

At term, the infant must be born by laparotomy (Rahaman et al., 2004). The placenta is often difficult to remove after birth if it is implanted on an abdominal organ such as the intestine. It may be left in place, therefore, and allowed to absorb spontaneously in 2 or 3 months. A follow-up sonogram can be used to detect whether this has occurred, or a woman can be treated with methotrexate to help the placenta absorb. This therapy may not be effective because the remaining trophoblasts are no longer fast-growing.

Checkpoint Question 2

Suppose Beverly Muzuki was discovered to have an ectopic pregnancy. What advice would you give her?

a. Most ectopic pregnancies go to completion, although the newborn is small.

b. If she must have a fallopian tube removed, she will be sterile afterward.

c. She will have a continuous nagging pain through the rest of pregnancy.

d. Ectopic pregnancy can be either medically or surgically treated.

CONDITIONS ASSOCIATED WITH SECOND-TRIMESTER BLEEDING

There are two main causes of bleeding during the second trimester: gestational trophoblastic disease and premature cervical dilatation.

Gestational Trophoblastic Disease (Hydatidiform Mole)

Gestational trophoblastic disease is abnormal proliferation and degeneration of the trophoblastic villi (ACOG, 2004). As the cells degenerate, they become filled with fluid and appear as clear fluid-filled, grape-sized vesicles. With this condition, the embryo fails to develop beyond a primitive start. Such structures must be identified because they are associated with choriocarcinoma, a rapidly metastasizing malignancy (Fig. 15.3).

The incidence of gestational trophoblastic disease is approximately 1 in every 1,500 pregnancies. The condition tends to occur most often in women who have a low protein intake, in women older than age 35 years, and in women of Asian heritage (Li & Karlan, 2003).

Two types of molar growth can be identified by chromosome analysis. With a *complete mole,* all trophoblastic villi swell and become cystic. If an embryo forms, it dies early at only 1 to 2 mm in size, with no fetal blood present in the villi. On chromosomal analysis, although the karyotype is a normal 46XX or 46XY, this chromosome com-

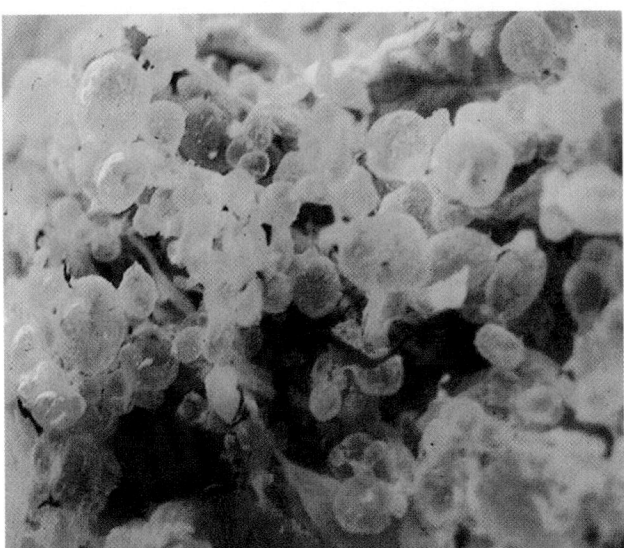

FIGURE 15.3 Gestational trophoblastic disease (hydatidiform mole). (From Rubin, E. & Farber, J. L. [1994]. Pathology, 2/e. Philadelphia: J. B. Lippincott.)

ponent was contributed only by the father or an "empty ovum" was fertilized and the chromosome material was duplicated (Fig. 15.4A).

With a *partial mole*, some of the villi form normally. The syncytiotrophoblastic layer of villi, however, is swollen and misshapen. A macerated embryo of approximately 9 weeks' gestation may be present and fetal blood may be present in the villi. A partial mole has 69 chromosomes (a triploid formation in which there are three chromosomes instead of two for every pair, one set supplied by an ovum that apparently was fertilized by two sperm or an ovum fer-

A

Sperm (23) + Ovum + Duplication = (46)

B

Sperm (46) + Ovum (23) = (69)

or

(23) + (23) = (69)
(23)

FIGURE 15.4 Formation of gestational trophoblastic disease (hydatidiform mole). (**A**) Complete mole. (**B**) Partial mole.

tilized by one sperm in which meiosis or reduction division did not occur). This could also occur if one set of 23 chromosomes was supplied by one sperm and an ovum that did not undergo reduction division supplied 46 (see Fig. 15.4B).

In contrast to complete moles, partial moles rarely lead to choriocarcinoma. Although still above average, hCG titers are lower in partial than in complete moles; titers also return to normal faster after mole evacuation.

Assessment

Because proliferation of the trophoblast cells occurs so rapidly with this condition, the uterus tends to expand faster than normally. This causes the uterus to reach its landmarks (just over the symphysis brim at 12 weeks, at the umbilicus at 20 to 24 weeks) before the usual time. This rapid development is also diagnostic of multiple pregnancy or a miscalculated due date, however, so this finding must be evaluated carefully. No fetal heart sounds are heard because there is no viable fetus. Because hCG is produced by the trophoblast cells that are overgrowing, a serum or urine test of hCG for pregnancy will be strongly positive (1 to 2 million IU compared with a normal pregnancy level of 400,000 IU).

Results continue to be strongly positive after day 100 of pregnancy, when the level of hCG normally would begin to decline. This fact must be evaluated carefully also, however, because highly positive test results can be characteristic of multiple pregnancies with more than one placenta. The nausea and vomiting of early pregnancy is usually marked, probably due to the high hCG level present. Symptoms of pregnancy-induced hypertension (i.e., hypertension, edema, and proteinuria) are ordinarily not present before week 20 of pregnancy. With gestational trophoblastic disease, they may appear before this time. A sonogram will show dense growth (typically a snowflake pattern) but no fetal growth in the uterus.

At approximately week 16 of pregnancy, if the structure was not identified earlier by sonogram, it will identify itself with vaginal bleeding. This may begin as vaginal spotting of dark-brown blood or as a profuse fresh flow. As the bleeding progresses, it is accompanied by discharge of the clear fluid-filled vesicles. This is why it is important for any woman who begins to miscarry at home to bring any clots or tissue passed to the hospital with her. The presence of clear fluid-filled cysts changes the diagnosis from miscarriage to gestational trophoblastic disease.

Therapeutic Management

Therapy for gestational trophoblastic disease is suction curettage to evacuate the mole. After surgery, hCG levels remain high. Half of women still have a positive reading at 3 weeks; one fourth still have a positive test result at 40 days.

Following mole extraction, women should have a baseline pelvic examination, a chest x-ray, and a serum test for the beta subunit of hCG. The hCG is then analyzed every 2 weeks until levels are again normal. Thereafter, serum hCG levels are assessed every 4 weeks for 6 to 12 months. Gradually declining hCG titers suggest no complication.

Levels that plateau for three times or increase suggest that malignant transformation has occurred (ACOG, 2004). A woman should be instructed to use a reliable contraceptive method such as an oral contraceptive agent for 12 months so that a positive pregnancy test (the presence of hCG) resulting from a new pregnancy will not be confused with increasing levels and a developing malignancy. After 6 months, if hCG levels are still negative, a woman is theoretically free of the risk of a malignancy developing. By 12 months, she could plan a second pregnancy. Although the development of gestational trophoblastic disease means that a pregnancy never materialized and that a fetus never formed, a woman may experience the same feeling of loss after its evacuation that she would have experienced after the loss of a true pregnancy: she did, after all, believe she was pregnant. In addition, she is faced with the possibility that a malignancy may develop. She also must delay her childbearing plans for a year. If she had already put off having a child for some time, this may seem to be an unbearably long time.

Some physicians give women who have had gestational trophoblastic disease a prophylactic course of methotrexate, the drug of choice for choriocarcinoma. However, because the drug interferes with white blood cell formation (leukopenia), prophylactic use must be weighed carefully. If malignancy should occur, it can be treated effectively in most instances with methotrexate at that time. Dactinomycin is added to the regimen if metastasis occurs.

Women need the opportunity to express their anger and sense of unfairness at this type of event. They may feel inadequate because something went wrong with the pregnancy. They may wonder whether it will happen again, or whether they will ever be able to have children. Unfortunately, women who have one incidence of gestational trophoblastic disease have an increased risk of a second molar pregnancy (Li & Karlan, 2003). They need early screening with ultrasound during a second pregnancy to be certain this is not happening again.

What if... Beverly Muzuki told you, after having had a gestational trophoblastic disorder, that she didn't believe in birth control so did not intend to take the oral contraceptives prescribed following her mole evacuation? How would you advise her?

Premature Cervical Dilatation

Premature cervical dilatation, previously termed an *incompetent cervix,* refers to a cervix that dilates prematurely and therefore cannot hold a fetus until term (Branch & Scott, 2003). It occurs in about 1% of women. The dilatation is usually painless. Often the first symptom is show (a pink-stained vaginal discharge) or increased pelvic pressure, which may be followed by rupture of the membranes and discharge of the amniotic fluid. Uterine contractions begin, and after a short labor the fetus is born. Unfortunately, this commonly occurs at approximately week 20 of pregnancy, when the fetus is still too immature to survive.

It is often difficult to explain in a particular instance what causes premature dilatation. It is associated with increased maternal age, congenital structural defects, and trauma to the cervix, such as might have occurred with a cone biopsy or repeated D&Cs. Although it may be diagnosed by an early sonogram before symptoms occur, it is usually diagnosed only after the pregnancy is lost.

After the loss of one child due to premature cervical dilatation, a surgical operation termed **cervical cerclage** can be performed to prevent this from happening again. As soon as a sonogram confirms that the fetus of a second pregnancy is healthy, at approximately weeks 12 to 14, purse-string sutures are placed in the cervix by the vaginal route under regional anesthesia. This procedure is called a McDonald or a Shirodkar procedure after the surgeons who perfected the technique. The sutures serve to strengthen the cervix and prevent it from dilating (Fig. 15.5).

In a McDonald procedure, nylon sutures are placed horizontally and vertically across the cervix and pulled tight to reduce the cervical canal to a few millimeters in diameter. With a Shirodkar technique, sterile tape is threaded in a purse-string manner under the submucous layer of the cervix and sutured in place to achieve a closed cervix. Although routinely accomplished by a vaginal route, sutures may be placed by a transabdominal route.

With these procedures, the sutures are then removed at weeks 37 to 38 of pregnancy so the fetus can be born vaginally. When a transabdominal approach is used, the sutures may be left in place and a cesarean birth performed.

Women who are discovered to have cervical dilatation but with membranes still intact at a prenatal visit may have emergent cerclage sutures placed in the cervix even at that point as prophylaxis against preterm birth. The success of this procedure is limited, however, compared to preventive suturing.

Still newer techniques allow purse-string sutures to be set before a woman becomes pregnant, providing added assurance that she will not begin miscarrying before week 14 of pregnancy.

Be certain to ask women who are reporting painless bleeding (the symptoms of spontaneous miscarriage also) whether they have had past cervical operations to remind them they may have sutures in place.

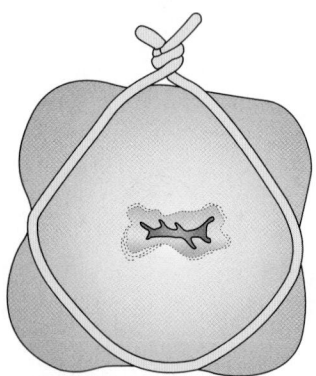

FIGURE 15.5 Shirodkar suture for cervical cerclage.

Team Member Responsible	Assessment	Intervention	Rationale	Expected Outcome
Nutrition				
Nurse	Obtain hematocrit and serum electrolyte levels every 4 hours or as ordered. Monitor IV fluid total every hour during infusion, keeping intake to 100 mL/hour or less.	Assist with or insert an IV line. Begin IV fluid therapy as ordered.	Hematocrit, electrolyte levels, and IV intake measures the client's fluid volume status. If fluid intake is greater than 100 mL/hour, overload may occur, placing the client at risk for pulmonary edema.	IV fluid improves hydration, which may help to minimize contractions.
Patient/Family Education				
Nurse	Assess client's knowledge of preterm labor.	Instruct client about preterm labor and about steps to be taken to counteract the process.	A well-informed client can participate more fully in her own care.	Client states the cause of preterm labor cannot always be identified; describes the part she can play in halting process.
Psychosocial/Spiritual/Emotional Needs				
Nurse	Assess anxiety level of client over preterm labor. Assess for possible feelings of guilt related to cause of preterm labor.	Assist client with using relaxation techniques, such as muscle relaxation, breathing, and music. Provide frequent updates about progress. Allow client to verbalize feelings and concerns.	Relaxation techniques help to decrease anxiety and fear, enhancing feelings of control. Frequent updates about progress help to minimize fear about the unknown. Client may feel responsible for preterm labor because of UTI.	Client verbalizes her feelings about this crisis in her life. Demonstrates anxiety but at a level that allows her to cooperate with caretakers.
Nurse	Determine whether client wants a support person to be with her.	Contact support person as necessary.	The presence of a support person can offer additional comfort to a client.	Client names a support person she wants notified about hospital admission.
Discharge Planning				
Nurse	Assess client's home surroundings to determine whether they are appropriate for bed rest and continuing monitoring at home.	Change tocolytic therapy to oral form as prescribed, administering first oral dose 30 minutes before discontinuing IV infusion. Contact home care nurse service to provide monitoring at home.	Administering oral dose prior to discontinuation of IV infusion maintains consistent serum drug concentrations for effective control. Home monitoring requires professional supervision.	Client states that she feels her home and support system will be adequate for home care with self-monitoring. Agrees on appointment for first home visit with home care nurse service.

Terbutaline may also be administered subcutaneously by continuous pump. This allows for home drug administration using lower doses of medicine. Oral terbutaline therapy has the potential of prolonging labor an average of 2 weeks. With subcutaneous pump infusions, labor can be delayed an average of 8 to 9 weeks. Similar to an insulin pump, a terbutaline pump contains a syringe filled with the drug. A small polyethylene catheter leads from the pump to a subcutaneous needle. When the needle is inserted into the subcutaneous tissue of the abdomen or the thigh, the pump automatically injects a continuous low dose of medication subcutaneously. The pump can be set to "bolus" an injection of the drug at the time of day when contractions tend to occur the most. A woman could manually trigger the pump to inject extra medicine (within set limits) if she should begin to feel contractions. Like insulin pumps, the pump can be carried in a sash around the waist or kept in a pocket of clothing. Pumps should never get wet, so the syringe should be removed from the pump while a woman showers. For tub bathing, she should remove both the pump and needle and replace the needle immediately afterward.

Fetal Assessment

In addition to supervising tocolytic therapy, be certain to assess overall fetal welfare daily in a woman trying to delay preterm labor. A woman may be instructed to use a daily fetal movement count or "count to 10" test. Teach her how to do this before hospital discharge and then continue it when she is at home. The typical fetus moves 10 times in an hour. To evaluate fetal movement, a woman lies down on her left side and times the number of minutes it takes for her to feel 10 fetal movements (about an hour) or counts the number of fetal movements she feels in 1 hour (the average is 10 to 12). If the time it takes to feel 10 fetal movements is twice what it was the day before or if she feels fewer than 5 movements during an hour (half of what she should feel), she monitors again for a second hour. If at the end of this second hour fetal activity is still under 10 per hour, she should report it immediately. Because of the variation of movements among normal, healthy fetuses, different perinatal centers use different protocols for counting fetal movements. What standard is accepted as normal also varies.

Labor That Cannot Be Halted

In some women, preterm labor is too far advanced when they are first seen in a health care facility for it to be halted. Usually, if membranes have ruptured or the cervix is more than 50% effaced and more than 3 to 4 cm dilated, it is unlikely labor can be halted. The rupturing of membranes, especially, can be thought of as a "point of no return" in stopping or delaying labor because of the increased risk of infection that begins from that point.

If the fetus is very immature at the time labor cannot be halted, a cesarean birth may be planned to reduce pressure on the fetal head and reduce the possibility of subdural or intraventricular hemorrhage from a vaginal birth.

Most women assume that if a fetus is preterm, labor will be shorter than normal because the infant is still so small. This is not necessarily true because the first stage of labor, the longest stage, proceeds exactly as it would with a term pregnancy. The second stage of labor may be shorter because a small infant can be pushed through the dilated cervix and the birth canal much more easily. Because the second stage takes at most 1 hour, however, this means the difference will not be more than 30 minutes to 1 hour. Unless a woman is given this explanation, she may worry not only that her labor is preterm but also that something is going wrong because it is lasting so long.

Because of the increased risk for prolapse of the cord around a small head, artificial rupture of the membranes is not done as a rule in preterm labor until the fetal head is firmly engaged. Delaying rupture of the membranes is another factor that may prolong the first stage of labor.

Analgesic agents are administered with caution during preterm labor because of the immaturity of the fetus. The immature infant will have enough difficulty breathing at birth without the additional burden of being sedated from a drug such as meperidine (Demerol). If a woman wants pain relief, an epidural is preferable.

Continuously monitor uterine contractions and fetal heart sounds during preterm labor. A woman can feel reassured by the evidence of the monitor screen or graph or the projected sound that although her infant is likely to be small, heart tones seem to be of good quality and the infant is reacting well to labor.

A woman may assume that because the infant's head is small, an episiotomy will not be needed for birth, and she will be able to avoid the discomfort of postpartum stitches. Although the head of a preterm infant is smaller than that of a mature infant, it is also more fragile. Excessive pressure could result in a subdural or intraventricular hemorrhage that could be fatal. That means a woman may actually need an episiotomy incision larger than usual. Forceps are another measure that may be used at birth to reduce pressure on the fetal head.

Following birth, the cord of the preterm infant is usually clamped immediately rather than waiting for pulsations to stop. This is because an immature infant has a difficult time excreting the large amount of bilirubin that will be formed if this extra blood is added to the circulation. The extra amount of blood could also overburden the circulatory system.

NURSING DIAGNOSES AND RELATED INTERVENTIONS

Examples of nursing diagnoses for a woman with preterm labor that cannot be halted include:

- Fear related to uncertain outcome of pregnancy
- Pain related to labor contractions
- Situational low self-esteem related to inability to carry pregnancy to term
- Risk for fetal injury related to preterm birth

Be certain that the outcomes established for care are realistic. Although many measures are available to help the preterm baby adjust to birth, a baby born preterm will be at risk for a variety of medical problems (see Chapter 26).

Nursing Diagnosis: Situational low self-esteem related to feelings of responsibility for preterm labor

Outcome Evaluation: Client expresses feelings and worries to nurse; states it is unknown why labor began, but she knows she is not responsible for her labor beginning prematurely.

A woman in preterm labor is undergoing an extreme crisis situation. She cannot help asking herself, "What did I do to cause this?" Time spent taking the initial history or timing contractions presents an opportunity to bring the concern out in the open: "Did Dr. Smith explain to you labor sometimes begins early this way without any reason? Some women worry they did something to bring on preterm labor. Have you had any thoughts like that?"

A woman in preterm labor that cannot be halted needs a support person with her because she is apt to be more concerned than the average person about labor. She needs frequent assurance during labor that she is breathing well with contractions or just that she is "doing well." She may not be mentally prepared for labor because it has come unexpectedly. During the postpartum period, she may need continued reassurance. Helping rebuild self-esteem this way can better prepare her to be a parent to her preterm infant.

Checkpoint Question 4

Beverly Muzuki is in preterm labor. When you see her in the emergency room, what should be your first action?

a. Keep her walking so the fetal head puts harder pressure on the cervix.
b. Ask her to lie down in a side-lying position and assess her contractions.
c. Obtain blood for a human chorionic gonadotropin hormone assessment.
d. Caution her to not allow anyone to start IV fluid; dehydration halts contractions.

PRETERM RUPTURE OF MEMBRANES

Preterm rupture of membranes is rupture of fetal membranes with loss of amniotic fluid during pregnancy before 37 weeks (Gibbs, 2003). The cause of preterm rupture is unknown, but it is associated with infection of the membranes (chorioamnionitis). It occurs in 5% to 10% of pregnancies. If rupture occurs early in pregnancy, it poses a major threat to the fetus. After rupture, the seal to the fetus is lost and uterine and fetal infection may occur. A second complication that can result from preterm membrane rupture is increased pressure on the umbilical cord from the loss of amniotic fluid, inhibiting the fetal nutrient supply, or cord prolapse (extension of the cord out of the uterine cavity into the vagina), a condition that could also interfere with fetal circulation. Cord prolapse is most apt to occur when the fetal head is still too small to fit the cervix firmly. Yet another risk to the fetus of remaining in a non-fluid-filled environment is the development of a Potter-like syndrome or distorted facial features and pulmonary hypoplasia from pressure. Preterm labor may follow rupture of the membranes. Inhibition of labor is rarely used after rupture of membranes because of the increased possibility of fetal infection after this point.

Assessment

Rupture of the membranes is suggested by the history. A woman usually describes a sudden gush of clear fluid from the vagina, with continued minimal leakage. Occasionally,

a woman mistakes urinary incontinence caused by exertion for rupture of membranes. Amniotic fluid cannot be differentiated from urine by appearance, so a sterile vaginal speculum examination is done to observe for vaginal pooling of fluid. If the fluid is tested with Nitrazine paper, amniotic fluid causes an alkaline reaction on the paper (appears blue) and urine an acidic reaction (remains yellow). The fluid can also be tested for ferning, or the typical appearance of a high-estrogen fluid on microscopic examination (amniotic fluid shows this; urine does not). If there is still a question as to whether the membranes have ruptured, a sonogram may be ordered to assess the amniotic fluid index. Because preterm rupture of membranes is associated with vaginal infection, cultures for *Neisseria gonorrhoeae*, streptococcus B, and *Chlamydia* are usually taken. Blood is drawn for white blood count and C-reactive protein. Avoid doing routine vaginal examinations because the risk of infection rises significantly when digital examinations are performed after preterm rupture of membranes.

If the fetus is estimated to be mature enough to survive in an extrauterine environment at the time of rupture and labor does not begin within 24 hours, labor contractions are usually induced by intravenous administration of oxytocin.

Therapeutic Management

If labor does not begin and the fetus is near a point of viability, a woman is placed on bed rest either in the hospital or at home and administered a corticosteroid to hasten fetal lung maturity. Prophylactic administration of broad-spectrum antibiotics during this period may delay the onset of labor and reduce the risk of infection in the newborn enough to allow the corticosteroid to have its effect. Women positive for streptococcus B need intravenous administration of penicillin or ampicillin to reduce the possibility of this infection in the newborn.

Following endoscopic intrauterine procedures, membranes can be resealed by use of a fibrin-based commercial sealant so they are again intact (Young et al., 2004). This is a future possibility for premature rupture of the membranes also.

NURSING DIAGNOSES AND RELATED INTERVENTIONS

Nursing Diagnosis: Risk for infection related to preterm rupture of membranes without accompanying labor

Outcome Evaluation: Maternal white blood cell count remains below 20,000/mm³; maternal temperature is less than 100.4°F (38.0°C).

An infection can be dangerous for both the mother and fetus. If at home, a woman is asked to take her temperature twice a day and to report a fever (a temperature greater than 100.4∞F [38.0∞C]), uterine tenderness, or odorous vaginal discharge. She should refrain from tub bathing, douching, and coitus because of the danger of introducing infection. The white cell count will need to be assessed frequently, perhaps as often as daily. A count of more than 18,000 to 20,000/mm3 suggests infection.

Before a woman is discharged to home care, be certain she knows how to read a thermometer, she has specific instructions as to what degree of temperature she should report, and she understands bed rest should be strictly followed. Help her make arrangements for a daily white blood cell count through a laboratory service or home care nurse.

Intrauterine amnioinfusion may be used to supply additional uterine fluid and help protect the umbilical cord from compression and the fetus from compression deformities or pulmonary hypoplasia (see Chapter 18).

Many misconceptions about the difficulty of labor after preterm rupture of the membranes (dry labor) exist. Every day, a woman hopes the fetus is ready to be born, ending the long wait, yet she is also afraid to begin labor because of these stories. You can reassure her that because amniotic fluid is always being formed, there is no such thing as a "dry labor."

PREGNANCY-INDUCED HYPERTENSION (PIH)

Pregnancy-induced hypertension (PIH) is a condition in which vasospasm occurs during pregnancy in both small and large arteries. Signs of hypertension, proteinuria, and edema develop. It is unique to pregnancy and occurs in 5% to 7% of pregnancies in the United States (Moldenhauer & Sibai, 2003). Despite years of research, the cause of the disorder is still unknown. Originally it was called toxemia because researchers pictured a toxin of some kind being produced by a woman in response to the foreign protein of the growing fetus, the toxin leading to the typical symptoms. No such toxin has ever been identified.

A condition separate from chronic hypertension, PIH tends to occur most frequently in women of color or with a multiple pregnancy, primiparas younger than 20 years of age or older than 40 years, women from low socioeconomic backgrounds (perhaps because of poor nutrition), those who have had five or more pregnancies, those who have hydramnios, or those who have an underlying disease such as heart disease, diabetes with vessel or renal involvement, and essential hypertension.

Pathophysiologic Events

The symptoms of PIH affect almost all organs. The vascular spasm may be caused by increased cardiac output that injures the endothelial cells of the arteries and the action of prostaglandins (notably decreased prostacyclin and increased thromboxane). Normally, blood vessels during pregnancy are resistant to the effects of pressor substances such as angiotensin and norepinephrine, so blood pressure remains normal during pregnancy. With PIH, this reduced responsiveness to blood pressure changes appears to be lost. Vasoconstriction occurs and blood pressure increases dramatically (Peters & Flack, 2004).

With hypertension, the cardiac system can become overwhelmed because the heart is forced to pump against rising peripheral resistance. This reduces the blood supply to organs, most markedly the kidney, pancreas, liver, brain, and placenta. Poor placental perfusion may reduce the fetal nutrient and oxygen supply. Ischemia in the pancreas may result in epigastric pain and an elevated amylase–creatinine ratio. Spasm of the arteries in the retina leads to vision changes. If retinal hemorrhages occur, blindness can result.

Vasospasm in the kidney increases blood flow resistance. Degenerative changes develop in kidney glomeruli because of back-pressure. This leads to increased permeability of the glomerular membrane, allowing the serum proteins albumin and globulin to escape into the urine (proteinuria). The degenerative changes also result in decreased glomerular filtration, so there is lowered urine output and clearance of creatinine. Increased kidney tubular reabsorption of sodium occurs. Because sodium retains fluid, edema results. Edema is further increased because as more protein is lost, the osmotic pressure of the circulating blood falls and fluid diffuses from the circulatory system into the denser interstitial spaces to equalize the pressure (edema; Fig. 15.8). Extreme edema can lead to cerebral and pulmonary edema and seizures (**eclampsia**).

Yet another effect is that arterial spasm causes the bulk of the blood volume in the maternal circulation to be pooled in the venous circulation, so a woman has a deceptively low arterial intravascular volume. In addition, thrombocytopenia or a lowered platelet count occurs as platelets cluster at the sites of endothelial damage. Measuring hematocrit levels helps to assess the extent of plasma loss to the interstitial space or the extent of the edema (the higher the hematocrit, the more is being lost). A hematocrit level above 40% suggests significant fluid loss into interstitial spaces.

Assessment

Although women may have additional symptoms such as vision changes, typically hypertension, proteinuria, and edema are considered the classic signs of PIH. Of the three, hypertension and proteinuria are the most significant as extensive edema occurs only after the other two are present. Symptoms rarely occur before 20 weeks of pregnancy (Box 15.11).

PIH is classified as gestational hypertension, mild preeclampsia, severe preeclampsia, and eclampsia, depending on how far development advances (Table 15.6). Any woman who falls into one of the high-risk categories for PIH should be observed carefully for symptoms at prenatal visits. She needs instructions about what symptoms to watch for so she can alert her clinician if additional symptoms occur between visits.

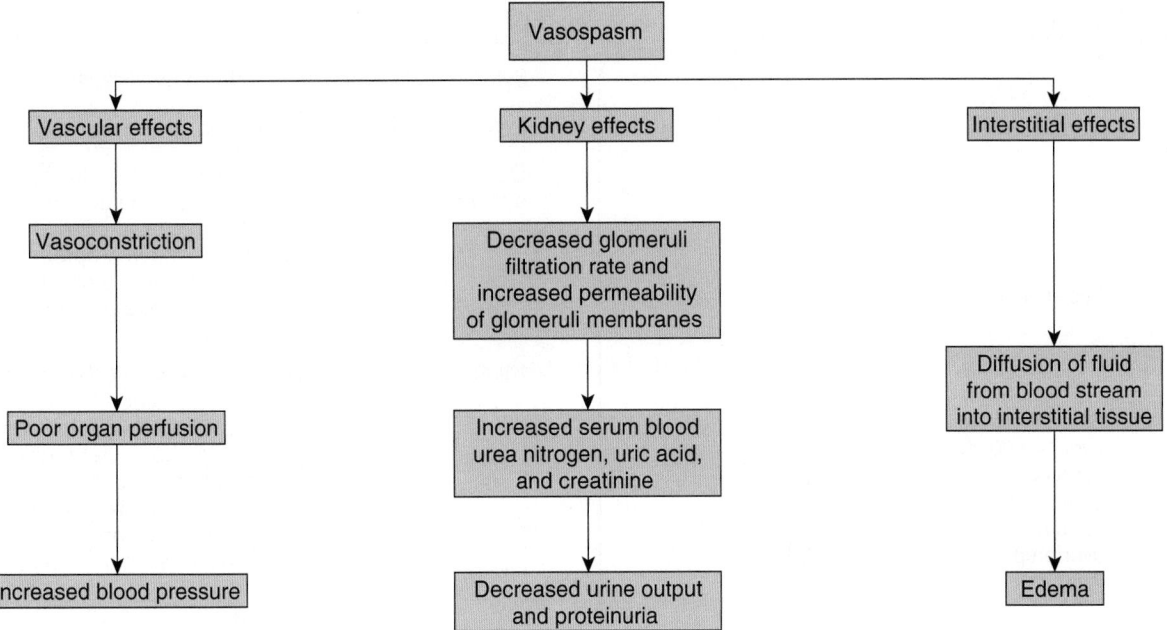

FIGURE 15.8 Physiologic changes with pregnancy-induced hypertension.

Gestational Hypertension

A woman is said to have gestational hypertension when she develops an elevated blood pressure (140/90 mm Hg) but has no proteinuria or edema. Perinatal mortality is not increased with simple gestational hypertension, so no drug therapy is necessary.

Mild Preeclampsia

If a seizure from PIH occurs, a woman has eclampsia, but any status above gestational hypertension and below a point of seizures is **preeclampsia.** A woman is said to be mildly preeclamptic when her blood pressure rises to 140/90 mm Hg, taken on two occasions at least 6 hours apart. The diastolic value of blood pressure is extremely important to document because it is this pressure that best indicates the degree of peripheral arterial spasm present.

A second criterion is systolic blood pressure greater than 30 mm Hg and diastolic pressure greater than 15 mm Hg above prepregnancy values. This rule is helpful, but the value of 140/90 mm Hg is a more useful cutoff point when there are no baseline data available, such as when a woman seeks prenatal care late in pregnancy.

Average blood pressures in American women are shown in Appendix G. According to these averages, a woman younger than age 20 could have a blood pressure of 98/61 and still be within normal limits. If her blood pressure were elevated 30 mm Hg systolic and 15 mm Hg diastolic, it would be only 128/76. This is well beneath the traditional warning point of 140/90 but would represent hypertension for her.

With mild preeclampsia, in addition to the hypertension a woman has proteinuria (1+ or 2+ on a reagent test strip on a random sample). Many women show a trace of protein during pregnancy. Actual proteinuria is said to

exist when it registers as at least 1+ or more (this represents a loss of 1 g/L).

Occasionally women have orthostatic proteinuria (on long periods of standing, they excrete protein; at bed rest, they do not). If proteinuria is present without other signs of PIH (no hypertension and no edema), check to see when the specimen was tested. Ask her to bring in a first morning urine sample. This may reveal that orthostatic proteinuria, not preeclampsia, may be the cause of protein in her urine.

Edema develops, as mentioned, because of the protein loss, sodium retention, and lowered glomerular filtration rate. Edema begins to accumulate in the upper part of the body, rather than just the typical ankle edema of pregnancy. A weight gain of more than 2 lb/wk in the second trimester or 1 lb/wk in the third trimester usually indicates abnormal tissue fluid retention. This is likely to be the first symptom a woman notices, or it may be discovered when a woman is weighed at a prenatal visit. Noticeable edema may or may not be present when this sudden increase in weight first occurs.

Severe Preeclampsia

A woman has passed from mild to severe preeclampsia when her blood pressure has risen to 160 mm Hg systolic and 110 mm Hg diastolic or above on at least two occasions 6 hours apart at bed rest (the position in which blood pressure is lowest) or her diastolic pressure is 30 mm Hg above her prepregnancy level. Marked proteinuria, 3+ or 4+ on a random urine sample or more than 5 g in a 24-hour sample, and extensive edema are also present.

With severe preeclampsia, the extreme edema will be noticeable as puffiness in a woman's face and hands. It is most readily palpated over bony surfaces, such as over the tibia on the anterior leg, the ulnar surface of the forearm,

BOX 15.11 ASSESSMENT

Assessing the Woman With Pregnancy-Induced Hypertension

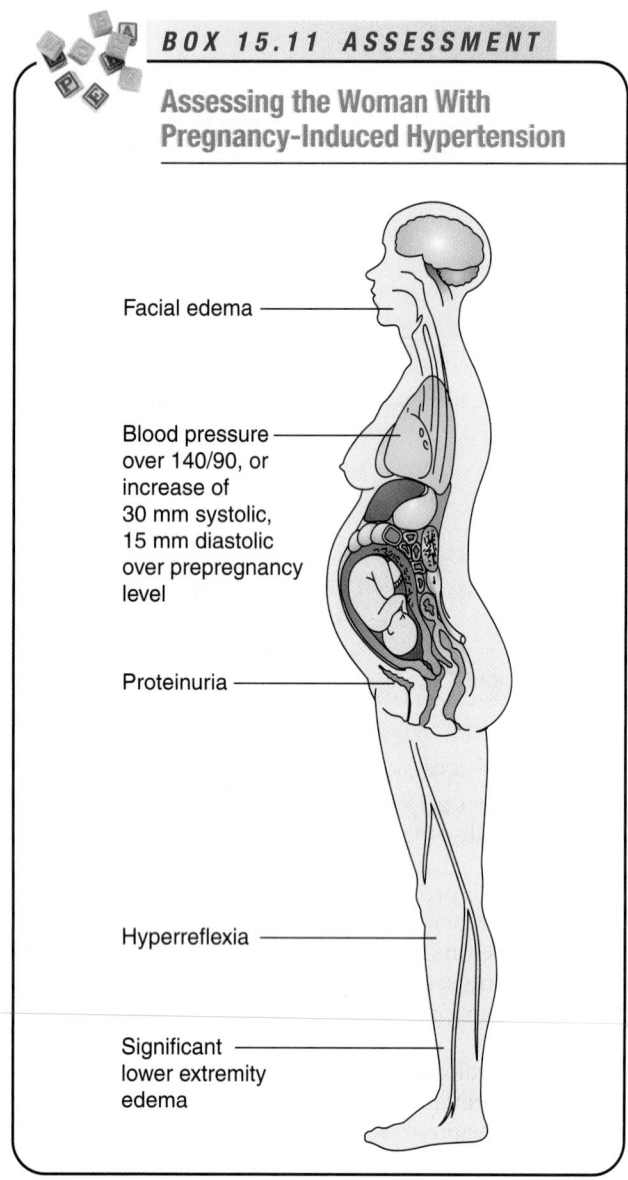

Facial edema

Blood pressure over 140/90, or increase of 30 mm systolic, 15 mm diastolic over prepregnancy level

Proteinuria

Hyperreflexia

Significant lower extremity edema

TABLE 15.6

Symptoms of Pregnancy-Induced Hypertension

Hypertension Type	Symptoms
Gestational hypertension	Blood pressure 140/90 or systolic pressure elevated 30 mm Hg or diastolic pressure elevated 15 mm Hg above prepregnancy level; no proteinuria or edema; blood pressure returns to normal after birth
Mild preeclampsia	Blood pressure 140/90 or systolic pressure elevated 30 mm Hg or diastolic pressure elevated 15 mm Hg above prepregnancy level; proteinuria of 1–2+ on a random sample; weight gain over 2 lb per wk in second trimester and 1 lb per wk in third trimester; mild edema in upper extremities or face
Severe preeclampsia	Blood pressure of 160/110; proteinuria 3–4+ on a random sample and 5 g on a 24-hour sample; oliguria (500 mL or less in 24 hours or altered renal function tests; elevated serum creatinine more than 1.2 mg/dL); cerebral or visual disturbances (headache, blurred vision); pulmonary or cardiac involvement; extensive peripheral edema; hepatic dysfunction; thrombocytopenia; epigastric pain
Eclampsia	Seizure or coma accompanied by signs and symptoms of preeclampsia

and the cheekbones, where the sponginess of fluid-filled tissue can be palpated against bone. If there is swelling or puffiness at these points to a palpating finger but the swelling cannot be indented with finger pressure, the edema is nonpitting. If the tissue can be indented slightly, this is 1+ pitting edema; moderate indentation is 2+; deep indentation is 3+; and indentation so deep it remains after removal of the finger is 4+ pitting edema.

Further assess edema by asking a woman if she has noticed any swelling anywhere in her body. Most women at the end of pregnancy have edema of the feet at the end of the day. They report this as difficulty fitting into their bedroom slippers, or kicking off their shoes at dinnertime and then not being able to put them back on again. This is a normal discomfort of pregnancy. However, edema that has progressed to the upper extremities or the face is abnormal. Women report upper extremity edema as "my rings are so tight I can't get them off" and facial edema as "when I wake in the morning, my eyes are swollen shut" or "I can't talk until I walk around awhile." This accumu-

lating edema will reduce their urine output to approximately 400 to 600 mL per 24 hours.

Some women have severe epigastric pain and nausea and vomiting, possibly due to abdominal edema or ischemia to the pancreas and liver. If pulmonary edema develops, a woman may report feeling short of breath. If cerebral edema occurs, reports may be voiced of visual disturbances such as blurred vision or seeing spots before the eyes. Cerebral edema also produces symptoms of severe headache and marked hyperreflexia and perhaps ankle clonus.

Eclampsia

This is the most severe classification of PIH. A woman has passed into this stage when cerebral edema is so acute that a seizure or coma occurs. With eclampsia, the maternal mortality rate is as high as 20% from causes such as cerebral hemorrhage, circulatory collapse, or renal failure (Moldenhauer & Sibai, 2003).

The fetal prognosis in eclampsia is poor because of hypoxia and consequent fetal acidosis. If premature separation of the placenta from vasospasm occurs, the fetal prognosis is even graver. If a fetus must be delivered before term, all the risks of immaturity will be faced. In preeclampsia, the fetal mortality rate is approximately 10%. If eclampsia develops, the mortality rate increases to as high as 25% (Moldenhauer & Sibai, 2003).

Nursing Diagnoses

The nursing diagnoses used with PIH are numerous because the disease has such wide-ranging effects. Some possible nursing diagnoses are:

- Ineffective tissue perfusion related to vasoconstriction of blood vessels
- Deficient fluid volume related to fluid loss to subcutaneous tissue
- Risk for fetal injury related to reduced placental perfusion secondary to vasospasm
- Social isolation related to prescribed bed rest

Nursing Interventions for a Woman With Mild PIH

Clients with mild preeclampsia can be managed at home with frequent follow-up care (see Chapter 16). Regardless of the setting, the care is similar.

Promote Bed Rest. When the body is in a recumbent position, sodium tends to be excreted at a faster rate than during activity. Bed rest, therefore, is the best method of aiding increased evacuation of sodium and encouraging diuresis. Rest should always be in a lateral recumbent position to avoid uterine pressure on the vena cava and prevent supine hypotension syndrome.

Promote Good Nutrition. A woman needs to continue her usual pregnancy diet. At one time, stringent restriction of salt was advised to reduce edema. This is no longer true because stringent sodium restriction may activate the renin-angiotensin-aldosterone system and result in increased blood pressure, compounding the problem.

Provide Emotional Support. It is difficult for a woman with preeclampsia to appreciate the potential seriousness of symptoms because they are still so vague. Neither high blood pressure nor protein in urine is something she can see or feel. She may be aware that edema is present, but it seems unrelated to the pregnancy: it is her hands that are swollen, not a body area near her growing child.

Women are also used to having severe disorders treated with some form of medication. With mild preeclampsia, no medication is prescribed. This can make a woman underestimate the severity of the situation. She may take instructions such as getting rest lightly. In addition, it is not always easy to comply with an instruction such as to get additional rest during the day. Ninety percent of women of childbearing age work outside the home at least part time. Most women with PIH, therefore, are being asked to take a leave of absence from work. Most working women contribute financially to the running of their household, such as providing a part of the mortgage or rent or car payments. If a woman is unmarried, her income is probably her sole support, and it will seem difficult to leave

work on the basis of a few vague symptoms—a little swelling or a little headache.

Health care providers cannot solve financial problems, but be certain to ask enough questions at health care visits so that financial need, if present, can be documented. Questions such as, "What will it mean to your family if you have to be on bed rest?" and "How long a maternity leave does your work allow?" bring concerns out into the open.

A woman with small children must usually make child care arrangements so she can get sufficient rest when receiving home care. The mother who spends considerable time chauffeuring school-age children to activities may need to investigate car pooling as an alternative. Another may need to discontinue being a volunteer leader or ask her family for more help around the house, such as cleaning or cooking. Ask, "What will it mean to your other children or your husband if you have to rest?" to allow her to begin to face these problems. Remember that having a wife or mother on bed rest is a stress on the total family, so other family members may need support as well.

Women with beginning signs of hypertension will be seen approximately weekly or more frequently for the remainder of pregnancy. Be certain a woman understands that if symptoms worsen before her next health care visit, she should call and report them immediately. Because there is no cure for preeclampsia, adherence to bed rest and attempts to reduce symptoms early are crucial.

Nursing Interventions for a Woman With Severe PIH

If the preeclampsia is severe (i.e., systolic blood pressure of more than 160 mm Hg, diastolic blood pressure of more than 110 mm Hg, or both on two occasions 6 hours apart after a woman has been on bed rest; extensive edema; marked proteinuria [3+ to 4+]; cerebral or visual disturbances; marked hyperreflexia; or oliguria [500 mL per 24 hours or less]), a woman may be admitted to the health care facility. If the pregnancy is 36 weeks or further along or fetal lung maturity can be confirmed by amniocentesis, labor can be induced to end the pregnancy at this point. If the pregnancy is less than 36 weeks or amniocentesis reveals immature lung function, interventions will be instituted to attempt to alleviate the severe symptoms and allow the fetus to come to term.

Support Bed Rest. With severe preeclampsia, most women are hospitalized so that bed rest can be enforced and the woman can be observed more closely than she can be on home care. Visitors are usually restricted to support people (e.g., husband, father of the child, mother, or older children). Because a loud noise such as a crying baby or a dropped tray of equipment may be sufficient to trigger a seizure initiating eclampsia, a woman with severe preeclampsia should be admitted to a private room so she can rest as undisturbed as possible. Raise side rails to help prevent injury if a seizure should occur.

Darken the room if possible because a bright light can trigger seizures. However, the room should not be so dark that caregivers need to use a flashlight to make assessments. Shining a flashlight beam into a woman's eyes is the kind of sudden stimulation to be avoided.

Stress is another stimulus capable of increasing blood pressure and evoking seizures in a woman with severe preeclampsia. Be certain a woman receives clear explanations of what is happening and what is planned. Clear explanations help her accept the need for visitor restrictions and not to "cheat" on bed rest. Allow her opportunities to express her feelings about what is happening or how bewildered she is because the few simple symptoms she noticed 2 weeks ago (increase in weight or increasing edema) have now developed into a syndrome that may be lethal to her baby and possibly even to her.

Monitor Maternal Well-Being. Take blood pressure frequently (at least every 4 hours) or with a continuous monitoring device to detect any increase, which is a warning that a woman's condition is worsening. Obtain blood studies as ordered (i.e., complete blood count, platelet count, liver function, blood urea nitrogen, and creatine and fibrin degradation products) to assess for renal and liver function and the development of DIC, which often accompanies severe vasospasm. Because she is at high risk for premature separation of the placenta and resulting hemorrhage, a blood sample for type and cross-match is usually also drawn.

Obtain daily hematocrit levels as ordered to monitor blood concentration. This level will rise if increased fluid is leaving the bloodstream for interstitial tissue (edema). Also, anticipate the need for frequent plasma estriol levels (a test of placenta function) and electrolyte levels. A woman's optic fundus is assessed daily for signs of arterial spasm, edema, or hemorrhage.

Obtain daily weights at the same time each day to evaluate tissue fluid retention. Ensure that a woman is wearing approximately the same amount of clothing at each weighing so any change in weight is not influenced by a change in the weight of her clothing.

An indwelling urinary catheter may be inserted to allow accurate recording of output and comparison with intake. Urinary output should be more than 600 mL per 24 hours (more than 30 mL/hour); an output lower than this suggests oliguria. Urinary proteins and specific gravity should be measured and recorded with voiding or hourly if an indwelling catheter is present. A 24-hour urine sample may be collected for protein and creatinine clearance determinations to evaluate kidney function. A woman with mild preeclampsia spills between 0.5 g and 1 g of protein every 24 hours (1+ on a random sample); a woman with severe preeclampsia spills approximately 5 g per 24 hours (3+ to 4+ on an individual specimen).

Monitor Fetal Well-Being. Generally, single Doppler auscultation at approximately 4-hour intervals is sufficient at this stage of management. However, the fetal heart rate may be assessed continuously with an external fetal monitor. A woman may have a nonstress test or biophysical profile done daily to assess uteroplacental sufficiency (see Chapter 8). Oxygen administration to the mother may be necessary to maintain adequate fetal oxygenation and prevent fetal bradycardia.

Support a Nutritious Diet. A woman needs a diet moderate to high in protein and moderate in sodium to compensate for the protein she is losing in urine. An intravenous fluid line should be initiated and maintained to serve as an emergency route for drug administration as well as to administer fluid to reduce hemoconcentration and hypovolemia.

Administer Medications to Prevent Eclampsia. A hypotensive drug such as hydralazine (Apresoline) or labetalol (Normodyne) may be prescribed to reduce hypertension. These drugs act to lower blood pressure by peripheral dilatation and thus do not interfere with placental circulation. They can cause tachycardia. Therefore, assess pulse and blood pressure after administration. Diastolic pressure should not be lowered below 80 to 90 mm Hg or inadequate placental perfusion could occur.

Despite these new drugs, magnesium sulfate remains the drug of choice to prevent eclampsia (Table 15.7). This drug, classified as a cathartic, reduces edema by causing a shift in fluid from the extracellular spaces into the intestine. It also has a central nervous system depressant action (it blocks peripheral neuromuscular transmissions), which lessens the possibility of seizures (Karch, 2004).

To achieve immediate reduction of the blood pressure, magnesium sulfate is first given intravenously in a loading or bolus dose. Given intravenously over 15 minutes, the drug acts almost immediately; unfortunately, the effect lasts only 30 to 60 minutes, so administration must be continuous.

For magnesium sulfate to act as an anticonvulsant, blood serum levels must be maintained at 5 to 8 mg/100 mL. If the blood serum level rises above this, respiratory depression, cardiac arrhythmias, and cardiac arrest can occur. The importance of different serum levels is shown in Box 15.9.

The most evident symptoms of overdose from magnesium sulfate administration include decreased urine output, depressed respirations, reduced consciousness, and decreased deep tendon reflexes (Nick, 2004). Because magnesium is excreted from the body almost entirely through the urine, urine output must be monitored closely to ensure adequate elimination. If severe oliguria should occur (less than 100 mL in 4 hours), excessively high serum levels of magnesium can result. Before you administer further magnesium sulfate, therefore, ensure that urine output is above 25 to 30 mL/hour, with a specific gravity of 1.010 or lower. Respirations should be above 12 per minute, a woman should be able to answer questions asked of her, **ankle clonus** (a continued motion of the foot) should be minimal, and deep tendon reflexes should be present. Make these assessments every hour if a continuous intravenous infusion is being used.

The easiest deep tendon reflex to assess is the patellar reflex (knee jerk). Instructions for initiating this reflex and ankle clonus are shown in Box 15.12. If an epidural block has been given for labor anesthesia, assess the biceps or triceps reflex (see Chapter 33).

In addition to making the above assessments when magnesium sulfate is being given, a solution of 10 mL of a 10% calcium gluconate solution (1 g) should be kept ready nearby for immediate intravenous administration should a woman develop signs and symptoms of magnesium toxicity, as calcium is the specific antidote for magnesium toxicity. Severe oliguria may be treated by the intravenous infusion of salt-poor albumin. This high-colloid solution

TABLE 15.7

Drugs Used in Pregnancy-Induced Hypertension

Drug	Indication	Dosage	Comments
Magnesium sulfate Pregnancy risk category B	Muscle relaxant; prevents seizures	Loading dose 4–6 g Maintenance dose 1–2 g/h IV	Infuse loading dose slowly over 15–30 min.
			Always administer as a piggyback infusion
			Assess respiratory rate, urine output, deep tendon reflexes, and clonus every hour.
			Keep in mind that urine output should be over 30 mL/hour and respiratory rate over 12/min. Serum magnesium level should remain below 7.5 mEq/L.
			Observe for CNS depression and hypotonia in infant at birth.
Hydralazine (Apresoline) Pregnancy risk category C	Antihypertensive (peripheral vasodilator); used to decrease hypertension	5–10 mg/IV	Administer slowly to avoid sudden fall in blood pressure.
			Maintain diastolic pressure over 90 mm Hg to ensure adequate placental filling.
Diazepam (Valium) Pregnancy risk category D	Halt seizures	5–10 mg/IV	Administer slowly. Dose may be repeated q 5–10 min (up to 30 mg/hour).
			Observe for respiratory depression or hypotension in mother and respiratory depression and hypotonia in infant at birth.
Calcium gluconate Pregnancy risk category C	Antidote for magnesium intoxication	1 g/IV (10 mL of a 10% solution)	Have prepared at bedside when administering magnesium sulfate.
			Administer at 5 mL/min.

Karch, A. M. (2004). *Lippincott's nursing drug guide.* Philadelphia: Lippincott Williams & Wilkins.

will call fluid into the bloodstream from interstitial tissue by osmotic pressure; the kidneys will then excrete the extra fluid along with magnesium sulfate levels.

On the day of birth, the anesthesiologist must be alerted to the fact that a woman has been receiving magnesium sulfate. If magnesium sulfate is given intravenously within 2 hours of the baby's birth, the baby may be born with respiratory depression because the drug crosses the placenta. A fetal heart rate monitor may show loss of variability of heartbeat immediately after magnesium therapy; the sonogram may reveal reduced fetal breathing movements. Observe carefully for other signs of fetal effects, such as late deceleration with labor contractions. Magnesium sulfate is continued for 12 to 24 hours after birth to prevent eclampsia during this period. The dose is then tapered and discontinued. Breast-feeding usually is delayed until the medication is discontinued. A long-term effect of magnesium sulfate therapy is osteoporosis. A woman may be started on a course of calcium to decrease the problem (Hung et al., 2005).

Nursing Interventions for a Woman With Eclampsia

Degeneration of a woman's condition from severe preeclampsia to eclampsia occurs when cerebral irritation from increasing cerebral edema becomes so acute that a seizure occurs. This usually happens late in pregnancy but can happen up to 48 hours after childbirth. Immediately before a seizure, a woman's blood pressure rises suddenly from additional vasospasm. Her temperature rises sharply to 103° to 104°F (39.4° to 40°C) from increased cerebral pressure. She notices blurring of vision or severe headache (from the increased cerebral edema) and her reflexes become hyperactive. She may experience a premonition that "something is happening." Vascular congestion of the liver or pancreas can lead to epigastric pain and nausea. Urinary output may decrease abruptly to less than 30 mL/hour. Eclampsia has actually occurred, however, only when a woman experiences a seizure.

Tonic-Clonic Seizures. An eclamptic seizure is a tonic-clonic type that occurs in stages. After the preliminary signal or aura that something is happening, all the muscles of the woman's body contract. Her back arches, her arms and legs stiffen, and her jaw closes abruptly. She may bite her tongue from the rapid closing of her jaw. Respirations halt because her thoracic muscles are held in contraction. This phase of the seizure, called the tonic phase, lasts approximately 20 seconds. It may seem longer because a woman may grow slightly cyanotic from the cessation of respirations.

The priority care for a woman with a seizure is to maintain a patent airway. Don't put a tongue blade between a woman's teeth: doing so can cause broken teeth, which

BOX 15.12

Eliciting A Patellar Reflex And Ankle Clonus

Patellar Reflex

With the woman in a supine position, ask her to bend her knee slightly. Place your hand under her knee to support the leg. Locate the patellar tendon in the midline just below the kneecap. Strike it firmly and quickly with a reflex hammer or the side of your hand. If the leg and foot move, a patellar reflex is present. The reflex is scored as:

0	=	No response; hypoactive; abnormal
1+	=	Somewhat diminished response but not abnormal
2+	=	Average response
3+	=	Brisker than average but not abnormal
4+	=	Hyperactive; very brisk; abnormal

Ankle Clonus

To elicit ankle clonus, dorsiflex the woman's foot three times in rapid succession. As you take your hand away, observe the foot. If no further motion is present, no ankle clonus is present. If the foot continues to move involuntarily, clonus is present. Although usually just rated as present or absent, it can be rated as:

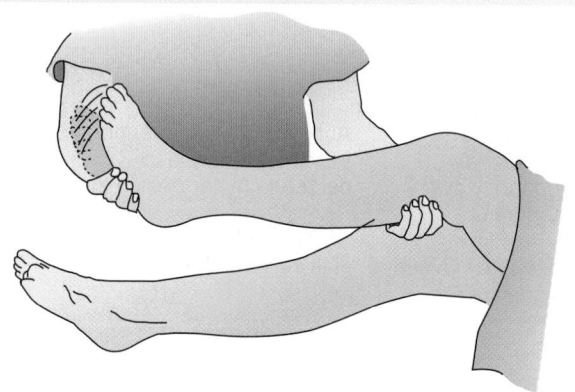

Mild (2 movements)
Moderate (3–5 movements)
Severe (over 6 movements)

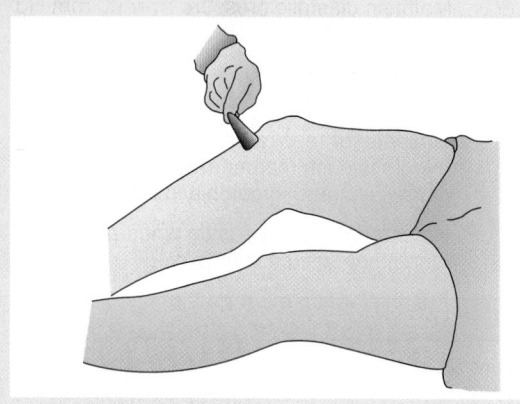

could then be aspirated. Administer oxygen by face mask to protect the fetus during this interval. Assess oxygen saturation via a pulse oximeter. Apply an external fetal heart monitor if one is not already in place to assess the condition of the fetus. To prevent aspiration, turn a woman on her side to allow secretions to drain from her mouth.

After the tonic phase of the seizure, all the muscles of the body contract and relax repeatedly, causing a woman's extremities to flail wildly (clonic phase). She inhales and exhales irregularly as her thoracic muscles contract and relax. She may aspirate the saliva that collected in her mouth during the tonic phase if she was not placed on her side.

Her bladder and bowel muscles contract and relax; incontinence of urine and feces may occur. Although a woman begins to breathe during this stage, the breathing is not entirely effective. She may remain cyanotic and may need continued oxygen therapy, not for herself but for the fetus. The clonic stage of a seizure lasts up to 1 minute. Magnesium sulfate or diazepam (Valium) may be administered intravenously as an emergency measure at this time.

The third stage of the seizure is the postictal state. During this stage, a woman is semicomatose and cannot be roused except by painful stimuli for 1 to 4 hours. Extremely close observation is as important during the post-

ictal stage as it was during the first two stages, because if the seizure caused premature separation of the placenta, labor may begin during this period and a woman will be unable to report the sensation of contractions. Also, the painful stimulus of contractions may initiate another seizure. Keep a woman on her side so secretions can drain from her mouth. Give her nothing to eat or drink by mouth. In coma, hearing is the last sense lost and the first one regained, so remember when talking at her bedside that she may be able to hear even though she does not respond. Continuously assess fetal heart sounds and uterine contractions. Check for vaginal bleeding every 15 minutes. Evidence that placental separation may have occurred will appear first on the fetal heart record; vaginal bleeding will strengthen the presumption.

Birth. If the pregnancy is more than 24 weeks along, a decision about birth will be made as soon as a woman's condition stabilizes, usually 12 to 24 hours after the seizure. There is some evidence that the fetus does not continue to grow after eclampsia occurs, so terminating the pregnancy at this point is appropriate for both mother and child. For an unexplained reason, fetal lung maturity appears to advance rapidly with PIH (possibly from the intrauterine stress), so even though the fetus is younger than 36 weeks, the lecithin–sphingomyelin ratio may indicate fetal lung maturity.

Cesarean birth is always more hazardous for the fetus because of the association of retained lung fluid (see Chapter 26). Further, a woman with eclampsia is not a good candidate for surgery. Because her vascular system is low in volume, she may become hypotensive with regional anesthesia, such as an epidural block. The preferred method for birth, therefore, is vaginal. If labor does not begin spontaneously, rupture of the membranes or induction of labor with intravenous oxytocin may be instituted. If this is ineffective and the fetus appears to be in imminent danger, cesarean birth is indicated.

Postpartum Hypertension. Postpartum hypertension may occur up to 10 to 14 days after birth, although it usually occurs in the first 48 hours after birth. Monitoring blood pressure in the postpartum period is essential to detect residual hypertensive or renal disease. Urge women who had an elevation of blood pressure during pregnancy to return for a postpartum checkup to have their blood pressure evaluated to be certain it has returned to normal.

Checkpoint Question 5

If Beverly Muzuki had developed severe preeclampsia, what would be the drug you would expect to administer?

a. Magnesium sulfate
b. Ranitidine (Zantac)
c. A nonsteroidal inflammatory agent
d. A loop diuretic

HELLP SYNDROME

HELLP syndrome is a variation of PIH named for the common symptoms that occur: *h*emolysis, *e*levated *l*iver enzymes, and *l*ow *p*latelets. The syndrome occurs in 4% to 12% of patients with PIH, or approximately 1 in every 150 births. It is a serious syndrome because it results in a maternal mortality rate as high as 24% and an infant mortality rate as high as 35% (Moldenhauser & Sibai, 2003).

Why some women with severe preeclampsia also develop the HELLP syndrome is unknown. It occurs in both primigravidas and multigravidas. The first symptoms are usually nausea, epigastric pain, general malaise, and right upper quadrant tenderness from liver inflammation. Laboratory studies reveal hemolysis of red blood cells (they appear fragmented on a peripheral blood smear), thrombocytopenia (a platelet count below 100,000/mm³), and elevated liver enzyme levels (alanine aminotransferase [ALT] and serum aspartate aminotransferase [AST]). The liver enzyme levels are elevated from hemorrhage and necrosis of the liver. Women with the HELLP syndrome need close observation for bleeding, in addition to the observations necessary for preeclampsia.

Therapy for the condition is to improve the platelet count by transfusion of fresh-frozen plasma or platelets. Complications associated with the syndrome are subcapsular liver hematoma, hyponatremia, renal failure, and hypoglycemia. If hypoglycemia is present, this is corrected by an intravenous dextrose infusion. The infant is delivered as soon as feasible by either vaginal or cesarean birth. Maternal hemorrhage may occur at birth because of poor clotting ability. Epidural anesthesia may not be possible because of the low platelet count and the high possibility of bleeding at the epidural site. Laboratory results return to normal after birth, the same as preeclamptic symptoms generally fade, but the experience of developing a HELLP syndrome is frightening (Kidner & Flanders-Stepans, 2004).

MULTIPLE PREGNANCY

Multiple gestation is considered a complication of pregnancy because a woman's body must adjust to the effects of more than one fetus. The incidence of multiple births has increased dramatically because of the use of in vitro fertilization. The rate of twinning in the United States is 1 in 40 births; triplets, 1 in 500 (Newman, 2003).

Identical (monozygotic) twins begin with a single ovum and spermatozoon. In the process of fusion, or in one of the first cell divisions, the zygote divides into two identical individuals. Single-ovum twins usually have one placenta, one chorion, two amnions, and two umbilical cords. The twins are always of the same sex. Fraternal (dizygotic, nonidentical) twins are the result of the fertilization of two separate ova by two separate spermatozoa (possibly not from the same sexual partner). Double-ova twins have two placentas, two chorions, two amnions, and two umbilical cords. The twins may be of the same or different sex (Fig. 15.9). Two thirds of twins are dizygotic. It is sometimes difficult to determine by sonogram or at birth whether twins are identical or fraternal because the two fraternal placentas may fuse and appear as one large placenta.

Multiple pregnancies of three, four, five, six, or seven children may be single-ovum conceptions, multiple-ova conceptions, or a combination of the two types. Most today occur from multiple ova being implanted as an in vitro fertility process. Naturally occurring multiple pregnancies are more frequent in nonwhites than in whites. The higher a woman's parity and age, the more likely she is to have a multiple gestation. Inheritance appears to play a role in natural dizygotic twinning; this has a familial maternal pattern of occurrence (Newman, 2003).

Assessment

Multiple gestation is suspected early in pregnancy, when the uterus begins to increase in size at a rate faster than usual. Alpha-fetoprotein levels are elevated. At the time of quickening, a woman may report flurries of action at different portions of her abdomen rather than at one consistent spot (where the feet are located). On auscultation of the abdomen, multiple sets of fetal heart sounds may be heard, but if one or more fetuses has his or her back positioned toward a woman's back, only one fetal heart sound may be heard.

A sonogram can reveal multiple gestation sacs early in pregnancy. In some instances, early ultrasound examinations reveal multiple amniotic sacs but then later in

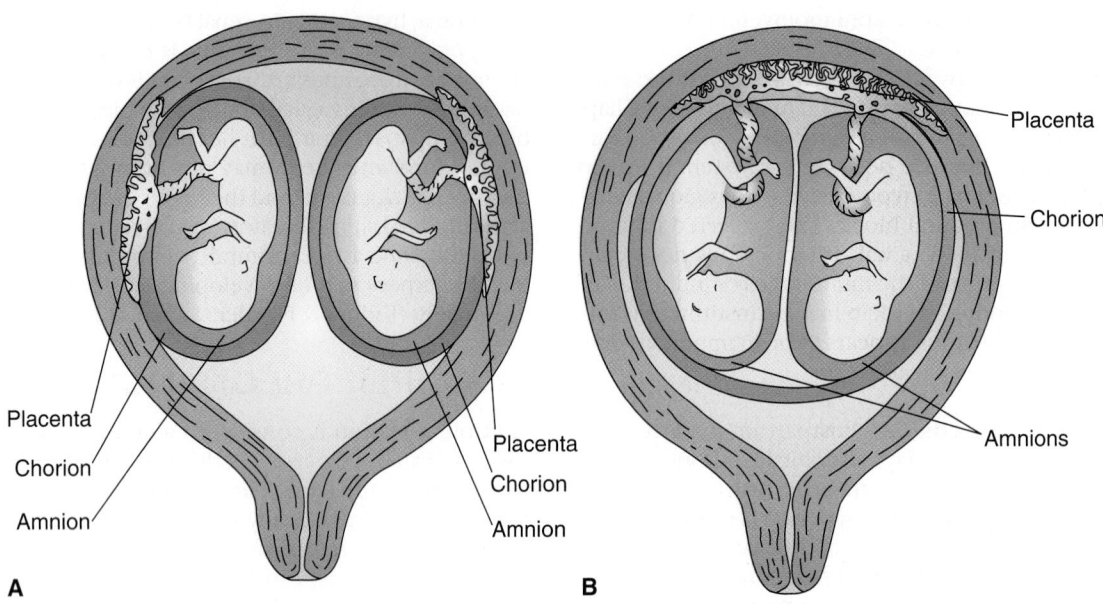

FIGURE 15.9 Multiple gestations. (**A**) Dizygotic twins showing two placentas, two chorions, and two amnions. (**B**) Monozygotic twins with one placenta, one chorion, and two amnions.

pregnancy, in as many as 30% of women, only one fetus remains (vanishing twin syndrome) (Briscoe & Street, 2003). Women may grieve for a vanished twin as much as if the baby had died at birth, a feeling that could disrupt pregnancy bonding work.

Therapeutic Management

Women with a multiple gestation are more susceptible to complications of pregnancy such as PIH, hydramnios, placenta previa, preterm labor, and anemia than are women carrying one fetus. They also are more prone to postpartum bleeding because of the additional uterine stretching. Because a multiple pregnancy usually ends before the normal term, 25% of low-birthweight babies are from multiple pregnancies. Because of this immaturity, the chance of an infant from a multiple birth developing cerebral palsy may be 12 times more than that with a single birth (Newman, 2003). There is also a higher risk of congenital anomalies in twins, such as spinal cord defect, than with single births. There is a higher incidence of velamentous cord insertion (the cord inserted into the fetal membranes) with twins than with single births, so the risk of bleeding at the time of birth from a torn cord is increased. With monozygotic twins, the fetuses can share vascular communication, possibly leading to overgrowth of one fetus and undergrowth of the second (a twin-to-twin transfusion), resulting in discordant infants (Machin, 2004) (see Chapter 26). If a single amnion is present, there can be knotting and twisting of umbilical cords, causing fetal distress or difficulty with birth. Because of the possibility of these complications, a woman with a twin pregnancy needs closer prenatal supervision than a woman with a single gestation to detect these problems as early as possible. A woman carrying more than two fetuses has even greater risks (Blickstein, 2004).

NURSING DIAGNOSES AND RELATED INTERVENTIONS

Nursing Diagnosis: Fatigue related to increased stress on body functioning secondary to multiple gestation

Outcome Evaluation: Client states she is tired but identifies steps she has taken to minimize fatigue.

Spend time at health care visits reviewing with a woman with a multiple pregnancy her need for extra rest, especially in a side-lying position during the day, to increase placental perfusion.

Because a woman is carrying a double weight during pregnancy, she may notice extreme fatigue and backache. She may have more difficulty resting or sleeping than the average woman because of this greater discomfort and increased fetal activity. As the growing uterus compresses her stomach, she may find her appetite decreasing and her intake falling. To compensate and maintain nutrition, a woman may need to eat six small meals a day rather than three large ones. She must be sure to take her iron, folic acid, and vitamin supplement.

Toward the end of pregnancy, a woman may have extreme difficulty ambulating because of her excess weight. Her abdomen may become so stretched that she feels as if she is going to burst.

Although there is little documentation that it makes a difference, many women with a multiple pregnancy are prescribed bed rest at home during the last 2 or 3 months of pregnancy in an attempt to decrease the risk of preterm labor and increase the possibility the pregnancy will come to term, or at least pass week 34, when the chances for survival of the fetuses rise markedly. Beginning with week 28 of pregnancy, a woman may be asked to come to a health care facility for monthly ultrasound examinations or weekly nonstress tests to document normal fetal growth, although this may not be necessary if the pregnancy is going well and the fetuses are growing consistently. If these tests are necessary, be certain appointments are scheduled to conserve her energy as much as possible.

Nursing Diagnosis: Parental role conflict related to recent discovery of multiple (as opposed to single) pregnancy

Outcome Evaluation: Client states she is looking forward to multiple infants (may express concern about her ability to manage their arrival); client identifies changes she is making in preparation now that more than one baby is expected.

A woman with a multiple pregnancy has to work through an additional role change during pregnancy. First, she completes the work to accept she is pregnant. Then she is having a baby. Then suddenly, at a routine office visit, two or more gestational sacs are seen on ultrasound or two or more sets of heart sounds are heard. She is told she has a multiple pregnancy. Now she has to work through a second role change—for example, becoming a mother of two, not of one, or a mother of four or five. This role change may be difficult to complete, especially if the pregnancy ends early. A woman may need extra help after birth to form a close mother–child relationship with her newborns.

Nursing Diagnosis: Fear concerning her own and the babies' health related to risks of multiple pregnancy

Outcome Evaluation: Client accurately states risks of multiple pregnancy; expresses confidence in health care team's ability to care for her and her babies through pregnancy and birth.

In addition to having to work through a role change, a woman with a multiple pregnancy has more reason to fear for her life and the life of her babies than does the average woman. Every woman has heard stories about twins being born so prematurely they did not survive, and about the special danger for the last infant born. If she has not already heard these stories, someone will mention them to her before her due date. Unfortunately, all these risks cannot simply be filed away under the heading of untrue stories: both prematurity and high risk to the last-born infant are real hazards in multiple gestation. Help a woman deal with her fears as positively as possible. It is helpful to tell her there is no indication so far that her babies are in any danger, so right now it is best to continue doing the things that have to be done; if any prob-

lems should arise, the health care team and a woman's family will be there to support her.

Sometimes a woman is so fearful her infants will be born too small to survive that she makes no preparations for the infants. She lacks confidence in herself or cannot imagine she will be lucky enough or "good" enough to be able to carry a multiple pregnancy to term. Give her assurance during pregnancy that she is managing well so her self-esteem is maintained at as high a level as possible. When her babies are born and all are healthy, the proof she needs that she "deserved" this or was capable of it will be present in her arms.

Nursing care at the birth of multiple infants is discussed in Chapter 21.

Checkpoint Question 6

If a patient developed a HELLP syndrome, what symptoms would be most important to assess for?

a. Rapid, anxious breathing
b. Ecchymosis or petechiae
c. Blink reflex
d. Enlarged thyroid

HYDRAMNIOS

Usually the amniotic fluid volume is 500 to 1,000 mL at term. Excess fluid more than 2,000 mL or an amniotic fluid index above 24 cm is considered **hydramnios** (Pauer et al., 2003). Too much amniotic fluid can cause fetal malpresentation because the additional uterine space allows the fetus to turn. It also can lead to premature rupture of the membranes from the increased pressure and possible prostaglandin release. Preterm rupture of the membranes adds the additional risks of infection, prolapsed cord, and preterm birth.

Assessment

Amniotic fluid is formed by the cells of the amniotic membrane and from fetal urine. It is swallowed by the fetus, absorbed across the intestinal membrane into the fetal bloodstream, and transferred across the placenta. Although hydramnios can occur separate from fetal involvement, accumulation of amniotic fluid suggests difficulty with the fetus's ability to swallow or absorb or else excessive urine production. Inability to swallow occurs in infants who are anencephalic or who have tracheoesophageal fistula with stenosis or intestinal obstruction (Kalish et al., 2003). Excessive urine output occurs in the fetuses of diabetic women (hyperglycemia in the fetus causes increased urine production).

The first sign of hydramnios may be an unusually rapid enlargement of the uterus. The small parts of the fetus are difficult to palpate because the uterus is unusually tense. Auscultating the fetal heart rate is difficult because of the increased amount of fluid surrounding the fetus.

A woman may begin to notice extreme shortness of breath as the overly distended uterus pushes up against her diaphragm. She may develop lower extremity varicosities and hemorrhoids because of poor venous return from the extensive uterine pressure. She will have increased weight gain. Generally, a sonogram is ordered to document the presence of hydramnios and to discover a reason for the excessive amount of fluid.

Therapeutic Management

Women with severe hydramnios may be admitted to the hospital for bed rest and further evaluation or may be cared for at home. Regardless of the setting, maintaining bed rest helps to increase uteroplacental circulation and reduces pressure on the cervix, which may help prevent preterm labor. Teach a woman to report any sign of ruptured membranes or uterine contractions. Although not common, there is a possibility that straining to defecate could increase uterine pressure and cause rupture of membranes. Help her avoid constipation, therefore, by encouraging her to eat a high-fiber diet. Suggest a stool softener be prescribed if diet alone is ineffective.

Assess vital signs and lower extremity edema frequently, because the extremely tense uterus puts unusual pressure on both the diaphragm and the vessels of the pelvis.

It is possible for amniocentesis to be performed to remove some of the extra amniotic fluid. Because amniotic fluid is replaced rapidly, however, this is only a temporary measure unless it is repeated daily. If contractions begin, tocolysis with magnesium sulfate may be begun to prevent or halt preterm labor.

In most instances of hydramnios, there will be preterm rupture of the membranes due to excessive pressure, followed by preterm labor. To prevent the sudden loss of fluid and the accompanying danger of a prolapsed cord, membranes can be "needled" (a thin needle is inserted vaginally to pierce them) to allow a slow, controlled release of fluid. After birth, the infant must be assessed carefully for factors that may have interfered with the ability to swallow in utero.

POST-TERM PREGNANCY

A term pregnancy is 38 to 42 weeks long. A pregnancy that exceeds these limits is prolonged (**post-term pregnancy,** *postmature,* or *postdate*). The infant of such a pregnancy is considered postmature, or dysmature, if there is evidence that placental insufficiency has interfered with fetal growth. Post-term pregnancy occurs in 3% to 12% of all pregnancies (Moore & Martin, 2003).

Included in this group are some pregnancies that appear to extend beyond the due date set for them because of a faulty due date. Women who have long menstrual cycles (40 to 45 days, for example) do not ovulate on day 14 as in a typical menstrual cycle. Because they ovulate 14 days from the end of their cycle, or on day 26 or 31, their children will be "late" by 12 to 17 days.

In other instances, the pregnancy is truly overdue. For some reason, the trigger that initiates labor did not turn on. Prolonged pregnancy can occur in a woman receiving a high dose of salicylates (for severe sinus headaches or rheumatoid arthritis) because salicylate interferes with the synthesis of prostaglandins, which may be responsible for the initiation of labor. It is also associated with myometrial quiescence, or a uterus that does not respond to normal labor stimulation.

Remaining in utero for more than 2 weeks beyond term creates a danger to a fetus for a number of reasons. Meconium aspiration is more apt to occur as fetal intestinal contents are more likely to reach the rectum. If the fetus continues to grow, macrosomia could create a birth problem. However, the usual effect of being post-term is lack of growth. A placenta seems to have adequate functioning ability for only 40 to 42 weeks. After that time, it acquires calcium deposits (becomes grade 3). A fetus is exposed to decreased blood perfusion. Such a fetus may suffer from a lack of oxygen, fluid, and nutrients (Caughey & Musci, 2004). Oligohydramnios (a decreased amount of amniotic fluid from lessened urine production in the fetus) can lead to variable decelerations from cord compression.

If labor has not begun by 41 weeks, a maternal vaginal fibronectin level, a nonstress test, and/or a biophysical profile may be ordered to document the state of placental perfusion and the amount of amniotic fluid present. If these are normal, it suggests the due date was miscalculated. If the test results are abnormal or the physical examination or biparietal diameter measured on sonography suggests the fetus is term size, labor will be induced (Sanchez-Ramos et al., 2003). Prostaglandin gel or misoprostol (Cytotec) applied to the cervix to initiate ripening, or stripping of membranes followed by an oxytocin infusion is a common method used to begin labor. If oxytocin is ineffective, cesarean birth will be necessary. Monitor the fetal heart rate closely during labor to be certain placental insufficiency is not occurring from aging of the placenta. Nursing care for the post-term infant at birth is discussed in Chapter 26.

PSEUDOCYESIS

In **pseudocyesis** (false pregnancy), nausea and vomiting, amenorrhea, and enlargement of the abdomen occur in a nonpregnant woman. This can also be seen in men (Berga & Parry, 2005). There are a number of theories as to why the phenomenon occurs: wish-fulfillment theory suggests a woman's desire to be pregnant actually causes physiologic changes to occur; conflict theory suggests a desire for and fear of pregnancy create an internal conflict leading to physiologic changes; and depression theory attributes the cause to major depression. In any event, a woman's body responds with physiologic symptoms such as breast tenderness and an enlarging abdomen. Her abdomen can become so enlarged that she appears to be 7 or 8 months pregnant. On physical examination, however, it is obvious only the abdomen, not the uterus, is enlarged. Sonographic imaging will rule out pregnancy. Both men and women with the disorder need psychological counseling to help them better handle their needs.

ISOIMMUNIZATION (RH INCOMPATIBILITY)

Approximately 15% of whites and 10% of African Americans in the United States are missing the Rh (D) factor in their blood or have an Rh-negative blood type. **Rh incom-**

patibility occurs when an Rh-negative mother (one negative for a D antigen or one with a dd genotype) is carrying a fetus with an Rh-positive blood type (DD or Dd genotype). For such a situation to occur, the father of the child must either be homozygous (DD) or heterozygous (Dd) Rh positive. If the father of the child is homozygous (DD) for the factor, 100% of the couple's children will be Rh positive (Dd). If the father is heterozygous for the trait, 50% of their children can be expected to be Rh positive (Dd). Although this is basically a problem that affects the fetus, it causes such concern and apprehension in a woman during pregnancy that it becomes a maternal problem as well (Porter, Peltier, & Branch, 2003).

Because people who have Rh-positive blood have a protein factor (the D antigen) that Rh-negative people do not, when an Rh-positive fetus begins to grow inside an Rh-negative mother who is sensitized, it is as though her body is being invaded by a foreign agent. Her body reacts in the same manner it would if the invading factor were a substance such as a virus: she forms antibodies against the invading substance. The Rh factor exists as a portion of the red blood cell, so these maternal antibodies cross the placenta and cause red blood cell destruction (hemolysis) of fetal red blood cells (Fig. 15.10). A fetus can become so deficient in red blood cells that sufficient oxygen transport to body cells cannot be maintained. This condition is termed **hemolytic disease of the newborn** or **erythroblastosis fetalis.** Management of the infant born with this condition is discussed in Chapter 26.

Theoretically, there is no connection between fetal blood and maternal blood during pregnancy, so the mother should not be exposed to fetal blood. It is well documented, however, that an occasional villus ruptures, allowing a drop or two of fetal blood to enter the maternal circulation. Procedures such as amniocentesis or percutaneous umbilical blood sampling can also cause this. During a first pregnancy this effect is small. As the placenta separates after birth of the child, there is an active exchange of fetal and maternal blood from damaged villi. Therefore, most of the maternal antibodies formed against the Rh-positive blood are not formed during pregnancy but in the first 72 hours after birth, making them a threat to a second pregnancy.

Assessment

All women with Rh-negative blood should have an anti-D antibody titer done at a first pregnancy visit. If the results are normal or the titer is minimal (normal is 0; a ratio below 1:8 is minimal), the test will be repeated at week 28 of pregnancy. If this is also normal, no therapy is needed.

If a woman's anti-D antibody titer is elevated at a first assessment (1:16 or greater), showing Rh sensitization, the well-being of the fetus in this potentially toxic environment will be monitored every 2 weeks (or more often) by Doppler velocity of the fetal middle cerebral artery, a technique that can predict when anemia is present (Segata & Mari, 2004).

If the artery velocity remains high, a fetus is not developing anemia and most likely is an Rh-negative fetus. If the reading is low, a fetus is in danger, and immediate birth will be carried out or intrauterine transfusion or intrauterine exchange transfusion will begin (Porter, Peltier, & Branch, 2003). If a spectrophotometer reading of amniotic fluid is moderate (zone 2), preterm birth by induction of labor at fetal maturity is indicated.

Therapeutic Management

To reduce the number of Rh (D) antibodies being formed, Rh (D) immune globulin (RhIG), a commercial preparation of passive Rh (D) antibodies against the Rh factor, is administered to women at 28 weeks of pregnancy. These cannot cross the placenta and destroy fetal red blood cells because the antibodies are not the IgG class, the only type that crosses the placenta. If RhIG is given again by injection to the mother in the first 72 hours after delivery of an Rh-positive child, it prevents the mother from forming natural antibodies. Because RhIG is passive antibody protection, it is transient, and in 2 weeks to 2 months, the

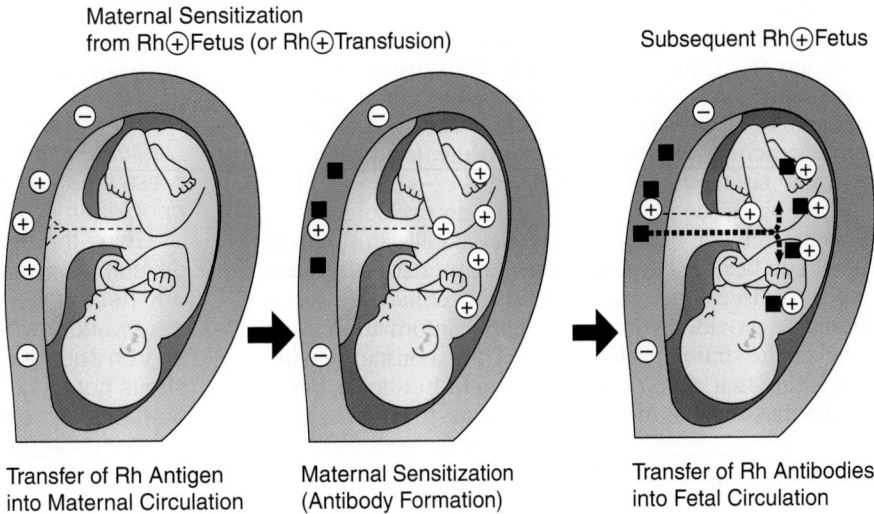

Maternal Sensitization
from Rh⊕Fetus (or Rh⊕Transfusion)

Subsequent Rh⊕Fetus

Transfer of Rh Antigen
into Maternal Circulation

Maternal Sensitization
(Antibody Formation)

Transfer of Rh Antibodies
into Fetal Circulation

FIGURE 15.10 Maternal antibody formation against the Rh antigen.

Key: ⊕ Rh Postive   ⊖ Rh Negative   ■ Rh Antibody

passive antibodies are destroyed. Only those few antibodies that were formed during pregnancy are left. For this reason, every pregnancy is like a first pregnancy in terms of the number of antibodies present, ensuring a safe intrauterine environment for any future pregnancies.

After birth, the infant's blood type will be determined from a sample of the cord blood. If it is Rh positive—Coombs' negative, indicating that a large number of antibodies are not present in the mother—the mother will receive the RhIG injection. If the newborn's blood type is Rh negative, no antibodies have been formed in the mother's circulation during pregnancy and none will form, so passive antibody injection is unnecessary.

Although in future years the problem of Rh sensitization will be greatly reduced, it currently remains a complication of pregnancy, particularly in women who gave birth to a first child in an undeveloped nation. Any woman who does not receive a RhIG injection after an induced abortion, miscarriage, ectopic pregnancy, or amniocentesis can have had antibody formation begin. Women may be administered high doses of gamma globulin (IVIG) to help reduce their antibody count and the chance of fetal involvement.

Intrauterine Transfusion. To restore fetal red blood cells, blood transfusion can be performed on the fetus in utero. This is done by injecting red blood cells directly into a vessel in the fetal cord or depositing them in the fetal abdomen using amniocentesis technique.

Blood used for transfusion in utero is either the fetus's own type (determined by percutaneous blood sampling) or group O negative if the fetal blood type is unknown. From 75 to 150 mL of washed red cells are used, depending on the age of the fetus. After deposition of the blood in the cord, the cannula is withdrawn and a woman is urged to rest for approximately 30 minutes while fetal heart sounds and uterine activity are monitored.

Obviously, intrauterine transfusion is not without risk. A cord blood vessel may be lacerated by the needle, or the uterus may be so irritated by the invasive procedure that labor contractions begin. For the fetus who is severely affected by isoimmunization, however, such a risk is no greater than that of leaving the fetus untreated in a destructive intrauterine environment. The mother receives an RhIG injection after the transfusion to help reduce increased sensitization from the amniocentesis. Transfusion is sometimes done only once during pregnancy, or it may be repeated as often as every 2 weeks. As soon as fetal maturity is reached, as shown by a mature lecithin–sphingomyelin ratio, birth will be induced.

After birth, the infant may require an exchange transfusion to remove hemolyzed red blood cells and replace them with healthy blood cells (see Chapter 26). A woman needs to discuss her plans for further childbearing and should be provided with contraceptive information if she believes the strain of this pregnancy, the constant feeling of wishing that everything was all right but never being certain that it was, is more than she wants to endure again.

FETAL DEATH

Obviously, one of the most severe complications of pregnancy is fetal death. The most likely causes include chromosomal abnormalities, congenital malformations, infections such as hepatitis B, immunologic causes, and complications of maternal disease. If fetal death happens before the time of quickening, a woman will not be aware the fetus has died because she was not able to feel fetal movements. This type of fetal death may be discovered at a routine prenatal visit when no fetal heartbeat can be heard. A real-time sonogram will reveal no fetal heartbeat is present.

That a fetus has died early in intrauterine life may first be revealed by the natural miscarriage that occurs. A woman begins painless spotting, gradually accompanied by uterine contractions with cervical effacement and dilatation. The fetus is born lifeless and emaciated. Carefully observe all women who deliver a dead fetus for excess bleeding because if the fetus has been dead in utero for any length of time, the risk for the development of DIC increases.

If a fetus dies in utero past the point of quickening, a woman becomes aware that fetal movements are suddenly absent. She may lie down or sit in a position that she knows usually causes fetal movement. Unable to believe that something could have happened, she may attribute the lack of movement to "sleeping" or "saving enough strength to be born." Because she is denying what is happening, it may be a full 24 hours before she telephones the health care facility to report the apparent lack of fetal movement. On assessment, no fetal heartbeat can be heard. A sonogram will confirm the absence of a fetal heartbeat.

If labor does not begin spontaneously, it will be induced through a combination of prostaglandin gel such as misoprostol (Cytotec) applied to the cervix to effect cervical ripening and oxytocin administration to begin uterine contractions. Blood for coagulation studies to detect DIC should be obtained.

NURSING DIAGNOSES AND RELATED INTERVENTIONS

Nursing Diagnosis: Powerlessness related to fetal death

Outcome Evaluation: Client and support person express meaning of pregnancy loss; identify support people/family with whom they can share grief.

Going through labor knowing a fetus is dead is difficult. A woman grieves for both her dead child and her inability to carry a pregnancy to term. She may wonder what she did to cause this (e.g., forgot an iron supplement or painted a crib) or may worry she is not as good a woman as others. Give her opportunities to express how she feels about this loss. "This must be a very difficult day for you" is the kind of statement that opens up the topic for discussion. If there are older children, it might be a help to explore how a woman plans to explain the fetal death to them.

Ask a couple about their desire for clergy or religious rites, such as baptism. Encourage a support person to remain with a woman during labor, but remember the support person is grieving too. Although this is a difficult time, expressing grief makes the birth real, ends the pregnancy, and allows the couple to begin rebuilding their life.

Labor involving a dead fetus is the same as for a live fetus because every fetus is basically a passive participant during labor. It may be difficult for a woman to use controlled breathing exercises, although encouraging her to use them is helpful in making the experience one of controllable pain. If a woman wishes a high level of analgesia, she may have it because there is no fetus to protect from narcotic effects, although too much may lead to poor uterine involution in the postpartum period.

Ask if the parents wish to see the child. If they do, wash away obvious blood, swaddle the baby as if he or she were a well newborn, and bring the baby to them. Point out particularly endearing features of the child that may provide a focus for memories. Some parents want to keep a lock of the child's hair. Others want to keep the hospital identification bracelet or to take a photograph. Parents may want to name the child. All of these measures help to make the death real to parents and let them begin the healthy process of grieving.

If the child has a congenital anomaly that led to the death, prepare them for this before bringing the child to them, and explain how the anomaly affected the child. Explain hospital procedures such as when the body will be released or what additional permission for autopsy is needed. Different communities have different laws concerning whether burial for an immature fetus is necessary. Consult local health department regulations so you can serve as a resource person for parents concerning this.

A woman needs to remain for only a short stay in the hospital, assuming no complications with labor developed. Many couples ask how soon it will be safe for them to have another child. For the answer to this, they need to consult with their obstetrician or nurse-midwife about why this fetal death occurred. For some couples, beginning a second pregnancy immediately is a good recommendation. For others, waiting for an interval of time (perhaps 6 months) is better as this gives them more time to work through their grief before starting a new pregnancy. This helps prevent the new baby from becoming a "replacement baby" or someone to take the place of the dead infant rather than a unique individual in his or her own right. This is important in years to come because replacement children are rarely able to live up to the image of what the dead baby would have been if only she or he had lived.

Prepare the couple for the possibility they may feel sad on the day the infant would have been born if the pregnancy had been carried to term, or if they visit a friend's child of the age their child would have been. Be certain before a woman is discharged from the hospital that she has a support person she can rely on during the following week or month, when the full impact of the fetal loss registers. Be certain she has a return appointment for a gynecologic checkup so her physiologic and psychological health can be evaluated at that time.

Checkpoint Question 7

Suppose Beverly Muzuki was Rh negative. Under what circumstance would she be eligible for Rh (D) immune globulin (RhIG)?

a. If she were having a multiple pregnancy
b. If her fetus were found to be Rh negative
c. If her fetus's heartbeat became tachycardic
d. If her fetus's blood type was Rh positive

Key Points

Vaginal bleeding during pregnancy is always serious until ruled otherwise because it has the potential to diminish the blood supply of both the mother and fetus.

The bleeding evident may not be indicative of the actual amount of bleeding occurring because so much internal bleeding may be happening. As a rule, women with bleeding during pregnancy should be positioned on their side to improve placental circulation.

Spontaneous miscarriage is the loss of a pregnancy before viability of the fetus (20 to 24 weeks). The majority of these early pregnancy losses are attributed to chromosomal abnormality. Miscarriages are classified as threatened, imminent, complete, incomplete, missed, or recurrent pregnancy loss. Women who have a spontaneous miscarriage at home should bring any tissue passed to the hospital for an analysis for gestational trophoblastic disease.

Ectopic pregnancy is pregnancy implantation outside the uterus, usually in a fallopian tube. If discovered before the tube ruptures, this can be treated with methotrexate or mifepristone. If not discovered early, it produces sharp lower quadrant pain at about 6 to 12 weeks as the tube ruptures. Surgery is done to remove the conceptus and repair the tube to halt bleeding.

Gestational trophoblastic disease is abnormal overgrowth of the trophoblast tissue. If not discovered by a sonogram before this, bleeding usually occurs at about the 16th week of pregnancy. Women need close follow-up after this because it can lead to choriocarcinoma, a malignancy.

Premature cervical dilatation occurs when the cervix dilates early in pregnancy, before viability of the fetus. Sutures (cervical cerclage) can be placed to prevent the cervix from dilating prematurely this way again in a second pregnancy.

Placenta previa is low implantation of the placenta so that it crosses the cervical os. If it is not discovered before labor, cervical dilatation may cause the placenta to tear, causing severe blood loss. Women who have symptoms of placenta previa (painless vaginal bleeding in the third trimester) should not have vaginal examinations done to prevent disruption of the low-implanted placenta.

Premature separation of the placenta (abruptio placentae), placental separation from the uterus before the fetus is born, usually occurs late in pregnancy. This separation immediately cuts off blood supply to the fetus. Women with increased parity, those with previous uterine surgery, and those who use cocaine are at highest risk for this. Often it is manifested by sudden, sharp fundal pain, then a continuing dull pain and vaginal bleeding.

Disseminated intravascular coagulation is a blood disorder that may occur with any trauma, so it can accompany such conditions as premature separation of the placenta and pregnancy-induced hypertension. Blood coagulation is so extreme at one point in the circulatory system that clotting factors are used up, resulting in their absence in the remainder of the system. Beginning symptoms of this include easy bruising, petechiae, and oozing from intravenous sites. Heparin is used to stop the local coagulation and free up clotting factors for systemic use.

Preterm labor is labor that occurs after 20 weeks and before the end of the 37th week of pregnancy. A woman is said to be in preterm labor when she has had uterine contractions every 10 minutes for 1 hour and cervical dilatation begins. Common tocolytics, drugs that can halt labor, are magnesium sulfate and beta-sympathomimetic agents such as terbutaline (Brethine).

Preterm rupture of the membranes is tearing of the fetal membranes with loss of amniotic fluid before the pregnancy is at term. After rupture, there is a high risk of fetal and uterine infection (chorioamnionitis) and preterm birth.

Pregnancy-induced hypertension is a unique disorder that occurs with pregnancy with three classic symptoms: hypertension, edema, and proteinuria. It is categorized as preeclampsia or eclampsia. If mild (blood pressure not over 140/90), treatment is bed rest. If severe (blood pressure over 160/110), bed rest plus administration of magnesium sulfate is necessary. If a seizure occurs, the condition becomes eclampsia. Helping prevent the disease from progressing to this stage is an important nursing responsibility.

The HELLP syndrome is a unique form of pregnancy-induced hypertension marked by hemolysis of red blood cells, elevated liver enzymes, and a low platelet count.

Multiple gestation puts an additional strain on a woman's physical resources and may lead to preterm birth with immaturity of the infants. Helping a woman obtain adequate nutrition and rest during pregnancy are nursing responsibilities.

Post-term pregnancy is pregnancy that extends beyond 42 weeks. As the placenta deteriorates at this time, it causes a fetus to receive decreased nutrients.

Hydramnios is overproduction of amniotic fluid (above 2,000 mL), a condition that can lead to ruptured membranes and premature birth because of increased intrauterine pressure.

Isoimmunization (Rh incompatibility) is a possibility when a woman who is Rh negative is sensitized and carrying a fetus who is Rh positive. Maternal antibodies form and destroy fetal red blood cells, leading to anemia, edema, and jaundice in the newborn. Being certain women are screened for blood type and antibody titer early in pregnancy is a nursing responsibility.

Critical Thinking Exercises

1. Beverly Muzuki is the woman you met at the beginning of the chapter who was in preterm labor at 30 weeks of pregnancy. Beverly discounted the symptoms she was having because she didn't think they could be early labor. What are the signs of early labor that you would have liked her to have been more aware of?

2. Suppose Beverly is bleeding because of placenta previa; everyone else on the unit is at lunch, and you are alone. You know you should not do a pelvic examination with a placenta previa. How would you estimate the amount of blood she has lost? How would you determine that blood loss was not affecting the fetus?

3. Suppose Beverly is placed on bed rest at home after preterm rupture of membranes at 30 weeks of pregnancy. What assessments would you want to do to ensure she is not developing chorioamnionitis? Suppose she tells you she is too busy to stay on bed rest. What suggestions would you give her so she could best achieve bed rest? Does she have an ethical obligation to her fetus to rest? What about a legal obligation?

4. Examine the National Health Goals related to complications of pregnancy. Most government-sponsored money for nursing research is allotted based on these goals. What would be a possible research topic to explore pertinent to these goals that would be applicable to the Muzuki family and also advance evidence-based practice?

PIH _____   GDM _____   IDDM _____   Eclampsia _____

No. of children living with her, and their ages: _____

_____

Any children in foster care, or living elsewhere: _____

_____

_____

II. Current State of Health:
   1. Physical
   2. Mental
   3. Emotional
   4. Social
   5. Hospitalizations/Surgeries
   6. Diet/Nutrition/weight prior to pregnancy; weight gain so far
   7. Activity
   8. Physical limitations
   9. Support systems
  10. Limitations
  11. Medications—Time, Frequency, Amount, Purpose, Side effects

  12. Teaching Needed

    __ Transportation   __ Self-treatment

    __ Changes during pregnancy

    __ Nutrition   __ Home Safety   __ Community Resources

                                __ utilities

                                __ phone

                                __ housing

                                __ cooking

                                __ water

                                __ respite

                                __ ref.

                                __ others

   __ Growth/Dev.

   __ Parenting Education

   __ Budgeting of financial resources

   __ Parenting skills   __ Parenting education

   __ Gestational diabetes   __ Premature labor

   __ Rupture of membranes   __ Signs/Symptoms of Labor

  13. Referrals already made: _____

  14. Referrals needed: _____

    __ WIC   __ Wheels

FIGURE 16.1 (continued)

IV. Family Data/Support Network:
1. Other household members (name, age, medical issues)
2. Other significant others/extended family members
   Are they available to assist with care of child—when delivered?
3. Summary of household function—Do people work together?
   Do they get along? Who is in charge?
4. Evidence of drug/ETOH use
5. Smoker

Housing Information
1. Current residence __ Permanent __ Temporary

2. Type of residence __ House __ Apt. __ Shelter __ Other explain _____

3. Length of time in current residence _____

4. Are there Plans to Move? __ Yes __ No __ When? _____

   New Address: _____

5. Layout of House:

   no. of bedrooms _____ no. of bathrooms _____

   __ Kitchen __ Dining area __ Living area __ Furniture

   Condition of House: _____

   Safety Issues at House:

   Outlets: __ 2 Prong __ 3 Prong __ Adeq. nos.
   __ Inadeq. nos.

   Smoke alarms: __ Yes __ No no. of alarms: _____

   Stable railings: __ Yes __ No

   Adequate lighting: __ Yes __ No (specify)

   Emergency nos. Posted: __ Yes __ No

   Sanitation: no. of Bathrooms: __

   A. Is kitchen sanitary? __ Yes __ No (specify)

   B. Pest Control: Are the following present:

      __ Roaches __ Rats/Mice __ Flies

   C. Plumbing problems _____

      Medication storage: Specify plan for storage, if refrigeration needed

      Infection control needs surrounding care:

      Summary of client home needs assessment

      _____

      Problem list—Preliminary

      _____

      Plan

FIGURE 16.1 (continued)

with their families. Because home care provides only intermittent visits, however, there is the possible disadvantage of not being constantly supervised by health care personnel. Reassure the woman and her family after assessment that her condition has not changed and it is safe for her to remain at home on the present program. If changes have occurred, introduce new interventions and evaluate their effectiveness.

Low birthweight occurs in newborns when preterm labor cannot be halted. Nurses can be instrumental in seeing that women who are candidates for home care receive enough orientation and support that they are able to remain on home care and possibly prevent low birthweight. They can be instrumental in seeing that time spent during home care is not wasted time for a woman, but a time of preparation for birth and childrearing.

Interventions performed for the pregnant client at home are little different from those performed in an acute care facility. They can range from teaching and counseling to hands-on care. The only difference is that they are done in the client's home. This means home care nurses need to have the same background and level of expertise as acute care nurses. In addition, they may need to be more flexible and adaptable because each home visit may be very different from the one just before or after.

● *Outcome Evaluation*

Outcome evaluation for the pregnant woman receiving home care includes determining whether a woman and fetus are remaining well at home and whether a woman feels comfortable and secure with the arrangement. For many women, successful home care can mean the difference between too early a birth and a successful term pregnancy.

Examples of outcome criteria include:

• Client demonstrates adequate skill at performing home monitoring procedures.
• Client verbalizes changes in condition she will need to report to her health care provider.
• Client participates as a member of the family within limitations imposed by pregnancy complication.
• Family members state they have adjusted to home care of mother.
• Client states she is able to maintain contact with friends and family despite complete bed rest at home.

HOME CARE

Discharge planners in acute care settings can be instrumental in setting the stage for home care by discussing the need for continued health supervision with women and helping them to begin establishing personal goals for home care. A number of steps are then necessary for the actual home visit to be successful (Box 16.2). These steps can be divided into previsit, visit, and postvisit phases.

BOX 16.2 FOCUS ON . . .

DIVERSITY OF CARE

Because the structure of families is culturally determined, home care of a woman during pregnancy will be easier for some than for others. If the family is extended, for example, a woman may be so involved in the care of other family members, such as an older adult, that she is unable to rest adequately at home. On the other hand, in such a family, there may be many people to offer care and support, so rest at home is ideal.

In some cultures, males are very dominant, so the thought of the man giving care to his wife contradicts a usual pattern. If a woman is the dominant member of the household, becoming a passive, cared-for partner may be extremely difficult for her.

Some cultures stress that women must be active during pregnancy to help ensure a small baby and therefore an easier birth. The culture of a particular community might oppose the use of technology, so a woman living there might not like having to use home monitoring equipment. Assess each family individually to determine how home care may affect that particular family.

Preparing for a Home Visit

Typically, a first home visit is made within 24 hours of discharge from an acute care facility or after notice from the ambulatory care facility. Be certain to obtain a copy of the client's referral form to familiarize yourself with her treatment course and her plan of care. Obtain any supplies that may be needed for the visit. Keep in mind that you are going to be a guest in the client's home, so respect for the client's and family's privacy, beliefs, lifestyles, routines, culture, and requests is crucial. As a part of this, it is best to telephone a client in advance to arrange a time for a visit so it will be convenient for her and her family. Obtain necessary instructions to reach the home. To avoid disrupting family routines, try not to visit at mealtime unless observing what a woman is eating for a typical meal is necessary for assessment. Be alert to possible environmental, social, and cultural factors identified on the referral form that may require nursing creativity. Keep in mind that the ethical and legal aspects of nursing care, such as confidentiality, informed consent, decision making, and client rights, commonly associated with acute care nursing are also applicable to home care. Remember this when transporting a chart or notes or when discussing the visit with others.

Ensuring Personal Safety

Because home care nurses work alone, they should take measures to ensure their personal safety on the way to a client's home, during a visit, and afterward. Safety tips for traveling in an unfamiliar community are shown in Box 16.3.

> ### Checkpoint Question 1
>
> You need to schedule a first home visit for Lee Puente. When is a first home-care visit typically made?
>
> a. Within 1 hour after discharge
> b. Within 24 hours after discharge
> c. Within 4 days after discharge
> d. Within 1 week of discharge

Making the Visit

Depending on the location of a client's home, the facilities and resources available may vary. The setting may be a house, apartment, mobile home, or shelter. On arrival at the client's home, knock or ring the bell and wait for someone to let you in. Greet the client and any other family members present. Greet family pets if they come to greet you (but don't pet strange dogs). Dogs typically serve a guard function, and you want them to view you as a friendly, not a threatening, visitor. Sometimes special advance arrangements, such as having a neighbor let you in, may be necessary if the client is alone and cannot walk down a stairway or a long hallway to answer the door.

As in any health care setting, wash your hands before touching a client for assessment, and follow standard precautions while caring for a client. Ask permission to use the kitchen or bathroom sink to wash. Many home care nurses carry liquid soap and paper towels or disposable wipes

---

> **BOX 16.3**
>
> #### Safety Tips for Home Health Care Travel
>
> - Plan your trip in advance using a reliable map of the area.
> - Let someone know where you are going and when you expect to return.
> - Keep your automobile in good repair and filled with gasoline so you can avoid having to make stops at unfamiliar service stations.
> - Lock any valuables in the trunk of your car *before* you leave the health care agency, not after you park in front of a home to visit.
> - Learn the location of public phones in the area, or keep a cellular phone with you.
> - If you suspect that someone is following you in your car, drive to the nearest police or fire station.
> - If you suspect that someone is following you while you are walking, walk into a business establishment.
> - Carry only minimal supplies so your hands are free and your appearance does not suggest that you carry drugs or valuables.
> - Drive or walk on main or busy streets; avoid shortcuts through alleys or unoccupied areas.
> - Walk determinedly, as if you have a purpose and are in charge of your environment and situation.

---

with them for handwashing if the client's facilities are inconvenient or unavailable.

What if... Lee Puente lives in a shelter for abused women? How would you anticipate your visit would differ from visiting her at home?

Assessing the Client

Typically, on a first visit, a thorough health assessment is necessary, including a review of systems and evaluation of the social environment, medications, nutrition, safety, and adherence to treatment this far. In addition, a consent for treatment and release of information form may need to be signed by the client (Fig. 16.2).

Provide privacy and confidentiality when obtaining the health history and performing a physical examination in the home. Some homes may be too cool early in the morning for physical assessment because the heat has been turned down during the night. Arranging for a visit later in the day may alleviate this problem. If a home has few rooms, finding a private location can be difficult. Include assessment not only of physical aspects but of mental or psychosocial ones as well. Women receiving home care are usually anxious to have a nurse confirm that they are well and that the self-assessments they have been making have been accurate.

If a woman is on bed rest, ask how she occupies her time. A woman is not really resting if she is concerned about her family or finances, is caring for older children, or is bored. Evaluate her carefully for depression (Jesse & Graham, 2005). Also evaluate her understanding of her condition and make sure she knows the danger signs to report immediately. Be certain that a woman has a means of obtaining refills on prescriptions and knows what measures to take if her condition should worsen, such as telephoning 911, a hospital, or her primary care provider. Be certain that she knows the importance of keeping health care appointments and has transportation to them. At all times, despite the informality of the setting, good interviewing and physical assessment skills are important (Box 16.4). Throughout the assessment, evaluate the client's needs and provide instructions and reinforcement about any specific areas that are necessary.

Assessing the Environment

During a visit, observe whether the house is safe for home care. This means adequate water, electricity, heat, and refrigeration. Are there smoke detectors in the home? Are they in working order? Are there drafts or broken windows? Are there rodents or insects in the house that will make the environment unsafe for a new baby? Is the room that will be the new baby's free of lead-based paint?

If a woman is on bed rest, do the arrangements seem adequate or is it likely that she will be getting up every few minutes to care for small children or answer the telephone? Evaluate how far the bathroom is from a woman's bed. A bedside commode may be necessary to avoid a long walk. Check that there is a telephone nearby the

Client Name: _____

Address: _____

City: _____ State: _____ Zip: _____ Phone: ( )_____

Insurance Company:_____ Insurance I.D.#

I, the _____ (of the patient), intending to be legally bound, hereby:

1. Consent to such care and treatment by _____, and its employees and agents (collectively, the "Agency"), as prescribed by the client's physician or dictated by the client's condition.

2. Authorize the Agency to release any medical records in its possession concerning the client as may be required by law or to pay benefits on the client's behalf. I authorize the client's physicians, insurors, and hospitals to release such medical records to the Agency at the Agency's request.

3. Authorize my insuror to disclose to the Agency the terms and extent of my coverage, and the amount of payments made to me for services provided by the Agency.

4. Assign, transfer and set over to the Agency all of my or the client's rights to insurance proceeds or other funds to which I am or the patient is or will become entitled as a result of the services rendered by the Agency.

5. Consent to and authorize payment, which would otherwise be payable to me or the client, to be made directly to the Agency. The Agency may issue a receipt for such payment which shall discharge the insurance company of its obligations under the policy to the extent of such payment.

6. Agree that I remain individually responsible to pay the Agency for all charges not paid for any reason by the insurer or other third-party payor. I understand that payment in full is due upon receipt of my bill. If payment for the Agency's service is made directly to me by my insuror, I agree to endorse the check to _____ and forward it to the Agency within three days of receipt.

A photocopy of this document, if executed, shall be considered as effective and valid as the original.

The effect of this form and the Client's Rights and Responsibilities on the back of this form have been explained to me by the Agency and I understand its content and significance.

Date: _____ Signature: _____

Name: _____

(Please Print)

FIGURE 16.2 A form for consent for treatment, release of information, assignment of benefits, and notice of client rights.

BOX 16.4 FOCUS ON . . .

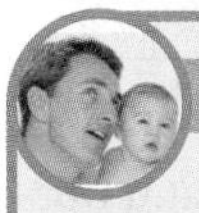

COMMUNICATION

Lee Puente is receiving home care because of preterm labor and hyperemesis of pregnancy. She lost 15 pounds at the beginning of pregnancy but now, at 20 weeks, has gained back the lost pounds, plus 2 extra, since beginning supplemental enteral feedings every day. A home health aide visits her three times a week to supervise her nutrition. She always seems pleased to be visited by a home care nurse once a week.

Less Effective Communication

Nurse: Hello, Lee. Is everything going all right?
Lee: Good.
Nurse: Are you eating everything you're supposed to?
Lee: Sure.
Nurse: Not throwing up any more, are you?
Lee: No.
Nurse: Good. I'm glad you're doing so well.

More Effective Communication

Nurse: Hello, Lee. How is everything?
Lee: All right.
Nurse: What did you eat for breakfast?
Lee: A slice of toast.
Nurse: What happened afterward?
Lee: I threw it up. I do that about once—maybe twice—a day.
Nurse: I need to do a more thorough assessment.

Because home settings are more informal than those of health care agencies, it is easy to forget that a home is a health care setting and to let a relationship become more relaxed than therapeutic. In the first scenario, the nurse lapsed into using leading questions rather than structured ones for a health interview. Lee responded to the leading questions by supplying answers she thought the nurse wanted to hear, not necessarily the true answers.

client so she has a means of calling someone, both to prevent loneliness and to secure emergency help. If a woman needs assistance with personal hygiene, evaluate the need for a referral for a home health aide to help her.

Effective home care requires a team of health care providers, including the supervising physician, home care nurses, health equipment suppliers, home care aides, and participating, informed clients. Home health aides are an invaluable help in providing home health care because they can supply the bulk of personal care services, such as assisting with or providing hygiene, assisting with ambulation, and providing adequate nutrition. Home health aides have varied levels of education depending on the home health care or community health care agency policies and the level of care they are being asked to provide. Assigning unlicensed assistive personnel to make home visits in place of nurses is cost-effective but the outcomes may not be as effective.

When working with unlicensed assistive personnel:

- Be sure you are familiar with their level of ability and education so you do not assign a task to them that is above their ability or one that prevents them from using their full potential.
- When making assignments, be certain they understand that making an assessment (e.g., recording a blood pressure) is not the same as evaluating the meaning of the assessment. That requires professional expertise.
- When they are in a client's house, remind them that they are a guest in the house and need to respect the values and patterns of that household.
- When a client no longer needs home care and the time comes to terminate the relationship, know that they may need your help with ending the relationship and saying good-bye because, often, their services have been of such a personal nature.

Before leaving the home, set the date and time of the next visit and review any signs and symptoms that a woman should report immediately to the agency or health care provider rather than waiting for the next visit. Be sure she has the home care agency's and health care provider's phone numbers. Many clients feel more comfortable calling the home care agency rather than the primary care provider's office if the agency has nurses on call around the clock. The nurse on call can then help the client determine what action would be best to take.

What if... when you're visiting Lee Puente, you discover large mouse holes in the bedroom that will be used by her new baby? What would you do?

Maintaining Personal Safety

Evaluation as to whether a home is a safe place to visit needs to be ongoing during a visit. Safety tips to keep in mind during home care visits are shown in Box 16.5.

Postvisit Planning

Postvisit planning consists of documenting all information gained from the visit in relation to the client's condition,

---

BOX 16.5

Safety Tips During Home Care Visits

- Do not carry a purse or backpack that suggests you are carrying a large sum of money or other valuables.
- Park your car in a well-lighted, busy area. Lock the car door.
- Do not leave valuable objects such as an expensive CD player in your car, so it is not a target for car thieves.
- Avoid approaching homes by a dark back alley; use the front door or a busy hallway.
- Use special caution in stairwells and elevators. Leave a stairwell or elevator if a potentially threatening person enters, with an excuse such as, "I've forgotten my red pen."
- When you first enter the home, assess it for personal safety. Ask who is at home. If there are animals in the house, ask if they are friendly.
- If there are animals, take precautions to avoid getting flea bites (sit on a kitchen chair, not an upholstered chair).
- Be cautious about accepting food or drink if you are not certain about the hygiene of the dishes or food. Decline it gracefully with an excuse such as, "I'm trying to cut down on the amount of coffee I drink," or "It's against my agency's rules."
- Leave a home immediately if you feel threatened or unsafe.
- Have your car keys in your hand when you leave the house so you can unlock and enter your car rapidly.
- Look under your car when approaching it and in the back seat of your car before entering it to be certain no one is there. Relock your car door immediately once inside.
- If both you and the client are in personal danger, call the community emergency number, such as 911, for help.

---

completing agency forms so billing for supplies and nursing time can be accurate, and evaluating the client's current status and future needs. It may include communicating a change in status to the primary health care provider, asking for a renewal of orders, or updating and revising the plan of care. Accurate documentation is essential. Although the forms may vary, the rules for documentation in home care are the same as for any health care facility.

Follow-Up Visits

Subsequent home visits are planned depending on a woman's circumstances and the amount of health education and supervision needed. A second visit could be scheduled as often as the next day or as infrequently as once a month. Frequent assessments accomplished at subsequent visits include vital signs, FHR, nutrition assessment, assessment of the possibility of beginning labor, and nursing care actions such as health education or medication adherence.

Checkpoint Question 2

What should you do if, in the middle of visiting Lee Puente at home, her former boyfriend arrives and threatens you and Lee? What would you do?

a. Tell him threatening someone is not mature behavior and he should stop.
b. Suggest that Lee change all of her home locks so this man can't visit again.
c. Leave the home and notify your agency that you were in unsafe circumstances.
d. Telephone 911 and report that you and a client are being threatened.

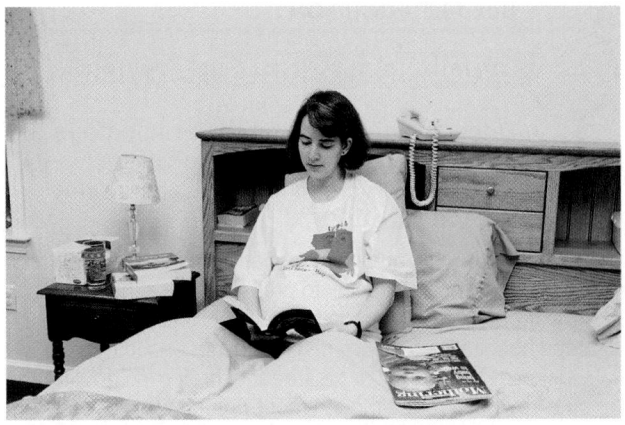

FIGURE 16.3 Bedrest can be stressful. Helping a woman who is on bedrest identify enjoyable and productive activities to pass the time can help ease stress.

NURSING RESPONSIBILITIES FOR HOME CARE

Nursing responsibilities for women receiving home care during pregnancy vary because the reason for home care during pregnancy also varies. Typical actions or interventions carried out in homes are discussed below.

Promoting a Therapeutic Environment

Home care is most successful if there are effective support people to help the client. Otherwise, a woman can experience loneliness and low self-esteem that may interfere with her ability to remain on continuous bed rest long enough to sustain a pregnancy.

Women on bed rest during pregnancy can react in a number of ways, but many report feeling "tied down," "like a prisoner," and "like I'm missing out." One way women can cope with the stress of the experience is by keeping busy or using their time to learn a new skill. Most women can identify activities for stimulation by themselves. A few may need a stimulation program to prevent them from passing the time simply by watching television or napping. For example, if a woman likes to read but doesn't always have the time to do so, bed rest at home may provide an ideal time for her to catch up on her reading (Fig. 16.3). If she has other children, she can spend part of her time reading to them. She could also use the time to take a home-study course, learn a new hobby, write a short story, or study for a certifying examination related to her work. In any event, helping her plan meaningful activities such as these can help her view home care not as wasted time, but as time invested in her family or career (Box 16.6).

Promoting Healthy Family Functioning

Many women fulfill multiple roles in their family, such as financial manager, peacemaker, problem solver, nurturer, and decision maker. Even when a woman is on bed rest, help her to continue in these roles to ensure the family's usual functioning, because support people often have great

BOX 16.6 FOCUS ON . . .

FAMILY TEACHING

Suggestions for Best Use of Time While on Bed Rest

Q. Lee Puente tells you, "I feel like I'm wasting my time just being home this way. What can I do to keep busy?"

A. Try these suggestions:

- Renew an old hobby or begin a new one.
- Ask someone to bring you books on newborn care from the library so you can pass the time reading.
- Telephone your friends. Rest next to a telephone so friends know they won't be disturbing you when they return calls.
- Catch up on your correspondence. Friends and family will be surprised and delighted to hear from you.
- Investigate whether there is a local community project (e.g., telephoning for a political campaign, urging neighbors to write letters of support for a new playground) you could work on while on bed rest.
- If you worked outside your home prior to bed rest, ask your employer if there is a project you could work on from home while on bed rest.
- If you have Internet access, spend time online looking for information about pregnancy, childbirth, or childrearing or just chatting with friends or others (if you have a dial-up connection, be conscious of the telephone bill that might result).
- Learn a second language; many books are available on this.
- Take a mail-order course on something you want to learn more about (e.g., creative writing; learning to be a paralegal).
- Ask your home care nurse about preparation-for-childbirth information. By conscientiously practicing breathing exercises while on bed rest, you can become well prepared for labor and birth.

Box 16.7 FOCUS ON . . .

EVIDENCE-BASED PRACTICE

Does allowing women to participate in decision making during a high-risk pregnancy make a difference in their satisfaction with prenatal care?

To answer this question, researchers interviewed 47 women who had received prenatal care at home from a nurse in a community health program or had been hospitalized. All women had experienced hypertension of pregnancy or the threat of preterm birth. Results revealed that although most women want to be actively involved in health care decision making, during a high-risk pregnancy some prefer a more passive role. The researchers concluded that the setting of prenatal care—community-based or in-hospital—was less important than the ability of nurses and physicians to support a woman in her preferred role in decision making.

This is an important study for nurses because it documents that women approach crisis situations with different expectations of how much decision making they should be asked to do. Helping to match the degree of decision making a woman wants to do with the degree of decision making asked of her by health care personnel is a nursing role.

Harrison, M. J., et al. (2003). Women's satisfaction with their involvement in health care decisions during a high-risk pregnancy. *Birth, 30*(2), 109–115.

difficulty assuming these roles in her place (Box 16.7). As a rule, support people can be supportive only if they understand the need for the home care program and the importance of their role. Arranging for a homemaker service to care for children or an aging parent or to help with light housework may be necessary to prevent support people from feeling stretched so thin they cannot function. Often support people are not present at the time of a home visit because they work during the day. Ask a woman at home visits how her support people are coping and if there are ways this experience could be made easier for them as well as for her. Ability to make decisions about her own care can make a significant difference in whether a woman thinks her home care experience is satisfactory or not (Harrison, 2003).

Health Teaching

A home care visit can provide many more opportunities for one-on-one health teaching than a health care agency setting. An important aspect of teaching may be providing childbirth education, because a woman on bed rest will not be able to attend formal classes.

Medicine Administration

Many pregnant women receiving home care need to take some type of medicine, such as a tocolytic to halt preterm labor or an antibiotic to prevent a uterine infection, in ad-

dition to the usual prenatal vitamin supplements. They may be taking an antihypertensive for hypertension of pregnancy (Moldenhauer & Sibai, 2003).

Review the rules of safe medication administration to minimize mistakes such as taking the medicine more frequently than prescribed or forgetting to take it. (Common safeguards for home administration of medicine are shown in Chapter 37.) If a woman does not have a support person who will remind her to take medicine, help her make out a written schedule or calendar for administration so she can remind herself. Encourage a woman to use this schedule as a practical tool, crossing off each time she has taken the medication. It helps to eliminate confusion and allows a home care nurse to evaluate whether medication is being taken.

Providing for Adequate Nutrition and Hydration

A woman who is on home care often needs help maintaining adequate nutrition. She may be the person who plans menus, shops for food, and cooks for the family. With her on bed rest, other family members must assume these roles; otherwise, the entire family, including the pregnant woman, will not eat enough healthy foods. Instruct family members about healthy nutrition practices. Assist with meal planning and suggestions for healthy snacks.

All women during pregnancy should drink six to eight full glasses of fluid a day to obtain adequate fluid for effective kidney function and placental exchange (Katz, 2003). Be certain women on bed rest have a supply of fluid close to their bed so they can do this easily.

Intravenous Administration

Pregnant women may be receiving intravenous therapy as a means of medication administration or, especially for women with hyperemesis gravidarum, as a means of hydration (Koren & Maltepe, 2004). Women with sickle cell anemia may receive blood transfusions in the home.

Intravenous medication and fluid administration is accomplished using either a peripheral or central insertion site. Because peripheral intravenous lines frequently become dislodged, in the home setting intravenous fluid is often administered by a central line or a peripherally inserted catheter threaded to a central blood vessel (a PICC line). Specially pressurized fluid containers allow for fast and easy administration of special solutions. To help women infuse large amounts of fluid slowly and accurately, an intravenous infusion pump is strongly recommended. Women can receive antibiotics through "piggyback" infusions they keep frozen until the time of administration. Be certain a woman knows how to monitor intravenous insertion sites for inflammation and infiltration, how to protect the site from becoming infected (e.g., cover it with plastic rather than letting it get wet), and how to monitor the amount and kind of fluid or medication infused.

Home Enteral Nutrition

Women who have hyperemesis gravidarum may also receive nutrition by a nasogastric tube. The supplies necessary for enteral feedings, such as feeding tubes and enteral pumps, are available for rent or purchase through pharmacies or medical supply houses or the home care agency. Such tubes are usually changed every 2 to 4 weeks. The home care nurse will most likely be the person responsible for changing the tube, but this depends on the home care agency's policies. In addition to assessing the client, be sure a woman is familiar with all aspects of care for the tube, equipment, and administration of the feeding. Encourage a woman to monitor the supply of formula for the feedings so it doesn't run out, especially over weekends. She probably will need to weigh herself daily and record the weight. Be certain she knows when to call for advice if she is having difficulty or is unsure if her weight is remaining adequate.

Total Parenteral Nutrition

Total parenteral nutrition (TPN) may be used to supply complete nutrition and fluid to women with hyperemesis gravidarum on home care. Usually the home care agency or a separate private vendor will furnish and deliver the formula, tubing, clean dressings, and an infusion pump. The formula, which consists of amino acids, hypertonic glucose, vitamins, and minerals in solution, should be stored in the client's refrigerator until 1 to 2 hours before use; it is then removed from the refrigerator and allowed to warm to room temperature. Women requiring this type of intravenous nutritional therapy usually have a central venous access device such as a central venous catheter or PICC inserted. The catheter may be inserted before a woman is discharged from the acute care facility or as an outpatient procedure if a woman is already at home. The home care nurse plays a key role in teaching a woman about the therapy and also in assessing her response to therapy.

Throughout the therapy, the client needs instruction about monitoring the infusion of the solution and the patency of the tube. She needs to know the correct frequency of feedings (whether continuous or intermittent) and the interval at which she should have blood work scheduled. She also needs to be taught to change dressings, observe the insertion site, and assess her temperature for signs of possible infection. She must be aware of any restrictions she should adhere to (e.g., no baths if the water level will rise above the catheter insertion site). Because TPN solutions are hypertonic, instruct a woman how to obtain fingerstick blood glucose levels as necessary, usually every 6 hours. Encourage her to record these findings so they can be evaluated on the next visit. Be sure she knows what findings should be reported immediately.

Promoting Elimination

Promoting elimination in a woman receiving home care can call for advance planning. The site where a woman is going to rest is often determined by the location of a bathroom. If strict bed rest is required, a bedside commode may be necessary.

Constipation occurs at a high rate during pregnancy and may occur even more frequently in women on bed rest from lack of exercise. Encourage women to eat a diet high in fiber and to drink at least eight glasses of fluid daily in an attempt to minimize this problem.

Teaching Self-Monitoring of Vital Signs

Monitoring vital signs in the home does not differ from monitoring them in a health care agency. Mercury thermometers may be used in place of electronic thermometers. If a woman will be using a mercury/glass thermometer, caution her that mercury is a toxic contaminant if the thermometer breaks. Remind women that this type of thermometer takes a full 3 minutes to register rather than the more convenient few seconds needed by electronic thermometers. For consistency, a woman should take her blood pressure in the same position (lying down or sitting up) and on the same arm. Encourage her to keep a record of the readings so you can evaluate them on your next visit. Using an automated cuff simplifies taking blood pressure. Results obtained by self-monitoring are as predictive of hypertension of pregnancy as those taken by health care providers in a clinic setting (Box 16.8).

Teaching Self-Monitoring of Uterine Height, Contractions, and Fetal Heart Rate

Fundal height is measured by using a paper tape measure according to McDonald's rule (see Chapter 8). If a woman is asked to record serial fundal height measurements, demonstrate the correct technique and have her give a return demonstration, as this measurement varies greatly depending on where the tape measure is placed. Be sure the client is measuring the height in the same location each time. It may be necessary to mark the points with an indelible pen to ensure consistent and accurate measurements.

Many women conduct count-to-10 assessments daily (count the number of fetal movements they feel in a designated time period; see Chapter 8) to help assess fetal well-being (Spong, 2003). FHR is usually recorded at each home visit. In addition, a client may be taught how to obtain this herself. FHR can be recorded by listening with a Doppler, a fetoscope, a regular stethoscope (although FHR may be very difficult to hear), or an electronic monitoring device supplied as part of her home care program.

The client can self-monitor uterine contractions using a uterine monitor, the same as in a health care facility, or by palpation. Instruct her to measure the time from the beginning to the end of each contraction and determine the interval between contractions (from the beginning of one contraction to the beginning of the next). Advise her to count and time contractions for 30 to 60 minutes. As a general rule, tell her to call the home care agency or health care provider if contractions are 10 minutes apart or less, or if they last 30 seconds or more.

A rhythm strip or nonstress test can be conducted using a portable monitor approximately the size of a transistor radio. A woman straps this device to her abdomen, positioning the sensor approximately 2 to 3 fingerbreadths below the umbilicus or at the top of the fundus, for 20 to

BOX 16.8: Focus on Nursing Care Planning

A Multidisciplinary Care Map for A Pregnant Woman at Home on Bed Rest

●

Lee Puente, a 20-year-old woman who is 20 weeks pregnant, has been vomiting at least four times daily since the beginning of pregnancy. She was admitted to the hospital for 3 days at 14 weeks of her pregnancy and placed on a program of total parental nutrition. She managed well on this until last week, when her blood pressure rose to 160/90 and she was diagnosed with hypertension of pregnancy. Bed rest with fetal and uterine surveillance at home was added to her care. She tells you it's impossible for her to rest at home: she has two preschool children who constantly need her care and interrupt her rest. She has missed three doses of her hypotensive agent because she forgot to take them. She wants to be hospitalized instead for care.

Family Assessment

Client is primary wage earner in the family; works full time as a travel agent. Lives with husband and 2 children, 2 years and 4 years of age, in a two-story home. Client's bedroom is on second floor with bathroom located next to bedroom, approximately 20 feet from client's bed. She asks, "We just bought this house over a year ago. How are we going to make the mortgage payments?" Husband is full-time doctoral student receiving only a student stipend. He stays home until noon daily. Four-year-old child goes to half-day nursery school 3 days a week. Two-year-old home with mom, currently being potty trained.

Client Assessment

Vital signs: Temperature 98.4°F; pulse 76; respirations 22; blood pressure 144/94; FHR 148. Mild facial edema; +1 protein in urine; 2-pound weight gain in 1 week.

Nursing Diagnosis

Anxiety related to need for bed rest and interference with family and financial responsibilities secondary to hypertension of pregnancy

Outcome Criteria

Client identifies methods to participate in work and child care while maintaining bed rest; expresses increased satisfaction with imposed bed rest; maintains bed rest until fetal maturity. Blood pressure remains 140/90 or less; FHR within acceptable parameters; urine for protein remains +1 or less; weight gain limited to 1 lb/week; edema limited and without increase for the duration of her pregnancy.

Team Member Responsible	Assessment	Intervention	Rationale	Expected Outcome
Activities of Daily Living				
Nurse	Assess vital signs, including heart rate, BP, and FHR at every visit.	Instruct client how to take own vital signs and monitor FHR. Instruct how to do a "count-to-ten" assessment.	Assessment of vital signs, especially BP, FHR, and fetal activity, provides a baseline for future comparison and evidence of the client's and fetus's status.	Client demonstrates she is able to accurately obtain own pulse, BP, and FHR. Findings compare with nurse's weekly findings.

(continued)

Team Member Responsible	Assessment	Intervention	Rationale	Expected Outcome
Consultations				
Physician/ nurse	Investigate whether hospital's home care team services the area in which client lives.	Arrange for home care visiting by hospital home care team. Care aide: daily; RN 1X week.	Home visiting can function best when it is part of a "seamless" service.	Client agrees to services of hospital home care team.
Procedures/Medications				
Nurse	Assess random urine specimen for protein at each home visit. Assess what client interprets home bed rest to mean.	Instruct client to assess urine specimen daily and report any values above +1. Instruct client to weigh herself every day at the same time, wearing the same amount of clothing. Teach her how to measure and record intake and output. Review concept of complete bed rest. Arrange for a bedside commode if necessary.	Proteinuria +3 indicates severe edema. Weight and intake and output provide evidence of tissue fluid retention. Varying degrees of bed rest may be necessary to reduce symptoms of hypertension of pregnancy.	Client voices an understanding of need for bed rest and adheres to restrictions. Demonstrates ability to carry out procedures accurately.
Nutrition				
Nutritionist/ nurse	Obtain a 24-hour recall pattern to determine usual diet.	Encourage a diet high in protein and adequate fluid intake.	Protein may affect the degree of hypertension of pregnancy.	Client lists a 24-hour intake that is adequate for pregnancy.
Patient/Family Education				
Social worker/ nurse	Assess what client feels are her chief needs to allow her to remain on bed rest at home.	Assist client with planning effective child care; discuss possible sources of help from friends and family. Arrange for a home health care aide to assist with household management and child care.	Planning methods for child care and home management helps to alleviate stress. Personnel policies should allow for financial compensation during pregnancy.	Client demonstrates ways she has adapted to bed rest restrictions. Voices plan for child care and creative uses of her time.
		Have client check with employer about personnel policies regarding pregnancy problems. Review with client possible work activities she could continue at home.	Continuing some work from home may help to relieve financial stress.	Client describes her discussion with employer about pregnancy benefits and possible ways she could continue to contribute at work.
		Urge couple to arrange for telephone jack next to client's bed and a computer connection to continue work activities.	Helping establish a means of communication provides stimulation and the possibility of continuing work.	Client demonstrates how she will use telephone, computer, and fax machine to continue to communicate with work and friends.

(continued)

Team Member Responsible	Assessment	Intervention	Rationale	Expected Outcome
Psychosocial/Spiritual/Emotional Needs				
Nurse	Discuss with client areas of concern about finances, roles, home management, and child care.	Encourage the client to plan frequent periods of quiet time for herself. Suggest activities such as reading and listening to music.	Discussion provides baseline information to identify client's needs, beliefs, and responsibilities.	Client describes any areas of concern that could interfere with bed rest. Client lists at least three restful activities that she can use to occupy her day.
		Suggest that client allow for time each day to spend with children in quiet activities, such as reading to them or playing a game.	Planning quiet activities helps prevent the client from overdoing work-related activities and enhances the effectiveness of bed rest.	Client describes her plan for child care and activities she will use to encourage quiet activities with the children.
			Quiet activities with the children enhance family bonding and decrease feelings of isolation in the children while still allowing the client to maintain bed rest.	
Discharge Planning				
Nurse	Assess for readiness to participate in home monitoring.	Instruct client and family members in signs and symptoms of increased hypertension, such as increased edema, increased protein in urine, headache, dizziness, blurred vision, increased weight gain, or decreased urine output. Advise client to call the home care agency or primary health care provider if any occur.	Knowledge of danger signs and symptoms allows for early identification and prompt intervention to prevent threats to the mother and fetus.	Client lists signs and symptoms of elevated blood pressure and telephone number she will call if pressure is over 140/80.

30 minutes at a set time every day, or at any time she feels contractions or is concerned about the lack of fetal movement (Fig. 16.4). The monitor records both uterine contractions and FHR. At the conclusion of the monitoring period, the monitor is held next to a telephone and the tracing is transmitted to a central facility for evaluation. In this way, home monitoring can provide ready evaluation of contractions, possibly resulting in improved pregnancy outcomes and therefore decreasing the need for neonatal intensive care (Morrison & Chauhan, 2003).

Teaching Self-Monitoring by Serum or Urine Testing

Women who develop diabetes mellitus during pregnancy may be required to monitor their serum glucose levels using a test strip and glucometer at least once daily (typically, four times a day) (Reece & Homko, 2003). Many women are reluctant to learn this procedure because they don't like the thought of having to pierce the skin of a finger to draw

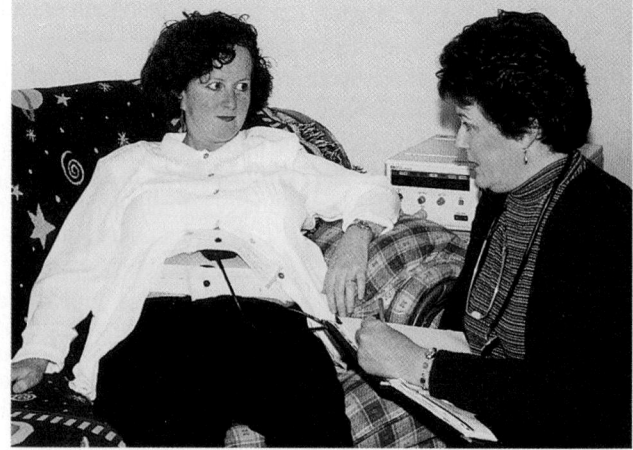

FIGURE 16.4 Fetal heart rate and uterine contractions can be recorded successfully by women at home. Photo by Melissa Olson, with permission of Healthy Home Coming, Inc., Bensalem, PA.

blood. Automated lancet devices and even skin sensors are available to help with this. Pregnant women can be taught to perform this procedure effectively and successfully in their homes.

Checkpoint Question 3

Lee Puente is developing constipation from being on bed rest. What measure would you suggest she take to help prevent this?

a. Drink more milk, as increased calcium intake prevents constipation.
b. Walk for at least half an hour daily to stimulate peristalsis.
c. Drink eight full glasses of a fluid such as water daily.
d. Eat more frequent small meals instead of three large ones daily.

Key Points

Home care can be more cost-effective than hospital care for women with a pregnancy complication or women considered at high risk for complications.

Home care, like hospital care, can be costly for people without health insurance. However, it has the advantage of preventing extensive disruption of a family.

Home care requires careful planning and a combined effort between a home care agency and a health care provider to ensure collaboration and continuity.

Frequent conditions for which women may require home care are preterm labor, hyperemesis gravidarum, diabetes mellitus, and hypertension of pregnancy.

Critical Thinking Exercises

1. Lee Puente is the woman you met at the beginning of the chapter. Was she a good candidate for home care? What additional interventions would she need to make home care more successful for her?
2. When you are visiting Lee in her home, do standard precautions to prevent the spread of infection apply? Explain your answer.
3. Lee Puente has two preschoolers. Her husband stays home from work until noon. An old school friend visits in the afternoon. Her mother comes over in the evening until Lee's husband gets home from work. What would be the best time of the day to schedule a home visit?
4. Examine the National Health Goals related to home care during pregnancy. Most government-sponsored money for nursing research is allotted based on these goals. What would be a possible research topic to explore pertinent to these goals that would be applica-

ble to the Puente family and also advance evidence-based practice?

References

Crowther, C. A. (2005). Hospitalization and bed rest for multiple pregnancy. *The Cochrane Library (Oxford) (2)* (CD000110).
Department of Health and Human Services. (2000). *Healthy people 2010.* Washington, DC: DHHS.
Fetrick, A., Christensen, M., & Mitchell, C. (2003). Does public health nurse home visitation make a difference in the health outcomes of pregnant clients and their offspring? *Public Health Nursing, 20*(3),184-189.
Harrison, M. J., et al. (2003). Women's satisfaction with their involvement in health care decisions during a high-risk pregnancy. *Birth, 30*(2), 109-115.
Jesse, D. E., & Graham, M. (2005). Are you often sad and depressed? Brief measures to identify women at risk for depression in pregnancy. *MCN: The American Journal of Maternal/Child Nursing, 30*(1), 40-45.
Katz, V. L. (2003). Prenatal care. In J. R. Scott et al. (Eds.), *Danforth's obstetrics and gynecology.* Philadelphia: Lippincott Williams & Wilkins.
Koniak-Griffin, D., et al. (2003). Nurse visitation for adolescent mothers: two-year infant health and maternal outcomes. *Nursing Research, 52*(2), 127-136.
Koren, G., & Maltepe, C. (2004). Pre-emptive therapy for severe nausea and vomiting of pregnancy and hyperemesis gravidarum. *Journal of Obstetrics & Gynaecology, 24*(5), 530-533.
Mackey, M. C., & Alexander, J. W. (2003). Program management of high-risk pregnancy: Outcomes and costs. *Disease Management & Health Outcomes, 11*(1), 1-6.
Moldenhauer, J. S., & Sibai, B. M. (2003). Hypertensive disorders of pregnancy. In J. R. Scott (Eds.), *Danforth's obstetrics and gynecology* (9th ed.). Philadelphia: Lippincott Williams & Wilkins.
Morrison, J. C., & Chauhan, S. P. (2003). Current status of home uterine activity monitoring. *Clinics in Perinatology, 30*(4), 757-801.
Reece, E. A., & Homko, C. J. (2003). Diabetes mellitus and pregnancy. In J. R. Scott et al. (Eds.), *Danforth's obstetrics and gynecology.* Philadelphia: Lippincott Williams & Wilkins.
Spong, C. Y. (2003). Fetal monitoring. In J. R. Scott et al. (Eds), *Danforth's obstetrics and gynecology* (9th ed.). Philadelphia: Lippincott Williams & Wilkins.

Suggested Readings

Brooten, D., et al. (2005). APN–physician collaboration in caring for women with high-risk pregnancies. *Journal of Nursing Scholarship, 37*(2), 178-184.
Humenick, S. S., & Howell, O. S. (2003). Perinatal experiences: the association of stress, childbearing, breastfeeding, and early mothering. *Journal of Perinatal Education, 12*(3), 16-41.
Lee, B. (2003). Caring for the emotions in pregnancy, birth and beyond. *RCM Midwives Journal, 6*(11), 472-475.
Logsdon, M. C., & Davis, D. W. (2003). Social & professional support for pregnant and parenting women. *MCN: The American Journal of Maternal/Child Nursing, 28*(6), 371-376.

Malcus, P. (2004). Antenatal fetal surveillance. *Current Opinion in Obstetrics & Gynecology, 16*(2), 123–128.

Olds, D.L., et al. (2004). Effects of home visits by paraprofessionals and by nurses: age 4 follow-up results of a randomized trial. *Pediatrics, 114* (6), 1560–1568.

Olsen, O. & Jewell, M.D. (2005). Home versus hospital birth. *The Cochrane Library (Oxford) (2)* (CD000352).

Pearce, L. (2005). Maternal instinct. *Nursing Standard, 19*(7), 18.

Persily, C. A. (2003). Lay home visiting may improve pregnancy outcomes. *Holistic Nursing Practice, 17*(5), 231–238.

Salvador, A., et al. (2003). Program evaluation of hospital-based antenatal home care for high-risk women. *Hospital Quarterly, 6*(3), 67–73.

Shilling, T. & DiFranco, J. (2004). Care practices that promote normal birth #2: freedom of movement throughout labor. *Journal of Perinatal Education, 13*(2), 11–15.

CHAPTER 17

High-Risk Pregnancy: A Woman With Special Needs

Key Terms

autonomic dysreflexia
emancipated minor
substance dependent

Objectives

After mastering the contents of this chapter, you should be able to:

1. Identify the characteristics of a pregnant woman who has special needs.
2. Describe the risks of pregnancy for a woman with special needs.
3. Assess a woman with special needs during pregnancy.
4. Formulate nursing diagnoses related to pregnancy for a woman with special needs.
5. Identify expected outcomes for a pregnant woman with special needs.
6. Plan nursing care to address the special growth and development needs of the adolescent and a woman over age 40, and the specific strengths and weaknesses of women who are physically or cognitively challenged or drug dependent during pregnancy.
7. Implement nursing care for a woman with special needs.
8. Evaluate outcomes to ensure that goals for care have been achieved.
9. Identify National Health Goals related to a woman with a special need that nurses can be instrumental in helping the nation achieve.
10. Identify areas related to care of a woman with special needs during pregnancy that would benefit from additional nursing research or application of evidence-based practice.
11. Use critical thinking to analyze ways that nursing care of the pregnant woman with a special need can be optimally family-centered.
12. Integrate knowledge of the risks of pregnancy with age extremes, drug use, and physical or cognitive challenges with the nursing process to achieve quality maternal and child health nursing care.

*M*indy Carson, a 16-year-old girl, is 15 weeks pregnant. The father of Mindy's baby is a college student. He doesn't want Mindy to keep her baby after the birth because he doesn't want to get married until he finishes graduate school. Mindy insists she is old enough to be a parent and wants to keep her baby. Mindy's mother accuses the father of sharing methamphetamines with Mindy. She's worried Mindy has been working as a prostitute to support her drug habit. They both turn to you and ask you what you would recommend.

Typically, many women seen in a prenatal care setting do not fit the description of the average pregnant woman—a well young adult who maintains healthy patterns of living. Previous chapters discussed high-risk pregnancies for women who are ill when they become pregnant and for those who develop an illness while pregnant. This chapter presents information to add to your knowledge base about high-risk pregnancy in women with other special needs—very young adolescents and women who have waited until midlife to have their first child; those who are physically or cognitively challenged and those who are drug dependent.

Is Mindy old enough to be a parent? What qualities would you look for in her to discover if she is ready to parent? What type of referral does Mindy need?

After you've studied this chapter, access the accompanying website. Read the patient scenario and answer the questions to further sharpen your skills, grow more familiar with RN-CLEX types of questions, and reward yourself with how much you have learned.

Pregnancy and childbirth are leading causes of death in adolescents in developing countries (Mayor, 2004). In the United States, the adolescent pregnancy rate has decreased slightly to about 41/1,000 teenagers (NCHS, 2005). In contrast, the birth rate for women over age 40 is steadily increasing; it is currently about 10/1,000 (NCHS, 2005). Adolescents require special consideration during pregnancy because they are physically and psychosocially immature. Women over age 40 may need special consideration also because they can have difficulty adjusting psychosocially to a first pregnancy and the family changes that are required.

The pregnancy rate also is increasing among women who are physically or cognitively challenged, including those with conditions such as cerebral palsy that might have precluded pregnancy a few years ago. Physical and cognitive conditions present a challenge to childbearing and childrearing but do not necessarily prevent women from establishing their own families. Supportive nursing care that considers the limitations imposed by a particular disability, while focusing on the normal aspects of childbearing and childrearing and a woman's strengths, is vital.

Women who are drug dependent are yet another category of high-risk women who require a great deal of nursing support and care. Ideally, a woman would give up substance abuse for the health of a fetus, but that may not be possible. When this doesn't happen, every effort must be made to provide enough prenatal care and attention to protect the fetus in other ways.

These women with special needs have become a focus of attention, as evidenced by the National Health Goals (Box 17.1). The Department of Health and Human Services (DHHS) has initiated a special program to help reduce teenage pregnancy (*www.girlpower.gov*).

Nursing Process Overview

For Care of a Pregnant Woman With Special Needs

● *Assessment*
Assessing the strengths and weaknesses of individual clients is always crucial to establishing accurate nursing diagnoses and realistic outcomes as well as planning effective nursing interventions. When a client has a special need, this part of the assessment becomes even more important. Establishing as thorough a database as possible early in pregnancy helps to predict the risks a woman may be exposed to when pregnancy is affected by age extremes, physical or cognitive challenges, or an unhealthy lifestyle.

When caring for a woman who is physically challenged, keep in mind that physical disabilities occur in degrees; therefore, first establish the impact of the disability on a woman's life before offering any guidance for care measures during pregnancy. The capacity of a woman with special needs to adapt to pregnancy depends both on her physical capabilities and on her ability to persevere against odds and overcome what the average woman might think of as insurmountable obstacles. Be certain to assess physical strengths as well

BOX 17.1 FOCUS ON . . .

NATIONAL HEALTH GOALS

A number of National Health Goals have been formulated to improve the health of women with special needs during pregnancy. These are:

- Reduce the pregnancy rate among adolescent females to no more than 43/1,000 adolescents, from a baseline of 68/1,000.
- Increase abstinence from alcohol, cigarettes, and illicit drugs among pregnant women to 100%, from baselines of 86% (alcohol), 99% (binge drinking), and 98% (illicit drugs) (DHHS, 2000).

Nurses can help the nation achieve these goals by teaching adolescents about the dangers of substance abuse and the complications, both psychological and physical, of teenage pregnancy. Nurses can add to this knowledge base by being active research investigators. Topics for possible investigation and areas of evidence-based practice may include the most effective way to impress adolescents about the dangers of substance abuse, and the ideal birth control measure for adolescents (ie., one that would actually be used). As more and more women over age 40 are becoming pregnant, the effects of pregnancy on this age group and their adjustment to it also must be investigated.

as limitations and psychosocial strengths as well as challenges. A woman with a spinal cord injury, for example, is likely to have developed ways of coping in daily life that may never occur to someone who has not experienced that disability.

For some drug-dependent women, pregnancy may be the impetus they need to break a drug habit. All that other women can accomplish is to reduce their drug use. In both instances, encourage a woman to keep coming for prenatal care. As long as she feels comfortable with you during regular visits, you may be able to establish a trusting relationship that could eventually provide her with the confidence to try a more healthful pattern of living.

● *Nursing Diagnosis*
Nursing diagnoses established for pregnant women with special needs differ in degree, but not in substance, from the nursing diagnoses established for all pregnant women. For example, if a pregnant adolescent is still growing, nutrition is an important issue for both her and her fetus. Examples of appropriate nursing diagnoses are:

- Risk for imbalanced nutrition related to combined needs of adolescence and pregnancy
- Risk for fetal injury related to drug and alcohol use
- Impaired physical mobility related to physical disability
- Risk for injury related to unstable balance
- Impaired verbal communication related to spastic muscle functioning

NURSING DIAGNOSES AND RELATED INTERVENTIONS

———●———

Nursing Diagnosis: Health-seeking behaviors related to special care necessary for healthy adolescent pregnancy

Outcome Evaluation: Client states she feels confident in her ability to take care of herself and avoid pregnancy complications, and asks questions about her pregnancy.

Prenatal Health Teaching. Adolescents need a great deal of health teaching during pregnancy because they do not know many common measures of care that an older woman has learned from experience. They are often unwilling to follow health care advice, however, that makes them different in any way from their peers. On the other hand, adolescents often do not have well-established health practices, so they are adaptable.

Adolescent girls may respond to health teaching that is directed to their own health more than to that of a fetus inside them: "Eat a high-protein diet because protein makes your hair shiny (or prevents split fingernails)" often leads to better adherence than a statement such as "Protein is good for your baby." "Taking the iron supplement should make you feel less tired" is better than "It will help build the baby's blood supply," for the same reason. These are truthful statements and they appeal to an adolescent's preoccupation with self. In addition, this type of health teaching is the only form to which an adolescent who is denying her pregnancy can respond.

Be certain to include information on the effects of drugs on fetal welfare, including over-the-counter medications, herbal preparations, and recreational drugs. Pregnancy can become an important growth experience if it provides the motivation some adolescents need to withdraw from recreational drug use.

Adolescents also need instructions about possible discomforts and changes associated with pregnancy, and measures to relieve them. (See Chapter 11 for a complete discussion.) Many adolescents develop hemorrhoids during pregnancy because the disproportion of their body size to a fetus puts extra pressure on pelvic vessels, causing blood to pool in rectal veins. Reassure girls that this is a pregnancy-related phenomenon that will resolve when the pregnancy is over.

Adolescents may also develop many striae across the sides of their abdomens because so much stretching of the abdominal skin occurs. Assure them again that, because of skin elasticity, these marks will probably fade after pregnancy. Chloasma, excess pigment deposition on the face and neck, appears at the same rate in adolescents as in older women. Adolescents, however, may be more conscious of this pigment because overall they are more conscious and concerned about their facial appearance. Suggesting a cover makeup and offering reassurance the pigmentation will fade after pregnancy may help.

Nutrition. Good nutrition is a major problem during adolescent pregnancy because many girls enter pregnancy with poor nutritional stores from years of eating a less-than-optimal diet. Lack of good nutrition can result in low-birthweight newborns and preterm births. The younger the girl is, the more likely she is to have a low-birthweight infant. To prevent these complications, the girl's diet must be sufficient to allow for the growth of a fetus and also provide for the needs of her own growing body. This means she may need to gain more weight than the mature woman does during pregnancy. Protein, iron, folic acid, and vitamin A and C deficiencies may become acute. Besides eating larger amounts of food, a pregnant adolescent should be sure to eat proper foods, possibly abandoning the food fads she has been following. Some girls are so peer-oriented they balk at substituting a glass of orange juice for a cola beverage because no one else they know drinks orange juice. The best you may be able to accomplish is to secure her agreement to switch to non-caffeinated soft drinks.

Many adolescent girls eat poorly during pregnancy because they simply do not know what constitutes a good diet. Some girls have little choice in what foods are prepared at home. To change a dietary pattern, you may have to talk to the person who does the cooking in the family.

Many adolescents eat at least one meal a week at a fast-food restaurant. Remember that if the girl is attending school, she eats at least one meal away from home each day. If she travels by school bus, she may have to leave by 6:00 or 7:00 in the morning, so she needs suggestions on how to construct a quick but healthy breakfast. If she leaves home this early, she will have a long wait until lunchtime. Suggest midmorning snacks, such as fruit, that are not just empty calories. Be certain nutrition education includes how to "brown-bag" or buy a nutritious cafeteria lunch (type A school lunches are discussed in Chapter 31).

> *What if...* Mindy Carson tells you her daily nutrition consists of a liquid diet beverage for breakfast and lunch and pizza for dinner? Will this typical teenage diet be adequate for her during pregnancy?

Adolescents traditionally do not take medicine conscientiously, so they may need frequent reminders that vitamin and iron supplements during pregnancy must not only be purchased but also must be taken. Be sure a girl posts a medication reminder chart at home or in her school locker to help increase adherence.

Activity and Rest. Adolescents vary greatly in their preferred level of activity. Assess a girl's participation in sports and determine which ones (if any) should be discontinued during pregnancy (diving, gymnastics, touch football). Many girls practice sports not for the enjoyment of the sport but for the feeling of "team" or companionship. You may need to suggest alternative activities (joining the drama or language club, inviting friends over once a week to watch a movie) so they don't suffer from the loss of companionship.

Adolescent girls may not plan enough rest time during pregnancy, especially if they are acting as if nothing is happening to them. It may help to explore a typical day and suggest ways to rest without compromising social relationships.

Pregnancy Information. A young girl may have distorted beliefs about her body. Despite all the health information given to children in school, it is not uncommon to find an adolescent who thinks her baby is growing in her stomach. Such a girl may be unwilling to eat large meals during pregnancy for fear of suffocating the fetus. All adolescent girls need substantial education on the physiologic changes that occur during pregnancy. In addition, specific information about labor and delivery is essential to counteract all the "scare stories" they may be hearing from their peers. Gaining knowledge is another way that pregnancy can be a growth experience. At the end of the pregnancy, this adolescent will know a great deal more about her body and her ability to monitor her health than her average classmate.

Childbirth Preparation. Adolescents have a strong need for peer companionship. When they become pregnant, they often are cut off from fellow adolescents. This makes them "ripe," therefore, to join a class of adolescents in preparation for childbirth. They are excellent students because being a student is age-appropriate for them. They have enough childish magical belief operating that they are not skeptical about whether prepared childbirth will work. In fact, believing that prepared childbirth will work is an important component in a successful prepared childbirth experience, so this becomes a self-fulfilling prophecy.

Birth Decisions. Pelvic measurements should be taken early and carefully in adolescent girls as cephalopelvic disproportion is a real possibility because of the girl's incomplete pelvic growth. Most girls who are told their baby will have to be born by cesarean birth respond well to the news, and many are relieved, because surgery seems controlled and simple compared with the agonies of labor they imagine. The decision on the method of birth should be shared with the girl and her parents when the health care team first reaches it. This is part of being honest with the girl. Adolescents, for the most part, want to know the truth. They tend to regard the withholding of information not as protection but as an indication they are being treated as children.

Plans for the Baby. Adolescents may need additional time at prenatal visits to talk to a good listener about how they feel about being pregnant and becoming a mother. Scared? Bewildered? Numb? Happy? Be certain they know all the options available to them: keeping the baby, or placing the baby in a temporary foster home or for adoption. Adolescents, like all women, should be encouraged to breast-feed (Sikorski et al., 2005). Breast tissue matures with pregnancy, so even the very young adolescent is physically capable of breast-feeding.

Complications of Adolescent Pregnancy

Adolescent pregnancy carries an increased incidence of pregnancy-induced hypertension, iron-deficiency anemia,

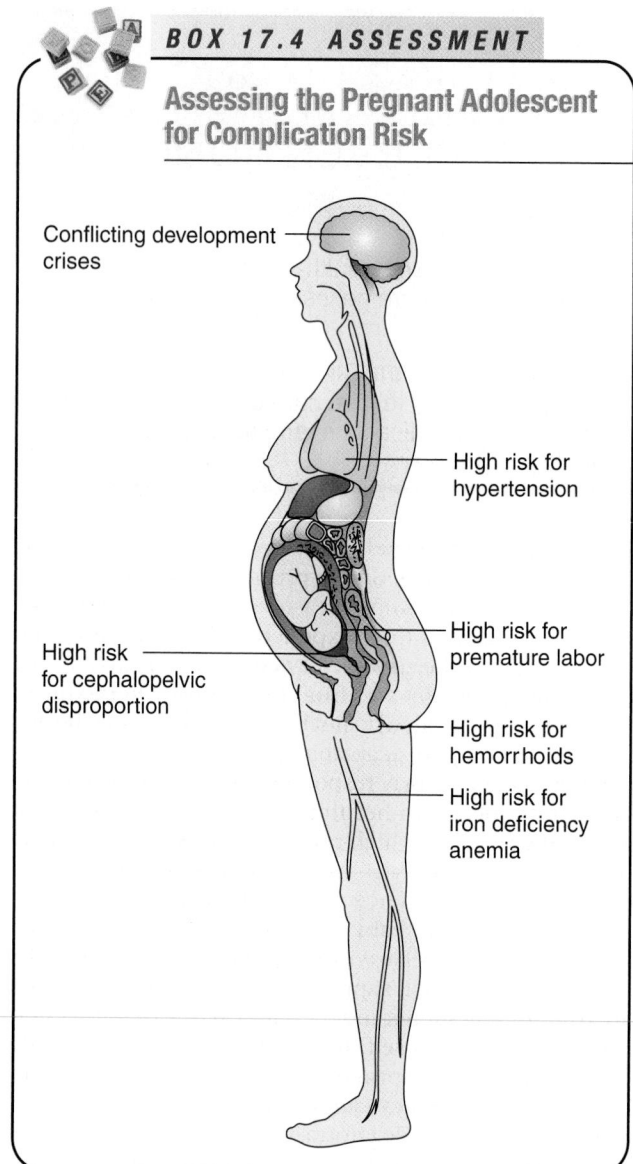

BOX 17.4 ASSESSMENT

Assessing the Pregnant Adolescent for Complication Risk

Conflicting development crises

High risk for hypertension

High risk for premature labor

High risk for hemorrhoids

High risk for iron deficiency anemia

High risk for cephalopelvic disproportion

preterm labor, and cephalopelvic disproportion (Box 17.4). Cephalopelvic disproportion leads to an increased incidence of cesarean birth. Fortunately, with conscientious prenatal care, these complications can be minimized.

Pregnancy-Induced Hypertension

Because adolescents are more prone to pregnancy-induced hypertension than the average woman (see Chapter 15), establishing a baseline blood pressure is important. This is particularly important if an adolescent has not had her blood pressure measured since a preschool or school-age checkup as long as 10 years earlier.

The best intervention for reducing an increasing blood pressure during pregnancy is bed rest, preferably in a side-lying position. Bed rest may be difficult for a teenager because she easily grows bored and being confined to bed limits her interactions with peers and school activities. Many girls on bed rest at home may rest better if they are lying on the living room couch, where they can be aware of household activity, rather than in an upstairs bedroom where they have to get up time and again to see what is happening. Also, it is easier for a parent to encourage bed rest if a girl is within eyesight. If called too many times to the distant bedroom for small tasks, a parent tends to say, "Get up and get it yourself this time."

Help to establish a specific routine of bed rest—does it mean being strictly confined to bed or sitting up part of the day in a lounge chair with legs elevated? Can she take a shower once a day? Use the bathroom? Knowing the exact rules from the beginning helps prevent misunderstandings and hurt feelings.

Girls on bed rest need activities to keep them busy. These can include homework or listening to music. If the end of the pregnancy is near, a girl may be able to have a friend bring her homework assignments. If the bed rest period will be longer than 2 weeks, however, she may need to make arrangements for home tutoring. You may need to advocate for her with the school system for this service (remembering that only rarely can it be denied on the basis of pregnancy). "Assignments" from the health care agency, such as reading about appropriate toys and games for infants, is also a way to occupy time. Frequent telephone calls from the health care facility show concern and offer an opportunity to enforce health teaching points. Be certain a girl does not interpret being placed on bed rest as being ill. This can cause her to reduce her nutritional intake or to curtail body hygiene.

Low-dose aspirin therapy may be prescribed to help reduce symptoms of hypertension of pregnancy. Keep in mind adolescents often are not reliable at taking daily medicine, particularly if it seems as unimportant as aspirin. Help a girl make a medicine reminder chart to promote adherence to this aspect of care.

If the hypertension continues after a period of bed rest at home (or if the symptoms of pregnancy-induced hypertension are acute when they are first discovered), a girl may be admitted to the hospital so bed rest can be better enforced. As soon as the fetus is mature, labor is induced.

Iron-Deficiency Anemia

Many adolescent girls are deficient in iron because their low protein intake cannot balance the amount of iron lost with menstrual flows. Deficiency is revealed by chronic fatigue, pale mucous membranes, and a hemoglobin level less than 11 g/dL. As if the girl's body has identified a mineral lack, iron-deficiency anemia is associated with pica, or the ingestion of inedible substances. Cravings for ice cubes or candy bars may develop because of this.

A pregnancy compounds iron-deficiency anemia because a girl must now supply enough iron for fetal growth and her increasing blood volume. All pregnant women should take an iron and folic acid supplement (folic acid is important for red blood cell growth and prevention of neural tube defects). This is especially important for the adolescent.

Help a girl plan a daily time for taking her iron supplement. Review with her how many iron-rich foods she needs to eat daily in addition to this. An iron supplement is not a supplement until her dietary intake is already strong in iron-rich foods.

As soon as the body has iron, it will begin forming immature red blood cells (reticulocytes) rapidly. A reticulocyte count may be obtained in 2 weeks to evaluate these levels and provide evidence that the iron supplement is being taken. If the reticulocyte count is not elevated by 2 weeks, it implies a girl did not take the supplement. Taking a stool swab and assessing it for the black tinge of an iron supplement or reassessing her serum iron level are other methods of assessing for adherence.

Preterm Labor

Adolescents are at high risk for preterm labor, probably because their uteruses are not fully grown. Review the signs of labor with them by the 3rd month of pregnancy. Stress that labor contractions begin as only a sweeping contraction no more intense than menstrual cramps. Also, any vaginal bleeding is suspicious of labor and should be reported. Adolescent girls have gained much of their knowledge of labor from television (where a woman suddenly announces she is in labor and within 15 minutes gives birth). Therefore, they may dismiss light contractions as simple discomfort, not realizing they might be the start of labor. Adolescents who recognize labor contractions early on can seek care to have premature labor halted.

Complications and Concerns of Labor, Birth, and the Postpartum Period
Cephalopelvic Disproportion

Because their own development is still immature, adolescents are prone to cephalopelvic disproportion. Cephalopelvic disproportion is suggested by lack of engagement at the beginning of labor, a prolonged first stage of labor, and poor fetal descent. Adolescent labor does not differ from labor in the older woman if cephalopelvic disproportion is absent. Graphing labor progress is a good way to detect labor that is becoming abnormal. Be certain the adolescent has a support person with her in labor so she can relax and breathe effectively with contractions. If this person is also an adolescent, you may need to serve as the true support person, or at least spend considerable time coaching so he or she can support the girl in labor.

Postpartum Hemorrhage

Young adolescents are more prone to postpartum hemorrhage than the average woman because if a girl's uterus is not yet fully developed, it becomes overdistended by pregnancy. An overdistended uterus does not contract as readily as a normally distended uterus in the postpartum period. Adolescents also may have more frequent or deeper perineal and cervical lacerations than older women because of the size of the infant in relation to their body. On the other hand, young adolescents are generally healthy and have supple body tissue that allows for adequate perineal stretching. If a laceration does occur, it usually heals readily without complication.

Inability to Adapt Postpartally

The immediate postpartum period may be an almost unreal time for an adolescent. Giving birth is such a stress and a major crisis that all women have difficulty integrating it into their life. It may be particularly difficult for the adolescent. The girl may "block out" the hours of labor as if they didn't happen. If she was particularly frightened by labor, she may have received a narcotic, so her memory of the labor hours may not be clear. Urge her to talk about labor and birth to make the happening real to her; otherwise, postpartum depression can occur.

Lack of Knowledge About Infant Care

Adolescents show the same positive bonding behavior with their infants as their more mature counterparts (Fig. 17.1). They may, however, lack knowledge of infant care. Although they may consider themselves to be knowledgeable in child care because they baby-sat for a neighbor's child or a younger sibling, they can be overwhelmed in the postpartum period to realize that when the baby is their own, child care is not as simple as it once seemed. When the child cries, they cannot hand it to someone else; at the end of 4 hours, when they are tired of caring for the baby, they cannot leave and walk away. Although these things were most likely discussed with an adolescent during pregnancy, these feelings may not arise until the child is actually born. Spend time with a girl observing how she handles her infant. Demonstrate bathing and changing the baby as appropriate. Model good parenting behaviors whenever possible by being aware of how you hold and care for the child.

Unfortunately, most adolescent mothers do not breastfeed. This is related to their perception of breast-feeding as something that will "tie me down" and the reality (in many instances) that they will be returning to school full-time soon after birth. Education about the importance of breast-feeding and tips for how to incorporate it into a busy lifestyle can increase the number of adolescents who breast-feed (see Chapter 25). Help young mothers who do not choose to breast-feed to find a feeding method that is satisfying to them and safe for the infant.

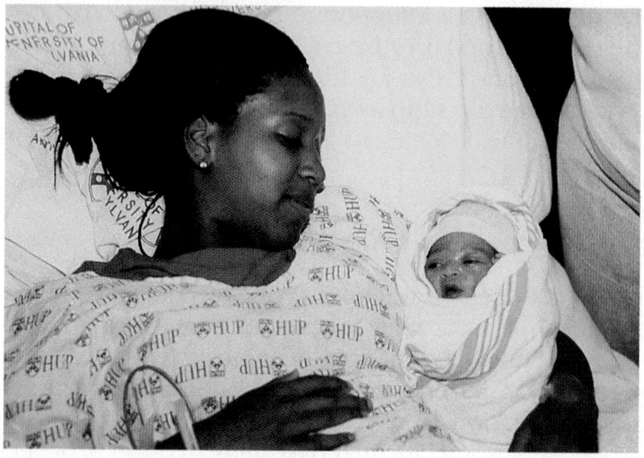

Checkpoint Question 2

Mindy Carson was placed on an iron supplement because her hemoglobin level was below normal. What is a usual test to demonstrate adherence to an iron supplement?

a. Assessing if her skin appears darker
b. Assessing her blood reticulocyte count
c. Analyzing her urine for iron deposits
d. Measuring if she has grown in height

THE PREGNANT WOMAN OVER AGE 40

The incidence of women delaying their first pregnancy until their late 30s or early 40s is increasing (Box 17.5). Eight percent of births in the United States today are to women over age 35; 3% to 4% are to women over age 40 (NCHS, 2005). In the past, it was assumed a woman of this age was past the optimal age for childbearing and was at risk for many complications. Today, with the exception of a greater incidence of chromosomal abnormality, there is little evidence of increasing complications in women older than age 35 as long as prenatal care is begun early in the pregnancy.

A woman over age 40 is more likely than a younger woman to have a previously diagnosed condition, such as hypertension, varicosities, or hemorrhoids. In addition, by age 40 a woman usually has a major role change to undertake during pregnancy, because she often is well established in a career or has an accustomed routine at home or in her community. She needs to think through how this

FIGURE 17.1 A new adolescent mother begins to bond with her infant. (Photo by John Gallagher, with permission of University of Pennsylvania Medical Center, Philadelphia, PA.)

BOX 17.5 FOCUS ON . . .

DIVERSITY OF CARE

What is perceived as the best time in life to have children is culturally influenced. In developing countries, many people believe having children young allows parents to grow with children. In other cultures, such as the United States, many believe delaying childbirth until a family is financially secure is best. What you believe, therefore, may not be the belief of a family for whom you provide care. What may be a catastrophe to you may seem like a blessing to someone else (and vice versa). Assess couples by history and observation to determine if childbearing appears to be timed correctly for them. If not, they may need extra time to accept a pregnancy and adapt to becoming parents.

pregnancy and childrearing are going to fit into and change her life. Although she may feel rich in the number of support people she perceives around her, she may discover she has few "pregnancy support" people because she does not have many friends her age who are also having babies—some may be close to becoming grandmothers. The only things these friends remember of pregnancy and labor are their particular highs and lows, and the care they received may not reflect current practice. This may leave a woman without access to the daily "shop talk" of other pregnant women, or someone to turn to with questions such as whether the backache she is experiencing or frequent need to urinate is normal. On the other hand, because many women delay childbearing today, she may be one of a sizable group of women in the community experiencing pregnancy at this stage of life.

Childbirth education classes oriented toward the older woman provide important information on pregnancy and can bring these women and their support people together. A woman over age 40, like any other pregnant woman, needs access to health care personnel who can supply her with factual information during a pregnancy. She also needs additional support while she works through this role change in her life.

Developmental Tasks and Pregnancy

The developmental challenge of the over-40 age group is to expand their awareness or develop generativity—that is, a sense of moving away from themselves and becoming involved with the world or community (Erikson, 1963). Some people assume that once they reach adulthood, the way they are is the way they will always be. They are amazed to find that their bodies change (e.g., men may lose their hair; women and men both gain weight) and so do their interests. They find themselves joining committees and clubs, coaching Little League teams, or organizing fundraising or community events.

A woman in this age group who is pregnant may begin to feel ambivalent during pregnancy, because she may want to continue with community activities, yet also wants to concentrate on the baby inside her. You may need to help her balance her life so she can manage crossing two life phases this way.

Many adults over the age of 40 are caring for aging parents. This additional responsibility may make it difficult for a woman to complete the psychological work of pregnancy. It also may create extra strain on her finances and time.

Prenatal Assessment

A woman over age 40, like all women, should begin prenatal care early in pregnancy. Fortunately, most women of this age group are well informed about the advisability of early prenatal care and have adequate health insurance, so they do seek an early appointment. A few mistakenly believe their lack of menstruation is the result of early menopause and do not seek an early health care consultation.

Health History

Ask women in this age group about their present symptoms of pregnancy, how they feel about the pregnancy, and how it fits into their lifestyle. If a woman did not realize she was pregnant, she may have self-medicated. Ask if she has been taking any medication or herbal remedies to relieve reported symptoms, such as nausea or fatigue. Because a woman is functioning well in a business world does not mean she has a healthy pregnancy lifestyle. Don't accept answers such as "I drink socially" or "I take the usual drugs" without exploring what those phrases mean specifically.

Family Profile. Some women over age 40 who are pregnant for the first time have recently changed their life pattern (married or became involved in a long-term sexual relationship) or have decided to have a child, perhaps through in vitro fertilization, without a spouse before they are no longer able to conceive. Whereas a younger woman often waits a while after marrying to become pregnant, a woman over age 40 often plans to become pregnant immediately after marriage because she senses her reproductive years are running out. Because of this, she may find herself making many adjustments at once (not only to a new life partner, house or apartment, and perhaps community, but also to a pregnancy).

Identify a woman's source of income. If she has a well-paying job, stopping work because of a pregnancy complication may reduce her family's income greatly. Also evaluate how many people are financially or emotionally dependent on her (such as children from a former marriage, elderly parents, an elderly neighbor, or fellow workers who count on her). During pregnancy, when a woman often needs extra emotional support, feeling responsible for so many people can be difficult (Box 17.6).

Day History. Ask specifically about a woman's job and estimate the amount of walking or back strain it entails. Ask about recent diet or exercise programs. If a woman belongs to a health club, remind her that the use of saunas and hot tubs for longer than 10 minutes at a time is contraindicated during pregnancy because of possible hyperthermia and teratogenic effects of extreme heat on the developing fetus. Identify personal habits, such as cigarette smoking and alcohol consumption, that may be detrimental to a fetus to determine if counseling to halt or decrease these habits could be effective.

Physical Examination

A woman over age 40 needs a thorough physical examination at her first prenatal visit to establish her general health and to identify any problems, particularly circulatory disturbances. Inspect her lower extremities thoroughly for varicosities, because these are more common in women over age 40. Obtain a urine specimen and test it for specific gravity, glucose, and protein to evaluate overall renal function and the possibility of gestational or type 2 diabetes, because older women are more prone than younger women to develop these conditions.

Assess a woman's breasts for any abnormalities, as women over age 40 are in a higher-risk group for breast cancer than are younger women. Ask if she has had yearly mammograms. In addition, assess for fetal heart sounds

BOX 17.6 FOCUS ON . . .

COMMUNICATION

Mindy Carson is 16 years old and pregnant. You talk to her at a prenatal clinic.

Less Effective Communication

Nurse: Hello, Mindy. How are you feeling?
Mindy: Good, but always tired. You know.
Nurse: You should try and rest more.
Mindy: Right.
Nurse: Why don't you ask your boyfriend to help you more?
Mindy: I'll do that.
Nurse: Or stop work. That'll leave you time to rest more.
Mindy: Right. Great solution.
Nurse: Glad I could be of help.

More Effective Communication

Nurse: Hello, Mindy. How are you feeling?
Mindy: Good, but always tired. You know.
Nurse: Are you getting enough sleep?
Mindy: How can I? I have to work every day after school.
Nurse: Is there anyone who could help you out more? Your boyfriend? A friend?
Mindy: I'm pretty much alone since I got pregnant.
Nurse: As long as you're coming to this clinic, you're not alone. Tell me about a typical day and let's investigate together what could be done.

In the first scenario, the nurse was so intent on problem solving she forgot the first step of effective problem solving—identify the exact problem that needs solving. In the second scenario, when the nurse continues to assess rather than offer advice, she is able to identify the problem.

and fetal movement at prenatal visits because gestational trophoblastic disease (hydatidiform mole) is more common in women over age 40 (see Chapter 15).

Chromosomal Assessment

Women over 40 are offered a triple-screen (alpha-fetoprotein [AFP], human chorionic gonadotropin, and unconjugated estriol levels) drawn on blood serum at the 15th week of pregnancy to detect whether an open spinal cord or chromosomal defect could be present in the fetus, because their risk for Down syndrome is so much higher than it is in younger women (Egan et al., 2004). If this test is positive, an amniocentesis will be scheduled at the 16th week of pregnancy. Be certain a woman is prepared for these studies and receives support during them. Alert her about the possibility of false-positive results with AFP testing. Many women of this age group do not begin nest-building until these tests confirm that the child will be healthy.

NURSING DIAGNOSES AND RELATED INTERVENTIONS

Nursing Diagnosis: Health-seeking behaviors related to special care necessary for healthy pregnancy

Outcome Evaluation: Client states she feels confident in self-care and her ability to decrease possible complications of pregnancy.

Be certain to adapt prenatal teaching to fit a woman's lifestyle. If she had not planned on ever being pregnant, she may have isolated herself through the years from "mothering" activities and so, despite her years, may know little about pregnancy and newborn care. In terms of knowledge, this puts her at the same level as the adolescent. Others have read so extensively that they may know more theoretical information than a woman who has already given birth. Be certain to review information about possible discomforts of pregnancy (see Chapter 11). A pregnant woman over age 40 is prone to hemorrhoids because she may have some rectal varicosities present at the beginning of pregnancy. Pain from rectal distention may, in fact, be one of the primary symptoms she reports at a first visit. Review measures to increase comfort.

Varicosities, like hemorrhoids, develop readily in a woman over age 40 because she may have had some tendency toward them even before the pregnancy. As with hemorrhoids, her best approach during pregnancy is to prevent varicosities (Box 17.7).

Record on a woman's chart any degree of varicosity formation during pregnancy so nurses caring for her during the postpartum period can take special precautions to prevent thrombophlebitis. With venous stasis present after birth, a woman is even more prone to develop this complication.

Nutrition. Assess the number of meals a woman eats outside her home each week, including those she packs for lunch or eats in restaurants. She may need tips on how to adjust pregnancy nutrition so she can obtain the same nutrition whether she prepares meals at home or eats them at an office or community function. Urge her to substitute a caffeine-free soft drink in place of an alcoholic beverage. In some offices, large amounts of coffee are consumed. Urge her to substitute milk or juice or decaffeinated coffee. Many women this age normally drink little milk. Rather than getting used to milk again, a woman may appreciate suggestions on other ways to ingest calcium, such as puddings or yogurt.

Prenatal Classes. Because a pregnant woman over age 40 may be unique in her circle of friends, she may feel shut out of her usual group because of the pregnancy. This

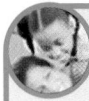

BOX 17.7 FOCUS ON . . .

FAMILY TEACHING

Tips on Preventing Varicose Veins

Q. Mindy says to you, "My mother developed terrible varicose veins when she was pregnant. Is there anything that I can do so this won't happen to me?"

A. Although the following activities aren't foolproof, incorporate them in your day to help prevent the development of varicose veins:

- Find opportunities during the day, such as a coffee or lunch break, to elevate your legs.
- Be certain your diet includes vitamin C, because this is important to strengthen vein walls.
- Rest in a side-lying position with your body tipped slightly forward (Sims' position). This allows leg veins to drain and empty.
- Avoid long periods of standing in one place by taking "walk breaks"; active muscle contraction helps venous return.
- Avoid sitting with your legs crossed.
- Don't wear anything constricting, such as knee-high stockings, on your lower legs.
- If you wear support hose, put them on before you get out of bed in the morning, before veins become swollen, for best results.

makes her ready, therefore, to join a childbirth preparation or prenatal exercise class where she is "one of the group" (Fig. 17.2).

Be certain a woman plans (or the couple plans together) to set aside a specific time every day to do breathing exercises in preparation for labor. Otherwise, a busy woman may never find time to get to them and will be unprepared in labor.

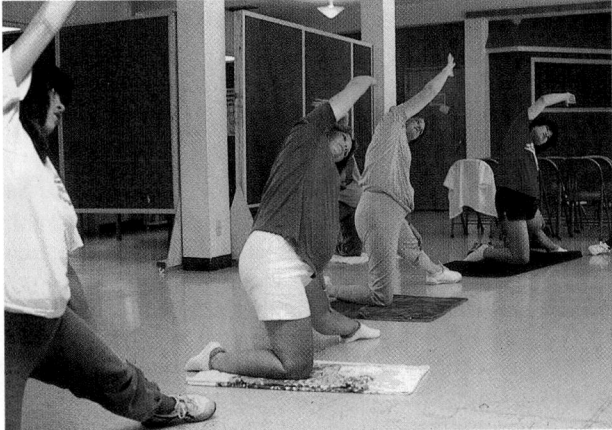

FIGURE 17.2 Exercise classes during pregnancy provide women with an opportunity to interact with other pregnant women while benefiting from a carefully monitored work-out. (© Kathy Sloane.)

Complications of Pregnancy for a Woman Over Age 40

The complications of pregnancy most likely to occur in a woman over age 40—hypertension of pregnancy, preterm or post-term birth, and cesarean birth—are related to the fact that the woman's circulatory system may not be as competent as when she was younger or her body tissues may not be as elastic as they once were (Box 17.8; Malee, 2003; Porter & Scott, 2003).

Pregnancy-Induced Hypertension

A woman over age 40 may have a higher incidence of pregnancy-induced hypertension than a younger woman, possibly related to blood vessel inelasticity or because hypertension tends to occur more frequently in nulliparas than multiparas or those with already elevated blood pressure. At any age, the best way to reduce the symptoms of

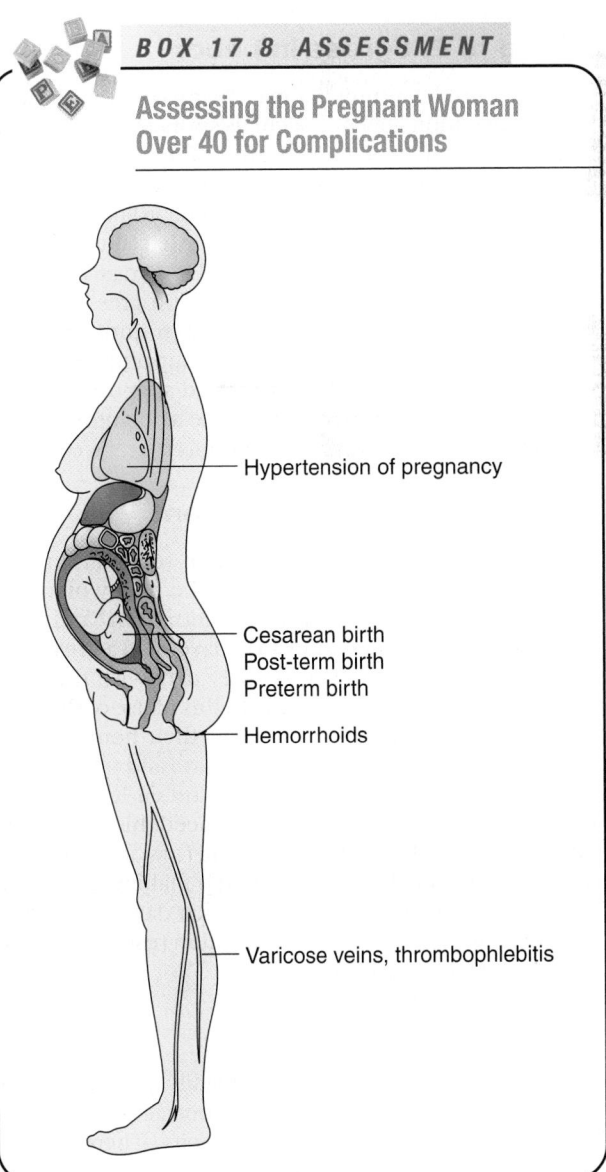

BOX 17.8 ASSESSMENT

Assessing the Pregnant Woman Over 40 for Complications

- Hypertension of pregnancy
- Cesarean birth
- Post-term birth
- Preterm birth
- Hemorrhoids
- Varicose veins, thrombophlebitis

pregnancy-induced hypertension is for a woman to rest for a good portion of each day. If a woman works full-time, stopping work may be difficult or impossible for her, not only because she believes she may miss out on a promotion or risk losing her job, but also because her income is important to her family and she is used to being productive, not merely resting all day. To allow her to rest effectively, you may need to help her plan activities she can accomplish on bed rest, such as reworking a school course outline, restructuring her office filing system, or working at a hobby she has wanted to pursue but never had time for before.

Complications and Concerns of Labor, Birth, and the Postpartum Period

Complications that occur with a woman over age 40 related to birth or the immediate period after birth also are the results of a body that may not be as elastic as it was when the woman was younger.

Failure to Progress in Labor

Labor in an older primipara may be prolonged because cervical dilatation may not occur as spontaneously as in a younger woman, probably because of decreased elasticity in cells. Graphing labor progress is a good method to use to determine when labor is becoming prolonged. Many women this age may need a cesarean birth if labor is overly prolonged and places the fetus at risk. Encourage a woman to verbalize how she is feeling about her progress throughout labor to allow for reassurance and prompt intervention should problems arise. Urge her support person to be present for the birth to offer needed support. Keep in mind that some older men may not be as comfortable in a birthing room as their younger counterparts would be.

Difficulty Accepting the Event

Women over age 40 may begin to have second thoughts about childbearing this late in life as the reality of a new baby registers with them during the intrapartal and postpartum period. Although they may have read a great deal about babies during pregnancy, they may wish they had read more or were as confident with this phase of their life as they are about other areas such as their home, office, or classroom. Review plans for child care and postpartum rest, with an emphasis on helping women learn to balance their lives. They most likely will need this help, especially if they are planning on returning to work soon after the birth. They might appreciate help making child care arrangements. You can assure them that day care for preschool children has positive socialization results (Zoritch, Roberts, & Oakley, 2005).

Postpartum Hemorrhage

Just as the cervix may not dilate as readily during an older woman's labor, the uterus may not contract as readily in the postpartum period due to inelasticity. Therefore, an older woman is at higher risk for postpartum hemorrhage.

Close observation is essential. Because a woman over age 40 may be an independent woman who is interested in self-care, she may ask for little help. Be sure to assess the amount of lochial flow to detect this complication.

Checkpoint Question 3

Women over 40 are at increased risk for developing pregnancy-induced hypertension. The reason for this is:

a. Many are overweight before they enter pregnancy.
b. They drink more fluids daily than younger women.
c. They do not exercise much, so edema fluid accumulates.
d. Their blood vessels are not as elastic as those of younger women.

THE PREGNANT WOMAN WHO IS PHYSICALLY OR COGNITIVELY CHALLENGED

In the past, women with conditions such as vision, hearing, cognitive, spinal cord, or orthopedic challenges were sheltered by their families to such an extent that women with even moderately physically challenging conditions did not meet potential sexual or marriage partners and so did not become pregnant. In addition, most people believed these individuals should not become pregnant. Today, women with varying degrees of disability attend public schools, work in offices, join community organizations, establish sexual relationships, marry, and plan pregnancies. Because these women (and in some instances their support persons also) face special problems related to their conditions, nursing care during pregnancy must be designed with these special concerns in mind so a woman's and family's problems and needs can be addressed and met.

Table 17.1 lists general areas of care that are important in planning for the physically or cognitively challenged woman who is pregnant.

Rights of the Physically or Cognitively Challenged Person

There are always ethical considerations related to women with disabilities and pregnancy (Scott, 2005). By federal law, physically disabled persons must have freedom of access to public buildings by means of ramps or handrails. All public health care facilities must be in compliance with these laws both in terms of physical facilities and in the true spirit of the law: that is, people should be made to feel psychologically welcome as well as physically able to reach the inside of the building. Under the same law, a hospital cannot deny care to a person with a disability even though the disabling condition complicates treatment considerably, possibly requiring extra personnel and time. A woman with a disability has full rights to her child, so the baby cannot be taken from her at birth without her full consent. Likewise, she cannot be forced to terminate the pregnancy or undergo sterilization unless that is her informed decision.

TABLE 17.1

Areas of Planning With Physically or Cognitively Challenged Women During Pregnancy

Area	Assessment and Planning Guidelines
Transportation	Ask if a woman has transportation for prenatal care and for emergencies.
Pregnancy counseling	Assess the special modifications of care that will need to be made depending on a woman's special challenge. Use additional visual or auditory aids to make your teaching points clear.
Support person	Determine who is the woman's support person. In some instances, a woman's condition requires so much assistance during pregnancy that one support person will not be enough. If necessary, contact community agencies to lend additional support, with her consent.
Health	Don't lose track of a woman's primary health problem. For example, a woman with cerebral palsy needs to continue an active muscle exercise program during pregnancy for her primary illness.
Work	Assess whether a woman works outside her home and, if work is discontinued during pregnancy, what she could substitute for a social contact activity. Women with physical or cognitive challenges may be lonely because they do not have a wide range of friends or social contacts.
Recreation	Assess whether her level of activity is adequate, and make concrete suggestions within her limitations for increasing it. Many women with a physically challenging condition lead a rather sedentary life (partly because they do not have many social contacts).
Self-esteem	Assess a woman's level of self-esteem: it may be low because of repeated failures in her life. Give praise at prenatal visits and help her make pregnancy a growth experience.

Modifications for Pregnancy

Most women with some degree of challenge need modifications of their care during pregnancy. Explore with them at a first prenatal visit the exact nature of their disability and their general self-image. Some women who are physically or cognitively challenged maintain high self-esteem despite severe limitations and are able to modify, grow, and learn with a pregnancy, whereas others have a poor sense of self-esteem that will make this particularly difficult for them. For many of them, pregnancy will become a special event, a 9-month announcement to everyone that, despite their seeming limitations, they are equal to other women and capable of participating in one of life's miracles (McKay-Moffat, 2003).

Safety Measures to Explore

Safety is a key area of concern when caring for the pregnant woman who is physically or cognitively challenged. Be sure to assess areas such as emergency contact persons, suppliers of transportation, and individual considerations such as mobility, elimination, and possible autonomic responses.

Emergency Contacts. Evaluate the client's ability to contact someone in case of an emergency. Does a woman have a telephone she can reach readily? Does she know how to activate the emergency medical system (911) in her community? If a woman's speech is not clear, evaluate whether she will be understood while using the telephone to call for help in an emergency. Some women with limited mobility, such as those with spinal cord injury or cerebral palsy, have a specially designed telephone contact system in their home that connects to a paramedic or hospital emergency service through a beeper system. Check that they intend to maintain this throughout pregnancy. Women who are

hearing challenged use a specially equipped telephone (a TDD device) that prints out messages for them.

Transportation. Assess a client's ability to come for prenatal care. If a woman depends on a support person for transportation to a health care facility, appointments may have to be arranged according to that person's schedule to prevent missed appointments. If a woman does not drive, who would transport her if a pregnancy emergency should occur? Women with cognitive or vision challenges, for example, may not qualify for a driver's license and so may need someone, such as a family member or friend, to drive. Women with spinal cord injury may have difficulty transferring into the specially equipped, hand-controlled car they usually drive as pregnancy progresses.

Mobility. All women who use wheelchairs are taught to press with their hands against the armrests and lift their buttocks up off the wheelchair seat for 5 seconds every hour. This prevents the formation of pressure ulcers on the buttocks and posterior thighs. Encourage the pregnant woman to continue to perform this maneuver during pregnancy as the increased weight of a fetus increases her risk for pressure ulcer formation from compression. In addition, severe hip flexion from sitting in a wheelchair limits venous return from the lower extremities. For at least 1 hour every morning and afternoon, encourage women who ambulate by wheelchair to decrease the sharp bend at the knees that results from sitting in the chair, to promote venous return and help prevent varicosities and thrombi formation. Adjusting the footrests of the wheelchair so a woman's legs are not sharply bent at the knees is helpful.

If balance is a problem, a woman may need reevaluation at the midpoint of pregnancy as the weight of her abdomen increases. This may necessitate the use of crutches if she did not use them before, or use of a wheelchair if she was ambulatory with crutches or a walker before pregnancy. Keep in mind that a woman who is physically challenged achieved the degree of ambulation that she first presents with usually after years of physical therapy and strengthening of leg and arm muscles. Help her see that reducing her degree of independence during pregnancy is not a step backward for her but a step forward, allowing her to have a safe pregnancy without the danger of falling (Fig. 17.3).

Elimination. When mobility is an effort, a woman may not drink as much as usual or use a bathroom as frequently as she would if those actions were effortless. Encourage a high fluid intake and frequent voiding to prevent urinary tract infections. Women with spinal cord injury who use an indwelling catheter are at especially high risk for contracting urinary tract infections during pregnancy. Women who perform self-catheterization or change their own indwelling catheter may be unable to continue to do this late in pregnancy because the increasing size of their abdomen interferes with their ability to see or reach the perineum comfortably. If this happens, it may be necessary for her to arrange for a support person, a home care nurse, or a home health aide to do this for her.

Autonomic Responses. In a woman who has a high spinal cord injury (cervical or high thoracic), observe for **autonomic dysreflexia** during pregnancy, labor, and the immediate postpartum period. This is an exaggerated autonomic response to stimuli. Any irritating condition, such as a distended bladder, increasing uterine size, labor contractions, or breast-feeding, may initiate the response (Malee, 2003). Without upper motor neuron control to reverse the phenomenon, extreme symptoms such as severe hypertension (300/160 mm Hg), throbbing headache, flushing of the skin and profuse diaphoresis above the level of the spinal lesion, nausea, and bradycardia may occur. Immediate action is necessary to protect against cerebrovascular accident or intraocular damage. Elevate a woman's head to reduce cerebral pressure and locate the irritating

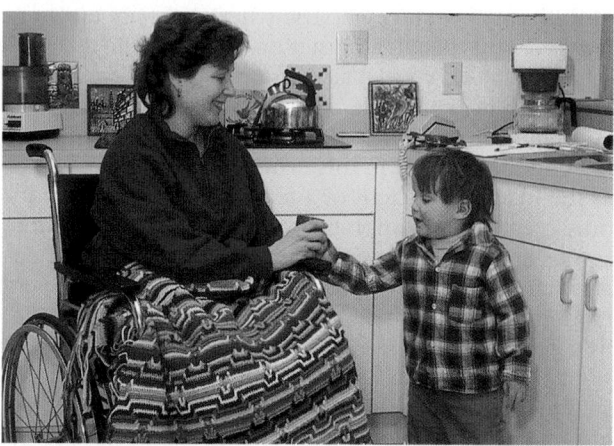

FIGURE 17.3 During pregnancy, a woman who is physically challenged may need to use a wheelchair to help safeguard against injury. Assure her that she may still enjoy her independence and daily activities, such as caring for an older child. (© Keith/Custom Medical Stock Photo.)

stimulus (usually a distended bladder or bowel). If bladder distention is the cause, remove the bladder pressure by catheterization if an indwelling catheter is not in place. If a catheter is in place, check to see why it is not draining, then encourage it to drain by unkinking or flushing to allow urine to flow freely again. Anticipate the need for an antihypertensive agent to alleviate the extreme hypertension, although as soon as the source of irritation is removed, symptoms typically fade quickly.

Prenatal Care Modifications to Meet Specific Needs

The physical examination may need to be modified depending on individual circumstances. Although women with disabilities have been followed by health care providers most of their life, they may never have had a pelvic examination before and so need clear instructions about why it is needed and what it will consist of. Many obstetric examining tables are built for the comfort of the examiner and are too high for a woman to transfer to from a wheelchair by simply sliding onto the table. To help a woman move to the table, a ramp from the physical therapy department may be necessary so the wheelchair can be elevated to the level of the table. Woman with spinal cord injury or cerebral palsy may be unable to maintain their legs in a lithotomy position because of either hip flexion contracture or laxness of leg support. This means a dorsal recumbent, rather than a lithotomy, position may be required for a pelvic examination.

Women who are cognitively challenged may not be aware how they became pregnant. If a woman became pregnant because she was taken advantage of sexually, she may need some time to talk and work through this experience before she can allow a pelvic examination.

If a visually challenged woman brings a guide dog with her to a health care visit, remember that although the dog's chief function is to offer direction, its instinct causes it to become a woman's protector. In this role, the dog may feel threatened by people who try to pet it. Petting a guide dog also distracts it from safeguarding its owner. When interviewing or teaching visually challenged women, do not use your hands to illustrate points ("I'll need a urine sample of at least this much urine [measured with your fingers]"). Do not use colors as descriptions of objects ("put on the blue gown"). Use demonstration aids that allow a woman to feel or touch. When helping with or performing physical assessment, let the woman know you are closing the door or drawing a curtain to ensure privacy. Always alert a woman when you are going to touch her, so as not to startle her. Otherwise, you may find yourself facing a growling guide dog that rises to protect her.

If a woman is hearing impaired, she may not be able to see the examiner's face during a pelvic examination. This means any question asked of her during this time will not be understood because she cannot see the examiner's lips to lip read (Josiah, 2004).

Pregnancy Education

Modify health teaching to meet a woman's specific needs. As stated previously, avoid references to colors or using your hands when explaining something to a visually challenged woman. Enlist the aid of her other senses, such as touch (McGuire, 2003). For a woman who is cognitively challenged, instructions about pregnancy may need to be limited to those few items crucial for safety, such as "do not drink alcohol or take any medicine."

If a woman and her support person are both visually challenged, pamphlets about pregnancy care will not be useful. If the support person can see, offer the pamphlets to him or her, suggesting he or she read them to her as a shared activity. This will be helpful for her and also makes the partner a more informed support person. Many visually challenged women have tape recorders supplied by Recording for the Blind and Dyslexic (*www.rfbd.org*), a national, nonprofit, voluntary organization. Telephone the local association and ask if they have any material already recorded on pregnancy or breast-feeding they could supply. If not, make a tape recording of any information you particularly want a woman to remember or she seems concerned about. Supply the health care facility telephone number at the beginning of the tape for an easy reminder in an emergency, and perhaps the date of her next visit as well.

Plan nutritional education based on each client's specific challenges and usual routine. Ask what a woman normally eats. A visually challenged woman or one who ambulates by wheelchair, for example, may prepare her own breakfast and lunch, meals that may not require a stove. The only hot meal a woman may eat is one a support person cooks in the evening. Nutrition counseling for two meals daily, therefore, needs to center on foods that can be prepared without cooking.

Activity and exercise, important for any pregnant woman, are crucial for a woman who is physically challenged. Evaluate the amount of exercise a woman gets daily. If mobility is a concern, exercise can be very reduced in bad weather. In this case, be sure a woman understands that walking around her home or apartment can provide the same level of exercise as if she were walking around the block or exercising in a health club.

Although labor and the child's birth may be modified somewhat because of a woman's physical condition, gaining general knowledge about labor and birth and participating in a shared experience with her partner are still valuable. Urge women who are challenged in some way to attend childbirth preparation classes. If a woman is not working outside her home, she may have more time than others to practice breathing exercises and enter labor more adept at using such a method to control pain in labor than other women.

If a woman is severely hearing challenged, she may not have heard the many spot television announcements on not smoking or drinking alcohol during pregnancy; she may need more time at prenatal visits so this can be discussed. In addition, lip reading is a difficult skill to learn, so many hearing-challenged persons cannot do this with ease. Even if a woman is skilled at this, she may not be able to decipher new words such as amniotic, gestation, or edema. Show her the printed words so she can see what your lip motion represents when presenting new pregnancy terms. If a woman uses sign language, she may bring an interpreter with her to translate. Be certain to talk to her, not the interpreter, when interviewing.

Modifications for Labor and Birth Preparation

Women who are physically or cognitively challenged will need adaptations in preparation for labor and birth. Helpful suggestions are:

- A woman with a spinal cord injury may not be able to feel uterine contractions. Late in pregnancy, she will need to palpate her abdomen periodically for tightening or the presence of contractions so she is aware of beginning labor.
- Women with muscle spasticity or spinal cord injury may not be able to push effectively for the second stage of labor and so may need cesarean birth or forceps birth.
- If a woman cannot assume a lithotomy position because of hip contracture, vaginal delivery from a Sims' or dorsal recumbent position can be used.
- Braille watches used by visually challenged persons may not have second hands. They may need to time the length of contractions by counting rather than timing them by a watch.
- During labor, the hearing-challenged woman cannot hear information on how she is progressing if you are not directly facing her. If she needs to communicate with her support person in sign language, act as an advocate to keep her hands unencumbered by equipment such as intravenous lines. Remember she cannot hear the infant cry at birth. Hand the infant to her as soon as possible after birth so she can see and feel the baby is crying and breathing well.
- Be certain to identify the usual sounds of birthing rooms (the beeping of a monitor, the swish of a central supply routing system, and so forth) for the visually challenged woman. Hearing sounds and not being able to identify them is frightening.

Modifications for Postpartum Care

After birth, be sure to assess and teach.

- Ask whether a woman desires contraceptive information.
- Support her attempts to breast-feed.
- Be certain a woman has a return appointment for both herself and her infant for follow-up care and that the arrangements are within her capabilities, transportation, and understanding.

Modifications for Planning Child Care

Allow for extra time during the first days after birth for mother–child interaction. For example, after birth, a woman who is cognitively challenged may need extra time to understand the transition from "being pregnant" to "having a baby." She may have difficulty learning to judge when her infant is hungry. She may need extra supervision to be certain she doesn't leave the baby unprotected on a bed. A woman with a spinal cord disability may be particularly interested in inspecting her baby's back. A visually challenged woman will probably want to reassure herself her baby can see. Be sure to give the baby to her as soon as possible so she can touch the baby and feel for intact body parts. If the birthing room is cold, explain to her that you want to rewrap the baby to prevent chilling, not because her touching is wrong or because you are trying to hide an imperfection in the baby.

Breast-feeding has special advantages for women who are physically or cognitively challenged because it is the method of feeding that is not only best for the baby, but also requires the least preparation effort on the mother's part. For a woman who is visually challenged and unable to read printed instructions, for example, breast-feeding eliminates formula errors. For a woman who uses a wheelchair, it eliminates trips to the refrigerator. However, breast-feeding may not be possible for a woman with muscle spasticity because the let-down reflex, which depends on muscle relaxation, may not occur. Be certain that women who are cognitively challenged understand they need to feed until the infant is satisfied, not until they are tired of feeding.

Encourage women to think through what baby care equipment will be best for them. Some infant crib rails lower by pressure on a foot pedal. Others use a waist-high lever. A woman who ambulates by wheelchair usually finds the waist-high lever most convenient because she can reach this most easily. Also review with a woman any special steps she will need to use for safe child care. Many women need a referral for home care follow-up and possibly the use of a home health aide for child care.

If a woman has difficulty with mobility, ask how she anticipates carrying her infant. Using an anterior baby sling is usually effective with a wheelchair. Women who are mobile by crutches or a walker can place the baby in a small wagon and pull it. Some women lie on their back on the floor, place the baby on their chest, and scoot across the floor. The important point is not how a woman carries her baby, but that she has thought through a safe and comfortable way to do this.

Urge a visually challenged woman to make eye contact when talking to her infant. Many visually challenged people do not turn on lights in their home because they do not perceive the difference between light and dark. Encourage a woman to develop a habit of turning on lights after dinner because her infant will need light to develop vision. If her support person also is visually challenged, suggest she check with a close friend or neighbor monthly to see that light bulbs have not burned out.

One of the biggest worries for the hearing-impaired woman is that she will not be able to hear her baby crying. Help her plan to bring the infant's crib or bassinet close to her bed so she can feel the vibration of the baby's stirring and waking. Urge her to talk to the infant as she gives care so the infant is introduced to sounds and words. Some women whose speech is severely affected by their hearing disorder are reluctant to speak to strangers. Assure her that her infant is not a stranger and will quiet readily to the sound of her voice. The child may develop her speech pattern because of this. Being spoken to and sung to during the first year is important for overall development, however, so this is still preferable to living in a world of silence.

Some women who are cognitively challenged may have been raised in a group home and only recently moved to their own apartment. Unlike those raised at home, these women may have unusual difficulty making plans for child care because they have never seen the care of young children. You have a legal obligation to investigate whether a newborn will receive safe care before hospital discharge. Be certain to ask enough questions so that you are sure a woman who is severely cognitively challenged, for example, has a responsible friend or partner to help her with child care.

Checkpoint Question 4

Women with high thoracic spinal cord injury can develop autonomic dysreflexia during labor. The best action to take for this would be:

a. Ask her to lie flat and take deep breaths.
b. Elevate her legs to restore her blood pressure.
c. Give a prescribed hypotensive medicine.
d. Talk to her calmly to reduce her anxiety.

A WOMAN WHO IS SUBSTANCE DEPENDENT

Substance dependence is a growing health problem in women of childbearing age, so its incidence during pregnancy is increasing. As many as 10% to 20% of pregnant women use illegal drugs during pregnancy (DHHS, 2000). The use of cocaine, amphetamines, and multiple drugs has increased dramatically in recent years. Adolescents have an increased rate of inhalant abuse and binge drinking.

Substance abuse is defined as the inability to meet major role obligations, legal problems, or an increase in risk-taking behavior or exposure to hazardous situations because of an addicting substance. A person is **substance dependent** when he or she has withdrawal symptoms following discontinuation of the substance, combined with abandonment of important activities, spending increased time in activities related to substance use, using substances for a longer time than planned, and continued use despite worsening problems due to substance use (Jaffe & Anthony, 2005).

Typically, substance-dependent women are thought to be in the younger age group, as the overall incidence of drug use is highest in this group. However, any woman could be substance dependent. Therefore, all pregnant women need to be assessed for the possibility of substance abuse.

A mark of a woman with a substance abuse problem is that she may come late in the pregnancy for prenatal care because she is afraid her drug use will be discovered and she will be reported to authorities (Brady et al., 2003). She may have difficulty following prenatal instructions for proper nutrition because although she may desire to eat well, she may lack sufficient money for both drugs and nutritious food, and choosing drugs will make her nutrition inadequate. She may not have money for supplemental vitamins or iron preparations for the same reason. If she is using a drug that sustains her for only a few hours, she cannot wait long at a health care facility to be seen for an appointment.

Illicit drugs tend to be of small molecular weight, so they cross the placenta readily. As a result, a fetus of an addicted mother has a drug concentration of about 50% that of the mother. Because this can lead to fetal effects, drug abuse can account for fetal abnormalities or preterm birth (Higley & Morin, 2004). If a woman uses injected drugs, the risk for hepatitis B or human immunodeficiency virus (HIV) infection increases. Additionally, a woman may earn money to buy drugs through prostitution, which increases the risk for sexually transmitted infection and poses an additional threat to a fetus.

NURSING DIAGNOSES AND RELATED INTERVENTIONS

———●———

Nursing Diagnosis: Risk for injury to self and fetus related to chronic substance abuse

Outcome Evaluation: Client states she has enrolled in a substance abuse treatment program and consequently has reduced or is no longer abusing drugs.

Women who are substance dependent need anticipatory guidance and nursing support all during pregnancy, as this is a long time to change a lifestyle. Often, women who abuse substances have few effective support people with whom they feel free to discuss their problems or concerns or who can answer their questions about pregnancy. Because of their numerous needs, they require a multidisciplinary team approach as offered by formal substance abuse treatment programs. Fortunately, with good support and active participation in a treatment program, pregnancy can become a stimulus for drug withdrawal and a maturing and growth experience for a woman.

If a woman is still abusing a drug by the time she begins labor, her infant may experience drug withdrawal symptoms after birth (usually nervousness, irritability or lethargy, and possibly seizures; see Chapter 26). Breast-feeding is usually not encouraged for women with substance abuse because, just as all drugs cross the placenta to some extent, they also are all excreted into breast milk. A woman who is still abusing a drug at this time needs additional referral so she can secure help. In some states, women who test positive for drug abuse, either during pregnancy or at the time of birth, are reported to state child protective agencies; they may be accused of child abuse and jailed, and their infant may be placed in foster care. Be certain you are familiar with agency and state policy concerning these directives (Kang, 2003).

? *What if...* Mindy Carson tells you she is not using drugs during pregnancy, but when she opens her purse, you notice several packets of white powder inside? What would you do?

Drugs Commonly Used During Pregnancy

Recreational drugs commonly used in pregnancy are those commonly used by women in their childbearing years: cocaine, amphetamines, marijuana, phencyclidine, inhalants, opiates, and alcohol.

Cocaine

Cocaine is derived from *Erythroxylum coca,* a plant grown almost exclusively in South America. When sniffed into the nose or smoked in a pipe, cocaine is absorbed across the mucous membranes, affecting the central nervous system. As a result, sudden vasoconstriction occurs. Respiratory and cardiac rates and blood pressure increase rapidly in response to the vasoconstriction. Immediate death may result from cardiac failure. Alkaloidal cocaine (crack), a concentrated mixture, produces an even more rapid and intense "high" when inhaled.

Cocaine has become one of the most frequently abused drugs during pregnancy, and its use is exceptionally harmful during pregnancy because the extreme vasoconstriction that occurs can severely compromise placental circulation, leading to abruptio placentae, or a tearing loose of the placenta, which then results in preterm labor or fetal death (Box 17.9). Infants born to cocaine-dependent women may suffer the immediate effects of intracranial hemorrhage and a withdrawal syndrome of tremulousness, irritability, and muscle rigidity. Long-term effects are not well documented, but learning defects are suspected (Higley & Morin, 2004; Lewis et al., 2004).

Counseling women to discontinue cocaine use during pregnancy is often disappointing. The effects of the drug are so intense that it is difficult for addicted women to withdraw. Cocaine use can be detected by urinalysis because the metabolites of cocaine can be detected in urine up to 1 week after use.

Amphetamines

Methamphetamine (speed) has a pharmacologic effect similar to cocaine. Its use is becoming more common because it is easily and cheaply manufactured. Ice, a rock type of methamphetamine that is smoked, can produce high concentrations of drug in the maternal circulation. Newborns whose mothers used the drug show jitteriness and poor feeding at birth and may be growth restricted (Smith et al., 2003).

Marijuana and Hashish

Both marijuana and hashish are obtained from the hemp plant, cannabis. When smoked, they produce tachycardia

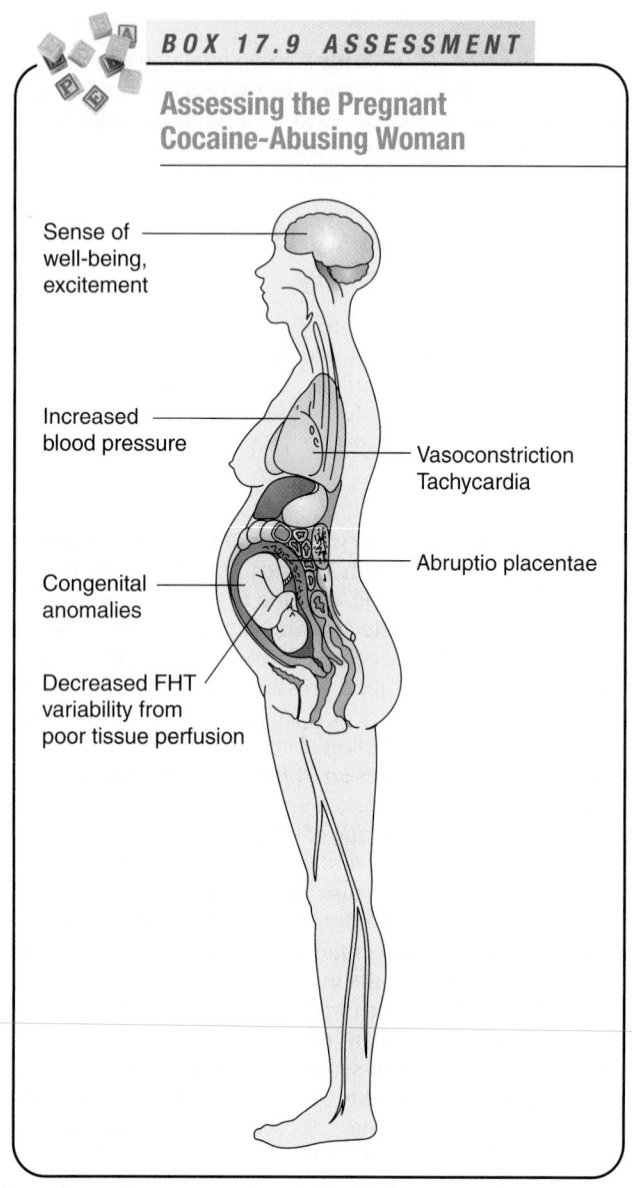

BOX 17.9 ASSESSMENT

Assessing the Pregnant Cocaine-Abusing Woman

Sense of well-being, excitement

Increased blood pressure

Vasoconstriction Tachycardia

Abruptio placentae

Congenital anomalies

Decreased FHT variability from poor tissue perfusion

Narcotic Agonists

Narcotic agonists, used for the treatment of pain (e.g., morphine or meperidine [Demerol]) and cough suppression (codeine), are also widely abused because of their potent analgesic and euphoric effect. Heroin, a raw opiate, is the main opiate used recreationally to the point of dependence, and its use is increasing in incidence in young adults. A short-acting narcotic, heroin is inactive until it crosses the blood–brain barrier (which it does more quickly than morphine). It may be administered intradermally ("skin popping"), through inhalation ("snorting"), or intravenously ("shooting"). It produces an immediate and short-lived feeling of euphoria followed by sedation. Pregnancy complications related to its use include pregnancy-induced hypertension and, because narcotics are often injected with shared needles, phlebitis, subacute bacterial endocarditis, and hepatitis B and HIV infection.

Withdrawal symptoms include nausea, vomiting, diarrhea, abdominal pain, hypertension, restlessness, shivering, insomnia, body aches, and muscle jerks. Withdrawal symptoms may begin as soon as 6 hours after the last drug dose and can continue for several days. Their severity and duration depend on the amount of drug used daily and the length of the dependence period.

Heroin abuse in the pregnant woman can result in fetal opiate dependence and severe withdrawal symptoms in the infant after birth. Infants of opiate-abusing women tend to be small for gestational age and have an increased incidence of fetal distress and meconium aspiration. They will have the same withdrawal symptoms after birth as the mother would if she abruptly stopped taking the drug.

Because a fetus is exposed to drugs that must be processed by the liver during pregnancy, the fetal liver is forced to mature faster than normal. For this reason, newborns of substance-abusing women seem better able to cope with bilirubin at birth than other babies; hyperbilirubinemia is therefore rarely a problem. Fetal lung tissue also appears to mature more rapidly than normal, apparently from the stress of intrauterine drug exposure. Therefore, although the infant is born preterm, the chance that he or she will develop a condition such as respiratory distress syndrome is less than average.

If possible, an opiate-dependent woman should be enrolled in a methadone maintenance program during pregnancy. Infants of women taking methadone do not escape withdrawal symptoms, and some infants appear to have more severe reactions to methadone withdrawal than to heroin withdrawal (Berghella et al., 2003). Because a woman is being provided an oral drug legally, however, a fetus is at least ensured better nutrition, better prenatal care, and less exposure to pathogens such as hepatitis B and HIV. If a methadone program is not available, women may be treated with buprenorphine (Comer & Annitto, 2004). Drug withdrawal symptoms of the newborn and accompanying nursing care are discussed in Chapter 26.

and a sense of well-being. Some women have begun to use marijuana to counteract nausea in early pregnancy (Westfall, 2004). These drugs are frequently part of polydrug abuse, so their effects are not well documented. They are associated with loss of short-term memory and an increased incidence of respiratory infection in adults. A frequent user may not be able to breast-feed because of reduced milk production and the risk to the newborn from excretion of the drug in the milk.

Phencyclidine

Phencyclidine (PCP) is an animal tranquilizer that is a frequently used street drug in polydrug abuse. It causes increased cardiac output and a sense of euphoria. It has the potential for causing long-term hallucinations (flashback episodes). PCP tends to leave the maternal circulation and concentrate in fetal cells, so it may be particularly injurious to a fetus.

Inhalants

Inhalant abuse refers to the "sniffing" or "huffing" of aerosol drugs. Frequently abused substances include airplane glue, cooking sprays, or computer keyboard cleaner. Most of these substances contain Freon as a propellant and can lead to severe respiratory and cardiac irregularities. The effect of these drugs during pregnancy is not well documented, but the respiratory depression they can cause could be enough to limit the fetal oxygen supply to a serious level.

Alcohol

Although alcohol can be legally purchased and is served generously at social functions, it is just as detrimental to fetal growth as illegal drugs. There is little documentation as to how much alcohol must be ingested before fetal alcohol syndrome, a syndrome with significant facial features and cognitive challenge, occurs, so women are advised to drink no alcohol during pregnancy (Burd, Klug, & Martsolf, 2004). When discussing alcohol ingestion with young adults, be certain to talk about binge drinking (five or more alcohol drinks on one occasion) to be certain a woman doesn't believe this type of occasional drinking is safe during pregnancy (Bailey et al., 2004).

Checkpoint Question 5

Mindy Carson tells you she takes methamphetamine almost daily. A fetus of a drug-addicted mother receives approximately what percentage of the mother's drug concentration?

a. 20%
b. 50%
c. 70%
d. 100%

Key Points

Adolescent pregnancy is a major concern, because although it is decreasing in incidence, it still occurs at a high rate and can interfere with the development of both an adolescent and fetus. Nursing care needs to be individualized to meet the prepartal, intrapartal, and postpartum needs of this age group. Helping adolescents view a pregnancy as a growth experience can help them mature in their ability to parent.

Women who delay childbearing until age 40 may need additional discussion time at prenatal visits to help them incorporate a pregnancy into their lifestyle. They may need reminders to save time during the day for rest, particularly if at risk for pregnancy-induced hypertension or varicosities.

Women who are physically, cognitively, visually, or hearing challenged or who have a spinal cord injury are apt to have special needs during pregnancy that must be addressed by health care providers. Providing time for discussion early in pregnancy so these needs can be identified and anticipated is an important role for nurses.

Women who are physically or cognitively challenged may need help in adjusting their usual regimen to pregnancy. Be certain they are aware of how to contact help in an emergency. Ensure that all medications they are taking for their primary disorder are safe for use during pregnancy.

A woman who is substance dependent presents a unique challenge during pregnancy. Encouraging her to decrease or halt her drug intake to safeguard the health of a fetus is a short-term goal. Addressing her need to decrease drug intake for the remainder of her life so she can be a quality parent is a long-term goal.

A fetus of a woman who is substance dependent is at high risk because of the direct effects of the drug and the indirect effects of an unhealthy lifestyle. Women addicted to opiates should be encouraged to join drug reduction maintenance programs if possible to reduce fetal risk.

Critical Thinking Exercises

1. Mindy, the 16-year-old girl you met at the beginning of the chapter who is 15 weeks pregnant, tells you she is old enough to be a responsible parent and plans to keep her baby. What clues would you look for to see if her self-evaluation is correct?
2. Mindy makes friends with Clara, a 44-year-old woman, at the prenatal clinic. Clara works at a desk job as a stockbroker. She eats most of her meals at restaurants. Mindy lives at home and attends school. Both have inactive lifestyles. How would your teaching to prevent pregnancy complications differ for these two clients?
3. Mindy is dependent on methamphetamine. You suspect she supports her drug habit by prostitution. Describe modifications to her plan of care that would be necessary to ensure consistent prenatal care. What specific advice would you want to stress with her to avoid complications of pregnancy?
4. Examine the National Health Goals related to women with special needs. Most government-sponsored money for nursing research is allotted based on these goals. What would be a possible research topic to explore pertinent to these goals that would be applicable to the Carson family and also advance evidence-based practice?

References

Bailey, B. N., et al. (2004). Prenatal exposure to binge drinking and cognitive and behavioral outcomes at age 7 years. *American Journal of Obstetrics and Gynecology, 191*(3), 1037–1043.

Berghella, V., et al. (2003). Maternal methadone dose and neonatal withdrawal. *American Journal of Obstetrics & Gynecology, 189*(2), 312–327.

Brady, T. M., et al. (2003). Maternal drug use and the timing of prenatal care. *Journal of Health Care for the Poor and Underserved, 14*(4), 588–607.

Bunting, L., & McAuley, C. (2004). Research review: teenage pregnancy and parenthood: the role of fathers. *Child and Family Social Work, 9*(3), 295–303.

Burd, L., Klug, M., & Martsolf, J. (2004). Increased sibling mortality in children with fetal alcohol syndrome. *Addiction Biology, 9*(2), 179–186.

Comer, V. G., & Annitto, W. J. (2004). Buprenorphine: a safe method for detoxifying pregnant heroin addicts and their unborn. *American Journal on Addictions, 13*(3), 317–318.

Davis, A. J. (2003). Pediatric and adolescent gynecology. In J. R. Scott et al. (Eds.), *Danforth's obstetrics and gynecology* (9th ed.). Philadelphia: Lippincott Williams & Wilkins.

Department of Health and Human Services. (2000). *Healthy people 2010.* Washington, DC: Author.

Egan, J. F. X., et al. (2004). Down syndrome births in the United States from 1989 to 2001. *American Journal of Obstetrics and Gynecology, 191*(3), 1044–1048.

Erikson, E. (1963). *Childhood and society.* New York: Norton.

Grady, M. A., & Bloom, K. C. (2004). Pregnancy outcomes of adolescents enrolled in a CenteringPregnancy program. *Journal of Midwifery & Women's Health, 49*(5), 412–420.

Higley, A. M., & Morin, K. H. (2004). Behavioral responses of substance-exposed newborns: a retrospective study. *Applied Nursing Research, 17*(1), 32–40.

Jaffe, J. H., & Anthony, J. C. (2005). Substance-related disorders: introduction and overview. In B. J. Sadock & V. A. Sadock (Eds.), *Kaplan & Sadock's comprehensive textbook of psychiatry* (8th ed.). Philadelphia: Lippincott Williams & Wilkins.

Josiah, B. (2004). Hearing the needs of deaf mothers-to-be. *Practising Midwife, 7*(3), 22–23.

Kang, H. (2003). Comparative analysis of state statutes: reporting, assessing, and intervening with prenatal substance abuse. *Social Policy Journal, 2*(4), 71–86.

Koniak-Griffin, D., et al. (2003). Nurse visitation for adolescent mothers: two-year infant health and maternal outcomes. *Nursing Research, 52*(2), 127–136.

Lewis, B. A., et al. (2004). Four-year language outcomes of children exposed to cocaine in utero. *Neurotoxicology & Teratology, 26*(5), 617–627.

Malee, M. P. (2003). Medical and surgical complications of pregnancy. In J. R. Scott, et al. (Eds.). *Danforth's obstetrics and gynecology* (9th ed.). Philadelphia: Lippincott Williams & Wilkins.

Mayor, S. (2004). Pregnancy and childbirth are leading causes of death in teenage girls in developing countries. *British Medical Journal, 328*(7449), 1152.

McGuire, K. (2003). Second-class service: a visually impaired mother's story. *Practising Midwife, 6*(7), 18–20.

McKay-Moffat, S. (2003). Meeting the needs of mothers with disabilities. *Practising Midwife, 6*(7), 12–15.

Moldenhauer, J. S., & Sibai, B. M. (2003). Hypertensive disorders of pregnancy. In J. R. Scott et al. (Eds.), *Danforth's obstetrics and gynecology* (9th ed.). Philadelphia: Lippincott Williams & Wilkins.

National Center for Health Statistics (2005). *Trends in the health of Americans.* Hyattsville, MD: NCHS.

Porter, T. F., & Scott, J. R. (2003). Cesarean delivery. In J. R. Scott, et al. (Eds.), *Danforth's obstetrics and gynecology* (9th ed.). Philadelphia: Lippincott Williams & Wilkins.

Scott, R. (2005). Prenatal testing, reproductive autonomy, and disability interests. *Cambridge Quarterly of Healthcare Ethics, 14*(1), 65–82.

Sikorski, J., et al. (2005). Support for breastfeeding mothers. *The Cochrane Library (Oxford) (1)* (CD001141).

Smith, L., et al. (2003). Effects of prenatal methamphetamine exposure on fetal growth and drug withdrawal symptoms in infants born at term. *Journal of Developmental & Behavioral Pediatrics, 24*(1), 17–23.

Westfall, R. E. (2004). Use of anti-emetic herbs in pregnancy: women's choices, and the question of safety and efficacy. *Complementary Therapies in Nursing & Midwifery, 10*(1), 30–36.

Zoritch, B., Roberts, I., & Oakley, A. (2005). Day care for preschool children. *The Cochrane Library (Oxford)(2)* (CD000564).

Suggested Readings

Crow, L. (2003). Viewpoint. Invisible and centre stage: a disabled woman's perspective on maternity services. *RCM Midwives Journal, 6*(4), 158–161.

Gomez, C., et al. (2005). Expired air carbon monoxide concentration in mothers and their spouses above 5 ppm is associated with decreased fetal growth. *Preventive Medicine, 40*(1), 10–15.

Hughes, R. B. et al. (2005). Stress and women with physical disabilities: identifying correlates. *Women's Health Issues, 15*(1), 14–20.

Kovalesky, A. (2004). Women with substance abuse concerns. *Nursing Clinics of North America, 39*(1), 205–217.

Low, L. K., et al. (2003). Adolescents' experiences of childbirth: contrasts with adults. *Journal of Midwifery & Women's Health, 48*(3), 192–198.

Merewood, A., & Philipp, B. L. (2003). Promoting breastfeeding in an inner-city hospital: how to address the concerns of the maternity staff regarding illicit drug use. *Journal of Human Lactation, 19*(4), 418–420.

Marcellus, L. (2003). Critical social and medical constructions of perinatal substance misuse: truth in the making. *Journal of Family Nursing, 9*(4), 438–452.

Prilleltensky, O. (2003). A ramp to motherhood: the experiences of mothers with physical disabilities. *Sexuality and Disability, 21*(1), 21–47.

Russell, S. T., & Lee, F. C. H. (2004). Practitioners' perspectives on effective practices for Hispanic teenage pregnancy prevention. *Perspectives on Sexual and Reproductive Health, 36*(4), 142–149.

Saewyc, E. M., Magee, L. L., & Pettingell, S. E. (2004). Teenage pregnancy and associated risk behaviors among sexually abused adolescents. *Perspectives on Sexual and Reproductive Health, 36*(3), 98–105.

Savage, C. (2003). Screening for alcohol use in women of childbearing age. *Journal of Addictions Nursing, 14*(2), 63–64.

Spear, H. J. (2004). Personal narratives of adolescent mothers-to-be: contraception, decision making, and future expectations. *Public Health Nursing, 21*(4), 338–346.

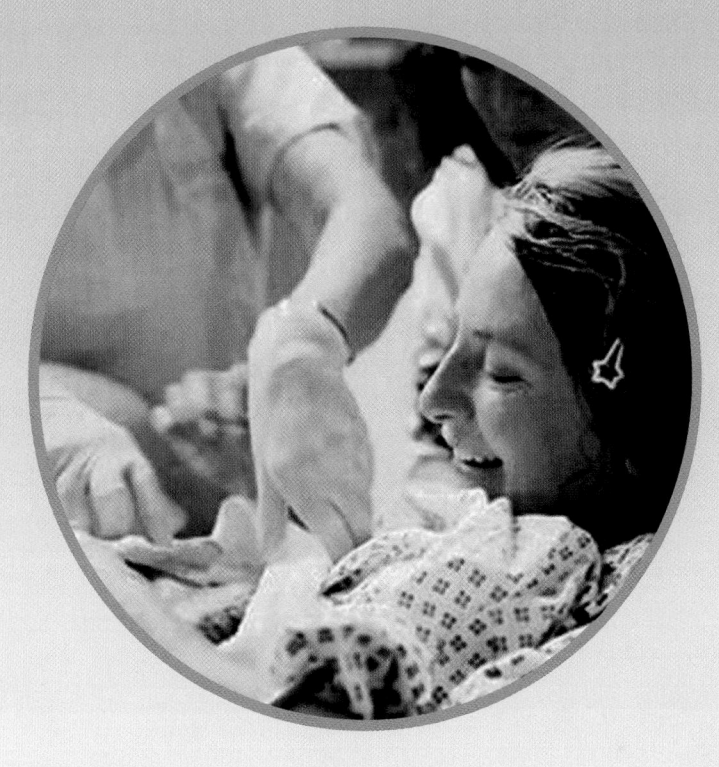

The Nursing Role in Caring for the Family During Labor and Birth

CHAPTER 18

Caring for a Woman During Vaginal Birth

Key Terms

amnioinfusion
attitude
breech presentation
cardinal movements of labor
cephalic presentation
crowning
dilatation
effacement
engagement
episiotomy
fetal descent
Leopold's maneuvers
lie
molding
pathologic retraction ring
physiologic retraction ring
position
ripening
station
transition

Objectives

After mastering the contents of this chapter, you should be able to:

1. Describe common theories explaining the onset of labor.
2. Discuss the role of the components of labor: passenger, passage, and powers.
3. Assess a woman in labor, identifying her stage and progression.
4. Formulate nursing diagnoses related to the physiologic and psychological aspects of labor.
5. Establish expected outcomes to meet the needs of a woman throughout the labor process.
6. Implement nursing care for a family during labor.
7. Evaluate expected outcomes for achievement and effectiveness of nursing care.
8. Identify National Health Goals related to safe labor and birth that nurses can help the nation achieve.
9. Identify areas related to labor and birth that could benefit from additional nursing research or application of evidence-based practice.
10. Use critical thinking to analyze the effectiveness of nursing care measures to meet the needs of women and their families so that labor is family centered.
11. Integrate knowledge of nursing care in labor with nursing process to achieve quality maternal and child health nursing care.

Celeste Bailey is a 26-year-old you admit to a birthing room. She's been having contractions 45 seconds long and 3 minutes apart for the last 6 hours. She tells you she wants to have her baby "naturally" without any analgesia or anesthesia. Her husband is in the Army and assigned overseas, so he is not with her. Although her sister lives only two blocks from the hospital, Celeste doesn't want her called. She asks if she can talk to her mother on the telephone instead. As you finish assessing contractions, she screams with pain and shouts, "I'm doing everything I'm supposed to do! How much longer does this go on?"

Previous chapters described the anatomic and physiologic changes that occur in pregnancy as well as effective steps women can take to prepare for labor. This chapter adds information about the labor process and how to explain what is happening during labor to a woman and give support. This is important information, because labor can be a frightening process if support people are not present.

What teaching does Celeste need about labor and birth?

After you've studied this chapter, access the accompanying website. Read the patient scenario and answer the questions to further sharpen your skills, grow more familiar with RN-CLEX types of questions, and reward yourself with how much you have learned.

abor is the series of events by which uterine contractions and abdominal pressure expel a fetus and placenta from a woman's body. Regular contractions cause progressive dilatation of the cervix and sufficient muscular force to allow the baby to be pushed to the outside. It is a time of change, both an ending and a beginning, for a woman, a fetus, and her family.

Labor and birth require a woman to use all the psychological and physical coping methods she has available. Regardless of the amount of childbirth preparation or the number of times she has been through the experience before, family-focused nursing care is needed to support the family as they mark the beginning of a new family structure. This need is further emphasized by National Health Goals (Box 18.1).

Nursing Process Overview

For a Woman in Labor

Labor and birth are enormous emotional and physiologic accomplishments, not only for a woman but for her support person as well. For this reason, support persons should be treated with respect and included in all phases of the process whenever possible. Interventions that make the experience more positive and memorable for them help to contribute to future family interactions.

● Assessment

Assessment of a woman in labor must be done quickly yet thoroughly and gently. A woman is keenly aware of words spoken around her and the manner with which procedures are carried out. Because of this sensitivity, she may perceive a venipuncture as a very painful experience. She may have difficulty relaxing for a vaginal examination if she fears that pressure on the fetal head will cause her pain. Remember that pain is a subjective symptom. Only the woman can evaluate how much she is experiencing or how much she will be able to endure.

Assess how much discomfort a woman in labor is having, not only by what she scores on a pain scale, but also by subtle signs of pain such as facial tenseness, flushing or paleness of the face, hands clenched in a fist, rapid breathing, or rapid pulse rate. Knowing the extent of a woman's discomfort helps guide the choice of comfort interventions she may need.

● Nursing Diagnosis
Common nursing diagnoses used during labor include the following:

- Pain related to labor contractions
- Anxiety related to process of labor and birth
- Health-seeking behaviors related to management of discomfort of labor
- Situational low self-esteem related to inability to use prepared childbirth method

Although the discomfort of labor is commonly referred to as "contractions" rather than "pain," do not omit the word "pain" from a nursing diagnosis, because the term strengthens an understanding of the problem.

● Outcome Identification and Planning
When establishing expected outcomes for a woman in labor and her partner, be certain they are realistic. Because labor usually takes place over a relatively short time frame (average, 12 hours), outcomes must be met within this period. On the other hand, it is important not to project a definite time limit for labor to be completed, because the length of labor can vary greatly from person to person and still be within normal limits. It is necessary also to appreciate the magnitude of labor. It is unlikely that all the fear or anxiety experienced during a woman's labor can be alleviated. Often, because it is such an unusual and significant experience, an average couple may need assistance with using additional coping measures.

Be certain to incorporate both the woman and her support person in planning, so that the experience is a shared one. Planning may include review and education about the normal labor process. Although a couple may have learned this information during pregnancy, the reality of labor may seem much different from what they imagined. Planning also must be flexible, changing with the progress of labor, and individualized, allowing a woman to experience the significance of the event for herself.

BOX 18.1 FOCUS ON . . .

NATIONAL HEALTH GOALS

Because labor and birth are high-risk times for both the fetus and the mother, a number of National Health Goals speak directly to them (DHHS, 2000):

- Reduce the rate of maternal deaths to no more than 3.3/100,000 live births, from a baseline of 7.1/100,000.
- Reduce the rate of fetal deaths at 20 or more weeks' gestation to no more than 4.1/1000 live births, from a baseline of 6.8/1000.
- Reduce the rate of fetal and infant deaths during the perinatal period (28 weeks' gestation to 7 days after birth) to no more than 4.5/1,000 live births, from a baseline of 7.5/1,000 live births.

Nurses can help the nation achieve these goals by closely monitoring women during labor and birth and by teaching women as much as possible about labor, so that they are able to use as little analgesia and anesthesia as possible. The less anesthesia and analgesia used, the fewer the complications that can result in fetal or maternal death.

Topics that could benefit from additional nursing research in this area are advantages and disadvantages of various birthing settings; the best way to teach unprepared women the breathing patterns for labor; how support people can best be prepared for their role; and advantages and disadvantages of various birthing or labor positions.

Comfort promotion is vital. A plan that addresses the discomforts of labor includes planning for education, validation, and response to a woman's pain to help her maintain realistic perceptions about it. Be certain to include nonpharmacologic comfort measures such as changing a wet sheet or offering a moisturizing cream for dry lips.

● *Implementation*

Interventions in labor must always be carried out between contractions if possible, so that the woman is free to use a prepared childbirth technique to limit the discomfort of contractions. This calls for good coordination of care among health care providers and planning with the woman and her support person. The person a woman chooses to stay with her during childbirth can be a husband, the father of the child, a sister or parent, or a close friend. Which of these persons a woman chooses is somewhat culturally determined.

It is important for women to be able to understand what is happening to them during labor. If the woman is not proficient in English, make arrangements to locate an interpreter. If she is hearing challenged, it is the hospital's responsibility to provide an interpreter for her so that she can receive adequate explanations of her progress. Remember that whether a woman enjoys being touched or not during labor is in part culturally determined. Assess early in a woman's labor whether she might benefit from such caring measures as having her hand held or her back rubbed.

● *Outcome Evaluation*

During labor, evaluation must be ongoing to preserve the safety of the woman and her new child. After birth, evaluation helps to determine a woman's opinion of her experience with labor and birth. Ideally, the experience should be not only one that she was able to endure but one that allowed her self-esteem to grow and the family to grow through a shared experience. It is advantageous to talk to women in the early postpartum period about their labor experience. Doing so serves as a means of evaluating nursing care during labor. It also provides a woman the chance to "work through" this experience and incorporate it into her self-image. Examples of possible outcome criteria include the following:

• Client states that pain during labor was tolerable because of her advance preparation.
• Client verbalizes that her need for additional comfort measures was met.
• Client and family members state that the labor and birth experience was a positive growth experience for them, both individually and as a family.

THEORIES OF LABOR ONSET

Labor normally begins when a fetus is sufficiently mature to cope with extrauterine life yet not too large to cause mechanical difficulty with birth. The trigger that converts the random, painless Braxton Hicks contractions into strong, coordinated, productive labor contractions is unknown. In some instances, labor begins before a fetus is mature (preterm birth). In others, labor is delayed until the fetus and the placenta have both passed beyond the optimal point for birth (postterm birth).

Although a number of theories have been proposed to explain why labor begins, it is believed that labor is influenced by a combination of factors originating from the mother and the fetus (Katz, 2003). These factors include the following:

• Uterine muscle stretching, which results in release of prostaglandins
• Pressure on the cervix, which stimulates the release of oxytocin from the posterior pituitary
• Oxytocin stimulation, which works together with prostaglandins to initiate contractions
• Change in the ratio of estrogen to progesterone (increasing estrogen in relation to progesterone stimulates uterine contractions)
• Placental age, which triggers contractions at a set point
• Rising fetal cortisol levels, which reduce progesterone formation and increase prostaglandin formation
• Fetal membrane production of prostaglandin, which stimulates contractions

SIGNS OF LABOR

Preliminary Signs of Labor

Before labor, a woman often experiences subtle signs that signal the onset of labor. All pregnant women should be taught these signs so that they can recognize when labor is beginning.

Lightening

In primiparas, lightening, or descent of the fetal presenting part into the pelvis, occurs approximately 10 to 14 days before labor begins. This changes a woman's abdominal contour, because the uterus becomes lower and more anterior. Lightening gives a woman relief from the diaphragmatic pressure and shortness of breath that she has been experiencing and in this way "lightens" her load. Lightening probably occurs early in primiparas because of tight abdominal muscles. In multiparas, it is not as dramatic and usually occurs on the day of labor or even after labor has begun. As the fetus sinks lower in the pelvis, the mother may experience shooting leg pains from the increased pressure on the sciatic nerve, increased amounts of vaginal discharge, and urinary frequency from pressure on the bladder.

Increase in Level of Activity

A woman may awaken on the morning of labor full of energy, in contrast to her feelings of chronic fatigue during the previous month. This increase in activity is related to an increase in epinephrine release that is initiated by a decrease in progesterone produced by the placenta. Additional epinephrine prepares a woman's body for the work of labor ahead.

Braxton Hicks Contractions

In the last week or days before labor begins, a woman usually notices extremely strong Braxton Hicks contractions, which she may interpret as true labor contractions. Table 18.1 summarizes the ways in which these contractions can be differentiated from true labor.

Primiparas may have great difficulty in distinguishing between the two forms of contractions. A woman may be admitted to the labor unit of a hospital or birthing center because false contractions so closely simulate true labor. It is discouraging for a woman who is having what seem like contractions (and strong Braxton Hicks contractions cause real discomfort) to be told she is not in true labor and should return home. When this happens, the woman needs sympathetic support. She can be reassured that misinterpreting labor signals is common. Remind her that if false contractions have become strong enough to be mistaken for true labor, true labor must not be far away.

Ripening of the Cervix

Ripening of the cervix is an internal sign seen only on pelvic examination. Throughout pregnancy, the cervix feels softer than normal, similar to the consistency of an earlobe (Goodell's sign). At term, the cervix becomes still softer (described as "butter-soft"), and it tips forward. Ripening is an internal announcement that labor is very close at hand.

Signs of True Labor

Signs of true labor involve uterine and cervical changes. The more a woman knows about true labor signs, the better, because then she will be better able to recognize them. This is helpful both to prevent preterm birth and for the woman to feel secure knowing what is happening during labor.

Uterine Contractions

The surest sign that labor has begun is productive uterine contractions. Because contractions are involuntary and come without warning, their intensity can be frightening in early labor. Helping a woman appreciate that she can predict her pattern and therefore can control the degree of discomfort she feels by using breathing exercises offers her a sense of control.

Show

As the cervix softens and ripens, the mucus plug that filled the cervical canal during pregnancy (operculum) is expelled. The exposed cervical capillaries seep blood as a result of pressure exerted by the fetus. The blood, mixed with mucus, takes on a pink tinge and is referred to as "show" or "bloody show." Women need to be aware of this event so that they do not think they are bleeding abnormally.

Rupture of the Membranes

Labor may begin with rupture of the membranes, experienced either as a sudden gush or as scanty, slow seeping of clear fluid from the vagina. Some women may worry if their labor begins with rupture of the membranes, because they have heard that labor will then be "dry" and that this will cause it to be difficult and long. Actually, amniotic fluid continues to be produced until delivery of the membranes after the birth of a fetus, so no labor is ever "dry." Early rupture of the membranes can be advantageous if it causes the fetal head to settle snugly into the pelvis; this can actually shorten labor.

Two risks associated with ruptured membranes are intrauterine infection and prolapse of the umbilical cord, which can cut off the oxygen supply to the fetus. In most instances, if labor has not spontaneously occurred by 24 hours after membrane rupture and the pregnancy is at term, labor is induced to help reduce these risks.

TABLE 18.1	
Differentiation Between True and False Labor Contractions	
False Contractions	**True Contractions**
Begin and remain irregular.	Begin irregularly but become regular and predictable.
Felt first abdominally and remain confined to the abdomen and groin.	Felt first in lower back and sweep around to the abdomen in a wave.
Often disappear with ambulation and sleep.	Continue no matter what the woman's level of activity.
Do not increase in duration, frequency, or intensity.	Increase in duration, frequency, and intensity.
Do not achieve cervical dilatation.	Achieve cervical dilatation.

Checkpoint Question 1

Celeste Bailey didn't recognize for over an hour that she was in labor. A sign of true labor is:

a. Sudden increased energy from epinephrine release.
b. "Nagging" but constant pain in the lower back.
c. Urinary urgency from increased bladder pressure.
d. "Show" or release of the cervical mucus plug.

COMPONENTS OF LABOR

A successful labor depends on four integrated concepts: (1) the woman's pelvis (the *passage*) is of adequate size and contour; (2) the *passenger* (the fetus) is of appropriate size and in an advantageous position and presentation; (3) the *powers* of labor (uterine factors) are adequate; and (4) a woman's *psyche* is preserved, so that afterward labor can be viewed as a positive experience.

Passage

The passage refers to the route a fetus must travel from the uterus through the cervix and vagina to the external perineum. Because the cervix and vagina are contained inside the pelvis, a fetus must also pass through the bony pelvic ring. (Pelvic anatomy is discussed in Chapter 4; see Figs. 4.12 and 4.13.) For a fetus to pass through the pelvis, the pelvis must be of adequate size. Two pelvic measurements are important to determine the adequacy of the pelvic size: the diagonal conjugate (the anterior-posterior diameter of the inlet) and the transverse diameter of the outlet (see Figs. 10.10 and 10.11 in Chapter 10). At the pelvic inlet, the anteroposterior diameter is the narrowest diameter; at the outlet, the transverse diameter is the narrowest (Fig. 18.1).

In most instances, if a disproportion between fetus and pelvis occurs, the pelvis is the structure at fault. If the fetus is causing the problem, it is often because the fetal head is presented to the birth canal at less than its narrowest diameter, not because the head is actually too large. Keep this in mind when discussing with parents why an infant cannot be born vaginally. In this situation, emphasize that it is the pelvis that is too small, not that the head is too big. For parents to learn that a child cannot be born vaginally because the mother's pelvis is too small can be upsetting. It can be much more upsetting, however, to think that their infant's head is too large, because it implies that something is seriously wrong with the baby (which usually is not the case). Avoiding this type of negative thought helps promote good parent–child bonding.

Passenger

The passenger is the fetus. The body part of the fetus that has the widest diameter is the head, so this is the part least likely to be able to pass through the pelvic ring. Whether a fetal skull can pass or not depends on both its structure (bones, fontanelles, and suture lines) and its alignment with the pelvis.

Structure of the Fetal Skull

The cranium, the uppermost portion of the skull, comprises eight bones. The four superior bones—the frontal (actually two fused bones), the two parietal, and the occipital—are the bones that are important in childbirth. The other four bones of the skull (sphenoid, ethmoid, and two temporal bones) lie at the base of the cranium; they are of little significance in childbirth because they are never presenting parts. The chin, referred to by its Latin name *mentum,* can be a presenting part.

The bones of the skull meet at suture lines. The sagittal suture joins the two parietal bones of the skull. The coronal suture is the line of juncture of the frontal bones and the two parietal bones. The lambdoid suture is the line of juncture of the occipital bone and the two parietal bones. The suture lines are important in birth because, as membranous interspaces, they allow the cranial bones to move and overlap, molding or diminishing the size of the skull so that it can pass through the birth canal more readily.

Significant membrane-covered spaces called the fontanelles are found at the junction of the main suture lines. The anterior fontanelle (sometimes referred to as the bregma) lies at the junction of the coronal and sagittal sutures. Because the frontal bone consists of two fused bones, four bones (counting the two parietal bones) are actually involved at this junction, making the anterior fontanelle diamond-shaped. Its anteroposterior diameter measures approximately 3 to 4 cm; its transverse diameter, 2 to 3 cm.

The posterior fontanelle lies at the junction of the lambdoidal and sagittal sutures. Because the two parietal bones and the occipital bone are involved at this junction, the posterior fontanelle is triangular. It is smaller than the anterior fontanelle, measuring approximately 2 cm across its widest part. Fontanelle spaces compress during birth to aid in molding of the fetal head. Their presence can be assessed manually through the cervix after it has dilatated during labor. This helps to establish the position of the fetal head and whether it is in a favorable position for birth. The space between the two fontanelles is referred to as the vertex (Fig. 18.2). The area over the frontal bone

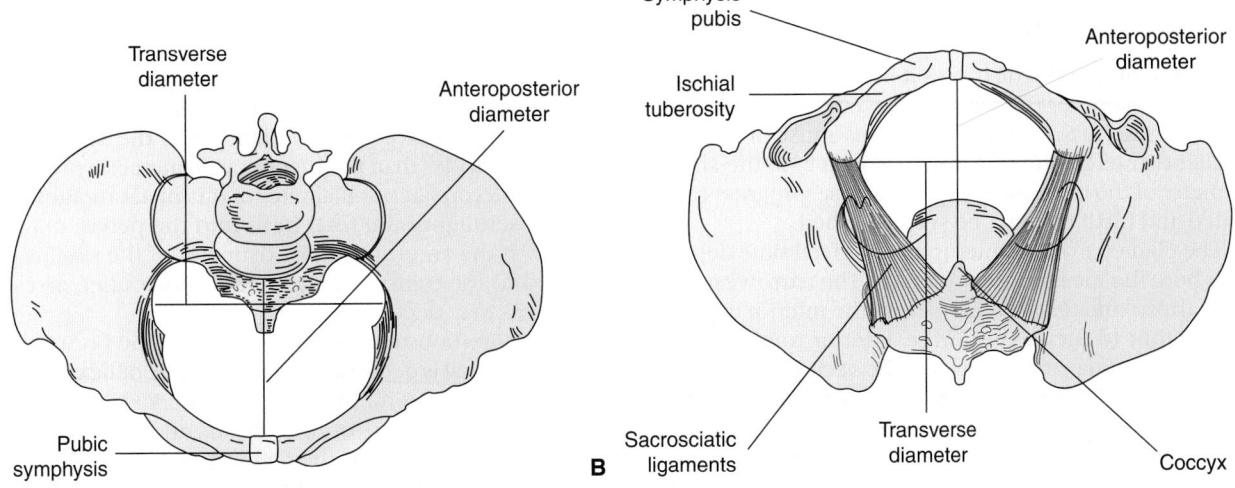

FIGURE 18.1 Views of the pelvic inlet and outlet: (**A**) pelvic inlet; (**B**) pelvic outlet.

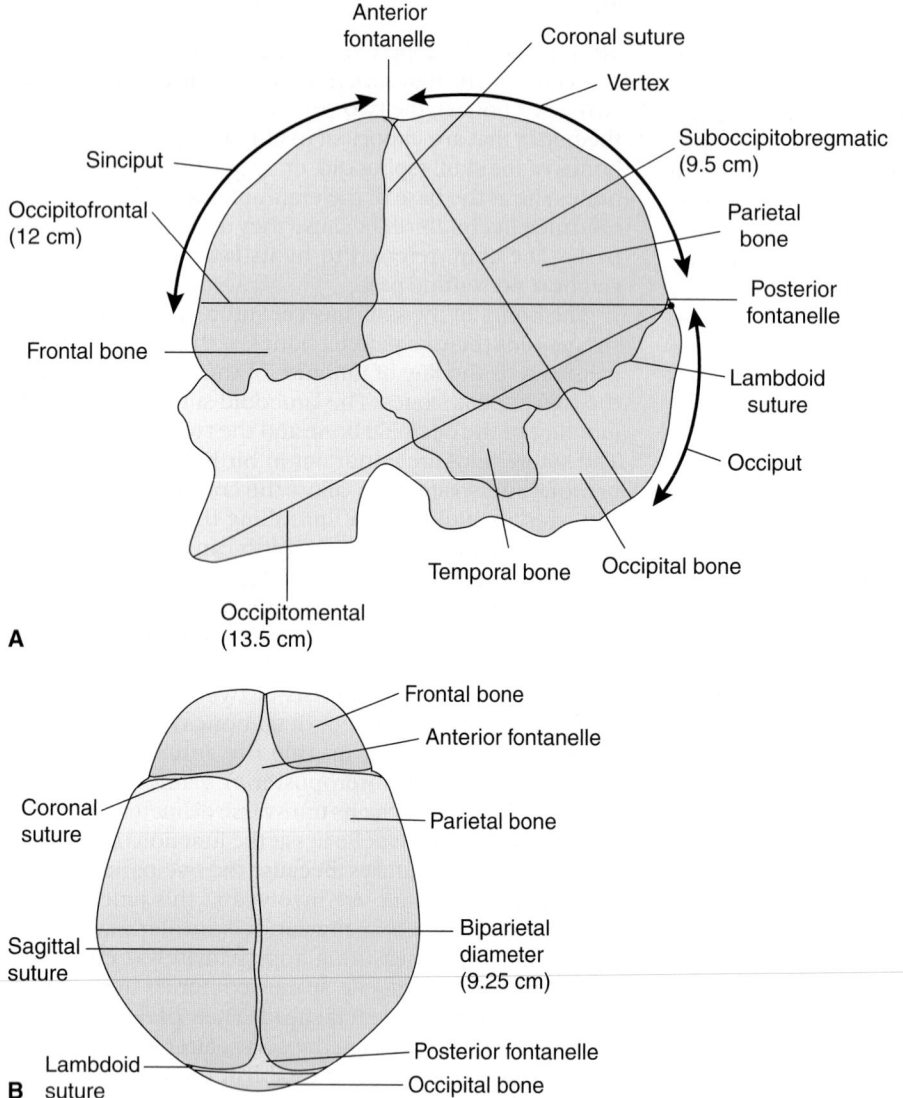

A

B

FIGURE 18.2 The fetal skull: (**A**) lateral view; (**B**) vertex view.

is referred to as the sinciput. The area over the occipital bone is referred to as the occiput.

Diameters of the Fetal Skull

The shape of a fetal skull causes it to be wider in its anteroposterior diameter than in its transverse diameter. To fit through the birth canal best, a fetus must present the smaller diameter (the transverse diameter) to the smaller diameter of the maternal pelvis; otherwise, progress can be halted and birth may not be accomplished.

The diameter of the anteroposterior fetal skull depends on where the measurement is taken. The narrowest diameter (approximately 9.5 cm) is from the inferior aspect of the occiput to the center of the anterior fontanelle (the suboccipitobregmatic diameter). The occipitofrontal diameter, measured from the bridge of the nose to the occipital prominence, is approximately 12 cm. The occipitomental diameter, which is the widest anteroposterior diameter (approximately 13.5 cm), is measured from the chin to the posterior fontanelle.

Because the anteroposterior diameter of the pelvis, a space approximately 11 cm wide, is the narrowest pelvic inlet diameter, a fetus must present the biparietal diameter, the narrowest fetal head diameter (approximately 9.25 cm), to this inlet (see Fig. 18.2A). At the outlet, this narrowest fetal head diameter must be presented to the maternal transverse diameter, a space approximately 11 cm wide. If the anteroposterior diameter of the skull (a measurement wider than the biparietal diameter) is presented to the anteroposterior diameter of the inlet, **engagement,** or the settling of the fetal head into the pelvis, may not occur. If the anteroposterior diameter of the skull is presented to the transverse diameter of the outlet, arrest of progress may occur.

The anteroposterior diameter that will be presented to the birth canal is determined by the degree of flexion of the fetal head (Fig. 18.3). In full flexion, a fetal head flexes so sharply the chin rests on the thorax, and the smallest anteroposterior diameter, the suboccipitobregmatic, is presented to the birth canal. If the head is held in moderate flexion, the occipitofrontal diameter will be presented. In

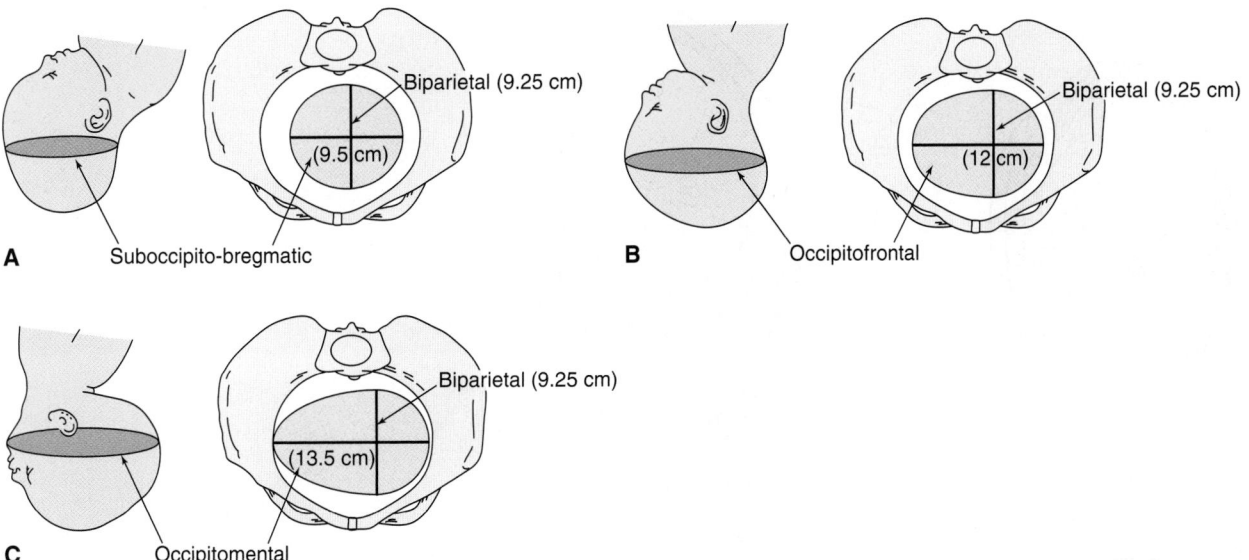

FIGURE 18.3 (A) Complete flexion allows the smallest diameter of the head to enter the pelvis. **(B)** Moderate flexion causes a larger diameter to enter the pelvis. **(C)** Poor flexion forces the largest diameter against the pelvic brim, but the head is too large to enter the pelvis.

poor flexion (the head hyperextended), the largest diameter (the occipitomental) will present.

These wider fetal head diameters must fit through the transverse diameter of the pelvic inlet, a space of approximately 12.4 to 13.5 cm; and at the outlet, through the anteroposterior diameter of the pelvis, a space of 9.5 to 11.5 cm. Good head flexion is important because it follows that a fetal head presenting a diameter of 9.5 cm will fit through a pelvis much more readily than if the diameter is 12.0 or 13.5 cm.

Molding

Molding is the change in shape of the fetal skull produced by the force of uterine contractions pressing the vertex of the head against the not-yet-dilatated cervix. Because the bones of the fetal skull are not yet completely ossified and therefore do not form a rigid structure, pressure causes them to overlap and cause the head to become narrower and longer, a shape that facilitates passage through the rigid pelvis. Molding is commonly seen in infants just after birth. The overlapping of the sagittal suture line and, generally, the coronal suture line can be easily palpated in the newborn skull. Parents can be reassured that molding only lasts a day or two and is not a permanent condition. There is little molding when the brow is the presenting part (described later), because frontal bones are fused. No skull molding occurs when a fetus is breech, because the buttocks, not the head, are presented first.

Fetal Presentation and Position

Two other factors play a part in whether a fetus is lined up in the best position to be born: fetal presentation and position.

Attitude. **Attitude** describes the degree of flexion a fetus assumes during labor or the relation of the fetal parts to each other (Fig. 18.4). A fetus in *good* attitude is in complete flexion: the spinal column is bowed forward, the head is flexed forward so much that the chin touches the sternum, the arms are flexed and folded on the chest, the thighs are flexed onto the abdomen, and the calves are pressed against the posterior aspect of the thighs (see Fig. 18.4*A*). This normal "fetal position" is advantageous for birth because it helps a fetus present the smallest anteroposterior diameter of the skull to the pelvis and also because it puts the whole body into an ovoid shape, occupying the smallest space possible.

A fetus is in *moderate* flexion if the chin is not touching the chest but is in an alert or "military position" (see Fig. 18.4*B*). This position causes the next-widest anteroposterior diameter, the occipital frontal diameter, to present to the birth canal. A fair number of fetuses assume a military position during the early part of labor. This does not usually interfere with labor, because during later mechanisms of labor (descent and flexion) the fetus is forced to flex the head fully.

A fetus in partial extension presents the "brow" of the head to the birth canal (see Fig. 18.4*C*). If a fetus is in poor flexion, the back is arched, the neck is extended, and a fetus is in complete extension, presenting the occipitomental diameter of the head to the birth canal (face presentation; see Fig. 18.4*D*). This unusual position presents too wide a skull diameter to the birth canal for normal birth. Such a position may occur if there is less than the normal amount of amniotic fluid present (oligohydramnios), which does not allow a fetus adequate movement. It also may reflect a neurologic abnormality causing spasticity.

Engagement. Engagement refers to the settling of the presenting part of a fetus far enough into the pelvis to be at the level of the ischial spines, a midpoint of the pelvis.

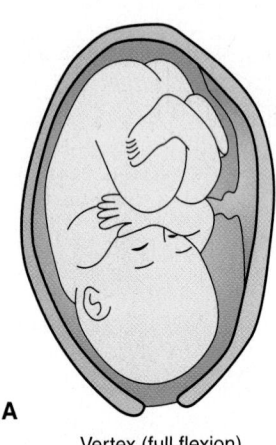

A
Vertex (full flexion)

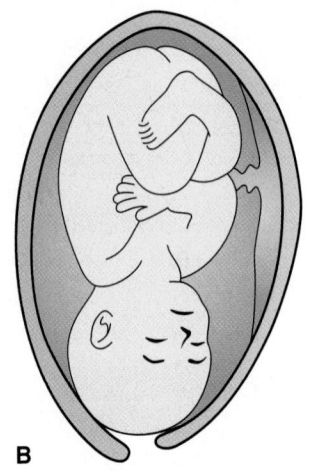

B
Sinciput (moderate flexion [military attitude])

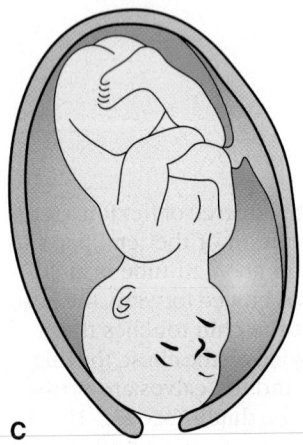

C
Brow (partial extension)

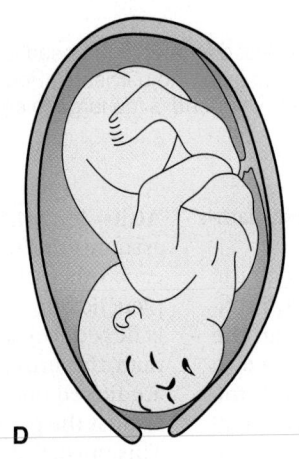

D
Face (poor flexion, complete extension)

FIGURE 18.4 Fetal attitude. (**A**) Fetus in full flexion presents smallest (suboccipito-bregmatic) anteroposterior diameter of skull to inlet in this good attitude (vertex presentation). (**B**) Fetus is not as well flexed (military attitude) as in A and presents occipitofrontal diameter to inlet (sinciput presentation). (**C**) Fetus in partial extension (brow presentation). (**D**) Fetus in complete extension presents wide (occipitomental) diameter (face presentation).

Descent to this point means that the widest part of the fetus (the biparietal diameter in a cephalic presentation; the intertrochanteric diameter in a breech presentation) has passed through the pelvis or the pelvic inlet is proven adequate for birth. In a primipara, nonengagement of the head at the beginning of labor indicates a possible complication, such as an abnormal presentation or position, abnormality of the fetal head, or cephalopelvic disproportion. In multiparas, engagement may or may not be present at the beginning of labor. The degree of engagement is assessed by vaginal and cervical examination. A presenting part that is not engaged is said to be "floating." One that is descending but has not yet reached the ischial spines is said to be "dipping."

Station. **Station** refers to the relationship of the presenting part of a fetus to the level of the ischial spines (Fig. 18.5). When the presenting part is at the level of the ischial spines, it is at a 0 station (synonymous with engagement). If the presenting part is above the spines, the distance is measured and described as minus stations, which range from −1 to −4 cm. If the presenting part is below the ischial spines, the distance is stated as plus stations (+1 to +4 cm). At a +3 or +4 station, the presenting part is at the perineum and can be seen if the vulva is separated (i.e., it is crowning).

Fetal Lie. **Lie** is the relationship between the long (cephalocaudal) axis of the fetal body and the long (cephalocaudal) axis of a woman's body; in other words, whether the fetus is lying in a horizontal (transverse) or a vertical (longitudinal) position. Approximately 99% of fetuses assume

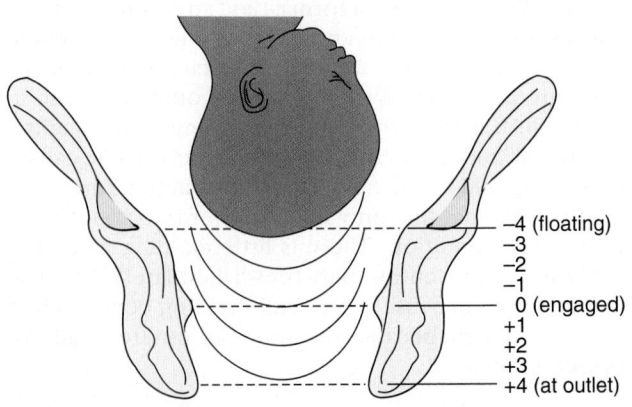

FIGURE 18.5 Station (anteroposterior view). Station, or degree of engagement, of the fetal head is designated by centimeters above or below the ischial spines. At −4 station, head is "floating." At 0 station, head is "engaged." At +4 station, head is "at outlet."

a longitudinal lie (with their long axis parallel to the long axis of the woman). Longitudinal lies are further classified as cephalic, which means the head will be the first part to contact the cervix, or breech, with the breech, or buttocks, as the first portion to contact the cervix.

Types of Fetal Presentation

Fetal presentation denotes the body part that will first contact the cervix or be born first. This is determined by a combination of fetal lie and the degree of fetal flexion (attitude).

Cephalic Presentation. A **cephalic presentation** is the most frequent type of presentation, occurring as often as 95% of the time. With this type of presentation, the fetal head is the body part that will first contact the cervix. The four types of cephalic presentation (vertex, brow, face, and mentum) are described in Table 18.2. The vertex is the ideal presenting part, because the skull bones are capable of molding so effectively to accommodate the cervix. It also may actually aid in cervical dilatation and prevents complications such as a prolapsed cord (i.e., a portion of the cord passing between the presenting part and the cervix and entering the vagina before the fetus does) (Cruikshank, 2003). During labor, the area of the fetal skull that contacts the cervix often becomes edematous from the continued pressure against it. This edema is called a caput succedaneum. In the newborn, the point of presentation can be analyzed from the location of the caput.

Breech Presentation. A **breech presentation** means that either the buttocks or the feet are the first body parts that will contact the cervix. Breech presentations occur in approximately 3% of births and are affected by fetal attitude. A good attitude brings the fetal knees up against the umbilicus; a poor attitude means that the knees are extended. Breech presentations can be difficult births, with the presenting point influencing the degree of difficulty. Three types of breech presentation (complete, frank, and footling) are possible (Table 18.3).

Shoulder Presentation. In a transverse lie, a fetus lies horizontally in the pelvis so that the longest fetal axis is perpendicular to that of the mother. The presenting part is usually one of the shoulders (acromion process), an iliac crest, a hand, or an elbow (Fig. 18.6).

Fewer than 1% of fetuses lie transversely. This presentation may be caused by relaxed abdominal walls from grand multiparity, which allow the unsupported uterus to fall forward. Another cause is pelvic contraction, in which the horizontal space is greater than the vertical space. Placenta previa (in which the placenta is located low in the uterus, obscuring some of the vertical space) may also limit a fetus' ability to turn, resulting in a transverse lie. With a transverse lie, the usual contour of the abdomen at term is distorted or is fuller side to side rather than top to bottom.

If an infant is preterm and smaller than usual, an attempt to turn the fetus to a horizontal lie may be made. Most infants in a transverse lie must be born by cesarean birth, however, because they cannot be turned and cannot be born normally from this "wedged" position. Discovering a shoulder presentation is an important assessment, because it almost always identifies a birth position that puts both mother and child in jeopardy unless skilled health care personnel are available to complete a cesarean birth.

Types of Fetal Position

Position is the relationship of the presenting part to a specific quadrant of a woman's pelvis. For convenience, the maternal pelvis is divided into four quadrants according to the mother's right and left: (1) right anterior, (2) left anterior, (3) right posterior, and (4) left posterior.

Four parts of a fetus have been chosen as landmarks to describe the relationship of the presenting part to one of the pelvic quadrants. In a vertex presentation, the occiput is the chosen point; in a face presentation, it is the chin (mentum); in a breech presentation, it is the sacrum; in a shoulder presentation, it is the scapula or the acromion process.

TABLE 18.2

Types of Cephalic Presentation

Type	Lie	Attitude	Description
Vertex	Longitudinal	Good (full flexion)	The head is sharply flexed, making the parietal bones or the space between the fontanelles (the vertex) the presenting part. This is the most common presentation and allows the suboccipitobregmatic diameter to present to the cervix.
Brow	Longitudinal	Moderate (military)	Because the head is only moderately flexed, the brow or sinciput becomes the presenting part.
Face	Longitudinal	Poor	The fetus has extended the head to make the face the presenting part. From this position, extreme edema and distortion of the face may occur. The presenting diameter (the occipitomental) is so wide that birth may be impossible.
Mentum	Longitudinal	Very poor	The fetus has completely hyperextended the head to present the chin. The widest diameter (occipitomental) is presenting. As a rule, the fetus cannot enter the pelvis in this presentation.

TABLE 18.3

Types of Breech Presentation

Type	Lie	Attitude	Description
Complete	Longitudinal	Good (full flexion)	The fetus has thighs tightly flexed on the abdomen; both the buttocks and the tightly flexed feet present to the cervix.

Frank	Longitudinal	Moderate	Attitude is moderate because the hips are flexed but the knees are extended to rest on the chest. The buttocks alone present to the cervix.

Footling	Longitudinal	Poor	Neither the thighs nor lower legs are flexed. If one foot presents, it is a single-footling breech; if both present, it is a double-footling breech.

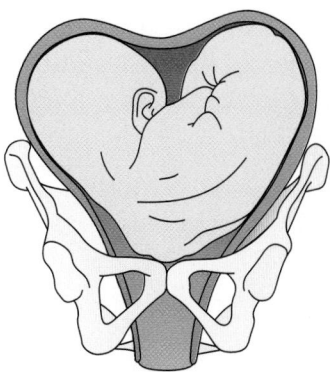

FIGURE 18.6 Transverse or shoulder presentation.

Position is indicated by an abbreviation of three letters. The middle letter denotes the fetal landmark (O for occiput, M for mentum or chin, Sa for sacrum, and A for acromion process). The first letter defines whether the landmark is pointing to the mother's right (R) or left (L). The last letter defines whether the landmark points anteriorly (A), posteriorly (P), or transversely (T).

If the occiput of a fetus points to the left anterior quadrant in a vertex position, for example, this is a left occipitoanterior (LOA) position. If the occiput points to the right posterior quadrant, the position is right occipitoposterior (ROP). LOA is the most common fetal position, and right occipitoanterior (ROA) the second most frequent. Box 18.2 summarizes the possible positions. Six common positions in cephalic presentations are depicted in Figure 18.7.

Position is important, because it influences the process and efficiency of labor. Typically, a fetus is born fastest from an ROA or LOA position. Labor is considerably extended if the position is posterior (ROP or LOP). Posterior positions may also be more painful for the mother, because the rotation of the fetal head puts pressure on the sacral nerves, causing sharp back pain.

Checkpoint Question 2

Celeste asks you which fetal position and presentation are ideal. Your best answer would be:

a. Right occipitoanterior with full flexion.
b. Left transverse anterior in moderate flexion.
c. Right occipitoposterior with no flexion.
d. Left sacroanterior with full flexion.

Mechanisms (Cardinal Movements) of Labor

Passage of a fetus through the birth canal involves a number of different position changes to keep the smallest diameter of the fetal head (in cephalic presentations) always presenting to the smallest diameter of the birth canal. These position changes are termed the **cardinal movements of labor:** descent, flexion, internal rotation, extension, external rotation, and expulsion (Fig. 18.8).

BOX 18.2

Possible Fetal Positions

Vertex Presentation (occiput)
LOA, left occipitoanterior
LOP, left occipitoposterior
LOT, left occipitotransverse
ROA, right occipitoanterior
ROP, right occipitoposterior
ROT, right occipitotransverse

Breech Presentation (sacrum)
LSaA, left sacroanterior
LSaP, left sacroposterior
LSaT, left sacrotransverse
RSaA, right sacroanterior
RSaP, right sacroposterior
RSaT, right sacrotransverse

Face Presentation (mentum)
LMA, left mentoanterior
LMP, left mentoposterior
LMT, left mentotransverse
RMA, right mentoanterior
RMP, right mentoposterior
RMT, right mentotransverse

Shoulder Presentation (acromion process)
LAA, left scapuloanterior
LAP, left scapuloposterior
RAA, right scapuloanterior
RAP, right scapuloposterior

Descent. Descent is the downward movement of the biparietal diameter of the fetal head to within the pelvic inlet. Full descent occurs when the fetal head extrudes beyond the dilated cervix and touches the posterior vaginal floor. Descent occurs because of pressure on the fetus by the uterine fundus. The pressure of the fetal head on the sacral nerves at the pelvic floor causes the mother to experience a pushing sensation. Full descent may be aided by abdominal muscle contraction as the woman pushes.

Flexion. As descent occurs and the fetal head reaches the pelvic floor, the head bends forward onto the chest, making the smallest anteroposterior diameter (the suboccipitobregmatic diameter) the one presented to the birth canal. Flexion is also aided by abdominal muscle contraction during pushing.

Internal Rotation. During descent, the head enters the pelvis with the fetal anteroposterior head diameter (suboccipitobregmatic, occipitomental, or occipitofrontal, depending on the amount of flexion) in a diagonal or transverse position. The head flexes as it touches the pelvic floor, and the occiput rotates until it is superior, or just below the symphysis pubis, bringing the head into the best relationship to the outlet of the pelvis (the anteroposterior diameter is now in the anteroposterior plane of the pelvis). This movement brings the shoulders, coming next, into the optimal position to enter the inlet, putting

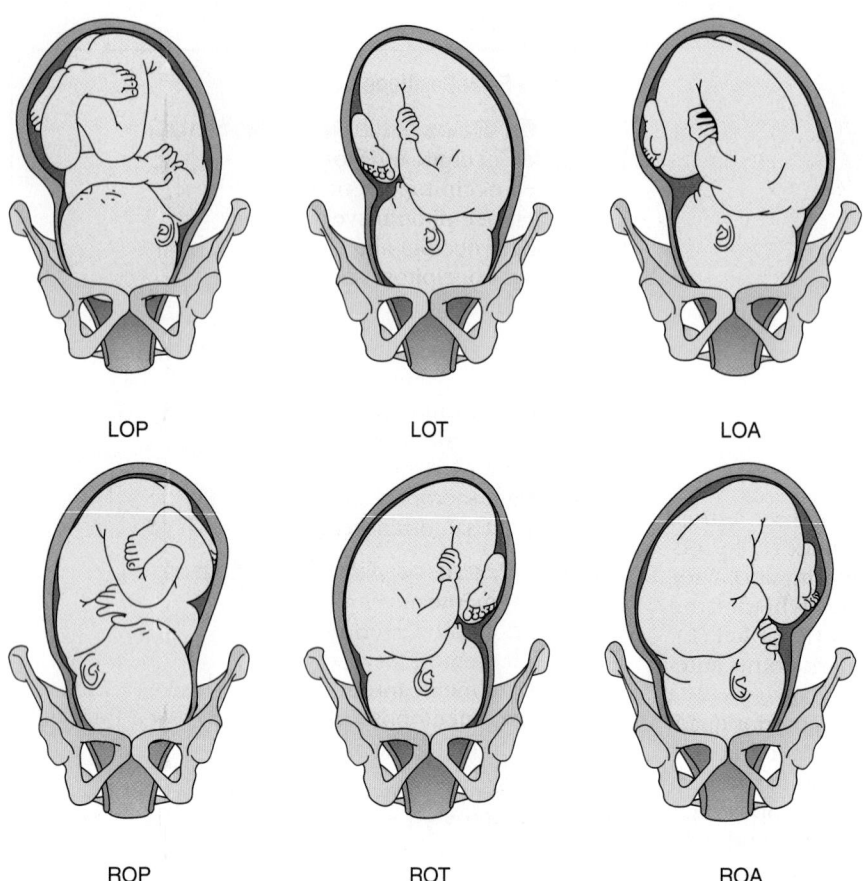

LOP   LOT   LOA

ROP   ROT   ROA

FIGURE 18.7 Fetal position. All are vertex presentations. A = anterior; L = left; O = occiput; P = posterior; R = right; T = transverse.

the widest diameter of the shoulders (a transverse one) in line with the wide transverse diameter of the inlet.

Extension. As the occiput is born, the back of the neck stops beneath the pubic arch and acts as a pivot for the rest of the head. The head extends, and the foremost parts of the head, the face and chin, are born.

External Rotation. In external rotation, almost immediately after the head of the infant is born, the head rotates (from the anteroposterior position it assumed to enter the outlet) back to the diagonal or transverse position of the early part of labor. This brings the aftercoming shoulders into an anteroposterior position, which is best for entering the outlet. The anterior shoulder is born first, assisted perhaps by downward flexion of the infant's head.

Expulsion. Once the shoulders are born, the rest of the baby is born easily and smoothly because of its smaller size. This movement, called expulsion, is the end of the pelvic division of labor.

For a view of the complete birth sequence, see Figure 18.9.

Importance of Determining Fetal Presentation and Position

It is important to document presentation and position, because the presentation of a body part other than the vertex could put a fetus at risk: it implies a proportional difference between the fetus and the pelvis (perhaps the pelvis is too narrow to allow the fetus to pass through), making

a cesarean birth necessary. The membranes also are more apt to rupture early, increasing the possibility of infection. The risk for fetal anoxia and meconium staining, complications that lead to respiratory distress at birth, are also increased.

If a body part other than the vertex presents to the cervix, labor is invariably longer due to ineffective descent of the fetus, ineffective dilatation of the cervix, or irregular and weak uterine contractions.

The less effective labor is, the longer it is, tiring the mother and reducing the excitement of the experience. If an operative birth is necessary and postoperative complications occur, the mother may require a longer hospital stay and have more pain and disability after the birth. If the fetus is born vaginally after a complicated labor, there is an increased risk for perineal tears or cervical lacerations, which may also increase a woman's disability and possibly interfere with her future childbearing. If labor is threatening and unsatisfactory, it can also interfere with maternal–child bonding.

Four methods are used to determine fetal position, presentation, and lie: (1) combined abdominal inspection and palpation, called Leopold's maneuvers; (2) vaginal examination; (3) auscultation of fetal heart tones; and (4) sonography.

Powers of Labor

The powers of labor, supplied by the fundus of the uterus, are implemented by uterine contractions, a process that

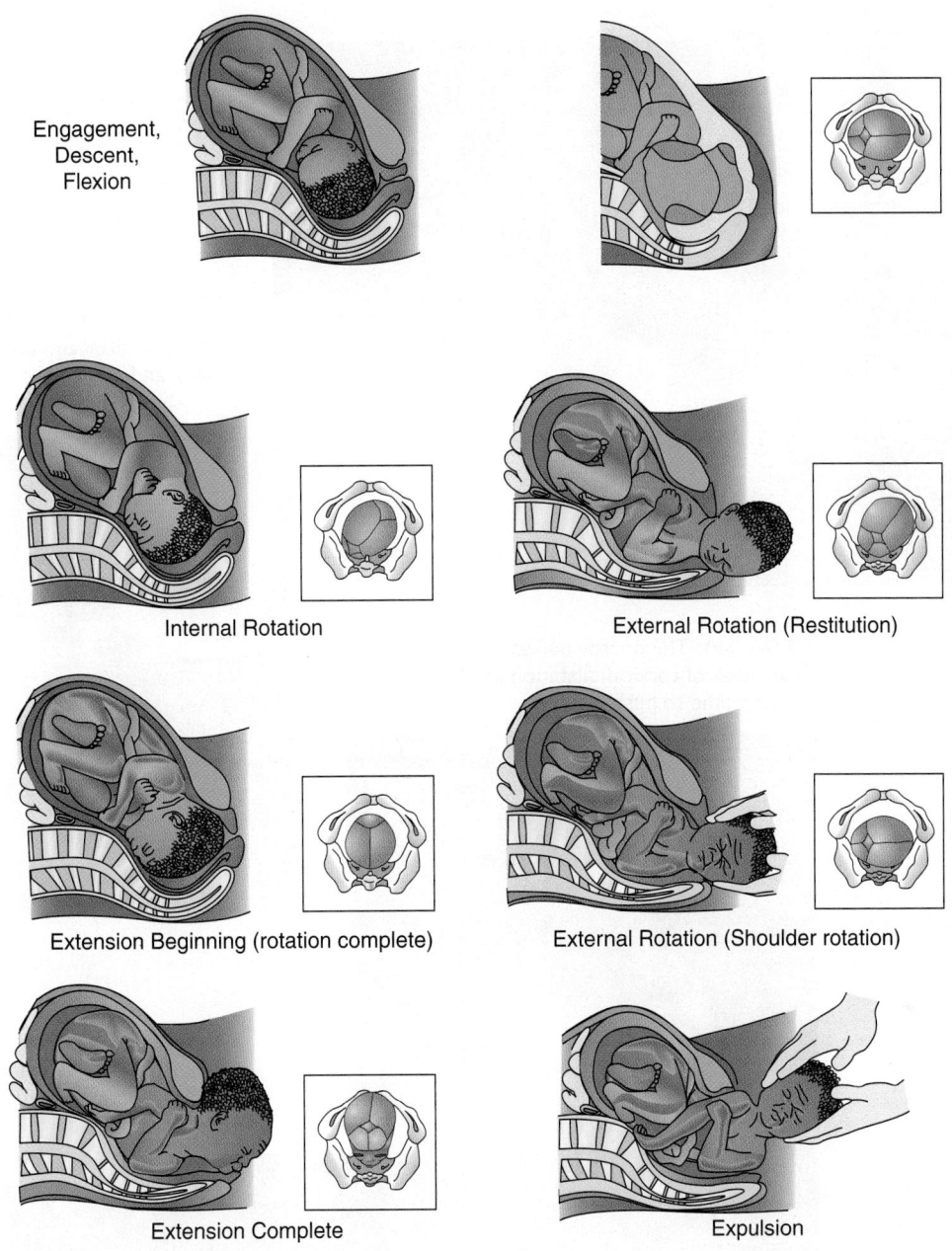

Engagement, Descent, Flexion

Internal Rotation

External Rotation (Restitution)

Extension Beginning (rotation complete)

External Rotation (Shoulder rotation)

Extension Complete

Expulsion

FIGURE 18.8 Mechanism of normal labor and cardinal positions of the fetus from a left occipitoanterior position.

causes cervical dilatation and then expulsion of the fetus from the uterus. After full dilatation of the cervix, the primary power is supplemented by use of the abdominal muscles. It is important for women to understand they should not bear down with their abdominal muscles until the cervix is fully dilatated. Doing so impedes the primary force and could cause fetal and cervical damage.

Uterine Contractions

The mark of effective uterine contractions is rhythmicity and progressive lengthening and intensity.

Origins. Like cardiac contractions, labor contractions begin at a "pacemaker" point located in the myometrium near one of the uterotubal junctions. Each contraction begins at that point and then sweeps down over the uterus as a wave. After a short rest period, another contraction is initiated and the downward sweep begins again.

In early labor, the uterotubal pacemaker may not be working in a synchronous manner. This makes contractions sometimes strong, sometimes weak, and irregular. This mild incoordination of early labor improves after a few hours as the pacemaker becomes more attuned to calcium concentrations in the myometrium and begins to function smoothly.

In some women, contractions appear to originate in the lower uterine segment rather than in the fundus. These are reverse, ineffective contractions, and they may actually cause tightening rather than dilatation of the cervix.

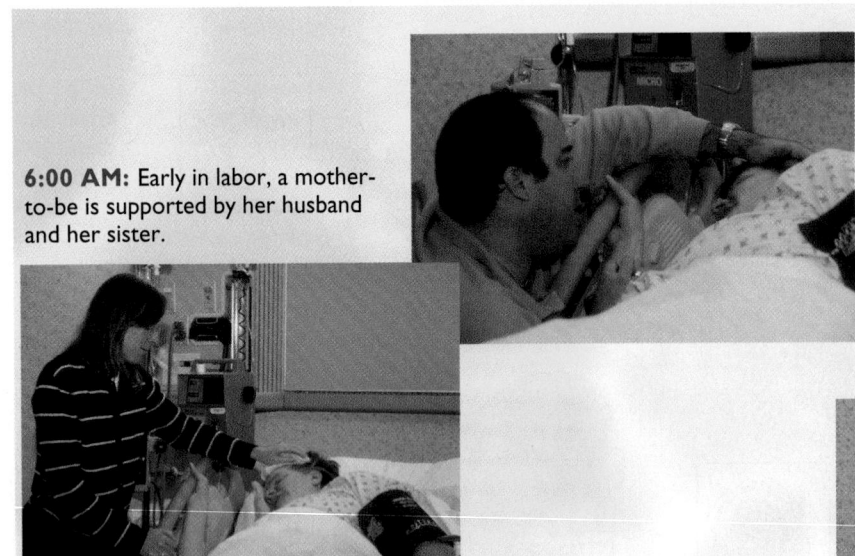

6:00 AM: Early in labor, a mother-to-be is supported by her husband and her sister.

9:00 AM: The nurse checks the fetal monitor and documents fetal and maternal status.

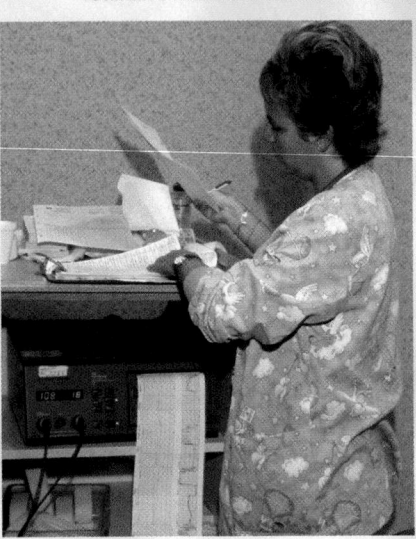

10:00 AM: The doctor makes a final check of cervical dilatation and says it's time to push.

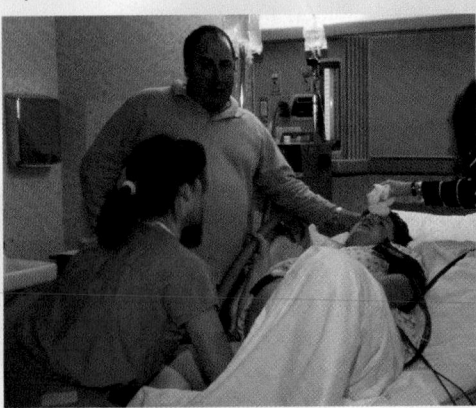

11:15 AM: She pushes from an alternative position, using a support bar.

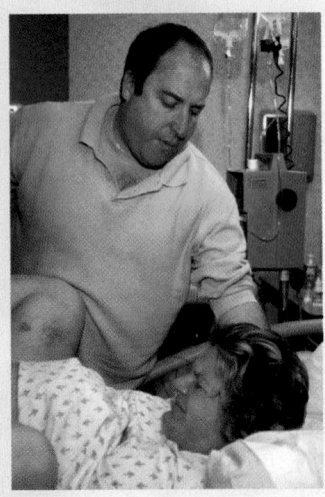

10:30 AM: The mother pushes in the lithotomy position, with her coach.

FIGURE 18.9 A day in the life of a new family.

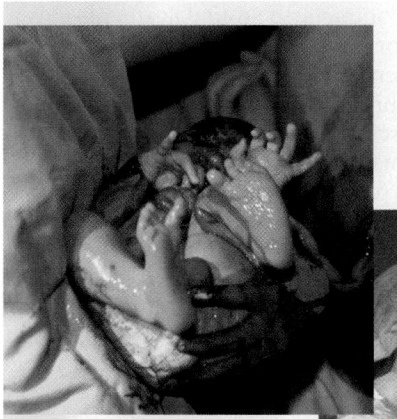

12:12 PM: Welcome to the world! Dad cuts the cord.

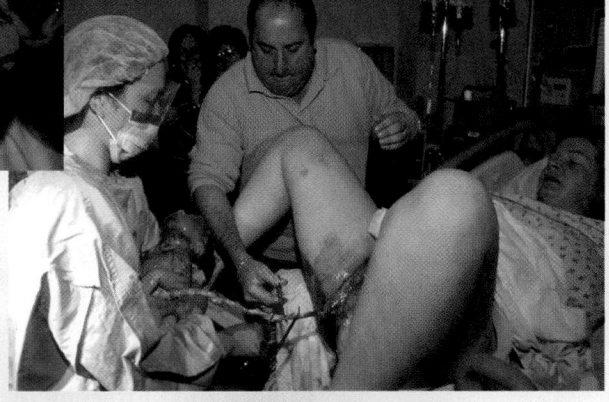

12:15 PM: Mom holds her son for the first time. Her mother and sister (now a grand-mother and aunt!) look on.

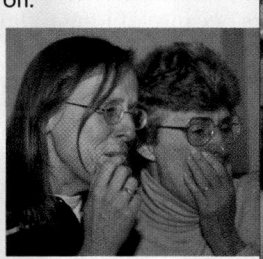

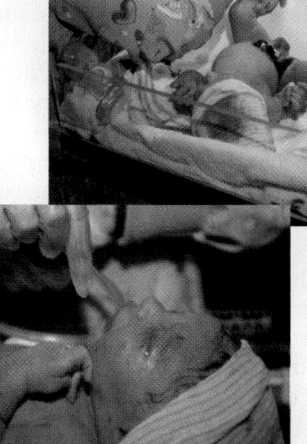

12:30 PM: The nurse suctions to clear the airway and takes the baby's footprints.

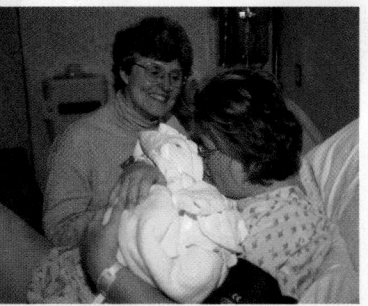

1:15 PM: Cleaned and swaddled, the newborn gets a kiss from Mom.

3:00 PM: The new mom-gives Stephen his first feeding, with support from the nurse.

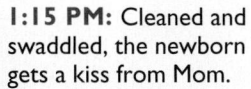

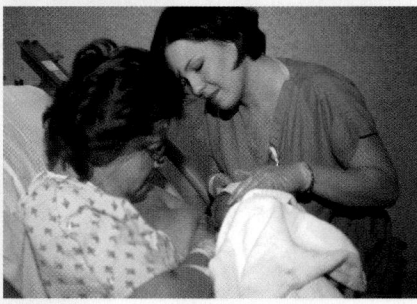

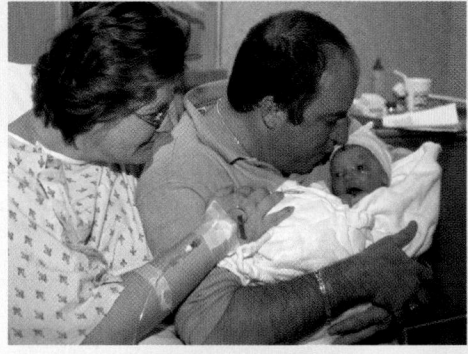

5:00 PM: New parents bond with the new member of their family.

FIGURE 18.9 (continued)

That contractions are being initiated in a reverse pattern is difficult to tell from palpation. It can be suspected if the woman tells you she feels pain in her lower abdomen before the contraction is readily palpated at the fundus. It is truly revealed only when cervical dilatation does not occur.

Some women seem to have additional pacemaker sites in other portions of the uterus. If so, contractions can be uncoordinated. Uncoordinated contractions may slow labor and can lead to failure to progress and fetal distress if they do not allow for adequate placental filling. All of these possibilities make evaluating the rate, intensity, and pattern of uterine contractions an important nursing responsibility.

Phases. A contraction consists of three phases: the increment, when the intensity of the contraction increases; the acme, when the contraction is at its strongest; and the decrement, when the intensity decreases (Fig. 18.10). Between contractions the uterus relaxes. As labor progresses, the relaxation intervals decrease from 10 minutes early in labor to only 2 to 3 minutes. The duration of contractions also changes, increasing from 20 to 30 seconds to a range of 60 to 90 seconds.

Contour Changes. As labor contractions progress and become regular and strong, the uterus gradually differentiates itself into two distinct functioning areas. The upper portion becomes thicker and active, preparing it to be able to exert the strength necessary to expel the fetus when the expulsion phase of labor is reached. The lower segment becomes thin-walled, supple, and passive, so that the fetus can be pushed out of the uterus easily. As these events occur, the boundary between the two portions becomes marked by a ridge on the inner uterine surface, the **physiologic retraction ring.**

The contour of the overall uterus also changes from a round, ovoid structure to an elongated one whose vertical diameter is markedly greater than its horizontal diameter. This lengthening serves to straighten the body of the fetus, placing it in better alignment with the cervix and pelvis. As the uterus contracts, the round ligaments move, keeping the fundus forward, again to assist in placing the fetus in good alignment with the cervix. The elongation of the uterus exerts pressure against the diaphragm and causes the often-expressed sensation that a uterus is "taking control" of a woman's body.

In a difficult labor, particularly if the fetus is larger than the birth canal, the round ligaments of the uterus become tense and may be palpable on the abdomen. The normal physiologic retraction ring may become prominent and observable as an abdominal indentation. Termed a **pathologic retraction ring** or Bandl's ring, it is a danger sign that signifies impending rupture of the lower uterine segment if the obstruction to labor is not relieved (Malee, 2003).

Cervical Changes

Even more marked than the changes in the body of the uterus are two changes that occur in the cervix: effacement and dilatation.

Effacement. Effacement is shortening and thinning of the cervical canal. Normally, the canal is approximately 1 to 2 cm long. With effacement, the canal virtually disappears (Fig. 18.11). This occurs because of longitudinal traction from the contracting uterine fundus.

In primiparas, effacement is accomplished before dilatation begins. Be sure to inform the woman of this fact. Otherwise, she may become discouraged if, for example, at noon after a cervical examination she is told she is 2 cm dilated and then at 4 PM is told she is still 2 cm dilated. This type of report makes it seem to her that absolutely nothing has happened in 4 hours. However, effacement will have been occurring, and when it is complete, dilatation will then progress rapidly.

In multiparas, dilatation may proceed before effacement is complete. Effacement must occur at the end of dilatation, however, before the fetus can be safely pushed

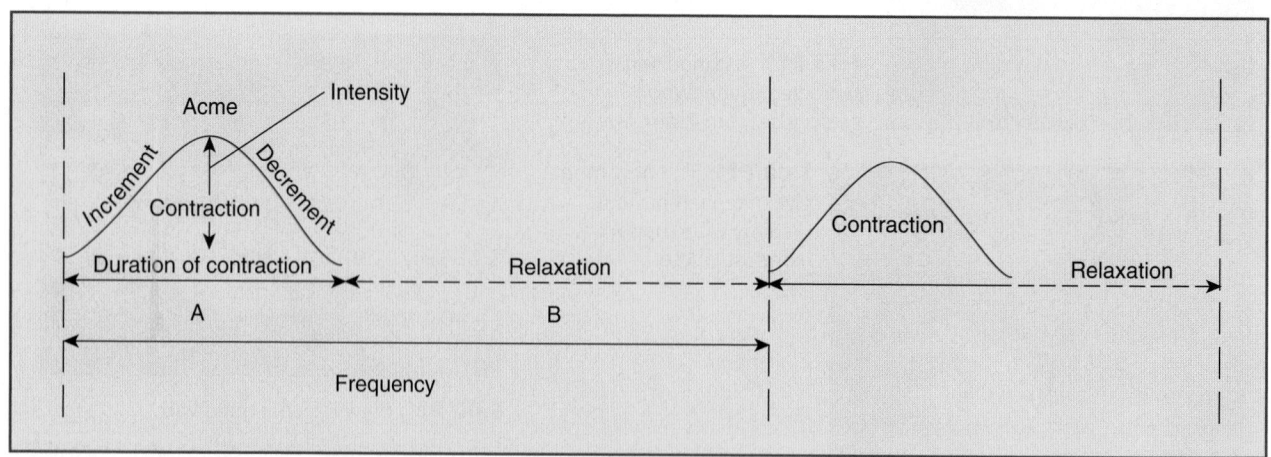

FIGURE 18.10 The interval and duration of uterine contractions. The frequency of contractions is the time from the beginning of one contraction to the beginning of the next contraction. It consists of two parts: (**A**) the duration of the contraction and (**B**) the period of relaxation. The broken line indicates an indeterminate period because the relaxation time (**B**) is usually of longer duration than the actual contraction (**A**).

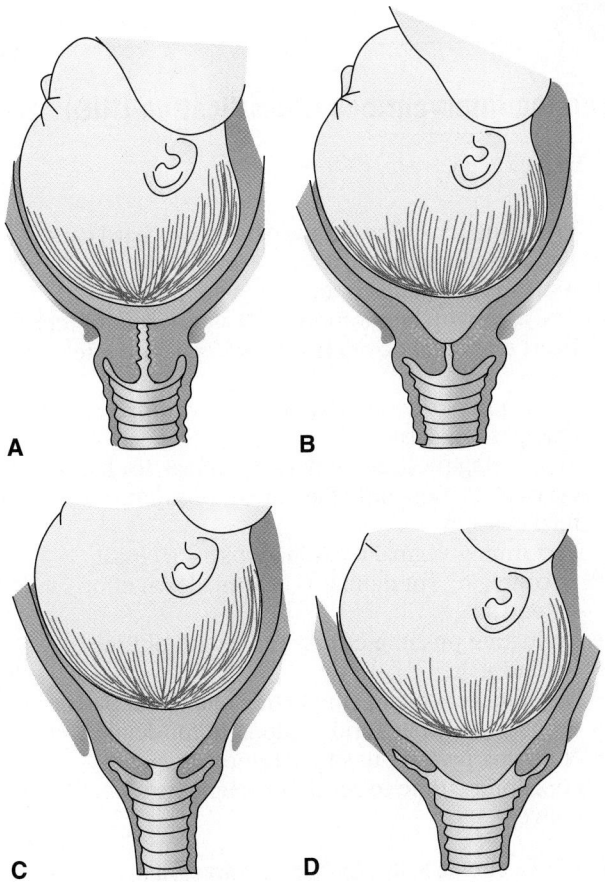

FIGURE 18.11 Effacement and dilation of cervix.
(A) Beginning labor. **(B)** Effacement is beginning; dilation is not apparent yet. **(C)** Effacement is almost complete. **(D)** After complete effacement, dilation proceeds rapidly.

through the cervical canal; otherwise, cervical tearing could result.

Dilatation. **Dilatation** refers to the enlargement or widening of the cervical canal from an opening a few millimeters wide to one large enough (approximately 10 cm) to permit passage of a fetus (see Fig. 18.11).

Dilatation occurs for two reasons. First, uterine contractions gradually increase the diameter of the cervical canal lumen by pulling the cervix up over the presenting part of the fetus. Second, the fluid-filled membranes press against the cervix. If the membranes are intact, they push ahead of the fetus and serve as an opening wedge. If they are ruptured, the presenting part serves this same function.

As dilatation begins, there is an increase in the amount of vaginal secretions (show), because the last of the operculum or mucus plug in the cervix is dislodged and minute capillaries in the cervix rupture.

Psyche

The fourth "P," or "psyche," refers to the psychological state or feelings that a woman brings into labor. For many women, this is a feeling of apprehension or fright. For almost everyone, it includes a sense of excitement or awe.

Women who manage best in labor typically are those who have a strong sense of self-esteem and a meaningful support person with them. These factors allow women to feel in control of sensations and circumstances that they have not experienced previously and that may not be at all what they pictured as happening. Women without adequate support can have an experience so frightening and stressful they can develop a posttraumatic stress syndrome (Beck, 2004).

Encouraging women to ask questions at prenatal visits and to attend preparation for childbirth classes helps prepare them for labor. Encouraging them to share their experience after labor serves as "debriefing time" and helps them integrate the experience into their total life.

STAGES OF LABOR

In nursing literature, labor is traditionally divided into three stages: a first stage of dilatation, which begins with the initiation of true labor contractions and ends when the cervix is fully dilatated; a second stage, extending from the time of full dilatation until the infant is born; and a third or placental stage, lasting from the time the infant is born until after the delivery of the placenta. The first 1 to 4 hours after birth of the placenta is sometimes termed the "fourth stage" to emphasize the importance of the close observation needed at this time. These designations are helpful in planning nursing interventions to ensure the safety of both the mother and the fetus. Box 18.3 highlights appropriate outcomes and interventions related to labor using the terminology identified by the Nursing Outcomes Classification (NOC) and Nursing Interventions Classification (NIC).

Friedman (1978), a physician who studied the process of labor extensively, used data to identify two phases of labor: latent and active phases. He further divided the active phase into three parts. His data, when plotted in graph form, are useful in monitoring an individual woman's labor progress (Fig. 18.12). Table 18.4 lists clinical features of the divisions of labor, as described by Friedman. Friedman's terms—preparatory division, dilatational division, and pelvic division—correspond to the first and second stages of labor. Because his "norms" refer to averages, an individual woman's labor can vary greatly from the ideal projected course of labor and still be normal for that woman. With the use of less analgesia in labor today, Friedman's norms may need to be reevaluated (Cesario, 2005).

Typically, a labor progress graph is labeled as follows:

- Left side numbered from 1 to 10 (representing the centimeters of cervical dilatation)
- Bottom line numbered to represent the number of hours of labor
- Right side numbered from −4 to +4 (representing the station of the presenting part)

After each cervical examination, cervical dilatation and **fetal descent** are plotted on the graph. The pattern of cervical dilatation usually plots as an S-shaped curve. The fetal descent pattern forms a downward curve. Both lines cross at the point of maximum cervical dilatation. A typical labor graph is shown in Figure 18.13.

BOX 18.3

Nursing Outcomes Classification (NOC) and Nursing Interventions Classification (NIC)

Intrapartal Period

NOC: Maternal Status, Intrapartum

Maternal status, intrapartum, is defined as the conditions and behaviors indicating maternal well-being from the onset of labor to delivery (Johnson, Maas, & Moorhead, 2000). Some specific indicators that suggest that this outcome has been achieved include demonstration of the following:

- Coping mechanisms
- Techniques to facilitate labor
- Uterine contraction frequency, duration, and intensity within expected range
- Physiologic parameters such as vital signs, neurologic reflexes, urine output, and blood glucose levels within expected range
- Progressive cervical dilation

NOC: Fetal Status, Intrapartum

Fetal status, intrapartum, is defined as the conditions and behaviors indicating fetal well-being from the onset of labor to delivery (Johnson, Maas, & Moorhead, 2000). Some specific indicators that suggest that this outcome has been achieved include demonstration of the following:

- Fetal heart rate between 120 and 160 beats per minute
- Fetal position, presenting part, heart rate, and scalp blood pH within expected range
- Amniotic fluid color and amount within expected range
- Deceleration patterns and variability findings without deviation from expected

NIC: Intrapartal Care

Intrapartal care is defined as the monitoring and management of stages one and two of the birth process (McCloskey & Bulechek, 2000). Some important activities involved when implementing this intervention include:

- Admitting client to birthing area after determining that client is in labor
- Determining if client's membranes have ruptured
- Encouraging family participation as appropriate with the labor process
- Performing Leopold maneuver and vaginal exams as appropriate
- Monitoring maternal vital signs and fetal heart rate and patterns, reporting any deviations or abnormalities
- Applying electronic fetal monitor as appropriate (see next NIC)
- Assessing pain level, instituting positioning, breathing, relaxation, and other methods for pain control; administering analgesics as ordered

- Providing ice chips, wet washcloth, or hard candy
- Encouraging voiding at least every 2 hours
- Assisting with anesthetic administration
- Assisting with amniotomy with assessment of fetal heart rate, fetal positioning, and fetal cord after amniotomy
- Cleansing perineum and assisting with pad changes regularly
- Monitoring progress including vaginal discharge, cervical dilation and effacement, position, and fetal descent
- Performing vaginal examinations as necessary
- Encouraging spontaneous bearing-down efforts for second stage
- Evaluating pushing efforts and length of time in second stage
- Assisting coach and supporting client and partner
- Preparing supplies and equipment for delivery
- Notifying primary health care provider at appropriate time to scrub for attending delivery

NIC: Electronic Fetal Monitoring, Intrapartum

Electronic fetal monitoring, intrapartum, is defined as electronic evaluation of the fetal heart rate response to uterine contractions during intrapartal care (McCloskey & Bulechek, 2000). Some important activities involved when implementing this intervention include:

- Verifying maternal and fetal heart rate response to uterine contractions during intrapartal care
- Instructing client and partner about reasons for electronic monitoring
- Applying tocotransducer snugly after determining fetal position via Leopold maneuver
- Palpating to determine contraction intensity with tocotransducer use
- Differentiating among multiple fetuses by documenting on tracing and comparing data when simultaneous tracings are being used
- Discussing appearance of rhythm strip with client and support person
- Reassuring client about normal fetal heart rates
- Adjusting monitor to achieve and maintain clear tracing
- Interpreting rhythm strips when at least a 10-minute tracing has been obtained
- Documenting elements of external tracing and relevant intrapartal care
- Initiating fetal resuscitation interventions (see below) to treat abnormalities
- Documenting changes in fetal heart patterns after resuscitation

tinual variations of heart rate that occur with labor—a slight slowing and then a return to normal (baseline) levels. During a contraction, the arteries of the uterus are sharply constricted and the filling of cotyledons almost completely halts. The amount of nutrients, including oxygen, exchanged during this time is reduced, causing a slight but inconsequential fetal hypoxia. Increased intracranial pressure caused by uterine pressure on the fetal head serves to keep circulation from falling below normal during the duration of a contraction.

Integumentary System

The pressure involved in the birth process is often reflected in minimal petechiae or ecchymotic areas on a fetus (particularly the presenting part). There may also be edema of the presenting part (caput succedaneum).

Musculoskeletal System

The force of uterine contractions tends to push a fetus into a position of full flexion, the most advantageous position for birth.

Respiratory System

The process of labor appears to aid in the maturation of surfactant production by alveoli in the fetal lung. The pressure applied to the chest from contractions and passage through the birth canal helps to clear it of lung fluid. For this reason, an infant born vaginally is usually able to establish respirations more easily than a fetus born by cesarean birth.

Danger Signs of Labor

Wide variation exists among individuals in their patterns of labor contractions and in maternal responses to labor and birth. Certain signs, however, indicate that the course of events is deviating too far from normal. These signs, both fetal and maternal, are described in Box 18.6. Nursing care of a woman who is experiencing a complication during labor or birth is addressed in Chapter 21.

Fetal Danger Signs

High or Low Fetal Heart Rate. As a rule, an FHR of more than 160 bpm (fetal tachycardia) or less than 110 bpm (fetal bradycardia) is a sign of possible fetal distress. An equally important sign is a late or variable deceleration pattern (described later) on the fetal monitor. The FHR may return to a normal range in between these irregular patterns, giving a false sense of security if FHR is assessed only between contractions.

Meconium Staining. Meconium staining, a green color in the amniotic fluid, is not always a sign of fetal distress but is highly correlated with its occurrence. It reveals that the fetus has had an episode of loss of sphincter control, allowing meconium to pass into the amniotic fluid. It may indicate that the fetus has or is experiencing hypoxia, which stimulates the vagal reflex and leads to increased

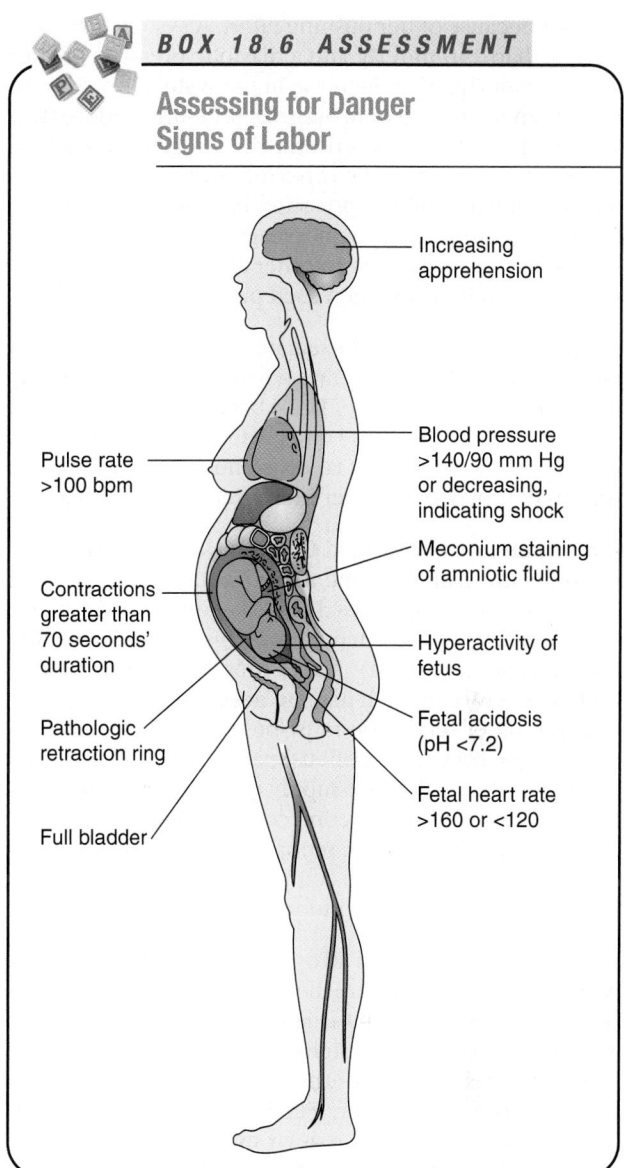

BOX 18.6 ASSESSMENT

Assessing for Danger Signs of Labor

- Increasing apprehension
- Blood pressure >140/90 mm Hg or decreasing, indicating shock
- Meconium staining of amniotic fluid
- Hyperactivity of fetus
- Fetal acidosis (pH <7.2)
- Fetal heart rate >160 or <120
- Pulse rate >100 bpm
- Contractions greater than 70 seconds' duration
- Pathologic retraction ring
- Full bladder

bowel motility. Although meconium staining may be normal in a breech presentation, because pressure on the buttocks causes meconium loss, it should always be reported immediately so that its cause can be investigated.

Hyperactivity. Ordinarily, a fetus is quiet and barely moves during labor. Fetal hyperactivity may be a sign that hypoxia is occurring, because frantic motion is a common reaction to the need for oxygen.

Fetal Acidosis. If blood analyses are made on a fetus during labor by use of a scalp capillary technique, the finding of acidosis (blood pH lower than 7.2) is a certain sign that fetal well-being is becoming compromised.

Maternal Danger Signs

Rising or Falling Blood Pressure. Normally, a woman's blood pressure rises slightly in the second (pelvic) stage of labor because of her pushing effort. A systolic pressure greater than 140 mm Hg and a diastolic pressure greater than 90 mm Hg, or an increase in the systolic pressure of more than 30 mm Hg or in diastolic pressure of more than 15 mm Hg (the basic criteria for pregnancy-induced hypertension), should be reported. Just as important to report is a falling blood pressure, because it may be the first sign of intrauterine hemorrhage. A falling blood pressure is often associated with other clinical signs of shock, such as apprehension, increased pulse rate, and pallor.

Abnormal Pulse. Most pregnant women have a pulse rate of 70 to 80 bpm. This rate normally increases slightly during the second stage of labor because of the exertion involved. A maternal pulse rate greater than 100 bpm during the normal course of labor is unusual and should be reported. It may be another indication of hemorrhage.

Inadequate or Prolonged Contractions. Uterine contractions normally become more frequent, intense, and longer as labor progresses. If they become less frequent, less intense, or shorter in duration, this may indicate uterine exhaustion (inertia). If this problem cannot be corrected, a cesarean birth may be necessary.

A period of relaxation must be present between contractions so that the intervillous spaces of the uterus can fill and maintain an adequate supply of oxygen and nutrients for the fetus. As a rule, uterine contractions lasting longer than 70 seconds should be reported, because contractions of this length may begin to compromise fetal well-being by interfering with adequate uterine artery filling.

Pathologic Retraction Ring. An indentation across a woman's abdomen, where the upper and lower segments of the uterus join, may be a sign of extreme uterine stress and possible impending uterine rupture. For this reason, it is important to observe the contours of the abdomen periodically during labor. Fetal heartbeat auscultation automatically provides a regular opportunity to assess a woman's abdomen. If an electronic monitor is in place, it is necessary to make this observation deliberately.

Abnormal Lower Abdominal Contour. If a woman has a full bladder during labor, a round bulge on her lower anterior abdomen may appear. This is a danger signal for two reasons: first, the bladder may be injured by the pressure of a fetal head; second, the pressure of the full bladder may not allow the fetal head to descend.

Increasing Apprehension. Warnings of psychological danger during labor are as important to consider in assessing maternal well-being as are physical signs. A woman who is becoming increasingly apprehensive despite clear explanations of unfolding events may only be approaching the second stage of labor. She may, however, not be "hearing" because she has a concern that has not been met. Using an approach such as, "You seem more and more concerned. Could you tell me what is worrying you?" may be helpful. Increasing apprehension also needs to be investigated for physical reasons, because it can be a sign of oxygen deprivation or internal hemorrhage.

Checkpoint Question 3

Celeste is having long and hard uterine contractions. What length of contraction would you report as abnormal?

a. Any length over 30 seconds.
b. A contraction over 70 seconds in length.
c. A contraction that peaks at 20 seconds.
d. A contraction shorter than 60 seconds.

MATERNAL AND FETAL ASSESSMENT DURING LABOR

Nursing assessment is instrumental to keep women safe during labor.

Immediate Assessment of a Woman in Stage One

A number of immediate assessment measures are necessary to safeguard maternal and fetal health when a woman first arrives at a birthing facility. Encourage every woman to bring a support person with her into labor (Hodnett et al., 2005). After she and her support person are oriented to the area, focus on obtaining vital assessment data (Box 18.7).

Initial Interview and Physical Examination

Important data that need to be obtained include a description of labor thus far, the woman's general physical condition, and her preparedness for labor and birth.
Obtain information about the following areas:

- Expected date of birth
- Frequency, duration, and intensity of contractions

BOX 18.7 FOCUS ON . . .

FAMILY TEACHING

Admission Procedures for the Laboring Client

Q. Celeste Bailey asks you, "What will happen when I arrive at a birthing center?"
A. Every setting differs, but actions you can expect include the following:

- Orientation to a birthing room
- Baseline assessment of your temperature, pulse, respirations, and blood pressure
- Recording of your pregnancy history and physical examination
- Assessment of fetal heart rate
- A vaginal examination
- Urine and necessary blood samples obtained
- Explanation of fetal or uterine monitoring equipment to be used and connection of this equipment

- Amount and character of show
- Whether rupture of membranes has occurred
- Vital signs—temperature, pulse, respirations, and blood pressure (assessed between contractions)
- Time the woman last ate
- Any known drug allergies
- Past pregnancy and previous pregnancy history
- Her birth plan or what individualized measures she has planned, such as no analgesia or who will cut the umbilical cord

This amount of information is scant but helps to establish whether the woman is in active labor and needs intense care or whether she has arrived at the hospital or birthing center at an early stage of labor and therefore can benefit most from paced interventions.

After these initial assessment procedures, the woman is categorized as to her risk for having difficulty in labor or fetal risk for needing special care at birth.

Detailed Assessment During the First Stage of Labor

If the woman is in active labor, the history taken on arrival may be the only history obtained until after the baby is born. If birth is not imminent, a more extensive history and physical examination can be completed.

History

The full history should include a review of a woman's pregnancy, including both physical and psychological events, and a review of past pregnancies, her general health, and family medical information—all data necessary to plan nursing care.

Performing a detailed interview of a woman in labor can be difficult because of the constant interruptions caused by labor contractions. Be patient. Remember that the longest contraction is rarely more than 60 seconds. If a woman concentrates so intently on a breathing exercise she completely forgets a question asked just before the contraction, repeat the question as the contraction subsides, as if it had not been asked before, or act as if it is no trouble to ask it again.

Current Pregnancy History. Important information needed for a complete history includes documentation of gravida and para status; a description of this pregnancy (planned or not, pattern and place of prenatal care, adequacy of nutrition, whether any complication such as spotting, falls, hypertension of pregnancy, infection, or alcohol or drug ingestion has occurred); plans for labor (does she want medication for pain, will she use breathing exercises, will she have a support person with her); and future childcare (will she breast-feed or bottle-feed, has she chosen a pediatrician).

Past Pregnancy History. Document prior pregnancies, including number, dates, types of birth, any complications, and outcomes, including sex and birthweights of children. What is the current health status of the children?

Past Health History. Document any previous surgeries (surgical adhesions might interfere with free fetal pas-

sage); heart disease or diabetes (special precautions are required during labor and birth); anemia (blood loss at birth may be more important than it is normally); tuberculosis (lung lesions may be reactivated at birth by changes in lung contour); kidney disease or hypertension (blood pressure must be monitored even more carefully than it is normally); or a sexually transmitted infection such as herpes (the infant may be exposed to the disease by vaginal contact if the disease is still active). Determine also whether the woman's lifestyle places her at high risk for human immunodeficiency virus (HIV) exposure.

Family Medical History. Ask if any family member is cognitively challenged or has a condition such as heart disease, a blood dyscrasia, diabetes, kidney disease, cancer, allergies, seizures, or a congenital disorder. Adequate preparation can then be made for a child who might have special needs.

Physical Examination

After history taking, perform a thorough physical examination, including a pelvic examination, to confirm the presentation and position of the fetus and the stage of cervical dilatation.

Physical assessment during labor begins, as does all physical assessment, with the woman's overall appearance and is similar to that for any woman. However, be prepared to adapt examination techniques to the client's stage of labor and its progression. Does she appear tired? Pale? Ill? Frightened? Is there obvious edema or dehydration? Does she have open lesions anywhere?

Palpate for enlargement of lymph nodes to detect the possibility of infection. Inspect the mucous membrane of the mouth and the conjunctiva of the eyes for color. Does the color (paleness) suggest anemia? What is the condition of the woman's teeth? Are there any caries? Do any teeth appear abscessed (such a condition needs to be documented because it might account for a postpartal fever)? Examine the outer and inner surfaces of her lips carefully. Does she have herpes lesions (pinpoint vesicles on an erythematous base)? Type II (genital) virus can be lethal to newborns. If herpetic lesions are present anywhere, a woman will probably be isolated from her child until the lesions crust.

Assess the lungs to be certain they are clear to auscultation. Listen for normal heart sounds and rhythms. Many pregnant women at term have a grade II to III systolic ejection murmur because of the extra volume of blood that must cross the heart valves. Inspect and palpate her breasts. Are they free of cysts and lumps? Mark the chart of a woman who has a palpable mass in her breasts for reexamination after labor and birth. This is probably an enlarged milk gland but needs further evaluation.

Abdominal Assessment. Assessing a woman's abdomen is important to estimate fetal size by fundal height (should be at the level of the xiphoid process at term). Assess presentation and position by Leopold's maneuvers (see later discussion). Palpate and percuss the bladder area (over the symphysis pubis) to detect a full bladder. Assess for abdominal scars, because abdominal or pelvic surgery can leave adhesions.

Finally, inspect lower extremities for skin turgor to assess hydration, and also for edema and varicose veins. Women with large varicosities are more prone to thrombophlebitis after birth than other women are. Some physicians prefer not to use birth room stirrups if varicosities are prominent during labor, because the stirrups may press against them. Severe edema suggests hypertension of pregnancy, so the extent and intensity of edema must be assessed and correlated with the woman's blood pressure.

Leopold's Maneuvers

Leopold's maneuvers are a systematic method of observation and palpation to determine fetal presentation and position. They are described in Box 18.8.

Assessing Rupture of Membranes

One of every four labors begins with spontaneous rupture of the fetal membranes. When this occurs, the woman may feel a sudden gush of amniotic fluid from her vagina. This is a startling sensation because it feels as if she has lost bladder control. She may feel embarrassed before she realizes the warm fluid on her perineum and legs is not urine but a sudden announcement that labor is beginning. In other women, rupture of membranes is more subtle, occurring as a slow loss of fluid. In such cases, there may be a question whether the membranes have ruptured.

A sterile vaginal examination using a sterile speculum usually reveals whether amniotic fluid is present in the vagina. After vaginal secretions are obtained (usually with the use of a sterile, cotton-tipped applicator), test them with a strip of Nitrazine paper. Vaginal secretions are usually acid; amniotic fluid, in contrast, is alkaline. If amniotic fluid has passed through the vagina recently, the pH of the vaginal fluid will probably be alkaline (greater than 6.5) when tested by Nitrazine paper (appears blue-green or gray to deep blue). A false reading may occur in a woman with intact membranes who has a heavy, bloody show, because blood is also alkaline. An additional test is the fern test (examination of vaginal secretions under a microscope). Because of its high estrogen content, amniotic fluid will show a fern pattern (see Fig. 4.16 in Chapter 4) when dried and examined in this way; urine will not.

If the woman's membranes ruptured at home, ask her to describe the color of the amniotic fluid. It should be as clear as water. Yellow-stained fluid may indicate a blood incompatibility between mother and fetus (the amniotic fluid is bilirubin-stained from the breakdown of red blood cells). Green fluid indicates meconium staining. Although meconium staining is normal in breech births because of buttocks compression, in a vertex presentation it may indicate fetal anoxia. A fetus with meconium staining needs immediate assessment to safeguard well-being. The infant will need continuing close assessment after birth because of possible meconium aspiration.

Vaginal Examination

A vaginal examination is necessary to determine the extent of cervical effacement and dilatation and to confirm the fetal presentation, position, and degree of descent. The technique for a vaginal examination during labor is shown in Box 18.9.

Vaginal examinations may be done either between contractions or during contractions. More of the fetal skull may be palpated during a contraction, because the cervix retracts more at that time. However, examination during a contraction is more painful and rarely is justified by the additional amount of information gained. Palpation of membranes during a contraction, when they are under pressure, may cause them to rupture.

Women are anxious to have frequent progress reports during labor, to reassure them everything is progressing well. Tell the woman immediately after an examination about her progress. Most women are aware of dilatation but not the word effacement. Just saying, "no further dilatation" is a depressing report. "You're not dilatated a lot more, but a lot of thinning is happening and that's just as important" is the same report given in a positive manner. After finishing a vaginal examination, plot the new degree of dilatation and descent of the presenting part on a labor progress graph, as described earlier.

Do not do vaginal examinations in the presence of fresh bleeding, because this may indicate a placenta previa (implantation of the placenta so low in the uterus that it encroaches on the cervical os). Performing a vaginal examination in this instance might tear the placenta and cause hemorrhage, resulting in danger to both mother and fetus. If in doubt, err on the side of postponing a vaginal examination.

Assessment of Pelvic Adequacy

Evaluating pelvic adequacy using internal conjugate and ischial tuberosity diameters is generally done during pregnancy, so that, by weeks 32 to 36 of pregnancy, the nurse-midwife or physician is alerted that a cephalopelvic disproportion could occur. Women with this potential problem are cautioned not to attempt a home birth or use a birthing center without nearby hospital facilities available.

Whether the pelvis is wide enough to allow the fetus to pass through the internal diameters can be reassessed during early labor. Because these procedures involve vaginal manipulation and discomfort (and the diameters obtained during pregnancy have not changed), they are not retaken routinely. However, if the woman did not receive prenatal care, they need to be estimated at this time. (These procedures are described in Chapter 10.)

The suprapubic angle may be estimated early in labor to determine how readily the fetal head will be born (if the angle is too steep, the fetal head can lock behind it and perineal tissue may tear during birth as the fetal head is pushed posteriorly). To estimate this angle, place the fingers vaginally and press up against the pubic arch. If the fingers cannot be separated in this position, the angle is unusually steep (less than 90 degrees).

Sonography

Sonography may be used at term to determine the diameters of the fetal skull and to determine presentation, pre-

BOX 18.8 NURSING PROCEDURE

Leopold's maneuvers

Purpose

Systematically observing and palpating the abdomen to determine fetal presentation and position.

PROCEDURE	PRINCIPLE

1. Prepare the client.
  a. Explain the procedure.
 	
  b. Instruct the client to empty her bladder.
 	
  c. Position the woman supine with knees slightly flexed. Place a small pillow or rolled towel under one side.
 	
  d. Wash your hands using warm water.
 	
  e. Observe the woman's abdomen for longest diameter and where fetal movement is apparent.
 	
2. Perform the first maneuver.
 	
  a. Stand at the foot of the client, facing her, and place both hands flat on her abdomen.
  b. Palpate the superior surface of the fundus. Determine consistency, shape, and mobility.
	a. Explanation reduces anxiety and enhances cooperation.
	  b. Doing so promotes comfort and allows for more productive palpation because fetal contour will not be obscured by a distended bladder.
	  c. Flexing the knees relaxes the abdominal muscles. Using a pillow or towel tilts the uterus off the vena cava, thus preventing supine hypotension syndrome.
	  d. Handwashing prevents the spread of possible infection. Using warm water aids in client comfort and prevents tightening of abdominal muscles.
	  e. The longest diameter (axis) is the length of the fetus. The location of activity most likely reflects the position of the feet.
	2. This maneuver determines whether fetal head or breech is in the fundus.
	  a. Proper positioning of hands ensures accurate findings.
	  b. When palpating, a head feels more firm than a breech. A head is round and hard; the breech is less well defined. A head moves independently of the body; the breech moves only in conjunction with the body.

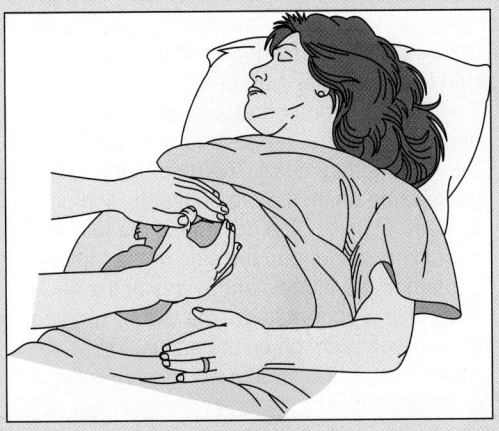

3. Perform the second maneuver.
  a. Face the client and place the palms of each hand on either side of the abdomen.
  b. Palpate the sides of the uterus. Hold the left hand stationary on the left side of the uterus while the right hand palpates the opposite side of the uterus from top to bottom. Then hold the right hand steady, and repeat palpation using the left hand on the left side.
	3. This maneuver locates the back of the fetus.
	  a. Proper positioning of hands ensures accurate findings.
	  b. This method is most successful to determine the direction the fetal back is facing. One hand will feel a smooth, hard, resistant surface (the back), while on the opposite side, a number of angular nodulations (the knees and elbows of the fetus) will be felt.

(continued)

PROCEDURE	PRINCIPLE

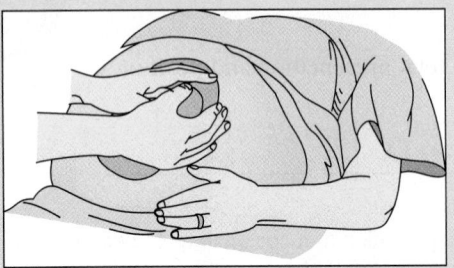

4. Perform the third maneuver.

   a. Gently grasp the lower portion of the abdomen just above the symphysis pubis between the thumb and index finger and try to press the thumb and finger together. Determine any movement and whether the part is firm or soft.

4. This maneuver determines the part of the fetus at the inlet and its mobility.

   a. If the presenting part moves upward so an examiner's hands can be pressed together, the presenting part is not engaged (not firmly settled into the pelvis). If the part is firm, it is the head; if soft, then it is the breech.

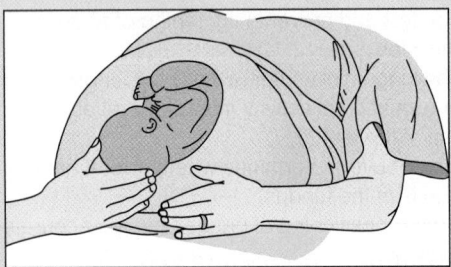

5. Perform the fourth maneuver.

   a. Place fingers on both sides of the uterus approximately 2 inches above the inguinal ligaments, pressing downward and inward in the direction of the birth canal. Allow fingers to be carried downward.

5. This maneuver determines fetal attitude and degree of fetal extension into the pelvis; it should be done only if the fetus is in cephalic presentation. Information about the infant's anteroposterior position may also be gained from this final maneuver.

   a. The fingers of one hand will slide along the uterine contour and meet no obstruction, indicating the back of the fetal neck. The other hand will meet an obstruction an inch or so above the ligament—this is the fetal brow. The position of the fetal brow should correspond to the side of the uterus that contained the elbows and knees of the fetus. If the fetus is in a poor attitude, the examining fingers will meet an obstruction on the same side as the fetal back. That is, the fingers will touch the hyperextended head. If the brow is very easily palpated (as if it lies just under the skin), the fetus is probably in a posterior position (the occiput is pointing toward the woman's back).

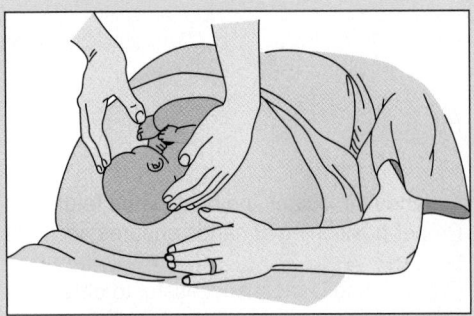

BOX 18.9 NURSING PROCEDURE

Vaginal Examination

Purpose
Determine cervical readiness and fetal position and presentation.

PROCEDURE	PRINCIPLE
1. Wash your hands; explain procedure to client. Provide privacy.	1. Handwashing helps prevent spread of microorganisms; explanations ensure client cooperation and compliance. Privacy enhances self-esteem.
2. Assess client status and adjust plan to individual client need.	2. Care is always individualized according to a client's needs.
3. Assemble equipment: sterile examining gloves, sterile lubricant, antiseptic solution. Ask the woman to turn onto her back with knees flexed (a dorsal recumbent position). Put on sterile examining gloves.	3. Organization and planning improve efficiency. Positioning in this manner allows for good visualization of perineum. Use of a sterile glove prevents contamination of birth canal.
4. Discard one drop of clean lubricating solution and drop an ample supply on tips of gloved fingers.	4. Discarding the first drop ensures that quantity used will not be contaminated.
5. Pour antiseptic solution over vulva using nondominant hand.	5. This prevents the spread of organisms from perineum to birth canal.
6. Place nondominant hand on the outer edges of the woman's vulva and spread her labia while inspecting the external genitalia for lesions. Look for red, irritated mucous membranes; open, ulcerated sores; clustered, pinpoint vesicles.	6. Positioning hands in this way allows for good perineal visualization. Presence of any lesions may indicate an infection and possibly preclude vaginal birth.
7. Look for escaping amniotic fluid or the presence of umbilical cord or bleeding.	7. Amniotic fluid implies membranes have ruptured and umbilical cord may have prolapsed. Bleeding may be a sign of placenta previa. *Do not do a vaginal examination if a possible placenta previa is present.*
8. If there is no bleeding or cord visible, introduce your index and middle fingers of dominant hand gently into the vagina, directing them toward the posterior vaginal wall.	8. The posterior vaginal wall is less sensitive than the anterior wall. Stabilize the uterus by placing your nondominant hand on the woman's abdomen.

9. Touch the cervix with your gloved examining fingers.
   a. Palpate for cervical consistency and rate if *firm* or *soft*.
 	
   b. Measure the extent of dilatation; palpate for an anterior rim or lip of cervix.
	9. a. The cervix feels like a circular rim of tissue around a center depression. Firm is similar to the tip of a nose; soft is as pliable as an earlobe. The anterior rim is usually the last portion to thin.
	   b. The width of the fingertip helps to estimate the degree of dilatation. An index finger averages about 1 cm; a middle finger about 1½ cm. If they can both enter the cervix, the cervix is dilated 2½ to 3 cm. If there would be room for double the width of your examining fingers in the cervix, the dilatation is about 5 to 6 cm. When the space is four times the width of your fingertips, dilatation is complete—10 cm. Measure the width of your fingertips on a centimeter scale if you are going to do a vaginal examination, so you know how wide your index and middle fingers are at the tip.

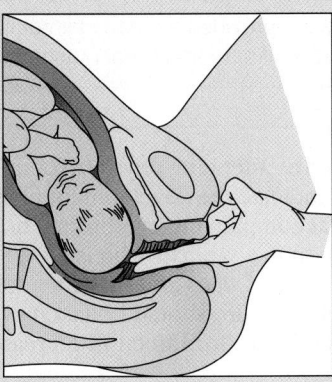

(continued)

PROCEDURE	PRINCIPLE
10. Estimate the degree of effacement.	**10.** Effacement is estimated in percentage depending on thickness. A cervix before labor is 2 to 2½ cm thick. If it is only 1 cm thick now, it is 50% effaced. If it is tissue paper thin, it is 100% effaced. With a 100% effaced cervix, dilatation is difficult to feel for because the edges of the cervix are so thin.
11. Estimate whether membranes are intact.	**11.** The membranes (with a slight amount of amniotic fluid in front of the presenting part) are the shape of a watch crystal. With a contraction, they bulge forward and become prominent and can be felt much more readily.
12. Locate the ischial spines. Rate the station of the presenting part. Identify the presenting part.	**12.** Ischial spines are palpated as notches at the 4 and 8 o'clock positions at the pelvic outlet. Station is the number of centimeters above or below the spines where the presenting part is. Identifying the presenting part confirms findings obtained with Leopold's maneuvers. Differentiating a vertex from a breech may be more difficult than would first appear. A vertex has a hard, smooth surface. Fetal hair may be palpable but massed together and wet; it may be difficult to appreciate through gloves. Palpating the two fontanelles, one diamond-shaped and one triangular, helps the identification. Buttocks feel softer and give under fingertip pressure. Identifying the anus may be possible because the sphincter action will "trap" the index finger.
13. Establish the fetal position.	**13.** The fontanelle palpated is invariably the posterior one because the fetus maintains a flexed position, presenting the posterior not the anterior fontanelle. In an ROA position, the triangular fontanelle will point toward the right anterior pelvic quadrant. In an LOA position, the posterior fontanelle will point toward the left anterior pelvis. In a breech presentation, the anus can serve as a marker for position. When the anus is pointing toward the left anterior quadrant of the woman's pelvis, the position is LSA.
14. Withdraw your hand. Wipe the perineum front to back to remove secretions or examining solution. Leave client comfortable and turned to side.	**14.** Use as gentle a technique with withdrawal as with insertion. Wiping front to back prevents moving rectal contamination forward to the vagina. Side-lying is the best position to prevent supine hypotension syndrome in labor.
15. Document procedure and assessment findings and how client tolerated procedure.	**15.** Documentation provides a means for communication and evaluation of care and client outcomes.

senting part, position, flexion, and degree of descent of a fetus. If the woman is going to be transported to another department to have this done, be sure someone accompanies her, so that, if labor should become more active, she can be returned quickly to the labor and birth service.

Vital Signs

Vital signs are taken at the beginning and then periodically during labor, as summarized in Table 18.5.

Temperature. Temperature is usually obtained every 4 hours during labor. Report a temperature greater than 37.2°C (99°F) to the attending physician or nurse-midwife, because it may indicate the development of infection. Unless there are accompanying symptoms, however, temperature elevation in a woman who is taking no fluids by mouth usually reflects dehydration. After rupture of the membranes, temperature should be taken every 2 hours, because the possibility for infection increases markedly after this time.

Pulse and Respiration. Pulse and respiration rate should be measured and recorded every 4 hours during labor. A woman's pulse may be rapid on admission because she is nervous and anxious. After she has become better

TABLE 18.5

Time Intervals for Nursing Interventions During First Stage of Labor

Intervention	Assessment on Admission	Continued Assessments
Assess and Record		
Temperature	X	q4h (unless membranes are ruptured, then q2h)
Pulse	X	q4h
Respirations	X	q4h
Blood pressure	X	q4h
Voiding	X	q2–4h
Fetal heart rate	X	Continuously by monitor or q30min
Contractions	X	Continuously by monitor or q30min
Provide		
Ambulation	X	Until membranes rupture
Support	X	Continuously

acquainted with her surroundings and has been assured that everything is going well, her pulse usually ranges between 70 and 80 bpm. A persistent pulse rate of more than 100 bpm suggests tachycardia from dehydration or hemorrhage. Respiratory rate during labor is usually 18 to 20 breaths per minute. Do not count respirations during contractions, because women tend to breathe rapidly from pain. Conversely, if a woman is using controlled breathing to decrease pain in labor, her respirations could be abnormally slow.

Observe for hyperventilation (rapid, deep respirations). Prolonged hyperventilation leads to the "blowing off" of carbon dioxide and accompanying symptoms of dizziness and tingling of hands and feet. Rebreathing into a paper bag and reassurance help to reverse this process.

Blood Pressure. Blood pressure is usually measured and recorded every 4 hours during labor. Measure blood pressure between contractions, both for the woman's comfort and for accuracy, because blood pressure tends to rise 5 to 15 mm Hg during a contraction. An increase in blood pressure may indicate the development of pregnancy-induced hypertension. A decrease in blood pressure or a decrease in the pulse pressure (the difference between the systolic and diastolic pressures) may indicate hemorrhage. If the woman receives an analgesic agent (such as meperidine) that tends to be hypotensive, check her blood pressure approximately 15 minutes after administration to be certain that extreme hypotension is not occurring.

Laboratory Analysis

Most women have some preliminary laboratory studies done in early labor.

Blood. Blood is drawn for hemoglobin and hematocrit, a serologic test for syphilis (VDRL), hepatitis B antibodies, and blood typing to determine the woman's baseline level of health. These findings can be used to alert the laboratory that a woman with a certain blood type is in labor and to help predict whether a blood incompatibility is likely to exist in the newborn.

Urine. Obtain a clean-catch urine specimen and test it immediately for protein and glucose; then send it to the laboratory for a complete or dipstick urinalysis. If the woman reports any symptoms that suggest a urinary tract infection (e.g., burning on urination, blood in urine, extreme frequency, flank pain), obtain a clean-catch specimen for culture. A woman in labor is able to void most easily if she is allowed to use a bathroom. However, if the woman has ruptured membranes, do not allow her to ambulate to a bathroom until it is confirmed that the fetal head is engaged, so that gravity does not cause a prolapsed cord. A bedpan or receptacle placed on a commode allows for collection of any material passed from the vagina.

Assessment of Uterine Contractions

Uterine contractions may be monitored intermittently by hand or continuously by an internal or external system. Most women are monitored for a short period in early labor to screen for fetal well-being. Continuing to monitor the duration, strength, and interval between contractions can aid in tracking the progress of labor (Thacker et al., 2005).

Length of Contractions. To determine the length of a contraction with a monitor in place, simply observe the rhythm strip and count the time interval of the contraction. To determine the beginning of a contraction without a monitor, rest a hand on a woman's abdomen at the fundus of the uterus very gently to sense the gradual tensing and upward rising of the fundus that accompanies a contraction (Fig. 18.15). It is possible to palpate this tensing approximately 5 seconds before the woman is able to feel the contraction. (Contractions are palpable when the intrauterine pressure reaches approximately 20 mm Hg. The pain of a contraction is not usually felt until pressure reaches approximately 25 mm Hg.) Time the duration of a contraction from the moment the uterus first tenses until it has relaxed again.

Intensity of Contractions. In addition to observing the duration of contractions, estimate the intensity or strength of the contraction. On a monitor, this is the height of the contraction. If you are assessing manually, rate a

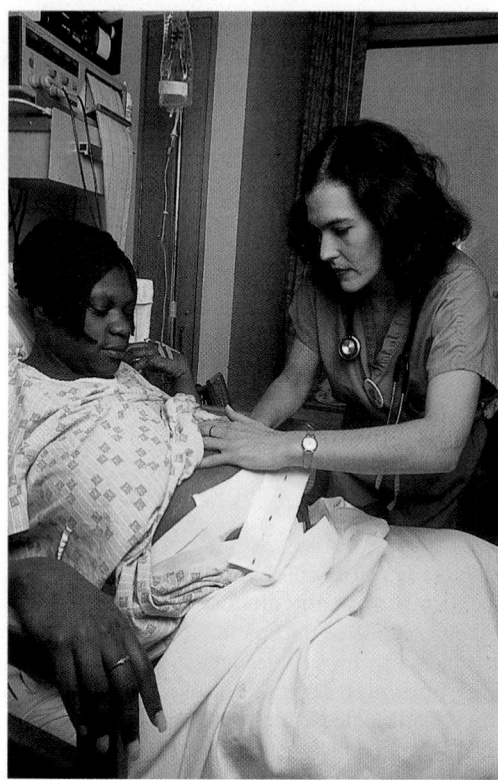

FIGURE 18.15 Contractions can be assessed by very gently placing the hand over the fundus of the uterus.

contraction as mild if the uterus does not feel more than minimally tense; as moderate if the uterus feels firm; and as strong if the uterus feels as hard as a wooden board at the peak of the contraction. With a strong contraction, you will also not be able to indent the uterus with your fingertips.

After estimating the intensity and duration of a contraction, recheck the fundus at the conclusion of the contraction, to be certain that it is relaxing and becoming soft to the touch again. This demonstrates that the uterus is not in continuous contraction but is providing a relaxation time during which blood vessels can fill to supply the fetus with adequate oxygen.

Frequency of Contractions. Next, time the frequency of contractions. The frequency is timed from the beginning of one contraction to the beginning of the next (see Fig. 18.10).

Use as light a touch as possible on a woman's abdomen while timing contractions or estimating their strength manually. The fundus of the uterus becomes tender if it has to push against the extra weight of a hand with each contraction. This is an unnecessary discomfort for a woman in labor.

Initial Fetal Assessment

Although passive in labor, a fetus is subjected to extreme pressure by uterine contractions and passage through the birth canal, so it is important to ascertain that the FHR remains within normal limits despite these pressures.

Auscultation of Fetal Heart Sounds

Fetal heart sounds are transmitted best through the convex portion of a fetus, because that is the part that lies in closest contact with the uterine wall. In a vertex or breech presentation, fetal heart sounds are usually best heard through the fetal back; in a face presentation, the back becomes concave so the sounds are best heard through the more convex thorax. In breech presentations, fetal heart sounds are heard most clearly high in the uterus, at the woman's umbilicus or above. In cephalic presentations, they are heard loudest low in the abdomen. In an ROA position, the sounds are heard best in the right lower quadrant; in an LOA position, in the left lower quadrant. In posterior positions (LOP or ROP), heart sounds are loudest on a woman's side. Figure 18.16 shows how to locate heart sounds for various fetal positions.

Hearing fetal heart sounds in these positions provides confirmatory information about fetal position. Conversely, recognizing fetal position aids in locating fetal heart sounds.

Determine the FHR every 30 minutes during beginning labor, every 15 minutes during active labor, and every 5 minutes during the second stage of labor. This can be done by viewing the FHR monitoring strip or by periodic auscultation.

To auscultate fetal heart sounds, use either a stethoscope or a fetoscope (a modified stethoscope attached to a headpiece), or obtain them with a Doppler unit, which uses ultrasound waves that bounce off the fetal heart to produce echoes or clicking noises (Fig. 18.17). These clicks reflect the FHR.

Electronic Monitoring

In most settings, FHR is screened at least for a short time in early labor by an external electronic monitoring system. The monitor is left in place for continuous monitoring on women who are categorized as high risk for any reason or who have oxytocin stimulation.

The use of fetal monitors has provoked one of the biggest controversies in modern obstetric health care. Monitors were widely adopted in the mid-1970s as a means of immediately detecting variations in FHR. However, prepared childbirth advocates have long criticized the overuse of monitoring devices, arguing that they intrude on the childbirth experience, causing needless discomfort and distraction to the mother. The medical profession readily admits that monitors contribute to the growing number of cesarean births (National Center for Health Statistics, 2005). Advocates of monitoring would say that the prevention of complications in even one baby is worth this increase. However, others believe that monitors often point to a problem where none exists, resulting in unnecessary cesarean births (which carries its own set of risks) and unnecessary frightening of parents (which could adversely affect early parent–infant bonding).

Monitoring does offer many advantages from a health care provider's standpoint. Observing the FHR on a monitor is easier than listening with a stethoscope or fetoscope. In addition, most health care providers have grown accustomed to monitors and may feel insecure without them. Few people advocate a return to the use of stethoscopes

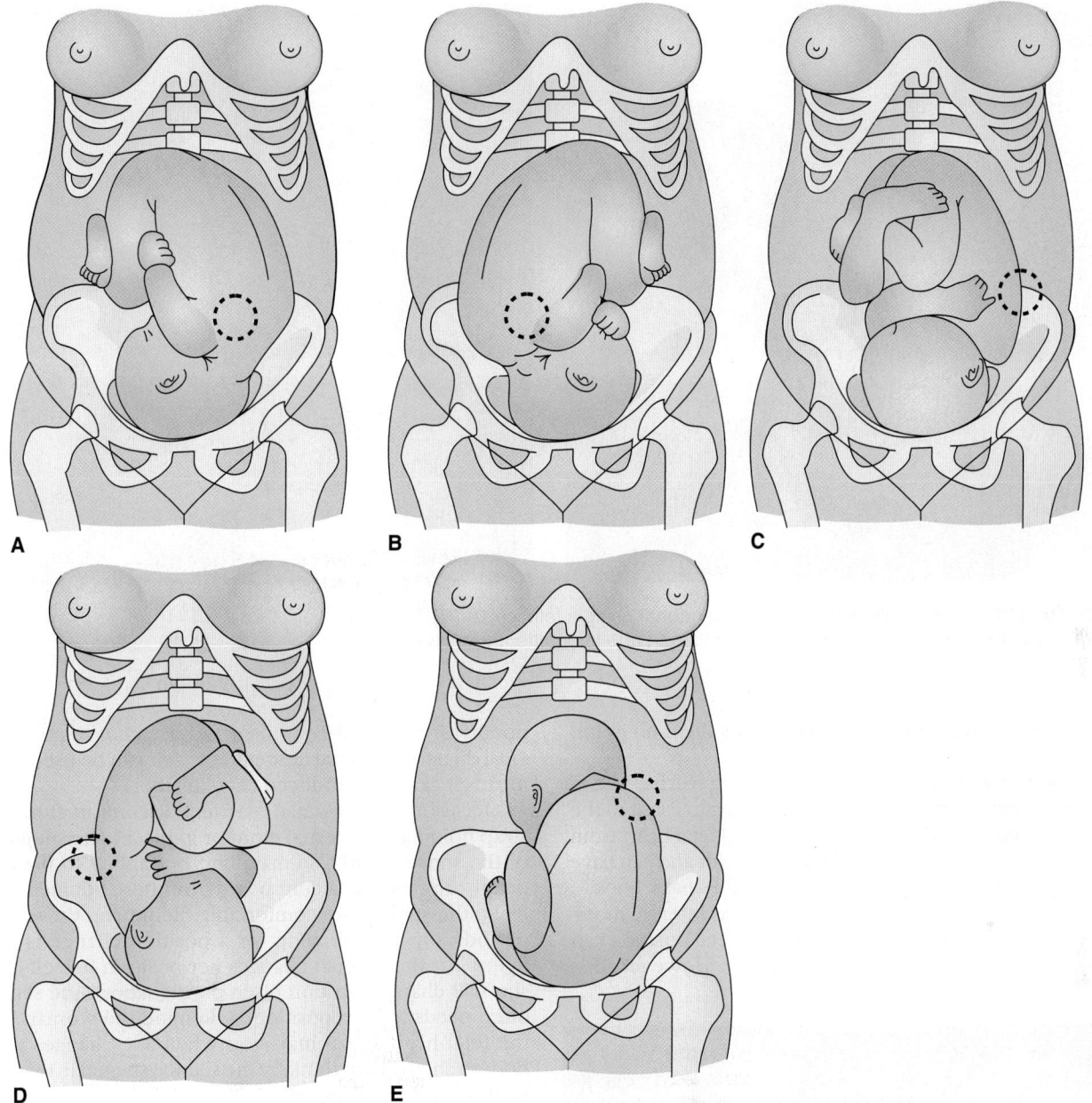

FIGURE 18.16 Locating fetal heart sounds by fetal position. (**A**) LOA, (**B**) ROA, (**C**) LOP, (**D**) ROP, (**E**) LSA.

for total assessment; use of monitors for periodic assessment rather than continuous monitoring is a compromise solution.

Be certain to tell parents that the FHR can vary greatly during labor and that the monitor is only an aid and should not be the focus of their attention. Parents can become so focused on what is happening on the monitor that they lose the ability to concentrate on previously learned relaxation and breathing techniques.

External Electronic Monitoring

External electronic monitoring is useful for monitoring both uterine contractions and FHR continuously or inter-

mittently. The information is obtained from sensors strapped to the woman's abdomen (Fig. 18.18).

Contractions are monitored by means of a pressure transducer or tocodynamometer (*toko* is Greek for contraction). Place the transducer over the uterine fundus or the area of greatest contractility. Verify that it is securely held in place by an adjustable strap or stockinette girdle (Fig. 18.19*A*). The transducer converts the pressure registered by the contraction into an electronic signal that is recorded on graph paper.

The FHR is monitored with the use of an ultrasonic sensor or monitor (see Fig. 18.19*A*) also strapped against a woman's abdomen at the level of the fetal chest. The small Doppler unit converts fetal heart movements into

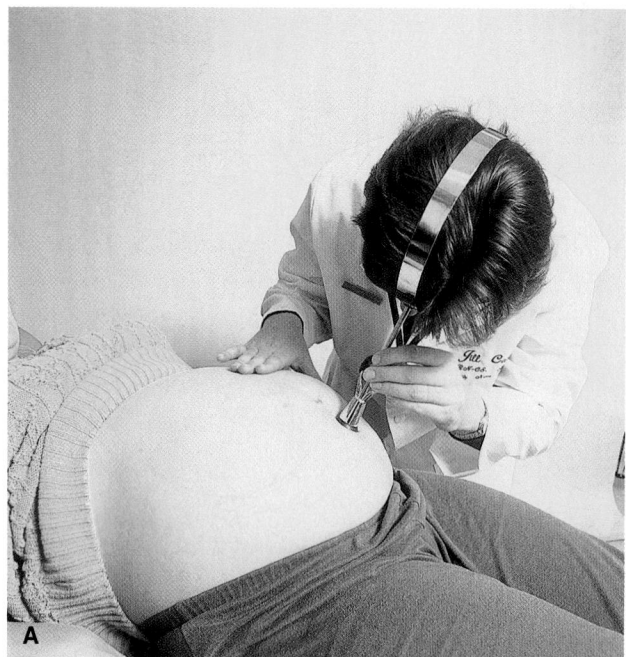
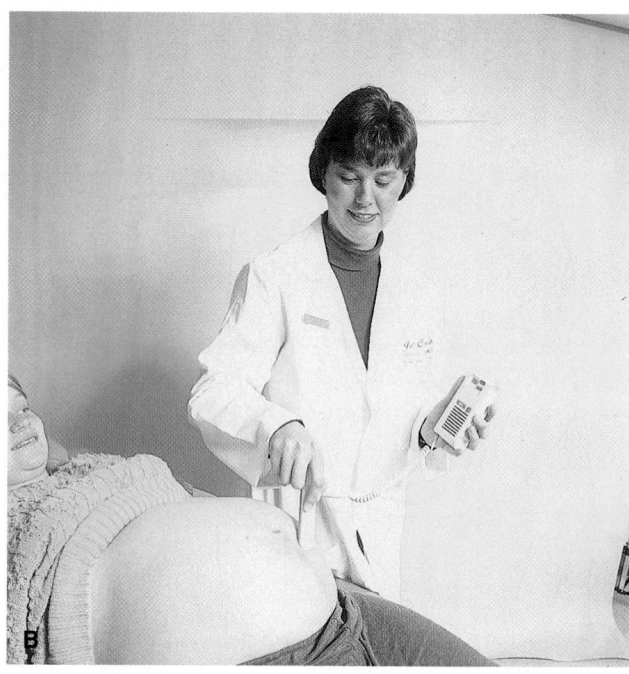

FIGURE 18.17 (**A**) Auscultation of the fetal heartbeat using a fetoscope. (**B**) A Doppler ultrasound device can be used to monitor fetal heart rate intermittently in low-risk labor. (Photos by Kieth Cotton.)

audible beeping sounds and also records them on graph paper.

A woman who is worried that something will happen to her child during labor will find it reassuring to listen to the regular beeping sound of the undistressed fetal heart from a fetal heart transducer. Many women ask for and can have a short graph tracing to save for their child's baby book.

External monitoring is not as reliable as internal monitoring, because a change in maternal or fetal position can interfere with the quality of the tracing. However, it is noninvasive and easily applied and does not require cervical dilatation or fetal descent before it can be used. This means it can be introduced early in labor.

Occasionally, a woman may feel discomfort from the strap holding an external monitor in place. The snugness of the sensor head also may limit her ability to breathe deeply. Spreading talcum powder on her abdomen may make the strap more comfortable. Removing the sensor periodically and allowing for a position change is also helpful. If the woman changes her position herself (and she will change position often during labor), the sensor often needs to be repositioned. Remind the woman that the fetal heart signal may stop when she changes position, so she will not think by the silence she hears that her baby's heart has stopped.

Women do not need to lie on their backs for monitoring, so the likelihood of supine hypotension syndrome is not increased. When giving care, be sure not to focus solely on the equipment; continue to communicate and offer support to the woman and her partner as needed.

What if... you enter Celeste Bailey's room while she has an electronic monitor in place and discover that she is lying on her back, seemingly frozen in one position? Would you urge her to turn or let her lie in a position that is comfortable for her?

Internal Electronic Monitoring

Internal electronic monitoring is the most precise method for assessing FHR and uterine contractions. A pressure-sensing catheter is passed through the vagina, into the uterine cavity and alongside the fetus, after the mem-

FIGURE 18.18 External electronic monitoring in place. Two devices (a transducer for the uterus and an ultrasound sensor for the fetus) are strapped to the woman's abdomen. (© Caroline Brown, RNC, MS, DEd.)

branes have ruptured and the cervix has dilatated to at least 3 cm (see Fig. 18.19*B*). The end of the catheter extending from the vagina is attached to a pressure recorder. As each contraction puts pressure on the uterine contents, the pressure exerted on the catheter is recorded. When uterine contractions are monitored by an internal pressure gauge in this way, the frequency, duration, baseline strength, and peak strength of contractions can all be evaluated. Strength of contractions is evaluated by the height of the peak of the contraction on the tracing. Equally important to evaluate is the return of the uterine tone to baseline strength between contractions. This ensures placental filling between contractions.

With contractions during the latent phase, the baseline level is usually less than 5 mm Hg; with active contractions, it is about 12 mm Hg. During the second stage of labor, the baseline may be as high as 20 mm Hg. Baseline readings that do not return to 20 mm Hg or less indicate uterine hypertonia and a possible compromise of fetal well-being.

The FHR recording is obtained from a fetal scalp electrode. Once the fetal head is engaged, the electrode is inserted vaginally and attached to the fetal scalp. A fetal electrocardiograph signal is obtained, amplified, and then fed into a cardiotachometer. The output from the cardiotachometer is recorded on permanent graph paper.

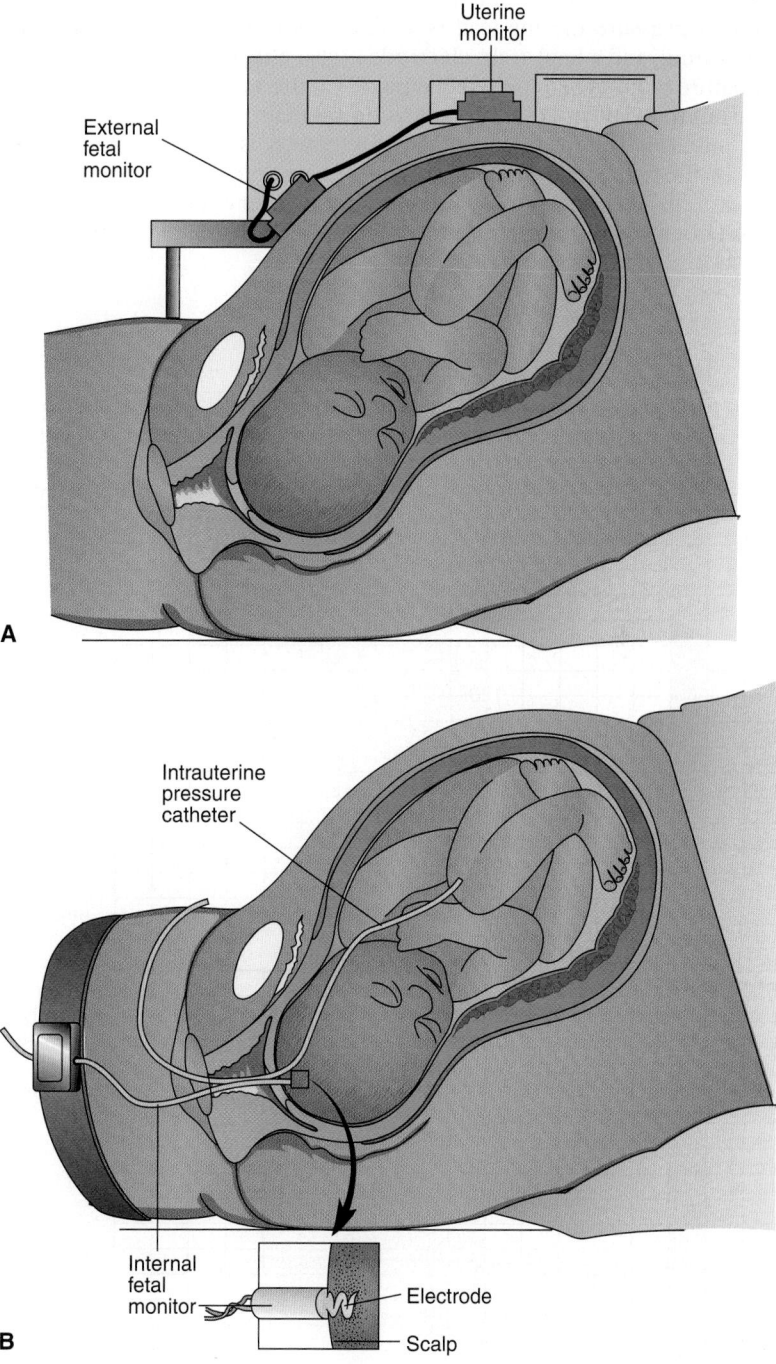

FIGURE 18.19 Placement of electronic monitoring leads. (**A**) External leads to monitor for FHR and uterine contractions. (**B**) An internal fetal heart rate lead in place on the fetal scalp. Uterine contractions are monitored by the intrauterine catheter.

The level of information obtained by internal monitoring cannot be matched by external monitoring, which records only the frequency and duration of contractions. The detail on fetal heartbeats is also clearer with internal monitoring (described later). On the other hand, internal monitoring is invasive, carries the risk of uterine infection, and limits a woman's movement. Because of these drawbacks, it is not used as routinely as external monitoring but is reserved for women who are at high risk during labor.

Telemetry

Telemetry allows monitoring of both FHR and uterine contractions to be carried out free of connecting wires that could hamper the woman's movements in labor. An internal pressure uterine lead is inserted, as in internal monitoring, and a fetal scalp electrode is also attached. A miniature radio transmitter is then placed in the vagina to transmit the FHR and uterine contraction signals to a distant monitor. The major advantage of telemetry is that it allows the woman to ambulate while being internally monitored. Because it is more expensive than other equipment, not all birth settings use telemetry.

Fetal Heart Rate and Uterine Contraction Records

Traditional abdominal monitors trace both the FHR and the duration and interval of uterine contractions onto paper rolls (Fig. 18.20). Uterine contraction information is recorded on the bottom half of the paper, FHR on the top half. Time can be calculated by counting the number of bold vertical lines on the paper (the space between two bold lines represents 60 seconds).

Fetal Heart Rate Patterns

Assessing and interpreting FHR patterns involves evaluating three parameters: the baseline rate, variabilities in the baseline rate (long-term and short-term), and periodic changes in the rate (acceleration and deceleration) (Spong, 2003).

Baseline Fetal Heart Rate

A baseline FHR is determined by analyzing the range of fetal heartbeats recorded on a 10-minute tracing that was obtained between contractions. A normal rate is 120 to 160 bpm. The rate fluctuates slightly (5 to 15 bpm) when

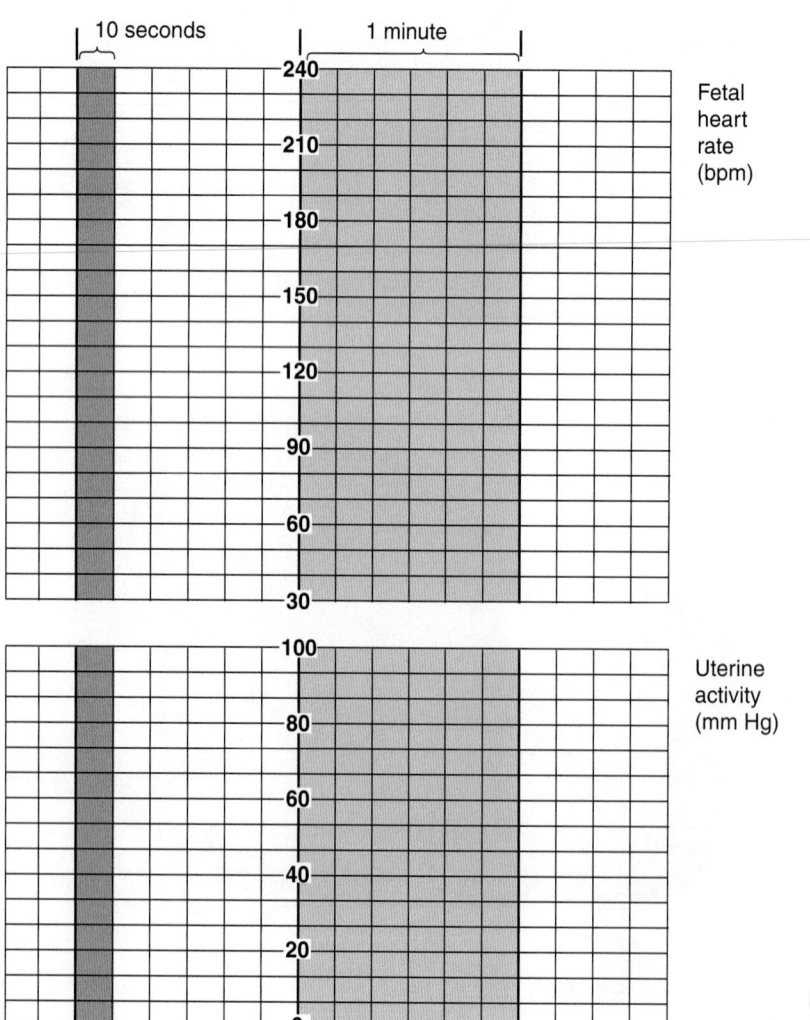

FIGURE 18.20 Paper strip for recording electronic fetal monitoring data.

a fetus moves or sleeps. If an increase or decrease occurs and is sustained for a 10-minute period, then a new baseline or a baseline change is established. Abnormal patterns in the baseline rate include fetal bradycardia and fetal tachycardia.

Fetal bradycardia occurs when the FHR is lower than 120 bpm for 10 minutes. A moderate bradycardia of 100 to 119 bpm is not considered serious and is probably due to a vagal response elicited by compression of the fetal head during labor. Marked bradycardia (less than 100 bpm) is a sign of possible hypoxia and is considered dangerous.

Fetal tachycardia occurs when the rate is 160 bpm or faster (for a 10-minute period). Moderate tachycardia is 161 to 180 bpm. Marked tachycardia is a rate greater than 180 bpm. Marked fetal tachycardia may be caused by fetal hypoxia, maternal fever, drugs, fetal arrhythmia, or maternal anemia or hyperthyroidism. In all instances, the cause needs to be investigated.

Variability

FHR variability is one of the most reliable indicators of fetal well-being. Baseline variability is the variation or differing rhythmicity in the heart rate over time and is reflected on the FHR tracing as a slight irregularity or "jitter" to the wave. The degree of baseline variability increases when the fetus is stimulated and slows when the fetus sleeps. If no variability is present, it indicates that the natural pacemaker activity of the fetal heart (effects of the sympathetic and parasympathetic nervous systems) has been affected. This may occur as a response to narcotics or barbiturates administered to a woman in labor, but the possibility of fetal hypoxia and acidosis must be investigated. Very immature fetuses show diminished baseline variability because of reduced nervous system response to stimulation and immature cardiac node function.

Baseline variability is defined as being either long-term or short-term (beat-to-beat) (Fig. 18.21). Long-term variability is seen on a broad view of the recording and results from fluctuations in the FHR, of 6 to 10 bpm, that occur 3 to 10 times per minute. Short-term or beat-to-beat variability refers to the difference between successive heartbeats, usually about 3 to 5 bpm. These changes are very subtle and can be picked up only with internal electronic

monitoring. Beat-to-beat variability can be rated as "present," "decreased," or "absent." Decreasing variability indicates the development of fetal distress. Absent variability is considered a severe sign, indicating that serious fetal compromise must be present.

Periodic Changes

Periodic changes or fluctuations in FHR occur in response to contractions and fetal movement and are described in terms of accelerations or decelerations. Periodic changes are short-term changes in rate rather than baseline; they last from a few seconds to 1 or 2 minutes. Four such responses are acceleration, early deceleration, late deceleration, and variable deceleration.

Accelerations. Accelerations are temporary normal increases in FHR caused by fetal movement or compression of the umbilical vein during a contraction.

Early Decelerations. Early decelerations are periodic decreases in FHR resulting from pressure on the fetal head during contractions. Parasympathetic stimulation in response to vagal nerve compression brings about a slowing of FHR. Early deceleration follows the pattern of the contraction, beginning when the contraction begins and ending when the contraction ends. However, the waveform of the FHR change is the inverse of the contraction waveform, with the lowest point of the deceleration occurring with the peak of the contraction. In this way, it serves as a mirror image of the contraction. The rate rarely falls below 100 bpm, and it returns quickly to between 120 and 160 beats at the end of the contraction (Fig. 18.22).

Early decelerations normally occur late in labor, when the head has descended fairly low. As such, they are viewed as a normal pattern. However, if they occur early in labor, before the head has fully descended, the head compression causing the waveform change could be the result of cephalopelvic disproportion and is a cause for concern.

Late Decelerations. Late decelerations are those that are delayed until 30 to 40 seconds after the onset of a contraction and continue beyond the end of the contraction (see Fig. 18.22). This is an ominous pattern in labor, be-

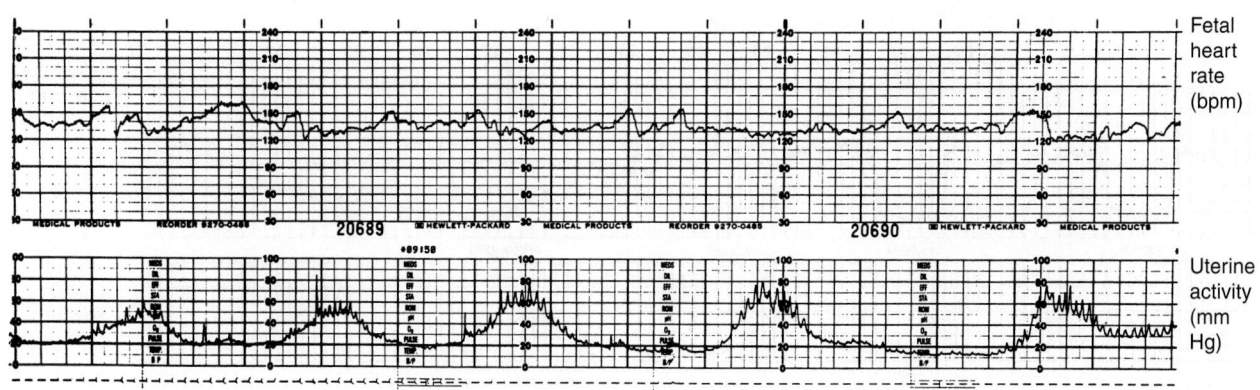

FIGURE 18.21 Fetal monitoring strip showing both long-term and short-term (beat-to-beat) variability.

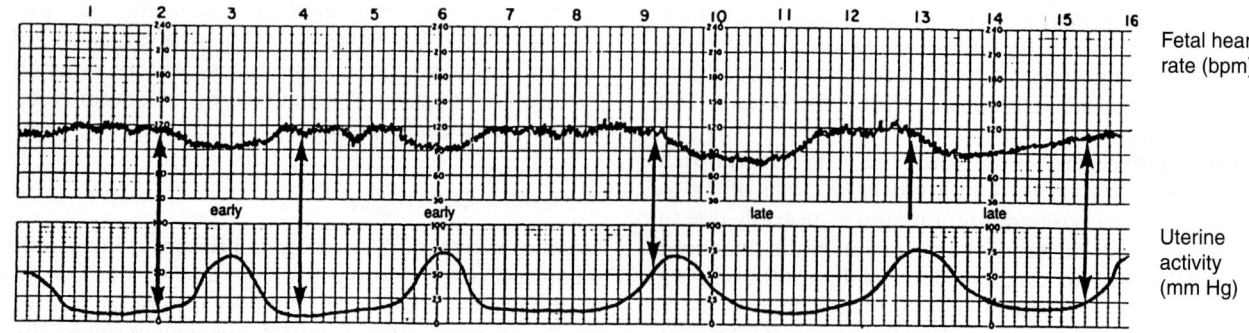

FIGURE 18.22 Schematic drawing of periodic FHR changes. Although the shape and depth of early and late decelerations are similar, note the differences in the onset of the decelerations and the recovery time to the baseline rate.

cause it suggests uteroplacental insufficiency or decreased blood flow through the intervillous spaces of the uterus during uterine contractions. The lowest point of the deceleration (nadir) occurs near the end of the contraction instead of at its peak. This pattern may occur with marked hypertonia or with abnormal uterine tone caused by the administration of oxytocin. Immediate steps to correct the situation must be initiated. If oxytocin is being used, stop or slow the rate of administration. Change the woman's position from supine to lateral (to relieve pressure on the vena cava and supply more blood to the uterus). Administer intravenous fluids or oxygen as prescribed. Prepare for possible prompt birth of the infant if the late decelerations persist or if FHR variability becomes abnormal (absent or decreased).

Prolonged decelerations are decelerations that last longer than 2 to 3 minutes but less than 10 minutes. They generally reflect an isolated occurrence, but they may signify a significant event, such as cord compression or maternal hypotension. For this reason, they must be reported and documented (Spong, 2003).

Variable Decelerations. The pattern of variable decelerations refers to decelerations that occur at unpredictable times in relation to contractions. They indicate compression of the cord, which can be an ominous development in terms of fetal well-being (Fig. 18.23). Cord compression may occur because of a prolapsed cord, but it also may occur because the fetus is lying on the cord. It tends

to occur more frequently after rupture of the membranes than when membranes are intact, or with oligohydramnios (the presence of less than a normal amount of amniotic fluid), such as occurs in postterm pregnancy or with intrauterine growth restriction. Because the pattern this produces is variable, often exhibited as U-, V-, or W-shaped waves, it can be completely missed if monitoring is not continuous. If this pattern is recognized on the monitor, change the woman's position from supine to lateral or to a Trendelenburg position to relieve pressure on the cord. Administer fluids and oxygen as prescribed. If variable decelerations are not relieved by these measures, amnioinfusion may be prescribed.

Amnioinfusion. **Amnioinfusion** is the addition of a sterile fluid into the uterus to supplement the amniotic fluid. The technique neither shortens nor prolongs labor; it just prevents additional cord compression. A sterile catheter is introduced through the cervix into the uterus after rupture of the membranes. It is attached to intravenous tubing, and a solution of warmed normal saline or lactated Ringer's solution is rapidly infused. Initially, approximately 500 mL is infused, and then the rate is adjusted to infuse the least amount necessary to maintain a monitor pattern without variable decelerations. Throughout the procedure, urge the woman to lie in a lateral recumbent position to prevent supine hypotension syndrome.

Help maintain strict aseptic technique during insertion and while caring for the catheter. Continuously monitor

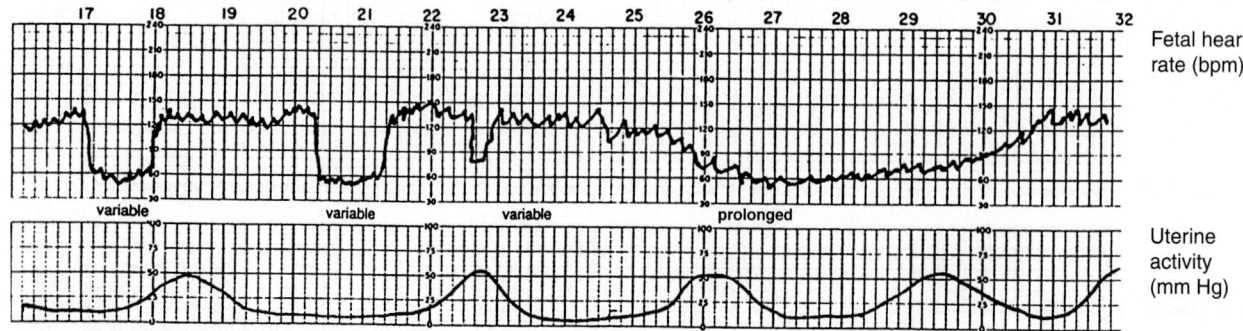

FIGURE 18.23 Schematic drawing of variable and prolonged decelerations. Note the abrupt drop in FHR in both types of decelerations. The variable decelerations return to baseline more quickly than the prolonged deceleration at 26–31 minutes, however.

FHR and uterine contractions internally during the infusion. Record maternal temperature hourly to detect infection. Be sure the solution is warmed to body temperature before the infusion, to prevent chilling of the mother and fetus. This can be done by placing the bag of fluid on a radiant heat warmer or by using a blood/fluid warmer before administration.

Because there will be a continuous flow of the infusing solution out of the woman's vagina during the procedure, change her bed frequently. Also assess that there is constant drainage. If vaginal leakage should stop, it usually means that the fetal head is firmly engaged and all fluid being infused is being held in the uterus. This is dangerous because it could lead to hydramnios (presence of excessive amniotic fluid) and possibly uterine rupture.

Sinusoidal Fetal Heart Rate Pattern

In a fetus who is severely anemic or hypoxic, central nervous system control of heart pacing may be so impaired that the FHR pattern resembles a frequently undulating wave. Long-term variability consists of 5 to 15 bpm every 3 to 5 minutes; beat-to-beat variability is minimal or absent; and there is a lack of specific responses to contractions. Although the cause of this pattern is poorly understood, it is recognized to be as ominous as a late deceleration or variable deceleration pattern.

Nonperiodic Changes

Nonperiodic changes are deceleration or acceleration changes that occur at times other than when the uterus is contracting. They are the result of events such as fetal movement, a change in maternal position, or administration of analgesia. Treatment may not be necessary and depends on the causative factor.

Other Assessment Techniques

Scalp Stimulation

If FHR variability is depressed, the welfare of the fetus can be further assessed by scalp stimulation. This is done by applying pressure with the fingers to the fetal scalp through the dilated cervix (Fig. 18.24). This causes a tactile response in the fetus that momentarily increases the FHR. If the fetus is in distress and becoming acidotic, FHR acceleration will not occur. Scalp stimulation, therefore, is an assessment of acid–base balance in a fetus.

Fetal Blood Sampling

Monitoring of the fetal blood composition may reveal hypoxia in a fetus before it becomes apparent on an electrocardiogram or external monitoring system. This is because changes in blood composition lead to alterations in FHR. It is unnecessary and impractical to monitor all fetuses by blood sampling during labor. The procedure is reserved for high-risk fetuses.

The oxygen saturation, partial pressures of oxygen (P_{O_2}) and carbon dioxide (P_{CO_2}), pH, bicarbonate excess, and hematocrit of fetal blood may all be determined during labor if a sample of capillary blood is taken from the

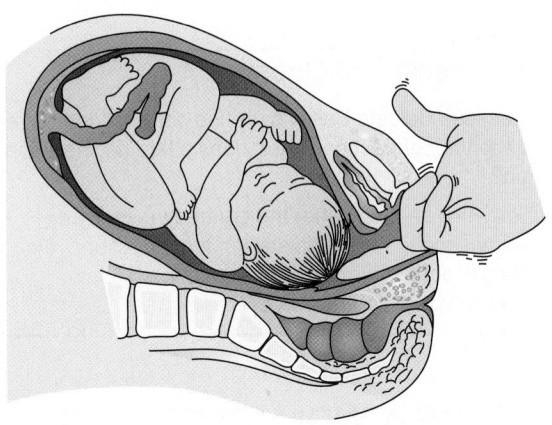

FIGURE 18.24 Technique for scalp stimulation. (Redrawn from *Journal of Perinatal and Neonatal Nursing, 1,* 16; with permission from Aspen Publishers, Inc.)

fetal scalp as it presents at the dilated cervix. After cervical dilatation of 3 to 4 cm and rupture of the membranes, the fetal head is visualized by the use of an amnioscope—a small, cone-shaped instrument with a light source at the far end. The scalp is cleaned with povidone-iodine and sprayed with silicon. A small scalpel is introduced vaginally into the cervix, and the fetal scalp is nicked. The silicon causes blood to form in beads, which are caught by a capillary tube. The incision is then compressed until the bleeding has stopped. After the procedure, the woman must be observed after two or three contractions to be certain that no new scalp bleeding occurs.

Although a blood sample obtained in this way may be analyzed for many parameters, usually only the pH results are necessary. If the fetus is hypoxic, the pH will fall (become acidotic). A scalp blood pH greater than 7.25 is considered normal for a fetus during labor. A pH between 7.21 and 7.25 should be remeasured in 30 minutes. A scalp blood pH lower than 7.20 is acidotic and signifies a level of fetal distress. This technique may be used to verify a heart rate pattern on a monitor that is becoming ominous. It can also be used to verify that no acidosis is occurring, even if a monitor rate is showing decreased variability. Fetal scalp sampling is becoming less popular because it has been found that firm pressure against the fetal head by a finger inserted vaginally increases monitor strip variability. If a variability increase occurs by this method, blood sampling is not necessary.

Fetal blood sampling involves no pain for the woman, but it may involve an uncomfortable sensation of pressure because of the examining hand in the vagina. Infants who have had internal scalp blood samples taken should not be born by vacuum extraction, because this procedure can lead to renewed bleeding at the puncture site.

Acoustic Stimulation

Acoustic stimulation, or instrumentally producing a sharp sound next to the woman's abdomen, is used with nonstress tests during pregnancy to produce FHR acceleration (see Chapter 8). It can also be used during labor to demonstrate that the fetus is reactive.

Checkpoint Question 4

You assess Celeste Bailey's uterine contractions. In relation to the contraction, when does a late deceleration begin?

a. Forty-five seconds after the contraction is over.
b. Thirty seconds after the start of a contraction.
c. After every tenth or more contraction.
d. After a typical contraction ends.

CARE OF A WOMAN DURING THE FIRST STAGE OF LABOR

Six major concepts to make labor and birth as natural as possible are currently stressed by childbirth educators: (1) labor should begin on its own, not be artificially induced; (2) women should be able to move about freely throughout labor, not be confined to bed; (3) women should receive continuous support during labor; (4) no interventions such as intravenous fluid should be used routinely; (5) women should be allowed to assume a non-supine (e.g., upright, side-lying) position for birth; and (6) mother and baby should be housed together after the birth, with unlimited opportunity for breast-feeding (Curl et al., 2004).

The first stage of labor begins with the beginning of uterine contractions and ends when the cervix has reached full dilatation. Most women have had labor contractions for hours before they arrive at a birthing center, because they deliberately stay at home until they are well into the first stage. Most likely, they have been experiencing pain and relying on their own judgment that everything is going well for a long time. One of their chief needs when they arrive at the birthing center, therefore, is to be reassured that everything is going well. For a woman who has been unable to manage pain by breathing exercises, pain relief is a priority need.

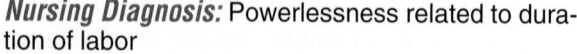

NURSING DIAGNOSES AND RELATED INTERVENTIONS

Nursing Diagnosis: Powerlessness related to duration of labor

Outcome Evaluation: Client expresses preferences for position and techniques to control pain; asks questions about her progress and states feelings about what is happening.

Care during the first stage of labor centers on helping the woman feel confident in her ability to control the pain and progress of labor and maintain physiologic stability. At first, it is exciting for a woman to feel labor contractions. They are little more than menstrual cramps and project a "this-is-really-happening" quality. Soon, however, if the woman is not concentrating on controlled breathing exercises, the contractions become biting in their intensity. Despite the fact that she is becoming more and more uncomfortable, however, nothing seems to be happening. A couple can begin to worry that something is going wrong; they may think that because the 9 months are over victory is near, yet it is eluding them. Give couples frequent progress reports during labor, so they do not become discouraged or fearful at this seeming lack of progress (Box 18.10).

A woman wants to feel that she has some control over her situation during labor. Most women accomplish this by stating their preferences, breathing with contractions, and changing their position to the one that makes them most comfortable. In contrast, some women handle the stress of labor by becoming extremely quiet. Others feel most comfortable when they can show their emotions by shouting or crying. Help a woman express her feelings in her own way, one that works the best for her.

Respect Contraction Time. Do not interrupt a woman who is in the middle of breathing exercises during labor because, once her concentration is disrupted, she will feel the extent of the contraction. If she has been successfully using breathing exercises to reduce pain, suddenly feeling the full force of a contraction can be frightening. She tenses, the pain becomes worse, and she may doubt her ability to breathe constructively in the face of such sharp pain with the next contraction. Instead of interrupting, allow her to finish breathing with her contraction, then ask questions or announce what procedure needs to be done next, or ask the question but wait patiently for the answer. (See Chapter 19 for a discussion of pain management techniques during labor.)

Promote Change of Positions. Because the bed is the main piece of furniture in a birthing room, most women assume that they are expected to lie quietly in bed during labor. In early labor, however, a woman may be out of bed walking or sitting up in bed or in a chair, kneeling, squatting, or in whatever position she prefers (Shilling & DiFranco, 2004) (Fig. 18.25). Reassure the woman that she may move about as needed (Box 18.11).

A woman whose membranes have ruptured should lie on her side until a fetal monitor shows good baseline variability and no variable decelerations or until she has been checked by a physician or nurse-midwife, because, unless the head of the fetus is well engaged (firmly fitting into the pelvic inlet), the umbilical cord may prolapse into the vagina if she walks.

If medication such as a narcotic is given, educate the woman to remain in bed for approximately 15 minutes afterward to avoid a fall if she should become dizzy from the medication. As labor becomes advanced, remaining in bed and assuming a

BOX 18.10: Focus on Nursing Care Planning

A Multidisciplinary Care Map for
A Woman Who Requires Comfort Measures
During Labor and Birth

•

Celeste Bailey is a 26-year-old you admit to a birthing room. She tells you she wants to have her baby "naturally" without any analgesia or anesthesia. Her husband is in the Army and assigned overseas, so he is not with her. Although her sister lives only two blocks from the hospital, Celeste doesn't want her called. She asks if she can talk to her mother on the telephone instead. As you finish assessing contractions, she screams with pain and shouts, "I'm doing everything I'm supposed to! How much longer does this go on?"

Family Assessment

Client lives with husband in Marine Base apartment. Husband currently assigned overseas. Finances rated as "horrible. If you want to be rich, don't marry a Marine." Both her mother and her married sister live nearby.

Client Assessment

Gravida 1, para 0. Contractions of moderate intensity, 45 seconds' duration, 3 minutes apart. Cervix dilated 3 cm, 60% effaced. Membranes intact. FHR 148; fetus in ROA position. Attended childbirth education classes, but is using breathing exercises ineffectively without coach. Brought a red rose to use as a focusing object.

Nursing Diagnosis

Pain related to uterine contractions and pressure on pelvic structures during labor

Outcome Criteria

Client confirms that her discomfort is controlled with nonpharmacologic or pharmacologic methods; responds to questions and instructions; identifies need for additional pain relief measures if needed as labor progresses.

Team Member Responsible	Assessment	Intervention	Rationale	Expected Outcome
Activities of Daily Living				
Nurse	Inspect the client's suprapubic area and palpate for bladder distention.	Encourage client to void every 2 hours.	A full bladder contributes to the client's discomfort and impedes fetal descent, possibly prolonging labor.	Client has no signs of bladder distention; voids every 2 hours during labor.
Nurse	Assess level of pain from uterine contractions and pelvic pressure by both verbal and nonverbal indicators; use 1 to 10 pain score.	Review and observe Lamaze breathing patterns with client to be certain she is obtaining maximum relief. Inform client about possible pharmacologic relief methods available to her if labor should be different than anticipated.	Pain is a subjective symptom, so only the client can determine her degree of pain or need for analgesia.	Client rates her level of pain from labor contractions as good to tolerable.

(continued)

Team Member Responsible	Assessment	Intervention	Rationale	Expected Outcome
Consultations				
Physician/ Nurse	Determine what personnel are available to prescribe or administer pharmacologic pain relief during labor, such as an epidural block.	Consult with nurse anesthetist about client's wish to not receive any pharmacologic pain relief.	Respecting client's wishes is a prime mode of encouraging self-efficacy.	Pain management team supports client's wish for no pharmacologic interventions; will be prepared to administer pain relief if client's wishes change or an emergency should change the client's goal.
Procedures/Medications				
Nurse	Assess what particular care measures, if any, client desires during labor (e.g., walking or not, birth position).	Establish a birth plan with client so all staff members can be aware of her individual preferences.	Respecting a client's choice helps to maintain self-esteem and a feeling of control.	Client expresses her preferences during labor.
Nutrition				
Nurse	Assess when client last ate. Ask about preferences for fluid during labor.	Provide client with ice chips or hard candy as desired.	Ice chips or hard candy can relieve mouth dryness from breathing exercises.	Client states she has no mouth discomfort and does not feel hungry.
Patient/Family Education				
Nurse	Assess what client knows about the usual process and time intervals of labor.	Provide information to supplement client's knowledge of labor; update client frequently on labor progress.	Teaching is most efficient if it is based on prior knowledge. Frequent updates about client's progress help to alleviate anxiety.	Client states that she understands the process of usual labor; indicates progress reports are helpful.
Psychosocial/Spiritual/Emotional Needs				
Nurse	Assess if physical environment seems conducive to labor without pharmacologic support.	Provide a comfortable environment (e.g., change sheets frequently, adjust room temperature, offer cool washcloths to forehead).	A comfortable environment aids in relaxation and minimizes distractions, promoting effective coping to manage discomfort.	Client reports that environment is comfortable and she feels secure. Client assumes a variety of positions during labor as desired. Client expresses that she is able to focus during contractions unimpaired by health care providers.
		Encourage client to assume different positions and to change them regularly. Allow client to walk or sit in chair, if not contraindicated.	Position changes promote comfort, reduce muscle tension, relieve pressure, and promote fetal descent.	
		Respect the need for focusing during contractions. Refrain from intervening with client during a contraction.	Interrupting client's focusing can be distracting, making the technique ineffective as a pain relief measure.	
Nurse	Assess if client would like to have a support person with her.	Help client locate a suitable support person (mother?). If none is available, serve as primary support person.	A support person can play a major role in making labor a tolerable experience.	Client names a person she wants as her support person. Person or nurse serves as a support person during labor.

(continued)

Team Member Responsible	Assessment	Intervention	Rationale	Expected Outcome
Discharge Planning				
Nurse	Assess how client evaluates her labor experience.	Help client voice her satisfaction or dissatisfaction with her labor experience.	Reviewing a possibly traumatic experience helps debrief (put it into perspective among life events).	Client states that labor and birth was at worst a tolerable experience; at best, a highlight of her life.

position of comfort may be best, so that, if the birth is precipitous, the infant will not be born while the woman is walking and suffer an injury.

While the woman is in bed, encourage her to lie on her side, preferably the left side. This position causes the heavy uterus to tip forward, away from the vena cava, allowing free blood return from the lower extremities and adequate placental filling and circulation. Most women are comfortable in this posi-

tion and adjust to it readily. Position the chair for the support person facing the laboring woman. Otherwise, she will keep turning to her back to talk.

Some women have learned to do breathing exercises in a supine position and may need additional coaching to do them in a side-lying position. If the woman must turn to her back during a contraction to make her breathing exercises effective, help her to remember to return to her side between

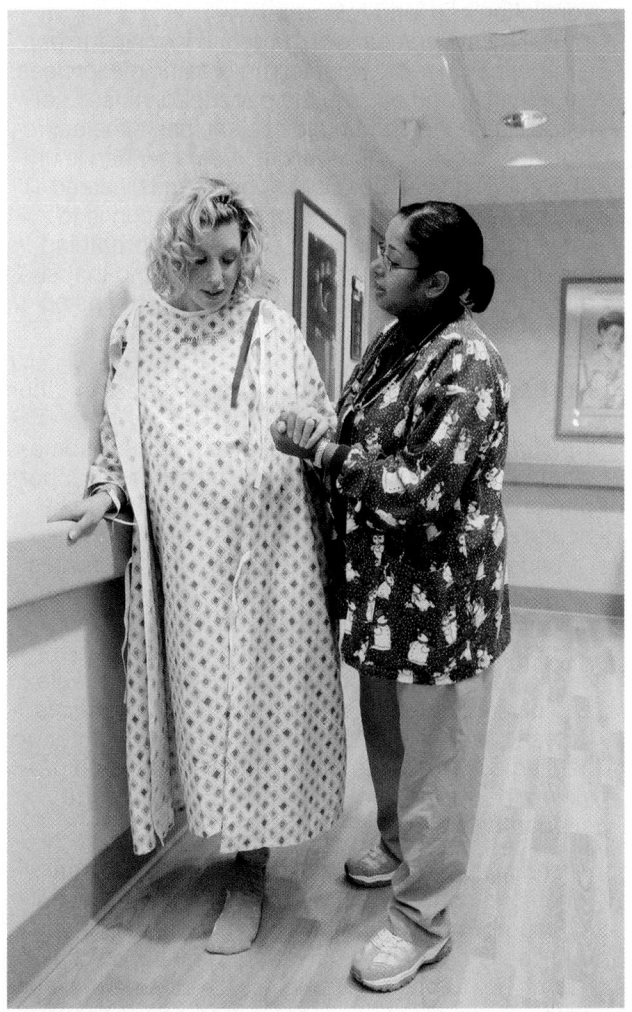

FIGURE 18.25 Finding a comfortable position during early labor is important. Here, a nurse assists a woman with walking during labor.

BOX 18.11 FOCUS ON . . .

COMMUNICATION

Celeste Bailey's baby is in an occiput posterior position, so she has had extensive back pain since labor began.

Less Effective Communication

Nurse: You don't look very comfortable, Celeste. Would you feel better if you sat in the rocking chair rather than staying in bed?

Celeste: Can I do that?

Nurse: I told you on admission. You can do whatever is most comfortable for you.

Celeste: Would it be all right if I walk over to the window?

Nurse: I told you on admission. Do whatever is most comfortable for you.

Celeste: I guess I'm not being a very good patient.

More Effective Communication

Nurse: You don't look very comfortable, Celeste. Would you feel better if you sat in the rocking chair rather than staying in bed?

Celeste: Can I do that?

Nurse: You can use any position that is comfortable for you.

Celeste: Would it be all right if I walk over to the window?

Nurse: Whatever is most comfortable for you.

Celeste: Thank you. You're very understanding.

Most women in labor are enduring so much pain and are under so much stress they don't "hear" or process instructions well. Reminding them that they have not processed information well is not therapeutic, because it can lower their self-esteem and sense of self-control.

contractions. A squatting position is very effective for birth because it helps to align the fetal presenting part with the cervix and also uses the fetal weight to help bring about cervical dilatation.

Promote Voiding and Provide Bladder Care. A full bladder or bowel can impede fetal descent, so encourage the woman to void, if possible, at least every 2 to 4 hours. The way a full bladder can impede descent of a fetus is shown in Figure 18.26. You need to remind the woman to do this during labor, because she may mistakenly interpret the discomfort of a full bladder as part of the sensations of labor. Assess for a full bladder by percussion (an empty bladder sounds dull; a full one sounds resonant). If she cannot void and the bladder becomes distended, she may need to be catheterized. Catheterizing a woman in labor is uncomfortable for her and difficult for you: the vulva is edematous from the pressure of the fetal presenting part,

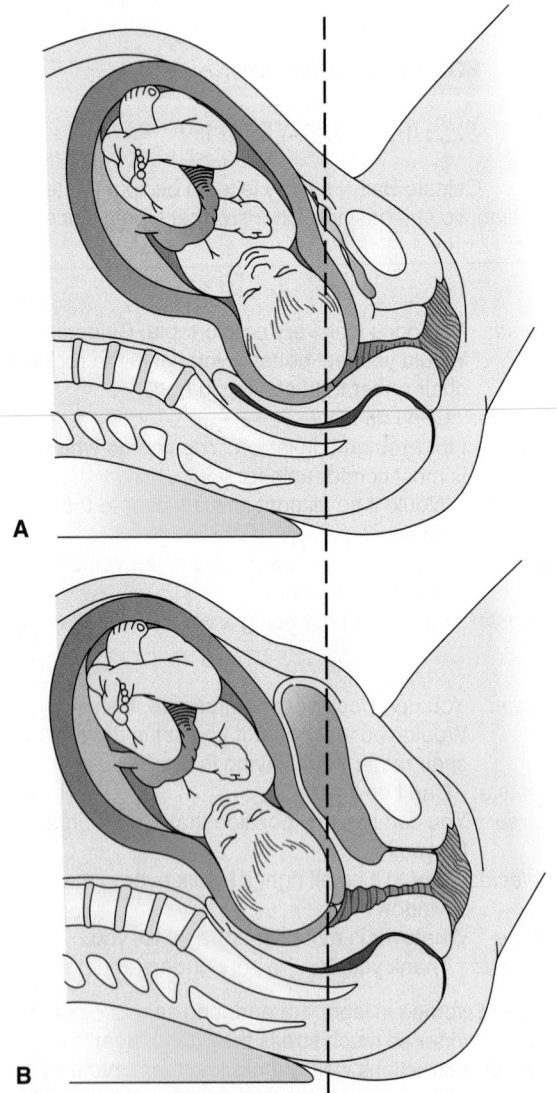

FIGURE 18.26 Effect of a full bladder on fetal descent. (**A**) Bladder is empty. (**B**) A full bladder impedes fetal progress.

stretching the urethral canal downward and making the urethra difficult to locate. For best results, use a small catheter (No. 12–14F), and insert it between contractions. Use extremely careful aseptic technique to avoid introducing any microorganisms that might result in a urinary tract infection.

Nursing Diagnosis: Risk for ineffective breathing pattern related to breathing exercises

Outcome Evaluation: Client's respiratory rate is within normal limits; skin is normal color, cool, and dry. No reports of lightheadedness or tingling/numbness in extremities.

Hyperventilation (an accelerated rate of respiration) occurs when a woman exhales more deeply than she inhales. As a result, extra carbon dioxide is blown off and respiratory alkalosis results. This can occur when a woman is practicing breathing exercises in preparation for labor, but it is most apt to occur during actual labor. The woman feels lightheaded and may have tingling or numbness in her toes and fingertips. If allowed to progress, hyperventilation can lead to coma.

To halt hyperventilation, urge the woman to keep a paper bag nearby when doing breathing exercises. Breathing in and out into the paper bag causes her to rebreathe the carbon dioxide she has exhaled, replacing the carbon dioxide lost. If a paper bag is unavailable, she can use her cupped hands instead.

The best way to handle hyperventilation is to prevent it. Be certain when a woman is breathing rapidly that she is not hyperventilating and that she ends all breathing sessions with a long cleansing breath to help restore carbon dioxide balance.

Nursing Diagnosis: Anxiety related to stress of labor

Outcome Evaluation: Client states she feels somewhat in control of her situation; she and her support person express confidence in themselves and in health care personnel.

Labor is such an intense process that it creates a high level of emotional stress for both a woman and her support person. Ability to tolerate stress (to cope adequately) depends on a person's perception of the event, the support people available, and past experience in using coping mechanisms. Ways to reduce stress in labor, therefore, center on helping a woman to perceive labor clearly and providing the opportunity for her partner to provide support as well.

Offer Support. There is no substitute for personal touch and contact as a way to provide support during labor. Patting a woman's arm while telling her that she is progressing in labor, brushing a wisp of hair off her forehead, wiping her forehead with a cool cloth—these are indispensable methods of conveying concern. This caring attitude has several benefits. First, it may make the difference in helping a woman feel safe and able to continue in control. In addition, a woman who is touched, who experiences the warmth and friendliness of human contact during labor—a time when she is physically dependent—may handle her newborn (who is also physically dependent and undergoing an adjustment not unlike the one she has just gone through) more warmly and affectionately. On the other hand, not all women care for physical contact during labor, and enjoyment of touch can be culturally determined.

Respect and Promote the Support Person's Activities. Admit a woman's support person to the birthing area and allow him or her to remain with the woman throughout the birth. Having someone with her during labor is important, because everything is new and a woman may not be used to the sensation of contractions. Acquaint the woman and her support person with the physical facilities, and point out where supplies such as towels, washcloths, and ice chips are stored, so the support person can get them when necessary. Review procedures and reassure the support person early in labor that he or she is welcome there. Also, be sure that all health care personnel are aware of who the support person is and make him or her feel welcome.

Often the support person will be acting as a labor coach. Ask both the woman and the support person whether they have been to prepared childbirth classes and whether the support person plans to help the woman with her breathing. If so, support this person's role. If he or she is hesitant, it is better to review techniques than to take over. Offer praise not only for the woman but for the support person as well. Relieve the support person as necessary, so that he or she can take a break and get something to eat or visit with older children (Fig. 18.27). If older children will view the birth, be certain that they are oriented and have a child care provider.

In addition to having the father of their baby present, many women choose a doula or another woman to be with them in labor (Pascali-Bonaro & Kroeger, 2004). Fathers may find it hard to provide doula-type support during labor because of their own emotional involvement in the birth. Having such a person present frees the father to enjoy the birth rather than feel occupied with coaching instructions. Although research in the subject is not extensive, there are suggestions that rates of oxytocin augmentation, epidural anesthesia, and cesarean birth can be reduced by doula support.

What if... a doula and Celeste Bailey's mother disagree on whether Celeste needs additional medication for pain while in labor? Whose suggestion would you pay most attention to? How could you resolve the issue?

Support a Woman's Pain Management Efforts. Some women believe that using a prepared childbirth method will create a pain-free, effortless labor. When they realize this is untrue, they may panic

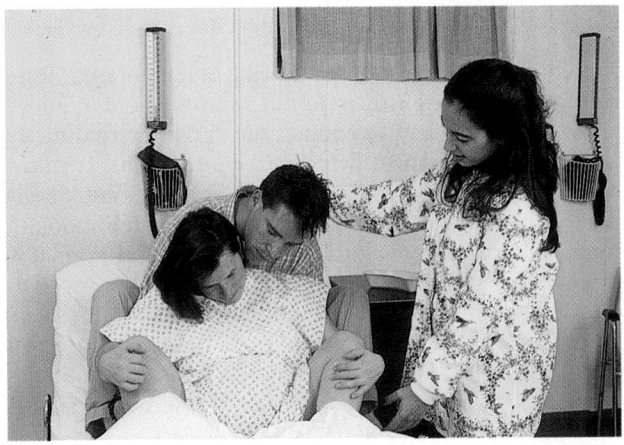

FIGURE 18.27 Encouraging the support person, so he can continue to give support, is an important nursing role. (© Barbara Proud.)

and lose the ability to use prepared breathing. Some support people are more nervous than they anticipated and have difficulty being supportive, leaving the woman to manage her anxiety on her own. In these instances, administering an analgesic might be effective in reducing anxiety or taking the edge off contractions. With this degree of relaxation, the woman may be able to return to effective breathing techniques. Sometimes, simply the support of a person, such as a nurse, who is confident that breathing can be effective in reducing the discomfort of labor is all a woman needs to resume her breathing exercises with success.

Many women plan on using nonpharmacologic pain relief measures such as aromatherapy during labor; ask what the woman has planned and what your role should be.

Nursing Diagnosis: Risk for fluid volume deficit related to prolonged lack of oral intake and diaphoresis from the effort of labor

Outcome Evaluation: Client states she does not feel thirsty; voids at least 30 mL/hour every 2 to 4 hours.

How much fluid or food a woman should ingest during labor is controversial. Most hospitals limit the amount of oral fluid or food intake during labor to ice chips or lollipops, to prevent aspiration if, in an emergency, administration of general anesthesia should be necessary. Because of this, a woman's mouth and lips may become uncomfortably dry from mouth breathing. Applying a cream to her lips or suggesting that she suck on hard candy or ice chips to relieve this discomfort can be helpful. Women in prolonged labor may need isotonic sports drinks to prevent secondary uterine inertia (a cessation of labor contractions) as well as generalized dehydration and exhaustion. If all oral fluids are contraindicated by the birth plan, intravenous glucose solutions may be administered to maintain caloric reserve.

Amniotomy

Amniotomy is the artificial rupturing of membranes. Rupturing membranes if they do not rupture spontaneously allows the fetal head to contact the cervix more directly and may increase the efficiency of contractions. For this, a woman's cervix must be dilated at least 3 cm. She is placed in a dorsal recumbent position; an amniohook (a long, thin instrument) or a hemostat is passed vaginally. The membranes are torn, and amniotic fluid is allowed to escape. This puts a fetus momentarily at risk for cord prolapse, because there is a possibility that a loop of cord will escape with the fluid. Always measure the FHR immediately after the rupture of membranes to determine that this did not happen (Katz, 2003).

Checkpoint Question 5

Celeste has an amniotomy (artificial rupture of the membranes). After this procedure, which of the following would be an important nursing assessment?

a. Ask her if her pain level is tolerable postprocedure.
b. Assess maternal heart rate to detect possible bleeding.
c. Assess fetal heart rate to detect possible cord prolapse.
d. Document the amount of amniotic fluid that has been lost.

CARE OF A WOMAN DURING THE SECOND STAGE OF LABOR

The second stage of labor is the time from full cervical dilatation to birth of the newborn. Even women who have taken childbirth education classes are surprised at the intensity of the contractions in this phase of labor. Because the feeling to push is so strong, some women react to this change in contractions by growing increasingly argumentative and angry, or by crying and screaming. Other women react by tensing their abdominal muscles and trying to resist, making the sensation even more painful and frightening.

The support person plays a vital role during this time, because all of the preparations done up to this point may still not be enough to sustain a woman during these final contractions unless she feels well supported. This participation also creates an important sharing time later, after the birth, that gives a couple a sense of family for the first time.

Women need to have an experienced health care person with them as well as they enter this stage of labor, to reassure them that the change in contractions is normal and to give knowledgeable support that everything is all right.

Assess fetal heart sounds at the beginning of the second stage of labor to be certain that the start of the baby's passage in the birth canal is not occluding the cord and interfering with fetal circulation. A general timetable for second-stage interventions is shown in Table 18.6.

Preparing the Place of Birth

At one time, women had little say as to the setting where their baby would be born, but today women are allowed a multitude of options. Some choose their own home. In the past, hospitals provided different rooms for labor (labor rooms), for birth (delivery rooms), and for recuperation (postpartal rooms). Today, these rooms are combined into labor-delivery-recovery-postpartal rooms (LDRP or LDR rooms).

Birthing Room

For a multipara, convert the birthing room into a birth room by opening the sterile packs of supplies on waiting tables when the cervix has dilatated to 7 to 9 cm. For a primipara, this can be delayed until the head has crowned to the size of a quarter or half-dollar (full dilatation and descent). A table set with equipment such as sponges, drapes, scissors, basins, clamps, bulb syringe, vaginal packing, and sterile gowns, gloves, and towels, can be left, covered, for up to 8 hours. Be certain that drapes and materials used for birth are sterile, so that no microorganisms can be accidentally introduced into the uterus.

To provide for baby care, open the partition at the end of the room to reveal the "baby island," or newborn care

---

TABLE 18.6

Time Intervals for Nursing Interventions During Second Stage of Labor

Intervention	Beginning of Second Stage	Continued Frequency	After Birth of Infant	After Delivery of Placenta
Assess and Record				
Temperature	X	q2h		X
Pulse	X	q1h	X	X
Respirations	X	q1h	X	X
Blood pressure	After anesthetic administration	q1h	X	X
Fetal heart rate	X	Continuously by monitor or q5min		
Contractions	X	Continuously by monitor or q5min		
Provide				
Support	X	Continuously	Continuously	Continuously

area. Such areas include a radiant heat warmer, equipment for suction and resuscitation, and supplies for eye care and identification of the newborn. Turn on the radiant heat warmer in advance, so that the bottom mattress is pleasantly warm to the touch at the time of birth. Place sterile towels and a blanket on the warmer, so that they will also be warm to use to dry and cover the infant.

Positioning for Birth

A variety of positions can be used for birth. At one time, the lithotomy position was the major position for birth, but it is no longer the position of choice in birthing rooms or alternative birth centers—although the labor beds in these locales usually have attached stirrups to allow birth in a lithotomy position. Alternative birth positions include the lateral or Sims' position, the dorsal recumbent position (on the back with knees flexed), semisitting, and squatting (Keen et al., 2004).

Nurse-midwives tend to favor these alternative birth positions for their clients because they seem to place less tension on the perineum, resulting in fewer perineal tears. An episiotomy can be made in alternative positions, although suturing is more difficult than in a lithotomy position.

If the physician prefers a lithotomy position for birth, position the woman into the table stirrups while the physician is scrubbing and donning a sterile mask, gown, and gloves. Raise both of the woman's legs at the same time to prevent strain on her back and lower abdominal muscles. The strap holding the leg in the stirrups should be secured snugly but not so tightly that it causes constriction. Many women perceive stirrups as an unnatural position for birth, but they provide the best position for performing an episiotomy or a forceps-assisted birth or for viewing the perineum to detect lacerations or other problems at birth, and they are generally not uncomfortable. Pad the stirrups with abdominal pads if a woman has ankle edema; to prevent thrombophlebitis, be certain that there is no pressure on her calves.

Because pushing becomes less effective in a lithotomy position, the top portion of the table can be raised to a 30- to 60-degree angle, so that the woman can continue to push effectively. Lying for longer than 1 hour in a lithotomy position leads to intense pelvic congestion, because blood flow to the lower extremities is impeded. Pelvic congestion may lead to an increase in thrombophlebitis in the postpartal period. It may also contribute to excessive blood loss with birth and placental loosening. For these reasons, place the woman's legs in a lithotomy position only at the last moment.

Once a woman is in a lithotomy position, the table's lower half is folded downward ("broken") so the physician can be in close proximity to the birth outlet. Make sure there is always someone at the foot of a broken birthing room table so that, if birth should occur precipitously, the infant will not fall and be injured.

Promoting Effective Second-Stage Pushing

For the most effective pushing during the second stage of labor, a woman must push with contractions and rest between them. The best approach is to allow her to push when she feels the urge and to use the position and technique she feels are best for her. Pushing is usually best done from a semi-Fowler's, squatting, or "all-fours" position rather than lying flat, to allow gravity to aid the effort (Fig. 18.28). A woman can use short pushes or long, sustained ones, whichever are more comfortable. Holding the breath during a contraction could cause a Valsalva maneuver or temporarily impede blood return to the heart because of increased intrathoracic pressure. This could also interfere with blood supply to the uterus. To prevent her from holding her breath during pushing, urge her to breathe out during a pushing effort.

In a multipara, to keep the second stage of labor from moving too fast, it may be necessary to prevent the woman from pushing. To accomplish this, ask her to pant with contractions. Because it is difficult to push effectively when she is using her diaphragm for panting, this limits pushing. Remember that pushing is involuntary. Regardless of how much a woman wants to cooperate, stopping this overwhelming urge to push is almost beyond her power. Demonstrating "panting like a puppy" and panting with her may be most effective. Be sure she is inhaling adequately. Otherwise, she might hyperventilate and become lightheaded while panting. Have her take deep cleansing breaths between contractions to prevent this.

Perineal Cleaning

Clean the perineum with a warmed antiseptic (cold solution causes cramping), and then rinse it with a designated solution before birth, according to the policy of the physician, nurse-midwife, or agency. Always clean from the vagina outward (so that microorganisms are moved away from the vagina, not toward it), using a clean compress for each stroke. Be sure and include a wide area (vulva, upper inner thighs, pubis, and anus). Figure 18.29 shows a typical pattern for cleaning. After cleaning, help place sterile drapes around the perineum.

As the woman pushes, the pressure of the fetal head on the bowel may cause fecal material to be expelled from the rectum. The physician or nurse-midwife will sponge this away as it occurs, to prevent contamination of the birth canal.

Episiotomy

An **episiotomy** is a surgical incision of the perineum that is made both to prevent tearing of the perineum and to release pressure on the fetal head with birth (Carroli & Belizan, 2005).

An episiotomy incision is made with blunt-tipped scissors in the midline of the perineum (a midline episiotomy) or is begun in the midline but directed laterally away from the rectum (a mediolateral episiotomy) (Fig. 18.30). Mediolateral episiotomies have the advantage over midline cuts in that, if tearing occurs beyond the incision, it will be away from the rectum, creating less danger of complication from rectal mucosal tears. However, midline episiotomies appear to heal more easily, cause less blood loss, and result in less postpartal discomfort.

Obstetric practice varies as to which type of episiotomy is done and how often. At one time this procedure

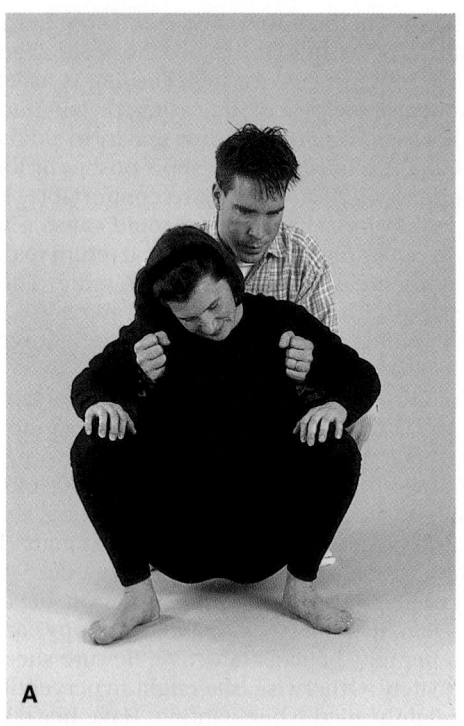

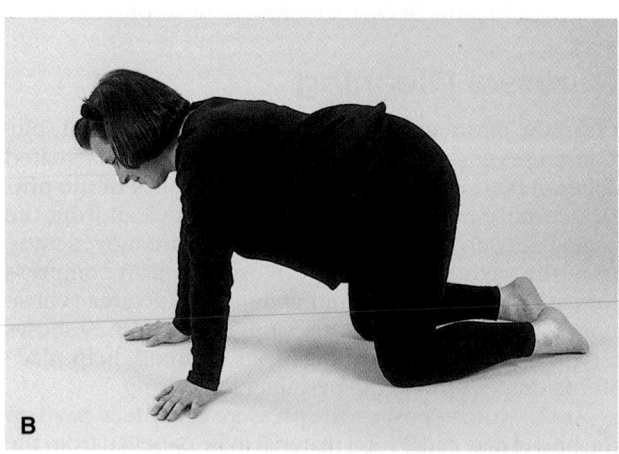

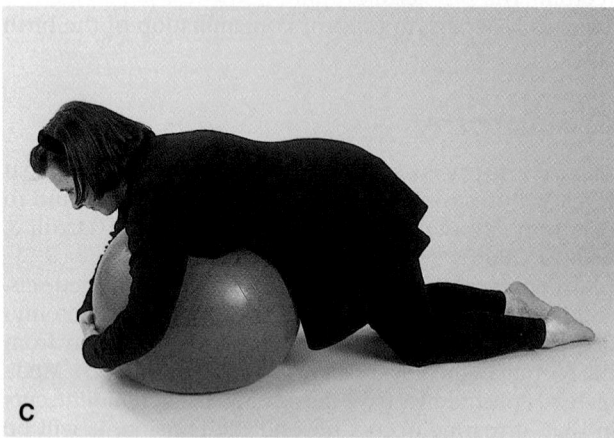

FIGURE 18.28 Positions for pushing during second stage labor: (**A**) squatting with support person; (**B**) all-fours; (**C**) all-fours with chest support. (© Barbara Proud.)

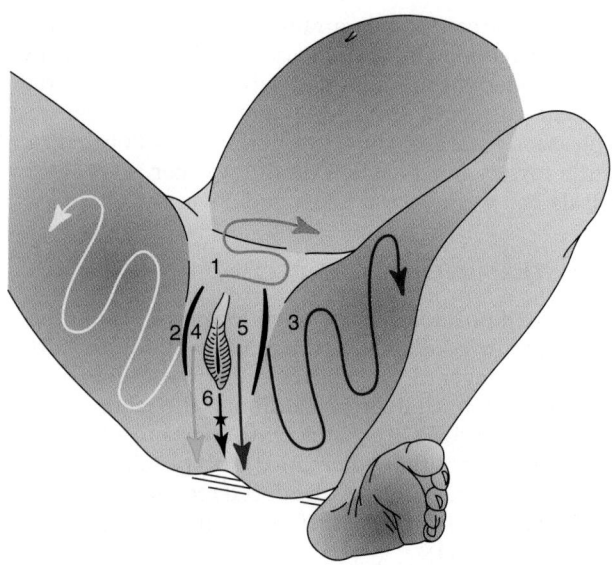

FIGURE 18.29 Pattern for cleaning perineum before birth. Cleaning from the birth canal outward moves bacteria away from, not into, the vagina. Numbers refer to steps of the procedure.

was done only if tearing seemed imminent; later, it was considered routine with a normal birth; and now it is used less frequently, again. The advantage of an episiotomy is that it substitutes a clean cut for a ragged tear, minimizes pressure on the fetal head, and may shorten the last portion of the second stage of labor.

The pressure of the fetal presenting part against the perineum is so intense that the nerve endings in the perineum are momentarily deadened. This lack of sensation allows an episiotomy to be done without anesthesia. For some women, a pudendal block may be done beforehand to ensure that there is no pain; lidocaine is injected via a long needle through the vaginal wall near the ischial spine, numbing the lower vaginal area and the perineum.

At the time of the episiotomy incision, there is a slight loss of blood, but the pressure of the presenting part im-

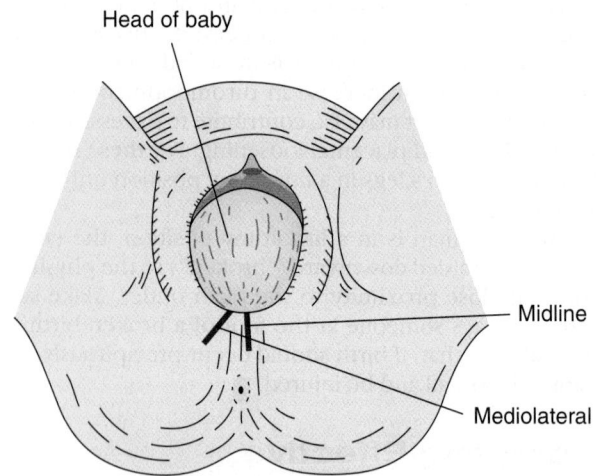

FIGURE 18.30 Position of episiotomy incision in a woman during second stage of labor. Baby's head is presenting to vagina outlet (crowning).

mediately seals the cut edges and minimizes bleeding. The fetal head usually moves forward considerably once the tension on the perineum is relieved.

Birth

As soon as the head of a fetus is prominent (approximately 8 cm across) at the vaginal opening, the physician or nurse-midwife may place a sterile towel over the rectum and press forward on the fetal chin while the other hand is pressed downward on the occiput (a Ritgen maneuver) (Fig. 18.31). This helps a fetus achieve extension, so that the head is born with the smallest diameter presenting. This also controls the rate at which the head is born. Pressure should never be applied to the fundus of the uterus to effect birth, because uterine rupture may occur.

The woman is asked to continue pushing until the occiput of the fetal head is firmly at the pubic arch. Then the head is born between contractions. This helps to prevent the head from being expelled too rapidly. It also helps to avoid perineal tears and a rapid change in pressure in the infant's head (which could rupture cerebral blood vessels). The woman may be asked to pant deliberately, so that she does not push during a contraction. She may be asked to push again without a contraction present to deliver the shoulders. Instructions should be repeated as necessary, because often the woman is so involved with the coming birth that she does not hear. Offer guidance and support to the partner as well, because he or she may be almost as overwhelmed by the birth process as the mother.

A woman who has not had anesthesia experiences the birth of the head as a flash of pain or a burning sensation, as if someone had momentarily poured hot water on her perineum. It is a fleeting sensation and is not particularly uncomfortable.

Immediately after birth of the baby's head, the physician or nurse-midwife suctions out the infant's mouth with a bulb syringe and then passes his or her fingers along the occiput to the newborn's neck, to determine whether a loop of umbilical cord is encircling the neck. It is not uncommon for a single loop of cord to be positioned this way (termed a nuchal cord). If such a loop is felt, it is gently loosened and drawn down over the fetal head. If it is too tightly coiled to allow this, it must be clamped and cut before the shoulders are born. Otherwise, it could tear and interfere with the fetal oxygen supply.

After expulsion of the fetal head, external rotation occurs. Gentle pressure is exerted downward on the side of the infant's head, and the anterior shoulder is born. Slight upward pressure on the side of the head allows the anterior shoulder to nestle against the symphysis as the posterior shoulder is born. The remainder of the body then slides free without any further difficulty.

A child is considered born when the whole body is born. This is the time that should be noted and recorded as the time of birth—a nursing responsibility. (Most physicians and nurse-midwives regard it as their responsibility or pleasure to announce the sex of the infant.) With the birth of the infant, the second stage of labor is complete (Fig. 18.32).

Cutting and Clamping the Cord

While the newborn is held with his or her head in a slightly dependent position, to allow secretions to drain from the nose and mouth, the mouth may be gently aspirated by a bulb syringe to remove additional secretions. The infant is then laid on the abdominal drape of the mother while the cord is cut. The cord continues to pulsate for a few minutes after birth, and then the pulsation ceases. There are a number of theories about the best time for cutting the cord. Delaying the cutting until pulsation ceases and maintaining the infant at a uterine level allows as much as 100 mL of blood to pass from the placenta into the fetus; this helps ensure an adequate red blood cell count in the newborn. On the other hand, late clamping of the cord could cause overinfusion with placental blood and the possibility of polycythemia and hyperbilirubinemia,

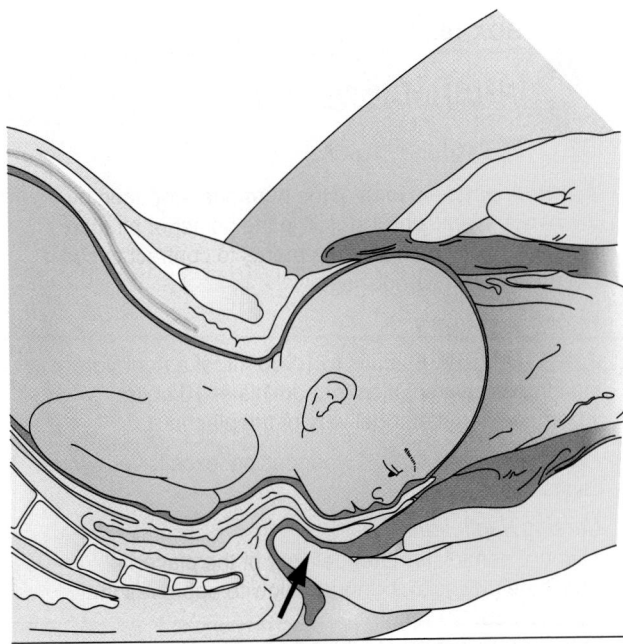

FIGURE 18.31 Ritgen's maneuver. The arrow shows direction of pressure.

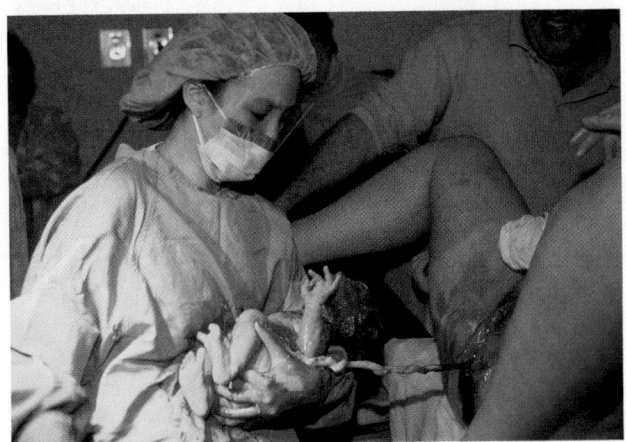

FIGURE 18.32 A child is considered born when the whole body is delivered. (© B. Proud.)

a particular concern in preterm infants. The timing of cord clamping, therefore, varies depending on the physician's or nurse-midwife's preference and the maturity of the infant. Placing the infant on the mother's abdomen may modify the amount of blood infused as well as allowing the parents a free, unobstructed view of their new child.

The cord is clamped with two Kelly hemostats placed 8 to 10 inches from the infant's umbilicus and then is cut between them. A cord blood sample is obtained to provide a ready source of infant blood if blood typing or other emergency measures need to be done. An umbilical clamp is then applied (Fig. 18.33). The vessels in the cord are counted to be certain that three are present. In most births, the woman's partner may have the privilege of cutting the cord.

Cutting the cord is part of the stimulus that initiates a first breath. With this, the infant's most important transition to the outside world, the establishment of independent respirations, has begun.

Introducing the Infant

After the cord is cut, it is time for the new parents to spend some time with their newborn. Take the infant from the physician or nurse-midwife and wrap him or her in a sterile blanket. Be sure to hold newborns firmly, because they are covered with slippery amniotic fluid and vernix. Lay the infant on a radiant heat warmer and dry him or her well with a warmed towel. Rewrap the infant snugly and cover the head with a wrapped towel or cap. Assuming that his or her respirations are good, take the infant to the head of the table to visit with the new parents.

Both the mother and her partner usually want to see and touch their newborn immediately; this assures them the baby is well and is an important step in establishing a parent–child relationship. Do not administer prophylactic eye ointment to the infant until after the parents have had this chance to see their infant (and the infant has had a chance to see them). (See Chapter 24 for infant care after birth.) If the woman wishes to breast-feed, this is an optimal time for her to begin. An infant sucking at the breast stimulates the release of endogenous oxytocin, encouraging uterine contraction and involution, or the return of the uterus to its prepregnant state.

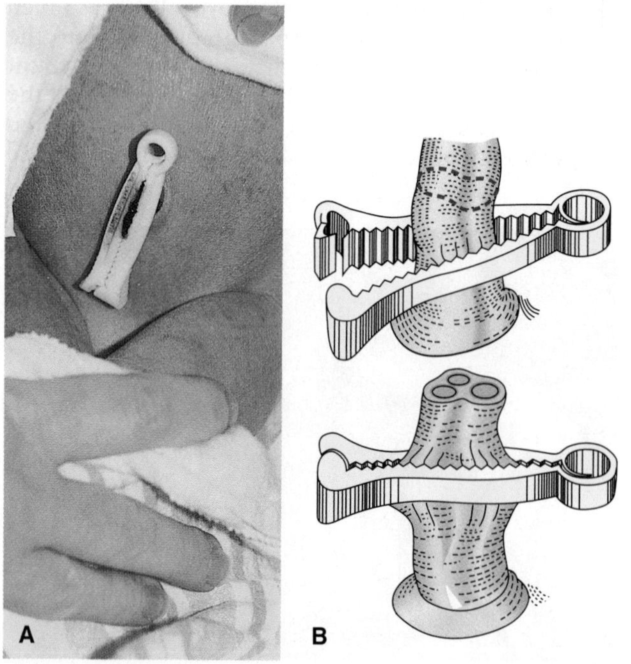

CARE OF A WOMAN DURING THE THIRD AND FOURTH STAGES OF LABOR

The third stage of labor is the time from the birth of the baby until the placenta is delivered. For most women, this is a time of excitement, because the infant has safely been born, but also a time of feeling anticlimactic, because the infant has finally arrived after being expected for so long. The fourth stage includes the first few hours after birth. It signals the beginning of dramatic changes because it marks the beginning of a new family.

Oxytocin

Once the placenta is delivered, oxytocin is usually ordered to be administered intramuscularly or intravenously to the mother. Such medication increases uterine contractions and thereby minimizes uterine bleeding (Elbourne et al., 2005).

Oxytocin (Pitocin) may be added to an existing intravenous line (20 to 40 U/L in intravenous fluid) or given as 10 U intramuscularly (Karch, 2004) (Box 18.12).

The administration of this drug is a nursing responsibility in most health care facilities. Do not administer it until the physician or nurse-midwife indicates it is appropriate. Although the agent may be given as early as the

FIGURE 18.33 **(A)** Umbilical clamp applied to cord. (© Caroline Brown, RNC, MC, DEd.) **(B)** Placing clamp; locking clamp.

BOX 18.12 FOCUS ON . . .

PHARMACOLOGY

Oxytocin (Pitocin)

Action: A synthetic form of the hormone produced by the hypothalamus and stored in the posterior pituitary. An oxytocic, it stimulates the uterus to contract to control postpartum hemorrhage.

Pregnancy Category: X

Dosage: Add 10–40 units to 1,000 mL of a nonhydrating intravenous solution, or administer 10 units intramuscularly after delivery of the placenta.

Possible Adverse Effects: Hypertension, excessive uterine contractility.

Nursing Implications
- Do not administer after delivery of the placenta until the physician or nurse-midwife approves the drug's use.
- Monitor the woman for blood pressure, because hypertension can occur.

birth of the fetal anterior shoulder, the physician or nurse-midwife may want to inspect the placenta first to ensure that it is intact and without gross abnormalities and that none of its cotyledons remains in the uterus. Because oxytocin causes hypertension by vasoconstriction, be sure to obtain a baseline blood pressure measurement before administration. Question the use of such a drug with women who have elevated blood pressure.

Intravenous administration of oxytocin may be continued for up to 8 hours after birth to ensure uterine contraction. Continue to monitor blood pressure during this time.

Placenta Delivery

If the placenta does not deliver spontaneously, the physician or nurse-midwife will need to remove it manually. After delivery, the placenta is inspected to be certain that it is intact and normal in appearance and weight. Normally, a placenta is one-sixth the weight of the infant. If it is unusually large or small, you may be asked to weigh it.

Perineal Repair

After delivery of the placenta, any necessary perineal stitching is performed. This process can be a long, tedious one from the mother's perspective. She must lie on her back and wait for the procedure to be completed, while the attention of others is riveted on the newborn lying in the warmer off to one side. It is important to be sensitive to the mother's needs at this time. Be certain to include her in explanations and appreciate how anticlimactic she may feel at this time.

Theoretically, if suturing of an episiotomy is done immediately after the birth of the placenta, a woman who gave birth without anesthesia will still have so much natural-pressure anesthesia of the perineum that she will not require an anesthetic. In actuality, by the time the placenta is delivered (approximately 5 minutes), enough sensation has returned to the perineum that the woman will probably need some type of medication for comfort. Women who received a regional anesthetic during labor (e.g., pudendal block) and those who have had epidural anesthesia will probably not need additional medication during episiotomy repair.

Immediate Postpartum Assessment and Nursing Care

Once the episiotomy repair is complete, the drapes are removed and the woman's legs are simultaneously and carefully lowered from the stirrups, if they were used, to prevent back injury.

Obtain vital signs (i.e., pulse, respirations, and blood pressure) every 15 minutes for the first hour and then according to the agency's policy. Pulse and respirations may be fairly rapid immediately after birth (80 to 90 bpm and 20 to 24 respirations per minute), and blood pressure slightly elevated due to the excitement of the moment and recent oxytocin administration. Palpate the woman's fundus for size, consistency, and position and observe the amount and characteristics of lochia. Perform perineal care, and apply a perineal pad.

If the birth was in a birthing room, return the birthing bed to its original position. Offer a clean gown and a warmed blanket, because a woman often experiences a chill and shaking sensation 10 to 15 minutes after birth. This may be due in part to the low temperature of the birthing room, but may also be a result of the sudden release of pressure on pelvic nerves or of excess epinephrine production during labor. In any event, it is a normal phenomenon but can be frightening to the mother. She may associate the shaking chill with fever or infection and worry she will be ill at a time when she most wants to be well to care for her new child. You can reassure her this is a normal, transitory sensation.

Aftercare

This is the beginning of the postpartal period or the fourth stage of labor. Because the uterus may be so exhausted from labor that it cannot maintain contraction, there is a high risk for hemorrhage. In addition, a woman often is so exhausted that she may be unable to assess her own condition or report any changes. Specific assessments done during this time are continued throughout the postpartal period. These assessments are discussed in Chapter 22.

UNIQUE CONCERNS OF A WOMAN IN LABOR

A Woman Without a Support Person

Some women have chosen to reject or want to labor without the infant's father, who is the usual support person during labor. Such women may appreciate having a family member or close friend act as their support person. A woman who has no support person needs a supportive nurse to be with her.

A woman whose acceptance of her pregnancy was slow to develop due to lack of adequate support people may not have completed the psychological tasks of pregnancy by the time she is in labor. This could make her more apprehensive about a new life role and calls for increased assessment of parent–child bonding in the immediate postpartal period.

A Woman Who Will Be Placing Her Baby for Adoption

Even if a woman has decided to place her baby for adoption, she needs to be an active participant in her labor and birth experience. She should watch the baby being born and be allowed to hold it as desired. Each state has a set number of days in which a mother must decide whether to keep her baby. Although this decision may have seemed easy to make during pregnancy, once she holds the baby in her arms, the prospect of giving up the child may be more painful than she realized. She needs support no matter what decision she eventually makes. Be certain you do not offer influencing advice, because the woman is the only person who knows whether keeping this child is right for her.

Vaginal Birth After Cesarean Birth

Women who have had a previous cesarean birth that involved a low transverse uterine incision are usually candidates for vaginal birth with their next pregnancy (Horey et al., 2005). The length of labor for vaginal birth after cesarean birth (VBAC) is usually comparable to that of primiparas, not multiparas, because it is their first vaginal birth. Most women are anxious for vaginal birth to be successful so that they do not have to undergo surgery again. At the same time, they may be surprised and dismayed at the length and discomfort of labor and wish that they could have another cesarean. Keep the woman well informed, and urge her to breathe with contractions and to push effectively to make the experience a positive one for her. Afterward, many women are relieved to realize that, although they did have more discomfort before birth, they have appreciably less pain afterward.

If during the previous labor a complication occurred that necessitated the cesarean birth, a woman cannot help but worry that this will happen again. She needs a support person with her and health care providers who are aware of her possible level of apprehension. Women having a VBAC usually have external electronic monitoring because of the risk for uterine rupture.

The outcome of VBAC is usually without complication. If necessary, oxytocin augmentation (see Chapter 21) can be used to strengthen uterine contractions; vacuum extraction and forceps birth can be used as necessary.

Key Points

Labor is the series of events by which uterine contractions expel a fetus and placenta from a woman's body.

The exact reason why labor begins is unknown. It most likely occurs because of an interplay between fetal and uterine factors.

Effective labor depends on interactions between the passage, the passenger, the power of contractions, and a woman's psychological readiness ("psyche").

Labor is an almost overwhelming experience because it involves such intense sensations and emotions. Women need a support person with them to help them cope with this experience.

Fetal presentation (the fetal body part that will initially contact the cervix) and position (the relationship of the fetal presenting part to a specific quadrant of the woman's pelvis) are both important in determining the success of labor.

The first stage of labor lasts from the onset of cervical dilatation until dilatation is complete (10 cm). The second stage extends from the time of full dilatation until the infant is born. A third or placental stage lasts from the time the infant is born until after delivery of the placenta. A fourth stage comprises the first few hours after birth.

Danger signs of labor include an abnormal FHR, meconium staining of amniotic fluid, abnormal maternal pulse or blood pressure, inadequate or prolonged contractions, formation of a pathologic retraction ring, development of an abnormal lower abdomen contour, and increasing apprehension.

Monitoring of uterine contractions and FHR is an important nursing responsibility. Fetal bradycardia, tachycardia, and late and variable decelerations are important observations to make. Interventions such as keeping the woman on her left side and promoting voiding help to prevent fetal distress. Offering psychological support is crucial to maternal well-being.

Pushing during the second stage of labor should be guided by the woman's need to push. Urge her to breathe out while pushing, if possible.

The placental stage follows birth and consists of placental separation and expulsion. Observe for excessive bleeding during this time. Do not pull on the cord to hasten separation, because this can lead to uterine inversion.

A fetus is in potential danger when the membranes rupture because of the possibility of cord prolapse. Always assess FHR at this point to safeguard the fetus.

A woman is at potential risk for hemorrhage throughout labor because of the possibility that the placenta could be dislodged. Assess for vaginal bleeding and vital signs to be sure this is not occurring.

Critical Thinking Exercises

1. Celeste Bailey, the woman you met at the beginning of the chapter, was certain her labor was not normal because it had lasted for 6 hours. Is this an unusually long time for a first stage of labor? Do you think she would have been comforted by learning the usual length?

2. Suppose that, when Celeste is admitted to a birthing room, she states she has read nothing during her pregnancy about labor and so has no idea what to expect. Would it be better to educate her or to let her proceed with not knowing? If you decide to teach her, what would you tell her early in labor? Midway in labor? Why might a woman enter labor without having read about it?

3. Most women today accept fetal monitoring equipment as an expected part of labor care. What would you do if Celeste Bailey tells you she does not want this type of fetal monitoring?

4. Examine the National Health Goals related to labor process. Most government-sponsored money for nursing research is allotted based on these goals. What would be a possible research topic to explore pertinent to these goals that would be applicable to the Bailey family and also advance evidence-based practice?

A B C
X Y Z
References

Beck, C. T. (2004). Post-traumatic stress disorder due to child-birth: The aftermath. *Nursing Research, 53*(4), 216-224.

Carroli, G., & Belizan, J. (2005). Episiotomy for vaginal birth. *The Cochrane Library (Oxford)(1)* (CD000081).

Cesario, S. K. (2005). Reevaluation of Friedman's labor curve: A pilot study. *JOGNN: Journal of Obstetric, Gynecologic and Neonatal Nursing, 33*(6), 713-722.

Cheng, Y. W., Hopkins, L. M., & Caughey, A. B. (2004). How long is too long: Does a prolonged second stage of labor in nulliparous women affect maternal and neonatal outcomes? *American Journal of Obstetrics and Gynecology, 191*(3), 933-938.

Cruikshank, D. P. (2003). Breech, other malpresentations and umbilical cord complications. In Scott, J. R., et al. *Danforth's obstetrics and gynecology* (9th ed.). Philadelphia: Lippincott Williams & Wilkins.

Curl, M., et al. (2004). Overview: Childbirth educators, doulas, nurses, and women respond to the six care practices for normal birth. *Journal of Perinatal Education, 13*(2), 42-50.

Department of Health and Human Services. (2000). *Healthy people 2010.* Washington, D.C.: DHHS.

Elbourne, D. R., et al. (2005). Prophylactic use of oxytocin in the third stage of labour. *The Cochrane Library (Oxford), (1)* (CD001808).

Friedman, E. (1978). *Labor, clinical evaluation and management* (2nd ed.). New York: Appleton-Century-Crofts.

Hodnett, E. D., et al. (2005). Continuous support for women during childbirth. *The Cochrane Library (Oxford) (4)* (CD003766).

Horey, D., Weaver, J., & Russell, H. (2005). Information for pregnant women about caesarean birth. *The Cochrane Library (Oxford) (4)* (CD003858).

Johnson, M., Maas, M., & Moorhead, S. (2000). *Nursing outcomes classification* (2nd ed.). St. Louis: Mosby.

Karch, A. M. (2004). *Lippincott's nursing drug guide.* Philadelphia: Lippincott Williams & Wilkins.

Katz, V. L. (2003). Prenatal care. In Scott, J. R., et al. (Eds.) *Danforth's obstetrics and gynecology* (9th ed.). Philadelphia: Lippincott Williams & Wilkins.

Keen, R., DiFranco, J., & Amis, D. (2004). Care practices that promote normal birth #5: Non-supine (e.g., upright or side-lying) positions for birth. *Journal of Perinatal Education, 13*(2), 30-34.

Malee, M. P. (2003). Medical and surgical complications of pregnancy. In Scott, J. R., et al. (Eds.) *Danforth's obstetrics and gynecology* (9th ed.). Philadelphia: Lippincott Williams & Wilkins.

Matthews, R., & Callister, L. C. (2004). Childbearing women's perceptions of nursing care that promotes dignity. *JOGNN: Journal of Obstetric, Gynecologic, and Neonatal Nursing, 33*(4), 498-507.

McCloskey, J., & Bulechek, G. (2000). *Nursing interventions classification* (3rd ed.). St. Louis: Mosby.

National Center for Health Statistics (2005). *Trends in the health of Americans.* Hyattsville, MD: NCHS.

Pascali-Bonaro, D., & Kroeger, M. (2004). Continuous female companionship during childbirth: A crucial resource in times of stress or calm. *Journal of Midwifery and Women's Health, 49*(4S), 19-27.

Rouse, D. J. & St. John, E. (2003). Normal labor, delivery, newborn care and puerperium. In Scott, J. R., et al. *Danforth's obstetrics and gynecology* (9th ed.). Philadelphia: Lippincott Williams & Wilkins.

Shilling, T., & DiFranco, J. (2004). Care practices that promote normal birth #2: Freedom of movement throughout labor. *Journal of Perinatal Education, 13*(2), 11-15.

Spong, C. Y. (2003). Fetal monitoring. In Scott, J., R., et al. *Danforth's obstetrics and gynecology* (9th ed.). Philadelphia: Lippincott Williams & Wilkins.

Thacker, S. B., Stroup, D., & Chang, M. (2004). Continuous electronic heart rate monitoring for fetal assessment during labor. *The Cochrane Library (Oxford) (4)* (CD000063).

A B C
X Y Z
Suggested Readings

Amis, D. (2004). Care practices that promote normal birth #1: Labor begins on it own. *Journal of Perinatal Education, 13*(2), 6-10.

Callister, L. C. (2004). Making meaning: women's birth narratives. *JOGNN: Journal of Obstetric, Gynecologic, and Neonatal Nursing, 33*(4), 508-518.

Goodman, P., Mackey, M. C., & Tavakoli, A. S. (2004). Factors related to childbirth satisfaction. *Journal of Advanced Nursing, 46*(2), 212-219.

Joseph, S., & Bailham, D. (2004). Traumatic childbirth: What we know and what we can do. *RCM Midwives Journal, 7*(6), 258-261.

Kelly, A. J., Kavanagh, J., & Thomas, J. (2005). Vaginal prostaglandin (PGE2 and PGF2a) for induction of labour at term. *The Cochrane Library (Oxford) (4)* (CD003101).

Kennedy, H. P., & Shannon, M. T. (2004). Keeping birth normal: Research findings on midwifery care during childbirth. *JOGNN: Journal of Obstetric, Gynecologic, and Neonatal Nursing, 33*(5), 554-560.

Maternity Center Association. (2004). Recommendations from Listening to Mothers: The First National U.S. Survey of Women's Childbearing Experiences. *Birth, 31*(1), 61-67.

Prendiveille, W. J., Elbourne, D., & McDonald, S. (2005). Active versus expectant management in the third stage of labour. *The Cochrane Library (Oxford) (1)* (CD000007).

Shibli, M. (2005). What are the special needs of Arab birthing women? *Midwifery Today, 73* (1), 55-56.

Weiss, M., et al. (2005). Length of stay after vaginal birth: Sociodemographic and readiness-for-discharge factors. *Birth, 31*(2), 93-101.

CHAPTER 19

Providing Comfort During Labor and Birth

Key Terms

analgesia
anesthesia
doula
endorphins
epidural anesthesia
pain
pressure anesthesia
pudendal nerve block
transcutaneous electrical
   nerve stimulation (TENS)

Objectives

After mastering the contents of this chapter, you should be able to:

1. Describe the physiologic basis of contractions during labor and birth and how they relate to theories of pain relief.
2. Identify complementary and alternative therapies that may be used to promote a woman's comfort during labor and birth.
3. Discuss the pharmacologic agents commonly used to provide pain relief during labor and birth.
4. Assess the degree and type of discomfort a woman is experiencing, including her ability to cope with it effectively during labor and birth.
5. Formulate nursing diagnoses related to the effect of pain or pain relief during labor and birth.
6. Establish expected outcomes to meet the needs of a woman experiencing discomfort during labor and birth.
7. Plan nursing interventions to promote comfort during labor and birth.
8. Implement common complementary and pharmacologic measures for pain relief during labor and birth.
9. Evaluate expected outcomes for effectiveness of nursing care and achievement of a satisfying labor experience for a woman and her family.
10. Identify National Health Goals, related to analgesia and anesthesia, that nurses can help the nation achieve.
11. Identify areas related to promoting comfort during labor that could benefit from additional nursing research or application of evidence-based practice.
12. Use critical thinking to analyze ways to maintain family-centered care when analgesia and anesthesia are used in childbirth.
13. Integrate knowledge of pain relief measures during labor and birth with the nursing process to achieve quality maternal and child health nursing care.

Jonny Baranca is a primipara in early labor whom you admit to a birthing unit. Her cervix is 4 cm dilated. She tells you her sister had epidural anesthesia for the birth of her baby 3 months ago. She told Jonny that an epidural block completely obliterated her pain in labor. Based on her sister's experience, Jonny expected to be given an epidural block as soon as she arrived at the hospital. When you enter her room, you find her lying on her back in a birthing bed, crying. Her husband is shouting that his wife deserves better care than this.

Previous chapters discussed the process of labor and care for a woman in labor. This chapter adds information to your knowledge base about how to promote comfort during labor. This is important information, because it can help change labor from an experience so negative that it can result in post-traumatic stress syndrome to a positive, forward-moving experience.

Was the advice Jonny received from her sister realistic?
What are some immediate interventions you could do to help her better manage her pain?

After you've studied this chapter, access the accompanying website. Read the patient scenario and answer the questions to further sharpen your skills, grow more familiar with RN-CLEX types of questions, and reward yourself with how much you have learned.

Concerns about the discomfort and pain that accompany labor and birth can dominate a pregnant woman's or couple's thoughts about childbirth, particularly as the baby's due date approaches. Providing information during prenatal visits about the numerous methods of comfort promotion and pain control available to women can help allay some of these fears. As discussed in Chapter 13, prepared childbirth classes can provide couples with an opportunity to learn and practice a variety of techniques, such as prepared childbirth breathing patterns, to help reduce the pain of labor. Often, however, the labor experience is so overwhelming, or so much greater than the couple expected, that administration of an analgesic or a regional anesthetic is necessary to reduce discomfort sufficiently to allow the woman to regain control over her labor process. If the result is to make labor a satisfying, positive experience, this intervention can ultimately promote the entire family's health (Goodman et al., 2004). In other instances, a woman may feel that she has failed because she required medication for pain relief. She needs to be reassured that labor is not a contest with winners and losers, only different routes to becoming new parents.

Much has been written in nursing literature about using the neutral term *contractions* instead of *labor pains,* to keep from reminding a woman how painful contractions can be. The theory is a sound one, not only because a woman is experiencing a *contracting* sensation but also because calling it *pain* could magnify her fear and tension. Tension, in turn, magnifies pain. Remember, however, that renaming it will not change its basic nature. By any name, discomfort accompanies labor. Fortunately, many nursing interventions can help reduce pain, so that labor is as fulfilling and rewarding an experience as a woman hoped it would be.

Making labor and birth a memorable experience for families is so important that National Health Goals have been established to address this topic. These are shown in Box 19.1.

Nursing Process Overview

For Pain Relief During Childbirth

● **Assessment**

Pain, the sensation of discomfort, is a subjective, personal symptom; it is what the person says it is and present when the person says it is (Pasero & McCaffery, 2004). It is unique to each individual, so a woman is the only person who can describe or know the extent of her pain. To assess the amount of discomfort a woman is having in labor, listen carefully to what she is saying. Also look for subtle signs such as facial tenseness, flushing or paleness, hands clenched in fists, rapid breathing, or rapid pulse rate (Box 19.2).

● **Nursing Diagnosis**

Although pain related to labor contractions is the most obvious nursing diagnosis applicable to labor, it is not the only relevant one during this time. Pain can create

BOX 19.1 FOCUS ON . . .

NATIONAL HEALTH GOALS

Because administration of either analgesia and anesthesia during labor can increase both maternal and fetal mortality, several National Health Goals are related to the types of pain relief used in labor. Examples include the following:

- Reduce the maternal mortality rate to no more than 3.3 per 100,000 live births, from a baseline of 7.1 per 100,000.
- Reduce the fetal death rate during the perinatal period (28 weeks of gestation to 7 days after birth) to no more than 4.5 per 1000 live births, from a baseline of 7.5 per 1000 (Department of Health and Human Services, 2000).

Nurses can help the nation achieve these goals by educating women about the advantages of preparing for childbirth, helping them to use breathing patterns or other complementary and alternative therapies and techniques during labor so that they need a minimum of analgesia and anesthesia, and conscientiously monitoring women who receive analgesics and anesthesia during labor and birth.

Areas that could benefit from additional nursing research include satisfaction with complementary or alternative therapy comfort measures, women's satisfaction with regional anesthesia in labor, and reasons that childbirth methods women prepare and use turn out to be inadequate.

other problems for the laboring woman that can negatively affect the childbirth experience. If not resolved, these problems can intensify pain. Some women may become more concerned with their reaction to the pain than to the pain itself. Applicable nursing diagnoses include the following:

- Pain related to labor contractions
- Powerlessness related to duration and intensity of labor
- Anxiety related to lack of knowledge about "normal" labor process
- Risk for situational low self-esteem related to ineffectiveness of prepared childbirth breathing exercises
- Decisional conflict related to use of analgesia or anesthesia during labor

● **Outcome Identification and Planning**

When developing outcomes and planning interventions to manage discomfort, consider the woman's perceptions about childbirth, her past childbirth experiences (if any), and the amount and type of childbirth preparation she and her partner have had to make the expected outcomes realistic for her. For example, an expectation that no medication will be used might be inappropriate.

Be aware that pharmacologic agents used during labor and birth may pose risks for both the mother (e.g., hypotension) and the fetus (e.g., bradycardia).

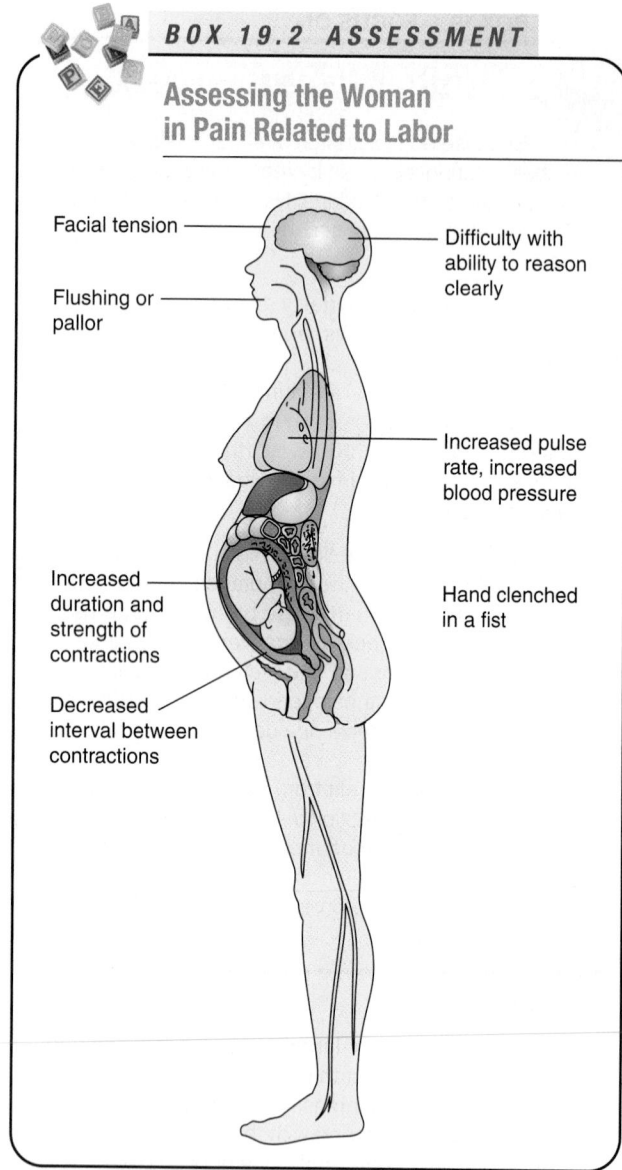

BOX 19.2 ASSESSMENT

Assessing the Woman in Pain Related to Labor

Facial tension

Flushing or pallor

Difficulty with ability to reason clearly

Increased pulse rate, increased blood pressure

Increased duration and strength of contractions

Hand clenched in a fist

Decreased interval between contractions

● *Outcome Evaluation*

Evaluation is ongoing and typically must occur within a short time frame. The following are examples of expected outcomes to indicate successful achievement of outcomes:

- Client states that pain during labor was within a tolerable level for her.
- Couple report that they felt in control throughout the labor process.
- Client states that she does not feel intimidated by thoughts of pain during labor.

Long-term evaluation should reveal that the woman found labor and birth to be an experience that was not only endurable but allowed her to grow in self-esteem and the family to grow through a shared experience. Asking a woman to describe her labor experience afterward in relation to pain not only aids evaluation but helps her work through this emotional period of life and integrate it into her previous experiences.

EXPERIENCE OF PAIN DURING CHILDBIRTH

Pain accompanies labor contractions for a number of different reasons.

Etiology of Pain During Labor and Birth

Normally, contractions of involuntary muscles, such as the heart, stomach, and intestine, do not cause pain. This concept makes uterine contractions unique because they do cause it. Several explanations exist for why this happens. During contractions, blood vessels constrict, reducing the blood supply to uterine and cervical cells, resulting in anoxia to muscle fibers. This anoxia can cause pain in the same way that blockage of the cardiac arteries causes the pain of a heart attack. As labor progresses and contractions become longer and harder, the ischemia to cells increases, the anoxia increases, and the pain intensifies.

Pain also probably results from stretching of the cervix and perineum. This phenomenon is the same as that causing intestinal pain when accumulating gas stretches the intestines. At the end of the transitional phase in labor, when stretching of the cervix is complete and the woman feels she has to push, pain from the contractions often disappears as long as the woman is pushing, until the fetal presenting part causes the final stretching of the perineum.

Additional discomfort in labor may stem from the pressure of the fetal presenting part on tissues, including pressure on surrounding organs, such as the bladder, the urethra, and the lower colon. Pain at birth largely results from stretching of the perineal tissue.

Physiology of Pain

Pain is a basic protective mechanism that alerts a person that something harmful is happening somewhere in the

Therefore, their use must always be weighed against the alternative risk to the mother (enduring a painful labor). The decision may also affect family functioning if the method chosen limits the partner's participation in the birth.

● *Implementation*

Many different interventions to promote comfort and relieve pain are available. Keeping a woman and her support person informed about their options as labor progresses is important. Simply knowing that birth is getting even a little closer can make the next few contractions easier to withstand. Supporting and encouraging a woman to use methods of complementary and alternative therapies for pain management (e.g., relaxation) also are helpful. Offering analgesia or assisting with anesthesia administration during labor or birth requires nursing judgment and a caring presence to help one woman accept analgesia when she needs it and to encourage another to experience childbirth without heavy sedation.

body. Pain sensation begins in nociceptors, the end points of afferent nerves, when they are activated by mechanical, chemical, or thermal stimuli. Nociceptors are located predominantly in the skin, bone periosteum, joint surfaces, and arterial walls. When end terminals are stimulated, chemical mediators such as prostaglandins, histamine, bradykinin, and serotonin are synthesized and sensitize the nociceptors. The pain impulse is transmitted along small, unmyelinated C fibers and large, myelinated A-delta fibers to the spinal cord. The more numerous C fibers conduct slowly and apparently carry dull, low-level pain; the fewer A-delta fibers apparently carry sharp, well-localized pain such as labor contractions.

In the dorsal horn of the spinal cord, somatostatin, cholecystokinin, and substance P serve as neurotransmitters or assist the pain impulse across the synapse between the peripheral nerve and the spinal nerve. The pain impulse then ascends the spinal cord to the brain cortex, where it is interpreted as pain.

The Melzack-Wall gate control theory of pain control (Melzack & Wall, 1965), the most widely accepted theory of pain response today, proposes that pain can be halted at three points: the peripheral end terminals, the synapse points in the dorsal horn, or the point at which the impulse is interpreted as pain in the brain cortex.

Pain in peripheral terminals is automatically reduced by the production of endorphins and enkephalins, naturally occurring opiates that limit transmission of pain from the end terminals. Pain can be reduced further by mechanically irritating nerve fibers by an action such as rubbing the skin. This technique blocks nerve transmission.

A major action of pain medications is to block spinal cord neurotransmitters, never allowing the pain impulse to cross to a spinal nerve. The brain cortex can be distracted from sensing impulses as pain by such techniques as imagery, thought stopping, aromatherapy, or yoga.

Sensory impulses from the uterus and cervix synapse at the spinal column at the level of T10 through T12 and L1. Pain relief measures for the first stage of labor, therefore, must block these upper synapse sites. For the elimination of pain during cesarean birth, receptors at the level of T6 through T8 must be blocked, so that both the upper and lower uterus are blocked.

Sensory impulses from the perineum are carried by the pudendal nerve to join the spinal column at S2, S3, and S4. When the perineum is initiating the pain, pain relief must block these lower receptor sites. This is an important point to remember when talking to a woman in labor about pain relief. Some interventions relieve pain for both the first and second stages of labor, whereas others work for one stage but not both.

Perception of Pain

The amount of discomfort a woman experiences during contractions differs according to her expectations of and preparation for labor, the length of her labor, the position of her fetus, and the availability of support people around her (Fig. 19.1). The discomfort she experiences can become compounded when fear and anxiety are also present.

Pain is perceived differently by different individuals because of psychosocial, physiologic, and cultural responses

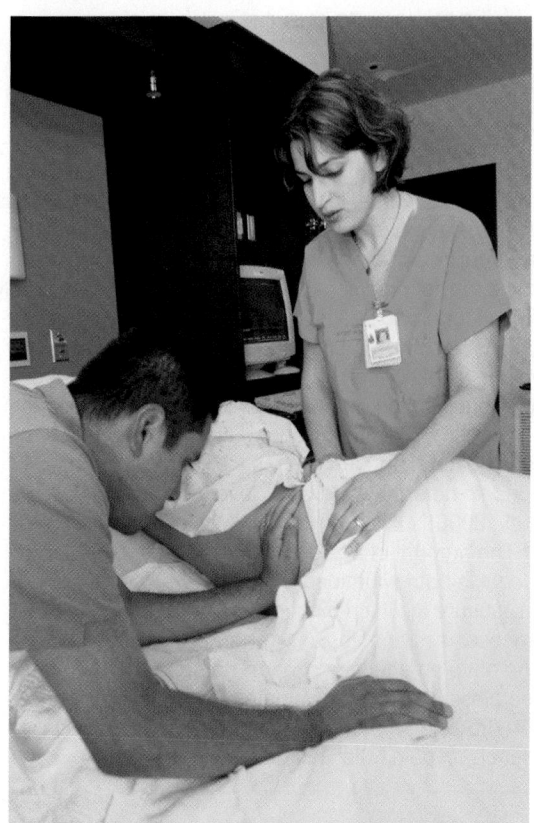

FIGURE 19.1 The discomfort a woman experiences during childbirth may be related to the amount of support she receives from her family or health care providers. Here, the woman's support person uses the palm of his hand to apply counterpressure to the woman's lower back, helping to ease back pain, while the nurse assists.

(Box 19.3). The body's ability to produce and maintain **endorphins** (naturally occurring opiate-like substances) may influence a person's overall pain threshold and the amount of pain a person perceives at any given time. Women who come into labor believing the pain will be horrible are usually surprised afterward to realize that the agony they expected never materialized. On the other hand, expectations of pain may make a woman so tense during labor that her pain is worse than it would have been if she had been relaxed. A woman cannot relax simply because she is instructed to do so by another person, however. Some additional interventions must be used.

Factors Influencing Pain Perception

Fetal position is a physical variable that can influence the degree of pain a woman experiences. If the fetus is in an occiput posterior position, for example, the woman often reports intense or nagging back pain, even between contractions.

Psychological factors that can influence pain include fear, anxiety, worry, expectation of pain, body image, and self-efficacy. Women who believe that they can control their situation (have self-efficacy) are more apt to report a satisfactory birth experience than those who do not feel in control (Goodman et al., 2004).

BOX 19.3 FOCUS ON . . .

DIVERSITY OF CARE

Responses to pain are, in part, culturally determined. Based on this, some women believe that being stoic and nonverbal is what is expected of them. Others believe that expressing their discomfort by screaming or verbalizing their feelings will best reduce pain. If a woman is not proficient in English, it may be particularly difficult for her to describe her level of discomfort. Assess each woman individually to determine not only what level of comfort she feels is right for her during labor but also the manner in which she feels most able to express discomfort. Depend on facial expression, body posture, and tension, as well as voiced expressions, to determine a client's level of comfort (Callister et al., 2003).

The amount of analgesia that women desire or will accept is both situationally and culturally determined. In a culture in which birth is seen as a "natural" process, less analgesia is generally desired. Women who have an effective support person with them may need less pharmacologic pain relief than those who do not. Providing nursing support can have a positive influence on pain relief in labor.

COMFORT AND PAIN RELIEF MEASURES

The pattern of interventions to promote comfort and manage pain in labor has swung from a philosophy of no intervention (none given), to a philosophy of drug intervention as an essential element (too much given), to a modern approach of empowering women and their partners with information so that they can choose how to best relieve pain during labor, within the limits of medical safety. For centuries, in Western civilization, offering pain relief in labor was thought to be amoral because, according to the Biblical account, God commanded Eve, "I will greatly multiply thy sorrow and thy conception; in sorrow thou shalt bring forth children. . . ." (Genesis 3:16). In the witch-burning period of American history, the concept that childbirth should be painful was so strongly ingrained that women were burned as witches for providing comfort to other women in labor.

With the discovery of ether and chloroform in the 1800s, it became apparent that childbirth could be managed completely pain free. Unfortunately, this goal was achieved by means of complete anesthesia or unconsciousness during labor and birth. Women, afterward, had difficulty realizing that the birth was over and they were a new parent.

Current philosophy centers on informed decision making. Nurses play a key role in educating women and their support persons about the numerous comfort and pain relief strategies available and making sure couples understand the choices available to them along with the benefits and risks. Throughout their decision-making process, couples need support for their choices so that they can feel confidence in the method chosen.

Support From a Doula or Coach

A woman's husband or the father of her child has traditionally served as the chief support person in labor. However, some husbands or fathers find it difficult to provide effective coaching or support in labor because of their own emotional involvement in the birth. Women who are aware that they may not have effective one-to-one support in labor from their baby's father should be encouraged to identify an additional person who could come with them and provide this support. A **doula** is a woman who is experienced in childbirth, but without professional credentials, who guides and assists women in labor (Rosen, 2004). Having a doula can increase a woman's self-esteem as well as decrease rates of oxytocin augmentation, epidural anesthesia, and cesarean birth.

Checkpoint Question 1

Jonny asks you what is the purpose of a doula in labor. Your best answer would be:

a. She times contractions and keeps them from becoming too lengthy.
b. She can cook for a woman in labor to keep her from becoming dehydrated.
c. She can serve as a support person and coach during labor.
d. She replaces the husband as a woman's support person.

Complementary and Alternative Therapies for Pain Relief

Complementary and alternative therapies for pain relief involve nonpharmacologic measures that may be used either as a woman's total pain management program or to complement pharmacologic interventions. Most of these interventions are based on the gate control theory concept that distraction can be effective in preventing the brain from processing pain sensations coming into the cortex.

Relaxation

The technique of relaxation, as discussed in Chapter 13, is taught in most preparation for childbirth classes. Relaxation keeps the abdominal wall from becoming tense, allowing the uterus to rise with contractions without pressing against the hard abdominal wall. It also serves as a distraction technique because, while concentrating on relaxing, a woman cannot concentrate on pain. In addition to conscious relaxation, having a woman shift position or find the position in labor that is most comfortable for her can be helpful. Asking a woman to bring favorite music tapes or aromatherapy with her to enjoy in the birthing room is a good way to aid relaxation.

Focusing and Imagery

Concentrating intently on an object is another method of distraction, or another method of keeping sensory input from reaching the cortex of the brain. For this technique, a woman uses a photograph of someone important to her or some image she finds appealing. She concentrates on it during contractions (focusing). Other women concentrate on a mental image, such as waves rolling onto a beach (imagery). Do not ask questions or talk to a woman while she is using imagery or focusing, because it breaks her concentration.

Breathing Techniques

Breathing patterns are also taught in most preparation for childbirth classes (see Chapter 13). They are advantageous because they help to relax a woman's abdomen. They are largely distraction techniques, because a woman concentrating on slow-paced breathing cannot concentrate on pain. Breathing strategies can be taught to a woman in labor if she is not familiar with their advantages before labor.

Herbal Preparations

Several herbal preparations have traditionally been used to reduce pain with dysmenorrhea or labor, although there is little factual support for their effectiveness. Examples include raspberry leaves, fennel, and life root. Blue cohosh (squaw root), used to induce uterine contractions, is not recommended because of the risk of acute toxic effects (e.g., cerebrovascular accident) to the mother or fetus (Finkel & Zarlengo, 2004).

Aromatherapy and Essential Oils

Aromatherapy is the use of aromatic oils to complement emotional and physical well-being. Their use is based on the principle that the sense of smell plays a significant role in overall health. When an essential oil is inhaled, its molecules are transported via the olfactory system to the limbic system in the brain. The brain responds to particular aromas with emotional responses. When applied externally, they are absorbed by the skin and then carried throughout the body. The oils used may be able to penetrate cell walls and transport nutrients or oxygen to the inside of cells. Jasmine and lavender are oils thought to be responsible for an easier labor. When a drop of oil, such as lavender, is placed on the skin, a woman is able to taste it within 15 seconds.

Heat or Cold Application

Heat and cold have always been used for pain relief after injuries such as minor burns or strained muscles. It is only lately that they have been investigated as effective ways to help relieve the pain of labor contractions. Women who are having back pain may find application of heat to the lower back by a heating pad or a moist compress very comforting.

Women who become warm from the exertion of labor find a cool washcloth to the forehead comforting. Ice chips to suck on to relieve mouth dryness are also refreshing.

Bathing or Hydrotherapy

Standing under a warm shower or soaking in a tub of warm water, jet hydrotherapy tub, or whirlpool is another way to apply heat to help reduce the pain of labor (Cluett et al., 2005). The temperature of water used should be between 95°F and 100°F (35.0°C and 37.8°C) to prevent hyperthermia. This type of pain relief measure usually is not recommended for women whose membranes have ruptured because of the risk of infection.

Therapeutic Touch and Massage

Therapeutic touch is the use of touch to comfort and relieve pain. It is based on the concept that the body contains energy fields that, when plentiful, lead to health and, when in less supply, result in ill health. Krieger (1990), in a classic work, defined therapeutic touch as the laying on of hands to redirect the energy fields that lead to pain. Although the action is not well documented, touch and massage probably work to relieve pain by increasing the release of endorphins. It also is a form of distraction. Effleurage, the technique of gentle abdominal massage often taught with Lamaze preparation for childbirth classes, is a form of therapeutic touch (Fig. 19.2).

Yoga

Yoga, a term derived from the Sanskrit word for union, denotes a series of exercises that were originally designed to bring people who practice it closer to their God. It offers a significant variety of proven health benefits, including increasing the efficiency of the heart, slowing the respiratory rate, improving fitness, lowering blood pressure, promoting relaxation, reducing stress, and allaying anxiety. Exercises consist of deep breathing exercises, body postures to stretch and strengthen muscles, and meditation to focus the mind and relax the body. It may be helpful in reducing the pain of labor through its ability to relax the body and possibly through the release of endorphins that may occur.

Reflexology

Reflexology is the practice of stimulating the hands, feet, and ears as a form of therapy (Martin, 2004). Professional

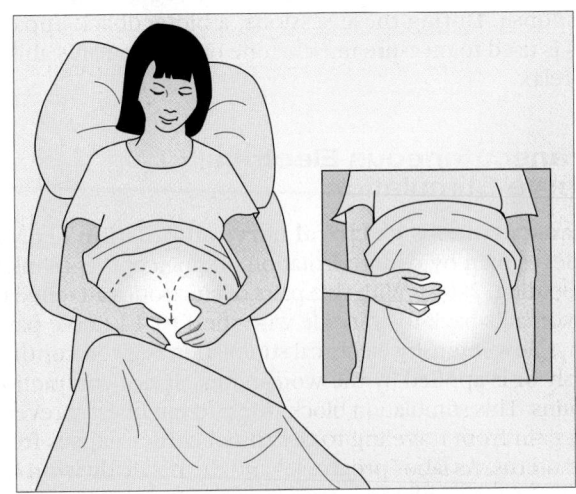

FIGURE 19.2 Effleurage is light massage that can distract a woman from discomfort during labor.

reflexologists apply pressure to specific areas of the hands, feet, and ears to alleviate common ailments such as headaches, back pain, sinus colds, and stress. The theory behind reflexology is that each of the body's organs and glands are linked to corresponding areas of the hands and feet. The body is divided into 10 zones that run in longitudinal lines from the top of the head to the tips of the toes. Application of pressure to the specific area aims to restore energy to the body and improve the overall condition.

Crystal or Gemstone Therapy

Some gemstones or crystals are thought to have healing powers, and women may bring these into a birthing room to use during labor. A woman who uses crystals or gemstones may believe that their healing power is magnified when they are positioned around her body. Be especially careful when changing bedding or rearranging equipment in a birthing room to respect the position of these crystals. A woman may feel that they do not work their healing powers in an altered position.

Hypnosis

Hypnosis is yet another method of pain relief for labor. A woman who wants to use this modality needs to meet with her hypnotherapist during pregnancy. At these visits, she is evaluated for and further conditioned for susceptibility to hypnotic suggestion. At the last prenatal visit, she is given the posthypnotic suggestion that she will experience reduced pain or absence of pain during labor. For a woman who is susceptible to hypnotic suggestion, the method can provide a very satisfactory drug-free method of pain relief (Cyna et al., 2004).

Biofeedback

Biofeedback is based on the belief that people have control and can regulate internal events such as heart rate and pain response. Women who are interested in using biofeedback for pain relief in labor must attend several sessions during pregnancy to condition themselves to regulate their pain response. During these sessions, a biofeedback apparatus is used to measure muscle tone or the woman's ability to relax.

Transcutaneous Electrical Nerve Stimulation

Transcutaneous electrical nerve stimulation (TENS) relieves pain by counterirritation on nociceptors (Simkin & Bolding, 2004). With two pairs of electrodes attached to a woman's back to coincide with the T10–L1 nerve pathways, low-intensity electrical stimulation is given continuously or is applied by the woman herself as a contraction begins. This stimulation blocks the afferent fibers, preventing pain from traveling to the spinal cord synapses from the uterus. As labor progresses and the pelvic division begins, the electrodes are moved to stimulate the S2–4 level. High-intensity stimulation is generally needed to control the pain at this stage.

TENS can be as effective as epidural anesthesia for pain relief in labor, but some women may object to being "tied down" to the equipment. Women with extreme back pain during labor may benefit the most from a TENS unit, because this type of pain is difficult to relieve with controlled breathing exercises. TENS is also discussed in Chapter 20 as it applies to the postoperative pain of a cesarean birth.

Acupressure and Acupuncture

Acupuncture is based on the concept that illness results from an imbalance of energy. To correct the imbalance, needles are inserted into the skin at designated susceptible body points (*tsubos*) located along meridians that course throughout the body to supply the organs of the body with energy. These points are not necessarily near the affected organ. Activation of these points apparently results in release of endorphins, so the system can be helpful, especially in the first stage of labor (Chung et al., 2003).

Acupressure, in contrast, is the application of pressure or massage at these points. A common point used for a woman in labor is Co4 (Hoku or Hegu point) located between the first and second metacarpal bones on the back of the hand. When a support person holds and squeezes a woman's hand in labor, he or she may be accidentally triggering this point.

Intracutaneous Nerve Stimulation

Intracutaneous nerve stimulation (INS) is a technique of counter-irritation involving the intradermal injection of sterile water or saline along the borders of the sacrum to relieve low back pain during labor (Leeman et al., 2003). Some women find the technique helpful; others prefer to bear back pain rather than submit to injections.

Checkpoint Question 2

Jonny asks you if she could use warm-water tub bathing during labor. Your best answer would be:

a. No. No one is allowed to tub bathe during labor.
b. Yes, as long as her membranes are not ruptured.
c. No, because warm water can diminish labor contractions.
d. Yes, as long as the warm water doesn't raise her temperature.

Pharmacologic Pain Relief During Labor

Pharmacologic management of pain during labor and birth includes **analgesia,** which reduces or decreases awareness of pain, and **anesthesia,** which causes partial or compete loss of sensation. Many choices are available today. For the best results, be sure women are included in a selection that is right for them.

Virtually all medication given during labor crosses the placenta and has some effect on the fetus, which makes it important for a woman to receive as little systemic medication as possible. On the other hand, labor should not test a woman to the limit of her endurance, especially since local anesthesia is available. Be sure to caution women not to take acetylsalicylic acid (aspirin) for pain in labor. Aspirin interferes with blood coagulation, increasing the risk for bleeding in the newborn or mother.

Goals of Pharmacologic Management of Pain During Labor

Medication effectively used during labor must relax a woman and relieve her discomfort, yet have minimal systemic effects on her uterine contractions, her pushing effort, or her fetus. Whether a drug affects a fetus depends on its ability to cross the placenta. Drugs with a molecular weight of more than 1,000 cross poorly, whereas those with a molecular weight of less than 600 cross very readily. Drugs with highly charged molecules or molecules strongly bound to protein cross more slowly than others. Fat-soluble drugs cross most easily. A preterm fetus, which has an immature liver and is unable to metabolize or inactivate drugs, is generally more affected by drugs than a term fetus. If a drug causes a systemic response, such as hypotension, in a woman, it can result in a decreased oxygen (PO_2) gradient across the placenta and fetal hypoxia. If it causes confusion or disorientation, she may be unable to work effectively with contractions, prolonging labor. If a medication causes changes in a fetus, such as a decreased heart rate or central nervous system (CNS) depression, it may be difficult for the newborn infant to initiate respirations at birth, severely compromising the infant in the important first minutes of life.

Because pain is a subjective sensation, women experience different levels of pain during labor. Some women are most aware of pain early in labor, whereas some report the second stage of labor as the most difficult. The point at which pain medication is needed, therefore, differs from one individual to another. Once labor is well underway, medication to relieve discomfort can speed its progress: with pain gone, the woman can relax and work with, not against, her contractions (Camann, 2005). The American College of Obstetricians and Gynecologists (ACOG) currently recommends that women receive pain relief at the point they request it, regardless of cervical dilatation, even though medication given too early tends to slow labor contractions (ACOG, 2002). Unfortunately, no perfect analgesic agent exists for labor or birth that has no effect on labor, the mother, and the fetus.

Preparation for Medication Administration

The type of medication used during labor varies among different health care agencies and also changes based on new research as the effectiveness and safety of new drugs for use during labor are tested. To be safe, remember the criteria that a drug must fulfill to be used in pregnancy, or expand the rule of basic medication administration from "Never give any drug unless you know it is safe for your individual client" to "Never give a drug during labor without knowing it is safe for both of your clients: the mother and the fetus."

Medicines frequently used in labor and birth are shown in Table 19.1. Prepare the woman for the type of agent to be given, how it will be administered (e.g., "You'll need to lie on your side"), and what she can expect to happen after administration (e.g., "I'll be taking your blood pressure frequently"). Women in labor are under stress. Experiencing surprising body sensations from a drug without preparation can be so frightening that it can defeat their individual coping abilities. When a person struggles against medication administration because she does not understand the strange feeling it is causing, the risk of inadvertent problems increases.

What If... Jonny tells you she wants something for pain in labor but has no idea what to ask for? How would you advise her? You notice that Jonny's sister grips her hand very tightly during contractions. What possible pain relief measure is her sister's tight pressure providing for her?

Narcotic Analgesics

Narcotics are often given during labor because of their potent analgesic effect (Hawkins, 2003). All drugs in this category cause fetal CNS depression to some extent. Be sure to question an order for a narcotic if a woman is in preterm labor. Because of possible lung immaturity, a preterm infant may have extreme difficulty coping with the added insult of respiratory depression at birth.

Narcotic analgesics commonly used include meperidine hydrochloride (Demerol), morphine sulfate, nalbuphine (Nubain), fentanyl (Sublimaze), and butorphanol tartrate (Stadol). Meperidine is advantageous as an analgesic in labor because it has additional sedative and antispasmodic actions; these make it effective not only for relieving pain but also for helping to relax the cervix and providing a feeling of euphoria and well-being. It may be given either intramuscularly or intravenously. The dose is 25 to 100 mg, depending on a woman's weight and the route of administration. The drug begins to act about 30 minutes after intramuscular (IM) injection and about 5 minutes after intravenous (IV) administration. Its duration of action is 2 to 3 hours (Karch, 2004).

Demerol also may be self-administered by a patient-controlled analgesic (PCA) pump for low-dose but frequent administration during labor (Chang et al., 2004). Intrathecal administration (injection into the cerebral spinal fluid) is used less frequently.

Because Demerol crosses the placenta, it can cause respiratory depression in a fetus. The drug crosses the placenta minutes after either IV or IM administration to the mother. However, because the fetal liver takes 2 to 3 hours to activate the drug into the fetal system, the effect will not be registered in the fetus for 2 to 3 hours after maternal administration. For this reason, Demerol is given when the mother is more than 3 hours away from birth. This allows the peak action of the drug in the fetus to have passed by the time of birth.

It may be puzzling to see a sleepy baby delivered to a woman who was given Demerol 2 hours before birth and an alert baby delivered to a woman who had Demerol

TABLE 19.1

Analgesics and Anesthetics Commonly Used in Labor and Birth

Type	Drug	Usual Dosage/Route	Effect on Mother	Effect on Labor Progress	Effect on Fetus or Newborn
Narcotic analgesic	Meperidine (Demerol)	25 mg IV, 50–100 mg IM q3–4 h; also epidurally	Effective analgesic; feeling of well-being	Relaxation, possibly aiding progress during cervical relaxation. Slows labor contractions if given early.	Should be given 3 h before birth to avoid respiratory depression in newborn. Decreases beat-to-beat variability in FHR.
	Nalbuphine (Nubain)	10–20 mg IM q3–6 h, 0.3–3 mg/kg over 10–15 min IV	Slowing of respiratory rate; effective analgesic	Mild maternal sedation	Results in some respiratory depression
	Butorphanol (Stadol)	1–2 mg IM or IV q3–4 h	Withdrawal symptoms if woman is opiate-dependent	Possible slowing of labor if given early	Results in some respiratory depression
	Morphine sulfate	Intrathecally 0.2–1 mg; 5 mg epidurally	Pruritus; effective analgesia	Possible slowing of labor contractions.	Has minimal effect
	Fentanyl (Sublimaze)	50–100 µg IM or 25–50 µg IV; also epidurally	Hypotension; respiratory depression	Slowing of labor if given early	May result in respiratory depression
Lumbar epidural block	Local anesthetic Bupivacaine (Marcaine), Ropivacaine (Naropin)	Administered for first stage of labor; with continuous block, anesthesia will last through birth; injected at L3–4; Fentanyl or morphine possibly added	Rapid onset, in minutes; lasting 60–90 min; loss of pain perception for labor contractions and birth; possible maternal hypo-tension	Slowing of labor if given early; pushing feeling obliterated, resulting in possible prolonged second stage	May be some differences in response in first few days of life
Pudendal block	Local anesthetic Lidocaine (Xylocaine)	Administered just before birth for perineal anesthesia; injected through vagina	Rapid anesthesia of perineum	None apparent	None apparent
Local infiltration of perineum	Local anesthetic Lidocaine (Xylocaine)	Injected just before episiotomy incision	Anesthesia of perineum almost immediately	None apparent	None apparent
General intravenous anesthetic	Thiopental	Administered IV by anesthesiologist or nurse-anesthetist	Rapid anesthesia; also rapid recovery	Forceps required because abdominal pushing is no longer possible	Results in infant being born with CNS depression

Karch, A. M. (2004). *Lippincott's nursing drug guide*. Philadelphia: Lippincott Williams & Wilkins.

within 1 hour of birth. In the second instance, the peak action or peak effect has not yet occurred in the infant. This newborn needs careful assessment for the next 4 hours until the drug reaches its peak.

Nalbuphine hydrochloride (Nubain), butorphanol tartrate (Stadol), and remifentanil (Ultiva) are synthetic narcotic analgesics. The action of these agents is comparable to that of Demerol. Like Demerol, they may also leave a degree of respiratory depression in the newborn.

Whenever a narcotic is given during labor, a narcotic antagonist such as naloxone (Narcan) should be available for administration to the infant at birth (Box 19.4). Carefully

BOX 19.4 FOCUS ON . . .

PHARMACOLOGY

Naloxone Hydrochloride (Narcan)

Action: Naloxone hydrochloride is a narcotic antagonist that counteracts the effect of narcotic analgesics (Karch, 2004).

Pregnancy category: B

Dosage: 0.01 mg/kg, administered either IV via umbilical vein, SC, or IM; repeated at 2- to 3-minute intervals until response is obtained.

Possible adverse effects: Hypotension, hypertension, tachycardia, diaphoresis, tremulousness

Nursing Implications
- Anticipate the need for resuscitative measures; have resuscitative equipment and emergency drugs readily available.
- If no IV access is available, prepare for possible administration via endotracheal tube.
- If no response is seen after two or three doses, question whether respiratory depression is caused by narcotics.
- Continuously monitor all vital signs for changes.
- Remember that the pain-relieving effect of narcotics will be reversed; assess for pain in the neonate.

observe an infant who receives naloxone in the immediate postpartum period, because the infant's respirations may become severely depressed again when the drug's effect wears off. If severe infant respiratory depression is anticipated, Narcan can be given to the mother just before birth. It readily crosses the placenta and, because it interferes with or competes for narcotic binding sites, may increase the chance for spontaneous respiratory activity in the newborn.

What If... Jonny receives no narcotics during labor, yet her newborn is born very sleepy? Would you administer naloxone? Would asking Jonny if she used recreational drugs be warranted?

Intrathecal Narcotics. *Intrathecal* administration refers to injection into the spinal cord. With intrathecal narcotic injection, a catheter is introduced into the spinal canal (the subarachnoid space), and a narcotic such as morphine or fentanyl citrate is injected into the canal by way of the catheter. Both drugs provide excellent pain relief for labor pain. They take effect in 15 to 30 minutes, and pain relief lasts 4 to 7 hours. The woman is able to feel the urge to push at the second stage of labor, allowing her to actively participate in the birth. Because intrathecal injections are not as effective in reducing the pain of the actual birth, they may be supplemented with a pudendal block in late labor. Possible side effects of intrathecal morphine are intense pruritus, nausea, and vomiting. The pruritus can be

treated with IV diphenhydramine (Benadryl) if it becomes too uncomfortable.

Additional Drugs

Additional drugs, such as tranquilizers, may be administered during labor to reduce anxiety or potentiate the action of a narcotic. Examples include hydroxyzine hydrochloride (Vistaril) or a phenothiazine derivative such as promethazine (Phenergan). These drugs do not relieve pain, so the woman in labor needs pain management measures in addition to these drugs.

Regional Anesthesia

Regional anesthesia is the injection of a local anesthetic such as chloroprocaine (Nesacaine) or bupivacaine (Marcaine) to block specific nerve pathways. It achieves pain relief by blocking sodium and potassium transport in the nerve membrane, thereby stabilizing the nerve in a polarized resting state, so that it is unable to conduct sensations.

Depending on the region anesthetized, the woman may or may not continue to be aware of contractions. Various regional anesthetic injection sites are shown in Figure 19.3. Women with preeclampsia may have associated bleeding defects and need to be assessed carefully before regional anesthesia is administered.

Because regional anesthetics are not introduced into the maternal circulation, it was once believed that they had no effect on a fetus. However, research has demonstrated that there is some uptake of these drugs by a fetus, possibly resulting in FHR decelerations and symptoms of flaccidity, bradycardia, and hypotension in the newborn (Karch, 2004). Effects are minimal when compared with those of systemic anesthetic agents, however. Most importantly, regional anesthesia allows a woman to be completely awake and aware of what is happening during birth. They do not depress uterine tone, so the uterus remains capable of optimal contraction after birth, thereby helping to prevent postpartal hemorrhage.

It is rare that an infant is born with symptoms of toxicity from a regional anesthetic. If this occurs, however, an exchange transfusion at birth will remove the anesthetic from the infant's bloodstream. Gastric lavage also will remove a great deal of anesthetic, because anesthetics have a strong affinity for acid media such as stomach acid.

Epidural Anesthesia (Peridural Block). The nerves in the spinal cord are protected by several tissue layers. The pia mater is the membrane adhering to the nerve fibers. Surrounding this is the *cerebrospinal fluid* (CSF). Next comes the arachnoid membrane and outside that, the *dura mater.* Outside the dura mater is a vacant space (the *epidural space*). Beyond it is the *ligamentum flavum,* yet another protective shield for the vulnerable spinal cord.

An anesthetic agent introduced into the CSF in the subarachnoid space is called a spinal injection or spinal anesthesia. An anesthetic agent placed just inside the ligamentum flavum in the epidural space is **epidural anesthesia** (see Fig. 19.3). Anesthetic agents placed in the epidural space at the L4-5, L3-4, or L2-3 interspace block

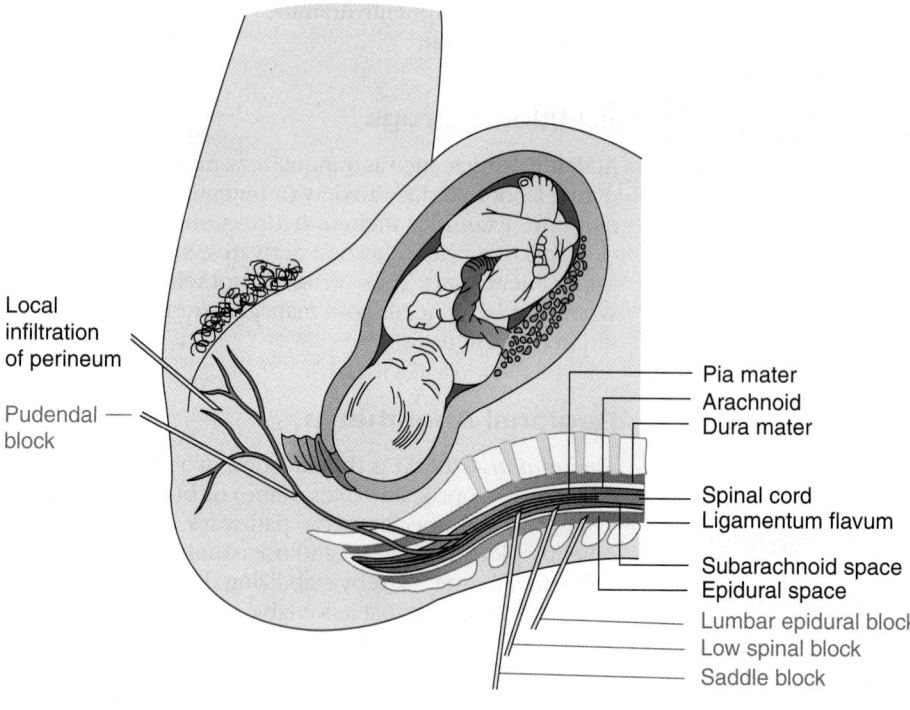

Local infiltration of perineum

Pudendal block

Pia mater
Arachnoid
Dura mater

Spinal cord
Ligamentum flavum

Subarachnoid space
Epidural space

Lumbar epidural block
Low spinal block
Saddle block

FIGURE 19.3 Anatomy of the spinal canal and sites of injection for regional anesthesia.

not only spinal nerve roots in the space but also the sympathetic nerve fibers that travel with them. Therefore, these blocks provide pain relief for both labor and birth. Such a block may actually increase contraction strength and blood flow to the uterus. Because the woman no longer experiences pain, the release of catecholamines (epinephrine) with a β-blocking effect from a pain response is decreased, making this a very effective pain relief measure for labor (Nystedt et al., 2004).

"Spinal headaches" occur only rarely after epidural anesthesia. These headaches are apparently caused by leakage of CSF or instillation of air into the CSF. With epidural anesthesia, the CSF space is not entered, so these problems do not occur. Because the injection technique is potentially frightening, women need continuous support during the process.

Epidural blocks, administered by an anesthesiologist or nurse-anesthetist, are suitable for almost all women. They are advantageous for women with heart disease, pulmonary disease, diabetes, and sometimes severe pregnancy-induced hypertension, because they make labor virtually pain free and thereby reduce stress from the discomfort of labor to a minimum. Because the woman does not feel contractions, her physical energy is preserved. Epidural blocks are acceptable for use in preterm labor because the drug has scant effect on a fetus and allows for a controlled and gentle birth with less trauma to an immature fetal skull. Because the woman receives no systemic medication, the infant responds more quickly after birth than if systemic narcotic analgesics were used.

The chief concern with epidural anesthesia is its tendency to cause hypotension because of its blocking effect on the sympathetic nerve fibers in the epidural space. This blocking leads to decreased peripheral resistance in the woman's circulatory system. Decreased peripheral resistance causes blood to flow freely into peripheral ves-

sels, and a pseudohypovolemia develops, registering as hypotension. The combined use of fentanyl and bupivacaine can lower the risk for hypotension. In addition, the risk also can be reduced by being sure the woman is well hydrated with 500 to 1,000 mL of IV fluid, such as Ringer's lactate, before the anesthetic is given. Ringer's lactate is preferable to a glucose solution, because too much maternal glucose can cause hyperglycemia with rebound hypoglycemia in the newborn. Be certain that the woman does not lie supine but remains on her side after an epidural block, to help prevent supine hypotension syndrome.

If hypotension does occur, raising the woman's legs and administering oxygen and additional IV fluid, along with an agent such as ephedrine to elevate blood pressure, may be necessary to stabilize cardiovascular status.

In rare instances, the anesthetic does enter the blood circulation (Jenkins, 2005). This occurrence is manifested as drowsiness, a metallic taste on the tongue, slurred speech, blurred vision, unconsciousness, and seizure leading to cardiac arrest. If such symptoms occur, it is an emergency situation. The woman needs oxygen and an anticonvulsant such as diazepam (Valium) or thiopental (Pentothal) IV, followed by prompt birth of the fetus.

The use of an epidural block tends to prolong the second stage of labor, but whether this leads to an increase in cesarean births is controversial (Howell, 2005). Descent can slow, for example, taking 3 hours rather than 2 hours, but if there is no indication that this is detrimental to the fetus, it should not lead to a greater need for vacuum extraction or cesarean birth. Relaxation of the levator ani muscle may impede internal rotation of the fetal head, further slowing labor or making the use of forceps necessary to effect rotation. This occurs primarily when the fetus is in an occiput-posterior position. Oxytocin may be given to shorten labor. Allowing an epidural to wear off by the second stage of labor, so that the woman can push with contractions, is another option. However, experiencing contractions at this point can be overwhelming for a woman and counteracts the original reason for giving the anesthetic: to reduce pain in labor.

Technique for Administration. Epidural anesthesia is begun when the cervix is dilatated 5 to 6 cm. An IV infusion and equipment for blood pressure monitoring should be in place. Help position the woman on her side or sitting upright. Her back should not be flexed, because this increases the possibility of puncturing the dura and accidentally giving the anesthetic as a spinal, not epidural, injection. The lumbar area of the back is cleaned with an antiseptic solution. A local anesthetic is injected into the skin to form a wheal over the L3 and L4 vertebrae. A special 3- to 5-inch needle is then passed through the L3–4 interspace into the epidural space. After needle placement, a polyethylene catheter is passed through the needle into the space, and the needle is then withdrawn, leaving the catheter to be taped in place. A closed system (a syringe is attached) is established to prevent infection through the catheter (Fig. 19.4).

The anesthetist then injects a small test dose of a local anesthetic solution into the catheter. Five minutes later, the woman's legs are inspected for flushing and warmness, evidence that the anesthetic is in the epidural space (peripheral dilatation is beginning). Assess the woman's pulse and blood pressure at this time. If the anesthetic was accidentally placed in a blood vessel, toxic symptoms of hypotension, slurred speech, and rapid pulse will be present. After assurance that the anesthetic is epidural, the initial dose of anesthetic is given through the catheter. This produces anesthesia up to the level of the umbilicus in 10 to 15 minutes. The effect of epidural anesthesia is short lived (40 minutes to 2 hours). To keep a woman free from discomfort during the duration of labor, another dose of anesthetic, termed a top-up, must be added, or anesthetic must be continually infused by an infusion pump.

Before an additional top-up dose is administered, ask the woman to both write and say out loud a phrase such as "I can do it" three times. If she is unable to do this, question the dose: lack of fine motor coordination and slurred speech indicate a slowly occurring toxic reaction.

Epidural anesthesia may also be given in a "segmented" fashion. With this technique, after the test dose, only a small dose (about 4 mL) is given. This provides anesthesia for uterine contractions but not perineal relaxation. Close to birth, if the woman sits up and an additional dose is given, perineal anesthesia will result. Leaving the lower anesthesia for late in labor in this way allows for better internal rotation of the fetal head, because the perineal muscle is not lax and there is less chance that forceps for rotation will be necessary.

A nurse should be in continuous attendance while an epidural anesthetic is given. Epidural anesthesia can cause a temporary elevation in temperature, so keep this in mind when evaluating a woman's temperature. To detect hypotension, continuously monitor blood pressure for the first 20 minutes after each new injection of anesthetic. Continue to monitor blood pressure throughout the time the anesthetic is in effect, to be certain that the systolic pressure does not fall to less than 100 mm Hg or decrease by 20 mm Hg or more in a hypertensive woman. A drop greater than this could be life-threatening to a fetus unless prompt, effective corrective measures are taken, such as repositioning and administering an antihypotensive agent. If such measures are instituted quickly, fetal outcome will not be compromised.

With an epidural block, the woman loses sensation of her bladder filling. Remind her to void every 2 hours, monitor intake and output, and observe and palpate for bladder distention to avoid overfilling. Be aware of the standards

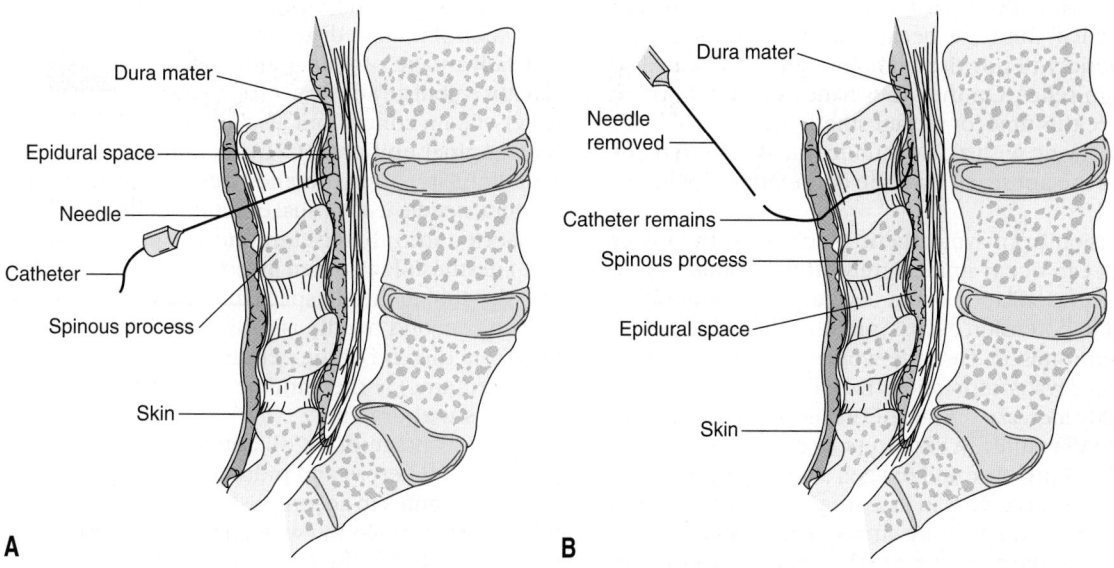

A **B**

FIGURE 19.4 Epidural anesthesia. (**A**) A needle is inserted into the epidural space. (**B**) A catheter is threaded into the epidural space; the needle is then removed. The catheter allows medication to be administered intermittently or continuously to relieve pain during labor and childbirth.

and policies of the health care agency related to adding additional anesthesia and removal of the catheter.

Yet another technique used with epidural anesthesia is self-administration or patient-controlled epidural analgesia (PCEA). With this technique, an epidural catheter delivers an analgesic mixture whenever the client presses a button on a special pump. A lockout period follows each self-administration, to avoid overdosage. This method of administration is advantageous because less anesthetic is required, compared with continuous epidural infusion (CEI).

Spinal (Subarachnoid) Anesthesia.

Spinal anesthesia is used less frequently today, in preference to lumbar epidural blocks. It may be used in an emergency, however, because the administration technique is simpler than that of an epidural and can be accomplished more rapidly.

For spinal anesthesia, a local anesthetic agent such as bupivacaine (Marcaine) or ropivacaine (Naropin) is injected using lumbar puncture technique into the subarachnoid space (into the CSF) at the third or fourth lumbar interspace. A narcotic agonist such as morphine or fentanyl may be added for additional pain relief. For administration, the woman is placed in a sitting position on the side of the birthing bed, with legs dangling and head bent. She is asked to bend her head forward so that her back curves and the intravertebral spaces open. Be sure to support her in this position, because she is "front-heavy" as a result of her pregnancy and could easily fall forward if not well supported.

After injection, the anesthetic normally rises to the level of T10. Anesthesia up to the umbilicus and including both legs will be achieved.

Spinal anesthetic agents may be "loaded" or "weighted" with glucose to make them heavier than CSF. This helps prevent them from rising too high in the spinal canal and interfering with the motor control of the uterus or with respiratory muscles.

After injection of the anesthetic, the anesthesiologist asks the woman to lie down again. It is important that she does lie down at this time, because if she sits up too long, the anesthetic will not rise high enough in the canal to achieve pain relief. On the other hand, she must not lie down before this time, or the anesthetic will rise too high in the canal. Lying with a pillow under the head also helps ensure that the anesthesia will be confined to the lower spinal canal.

Hypotension from sympathetic blockage in the lower extremities can occur immediately after administration. This leads to vasodilation and a decrease in central blood pressure. If hypotension occurs, placental blood perfusion will be compromised. Turn the woman to her left side to reduce vena cava compression. Expect the anesthesiologist to quickly increase the rate of IV fluid administration to increase blood volume. A vasopressor (e.g., ephedrine) to increase blood pressure and oxygen also may be administered. Never place a woman in a Trendelenburg position to help restore blood pressure after spinal anesthesia. This could make the anesthetic rise high in her spinal column, causing uterine or respiratory function to cease.

To guard against hypotension, IV fluids such as lactated Ringer's solution are usually given before the injection to ensure hydration. Be certain the fluid is infusing well before the anesthesia is administered.

A late complication of spinal anesthesia is a postpartal dural puncture headache (PDPH) or "spinal headache." This occurs because of continuous leakage of CSF from the needle insertion site and possibly from the irritation of a small amount of air that enters at the injection site. The shift in pressure of the CSF causes strain on the cerebral meninges, initiating the pain. The incidence of such headaches is reduced if a small-gauge needle is used for the injection and the woman drinks a quantity of fluid afterward, because a high fluid intake rapidly provides replacement of spinal fluid. Although it is usually encouraged, asking a woman to remain flat may not be necessary because of the routine use of small needles in most settings.

If a headache does occur, it can be relieved by having the woman lie flat and administering an analgesic. Some women find a cold cloth applied to the forehead helpful. If a headache is incapacitating, it can be treated with a blood patch technique. For this, 10 mL of blood is withdrawn from an accessible vein and then immediately injected into the epidural space over the spinal injection site. The injected blood clots and seals off any further leakage of CSF.

Checkpoint Question 3

Jonny chooses to have epidural anesthesia. What are two risks associated with this?

a. Hypotension and prolonged second stage of labor.
b. Severe headache and coldness of all extremities.
c. Continued back pain and short first stage of labor.
d. Hypertension and a reduced red blood cell count.

Combined Spinal Epidural Technique.

Spinal anesthesia has an advantage over epidural anesthesia in that the pain control is immediate after injection of the anesthetic. A disadvantage of spinal anesthesia is that the woman can not ambulate afterward. To take advantage of the rapid onset of pain control but also allow for ambulation, combined spinal epidural (CSE) technique was originated. To administer this, the anesthesiologist first inserts an epidural needle using usual epidural technique. A catheter is inserted into the epidural needle and taped in place. The anesthesiologist then inserts a very fine spinal needle into the subarachnoid space and the CSF. It is confirmed that the second needle is into the CSF if a drop of fluid falls from the end of the needle. A small dose of narcotic (e.g., fentanyl) is then added to the CSF, and the spinal needle is withdrawn.

The advantage of a CSE administration is immediate pain relief, whereas an epidural block alone would take 20 to 30 minutes to accomplish this (Hughes et al., 2005). In addition, it allows the woman to be ambulatory, because the drug added to the CSF is a narcotic, not a local anesthetic. Possible complications that can occur from the CSE method include hypotension, pruritus, urinary retention, nausea and vomiting, and a PDPH (although all of these are rare). Additional anesthesia for the duration of labor is achieved by the epidural route.

Medication for Pain Relief During Birth

Stretching of the perineum causes the pain during birth. The simplest form of pain relief for birth is the natural **pressure anesthesia** that results from the fetal head pressing against the stretched perineum. This natural anesthesia is often adequate to allow an episiotomy to be performed without a woman feeling the cut. The pain she experiences as the fetal head is born, although intense and hot, occurs suddenly and is over quickly. Often, after the hours of hard contractions a woman has come through, this flash of pain seems almost nothing. For some women, however, additional medication may be needed to reduce the pain of birth.

Local Anesthetics

Local Infiltration. Local infiltration is the injection of an anesthetic such as lidocaine (Xylocaine) into the superficial nerves of the perineum. It is used when the fetal head is too low to allow for a pudendal block. The anesthetic is placed along the borders of the vulva. The effect lasts for approximately 1 hour, allowing for suturing of an episiotomy without additional anesthetic.

Pudendal Nerve Block. A **pudendal nerve block** (Fig. 19.5) is the injection of a local anesthetic such as chloroprocaine (Nesacaine) or bupivacaine (Marcaine) near the right and left pudendal nerves at the level of the ischial spine. The injection, made through the vagina with the woman in a lithotomy or dorsal recumbent position, provides relief of perineal pain in 2 to 10 minutes that lasts for approximately 1 hour. Anesthesia achieved with this method is sufficiently deep to allow the use of low forceps

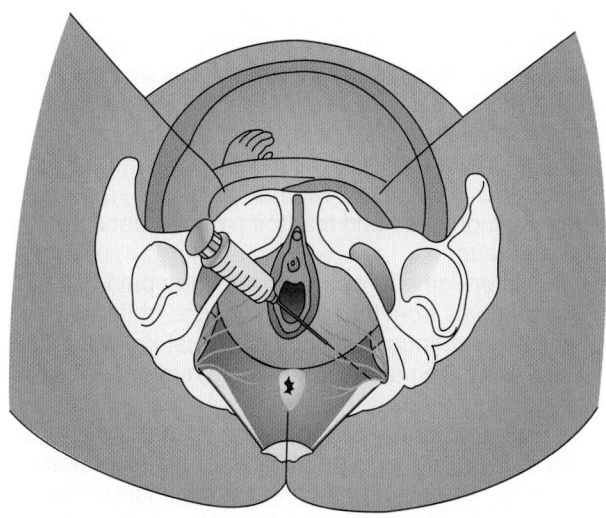

FIGURE 19.5 Pudendal nerve block.

during birth and an episiotomy repair. Although the injection is only local, the FHR and the mother's blood pressure should be checked immediately after the injection, in case maternal hypotension occurs.

General Anesthesia

General anesthesia is never preferred for childbirth, because it carries the dangers of hypoxia and possible inhalation of vomitus during administration. Pregnant women are particularly prone to gastric reflux and aspiration because of increased stomach pressure from the weight of the full uterus beneath it. The gastroesophageal valve also may be displaced and possibly functioning improperly. Despite these risks, general anesthesia may be necessary in emergency situations (e.g., abruptio placentae) when an immediate cesarean birth is required.

For complete and rapid anesthesia during childbirth, thiopental sodium (Pentothal), a short-acting barbiturate, is usually the drug of choice. It causes rapid induction of anesthesia and, because it has a short half life, allows for good uterine contraction afterward, with minimal postpartal bleeding. After induction with thiopental sodium, the woman is intubated, and anesthesia is then maintained by administration of nitrous oxide and oxygen. Thiopental sodium crosses the placenta rapidly. Infants born of a woman anesthetized by this method may be slow to respond at birth and may need resuscitation. However, in view of the degree of barbiturate intoxication demonstrable in these infants, their ability to respond and alertness at birth are always surprising.

All women who receive a general anesthetic must be observed closely in the postpartal period, because most gases used for general anesthesia cause uterine relaxation, opening the possibility of uterine atony and postpartal hemorrhage. Some women comment that their throat feels raw or sore afterward from insertion of an endotracheal tube. Using an anesthetic throat spray or gargle, sipping cold liquids, or sucking on ice chips (as soon as this is safe after general anesthesia) may help to relieve the discomfort.

Preparation for the Safe Administration of General Anesthesia. To ensure safe anesthesia administration, an anesthesiologist or nurse anesthetist needs a minimum of six drugs readily available: (1) ephedrine, to use in the event blood pressure falls; (2) atropine sulfate, to dry oral and respiratory secretions to prevent aspiration; (3) thiopental sodium (Pentothal), for rapid induction of a general anesthetic; (4) succinylcholine (Anectine), to achieve laryngeal relaxation for intubation; (5) diazepam (Valium), to control seizures, a possible reaction to anesthetics; and (6) isoproterenol (Isuprel), to reduce bronchospasm should aspiration occur. In addition to these medications, an adult laryngoscope, an endotracheal tube, a breathing bag with a source of 100% oxygen, and a suction catheter and suction source should be at hand.

Aspiration of Vomitus. Inhalation of vomitus from pressure of the uterus on the stomach can be fatal if a woman's airway becomes occluded by the foreign matter. In addition, stomach contents have an acid pH that can cause chemical pneumonitis and secondary infection of the respiratory tract.

Some anesthesiologists may order IV ranitidine (Zantac) or an oral antacid such as sodium citrate to be given before general anesthesia is administered, to reduce the level of acid in stomach contents should aspiration occur. Metoclopramide (Reglan) increases gastric emptying and may also be prescribed.

For general anesthesia administration, a woman should be placed on her back with a wedge under her right hip to displace the uterus from the vena cava. To reduce the occurrence of hypotension and to establish a line for emergency medications, IV fluid administration is begun. The woman is given a rapid-induction IV agent and is then intubated with a cuffed endotracheal tube. To prevent gastric reflux and aspiration before intubation is achieved, cricoid pressure (which seals off the esophagus by compressing it between the cricoid cartilage and the cervical vertebrae) must be applied as soon as the IV agent is begun until the cuff on the tube is in place.

The moments of induction of general anesthesia before the endotracheal tube is safely in place are critical ones for the anesthesiologist. Respect his or her need to concentrate until the task is achieved.

If aspiration of vomitus occurs in the delivery room, prompt attention is essential. The anesthesiologist suctions the woman's trachea to remove as much foreign material as possible. The woman is intubated, if she was not previously, and given 100% oxygen. IV isoproterenol to reduce bronchospasm and a corticosteroid to reduce inflammation may be given. Positive-pressure ventilation may be started. Blood gas analysis and a chest radiograph usually are obtained to determine the degree of aeration of which the woman is still capable.

Usually, the woman will receive mechanical ventilation until her overall clinical condition improves, as shown by the x-ray films and blood gas concentrations. She is critically ill at the time of aspiration and often will be transferred to an intensive care unit for the special care she needs to survive this emergency.

Checkpoint Question 4

There is no reason to think that Jonny will need a general anesthetic. If she did, what type of drug is usually prescribed to minimize the risk of aspiration of vomitus?

a. An anticonvulsant such as diazepam (Valium).
b. A nerve relaxant such as phenobarbital.
c. Metoclopramide (Reglan) to speed gastric emptying.
d. Oxytocin to increase the effectiveness of labor.

NURSING CARE TO PROMOTE THE COMFORT OF A WOMAN DURING LABOR

The best approach to pain management for women in labor combines both pharmacologic and complementary and alternative therapy measures.

NURSING DIAGNOSES AND RELATED INTERVENTIONS

Nursing Diagnosis: Anxiety related to lack of knowledge about labor experience

Outcome Evaluation: Client identifies beginning and ending of contractions; expresses confidence rather than confusion about ongoing process.

In addition to causing local discomfort, pain can evoke a general stress response (fight-or-flight syndrome). This releases epinephrine, which causes peripheral and uterine vasoconstriction. The degree of pain experienced may increase because of the resulting increase in tissue anoxia. Reducing anxiety through relaxation techniques such as planned breathing exercises, or through administration of medication to reduce anxiety, can reduce vasoconstriction and help reduce pain.

Reduce Anxiety With Explanations of the Labor Process. Planning with women about their options for pain relief during labor should begin prenatally (Box 19.5). During labor, use a standard method of pain assessment, such as a scale of 1 to 10, so that the woman can rate her pain. Evaluate whether pain relief is adequate—not only whether pain relief was offered, but whether it was effective (Pasero & McCaffery, 2004).

Help women use natural methods based on the gate control theory (see Chapter 13) as well as pharmacology relief. Be sure to offer careful explanations of what is happening or what will happen during labor, because this can help alleviate anxiety and thereby reduce some discomfort.

Be sure to explain the characteristics of contractions and reinstruct as necessary (e.g., that labor contractions are rhythmic in nature and come and go repeatedly). Do not assume that a woman is aware of this simply because she is experiencing the contractions. Her pain may be so intense that she is unaware of any relief between contractions (Box 19.6). She may fear that things will worsen as labor progresses and that the pain will become continuous.

This on–off effect differentiates the pain of labor contractions from that of a toothache or headache, which is continuous. Sometimes, just knowing this can help a woman tolerate the pain even as it increases in intensity.

Do not assume everyone knows that the rupturing of membranes is painless, that a pink-stained show is normal, or that contractions change in character during the pelvic division of labor. A woman having her first child probably does not know these things. A woman having her second child may not

Team Member Responsible	Assessment	Intervention	Rationale	Expected Outcome
Psychosocial/Spiritual/Emotional Needs				
Nurse	Assess what nonpharmacologic measures (e.g., music, room temperature) client thinks would help complement epidural block and aid comfort.	Provide a comfortable environment: clean sheets, comfortable room temperature, cool washcloth to forehead, closed room door. Refrain from intervening with client during a contraction.	A comfortable environment aids in relaxation, promoting effective coping. Interrupting the client's breathing can make the technique ineffective as a pain relief measure.	Client reports she feels environment is comfortable and complements other pain relief measures.
Discharge Planning				
Nurse	Ask client and husband to evaluate their labor experience.	Review with client pain relief measures used and determine which were most effective.	Reviewing a possibly traumatic event experience helps to put it into perspective among life events.	Client and support person state that labor and birth was at worst a tolerable experience; at best, a highlight of their lives.

be given requires an in-depth understanding of the available drugs, their effects on the mother and the fetus, and their mechanism and duration of action. It also requires sympathetic listening and counseling skills. Many women come into labor wishing to avoid drugs entirely. Once in labor, they may change their minds but hesitate to say so, especially if their partners also believe that a birth without the use of drugs is ideal. Other women come into labor asking to receive something immediately to avoid experiencing any pain. In both instances, provide information about the use of drugs and their ultimate effects. Maintain a supportive presence to help a woman make the best decision for herself and her baby. Some women require analgesia or anesthesia because of a complication. Helping these women and their support persons understand why the medication is necessary calls for equal care and skill. As a rule, record a baseline FHR and maternal blood pressure and pulse before administering medication; reassess 15 minutes later for fetal and maternal safety.

Checkpoint Question 5

Jonny reports in early labor she isn't having much pain. You assess that her contractions are also not strong. What position usually promotes efficient uterine contractions in early labor?

a. Sitting or standing.
b. Lying supine.
c. Lying prone.
d. Side-lying.

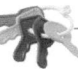

Key Points

Pain in labor occurs because of anoxia to uterine cells, stretching of the cervix and perineum, and pressure of the presenting part of the fetus on maternal tissues.

Each person perceives pain differently. Only a woman herself can describe the extent of her pain.

Usually, the better prepared a woman is for childbirth, the less analgesia and anesthesia is necessary.

Encourage complementary and alternative therapies such as reducing anxiety, providing changes in position, increasing knowledge, and supporting prepared childbirth exercises in conjunction with prescribed analgesics.

Be certain to ask about allergy to a medication before administering it during labor. Women under stress may omit mentioning this unless directly asked.

Women may lose their ability to use controlled breathing after systemic narcotic administration because of a "lightheaded" feeling. They may need additional support during this time to be able to continue with a breathing technique until the analgesic agent begins to have an effect.

Regional anesthesia (e.g., epidural anesthesia) can be extremely effective in relieving labor pain. Be certain the woman is well hydrated with IV fluid and that her blood pressure is within normal limits before administration of the anesthetic agent.

During regional or general anesthesia administration, if the woman must lie supine, she should have a wedge positioned under her right buttock to help prevent supine hypotension syndrome. If hypotension should occur after epidural anesthesia administration, elevating a woman's legs is an emergency measure to help relieve hypotension.

If a narcotic analgesic is used, naloxone (Narcan) must be available for possible newborn resuscitation.

General anesthesia is rarely administered for an uncomplicated labor, because it has risks for both the mother and the infant, but may still be used in an emergency.

Critical Thinking Exercises

1. Jonny, the patient you met at the beginning of the chapter, did not attend any preparation for childbirth classes because she planned to rely totally on a regional block for pain relief. If you had met her during pregnancy, instead of when she was beginning labor, would you have supported this plan? Are there any complementary and alternative therapies that she could have planned for in addition to relying on a regional block?

2. Suppose Jonny says she wants a general anesthetic for labor or she will leave the hospital. Her physician has said that he cannot justify a general anesthetic for uncomplicated labor. You find Jonny crying because her doctor won't give her anything for pain. How would you handle this situation?

3. Suppose Jonny seems well prepared for labor but, after an injection of meperidine early in labor, grows angry with her husband and refuses to use breathing exercises because she feels "so lightheaded" from the medicine. How would you help her at this point?

4. Examine the National Health Goals related to comfort in labor. Most government-sponsored money for nursing research is allotted based on these goals. What would be a possible research topic to explore pertinent to these goals that would be applicable to the Baranca family and also advance evidence-based practice?

References

American College of Obstetricians and Gynecologists. (2002). Analgesia and cesarean delivery rates. *Obstetrics and Gynecology, 99*(2), 369–370.

Callister, L. C., et al. (2003). The pain of childbirth: Perceptions of culturally diverse women. *Pain Management Nursing, 4*(4), 145–154.

Camann, W. (2005). Pain relief during labor. *New England Journal of Medicine, 352*(7), 718–720.

Chang, A. M., Ip, W. Y., & Cheung, T. H. (2004). Patient-controlled analgesia versus conventional intramuscular injection: A cost effectiveness analysis. *Journal of Advanced Nursing, 46*(5), 531–541.

Chung, U., et al. (2003). Effects of LI4 and BL67 acupressure on labor pain and uterine contractions in the first stage of labor. *Journal of Nursing Research, 11*(4), 251–260.

Cluett, E. R., et al. (2004). Immersion in water in pregnancy, labour and birth. *The Cochrane Library (Oxford) (4)* (CD000111).

Cyna, A. M., McAuliffe, G. L., & Andrew, M. I. (2004). Hypnosis for pain relief in labour and childbirth: A systematic review. *British Journal of Anaesthesia, 93*(4), 505–511.

Department of Health and Human Services. (2000). *Healthy people 2010.* Washington, D.C.: Author.

Escott, D., et al. (2004). The range of coping strategies women use to manage pain and anxiety prior to and during first experience of labour. *Midwifery, 20*(2), 144–156.

Finkel, R. S., & Zarlengo, K. M. (2004). Blue cohosh and perinatal stroke. *New England Journal of Medicine, 351*(3), 302–303.

Goodman, P., Mackey, M. C., & Tavakoli, A. S. (2004). Factors related to childbirth satisfaction. *Journal of Advanced Nursing, 46*(2), 212–219.

Hawkins, J. L. (2003). Obstetric analgesia and anesthesia. In Scott, J. R., et al. *Danforth's obstetrics and gynecology* (9th ed.). Philadelphia: Lippincott Williams & Wilkins.

Howell, C. J. (2005). Epidural versus non-epidural analgesia for pain relief in labour. *The Cochrane Library (Oxford) (4)* (CD000331).

Hughes, D., et al. (2004). Combined spinal-epidural versus epidural analgesia in labour. *The Cochrane Library (Oxford) (4)* (CD003401).

Jenkins, J. G. (2005). Some immediate serious complications of obstetric epidural analgesia and anaesthesia: a prospective study of 145,550 epidurals. *International Journal of Obstetric Anesthesia, 14* (1), 37–42.

Karch, A. M. (2004). *Lippincott's nursing drug guide.* Philadelphia: Lippincott Williams & Wilkins.

Krieger, D. (1990). Therapeutic touch: Two decades of research, teaching, and clinical practice. *Imprint, 37*(3), 83–89.

Leeman, L., et al. (2003). The nature and management of labor pain: Part I. Nonpharmacologic pain relief. *American Family Physician, 68*(6), 1109–1112.

Martin, M. (2004). The art and science of reflexology: Touch as a therapeutic tool. *Positive Health, 1*(100), 20.

Melzack, R., & Wall, P. (1965). Pain mechanisms: A new theory. *Science, 150*(2), 971–982.

Nystedt, A., Edvardsson, D., & Willman, A. (2004). Epidural analgesia for pain relief in labour and childbirth: A review with a systematic approach. *Journal of Clinical Nursing, 13*(4), 455–466.

Pasero, C., & McCaffery, M. (2004). Pain control. Comfort-function goals: A way to establish accountability for pain relief. *American Journal of Nursing, 104*(9), 77–81.

Rosen, P. (2004). Supporting women in labor: Analysis of different types of caregivers. *Journal of Midwifery and Women's Health, 49*(1), 24–31.

Simkin, P., & Bolding, A. (2004). Update on nonpharmacologic approaches to relieve labor pain and prevent suffering. *Journal of Midwifery and Women's Health, 49*(6), 489–504.

Suggested Readings

Baston, H. (2003). Midwifery basics: Care during labour. Non-pharmacological methods of pain relief. *Practising Midwife, 6*(10), 33–37.

Florence, D. J., & Palmer, D. G. (2003). Therapeutic choices for the discomforts of labor. *Journal of Perinatal and Neonatal Nursing, 17*(4), 238–251.

Huntley, A. L., Coon, J. T., & Ernst, E. (2004). Complementary and alternative medicine for labor pain: A systematic review. *American Journal of Obstetrics and Gynecology, 191*(1), 36-44.

Kao, B. C., et al. (2004). A comparative study of expectant parents' childbirth expectations. *Journal of Nursing Research, 12*(3), 191-202.

Leeman, L., et al. (2003). The nature and management of labor pain: Part II. Pharmacologic pain relief. *American Family Physician, 68*(6), 1115-1120.

Pascali-Bonaro, D., & Kroeger, M. (2004). Continuous female companionship during childbirth: A crucial resource in times of stress or calm. *Journal of Midwifery and Women's Health, 49*(4Suppl), 19-27.

Pasero, C. (2004). Pain and comfort issues. *Journal of PeriAnesthesia Nursing, 19*(3), 135-137.

Radzyminski, S. (2003). The effect of ultra low dose epidural analgesia on newborn breastfeeding behaviors. *JOGNN: Journal of Obstetric, Gynecologic, and Neonatal Nursing, 32*(3), 322-331.

Smith, C. A., et al. (2004). Complementary and alternative therapies for pain management in labour. *The Cochrane Library (Oxford) (4)* (CD00352).

Waldenstrom, U., et al. (2004). A negative birth experience: Prevalence and risk factors in a national sample. *Birth, 31*(1), 17-27.

CHAPTER 20

Cesarean Birth

Key Terms

cesarean birth
classic cesarean incision
dehiscence
low segment incision
no-indicated-risk cesarean
birth

Objectives

After mastering the contents of this chapter, you should be able to:

1. Describe the indications for cesarean birth.
2. Assess a woman scheduled for cesarean birth for effective preoperative, intraoperative, and postoperative needs.
3. Formulate nursing diagnoses related to women undergoing cesarean birth.
4. Establish outcomes that meet the needs of a woman requiring a cesarean birth.
5. Plan appropriate nursing care to ensure family-centered care for a woman requiring a cesarean birth.
6. Implement common preoperative and postoperative care measures for cesarean birth.
7. Evaluate expected outcomes related to cesarean birth for achievement and effectiveness of nursing care.
8. Identify National Health Goals related to cesarean birth that nurses can help the nation achieve.
9. Identify areas related to cesarean birth that could benefit from additional nursing research or application of evidence-based practice.
10. Use critical thinking to analyze common complications of cesarean birth in order to develop preventive strategies and keep it family centered.
11. Integrate knowledge of cesarean birth with the nursing process to achieve quality maternal and child health nursing care.

*M*oja Hamma is a 29-year-old woman who is pregnant with her first baby. Her labor began with ruptured membranes and dark green meconium-stained amniotic fluid. Moja telephoned her nurse-midwife, who asked her to come to the hospital immediately. Moja drove herself to the birthing center and arrived in 20 minutes. Fetal heart rate was 100 bpm. An obstetrician was consulted, and she scheduled Moja for an immediate cesarean birth. Moja reacted calmly to the news that she needed surgery until she realized her boyfriend would not be able to get to the hospital until her surgery was over. She refused to sign for permission, saying, "I can't. I just can't go through this alone."

Previous chapters described the normal anatomy and physiology of labor and the sequence of usual birth. This chapter adds information about cesarean birth as a way to help a woman ensure a healthy outcome for both herself and her child.

Is Moja's response typical of a woman who is told she needs a surgical procedure for the birth of her baby? What action by a nurse would be best to help her accept this procedure without feeling so alone?

After you've studied this chapter, access the accompanying website. Read the patient scenario and answer the questions to further sharpen your skills, grow more familiar with RN-CLEX types of questions, and reward yourself with how much you have learned.

Cesarean birth, or birth accomplished through an abdominal incision into the uterus, is one of the oldest types of surgical procedures known. It is a procedure always slightly more hazardous than vaginal birth. However, when compared with other surgical procedures, it is one of the safest types of surgeries and one with few complications (Porter & Scott, 2003).

The word "cesarean" is derived from the Latin *caedore,* which means "to cut." At one time, there was a popular belief that Julius Caesar was born by a cesarean birth and the procedure was named for him. However, because Caesar was born before antibiotics and sterile surgical technique, it seems unlikely that his mother (who is known to have been alive in his adult years) would have survived such a procedure. Currently, cesarean birth is used most often as a prophylactic measure, to alleviate problems of birth for conditions such as those listed in Box 20.1. It is generally contraindicated when there is a documented dead fetus (labor can be induced to avoid a surgical procedure).

The term *cesarean birth,* rather than *cesarean delivery,* is used to accentuate that this is a birth more than a surgical procedure. A major concern in maternal and child health nursing is the increasing number of cesarean births being performed annually (Box 20.2). In 1970, only 5.5% of women in the United States had infants born by cesarean birth. Currently, the incidence of primary cesarean births is 26% (NCHS, 2005). This increased rate results from a combination of the increasing safety of cesarean birth, the use of fetal monitors (which provide for early detection of fetal problems), and elective cesarean births chosen by women to prevent potential urinary or anal incontinence later in life (Handa et al., 2004; Wu et al., 2005).

BOX 20.1

Selected Indications for Cesarean Birth

Maternal Factors
Active genital herpes or papilloma
AIDS or HIV-positive status
Cephalopelvic disproportion
Cervical cerclage
Disabling conditions, such as severe hypertension of pregnancy, that prevent pushing to accomplish the pelvic division of labor
Failed induction or failure to progress in labor
Obstructive benign or malignant tumor
Previous cesarean birth by classic incision
Elective—no indicated risks

Placenta Factors
Placenta previa
Premature separation of the placenta
Umbilical cord prolapse

Fetal Factors
Compound conditions such as macrosomic fetus in a breech lie
Extreme low birth weight
Fetal distress
Major fetal anomalies, such as hydrocephalus
Multigestation or conjoined twins
Transverse fetal lie

BOX 20.2 FOCUS ON . . .

NATIONAL HEALTH GOALS

Two National Health Goals speak directly to cesarean birth:

- Reduce the rate of cesarean births among low-risk (full-term, singleton, vertex presentation) women having their first child to 15% of live births, from a baseline of 18%.
- Reduce the rate of cesarean births among women who have had a prior cesarean birth to 63% of live births, from a baseline of 72% (DHHS, 2000).

Nurses can help the nation achieve these goals by encouraging women who fulfill the criteria for vaginal birth after cesarean (VBAC) to attempt a vaginal birth with a second child.

Additional nursing research in this area could include studies and application of evidence-based practice on the effect of nursing practice and the cesarean birth rate, effective pain management for cesarean birth, and measures to help the family adjust smoothly from the hospital to the home setting after a cesarean birth.

Its increase may also be related to physicians' fears of malpractice suits should a fetus be allowed to be born vaginally and then be discovered to have suffered anoxia. Although the present incidence of cesarean births is a concern, this concern must be weighed against the potential for the procedure to reduce the incidence of infants who are born cognitively or physically challenged or who die at birth. Few parents insist that giving birth vaginally is more important than ensuring the birth of a healthy baby by cesarean birth.

A number of legal and ethical issues have arisen in recent years when women have refused to undergo cesarean birth after being advised that they need one. Because women do have a right to decide whether they will undergo surgery, the right to refuse the procedure is respected. In some instances, however, a court order for the procedure has been obtained to save a fetus. Most circumstances do not come to this point of conflict with health care providers. Maternal child care nurses should be aware of the opinion of their agency's ethics committee on this issue. As a rule, nurse-midwifery birthing services have a lower incidence of cesarean births than hospital services do. Continuous support during labor also appears to decrease the incidence (Hodnett et al., 2005).

Nursing Process Overview

For a Woman Having a Cesarean Birth

● *Assessment*

Many women with smaller than usual pelvic diameters are told during pregnancy that a cesarean birth may be necessary. Others learn only during labor that a cesarean birth will be likely. Assessment as to whether a woman will be a good candidate for surgery is sometimes done throughout pregnancy and sometimes done very quickly in an emergency. Either way, assessment must include both physiologic and psychological status and preparedness.

● *Nursing Diagnosis*
Nursing diagnoses specific to cesarean birth are often related to prevention of common complications from surgery or patient/family concerns about surgical birth. Specific examples include the following:

- Risk for infection related to a surgical incision
- Fear related to impending surgery
- Pain related to a surgical incision
- Deficient fluid volume related to blood loss from surgery
- Powerlessness related to medical need for cesarean birth

● *Outcome Identification and Planning*
The same outcome applies to a woman giving birth by cesarean as a woman giving birth vaginally: a healthy mother and a healthy child. Because cesarean birth decisions can be made suddenly, planning can be limited to only a few minutes. This means you have only a few minutes to organize presurgery steps such as gastrointestinal or anesthesia preparation. Plans must include discharge instructions and home care, because a woman will remain in the health care facility only 2 or 3 days.

● *Implementation*
Every woman is aware that childbirth poses some risk to her health. When major surgery is superimposed on top of this, it is imperative that the woman and her support person feel confidence in the health care personnel who care for them. Otherwise, they could have difficulty coping with the insult of surgery. When giving care to any woman during labor, be certain to establish a helping relationship with both the woman and her support person, because this relationship becomes especially advantageous should the birth method need to be altered. For a woman who knows in advance that she will have a cesarean birth, the following organization can be helpful: International Cesarean Awareness Network (*www.ICAN-ONLINE.org*).

Many interventions focus on teaching and support, because the more a woman understands about what is happening to her, the more she can accept and cooperate with the procedure. During surgery, sterile technique is essential. A postpartal infection can be devastating to a woman who already has made many other physical adaptations. After the procedure, be sure to provide adequate "talk time" to allow a woman time to review what has happened and integrate it into what she and her partner expected.

Another important intervention includes coordination of health care team members (i.e., anesthesiologist, surgeon, pediatrician or neonatologist, and recovery room or nursery personnel). This is particularly important if the surgery will be performed in a hospital surgery department rather than in a labor and birthing suite, or if the infant will be transferred to an intensive care nursery or a distant site for intensive care after the birth.

● *Outcome Evaluation*
Evaluation of expected outcomes is important in the care of a woman after cesarean birth to ensure she is not developing a complication. Such evaluation is sometimes difficult to do because of shortened hospital stays. It is especially important to consider the overall goals of a healthy baby and a healthy mother and the development of a positive mother–infant (or parent– or family–infant) relationship. The following are examples that demonstrate successful achievement of outcomes:

- Patient states that she understands the reason for a cesarean birth.
- Patient states that she felt well prepared for cesarean birth even in light of an emergency.
- Couple states that they feel able to cope with newborn care even with mother recovering from surgery.
- Patient remains free of signs and symptoms of infection after cesarean birth.
- Patient states that incisional pain is controlled and tolerable.

CESAREAN BIRTH

There are two types of cesarean birth: scheduled and emergency. In the first instance, there is time for thorough preparation for the experience throughout the antepartal period. Some women even take a childbirth preparation class specifically for cesarean birth. With the second type of cesarean birth, preparation must be done much more rapidly but with the same concern for fully informing a woman and her support person about what circumstances created the need for a cesarean birth and how the birth will proceed. Cesarean birth is mentioned in most childbirth classes, so any woman who has taken such a class may at least understand that cesarean births are sometimes necessary. Box 20.3 highlights appropriate outcomes and interventions for cesarean birth using the terminology identified by the Nursing Outcomes Classification (NOC) and Nursing Interventions Classification (NIC).

Scheduled Cesarean Birth

In the 1950s, cesarean birth became a status symbol when Hollywood stars asked to have cesarean births to save themselves the strain of labor and in some instances to schedule the birth conveniently between movie contracts. The average woman came to think of cesarean birth not as a surgical procedure but as an easy method of painless childbirth. Because the risk of injury from cesarean birth is higher than that from vaginal birth, this philosophy put both mothers and fetuses at greater risk than necessary. Scheduling cesarean births this freely also resulted in preterm births.

Today, a physical indication for a cesarean birth, such as a transverse presentation, genital herpes, cephalopelvic disproportion, or avoidance of postprocedure stress incontinence, must be documented before a cesarean pro-

BOX 20.3

Nursing Outcomes Classification (NOC) and Nursing Interventions Classification (NIC)

Cesarean birth

NOC: Knowledge, Labor and Delivery

Knowledge, labor and delivery, is defined as the extent of understanding conveyed about labor and delivery (Johnson, Maas, & Moorhead, 2000). Some specific indicators suggesting that this outcome has been achieved may include the woman's ability to describe the following:

* Birthing options
* Role of support person
* Stages and phases of labor and delivery
* Methods of pain control
* Effective breathing techniques
* Potential complications

NIC: Cesarean Section Care

Cesarean birth care is defined as the preparation and support of the client delivering a baby by cesarean birth (McCloskey & Bulechek, 2000). Some important activities when implementing this intervention include:

* Determining client's perception and preparation
* Explaining reasons for unplanned cesarean birth
* Encouraging client to express feelings and urging support person to be present
* Setting up equipment for the procedure
* Providing information about the procedure and sensations afterward, progress during the procedure, and status of infant throughout the procedure
* Inspecting incisional site
* Encouraging early ambulation
* Administering pain medication as needed
* Discussing client's and support person's feelings about the procedure after birth

---

cedure can be performed. The rate of cesarean births performed to avoid stress incontinence (**no-indicated-risk cesarean birth**) is increasing in some areas, but this practice is controversial. Cesarean birth may reduce the transfer of the human immunodeficiency virus (HIV), hepatitis C, or herpes type 2 from mother to newborn, so it is recommended for women who are HIV positive (Brown, 2004; Panburana et al., 2004). It can reduce mortality among infants presenting breech (Gilbert et al., 2004). With new surgical techniques, particularly the use of a low cervical incision, "once a cesarean, always a cesarean" no longer applies. Most women who have had a cesarean birth within the past 10 years are eligible to give birth vaginally in subsequent pregnancies if the circumstances otherwise are appropriate for vaginal birth. About 60% of women today have a vaginal birth after a cesarean birth (VBAC) (Horey et al., 2005). For more information on VBAC, see Chapter 18.

Emergency Cesarean Birth

Emergency cesarean births are done for reasons such as placenta previa, abruptio placentae, fetal distress, or failure to progress in labor. An emergency cesarean birth carries with it the risk of any emergency surgery: the woman may not be a prime candidate for anesthesia and is psychologically unprepared for the experience. In addition, the woman may have a fluid and electrolyte imbalance and be both physically and emotionally exhausted from a long labor.

Effects of Surgery on a Woman

Cesarean birth, like any surgical procedure, has systemic effects.

Stress Response

Whenever the body is subjected to stress, either physical or psychosocial, it responds with measures to preserve the function of major body systems. This results in release of epinephrine and norepinephrine from the adrenal medulla. Epinephrine causes an increased heart rate, bronchial dilatation, and elevation of the blood glucose level. It also leads to peripheral vasoconstriction, which forces blood to the central circulation and increases blood pressure. These normally positive responses (the person is tensed or ready for action with good heart and lung function and glucose for energy) may antagonize anesthetic action, which is aimed at minimizing body activity. In the pregnant woman, such responses may minimize blood supply to the lower extremities. The woman is already prone to thrombophlebitis from stasis of blood flow, and these responses compound or greatly increase the risk of thrombophlebitis. Combined with interferences to major body systems, these effects can add to the risks of surgery.

Interference With Body Defenses

The skin serves as the primary line of defense against bacterial invasion. When skin is incised for a surgical procedure, this important line of defense is lost. Strict adherence to aseptic technique during surgery and in the days following the procedure are necessary to compensate for this impaired defense. If cesarean birth is performed hours after the membranes ruptured, a woman's risk for infection will be higher than if the membranes were intact. Many women receive prophylactic antibiotics, such as ampicillin (Omnipen), to ensure protection against postsurgical endometritis, even if the membranes were intact (Porter & Scott, 2003).

Interference With Circulatory Function

Although vessels that must be cut for surgery are immediately clamped and ligated, some blood loss always occurs with surgery. Extensive blood loss can lead to hypovolemia and lowered blood pressure. This could lead to ineffective perfusion of all body tissues if the problem is not quickly recognized and corrected. The amount of blood lost in cesarean birth is comparatively high, because pelvic vessels are congested with blood waiting to supply the placenta. During a vaginal birth, a woman loses 300 to 500 mL of blood. This loss increases to 500 to 1,000 mL with a cesarean birth.

Interference With Body Organ Function

When any body organ is handled, cut, or repaired in surgery, it may respond with a temporary disruption in function. Pressure from edema or inflammation as fluid moves into the injured area further impairs function of the primary organ involved, as well as that of surrounding organs. If blood vessels become compressed as a result of edema, distant organs may be deprived of blood flow, leading to reduced function in those organs. Postoperatively, close assessment, not only of the primary organ involved but of total body function, is necessary to determine the total degree of disruption.

Because the uterus is handled during cesarean birth, it may not contract well afterward, which can lead to postpartum hemorrhage. For a surgeon to reach the uterus, the bladder must be displaced anteriorly. As a result of this handling, the bladder may not sense filling as well as usual after the procedure (Phipps et al., 2005). Lower-extremity circulation may be compromised due to edema. Surgery also puts pressure on the intestine, so a paralytic ileus or halting of intestinal function is yet another possibility. After a cesarean birth, therefore, uterine, bladder, intestinal, and lower circulatory function must all be carefully assessed.

Interference With Self-Image or Self-Esteem

Surgery always leaves an incisional scar that will be noticeable to some extent afterward. Fortunately, the scar resulting from cesarean birth (a horizontal one across the lower abdomen) is not overly noticeable, but its appearance may cause a woman to feel self-conscious later. Although most women accept cesarean birth well, a woman may feel a loss of self-esteem if she believes it marks her as a woman less than others because she was unable to give vaginal birth.

Checkpoint Question 1

Moja Hamma is concerned she may lose an excessive amount of blood with cesarean surgery. What is the usual amount of blood lost with cesarean birth?

a. 100–220 mL
b. 250–350 mL
c. 300–500 mL
d. 500–1,000 mL

NURSING CARE OF A WOMAN ANTICIPATING A CESAREAN BIRTH

A woman who is admitted to the hospital for an anticipated cesarean birth may be more worried about the procedure, because she has had more time to worry, than a woman who is told during labor that an emergency cesarean is necessary. After the woman is admitted to the health care facility, allow her time to talk about any fears she has. Encourage her to do as much as possible for herself preoperatively, to help her feel in control and diminish her fear.

A woman undergoing surgery cannot begin to relax as long as her support person is nervous and worried. Make a point of including this person in all explanations and admission routines, to keep his or her anxiety under control as well.

Preoperative Interview

Both the physician and the anesthesiologist or nurse-anesthetist will interview the woman preoperatively to obtain a health history and make an assessment and decision for safe use of anesthesia. A nursing assessment is also essential. Be sure to ask about any past surgeries, secondary illnesses, allergies to foods or drugs, and current medications, to help establish surgical risk. In addition, include the following information:

- The woman's knowledge about the procedure
- The length of hospitalization anticipated
- Any postsurgical equipment to be used, such as an indwelling catheter or intravenous fluid line
- Any special precautions that will be necessary for her infant

Operative Risk for a Woman

For any surgery to be performed safely, a person must be in the best possible physical and psychological state. People who are in less than optimal physical or psychological health are at risk for a complicated surgical outcome unless the risk factor is identified and special precautions are taken (Hager et al., 2004).

Poor Nutritional Status

A woman who is obese is at risk because such a condition interferes with wound healing. Tissue that contains an abundance of fatty cells is difficult to suture, so the incision may take longer to heal. A prolonged healing period increases the risk for infection and rupture of the incision (**dehiscence**). The person's heart may also have an increased workload. Therefore, the physiologic shock of surgery may place greater stress on an already overworked organ. In addition, an obese person often has more difficulty turning and ambulating postoperatively than does a person of normal weight and therefore has an increased risk for development of respiratory or circulatory complications such as pneumonia or thrombophlebitis (Ehrenberg et al., 2004).

A woman with a protein or vitamin deficiency is also at risk for poorer healing, because protein and vitamins C and

D are necessary for new cell formation at the incision site. In addition, vitamin K is necessary for blood clotting after surgery. Although most pregnant women follow sound nutritional practices and take iron supplements, some may still be iron deficient (particularly women with a multiple gestation or women who have not taken supplements). This places them at high risk for extreme fatigue after surgery, which could interfere with parent–child bonding.

Age Variations

Age affects surgical risk because it can cause decreased circulatory and renal function. Fortunately, most pregnant women fall within the young adult age group, so they are excellent candidates for surgery. A woman older than 40 years of age falls into a category of slightly higher risk.

Altered General Health

A woman who has a secondary illness (e.g., cardiac disease, diabetes mellitus, anemia, kidney or liver disease) is at greater than usual surgical risk, depending on the extent of disease, because the pathology from the secondary illness may interfere with the woman's ability to adjust physically to the demands of surgery. A woman with a secondary illness may also have an accompanying nutritional or electrolyte imbalance related to her primary illness.

Therefore, asking about any secondary illnesses is an essential component of the preoperative nursing history. While waiting for surgery, people are under stress, a condition that can limit their reasoning and decision-making abilities. For example, it is not unusual for people admitted for any type of surgery to state that they are generally healthy and, minutes later, request insulin on the day of surgery because they are diabetic.

A medication history also is important, because some drugs increase surgical risk by interfering with the effect of an anesthetic or with healing of tissue. Several drugs that pregnant women might be taking and their potential complications are shown in Table 20.1.

Fluid and Electrolyte Imbalance

A woman who enters surgery with a lower than normal blood volume will feel the effect of surgical blood loss more than a woman who has a normal blood volume. A woman who began labor and later was told that she is to have a cesarean birth may fall into this category, because she may have had nothing to eat or drink for almost 24 hours. Recent vomiting, diarrhea, or a chronic poor fluid intake can compound her risk. Intravenous fluid replacement usually is initiated preoperatively and continued postoperatively to prevent fluid and electrolyte imbalances.

Fear

Women who are extremely worried need a very detailed explanation of the procedure before they can enter surgery without intense fear. Most cesarean births currently are performed under epidural anesthesia, so they are less frightening for women than when general anesthesia was used. If general anesthesia is used, a person who is fright-

TABLE 20.1

Drugs That May Result in Complications of Surgery

Type of Drug	Action
Antibiotics	Specific antibiotics may predispose to renal insufficiency or increase neuromuscular blockage; can lead to opportunistic infections
Anticoagulants	May cause hemorrhage due to lack of hemostasis during surgery
Anticonvulsants	May increase liver action and metabolism of anesthetic agent
Antihypertensives	May result in hypotension after anesthesia
Corticosteroids	May block body's response to shock and lead to lack of adrenal function
Insulin	May lead to hypoglycemia during labor or hyperglycemia if a dextrose solution is administered
Antianxiety agents	May cause hypotension after anesthesia

ened is at a greater risk for cardiac arrest during anesthesia administration than a person who is calm and relaxed.

In many instances, just helping a woman acknowledge that her fear of surgery is normal may be helpful. This does not make the procedure any less traumatic, but the woman can view her feelings as "normal" and expected, which helps to enhance her self-esteem.

Operative Risk to the Newborn

Cesarean birth places a newborn at a greater risk than does a vaginal birth. When a fetus is pushed through the birth canal, pressure on the chest helps to rid the lungs of lung fluid. Therefore, respirations are more likely to be adequate at birth than if the fetus had not been subjected to this pressure. For this reason, more infants born by cesarean birth develop some degree of respiratory difficulty for a day or two after birth than those born vaginally. See Chapter 26 for a discussion of this condition, which is often referred to as transient tachypnea of the newborn.

Preoperative Diagnostic Procedures

For surgery to be performed safely, adequate circulatory and renal function must be documented immediately preoperatively. Preoperative diagnostic procedures for a woman who is to have a cesarean birth usually include the following:

- Vital sign determination
- Urinalysis
- Complete blood count

- Coagulation profile (prothrombin time [PT], partial thromboplastin time [PTT])
- Serum electrolytes and pH
- Blood typing and cross-matching
- Sonogram to determine fetal presentation and maturity

During pregnancy, a woman, and particularly one who was in prolonged labor, may have an elevated leukocyte count (up to 20,000/mm^3), so this finding is not as helpful an indicator for the presence of infection in the pregnant woman as it is in others.

Preoperative Teaching

Fear of the unknown is one of the hardest fears to conquer. Preoperative teaching is aimed at acquainting a woman with cesarean procedure and any special equipment to be used, to make her as informed as possible. Activities that help maintain respiratory and skeletal muscle function, to prevent postsurgical complications, should also be included in teaching.

Before beginning teaching, assess how much the woman already knows about the surgery. A woman who has had a cesarean birth for her first child and now is being admitted for a second procedure already knows many details. Even so, she will undoubtedly appreciate having her memory refreshed and recall confirmed. Answer all specific questions, and fill in gaps in knowledge. Ensure that all information offered is accurate. It is confusing and potentially frightening for a woman to be told, for instance, that she will not have intravenous fluid after the surgery and then discover that an intravenous line will be placed. Be certain not to use hospital jargon such as "NPO." People under stress do not process new information well. They cannot process information at all if they do not understand the terminology. Have the woman return demonstrate activities, such as deep breathing, to show that she understands the information and can do this well.

Explain the preoperative measures that will be necessary, such as surgical skin preparation, eating nothing before the time of surgery, premedication (if this will be used), and method of transport to surgery. Review the necessity for an indwelling catheter, intravenous fluid administration, placement of an epidural catheter (if used for postprocedural pain relief), and the advantage of early ambulation afterward.

Throughout teaching, use visual aids as necessary. Draw pictures or show illustrations of anatomy, if necessary. Be careful not to leave textbooks about cesarean procedure techniques with the patient. Typically, these books also describe complications, and, although knowledge of possible complications is necessary for informed consent, reading about complications complete with color illustrations can be overwhelming.

Teaching to Prevent Complications

Women who work to maintain good respiratory and circulatory function postoperatively will probably experience fewer postoperative respiratory and circulatory complications than those who do not. These preventive measures are best taught during the preoperative period, when the woman is free of pain and can concentrate on the teaching. Such teaching also gives a woman a positive outlook about surgery and a sense of control over the situation. By teaching about postoperative care, you are saying, "I'll see you and your new child safely back here in your room afterward"—a communication with a comforting subliminal message for a woman who has serious doubts that there will be an afterward, or at least not one with a healthy newborn.

Deep Breathing. Periodic deep breathing exercises fully aerate the lungs and help to prevent stasis of lung mucus, which tends to occur because of the prolonged time spent in the supine position during surgery. Because stasis always has the potential to cause infection, it must be prevented as much as possible.

Taking 5 to 10 deep breaths every hour postoperatively helps to increase lung function. Teach a woman to do this simply by inhaling as deeply as possible, holding her breath for a second or two, and then exhaling as deeply as possible. Be certain she inhales and exhales fully. Otherwise, she might experience lightheadedness from hyperventilation.

Incentive Spirometry. A common device used postoperatively to encourage deep breathing is an incentive spirometer. These devices are not only easy and fun to operate but give a patient a sense of reward for her effort. The initial impression of most people is that the device works by blowing into it. Because its purpose is to fully aerate lung spaces, though, most models are triggered by *inhalation,* not exhalation.

Turning. Women do not need to practice turning side to side before surgery, because this activity is tiring for them to do while pregnant. They should understand, however, that turning postoperatively is important to prevent both respiratory and circulatory stasis.

Ambulation. The most effective way to stimulate lower-extremity circulation after a cesarean birth is with early ambulation. For this reason, most surgeons prefer a woman to be out of bed and walking by 4 hours after surgery (as soon as the effect of the epidural anesthesia has worn off). Helping a woman ambulate this early can be difficult, because she is both fatigued and in pain. Help her to understand that ambulation is extremely important after cesarean birth, because the edema of the low pelvic surgery compresses circulation to the lower extremities, increasing the risk for lower-extremity circulatory stasis. Some women may be prescribed antiembolic stockings (TEDS) to support and encourage venous return.

Immediate Preoperative Care Measures

A number of measures must be taken immediately before surgery to ensure a safe outcome.

Informed Consent

Obtaining operative consent is the surgeon's responsibility, but seeing that it is obtained is everyone's responsibility. You may be asked to witness a woman's signature on such a form. Before signing as a witness, be certain that it was *informed* consent, or one in which the risks and benefits of the procedure were explained in terms the woman could easily understand.

The law differs from state to state regarding emancipated minors (girls under legal age who are pregnant or already the mother of a previous child). Emancipated minors can sign their own surgical permission, even though they are legally underage.

Overall Hygiene

Most women who are having a planned cesarean birth are admitted to the facility on the morning of surgery and have showered or bathed at home. On admission, provide a clean hospital gown. If the woman's hair is long, encourage her to braid it or put it into a ponytail so that it will more easily fit under the surgical cap she will wear. Hair contained by a cap that way is less likely to spread microorganisms during surgery. Follow institutional procedure about removing nail polish, jewelry, contact lenses, or hair ornaments before surgery. A growing number of women wear acrylic fingernails and are reluctant to remove them for surgery. In such cases, ensure that the woman's toenails are free of polish and use the toenails to assess capillary refill.

What if... Moja Hamma, who is going to have epidural anesthesia, refuses to remove her contact lenses for surgery even though it is hospital policy for anyone receiving anesthesia? She says, "Without them, I won't be able to see my baby being born." Would you ask the nurse anesthetist whether removing them is absolutely necessary, or would you insist that she follow procedure without question?

Gastrointestinal Tract Preparation

A physician may order an enema before surgery to empty the woman's bowel for surgery and allow the bowel to rest for a few days postsurgery. If an enema is ordered, be certain to administer it using gentle, gravity-only pressure. Provide a bedpan for the woman to expel the enema, or remain with her and accompany her to the bathroom, so that she does not fall as a result of hurrying to reach the bathroom.

A gastric emptying agent such as metoclopramide (Reglan) to speed stomach emptying or a histamine blocker such as ranitidine (Zantac) to decrease stomach secretions may be prescribed. Yet another possibility is an oral antacid such as sodium citrate (Bicitra), which acts to neutralize acid stomach secretions. These precautions are necessary because the woman will be lying on her back during the procedure, making esophageal reflux and aspiration highly possible.

Baseline Intake and Output Determinations

To reduce bladder size and keep the bladder away from the surgical field, an indwelling urinary catheter may be prescribed before transport for surgery or after arrival in the surgical suite. Catheterizing a pregnant woman is more difficult than catheterizing a nonpregnant woman, because the pressure of the fetal head puts pressure on the urethra and distorts anatomic landmarks. In addition, the vulva may be swollen and distorted from vulval varicosities or edema. Use good lighting so that the perineum is clearly revealed. After catheter insertion, be certain that urine is draining freely, because fetal pressure on the urethra may reduce the flow of urine considerably. During transport, keep the drainage bag below the level of the woman's bladder, to prevent urine backflow and the possible introduction of microorganisms into the bladder.

If catheterization is difficult before surgery, do not traumatize the urethra by repeated attempts. Catheterization can be done in the birthing or delivery room after the anesthetic agent is given. If there is a delay between the catheter insertion time and surgery, mark the drainage bag just before surgery with the amount in the bag, or empty it, so that presurgery urine output can be differentiated from postsurgery urine output. One of the gravest dangers of any surgical procedure is kidney failure from the physiologic stress of surgery or lack of blood flow to the kidneys due to decreased blood pressure. All reproductive tract surgery puts ureter flow as well as kidney function at risk, because of collecting edema in the surgery area that presses on the ureters.

Hydration

Most women have an intravenous fluid line begun before surgery with a fluid such as lactated Ringer's solution. Doing so helps to ensure that the woman is fully hydrated and will not experience hypotension from epidural anesthesia administration, temporary use of a supine position, or blood loss at birth. Be certain that this line is started in the woman's nondominant hand, so that she can hold her newborn after surgery without interference. Use a large-size catheter or needle (18 or 20 gauge), so that blood replacement therapy can be administered, if needed, by the same line.

Preoperative Medication

A minimum of preoperative medication is used with a woman having a cesarean birth, to prevent compromising the fetal blood supply and to ensure that the newborn is wide awake at birth and can initiate respirations spontaneously.

Patient Chart and Presurgery Checklist

Documentation of nursing care up until the time the woman leaves the nursing care unit or labor room must be completed before the woman leaves for the surgical suite. Many hospitals use an additional preoperative checklist, such as that shown in Figure 20.1, as a reminder of all necessary measures to be taken. Checking and signing such a form indicates that the specific measures are complete.

Transport to Surgery

A woman may be transferred to surgery in her bed, or she may be helped to move to a stretcher. If a stretcher is used, be certain to hold it tightly against the side of the woman's

Patient concerns   Completed
   Skin preparation   _____
   Identification in place   _____
   Temperature, pulse, respiration _____   _____
   Blood pressure _____   _____
   Height _____ Weight _____   _____
   Voided _____ Time _____ Amount _____   _____
   NPO after _____   _____
   Hospital gown   _____
   Hairpins removed   _____
   Nail polish removed   _____
   Jewelry removed   _____
   Preoperative medication _____   _____
   Dentures removed _____ In place _____   _____
   Contact lenses removed _____   _____
   Prosthetic devices removed _____   _____

Chart concerns
   Addressograph plate attached   _____
   Operative permit obtained   _____
   Urinalysis   _____
   Hematocrit or CBC   _____
   Blood order of _____
             Signature _____ R.N.

FIGURE 20.1 Preoperative checklist for cesarean birth. Checklists vary from hospital to hospital.

bed for safe transfer. A woman is awkward in her movements at term and could easily slip and fall if the stretcher moves. Urge her to lie on her left side during transport, to prevent supine hypotension syndrome. Ensure additional safety by raising the side rails on the bed or stretcher. Cover her with a blanket or sheet to avoid her feeling chilled. Check that her identification is secure before she leaves the patient unit. Make sure that her chart with the surgical checklist accompanies her.

Role of the Support Person

In most instances, a woman's family can be as involved in the cesarean birth as they would be for a vaginal birth. A support person may need more encouragement to watch a cesarean birth than a vaginal one, because he or she may believe that the surgery will be much bloodier than it actually is. Helping family members realize that cesarean birth is little different from vaginal birth not only allows them to watch the procedure but helps them progress to bonding with the infant and incorporating a new member into the family.

Checkpoint Question 2

What is an important measure to reduce the size of the bladder and keep it away from the surgical field during a cesarean birth?

a. Restrict fluids in the woman for 4 hours before surgery.
b. Insert a urinary catheter to drain the bladder and decrease its size.
c. Administer an oxytocic to contract the bladder.
d. Give a diuretic to reduce the bladder to its smallest size.

NURSING CARE OF A WOMAN HAVING AN EMERGENCY CESAREAN BIRTH

Many women who will have a cesarean birth have no warning during pregnancy that this will be necessary. Suddenly, during labor, they develop a complication such as prolapsed cord or fetal distress, and it becomes necessary.

A woman who was having severe pain with labor and is told an emergency procedure is necessary actually may be relieved that surgery has been suggested, because the surgery will alleviate the pain. In contrast, another woman might feel great disappointment when told her baby must be born by cesarean birth. In many women, both emotions are present.

Surgical risk in an emergency situation is determined from the baseline history and physical examination information previously obtained at the beginning of labor. Preoperative preparation measures such as vital signs, urinalysis, and blood work have also been obtained. Immediate preparation concerns such as informed consent, application of elastic stockings (if appropriate), gastrointestinal tract preparation, bladder catheterization, and establishment of an intravenous line will be the same. Because most institutions try to achieve a cesarean birth within 30 minutes of the time it is documented to be necessary, there is little or no time for postoperative teaching (Nasrallah et al., 2004).

Available time must be spent explaining the immediate procedures to the woman (e.g., transfer, abdominal preparation, anesthesia). Document carefully what was taught, so that the nurse caring for the woman postoperatively will be aware of the need for additional teaching (Box 20.4).

BOX 20.4 FOCUS ON . . .

COMMUNICATION

Moja Hamma has been told she will need a cesarean birth because of cephalopelvic disproportion that has led to meconium staining.

Less Effective Communication

Nurse: Moja. Can I answer any questions for you?

Moja: I guess I want something to put me to sleep so I won't know what's happening.

Nurse: Most women want an epidural.

Moja: That won't be good enough. I want to be so sound asleep I won't know what's happening.

Nurse: Most people . . .

Moja: . . . don't have cesarean births, so what applies to them doesn't apply to me.

Nurse: I'll tell the anesthesiologist you want general anesthesia.

More Effective Communication

Nurse: Moja. Can I answer any questions for you?

Moja: I guess I want something to put me to sleep so I won't know what's happening.

Nurse: Most women want an epidural.

Moja: That won't be good enough. I want to be so sound asleep I won't know what's happening.

Nurse: You're not interested in seeing your baby born?

Moja: I'm not interested in seeing him born dead.

Nurse: Let me find your doctor to explain to you again that you need surgery to prevent something going wrong, not because something is wrong.

Most women appreciate that cesarean births are done to prevent their infant from being harmed. Others interpret a cesarean birth as being done because the harm has already occurred. Some women interpret a cesarean birth as an announcement they are somehow not as competent as other women. Still others are relieved that labor is over. Be certain to ask enough questions so that you can learn the importance or meaning of the event to an individual woman.

INTRAOPERATIVE CARE MEASURES

Cesarean birth is most similar to vaginal birth if the woman is awake during the surgery; therefore, the anesthesia chosen is usually a regional block.

Administration of Anesthesia

The surgical nurse will assist the woman to move from the transport stretcher or bed to the operating room table and will remain with her while anesthesia is administered. If the woman has an epidural catheter in place from labor, be careful not to dislodge it while she is being moved. During transport or in surgery, encourage the woman to remain on her side, or insert a pillow under her right hip to keep her body slightly tilted to the side, to prevent supine hypotension syndrome. If a spinal anesthetic (which may be used in an emergency) is to be administered, the anesthesiologist usually will do this with the woman sitting up. The anesthesiologist may ask you to help the woman curve her back to separate the vertebrae and facilitate entry of the spinal needle. It is difficult for a woman having uterine contractions to remain in this position for long. Talking to her while gently restraining her and letting her lean against you is the most effective means of helping her maintain this position. Epidural anesthesia is usually administered with the woman lying on her side. Either method achieves good results for both the mother and infant (Ng et al., 2005).

Skin Preparation

Reducing the number of bacteria on the skin before surgery automatically reduces the possibility of bacteria entering the incision at the time of surgery. Shaving away abdominal hair, if indicated, and washing the skin area over the incision site with soap and water accomplishes this.

The skin preparation area for a cesarean birth varies among agencies. Some require extensive skin preparation, from above the umbilicus to below the pubic hair, whereas others require only a limited preparation of the immediate incisional area.

Surgical Incision

After anesthetic administration, a woman is positioned with a towel under her right hip to move abdominal contents away from the surgical field and to lift her uterus off the vena cava. A screen may be placed at her shoulder level and covered with a sterile drape to block the flow of bacteria from her respiratory tract to the incision site. This also helps block the patient's and support person's lines of vision, preventing additional anxiety caused by the sight of the incision. Be sure the support person is positioned at the patient's head to provide support.

The incision area on the woman's abdomen is then scrubbed with an antiseptic (e.g., iodine), and appropriate drapes are placed around the area of incision, so that only a small area of skin is left exposed. Watching a cesarean birth is usually the first time a father or support person has ever witnessed surgery. Because of this, the person may be too overwhelmed by and interested in the procedure to be of optimum support. He or she may become concerned about the amount of manipulation and cutting that occurs before the uterus itself is cut (assuming fetal distress is not extreme). Prepare the patient and support person for the sights they might see, or help talk them through them as they occur.

Types of Cesarean Incision

There are two types of cesarean incision. The type chosen depends on the presentation of the fetus and the speed with which the procedure will be performed (Fig. 20.2). In a **classic cesarean incision,** the incision is made vertically through both the abdominal skin and the uterus. It is made high on the uterus so that it can be used with a placenta previa, to avoid cutting the placenta. A disadvantage of this type of incision is that it leaves a wide skin scar and

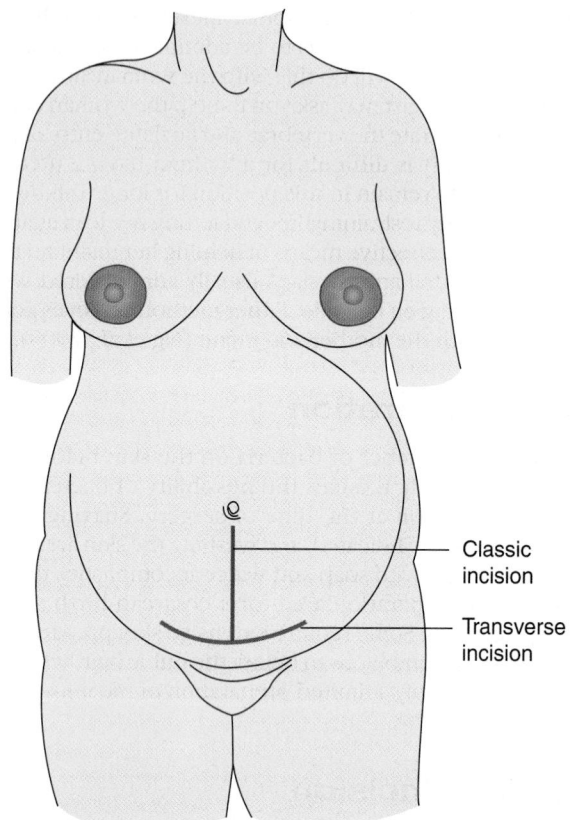

Classic incision

Transverse incision

FIGURE 20.2 Types of cesarean incisions.

also runs through the active contractile portion of the uterus. Because this type of scar could rupture during labor, it is likely, if this type of incision is used, that the woman will not be able to have a subsequent vaginal birth.

A **low segment incision** is one made horizontally across the abdomen just over the symphysis pubis and also horizontally across the uterus just over the cervix. This is the most common type of cesarean incision currently used. It is also referred to as a Pfannenstiel incision or a "bikini" incision, because even a low-cut bathing suit would cover it. Because this type of incision is through the nonactive portion of the uterus (the part that contracts minimally with labor), it is less likely to rupture in subsequent labors, making it possible for the woman to have a VBAC with a future pregnancy. It also results in less blood loss, is easier to suture, decreases postpartal uterine infections, and is less likely to cause postpartum gastrointestinal complications. The major disadvantage of this incision is that it takes longer to perform, possibly making it impractical for an emergency cesarean birth. In a few instances, the skin incision is made horizontally and then the uterine incision is made vertically, or vice versa. For this reason, during a future pregnancy, do not assume that a woman who has had a small skin incision also has had a small uterine incision.

Birth of the Infant

Once the surgical incision is complete, retractors (long, curved, metal instruments) are slipped into the incision. Gentle traction on the handles by an assistant keeps the incision spread apart, allowing good visualization of the uterus and the internal incision. Sterile towels may be placed in the incision to separate the uterus from other organs. The uterus is then cut, and the child's head may be born manually or by the application of forceps (Fig. 20.3). The mouth and nose of the baby are suctioned by a bulb syringe, the same as in a vaginal birth, before the remainder of the child is born. Oxytocin is administered intravenously by the anesthesiologist as the child or placenta is delivered, to increase uterine contraction and reduce blood loss. In many instances, a woman's partner may be allowed to cut the umbilical cord. After full birth, the uterus is pulled forward onto the abdomen and covered with moist gauze. The internal cavity of the uterus is then inspected, and the membranes and placenta are manually removed. If the woman wishes to have a tubal ligation, it can be done at this time. The uterus, subcutaneous tissues, and skin incisions are then closed. Be sure to remind the woman and her support person that closing the incision can be a long process, so they do not become concerned that something is going wrong. Metal staples are usually used on the exterior skin, because they leave the least amount of scarring.

Observing the amount of abdominal manipulation that is accomplished during surgery increases understanding of how tender a woman's abdomen will be afterward. This also helps to explain why a patient who has undergone cesarean birth often has an overall "aching" feeling after surgery.

Introduction of the Newborn

Once it is determined that the newborn is breathing spontaneously, he or she is shown to the mother and support person, just as is done after a vaginal birth. The support person may hold the baby immediately. The mother may have difficulty doing this if she has intravenous fluid infusing into one hand and the surgical drapes are still in place. Assist her as necessary. Visiting with the newborn lays a foundation for bonding and also distracts the couple from the tedious process of incision closure. Women are able to breast-feed after cesarean births the same as after vaginal births, but initial breast-feeding is usually delayed until the woman has been moved to a recovery room, because breast-feeding initiates uterine contractions and that may interfere with suture placement. Breast-feeding also may be awkward with the anesthesia screen in place and because of the lack of privacy.

Checkpoint Question 3

Moja Hamma asks you how big her scar will be after cesarean birth. Your best answer would be:

a. The incision is big and runs vertically across your abdomen.

b. The incision is made through the vagina so doesn't leave a scar.

c. Most cesarean-birth incisions are so low they don't show over a bikini.

d. It is so large that it will always show, but think of it as a mark of pride.

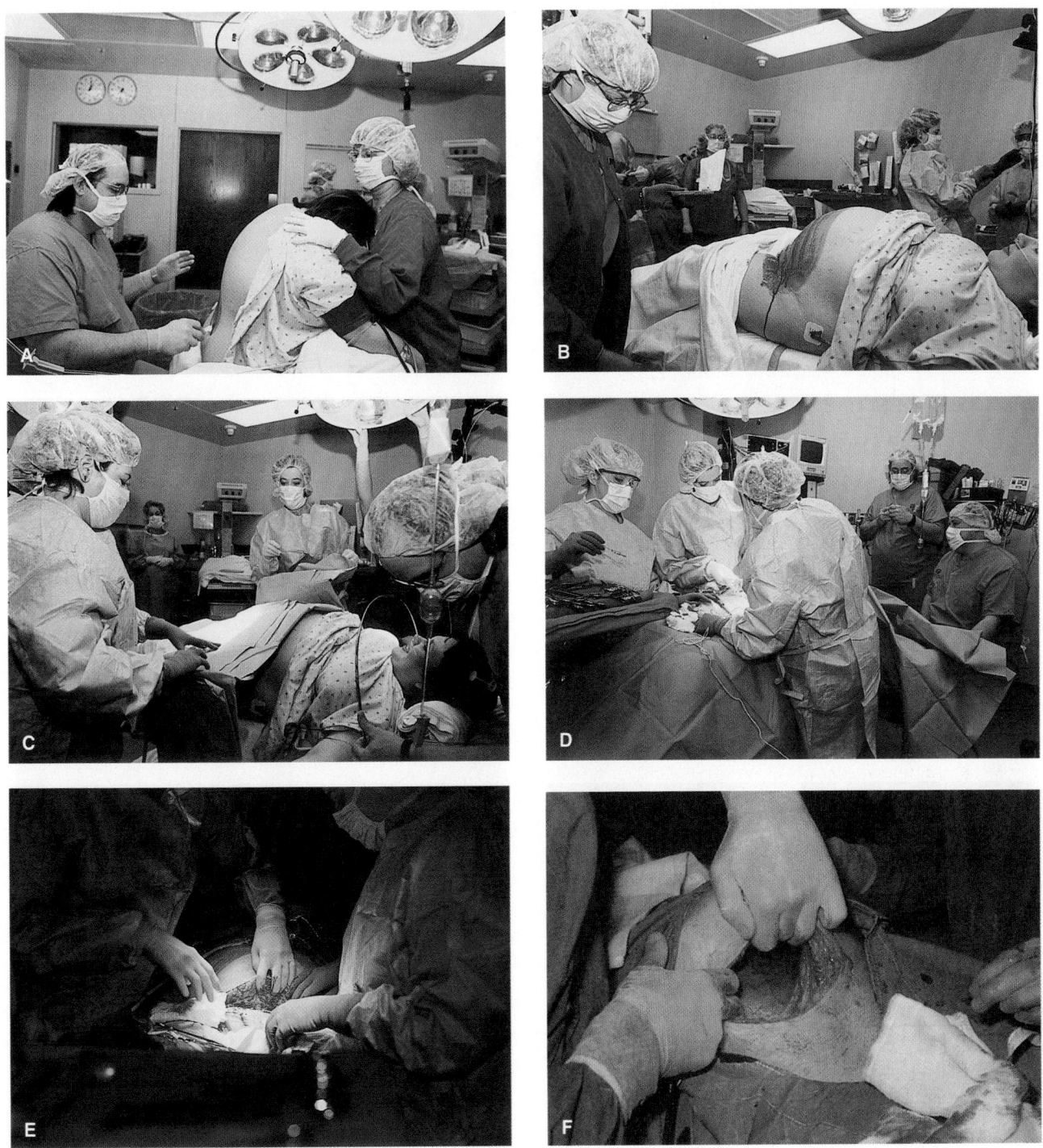

FIGURE 20.3 Cesarean birth. (**A**) Preparation for anesthesia. (**B**) Abdominal skin preparation. (**C**) Draping of operative site. (**D**) Preparation for initial incision. (**E**) Initial incision. (**F**) Opening of the peritoneum. *(continued)*

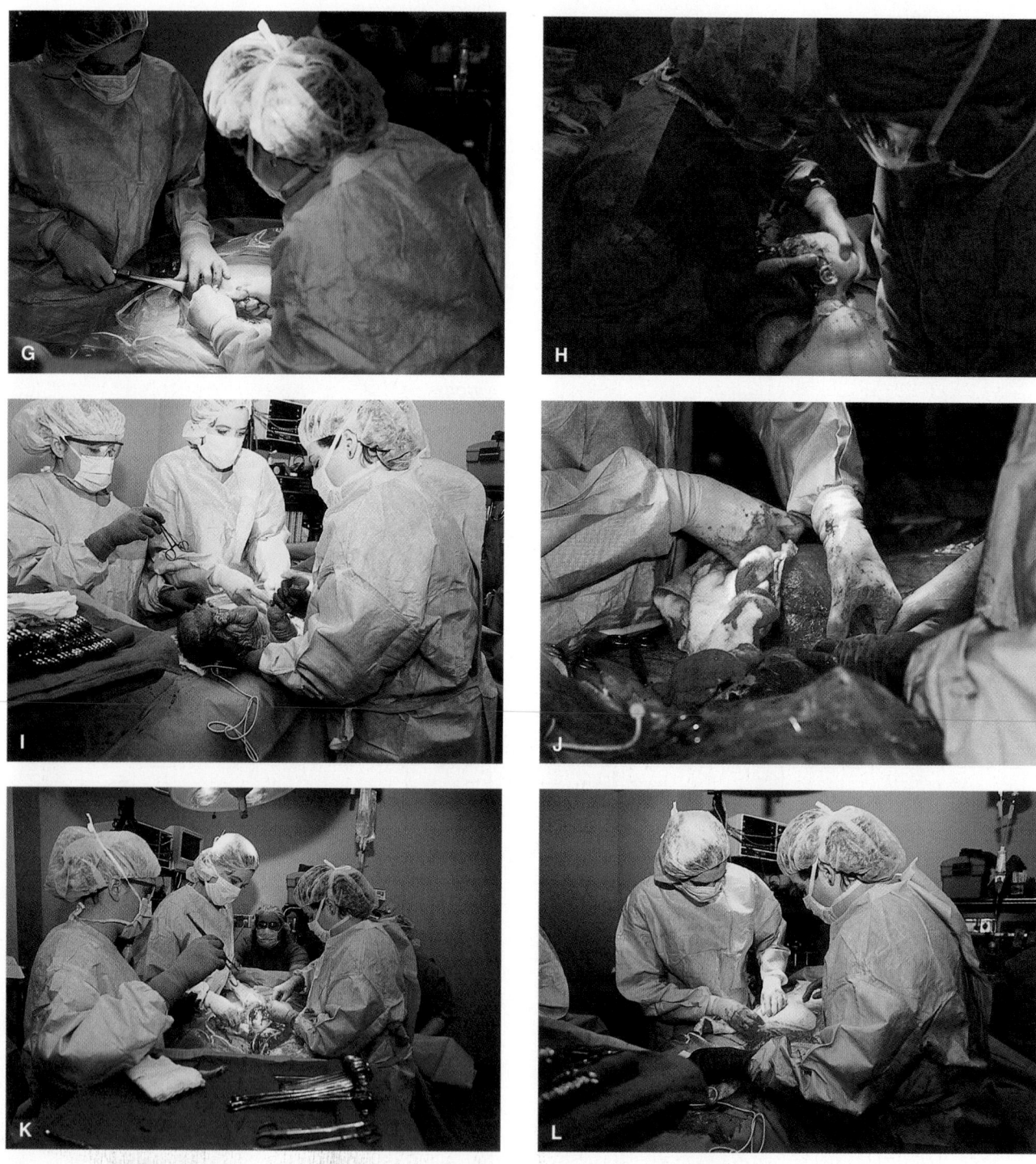

FIGURE 20.3 (continued) (**G**) Retractors in place. (**H**) Birth of head and posterior shoulder. (**I**) Infant born. (**J**) Suturing of uterus complete. (**K**) Suturing of abdominal layers. (**L**) Skin closure.

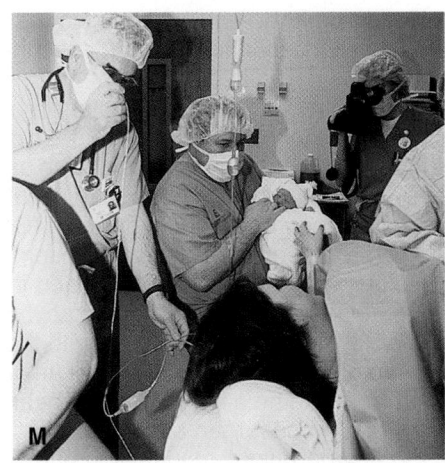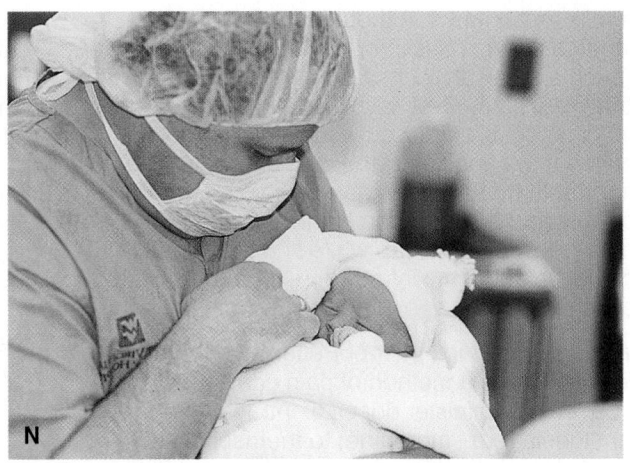

FIGURE 20.3 (continued) (**M**) Family bonding with mother's first touch. (**N**) Father bonding with newborn. (© Caroline Brown, RNC, MS, DEd.)

POSTPARTAL CARE MEASURES

Women who have infants by cesarean birth develop an additional care concern in the immediate postpartal period. They are not only postpartal patients but postsurgical ones as well. Due to the strain of the unexpected procedure, they may have increased difficulty bonding with their new infant. There is little time for teaching because of shortened hospital stays. As with all postpartal women, the postpartal phase for a woman who has her child by cesarean birth can be divided into an immediate recovery period (the so-called fourth stage of labor) and an extended postpartal period.

NURSING DIAGNOSES AND RELATED INTERVENTIONS DURING THE IMMEDIATE POSTPARTAL PERIOD

●

Immediately after surgery, the woman is transferred by stretcher from the operating room table to the postanesthesia care unit (PACU) or postpartal room. If spinal anesthesia was used, remember that her legs are fully anesthetized and she will not be able to help move them.

Nursing Diagnosis: Pain related to surgical incision

Outcome Evaluation: Patient verbalizes extent of pain (from 1 to 10) and need for relief; states that level of pain is tolerable.

In the past, pain control was a major problem after cesarean birth. Pain was so intense from the uterine or abdominal incision that it interfered with a woman's ability to move and deep breathe. This led to surgical complications such as pneumonia or thrombophlebitis. It also impaired a woman's ability to bond with her newborn, because holding the infant was so painful. Today, a number of effective types of pain management are available. Use a pain rating scale to allow the woman to rate her pain. Without the use of a specific tool, assessment can be unreliable, because the woman's overall excitement at having a new child may interfere with the accuracy of the assessment.

A woman who is concerned about her infant may experience more pain than a woman who feels confident that her infant is doing well, because anxiety and fear heighten the pain response, and a tense body posture causes pressure on sutures. Be certain the woman understands that her infant has survived the surgical birth well (assuming this is true) or what steps are being taken to make the infant well.

No matter what system of pain relief is used, when administering analgesics after surgery, be sure to supplement them with other comfort measures, such as change of position or straightening of bed linen. Check for abdominal distention, which suggests the pain may be caused by intestinal gas rather than incision pain. If so, ambulation is often the most effective method to relieve this type of pain. Always ask the woman what type of pain she is experiencing before administering a new dose of analgesia, to be certain that she is describing incisional or uterine pain and not pain in a leg or some other body part that would suggest a complication of surgery.

Urge the woman to continue to take adequate analgesia to effectively manage her pain after she returns home, so she is not so distressed that she cannot nurse her infant. Be certain she understands not to use acetylsalicylic acid (aspirin), because this can interfere with blood clotting and healing. Many women who are breast-feeding are reluctant to accept any type of analgesic, especially just before breast-feeding, for fear that it will pass in breast milk to the infant. Although it is true that most analgesics do pass in breast milk, the infant takes such a small amount of breast milk (mainly colostrum) during the first days after surgery that the amount of analgesia received would be negligible. Also, without the analgesic, the woman may be so uncomfortable that she is unable to hold her infant comfortably and enjoy having the infant with her. Placing a pillow over her lap while she feeds can deflect the weight of the infant from her suture line and lessen pain.

Patient-Controlled Analgesia. Patient-controlled analgesia (PCA) is a method of pain control in which patients administer doses of intravenous narcotic analgesia (e.g., morphine) to themselves as needed. Although the technique may be used during labor, it is most frequently used to control post-surgical pain. With a solution such as Ringer's lactate or 5% dextrose infusing intravenously, a PCA pump containing a locked syringe of narcotic (meperidine or morphine) is attached to the intravenous line at a port close to the patient. To receive a dose of analgesia, the patient pushes a button similar to a call bell. This alerts the automatic pump to deliver a set amount of narcotic into the intravenous line. The pump has a "lock-out" setting that prevents a patient from administering a larger dose or doses more frequently than would be safe (e.g., every 8 minutes) (Fig. 20.4).

With PCA, a fairly constant level of pain relief can be maintained, and the pain and fear of injections are eliminated. Overall, women tend to use less analgesia with a PCA system than they would with intramuscular injections. PCA works well with postcesarean patients because they feel well enough to be interested in self-care and self-administration of analgesia.

Epidural Analgesia. Today, women who have epidural anesthesia for cesarean birth can have mor-

phine (Duramorph) or fentanyl added to the epidural catheter immediately after surgery, a technique that keeps them pain free for the next 24 hours (see Chapter 19). Although epidural analgesia provides effective pain relief after cesarean birth, side effects of epidural morphine administration, such as intense itching and nausea and vomiting, can occur. An antihistamine such as diphenhydramine (Benadryl) may be given to reduce pruritus; an antiemetic such as metoclopramide (Reglan) may be administered to counteract nausea. The use of fentanyl reduces the risk for these side effects. Even with these annoying side effects, however, epidural analgesia with morphine can be a very effective means of pain control after cesarean birth.

On the postpartal unit, an infusion pump is connected to the woman's epidural catheter and the woman can infuse a bolus of narcotic as additional pain relief is needed. This patient-controlled epidural anesthesia (PCEA) not only is an effective means of relieving pain but omits the problem of infiltration of an intravenous infusion, which can occur with intravenous PCA (Yost et al., 2004).

Transcutaneous Electrical Nerve Stimulation. Transcutaneous electrical nerve stimulation (TENS) is, as the name implies, the transmission of an electrical current across the skin. Small electrodes are attached to the woman's skin; when she feels pain, she pushes a transformer button. Irritation or stimulation of large afferent nerve fibers by the electrical stimulation blocks the ability of the smaller, pain-carrying nerve fibers to transmit impulses (as predicted by gating control theory). This is the same phenomenon that rubbing or scratching skin at the point of pain achieves (see also Chapter 13). The use of TENS can provide important pain relief after a cesarean birth, because it gives a woman a sense of control over her situation, as does PCA or PCEA.

? *What if...* Moja Hamma refuses to allow you to assess her fundal height after her cesarean birth because she has so much pain? How would you approach this situation?

Nursing Diagnosis: Risk for deficient fluid volume related to blood loss during surgery

Outcome Evaluation: Patient's blood pressure is 100/60 mm Hg or higher; pulse remains between 60 and 100 bpm; scant to no bleeding on surgical dressing is apparent.

The potential always exists for deficient fluid volume because of blood loss from surgery until all blood vessels that were cut and ligated during surgery have thrombosed, sclerosed, and permanently sealed closed. The risk of heavy bleeding doubles for the postpartum woman, because she may hemorrhage vaginally from an uncontracted uterus as well as internally from blood vessels that

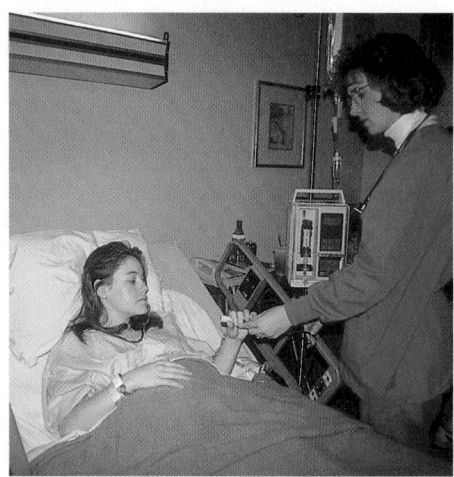

FIGURE 20.4 Patient-controlled analgesia (PCA) pump. By pushing the button, a client delivers a bolus of narcotic to herself. (© Caroline Brown, RNC, MS, DEd.)

were not securely ligated. This danger is most acute during the first hour after surgery, but it remains an acute problem for the first 24 hours.

To detect the earliest signs of bleeding, monitor blood pressure, pulse, and respiratory rate approximately every 15 minutes for the first hour after surgery, every 30 minutes for the next 2 hours, every hour for the next 4 hours, or as specifically ordered. Signs indicative of possible hemorrhage include the following:

- Falling blood pressure (more than 20 mm Hg), or a systolic blood pressure less than 80 mm Hg, or a drop of 5 to 10 mm Hg over several readings
- A change in pulse rate (greater than 110 bpm or less than 60 bpm)
- Rapid respirations
- Restlessness and a sense of thirst

Inspect the dressing over the surgical incision for blood staining at the same time vital signs are assessed. Observe the perineal pad for lochia flow, and palpate the fundal height each time. Lochial discharge may be decreased in a woman after a cesarean birth because the uterus was cleaned during surgery, but some lochia will always be present, and it follows a typical rubra, serosa, alba pattern. Be certain to help the woman turn so you can look under her body for bleeding. Blood oozing from a surgical wound or vaginally can pool considerably under a patient before it is visible.

Oxytocin may be ordered to be added to the first 1 or 2 L of intravenous fluid after surgery to ensure firm uterine contraction. If the rate of fluid administration gets behind, be careful about "catch-up" administration. Oxytocin can elevate blood pressure by causing vasoconstriction. It may be safer to allow the fluid to remain behind for a time, rather than risk dangerously elevating blood pressure. Be aware that a woman is very prone to hemorrhage when the oxytocin is discontinued, because this is the first time her uterus is being asked to maintain contraction on its own. Notify the surgeon of any changes in vital signs that might indicate hemorrhage, so that prompt action can be taken. Remember that a minimal but continued change in vital signs (pulse steadily increasing, blood pressure steadily declining) is as ominous a sign of hemorrhage as is a sudden alteration in these measurements.

A woman who has had either spinal or epidural anesthesia usually will not experience pain on uterine palpation until the anesthesia has worn off, approximately 4 to 24 hours. Therefore, uterine palpation should not increase her pain. Once the effect of the anesthesia or analgesia has decreased, always palpate gently but thoroughly enough to determine uterine consistency.

At the same time the uterus is assessed for firmness, assess the remainder of the woman's abdomen for softness. A hard, "guarded" abdomen is one of the first signs of peritonitis (peritoneal infection), a complication that may occur with any abdominal surgical procedure.

NURSING DIAGNOSES AND RELATED INTERVENTIONS DURING THE EXTENDED POSTPARTAL PERIOD

The average woman whose child is born by cesarean birth remains in the hospital from 48 hours to 4 days, depending on her preferences and the regulations of her insurance carrier. During this period and until she returns to have her sutures or staples removed, several interventions are necessary to promote healing, prevent postoperative complications, and help the woman and her family establish bonding with the new child. Common concerns of women include pain, fatigue, interference with gastrointestinal function, and reduced activity level.

Nursing Diagnosis: Risk for deficient fluid volume related to postsurgical fluid restriction

Outcome Evaluation: Patient's urine specific gravity remains between 1.003 and 1.030; weight loss is not more than 5 to 10 lb; fluid intake equals 2 to 3 L/day.

Adequate fluid intake is important after surgery, to replace blood loss from surgery and to maintain blood pressure and renal function. Because the intestine is handled during surgery, it takes approximately 24 to 48 hours before full peristaltic function is restored and oral intake is possible. Administer intravenous fluids as prescribed during this time, at a rate that is not too rapid (which could lead to cardiac overload) or too slow (which could lead to inadequate circulatory compensation). Keep an accurate intake and output record for at least the first 24 hours, to ascertain whether an adequate fluid balance has been achieved.

Teach the woman to "guard" her intravenous fluid line, because she needs a high proportion of fluid during this time (all postpartal women undergo diuresis as a physiologic postpartal change). At the same time, do not urge such caution that she is afraid to turn or ambulate. Her risk for thrombophlebitis is high, so she must turn frequently when in bed and ambulate early in the postpartal period to reduce this risk.

Assess the woman's abdomen at least once every 8 hours for bowel sounds, small "pinging" sounds heard on auscultation at a rate of 5 to 10 per minute, which demonstrate that air and fluid are moving through the intestines. Passage of flatus is another indication that intestinal function is again active. As soon as these signs are present, intravenous fluid therapy is usually discontinued and the woman is allowed sips of fluid. After beginning oral intake, wait 1 hour before removing the intravenous line. Doing so ensures that the woman is not experiencing nausea and vomiting, which might require restarting intravenous therapy. Introduce oral fluid slowly—for example, with ice chips for the first hour, then sips of clear fluid such as ginger ale, Jello, tea, or flavored frozen ice. Gradually advance her diet to a soft and then a regular diet as ordered. Some women assume that they will not be allowed to eat for a long time and are surprised (and suspicious) to learn that they can have ice chips only hours after surgery. This is possible because ice chips dissolve so slowly that the woman receives little fluid from them; they feel cool, however, and quickly take away the dry, "cottony" feeling in her mouth caused by lack of fluid.

Teach women to continue to drink large quantities of fluid after they return home (at least six glasses daily), so that they have adequate body fluid to make breast-feeding successful.

Nursing Diagnosis: Constipation related to effects of abdominal surgery and anesthesia

Outcome Evaluation: Woman voices she has a bowel movement every 2 to 3 days or her usual pattern.

Note carefully the time of the woman's first bowel movement after surgery. If there has been no bowel movement by the time of hospital discharge, the physician may order a stool softener, a suppository, or an enema to facilitate stool evacuation. Reassure a woman who is not receiving much food yet that it is normal not to have bowel movements for 3 or 4 days postoperatively, especially if an enema was administered before surgery.

Teach women to eat a diet high in roughage and fluid and to attempt to move their bowels at least every other day to avoid constipation after they return home. Some women need a stool softener prescribed, because incisional pain interferes with their ability to use their abdominal muscles effectively. Caution them not to strain to pass stools, because this puts pressure on their incision.

Nursing Diagnosis: Risk for impaired urinary elimination related to surgical procedure

Outcome Evaluation: Urinary output is more than 30 mL/h; patient reports no pain, frequency, burning, or hesitancy on voiding.

Because the bladder was handled and displaced during surgery, its tone or ability to sense filling may be inadequate to initiate voiding after surgery. For this reason, the indwelling catheter placed before surgery is usually left in place for 4 to 24 hours to ensure good urine drainage. Assess that the catheter is draining (a postpartal woman has a urine output of 3,000 to 5,000 mL per 24 hours). Bladder distention will occur rapidly if the catheter becomes blocked.

Before catheter removal, a urine culture may be ordered to check for the possibility of a urinary tract infection. After removal of the catheter, the average woman voids in 4 to 8 hours. Assess for bladder filling at the end of this time by palpation, pressing lightly over the symphysis pubis to assess fullness (Fig. 20.5A), and by percussion. On percussion, an empty bladder sounds dull; a full bladder, resonant; and an extended bladder, hyperresonant (Figure 20.5B). If a bladder has filled to capacity but cannot empty properly, the woman may have "retention

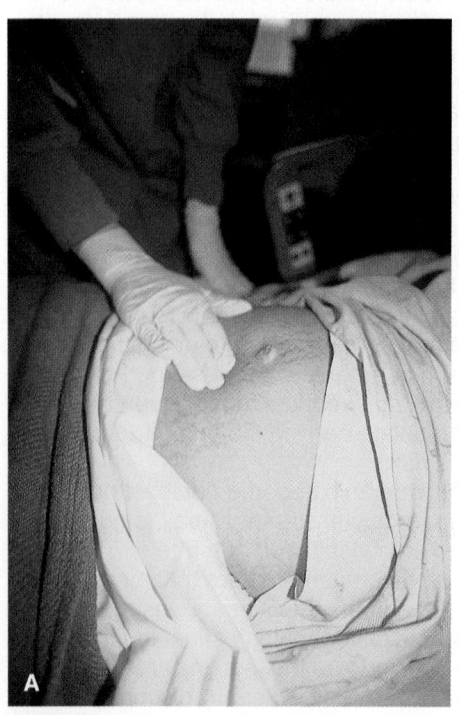
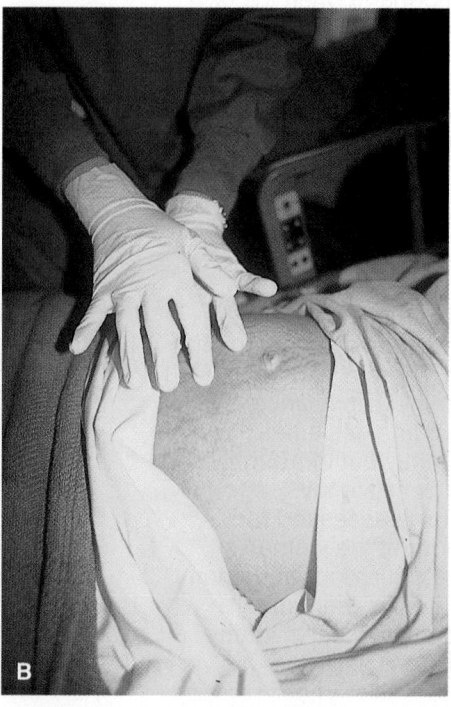

FIGURE 20.5 (A) Assessing bladder filling by palpation. **(B)** Assessing bladder filling by percussion. (© Caroline Brown, RNC, MS, DEd.)

with overflow," voiding 30 to 60 mL of urine every 15 to 20 minutes. This voiding pattern is potentially dangerous because it means that the woman's bladder is held continuously under tension. This can result in permanent bladder damage if the condition goes undetected. In addition, the constantly full bladder may prevent the uterus from contracting, possibly increasing the risk of postpartal hemorrhage.

To help a woman void, administer her prescribed analgesic, which helps to relax abdominal musculature. In addition, provide privacy for voiding, and offer a bedpan or assist the woman to walk to the bathroom at least every 2 hours. Other measures that might be effective include pouring warm water over her vulva (measure the amount of water used, so that it can be differentiated from urine) or running water from a tap within hearing distance.

Voiding after surgery provides evidence of adequate renal and circulatory function, because the kidneys must have adequate blood flow through them to function.

Teach women to continue to drink adequate fluid (at least five to six glasses daily) to ensure an adequate fluid output and help prevent urinary tract infection after they return home. Be certain they know to telephone their primary care provider if they should develop symptoms of a urinary tract infection, such as pain or frequency with voiding or blood in urine.

Nursing Diagnosis: Risk for ineffective peripheral tissue perfusion related to immobility during and after surgery

Outcome Evaluation: Capillary refill is less than 5 seconds; there is absence of calf pain, redness, edema, or areas of warmth on lower extremities.

Because a woman's abdominal muscles are lax from the stretching that occurred during pregnancy, abdominal contents tend to shift forward and put pressure on the suture line when she is sitting or standing, causing pain and an uncomfortable feeling often described as "everything falling out." A woman may feel more comfortable turning and sitting up if she supports her abdomen with one hand or splints the incision with a pillow.

Leg exercises (e.g., flexing and extending the knees) and early ambulation are a woman's best safeguards against lower-extremity circulatory problems. Thrombohemolytic stockings may be prescribed to help promote venous return and prevent venous stasis. Teach the woman to apply these before arising, while she is supine and venous distention is minimal. Always allow the woman to sit on the edge of the bed for a few minutes before helping her to a standing position, to prevent orthostatic hypotension (sudden low blood pressure that occurs with sudden position changes). Assessing blood pressure before the woman gets out of bed for the first time is an additional safeguard. Before ambulation, also assess

the lower extremities for pain in the calf on dorsiflexion of the foot (Homans' sign—which may or may not be reliable) or for pain, edema, warmth, or redness in the calf, to detect the possibility of a thrombus. It is dangerous for a patient to ambulate if signs of a thrombus are present. A thrombus could shift, becoming an embolus, a potentially lethal situation.

Often, it is difficult for women to understand the importance of turning and ambulating as soon as possible after surgery (Fig. 20.6). Still experiencing the "taking in" postpartal phase, a woman may prefer to spend the first days after surgery just resting quietly in bed. Encourage her to use adequate analgesia during this time, to enable her to move and ambulate with the least amount of pain. Reinforce the need for continued activity balanced with rest after discharge. Be certain she understands the signs and symptoms of complications, such as thrombophlebitis and pulmonary embolism.

Nursing Diagnosis: Risk for impaired parenting related to the emergency nature of birth or discomfort from surgery

Outcome Evaluation: Parents hold and feed child and voice positive comments about the infant.

When a cesarean birth is unscheduled, a woman does not have much time preoperatively to think about how she will feel after surgery. Most women are surprised to realize how well they feel overall but also how quickly they become fatigued and how painful a simple surgical incision can be. Being reassured they are recovering well but that surgery is a physiologic shock to the system helps them to accept temporary discomforts. It can help them bond with their newborn after a cesarean birth, just as women who give birth vaginally do. Encourage women to breast-feed even if this causes temporary uterine pain as the uterus contracts with breast-feeding.

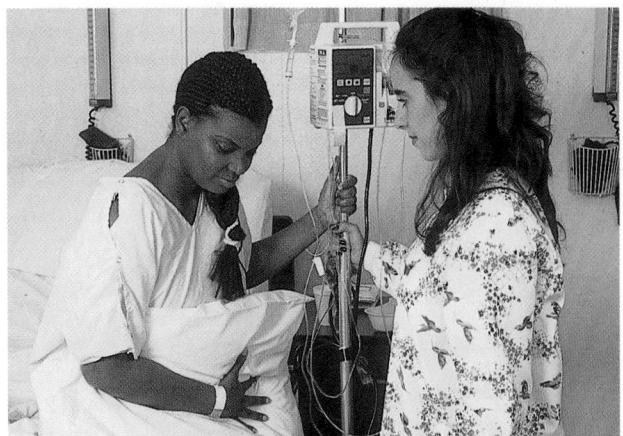

FIGURE 20.6 Encouraging women to be out of bed will help prevent complications from a cesarean birth. It is important to splint the incision area while getting up and ambulating. (© Barbara Proud.)

If the woman's baby was born with a complication or has been placed in an intensive care nursery or transferred to a distant hospital for tertiary care, the woman's postpartal course can be difficult because she experiences a sense of loss in addition to the pain and fatigue of surgery. Depression, which can slow all body functions and certainly her ability to "take hold" in the postpartal period, may occur.

Unless the baby was transferred to another site, be certain to provide the woman with ample time to hold and feed her child. Most women can breast-feed satisfactorily after cesarean birth. If intravenous lines or other devices are present, assist the woman with holding her newborn, so that the equipment does not interfere with the time spent with the infant. She may have some reason to think her baby is not quite perfect—after all, the baby was not born "perfectly"—so she may need additional time to inspect the baby and feel comfortable with him or her (Fig. 20.7) (Box 20.5).

Nursing Diagnosis: Fatigue related to effects of surgery

Outcome Evaluation: Patient states she is pleased with level of self-care; ambulates well by 24 hours, and sleeps restfully at night.

Although a woman needs activity and movement after surgery, she also needs adequate rest. Many women attempt to handle their own and their newborn's needs immediately after surgery, because their excitement over their baby and their new role makes them unaware of their underlying fatigue. Extreme fatigue interferes with healing and possibly increases the risk for infection. It also can eventually interfere with bonding. Help the woman plan a day that includes care of her new child as well as periods of rest for herself. Be certain she has adequate analgesic medication at bedtime to allow her to be pain free for the night. Provide a time in the middle of the morning and again in the afternoon for uninterrupted rest. Explore her plans for care at home to be certain that her plans for rest seem realistic for a postsurgical-postpartal woman (Box 20.6).

Once a woman returns home, rest is often best accomplished if it is scheduled for every time her newborn sleeps. Without adequate rest this way, she can notice increased uterine bleeding, which has the potential to lead to excessive loss of fluid and iron stores.

Nursing Diagnosis: Impaired skin integrity related to surgical incision

Outcome Evaluation: Incision line is clean, dry, and intact without erythema; oral temperature is less than 38°C.

Surgical incisions heal by primary intention, or by the gradual removal and replacement of dead or damaged cells at the wound site with new cells produced by the surrounding tissue. Assess the surgical incision once during each nursing shift while the woman is hospitalized, to ensure that the wound edges are approximated and there are no signs of infection, such as erythema. As soon as she can walk steadily, a woman can take a shower (after first removing the dressing), because warm, clean water on the incision is soothing. After this point, she can make a decision about whether to continue to wear a dressing. Lack of a dressing prevents moisture accumulation at the incision site and decreases the possibility of infection.

Teach women to continue to observe their incision daily at home. Instruct them in signs and symptoms of possible infection, including redness or the presence of a discharge, and to report any of these signs to their primary care provider. With a cesarean birth, healing will be adequate enough by day 4 or 5 that skin sutures or clamps can be removed, although many are left in place until the woman returns for a follow-up appointment in 2 weeks.

Discharge Planning

A woman being discharged after cesarean birth takes home not only her new baby but a fair amount of pain and discomfort. Be certain to discuss home care arrangements, emphasizing the need for adequate help with the newborn and other responsibilities at home, before discharge (Box 20.7). Be sure the woman is aware of any restrictions on exercise or activity that she needs to follow (as a rule, she should not lift any object heavier than 10 lb for the first 2 weeks or walk upstairs more than once a day). Also teach her to recognize signs of possible complications directly related to the surgery, such as the following:

- Redness or drainage at the incision line
- Lochia heavier than a normal menstrual period
- Abdominal pain
- Temperature greater than 38°C (100.4°F)
- Frequency or burning on urination

A woman can plan on resuming coitus as soon as the act is comfortable for her, possibly as early as 1 week after

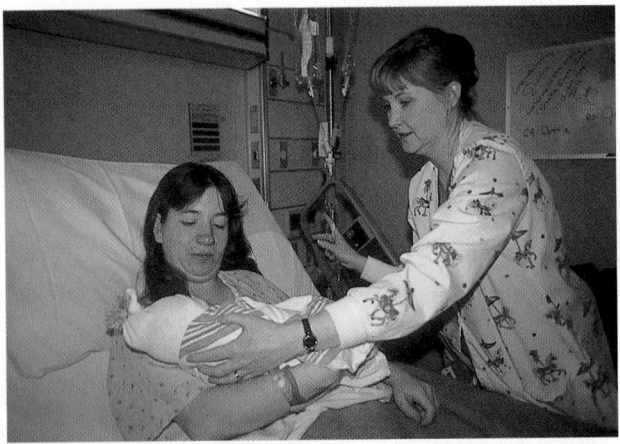

FIGURE 20.7 A nurse assists with holding the newborn and positioning the equipment so that the intravenous line does not interfere with mother–child interactions. (© Caroline Brown, RNC, MS, DEd.)

A Multidisciplinary Care Map for A Woman Following an Emergency Cesarean Birth

•

Moja Hamma is a 29-year-old primigravida who underwent an emergency cesarean birth with combined spinal-epidural anesthesia for fetal distress. Moja gave birth to a healthy 8 lb, 2 oz baby girl. She tells you, "I'm thirsty, and it hurts so much I can't move. Take the baby away. I can't hold her right now."

Family Assessment

Client lives with boyfriend in west-side apartment. Client worked before pregnancy as a clerk in a bridal salon. Boyfriend is currently unemployed. Borrowed money from a friend for hospital bill.

Client Assessment

Post-cesarean birth 4 hours ago. Estimated blood loss of 700 mL. Abdomen soft but tender with low transverse incision. No bowel sounds present. Incisional dressing clean, dry, and intact. Uterus firm, 1 fingerbreadth below umbilicus. Minimal lochia rubra vaginal drainage. Urine output 100 mL in last hour. Skin pink, warm, and dry. Skin turgor good. Ringer's Lactate infusing at 100 mL/hour. Intravenous site clean, dry, without signs of infiltration. Vital signs: temperature, 98.4°F; pulse, 78 bpm; respirations, 23 per minute; blood pressure, 130/76 mm Hg. Pulse, respirations, and blood pressure slightly elevated above baseline. Respirations shallow. States she has abdominal pain, especially at incisional area. Holding hands over abdomen; barely moving in bed. Client's mother at bedside holding her hand and stroking her forehead. PCEA pump in place but not being used by client. When asked why she wasn't using the PCEA pump, she answered, "I don't want to take the chance of being paralyzed forever."

Nursing Diagnosis

Pain related to tissue trauma from abdominal incision of cesarean birth

Outcome Criteria

Client identifies pain management measure of choice; reports a decrease in pain with analgesic administration; pulse, respirations, and blood pressure return to baseline. Client holds infant warmly; maintains eye contact with infant; makes positive statements about the newborn prior to discharge.

Team Member Responsible	Assessment	Intervention	Rationale	Expected Outcome
Activities of Daily Living				
Nurse	Assess client's ability to move in bed and breast-feed infant.	Stress the importance of getting out of bed and caring for infant.	Early ambulation helps prevent thrombophlebitis; early breast-feeding helps establish adequate milk supply.	Client feels well enough to be out of bed and feeding infant by 4 hours' time due to chosen pain relief method.

(continued)

Team Member Responsible	Assessment	Intervention	Rationale	Expected Outcome
Consultations				
Nurse	Investigate whether pain management team is available for consultation.	Ask pain management team to consult on more appropriate pain relief measures.	Client states she is afraid to use PCEA for pain relief.	Pain management team discusses options for pain relief with client and they agree on a suitable procedure by 2 hours.
Procedures/Medications				
Nurse	Assess what measures client feels would make her most comfortable.	Institute additional comfort measures, such as changing position, splinting incision, using pillows and blankets for support. Institute different pain management system if one is employed or assist with present system if client agrees with system.	Comfort measures reduce stress and anxiety, elevate mood, and raise the pain threshold, thus enhancing the therapeutic effectiveness of analgesics and the client's control over and ability to tolerate pain.	Client reports additional comfort measures aid pain relief. Client reports pain management system is operating effectively.
Nurse	Assess what measures client thinks would help her be more successful with breast-feeding.	Assist client with handling newborn. Support breast-feeding efforts.	Breast-feeding is a new skill for a first time mother.	Client breast-feeds the infant successfully with support from health care providers.
Nutrition				
Nurse	Assess bowel sounds to determine when oral fluid can be offered.	Offer ice cubes for dry mouth as soon as bowel sounds are present.	Client cannot drink full liquid until bowel sounds return.	Client states mouth discomfort is reduced by 1 hour after first fluid.
Patient/Family Education				
Pain management Team/nurse	Assess client's expectations of pain relief measures.	Review PCEA pump and technique with client. Stress that catheter is not in CSF.	Client cannot have realistic expectations unless she understands technique.	Client states that she will use PCEA pump on trial basis for 4 hours.
Psychosocial/Spiritual/Emotional Needs				
Nurse	Assess what additional measures client feels she needs to feel secure after frightening experience of emergency cesarean birth.	Provide reinforcement for positive coping mechanisms that client demonstrates.	Positive reinforcement enhances self-esteem and control. Praise promotes self-esteem and confidence to manage new situations.	Client states she feels her coping measures are reinforced by health care providers. Client states she feels health care providers provide her support equal to her level of pain and fatigue.
Nurse	Assess client's expectations of a newborn.	Praise the client for positive behaviors and interactions with the child in light of pain and fatigue level. Encourage the client to keep the newborn in the room with her for extended periods as she is able.	Extended contact within the client's ability to tolerate the activity encourages bonding while minimizing the risk for additional fatigue.	Client keeps newborn with her in room for the majority of daylight hours. Interacts actively with child.

(continued)

Team Member Responsible	Assessment	Intervention	Rationale	Expected Outcome
Discharge Planning				
Nurse	Assess the level of support client will have after she returns home.	Review with client importance of maintaining a level of pain relief at home so she can ambulate and care for new child.	Ambulation and child care are important for both maternal and child health. Keeping pain to a minimum helps the client achieve these activities.	Client states she will take enough pain relief at home to allow her to be active and care for newborn. She names at least one person to serve as support person.
Nurse	Assess whether client understands signs and symptoms she will need to report after discharge.	Teach signs of complications she should report to her health care provider.	Knowing signs and symptoms of complications adds to client's base of knowledge.	Client repeats danger signs that she will report to her health care provider.

BOX 20.6 FOCUS ON . . .

EVIDENCE-BASED PRACTICE

Do women who have cesarean births because of difficulty in second-stage labor breast-feed as often as those who have instrumental second-stage interventions?

For this study, 393 women who had had term, singleton, live, cephalic pregnancies and either a cesarean birth or an instrumental vaginal birth were mailed a questionnaire at 6 weeks and again at 1 year after birth of their children. Results of the questionnaires revealed the total rate of women who were breast-feeding exclusively at hospital discharge was 70%; at 6 weeks postpartum, this rate had already fallen to 44%. There was no significant difference in breast-feeding rates between women who had given birth by instrumental vaginal birth and those who had a cesarean birth. Women who had an extended inpatient stay after a cesarean birth were more likely than other women to have achieved exclusive breast-feeding by hospital discharge (78% vs. 66%). The researchers concluded that the method of operative delivery in the second stage of labor does not appear to influence initiation or duration of exclusive breast-feeding. A prolonged inpatient stay helps women who have had cesarean births to initiate breast-feeding.

This is an important study for nurses, because nurses are the health care providers most likely to discuss breast-feeding either during pregnancy or postpartal. Knowing that women who have had cesarean births can be as successful as other women at breast-feeding can help to remind nurses to include breast-feeding information in postpartal care.

Patel, R. R., Liebling, R. E., & Murphy, D. J. (2003). Effect of operative delivery in the second stage of labor on breastfeeding success. *Birth, 30*(4), 255–260.

discharge. Be sure that she has contraceptive information, if desired. Also ensure that she has an appointment for a return visit with her health care provider (usually in 2 weeks), for both herself and her newborn.

Unless the reason for the cesarean birth was cephalopelvic disproportion, a woman can probably have her

BOX 20.7 FOCUS ON . . .

FAMILY TEACHING

Measures to Regain Energy After a Cesarean Birth

Q. Suppose Moja Hamma tells you, "I feel so tired after my cesarean. What can I do to feel stronger?"

A. After a cesarean birth, women usually regain energy rapidly. This is because, unlike most people who have had surgery, you did not have it because you were ill, but because it was an alternative method to have a healthy baby. The following measures can help you regain your energy rapidly:

- Drink adequate fluid daily (at least six glasses). This helps prevent a urinary tract infection and also helps supply all the cells in your body with adequate nutrients.
- Rest twice a day for at least one-half hour each time. This helps because your baby will probably wake you at least once during the night.
- Don't hesitate to accept help from family and friends for tasks such as house cleaning or grocery shopping.
- Limit the number of stairs that you climb daily to one flight once a day. Also limit the amount of weight you lift to the weight of your new baby.
- Don't attempt to be the "perfect" new mom. Relax and enjoy your new baby.

next child by VBAC (see Chapter 18). Being certain the woman is aware of this not only makes her an informed consumer of health care but also can influence whether she plans an additional pregnancy.

Key Points

The term *cesarean birth* is preferred to *cesarean section* or *delivery,* because it puts the focus on the childbirth rather than surgical elements of the procedure.

Cesarean birth may be either a scheduled or an emergency procedure. Because it carries more risk for the mother and infant than does vaginal birth, it is usually undertaken only when medically necessary, although a current trend allows for elective procedures.

Establishing surgical risk includes assessment of nutritional status, age, general health, fluid and electrolyte balance, and psychological condition.

Assessment measures before surgery usually include vital sign determination; urinalysis; blood studies such as complete blood count, electrolytes, blood typing, and cross-matching; and sonography.

The skin incision may be vertical (a classic incision), although it is usually a horizontal one just above the pubic hair. The internal incision into the uterus is also usually a horizontal incision into the lower uterine segment.

The old saying, "Once a cesarean, always a cesarean," is no longer true, as long as cephalopelvic disproportion does not exist and the previous incision was a low transverse one.

Support people can lose a great deal of their ability to support if they feel intimidated and out of place in an operating room; offer them support as needed to make this a positive experience for them as well.

Cesarean birth is one of the safest types of surgery performed. To keep a woman safe after the procedure, remember that she is both a postsurgical and a postpartum patient. Make assessments to ensure that neither postpartum nor postsurgical complications occur.

Adequate pain management is important to allow a woman a sense of control and comfort and bonding with her newborn.

Women are physically exhausted after cesarean birth and may be psychologically exhausted because of the emergency nature of the experience. Provide rest time to relieve the physical strain and a chance to verbalize the experience to help relieve the psychological strain.

A major intervention after cesarean birth is early ambulation to prevent complications. Incisional pain may make this difficult, so strong nursing support and adequate pain management are necessary.

Critical Thinking Exercises

1. Moja, the woman you met at the beginning of this chapter, was afraid to have a cesarean birth because she didn't want to be alone. What actions could you take to make her situation easier to accept?

2. Suppose Moja is receiving PCEA after her cesarean birth. She tells you that she is not interested in PCEA and would rather have injections for pain. Describe and explain the action you might take. Would you advocate for use of PCEA or advocate with her physician for a changed order?

3. Moja's boyfriend tells you that he cannot possibly stay with her in the operating room while she has a cesarean birth. He's sure he will feel nauseated and probably faint. How would you intervene to promote family-centered care and meet the couple's needs?

4. Examine the National Health Goals related to cesarean birth. Most government-sponsored money for nursing research is allotted based on these goals. What would be a possible research topic to explore pertinent to these goals that would be applicable to the Hamma family and also advance evidence-based practice?

References

Brown, Z. (2004). Preventing herpes simplex virus transmission to the neonate. *Herpes, 11*(Suppl 3), 175A–186A.

Department of Health and Human Services. (2000). *Healthy people 2010.* Washington, D.C.: Author.

Ehrenberg, H. M., et al. (2004). The influence of obesity and diabetes on the risk of cesarean delivery. *American Journal of Obstetrics and Gynecology, 191*(3), 969–974.

Gilbert, W. M., et al. (2004). Vaginal versus cesarean delivery for breech presentation in California: A population-based study. *Obstetrics and Gynecology, 102*(5 Pt 1), 911–917.

Hager, R. M. E., et al. (2004). Complications of cesarean deliveries: Rates and risk factors. *American Journal of Obstetrics and Gynecology, 190*(2), 428–434.

Handa, V. L., et al. (2004). Parity and route of delivery: Does cesarean delivery reduce bladder symptoms later in life? *American Journal of Obstetrics and Gynecology, 191*(2), 463–469.

Hodnett, E. D., et al. (2005). Continuous support for women during childbirth. *The Cochrane Library (Oxford) (4)* (CD003766).

Horey, D., Weaver, J., & Russell, H. (2005). Information for pregnant women about caesarean birth. *The Cochrane Library (Oxford) (4)* (CD003858).

Johnson, M., Maas, M., & Moorhead, S. (2000). *Nursing outcomes classification* (2nd ed.). St. Louis: Mosby.

McCloskey, J., & Bulechek, G. (2000). *Nursing interventions classification* (3rd ed.). St. Louis: Mosby.

Nasrallah, F. K., et al. (2004). The 30-minute decision-to-incision interval for emergency cesarean delivery: Fact or fiction? *American Journal of Perinatology, 21*(2), 63–68.

National Center for Health Statistics (2005). *Trends in the health of Americans.* Hyattsville, Md.: NCHS.

Ng, K., et al. (2005). Spinal versus epidural anaesthesia for caesarean section. *The Cochrane Library (Oxford) (4)* (CD003765).

Panburana, P., et al. (2004). Elective cesarean delivery plus short-course lamivudine and zidovudine for the prevention of mother-to-child transmission of human immunodeficiency virus type 1. *American Journal of Obstetrics and Gynecology, 190*(3), 803–808.

Patel, R. R., Liebling, R. E., & Murphy, D. J. (2003). Effect of operative delivery in the second stage of labor on breast-feeding success. *Birth, 30*(4), 255–260.

Phipps, M. G., et al. (2005). Risk factors for bladder injury during cesarean delivery. *Obstetrics and Gynecology, 105*(1), 156–160.

Porter, T. F., & Scott, J. R. (2003). Cesarean delivery. In Scott, J. R., et al. *Danforth's obstetrics and gynecology* (9th ed.). Philadelphia: Lippincott Williams & Wilkins.

Wu, J. M., Hundley, A. F., & Visco, A. G. (2005). Elective primary cesarean delivery: Attitudes of urogynecology and maternal-fetal medicine specialists. *Obstetrics and Gynecology, 105*(2), 301–306.

Yost, N. P., et al. (2004). A hospital-sponsored quality improvement study of pain management after cesarean delivery. *American Journal of Obstetrics and Gynecology, 190*(5), 1341–1346.

Suggested Readings

Anderson, G. M. (2004). Making sense of rising caesarean section rates. *BMJ, 329*(7468), 696–697.

Cheng, Y. W., Hopkins, L. M., & Caughey, A. B. (2004). How long is too long: Does a prolonged second stage of labor in nulliparous women affect maternal and neonatal outcomes? *American Journal of Obstetrics and Gynecology, 191*(3), 933–938.

Foley, M. E., et al. (2004). The continuing effectiveness of active management of first labor, despite a doubling in overall nulliparous cesarean delivery. *American Journal of Obstetrics and Gynecology, 191*(3), 891–905.

Hannah, M. E., et al. (2004). Maternal outcomes at 2 years after planned cesarean section versus planned vaginal birth for breech presentation at term. *American Journal of Obstetrics and Gynecology. 191*(3), 917–927.

Heck, K. E., et al. (2003). Does postpartum length of stay affect breastfeeding duration? *Birth, 30*(3), 153–159.

Jackson, D. J., et al. (2003). Impact of collaborative management and early admission in labor on method of delivery. *JOGNN: Journal of Obstetric, Gynecologic, and Neonatal Nursing, 32*(2), 147–157.

Kim, S. Y., et al. (2003). Is the intrapartum biophysical profile useful? *Obstetrics and Gynecology, 102*(3), 471–476.

McKenna, D. S., Ester, J. B., & Fischer, J. R. (2003). Elective cesarean delivery for women with a previous anal sphincter rupture. *American Journal of Obstetrics and Gynecology, 189*(5), 1251–1256.

Richter, H. M. (2005). Elective cesarean section and midwifery care. *Journal of Midwifery and Women's Health, 50*(1), 65.

Rowe-Murray, H. J., & Fisher, J. R. W. (2003). Baby friendly hospital practices: Caesarean section is a persistent barrier to early initiation of breastfeeding. *Breastfeeding Review, 11*(1), 21–27.

Wax, J. R., et al. (2004). Patient choice cesarean: An evidence-based review. *Obstetrical and Gynecological Survey, 59*(8), 601–616.

Whyte, H., et al. (2004). Outcomes of children at 2 years after planned cesarean birth versus planned vaginal birth for breech presentation at term. *American Journal of Obstetrics and Gynecology, 191*(3), 864–871.

CHAPTER 21

The Woman Who Develops a Complication During Labor and Birth

Key Terms

amniotic fluid embolism
augmentation of labor
battledore placenta
dysfunctional labor
dystocia
external cephalic version
forceps birth
hypertonic uterine contractions
hypotonic uterine contractions
induction of labor
oxytocin
pathologic retraction ring
placenta accreta
placenta circumvallata
placenta marginata
placenta succenturiata
precipitate labor
umbilical cord prolapse
uterine inversion
vacuum extraction

Objectives

After mastering the contents of this chapter, you should be able to:

1. Define the terms *dystocia* and *dysfunctional labor.*
2. Describe the common deviations in the power (force of labor), the passage, or the passenger that can cause dystocia or dysfunctional labor.
3. Assess a woman in labor and during birth for deviations from the normal labor process.
4. Formulate nursing diagnoses related to deviations from normal in labor and birth.
5. Identify expected outcomes associated with deviations from normal labor and birth and resultant complications.
6. Plan nursing interventions to help the family meet expected outcomes when complications of labor occur.
7. Implement care related to complications of labor or birth.
8. Evaluate expected outcomes for achievement and effectiveness of care.
9. Identify National Health Goals related to complications of labor that nurses could help the nation achieve.
10. Identify areas related to complications of labor that could benefit from additional nursing research or application of evidence-based practice.
11. Use critical thinking to analyze ways to maintain family-centered nursing care when deviations from the normal in labor and birth occur.
12. Integrate the knowledge of deviations of normal in labor and birth with nursing process to achieve quality maternal and child health nursing care.

*R*oseann Bigalow, a 28-year-old woman about to give birth to her first baby, is admitted to a birthing room. Her contractions have been 5 minutes apart for 10 hours. She feels more pain in her back than in her abdomen, "like my spine is tearing apart." A contraction monitor shows contractions are hypotonic. A sonogram shows the fetus is above average in weight and in an occipitoposterior position. Her husband asks you if it is the posterior fetal position that is making his wife's labor so long.

Previous chapters discussed pregnancy and normal labor and birth. This chapter adds information about what happens when complications of labor occur. This information is important to know, because the sooner a complication in labor is recognized, the better the chance the situation can be corrected and both fetal and maternal health can be protected.

What would you tell the Bigalows?

After you've studied this chapter, access the accompanying website. Read the patient scenario and answer the questions to further sharpen your skills, grow more familiar with RN-CLEX types of questions, and reward yourself with how much you have learned.

Although labor usually proceeds without any deviation from the normal, many potential complications can occur. A difficult labor—**dystocia**—can arise from any of the three main components of the labor process: (1) the power, or the force that propels the fetus (uterine contractions); (2) the passenger (the fetus); or (3) the passageway (the birth canal). In addition, medical interventions used to prevent or manage certain complications can cause difficulties of their own.

Because complications can occur at any point in labor, continuous monitoring of a laboring woman and fetus and providing emotional support for her and her partner are essential. The hours of labor are stressful even when everything is proceeding normally. Be sure to reassure a woman in labor that everything is going smoothly and that both she and her fetus appear to be doing well. If a complication arises and assurances cannot be given as freely, the stress for the woman and her support person can increase tremendously.

A woman who is experiencing a complication in labor needs someone who is knowledgeable about the deviation and its treatment and understands her feelings of helplessness. Nurses play a key role in providing this type of skilled physical and emotional care.

National Health Goals related to attempts to decrease maternal complications and prevent infant injury are shown in Box 21.1.

BOX 21.1 FOCUS ON . . .

NATIONAL HEALTH GOALS

A number of National Health Goals speak directly to complications of labor (DHHS, 2000).

- Reduce the number of cesarean births among low-risk women to no more than 15 per 100 births, from a baseline of 18 per 100.
- Reduce the maternal mortality rate to no more than 3.3 per 100,000 live births, from a baseline of 7.1 per 100,000.
- Reduce the rate of maternal complications during hospitalized labor and birth to no more than 24 per 100 births, from a baseline of 31.2 per 100 births.

Nurses can help the nation achieve these goals by helping identify women in labor who are developing a complication; by assisting with cesarean births and uterine monitoring; and by being alert to the preliminary symptoms of uterine rupture, which accounts for a substantial number of maternal deaths during labor. Further nursing research is needed to explore whether breech and occipitoposterior positions can be effectively prevented by position changes during pregnancy.

Nursing Process Overview

For a Woman With a Labor or Birth Complication

● *Assessment*

One of the major assessments used to detect deviations from normal in labor and birth is fetal and uterine monitoring. Working with such apparatus involves explaining its importance to parents, winning their cooperation, and using judgment in reading the various patterns. Typically, monitoring women in labor entails problems not found in other high-risk areas such as an intensive care unit (ICU). In an ICU, the person being monitored has been admitted to the unit because he or she is seriously ill. The person lies still to prevent artifacts on the tracing. However, a woman in labor, who is well except for the complication of labor, may be less accepting of technologic or pharmacologic intervention. She moves about rather than lying still, because she is in pain. Her movement causes artifacts on tracings, requiring frequent adjustment of equipment to achieve a clear tracing. Understanding that this is a normal consequence of labor is essential for effective assessment and continued care.

● *Nursing Diagnosis*

Common nursing diagnoses specific to a woman experiencing a complication during labor or birth refer to specific problems. Some examples include the following:

- Fear related to uncertainty of pregnancy outcome
- Anxiety related to medical procedures and apparatus necessary to ensure health of mother and fetus
- Fatigue related to loss of glucose stores through work and duration of labor
- Risk for ineffective tissue perfusion related to excessive loss of blood with complication of labor
- Risk for injury (maternal or fetal) related to effect on mother and fetus of a labor complication and treatment required
- Risk for injury (maternal or fetal) related to labor involving a multiple-gestation pregnancy
- Anticipatory grieving related to nonviable monitoring pattern of fetus

● *Outcome Identification and Planning*

If a complication of labor or childbirth occurs, identification of expected outcomes can be difficult because the outcome that may occur is not what the woman desires. Encouraging the couple to clarify their priorities is helpful. For example, early in labor, the woman might say that her chief goal is to avoid monitoring equipment or an episiotomy. If fetal bradycardia occurs, however, monitoring and a cesarean birth may become necessary. If this happens, reminding the woman that her primary goal is really to have a healthy baby may help her accept the change, including whatever interventions are necessary to achieve her ultimate objective.

● *Implementation*

If a woman develops a complication of labor or birth, the situation is a priority, possibly an emergency. Interventions must be planned and performed efficiently and effectively, based on the individual circumstances.

Be certain to provide psychological reassurance to accompany actions to fully safeguard both the woman and her fetus.

● *Outcome Evaluation*

Evaluation of client outcomes may reveal unhappiness, because not every woman who experiences a deviation from the normal in labor and birth will be able to give birth to a healthy child. Some deviations will be too great. Some interventions will not be maximally effective because of individual circumstances. Some infants will die, a few women may be left unable to bear future children. Evaluation may lead to a new analysis that the couple's chief need at that point is to grieve for the child or for a lifestyle that can no longer be theirs. If the outcome is more positive, evaluate the couple for signs that they are able to begin interaction with the child after their harrowing experience.

Examples of outcome achievement include the following:

• Client voices confidence that she can cope with the fear she feels about her fetus' welfare.
• Client demonstrates adequate energy during course of labor to maintain effective breathing patterns.
• Client's blood pressure remains higher than 110/60 mm Hg despite excessive blood loss with delivery of the placenta.
• Client begins positive grieving behaviors in response to loss of newborn.

COMPLICATIONS WITH THE POWER (THE FORCE OF LABOR)

Inertia is a time-honored term to denote that sluggishness of contractions, or the force of labor, has occurred. A more current term is **dysfunctional labor.** Dysfunction can occur at any point in labor, but it is generally classified as primary (occurring at the onset of labor) or secondary (occurring later in labor). The risk of maternal postpartal infection and hemorrhage and infant mortality is higher in women who have a prolonged labor than in those who do not (Dudley, 2003). Therefore, it is vital to recognize and prevent dysfunctional labor to the extent possible.

Prolonged labor appears to result from several factors. It is likely to occur if the fetus is large. Hypotonic, hypertonic, and uncoordinated contractions all play roles (Box 21.2).

Ineffective Uterine Force

Uterine contractions are the basic force moving the fetus through the birth canal. Uterine contractions occur because of the interplay of the contractile enzyme adenosine triphosphate and the influence of major electrolytes such as calcium, sodium, and potassium, specific contractile proteins (actin and myosin), epinephrine and norepinephrine, oxytocin, estrogen, progesterone, and prostaglandins. About 95% of labors are completed with contractions that follow a predictable, normal course. Ab-

---

BOX 21.2

Common Causes of Dysfunctional Labor

Inappropriate use of analgesia (excessive or too early administration)
Pelvic bone contraction that has narrowed the pelvic diameter so that a fetus cannot pass (e.g., in a client with rickets)
Poor fetal position (posterior rather than anterior position)
Extension rather than flexion of the fetal head
Overdistention of the uterus, as with multiple pregnancy, hydramnios, or an excessively oversized fetus
Cervical rigidity (unripe)
Presence of a full rectum or urinary bladder that impedes fetal descent
Mother becoming exhausted from labor
Primigravida status

---

normal, ineffective contractions can lead to an ineffective labor.

Hypotonic Contractions

Figure 21.1*A* illustrates the appearance of normal uterine contractions. With **hypotonic uterine contractions,** the number of contractions is usually low or infrequent (not increasing beyond two or three in a 10-minute period). The resting tone of the uterus remains less than 10 mm Hg, and the strength of contractions does not rise above 25 mm Hg (Fig. 21.1*B*). Hypotonic contractions are most apt to occur during the active phase of labor. They may occur after the administration of analgesia, especially if the cervix is not dilatated to 3 to 4 cm or if bowel or bladder distention prevents descent or firm engagement. They may occur in a uterus that is overstretched by a multiple gestation, a larger-than-usual single fetus, or hydramnios, or in a uterus that is lax from grand multiparity. Such contractions are not exceedingly painful, because of their lack of intensity. Keep in mind, however, that the strength of a contraction is a subjective symptom. Some women may interpret these contractions as very painful (Box 21.3).

Hypotonic contractions increase the length of labor, because more of them are necessary to achieve cervical dilatation. This can cause the uterus to not contract as effectively during the postpartal period because of exhaustion, increasing a woman's chance for postpartal hemorrhage. With the cervix dilatated for a long period, both the uterus and the fetus are also at greater risk for infection.

For these reasons, after ultrasonic confirmation rules out cephalopelvic disproportion (CPD), an infusion of **oxytocin,** a synthetic form of the naturally occurring pituitary hormone, usually is started to augment labor by strengthening contractions and increasing their effectiveness. Membranes may be artificially ruptured (amniotomy) to further speed labor. In the first hour after birth, palpate the uterus and assess lochia every 15 minutes to ensure that postpartal contractions are not also hypotonic and therefore inadequate to halt bleeding.

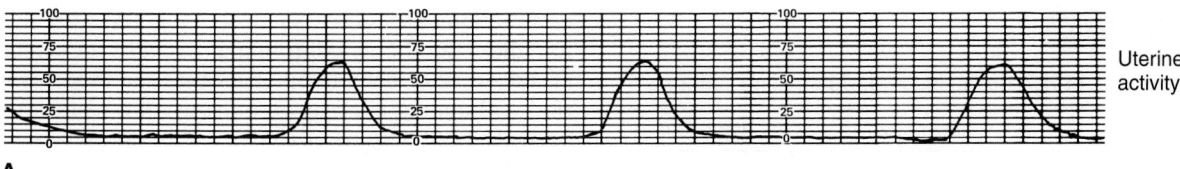

A

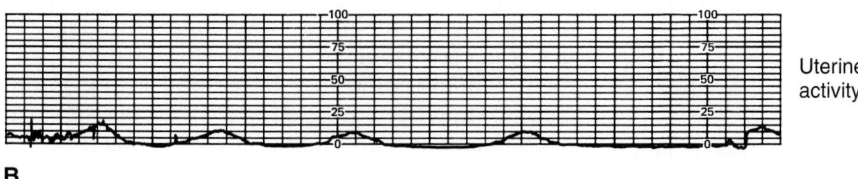

B

C

FIGURE 21.1 (**A**) Normal uterine contractions. (**B**) Hypotonic contractions; notice rise in pressure no more than 10 mm Hg. (**C**) Hypertonic contractions; notice the high resting pressure (35–40 mm Hg).

BOX 21.3 FOCUS ON . . .

EVIDENCE-BASED PRACTICE

Do some women perceive labor contractions better than others?

Some women report that they have been in labor for hours when their contractions finally reach a 5-minute interval and they are admitted to a birthing unit; others report a much shorter time interval before contractions become regular and spaced close to each other. To see if the reason for these different types of history could be that some women perceive uterine contractions better or earlier than others, researchers tested 7,808 women with singleton pregnancies to determine how many uterine contractions they perceived during a set period. Women's perceptions of the number of contractions that occurred were then compared with the number of contractions a uterine monitor had recorded during that same interval. The results revealed that some women do perceive contractions better than others, and that obese and nulliparous women have the greatest difficulty perceiving contractions.

This is an important study for nurses, because nurses are often the first persons who interview a woman when she arrives in labor at a birthing unit. Knowing that a woman having her first baby or a woman who is obese may not be able to detect contractions as well as others should alert nurses to carefully assess these women's progress in labor. Doing so could help prevent unattended precipitous birth.

Cottrill, H. M., et al. (2004). Factors influencing maternal perception of uterine contractions. *American Journal of Obstetrics and Gynecology, 190*(5), 1455–1457.

Hypertonic Contractions

Hypertonic uterine contractions are marked by an increase in resting tone to more than 15 mm Hg (see Fig. 21.1*C*). However, the intensity of the contraction may be no stronger than that associated with hypotonic contractions. In contrast to hypotonic contractions, hypertonic ones tend to occur frequently and are most commonly seen in the latent phase of labor. This type of contraction occurs because the muscle fibers of the myometrium do not repolarize or relax after a contraction, thereby "wiping it clean" to accept a new pacemaker stimulus. They may occur because more than one pacemaker is stimulating the contractions. They tend to be more painful than usual, because the myometrium becomes tender from constant lack of relaxation and the anoxia of uterine cells that results. A woman may become frustrated or disappointed with her breathing exercises for childbirth, because such techniques are ineffective with this type of contraction.

A danger of hypertonic contractions is that the lack of relaxation between contractions may not allow optimal uterine artery filling; this could lead to fetal anoxia early in the latent phase of labor. Any woman whose pain seems out of proportion to the quality of her contractions should have both a uterine and a fetal external monitor applied for at least 15 minutes to ensure that the resting phase of the contractions is adequate and that the fetal pattern is not showing late deceleration.

Management of hypertonic contractions involves rest and pain relief with a drug such as morphine sulfate. Changing the linen and the client's gown, darkening room lights, and decreasing noise and stimulation are also helpful. If deceleration in the fetal heart rate (FHR), an abnormally long first stage of labor, or lack of progress with pushing ("second-stage arrest") occurs, cesarean birth

TABLE 21.1

Comparison of Hypotonic and Hypertonic Contractions

Criteria	Hypertonic	Hypotonic
Phase of labor	Latent	Active
Symptoms	Painful	Painless
Medication		
Oxytocin	Unfavorable reaction	Favorable reaction
Sedation	Helpful	Little value

may be necessary. Both the woman and her support person need to understand that, although the contractions are strong, they are ineffective and are not achieving cervical dilatation. To help identify the difference, hypotonic and hypertonic contractions are compared in Table 21.1.

What if... Roseann's doctor tells her not to eat during labor because she may need general anesthesia for a cesarean birth, but you find her eating potato chips because she doesn't want general anesthesia? What would you do?

Uncoordinated Contractions

Normally, all contractions are initiated at one pacemaker point high in the uterus. A contraction sweeps down over the organ, encircling it; repolarization occurs; relaxation or a low resting tone is achieved; and another pacemaker-activated contraction begins. With uncoordinated contractions, more than one pacemaker may be initiating contractions, or receptor points in the myometrium may be acting independently of the pacemaker. Uncoordinated

contractions may occur so closely together that they do not allow good cotyledon filling. Because they occur so erratically (e.g., one on top of another and then a long period without any), it may be difficult for a woman to rest between contractions or to use breathing exercises with contractions.

Applying a fetal and a uterine external monitor and assessing the rate, pattern, resting tone, and fetal response to contractions for at least 15 minutes (or longer if necessary in early labor) reveals the abnormal pattern. Oxytocin administration may be helpful in uncoordinated labor to stimulate a more effective and consistent pattern of contractions with a better, lower resting tone.

Dysfunctional Labor and Associated Stages of Labor

As stated previously, dysfunctional or ineffective labor can occur at any point during labor. For a graphic illustration of these times, see Figure 21.2. Regardless of when dysfunctional labor occurs, the effect on a woman and her support person will be the same: anxiety, fear, or discouragement. A woman needs good explanations of what is happening: "We're going to take a sonogram to check the baby's position." "This is a drug to make your contractions stronger." "I know resting is the last thing you feel like doing, but that is what I want you to try to do."

Dysfunction With the First Stage of Labor

Prolonged Latent Phase. The major dysfunction that can occur in the first stage of labor is a prolonged latent phase. The normal parameters for the stages of labor are highlighted in Table 21.2. A prolonged latent phase, as defined by Friedman (1978), is a latent phase that is longer than 20 hours in a nullipara or 14 hours in a multipara. This may occur if the cervix is not "ripe" at the beginning of labor and time must be spent getting truly ready for labor. It may occur if there is excessive use of an analgesic early in labor. With a prolonged latent phase, the uterus

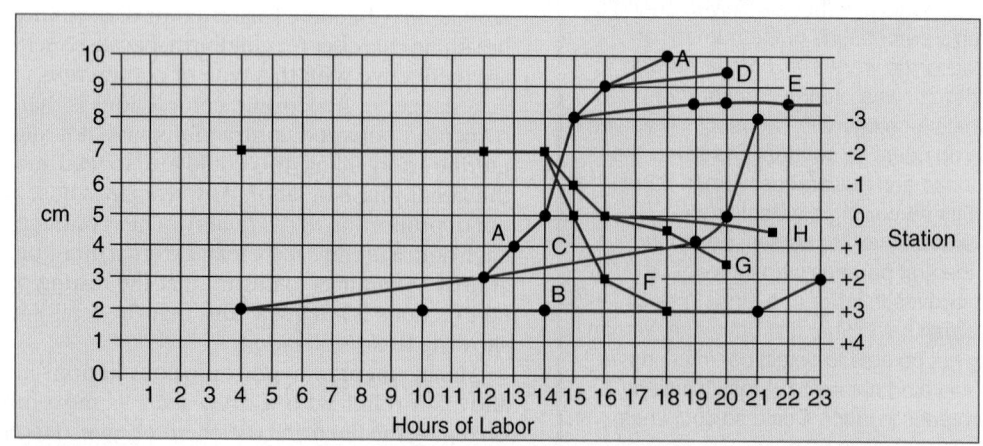

FIGURE 21.2 Graph showing types of abnormal labor. (**A**) Normal labor curve. (**B**) Prolonged latent phase. (**C**) Protracted active-phase dilatation. (**D**) Prolonged deceleration phase. (**E**) Secondary arrest of dilatation. (**F**) Normal descent. (**G**) Prolonged descent. (**H**) Arrest of descent.

TABLE 21.2

Lengths of Phases and Stages of Normal Labor in Hours

Phase	Nullipara		Multipara	
	Average	Upper Normal	Average	Upper Normal
Latent phase	8.6	20.0	5.3	14.0
Active phase	5.8	12.0	2.5	6.0
Second stage	1	1.5	0.25	—*

*There is no limit to the length of the second stage as long as progress is being made and fetal distress is not present.

tends to be in a hypertonic state. Relaxation between contractions is inadequate, and the contractions are only mild (less than 15 mm Hg on a monitor printout) and therefore ineffective. One segment of the uterus may be contracting with more force than another segment.

Management of a prolonged latent phase in labor includes helping the uterus to rest and administering adequate fluid to the woman to prevent dehydration. Administration of morphine may relax hypertonicity. This usually allows labor to become effective and begin to progress. If it does not, a cesarean birth or amniotomy and oxytocin infusion to assist labor may be necessary.

Protracted Active Phase. A protracted active phase is usually associated with CPD or fetal malposition, although it may reflect ineffective myometrial activity. This phase is prolonged if cervical dilatation does not occur at a rate of at least 1.2 cm/hour in a nullipara or 1.5 cm/hour in a multipara, or if the active phase lasts longer than 12 hours in a primigravida or 6 hours in a multigravida (see Fig. 21.2). If the cause of the delay in dilatation is fetal malposition or CPD, cesarean birth may be necessary. Dysfunctional labor during the dilatational division of labor tends to be hypotonic, in contrast to the hypertonic action at the beginning of labor. After a sonogram to show that CPD is not present, oxytocin may be prescribed to augment labor.

Prolonged Deceleration Phase. A deceleration phase has become prolonged when it extends beyond 3 hours in a nullipara or 1 hour in a multipara. Prolonged deceleration phase most often results from abnormal fetal head position. A cesarean birth is frequently required.

Secondary Arrest of Dilatation. A secondary arrest of dilatation has occurred if there is no progress in cervical dilatation for more than 2 hours.

Dysfunction at the Second Stage of Labor

Prolonged Descent. Prolonged descent of the fetus occurs if the rate of descent is less than 1.0 cm/hour in a nullipara or 2.0 cm/hour in a multipara.

With both a prolonged active phase of dilatation and prolonged descent, contractions have been of good quality and proper duration, and effacement and beginning dilatation have occurred, but then the contractions become infrequent and of poor quality and dilatation stops. If everything is normal except for the suddenly faulty contractions (i.e., CPD and poor fetal presentation have been ruled out by sonography), then rest and fluid intake, as advocated for hypertonic contractions, also apply. If the membranes have not ruptured, rupturing them at this point may be helpful. Intravenous (IV) oxytocin may be used to induce the uterus to contract effectively. A semi-Fowler's position, squatting, kneeling, or more effective pushing may speed descent.

Arrest of Descent. Arrest of descent results when no descent has occurred for 1 hour in a multipara or 2 hours in a nullipara. Failure of descent has occurred when expected descent of the fetus does not begin (i.e., engagement or movement beyond 0 station has not occurred). The most likely cause for arrest of descent during the second stage is CPD. Cesarean birth usually is necessary. If there is no contraindication to vaginal birth, oxytocin may be used to assist labor.

Checkpoint Question 1

Roseann Bigalow has prolonged labor. What is the most common cause for arrest of descent during the second stage of labor?

a. Cephalopelvic disproportion (CPD)
b. Maternal calcium deficiency
c. The fetus is asleep during labor
d. The maternal outlet is narrow

NURSING DIAGNOSES AND RELATED INTERVENTIONS FOR DYSFUNCTIONAL LABOR

It is impossible to prevent all dysfunctional labor, just as it is impossible to predict the functioning of any woman's hormonal system or individual response to labor. However, a number of nursing interventions can contribute to the progression of normal labor and help change a dysfunctional labor to a functional one.

Nursing Diagnosis: Fatigue and anxiety related to prolonged labor

Outcome Evaluation: Client states that she is able to continue active participation in labor; maintains effective breathing with contractions.

Because labor is work, it can cause a woman to deplete her glucose stores. On a client's admission to a birthing room, assess the likelihood of glucose depletion by asking the time of her last meal. If she ate breakfast at 8 AM and then began labor by 2 PM, she is only 6 hours away from a full meal. However, if she last ate at 5 PM the preceding evening and did not eat breakfast because she awoke with labor this morning, she is 11 hours away from a full meal. Alert the physician or nurse-midwife to this situation. If the client is still in early labor, she may be allowed to drink some high-carbohydrate fluid (e.g., orange juice) or to eat a light meal. IV fluid therapy also may be initiated to provide glucose for energy. Most physicians and nurse-midwives also allow women to have lolli-pops or hard candy to suck on during labor to supply additional glucose.

Although the effect of emotion on labor is difficult to document, it seems that the cervix dilatates more rapidly and therefore normal labor is shortened if a woman is neither tense nor frightened. Manage stress by making the transfer from home to the health care facility as untraumatic as possible. Ask directly whether the woman has any concerns. Offer explanations of all procedures. Make the support person feel just as welcome and comfortable as the woman herself. Asking a question such as, "Is labor what you thought it would be?" of both the woman and her support person often helps them to express their concerns.

Remember that pain is an exhausting phenome-non. Encourage the use of nonpharmacologic com-fort measures. Breathe with the woman, give back rubs, change sheets, use cool washcloths, and so forth. Complementary therapies such as aroma-therapy or music can also be helpful.

To increase the blood supply to the uterus and prevent hypotension, urge the woman to lie on her side so that the uterus is lifted off the vena cava. If a woman insists on lying supine, place a hip roll under one or the other of her buttocks to cause her pelvis to "tip" and, at least to some extent, move the uterus to the side.

A full bladder prevents descent of the fetus and may impede uterine contractions. Urge a woman in labor to void every 2 hours to keep the bladder empty and to aid progress.

Nursing Diagnosis: Risk for deficient fluid volume related to length and work of labor

Outcome Evaluation: Urine is free of ketones; spe-cific gravity is between 1.003 and 1.030; skin turgor and serum electrolyte levels are within acceptable parameters.

Low levels of serum electrolytes or body fluid can occur in labor for the same reason as a de-creased glucose level—a long interval between eating and the end of labor. Additionally, vomiting and diarrhea occasionally accompany labor and can increase fluid and electrolyte losses. Question a woman about any vomiting or diarrhea she has had to determine the extent (e.g., one episode of a small amount of diarrhea or vomiting that lasted on and off for less than 30 minutes). Profuse diaphore-sis and hyperventilation that occur with labor further increase fluid and electrolyte losses through insen-sible water loss.

Test voidings frequently during labor for glucose, protein, ketones, and specific gravity (place a urine collector container on the bathroom toilet if the woman is going to use the toilet). Ketones in the urine suggest starvation ketosis. A concentrated specific gravity suggests a lack of fluid. Extreme dehydration not only may slow labor but can lead to increased blood viscosity, possibly increasing the risk for thrombophlebitis during the postpartal period.

Many women react negatively to the idea of IV fluid therapy during labor to restore body fluid, possibly perceiving it as loss of control over their bodies or removal of the "naturalness" of labor and birth. Introduce the idea of IV fluid therapy, explaining its purpose before arriving with the bag of fluid and tubing. When inserting the IV catheter device, try to use an insertion site in the woman's nondominant hand and, if necessary, only a small "reminder" handboard. Assure the woman that she can be out of bed and walking, can turn freely, squat, sit, or use whatever position she prefers during labor with the IV line in place. None of these acts will interfere with the infusion (Fig. 21.3).

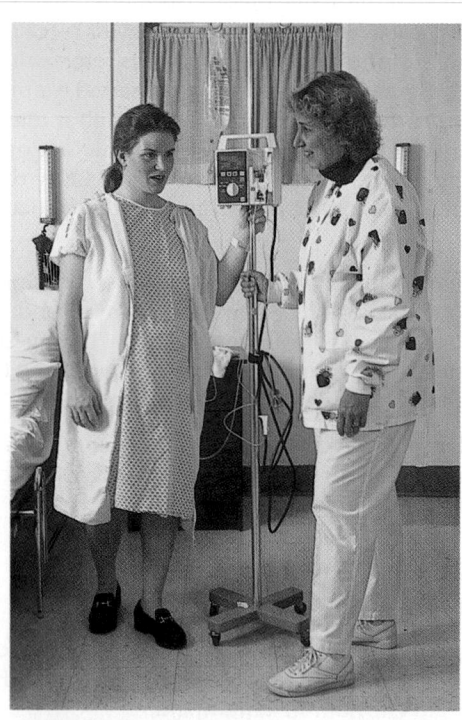

FIGURE 21.3 If intravenous fluid is used for women in labor, it does not need to limit mobility.

Contraction Rings

Two types of contraction rings can occur in a dysfunctional labor. A simple type is a constriction ring, which can occur at any point in the myometrium and at any time during labor. The most common form is a **pathologic retraction ring** (Bandl's ring) that occurs at the junction of the upper and lower uterine segments. The ring usually appears during the second stage of labor as a horizontal indentation across the abdomen (Fig. 21.4) and is a warning sign that severe dysfunctional labor is occurring. It is formed by excessive retraction of the upper uterine segment; the uterine myometrium is much thicker above than below the ring.

When a pathologic retraction ring occurs in early labor, it is usually caused by uncoordinated contractions. In the pelvic division of labor, it is usually caused by obstetric manipulation or by the administration of oxytocin. In either event, the fetus is gripped by the retraction ring and cannot advance beyond that point. The undelivered placenta will also be held at that point.

Contraction rings often can be identified by sonography. Such a finding is extremely serious and should be reported promptly. Administration of IV morphine sulfate or the inhalation of amyl nitrite may relieve a retraction ring. A tocolytic may be administered to halt contractions. If the situation is not relieved, uterine rupture and death of the fetus may occur. In the placental stage, massive maternal hemorrhage may result, because the placenta is loosened but then cannot be delivered, preventing the uterus from contracting (MacMullen et al., 2005).

Most likely, a cesarean birth will be necessary to ensure safe birth of the fetus. Manual removal of the placenta under general anesthesia may be required if the retraction ring does not allow the placenta to be delivered.

Precipitate Labor

Precipitate labor and birth occur when uterine contractions are so strong that the woman gives birth with only a few, rapidly occurring contractions. It is often defined as a labor that is completed in fewer than 3 hours (Dudley, 2003). Such rapid labor is likely to occur with grand multiparity, or it may occur after induction of labor by oxytocin or amniotomy. Contractions can be so forceful that they lead to premature separation of the placenta, placing the mother and fetus at risk for hemorrhage. Rapid labor also poses a risk to the fetus, because subdural hemorrhage may result from the sudden release of pressure on the head. A woman may sustain lacerations of the birth canal from the forceful birth. She also can feel overwhelmed by the speed of labor.

A precipitate labor can be predicted from a labor graph if, during the active phase of dilatation, the rate is greater than 5 cm/hour (1 cm every 12 minutes) in a nullipara or 10 cm/hour (1 cm every 6 minutes) in a multipara. In such cases, a tocolytic may be administered to reduce the force and frequency of contractions.

Caution a multiparous woman by week 28 of pregnancy that, because a past labor was so brief, her labor this time also may be brief. This allows her to plan for

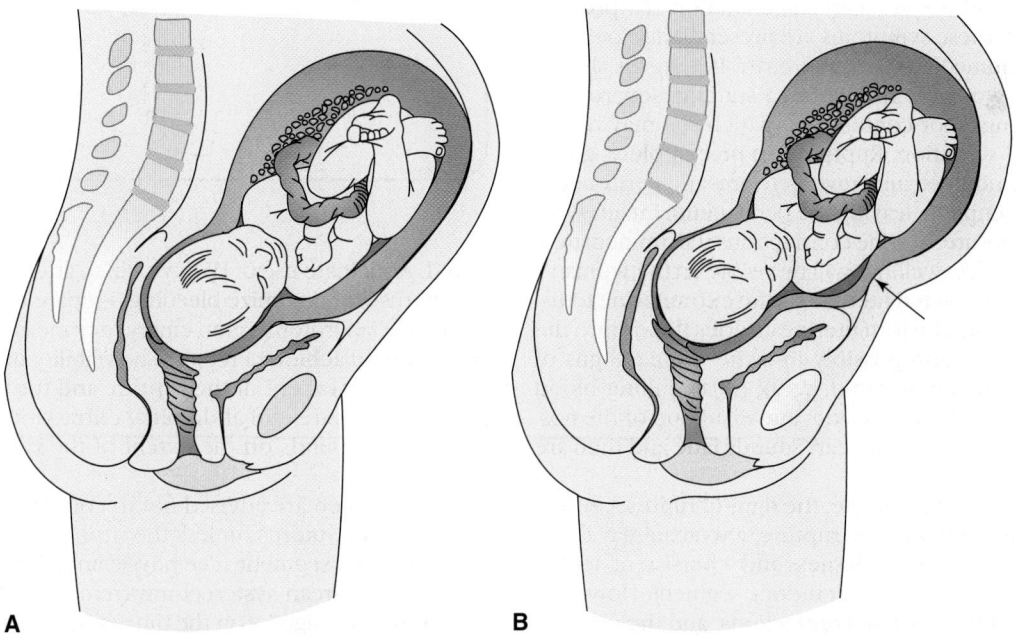

A   **B**

FIGURE 21.4 Pathologic retraction ring. (**A**) Uterus in the normal second stage of labor. Notice how the upper uterine segment is becoming thicker and the lower uterine segment is thinning. A physiologic retraction ring is normally formed at the division of the upper and lower uterine segments. (**B**) Uterus with a pathologic retraction ring (Bandl's ring). The wall below the ring is thin and the abdomen shows an indentation. This constriction is caused by obstructed labor and is a warning sign that if the obstruction is not relieved, the lower segment may rupture.

appropriately timed transportation to the hospital or alternative birthing center. Both grand multiparas and women with histories of precipitate labor should have the birthing room converted to birth readiness before full dilatation is obtained. Then, even a sudden birth can be accomplished in a controlled surrounding.

? What if... Roseann tells you that her sister was only in labor 1 hour when she had her baby, but Roseann is planning to spend the last days of this pregnancy in a mountain cabin 60 miles from the hospital? What would you do?

Uterine Rupture

Rupture of the uterus during labor, although rare (about 1 in 1,500 births), is always a possibility (Dudley, 2003). It is always serious, because it accounts for as many as 5% of all maternal deaths. Uterine rupture occurs when a uterus undergoes more strain than it is capable of sustaining. Rupture occurs most commonly when a vertical scar from a previous cesarean birth or hysterotomy repair tears (Guise et al., 2004). Contributing factors may include prolonged labor, abnormal presentation, multiple gestation, unwise use of oxytocin, obstructed labor, and traumatic maneuvers of forceps or traction. When uterine rupture occurs, fetal death will follow unless immediate cesarean birth can be accomplished. In these instances, fetal outcome can be optimal.

Impending rupture may be preceded by a pathologic retraction ring (see earlier discussion) and by strong uterine contractions without any cervical dilatation. To prevent rupture when these symptoms are present, anticipate the need for an immediate cesarean birth. If a uterus should rupture, the woman experiences a sudden, severe pain during a strong labor contraction, which she may report as a "tearing" sensation. Rupture can be complete, going through the endometrium, myometrium, and peritoneum layers, or incomplete, leaving the peritoneum intact. With a complete rupture, uterine contractions will immediately stop. Two distinct swellings will be visible on the woman's abdomen: the retracted uterus and the extrauterine fetus. Hemorrhage from the torn uterine arteries floods into the abdominal cavity and possibly into the vagina. Signs of shock begin, including rapid, weak pulse; falling blood pressure; cold and clammy skin; and dilatation of the nostrils from air hunger. Fetal heart sounds fade and then are absent.

If the rupture is incomplete, the signs of rupture are less evident. With an incomplete rupture, a woman may experience only a localized tenderness and a persistent aching pain over the area of the lower uterine segment. However, fetal heart sounds, a lack of contractions, and the changes in the woman's vital signs will gradually reveal fetal and maternal distress (Box 21.4).

Because the uterus at the end of pregnancy is such a vascular organ, uterine rupture is an immediate emergency situation, comparable to splenic or hepatic rupture. Administer emergency fluid replacement therapy as or-

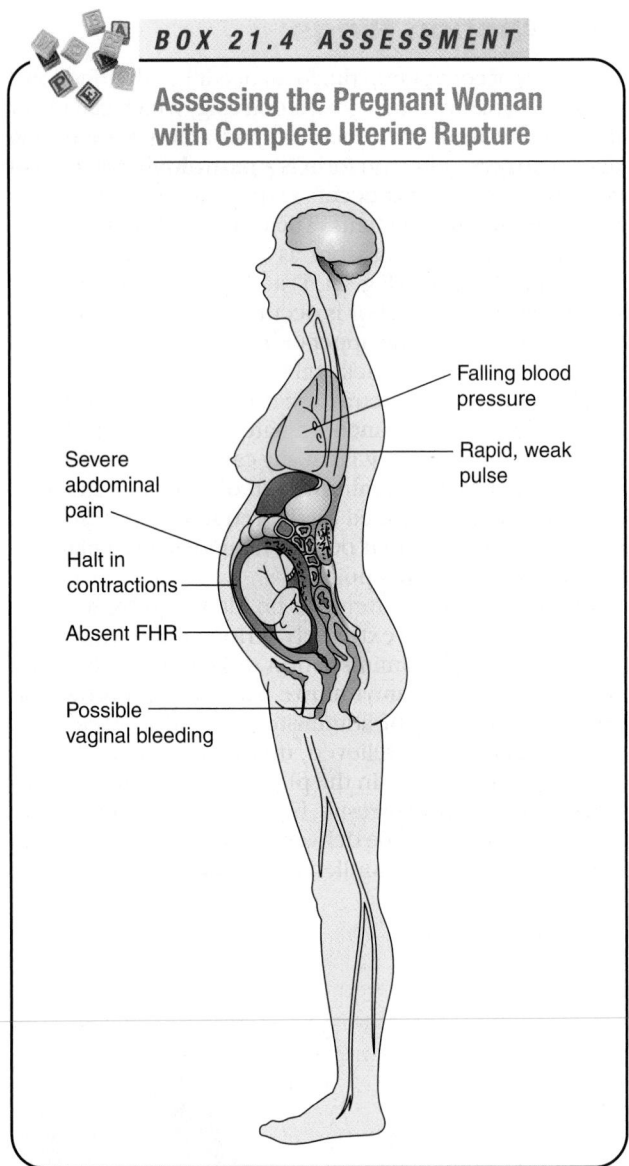

BOX 21.4 ASSESSMENT

Assessing the Pregnant Woman with Complete Uterine Rupture

- Falling blood pressure
- Rapid, weak pulse
- Severe abdominal pain
- Halt in contractions
- Absent FHR
- Possible vaginal bleeding

dered. Anticipate use of IV oxytocin to attempt to contract the uterus and minimize bleeding. Prepare the woman for a possible laparotomy as an emergency measure to control bleeding and achieve a repair. The viability of the fetus depends on the extent of the rupture and the time elapsed between rupture and abdominal extraction. A woman's prognosis depends on the extent of the rupture and the blood loss.

Most women are advised not to conceive again after a rupture of the uterus, unless the rupture occurred in the inactive lower segment. The physician, with consent, may perform a cesarean hysterectomy (removal of the damaged uterus) or tubal ligation at the time of the laparotomy; both procedures result in loss of childbearing ability. A woman may have difficulty giving her consent at this time, because it is unknown whether her present baby will live. If blood loss was acute, she may be nonresponsive because of decreased cerebral perfusion from hypotension. If this has happened, the woman's support person must be the one who gives this consent, relying on the information provided by the operating surgeon to decide whether a functioning uterus can be saved.

Be prepared to offer information to the support person and to inform him or her about fetal outcome, the extent of the surgery, and the woman's safety as soon as possible. Initially, a woman and her support person will probably be thankful that her life was saved. However, they may become almost immediately angry that the rupture occurred, especially if the fetus died and the woman will no longer be able to have children. Allow them time to express these emotions without feeling threatened. They are grieving for the loss of both the child and their fertility as a couple.

Inversion of the Uterus

Uterine inversion refers to the uterus' turning inside out with either birth of the fetus or delivery of the placenta. It is a rare phenomenon, occurring in about 1 in 15,000 births (Dudley, 2003). It may occur if traction is applied to the umbilical cord to remove the placenta or if pressure is applied to the uterine fundus when the uterus is not contracted. It may also occur if the placenta is attached at the fundus so that, during birth, the passage of the fetus pulls the fundus down.

Inversion occurs in various degrees. The inverted fundus may lie within the uterine cavity or the vagina, or, in total inversion, it may protrude from the vagina (Hatada, 2004). When an inversion occurs, a large amount of blood suddenly gushes from the vagina. The fundus is not palpable in the abdomen. If the loss of blood continues unchecked for longer than a few minutes, the woman will show signs of blood loss: hypotension, dizziness, paleness, or diaphoresis. Because the uterus is not contracted in this position, bleeding continues, and exsanguination could occur within a period as short as 10 minutes.

Never attempt to replace an inversion, because handling of the uterus may increase the bleeding. Never attempt to remove the placenta if it is still attached, because this only creates a larger surface area for bleeding. In addition, administration of an oxytocic drug only compounds the inversion or makes the uterus more tense and difficult to replace. An IV fluid line needs to be started, if one is not already present (use a large-gauge needle, because blood will need to be replaced). If a line is already in place, open it to achieve optimal flow of fluid to restore fluid volume. Administer oxygen by mask, and assess vital signs. Be prepared to perform cardiopulmonary resuscitation (CPR) if the woman's heart should fail from the sudden blood loss. The woman will immediately be given general anesthesia or possibly nitroglycerin or a tocolytic drug intravenously, to relax the uterus. The physician or nurse-midwife then replaces the fundus manually. Administration of oxytocin after manual replacement helps the uterus to contract and remain in its natural place. Because the uterine endometrium was exposed, a woman will need antibiotic therapy to prevent infection. She needs to be informed that cesarean birth will probably be necessary in any future pregnancy, to prevent the possibility of repeat inversion (Tank-Parikshit et al., 2004).

Checkpoint Question 2

Suppose a woman experiences a uterine inversion and the placenta is still attached. What would be your best action?

a. Remove the placenta manually so that the uterus contracts.
b. Attempt to replace the uterus so that it becomes compressed.
c. Increase the woman's intravenous fluid to help restore blood loss.
d. Give an emergency bolus of an oxytocin such as Pitocin IV.

Amniotic Fluid Embolism

Amniotic fluid embolism occurs when amniotic fluid is forced into an open maternal uterine blood sinus through some defect in the membranes or after membrane rupture or partial premature separation of the placenta (Perozzi & Englert, 2004). Previously, it was thought that particles such as meconium or shed fetal skin cells in the amniotic fluid entered the maternal circulation and reached the lungs as small emboli. Now, it is recognized that a humoral or anaphylactoid response is the more likely cause (Aurangzeb et al., 2004). This condition may occur during labor or in the postpartal period. The incidence may be as high as 1 in 8,000 births; it is not preventable because it cannot be predicted. Possible risk factors include oxytocin administration, abruptio placentae, and hydramnios.

The clinical picture is dramatic. A woman, in strong labor, sits up suddenly and grasps her chest because of sharp pain and inability to breathe (secondary to pulmonary artery constriction). She becomes pale and then turns the typical bluish gray associated with pulmonary embolism and lack of blood flow to the lungs. The immediate management is oxygen administration by face mask or cannula. Within minutes, she will need CPR. CPR may be ineffective, however, because these procedures (inflating the lungs and massaging the heart) do not relieve the pulmonary constriction. Therefore, blood still cannot circulate to the lungs. Death may occur within minutes.

A woman's prognosis depends on the size of the embolism, the speed with which the emergency condition was detected, and the skill and speed of emergency interventions. Even if the woman survives the initial insult, the risk for disseminated intravascular coagulation (DIC) is high, further compounding her condition. In this event, she will need continued management that includes endotracheal intubation to maintain pulmonary function and therapy with fibrinogen to counteract DIC. Most likely, she will be transferred to an ICU. The prognosis for the fetus is guarded, because reduced placental perfusion results from the severe drop in maternal blood pressure. Labor often begins or the fetus is born immediately by cesarean birth.

PROBLEMS WITH THE PASSENGER

Birth complications may arise if the maternal pelvis is undersized, such as in early adolescence or in women with altered bone growth (e.g., from rickets). It also can occur if the umbilical cord prolapses, if more than one fetus is present, or if a fetus is malpositioned or too large for the birth canal.

Prolapse of the Umbilical Cord

In **umbilical cord prolapse,** a loop of the umbilical cord slips down in front of the presenting fetal part (Fig. 21.5). Prolapse may occur at any time after the membranes rupture if the presenting part is not fitted firmly into the cervix. It tends to occur most often with the following conditions:

- Premature rupture of membranes
- Fetal presentation other than cephalic
- Placenta previa
- Intrauterine tumors preventing the presenting part from engaging
- A small fetus
- CPD preventing firm engagement
- Hydramnios
- Multiple gestation

The incidence is about 0.4% of births (Kahana et al., 2004).

Assessment

In rare instances, the cord may be felt as the presenting part on an initial vaginal examination during labor. It may also be identified in this position on a sonogram. In such cases, cesarean birth is necessary before rupture of the membranes occurs. Otherwise, membrane rupture would cause the cord to slide down into the vagina from the pressure exerted by the amniotic fluid. More often, however, cord prolapse is first discovered only after the membranes have ruptured, when a variable deceleration FHR pattern suddenly becomes apparent. The cord may be visible at the vulva.

To rule out cord prolapse, always assess fetal heart sounds immediately after rupture of the membranes occurring either spontaneously or by amniotomy.

Therapeutic Management

Cord prolapse automatically leads to cord compression, because the fetal presenting part presses against the cord at the pelvic brim. Management is aimed toward relieving pressure on the cord, thereby relieving the compression and the resulting fetal anoxia. This may be done by placing a gloved hand in the vagina and manually elevating the fetal head off the cord, or by placing the woman in a knee–chest or Trendelenburg position, which causes the fetal head to fall back from the cord. Administering oxygen at 10 L/min by face mask to the mother is also helpful to improve oxygenation to the fetus. A tocolytic agent may be prescribed to reduce uterine activity and pressure on the fetus.

If the cord has prolapsed to the extent that it is exposed to room air, drying will begin, leading to atrophy of the umbilical vessels. Do not attempt to push any exposed cord back into the vagina. This may add to the compression by causing knotting or kinking. Instead, cover any exposed portion with a sterile saline compress to prevent drying.

If the cervix is fully dilated at the time of the prolapse, the physician may choose to deliver the infant quickly, possibly with forceps, to prevent fetal anoxia. If dilatation is incomplete, the birth method of choice is upward pressure on the presenting part, applied by the practitioner's hand in the woman's vagina, to keep pressure off the cord until the baby can be born by cesarean birth. Prolapsed cord is always an emergency situation, because the reduced blood flow to the fetus can quickly cause fetal harm.

Multiple Gestation

A woman with a multiple gestation usually causes a flurry of excitement in a birthing room. Additional personnel are needed for the birth (as many nurses to attend to possibly immature infants as there are infants, plus additional pediatricians or neonatal nurse practitioners). In the mid-

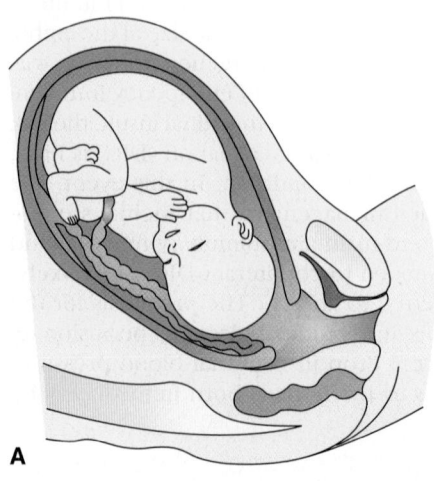
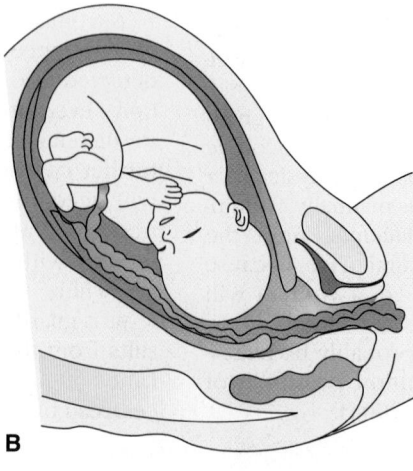

A   **B**

FIGURE 21.5 Prolapse of the umbilical cord. (**A**) The cord is prolapsed but still within the uterus. (**B**) The cord is visible at the vulva. In both instances the fetal nutrient supply is being compromised, although only a cord such as that shown in B would be visible. Both prolapses could be detected by fetal monitoring.

dle of all the preparatory activity, it is easy to forget that the woman may be more frightened than excited. Be sure to focus on her needs and those of the babies. Twins may be born by cesarean birth to decrease the risk that the second fetus will experience anoxia; this also is often the situation in multiple gestations of three or more, because of the increased incidence of cord entanglement and premature separation of the placenta (Wen et al., 2004).

Anemia and pregnancy-induced hypertension occur at higher-than-usual incidences during multiple gestations. Be certain to assess the woman's hematocrit level and blood pressure closely during labor or while waiting for cesarean surgery.

If a woman with a multiple gestation will be giving birth vaginally, she is usually instructed to come to the hospital early in labor. The first stage of labor does not differ greatly from that of a mother with a single-gestation pregnancy. Coming to a hospital this early in labor, however, will make labor seem long. Urge the woman to spend the early hours of labor engaged in an activity such as playing cards or reading, to make the time pass more quickly. Multiple pregnancies often end before full term, so the woman may not yet have practiced breathing exercises. The early hours of labor can be used for this as well. During labor, support the woman's breathing exercises to minimize the need for analgesia or anesthesia; this helps to minimize any respiratory difficulties the infants may have at birth because of their immaturity.

If possible, monitor each FHR by a separate fetal monitor during labor. Because the babies are usually small, firm head engagement may not occur, increasing the risk for cord prolapse after rupture of the membranes. Be-

cause of the multiple fetuses, abnormal fetal presentation may occur. Uterine dysfunction from a long labor, an overstretched uterus, and premature separation of the placenta after the birth of the first child may also be more common. Box 21.5 highlights appropriate outcomes and interventions for a woman at risk for injury related to multiple gestation using the terminology of the Nursing Outcomes Classification (NOC) and Nursing Interventions Classification (NIC).

With a multiple gestation, the first fetus usually presents vertex. After the first infant is born, both ends of the baby's cord are tied or clamped permanently, rather than with cord clamps, which could slip. This prevents hemorrhage through an open cord end if additional infants have shared the placenta. The first infant is identified as *A*, and newborn care is started for him or her. In singleton pregnancies oxytocin usually is given immediately to contract the uterus and minimize bleeding as an infant is born; in this case, however, it will not be given, to avoid compromising the circulation of the infants not yet born.

Most twin pregnancies present with both twins vertex. This is followed in frequency by vertex and breech, breech and vertex, and then breech and breech (Fig. 21.6). Multiple gestations of three or more fetuses have extremely varied presentations. After the birth of the first child, the lie of the second fetus is determined by external abdominal palpation and sonography. If the presentation is not vertex, external version may be attempted to make it so. If this is not successful, a decision for a breech delivery or cesarean birth must be made (Crowther, 2005). If the infant will be born vaginally, an oxytocin infusion may be begun at this point to assist uterine contractions, thereby shortening the

---

BOX 21.5

Nursing Outcomes Classification (NOC) and Nursing Interventions Classification (NIC)

Multiple Gestation

NOC: Maternal Status, Intrapartum
Maternal status, intrapartum is defined as the conditions and behaviors indicating maternal well-being from the initiation of labor through delivery (Johnson, Maas, & Moorhead, 2000). Some specific indicators suggesting that this outcome has been achieved include the following:

- Vital signs, neurologic status, and urine output are within expected range
- Frequency, duration, and intensity of uterine contractions are within expected range
- Cervical dilation is progressing as expected.
- Client demonstrates use of techniques to facilitate and cope with labor

NIC: Intrapartum Care, High-Risk Delivery
Intrapartum care, high-risk delivery is defined as assisting with the vaginal birth of multiple or

malpositioned fetuses (McCloskey & Bulechek, 2000). Some important activities involved when implementing this intervention for the woman with multiple gestation include:

- Informing the client and her support person about the additional procedures and techniques that may be necessary during the delivery process.
- Preparing additional equipment and personnel for delivery
- Assisting with amniotomy, ultrasonography, forceps or vacuum extraction application as needed
- Recording the time of birth for the first neonate and any subsequent neonates delivered
- Assisting with neonatal resuscitation, if necessary
- Explaining any newborn characteristics related to the high-risk birth, such as forcep marks or bruising
- Encouraging parental interaction with neonates immediately after delivery

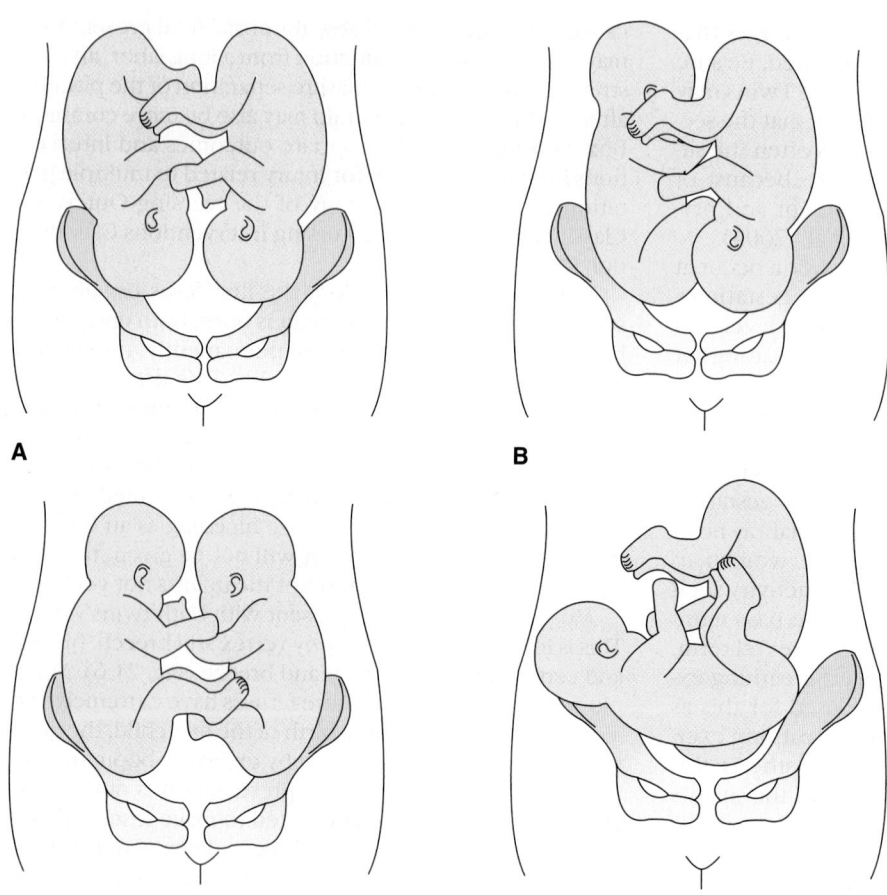

A

B

C

D

FIGURE 21.6 Four different twin presentations. (**A**) Both infants vertex. (**B**) One infant vertex and one breech. (**C**) Both infants breech. (**D**) One infant vertex and one in a transverse lie.

time span between births. Nitroglycerin may be administered to relax the uterus.

Occasionally, the placenta of the first infant separates before the second fetus is born, and there is sudden, profuse bleeding at the vagina. This creates a risk for the woman. The uterus cannot contract as it normally would, because it is still full with the second twin, so it is difficult to halt the bleeding. If the separation of the first placenta caused loosening of additional placentas, or if a common placenta is involved, the fetal heart sounds of the other fetuses will register distress immediately. They need to be born at once if they are to survive. For this reason, with most multiple gestations today, if all of the fetuses are not vertex presentations, they will be born by cesarean birth.

Parents usually want to inspect multiple-gestation infants thoroughly after birth. The time allowed for this inspection depends on the infants' weights and conditions. Some parents worry that the hospital will confuse their infants through improper identification. Review with them the measures used to ensure correct identification.

Even though women have known for months that they are having multiple infants, many have difficulty believing that this has really happened. They feel a need to recount over and over their surprise and to view all their infants together to prove to themselves that it is true. If parents are unable to inspect their infants thoroughly immediately after birth because of the infants' low birthweights and the danger of chilling, they need the opportunity to do so as soon as possible, to dispel any fears they had

throughout pregnancy that the babies would be born less than perfect.

Assess the mother carefully in the immediate postpartal period, because the uterus that has been overly distended due to the multiple gestation may have more difficulty contracting than usual, placing the mother at risk for hemorrhage from uterine atony. In addition, the risk for uterine infection increases if labor or birth was prolonged. The infants need careful assessment to determine their true gestational age and whether a phenomenon such as twin-to-twin transfusion could have occurred (see Chapter 26).

Problems With Position, Presentation, or Size

Occipitoposterior Position

In approximately one tenth of all labors, the fetal position is posterior rather than anterior. That is, the occiput (assuming the presentation is vertex) is directed diagonally and posteriorly, either to the right (ROP) or to the left (LOP). In these positions, during internal rotation, the fetal head must rotate, not through a 90-degree arc (Fig. 21.7), but through an arc of approximately 135 degrees (Fig. 21.8).

Posterior positions tend to occur in women with android, anthropoid, or contracted pelves. A posterior position is suggested by a dysfunctional labor pattern such as

version of fetal malpresentations. *Biological Research for Nursing, 6*(2), 126-140.

Aurangzeb, I., George, L., & Raoof, S. (2004). Amniotic fluid embolism. *Critical Care Clinics, 20*(4), 643-650.

Belfort, M. A. (2003). Operative vaginal delivery. In Scott, J. R., et al. *Danforth's obstetrics and gynecology* (9th ed.). Philadelphia: Lippincott Williams & Wilkins.

Bishop, E. H. (1964). Pelvic scoring for elective induction. *Obstetrics and Gynecology, 24*(2), 266-269.

Bolnick, J. M., et al. (2004). Randomized trial between two active labor management protocols in the presence of an unfavorable cervix. *American Journal of Obstetrics and Gynecology, 190*(1), 124-128.

Buhimschi, C. S., et al. (2003). Uterine contractility in women whose fetus is delivered in the occipitoposterior position. *American Journal of Obstetrics and Gynecology, 188*(3), 734-739.

Cottrill, H. M., et al. (2004). Factors influencing maternal perception of uterine contractions. *American Journal of Obstetrics and Gynecology, 190*(5), 1455-1457.

Crowther, C. A. (2005). Caesarean delivery for the second twin. *The Cochrane Library (Oxford), (4)*, CD000047.

Damron, D. P., & Capeless, E. L. (2004). Operative vaginal delivery: A comparison of forceps and vacuum for success rate and risk of rectal sphincter injury. *American Journal of Obstetrics and Gynecology, 191*(3), 907-910.

Demissie, K., et al. (2004). Operative vaginal delivery and neonatal and infant adverse outcomes. *BMJ, 329*(7456), 24-29.

Department of Health and Human Services. (2000). *Healthy people 2010.* Washington, D.C.: Author.

Dudley, D. J. (2003). Complications of labor. In Scott, J. R., et al. *Danforth's obstetrics and gynecology* (9th ed.). Philadelphia: Lippincott Williams & Wilkins.

Ehrenberg, H. M., Mercer, B. M., & Catalano, P. M. (2004). The influence of obesity and diabetes on the prevalence of macrosomia. *American Journal of Obstetrics and Gynecology, 191*(3), 964-968.

Foley, M. E., et al. (2004). The continuing effectiveness of active management of first labor, despite a doubling in overall nulliparous cesarian delivery. *American Journal of Obstetrics and Gynecology, 191*(3), 891-895.

Friedman, E. A. (1978). *Labor: Clinical evaluation and management* (2nd ed.). New York: Appleton.

Guise, J. M., et al. (2004). Systematic review of the incidence and consequences of uterine rupture in women with previous caesarean section. *BMJ, 329*(7456), 19-25.

Hatada, Y. (2004). Acute puerperal uterine inversion: Careful usage of oxytocic agents for the success of immediate replacement. *Journal of Obstetrics and Gynaecology, 24*(3), 320-321.

Hutton, E. K., et al. (2003). External cephalic version beginning at 34 weeks' gestation versus 37 weeks' gestation: A randomized multicenter trial. *American Journal of Obstetrics and Gynecology, 189*(1), 245-254.

Johnson, M., Maas, M., & Moorhead, S. (2000). *Nursing outcomes classification* (2nd ed.). St. Louis: Mosby.

Kahana, B., et al. (2004). Umbilical cord prolapse and perinatal outcomes. *International Journal of Gynaecology and Obstetrics, 84*(2), 127-132.

Karch, A. M. (2004). *Lippincott's nursing drug guide.* Philadelphia: Lippincott Williams & Wilkins.

Kelly, A. J., & Tan, B. (2005). Intravenous oxytocin alone for cervical ripening and induction of labour. *The Cochrane Library (Oxford) (4)* (CD003246).

MacMullen, N. J., Dulski, L. A., & Meagher, B. (2005). Red alert: Perinatal hemorrhage. *MCN: The American Journal of Maternal/Child Nursing, 30*(1), 46-51.

McCloskey, J., & Bulechek, G. (2000). *Nursing interventions classification* (3rd ed.). St. Louis: Mosby.

Mehta, S. H., et al. (2004). Is abnormal labor associated with shoulder dystocia in nulliparous women? *American Journal of Obstetrics and Gynecology, 190*(6), 1604-1609.

Perozzi, K. J., & Englert, N. C. (2004). Amniotic fluid embolism: An obstetric emergency. *Critical Care Nurse, 24*(4), 54-61.

Su, M., et al. (2004). Planned caesarean section decreases the risk of adverse perinatal outcome due to both labour and delivery complications in the Term Breech Trial. *BJOG: An International Journal of Obstetrics and Gynaecology, 111*(10), 1065-1074.

Tank-Parikshit, D., et al. (2004). Pregnancy outcome after operative correction of puerperal uterine inversion. *Archives of Gynecology and Obstetrics, 269*(3), 214-216.

Wen, S. W., et al. (2004). Maternal morbidity and obstetric complications in triplet pregnancies and quadruplet and higher-order multiple pregnancies. *American Journal of Obstetrics and Gynecology, 191*(1), 254-258.

Suggested Readings

Bricker, L., & Luckas, M. (2005). Amniotomy alone for induction of labour. *The Cochrane Library (Oxford) (4)* (CD002862).

Cargill, Y. M., et al. (2004). Guidelines for operative vaginal birth. *JOGC: Journal of Obstetrics and Gynaecology Canada, 26*(8), 747-761.

Cesario, S. K. (2005). Reevaluation of Friedman's Labor Curve: A pilot study. *JOGNN: Journal of Obstetric, Gynecologic, and Neonatal Nursing, 33*(6), 713-722.

Gurewitsch, E. D., et al. (2004). Episiotomy versus fetal manipulation in managing severe shoulder dystocia: A comparison of outcomes. *American Journal of Obstetrics and Gynecology, 191*(3), 911-916.

Hlibczuk, V. (2004). Spontaneous uterine rupture as an unusual cause of abdominal pain in the early second trimester of pregnancy. *Journal of Emergency Medicine, 27*(2), 143-145.

Luckas, M., & Bricker, L. (2004). Intravenous prostaglandin for induction of labour. *The Cochrane Library (Oxford) (4)* (CD002864).

Ofir, K., et al. (2004). Uterine rupture: Differences between a scarred and an unscarred uterus. *American Journal of Obstetrics and Gynecology, 191*(2), 425-429.

Ramsey, P. S., & Repke, J. T. (2003). Intrapartum management of multifetal pregnancies. *Seminars in Perinatology, 27*(1), 54-72.

Rudisill, P. T. (2004). Amniotic fluid embolism. *Critical Care Nursing Clinics of North America, 16*(2), 221-225.

Steer, P. (2004). The management of large and small for gestational age fetuses. *Seminars in Perinatology, 28*(1), 59-66.

Yarrow, C., Benoit, G., & Klein, M. C. (2004). Outcomes after vacuum-assisted deliveries: Births attended by community family practitioners. *Canadian Family Physician, 50*(5), 1109-1114.

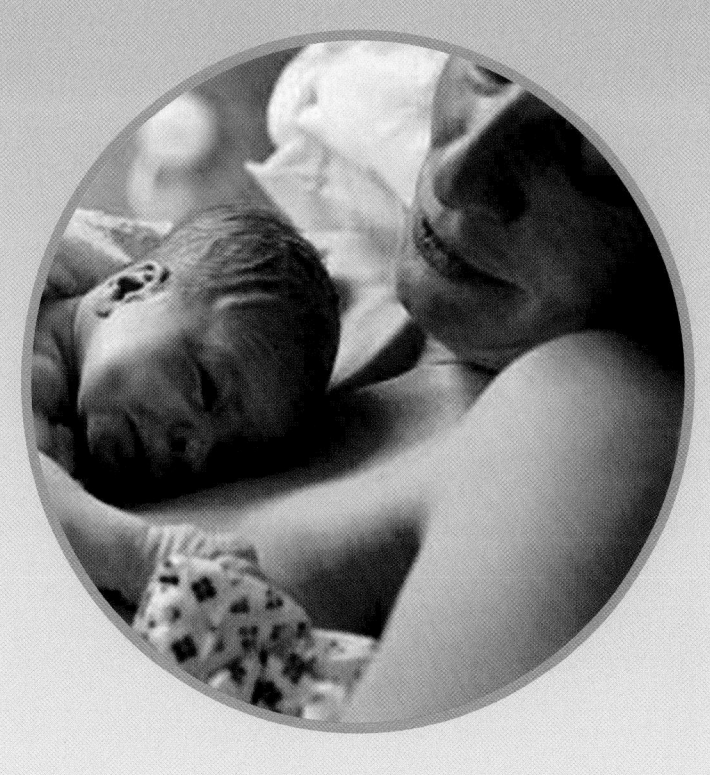

UNIT FIVE

The Nursing Role in Caring for the Family During the Postpartal Period

CHAPTER 22

Nursing Care of a Postpartal Woman and Family

Key Terms

afterpains
diastasis recti
en face position
engrossment
Homans' sign
involution
letting-go phase
lochia
lochia alba
lochia rubra
lochia serosa
postpartal depression
primary engorgement
rooming-in
sitz bath
taking-hold phase
taking-in phase
uterine atony

Objectives

After mastering the contents of this chapter, you should be able to:

1. Describe the psychological and physiologic changes that occur in a postpartal woman.
2. Assess a woman and her family for physiologic and psychological changes after childbirth.
3. Formulate nursing diagnoses related to physiologic and psychological transitions of the postpartal period.
4. Identify expected outcomes for a postpartal woman and family related to the changes during this period.
5. Plan nursing care such as measures to aid uterine involution or encourage bonding.
6. Implement nursing care to aid the progression of physiologic and psychological transitions occurring in a postpartal woman and family.
7. Evaluate expected outcomes to determine effectiveness of nursing care and achievement of outcomes.
8. Identify National Health Goals related to the postpartal period that nurses can help the nation achieve.
9. Identify areas related to care of the postpartal family that could benefit from additional nursing research or application of evidence-based practice.
10. Use critical thinking to analyze ways that postpartum nursing care can be more family centered.
11. Integrate knowledge of the physiologic and psychological changes of the postpartal period with the nursing process to achieve quality maternal and child health nursing care.

---

*A*s the nurse working in a postpartum unit, you are caring for *Mike and Joan Cooper, who have just become parents of an 8 lb, 2 oz baby girl. Mike will be taking a week off from work to spend time with Joan and the new baby. Joan is on maternity leave from her job as a court reporter.*

As you prepare them for discharge, you notice they seem overwhelmed with much of the information they have been provided. Joan says, trying to get the baby to nurse, "He's so big and my breasts are so small, maybe he can't get enough milk. I was hoping by breastfeeding I wouldn't have to worry about birth control for a while, but I'm having so much trouble maybe that won't work out." Mike pulls

you aside and says, "Sometimes, I see my wife crying for no reason. Isn't she as happy as I am?"

Previous chapters discussed caring for the pregnant woman and family during the antepartal and intrapartal periods. This chapter adds information about caring for a postpartal woman and family to your knowledge base. Many physiologic and psychological changes occur during this period, enabling nurses to play major roles in assessment, comfort promotion, and education.

What additional postpartal teaching does the Cooper family need?

After you've studied this chapter, access the accompanying website. Read the patient scenario and answer the questions to further sharpen your skills, grow more familiar with RN-CLEX types of questions, and reward yourself with how much you have learned.

The postpartal period, or *puerperium* (from the Latin *puer*, "child," and *parere*, "to bring forth"), refers to the 6-week period after childbirth. It is a time of maternal changes that are both retrogressive (involution of the uterus and vagina) and progressive (production of milk for lactation, restoration of the normal menstrual cycle, and beginning of a parenting role). Protecting a woman's health as these changes occur is important for preserving her future childbearing function and for ensuring that she is physically well enough to incorporate her new child into her family. The period is popularly termed the *fourth trimester of pregnancy*.

The physical care a woman receives during the postpartal period can influence her health for the rest of her life. The emotional support she receives can influence the emotional health of her child and family so much that it can be felt into the next generation. National Health Goals related to the postpartal period that nurses can help the nation achieve are shown in Box 22.1.

Nursing Process Overview

For a Postpartal Woman and Family

● *Assessment*

During the puerperium, assessment of a woman is accomplished by health interview, physical examination,

and analysis of laboratory data. Assessment of a woman's psychological adjustment begins with her reaction at birth (e.g., Was she disappointed or happy with the sex of her baby? Is she glad to be through with the pregnancy or still longing to be back in it?) and continues with every contact made with the family during and after the hospital stay. Assess the extent and quality of the woman's interaction with her child (Does she hold the infant and talk to him or her?), her overall mood (Do you observe her crying? Does she have long periods of staring into space or not talking?), and her ability to begin infant care. Observe also for self-care. A woman who feels good about herself, even though she is exhausted from childbirth, usually will try to maintain her appearance. If she is depressed, she probably has little energy to do things such as comb her hair or worry about her appearance.

It is also important to ensure that physical changes, such as uterine involution, are occurring by evaluating uterine size and consistency and lochia flow amount (Box 22.2).

BOX 22.1 FOCUS ON . . .

NATIONAL HEALTH GOALS

The first hour after birth is an extremely dangerous one for hemorrhage. It is also the optimal period when breast-feeding should begin. National Health Goals that involve this time period include the following (DHHS, 2000):

- Reduce the maternal mortality rate to no more than 3.3/100,000 live births, from a baseline of 7.1/100,000.
- Reduce the proportion of births occurring within 24 months of a previous birth to 6%, from a baseline of 11%.
- Increase to at least 75% the proportion of mothers who breast-feed their babies in the early postpartum period, from a baseline of 64%.

Nurses can help the nation achieve these goals by maintaining close observation in the immediate postpartal period to detect maternal hemorrhage, encouraging and supporting women who breast-feed, and ensuring that women receive reproductive life planning information.

Areas that could benefit from additional nursing research include discovering effective means to encourage women to maintain breast-feeding and effective ways to teach women to monitor their own health in the postpartal period, particularly because, due to early discharge, they may be at home when uterine hemorrhage occurs.

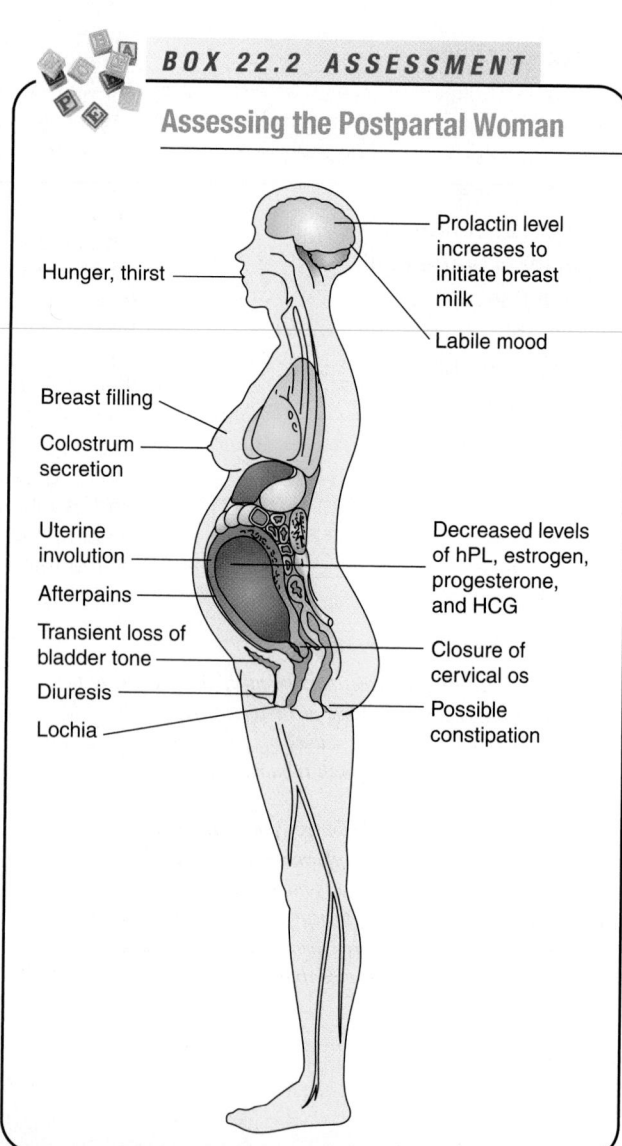

BOX 22.2 ASSESSMENT

Assessing the Postpartal Woman

Hunger, thirst

Breast filling

Colostrum secretion

Uterine involution

Afterpains

Transient loss of bladder tone

Diuresis

Lochia

Prolactin level increases to initiate breast milk

Labile mood

Decreased levels of hPL, estrogen, progesterone, and HCG

Closure of cervical os

Possible constipation

● *Nursing Diagnosis*

Nursing diagnoses during the postpartal period usually are concerned either with a family's inability to accept and bond with a new child or with physiologic considerations. Examples include the following:

- Health-seeking behavior related to care of newborn.
- Risk for impaired parenting related to disappointment in the sex of the child
- Fear related to lack of preparation for child care
- Risk for deficient fluid volume related to postpartal hemorrhage

● *Outcome Identification and Planning*

Be certain that outcomes established during this time are realistic in light of the woman's changed life pattern. Most postpartal families remain in the hospital for a relatively short time, about 48 to 72 hours. The postpartum stay in an alternative birth center can be as short as 4 hours. Outcomes must be devised that can be accomplished and evaluated during this short period of client contact. Inability to accomplish certain outcomes during this time may require follow-up home care.

When planning care in the postpartal period, try to arrange procedures to allow optimal time for family–infant interaction and yet adequate time for the woman to rest, to prevent exhaustion. Prevention of exhaustion can improve coping ability and plans for self-care. After adequate instruction, women should be prepared to monitor their own health after they return home.

Planning should also include ample time for health teaching. An important part of teaching related to care of the newborn is preparation for the unexpected and the need for flexibility, because parents do not yet know what their new life will be like (e.g., whether their child will sleep deeply or fitfully at night, whether their child will become hungry at long or short intervals) or how tired they will become after being awakened frequently during the night. Brainstorming—practicing to produce at least three different methods of reaching a particular goal—is excellent practice for parenting.

● *Implementation*

All interventions in the postpartal period should be family centered, to enhance family functioning and bonding.

Interventions also are geared toward increasing a woman's self-esteem and allowing her to view herself as a new mother and her new infant as part of her family. Teaching new mothers is important, but it is also important to explore what they already know about child care and what they think would be a sensible solution to a problem. Giving advice only solves an immediate problem; helping a woman learn good problem-solving technique improves her ability to handle the many challenges that will arise with child rearing.

● *Outcome Evaluation*

If a woman fails to make an adequate adjustment in the postpartal period, she may have difficulty integrating an infant into the family. This could affect the child's mental health, self-esteem, and ability to form a sense of trust. Follow-up evaluation can be done by telephone, during home visits, or during postpartal and well-child return visits.

Evaluation in the postpartal period involves being certain not only that the woman and her baby are safe but also that the woman knows how to maintain her own health.

Examples of expected outcomes include the following:

- Parents spontaneously make at least one positive comment about their child's characteristics before hospital discharge.
- Client states that she believes she will be able to manage newborn care with the support of her significant other.
- Client's lochial flow is no more than one saturated perineal pad (50 mL) every 3 hours.

PSYCHOLOGICAL CHANGES OF THE POSTPARTAL PERIOD

A transition is a movement or passage from one position or concept to another or a pause between what was and what is to be. It represents an internal process experienced by people when change occurs. In a classic presentation of what transition entails, Bridges (1994) stated that change is something that happens to people, and transition is how they respond to change.

People move through several predictable stages during transition: first is the act of ending old ways of thinking or believing (letting go); next, there is a neutral zone, during which the old way is gone but the new way is not yet comfortable; and finally, there is a new beginning, during which new ideas and concepts are put into action (Bridges, 1994). The postpartum period is a time of transition, during which a couple gives up concepts such as "childless" or "parents of one" and moves to the beginning of new parenthood. The immediate postpartal period is a neutral time during which a couple tries out the new role and attempts to "fit" their expectations for that role. Nurses can help couples acknowledge the extent of the change, so that they can gain closure on their previous lifestyle. Opening channels for communication, anticipating new needs, and highlighting potential gains that will occur because of the change are important actions.

Phases of the Puerperium

In her classic work on maternal behavior, Reva Rubin, a nurse, divided the puerperium into three separate phases (Rubin, 1977). She viewed the first of these as a **taking-in phase,** or a time when the new parents review their pregnancy and the labor and birth. The subsequent phases, called the **taking-hold phase** and the **letting-go phase,** are times of renewed action and forward movement. At the time these phases of the puerperium were identified, women were hospitalized for 5 to 7 days after childbirth and moved in a paced manner from one step to the next. Today, with hospitalization as short as a few hours, women appear to move through these phases much more quickly and may even be experiencing two different phases at once.

Taking-In Phase

The taking-in phase, the first phase experienced, is a time of reflection. During this 2- to 3-day period, the woman is largely passive. She prefers having a nurse minister to her (e.g., bringing her a bath towel or a clean nightgown) and make decisions for her, rather than do these things herself. This dependence results partly from her physical discomfort due to perineal stitches, afterpains, or hemorrhoids; partly from her uncertainty in caring for her newborn; and partly from the extreme exhaustion that follows childbirth.

As a part of thinking and pondering about her new role, the woman usually wants to talk about her pregnancy, especially about her labor and birth. She holds her new child with a sense of wonder and asks: Is birth really over? Could this child really have been inside me? Could I be this lucky? During the taking-in phase, she rests to regain her physical strength and to calm and contain her swirling thoughts. Encouraging her to talk about the birth helps her integrate it into her life experiences (Box 22.3).

Taking-Hold Phase

After a time of passive dependence, the woman begins to initiate action. She prefers to get her own washcloth and to make her own decisions. Women who give birth with-out any anesthesia may reach this second phase in a matter of hours after birth.

During the taking-in period, a woman may have expressed little interest in caring for her child. Now, she begins to take a strong interest. As a rule, therefore, it is always best to give a woman brief demonstrations of baby care and then allow her to care for her child herself—with watchful guidance.

Although a woman's actions suggest strong independence during this time, she often still feels insecure about her ability to care for her new child. She needs praise for the things she does well (e.g., supporting the baby's head, beginning breast-feeding) to give her confidence. This positive reinforcement begins in the health care facility and continues after discharge, at home, and at postpartum and well-baby visits.

Do not rush a woman through the phase of taking-in or prevent her from taking hold when she reaches that point. For many young mothers, learning to make decisions about their child's welfare is one of the most difficult phases of motherhood. It helps if the woman has practice in making such decisions in a sheltered setting, such as a hospital, rather than first taking on that level of responsibility after she is on her own.

Letting-Go Phase

In the third phase, called letting-go, the woman finally redefines her new role. She gives up the fantasized image of

---

BOX 22.3 FOCUS ON . . .

COMMUNICATION

Joan Cooper gave birth 6 hours ago. You want to assess her for postpartal pain, so you enter her hospital room. She is wearing a hospital gown and sitting in the chair by her bed.

Less Effective Communication

Nurse: How are you feeling, Mrs. Cooper?

Mrs. Cooper: Like I'm still rushing around. I called my husband as soon as my water broke. He hit a truck on the way home, though, so he couldn't get there in time. I tried to call—

Nurse: Do you have any pain?

Mrs. Cooper: It's not bad. I tried to call my mother, but she couldn't come over because she didn't have a car. Our neighbor—

Nurse: Okay, then let me check your stitches.

More Effective Communication

Nurse: How are you feeling, Mrs. Cooper?

Mrs. Cooper: Like I'm still rushing around. I called my husband as soon as my water broke. He hit a truck on the way home, though, so he couldn't get there in time. I tried to call—

Nurse: Do you have any pain?

Mrs. Cooper: It's not bad. I tried to call my mother, but she couldn't come over because she didn't have a car. Our neighbor—

Nurse: Go on. I didn't mean to interrupt.

Mrs. Cooper: Our neighbor said he'd drive me but then discovered his wife had his car keys. It was a three-ring circus of problems.

Nurse: A three-ring circus?

Mrs. Cooper: Finally, my husband made it home, but then there was such a bad accident on the freeway we had to drive all the way around the lake. I thought I'd have the baby in the middle of the bridge!

Nurse: That must have been terrifying for you.

Most women are interested in discussing their labor and birth experience in the days immediately after birth as a part of a "taking-in" phase. Repeating the story of how worried they were when labor started, how much pain they had, or how scared they were when their membranes broke helps them put these sensations into perspective and integrate them into their life experiences. Communication that encourages women to elaborate on a story is therapeutic; communication that discourages story-telling is not. Once you have talked about what concerned her most, returning to a discussion and assessment of her pain would be appropriate.

her child and accepts the real one; she gives up her old role of being childless or the mother of only one or two (or however many children she had before this birth). This process requires some grief work and readjustment of relationships, similar to what occurred during pregnancy. It is extended and continues during the child's growing years. A woman who has reached this phase is well into her new role.

Checkpoint Question 1

Which of the following actions would alert you that a new mother is entering a postpartal taking-hold phase?

a. She tells you she was in a lot of pain all during labor.
b. She sleeps as if exhausted from the effort of labor.
c. She urges the baby to stay awake so that she can breast-feed him or her.
d. She says that she has not selected a name for the baby as yet.

Development of Parental Love and Positive Family Relationships

During pregnancy, almost every woman worries about her ability to be a "good" mother, and this concern does not evaporate as soon as the baby is born. Some women seem able to recognize a newborn's needs immediately and to give care with confident understanding right from the start. More often, however, a woman enters into a relationship with her newborn tentatively and with qualms and conflicts that must be addressed before the relationship can be meaningful. This is because parental love is only partly instinctive. A major portion develops gradually, in stages such as planning the pregnancy, hearing the pregnancy confirmed, feeling the child move in utero, birthing, seeing the baby, touching the baby, and, finally, giving total care for the child. Factors such as a difficult labor or transport and separation from the newborn may lead to symptoms of a traumatic stress disorder that slows the process or interferes with the ability to bond warmly (Beck, 2004).

Many women may not experience maternal feelings for their infants until days or even weeks after giving birth. Some fathers admit they have difficulty "claiming" or bonding with an infant (feeling fatherly toward the new child) until as late as 3 months after the birth, when the child begins to smile or coo and interact more directly with them. The ability of both parents to reach out to their child can be strengthened by allowing them to touch and spend as much time as possible with the new child during the first few hours of life.

Forming a strong bond with a child is not a problem only for first-time parents. Experienced parents can have just as much difficulty—they know they love 4-year-old Johnny and 2-year-old Sue at home, but worry that their hearts may not be big enough to love a third child, too.

Because of these mixed feelings, parents may not show genuine warmth the first time they hold their infant. Although the woman carried the child inside her for 9 months, she now approaches her newborn as she would

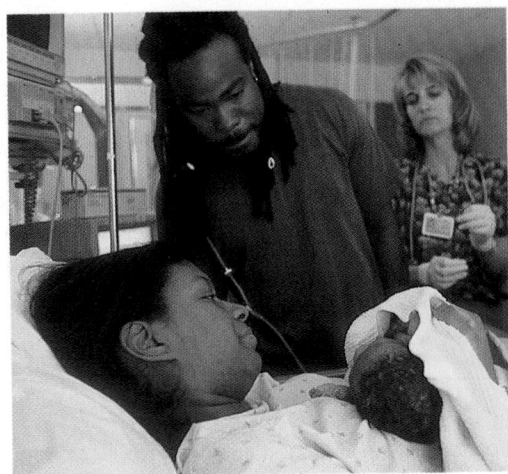

FIGURE 22.1 A mom and dad begin interaction with their newborn immediately after birth: a very special moment in their life. (© Kathy Sloane.)

a stranger. The first time she holds the infant, she may touch only the blanket and never make close physical contact. If she unfolds the blanket to examine the baby or count the fingers or toes, she may use only her fingertips for touch (Fig. 22.1).

Gradually, as the woman holds her child more, she begins to express more warmth, touching the child with the palm of her hand rather than with her fingertips. She smooths the baby's hair, brushes a cheek, plays with toes, and lets the baby's fingers clasp hers. Soon, she feels comfortable enough to press her cheek against the baby's or kiss the infant's nose or mouth; she has become a mother tending to her child. This identification process is termed *claiming* or *bonding*. Looking directly at her newborn's face, with direct eye contact (termed an **en face position**), is a sign a woman is beginning effective interaction. Many fathers can be observed staring at a newborn for long intervals in this same way. Often termed **engrossment,** this action alerts caregivers to how actively the father, as well as the mother, contributes to bonding (Fig. 22.2). The length

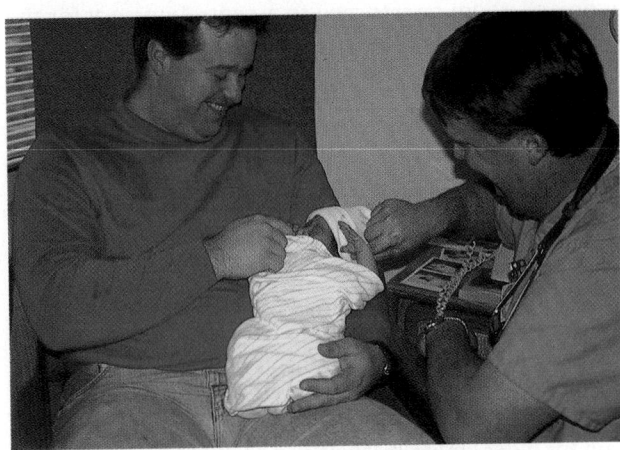

FIGURE 22.2 A nurse encourages a father as he interacts and bonds with his newborn. (© Caroline Brown, RNC, MS, DEd.)

of time parents take to bond with a child depends on the circumstances of the pregnancy and birth, the wellness and ability of the child to meet the parent's expectations, reciprocal actions by the newborn, and the opportunities the parents have to interact with the child. Freedom from stringent rules helps to develop good parent–child relationships. To help parents sort out their feelings about being a mother or father and about their new responsibility, provide a supportive presence and offer anticipatory guidance if necessary.

Checkpoint Question 2

You observe Joan Cooper holding her newborn. Which position would best reassure you that she is relating well to her newborn?

a. She looks directly at her infant's face and talks to him.
b. She holds the infant over her shoulder to burp him.
c. She sits in a rocking chair and rocks the new infant.
d. She lies in bed and places the infant on her stomach.

Rooming-In

The more time a woman has to spend with her baby, the sooner she may feel competent in child care, and the more likely she may be to form a sound mother–child relationship (Crenshaw, 2004). Because the average postpartal hospital stay ranges from 1 to 3 days, a woman has very little time to become acquainted with her newborn before going home. If her infant stays in the room with her (called **rooming-in**) rather than in a central nursery, she can become better acquainted with her child and begin to feel more confident in her ability to care for him or her after discharge. In many settings, the father can stay overnight in the room, or room-in, as well.

There are two types of rooming-in: complete, in which the mother and child are together 24 hours a day, and partial, in which the infant remains in the woman's room for most of the time, perhaps from 8:00 AM to 9:00 PM, but then he or she is taken to a small nursery near the woman's room or returned to a central nursery for the night. With both complete and partial rooming-in, the father and siblings can hold and feed the infant when they visit.

Rooming-in also may allow a couple to retain anticipatory guidance and instructions in newborn care better, because a nurse has demonstrated bathing, feeding, changing, and so forth on their own child.

Sibling Visitation

Separation from children is often as painful for a mother as it is for her children. Waiting at home, separated from their mother and listening only to telephone reports of what a new brother or sister looks like, can be very difficult for older children. They may picture the new baby as much older than he or she actually is. "He is eating well" may produce an image of a child sitting at a table using a fork and spoon. "He weighs 8 pounds" can be meaning-less information. A chance to visit the hospital and see the new baby and their mother reduces feelings that their mother cares more about the new baby than about them. It can help to relieve some of the impact of separation. It helps to make the baby a part of the family (Fig. 22.3).

Check to be sure that siblings are free of contagious diseases (e.g., upper respiratory tract illnesses, recent exposure to chickenpox) before they visit. Then, have them wash their hands and, if they choose, actually hold or touch the newborn with parental assistance. Some hospitals require siblings to wear a cover gown before holding a new brother or sister.

You may need to caution a woman that the opinions of a new brother or sister expressed by her older children may not be complimentary. This baby with little hair is not their idea of a "pretty baby." If they thought the new baby would be big enough to play with, they may not believe that he is a "big baby." However, seeing the baby, even if his or her appearance is not what the other children expected, is helpful in establishing strong relationships and should be encouraged.

Maternal Concerns and Feelings in the Postpartal Period

Traditionally, it is assumed that the bulk of a woman's concerns in the postpartal period center on the care of her new infant. Based on this, classes in the postpartal period have traditionally focused on teaching how to breast-feed and bathe infants. Although these acts are concerns for many mothers, they are not necessarily a new mother's chief concern. She has come through a tremendous psychological experience during pregnancy and the birth of a child. She is in the middle of a complete role change. It is only to be expected that some of her attention and in-

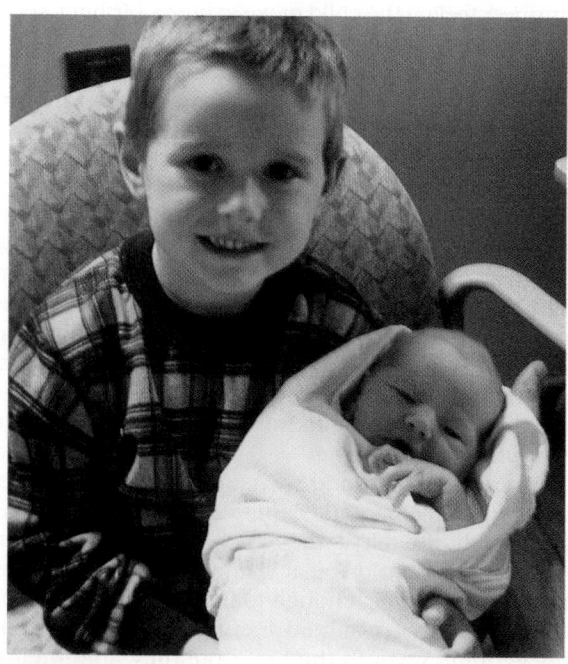

FIGURE 22.3 Sibling visiting is important to bring a family together.

terest during this time will be directed inward as she tries to view herself in this new role.

Typical issues identified by postpartal women include breast soreness; regaining their figure; regulating the demands of housework, their partner, and their children; coping with emotional tension and sibling jealousy; and fatigue.

Abandonment

Many mothers, if given the opportunity, admit to feeling abandoned and less important after giving birth. Only hours before, they were the center of attention, with everyone asking about their health and well-being. Now, suddenly, the baby seems to be everyone's chief interest. Relatives ask about the baby; the gifts are all for the baby. Even a woman's obstetrician, who has made her feel so important for the last 9 months, may ask during a visit, "How's that healthy 8-pound boy?" It can make a woman feel confused by a sensation very close to jealousy. And how can a good mother be jealous of her own baby?

You can help a woman move past these feelings by verbalizing the problem: "How things have changed! Everyone's asking about the baby today and not about you, aren't they? How does that make you feel?" These are welcome words for a woman to hear. It is reassuring to know that the sensation she is experiencing, although uncomfortable, is normal.

When a newborn comes home, a father may express much the same feelings. He may become resentful of the time the mother spends with the infant. Perhaps the two used to sit at the table after dinner and discuss their day or the future, and now she hurries away to feed the baby. She used to watch the late show with him at night; now she goes to bed earlier, because she knows she will be up again at 2:00 AM.

Examination of competitive feelings—both motherhood and fatherhood involve some compromise in favor of the baby's interests—should start during the pregnancy or early in the postpartal period. Making infant care a shared responsibility can help alleviate these feelings and make both partners feel equally involved in the baby's care.

Disappointment

Another common feeling parents may experience is disappointment in the baby. All during pregnancy, they pictured a chubby-cheeked, curly-haired, smiling girl or boy. They have instead a skinny baby, without any hair, who seems to cry constantly. It can be difficult for parents to feel positive immediately about a child who does not meet their expectations in this way. It can cause parents to remember their adolescence, when they felt gangly and unattractive, or to experience feelings of inadequacy all over again.

You can never change the sex, size, or look of a child, but in the short time you care for a postpartal family, you can help to change the feelings of the mother or father about their infant. Handle the child warmly, to show that you find the infant satisfactory or even special. Comment on the child's good points, such as long fingers, lovely eyes, and good appetite. During periods of crisis such as childbearing, it is possible for a key person (e.g., a nurse) to offer support that tips the scale toward acceptance or at least helps the person involved to take a clearer look at his or her situation and begin to cope with the new circumstances.

Postpartal Blues

During the postpartal period, as many as 50% of women experience some feelings of overwhelming sadness (St. John & Rouse, 2003). They may burst into tears easily or feel let down or irritable. This temporary feeling after birth has long been known as the "baby blues." This phenomenon may be caused by hormonal changes, particularly the decrease in estrogen and progesterone that occurs with delivery of the placenta. For some women, it may be a response to dependence and low self-esteem caused by exhaustion, being away from home, physical discomfort, and the tension engendered by assuming a new role, especially if the woman is not receiving support from her partner. The syndrome is evidenced by tearfulness, feelings of inadequacy, mood lability, anorexia, and sleep disturbance.

You can reassure a woman that sudden crying episodes are normal; otherwise, she may have difficulty understanding what is happening to her. Her support person also needs reassurance, or lest he think the woman is unhappy with him or with their new baby or is keeping some terrible secret about the baby from him.

Anticipatory guidance and individualized support from health care personnel are important to help the parents understand that this response is normal. It is also important to give the woman a chance to verbalize her feelings: "I know there's absolutely no reason for me to be crying, but I cannot stop." Allowing her to make as many decisions as possible can help give her a sense of control over her life.

Remember, however, that not all postpartal women cry because they have baby blues. A woman sometimes has other reasons to feel sad during this time. Perhaps problems at home have become overwhelming. Her husband may have been laid off from his job just when they most need the money. One of her parents may be ill, or her house may have been damaged in some way. Keeping the lines of communication open is important to help differentiate between problems that can be handled best with discussion and concerned understanding and those that should be referred to the social service department or a community health agency.

Thirty percent of women experience a more serious level of sadness after birth, termed **postpartal depression.** Serious depression requiring formal counseling or psychiatric care occurs in about 12% of women during this time (St. John & Rouse, 2003). Because they are complications of the puerperium, postpartal depression and psychosis are discussed in Chapter 23.

PHYSIOLOGIC CHANGES OF THE POSTPARTAL PERIOD

Retrogressive physiologic changes that occur during the postpartal period include those related specifically to the reproductive system as well as other systemic changes.

Reproductive System Changes

Involution is the process whereby the reproductive organs return to their nonpregnant state. A woman is in danger of hemorrhage from the denuded surface of the uterus until involution is complete (Ural, 2004).

The Uterus

Involution of the uterus involves two main processes. First, the area where the placenta was implanted is sealed off to prevent bleeding. Second, the organ is reduced to its approximate pregestational size.

The sealing of the placenta site is accomplished by rapid contraction of the uterus immediately after delivery of the placenta. This contraction pinches the blood vessels entering the 7-cm-wide area left denuded by the placenta and stops bleeding. With time, thrombi form within the uterine sinuses and permanently seal the area. Eventually, endometrial tissue undermines the site and obliterates the organized thrombi, covering and healing the area so completely that the process leaves no scar tissue within the uterus and does not compromise future implantation sites.

The same contraction process reduces the bulk of the uterus. Devoid of the placenta and the membranes, the walls of the uterus thicken and contract, gradually reducing the uterus from a container large enough to hold a full-term fetus to one the size of a grapefruit. A few cells of the uterine wall are broken down into their protein components by an autolytic process. These components are then absorbed by the bloodstream and excreted by the body in urine. The main mechanism that reduces the bulk of the uterus, however, is contraction, a phenomenon that can be compared with a rubber band which has been stretched for many months and now is regaining its normal contour. None of the rubber band is destroyed; the shape is simply altered. For this reason, the postpartal period, like pregnancy, is not a period of illness, of necrosing cells being evacuated, but primarily a period of healthy change.

Although the uterus will never completely return to its prepregnancy state, its reduction in size is dramatic. Immediately after birth, the uterus weighs about 1,000 g. At the end of the first week, it weighs 500 g. By the time involution is complete (6 weeks), it weighs approximately 50 g, similar to its prepregnant weight.

Because uterine contraction begins immediately after placental delivery, the fundus of the uterus may be palpated through the abdominal wall, halfway between the umbilicus and the symphysis pubis, within a few minutes after birth. One hour later, it will have risen to the level of the umbilicus, where it remains for approximately the next 24 hours. From then on, it decreases one fingerbreadth per day—on the first postpartal day, it will be palpable one fingerbreadth below the umbilicus; on the second day, two fingerbreadths below the umbilicus; and so on. Because a fingerbreadth is about 1 cm, this can be recorded as 1 cm below the umbilicus, 2 cm below it, and so forth. In the average woman, by the ninth or tenth day, the uterus will have contracted so much that it is withdrawn into the pelvis and can no longer be detected by abdominal palpation (Fig. 22.4). The uterus of a breast-feeding mother may

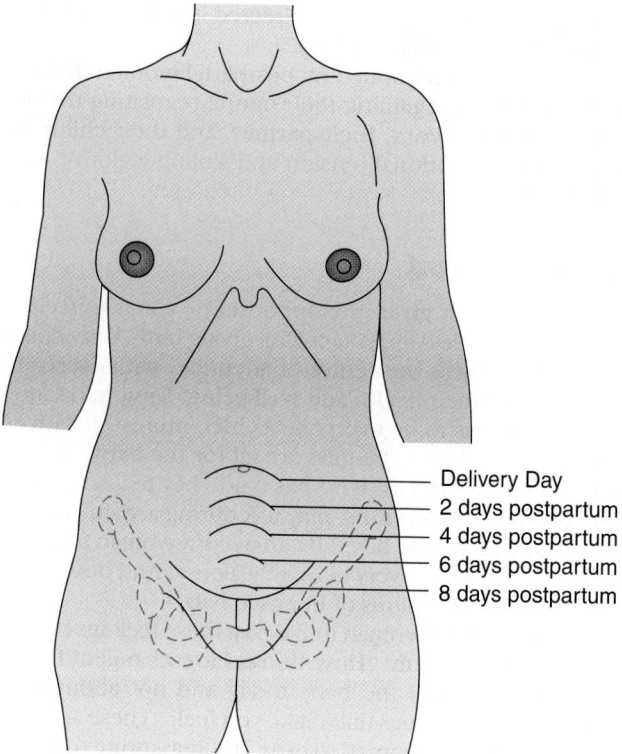

Delivery Day
2 days postpartum
4 days postpartum
6 days postpartum
8 days postpartum

FIGURE 22.4 Uterine involution. The uterus decreases in size at a predictable rate during the postpartal period. After 10 days, it recedes under the pubic bone and is no longer palpable.

contract even more quickly, because oxytocin, which is released with breast-feeding, stimulates uterine contractions. However, breast-feeding alone is not enough to protect against postpartum hemorrhage.

The fundus is normally in the midline of the abdomen. Occasionally, it is found slightly to the right, because the bulk of the sigmoid colon forces it to that side during pregnancy and it tends to remain in that position. Assess fundal height shortly after a woman has emptied her bladder for most accurate results, because a full bladder can keep the uterus from contracting, pushing it upward and possibly deviating it from the midline, due to the laxness of the uterine ligaments.

Uterine involution may be delayed by a condition such as birth of multiple fetuses, hydramnios, exhaustion from prolonged labor or a difficult birth, grand multiparity, or physiologic effects of excessive analgesia. Contraction may be difficult if there is retained placenta or membranes or a full bladder. Involution will occur most dependably in a woman who is well nourished and who ambulates early after birth (gravity may play a role).

An estimation of the consistency of the postpartal uterus is as important as measurement of its height. A well-contracted fundus feels firm. It can be compared with a grapefruit in both size and tenseness. Whenever the fundus feels boggy (soft or flabby), it is not as contracted as it should be, despite its position in the abdomen.

The first hour after birth is potentially the most dangerous time for a woman. If her uterus should become relaxed during this time (**uterine atony**), she will lose blood very rapidly, because no permanent thrombi have yet formed at the placental site.

In some women, contraction of the uterus after birth causes intermittent cramping similar to that accompanying a menstrual period. These cramps are termed **afterpains.** They tend to be noticed most by multiparas rather than primiparas and by women who have given birth to large babies or had an overdistended uterus for any other reason. In these situations, the uterus must contract more forcefully to regain its prepregnancy size and has difficulty maintaining a steady contracted state. These sensations are noticed most intensely with breast-feeding, when the infant's sucking causes a release of oxytocin from the posterior pituitary, increasing the strength of the contractions.

Lochia

The separation of the placenta and membranes occurs in the spongy layer or outer portion of the decidua basalis. By the second day after birth, the layer of decidua remaining under the placental site (an area 7 cm wide) and throughout the uterus differentiates into two distinct layers. The inner layer attached to the muscular wall of the uterus remains, serving as the foundation from which a new layer of endometrium will be formed. The layer adjacent to the uterine cavity becomes necrotic and is cast off as a uterine discharge similar to a menstrual flow. This uterine flow, consisting of blood, fragments of decidua, white blood cells, mucus, and some bacteria, is known as **lochia.**

The portion of the uterus where the placenta was not attached is so fully cleansed by this sloughing process it will be in a reproductive state in about 3 weeks' time. It takes approximately 6 weeks (the entire postpartal period) for the placental implantation site to be cleansed and healed.

For the first 3 days after birth, a lochia discharge consists almost entirely of blood, with only small particles of decidua and mucus. Because of its mainly red color, it is termed **lochia rubra.** As the amount of blood involved in the cast-off tissue decreases (about the fourth day) and leukocytes begin to invade the area, as they do with any healing surface, the flow becomes pink or brownish in color (**lochia serosa**). On about the tenth day, the amount of the flow decreases and becomes colorless or white (**lochia alba**). Lochia alba is present in most women until the third week after birth, although it is not unusual for a lochia flow to last the entire 6 weeks of the puerperium. Characteristics of lochia are summarized in Table 22.1. Several rules for judging whether lochia flow is normal are summarized in Box 22.4.

The Cervix

Immediately after birth, a cervix is soft and malleable. Both the internal and external os are open. Like contraction of the uterus, contraction of the cervix toward its prepregnant state begins at once. By the end of 7 days, the external os has narrowed to the size of a pencil opening; the cervix feels firm and nongravid again.

In contrast to the process of uterine involution, in which the changes consist primarily of old cells being returned to their former position by contraction, the process in the

TABLE 22.1

Characteristics of Lochia

Type of Lochia	Color	Postpartal Day	Composition
Lochia rubra	Red	1–3	Blood, fragments of decidua, and mucus
Lochia serosa	Pink	3–10	Blood, mucus, and invading leukocytes
Lochia alba	White	10–14 (may last 6 weeks)	Largely mucus; leukocyte count high

cervix involves the formation of new muscle cells. Like the fundus, the cervix does not return exactly to its prepregnant state. The internal os closes as before, but after a vaginal birth the external os usually remains slightly open and appears slitlike or stellate (star shaped), whereas previously it was round. Finding this pattern on pelvic examination suggests that childbearing has taken place.

The Vagina

After a vaginal birth, the vagina is soft, with few rugae, and its diameter is considerably greater than normal. The hymen is permanently torn and heals with small, separate tags of tissue. It takes the entire postpartal period for the vagina to involute (by contraction, as with the uterus) until it gradually returns to its approximate prepregnant state. Thickening of the walls also appears to depend on renewed estrogen stimulation from the ovaries. Because a woman who is breast-feeding may have delayed ovulation, she may continue to have thin-walled or fragile vaginal cells that cause slight vaginal bleeding during sexual intercourse until about 6 weeks' time. Like the cervix, the vaginal outlet remains slightly more distended than before. If a woman practices Kegel exercises, the strength and tone of the vagina will increase more rapidly (see Chapter 11). This may be important for the sexual enjoyment of both the woman and her partner.

The Perineum

Because of the great amount of pressure experienced during birth, the perineum develops edema and generalized tenderness. Ecchymosis from ruptured capillaries may show on the surface. The labia majora and labia minora typically remain atrophic and softened after birth, never returning to their prepregnant state.

Systemic Changes

The same body systems that are involved in pregnancy are also involved in postpartal changes as the body returns to its prepregnant state.

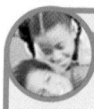

BOX 22.4 FOCUS ON . . .

FAMILY TEACHING

Evaluating Lochia Flow

Q. Joan Cooper asks you, "How do I know if my lochia is normal?"

A. A number of guidelines are helpful for evaluating lochia flow:

Evaluate the Amount: Lochia amount will vary from woman to woman. Mothers who breast-feed tend to have less lochial discharge than those who do not, because the natural release of the hormone oxytocin during breast-feeding strengthens uterine contractions. Conservation of fluid for lactation also may be a factor. Lochial flow increases on exertion, especially the first few times a woman is out of bed, but decreases again with rest. The increase in amount that occurs with ambulation is the result of vaginal discharge of pooled lochia, not a true increase in amount. However, lochia amount truly does increase with strenuous exercise, such as lifting a heavy weight or walking up stairs. Saturating a perineal pad in less than 1 hour is considered an abnormally heavy flow and should be reported.

Check the Consistency: Lochia should contain no large clots. Clots may indicate that a portion of the placenta has been retained and is preventing closure of the maternal uterine blood sinuses. In any event, large clots denote poor uterine contraction, which needs to be corrected.

Observe the Pattern: Lochia is red for the first 1 to 3 days (lochia rubra), pinkish-brown from days 4 to 10 (lochia serosa), and then white (lochia alba) for as long as 6 weeks after birth. The pattern of lochia (rubra to serosa to alba) should not reverse. A red flow after a pink or white flow may indicate that placental fragments have been retained or that uterine contraction is decreasing and new bleeding is beginning.

Assess the Odor: Lochia should not have an offensive odor. Lochia has the same odor as menstrual blood. An offensive odor usually indicates that the uterus has become infected. Immediate intervention is needed to halt postpartal infection.

Watch for Absence: Lochia should never be absent during the first 1 to 3 weeks. Absence of lochia, like presence of an offensive odor, may indicate postpartal infection. Lochia may be scant in amount after cesarean birth, but it is never altogether absent.

The Hormonal System

Pregnancy hormones begin to decrease as soon as the placenta is no longer present. Levels of human chorionic gonadotropin (hCG) and human placental lactogen (hPL) are almost negligible by 24 hours. By week 1, progestin, estrone, and estradiol are at prepregnancy levels. Estrol may be elevated for an additional week before it reaches prepregnancy levels. Follicle-stimulating hormone (FSH) remains low for about 12 days and then begins to rise as a new menstrual cycle is initiated.

The Urinary System

During pregnancy, as much as 2,000 to 3,000 mL excess fluid accumulates in the body. An extensive diuresis begins to take place almost immediately after birth to rid the body of this fluid. This easily increases the daily output of a postpartal woman from a normal level of 1,500 mL to as much as 3,000 mL/day during the second to fifth day after birth. This marked increase in urine production causes the bladder to fill rapidly.

During a vaginal birth, the fetal head exerts a great deal of pressure on the bladder and urethra as it passes on the bladder's underside. This pressure may leave the bladder with a transient loss of tone that, together with the edema surrounding the urethra, decreases a woman's ability to sense when she has to void. A woman who has undergone epidural, spinal, or general anesthesia can feel no sensation in the bladder area until the anesthetic has worn off.

To prevent permanent damage to the bladder from overdistention, assess the woman's abdomen frequently in the immediate postpartal period. On palpation, a full bladder is felt as a hard or firm area just above the symphysis pubis. On percussion (placing one finger flat on the woman's abdomen over the bladder and tapping it with the middle finger of the other hand), a full bladder sounds resonant, in contrast to the dull, thudding sound of non–fluid-filled tissue. Pressure on this area may make a woman feel as if she has to void, but she is then unable to do so. As the bladder fills, it displaces the uterus; uterine position is therefore a good gauge of whether a bladder is full or empty. If the uterus is becoming uncontracted or feels soft on palpation and is pushed to the side, the usual cause is an overfilled bladder.

The hydronephrosis or increased size of ureters that occurred during pregnancy remains present for about 4 weeks after delivery. The increased size of these structures, in conjunction with reduced bladder sensitivity, increases the possibility of urinary stasis and urinary tract infection in the postpartal period.

In the postpartal period, urine tends to contain more nitrogen than normal. This is probably due in part to a woman's increased muscle activity during labor and in part to the breakdown of protein in a portion of the uterine muscle that occurs during involution. Lactose levels in the urine are the same as during pregnancy, as the body prepares for breast-feeding. Diaphoresis (excessive sweating) is another way by which the body rids itself of excess fluid. This is noticeable in women soon after birth.

The Circulatory System

The diuresis that is evident between the second and fifth days after birth, as well as the blood loss at birth, act to reduce the added blood volume a woman has accumulated during pregnancy. This reduction occurs so rapidly, in fact, that the blood volume has returned to its normal prepregnancy level by the first or second week after birth.

Usual blood loss with a vaginal birth is 300 to 500 mL. With a cesarean birth, it is 500 to 1,000 mL. A four-point decrease in hematocrit (proportion of red blood cells to circulating plasma) and a 1-g decrease in hemoglobin value occurs with each 250 mL of blood lost. For example, if an average woman enters labor with a hematocrit of 37%, it will be about 33% on the first postpartal day, and hemoglobin will fall from 11 to 10 g/dL. If the woman was anemic during pregnancy, she can expect to continue to be anemic afterward. As excess fluid is excreted, the hematocrit gradually rises (due to hemoconcentration), reaching prepregnancy levels by 6 weeks after delivery.

Women usually continue to have the same high level of plasma fibrinogen during the first postpartal weeks as they did during pregnancy. This is a protective measure against hemorrhage. However, this high level also increases the risk of thrombus formation. There is also an increase in the number of leukocytes in the blood. The white blood cell count may be as high as 30,000 cells/mm³ (mainly granulocytes), particularly if labor was long or difficult. This, too, is part of the body's defense system, a defense against infection and an aid to healing.

Any varicosities that are present will recede, but they rarely return to a completely prepregnant appearance. Although vascular blemishes, such as spider angiomas, fade slightly, they may not disappear completely either.

The Gastrointestinal System

Digestion and absorption begin to be active again soon after birth. Almost immediately, the woman feels hungry and thirsty because of the long period of restricted fluid during labor and the beginning diaphoresis. Unless she has aftereffects of general anesthesia, she can eat without difficulty from nausea or vomiting during this time.

Hemorrhoids (distended rectal veins) that have been pushed out of the rectum due to the effort of pelvic-stage pushing often are present. Bowel sounds are active, but passage of stool through the bowel may be slow because of the still-present effect of relaxin on the bowel. Bowel evacuation may be difficult due to the pain of episiotomy sutures or hemorrhoids.

The Integumentary System

After birth, the stretch marks on the woman's abdomen (striae gravidarum) still appear reddened and may be even more prominent than during pregnancy, when they were tightly stretched. Typically, in a Caucasian woman, these will fade to a pale white over the next 3 to 6 months; in an African-American woman, they may remain as areas of slightly darker pigment. Excessive pigment on the face and neck (chloasma) and on the abdomen (linea nigra) will become barely detectable in 6 weeks' time. If **diastasis recti** (overstretching and separation of the abdominal musculature) is present, the area will appear slightly indented. If the separation is large, it will appear as a bluish area in the abdominal midline. Modified sit-ups help to strengthen abdominal muscles and return abdominal support to its prepregnant level. Both the abdominal wall and the ligaments that support the uterus, which were obviously stretched during pregnancy, usually require the full 6 weeks of the puerperium to return to their former state.

Effects of Retrogressive Changes

The overall effects of the postpartal changes discussed earlier are exhaustion and weight loss.

Exhaustion

As soon as birth is completed, a woman experiences total exhaustion. For the last several months of pregnancy, she probably has experienced some difficulty sleeping. Near the end of pregnancy, she probably was unable to find a comfortable position in bed because of the fetus' activity or the presence of back or leg pain. All during labor, she has eaten very little, if anything, and has worked very hard with little or no sleep. Now she has "sleep hunger," which may make it difficult for her to cope with new experiences and stressful situations.

Weight Loss

The rapid diuresis and diaphoresis during the second to fifth days after birth usually result in a weight loss of 5 lb (2 to 4 kg), in addition to the approximately 12 lb (5.8 kg) lost at birth. Lochia flow causes an additional 2- to 3-lb (1-kg) loss, for a total weight loss of about 19 lb. Additional weight loss is most dependent on the amount of pregnancy weight gain and whether the woman takes active measures to lose weight. It is also influenced by nutrition, exercise, and breast-feeding. The weight a woman reaches at 6 weeks after birth becomes her baseline postpartal weight. In many women, this baseline is higher than their prepregnancy weight, and this is one of the reasons that obesity has become a national health concern.

Vital Sign Changes

Vital sign changes in the postpartum period reflect the internal adjustments that occur as the woman's body returns to its prepregnant state.

Temperature

Temperature is always taken orally or tympanically (never rectally) during the puerperium, because of the danger of vaginal contamination and the discomfort involved in rectal intrusion.

A woman may show a slight increase in temperature during the first 24 hours after birth because of dehydration that occurred during labor. If she receives adequate fluid during the first 24 hours, this temperature elevation will return to normal. Most women are thirsty immediately after birth and are eager to take in fluid. This makes drinking a large quantity of fluid not a problem unless the woman is nauseated from a birth anesthetic.

Any woman whose oral temperature rises above 100.4°F (38°C), excluding the first 24-hour period, is considered by criteria of the Joint Commission on Maternal Welfare to be febrile. In such cases, a postpartal infection may be present.

Occasionally, when a woman's breasts fill with milk on the third or fourth postpartum day, her temperature rises for a period of hours because of the increased vascular activity involved. If the elevation in temperature lasts longer than a few hours, however, infection is a more likely reason. Infection is a major cause of postpartal mortality and morbidity. Because nurses play a major role in assessing postpartum temperature, they have the important role of being the health care providers who may first detect infection.

Pulse

A woman's pulse rate during the postpartal period is usually slightly slower than normal. During pregnancy, the distended uterus obstructed the amount of venous blood returning to the heart; after birth, to accommodate the increased blood volume returning to the heart, stroke volume increases. This increased stroke volume reduces the pulse rate to between 60 and 70 bpm. As diuresis diminishes the blood volume and causes blood pressure to fall, the pulse rate increases accordingly. By the end of the first week, the pulse rate will have returned to normal.

Evaluate pulse rate conscientiously in the postpartal period, because a rapid and thready pulse during this time could be a sign of hemorrhage. Be certain to compare a woman's pulse rate with the normal range of the postpartal period, not with the normal pulse rate in the general population. Otherwise, this important finding of hemorrhage may be missed.

Blood Pressure

Blood pressure should also be monitored carefully during the postpartal period, because a decrease can indicate bleeding. In contrast, an elevation above 140 mm Hg systolic or 90 mm Hg diastolic may indicate the development of postpartal pregnancy-induced hypertension, an unusual but serious complication of the puerperium (Matthys et al., 2004) (see Chapter 15).

To evaluate blood pressure, compare the woman's pressure with her prepregnancy level if possible, rather than with standard blood pressure ranges; otherwise, if her blood pressure rose during pregnancy, a significant postpartal decrease in pressure could be missed.

Oxytocics, drugs frequently administered during the postpartal period to achieve uterine contraction, cause contraction of all smooth muscle, including blood vessels. Consequently, these drugs can increase blood pressure. To prevent blood pressure from rising too high, always measure it before administering one of these agents. If the blood pressure is greater than 140/90 mm Hg, withhold the agent and notify the woman's physician or nurse-midwife to prevent hypertension and, possibly, cerebrovascular accident.

A major complication in women who have lost an appreciable amount of blood with birth is orthostatic hypotension, or dizziness that occurs on standing due to the lack of adequate blood volume to maintain nourishment of brain cells. To test whether a woman will be susceptible to orthostatic hypotension, assess her blood pressure and pulse while she is lying supine. Next, raise the head of the bed fully upright, wait 2 or 3 minutes, and reassess these values. If the pulse rate is increased by more than 20 bpm and blood pressure is 15 to 20 mm Hg lower than formerly, the woman might be susceptible to dizziness and fainting when she ambulates. Advise her to always sit up slowly and "dangle" on the side of her bed before attempting to walk. If she notices obvious dizziness on sitting upright, support her during ambulation to avoid the possibility of a fall. Caution her not to attempt to walk carrying her newborn until her cardiovascular status adjusts better to her blood loss. Inform the woman's physician or nurse-midwife of these findings.

What if... Joan Cooper, now 12 hours postpartum, has an oral temperature of 99°F (37.2°C) and is uncomfortable from profuse diaphoresis and extreme fatigue. What actions would you take?

Progressive Changes

Two physiologic changes that occur during the puerperium involve progressive changes, or the building of new tissue. Because building new tissue requires good nutrition, caution women against strict dieting that would limit cell-building ability during the first 6 weeks after childbirth.

Lactation

The formation of breast milk (lactation) begins in a postpartal woman whether or not she plans to breast-feed.

Early in pregnancy, the increased estrogen level produced by the placenta stimulates the growth of milk glands; breasts increase in size due to the larger glands, accumulated fluid, and some extra adipose tissue. For the first 2 days after birth, an average woman notices little change in her breasts from the way they were during pregnancy. Since midway through pregnancy, she has been secreting colostrum, a thin, watery, prelactation secretion. She continues to excrete this fluid the first 2 postpartum days. On the third day, her breasts become full and feel tense or tender as milk forms within breast ducts.

Breast milk forms in response to the decrease in estrogen and progesterone levels that follows delivery of the placenta (which stimulates prolactin production and, consequently, milk production). When breast milk first begins to form, the milk ducts become distended. The nipple secretion changes from the clear colostrum to bluish white, the typical color of breast milk. The woman's breasts become fuller, larger, and firmer. In many women, breast distention becomes marked, and this often is accompanied by a feeling of heat or throbbing pain. Breast tissue may appear reddened, simulating an acute inflammatory or infectious process. The distention is not limited to the milk ducts but occurs in the surrounding tissue as well, because blood and lymph enter the area to contribute fluid to the formation of milk. This feeling of tension in the breasts on the third or fourth day after delivery is termed **primary engorgement.** It fades as the infant begins effective sucking and empties the breasts of milk. Whether milk production continues depends on the sucking of the infant at the breasts or the use of a breast pump; both actions release oxytocin, contract milk ducts, and push milk forward to cause a let-down reflex. Whether women continue to breast-feed after hospital discharge is influenced by such factors as employment, personal habits, and how important they view breast-feeding to be (Dodgson et al., 2004). Postpartum care of breasts and breast-feeding are discussed in Chapter 25.

Return of Menstrual Flow

With the delivery of the placenta, the production of placental estrogen and progesterone ends. The resulting decrease in hormone concentrations causes a rise in production of FSH by the pituitary, which leads, with only a slight delay, to the return of ovulation. This initiates the return of normal menstrual cycles.

A woman who is not breast-feeding can expect her menstrual flow to return in 6 to 10 weeks after birth. If she is breast-feeding, menstrual flow may not return for 3 or 4 months (lactational amenorrhea) or, in some women, for the entire lactation period. However, the absence of a menstrual flow does not guarantee that the woman will not conceive during this time, because she may ovulate well before menstruation returns (Van der Wijden et al., 2005).

NURSING CARE OF A WOMAN AND FAMILY DURING THE FIRST 24 HOURS AFTER BIRTH

A woman usually remains in a birthing or recovery room for the first hour after birth for careful observation. After this initial hour, teach perineal care and encourage the woman to shower. She then remains in the room as a postpartal patient or is transferred to a separate postpartal room. The most dangerous hour in childbearing—the first hour after birth—has passed.

Hemorrhage is still a possibility for the first 2 or 3 days after birth, until the myometrial vessels have sclerosed. One of the worries for a woman giving birth at home is that she will not appreciate how dangerous a time this is. With attention focused more on the newborn than on the mother, postpartal hemorrhage could occur. In the hospital, various health care personnel may be involved in caring for the woman: be sure all members of the health care team are knowledgeable about this danger. Box 22.5 highlights appropriate outcomes and interventions for a postpartal woman, using the terminology from the Nursing Outcomes Classification (NOC) and Nursing Interventions Classification (NIC).

Assessment

Assessment of a postpartal woman includes history, physical examination, and analysis of laboratory findings.

BOX 22.5

Nursing Outcomes Classification (NOC) and Nursing Interventions Classification (NIC)

The Postpartal Woman

NOC: Maternal Status, Postpartum

Maternal status, postpartum is defined as the condition and behaviors indicating maternal well-being from delivery of the placenta to completion of involution (Johnson, Maas, & Moorhead, 2000). Some specific indicators suggesting that this outcome has been achieved include the following:

- Temperature, heart rate, and blood pressure within expected range
- Uterine fundal height and lochia characteristics as expected
- Urinary and bowel elimination status within expected range
- Evidence of perineal healing
- Physical activity and endurance within expected range

NIC: Postpartal Care

Postpartal care is defined as the monitoring and management of the patient who has recently given birth (McCloskey & Bulechek, 2000). Some important

activities involved when implementing this intervention include the following:

- Monitoring vital signs, lochia (character, amount, odor, and presence of clots), fundal height, and status of episiotomy
- Gently massaging fundus until firm, as needed
- Reinforcing appropriate perineal hygiene techniques
- Applying ice to perineum to minimize swelling
- Administering analgesics PRN
- Encouraging early ambulation and beginning postpartal exercises with resumption of normal activities as tolerated
- Monitoring for symptoms of postpartum depression
- Determining how patient feels about changes in body after delivery
- Providing anticipatory guidance about sexuality and family planning
- Scheduling follow-up examinations for newborn and mother
- Performing discharge teaching
- Arranging for follow-up home care if necessary

Health History

The technical aspects of a woman's pregnancy, labor, and birth can be learned from her pregnancy, labor, and birth charts. Most of this information is best obtained from the woman herself, however, because this supplies not only information on the events of her pregnancy and labor but also her emotions and impressions about them. If you previously cared for the woman during labor and birth and gained this information then, it is unnecessary to do so again.

Family Profile. Information for a family profile includes age, support persons, other children, type of housing and community setting, occupation, education level, and socioeconomic level or information necessary to evaluate the impact the new child will have on the woman and her family. This information also lays a foundation for teaching of self-care and child care specific to the woman's knowledge level and needs.

Pregnancy History. Information for a pregnancy history includes para and gravida status (and the reason for any discrepancy), expected date of birth, whether the pregnancy was planned, and any problems or complications such as spotting or pregnancy-induced hypertension that occurred. This information helps you to gauge the woman's potential for bonding, because an unplanned pregnancy or complications arising during pregnancy may interfere greatly with bonding.

Labor and Birth History. It is important to gather information on the length of labor, position of the fetus, type of birth, any analgesia or anesthesia used, problems during labor (e.g., fetal distress), supine hypotension syndrome, and the presence of perineal sutures. This information helps in planning for necessary procedures.

Infant Data. The sex and weight of the infant, any difficulty at birth (e.g., need for resuscitation), plans to breast-feed or formula-feed, and any congenital anomalies present are the major facts to obtain. This information helps in planning care for the infant and promoting bonding with the parents.

Postpartal Course. Ask about the woman's general health; her activity level since the birth; a description of lochia; the presence of perineal, abdominal, or breast pain; difficulty with elimination; success with infant feeding; and response of her support person to parenting. This information helps in planning what anticipatory guidance will be needed for home care.

Laboratory Data

Women routinely have their hemoglobin and hematocrit levels measured 12 to 24 hours after birth, to determine whether blood loss at birth has left them anemic. If the hemoglobin is lower than 10 g/100 mL, supplementary iron is usually prescribed. Take note of the laboratory reports on a postpartal woman, and make certain that any abnormal finding, such as low hemoglobin, is brought to the attention of the woman's physician or nurse-midwife. The responsibilities of being a new mother, coupled with the additional burden of an undetected low hemoglobin level, can severely tax a woman's energy levels.

If a woman required catheterization during labor or had a urinary tract infection during pregnancy, a urinalysis or urine culture may be ordered in the postpartal period. Obtain the urine specimen with a clean-catch technique, using a sterile cotton ball tucked in the vaginal introitus to prevent lochia from contaminating the specimen. In some women, it may be necessary to obtain a specimen by urinary catheterization to rule out urinary infection.

Physical Assessment

During early labor, a woman is given a fairly complete physical examination. During the immediate postpartal period, therefore, repetition of a complete examination is not necessary. Crucial assessments examining particular aspects of health, such as an estimation of nutrition and fluid state, energy level, presence or absence of pain, breast health, fundal height and consistency, lochia amount and character, perineal integrity, and circulatory adequacy, are required.

General Appearance. A woman's general appearance in the postpartal period reveals a great deal about her energy level, her self-esteem, and whether she is moving into the taking-hold phase of recovery. Before beginning assessment, ask the woman to void so that she has an empty bladder. Observe how much energy she uses when reaching for her robe or walking to the bathroom—does she struggle or move listlessly, or does she accomplish this task quickly? Observe for a cringing expression or hand pressure against her abdomen that suggests pain on movement. Observe whether she has combed her hair, applied makeup, and put on her own clothing or an agency gown. Many women choose to sleep in an agency gown to prevent lochia stains on their own clothing, but a woman who is pleased with herself, her pregnancy, and her birth experience is usually anxious to wear her own clothing and "fuss" with her appearance within an hour after birth. A woman who is extremely exhausted or depressed probably will not bother with her appearance this way. Keep in mind that a woman whose labor progressed so rapidly that she came to the health care agency as an emergency admission may not have had time to pack a comb and brush or her own clothing. Cultural variations also affect appearances (Box 22.6).

Hair. Palpate the woman's hair to determine its firmness and strength. Whenever a diet is deficient in nutrients, hair becomes listless and "stringy." A woman who had good nutritional intake during pregnancy has firm, crisp hair. Many women begin to lose a quantity of hair in the postpartal period. This is because, during pregnancy, metabolism was increased and hair growth was rapid, so many hairs reached maturity at the same time. As the woman's body returns to a normal metabolism level, this hair is lost. You may need to reassure the woman that hair loss is not a sign of illness but just another aspect of return to her prepregnant state.

Face. Assess the woman's face for evidence of edema, which is most apparent early in the morning if she has been lying supine with her head level during the night. Edema is manifested as puffy eyelids or a prominent fold

BOX 22.6 FOCUS ON . . .

DIVERSITY OF CARE

In the United States, the postpartal period is generally regarded as a time of wellness; early ambulation and eating a varied diet are encouraged. In other cultures, the period after childbirth may be regarded primarily as a time of rest. Cultural differences include restricting certain foods, reducing activity levels, or both; taboos and rituals are not uncommon (Maimbolwa et al., 2003; White, 2004).

Assessing women in the postpartal period for cultural variations is important, because such variations explain why a woman might be reluctant to ambulate or why she leaves a lunch of food she views as unacceptable uneaten although she said she was hungry.

of tissue inferior to the lower eyelid. Normally, this is negligible. However, in a woman who had pregnancy-induced hypertension and accumulated excessive fluid, it may be evident. It also will become evident in a woman who is developing postpartal pregnancy-induced hypertension, although this condition is rare.

Eyes. Inspect the color and texture of the inner conjunctiva. If a woman is dehydrated, the area will appear dry. A woman who is anemic from poor pregnancy nutrition or excessive blood loss at birth has a pale conjunctiva. Be alert to possible variations because of skin color, however. The conjunctiva always appears lightly shaded in fair-skinned women. Dark-skinned women may have a ruddy conjunctiva appearance even with anemia. Check the hemoglobin level of any woman with paler than usual conjunctivae to determine whether anemia is present.

Breasts. Breast tissue increases as breast milk forms, so a bra that was adequate during pregnancy may no longer be adequate by the second or third postpartal day. Use of a bra supports breast tissue that feels heavy because of increased fluid accumulation in preparation for breast-feeding and aids comfort. Advise a woman to buy a nursing bra for the postpartal period that is one to two sizes larger than her pregnancy size to allow for this increase. Properly fitted, the straps of a bra should not leave erythremic marks on a woman's shoulders. In addition, a bra should fit firmly and snugly, but not so tightly as to leave red marks on the skin.

To assess the breasts, ask the woman to remove her bra and cover her breasts with a towel or folded sheet to protect modesty. Ask her to raise her hands over her head and then tuck them under her head, because this stretches and thins breast tissue. Inspect and then palpate for breast size, shape, and color.

Breast tissue should feel soft on palpation on the first and second postpartal day. On the third day, it should begin to feel firm and warm (described as *filling*). On the third or fourth day, breasts appear large and reddened, with taut, shiny skin (engorgement). On palpation, they feel hard and tense and are painful. Normally, engorgement causes the entire breast to feel warm or appear reddened. If only one portion of a breast is warm or reddened, mastitis or in-

flammation or, possibly, infection of glands or milk ducts is suggested (Wambach, 2003).

Occasionally, a firm nodule is detected on palpation. Usually, this is only a temporarily blocked milk duct or milk contained in a gland that is not flowing forward to the nipple. However, the location of the nodule should be noted and reported to the woman's physician or nurse-midwife, so that it can be reassessed before discharge from the hospital. Such blocking of breast milk usually is relieved by the infant's sucking. Nevertheless, any nodule needs reassessment, because a fibrocystic or malignant growth unrelated to the pregnancy could be present.

Note whether the breast nipples are normally erect and not inverted. Assess for any cracks, fissures, or the presence of caked milk. Avoid squeezing the nipples, because this can be painful. Unnecessary nipple manipulation also may increase the risk of mastitis by providing a portal for infection.

Uterus. For uterine assessment, position the woman supine so that the height of the uterus is not influenced by an elevated position. Observe her abdomen for contour, to detect distention, and for the appearance of striae or a diastasis. If a diastasis is present (a slightly indented, possibly bluish-tinged groove in the midline of the abdomen), measure the width and length by fingerbreadths.

Palpate the fundus of the uterus by placing one hand on the base of the uterus, just above the symphysis pubis, and the other at the umbilicus. Press in and downward with the hand at the umbilicus until you "bump" against a firm globular mass in the abdomen: the uterine fundus (Fig. 22.5). For the first hour after birth, the height of the

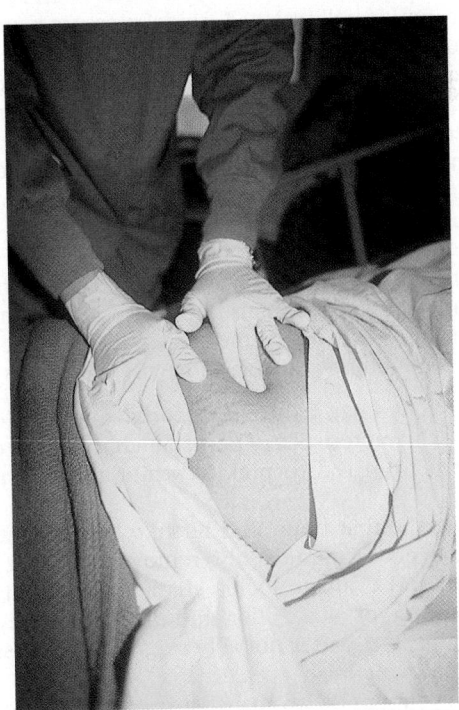

FIGURE 22.5 To palpate a uterus, be certain to place one hand at the base of the uterus. This fundus measures about 2 fingerbreadths below the umbilicus.

fundus is at the umbilicus or even slightly above it. Assess consistency (firm, soft, or boggy), location (midline), and height. Measure in fingerbreadths, such as "2 F↓ umbilicus" (2 cm beneath the umbilicus). Although this measurement seems less scientific than a measurement of the height of the uterus from the pubis might be, it is the most useful measurement because it shows the gradual decline in size or distance from the umbilicus.

Never palpate a uterus without supporting the lower segment, because the uterus potentially could invert if not stabilized (resulting in a massive hemorrhage).

Palpation of a fundus should not cause pain as long as the action is done gently. If the uterus is not firm on palpation, massage it gently with the examining hand. This usually causes the uterus to contract and become firm immediately. Use a gentle rotating motion, never a hard or forceful touch, so that you do not cause pain or cause the uterus to expend excess energy in contracting. If the uterine fundus does not grow firm with massage, extreme atony, possibly retained placenta fragments, or an excess amount of blood loss may be occurring. Notify the woman's physician or nurse-midwife. Administer PRN oxytocin as ordered. In addition, placing the woman's infant at breast will cause endogenous release of oxytocin and achieve the same effect as oxytocin administration.

A woman who received no oxytocin after birth to help her uterus contract is at greater risk for poor uterine contraction than other women are. In such cases, assess the uterine fundus every 10 to 15 minutes immediately after birth, to evaluate and assist the fundus to contract should it become soft or relaxed. If massage appears ineffective, a clot may be present in the cavity of the uterus. The clot may be expressed from the uterus by gentle pressure on the fundus, but only after the uterus has been massaged. If the uterus is totally relaxed, fundal pressure could cause inversion of the uterus, an extremely serious complication that leads to rapid hemorrhage, possibly necessitating an emergency hysterectomy to save the woman's life. Another reason the uterus may not be well contracted is that a rapidly filling bladder is preventing contraction. If contraction remains inadequate, a uterine sonogram may be ordered to help detect any abnormalities.

Once the first hour after birth has passed, a woman's uterus may be evaluated for height and consistency less frequently, depending on institutional policy. By the ninth or tenth day after delivery, the uterus will have become so small it is no longer palpable above the symphysis pubis.

Lochia. A woman can expect to have lochia for 2 to 6 weeks. Characteristics of normal lochia and the change in pattern from red to pink to white are described in Table 22.1.

During the first hour after birth, when the fundus is checked every 15 minutes, also remove the mother's perineal pad and evaluate lochia character, amount, color (rubra, serosa, or alba), odor, and presence of any clots. Be certain that a pad is not adhering to perineal stitches before removing it.

When you turn the woman to inspect her perineum, be sure to check under her buttocks to observe any blood that may be pooling beneath her. If you observe a constant trickle of vaginal flow or the woman is soaking through a pad every 60 minutes, she is losing more than the average amount of blood. She needs to be checked by a physician or nurse-midwife to be certain that there is no cervical or vaginal tear causing excessive bleeding.

While the woman is at the health care facility, inspect her lochia discharge once every 15 minutes for the first hour, and then according to the institution's policy. Make certain the woman understands that she must wash her hands after handling pads and must use only her own personal care equipment so that she does not contract or spread infection. Demonstrate good role modeling for handwashing and equipment use. Encourage the woman to change perineal pads frequently as she begins self-care, because lochia is an excellent medium for bacterial growth that could spread through the vagina to the uterus. The presence of constantly wet pads against an episiotomy suture line also slows healing. Often this is not a problem for a woman while she is at the health care facility, but if she is trying to save money, she may try to conserve on the number of pads she uses at home. Be certain she knows not to use tampons until after she returns for her postpartal checkup, to diminish the risk for infection and toxic shock syndrome (see Chapter 47). Ensure that women know the criteria for judging the amount and type of normal lochia (see Box 22.4), so they can do this accurately.

Perineum. While evaluating lochia, also inspect the perineum. Ask the woman to turn on her side, into a Sims' position with her back toward you. If a midline episiotomy was performed, position the mother on either side. If a mediolateral incision is present, turning her so that the incision is on the bottom buttock often causes less pain and offers better visibility. Gently lift the upper buttock and inspect the perineum. Observe for ecchymosis, hematoma, erythema, edema, intactness, and presence of drainage or bleeding from any episiotomy stitches.

An episiotomy is usually 1 or 2 inches long. However, if a laceration was involved, stitches may extend from the vagina back to the rectum. Rarely, they extend forward toward the urethra. An episiotomy incision is usually fused (edges sealed) by 24 hours after birth; if it is a midline incision, it may be almost invisible because the perineal fold obscures it. A hematoma (blood-filled, protruding sphere) could be present if surface capillaries were broken during the pressure of birth; this should be noted as a potential complication. If there is clotted lochia along the incision, review postpartal perineal care so that this does not continue to occur. Before discharge, teach the woman how to lie on her back and view her perineum with a handheld mirror, so that, once a day while at home, she can inspect the perineum for redness, sloughing of sutures, pus formation, or drainage at the suture line.

After perineal assessment, assess the rectal area for the presence of hemorrhoids. Document their number, appearance, and size in centimeters.

What if... Joan Cooper, at 18 hours postpartum, states that she has had to change her perineal pads twice in the last 30 minutes because they were saturated. She noticed two large clots on the last pad. What assessment should you first perform on her, and why?

NURSING DIAGNOSES AND RELATED INTERVENTIONS

Nursing Diagnosis: Pain related to uterine cramping (afterpains) or perineal sutures

Outcome Evaluation: Client states degree of pain is tolerable; demonstrates knowledge of measures for adequate pain relief.

Provide Pain Relief for Afterpains. Pain from uterine contractions can be intense, but you can assure the woman that this type of discomfort is normal and rarely lasts longer than 3 days. If necessary, either ibuprofen (e.g., Motrin), which has antiinflammatory properties, or a common analgesic such as acetaminophen (e.g., Tylenol) is effective for relief. As with any abdominal pain, heat to the abdomen should be avoided, because it could cause relaxation of the uterus and subsequent uterine bleeding.

Relieve Muscular Aches. Many women feel sore and aching after labor and birth because of the excessive energy they used for pushing during the pelvic division of labor. They describe feeling as if they had "run for miles." A woman may need a mild analgesic such as acetaminophen for the pain. A backrub is effective for relieving an aching back or shoulders. Carefully assess a woman who states that she has pain on standing. Pain in the calf of the leg on standing (a position that dorsiflexes the foot) is a sign similar to Homans' sign suggesting thrombophlebitis (see later discussion).

Give Episiotomy Care. Although the frequency of episiotomy is decreasing, as many as 50% of women may still receive one. Although relatively small in size, episiotomy sutures can cause considerable discomfort, because the perineum is an extremely tender area and the muscles of the perineum are involved in many activities (e.g., sitting, walking, stooping, squatting, bending, urinating, defecating).

Most women expect labor to be painful. However, they usually do not anticipate the pulling pain from perineal stitches in the postpartal period, discomfort that interferes with their rest and sleep, with eating, and with being able to sit and hold their baby comfortably.

Because the perineal area heals rapidly, you can assure a woman that this discomfort is normal and does not usually last longer than 5 or 6 days. Many physicians and nurse-midwives order a soothing cream or anesthetic spray to be applied to the suture line to reduce discomfort. A cortisone-based cream or sitz bath helps to decrease inflammation and relieve tension in the area. Because of their cooling effect, witch hazel preparations are a mainstay for relief of both perineal and hemorrhoidal discomfort.

A woman may worry that she will experience additional discomfort when the episiotomy sutures are removed. Explain that these sutures are made of an absorbable material and will not need to be removed. Sutures usually dissolve within 10 days.

Promote Perineal Exercises. Some women find that carrying out perineal exercises three or four times a day greatly relieves episiotomy discomfort. The exercise consists of contracting and relaxing the muscles of the perineum five to ten times in succession, as if trying to stop voiding (Kegel exercises). This aids comfort by improving circulation to the area and decreasing edema. When repeated frequently, Kegel exercises also help a woman regain her prepregnant muscle tone and form (Harvey, 2003).

Administer Cold and Hot Therapy. Applying an ice or cold pack to the perineum during the first 24 hours reduces perineal edema and the possibility of hematoma formation, thereby reducing pain and promoting healing and comfort. Be certain not to place ice or plastic directly on the woman's perineum. Wrap the ice bag first in a towel or disposable pad, to decrease the chance of a thermal burn (risk of injury increases because the perineum has decreased sensation from edema after birth). Commercial cold packs combined with perineal pads also are available. For a low-cost alternative, a rubber glove may be partially filled with ice chips, provided latex allergy is not a concern.

Ice to the perineum after the first 24 hours is no longer therapeutic. After this time, healing increases best if circulation to the area is encouraged by the use of heat. Dry heat in the form of a perineal hot pack or moist heat with a sitz bath is an effective way to increase circulation to the perineum, provide comfort, reduce edema, and promote healing.

Commercial hot packs are available, which grow warm after they are "cracked" and the chemicals in them combine. Caution women to use a washcloth or gauze square between the pack and their skin, to prevent a possible burn.

Administer Sitz Baths. A **sitz bath** is a portable basin that fits on a toilet seat. A reservoir filled with water provides a constant supply of swirling water to the basin. The movement of water soothes healing tissue, decreases inflammation by causing vasodilation in the area, and thereby effectively reduces discomfort and promotes healing.

Sitz baths usually use water that is maintained at 100°F to 105°F (38°C to 41°C). Be certain that the water in a sitz bath is not too hot before you help a woman to use it; it should feel pleasantly warm, not hot. The woman will not be sensitive to the temperature herself, because healing surfaces are not good indicators of temperature. This caution applies particularly to a woman who is using an analgesic cream or spray on her perineum or who has a great deal of generalized perineal edema. Both situations make her prone to burns from scalding water unless you act to protect her (Box 22.7).

Teach women to use a sitz bath three to four times a day for a maximum of 20 minutes each

BOX 22.7 NURSING PROCEDURE

Sitz baths

Purpose
To aid healing of the perineum through application of moist heat

PROCEDURE	PRINCIPLE
1. Wash your hands; identify client and explain procedure.	1. Handwashing prevents the spread of infection; identification ensures that procedure is performed on correct client, thereby promoting safety; explanation assists in alleviating any anxiety.
2. Assess client's condition; ascertain whether client is able to ambulate to bathroom; assist and modify as necessary.	2. A sitz bath can make a woman feel lightheaded, increasing her risk of injury. Fatigue and exhaustion may interfere with client's ability to ambulate or tolerate procedure, also increasing her risk for injury.
3. Assemble equipment, including sitz bath, clean towel, perineal pad.	3. Organization of equipment increases efficiency of the procedure.
4. Place sitz bath on toilet seat. Fill collecting bag with warm water at a temperature of 100°F to 105°F (38°C to 41°C). Hang the bag overhead so a steady stream of water will flow from the bag, through the tubing, and into the basin.	4. Using correct temperature of water (pleasantly warm) eliminates risk of thermal injury. Adequate flow of warm water increases circulation to the perineum, thereby reducing inflammation and aiding healing.

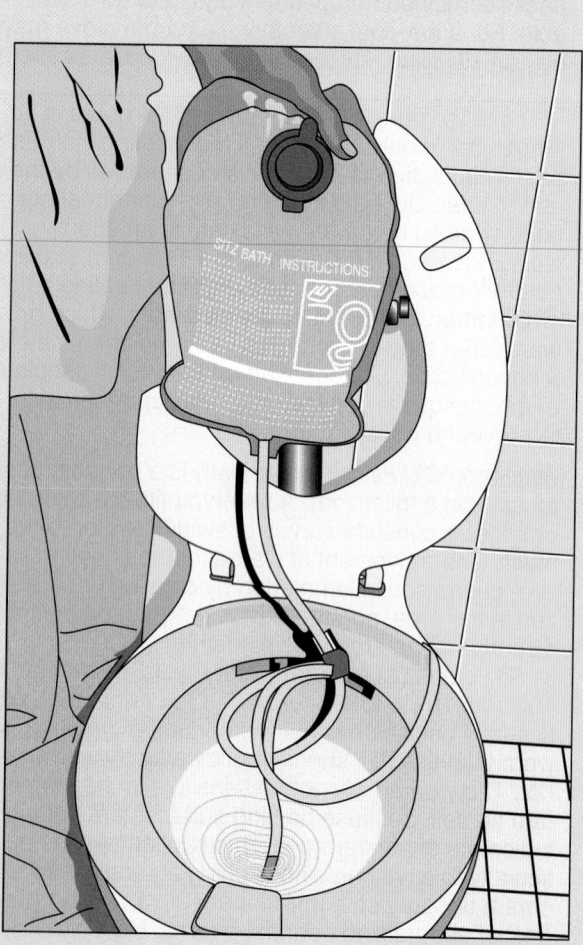

PROCEDURE	PRINCIPLE
5. Assist client with ambulating to bathroom; help with removal of perineal pad from front to back. Assist client to sit in basin.	5. Assisting ambulation minimizes risk of injury. Removing pad from front to back minimizes risk of infection transmission. Proper placement ensures effectiveness of treatment.
6. Instruct client to use clamp on tubing to regulate water flow; use robe or blankets to prevent chilling and provide for privacy. Have call bell within reach.	6. Continuous swirling water aids in reducing edema and promoting comfort. Privacy enhances self-esteem. Quick, easy access to call bell allows for prompt intervention should problems arise.
7. After 20 minutes, assist client with drying perineum and applying clean pad (holding pad by the bottom side or ends).	7. After 20 minutes, heat is no longer therapeutic because vasoconstriction occurs. Proper handling of pad prevents contamination and possible risk of infection.
8. Assist client with ambulating back to room.	8. Client may become fatigued from the procedure or lightheaded from the warm water, increasing her risk of falling.
9. Evaluate client's tolerance and response to procedure; ask client to report how she feels. Institute health teaching, such as continuing sitz baths when at home.	9. Evaluation assists with determining effectiveness of procedure and making any changes. Health teaching helps to promote continuity of care after discharge.
10. Record completion of procedure, condition of perineum, and client's condition and response.	10. Documentation provides additional means for evaluation of care and client outcomes.

time. Because of the soothing effect of the warm water and the sitting position, alert the woman that she may feel extremely tired and unsteady on her feet after using a sitz bath and may need help in getting back to bed.

Provide Pain Management. Several topical medications with lidocaine (Xylocaine) bases, such as gels or sprays, are available to relieve perineal pain. These are applied to the incision line with a clean gauze square or via a spray. Because of their anesthetic action, they instantly reduce incision line pain. Tucks, a commercial form of soft pads impregnated with witch hazel that can be tucked between the perineum and a sanitary pad, also are effective in relieving perineal pain. Some women doubt the efficacy of suture-line medications or worry that applying the cream will hurt more than not applying it. They may need extra encouragement to try these helpful aids.

In addition to local perineum creams or sprays, many women require an oral or parenteral analgesic to relieve their episiotomy discomfort. Most physicians and nurse-midwives order a moderate-strength analgesic such as propoxyphene/acetaminophen (Darvocet) or codeine for the first 24 hours, then a milder one such as acetaminophen for the remainder of the first week. Ibuprofen also is widely prescribed. Advise a woman not to use aspirin for pain relief during the postpartal period, because it interferes with blood clotting and may increase her risk for hemorrhage from the denuded placental site (Karch, 2004).

Nursing Diagnosis: Risk for infection (uterine) related to lochia and episiotomy

Outcome Evaluation: Client's temperature remains below 100.4°F; no redness or abnormal discharge is present at episiotomy line; lochia is present and without foul odor.

Provide Perineal Care. Postpartal women are particularly prone to perineal infection because lochia, if allowed to dry and harden on the vulva and perineum, furnishes a rich bed for bacterial growth. Because the vagina lies in close proximity to the rectum, there is also always the danger that bacteria will spread from the rectum to the vagina and cause uterine infection. Interruption in skin integrity from an episiotomy also increases the client's risk for infection.

Teach a woman to include perineal care as part of her daily bath or shower and after every voiding or bowel movement. If the woman is on bed rest during the first hour after birth, you will need to provide perineal care for her.

Before beginning perineal care, wash your hands and pull on clean gloves to prevent the risk of infection transmission. Place a plastic-covered pad under the woman's buttocks to protect the bed during the procedure. With the woman lying in a supine position, remove the perineal pad from the front to back; the direction is important to prevent the portion of the pad that was over her rectal area from sliding forward to contaminate the vaginal opening.

Perineal care is a clean but not a sterile procedure. Agencies differ as to the type of cleansing that is done and the articles and solutions used. If actual washing is to be done, use a clean gauze square or a clean portion of a washcloth with soap and water for each stroke, always washing from front to back, from the pubis toward the rectum. Rinse the area in the same manner, and dry it.

A second common method is to spray the perineum with clear tap water from a spray bottle. Direct the spray toward the front of the perineum, and allow it to flow from front to back. Be certain that none of the solution enters the vagina, as it could be a source of contamination. The labia have a tendency to close and cover the vaginal opening, which normally prevents solution from entering the vagina. Do not separate the labia; instead, allow them to perform this protective function. Spray gently to avoid splashing any blood-tinged solution on yourself (to guard against contacting body secretions).

It may be advantageous to have the woman turn on her side in a Sims' position, to permit better visualization of the episiotomy area. In some women, better cleaning of this area can also be done in this position.

Promote Perineal Self-Care. As soon as a woman is allowed to get up to go to the bathroom (if her infant was born without an anesthetic, this is within the first hour after birth), teach her how to carry out her own perineal care.

The bathroom should have an area close to the toilet where a woman can place the equipment she needs for care: a spray bottle, sponges to dry, her clean pad, and so forth. Instruct her on how to remove the soiled perineal pad and where to dispose of it. Remind her of the importance of using any cream or medication that has been prescribed. Caution her not to flush the toilet until she is standing upright. Otherwise, the flushing water might spray the perineum and cause infection.

If women are given a clear explanation as to why perineal care is important, they perform it well. However, self-care does not eliminate a nurse's responsibility for checking a woman's perineum to assess its condition and the amount and type of lochia flow present. By continuing with these assessments, a nurse remains a woman's first line of defense against postpartal complications such as infection and hemorrhage.

Nursing Diagnosis: Disturbed sleep pattern related to exhaustion from and excitement of childbirth

Outcome Evaluation: Client states she is able to sleep and feels rested during postpartal period.

After birth, a woman is a paradox. She is excited. She has a baby and she wants to hold and be with this new person in her life. She wants to talk to her support person about the experience, their child, and their future. At the same time, she is so exhausted that in most cases she falls asleep instantly.

Allow a woman to have time with her expanded family in the birthing room immediately after the baby's birth. If the father did not watch the birth for some reason, allow time for mother, father, and baby to be together as soon as possible. After this time, encourage a period of rest to help the woman regain energy.

Promote Rest in the Early Postpartal Period. Few women are prepared for the degree of fatigue they experience after childbirth (Box 22.8). Try to do all procedures swiftly yet gently, to allow as much time for sleep as possible. If a woman has discomfort from hemorrhoids, perineal stitches, or afterpains, be sure she has pain relief so that she can rest comfortably or sleep.

Some women experience shaking chills immediately or within a half-hour after birth. This is caused in part by the pressure changes in the abdomen that occur with reduction in the bulk of the uterus and temperature readjustment in response to the diaphoresis of labor. It also may result from the exhilaration the woman is feeling, combined with exhaustion. In any event, shaking chills at this point are common. Reassure the woman that chills are common, so that she will not attribute them to a developing cold or infection. Cover her with a warm blanket, offer her a warm drink if she is not nauseated from an analgesic, and assure her the occurrence is normal. These actions are usually enough to make the chill transient and allow the woman to fall into a sound, much-needed sleep of about an hour.

Although a woman may choose any position to sleep, she may enjoy being able to sleep on her stomach, something she was not able to do during pregnancy.

Promote Rest Throughout the Puerperium. The importance of rest throughout the entire puerperium cannot be stressed enough. As long as a woman is in the health care facility, reserve time for naps. Include

BOX 22.8 FOCUS ON . . .

EVIDENCE-BASED PRACTICE

Do Postpartal Mothers and Fathers Get Enough Rest?

To answer this question, researchers used wrist actigraphy and questionnaires to estimate sleep and fatigue in 72 couples during their last month of pregnancy and first month after birth. Results of the study showed that sleep patterns were related to the parents' work status and the type of infant feeding. Both husbands and wives experienced more sleep disruption at night during the postpartum period than during their last month of pregnancy. Mothers reported more sleep disturbance than did fathers, although there was no gender difference in ratings of fatigue. Mothers were found to have less sleep at night and more sleep during the day after the baby was born. The researchers recommended that interventions for improving sleep patterns of new parents need to be devised.

This is an important study for nurses, because nurses can help to see that women receive enough rest and sleep in the immediate postpartal period, so they can return home rested, and can help them plan for additional rest at home.

Gay, C. L., Lee, K. A., & Lee, S. (2004). Sleep patterns and fatigue in new mothers and fathers. *Biological Research for Nursing, 5*(4), 311–318.

suggestions for getting adequate rest while at home in discharge instructions, because rest may prove difficult. The newborn will wake at least twice a night, and relatives and friends will be coming to see the baby during the day.

Many women do not realize how long it will take to fully return to their previous level of functioning. When families were closely knit and neighborhoods were smaller, a new mother had someone in her family or neighborhood to look after the baby while she napped. Today, many couples do not have family or close friends nearby. If the parents have not thought through this problem before birth, you can help them look at their situation and see what is available to them. Perhaps the woman's mother, a sister, her partner's mother, or another relative could come and stay with them for the first week. Perhaps the father could take a week off from work or school to help out at home; many employment benefit programs provide for this time. If none of these solutions seems appropriate, the couple might appreciate being given the name of a community service agency that supplies homemakers on a short-term basis. A referral to a community health agency for an early home visit is yet another suggestion.

A woman without support has many demands for her new role—being a mother instead of a daughter; a mother as well as a wife; a mother of three, not two. If she is overcome by sleep hunger, her judgment and sense of balance may be blurred. Although it is not the only contributing factor, extreme fatigue is associated with the development of postpartal depression (St. John & Rouse, 2003).

Nursing Diagnosis: Risk for bathing/hygiene self-care deficit related to exhaustion from childbirth

Outcome Evaluation: Client takes daily responsibility for own hygiene. Client appears clean, dressed, and well groomed.

After childbirth, women often report that their hospital or birthing center room is being kept too warm; to prove it, they point out how heavily they are perspiring. Postpartal rooms often are kept warm so that newborns will be comfortable, but the profuse perspiration a woman is experiencing normally comes from her body's attempt to regulate fluid, not from the heat of the environment.

You can reassure the woman that sweating is a normal postpartal event that helps to bring her body back to its prepregnant state. If she has profuse diaphoresis, particularly at night, she usually prefers to wear a hospital gown rather than one of her own. She may need frequent gown changes during the day to be comfortable and not become chilled.

A daily shower is refreshing. Be certain to accompany the woman for a shower on her first postpartal day, because she often is more fatigued than she realizes. Standing under warm water may also make her dizzy, and she may need help to walk safely back to bed.

Formerly, women were not allowed to take tub baths after birth, for fear that bacteria from the bath water would enter the vagina and cause infection. There appears to be little evidence that this is a real danger, however, so if a woman wants to bathe instead of shower, she may do so.

Nursing Diagnosis: Imbalanced nutrition, less than body requirements, related to lack of knowledge about postpartal needs

Outcome Evaluation: Client ingests a 2,200- to 2,700-kcal diet and drinks 6 to 8 glasses of fluid daily.

Postpartal menu planning should include a diet of between 2,200 and 2,300 calories daily. Foods should be high in protein and in the vitamins and minerals needed for good tissue repair. An adequate supply of roughage is important to help restore the peristaltic action of the bowel. A woman who is breast-feeding needs an additional 500 calories (i.e., a 2700-kcal diet) and an additional 500 mL of fluid (these may be from the same source) each day to encourage the production of high-quality breast milk. Most mothers are hungry during the immediate postpartal period and consume an adequate diet without urging.

Teach a woman to continue to eat a nutritious diet after she returns home. This can be a problem, because some women become so fatigued during their first weeks at home that they feel unable to prepare adequate meals. Neglecting to eat properly leads to more fatigue and, ultimately, to an even less nutritious diet.

If a woman has any prenatal vitamins or supplementary iron preparations left over from pregnancy, she should, as a rule, continue to take them until her supply is used. If she needs further supplements, her physician or nurse-midwife will prescribe them for her, either on discharge or when she returns for her postpartum checkup.

Promote Adequate Fluid Intake. The rapid diuresis and diaphoresis that occur during the second to fifth postpartal days ordinarily result in a weight loss of 5 lb in addition to the approximately 12 lb lost at childbirth.

Women often feel thirsty during this period of rapid fluid loss and want additional fluid. It seems a paradox that while the body is ridding itself of unwanted fluid, it should also demand fluid. Part of this paradox stems from a woman's having had little to drink during labor. She may say immediately after the birth, "I don't think I'll ever get enough to drink again." Part of the need for fluid stems from the increased amount of nitrogen being released from catabolized uterine cells. A woman needs to increase her fluid intake to rid her body of these wastes.

You may need to encourage some women to drink adequate fluid during the first few postpartum days because they are restricting fluid in the hope of preventing their breasts from becoming engorged. Other mothers are beginning diets that they hope will bring their bodies more quickly back to their nonpregnant slim state. However, fluid restriction does little to deter breast engorgement, and unless a woman is extremely obese, this is not a good time for dieting. The postpartal period is a time of rebuilding and readjusting, for which a woman needs both ample nourishment and adequate fluid intake. Encourage her to drink at least three to four 8-oz glasses of fluid each day (six to eight glasses if breast-feeding).

Nursing Diagnosis: Risk for impaired urinary elimination or constipation related to loss of bladder and bowel sensation after childbirth

Outcome Evaluation: Client voids more than 30 mL/hour without urinary retention, beginning 1 hour after birth, and has a bowel movement by postpartum day 4. No urinary incontinence is noted.

Promote Urinary Elimination. Because the diuresis of the postpartal period begins almost immediately after birth, a woman's bladder begins filling almost immediately. A full bladder puts pressure on the uterus. An overdistended bladder may damage bladder function (Box 22.9).

BOX 22.9: Focus on Nursing Care Planning

A Multidisciplinary Care Map for A Postpartal Client

•

Joan Cooper is 6 hours postpartum after birth of an 8 lb, 2 oz baby girl. She states, "I haven't urinated since before the birth. What kind of mother am I going to be if I can't even manage my own care?" Her husband Mike pulls you aside and says, "Sometimes, I see my wife crying for no reason. Isn't she as happy as I am?"

Family Assessment
Couple has been married for 3 years. Husband works as a pharmacist. Will be taking a week off from work to spend time with Joan and the new baby. Joan is on maternity leave from her job as a court reporter.

Client Assessment
Labor and birth were without incident. Abdomen soft. Uterus ½ fingerbreadth above umbilicus, soft, and displaced to the right. Moderate lochia rubra. Midline episiotomy with intact sutures. Perineal edema present. Bladder firm on palpation above symphysis pubis. Resonant on percussion. Vital signs within acceptable parameters.

Nursing Diagnosis
Altered urinary elimination related to perineal edema and decreased bladder tone from fetal head pressure during labor and birth.

Outcome Criteria
Client attempts common measures to initiate voiding; voids more than 100 mL within 2 hours' time.

Team Member Responsible	Assessment	Intervention	Rationale	Expected Outcome
		Activities of Daily Living		
Nurse	Assess amount of urine voided during labor, and reassess fundal height and position.	Discuss importance of continuing to drink to help initiate bladder reflex. Also discuss importance of emptying bladder.	Assessing fundal height and position provides evidence about the degree of bladder filling. Retention of urine in the bladder predisposes to infection.	Client voids a minimum of 100 mL by 2 hours' time, and fundal height returns to 1 fingerbreadth below umbilicus after voiding.

(continued)

find commercial abdominal exercisers helpful to fully strengthen their abdominal wall.

Teach Methods to Promote Uterine Involution. All during the postpartal period, lying on the abdomen gives support to abdominal muscles and may aid involution, because it tips the uterus into its natural forward position. If this puts too much pressure on sore breasts, placement of a small pillow under the abdomen usually solves the problem.

It is dangerous for a woman to assume a knee–chest position until at least the third week after birth. In a knee–chest position, the vagina tends to open. Because the cervical os remains open to some extent until the third week, there is a danger that air will enter the vagina and the open cervix, penetrate the open blood sinuses inside the uterus, enter the circulatory system, and cause an air embolism (St. John & Rouse, 2003).

It is therefore good practice for a woman to avoid this position until she returns for a postpartal examination and is assured that her cervix has closed properly. Women who have used a knee–chest position during pregnancy to relieve the pressure of hemorrhoids need to be cautioned that a modified Sims' position, such as they used for a rest position during pregnancy, is better for them now.

Nursing Diagnosis: Risk for ineffective sexuality patterns related to physiologic changes of postpartal period

Outcome Evaluation: Client states she has a satisfactory sexual relationship with her partner; demonstrates understanding of both coital and noncoital methods of sexual expression.

At one time, women were cautioned not to resume sexual relations after the birth of a baby until after their medical checkup at 6 weeks. However, there is no apparent physiologic reason to delay sexual relations this long. For most couples, coitus may be resumed as soon as lochia serosa has stopped—about 1 to 2 weeks after birth.

Caution women, however, that sex may be somewhat uncomfortable if it is begun this early. Tissue at an episiotomy site may be sensitive. Because the vaginal epithelium is still thin, vaginal tenderness may be noticed. Use of a lubricant will help any mucosal dryness. A female-superior position can be suggested because it allows the woman to control the depth of penile penetration.

A woman who is breast-feeding may notice that milk is released from her nipples with sexual arousal. Women may already be aware that their degree of exhaustion can make them less receptive to sexual arousal than before.

Be sure that women receive adequate reproductive planning information, if desired, before they resume sexual relations (see Chapter 4).

Nursing Diagnosis: Risk for impaired parenting related to inadequate bonding behavior after childbirth

Outcome Evaluation: Parents hold and comfort their infant appropriately and voice positive characteristics of child.

To assess that bonding is occurring, listen to what parents say about their newborn in the immediate postpartal period. Do they make positive statements (e.g., "I'm glad he's a boy," "She's cute") or negative ones (e.g., "I really hoped it would be a girl," "She looks like a circus clown with no hair")? First impressions may not be lasting ones. However, negative comments need to be identified, so that extra discussion about things such as what it feels like to have four boys, or not to have the prettiest child in the nursery, can take place. If such discussion does not occur, a family may be discharged from the health care agency with their needs unmet. At home, away from health care personnel who are attuned to how disappointment can interfere with parent–child interaction, parents may have great difficulty adjusting to and relating to this new child. Some signs of good parent–child adaptation are shown in Box 22.11.

NURSING CARE OF A WOMAN AND FAMILY IN PREPARATION FOR DISCHARGE

The greatest need of a postpartal woman before discharge from a health care agency is education to prepare her to care for herself and her newborn at home. She must be aware of danger signs to look for and know whom to call if she notices any of them. She must understand safe baby care. Because of shortened lengths of stay, every contact with a woman should include some teaching information. At the same time, be aware that learning does not take place if the learner is overwhelmed and hurried. Use common sense to determine when it is time to teach and when it is time to observe or listen. Observation of mother–child or parent–child interactions and evaluation of a woman's support system at home are the basis for much of the teaching.

BOX 22.11

Signs of Good Parent–Child Adaptation

Good parent-child adaptation is demonstrated when a parent:

Speaks of infant as desirable and attractive

Is not upset by vomiting, drooling, and the like

Holds baby warmly

Makes eye contact with infant

Plays with and soothes infant

Talks or sings to baby

Expresses confidence that infant is well

Finds physical or psychological attributes to admire about baby

Is able to discriminate between baby's signs of hunger, sleep, and so on

Most women attend classes in newborn care during their pregnancies. They remember many points from these classes, but when they actually have a newborn they become worried that they will not remember enough. Many mothers say that child care did not seem real during pregnancy. The postpartal period is a time for teaching, reteaching, and offering anticipatory guidance to help in the new situations a family can expect when they go home.

During the taking-in phase of the puerperium, a woman may not show much interest in learning; she is more in need of the comfort of being taken care of. As she enters her taking-hold period, she grows increasingly receptive to advice and looks to the nurse for the information she needs. Some nurses assume that multiparas will react negatively to child care suggestions. They are, after all, veterans of child care. If you listen carefully, however, you may discover that a mother of two girls feels insecure about the care of her new baby boy. A woman whose next youngest child is 5 years old may admit that in 5 years she has completely forgotten how small newborns are. She yearns to have a nurse who is comfortable with such small human beings reassure her that she is holding her new baby correctly and giving proper care. All mothers, whether primiparas or multiparas, need to be evaluated individually and helped whenever they ask or you find that they need guidance.

Group Classes

Providing group classes on bathing infants, preparing formula, breast-feeding techniques, minimizing jealousy in older children, and maintaining health in the newborn can be helpful to mothers and fathers, because in these settings they can learn not only from the instructor but also from other parents. Be certain that a time for questions and answers is planned at these sessions, so parents can apply what is being taught to their individual circumstances. Urging fathers to attend classes is helpful, because many fathers give direct child care for at least part of every day. Including the father in teaching is also important, because the problems that arise with newborn care are, by their nature, family problems, and every effort should be made by nursing personnel to help both parents prepare to deal with them.

Individual Instruction

Every family needs some individual instruction in how to care for their infant and how the woman can care for herself after discharge. Rooming-in is an ideal setup for letting you observe and work with a family and their infant. How to bathe and feed the baby, how to care for the infant's cord and circumcision, a review of how much infants sleep during 24 hours, and how to fit a newborn into the family's pattern of living are topics parents like to discuss. Teaching does not have to be formal. You can teach without lecturing by making a comment such as, "Notice how large all newborns' heads seem" while you are showing the parents how to bathe the baby, or "Babies like to be bundled firmly" while you are helping dress the child, or "Notice how uneven newborn respirations are." This kind of instruction saves parents many anxious moments

when they are at home. Techniques for home care of the newborn are discussed in Chapter 24.

Discharge Planning

Before a postpartal family is discharged from the health care agency, the woman will be given instructions by her physician or nurse-midwife concerning her care at home. These instructions differ among health care providers but have common points that are summarized in Table 22.3.

Before discharge, make sure the woman is aware that she must return for an examination 4 to 6 weeks after birth, and that she should make an appointment to take her baby to a primary care provider for an examination at 2 to 4 weeks of age. If the woman does not have an adequate rubella antibody titer and anticipates further pregnancies, she may receive a rubella immunization before discharge. Women who are Rh negative and who have had an Rh-positive infant will receive RhIG or Rh antibodies to prevent problems in a future pregnancy (Crowther & Middleton, 2005).

Be certain that discharge instructions for the family are given both verbally and in writing. Getting ready to go home, dressing the baby, seeing him or her in new clothes for the first time, and experiencing the thrill of realizing the baby is really theirs to take home is so exciting that oral instructions may go unheard. On the other hand, parents should not simply be handed a list of instructions. Review the instructions with the parents to be sure they understand them.

Many health care agencies have a community liaison person, ideally a nurse, who telephones or makes a home visit to mothers after discharge. This person helps the mother assess her own health and that of her baby and answers questions from families who lose their instructions or are unable to interpret them after they have returned home.

Routinely, this type of follow-up is performed within 24 to 48 hours after the family's discharge. Follow-up visits are completed from 2 to 7 days after discharge. Making a telephone call to or visiting a family 24 hours after discharge is a helpful way to evaluate whether the family is able to continue self-evaluation and infant care and is able to integrate the new infant into the family. Such visits may also reduce the number of acute care visits and rehospitalizations for newborns.

NURSING CARE OF A WOMAN AND FAMILY AFTER DISCHARGE

Postpartal Home Visits

In today's health care climate of cost containment, most women are discharged from a health care facility 2 to 3 days after childbirth. Such a practice has the advantage of allowing the family unit to be interrupted as little as possible. A new mother may rest better at home than in a strange setting, and she may eat better if she has cultural preferences for specific foods. The infant can be more quickly exposed to family routines rather than a superficial facility schedule. However, early discharge has the disadvantage of not allowing a new family to have the ready support of health

TABLE 22.3

Postpartal Discharge Instructions

Area	Instructions
Work	All women should avoid heavy work (lifting or straining) for at least the first 3 weeks after birth. Women differ in their concept of heavy work, so it is a good idea to explore with a woman what she considers heavy work. If she plans to do too much, you can perhaps help her to modify her plans. It is usually advised that a woman not return to an outside job for at least 3 weeks (or better, 6 weeks), not only for her own health but also for enjoyment of the early weeks with her newborn.
Rest	A woman should plan at least one rest period each day and try to get a good night's sleep. She can rest during the day when her newborn is sleeping, unless she has other children or an aged parent to care for. If she has others dependent on her, explore the possibility of having a neighbor, another family member, or a person from a community health agency relieve her.
Exercise	A woman should limit the number of stairs she climbs to one flight/day for the first week at home. Beginning the second week, if her lochial discharge is normal, she may start to increase this activity. This limitation will involve some planning on her part, especially if her washing machine is in the basement and she must wash diapers every day, or if she must go up and down stairs to check on the baby. It is probably better to arrange for a place for the baby to sleep downstairs as well as upstairs, so he or she must be taken upstairs only at bedtime. She should continue with muscle-strengthening exercises, such as abdominal crunches.
Hygiene	A woman may take either tub baths or showers. She should continue to apply any cream or ointment as ordered for the perineal area and cleanse her perineum from front to back. Any perineal stitches will be absorbed within 10 days. She should not use vaginal douches until she returns for her postpartal checkup.
Coitus	Coitus is safe as soon as a woman's lochia has turned to alba and, if present, the episiotomy is healed (usually about the first week after birth). Vaginal cells may not be as thick as formerly because pre-pregnancy hormone balance has not yet completely returned. Use of a contraceptive foam or lubricating jelly will aid comfort. Be certain she knows safer sex precautions.
Contraception	If desired, a woman should begin a contraception measure with the initiation of coitus. If she wishes an IUD, this may be fitted immediately after birth or at her first postpartal checkup. Oral contraceptives are begun about 2–3 weeks after birth. A diaphragm must be refitted at a 6-week checkup. Until she returns for this checkup, an over-the-counter spermicidal jelly and condoms can provide protection.
Follow-up	A woman should notify her physician or nurse-midwife if she notices an increase, not a decrease, in lochial discharge, or if lochia serosa or lochia alba becomes lochia rubra. Delayed postpartal hemorrhage can occur in women who become extremely fatigued. Getting adequate rest during her first weeks at home will do much to prevent the possibility of this complication. Four to six weeks after birth, a woman should return to her physician or nurse-midwife for an examination. This visit is important to ensure that involution is complete and reproductive life planning, if desired, can be discussed further.

care personnel if they have questions about the newborn or about the woman's condition. Although home visits are helpful for everyone, they should especially be planned for high-risk newborns, including newborns who are preterm, those born with a congenital anomaly, infants of adolescent mothers, and infants of mothers who have abused drugs during pregnancy.

The purposes of a home visit for the well postpartum woman and her newborn are to help integrate the infant into the family and to provide the family with additional information on newborn care that they may not have been able to learn during a brief hospital stay. Such a visit also allows for physical examination of the woman and newborn and for newborn screening procedures or bilirubin testing, if these were not done during the hospital stay.

Because women need to preserve their energy during the postpartal period, try to arrange a home visit at the woman's convenience. Preparation for home visiting is discussed in Chapter 16, with other aspects of home care.

Important assessments to make at a postpartal home visit include the following:

Pregnancy History: Are there physical factors that could have interfered with pregnancy bonding, such as painful varicose veins or gestational diabetes? Are there psychosocial factors such as an unwelcome move or loss of an important support person? Ask the woman to describe her labor and birth at a home visit, both to determine whether any complications are present and to evaluate her reaction to the event.

Newborn History: Has the baby had a return visit for a physical examination, and what were the findings? Is there anything about her infant for which a woman is concerned? Is the baby eating well? Sleeping at spaced intervals? Constantly fretful? Is the baby voiding?

Postpartal Course: Does a woman still have pain? Are there any concerns about her health? Is she managing to obtain adequate rest? A woman may be unprepared for feelings of postpartal depression ("baby blues") that she is experiencing. Ask whether she feels "blue" or extremely fatigued.

Future Plans: Will the woman be returning to work outside her home? If so, what plans has she made for child care?

Family Assessment: How are the other children adapting? Does the client have adequate help with the new baby? How are her finances?

Physical Examination of the Mother: Assess temperature, pulse, and respiratory rate to detect possible infection or excessive blood loss. Assess uterine height and consistency (by the 10th day after delivery, the uterus should no longer be palpable as an abdominal organ). Assess the perineum to be certain there are no signs of infection in episiotomy stitches and that lochia color and odor are normal. Assess the breasts for engorgement or any sign of infection.

Physical Examination of the Infant: Assess temperature, pulse, respiratory rate, and skin turgor. Assess the abdomen for distention. Inspect for any ecchymotic marks. Assess for full range of motion of extremities and that the child follows a moving light. Assess for jaundice. Inspect for possible diaper rash. Check that the skin around the cord is not reddened. (Full assessment of a newborn is discussed in Chapter 24.)

Follow-Up Information: Be certain the family has made plans (or knows how to make plans) for continued care for both the infant and the mother. Be certain that they have the telephone number of a health care provider they can call if they have a concern before their next follow-up appointment.

Visiting a new family a few days after a hospital discharge is enjoyable, because most families have at least one question about their newborn that they are pleased to have answered. They are always pleased to be reassured that they are parenting well.

Postpartal Examination

Every newborn should have a health maintenance visit 2 to 4 weeks after birth (see Chapter 24). Every woman should have a checkup by her physician or nurse-midwife at 4 to 6 weeks after birth (the end of the postpartal period), to assure herself and her health care provider that she is in good health and has no residual problems from childbearing.

During this examination, the woman's abdominal wall is inspected for tone. Her breasts are inspected to see whether they have returned to their nonpregnant state if she is not breast-feeding, or to see that they are unfissured and free of complications if she is breast-feeding. Most important, a thorough internal examination is performed to be certain that involution is complete, the ligaments and the pelvic muscle supports have returned to good functional alignment, and any lacerations sustained during birth have healed (Table 22.4). Ask about the possibility of intimate partner abuse, because it can increase during the postpartal period due to the added stress.

If a woman has hemorrhoids or varicosities as a result of the pregnancy, her physician or nurse-midwife will discuss with her whether further management of these conditions is necessary. You should review the necessity of having a breast examination, Papanicolaou (Pap) smear, and pelvic examination every year as a means of screening for breast, cervical, and uterine cancer. If a woman is older than 40 years of age, include a discussion about the need for mammogram examinations at least every other year. Encourage women who have stopped smoking during pregnancy to continue to be smoke-free as yet another good health measure.

The postpartal examination should be a time for a woman to discuss any problems she had with childbearing and any she now has with childrearing, because these are a continuum. If reproductive life planning was not discussed immediately after birth, this visit is an opportune time for such a discussion. If the woman desires to use a diaphragm or a cervical cap, they can be fitted during this examination. Subcutaneous implanted hormonal contraception (Norplant) also can be inserted at this time.

Checkpoint Question 3

You care for Joan Cooper at a 6-week postpartum visit. What should her fundal height be at this time?

a. Six fingerbreadths below the umbilicus.
b. No longer palpable on her abdomen.
c. One centimeter above the symphysis pubis.
d. Inverted and palpable at the cervix.

NURSING CARE OF A POSTPARTAL WOMAN AND FAMILY WITH UNIQUE NEEDS

A Woman Who Chooses Not to Keep Her Child

Although the availability of birth control information and the ability of women to secure abortions have reduced the number of unwanted or unplanned children, some women still may complete a pregnancy and then give up their child for adoption. There are numerous reasons for this decision: a woman may be unmarried, or her marriage may be failing, and she does not want to raise a child alone. She may feel that her family is already complete. She may want to finish school before having a child, or she may want to pursue a career.

During pregnancy, most women decide whether they will keep their child. During labor, they express confidence in their decision, but with the actual birth of their child, they may find that their resolve wavers. A woman who was certain she was going to surrender her child for adoption may realize she wants to keep the child. A woman who was certain she was going to keep her child could become aware for the first time of the responsibility involved and decide that the best course for the child is adoption. In either event, a woman's feelings become confused.

For a woman who chooses not to keep her child, the wait in the birthing room for completion of perineal re-

TABLE 22.4

Six-Week Physical Assessment

Area of Assessment	Data Collection
History	Assess chief concern, family profile (support system, bonding, self-esteem, family integrity), interval history, and review of systems (urinary system for pain, frequency, or stress incontinence along with gastrointestinal tract and reproductive tract in particular). Assess maternal intake. Some new mothers are too fatigued to eat well, so they eat mainly carbohydrate snack foods or, at least, not a balanced diet.
Physical Examination	**Expected Findings**
General appearance	Alert; positive mood. If not, woman is probably still extremely fatigued
Weight	Achievement of prepregnant weight; if not, this will be her baseline postpregnant weight
Hair	Healthy, firm hair; excess loss of hair from early postpartal period has halted
Eyes	Pink and moist conjunctiva; if pallor persists, diet may be inadequate due to fatigue
Breasts	
Nursing women	Full and firm to palpation; blue veins prominent under skin; only slightly tender. No palpable nodules or lumps. If erythematous or tender, mastitis may be present. If fissures on nipples are present, the woman may need to expose her nipples to air or to apply additional cream. An occasional filled milk gland may present as a lump; reexamine after breast-feeding
Non-nursing women	Return to prepregnant size; no palpable nodules or lumps
Abdomen	Striae less prominent; linea nigra fading, muscle tone improving. No distended bowel from constipation. No distended bladder from retention. No history of pain, frequency, or blood on urination. (If lax abdominal muscle tone is present, women need to increase abdominal exercises. For constipation, increase fluid and fiber. Urinary symptoms probably reflect urinary infection that needs specific treatment.)
Perineum and uterus	No lochia; cervix closed; uterus has returned to prepregnant size. Pap test is normal. Ask woman to bear down during pelvic examination to observe for uterine prolapse, rectocele, or cystocele. If involution is not complete, reason for subinvolution must be investigated
Lower extremities	Varicosities barely noticeable
Rectum	Hemorrhoids receded to prepregnant size or are no longer observable
Laboratory Report	
Laboratory values	Hct: 37%; Hgb: 11–12 g/100 mL. If these are low, reassess diet; possibly iron supplement may be needed Rubella antibody titer: 1:8; if low, additional immunization is recommended before a second pregnancy

Hct, hematocrit; Hgb, hemoglobin.

pair and preparations for transfer of the baby to a nursery may seem unusually long. She may also be alone, with no partner or support person with her during this time. Every woman has a right to see, hold, and feed her child if she wishes. A woman who is not going to keep her child may feel proud that she has produced a healthy baby. The realization that the baby is well can provide a foundation on which to build a sound future so she does not have to make this choice again.

Do not attempt to change a woman's mind about keeping her child or placing the child for adoption during the postpartal period. She is extremely vulnerable to suggestion at this time, and such decisions are too long range and too important to be made at such an emotional time. Her earlier conclusions may be the sound ones. Instead, offer nonjudgmental support. Be especially aware of your own feelings about this issue, to avoid influencing a woman's decision making unnecessarily.

During the taking-in phase of the puerperium, be especially careful that you do not "lead" the woman's thinking. Women enjoy having decisions made for them during this time and may ask what you think is best. An answer such as, "You're the one who has to make this decision. What are your thoughts about it?" can help her begin to think through the problem.

It is not uncommon for women who surrender their infants for adoption to experience grief reactions, the same as those of women whose children have died. If a woman decides to surrender her child for adoption, refer her to an official adoption agency, if she has not contacted one already. An official agency gives a woman the best assurance that the parents chosen for her child will be appropriate. This assurance helps to relieve any misgivings or guilt she may have about surrendering the child and should reduce the moments of doubt that can come in future years, such as wondering whether the child is well cared for and is getting everything the mother could have given her.

Some women do not openly voice a wish to give up their child, but their actions demonstrate that they feel little attachment to him or her. A woman who wants to keep her baby has a tentative but eager approach to her newborn, whereas a woman who has doubts is slow to make contact, barely touching the baby even by the time of discharge, and asking few questions about newborn care. When this happens, the hospital social service department can be of assistance in helping the woman plan the child's future. A single mother or a married couple may place an infant for adoption or into a foster home, although for some couples family counseling may be a greater need.

It is a fallacy to assume that everything will work out once the woman and infant arrive home. The number of abused children seen in hospital emergency departments is proof of the harm that can follow when assessment to detect poor parent–child bonding is inadequate in the first few days of life.

A Woman Who Is Discharged But Whose Child Remains Hospitalized

Newborns who are ill at birth often are transported to a regional center or to a neonatal intensive care nursery for care, a move that automatically separates them from their parents. Many transport teams take an instant photograph of the baby and leave it with the mother. They also leave the nursery telephone number and the name of a nurse or doctor to contact for questions or information. Most transport teams telephone the mother after they arrive at the distant hospital to assure her that her infant managed the stress of transport well.

Maintaining communication with the nursery is important so that parents can begin to bond with their child. Urge them to telephone the nursery at least once daily to ask about their infant. If the infant is hospitalized in the same hospital, help the mother arrange visiting time with the infant. Transport her to the nursery, so that she can see and, ideally, hold her child. Without this assistance, some women will not telephone or visit, because they are afraid that this is an imposition or inconvenience for the nursery. Assure the mother that her telephone calls and visits are expected (the nursery wants to encourage bonding). Visiting in the intensive care nursery is further discussed in Chapter 26.

Some mothers whose infants are ill at birth feel uncomfortable sharing a hospital room with a postpartal roommate who is caring for a well baby. This is often a good time to arrange for a visit to the nursery, or to suggest that you and the woman take a walk in the hallway to increase her amount of ambulation.

A Family Who Is Adopting a Child

A family who is adopting an infant may come into the hospital or birthing center to meet their new infant for the first time. Such a couple needs the same introduction to newborn care as biologic parents do. Additional needs of adopting parents are discussed in Chapter 2.

Key Points

The postpartal period (puerperium) is the 6-week period after childbirth. This is an important period, because it marks the child's introduction to the family. Women move through an initial "taking-in" phase, in which they are dependent; a "taking-hold" phase, in which they manifest independence; and a "letting-go" phase, in which the mother role is finally defined.

Rooming-in is the preferred health care agency arrangement for postpartal families, because it allows a new family the best chance for quality interaction. The more time new parents spend with a newborn, the more likely it is that effective bonding will occur. Help parents to feel comfortable with their newborn by offering anticipatory guidance and role modeling infant care.

"Postpartal blues" are a normal accompaniment to childbirth. You can reassure a woman that her feelings are normal and offer supportive care until the emotion passes.

Uterine involution is the process whereby the uterus returns to its prepregnant state. A uterus decreases in size 1 fingerbreadth a day until it disappears under the pubic bone at about day 10. Lochia is the name of the vaginal flow after childbirth: the flow is lochia rubra (red) for the first 1 to 3 days; lochia serosa (pink to brown) on days 4 through 10; and lochia alba (white) until 2 to 6 weeks after the birth.

A woman is at great risk for hemorrhage in the postpartal period, so assessments done during this time are some of the most critical assessments made in nursing. Do not discount the importance of these assessments because the overall content of the postpartal period is so focused on wellness.

Lactation is the production of breast milk. Colostrum is present immediately after birth; milk forms on the third to fourth postpartal day. A feeling of fullness and firmness on this day is termed *filling;* if warmth and discomfort occur, it is termed *engorgement.*

Women may need various comfort measures to alleviate pain from sutures, uterine pain (afterpains), and breast tenderness. Application of cold or heat and administration of analgesics are important nursing interventions.

Women need to learn about self-care before health care agency discharge, so that they can maintain self-care at home. A follow-up telephone call or home visit is helpful. All women should conscientiously return for a visit at 6 weeks after childbirth, to be certain their reproductive organs have returned to normal. A menstrual flow should return within 6 to 10 weeks in the non–breast-feeding mother, or 3 to 4 months in the breast-feeding mother.

Critical Thinking Exercises

1. As the nurse working in a postpartum unit, you are caring for Mike and Joan Cooper, who have just become parents of an 8 lb, 2 oz baby girl. Mike will be taking a week off from work to spend time with Joan and the new baby. Joan is on maternity leave from her job as a court reporter. As you prepare them for discharge, you notice that they seem overwhelmed with much of the information they have been provided. Joan says, trying to get the baby to nurse, "He's so big and my breasts are so small, maybe he can't get enough milk. I was hoping by breast-feeding I wouldn't have to worry about birth control for a while, but I'm having so much trouble maybe that won't work out." Mike pulls you aside and says, "Sometimes, I see my wife crying for no reason. Isn't she as happy as I am?" What additional postpartal teaching does the Cooper family need?

2. Suppose Joan Cooper did not have an episiotomy incision, so you expect her to have little perineal discomfort. Instead, she states that her perineal pain is excruciating. You notice she has hemorrhoids. You overhear her tell her husband that he is acting selfishly for paying more attention to their new daughter than to her. You observe her handing her baby roughly to her husband. What could you suggest to make her more comfortable?

3. Suppose you are present at Joan's 6-week postpartal checkup. What would you include in an assessment plan to ensure that she has physically and emotionally adjusted well to childbirth?

4. Examine the National Health Goals related to the postpartal period. Most government-sponsored money for nursing research is allotted based on these goals. What would be a possible research topic to explore pertinent to these goals that would be applicable to the Cooper family and also advance evidence-based practice?

References

Beck, C. T. (2004). Post-traumatic stress disorder due to childbirth: The aftermath. *Nursing Research, 53*(4), 216-224.

Bridges, W. (1994). *Job shift: How to prosper in a workplace without jobs.* Menlo Park, Calif.: Addison-Wesley.

Crenshaw, J. (2004). Care practices that promote normal birth #6: No separation of mother and baby with unlimited opportunity for breastfeeding. *Journal of Perinatal Education, 13*(2), 35-41.

Crowther, C., & Middleton, P. (2005). Anti-D administration after childbirth for preventing Rhesus alloimmunisation. *The Cochrane Library (Oxford) (4)* (CD000021).

Department of Health and Human Services. (2000). *Healthy people 2010.* Washington, D.C.: Author.

Dodgson, J. E., Chee, Y., & Yap, T. S. (2004). Workplace breast-feeding support for hospital employees. *Journal of Advanced Nursing, 47*(1), 91-100.

Gay, C. L., Lee, K. A., & Lee, S. (2004). Sleep patterns and fatigue in new mothers and fathers. *Biological Research for Nursing, 5*(4), 311-318.

Harvey, M. A. (2003). Pelvic floor exercises during and after pregnancy: A systematic review of their role in preventing pelvic floor dysfunction. *JOGC: Journal of Obstetrics and Gynaecology Canada, 25*(6), 487-498.

Johnson, M., Maas, M., & Moorhead, S. (2000). *Nursing outcomes classification* (2nd ed.). St. Louis: Mosby.

Karch, A. M. (2004). *Lippincott's nursing drug guide.* Philadelphia: Lippincott Williams & Wilkins.

Maimbolwa, M. C., et al. (2003). Cultural childbirth practices and beliefs in Zambia. *Journal of Advanced Nursing, 43*(3), 263-274.

Matthys, L. A., et al. (2004). Delayed postpartum preeclampsia: An experience of 151 cases. *American Journal of Obstetrics and Gynecology, 190*(5), 1464-1466.

McCloskey, J., & Bulechek, G. (2000). *Nursing interventions classification* (3rd ed.). St. Louis: Mosby.

Rubin, R. (1977). Binding-in in the postpartum period. *Maternal Child Nursing Journal, 6*(2), 67-69.

St. John, E., & Rouse, D. J. (2003). Normal labor, delivery, newborn care and puerperium. In Scott, J. R., et al. *Danforth's obstetrics and gynecology* (9th ed.). Philadelphia: Lippincott Williams & Wilkins.

Ural, S. H. (2004). Management of catastrophic obstetrical hemorrhages: Review questions. *Hospital Physician, 40*(2), 35-36.

Van der Wijden, C., Kleijnen, J., & Van den Berk, T. (2005). Lactational amenorrhea for family planning. *The Cochrane Library (Oxford) (4)* (CD001329).

Wambach, K. A. (2003). Lactation mastitis: A descriptive study of the experience. *Journal of Human Lactation, 19*(1), 24-34.

White, P. M. (2004). Heat, balance, humors, and ghosts: Postpartum in Cambodia. *Health Care for Women International, 25*(2), 179-194.

Suggested Readings

Brown, S., et al. (2005). Early postnatal discharge from hospital for healthy mothers and term infants. *The Cochrane Library (Oxford) (4)* (CD002958).

Fredriksson, G. E. M., et al. (2003). Postpartum care should provide alternatives to meet parents' need for safety, active participation, and 'bonding.' *Midwifery, 19*(4), 267-276.

Levitt, C., et al. (2004). Systematic review of the literature on postpartum care: Methodology and literature search results. *Birth, 31*(3), 196-202.

Morse, C., et al. (2004). Improving the postnatal outcomes of new mothers. *Journal of Advanced Nursing, 45*(5), 465-474.

Murray, L., Woolgar, M., & Cooper, P. (2004). Detection and treatment of postpartum depression. *Community Practitioner, 77*(1), 13-17.

Ockleford, E. M., Berryman, J. C., & Hsu, R. (2004). Postnatal care: What new mothers say. *British Journal of Midwifery, 12*(3), 166-170.

Phillips, S. (2003). Psychological issues: Debriefing following traumatic childbirth. *British Journal of Midwifery, 11*(12), 725-727.

Shevell, T., & Malone, F. D. (2003). Management of obstetric hemorrhage. *Seminars in Perinatology, 27*(1), 86-104.

Stowe, Z. N., Hostetter, A. L., & Newport, D. J. (2005). The onset of postpartum depression: Implications for clinical screening in obstetrical and primary care. *American Journal of Obstetrics and Gynecology, 192*(2), 522-526.

Wolfberg, A. J., et al. (2004). Dads as breastfeeding advocates: Results from a randomized controlled trial of an educational intervention. *American Journal of Obstetrics and Gynecology, 191*(3), 708-712.

CHAPTER 23

Nursing Care of a Woman and Family Experiencing a Postpartal Complication

Key Terms

endometritis
mastitis
peritonitis
postpartal depression
postpartal psychosis
thrombophlebitis

Objectives

After mastering the contents of this chapter, you should be able to:

1. Describe common deviations from the normal that can occur during the puerperium.
2. Assess a woman and her family for deviations from the normal during the puerperium.
3. Formulate nursing diagnoses related to deviations from the normal during the puerperium.
4. Identify expected outcomes of a postpartal woman experiencing a complication.
5. Plan interventions that meet the special needs of a family with a postpartal complication, such as planning for an extended hospitalization.
6. Implement nursing care when a postpartal complication such as hemorrhage, infection, pregnancy-induced hypertension, or postpartal psychosis develops.

7. Evaluate expected outcomes for achievement and effectiveness of care.
8. Identify National Health Goals related to postpartal complications that nurses can help the nation achieve.
9. Identify areas related to care of women with postpartal complications that could benefit from additional nursing research or application of evidence-based practice.
10. Use critical thinking to analyze ways that promote family-centered nursing care when a postpartal complication occurs.
11. Integrate knowledge of postpartal complications with the nursing process to achieve quality maternal and child health nursing care.

*M*ary Blackhawk *is a 30-year-old woman who had a "textbook-perfect" pregnancy. You enter her room 4 hours after delivery, but, because she is sleeping and appears comfortable, you hesitate to awaken her. When you observe her more closely, however, you realize she appears abnormally pale. When you obtain her vital signs, you document her pulse as 90 bpm and her blood pressure as 96/50 mm Hg. When you fold back her bedclothes, you discover that her bed is soaked with blood. You suspect she is experiencing one of the most serious complications of pregnancy, postpartum hemorrhage. Yet because she was sleeping, she was totally unaware of it.*

In the previous chapter, you learned about caring for a woman during the normal postpartal period. In this chapter, you will add to your knowledge base information about how to care for a woman and her family when there is a complication during this time. This is important information, because it can help protect the health of both women and their families.

What emergency measures does Ms. Blackhawk need? What should be your first action?

After you've studied this chapter, access the accompanying website. Read the patient scenario and answer the questions to further sharpen your skills, grow more familiar with RN-CLEX types of questions, and reward yourself with how much you have learned.

Although the puerperium is usually a period of health, complications can occur. When they do, immediate intervention is essential to prevent long-term disability and interference with parent–child relationships. Box 23.1 describes National Health Goals related to this period.

A woman with a postpartal complication is at risk from three points of view: her own health, her future childbearing potential, and her ability to bond with her new infant. The family may be disrupted because of an extended hospital stay that removes the mother from other family members. Financial difficulties may arise because of the need for additional child care. Fortunately, most postpartal complications are preventable, and if they do occur, the majority can be treated effectively.

Nursing Process Overview

For a Woman Experiencing a Postpartal Complication

● *Assessment*

Assessment findings associated with a postpartal complication may be extremely subtle, such as tenderness in the calf of a leg, a slight increase in pain, a slight elevation in temperature, or a slight increase in the amount of lochia (Box 23.2). Because the average woman usually has no postpartal complications and the length of stay in a hospital is short, it is easy to overlook these subtle signs. Be alert to any findings

BOX 23.1 FOCUS ON . . .

NATIONAL HEALTH GOALS

The postpartal period is a time when women are very susceptible to hemorrhage and thrombophlebitis, and women with a complication after childbirth may choose not to breast-feed. Two National Health Goals directly relate to this period (DHHS, 2000):

- Reduce the maternal mortality rate to no more than 3.3 per 100,000 live births, from a baseline of 7.1 per 100,000.
- Increase to at least 75% the proportion of mothers who breast-feed their babies in the early postpartal period, from a baseline of 64%.

Nurses can help the nation achieve these goals by careful monitoring of uterine involution in the postpartal period and by encouraging women to breast-feed even in the face of a postpartal complication.

Areas related to complications of the postpartal period that could benefit from additional nursing research include methods to better identify risk factors for mastitis and endometritis; identifiable differences between women who stop breast-feeding and those who continue when a complication is present; and health teaching that is effective in preventing mastitis.

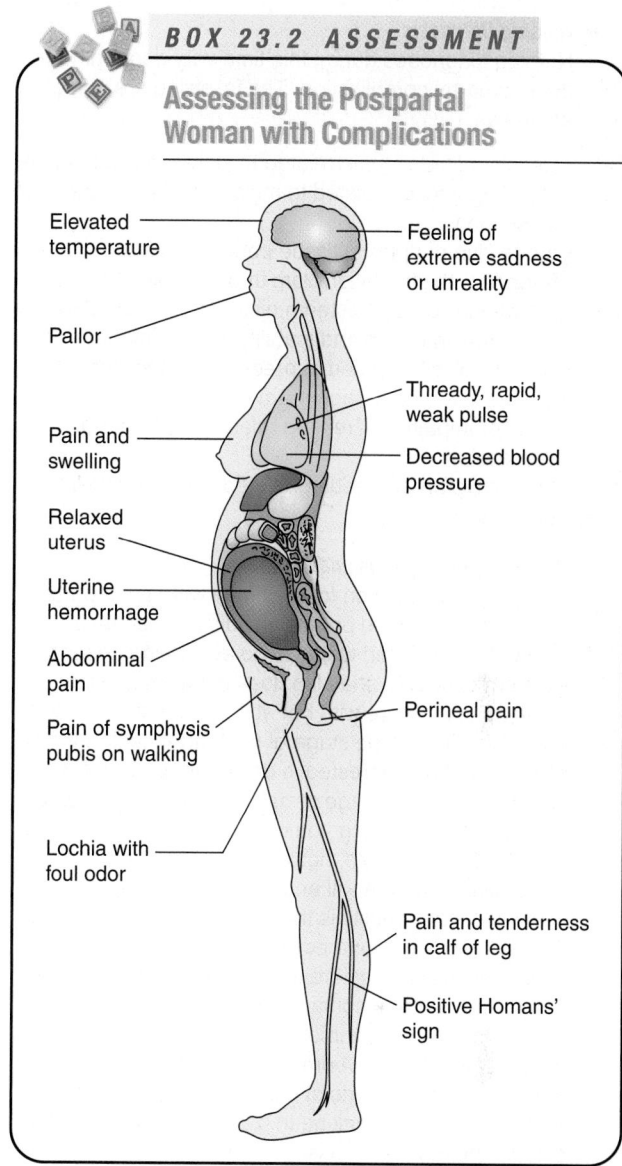

BOX 23.2 ASSESSMENT

Assessing the Postpartal Woman with Complications

- Elevated temperature
- Pallor
- Pain and swelling
- Relaxed uterus
- Uterine hemorrhage
- Abdominal pain
- Pain of symphysis pubis on walking
- Lochia with foul odor
- Feeling of extreme sadness or unreality
- Thready, rapid, weak pulse
- Decreased blood pressure
- Perineal pain
- Pain and tenderness in calf of leg
- Positive Homans' sign

that are "different from usual," because they may indicate a problem. To be certain, do not rely solely on a mother's report of perineal healing or amount of lochia. Always inspect her perineum yourself, because the report of "I feel fine" may be deceptive (e.g., she expected to have pain and so reports extreme pain as nothing out of the norm; she has no knowledge of "normal" lochia or fundal height against which to compare her own condition accurately).

An increased temperature during the first 24 hours after birth is an extremely serious finding. Women may try to "explain away" an increased temperature, because they know that if they have an elevated temperature they may not be allowed to go home or feed their infant. Do not be tempted to rationalize such a finding with explanations such as "The room was warm," or "She just drank some hot coffee." Although these factors may make a slight difference (part of one degree) in temperature level, they do not affect it enough to account for an oral temperature greater than 100.4°F (38.0°C).

● *Nursing Diagnosis*

Nursing diagnoses during this time vary depending on the postpartal complication. The following are some examples:

- Deficient fluid volume related to increased lochia flow
- Risk for infection related to microorganism invasion of episiotomy
- Ineffective peripheral tissue perfusion related to interference with circulation from thrombophlebitis
- Situational low self-esteem disturbance related to postpartal infection and inability to feed infant
- Social isolation related to precautions necessary to protect infant and others from infection transmission
- Risk for impaired parenting related to postpartal depression
- Ineffective breast-feeding related to development of mastitis

● *Outcome Identification and Planning*

Outcome identification for a woman with a postpartal complication may be particularly difficult because, although the woman wants to do everything necessary to return to health, she also does not want to allow anything to interfere with her ability to bond with her new child. During the stage of postpartal "taking-in," she may not be interested in doing things for herself; during the second stage of "taking-hold," she may not be interested in having you do procedures for her (see Chapter 22). As a rule, however, never underestimate how much a woman will endure to prepare to care for a new child. That quality is the essence of motherhood.

When planning for a postpartal family, provide for measures that will restore the woman most quickly to health and promote contact among her, her child, and her primary support person. If physical contact between a mother and her newborn is not possible, give the mother frequent reports of her infant's health and preferences. During her taking-in phase, have the nursery contact the mother at least once every nursing shift to update her on the infant's status; during her taking-hold phase, encourage her to contact the nursery. If the infant is being cared for in another facility, ask them to fax or e-mail photographs of the infant. This provides something concrete to which a new mother can relate. Many mothers respond well to notes written as if they were from the child, for example, "Hi, Mom. Just a note to say hello. I'm drinking well but I miss you and can't wait for you to get better and be allowed to take care of me. Love, Kelsey Marie." Such a note serves to relieve a mother's concern for her child (she is doing well) and also helps to increase the mother's self-esteem, which can promote bonding. As many as 1 woman in every 500 develops severe depression and even psychosis after childbirth (St. John & Rouse, 2003). This risk increases when a complication develops. A helpful national volunteer support group for women who are depressed after childbirth is Depression After Delivery (*www.depressionafterdelivery.com*).

● *Implementation*

Interventions for a woman with a postpartal complication should include instruction for both self-care and child care (if appropriate), emphasizing the transitory nature of the complication. Continuing to review well-child care in this way helps the woman accept her situation as temporary, reinforcing the idea she will be able to care for her infant when she is healthy again.

● *Outcome Evaluation*

Evaluation of a woman with a postpartal complication should address her and her family's health as well as her family's ability to bond with the new child. Evaluation may suggest the need for home care follow-up to assist the woman in coping with the responsibility of child care and integrating a new child into the family in the face of reduced energy from illness.

Examples of expected outcomes include the following:

- Oral temperature decreases to less than 100.4°F (38.0°C).
- Lochia is free of foul odor.
- Client maintains blood pressure higher than 110/60 mm Hg.
- Client demonstrates bonding behaviors with infant despite separation.
- Client demonstrates warm contact with her child while maintaining required bed rest.

POSTPARTAL HEMORRHAGE

Hemorrhage, one of the most important causes of maternal mortality associated with childbearing, poses a possible threat throughout pregnancy and is a major potential danger in the immediate postpartal period. Traditionally, postpartal hemorrhage has been defined as any blood loss from the uterus greater than 500 mL within a 24-hour period (St. John & Rouse, 2003). In specific agencies, the loss may not be considered hemorrhage until it reaches 1,000 mL. Hemorrhage may occur either early (i.e., within the first 24 hours), or late (anytime after the first 24 hours during the remaining days of the 6-week puerperium). The greatest danger of hemorrhage is in the first 24 hours because of the grossly denuded and unprotected area left after detachment of the placenta.

There are four main causes for postpartal hemorrhage: uterine atony, lacerations, retained placental fragments, and disseminated intravascular coagulation (Fig. 23.1).

Uterine Atony

Uterine atony, or relaxation of the uterus, is the most frequent cause of postpartal hemorrhage (Miller et al., 2004). The uterus must remain in a contracted state after birth to allow the open vessels at the placental site to seal. Factors that predispose to poor uterine tone and an inability to maintain a contracted state are summarized in Box 23.3. When caring for a client in whom any of these conditions are present, be especially cautious in your observations and be on guard for signs of uterine bleeding. This is especially important because many postpartal clients are discharged within 48 hours after birth.

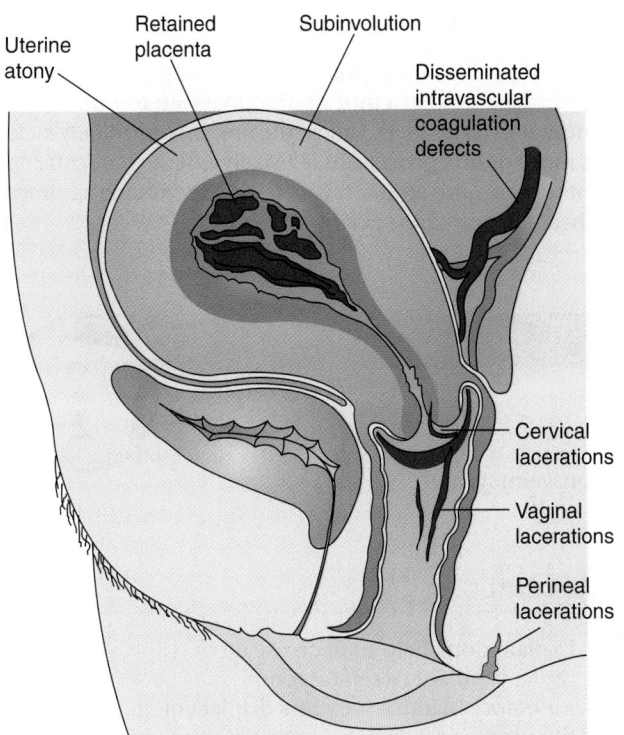

Uterine atony

Retained placenta

Subinvolution

Disseminated intravascular coagulation defects

Cervical lacerations

Vaginal lacerations

Perineal lacerations

FIGURE 23.1 Common causes of postpartal hemorrhage.

NURSING DIAGNOSIS AND RELATED INTERVENTIONS

Nursing Diagnosis: Deficient fluid volume related to excessive blood loss after birth.

Outcome Evaluation: Client's blood pressure remains higher than 100/60 mm Hg; pulse remains between 70 and 90 bpm; lochia flow is less than one saturated perineal pad per hour.

If the uterus suddenly relaxes, there will be an abrupt gush of blood vaginally from the placental site. Vaginal bleeding can be extremely copious, and the client may exhibit symptoms of shock and blood loss. This may occur immediately after birth or more gradually, over the first postpartum hour, as the uterus slowly becomes uncontracted. When the vaginal bleeding occurs gradually, it results in seepage, not a gush of blood. Over a period of hours, however, continued seepage can be as lethal as a sudden release of blood.

It is difficult to estimate the amount of blood a postpartal woman has lost, because it is difficult to estimate the amount of blood it takes to saturate a perineal pad. The amount is about 25 to 50 mL. By counting the number of perineal pads saturated in given lengths of time (e.g., such as half-hour intervals), you can form a rough estimate of blood loss.

BOX 23.3

Conditions That Increase A Woman's Risk For Postpartal Hemorrhage

Conditions That Distend the Uterus Beyond Average Capacity
Multiple gestation
Hydramnios (excessive amount of amniotic fluid)
Large baby (more than 9 lb)
Presence of uterine myomas (fibroid tumors)

Conditions That Could Have Caused Cervical or Uterine Lacerations
Operative birth
Rapid birth

Conditions With Varied Placental Site or Attachment
Placenta previa
Placenta accreta
Premature separation of the placenta
Retained placental fragments

Conditions That Leave the Uterus Unable to Contract Readily
Deep anesthesia or analgesia
Labor initiated or assisted with an oxytocin agent
Maternal age greater than 30 years
High parity
Previous uterine surgery
Prolonged and difficult labor
Possible chorioamnionitis
Secondary maternal illness (e.g., anemia)
Prior history of postpartum hemorrhage
Endometritis
Prolonged use of magnesium sulfate or other tocolytic therapy

Conditions That Lead to Inadequate Blood Coagulation
Fetal death
Disseminated intravascular coagulation

Five pads saturated in half an hour is obviously a different situation from five pads saturated in 8 hours. In either situation, however, a woman will have lost approximately 250 mL of blood, and if either scenario is allowed to continue unattended, she will be in grave danger. Be sure you differentiate between *saturated* and *used* when counting pads. Weighing perineal pads before and after use and then subtracting the difference is an accurate way to measure vaginal discharge: 1 g of weight is comparable to 1 mL of blood volume. Always be sure to turn a woman on her side when inspecting for blood loss, to be certain that a large amount of blood is not pooling undetected beneath her.

Palpate a woman's fundus at frequent intervals postpartally to ascertain that her uterus is remaining in a state of contraction. This is the best measure for preventing early hemorrhage. When palpating a uterine fundus, if you are unsure whether you have located it, the uterus is probably in a state of relaxation. Under normal circumstances, a well-contracted uterus is firm and easily recognized because it feels like no other abdominal structure. Frequent assessment of lochia and vital signs, particularly pulse and blood pressure, is equally important (Roman & Rebarber, 2003).

Therapeutic Management

In the event of uterine atony, the first step in controlling hemorrhage is to attempt uterine massage to encourage contraction (Box 23.4). Unless the uterus is extremely lacking in tone, this procedure is usually effective in causing contraction, and, after a few seconds, the uterus assumes its healthy, grapefruit-like feel.

BOX 23.4 NURSING PROCEDURE

Fundal Massage

Purpose
To stimulate uterine contraction, promote uterine tone and consistency, and minimize the risk of hemorrhage.

PROCEDURE	PRINCIPLE
1. Explain the procedure to the client and provide privacy.	1. Explanations help to decrease anxiety; providing privacy enhances self-esteem.
2. Ask the client to void (unless bleeding is extensive and more rapid action seems necessary).	2. An empty bladder prevents displacement of the uterus and ensures accurate assessment of uterine tone.
3. Place the client supine with her knees flexed and feet together.	3. Proper positioning enhances visualization and effectiveness of procedure.
4. a. Put on gloves. Place one hand on the abdomen just above the symphysis pubis.	4. a. This location anchors the lower uterine segment.
b. Place the other hand around the top of the fundus.	b. This location helps to assess and locate the fundus and determine height.

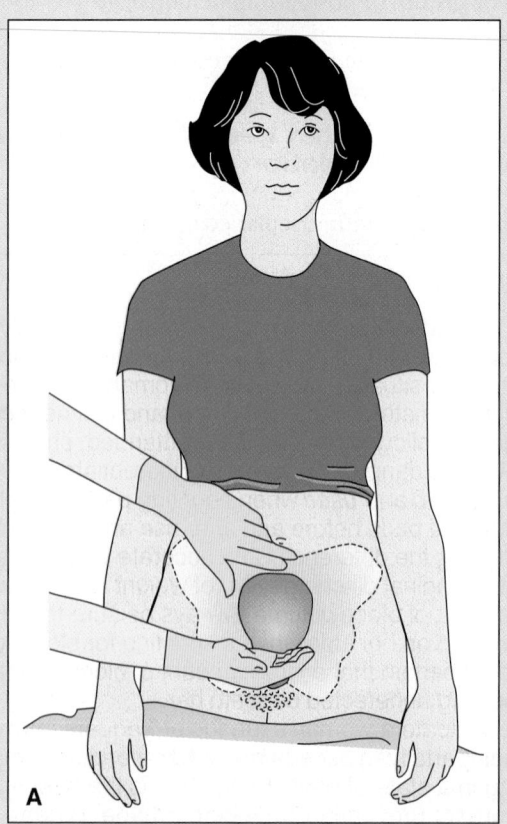

A

PROCEDURE	PRINCIPLE
5. Rotate the upper hand to massage the uterus until it is firm, being careful not to overmassage the uterus.	5. Massage should be done only when uterus is not firm; otherwise muscle fatigue and uterine relaxation may occur. Aggressive massage may lead to partial or complete uterine prolapse.

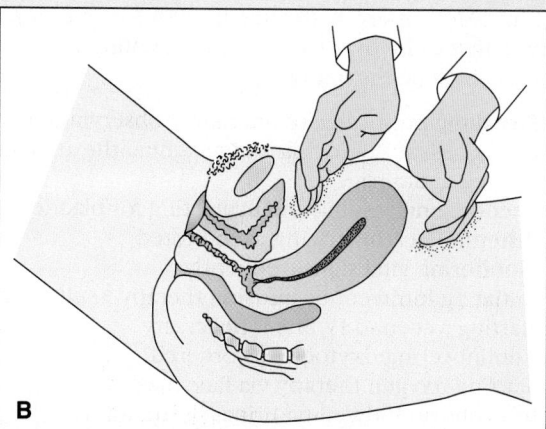

PROCEDURE	PRINCIPLE
6. When the uterus is firm, gently press the fundus between the hands using slight downward pressure against the lower hand.	6. Gently squeezing with downward pressure helps to expel blood or clots collected in the uterine cavity.
7. Remove the perineal pad. Observe the perineum for passage of clots and amount of bleeding.	7. This helps to assess the degree of bleeding.
8. When the uterus is again firm, cleanse the perineum and apply a clean perineal pad. Discard gloves and soiled pads according to agency policy.	8. This helps to promote comfort and hygiene while reducing the risk for infection.
9. Document results of procedure. Continue to assess fundus and lochia according to agency policy. Notify physician or nurse-midwife if fundus does not remain firm or bleeding continues.	9. Documentation provides a means for evaluation. Continued assessment allows for early identification and prompt intervention with additional measures, such as oxytocin, to prevent hemorrhage.

With uterine atony, even if the uterus responds well to massage, the problem may not be completely resolved. After you remove your hand from the fundus, the uterus may relax and the lethal seepage may begin again. Therefore, remain with the woman after massaging her fundus, to be certain the uterus is not relaxing again. Observe carefully, including fundal height and consistency and lochia, for the next 4 hours.

If a uterus cannot remain contracted, the physician or nurse-midwife probably will order a dilute intravenous infusion of oxytocin (Pitocin) to help the uterus maintain tone (see Box 18.12 in Chapter 18). Intramuscular methylergonovine (Methergine), an ergot compound, is a second possibility. Both drugs should be readily available for use on a hospital unit in the event of postpartal hemorrhage.

The usual dosage of oxytocin is 10 to 40 U per 1,000 mL of a 5% dextrose solution. When oxytocin is given intravenously, its action is immediate. However, be aware that oxytocin has a short duration of action, approximately 1 hour, so symptoms of uterine atony can recur quickly after administration of only a single dose. Box 23.5 highlights appropriate outcomes and interventions related to postpartum hemorrhage, using the terminology identified by the Nursing Outcomes Classification (NOC) and Nursing Interventions Classification (NIC).

Additional measure that can be helpful are the following:

- Offer a bedpan or assist the woman with ambulating to the bathroom at least every 4 hours to keep her bladder empty. A full bladder pushes an uncontracted uterus into an even more uncontracted state. To reduce bladder pressure, insertion of a urinary catheter may be ordered.
- If the woman is experiencing respiratory distress from decreasing blood volume, administer oxygen by face mask at a rate of 4 L/minute. Position her supine to allow adequate blood flow to her brain and kidneys.
- Obtain vital signs frequently and make sure to interpret them accurately, looking for trends. For example, a continuously rising pulse rate is an ominous pattern.

If a woman is losing enough blood to affect her systemic circulation, she will develop signs of shock, such as an increased, thready, and weak pulse; decreased blood pressure; increased and shallow respirations; pale, clammy skin; and increasing anxiety.

In the event of slow bleeding, there is little change in pulse and blood pressure at first because of circulatory

BOX 23.5

Nursing Outcomes Classification (NOC) and Nursing Interventions Classification (NIC)

Postpartum Hemorrhage

NOC: Circulation Status

Circulation status is defined as the extent to which blood flows unobstructed, unidirectionally, and at an appropriate pressure through large vessels of the systemic and pulmonary systems (Johnson, Maas, & Moorhead, 2000). Some specific indicators suggesting that this outcome has been achieved include the following:

- Vital signs, including systolic and diastolic blood pressure, pulse, and heart rate within expected ranges
- Central venous pressure and pulmonary wedge pressure within acceptable parameters
- Absence of orthostatic hypotension, abnormal heart sounds, bruits, and adventitious breath sounds
- Strong, symmetric peripheral pulses
- Balanced 24-hour intake and output
- Cognitive status within expected range

NIC: Bleeding Reduction: Postpartum Uterus

Bleeding reduction, postpartum uterus, is defined as limiting the amount of blood loss from the postpartum uterus (McCloskey & Bulechek, 2000). Some important activities involved when implementing this intervention include the following:

- Providing perineal care, including observing the characteristics of lochia and weighing the amount of vaginal drainage
- Encouraging voiding and evaluating for bladder distention; catheterizing as indicated
- Monitoring vital signs frequently
- Initiating intravenous infusion therapy, including starting a second IV line if necessary
- Administering oxytocics as ordered
- Starting oxygen therapy via face mask
- Inserting an indwelling urinary catheter to evaluate urinary output
- Administering blood products as appropriate
- Assisting with packing the uterus, evacuating hematoma, or suturing lacerations as indicated
- Preparing for an emergency hysterectomy as needed
- Keeping the client and family informed of condition and measures being performed

---

compensation. Suddenly, however, the system can compensate no more, and then the pulse rate rises rapidly. The pulse becomes weak and thready, and the blood pressure drops abruptly. The woman's skin becomes cold and clammy, and she shows obvious signs of shock. Consistent frequent assessments of uterine tone and vital signs help to detect blood loss before this point is ever reached.

When planning continuing care after sudden blood loss, understand that the woman may be so exhausted that she resents frequent uterine and blood pressure assessments. Explain that these measures, although disturbing, are important for her welfare. Obtain vital signs as quickly and gently as possible, so that the woman feels a minimum of discomfort and disruption, allowing her time to rest.

Bimanual Massage. If fundal massage and administration of oxytocin or methylergonovine are not effective in stopping uterine bleeding, the physician or nurse-midwife may attempt bimanual compression. With this procedure, the physician or nurse-midwife inserts one hand into a woman's vagina while pushing against the fundus through the abdominal wall with the other hand. If necessary, a sonogram may be done to detect possible retained placental fragments. The woman may be returned to the delivery or birthing room so that her uterine cavity can be explored manually. Uterine packing may be inserted during this procedure to help halt bleeding. Uterine manipulation is painful; anticipate the need for analgesia or anesthesia to provide comfort.

Prostaglandin Administration. Prostaglandins promote strong, sustained uterine contractions. Prostaglandin F may be injected intramuscularly to initiate uterine contractions. Watch for nausea, diarrhea, tachycardia, and hypertension, all of which are possible adverse effects of prostaglandin administration (Karch, 2004).

Blood Replacement. Blood transfusion to replace blood loss with postpartal hemorrhage may be necessary. Make sure that blood typing and cross-matching were done when the client was admitted and that blood is available. Some women donate blood during pregnancy so that they can be autotransfused if hemorrhage should occur postpartally.

The average woman takes the full postpartal period to regain her strength. Women who experience postpartal hemorrhage tend to have a longer than average recovery period, because the physiologic exhaustion of body systems may interfere with their recovery. Iron therapy may be prescribed to ensure good hemoglobin formation. Activity level, exertion, and postpartal exercise may be restricted somewhat. Discuss with the woman the possibility of having someone stay with her at home, at least for the first week, to help with the care of her new baby and to prevent exhaustion from turning childbearing into a less than satisfying event.

Extensive blood loss is one of the precursors of postpartal infection because of the general debilitation that results. Any woman who has experienced more than a normal loss of blood should be observed closely for changes in lochia discharge. Also, monitor her temperature closely in the postpartal period, to detect the earliest signs of developing infection. Make sure the patient knows how to check for normal lochia and temperature once she is discharged.

Hysterectomy. Usually, therapeutic management is effective in halting bleeding. In the rare instance of extreme uterine atony, ligation of the uterine arteries or a hysterectomy may be necessary (Shevell & Malone, 2003). These measures are done as a last resort only. In this emergency situation, provide comfort and support to the woman, because this is a totally unexpected outcome of childbearing for her and her support person.

After hysterectomy, a woman may want to talk about what happened, why surgery was necessary, or how she feels now that she can no longer bear children. She needs to discuss her feelings with a person who will listen quietly and help her sort through her feelings of "Why me?" She may have ambiguous feelings: she wanted to have more children (or at least have the ability to have more), but she also wants to live. She is thankful that her life was saved, but she may feel resentful that she has been left incapable of future childbearing. She may grieve for children who will not be born. If this child was born outside the hospital and the woman was brought there under emergency circumstances, she may have a need to talk about her choice of location for childbirth. She may feel guilty that she did not choose a more controlled place for childbirth.

Open lines of communication between the couple and the staff that allow the family to vent its feelings are most helpful to the couple in this crisis (Phillips, 2003). Grieving for future children who will not be born can interfere with bonding with the present child.

Lacerations

Small lacerations or tears of the birth canal are common and may be considered a normal consequence of childbearing. However, large lacerations are complications. They occur most often in the following circumstances:

- With difficult or precipitate births
- In primigravidas
- With the birth of a large infant (more than 9 lb)
- With the use of a lithotomy position and instruments

Either cervical, vaginal, or perineal lacerations may occur. After birth, any time a uterus feels firm but bleeding persists, suspect a laceration of one of these three sites.

Cervical Lacerations

Lacerations of the cervix are usually found on the sides of the cervix, near the branches of the uterine artery. If the artery is torn, the blood loss may be so great that blood gushes from the vaginal opening. Because this is arterial bleeding, it is brighter red than the venous blood lost with uterine atony. Fortunately, this bleeding ordinarily occurs immediately after delivery of the placenta, when the physician or nurse-midwife is still in attendance.

Therapeutic Management. Repair of a cervical laceration is difficult, because the bleeding can be so intense that it obstructs visualization of the area. Be certain that a physician or nurse-midwife has adequate space to work, adequate sponges and suture supplies, and a good light source. The woman is not always aware of what is happening at this point, but she senses quickly that something is seriously wrong. Try to maintain an air of calm and, if possible, stand beside the woman, at the head of the table. She may be worried that the extra activity in the room has something to do with her baby. Reassure her about her baby's condition and inform her about the need to stay in the birthing room a little longer than expected while the doctor or nurse-midwife places additional sutures. Remember that the protective attitude the woman has felt toward her body all during pregnancy is now turned toward the baby, so she usually is relieved to learn that any problem that may be occurring is hers, not her infant's.

If the cervical laceration appears to be extensive or difficult to repair, it may be necessary for the woman to be given a regional anesthetic to relax the uterine muscle and to prevent pain. Explain the need for an anesthetic and the procedures being carried out.

Vaginal Lacerations

Although they are rare, lacerations can also occur in the vagina. They are easier to assess than cervical lacerations, because they are easier to view.

Therapeutic Management. Because vaginal tissue is friable, vaginal lacerations are hard to repair. Some oozing often occurs after a repair, so the vagina may be packed to maintain pressure on the suture line. An indwelling urinary catheter (Foley catheter) may be placed at the same time, because the packing causes pressure on the urethra and can interfere with voiding. If packing is inserted, document in the client's nursing care plan when it was placed, so you can be sure it will be removed after 24 to 48 hours or before discharge. Packing that is left in place too long leads to stasis and infection similar to toxic shock syndrome (Golden, 2003).

Perineal Lacerations

Lacerations of the perineum usually occur when a woman is placed in a lithotomy position for birth, because this position increases tension on the perineum. Perineal lacerations are classified by four categories, depending on the extent and depth of the tissue involved. These categories are shown in Table 23.1.

Therapeutic Management. Perineal lacerations are sutured and treated as an episiotomy repair. Make certain that the degree of the laceration is documented, because afterward it is often difficult to distinguish a repaired perineal laceration from an episiotomy repair on inspection. Lacerations and episiotomies tend to heal in the same length of time. A diet high in fluid and a stool softener may be prescribed for the first week after birth to prevent constipation and hard stools, which could break the sutures. Any woman who has a third- or fourth-degree laceration should not have an enema or a rectal suppository prescribed or have her temperature taken rectally, because the hard tips of equipment could open sutures near to or in-

TABLE 23.1

Classification of Perineal Lacerations

Classification	Description of Involvement
First degree	Vaginal mucous membrane and skin of the perineum to the fourchette
Second degree	Vagina, perineal skin, fascia, levator ani muscle, and perineal body
Third degree	Entire perineum, and reaches the external sphincter of the rectum
Fourth degree	Entire perineum, rectal sphincter, and some of the mucous membrane of the rectum

cluding those of the rectal sphincter. Be sure that ancillary caregivers such as nurses' aides are informed of this, so that they understand why these measures are contraindicated. Unless a secondary complication such as infection occurs, even fourth-degree lacerations heal without long-term dyspareunia or incontinence or sexual dissatisfaction.

Retained Placental Fragments

Occasionally, a placenta does not deliver in its entirety; fragments of it separate and are left behind. Because the portion retained keeps the uterus from contracting fully, uterine bleeding occurs. Although this is most likely to happen with a succenturiate placenta—a placenta with an accessory lobe (see Chapter 21)—it can happen in any instance. Placenta accreta—a placenta that fuses with the myometrium because of an abnormal decidua basalis layer—may also be retained. To detect the complication of retained placenta, every placenta should be inspected carefully after birth to see that it is complete. A blood serum sample that contains human chorionic gonadotropin hormone (hCG) also reveals that part of a placenta is still present (Katz, 2003).

Assessment

If an undetected retained fragment is large, bleeding will be apparent in the immediate postpartal period, because the uterus cannot contract with the fragment in place. If the fragment is small, bleeding may not be detected until postpartum day 6 to 10, when the woman notices an abrupt discharge and a large amount of blood.

On examination, usually the uterus is not fully contracted. Retained placental fragments also may be detected by sonography.

Therapeutic Management

Removal of the placental fragment is necessary to stop the bleeding. Usually, a dilatation and curettage (D&C) is performed to remove the placental fragment. In some instances, placenta accreta is so deeply attached that it cannot be surgically removed. Methotrexate may be prescribed in these instances to destroy the retained placental tissue (Kay, 2003). Because the hemorrhage from retained fragments may be delayed until after a woman is at home, be certain the client knows to continue to observe the color of lochia discharge and to report any tendency for the discharge to change from lochia serosa or alba back to rubra.

Checkpoint Question 1

Suppose Mary Blackhawk has a retained placental fragment that is causing extensive postpartal bleeding. What hormone test would you anticipate being ordered to detect whether placenta is still present?

a. Placental and cord blood estrogen
b. Progesterone from the placenta
c. Human chorionic gonadotropin hormone
d. Systemic prolactin (a pituitary hormone)

Disseminated Intravascular Coagulation

Disseminated intravascular coagulation (DIC) is a deficiency in clotting ability caused by vascular injury. It may occur in any woman in the postpartal period, but it is usually associated with premature separation of the placenta, a missed early miscarriage, or fetal death in utero. DIC is discussed in Chapter 15.

Subinvolution

Subinvolution is incomplete return of the uterus to its prepregnant size and shape. With subinvolution, at a 4- or 6-week postpartal visit, the uterus is still enlarged and soft. Lochial discharge usually is still present. Subinvolution may result from a small retained placental fragment, a mild endometritis, or an accompanying problem (e.g., a myoma) that is interfering with complete contraction.

Therapeutic Management

Oral administration of Methergine, 0.2 mg four times daily, usually is prescribed to improve uterine tone and complete involution. If the uterus is tender to palpation, suggesting endometritis, an oral antibiotic also may be prescribed. Be certain a woman is able to recognize the normal process of involution and lochial discharge before she returns home, to help prevent delay in seeking health care. A chronic loss of blood from subinvolution will result in infection or anemia and lack of energy, conditions that possibly could interfere with bonding also.

Perineal Hematomas

A perineal hematoma is a collection of blood in the subcutaneous layer of tissue of the perineum. The overlying skin, as a rule, is intact with no noticeable trauma. Such blood collections may be caused by injury to blood vessels

CHAPTER 24

Nursing Care of a Newborn and Family

Key Terms

acrocyanosis	natal teeth
caput succeda-	neonatal
neum	period
cavernous	neonate
hemangioma	nevus
central	flammeus
cyanosis	physiologic
cephal-	jaundice
hematoma	pseudomen-
conduction	struation
convection	radiation
erythema	strawberry
toxicum	heman-
evaporation	gioma
hemangioma	subconjunc-
jaundice	tival
kangaroo care	hem-
kernicterus	orrhage
lanugo	thrush
meconium	transitional
milia	stool
mongolian spot	vernix
	caseosa

Objectives

After mastering the contents of this chapter, you should be able to:

1. Describe the normal characteristics of a term newborn.
2. Assess a newborn for normal growth and development.
3. Formulate nursing diagnoses related to a newborn or the family of a newborn.
4. Identify expected outcomes for a newborn and family during the first 4 weeks of life.
5. Plan nursing care to augment normal development of a newborn, such as ways to aid parent–child bonding.
6. Implement nursing care of a normal newborn, such as administering a first bath or instructing parents on how to care for their newborn.
7. Evaluate expected outcomes to determine effectiveness of nursing care and outcome achievement.
8. Identify National Health Goals related to newborns that nurses could help the nation achieve.
9. Identify areas related to newborn assessment and care that could benefit from additional nursing research or application of evidence-based practice.
10. Use critical thinking to analyze ways that the care of a term newborn can be more family centered.
11. Integrate knowledge of newborn growth and development and immediate care needs with the nursing process to achieve quality maternal and child health nursing care.

*C*arlotta Ruiz has just given birth to her second child, a 6-lb, 5-oz baby girl she named Beth. Newborn Apgar scores at 1 and 5 minutes were 6 and 8. Vital signs are: temperature (axillary), 98.2°F (36.8°C); heart rate, 136 bpm; respirations, 74 breaths per minute. She is 18.5 inches long, with a head circumference of 34 cm and a chest circumference of 32 cm. She has a small port-wine birthmark on her right thigh.

While Jose, Carlotta's husband, is in the room, Carlotta tells you she is a "veteran" at baby care. Jose adds, "Little Joe {their 3-year-old} will be so excited to see his new sister. That's all he's been talking about lately."

When Carlotta is alone, you notice she seems a little apprehensive about caring for her new daughter. She tells you, "She's so much smaller than Joe was. And why does it sound like she has a cold? And what is this rash all over her? Isn't it bad enough she has a birthmark?"

Previous chapters described the care of the pregnant woman and family during the antepartal, intrapartal, and postpartal periods. This chapter adds information about caring for a newborn and family to your knowledge base.

Does Carlotta know as much about newborns as she thought? What additional teaching does this family need?

After you've studied this chapter, access the accompanying website. Read the patient scenario and answer the questions to further sharpen your skills, grow more familiar with RN-CLEX types of questions, and reward yourself with how much you have learned.

Newborns undergo profound physiologic changes at the moment of birth (and, probably, psychological changes as well), as they are released from a warm, snug, dark, liquid-filled environment that has met all of their basic needs, into a chilly, unbounded, brightly lit, gravity-based, outside world.

Within minutes after being plunged into this strange environment, a newborn's body must initiate respirations and accommodate a circulatory system to extrauterine oxygenation. Within 24 hours, neurologic, renal, endocrine, gastrointestinal, and metabolic functions must be operating competently for life to be sustained.

How well a newborn makes these major adjustments depends on his or her genetic composition, the competency of the recent intrauterine environment, the care received during the labor and birth period, and the care received during the newborn or **neonatal period** (from birth through the first 28 days of life). National Health Goals related to the first days of life are shown in Box 24.1. Nurses can play a major role in achieving these goals.

Two thirds of all deaths that occur during the first year of life occur in the neonatal period. More than half occur in the first 24 hours after birth—an indication of how hazardous this time is for an infant. Close observation of a newborn for indications of distress is essential during this period (National Center for Health Statistics, 2005).

Nursing Process Overview

For Health Promotion of the Term Newborn

● *Assessment*

Assessment of a newborn or **neonate** (a baby in the neonatal period) includes a review of the mother's pregnancy history; physical examination of the infant; analysis of laboratory reports such as hematocrit and blood type, if indicated; and assessment of parent–child interaction for the beginning of bonding. Assessment begins immediately after birth and is continued at every contact during a newborn's hospital or birthing center stay, early home visits, and well-baby visits. Teaching parents to make assessments concerning their infant's temperature, respiratory rate, and overall health is crucial so that they can continue to monitor their infant's health at home (Box 24.2).

● *Nursing Diagnosis*

Nursing diagnoses associated with a newborn often center on the problems of establishing respirations, beginning nutrition, and assisting with parent–newborn bonding. Examples are the following:

• Ineffective airway clearance related to mucus in airway
• Ineffective thermoregulation related to heat loss from exposure in birthing room

BOX 24.1 FOCUS ON . . .

NATIONAL HEALTH GOALS

A number of National Health Goals deal directly with the newborn period (DHHS, 2000):

• Increase to at least 75% the proportion of mothers who breast-feed their babies in the early postpartal period, from a baseline of 64%.

• Increase to at least 50% the proportion of women who continue breast-feeding until their babies are 5 to 6 months old, from a baseline of 29%.

• Increase to 70% the percentage of healthy full-term infants who are put to sleep on their backs, from a baseline of 35%.

• Increase to at least 75% the proportion of parents and caregivers who use feeding practices that prevent baby-bottle tooth decay.

• Reduce the neonatal mortality rate to no more than 2.9 per 1,000 live births, from a baseline of 4.8 per 1,000 live births.

Nurses can help the nation achieve these goals, by encouraging women not only to begin breast-feeding but also to continue it through the first 6 months of life; by advising parents on the advantage of placing infants on their backs to sleep and on the danger of tooth decay from letting a baby drink from a bottle of milk or juice while falling asleep; and by discussing with parents who use formula the proper methods for preparation so that gastrointestinal illness does not occur.

Areas that could benefit from additional nursing research include identifying the reasons why some women end breast-feeding shortly after discharge from a health care agency and investigating common methods of encouraging sleep in infants other than by a bottle-feeding.

BOX 24.2 ASSESSMENT

Assessing the Average Newborn

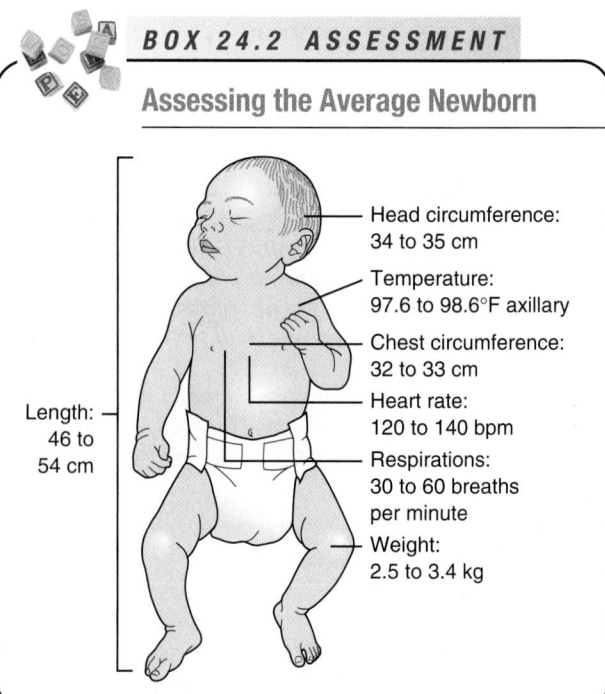

Length: 46 to 54 cm

Head circumference: 34 to 35 cm

Temperature: 97.6 to 98.6°F axillary

Chest circumference: 32 to 33 cm

Heart rate: 120 to 140 bpm

Respirations: 30 to 60 breaths per minute

Weight: 2.5 to 3.4 kg

- Imbalanced nutrition, less than body requirements, related to poor sucking reflex
- Readiness for enhanced family coping related to birth of planned infant
- Health-seeking behaviors related to newborn needs

If a minor deviation from the normal is present, such as a hemangioma, a diagnosis such as "Parental fear related to hemangioma on left thigh of newborn" might be relevant.

● *Outcome Identification and Planning*

Planning nursing care should take into account both the newborn's needs during this transition period and the mother's need for adequate rest during the postpartal period. Try to adapt teaching time to the schedules of the mother and her newborn. Although the woman must learn as much as possible about newborn care, she also must go home from the health care setting with enough energy to practice what she has learned. Important planning measures for newborns include helping them regulate their temperature and helping them grow accustomed to breast- or bottle-feeding.

● *Implementation*

A major portion of implementation in the newborn period is role modeling to help new parents grow confident with their newborn. Be aware how closely parents observe you for guidance in newborn care. Conserving newborn warmth and energy, to help prevent hypoglycemia and respiratory distress, should be an important consideration to accompany all interventions.

● *Outcome Evaluation*

Evaluation of expected outcomes should reveal that the parents are able to give beginning newborn care with confidence. Be certain parents make arrangements for continued health supervision for their newborn, so that evaluation can be continued and the family's long-term health needs can be met. Examples indicating achievement of outcomes are the following:

- Infant establishes respirations of 30 to 60 per minute.
- Infant maintains temperature at 97.8°F to 98.6°F (36.5°C to 37°C).
- Infant breast-feeds for a minimum of 10 minutes every 3 hours.

PROFILE OF A NEWBORN

It is not unusual to hear the comment "all newborns look alike" from people viewing a nursery full of babies. In actuality, every child is born with individual physical and personality characteristics that make him or her unique right from the start (Fig. 24.1).

Some newborns are born stocky and short, some large and bony, some thin and rangy. Some have a temperament that causes them to feed greedily, protest procedures loudly, and respond to their parent's inexperienced handling with restlessness and spitting up. Other newborns sleep soundly, make no protest over procedures or diaper changes, and seem passive in accepting this new step in life. With experience in working with newborns, it be-

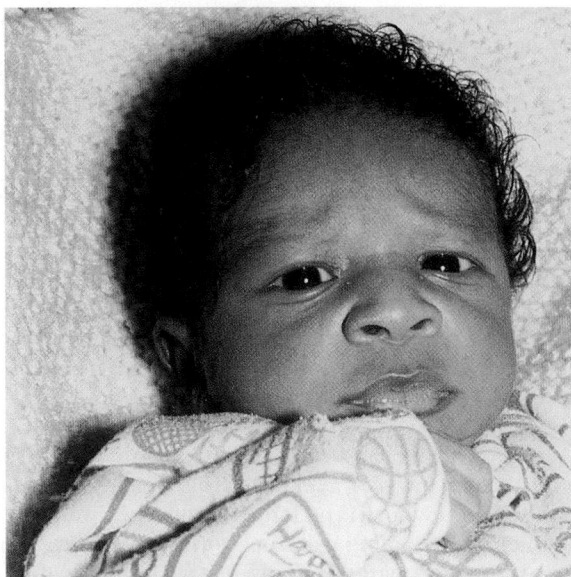

FIGURE 24.1 Personality is apparent in a newborn from the start. Note the alert, searching interest.

comes easier to differentiate newborns who are merely demonstrating the extremes of normal behavior from those whose behavior or appearance indicates a need for more skilled care than is available in typical rooming-in surroundings.

Vital Statistics

Vital statistics for a newborn include weight, length, and head and chest circumference. The technique for obtaining these is shown in Chapter 33, along with other aspects of health assessment. Be sure all health care providers involved with newborns are aware of safety issues specific to newborn care when taking these measurements (e.g., not leaving a newborn unattended on a bed or scale).

Weight

The birth weight of newborns varies depending on the racial, nutritional, intrauterine, and genetic factors that were present during conception and pregnancy. The weight in relation to the gestational age should be plotted on a standard neonatal graph, such as the one shown in Appendix E. Plotting weight helps identify newborns who are at risk because of their small size. This information also separates those who are small for their gestational age (newborns who have suffered intrauterine growth restriction) from preterm infants (infants who are healthy but small only because they were born early). These first measurements also establish a baseline for future evaluation.

Plotting weight in conjunction with height and head circumference is also helpful because it highlights disproportionate measurements (see Appendix E). All three of these measurements should fall near the same percentile in an individual child. For example, a newborn who falls within the 50th percentile for height and weight but whose head circumference is in the 90th percentile may have abnormal head growth. A newborn who is in the 50th percentile for weight and head circumference but in the 3rd percentile for height may have a growth problem.

Second-born children usually weigh more than first-borns. Birth weight continues to increase with each succeeding child in a family.

The average birth weight (50th percentile) for a white, mature female newborn in the United States is 3.4 kg (7.5 lb); for a white, mature male newborn, it is 3.5 kg (7.7 lb). Newborns of other races weigh approximately 0.5 lb less. The arbitrary lower limit of normal for all races is 2.5 kg (5.5 lb). Birth weight exceeding 4.7 kg (10 lb) is unusual, but weights as high as 7.7 kg (17 lb) have been documented. If a newborn weighs more than 4.7 kg, a maternal illness, such as diabetes mellitus, must be suspected (Katz, 2003).

A newborn loses 5% to 10% of birth weight (6 to 10 oz) during the first few days after birth. This weight loss occurs because the newborn is no longer under the influence of salt- and fluid-retaining maternal hormones. Diuresis begins to remove a part of the infant's high fluid load during the second to third day of life. A newborn also voids and passes stool, all measures that reduce weight, because approximately 75% to 90% of a newborn's weight is fluid. In addition, breast-fed newborns have a limited intake until about the third day of life because of the relatively low caloric content and amount of colostrum. If newborns are formula-fed, their intake during this time is also limited because of the time needed to establish effective sucking.

After this initial loss of weight, a newborn has 1 day of stable weight, then begins to gain weight. The breast-fed newborn recaptures birth weight within 10 days; a formula-fed infant accomplishes this gain within 7 days. After this, a newborn begins to gain about 2 lb/month (6 to 8 oz/week) for the first 6 months of life.

Length

The average birth length (50th percentile) of a mature female neonate is 53 cm (20.9 in). For mature males, the average birth length is 54 cm (21.3 in). The lower limit of normal length is arbitrarily set at 46 cm (18 in). Although rare, babies with lengths as great as 57.5 cm (24 in) have been reported.

Head Circumference

In a mature newborn, the head circumference is usually 34 to 35 cm (13.5 to 14 in). A mature newborn with a head circumference greater than 37 cm (14.8 in) or less than 33 cm (13.2 in) should be carefully investigated for neurologic involvement, although occasionally a well newborn falls within these limits. Head circumference is measured with a tape measure drawn across the center of the forehead and around the most prominent portion of the posterior head (the occiput; see Fig. 18.2 in Chapter 18).

Chest Circumference

The chest circumference in a term newborn is about 2 cm (0.75 to 1 in) less than head circumference. This is measured at the level of the nipples. If a large amount of breast tissue or edema of breasts is present, this measurement will not be accurate until the edema has subsided.

Vital Signs

Vital sign measurements begin to change from those present in intrauterine life at the moment of birth.

Temperature

The temperature of newborns is about 99°F (37.2°C) at birth because they have been confined in an internal body organ. The temperature falls almost immediately to below normal because of heat loss and immature temperature-regulating mechanisms. The temperature of birthing rooms, approximately 68°F to 72°F (21°C to 22°C), can add to this loss of heat.

Newborns lose heat by four separate mechanisms: convection, conduction, radiation, and evaporation (Fig. 24.2).

Convection is the flow of heat from the newborn's body surface to cooler surrounding air. The effectiveness of convection depends on the velocity of the flow (a current of air cools faster than nonmoving air). Eliminating drafts, such as from windows or air conditioners, reduces convection heat loss.

Conduction is the transfer of body heat to a cooler solid object in contact with a baby. For example, a baby placed on a cold counter or on the cold base of a warming unit quickly loses heat to the colder metal surface. Covering surfaces with a warmed blanket or towel helps to minimize conduction heat loss.

Radiation is the transfer of body heat to a cooler solid object not in contact with the baby, such as a cold window or air conditioner. Moving an infant as far from the cold surface as possible helps reduce this type of heat loss.

Evaporation is loss of heat through conversion of a liquid to a vapor. Newborns are wet, and they lose a great deal of heat as the amniotic fluid on their skin evaporates. To prevent this heat loss, dry newborns as soon as possible, especially their face and hair, which will not be covered by clothing. The head, a large surface area in a newborn, can be responsible for a great amount of heat loss. Covering the hair with a cap after drying it further reduces the possibility of evaporation cooling.

A newborn not only loses heat easily by the means just described but also has difficulty conserving heat under any circumstance. Insulation, an efficient means of conserving heat in adults, is not effective in newborns because they have little subcutaneous fat to provide insulation. Shivering, a means of increasing metabolism and thereby providing heat in adults, is also rarely seen in newborns.

Newborns can conserve heat by constricting blood vessels and moving blood away from the skin. *Brown fat,* a special tissue found in mature newborns, apparently helps to conserve or produce body heat by increasing metabolism. The greatest amounts of brown fat are found in the intrascapular region, thorax, and perirenal area. Brown fat is thought to aid in controlling newborn temperature similar to temperature control in a hibernating animal. In later life, it may influence the proportion of body fat retained.

Newborns exposed to cool air tend to kick and cry to increase their metabolic rate and produce more heat. This re-

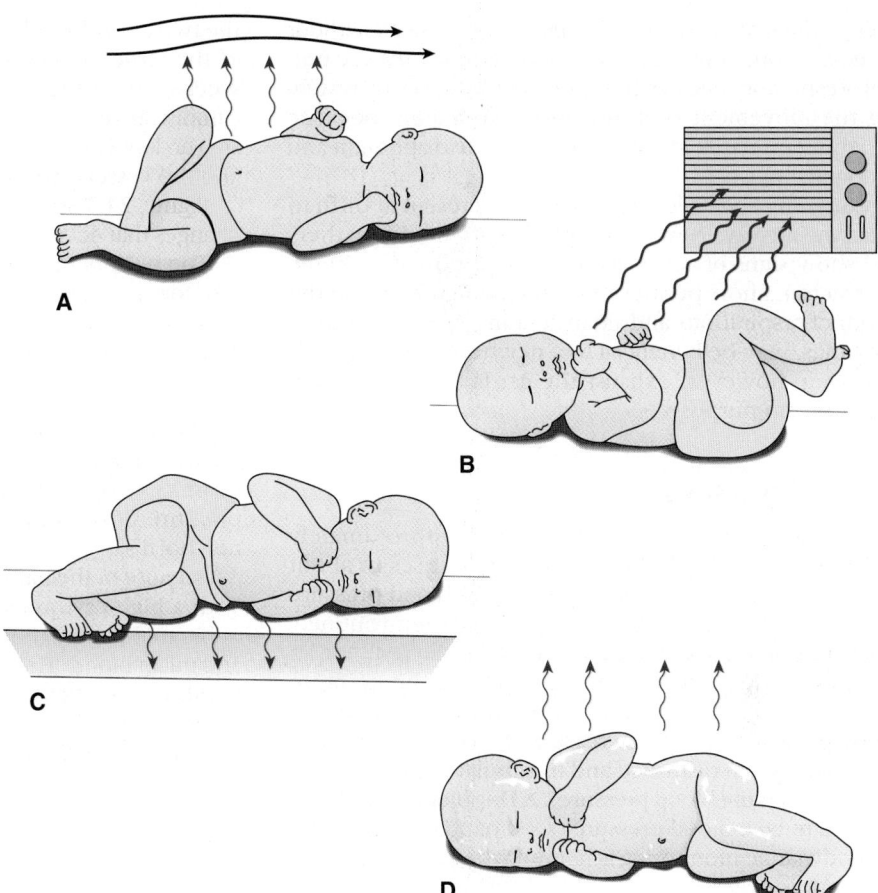

FIGURE 24.2 Heat loss in the newborn. (**A**) Convection. (**B**) Radiation. (**C**) Conduction. (**D**) Evaporation.

action, however, also increases their need for oxygen and their respiratory rate. An immature newborn with poor lung development has trouble making such an adjustment. Newborns who cannot increase their respiratory rate in response to increased needs will be unable to deliver sufficient oxygen to their systems. The resultant anaerobic catabolism of body cells releases acid. Every newborn is born slightly acidotic. Any new buildup of acid may lead to severe, life-threatening acidosis. In addition, a newborn becomes fatigued by rapid breathing, placing additional strain on an already stressed cardiovascular system.

Drying and wrapping newborns and placing them in warmed cribs, or drying them and placing them under a radiant heat source, are excellent mechanical measures to help conserve heat. In addition, placing a newborn against the mother's skin and then covering the newborn also helps to transfer heat from the mother to the newborn; this is termed **kangaroo care** (Anderson et al., 2005).

All early care of newborns should be done speedily to avoid exposing the newborn unnecessarily. Any procedure during which a newborn must be uncovered (e.g., resuscitation, circumcision) should be done under a radiant heat source to prevent damaging heat loss. If chilling is prevented, a newborn's temperature stabilizes at 98.6°F (37°C) within 4 hours after birth.

In contrast to an adult, a newborn with a bacterial infection may run a subnormal temperature. Therefore, if a newborn's temperature does not stabilize shortly after birth, the cause must be investigated so that corrective measures can be taken.

Pulse

The heart rate of a fetus in utero averages 120 to 160 bpm. Immediately after birth, as the newborn struggles to initiate respirations, the heart rate may be as rapid as 180 bpm. Within 1 hour after birth, as the newborn settles down to sleep, the heart rate stabilizes to an average of 120 to 140 bpm.

The heart rate of a newborn often remains slightly irregular because of immaturity of the cardiac regulatory center in the medulla. Transient murmurs may result from the incomplete closure of fetal circulation shunts. During crying, the rate may rise again to 180 bpm. In addition, heart rate can decrease during sleep, ranging from 90 to 110 bpm.

You should be able to palpate femoral pulses in a newborn, but the radial and temporal pulses are more difficult to palpate with any degree of accuracy. Therefore, a newborn's heart rate is always determined by listening for an apical heartbeat for a full minute, rather than assessing a pulse in an extremity. Always palpate for femoral pulses, because their absence suggests possible coarctation (narrowing) of the aorta, a cardiovascular abnormality.

Respiration

The respiratory rate of a newborn in the first few minutes of life may be as high as 80 breaths per minute. As respiratory activity is established and maintained, this rate settles to an average of 30 to 60 breaths per minute when the newborn is at rest. Respiratory depth, rate, and rhythm are likely to be irregular, and short periods of apnea (without cyanosis), sometimes called *periodic respirations,* are normal. Respiratory rate can be observed most easily by watching the movement of a newborn's abdomen, because breathing primarily involves the use of the diaphragm and abdominal muscles.

Coughing and sneezing reflexes are present at birth to clear the airway. Newborns are obligate nose-breathers and show signs of acute distress if their nostrils become obstructed. Short periods of crying, which increase the depth of respirations and aid in aerating deep portions of the lungs, may be beneficial to a newborn. Long periods of crying, however, exhaust the cardiovascular system and serve no purpose.

Blood Pressure

The blood pressure of a newborn is approximately 80/46 mm Hg at birth. By the 10th day, it rises to about 100/50 mm Hg. Because measurement of blood pressure in a newborn is somewhat inaccurate, it is not routinely measured unless a cardiac anomaly is suspected. For an accurate reading, the cuff width used must be no more than two thirds the length of the upper arm or thigh. Blood pressure tends to increase with crying (and a newborn cries when disturbed and manipulated by such procedures as taking blood pressure). A Doppler method may be used to take blood pressure (see Chapters 33 and 36). Hemodynamic monitoring is helpful when continuous assessment is necessary.

the two atria closes because of the pressure against the lip of the structure (permanent closure does not occur for weeks). With the remaining fetal circulatory structures (umbilical vein, two umbilical arteries, and ductus venosus) no longer receiving blood, the blood within them clots, and the vessels atrophy over the next few weeks.

Figure 24.3 shows the respiratory and cardiovascular changes that occur at birth, beginning with the first breath.

The peripheral circulation of a newborn remains sluggish for at least the first 24 hours. It is common to observe cyanosis in the infant's feet and hands (**acrocyanosis**) and for the feet to feel cold to the touch at this time.

Blood Values. A newborn's blood volume is 80 to 110 mL per kilogram of body weight, or about 300 mL total. The oxygen dissociation curve is shifted to the left; that is, the quantity of oxygen bound to hemoglobin and the partial pressure of oxygen are greater in fetal blood than in a newborn's.

Because of the nature of fetal circulation, a baby is born with a high erythrocyte count, about 6 million cells per cubic millimeter. Hemoglobin level averages 17 to 18 g/100 mL of blood. The hematocrit is between 45% and 50%. Capillary heel sticks may reveal a falsely high hematocrit or hemoglobin value because of sluggish peripheral circulation. Before obtaining a blood specimen from a heel, warm the foot by wrapping it in a warm cloth. This increases circulation and improves the accuracy of this value.

Once proper lung oxygenation has been established, the need for the high erythrocyte count diminishes. Therefore, within a matter of days, a newborn's red cells begin to

✔ Checkpoint Question 1

Beth Ruiz, like all newborns, can lose body heat by conduction. Under which condition is this most apt to occur?

a. If the nursery is cooled by air conditioning.
b. If the infant is wet from amniotic fluid.
c. If there is a breeze from an open window.
d. If Beth is placed in a cold bassinet.

Physiologic Function

Just as changes occur in vital signs after birth, so do changes occur in all the major body systems.

Cardiovascular System

Changes in the cardiovascular system are necessary after birth because now the lungs must oxygenate the blood that was formerly oxygenated by the placenta. When the cord is clamped, a neonate is forced to take in oxygen through the lungs. As the lungs inflate for the first time, pressure decreases in the chest generally, and in the pulmonary artery specifically (the artery leading to the lungs). This decrease in pressure in the pulmonary artery plays a role in promoting closure of the ductus arteriosus, a fetal shunt. As pressure increases in the left side of the heart from increased blood volume, the foramen ovale between

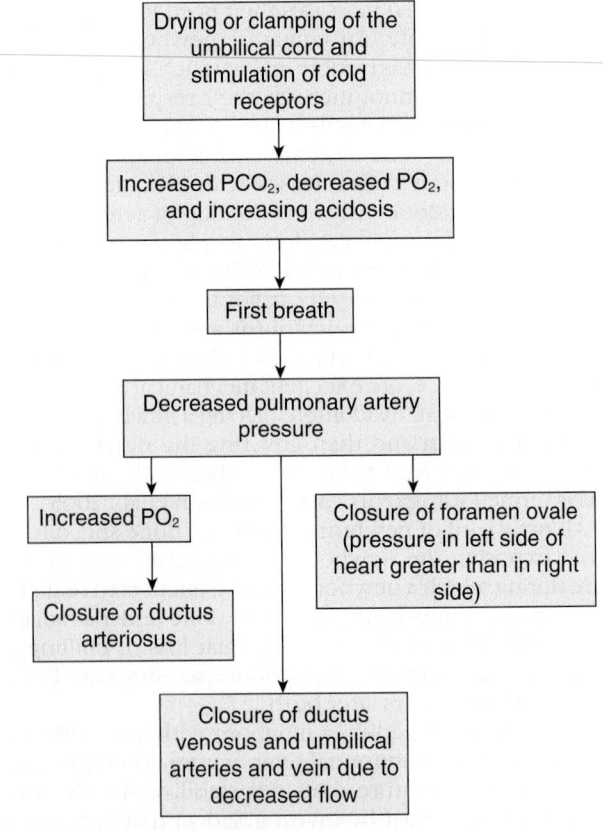

FIGURE 24.3 Circulatory events at birth.

deteriorate. An indirect bilirubin level at birth is 1 to 4 mg/100 mL. Any increase over this amount reflects the release of bilirubin as excessive red blood cells begin their breakdown (Boyd, 2004).

A newborn has an equally high white blood cell count at birth, about 15,000 to 30,000 cells/mm³. Values as high as 40,000 cells/mm³ may be seen if the birth was stressful. Polymorphonuclear cells (neutrophils) account for a large part of this leukocytosis, but by the end of the first month, lymphocytes become the predominant cell type. This leukocytosis is a response to the trauma of birth and is nonpathogenic; an increased white blood cell count should not be taken as evidence of infection. On the other hand, although the high white blood cell count makes infection difficult to prove in a newborn, infection must not be dismissed as a possibility if other signs of infection (e.g., pallor, respiratory difficulty, cyanosis) are present. Usual blood values in a newborn are summarized in Appendix F.

Blood Coagulation. Because most newborns are born with a lower than normal level of vitamin K, they have a prolonged coagulation or prothrombin time. Vitamin K, synthesized through the action of intestinal flora, is necessary for the formation of factor II (prothrombin), factor VII (proconvertin), factor IX (plasma thromboplastin component), and factor X (Stuart-Prower factor). Because a newborn's intestine is sterile at birth unless membranes were ruptured more than 24 hours before birth, it takes about 24 hours for flora to accumulate and for vitamin K to be synthesized. Because almost all newborns can be predicted to have this diminished blood coagulation ability, vitamin K (e.g., AquaMEPHYTON) is administered intramuscularly into the lateral anterior thigh, the preferred site for all injections in a newborn, immediately after birth.

Respiratory System

A first breath is a major undertaking because it requires a tremendous amount of pressure (about 40 to 70 cm H_2O). It is initiated by a combination of cold receptors; a lowered partial pressure of oxygen (PO_2), which falls from 80 to as low as 15 mm Hg before a first breath; and an increased partial carbon dioxide pressure (PCO_2), which rises as high as 70 mm Hg before a first breath. All newborns have some fluid in their lungs from intrauterine life that eases the surface tension on alveolar walls and allows alveoli to inflate more easily than if the lung walls were dry. About a third of this fluid is forced out of the lungs by the pressure of vaginal birth. Additional fluid is quickly absorbed by lung blood vessels and lymphatics after the first breath.

Once the alveoli have been inflated with a first breath, breathing becomes much easier for a baby, requiring only about 6 to 8 cm H_2O pressure. Within 10 minutes after birth, most newborns have established a good residual volume. By 10 to 12 hours of age, vital capacity is established at newborn proportions. The heart in a newborn takes up proportionately more space than in an adult, so the amount of lung expansion space available is proportionately limited.

A baby born by cesarean birth does not have as much lung fluid expelled at birth as one born vaginally and may have more difficulty establishing effective respirations, because excessive fluid blocks air exchange space. Newborns who are immature and whose alveoli collapse each time they exhale (because of the lack of pulmonary surfactant) have difficulty establishing effective residual capacity and respirations. If the alveoli do not open well, a newborn's cardiac system becomes compromised, because closure of the foramen ovale and ductus arteriosus depends on free blood flow through the pulmonary artery and good oxygenation of blood. Therefore, a newborn who has difficulty establishing respirations at birth should be examined closely in the postpartal period for a cardiac murmur or other indication that he or she still has patent cardiac structures, especially a patent ductus arteriosus.

Gastrointestinal System

Although the gastrointestinal tract is usually sterile at birth, bacteria may be cultured from the intestinal tract in most babies within 5 hours after birth and from all babies at 24 hours of life. Most of these bacteria enter the tract through the newborn's mouth from airborne sources. Others may come from vaginal secretions at birth, from hospital bedding, and from contact at the breast. Accumulation of bacteria in the gastrointestinal tract is necessary for digestion and for the synthesis of vitamin K. Because milk, the infant's main diet for the first year, is low in vitamin K, this intestinal synthesis is necessary for blood coagulation.

Although a newborn's stomach holds about 60 to 90 mL, a newborn has limited ability to digest fat and starch because the pancreatic enzymes, lipase and amylase, remain deficient for the first few months of life. A newborn regurgitates easily because of an immature cardiac sphincter between the stomach and esophagus. Immature liver functions may lead to lowered glucose and protein serum levels.

Stools. The first stool of a newborn is usually passed within 24 hours after birth. It consists of **meconium,** a sticky, tarlike, blackish-green, odorless material formed from mucus, vernix, lanugo, hormones, and carbohydrates that accumulated during intrauterine life. If a newborn does not pass a meconium stool by 24 to 48 hours after birth, the possibility of meconium ileus, imperforate anus, or bowel obstruction should be suspected.

About the second or third day of life, newborn stool changes in color and consistency, becoming green and loose. This is termed **transitional stool,** and it may resemble diarrhea to the untrained eye. By the fourth day of life, breast-fed babies pass three or four light yellow stools per day. They are sweet smelling, because breast milk is high in lactic acid, which reduces the amount of putrefactive organisms in the stool. A newborn who receives formula usually passes two or three bright yellow stools a day. These have a slightly more noticeable odor, compared with the stools of breast-fed babies.

A newborn placed under phototherapy lights as a treatment for jaundice has bright green stools because of increased bilirubin excretion. Newborns with bile duct obstruction have clay-colored (gray) stools, because bile pigments are not entering the intestinal tract. Blood-flecked stools usually indicate an anal fissure. Occasionally, a newborn has swallowed some maternal blood during birth and either vomits fresh blood immediately after birth or passes a black tarry stool after two or more days. Maternal blood may be differentiated from fetal blood by a dipstick Apt test. If the stools remain black or tarry, intestinal bleeding should be suspected. If mucus is mixed with stool or the stool is watery and loose, a milk allergy, lactose intolerance, or some other condition should be suspected.

Urinary System

The average newborn voids within 24 hours after birth. A newborn who does not take in much fluid for the first 24 hours may void later than this, but the 24-hour point is a good general rule. Newborns who do not void within this time should be examined for the possibility of urethral stenosis or absent kidneys or ureters.

The possibility of obstruction in the urinary tract can be assessed by observing the force of the urinary stream in both male and female infants. Males should void with enough force to produce a small projected arc; females should produce a steady stream, not just continuous dribbling. Projecting urine farther than normal also may signal urethral obstruction, because it indicates that urine is being forced through a narrow channel.

The kidneys of newborns do not concentrate urine well, making newborn urine usually light-colored and odorless. The infant is about 6 weeks of age before much control over reabsorption of fluid in tubules and concentration of urine becomes evident.

A single voiding in a newborn is only about 15 mL and may be easily missed in a thick diaper. Specific gravity ranges from 1.008 to 1.010. The daily urinary output for the first 1 or 2 days is about 30 to 60 mL total. By week 1, total daily volume rises to about 300 mL. The first voiding may be pink or dusky because of uric acid crystals that were formed in the bladder in utero; this is an innocent finding. A small amount of protein may be normally present in voidings for the first few days of life, until the kidney glomeruli are more fully mature. Diapers can be weighed to determine the amount and timing of voidings.

Immune System

Because they have difficulty forming antibodies against invading antigens until about 2 months of age, newborns are prone to infection. This inability to form antibodies is the reason that most immunizations against childhood diseases are not given to infants younger than 2 months of age. Newborns do have some immunologic protection, because they are born with passive antibodies (immunoglobulin G) from the mother that crossed the placenta. In most instances, these include antibodies against poliomyelitis, measles, diphtheria, pertussis, chickenpox, rubella, and tetanus. Newborns are routinely administered hepatitis B vaccine during the first 12 hours after birth to protect against this disease (American Academy of Pediatrics [AAP], 2005). Little natural immunity is transmitted against herpes simplex. Any health care personnel with herpes simplex eruptions (cold sores) should not care for newborns until the lesions have crusted. Once this occurs,

these personnel should use excellent handwashing technique, because, without antibody protection, herpes simplex infections can become systemic or create a rapidly fatal form of the disease in a newborn.

Neuromuscular System

Mature newborns demonstrate neuromuscular function by moving their extremities, attempting to control head movement, exhibiting a strong cry, and demonstrating newborn reflexes. Limpness or total absence of a muscular response to manipulation is never normal and suggests narcosis, shock, or cerebral injury. A newborn occasionally makes twitching or flailing movements of the extremities in the absence of a stimulus because of the immaturity of the nervous system. Newborn reflexes can be tested with consistency by using simple maneuvers.

Blink Reflex. A blink reflex in a newborn serves the same purpose as it does in an adult—to protect the eye from any object coming near it by rapid eyelid closure. It may be elicited by shining a strong light such as a flashlight or otoscope light on an eye. A sudden movement toward the eye sometimes can elicit the blink reflex.

Rooting Reflex. If the cheek is brushed or stroked near the corner of the mouth, a newborn infant will turn the head in that direction. This reflex serves to help a newborn find food: when a mother holds the child and allows her breast to brush the newborn's cheek, the reflex makes the baby turn toward the breast. The reflex disappears at about the sixth week of life. At about this time, newborn eyes focus steadily, so a food source can be seen, and the reflex is no longer needed.

Sucking Reflex. When a newborn's lips are touched, the baby makes a sucking motion. The reflex helps a newborn find food: when the newborn's lips touch the mother's breast or a bottle, the baby sucks and so takes in food. The sucking reflex begins to diminish at about 6 months of age. It disappears immediately if it is never stimulated (e.g., in a newborn with a tracheoesophageal fistula who cannot take in oral fluids). It can be maintained in such an infant by offering the child a non-nutritive sucking object such as a pacifier (after the fistula has been corrected by surgery and until oral feedings can be given).

Swallowing Reflex. The swallowing reflex in a newborn is the same as in the adult. Food that reaches the posterior portion of the tongue is automatically swallowed. Gag, cough, and sneeze reflexes also are present to maintain a clear airway in the event that normal swallowing does not keep the pharynx free of obstructing mucus.

Extrusion Reflex. A newborn extrudes any substance that is placed on the anterior portion of the tongue. This protective reflex prevents the swallowing of inedible substances. It disappears at about 4 months of age. Until then, the infant may seem to be spitting out or refusing solid food placed in the mouth.

Palmar Grasp Reflex. Newborns grasp an object placed in their palm by closing their fingers on it (Fig. 24.4). Mature newborns grasp so strongly that they can be raised from a supine position and suspended momentarily from an

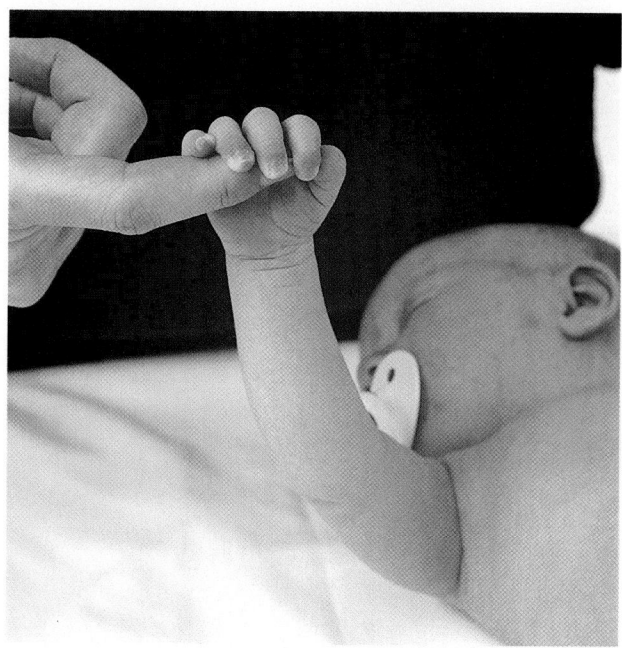

FIGURE 24.4 Palmar grasp reflex.

examiner's fingers. This reflex disappears at about 6 weeks to 3 months of age. A baby begins to grasp meaningfully at about 3 months of age.

Step (Walk)-in-Place Reflex. Newborns who are held in a vertical position with their feet touching a hard surface will take a few quick, alternating steps (Fig. 24.5). This reflex disappears by 3 months of age. By 4 months, babies can bear a good portion of their weight unhindered by this reflex.

Placing Reflex. The placing reflex is similar to the step-in-place reflex, except that it is elicited by touching the anterior surface of the newborn's leg against a hard surface such as the edge of a bassinet or table. The newborn makes a few quick lifting motions, as if to step onto the table, because of the reflex.

Plantar Grasp Reflex. When an object touches the sole of a newborn's foot at the base of the toes, the toes grasp in the same manner as the fingers do. This reflex disappears at about 8 to 9 months of age in preparation for walking. However, it may be present during sleep for a longer period.

Tonic Neck Reflex. When newborns lie on their backs, their heads usually turn to one side or the other. The arm and the leg on the side toward which the head turns extend, and the opposite arm and leg contract (Fig. 24.6). The movement is most evident in the arms but may also be observed in the legs. If you turn a newborn's head to the opposite side, he or she will often change the extension and contraction of legs and arms accordingly. This is also called a boxer or fencing reflex, because the position simulates that of someone preparing to box or fence. Unlike many other reflexes, the tonic neck reflex does not appear to have a function. It does stimulate eye coordination, because the extended arm moves in front of the face. It may signify handedness. The reflex disappears between the second and third months of life.

Moro Reflex. A Moro (startle) reflex (Fig. 24.7) can be initiated by startling a newborn with a loud noise or by jarring the bassinet. The most accurate method of eliciting the reflex is to hold newborns in a supine position and allow their heads to drop backward about 1 inch. In response to this sudden head movement, they abduct and extend their arms and legs. Their fingers assume a typical "C" position.

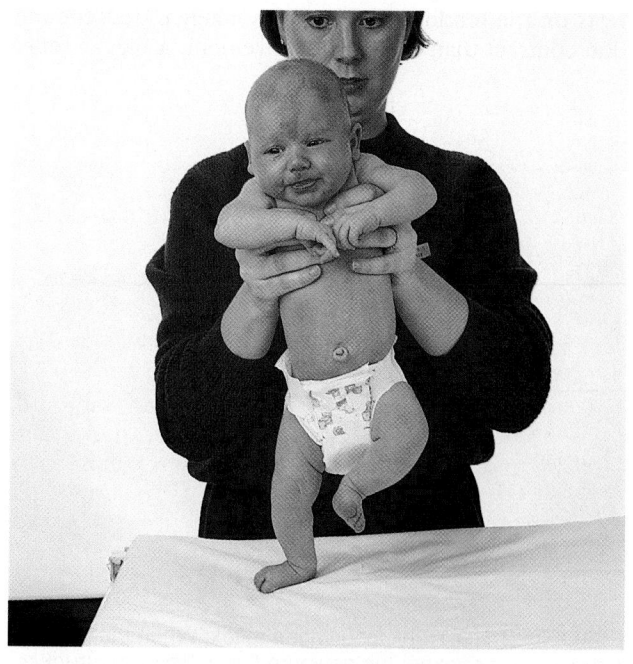

FIGURE 24.5 Step-in-place reflex.

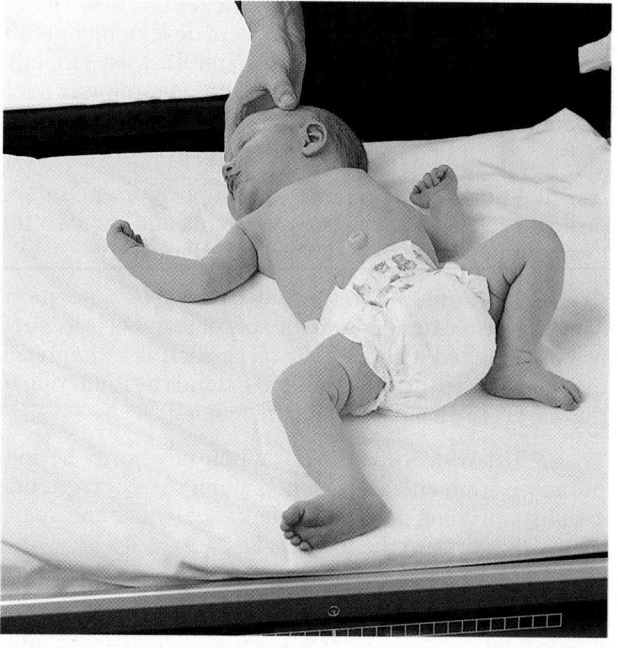

FIGURE 24.6 Tonic neck reflex.

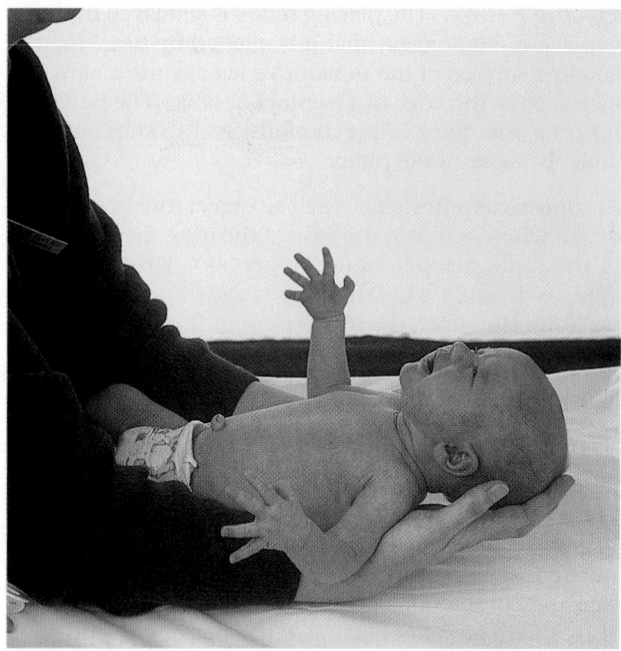

FIGURE 24.7 Moro reflex.

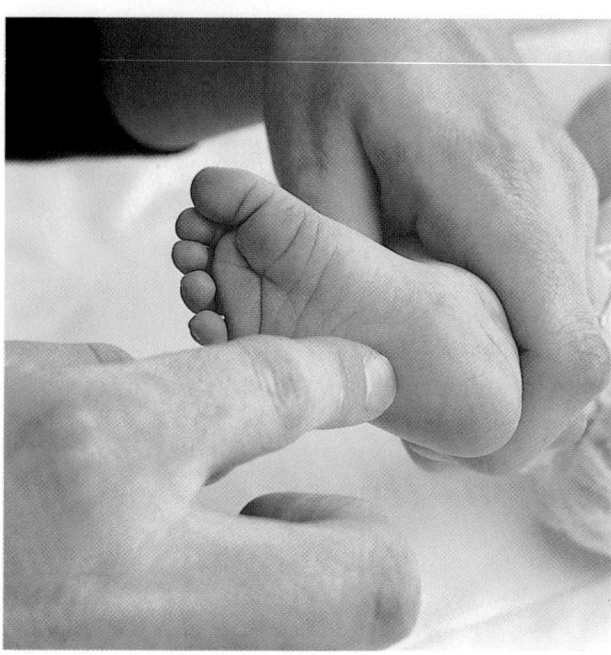

FIGURE 24.8 Babinski reflex. When the examiner moves her finger upward, the newborn's toes will fan outward.

Finally, they swing their arms into an embrace position and pull up their legs against their abdomen (adduction). The reflex simulates the action of someone trying to ward off an attacker, then covering up to protect himself. It is strong for the first 8 weeks of life and then fades by the end of the fourth or fifth month, at the same time an infant can roll away from danger.

Babinski Reflex. When the side of the sole of the foot is stroked in an inverted "J" curve from the heel upward, a newborn fans the toes (positive Babinski sign) (Fig. 24.8). This is in contrast to the adult, who flexes the toes. This reaction occurs because nervous system development is immature. It remains positive (toes fan) until at least 3 months of age, when it is supplanted by the down-turning or adult flexion response.

Magnet Reflex. If pressure is applied to the soles of the feet of a newborn lying in a supine position, he or she pushes back against the pressure. This and the two following reflexes are tests of spinal cord integrity.

Crossed Extension Reflex. If one leg of a newborn lying supine is extended and the sole of that foot is irritated by being rubbed with a sharp object, such as a thumbnail, the infant raises the other leg and extends it, as if trying to push away the hand irritating the first leg.

Trunk Incurvation Reflex. When newborns lie in a prone position and are touched along the paravertebral area by a probing finger, they flex their trunk and swing their pelvis toward the touch (Fig. 24.9).

Landau Reflex. A newborn who is held in a prone position with a hand underneath, supporting the trunk, should demonstrate some muscle tone. Babies may not be able to lift their head or arch their back in this position (as they

will at 3 months of age), but neither should they sag into an inverted "U" position. The latter response indicates extremely poor muscle tone, the cause of which should be investigated.

Deep Tendon Reflexes. A patellar reflex can be elicited in a newborn by tapping the patellar tendon with the tip of the finger. The lower leg moves perceptibly if the infant has an intact reflex. To elicit a biceps reflex, place the thumb of your left hand on the tendon of the biceps muscle on the inner surface of the elbow. Tap the thumb as it rests on the tendon. You are more likely to feel the tendon contract than to observe movement. A biceps reflex

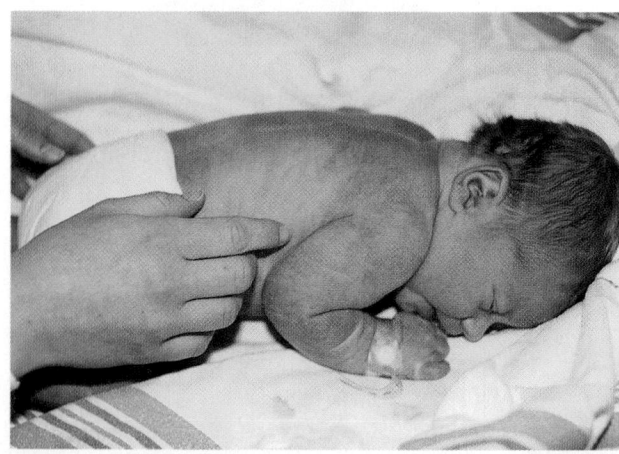

FIGURE 24.9 Trunk incurvation reflex. When the paravertebral area is stroked, the newborn flexes his or her trunk toward the direction of the stimulation.

is a test for spinal nerves C5 and C6; a patellar reflex is a test for spinal nerves L2 through L4.

Checkpoint Question 2

A Moro reflex is the single best assessment of neurologic ability in a newborn. What is the best way to test this reflex?

a. Observe the infant while she is on her abdomen to see whether she can turn her head.
b. Lift the infant's head while she is supine and allow it to fall back 1 inch.
c. Shake the infant's crib until the infant responds by flailing her arms.
d. Make a sharp noise, such as clapping your hands, to wake the infant.

The Senses

The senses in newborns are already developed at birth.

Hearing. A fetus is able to hear in utero even before birth. As soon as amniotic fluid drains or is absorbed from the middle ear by way of the eustachian tube—within hours after birth—hearing becomes acute. Newborns appear to have difficulty locating sound, however, and do not turn toward it consistently. Perhaps they must learn to interpret small differences among sounds arriving at their ears at different times. They respond with generalized activity to a sound such as a bell ringing a short distance from their ear. A newborn who is actively crying when the bell is rung stops crying and seems to attend. Similarly, newborns calm in response to a soothing voice and startle at loud noises. They recognize their mother's voice almost immediately, as if they have heard it in utero.

Vision. Newborns see as soon as they are born and possibly have been "seeing" light and dark in utero for the last few months of pregnancy, as the uterus and the abdominal wall were stretched thin. Newborns demonstrate sight at birth by blinking at a strong light (blink reflex) or by following a bright light or toy a short distance with their eyes. Because they cannot follow past the midline of vision, they lose track of objects easily. This is why parents sometimes think and report that their newborn does not see. Newborns focus best on black and white objects at a distance of 9 to 12 in. A pupillary reflex or ability to contract the pupil is present from birth.

Touch. The sense of touch is also well developed at birth. Newborns demonstrate this by quieting at a soothing touch and by positive sucking and rooting reflexes, which are elicited by touch. They also react to painful stimuli.

Taste. A newborn has the ability to discriminate taste, because taste buds are developed and functioning even before birth. A fetus in utero, for example, will swallow amniotic fluid more rapidly than usual if glucose is added to sweeten its taste. The swallowing decreases if a bitter flavor is added. A newborn turns away from a bitter taste such as salt but readily accepts the sweet taste of milk or glucose water.

Smell. The sense of smell is present in newborns as soon as the nose is clear of mucus and amniotic fluid. Newborns turn toward their mothers' breast partly out of recognition of the smell of breast milk and partly as a manifestation of the rooting reflex. Their ability to respond to odors can be used to document alertness.

Physiologic Adjustment to Extrauterine Life

All newborns seem to move through periods of irregular adjustment in the first 6 hours of life, before their body systems stabilize. These periods were first described by Desmond in 1963 and are termed periods of reactivity (Desmond, 1963). The first phase lasts about half an hour. During this time, the baby is alert and exhibits exploring, searching activity, often making sucking sounds. Heart beat and respiratory rate are rapid. This is called the *first period of reactivity.*

Next comes a quiet *resting period.* Heartbeat and respiratory rates slow, and the newborn typically sleeps for about 90 minutes. The *second period of reactivity,* between 2 and 6 hours of life, occurs when the baby wakes again, often gagging and choking on mucus that has accumulated in the mouth. He or she is again alert and responsive and interested in the surroundings.

These three periods are summarized in Table 24.1. Newborns who are ill or who had difficulty at birth may not pass through these typical stages; they may never have periods of alertness or periods of quiet. Their vital signs may not fall and rise again but remain rapid; their temperature may remain subnormal. Demonstration of this typical reactivity pattern, therefore, is an indication that the newborn is healthy and adjusting well to extrauterine life. The ability to transition from one period to another is an important indicator of neurologic status.

APPEARANCE OF A NEWBORN

Although all newborns have similar physical findings, there are individual differences.

Skin

General inspection of a newborn's skin reveals many characteristic findings.

Color

Most term newborns have a ruddy complexion because of the increased concentration of red blood cells in blood vessels and a decrease in the amount of subcutaneous fat, which makes the blood vessels more visible. This ruddiness fades slightly over the first month. Infants with poor central nervous system control may appear pale and cyanotic. A gray color in newborns generally indicates infection. Twins may be born with a twin transfusion phenomenon, in which one twin is larger and has good color and the smaller twin has pallor (Duncombe et al., 2003).

Cyanosis. Generalized mottling of the skin is common. A newborn's lips, hands, and feet are likely to appear blue

TABLE 24.1

Periods of Reactivity: Normal Adjustment to Extrauterine Life

Assessment	First Period (First 15–30 Min)	Resting Period (30–120 Min)	Second Period (2–6 H)
Color	Acrocyanosis	Color stabilizing	Quick color changes occur with movement or crying
Temperature	Temperature begins to fall from intrauterine temperature of about 100.6°F (38.1°C)	Temperature stabilizes at about 99°F (37.2°C)	Temperature increases to 99.8°F (37.6°C)
Heart rate	Rapid, as much as 180 bpm while crying	Slowing to 120–140 bpm	Wide swings in rate with activity
Respirations	Irregular; 30–90 breaths per min while crying; some nasal flaring, occasional retraction may be present	Slowing to 30–50 breaths per min; barreling of chest occurs	Becoming irregular again with activity
Activity	Alert; watching	Sleeping	Awakening
Ability to respond to stimulation	Vigorous reaction	Difficult to arouse	Becoming responsive again
Mucus	Visible in mouth	Small amount present while sleeping	Mouth full of mucus, causing gagging
Bowel sounds	Can be heard after first 15 min	Present	Often passage of first meconium stool

Desmond, M. N., et al. (1963). The clinical behavior of the newly born: The term infant. *Journal of Pediatrics, 62*(3), 307–309.

from immature peripheral circulation. Acrocyanosis (blueness of hands and feet) is so prominent in some newborns that it appears as if some stricture were cutting off circulation, with usual skin color on one side and blue on the other. Acrocyanosis is a normal phenomenon in the first 24 to 48 hours after birth; however, **central cyanosis,** or cyanosis of the trunk, is always a cause for concern. Central cyanosis indicates decreased oxygenation. It may be the result of a temporary respiratory obstruction or an underlying disease state.

Mucus obstructing a newborn's respiratory tract causes sudden cyanosis and apnea. Suctioning of the mucus relieves the condition. Always suction the mouth of a newborn before the nose, because suctioning the nose first may trigger a reflex gasp, possibly leading to aspiration if there is mucus in the posterior throat. Follow mouth suctioning with suction to the nose, because the nose is the chief conduit for air in a newborn.

What if... Ms. Ruiz inspects her new baby and says to you, "Her hands are cold and blue. Is something wrong with her hands?" How should you answer?

Hyperbilirubinemia. Hyperbilirubinemia leads to **jaundice,** or yellowing of the skin. This occurs on the second or third day of life in about 50% of all newborns, as a result of the breakdown of fetal red blood cells (**physiologic jaundice**). The infant's skin and the sclerae of the eyes appear noticeably yellow. This happens because the

high red blood cell count built up in utero is destroyed, and heme and globin are released. Globin is a protein component that is reused by the body and is not a factor in the developing jaundice. Heme is further broken down into iron (which is also reused and not involved in the jaundice) and protoporphyrin. Protoporphyrin is further broken down into indirect bilirubin. Indirect bilirubin is fat soluble and cannot be excreted by the kidneys in this state. For removal from the body, it is converted by the liver enzyme glucuronyl transferase into direct bilirubin, which is water soluble. This is incorporated into stool and then excreted in feces. Many newborns have such immature liver function that indirect bilirubin cannot be converted to the direct form; it therefore remains indirect. As long as the bilirubin remains in the circulatory system, the red coloring of the blood cells covers the yellow tint of the bilirubin. After the level of this indirect bilirubin has risen to more than 7 mg/100 mL, however, bilirubin permeates the tissue outside the circulatory system and causes the infant to appear jaundiced.

Observe infants who are prone to extensive bruising (large, breech, or immature babies) carefully for jaundice, because bruising leads to hemorrhage of blood into the subcutaneous tissue or skin. As this blood is broken down, jaundice can occur.

Cephalhematoma, a collection of blood under the periosteum of the skull bone, can lead to the same phenomenon. As the bruising heals and the red blood cells are hemolyzed, additional indirect bilirubin is released.

If intestinal obstruction is present and stool cannot be evacuated, intestinal flora may break down bile into its basic components, leading to the release of indirect bilirubin into the bloodstream again. Early feeding of newborns promotes intestinal movement and excretion of meconium and helps prevent indirect bilirubin buildup from this source.

The level of jaundice in newborns may be judged grossly by estimating the extent to which it has progressed on the surface of the infant's body, starting in the head and spreading to the rest of the body.

Various commercial devices (transcutaneous bilirubinometry devices) are available to measure skin tone for jaundice and help in estimating jaundice levels. Although use of these devices rarely replaces serum measurements, they can be used to identify infants who need serum bilirubin determinations. The technique for obtaining a serum bilirubin specimen by heel puncture is shown in Chapter 36.

Treatment for physiologic jaundice or the routine rise in bilirubin in newborns is rarely necessary, except for measures such as early feeding to speed passage of feces through the intestine and prevent reabsorption of bilirubin from the bowel.

Above-normal indirect bilirubin levels are potentially dangerous because, if enough indirect bilirubin (about 20 mg/100 mL) leaves the bloodstream, it can interfere with the chemical synthesis of brain cells, resulting in permanent cell damage, a condition termed **kernicterus.** If this occurs, permanent neurologic damage, including cognitive challenge, may result.

There is no set level at which indirect serum bilirubin requires treatment, because other factors, such as age, maturity, and breast-feeding status, affect this determination. If the level rises to more than 10 to 12 mg/100 mL, treatment is usually considered. Phototherapy (exposure of the infant to light to initiate maturation of liver enzymes) may be used (see Chapter 26). If this is necessary, the incubator and light source can be moved to the mother's room so that the mother is not separated from her baby. Some infants need continued therapy after discharge and receive phototherapy at home (Walls, 2004).

Compared with formula-fed babies, a small proportion of breast-fed babies may have more difficulty converting indirect bilirubin to direct bilirubin, because breast milk contains pregnanediol (a metabolite of progesterone), which depresses the action of glucuronyl transferase (Reiser, 2004). However, breast-feeding rarely causes enough jaundice to warrant therapy. The decision to stop nursing in the first 2 weeks of life must never be made lightly, because it could interfere with breast filling and the breast milk supply.

Pallor. Pallor in newborns is usually the result of anemia. This may be caused by (1) excessive blood loss when the cord was cut, (2) inadequate flow of blood from the cord into the infant at birth, (3) fetal–maternal transfusion, (4) low iron stores caused by poor maternal nutrition during pregnancy, or (5) blood incompatibility in which a large number of red blood cells were hemolyzed in utero. It also may be the result of internal bleeding. The baby should be watched closely for signs of blood in stool or vomitus.

Harlequin Sign. Occasionally, because of immature circulation, a newborn who has been lying on his or her side appears red on the dependent side of the body and pale on the upper side, as if a line had been drawn down the center of the body. This is a transient phenomenon; although startling, it is of no clinical significance. The odd coloring fades immediately if the infant's position is changed or the baby kicks or cries vigorously.

Birthmarks

Several common types of birthmarks occur in newborns. It is important to be able to differentiate the various types of hemangiomas that occur, so that you neither give false reassurance to parents nor worry them unnecessarily about these lesions.

Hemangiomas. The **hemangiomas** are vascular tumors of the skin. Three types of hemangiomas occur.

Nevus Flammeus. **Nevus flammeus** (Fig. 24.10*A*) is a macular purple or dark-red lesion (sometimes called a *port-wine stain* because of its deep color) that is present at birth. These lesions typically appear on the face, although they are often found on the thighs as well. Those above the bridge of the nose tend to fade; the others are less likely to fade. Because they are level with the skin surface (macular), they can be covered by a cosmetic preparation later in life or removed by laser therapy, although lesions may reappear after treatment (Waner, 2003).

Nevus flammeus lesions also occur as lighter, pink patches at the nape of the neck, known as *stork's beak marks* (see Fig. 24.10*B*). These do not fade, but they are covered by the hairline and therefore are of no consequence. They occur more often in females than in males.

Strawberry Hemangioma. **Strawberry hemangiomas** are elevated areas formed by immature capillaries and endothelial cells (see Fig. 24.10*C*). Most are present at birth in the term neonate, although they may appear up to 2 weeks after birth. Typically, they are not present in the preterm infant because of the immaturity of the epidermis. Formation is associated with the high estrogen levels of pregnancy. They may continue to enlarge from their original size up to 1 year of age. After the first year, they tend to be absorbed and shrink in size. By the time the child is 7 years old, 50% to 75% of these lesions have disappeared. A child may be 10 years old before the absorption is complete. Application of hydrocortisone ointment may speed the disappearance of these lesions by interfering with the binding of estrogen to its receptor sites.

Be certain parents understand that the mark may grow in their child's early years. Otherwise, they may confuse it with cancer (a skin lesion increasing in size is one of the seven danger signals of cancer). Be sure they also understand that the mark will eventually disappear, so that they do not think of their child as imperfect or disfigured. Surgery to remove strawberry hemangiomas is rarely recommended because it can lead to secondary infection, resulting in scarring and permanent disfigurement. Laser therapy may be used to remove the lesion (Waner, 2003).

Cavernous Hemangioma. **Cavernous hemangiomas** (see Fig. 24.10*D*) are dilated vascular spaces. They are usually raised and resemble a strawberry hemangioma in appearance. However, they do not disappear with time as

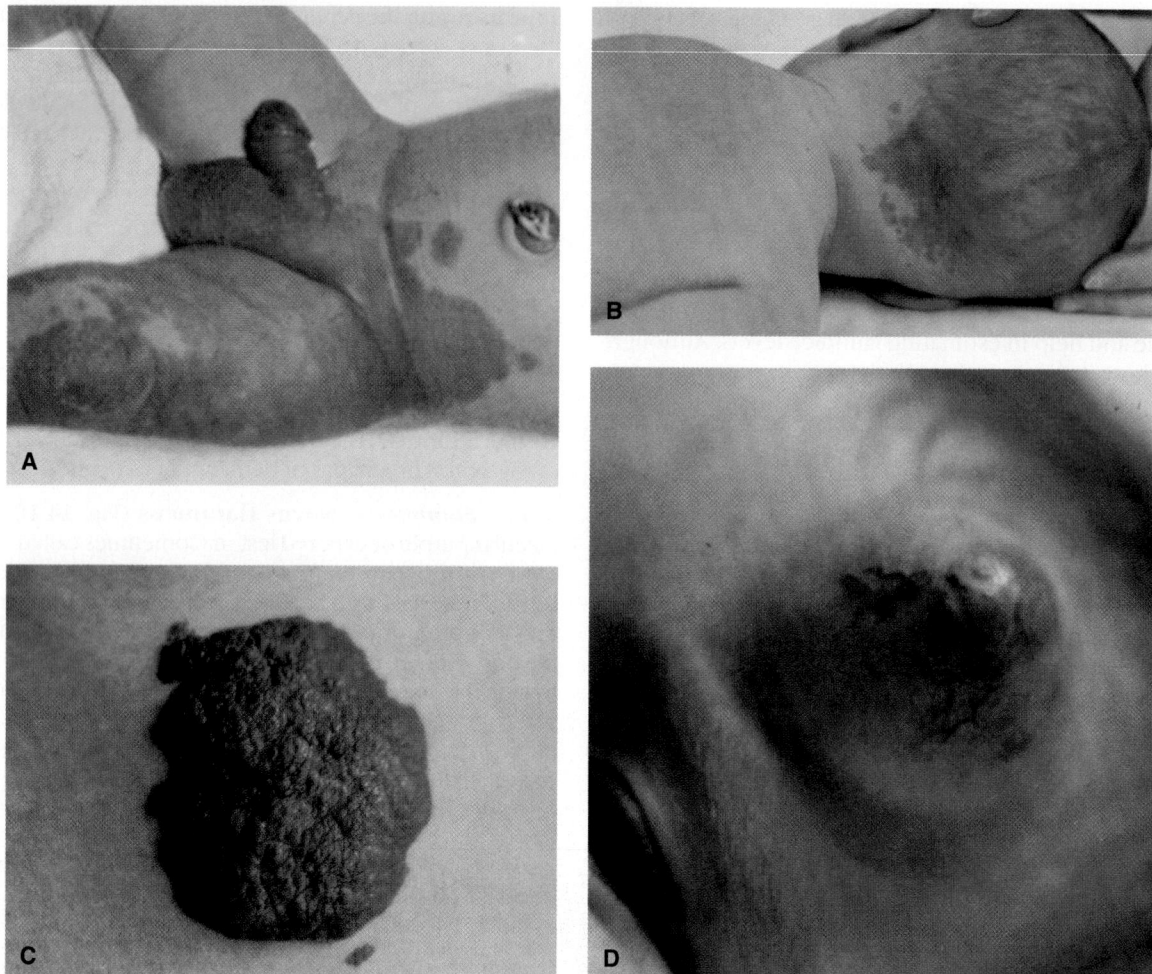

FIGURE 24.10 Types of hemangiomas found on a newborn. (**A**) Nevus flammeus (port-wine stain) formed of a plexus of newly formed capillaries in the papillary layer of the corium. It is deep red to purple, does not blanch on pressure, and does not fade with age. (**B**) A telangectasia or Stork's beak mark, commonly occurring on nape of neck. It blanches on pressure; although it does not fade, it is not noticeable as it becomes covered by hair. (**C**) Strawberry hemangiomas consist of dilated capillaries in entire dermal and subdermal layers. They continue to enlarge after birth but usually disappear by age 10 years. (**D**) Cavernous hemangiomas consist of a communicating network of venules in subcutaneous tissue and do not fade with age.

the strawberry hemangiomas do. Subcutaneous infusions of interferon-alfa-2a can be used to reduce these lesions in size (Greene et al., 2004), or they can be removed surgically. Children who have a skin lesion may have additional ones on internal organs. Blows to the abdomen, such as those from childhood games, can cause bleeding from internal hemangiomas. For this reason, children with cavernous hemangiomas usually have their hematocrit levels assessed at health maintenance visits, to evaluate for possible internal blood loss.

Mongolian Spots. **Mongolian spots** are collections of pigment cells (melanocytes) that appear as slate-gray patches across the sacrum or buttocks and possibly on the arms and legs. They tend to occur in children of Asian, Southern European, or African extraction (Constantinou, 2003). They disappear by school age without treatment. Be sure to inform parents that these are not bruises.

Otherwise, they may worry their baby sustained a birth injury.

Vernix Caseosa

Vernix caseosa is a white, cream cheese–like substance that serves as a skin lubricant. Usually, it is noticeable on a term newborn's skin, at least in the skin folds, at birth. Document the color of vernix, because it takes on the color of the amniotic fluid. For example, a yellow vernix implies that the amniotic fluid was yellow from bilirubin; green vernix indicates that meconium was present in the amniotic fluid.

Until the first bath, when vernix is washed away, handle newborns with gloves to protect yourself from exposure to body fluids. Never use harsh rubbing to wash away vernix. A newborn's skin is tender, and breaks in the skin caused by too vigorous attempts at removal may open portals of entry for bacteria.

Lanugo

Lanugo is the fine, downy hair that covers a newborn's shoulders, back, and upper arms. It may be found also on the forehead and ears. A baby born after 37 to 39 weeks of gestation has more lanugo than a newborn of 40 weeks' gestational age. Postmature infants (more than 42 weeks of gestation) rarely have lanugo. Lanugo is rubbed away by the friction of bedding and clothes against the newborn's skin. By 2 weeks of age, it has disappeared.

Desquamation

Within 24 hours after birth, the skin of most newborns has become extremely dry. The dryness is particularly evident on the palms of the hands and soles of the feet. This results in areas of peeling similar to those caused by sunburn. This is normal, however, and needs no treatment. Parents may apply hand lotion to prevent excessive dryness if they wish.

Newborns who are postmature and have suffered intrauterine malnutrition may have extremely dry skin, with a leathery appearance and cracks in the skin folds. This should be differentiated from normal desquamation.

Milia

All newborn sebaceous glands are immature. At least one pinpoint white papule (a plugged or unopened sebaceous gland) can be found on the cheek or across the bridge of the nose of every newborn. Such lesions, termed **milia** (Fig. 24.11), disappear by 2 to 4 weeks of age, as the sebaceous glands mature and drain. Teach parents to avoid scratching or squeezing the papules, to prevent secondary infections.

Erythema Toxicum

In most normal mature infants, a newborn rash called **erythema toxicum** can be observed (Fig. 24.12). This usually appears in the first to fourth day of life, but may appear up to 2 weeks of age. It begins with a papule, increases in severity to become erythema by the second day, and then disappears by the third day. It is sometimes called a *flea-bite rash* because the lesions are so minuscule. One of the chief characteristics of the rash is its lack of pattern. It occurs sporadically and unpredictably, and may last hours rather than days. It is caused by a newborn's eosinophils reacting to the environment as the immune system matures. It requires no treatment.

Forceps Marks

If forceps were used for birth, there may be a circular or linear contusion matching the rim of the blade of the forceps on the infant's cheek (Fig. 24.13). This mark disappears in 1 to 2 days, along with the edema that accompanies it. The mark is the result of normal forceps use and does not denote unskilled or too vigorous application of forceps. Closely assess the facial nerve while a newborn is at rest and during crying episodes, to detect any potential facial nerve compression requiring further evaluation.

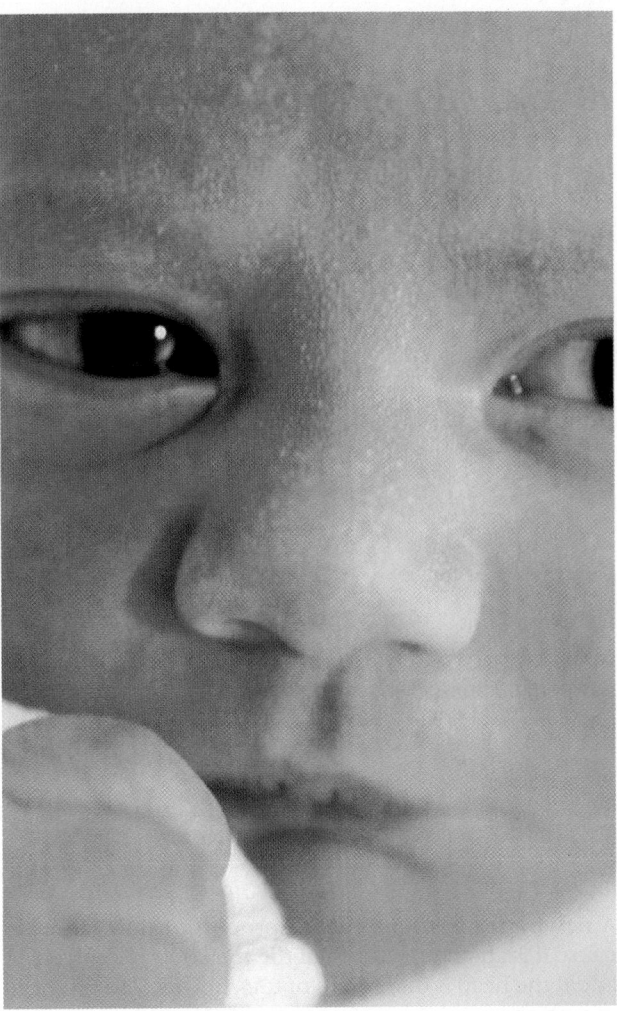

FIGURE 24.11 Milia are unopened sebaceous glands frequently found on the nose, chin, or cheeks of a newborn.

Skin Turgor

Newborn skin should feel resilient if the underlying tissue is well hydrated. If a fold of the skin is grasped between the thumb and fingers, it should feel elastic. When it is released, it should fall back to form a smooth surface. If severe dehydration is present, the skin will not smooth out again but will remain in an elevated ridge. Poor turgor is seen in newborns who suffered malnutrition in utero, who have difficulty sucking at birth, or who have certain metabolic disorders such as adrenogenital syndrome.

 Checkpoint Question 3

Beth Ruiz has milia on her nose. What is the necessary therapy for this?

a. Ice packs to reduce inflammation.
b. Warm heat to increase circulation.
c. No therapy is necessary for milia.
d. Lancing the lesions so they drain.

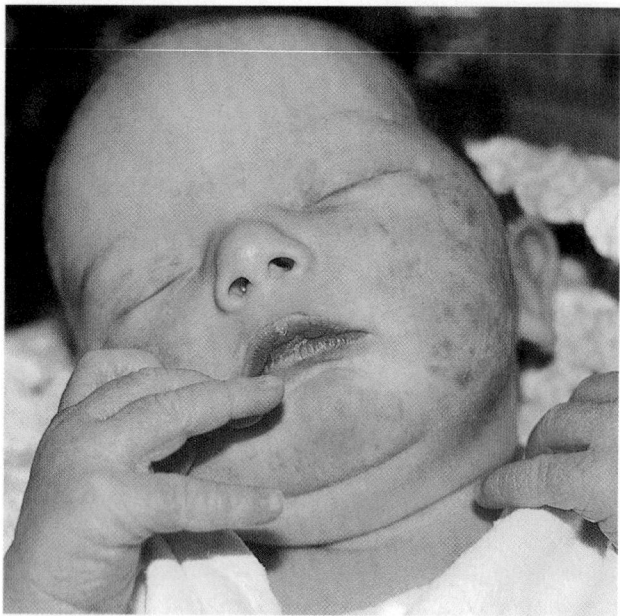

FIGURE 24.12 Erythema toxicum is found on almost all newborns. The reddish rash consists of sporadic pinpoint papules on an erythematous base. It fades spontaneously in a few days.

Head

A newborn's head appears disproportionately large because it is about one fourth of the total body length; in an adult, the head is one eighth of total height. The forehead of a newborn is large and prominent. The chin appears to be receding, and it quivers easily if the infant is startled or cries. Well-nourished newborns have full-bodied hair; poorly nourished and preterm infants have thin, lifeless hair. If internal fetal monitoring was used during labor, the newborn may exhibit a pinpoint ulcer at the point where the monitor was attached.

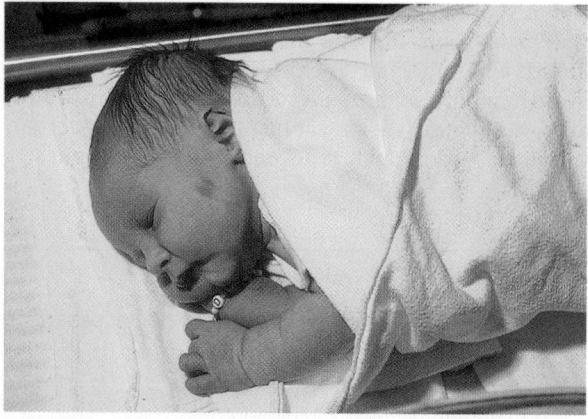

FIGURE 24.13 Forceps marks are commonly found in newborns born by forceps. Such marks are transient and disappear in a day or two.

Fontanelles

The fontanelles are the spaces or openings where the skull bones join. The anterior fontanelle is located at the junction of the two parietal bones and the two fused frontal bones. It is diamond shaped and measures 2 to 3 cm (0.8 to 1.2 in) in width and 3 to 4 cm (1.2 to 1.6 in) in length. The posterior fontanelle is located at the junction of the parietal bones and the occipital bone. It is triangular and measures about 1 cm (0.4 in) in length.

The anterior fontanelle can be felt as a soft spot. It should not appear indented (a sign of dehydration) or bulging (a sign of increased intracranial pressure) when the infant is positioned upright at an angle of 45° to 90°. The fontanelle may bulge if the newborn strains to pass a stool or cries vigorously or is lying supine. With vigorous crying, a pulse may additionally be seen in the fontanelle. The anterior fontanelle normally closes at 12 to 18 months of age.

In some newborns, the posterior fontanelle is so small that it cannot be palpated readily. The posterior fontanelle closes by the end of the second month.

Sutures

The skull *sutures,* the separating lines of the skull, may override at birth because of the extreme pressure exerted on the head during passage through the birth canal. If the sagittal suture between the parietal bones overrides, the fontanelles are less perceptible than usual. The overriding subsides in 24 to 48 hours.

Suture lines should never appear widely separated in newborns. Wide separation suggests increased intracranial pressure due to abnormal brain formation, abnormal accumulation of cerebrospinal fluid in the cranium (hydrocephalus), or an accumulation of blood from a birth injury (e.g., subdural hemorrhage). Fused suture lines also are abnormal; they require radiographic confirmation and further evaluation, because they will prevent the head from expanding with growth.

Molding

The part of the infant's head that engages the cervix (usually the vertex) is molded to fit the cervix contours. After birth, this area appears prominent and asymmetric. Molding may be so extreme in the baby of a primiparous woman that the baby's head looks like a dunce cap (Fig. 24.14). The head will be restored to its normal shape within a few days after birth.

Caput Succedaneum

Caput succedaneum (Fig. 24.15*A*) is edema of the scalp at the presenting part of the head. It may involve wide areas of the head, or it may be the size of a large egg. The edema, which crosses the suture lines, is gradually absorbed and disappears at about the third day of life. It needs no treatment.

Cephalhematoma

A *cephalhematoma* is a collection of blood between the periosteum of a skull bone and the bone itself; it is caused

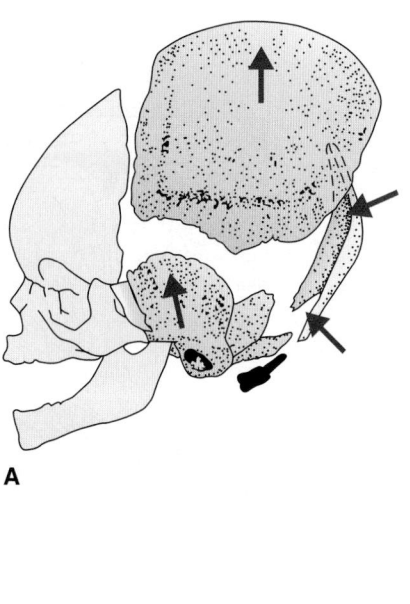

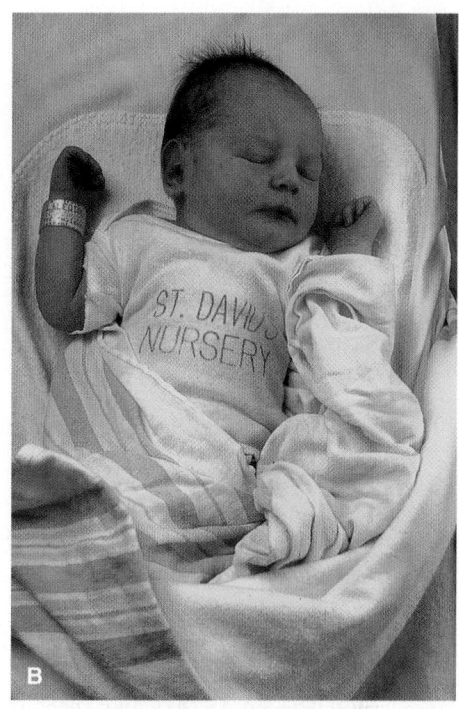

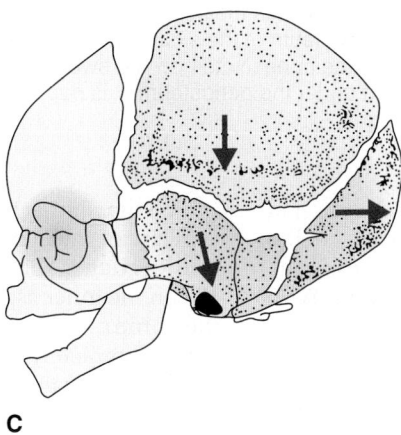

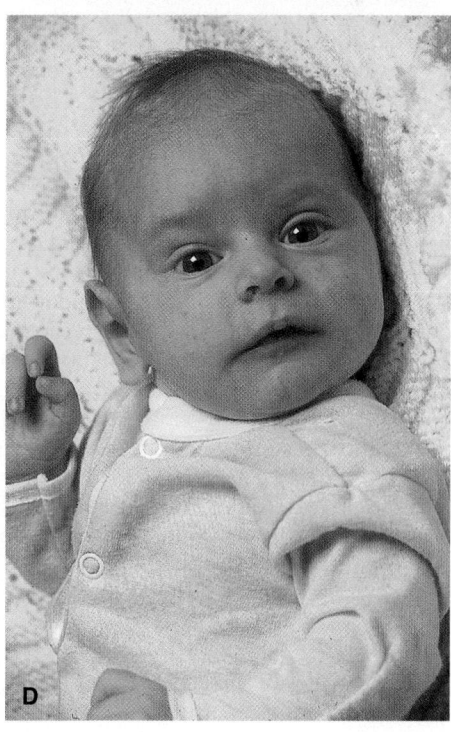

FIGURE 24.14 Molding. (**A, B**) The infant head molds to fit the birth canal more easily. On palpation, the skull sutures will be felt to be overriding. (**C, D**) The head shape returns to normal within 1 week.

by rupture of a periosteal capillary due to the pressure of birth (see Fig. 24.15*B*). It usually appears 24 hours after birth. Although the blood loss is negligible, the swelling is usually severe and is well outlined as an egg shape. It may be discolored (black and blue) because of the presence of coagulated blood. A cephalhematoma is confined to an individual bone, so the associated swelling stops at the bone's suture line.

It often takes weeks for a cephalhematoma to be absorbed. It might be supposed that the blood could be aspi-

rated to relieve the condition. However, such a procedure would introduce the risk of infection and is unnecessary, because the condition will subside by itself. As the blood captured in the space is broken down, a great amount of indirect bilirubin may be released, leading to jaundice.

Craniotabes

Craniotabes is a localized softening of the cranial bones that is probably caused by pressure of the fetal skull against

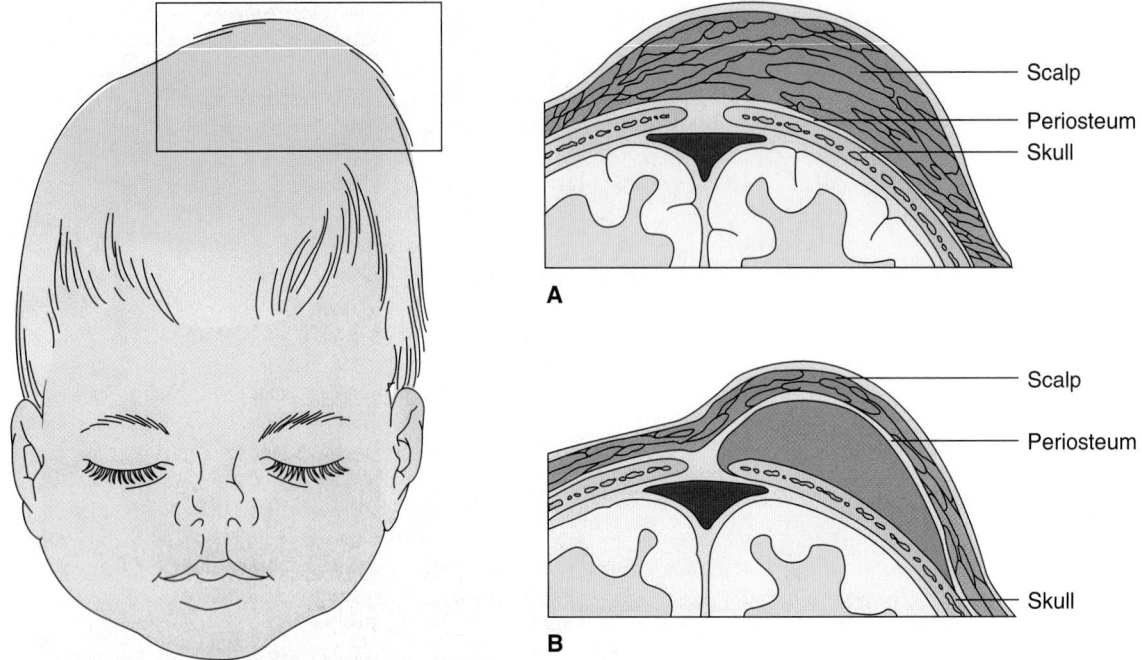

FIGURE 24.15 (A) Caput succedaneum. From pressure of the birth canal, an edematous area is present beneath the scalp. Note how it crosses the midline of the skull. **(B)** Cephalhematoma. A small capillary beneath the periosteum of the skull bone has ruptured, and blood has collected under the periosteum of the bone. Note how the swelling now stops at the midline. Because the blood is contained under the periosteum, it is necessarily stopped by a suture line.

the mother's pelvic bone in utero. It is more common in first-born infants than in infants born later, because of the lower position of the fetal head in the pelvis during the last 2 weeks of pregnancy in primiparous women. With craniotabes, the skull is so soft that the pressure of an examining finger can indent it. The bone returns to its normal contour after the pressure is removed. The condition corrects itself without treatment after a few months, as the infant takes in calcium in milk. It is an example of a condition that is normal in a newborn but would be pathologic in an older child or adult (in whom it probably would be the result of faulty metabolism or kidney dysfunction).

Eyes

Newborns usually cry tearlessly, because their lacrimal ducts do not fully mature until about 3 months of age. Almost without exception, the irises of the eyes of newborns are gray or blue; the sclera may be blue due to its thinness. Infant eyes assume their permanent color between 3 and 12 months of age.

To inspect the eyes, lay the newborn in a supine position and lift the head. This maneuver causes the baby to open his or her eyes. A newborn's eyes should appear clear, without redness or purulent discharge. Occasionally, the administration of an antibiotic ointment such as erythromycin at birth, to protect against *Chlamydia* infection as well as ophthalmia neonatorum (gonorrheal conjunctivitis), has caused a purulent discharge that lasts for the first 24 hours of life.

Pressure during birth sometimes ruptures a conjunctival capillary of the eye, resulting in a small **subconjunctival hemorrhage.** This appears as a red spot on the sclera, usually on the inner aspect of the eye, or as a red ring around the cornea. The bleeding is slight, requires no treatment, and is completely absorbed within 2 or 3 weeks. You can reassure the parents that these hemorrhages are normal variations. Otherwise, they may assume that their baby is bleeding from within the eye and that his or her vision will be impaired.

Edema is often present around the orbit or on the eyelids. This remains for the first 2 or 3 days, until the newborn's kidneys are capable of evacuating fluid more efficiently.

The cornea of the eye should appear round and proportionate in size to that of an adult eye. A cornea that appears larger than usual may be the result of congenital glaucoma. An irregularly shaped pupil or discolored iris may denote disease (see Chapter 33). The pupil should be dark. A white pupil suggests the presence of a congenital cataract.

Ears

A newborn's external ear is not as completely formed as it will be eventually, so the pinna tends to bend easily. In the term newborn, however, the pinna should be strong enough to recoil after bending.

The level of the top part of the external ear should be on a line drawn from the inner canthus to the outer canthus of the eye and back across the side of the head (see

Chapter 33). Ears that are set lower than this are found in infants with certain chromosomal abnormalities, particularly trisomy 18 and 13, syndromes in which low-set ears and other physical defects are coupled with varying degrees of cognitive challenge (see Chapters 7 and 54).

A small tag of skin is sometimes found just in front of an ear. Although these tags may be associated with chromosomal abnormalities or kidney disease, they usually are isolated findings that are of no consequence. They can be removed by ligation immediately or when the child is 1 week old. A preauricular dermal sinus may be present directly in front of the ear as well. Always inspect in front of newborns' ears for pinpoint-size openings that reveal these sinuses. The sinus is usually small and can be removed surgically without consequence when the child is near school age.

Visualization of the tympanic membrane of the ear in a newborn is difficult and usually is not attempted, because amniotic fluid and flecks of vernix still fill the canal, obliterating the drum and its accompanying landmarks.

A good practice is to test a newborn's hearing by ringing a bell held about 6 inches from each ear. A hearing infant who is crying will stop momentarily at the sound. If quiet, a newborn who can hear will blink the eyes, appear to attend to the sound, and possibly startle. Although this method of testing is not highly accurate, a negative response (lack of response) is unusual. Infants with negative responses should be retested later. In many health care facilities, all newborns are tested by a commercial standardized response to sound before discharge (Brennan, 2004).

Nose

A newborn's nose tends to appear large for the face. As the infant grows, the rest of the face grows more than the nose does, and this discrepancy disappears.

Test for choanal atresia (blockage at the rear of the nose) by closing the newborn's mouth and compressing one naris at a time with your fingers. Note any discomfort or distress with breathing. Also record any evidence of milia on the nose.

Mouth

A newborn's mouth should open evenly when he or she cries. If one side of the mouth moves more than the other, cranial nerve injury is suggested. A newborn's tongue appears large and prominent in the mouth. Because the tongue is short, the frenulum membrane is attached close to the tip of the tongue, creating the impression that the infant is "tongue tied." At one time, it was almost routine to snip a newborn's frenulum membrane to lengthen it. Now this procedure is regarded as harmful, because it leaves a portal of entry for infection, risks hemorrhage because of the low level of vitamin K in most newborns, and causes feeding difficulties by making the tongue sore and irritated. And is unnecessary because, as the tongue grows, the frenulum recedes to its adult placement.

Inspect the palate of a newborn to be sure it is intact. Occasionally, one or two small round, glistening, well-circumscribed cysts (Epstein's pearls) are present on the palate, a result of the extra load of calcium that was deposited in utero. Be sure to inform parents that these pearl-like cysts are insignificant, require no treatment, and will disappear spontaneously within 1 week. Otherwise, a parent may mistake them for **thrush,** a *Candida* infection, which usually appears on the tongue and sides of the cheeks as white or gray patches.

All newborns have some mucus in their mouths. Newborns delivered by cesarean birth usually have an increased amount. If a newborn is placed on the side, the mucus drains from the mouth and results in no distress. If the mouth is filled with so much mucus that the neonate seems to be blowing bubbles, a tracheoesophageal fistula is suspected. This must be confirmed or ruled out before the newborn is fed; otherwise, formula can be aspirated into the lungs from the inadequately formed esophagus.

Small, white epithelial pearls (benign inclusion cysts) may be present on the gum margins. No therapy is necessary for these.

It is unusual for a newborn to have teeth, but sometimes one or two (called **natal teeth**) will have erupted. Any teeth that are present must be evaluated for stability. If loose, they should be extracted to prevent possible aspiration during feeding. Also, any natal teeth not covered by the gum membrane should be removed, because they can loosen, increasing the risk for aspiration.

Neck

The neck of a newborn is short and often chubby, with creased skin folds. The head should rotate freely on it. If there is rigidity of the neck, congenital torticollis, caused by injury to the sternocleidomastoid muscle during birth, might be present (see Chapter 39). In newborns whose membranes were ruptured more than 24 hours before birth, nuchal rigidity suggests meningitis.

The neck of a newborn is not strong enough to support the total weight of the head. In a sitting position, a newborn should make a momentary effort at head control. When lying prone, newborns can raise the head slightly, usually enough to lift the nose out of mucus or spit-up formula. If they are pulled into a sitting position from a supine position, the head will lag behind considerably. Again, however, they should make some effort to control and steady the head as they reach the sitting position.

The trachea may be prominent on the front of the neck, and the thymus gland may be enlarged because of the rapid growth of glandular tissue (in comparison with other body tissues) early in life. The thymus gland will triple in size by 3 years of age; it remains at that size until the child is about 10 years old, and then shrinks. Although the thymus may appear to be bulging in a newborn, it is rarely a cause of respiratory difficulty, as was previously believed.

Chest

The chest in some newborns looks small because the head is large in proportion. Not until a child is 2 years of age does the chest measurement exceed that of the head.

In both female and male infants, the breasts may be engorged. Occasionally, the breasts of newborn babies secrete a thin, watery fluid popularly termed *witch's milk.* Engorgement develops in utero as a result of the influence of the mother's hormones. As soon as the hormones are cleared from the infant's system (about 1 week), the engorgement and any fluid that is present subside. Fluid should never be expressed from infants' breasts, because the manipulation could introduce bacteria and lead to mastitis.

The chest of a neonate is approximately 2 inches smaller in circumference than the head, and as wide in the anteroposterior diameter as it is across. The clavicles should be straight. A crepitus or actual separation on one or the other clavicle may indicate that a fracture occurred during birth and calcium is now being deposited at that point. As the area heals, it may be possible to palpate a lump on the clavicle caused by temporary calcium overgrowth. Overall, a newborn's chest should appear symmetric side to side. Respirations are normally rapid (30 to 60 breaths per minute) but not distressed. A supernumerary nipple (usually found below and in line with the normal nipples) may be present. If so, it may be removed later for cosmetic purposes.

Retraction (drawing in of the chest wall with inspiration) should not be present. An infant with retractions (Fig. 24.16) is using such strong force to pull air into the respiratory tract that he or she is pulling in the anterior chest muscle.

Because a newborn's lung alveoli open slowly over the first 24 to 48 hours and the baby invariably has mucus in the back of the throat, listening to lung sounds often reveals the sounds of rhonchi—the harsh, innocent sound of air passing over mucus. An abnormal sound, such as grunting, suggests respiratory distress syndrome; a high, crowing sound on inspiration suggests stridor or immature tracheal development.

Abdomen

The contour of a newborn abdomen looks slightly protuberant. A scaphoid or sunken appearance may indicate missing abdominal contents or a diaphragmatic hernia. Bowel sounds should be present within 1 hour after birth.

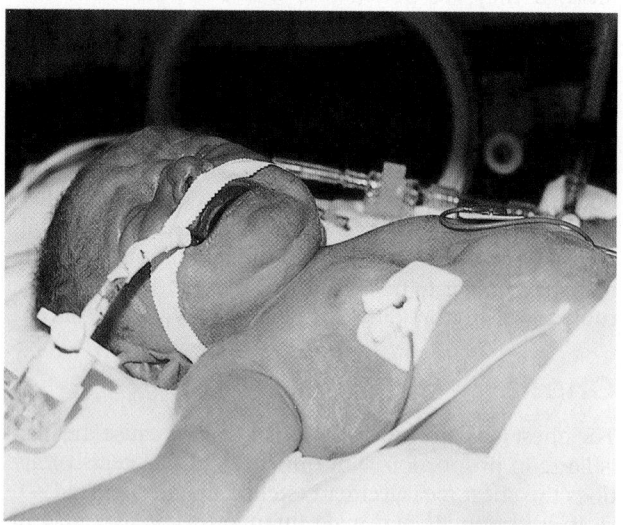

FIGURE 24.16 Sternal retractions are a sign of respiratory distress requiring immediate intervention, such as mechanical ventilation or increased oxygen.

The edge of the liver is usually palpable 1 to 2 cm below the right costal margin. The edge of the spleen may be palpable 1 to 2 cm below the left costal margin. Tenderness is difficult to determine in a newborn. If it is extreme, however, palpation will cause the infant to cry, thrash about, or tense the abdominal muscles to protect the abdomen.

For the first hour after birth, the stump of the umbilical cord appears as a white, gelatinous structure marked with the red and blue streaks of the umbilical vein and arteries. When the cord is first cut, the vessels are counted to be certain that one vein and two arteries are present. In 0.5% of births (3.5% of twin births), there is only a single umbilical artery, and in one third of such infants, this single artery is associated with a congenital heart or renal abnormality. Because these heart and kidney anomalies may not be readily apparent, any child with a single umbilical artery needs close observation and assessment until anomalies are ruled out.

Inspect the cord clamp to be certain it is secure. After the first hour of life, the cord begins to dry and shrink, and it turns brown like the dead end of a vine. By the second or third day, it has turned black. It breaks free by day 6 to 10, leaving a granulating area a few centimeters wide that heals during the following week.

There should be no bleeding at the cord site. Bleeding suggests that the cord clamp has become loosened or the cord has been tugged loose by the friction of the bedclothes. The base of the cord should appear dry. A moist or odorous cord suggests infection. If present, infection should receive immediate treatment or it may enter a newborn's bloodstream and cause septicemia. Moistness at the base of the cord also may indicate a patent urachus (a canal that connects the bladder and the umbilicus), which will drain urine at the cord site until it is surgically repaired.

Inspect the base of the cord to be sure no abdominal wall defect (e.g., umbilical hernia) is present. If there is a fascial (abdominal wall) defect smaller than 2 cm in diameter, it usually closes on its own by school age; a larger defect will probably require surgical correction. Taping or putting buttons or coins on the cord are home remedies that do not help defects to close. In fact, heavy taping may worsen the condition by preventing the development of good muscle tone in the abdominal wall. Tape also tends to keep the cord moist, making infection more likely than when it is dry (Box 24.3).

Because a newborn's voiding only demonstrates there is at least one kidney, not that there are two, attempt to verify the presence of kidneys by deep palpation of the right and left abdomen within the first few hours after birth. After this time, the intestines fill with air, making palpation more difficult. The right kidney (at least its lower pole) can usually be palpated, because it is located lower than the left; the left kidney is more difficult to locate, because the intestine is bulkier on the left side and the left kidney is higher in the retroperitoneal space. Nonetheless, try to locate it. Placing one hand behind the infant while you palpate offers a firmer base and helps when evaluating kidney size (newborn kidneys are about the size of a walnut). An enlarged kidney suggests a polycystic kidney or pooling of urine from a urethral obstruction.

To finish the abdominal assessment, elicit an abdominal reflex. Stroking each quadrant of the abdomen will

BOX 24.3 FOCUS ON . . .

DIVERSITY OF CARE

Newborn care is not universal but varies among cultures. For example, although it is usually a sound policy to point out the positive aspects of a child to parents to aid parent–child bonding, in some areas of the world, such as traditional Cambodia and Laos, newborns are not given compliments this way. It is believed that compliments will leave them vulnerable to evil spirits.

In the traditional Haitian culture, infants are not named immediately, but only after a full month. In some cultures, it is important for newborns to have an amulet (good-luck charm) tied around their neck or wrist. Respect these and leave them in place when bathing the infant. Oiling the infant's body and placing a belly band over the umbilical cord also are common care procedures. Being aware of cultural variations in newborn care such as these helps you plan care that is specific and meaningful to individual parents and can aid parent–child bonding.

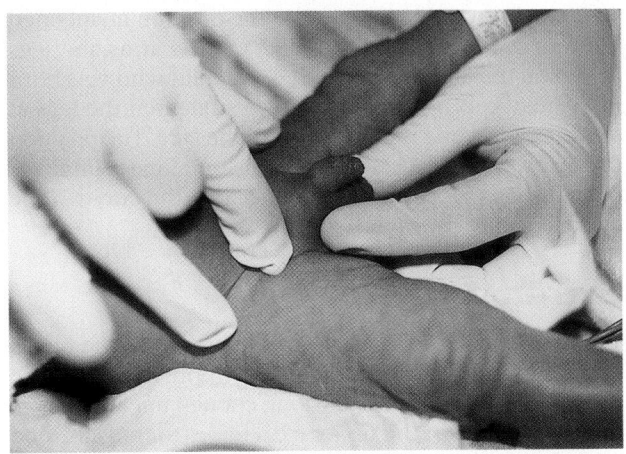

FIGURE 24.17 Press the nondominant hand against the inguinal ring when palpating testes.

cause the umbilicus to move or "wink" in that direction. This superficial abdominal reflex is a test of spinal nerves T8 through T10. The reflex may not be demonstrable in newborns until the 10th day of life.

Anogenital Area

Inspect the anus of the newborn to be certain it is present, patent, and not covered by a membrane (imperforate anus). Test for anal patency by gently inserting the tip of your little finger, gloved and lubricated. Also note the time after birth at which the infant first passes meconium. If a newborn does not do so in the first 24 hours, suspect imperforate anus or meconium ileus.

Male Genitalia

The scrotum in most male newborns is edematous and has rugae. It may be deeply pigmented in African-American or dark-skinned newborns.

Both testes should be present in the scrotum. If one or both testicles are not present (cryptorchidism), further referral is needed to establish the extent of the problem. This condition could be caused by agenesis (absence of an organ), ectopic testes (the testes cannot enter the scrotum because the opening to the scrotal sac is closed), or undescended testes (the vas deferens or artery is too short to allow the testes to descend). Newborns with agenesis of the testes are usually referred for investigation of kidney anomalies, because the testes arise from the same germ tissue as the kidneys. Make a practice of pressing your nondominant hand against the inguinal ring before palpating for testes, so they do not slip upward and out of the scrotal sac as you palpate (Fig. 24.17).

The cremasteric reflex is elicited by stroking the internal side of the thigh. As the skin is stroked, the testis on

that side moves perceptibly upward. This is a test for the integrity of spinal nerves T8 through T10. The response may be absent in newborns who are younger than about 10 days old.

The penis of newborns appears small, approximately 2 cm long. If it is less than this, the newborn should be referred for evaluation by an endocrinologist. Inspect the tip of the penis to see that the urethral opening is at the tip of the glans, not on the dorsal surface (epispadias) or on the ventral surface (hypospadias).

In most newborns, the prepuce (foreskin) slides back poorly from the meatal opening, so this should not be done. Although today most male newborns are circumcised, the necessity for this operation can be questioned unless it is for religious reasons, because it is rare to find an infant who physically requires it (i.e., has a foreskin so constricted that it interferes with voiding or circulation) (Katz, 2003). In addition, surgery this early in life poses the risk of hemorrhage and infection. Circumcision should not be done if hypospadias or epispadias is present, because the surgeon may want to use the foreskin as tissue when repairing these conditions (see later discussion).

Female Genitalia

The vulva in female newborns may be swollen because of the effect of maternal hormones. Some female newborns have a mucus vaginal secretion, which is sometimes blood-tinged (**pseudomenstruation**). Again, this is caused by the action of maternal hormones. The discharge disappears as soon as the infant's system has cleared the hormones. The discharge should not be mistaken for an infection or taken as an indication that trauma has occurred.

Back

The spine of a newborn typically appears flat in the lumbar and sacral areas. The curves seen in an adult appear only after the child is able to sit and walk. Inspect the base of a newborn's spine carefully to be sure there is no pinpoint opening, dimpling, or sinus tract in the skin, which would suggest a dermal sinus or spinal bifida occulta.

A newborn normally assumes the position maintained in utero, with the back rounded and the arms and legs flexed on the abdomen and chest. A child who was born in a frank breech position tends to straighten the legs at the knee and bring them up next to the face. The position of a baby with a face presentation sometimes simulates opisthotonos for the first week, because the curve of the back is deeply concave.

Extremities

The arms and legs of a newborn appear short. The hands are plump and clenched into fists. Newborn fingernails are soft and smooth, and usually long enough to extend over the fingertips. Test the upper extremities for muscle tone by unflexing the arms for approximately 5 seconds. If tone is good, the arm should return immediately to its flexed position after being released. Hold the arms down by the sides and note their length. The fingertips should cover the proximal thigh. Unusually short arms may signify achondroplastic dwarfism. Observe for unusual curvature of the little finger, and inspect the palm for a simian crease (a single palmar crease, in contrast to the three creases normally seen in a palm). Although curved fingers and simian creases can occur normally, they are commonly associated with Down syndrome (Chung, 2003).

A newborn's arms and legs should move symmetrically (unless the infant is demonstrating a tonic neck reflex). An arm that hangs limp and unmoving suggests possible birth injury, such as injury to a clavicle or to the brachial or cervical plexus or fracture of a long bone. Assess for webbing (syndactyly), extra toes or fingers (polydactyly), or unusual spacing of toes, particularly between the big toes and the others (this finding is present in certain chromosomal disorders, although it is also a normal finding in some families). Test to see whether the toenails fill immediately after blanching from pressure.

Normally, newborn legs are bowed as well as short. The sole of the foot appears flat because of an extra pad of fat in the longitudinal arch. The foot of a term newborn has many crisscrossed lines on the sole, covering approximately two thirds of the foot. If these creases cover less than two thirds of the foot or are absent, suspect immaturity.

Move the ankle through a range of motion to evaluate whether the heel cord is unusually tight. Check for ankle clonus by supporting the lower leg in one hand and dorsiflexing the foot sharply two or three times by pressure on the sole of the foot with the other hand. After the dorsiflexion, one or two continued movements are normal. Rapid alternating contraction and relaxation (clonus) is abnormal, suggesting neurologic involvement. The feet of many newborns turn in (varus deviation) because of their former intrauterine position. This simple deviation needs no correction if the feet can be brought into the midline position by easy manipulation. When the infant begins to bear weight, the feet will align themselves. If a foot does not align readily or will not turn to a definite midline position, a talipes deformity (clubfoot) may be present. This condition needs investigation, because congenital problems of this kind are best treated in the newborn period.

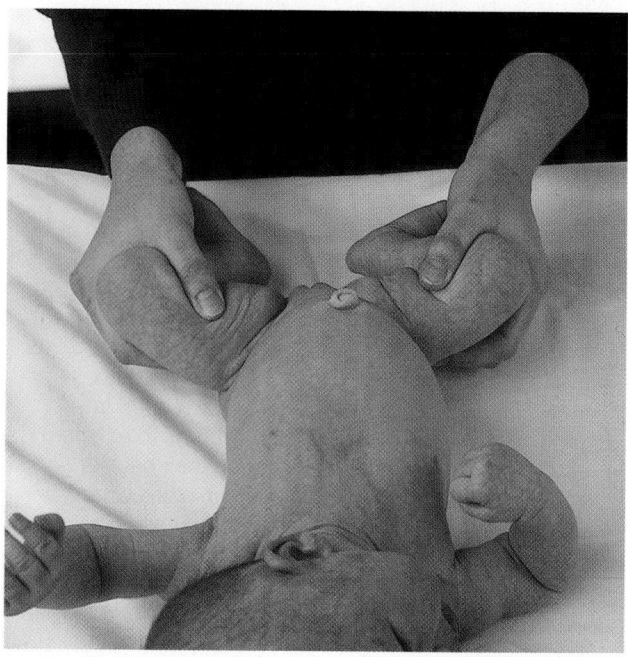

FIGURE 24.18 Hip abduction in a newborn—both hips should abduct so completely they lie almost flat against the mattress (180 degrees).

With a newborn in a supine position, both hips can be flexed and abducted to such an extent (180°) that the knees touch or nearly touch the surface of the bed (Fig. 24.18). If the hip joint seems to lock short of this distance (160° to 170°), hip subluxation (a shallow and poorly formed acetabulum) is suggested (Weinstein et al., 2003). Test for subluxation by holding the infant's leg with the fingers on the greater and lesser trochanters and then abducting the hip; if subluxation is present, a "clunk" of the femur head striking the shallow acetabulum can be heard (Ortolani's sign). If the hip can be felt to actually slip in the socket, this is Barlow's sign. Subluxated hip may be bilateral but is usually unilateral. It is important that hip subluxation be discovered as early as possible, because correction is most successful if it is initiated early.

When lying on the abdomen, newborns are capable of bringing their arms and legs underneath them and raising the stomach off the bed high enough for a hand to be slipped underneath. This ability helps to prevent pressure or rubbing at the cord site, because the cord does not actually touch the bedding when in this position. The preterm newborn does not have this ability, so it is an indication of maturity.

ASSESSMENT FOR WELL-BEING

There are a number of traditional standardized assessments to evaluate a newborn quickly at birth.

Apgar Scoring

At 1 minute and 5 minutes after birth, newborns are observed and rated according to an Apgar score, an assessment scale used as a standard since 1958 (Apgar et al., 1958). As shown in Table 24.2, heart rate, respiratory ef-

TABLE 24.2

Apgar Scoring Chart

Sign	Score		
	0	*1*	*2*
Heart rate	Absent	Slow (<100)	>100
Respiratory effort	Absent	Slow, irregular; weak cry	Good; strong cry
Muscle tone	Flaccid	Some flexion of extremities	Well flexed
Reflex irritability:			
Response to catheter in nostril, *or* Slap to sole of foot	No response No response	Grimace Grimace	Cough or sneeze Cry and withdrawal of foot
Color	Blue, pale	Body normal pigment, extremities blue	Normal skin coloring

Apgar, V., et al. (1958). Evaluation of the newborn infant: Second report. *JAMA: Journal of the American Medical Association, 16*(82), 1985–1988. Copyright 1958, American Medical Association.

fort, muscle tone, reflex irritability, and color of the infant are each rated 0, 1, or 2; the five scores are then added. A newborn whose total score is less than 4 is in serious danger and needs resuscitation. A score of 4 to 6 means that the infant's condition is guarded and the baby may need clearing of the airway and supplementary oxygen. A score of 7 to 10 is considered good, indicating that the infant scored as high as 70% to 90% of all infants at 1 to 5 minutes after birth (10 is the highest score possible).

The Apgar score standardizes infant assessment at birth and serves as a baseline for future evaluations. There is a high correlation between low 5-minute Apgar scores and mortality and morbidity, particularly neurologic morbidity (Katz, 2003). The following points should be considered in obtaining an Apgar rating.

Heart Rate. Auscultating a newborn heart with a stethoscope is the best way to determine heart rate; however, heart rate also may be obtained by observing and counting the pulsations of the cord at the abdomen if the cord is still uncut.

Respiratory Effort. Respirations are counted by watching respiratory movements. A mature newborn usually cries and aerates the lungs spontaneously at about 30 seconds after birth. By 1 minute, he or she maintains regular, although rapid, respirations. Difficulty with breathing might be anticipated in a newborn whose mother received large amounts of analgesia or a general anesthetic during labor or birth (Box 24.4).

Muscle Tone. Mature newborns hold their extremities tightly flexed, simulating their intrauterine position. Muscle tone is tested by observing their resistance to any effort to extend their extremities.

Reflex Irritability. One of two possible cues is used to evaluate reflex irritability in a newborn: response to a suction catheter in the nostrils and response to having the soles of the feet slapped. A baby whose mother was heavily sedated will probably demonstrate a low score in this category.

Color. All infants appear cyanotic at the moment of birth. They grow pink with or shortly after the first breath, which makes the color of newborns correspond to how well they are breathing. Acrocyanosis (cyanosis of the hands and feet) is so common in newborns that a score of 1 in this category can be thought of as normal.

Respiratory Evaluation

Good respiratory function obviously has the highest priority in newborn care, so assessment for it is ongoing at every newborn contact. The Silverman and Andersen index, originally devised in 1956 (Silverman & Andersen, 1956), can be used to estimate degrees of respiratory distress in newborns. For this assessment, a newborn is observed and then scored on each of five criteria (Fig. 24.19). Each item is given a value of 0, 1, or 2; the values are then added. A total score of 0 indicates no respiratory distress. Scores of 4 to 6 indicate moderate distress. Scores of 7 to 10 indicate severe distress. (The scores of this index run opposite to those of the Apgar: an Apgar score of 7 to 10 would indicate a well infant.)

Checkpoint Question 4

Beth Ruiz had Apgar scores of 6 and 8. The five areas assessed with Apgar scoring are:

a. Heart rate, respiratory effort, muscle tone, reflex irritability, and color.
b. Respiratory rate, abdominal tone, reflex irritability, color, head circumference.
c. Color, breathing rate, cry, amount of brown fat, response to an adult voice.
d. **A**bdominal tone, **p**ersistence, **g**astric acidity, **a**rterial pressure, **r**esponse to pain.

BOX 24.4: Focus on Nursing Care Planning

A Multidisciplinary Care Map for
A Term Newborn
●

Carlotta Ruiz has just given birth to her second child, a 6-lb, 5-oz baby girl. While Jose, Carlotta's husband, is in the room, Carlotta tells you she is a "veteran" at baby care. Jose adds, "Little Joe [their 3-year-old] will be so excited to see his new sister. That's all he's been talking about lately." When Carlotta is alone, you notice she seems a little apprehensive about caring for her new daughter. She tells you, "She's so much smaller than Joe was. And why does it sound like she has a cold? And what is this rash all over her? Isn't it bad enough she has a birthmark?"

Family Assessment
Family is composed of two parents, a 3-year-old sibling, and newborn. They live in a three-bedroom flat over a drycleaning store. Father clerks in a grocery store; mother works as a school bus driver. Finances rated as "Hanging in there."

Client Assessment
Apgar score: 6 at 1 minute; 8 at 5 minutes. Birth from LOA position. Breathed at 30 seconds after birth after administration of blow-by oxygen. Respiratory rate, 74 breaths per minute with mild substernal retractions; rhonchi in upper lobes bilaterally; no grunting or nasal flaring present. Vital signs: temperature (axillary), 98.2°F (36.8°C); heart rate, 136 bpm. Length, 18.5 inches; head circumference, 34 cm; chest circumference, 32 cm. She has a 2 × 3 cm red pigmented area on outer right thigh. Mother attempted breast-feeding in birthing room, but newborn had difficulty sucking because of rapid respirations. Remainder of physical examination within acceptable parameters.

Nursing Diagnosis
Risk for ineffective parenting related to infant's smaller than expected size and birthmark.

Outcome Criteria
Respiratory rate is decreased to 30 to 50 breaths per minute; retractions, nasal flaring, and grunting are absent; lungs are clear to auscultation.

Team Member Responsible	Assessment	Intervention	Rationale	Expected Outcome
Activities of Daily Living				
Nurse	Assess respiratory rate every 15 min. for 1 hr.	Report increase in rate, retractions, or development of nasal flaring or grunting.	Increases in respiratory rate and retractions, accompanied by nasal flaring and grunting, may indicate respiratory distress.	Infant gradually decreases respiratory rate to 30–50/min by 24 hr.
Nurse	Monitor newborn's temperature every hour.	Keep infant warm via radiant warmer. Wrap loosely in a blanket and place a cap on her head.	Newborns have difficulty conserving body heat. Exposure to cold increases metabolic rate, increasing need for oxygen and a higher respiratory rate.	Infant's temperature remains at 98.2°F axillary.

(continued)

Team Member Responsible	Assessment	Intervention	Rationale	Expected Outcome
Consultations				
Nurse/ Physician	Assess whether parents would like a dermatology consultation for child's birthmark.	Refer parents to dermatology consultant if desired.	A second opinion can help assure parents birthmark is no more than a birthmark.	Parents visit with consultant if desired; state they understand the prognosis for port-wine lesions.
Procedures/Medications				
Nurse	Assess whether infant's lung sounds reveal fluid.	Position newborn on her side with head slightly lower than body; suction mouth and then nose with bulb syringe as indicated.	Positioning facilitates drainage of secretions from airway. Gentle suctioning removes secretions. Suctioning mouth before nose prevents possible aspiration of oral secretions.	Infant appears comfortable in chosen position; need for suctioning becomes infrequent.
Nutrition				
Nurse	Assess mother's knowledge of breast-feeding techniques.	Assist mother with breast-feeding as needed; remind her that rapid respirations make sucking difficult.	Breast milk is the preferred milk for human newborns; a mother may need assistance if an infant sucks poorly.	Infant and mother establish mutually enjoyable breast-feeding by hospital discharge.
Patient/Family Education				
Nurse/ Physician	Review with parents what were their expectations of new child (bigger? prettier? more relaxed?)	Inform parents that a rapid respiratory rate is common in newborns because of unabsorbed lung fluid. Help them mold expectations with reality.	Providing information helps to allay parents' anxieties and fears.	Parents state they understand their infant's condition.
Psychosocial/Spiritual/Emotional Needs				
Nurse	Assess what is parents' greatest concern about taking newborn home.	Explain that the presence of a birthmark, rapid respirations, and smaller than expected size are normal variations of newborns.	Explanation of normal range of infant variation provides information to help allay parents' fears and concerns.	Parents state they were initially surprised by baby's appearance, but are adjusting to new image.
Nurse	Assess infant for general physical condition.	Point out positive attributes of newborn, such as pretty eyes, alert expression.	Pointing out positive areas helps parents focus attention on the unique and special qualities of their child.	Parents state they appreciate learning more about their newborn from health care professionals.
Discharge Planning				
Nurse	Assess whether parents have made plans for hospital discharge.	Remind parents about importance of car seat, falls, and aspiration.	Safety awareness plays a big role in preventing early-age accidents.	Parents state they feel ready to begin parenting their new infant.

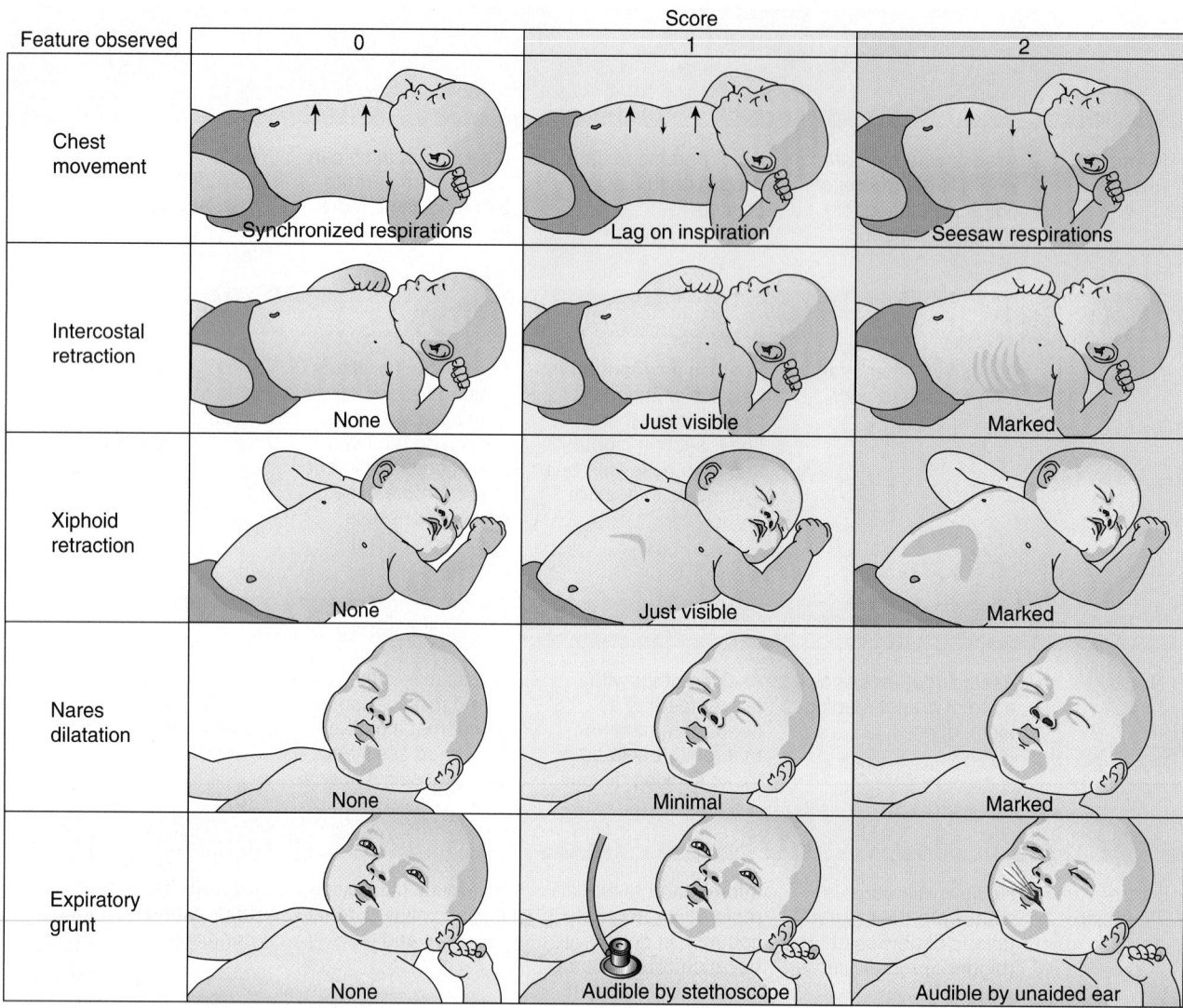

Feature observed	Score 0	Score 1	Score 2
Chest movement	Synchronized respirations	Lag on inspiration	Seesaw respirations
Intercostal retraction	None	Just visible	Marked
Xiphoid retraction	None	Just visible	Marked
Nares dilatation	None	Minimal	Marked
Expiratory grunt	None	Audible by stethoscope	Audible by unaided ear

FIGURE 24.19 Grading of neonatal respiratory distress based on Silverman-Andersen index. (Silverman, W. A., & Andersen, D. H. [1956]. A controlled clinical trial of effects of water mist on obstructive respiratory signs, death rate and necroscopy findings among premature infants. *Pediatrics, 17*[4], 1–9.)

Physical Examination

A newborn is given a preliminary physical examination immediately after birth, to establish gestational age and to detect any observable condition such as difficulty breathing, a congenital heart anomaly, meningocele, cleft lip or palate, hydrocephalus, a birthmark, imperforate anus, tracheo-esophageal atresia, or bowel obstruction (Table 24.3). This assessment may be the responsibility of the delivering physician, nurse practitioner, nurse-midwife, pediatrician, or nurse. This health assessment is done quickly, to prevent overexposing the newborn, yet not so swiftly that important findings are overlooked.

Height and Weight

Assuming newborns are breathing well, they are weighed nude and without a blanket immediately after birth in the birthing room (Fig. 24.20). Measurements such as body length and head, chest, and abdominal circumferences can be obtained in a newborn or transitional nursery. Performing these measurements while an infant is still damp only exposes the newborn unnecessarily to chilling.

Newborn weight helps to determine maturity and establishes a baseline against which other weights can be compared. An infant is weighed nude once a day, at approximately the same time every day, during a hospital or birthing center stay. Compare the weight obtained each day with that of the preceding day to be certain an infant is not losing more than the normal physiologic amount (5% to 10% of birthweight). Abnormal loss of weight may be the first indication that a newborn has an inborn error of metabolism, such as adrenogenital syndrome (salt-dumping type), or is becoming dehydrated.

TABLE 24.3

Congenital Anomaly Appraisal

Procedure	Abnormalities Considered
Inquire for hydramnios or oligohydramnios	Presence of hydramnios suggests congenital gastrointestinal obstruction. Oligohydramnios suggests genitourinary obstruction or extreme prematurity.
Appearance of abdomen	Distended abdomen suggests ascites or tumor. Empty abdomen suggests diaphragmatic hernia.
Passage of nasogastric tube (No. 8 feeding catheter) through nares into stomach	Failure to pass nasogastric tube through nares on either side establishes choanal atresia. Failure to pass it into the stomach confirms presence of esophageal atresia.
Aspiration of stomach with recording of color and amount of fluid obtained	With excess of 20 mL of fluid, or yellow fluid, duodenal or ileal atresia is suspected.
Insertion of rectal catheter	Failure to obtain meconium suggests imperforate anus or higher obstruction.
Counting of umbilical arteries	The presence of one artery suggests possible congenital urinary or cardiac anomalies or chromosomal trisomy (if other portions of examination are consistent).

Van Leeuwen, G. & Glenn, L. (1968). Screening for hidden congenital anomalies. *Pediatrics, 41*(6), 147–152. Copyright American Academy of Pediatrics, 1968.

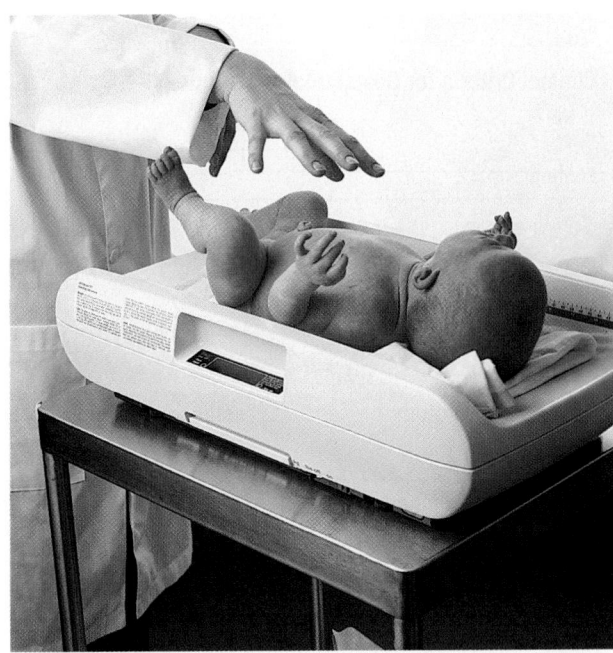

FIGURE 24.20 Weighing a newborn. Notice the protective hand held over the infant.

Laboratory Studies

After the first hour of undisturbed rest, depending on health agency policy, newborns may have heel-stick tests for hematocrit, hemoglobin, and hypoglycemia determinations. Heel-sticks require a minimum of blood, and, although not pain free, they cause minimal trauma to a baby. In some settings, these tests are not routine but are reserved only for newborns with symptoms of anemia, polycythemia, or hypoglycemia.

Hematocrit and hemoglobin determinations are done to detect newborn anemia, because it is difficult to appreciate that anemia is present by clinical observation alone. Anemia can be caused by hypovolemia due to bleeding from placenta previa or abruptio placentae or by a cesarean birth that involved incision into the placenta. Another condition as dangerous as anemia is the presence of an excess of red blood cells (polycythemia), probably caused by excessive flow of blood into an infant from the umbilical cord. A heel-stick hematocrit reveals both of these conditions, and treatment then can be instituted. A normal hematocrit at 1 hour of life is about 50% to 55%.

Hypoglycemia may also produce few symptoms, so it is determined by a heel-stick glucose measurement. If a blood glucose heel-stick reading is less than 40 mg/100 mL of blood (30 mg/100 mL in the first 3 days of life), hypoglycemia is present (Fischback, 2004). To correct this condition, the infant is prescribed oral glucose or infant formula to be given immediately. This elevates the infant's blood sugar to a safe level. It is important to treat hypoglycemia quickly because, if brain cells become completely depleted of glucose, brain damage can result. If a newborn exhibits symptoms of hypoglycemia (jitteriness, lethargy, seizures) in addition to the low laboratory test results, intravenous glucose probably will be prescribed. A continuous intravenous infusion of glucose may be necessary if the newborn is unable to maintain glucose levels higher than 40 mg/100 mL.

Assessment of Gestational Age

Specific findings on physical assessment provide clues to a newborn's gestational age. As early as 1966, Usher and colleagues (1966) proposed five criteria to evaluate gestational maturity (Table 24.4). These quick criteria can be used for assessment of all newborns.

Dubowitz Maturity Scale

Dubowitz and colleagues (1970) devised a gestational rating scale that uses more extensive criteria. All newborns appearing to be immature by Usher's criteria or who are light in weight at birth or early by dates should

TABLE 24.4

Clinical Criteria for Gestational Assessment

Finding	Gestation Age (wk)		
	0–36	*37–38*	*39 and Over*
Sole creases	Anterior transverse crease only	Occasional creases in anterior two thirds	Sole covered with creases
Breast nodule diameter (mm)	2	4	7
Scalp hair	Fine and fuzzy	Fine and fuzzy	Coarse and silky
Ear lobe	Pliable; no cartilage	Some cartilage	Stiffened by thick cartilage
Testes and scrotum	Testes in lower canal; scrotum small; few rugae	Intermediate	Testes pendulous, scrotum full; extensive rugae

Usher, R., et al. (1966). Judgment of fetal age. *Pediatric Clinics of North America, 13*(4), 835–840.

be assessed by means of these more definitive criteria. Although completing a Dubowitz assessment takes practice, it can yield important results; it can help determine whether a newborn needs immediate high-risk nursery intervention.

During the 1970s and again in the 1990s, Ballard modified the Dubowitz scale (Ballard et al., 1991) to an assessment scale that can be completed in 3 to 4 minutes. The assessment consists of two portions: physical maturity and neuromuscular maturity (Fig. 24.21). The first is a series of observations about skin texture, color, lanugo, foot creases, genitalia, ear, and breast maturity. Each designated body part is inspected and given a score of 0 to 5, as described in Figure 24.21A. This observational scoring should be done as soon as possible after birth, because skin assessment becomes much less reliable after 24 hours. Illustrations of mature and immature body features for Ballard scale use are shown in Chapter 26 as part of the discussion of the preterm infant.

To complete the second half of the gestational examination, observe or position a newborn as shown in Figure 24.21B. Again, score the child's response numerically from 0 to 5.

To establish a baby's gestational age, the total score obtained (on both sections) is compared with the rating scale in Figure 24.21C. An infant with a total score of 5 is at 26 weeks' gestational age; a total score of 10 reveals a gestational age of about 28 weeks; a total score of 40 points is found in infants at term or 40 weeks' gestation.

Using such a standard method to rate maturity is helpful in detecting infants who are small for gestational age (they are light in weight, but the neuromuscular and physical observation scales are adequate for their weeks in utero) and differentiating them from newborns who are immature because of a miscalculated due date. An infant who is found to be less than 35 weeks' gestation requires close observation, usually in a special care nursery.

Assessment of Behavioral Capacity

Term newborns are physically active and emotionally prepared to interact with the people around them. They are people oriented from the beginning—how much so can be demonstrated by the way they immediately attune to human voices or concentrate on their mother's face (Fig. 24.22).

Brazelton Neonatal Behavioral Assessment Scale

The *Brazelton Neonatal Behavioral Assessment Scale* is a rating scale devised by Brazelton in the early 1970s (Brazelton, 1973) to evaluate a newborn's behavioral capacity or ability to respond to set stimuli. Six major categories of behavior—habituation, orientation, motor maturity, variation, self-quieting ability, and social behavior—are assessed.

To perform an assessment using the scale requires training to ensure that it is used consistently from one individual to another. Unlike many assessment scales, the infant is scored on best performance rather than on average performance. A total evaluation takes 20 to 30 minutes to complete. It is useful for comparing different groups of infants, such as those exposed or not exposed to cocaine in utero (Myers et al., 2003).

The information supplied by this scale has provided concrete evidence that newborns are not passive, nonhearing, unseeing, unresponsive, or even all alike. An important finding from the scale is that newborns are able to quiet themselves after crying. Many of the items tested on the scale, such as how infants alert (eyes widen, head held as if listening) or orient to sound (turn toward the direction of the parent's voice or appear to listen to the sound of a voice) and how they naturally cuddle when held next to their parent, are excellent examples of newborn behavior to point out to parents. If parents perceive a newborn as passive and unresponsive, they are likely to talk or

prevent accidental bowel perforation. If the temperature is subnormal and the baby is in a bassinet, he or she should be placed in a heated bassinet or under a radiant warmer for additional heat. If the temperature is normal, a newborn can be bathed quickly to remove excess vernix caseosa and blood, then dressed in a shirt and diaper, reswaddled in a snug blanket (to give the baby a familiar feeling of the tight confines of the uterus), and placed in a bassinet or returned to the mother's side.

During the first day of life, a newborn's temperature is usually taken every 4 to 8 hours. Thereafter, unless the temperature is elevated or subnormal, or the infant appears to be in distress, measurement once a day while in the health care facility is enough.

Nursing Diagnosis: Risk for ineffective airway clearance related to presence of mucus in mouth and nose at birth

Outcome Evaluation: Neonate maintains a respiratory rate of 30 to 60 breaths per minute without evidence of retraction or grunting by 5 minutes after birth.

Promote Adequate Breathing Pattern and Prevent Aspiration. Mucus is suctioned from a newborn's mouth by a bulb syringe as soon as the head is born. As soon as the body is born, he or she should be held for a few seconds with the head slightly dependent, for further drainage of secretions. It is important that mucus be removed from the mouth and pharynx before the first breath this way to prevent aspiration of the secretions. If the infant continues to have an accumulation of mucus in the mouth or nose after these first steps, you may need to suction further after the baby is placed under a warmer (Fig. 24.27). Use a bulb syringe or a soft, small (no. 10 or 12) catheter to suction. Never suction vigorously, because this irritates the mucous mem-

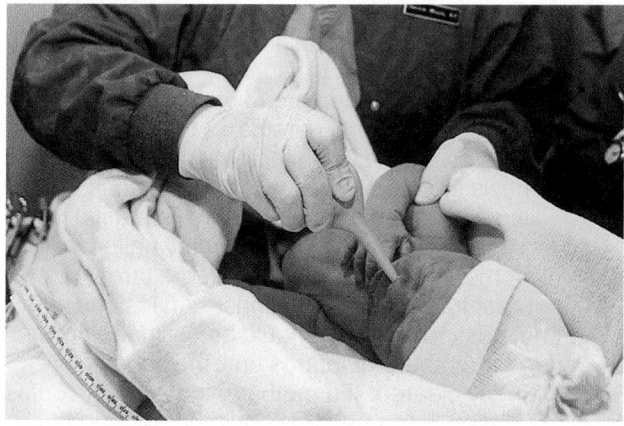

FIGURE 24.27 A newborn is suctioned by means of a bulb syringe to remove mucus from the mouth and nose. The head-down-and-to-the-side position facilitates drainage. Care is given with the infant under a radiant heat source.

brane and could leave a portal of entry for infection. Brisk suctioning also has been associated with bradycardia in newborns because of vagal nerve stimulation. If you use a bulb syringe, decompress the bulb before inserting it into the infant's mouth or nose; otherwise, the force of decompression will push secretions back into the pharynx or bronchi rather than remove them. Although the effectiveness of the procedure is not well documented, when an infant is born with meconium-stained amniotic fluid, intubation may be performed so that deep tracheal suction can be accomplished before the first breath, to help prevent meconium aspiration (Halliday & Sweet, 2005).

Record the First Cry. A crying infant is a breathing infant, because the sound of crying is made by a current of air passing over the larynx. The more lusty the cry, the greater the assurance the newborn is breathing deeply and forcefully. Vigorous crying also helps blow off the extra carbon dioxide that makes all newborns slightly acidotic, so helps to correct this condition. Although gentleness is necessary to make an infant's transition from intrauterine life to extrauterine life as untraumatic as possible, there is no need to completely halt the initial crying of a newborn.

A newborn who does not breathe spontaneously or who takes a few quick, gasping breaths but is unable to maintain respirations needs resuscitation as an emergency measure. An infant with grunting respirations needs careful observation for respiratory distress syndrome (see Chapter 26).

Nursing Diagnosis: Risk for infection related to newly clamped umbilical cord and exposure of eyes to vaginal secretions

Outcome Evaluation: Area around cord is dry and free of erythema. Eyes are free of inflammation and drainage. Axillary temperature is maintained between 97.6°F and 98.6°F (36.5°C and 37°C).

Inspect and Care for Umbilical Cord. The umbilical cord pulsates for a moment after an infant is born as a last flow of blood passes from the placenta into the infant. Two clamps are then applied to the cord about 8 inches from the infant's abdomen, and the cord is cut between the clamps. Some fathers choose to do this as their responsibility. The infant cord is then clamped again by a permanent cord clamp, such as a Hazeltine or a Kane clamp. The clamp on the maternal end of the cord should not be released after the cord is cut, to prevent blood still remaining in the placenta from leaking out. This loss is not important, because the mother's circulation does not connect to the placenta. It is messy, however, and that is why the clamp is left in place.

Every time you handle a newborn, inspect the cord to be certain it is clamped securely. If the clamp loosens before thrombosis obliterates the umbilical vessels, hemorrhage could result. As previously mentioned, the number of cord vessels should be counted and noted immediately after the cord is cut. Cords begin to dry almost immediately, and the vessels may be obscured by the time of the infant's first thorough physical examination in the nursery.

Within a few minutes after the cord is cut, apply antibiotic ointment or triple dye as required by agency policy to help reduce infection. Until the cord falls off, at about day 7 to 10 of life, it should be kept dry. The newborn should receive sponge baths rather than be immersed in a tub of water. Be certain that diapers are folded below the level of the umbilical cord, so that, when the diaper becomes wet, the cord does not become wet also.

Remind parents to continue to keep the cord dry until it falls off after they return home. The use of creams, lotions, and oils near the cord should be discouraged, because they tend to slow drying of the cord and invite infection. Some health care agencies recommend applying rubbing alcohol to the cord site once or twice a day to hasten drying. Others prefer the cord be left strictly alone, because manipulation could invite infection.

After the cord falls off, a small, pink, granulating area about a quarter of an inch in diameter may remain. This should also be left clean and dry until it has healed (about 24 to 48 more hours). If the ulcerous area has remained as long as 1 week, it may require cautery with silver nitrate to speed healing.

Administer Eye Care. Although the practice may shortly become obsolete (as it is in Europe), every U.S. state still requires that newborns receive prophylactic eye treatment against gonorrheal conjunctivitis (Katz, 2003). Such infections are usually acquired from the mother as the infant passes through the birth canal. Formerly, eye prophylaxis was applied immediately after birth. Many parents today prefer to visit with their infant before the procedure, to be certain their newborn can focus on them without blurry vision caused by ointment or drops. As long as it is completed as soon as possible after birth, either in the birthing room or on arrival in the nursery, the exact time the ointment is administered is unimportant. Silver nitrate was exclusively used for prophylaxis in the past; today, erythromycin ointment is the drug of choice. Erythromycin ointment has the advantage of eliminating not only the organism of gonorrhea but that of chlamydia as well (Box 24.7).

Always use a single-use tube or package of ointment, to avoid transmitting infection from one newborn to another. To instill the ointment, first dry the face of the newborn with a soft gauze square so that the skin is not slippery. The best procedure to open a newborn's eyes is to shade them from the overhead light and open one eye at a time by pressure on the lower and upper lids. Squeeze a line of ointment along the lower conjunctival sac, from the inner canthus outward, and then close the eye to allow the ointment to spread across the conjunctiva.

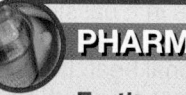

BOX 24.7 FOCUS ON . . .

PHARMACOLOGY

Erythromycin Ophthalmic Ointment

Classification: Erythromycin ointment is a topical antibiotic.

Action: Erythromycin is effective against gonorrhea and chlamydia organisms, making it the drug of choice for eye prophylaxis at birth (Karch, 2004).

Pregnancy Risk Category: B

Dosage: 0.5–1 cm each eye

Possible Adverse Effects: Mild irritation to conjunctiva; slight blurring of vision.

Nursing Implications
- Use a single-dose application tube.
- After gently pulling down on a newborn's lower eyelid, extrude a line of ointment the length of the lower eyelid from the inner canthus outward.
- Discard any remaining ointment to prevent its being used again.
- Close the child's eyes and count to about 5.
- Wipe away any excess ointment from the child's face.
- If desired, delay application for an hour after birth to allow the infant to view his or her parents for the first time with the clearest vision possible.

Credé, a German gynecologist, first proposed silver nitrate prophylaxis against gonorrheal conjunctivitis in 1884. For this reason, it is often referred to as the *Credé treatment* and may be listed that way on a health care agency form even though silver nitrate is no longer used. Babies born outside hospitals, in homes or in less orthodox settings such as a car or taxi, have the prophylactic treatment administered on admission to the hospital.

General Infection Precautions. Each newborn should have his or her own bassinet. Compartments in the bassinet should hold a supply of diapers, shirts, gowns, and individual equipment for bathing and temperature taking. Avoid sharing of these items, which could lead to the spread of infection.

Health care workers, parents, or siblings caring for newborns should wash their hands and arms to the elbows thoroughly with an antiseptic soap before handling an infant. Agency personnel are usually required to wear cover gowns or nursery uniforms.

Staff members with infections (sore throats, upper respiratory tract infections, skin lesions, or gastrointestinal upsets) should be excluded from caring for mothers or infants until the condition is completely cleared. If a mother might have a contagious illness, her newborn should be excluded from her room until there is no longer a possibility of contagion. An instant photograph can be taken of the baby and shown to the mother so that she can follow the baby's progress. If the infant is breast-fed, the mother should manually express milk during the time the infant is excluded, to maintain her milk supply. The milk, however, should be discarded. The mother can resume breast-feeding as soon as it is both possible and safe for her infant.

Any baby born outside a hospital or under circumstances conducive to infection (e.g., rupture of membranes more than 24 hours before birth) should be kept in a closed bassinet or in the mother's room until negative cultures show that the newborn is free of infection. Any newborn in whom symptoms of infection develop (e.g., skin lesions, fever) should be removed to an isolation nursery or housed in the mother's room to prevent the spread of infection to other babies. There is no reason for parents not to visit a baby housed in isolation care. In fact, they may have more need to hold a baby who is isolated than average parents do, because they have an extra reason to be worried that something is wrong with their child. To visit in isolation nurseries, parents should be required to use the same infection control techniques that staff members use.

What if... Beth Ruiz had been born by cesarean birth? Would you still administer eye prophylaxis? Or do newborns acquire eye infections only during their transit through the birth canal?

NURSING CARE OF A NEWBORN AND FAMILY IN THE POSTPARTAL PERIOD

Newborns are usually kept in either a birthing room or a transitional nursery for optimal safety in the first few hours of life. During this period of close observation, certain principles of care always apply.

Initial Feeding

A term newborn who is to be breast-fed may be fed immediately after birth. A baby who is to be formula-fed may receive a first feeding at about 2 to 4 hours of age. Both formula-fed and breast-fed infants do best on a demand schedule; many need to be fed as often as every 2 hours in the first few days of life. Chapter 25 covers the elements of breast-feeding and formula-feeding in detail.

Bathing

In most hospitals, newborns receive a complete bath to wash away vernix caseosa within an hour after birth. Thereafter, they are bathed once a day, although the procedure may be limited to washing only the baby's face, diaper area, and skin folds. Wear gloves when handling newborns until the first bath, to avoid exposing your hands to body secretions; babies of mothers with human immunodeficiency virus (HIV) infection should have a thorough bath immediately, to decrease the possibility of HIV transmission.

Bathing of an infant is best done by the parents under a nurse's supervision. Be sure the room is warm (about 75°F [24°C]), to prevent chilling. Bath water should be approximately 98°F to 100°F (37°C to 38°C), a temperature that feels pleasantly warm to the elbow or wrist. If soap is used, it should be mild and without a hexachlorophene base. Bathing should take place before, not after, a feeding, to prevent spitting up or vomiting and possible aspiration.

Equipment necessary for an infant's bath consists of a basin of water, soap, washcloth, towel, comb, and clean diaper and shirt. Assemble these items beforehand, so the baby is not left exposed or unattended while you go for more equipment.

Teach parents that bathing should proceed from the cleanest to the most soiled areas of the body—that is, from the eyes and face to the trunk and extremities and, last, to the diaper area. Wipe a newborn's eyes with clear water from the inner canthus outward, using a clean portion of the washcloth for each eye to prevent spread of infection to the other eye. Wash the face with clear water only (no soap) to avoid skin irritation; soap may be used on the rest of the body.

Teach parents to wash the infant's hair daily with the bath. The easiest way to do this is to first soap the hair with the baby lying in the bassinet. Then, hold the infant in one arm over the basin of water, as you would a football (Fig. 24.28). Splash water from the basin against the head to rinse the hair. Dry the hair well to prevent chilling.

Wash each area of the baby's body, rinse so no soap is left on the skin (soap is drying and newborns are susceptible to desquamation), and then dry the body part. When you wash the skin around the cord, take care not to soak the cord, because a wet cord remains in place longer than a dry one and furnishes a breeding ground for bacteria. Give particular care to the creases of skin, where milk tends to collect if the child spits up after feedings.

In male infants, the foreskin of the uncircumcised penis should not be forced back, or constriction of the penis may result. Wash the vulva of a female infant, wiping from front to back to prevent contamination of the vagina or urethra by rectal bacteria.

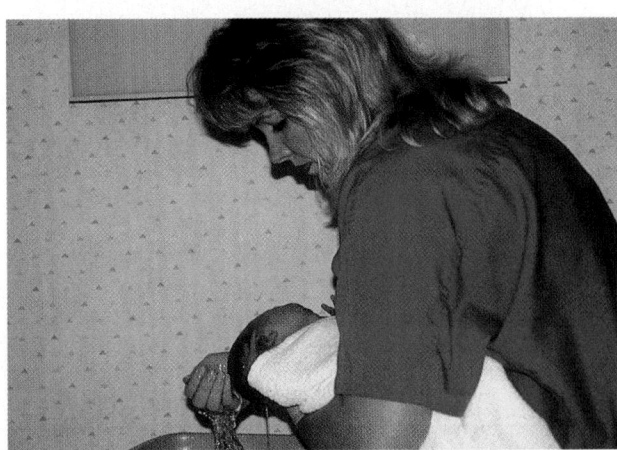

FIGURE 24.28 A football hold. Such a position supports the infant's head and back and leaves the nurse's or mother's other hand free for assembling or using equipment.

Most health care agencies do not apply powder or lotion to newborns, because some infants are allergic to these products. In addition, many adult talcum powders contain zinc stearate, which is irritating to the respiratory tract; such preparations should always be avoided. If a newborn's skin seems extremely dry and portals for infection are becoming apparent, a lubricant such as Nivea oil, added to the bath water or applied directly to the baby's skin, should relieve the condition.

Sleeping Position

Stress to parents that a newborn should be positioned on the back for sleep. Sudden infant death syndrome (SIDS) is the sudden, unexplained death of an infant younger than 1 year of age. Although the specific cause of SIDS cannot be explained, placing infants in a supine position has been shown to decrease the incidence of the syndrome (Box 24.8).

BOX 24.8 FOCUS ON . . .

EVIDENCE-BASED PRACTICE

Do Nurses Follow the Recommendation to Put Newborns to Sleep on Their Back?

The American Academy of Pediatrics (AAP) has recommended that all infants be positioned on their back for sleeping, because this position appears to lower the incidence of sudden infant death syndrome (SIDS). To discover what position nurses in newborn nurseries use when they put newborns to sleep, researchers distributed questionnaires to 96 hospital newborn nursery staff and 579 mothers of newborns at eight separate perinatal hospitals. Surprisingly, although 72% of sampled nursery staff identified the supine position as the placement that most lowers the risk for SIDS, only 30% reported most often placing infants to sleep in that position. The most common reason for not using the supine position was fear of aspiration. In addition, only 34% of staff reported advising exclusive supine infant positioning to mothers. When mothers were asked whether they used a supine position for their infant, only 36% reported using this placement exclusively. Mothers' rate of use was influenced by the advice they received as to infant position and the role modeling they observed. Those who used the position most had both received advice and observed role modeling. Nonwhite women used a supine position less often than white women did, and multiparas used it less than primiparas.

This study is important to nurses, because it reveals how important role modeling newborn care is to new mothers as well as how evidence-based interventions are not always used in practice.

Stastny, P. F., et al. (2004). Infant sleep positioning by nursery staff and mothers in newborn hospital nurseries. *Nursing Research, 53*(2), 122–129.

Diaper Area Care

Preventing diaper dermatitis is a practice that parents need to start from the very beginning with their newborns. With each diaper change, the area should be washed with clear water and dried well, to prevent the ammonia in urine from irritating the infant's skin and causing a diaper rash. After cleaning, a mild ointment (e.g., petroleum jelly, A and D ointment) may be applied to the buttocks. The ointment keeps ammonia away from the skin and also facilitates the removal of meconium, which is sticky and tarry. Wear gloves for diaper care as part of standard precautions.

Metabolic Screening Tests

By state law, every infant must be screened for phenylketonuria (PKU; a disease of defective protein metabolism), hypothyroidism, and cystic fibrosis. This is done by means of a simple blood test in which three drops of blood from the heel are dropped onto a special filter paper. Ideally, the baby should have received formula or breast milk for 24 hours (providing an intake of phenylalanine, an essential amino acid found in milk) before the test for PKU will be accurate. If the infant has not received adequate milk before the blood sample is taken, the results may be falsely negative (a child with PKU will test as if normal). If an infant is discharged before this 24-hour period, a second screening test is necessary. Many states require other metabolic tests at birth, such as screening for galactosemia and maple syrup urine disease, that also require filter paper blood tests.

If blood testing was not done before discharge, alert the parents that they must schedule the tests at an ambulatory visit in 2 to 3 days' time. Always assess at the first newborn health supervision visit whether this procedure was done. As with any heel-stick for blood, sampling of this nature is done best by a spring-activated lancet rather than a regular lancet, so that the skin incision is made as quickly and painlessly as possible. Allowing a newborn to suck on a pacifier during painful procedures may be helpful.

Hepatitis B Vaccination

All newborns receive a first vaccination against hepatitis B within 12 hours after birth; a second dose is administered at 1 month and a third at 6 months. Infants whose mothers are positive for the hepatitis B surface antigen (HBsAg) also receive hepatitis B immune globulin (HBIG) at birth (AAP, 2005).

Vitamin K Administration

Newborns are at risk for bleeding disorders during the first week of life because their gastrointestinal tract is sterile at birth and unable to produce vitamin K, which is necessary for blood coagulation. A single dose of 0.5 to 1.0 mg of vitamin K is administered intramuscularly within the first hour of life to prevent such problems (Box 24.9). Infants born outside a hospital also should receive this important protection.

BOX 24.9 FOCUS ON . . .

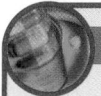

PHARMACOLOGY

Vitamin K (Phytonadione, AquaMEPHYTON)

Action: Vitamin K is used to prevent and treat hemorrhagic disease in newborns. It is a necessary component for the production of certain coagulation factors (II, VII, IX, and X) and is produced by microorganisms in the intestinal tract (Karch, 2004).

Pregnancy risk category: C

Dosage: Prophylaxis—0.5 to 1.0 mg IM one time immediately after birth; treatment of hemorrhagic disease—1 to 2 mg IM or SC daily.

Possible adverse reactions: Local irritation, such as pain and swelling at the site of injection.

Nursing Implications
- Anticipate the need for injection immediately after birth.
- Administer IM injection into large muscle, such as the anterolateral muscle of a newborn's thigh.
- If giving for treatment, obtain prothrombin time before administration (the single best indicator of vitamin K–dependent clotting factors).
- Assess for signs of bleeding, such as black, tarry stools (different from meconium stools, which have a greenish shade), hematuria, decreased hemoglobin and hematocrit levels, and bleeding from any open wounds or base of the cord. (These signs would indicate that more vitamin K is necessary, because bleeding control has not been achieved.)

Circumcision

Circumcision is the surgical removal of the foreskin of the penis. In only a few babies, constriction (phimosis) of the foreskin is so severe that it obstructs the urinary meatal opening; otherwise, there are few medical indications for circumcision of a male newborn. Circumcision is performed on Jewish boys on the eighth day of life as part of a religious requirement, in a ceremony called a *bris.* In the United States, from the 1920s to the 1960s, circumcision became so popular for aesthetic reasons that virtually all male infants were routinely circumcised at birth. The reasons supporting circumcision include easier hygiene because the foreskin does not have to be retracted during bathing, and possibly fewer urinary tract infections. There also may be an increased incidence of penile cancer in uncircumcised men, as well as increased cervical cancer in their sexual partners. However, because the procedure is not essential and does carry some risk, parents should be well informed about the procedure so they can evaluate carefully whether they wish to have it performed on their son.

Contraindications for circumcision include congenital abnormalities such as hypospadias or epispadias, because the prepuce skin may be needed when a plastic surgeon repairs the defect. Another contradiction is a history of a bleeding tendency in the family.

The procedure is not done immediately after birth, because at that time a newborn's level of vitamin K, which is necessary to prevent hemorrhage, is at a low point and the child would be exposed to unnecessary cold. It is best performed during the first or second day of life, after the baby has synthesized enough vitamin K to reduce the chance of faulty blood coagulation. If parents elect early discharge, they may be asked to return the infant to the hospital or to an ambulatory setting for the surgery. Parents should check that their health insurance plan will reimburse for the procedure if it is done on a return visit, after their newborn has been discharged from the hospital.

For the procedure, an infant is placed in a supine position and restrained either manually or with a commercial swaddling board. In the past the procedure was done without anesthesia, but today the trend is toward use of local or regional block anesthesia to reduce the pain as much as possible (Razmus et al., 2004). Application of EMLA cream (a *e*utectic *m*ixture of *l*ocal *a*nesthetics) is a popular choice for local anesthesia (Taddio et al., 2005).

A specially designed plastic bell (Plastibell) is fitted over the end of the penis. A suture is then tied around the rim of the bell and a circle of the prepuce is cut away so that the foreskin can be easily retracted and the glans will be fully exposed (Fig. 24.29). The rim of the bell, which remains in place for about 1 week and then falls off by itself, protects the healing penis from sticking to the diaper. The bell also helps protect against infection and bleeding. In the past, petrolatum ointment was applied to circumcision incisions. With the bell rim in place, this is no longer necessary, although it still may be applied if desired.

Complications that can occur from circumcision include hemorrhage, infection, and urethral fistula formation. To keep the risk of these complications to a minimum, observe infants closely for about 2 hours after circumcision. Check the infant for bleeding every 15 minutes for the first hour. Also, document that the infant is voiding after the procedure.

Parents should keep the area clean and covered with petrolatum (if used) for about 3 days, until healing is complete. If they see any redness or tenderness, or if the baby cries as if in constant pain, they should report it by telephone. Circumcision sites appear red but should never have a strong odor or discharge. A film of yellowish mucus often covers the glans (similar to a scab) by the second day after surgery. This should not be washed away. The yellow color is from accumulated serum, an innocent finding, and should not be mistaken for the yellow of a purulent exudate.

ASSESSMENT OF FAMILY'S READINESS TO CARE FOR A NEWBORN AT HOME

It is important to assess how prepared each family is to care for their newborn at home, to be sure the newborn remains safe (Box 24.10). Parents may need to make changes in their routine, such as shifting their usual dinner time or work schedule. Sleep schedules are certain to

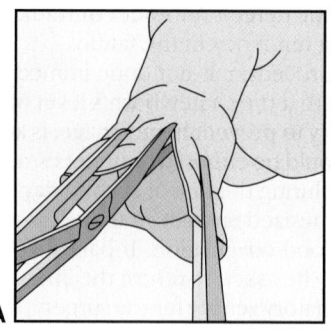

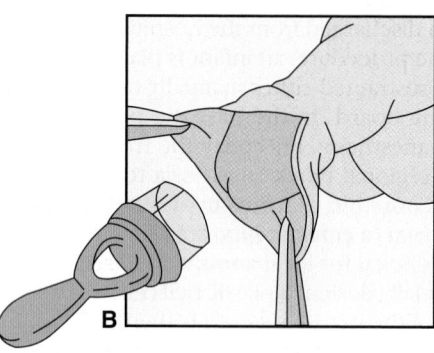

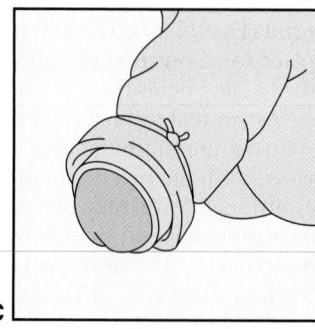

FIGURE 24.29 Technique for performing circumcision using a Plastibell. (**A**) An incision is made in the top of the foreskin. (**B**) The Plastibell is placed over the head of the penis, and the foreskin is pulled over the Plastibell. (**C**) A suture is tied around the foreskin over the tying groove in the Plastibell. Excess skin beyond the suture is trimmed away. The Plastibell falls off in 3 to 7 days. (Courtesy of Hollister Inc., Libertyville, IL.)

BOX 24.10 FOCUS ON . . .

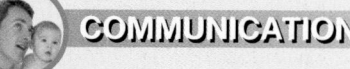

COMMUNICATION

When you enter Beth Ruiz's room, you notice her mother sitting on the side of the bed staring into Beth's face.

Less Effective Communication

Nurse: You seem concerned, Mrs. Ruiz. Is something wrong?

Mrs. Ruiz: Do you think she can tell how little I remember about babies?

Nurse: You're doing a great job. That's the important thing.

Mrs. Ruiz: How long will it take for me to feel like a great mother?

Nurse: You're worrying too much. Relax and enjoy your new baby.

More Effective Communication

Nurse: You seem concerned, Mrs. Ruiz. Is something wrong?

Mrs. Ruiz: Do you think she can tell how little I remember about babies?

Nurse: Is there something special you feel you don't know?

Mrs. Ruiz: My big problem is, I don't feel anything toward her yet. Why do I keep wondering if this whole thing is real?

Nurse: Let's talk about how maternal love develops. It isn't automatic.

Most new mothers have so many questions, it is easy to dismiss a very serious question as "just another question." Resist assuring women that they will be good mothers until you are certain their concern isn't something that could interfere with good mothering.

---

be disrupted, because infants wake during the night for one or more feedings for about the first 4 months of life.

The physical environment of the home to which a newborn will be discharged is a good subject to explore with parents. Questions and areas to consider include the following:

- Is it an apartment or a house?
- How many flights of stairs will the mother have to climb when she takes the baby home or when she takes the baby out in a stroller?
- How many other people live in the home? (Infections spread more rapidly in crowded homes.)

- Are there any pets in the home? Will a large dog, for example, be a safe pet around the baby?
- Is there a bed for the baby?
- Will the baby be sleeping alone in a room or with older children? Will the baby share a bed with a parent?
- Who will be the primary caregiver?
- Will grandparents or other persons offer support by visiting or helping with care of the child?
- Do the parents have anyone to turn to if they have questions about the baby?
- Is there a refrigerator in which formula or breast milk can be stored?
- Is there adequate heat? An infant needs a temperature of 70°F to 75°F during the day and 60°F to 65°F at night.
- Are the windows draft free and screened to keep out insects?
- If housing is in poor condition, is there a danger that rodents might attack the baby?
- Is there a danger of lead poisoning?
- Does the mother or do the parents have a source of income? If not, what sort of referral should be made so that money can be provided to care for this child?

These are not prying questions but means of determining whether the home will be adequate and safe. Good prenatal and postnatal care is wasted if an infant contracts pneumonia during the first week at home because no one at the hospital or a birthing center took the time to ask the right questions about the home environment. If the home environment is found to be unsafe, a referral to social services may be necessary before the newborn is discharged.

NURSING DIAGNOSES AND RELATED INTERVENTIONS

Nursing Diagnosis: Health-seeking behaviors related to needs of a normal newborn after discharge from the health care facility

Outcome Evaluation: Parents state ways in which they have already altered their home and lifestyle to accommodate their newborn and indicate that they are prepared for other changes; parents voice relative confidence in their ability to care for the newborn and state names of individuals within their family or community who can be resources to them when needed.

Before discharge, the parents should have thought through how they are going to care for their child at home. Many parents have been mulling over these questions throughout the pregnancy, whereas others may not yet have addressed some or any of these important issues. Box 24.11 highlights appropriate outcomes and interventions for safe parent–child attachment, using the terminology identified by the Nursing Outcomes Classification (NOC) and Nursing Interventions Classification (NIC).

Young, single mothers without family support and mothers who did not seek regular prenatal care in particular may be unprepared for the months ahead. With all parents, try to anticipate problems that may be relevant to them. If there are other children at home, discuss whether the parents are aware that sibling jealousy may occur. Pets in the home can cause similar problems with jealousy. Discuss with a mother who is not going to breast-feed what she will use to feed her baby until she has time to buy formula. Most hospitals supply or sell a discharge formula kit to help parents through the first day at home. Be sure the parents have decided when and where they will take their newborn for health supervision. Check the child's identification band against the mother's one final time before discharge, to help prevent the possibility of wrong identification of the infant.

Daily Home Care. Newborns thrive on a gentle rhythm of care, a sense of being able to anticipate

---

BOX 24.11

Nursing Outcomes Classification (NOC) and Nursing Interventions Classification (NIC)

Parents and the Neonate

NOC: Parent–infant Attachment
Parent–infant attachment is defined as the behaviors demonstrating an enduring affectionate bond between parents and infant (Johnson, Maas, & Moorhead, 2000). Some specific indicators suggesting that this outcome has been achieved include demonstration of the following behaviors by the parents:

- Verbalizing positive feelings toward the infant.
- Holding the infant close, touching, stroking, patting, and kissing the infant
- Talking to the infant in the en face position and maintaining eye contact
- Smiling, vocalizing, and playing with the infant
- Responding to cues, consoling, and feeding the infant

Also, some specific indicators suggesting achievement of this outcome include demonstration of the following behaviors by the neonate:

- Looking at parents
- Exploring the environment

- Responding to parental cues
- Seeking proximity with the parents

NIC: Environmental Management: Attachment Process
Environmental management, attachment process is defined as manipulation of the surroundings to facilitate development of the parent–infant relationship (McCloskey & Bulechek, 2000). Some important activities involved when implementing this intervention include the following:

- Creating a clean, homelike environment that fosters privacy and consistency of staff
- Individualizing daily routine to meet the family's needs
- Providing comfortable seating, such as a rocking chair, for parents
- Limiting the number of people in the environment, allowing for family visitation as desired
- Preventing and reducing interruptions from visitors, phone calls, and agency personnel
- Maintaining a low level of stimuli in the environment

what is to come next. Based on this, parents can decide what is the best daily at-home routine for them and their new child. There are no fixed rules. There is no set time at which an infant must be bathed, nor even a rule that requires a bath every day. All infants do not have to be in bed for the night by 8 PM. If the father works evenings, it may be important to have the baby awake at midnight so that he has time to spend with his child.

Your aim in helping parents plan their schedule of care is to arrive at one that does the following:

- Offers a degree of consistency (a mother cannot expect an infant to stay awake until midnight five nights a week, then go to sleep at 7 PM on the sixth night)
- Appears to satisfy the infant
- Gives the parents a sense of well-being and contentment with their child

Sleep Patterns. A newborn sleeps an average of 16 hours of every 24 during the first week home, an average of 4 hours at a time. By 4 months of age, an infant sleeps an average of 15 hours of every 24 and through the night.

It is exhausting for a parent who is already tired from labor and birth to have to awaken during the night to feed a newborn. For this reason, parents may try various methods to induce a baby to sleep through the night much earlier than 4 months. One approach is to introduce solid food (particularly cereal) in the first weeks of life, on the theory that the bulk will fill the infant's stomach so that he or she will not wake up crying to be fed. Actually, there is no correlation between the age at which solid food is introduced and a baby's capability for sustained sleep. Also, a newborn is not developmentally ready to deal with nonliquid food until about the end of the third month. There are also other reasons not to introduce solid food early: large protein molecules from solid foods can pass through a newborn's immature gastrointestinal tract, becoming antigens that may sensitize the newborn for possible allergic reactions. In breast-fed infants, too-early introduction of solid foods may interfere with the desire for breast milk, decrease the newborn's sucking, and subsequently decrease the mother's milk supply.

A baby probably wakes every 4, 5, 6, or 8 hours because of a physiologic need for fluid. Advise parents that, because of this fluid need, they should not try to eliminate night feedings. Knowing their baby is not sick, that you are concerned and willing to listen to their questions, and that every other parent of a newborn is also up at night does not solve the difficulty, but it is a help.

Encourage parents to position infants on the back. Infants should not sleep on the stomach, because there is an association between this sleeping position and SIDS (Livesey, 2005).

Crying. Many new parents are not prepared for the amount of time a newborn spends crying. When-

ever the mother saw the baby at the health care agency, the baby was sleeping; she woke the infant for feeding, and immediately he or she went back to sleep. Infants, however, typically cry an average of about 2 hours of every 24 during the first 7 weeks of life. The frequency seems to peak at age 6 or 7 weeks and then tapers off.

Almost all infants have a period during the day when they are wide awake and invariably fussy. New parents need to recognize this as normal and not worry that it means their child is ill. Parents might use this fussy time for bathing or playing with the infant, arranging their schedules accordingly. It is important to learn the infant's cues and to help the infant learn to self-quiet. The most typical time for wakefulness is between 6 PM and 11 PM, which, unfortunately, is when parents may be tired and least able to tolerate crying.

Whether to use pacifiers to reduce crying is a question parents must decide for themselves, depending on how they feel about them and their infant's needs. It is rare that infants have such a need for sucking they must have a pacifier in their mouth constantly. Discussing a few pros and cons with parents helps clarify the subject.

An infant who completes a feeding and still seems restless and discontented, who actively searches for something to put into the mouth, and who sucks on hands and clothes may need the increased sucking activity a pacifier provides. The major drawback of pacifiers is the problem of cleanliness. They tend to fall on the floor or sidewalk and are then put back into the infant's mouth. Attaching the pacifier to a string worn around the infant's neck prevents this problem but could cause strangulation. A big drawback to pacifier use is that they are associated with an increase in middle ear infections (Cinar, 2004). If parents use pacifiers, be certain they are of one-piece construction, so that loose parts cannot be aspirated.

Parental Concerns Related to Breathing. Some parents report that their newborns have stuffy noses or make snoring noises in their sleep and that they sneeze frequently. This occurs because most newborns continue to have some mucus in the upper respiratory tract and posterior pharynx for up to 2 weeks after birth. The snoring noise is a result of this mucus, not a cold. In addition, infants continue to breathe irregularly for about the first month. A new parent who did not room with her child at the hospital may wake at night, notice this breathing pattern, and grow alarmed that the child is in respiratory distress. If these are the only symptoms, this is a normal newborn respiratory pattern. If the child has rhinitis (nasal discharge) or a fever, he or she needs to be seen by a health care provider, because these symptoms suggest an upper respiratory tract infection.

Continued Health Maintenance for a Newborn. Parents do not need to continue to weigh a newborn or take his or her temperature at home. These practices

BOX 24.12 FOCUS ON . . .

FAMILY TEACHING

Determining If a Newborn Is Well

Q. Ms. Ruiz asks you, "Could you review with me how to know if a newborn is well?"

A. The following items are helpful to determine your newborn is well:

- Drinks as if she is hungry
- Possibly spits up a slight amount after feeding, but has no vomiting
- Moves bowels approximately three to four times per day (may be more often if breast-fed), with stools that are loose or semiformed but not runny and watery
- Appears happy overall (despite a fussy period during the day) and sleeps for 2 to 3 hours at a time
- Has a normal temperature
- Breathes more rapidly than an adult, but breathing is easy and not stressed
- Skin lacks appearance of a yellow or blue tone

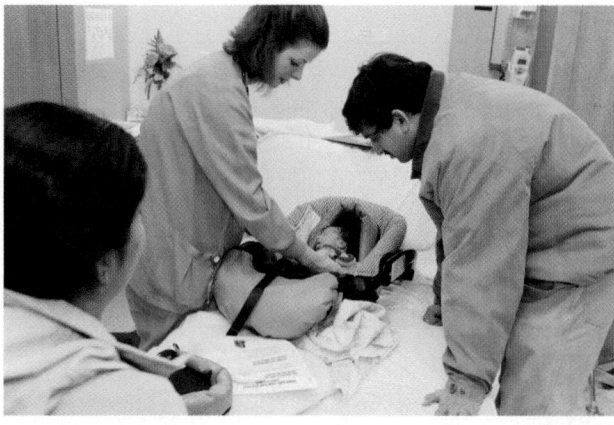

FIGURE 24.30 Most states require infants and children to ride in car seats. It is the nurse's responsibility to make sure that every parent planning to drive a child home from the health care facility is properly equipped.

only cause worry, because weight fluctuates day by day, and infant activity and clothing can influence temperature. Teach parents to judge their infant's state of health by overall appearance, eagerness to eat, general activity, and disposition, as well as weight gain (Box 24.12).

Make certain that parents make and keep a health care appointment for a first newborn assessment according to their primary care provider's schedule (2 to 6 weeks). The mother was conscientious throughout pregnancy to bring a well child into the world. Parents must now begin a health care program to keep the child well.

Car Safety. Automobile accidents are a safety problem all during childhood. For protection while in automobiles, newborns should always be transported in car seats (National Center for Health Statistics, 2005). Without this protection, if a car stops suddenly, an infant can be thrown onto the floor or, in a collision, thrown out of the car or through the windshield. In an accident, centrifugal force on an infant can be as much as 450 lb, making it impossible for a passenger to hold onto the child. At a speed of only 30 mph, an infant may hit the dashboard with a force equal to a fall from a three-story building. If an adult holding the infant is not wearing a seat belt, the adult can be thrown against the infant, killing the child.

When purchasing a car seat, parents should look at the label to be sure the seat meets federal guidelines. The local health department or Red Cross chapter should have a list of all the car seats available in a particular area as well as details of their comparable features and cost. The AAP web site (*www.aap.org*) lists these as well. Some hospitals

and Red Cross chapters loan infant car seats for temporary use, such as when visiting with grandparents or when first coming home from the hospital. New cars are mandated to be equipped with lower anchors and tethers for car seats.

The best location for a car seat is the back seat of the car; this is especially true if the car has a passenger seat air bag, because the force of an air bag expanding can kill an infant in the front seat. While the infant is less than 21 lb or 26 inches long, the best type of car seat is an "infant-only" seat that, when properly positioned, faces the back of the car (Fig. 24.30). The ideal model has a five-point harness with broad straps, which help spread the force of a collision over the chest and hips, and a shield, which cushions the head.

Parents should dress an infant in clothing with pant legs if he or she is to be placed in a car seat, because the harness crotch strap must pass between the legs for a snug and correct fit. Advise parents not to use a sack sleeper or papoose bunting; nor should they wrap the baby in a bulky blanket so that the straps do not fit securely while the baby is in the seat. To support the baby's head, parents can use a rolled-up receiving blanket, towel, or diaper on each side of the head or purchase commercial head supports. To provide extra warmth, they can cut holes in a blanket for the harness and crotch straps to pass through, place the baby in the seat, fasten the buckles, and then fold the blanket over the child for warmth. A second blanket can be draped over the seat if needed.

Infants should sit in a backward-facing seat until they are able to sit up without support, usually when they weigh about 21 lb. At that point, they are old enough for a toddler seat. Caution parents that plastic car seats grow extremely hot in the summer, so they need to test the temperature of the surface before placing an infant in one. Stress also that it is dangerous to use a car seat improperly, such as not fastening the harness or not securing the seat belt.

Checkpoint Question 5

Ms. Ruiz is preparing to take her new daughter home. On about what day of life can she expect her baby's umbilical cord to fall off?

a. Day 1.
b. Day 2 to 3.
c. Day 6 to 10.
d. Day 30.

Key Points

Converting from fetal to adult respiratory function is a major step in adaptation to extrauterine life. Newborns need particularly close observation during the first few hours of life to determine that this adaptation has been made.

Maintaining body heat is a second major problem of newborns. The temperature of the term baby's environment should be about 75°F (24°C). When procedures that require undressing an infant for an extended period are being carried out (e.g., circumcision), a radiant heat source should be used.

Newborns may suffer hypoglycemia in the first few hours of life because they use energy to establish respirations and maintain heat. Signs of jitteriness and a blood glucose level of less than 40 mg/100 mL by heel-stick help to identify hypoglycemia.

Identification bands should be attached securely to newborns; assess these bands carefully before hospital discharge. To help prevent the possibility of kidnapping, be certain of the identification of anyone to whom you give a newborn.

To feel confident with newborn care, parents need to hold and give care in the hospital. Encouraging them to spend as much time as possible with a newborn is a major nursing role.

Critical Thinking Exercises

1. Beth Ruiz is the newborn described at the beginning of the chapter. Her mother is concerned because Beth seems small, is covered by erythema toxicum, and has noisy respirations. You discover that the family has no car seat to transport the baby home. What would you teach the mother to make her feel more comfortable with her newborn? What would you do about the car seat—ask that they stay until they can arrange to rent or borrow one, or discharge them?

2. When you are assessing Beth in her mother's room, what newborn reflexes would you assess? Suppose it is cold in the room, so that you have time to test only one reflex. Which one would you test, and why?

3. Beth has a port-wine stain on her left thigh. Her father tells you he is not concerned about this because he knows that all birthmarks fade by school age. How would you respond to him?

4. Examine the National Health Goals related to newborn care. Most government-sponsored money for nursing research is allotted based on these goals. What would be a possible research topic to explore pertinent to these goals that would be applicable to the Ruiz family and also advance evidence-based practice?

References

American Academy of Pediatrics. (2005). *2004 immunization schedule.* Washington, D.C.: Author.

Anderson, G. C., et al. (2005). Early skin-to-skin contact for mothers and their healthy newborn infants. *The Cochrane Library (Oxford) (4)* (CD003519).

Apgar, V., et al. (1958). Evaluation of a newborn infant: Second report. *JAMA: Journal of the American Medical Association, 16*(82), 1985–1988.

Ballard, J. L., et al. (1991). The new Ballard Scale. *Journal of Pediatrics, 119*(3), 417–424.

Boyd, S. (2004). Treatment of physiological and pathological neonatal jaundice. *Nursing Times, 100*(13), 40–43.

Brazelton, T. B. (1973). Neonatal behavior assessment scale. *Clinics in Developmental Medicine, 50*(5), 1–15.

Brennan, R. A. (2004). A nurse-managed universal newborn hearing screen program. *MCN: American Journal of Maternal Child Nursing, 29*(5), 320–325.

Capitulo, K. L., & Cox, J. M. (2004). Does an electronic infant security system ensure a more secure hospital environment? Writing for the PRO position. *MCN: The American Journal of Maternal/Child Nursing, 29*(5), 280.

Cinar, N. D. (2004). The advantages and disadvantages of pacifier use. *Contemporary Nurse, 17*(1–2), 109–112.

Chung, E. K. (2003). Down (trisomy 21) syndrome. In Schwartz, M. W. (Ed.). *5-Minute pediatric consult* (3rd ed.). Philadelphia: Lippincott Williams & Wilkins.

Constantinou, J. (2003). Mongolian spots. *Neonatal Network: The Journal of Neonatal Nursing, 22* (2), 58.

Department of Health and Human Services. (2000). *Healthy people 2010.* Washington, D.C.: Author.

Desmond, M. N., et al. (1963). The clinical behavior of the newly born: The term infant. *Journal of Pediatrics, 62*(3), 307–309.

Dubowitz, L., et al. (1970). Clinical assessment of gestational age in a newborn infant. *Journal of Pediatrics, 77*(10), 1–12.

Duncombe, G. J., Dickinson, J. E., & Evans, S. F. (2003). Perinatal characteristics and outcomes of pregnancies complicated by twin-twin transfusion syndrome. *Obstetrics and Gynecology, 101*(6), 1190–1196.

Fischbach, F. T. (Ed.) (2004). *Manual of laboratory and diagnostic tests* (7th ed.). Philadelphia: Lippincott Williams and Wilkins.

Greene, A. K., Rogers, G. F., & Mulliken, J. B. (2004). Management of parotid hemangioma in 100 children. *Plastic & Reconstructive Surgery, 113*(1), 53–60.

Halliday, H. L., & Sweet, D. (2004). Endotracheal intubation at birth for preventing morbidity and mortality in vigorous, meconium-stained infants born at term. *The Cochrane Library (Oxford) (4)* (CD000500).

Johnson, M., Maas, M, & Moorhead, S. (2000). *Nursing outcomes classification* (2nd ed.). St. Louis: Mosby.

Karch, A. M. (2004). *Lippincott's nursing drug guide.* Philadelphia: Lippincott Williams & Wilkins.

Katz, V. L. (2003). Prenatal care. In Scott, J. R., et al. (Eds.). *Danforth's obstetrics and gynecology* (9th ed.). Philadelphia: Lippincott, Williams & Wilkins.

Livesey, A. (2005). A multiagency protocol for responding to sudden unexpected death in infancy: Descriptive study. *BMJ, 330*(7485), 227–228.

McCloskey, J., & Bulechek, G. (2000). *Nursing interventions classification* (3rd ed.). St. Louis: Mosby.

Myers, B. J., et al. (2003). Prenatal cocaine exposure and infant performance on the Brazelton Neonatal Behavioral Assessment Scale. *Substance Use and Misuse, 38*(14), 2065–2096.

National Center for Health Statistics. (2005). *Trends in the health of Americans.* Hyattsville, Md.: Author.

Razmus, I. S., Dalton, M. E., & Wilson, D. (2004). Practice applications of research: Pain management for newborn circumcision. *Pediatric Nursing, 30*(5), 414–417.

Reiser, D. J. (2004). Neonatal jaundice: Physiologic variation or pathologic process. *Critical Care Nursing Clinics of North America, 16*(2), 257–269.

Silverman, W. A., & Anderson, H. (1956). A controlled clinical trial of effects of water mist on obstructive respiratory signs, death rate and necroscopy findings among premature infants. *Pediatrics, 17*(4), 1–9.

Stastny, P. F., et al. (2004). Infant sleep positioning by nursery staff and mothers in newborn hospital nurseries. *Nursing Research, 53*(2), 122–129.

Taddio, A., Ohlsson, K., & Ohlsson, A. (2004). Lidocaine-prilocaine cream for analgesia during circumcision in newborn boys. *The Cochrane Library (Oxford) (4)* (CD000496).

Usher, R., et al. (1966). Judgment of fetal age. *Pediatric Clinics of North America, 13*(4), 835–840.

Van Leeuwen, G., & Glenn, L. (1968). Screening for hidden congenital anomalies. *Pediatrics, 41*(6), 147–152.

Walls, M., et al. (2004). Home phototherapy: A feasible, safe and acceptable practice. *Journal of Neonatal Nursing, 10*(3), 92–94.

Waner, M. (2003). Recent developments in lasers and the treatment of birthmarks. *Archives of Disease in Childhood, 88*(5), 372–374.

Weinstein, S. L., Mubarak, S. J., & Wenger, D. R. (2003). Developmental hip dysplasia and dislocation. *Journal of Bone and Joint Surgery (American), 85A*(9), 1824–1832.

Suggested Readings

Duhn, L. J., & Medves, J. M. (2004). A systematic integrative review of infant pain assessment tools. *Advances in Neonatal Care, 4*(3), 126–140.

Lund, C. H., & Osborne, J. W. (2004). Validity and reliability of the neonatal skin condition score. *JOGNN: Journal of Obstetric, Gynecologic, and Neonatal Nursing, 33*(3), 320–327.

Medves, J. M., & O'Brien, B. (2004). The effect of bather and location of first bath on maintaining thermal stability in newborns. *JOGNN: Journal of Obstetric, Gynecologic, and Neonatal Nursing, 33*(2), 175–182.

Pellowe, C. M., Macqueen, S., & Coe, L. (2004). Preventing healthcare associated infections in the neonatal unit: The use of evidence-based infection control guidelines. *Journal of Neonatal Nursing, 10*(5), 171–175.

Roberts, D., Neilson, J. P., Weindling, A. M. (2005). Interventions for the treatment of twin-twin transfusion syndrome. *The Cochrane Library (Oxford) (4)* (CD002073).

Ross, G., et al. (2004). Prevalence and characteristics of term infants readmitted to the hospital for hyperbilirubinemia. *Neonatal Intensive Care, 17*(4), 54–59.

Short, M. A. (2004). Guide to a systematic physical assessment in the infant with suspected infection and/or sepsis. *Advances in Neonatal Care, 4*(3), 141–157.

Stephen-Haynes, J. (2004). Care study. Vascular birthmarks: A care study of an infant with haemangioma. *British Journal of Nursing, 13*(2), 87–93.

Thompson, D. G. (2005). Utilizing an oral sucrose solution to minimize neonatal pain. *JSPN: Journal for Specialists in Pediatric Nursing, 10*(1), 3–10.

White-Traut, R. (2004). Providing a nurturing environment for infants in adverse situations: Multisensory strategies for newborn care. *Journal of Midwifery and Women's Health, 49*(4S), 36–41.

CHAPTER 25

Nutritional Needs of a Newborn

Key Terms

areola
bifidus factor
colostrum
engorgement
fore milk
hind milk
interferon
lactiferous sinuses
lactoferrin
let-down reflex
lysozyme
prolactin

Objectives

After mastering the contents of this chapter, you should be able to:

1. Describe nutritional requirements for a term newborn.
2. Assess nutritional intake of a newborn to determine adequate nutritional status.
3. Formulate nursing diagnoses related to newborn nutrition.
4. Identify outcomes for a newborn and parents related to nutrition.
5. Plan a method of infant feeding with a mother that will be satisfying for both her and her infant.
6. Implement or help parents implement feeding procedures with newborn infants.
7. Evaluate expected outcomes for achievement and effectiveness of care.
8. Identify National Health Goals related to newborn nutrition that nurses can help the nation achieve.
9. Identify areas related to nutrition and newborns that could benefit from additional nursing research or application of evidence-based practice.
10. Use critical thinking to assist parents with nutritional problem solving and make newborn nutrition more family-centered.
11. Integrate knowledge of normal newborn nutrition with nursing process to achieve quality maternal and child health nursing care.

*P*alaka Satir is a new mother of a term baby girl. During the pregnancy, she and her husband, Paul, both agreed Palaka would breast-feed. Palaka will be returning to work as an executive assistant after her 6-week maternity leave. She attempted to breast-feed her newborn in the birthing room with minimal success. As you offer to help her feed her baby for the second time, she says, "Do you think I made the right choice? Maybe I should bottle-feed her. Paul could help that way and I won't have to worry about what to do when I go back to work."

Previous chapters described the care of a woman and family during the antepartal, intrapartal, postpartal, and newborn periods. This chapter adds information about the nutritional needs of a newborn to your knowledge base. This knowledge is important because a newborn's nutritional needs are high due to rapid rates of growth and development. It fortifies you to play a key role in educating parents about how to provide adequate nutrition to meet both physiologic and psychological needs of their newborn.

How would you answer Palaka?

After you've studied this chapter, access the accompanying website. Read the patient scenario and answer the questions to further sharpen your skills, grow more familiar with RN-CLEX types of questions, and reward yourself with how much you have learned.

Proper nutrition is essential for optimal growth and development, especially in the first few months of life, because brain growth proceeds at such a rapid rate during this time. Providing adequate nutrition for a newborn extends beyond physiologic need, however; it also fulfills important psychological needs. During feeding, a parent is close to the infant, and a baby is apt to be particularly sensitive to the parent's demonstration of affection or lack of warmth. An infant who does not experience a warm relationship with a mother or primary caregiver may fail to thrive as surely as one who is denied sufficient protein or calories. National Health Goals related to newborn nutrition are shown in Box 25.1.

Nursing Process Overview

For Promoting Nutritional Health in a Newborn

- **Assessment**

Assessment of infant nutrition begins during pregnancy with assessment of the mother's and father's attitudes and choices about infant feeding. Breast-feeding is widely accepted as the preferred method of human newborn nutrition. However, if a mother chooses not to breast-feed because of her individual circumstances, it is important that she not be made to feel guilty for her choice, because formula-feeding can be substituted. Most importantly, parents need to feel comfortable with and confident about the feeding method they have chosen.

Teach parents how to recognize signs of hunger in a newborn, including restlessness, tense body posture, smacking lips, and tongue thrusting. Otherwise, they may wait for their infant to cry, and this is actually a late sign of newborn hunger. Once infant feeding begins, teach the mother to assess whether the amount the infant is receiving is adequate—not by how long the newborn breast-feeds at a time or by how much formula is taken at a feeding, but by a larger measure, such as whether the newborn is voiding, growing, and alert (Box 25.2). A bottle-fed newborn regains birthweight at about 10 days, a breast-fed infant at about 14 days.

- **Nursing Diagnosis**

Nursing diagnosis in relation to nutrition usually centers on a mother's choice regarding method of feeding or a newborn's nutritional intake and feeding patterns. It may be difficult to establish diagnoses during the first part of the newborn period, because the mother and infant are still getting used to each other. Examples of possible nursing diagnoses are the following:

- Effective breast-feeding related to well-prepared mother and healthy newborn
- Risk for ineffective breast-feeding related to nipple soreness

---

BOX 25.1 FOCUS ON . . .

NATIONAL HEALTH GOALS

Two National Health Goals address nutrition of a newborn (DHHS, 2000).

- Increase to at least 75% (from a baseline of 64%) the proportion of mothers who breast-feed their babies in the early postpartum period, to at least 50% (from a baseline of 29%) the proportion who continue breast-feeding until their babies are 5 to 6 months old, and to 25% (from a baseline of 16%) the proportion who continue breast-feeding until 1 year of age.
- Decrease the proportion of children with untreated dental decay in primary or permanent teeth to 21%, from a baseline of 29%.

Nurses can help the nation achieve these goals by educating women about breast-feeding during pregnancy and supporting the family during the postpartal period while the woman is breast-feeding. Home visits with postpartal families and well-child health assessments provide opportunities to advocate for continued breast-feeding. For the woman who will formula-feed her infant, education during pregnancy should include the fact that putting an infant to bed with a bottle of milk or juice is associated with tooth decay and should be avoided.

Areas that could benefit from additional nursing research include techniques parents use to initiate sleep without using a bedtime bottle; reasons women discontinue breast-feeding early in the postpartal period; and legislation or education necessary in the workplace to encourage women to continue breast-feeding after they return to work.

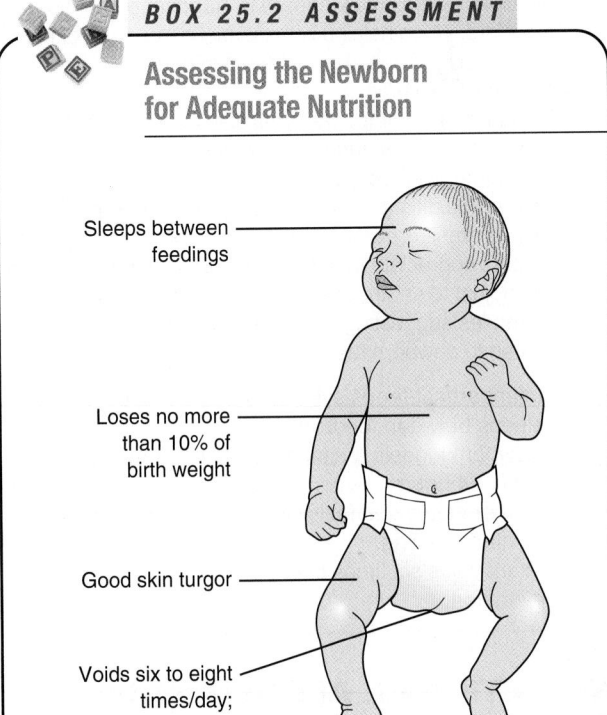

BOX 25.2 ASSESSMENT

Assessing the Newborn for Adequate Nutrition

Sleeps between feedings

Loses no more than 10% of birth weight

Good skin turgor

Voids six to eight times/day; two to three bowel movements

- Imbalanced nutrition, less than body requirements, related to poor newborn sucking response
- Impaired parenting related to ineffective coping secondary to father's feeling of resentment because mother is breast-feeding

● *Outcome Identification and Planning*

Planning begins while a woman is still pregnant, with the focus on providing her with the information necessary to permit an informed decision about breast-feeding or bottle-feeding. Once a decision is made, a teaching plan addressing the nutritional needs of both the woman and her newborn can be developed. Parents who expect to formula-feed can purchase supplies in advance. They can read about newborn care and plan ways to make feeding time special for both themselves and the baby.

● *Implementation*

A major intervention related to newborn nutrition is supporting a mother's choice of feeding method and helping her to trust her judgment as to whether her infant is full and content and the feeding method is as natural as possible. Referral to a support group such as the La Leche League (*www.lalecheleague.org*) or the International Lactation Consultant Association (*www.ilca.org*) might be appropriate. In addition to sponsoring classes on breast-feeding, a helpful service of La Leche League is its hotline, through which a breast-feeding woman who is discouraged or is having difficulty can contact a member and ask for advice. "The Womanly Art of Breast-feeding," published by the League (1997), is a comprehensive and informative book for both new mothers and fathers.

When assisting a new mother with breast-feeding, remember that breast milk can carry the human immunodeficiency virus (HIV). Adhere to standard precautions, therefore, when helping with manual expression of milk or disposing of soiled breast-feeding pads.

● *Outcome Evaluation*

Evaluation is an important final step to ensure that a newborn receives adequate nutrition, because unforeseen circumstances, such as an unsuspected milk allergy or mastitis (breast infection), may interfere and require drastic changes to reach desired outcomes. Help parents appreciate that newborns are very adaptive and can adjust to another feeding method if necessary. Examples suggesting successful expected outcomes related to newborn feeding are the following:

- Infant breast-feeds every 2 to 3 hours; is content and sleeps between feedings.
- Newborn ingests a total of 12 oz of formula with iron every 24 hours.
- Mother states she feels satisfied with chosen method of infant feeding.
- Infant voids six times daily as a measure of adequate hydration.

NUTRITIONAL ALLOWANCES FOR A NEWBORN

Nutritional allowances for a newborn need to take into account both total calories and total fluid intake.

Calories

Growth in the neonatal period and early infancy is more rapid than at any other period of life. Therefore, the caloric requirements exceed those at any other age. An infant up to 2 months of age requires 110 to 120 calories per kilogram of body weight (50 to 55 kcal/lb) every 24 hours to provide an adequate amount of food for maintenance and growth. After 2 months of age, the amount gradually declines until the requirement at 1 year is 100 kcal/kg (45 kcal/lb) per day. In contrast, the adult requirement is 42 kcal/kg (20 kcal/lb) per day.

The actual caloric requirement, of course, depends on an infant's individual activity level and growth rate. For example, an active infant, one who cries frequently and squirms constantly, needs more calories than one who is more passive, content to spend long hours playing quietly or just studying the environment. During growth spurts, more calories are needed to supply additional energy. Dietary intakes for newborns are shown in Table 25.1.

Commercial infant formulas simulate breast milk. They contain about 9% to 12% of their calories as protein and 45% to 55% of calories as lactose carbohydrate. The balance is fat, of which about 10% (4% of the calories) is linoleic acid.

Protein

Protein, necessary for the formation of new cells, has a high requirement during the newborn and infancy periods to provide for rapid growth of new cells as well as maintenance of existing cells. The nutritional allowance of protein for the first 2 months of life is 2.2 g per kilogram of body weight. Both human milk and commercial formulas provide all the essential amino acids necessary to form protein. Histidine, an amino acid that appears to be essential for infant growth but is not necessary for adult growth, is found in both milk forms.

Unaltered cow's milk is not recommended for newborns, because it contains about 16% of its calories as protein, whereas human milk contains about 8%. Cow's milk can create such a rich solute load (the amount of urea and electrolytes that must be excreted in the urine) that a newborn's kidneys could be overwhelmed by it. In addition, the protein in cow's milk, casein, differs from that in human milk, lactalbumin, both in composition and in amount. The amount of casein present in milk determines its curd tension. The curd in cow's milk is large, tough, and difficult to digest, whereas in human milk the curd is softer and easier to digest. This is the rationale for bottle-fed infants to be given a commercial formula containing albumin rather than cow's milk. Cow's milk products, such as yogurt and cottage cheese, should not be introduced until 9 to 12 months of age for the same reason.

Fat

Linoleic acid, an essential fatty acid necessary for growth and skin integrity in infants, is found in both human milk and commercial formulas. Use of fat-free milk for long periods (when other sources of food are not being offered)

- Breast-feeding may serve a protective function in preventing breast cancer.
- The release of oxytocin from the posterior pituitary gland aids in uterine involution.
- Successful breast-feeding can have an empowering effect, because it is a skill only a woman can master.
- Breast-feeding reduces the cost of feeding and preparation time.
- Breast-feeding provides an excellent opportunity to enhance a true symbiotic bond between mother and child. Although this does occur readily with breast-feeding, a woman who holds her baby to bottle-feed can form this bond as well.

Some women believe that breast-feeding, because it causes a delay in menstruation (lactational amenorrhea), is a foolproof contraceptive technique. It is not: 50% of women resume ovulating by the fourth week after delivery, even while breast-feeding (Van der Wijden et al., 2005).

Some women believe that breast-feeding will help them lose weight gained during pregnancy. This also is not true, and women who are breast-feeding need to concentrate on eating a well-balanced diet to ensure their milk will be rich in nutrients. Some women are reluctant to breast-feed because they fear that having to be available to feed the baby every 3 or 4 hours will tie them down. Like mothers who bottle-feed, however, they can leave a bottle (with expressed breast milk or formula) with the baby's father or a caregiver if they need to be away from their baby at the time of a feeding.

Advantages for a Baby

Breast-feeding has major physiologic advantages for a baby. Breast milk contains secretory immunoglobulin A (IgA), which binds large molecules of foreign proteins, including viruses and bacteria, keeping them from being absorbed from the gastrointestinal tract into the infant. **Lactoferrin** is an iron-binding protein in breast milk that interferes with the growth of pathogenic bacteria. The enzyme **lysozyme** in breast milk apparently actively destroys bacteria by lysing (dissolving) their cell membranes, possibly increasing the effectiveness of antibodies. Leukocytes in breast milk provide protection against common respiratory infectious invaders. Macrophages, responsible for producing **interferon** (a protein that protects against viruses), interfere with virus growth. The **bifidus factor** is a specific growth-promoting factor for the beneficial bacteria *Lactobacillus bifidus*. The presence of *L. bifidus* in breast milk interferes with the colonization of pathogenic bacteria in the gastrointestinal tract, reducing the incidence of diarrhea.

In addition to these antiinfective properties, breast milk contains the ideal electrolyte and mineral composition for human infant growth. It is high in lactose, an easily digested sugar that provides ready glucose for rapid brain growth. The protein in breast milk is easily digested, and the ratio of cysteine to methionine (two amino acids) in breast milk favors rapid brain growth in the early months. It contains nitrogen in compounds other than protein, so that an infant can receive cell-building materials from sources other than just protein.

Breast milk contains more linoleic acid, an essential fatty acid for skin integrity, and less sodium, potassium, calcium, and phosphorus than do many formulas. Breast milk also has a better balance of trace elements, such as zinc. These levels of nutrients are enough to supply the infant's needs, yet they spare the infant's kidneys from having to process a high renal solute load of unused nutrients. Women who have a familial history of allergy are usually encouraged to breast-feed to try and eliminate the possibility of exposing their infant to cow's milk protein, which could be allergenic this early in life.

Yet another advantage is that breast-fed newborns appear to be able to regulate their calcium/phosphorus levels better than infants who are bottle-fed. Decreased calcium levels in a newborn can lead to tetany (muscle spasm). The increased concentration of fatty acid in commercial formulas may bind calcium in the gastrointestinal tract, increasing the danger of tetany.

A great deal of discussion about the benefits of breast-feeding has centered on the effects of breast-feeding on the formation of the dental arch, because babies suck differently from a breast than from a bottle (Fig. 25.2). Babies pull their tongue backward as they suck from a breast. They thrust their tongue forward to suck from a rubber nipple (Charchut et al., 2003).

One disadvantage of breast milk is that it may carry microorganisms such as hepatitis B and cytomegalovirus, although the risk to infants is small. HIV is carried at a high enough level in breast milk that women who are HIV positive are advised not to breast-feed (Schilling-McCann, 2004). In addition, both illicit and prescription drugs as well as environmental contaminants can be carried via breast milk to the infant (AAP Committee on Drugs, 2002).

Checkpoint Question 2

How does breast milk help prevent infection in a newborn?

a. It is rich in fatty acid, so bacteria are destroyed by it.
b. It is always flowing forward in the breast, so it is not static.
c. It contains maternal antibodies and viral binding factors.
d. It is low in lactose, so it becomes a poor culture medium.

Preparing for Breast-Feeding

Ask all women during pregnancy whether they plan to breast-feed or formula-feed their newborn. Thinking about feeding in advance allows couples to make informed choices (Box 25.4). Some fathers experience jealousy at the thought of breast-feeding. Early discussion can help them work through this natural sensation, with the eventual realization that parenting involves more than simply feeding a child.

Physical preparation such as nipple rolling, advised in the past as a way of making a woman's nipples more protuberant, is no longer advised. It is unnecessary, because

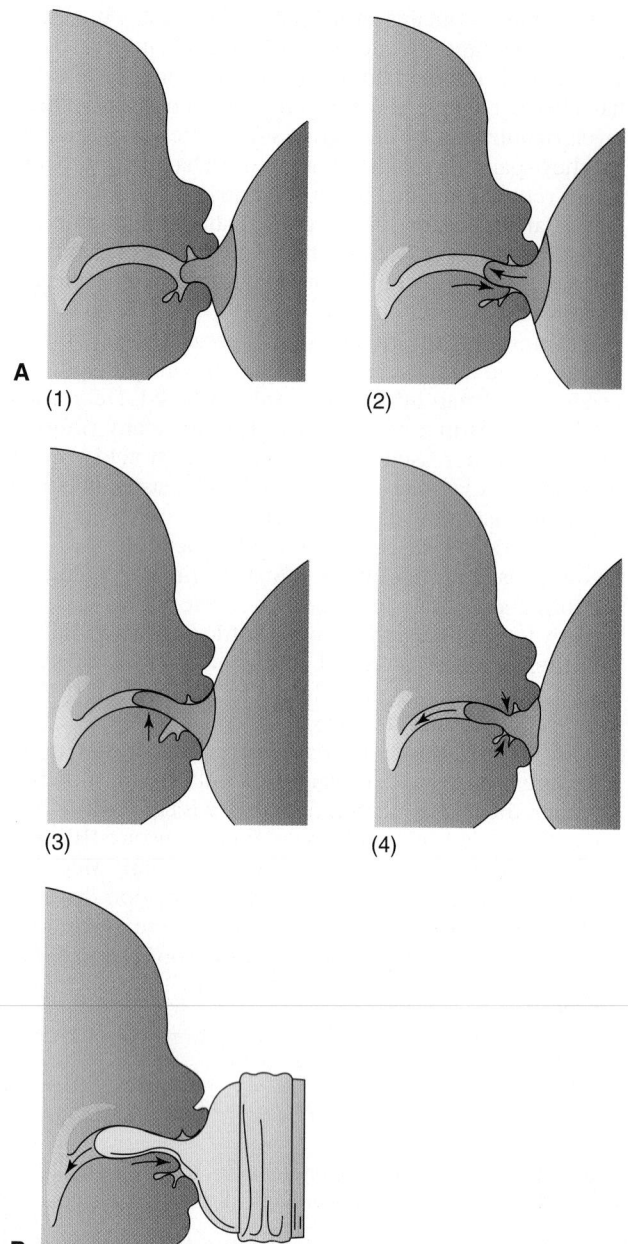

BOX 25.4 FOCUS ON . . .

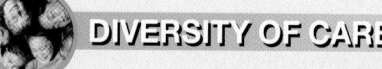

DIVERSITY OF CARE

Women are known as the "keepers of the culture," or the main people who transmit customs to the next generation. Chief among these customs is the method for feeding newborns. If a woman comes from a family where no one has ever breast-fed, she may be very interested in being a "pioneer" in her family. On the other hand, she may be more interested in following her family's tradition of formula-feeding.

How soon women want to begin breast-feeding after birth is also culturally determined. Although it is the usual practice in hospitals to begin immediately after birth, some cultures believe that colostrum is not appropriate for newborns and have a cultural preference not to begin breast-feeding until milk is present, at about 3 days of age. It is necessary to assess each family individually to recognize cultural preferences such as these.

FIGURE 25.2 Differences in sucking mechanism. **(A)** The breast. **(1)** Lips of the infant clamp in a C-shape. The cheek muscles contract. **(2)** The tongue thrusts forward to grasp nipple and areola. **(3)** The nipple is brought against the hard palate as the tongue pulls backward, bringing the areola into the mouth. **(4)** The gums compress the areola, squeezing milk into the back of the throat. **(B)** Bottle-feeding. The large rubber nipple of a bottle strikes the soft palate and interferes with the action of the tongue. The tongue moves forward against the gums to control the overflow of milk into the esophagus.

few women have inverted or nonprotuberant nipples. In addition, oxytocin, which is released by this maneuver, could lead to preterm labor (nipple rolling is used to create uterine contractions for stress tests). The occasional woman who has inverted nipples may need to wear a nip-

ple cup (a plastic shell) to help the nipples become more protuberant.

Practicing breast massage to move the milk forward in the milk ducts (manual expression of milk) may be helpful. This can help a woman who feels hesitant about handling her breasts grow accustomed to doing so, allowing her to assist with milk production in the first few days after birth. Manual expression consists of supporting the breast firmly, then placing the thumb and forefinger on the opposite sides of the breast, just behind the areolar margin, first pushing backward toward the chest wall and then downward until secretion begins to flow (Box 25.5). During the last months of pregnancy and immediately after birth, the fluid obtained will be colostrum. By the third day of infant life, milk will be obtained.

Teach women not to use soap on their breasts during pregnancy, because soap tends to dry and crack the nipples.

Beginning Breast-Feeding

Breast-feeding should begin as soon after birth as possible, ideally while the woman is still in the birthing room and while the infant is in the first reactivity period. The release of oxytocin by breast-feeding at this time begins the letdown of milk and also stimulates uterine contraction. However, if the woman is overly fatigued or extremely modest, trying to learn this new skill at this time may only convince her that breast-feeding is not for her.

Most women enjoy having an experienced nurse with them for a first feeding to offer suggestions (Box 25.6). It is important that infants open their mouths wide enough to grasp both the nipple and the **areola** (the pigmented circle surrounding the nipple) when sucking. This gives them effective sucking action and helps to empty the collecting sinuses completely.

Milk forms in response to being used. If the breasts are completely emptied, they completely fill again. If

ulate the nutritional content of breast milk. They all contain supplemental vitamins. Parents should be advised to purchase types with added iron to ensure that their newborn receives enough of this element to prevent iron-deficiency anemia (AAP Committee on Nutrition, 2000). Formulas for term newborns contain 20 cal/oz when diluted according to directions (the same number of calories as breast milk contains). Common brands are shown in Appendix B. Parents should plan on using formula for the first full year of their infant's life. Participation in a supplemental food program such as the Women, Infants, and Children (WIC) program helps low-income parents afford formula.

Four separate forms of commercial formulas are available:

- Powder that is combined with water
- Condensed liquid that is diluted with an equal amount of water
- Ready-to-pour type, which requires no dilution
- Individually prepackaged and prepared bottles of formula

The powder is the least expensive. A single bottle at a time is easy to prepare by vigorous shaking. The prepackaged type does not need refrigeration or preparation (simply remove the bottle cap and it is ready), but it is the most expensive type. Cost should not be the only basis for a parent's choice, however. Tolerance of the formula by the infant and convenience for the parents also are important.

Calculating a Formula's Adequacy

To calculate the adequacy of a formula, remember these two rules of thumb:

1. The total fluid ingested for 24 hours must be sufficient to meet the infant's fluid needs: 75 to 90 mL (2.5 to 3 oz) of fluid per pound of body weight (150 to 200 mL/kg) per day.
2. The number of calories required per day is 50 to 55 per pound of body weight (100 to 120 kcal/kg).

If an infant is taking a commercial formula, only total fluid needs to be calculated. For example, a 7-lb infant needs 17.5 to 21 oz (7 lb × 2.5 to 3 oz) per day. Commercial formula contains 20 cal/oz, so this amount supplies 350 to 420 cal/day. The total volume can be divided into six feedings of 3 to 3.5 oz each. A 9-lb infant would need 22.5 to 27 oz of fluid per day, supplying 450 to 540 cal/day as well as adequate protein, minerals, and vitamins.

A quick rule of thumb to determine how much an infant usually takes at a feeding is to add 2 or 3 to the infant's age in months. After initially taking 0.5 to 1 oz for the first 2 days, a newborn (0 age) will take 2 to 3 oz each feeding; a 3-month-old child, 5 to 6 oz; and a 6-month-old child, 8 oz. As infants change from six to five feedings a day (at about 4 months of age, when they begin to sleep through the night), they begin to take more at each feeding, keeping their total intake the same. Knowing the minimum requirements for fluid and calories per day, being able to calculate whether formula is adequate, and remembering to assess the infant's intake over 24 hours allow evaluation of the adequacy of an infant's intake.

NURSING DIAGNOSES AND RELATED INTERVENTIONS

Nursing Diagnosis: Health-seeking behaviors related to techniques of bottle-feeding

Outcome Identification: Client verbalizes knowledge of techniques of formula-feeding by hospital discharge.

Provide Information Regarding Supplies Needed. Most parents today do not prepare a full day's supply of formula at once but prepare it bottle by bottle, as needed. They can use glass, plastic, or disposable refill bottles. Women who breast-feed and use supplemental bottles can do the same. Caution parents to keep opened cans of liquid formula covered and refrigerated, discarding any unused formula within 24 hours.

The type of bottle used with the average baby makes no difference. A baby who develops colic (abdominal pain after feeding) may be pulling in too much air and would benefit from an angled or disposable liner bottle.

Nipples for bottles should be firm enough so the infant sucks vigorously. A soft, flabby nipple allows a baby to suck in milk so rapidly that the need for sucking may not be satisfied. A way to judge a nipple's adequacy is to hold a bottle of milk with nipple attached upside down. The milk should come out at a rate of about one drop a second. Bottle caps to cover nipples are helpful to keep nipples clean when outdoors or during transport.

Provide Information Regarding Formula Preparation. Infant formula of any type must be prepared with careful attention to cleanliness to prevent pathogenic microorganisms from growing in it.

When using presterilized formula, the parent need only do the following to prepare a full day's supply of formula:

- Wash off the top of the can with warm, soapy water and rinse.
- Open the can and pour the desired amount of formula and water into each previously cleaned bottle (cleaning in a dishwasher is best).
- Put on the nipples, taking care not to handle the nipple projection.
- Place the bottle caps over the nipples and refrigerate.

To prepare a single bottle, the parent simply combines clean water and liquid or powdered formula in a previously cleaned bottle, caps the bottle, and shakes it to mix the ingredients.

Provide Information Regarding Feeding Techniques. Whether to warm formula is a parental decision:

infants who are fed cooled formula directly from the refrigerator thrive as well as those who are fed warmed formula. Caution parents to use care when warming a bottle in a microwave oven, because the milk in the center of the bottle can become hotter than that near the sides. If parents do use a microwave, caution them to shake the bottle well after microwaving, to mix the cool and warm portions, and then test the temperature on their wrist before feeding.

Other ways to heat formula are setting the bottle into a pan of hot water, warming it in a pan of water on the stove, or holding it under a faucet of running hot water. Caution parents using a pan on the stove not to allow the pan to boil dry, or the bottle of milk will burst. They also must be certain to check the temperature of the formula by allowing a drop or two to fall onto the inside of a wrist, to make sure it is not hot enough to burn the baby's mouth. Disposable bottles with plastic liners should not be heated on the stove; they tend to melt and then leak during feeding.

With any type of bottle, any contents remaining after a feeding should be thrown away, not stored and reused. When sucking, an infant exchanges a small amount of saliva for milk. Because milk is a good growth medium for bacteria and the baby's mouth harbors many bacteria, the bacterial content in reused formula is likely to be very high.

Like breast-feeding, bottle-feeding an infant is a skill that must be learned. A parent needs a comfortable chair (as does a nurse who feeds babies) and adequate time (at least half an hour) to enjoy the process and not rush the baby (Fig. 25.9). Holding the baby with the head slightly elevated reduces the danger of aspiration and retention of air bubbles. A parent should be sure the nipple is kept filled so that the baby is sucking milk, not air. He or she can be assured a baby is sucking effectively if small bubbles rise in the bottle. Babies in the early weeks should be bubbled (burped) after every ounce of milk taken. The technique is the same as that used for breast-fed infants.

Remind parents not to prop up bottles, because babies are in danger of aspiration if a bottle is propped. In addition, an increased incidence of otitis media has been associated with bottle-propping, because the infant's head is not upright and formula may enter the eustachian tube. Propping also can limit the amount of parent–child interaction. Also remind parents not to put a baby to bed with a bottle of formula, because this can lead to "baby-bottle syndrome," or cavities of the lower teeth (see Chapter 28). Some common problems that can arise with formula-feeding are summarized in Table 25.6.

What If... Palaka tells you she is going to give her baby one supplemental bottle of formula daily in addition to breast-feeding while she works? She does not plan to refrigerate this bottle during the day. What questions would you want to ask her to be certain this approach is safe for her baby?

DISCHARGE PLANNING

With shortened lengths of stay in health care facilities, teaching a mother and her family about either breast- or formula-feeding is crucial. Be certain to review a mother's plans for feeding her baby just before discharge, so there is time to answer any remaining questions. If this is an early discharge, check to see that a home care referral or visit has been scheduled and that the new mother has a telephone number she can call if she has a question before the home visit occurs.

Review with the mother the criteria for adequate nutrition (wetting a diaper six to eight times a day, sleeping between feedings, no excessive crying). Supply the telephone number of the local La Leche League or Association of Lactation Consultants or any other local support group.

Be certain a woman has an appointment with a primary care provider for her infant or the telephone number of this person to call for an appointment. Remind her that infant nutrition is an important topic and one she should always feel free to discuss at health care visits. Babies experience growth spurts during the first year at about 3 months, 6 months, and 9 months; during these times, they need to be fed more frequently to meet their nutritional needs. No one can anticipate all of the questions or problems regarding feeding that will arise in the next few months. Empowering women to learn to make decisions regarding feeding and not be reluctant to ask for help when they need it will go a long way toward solving these problems.

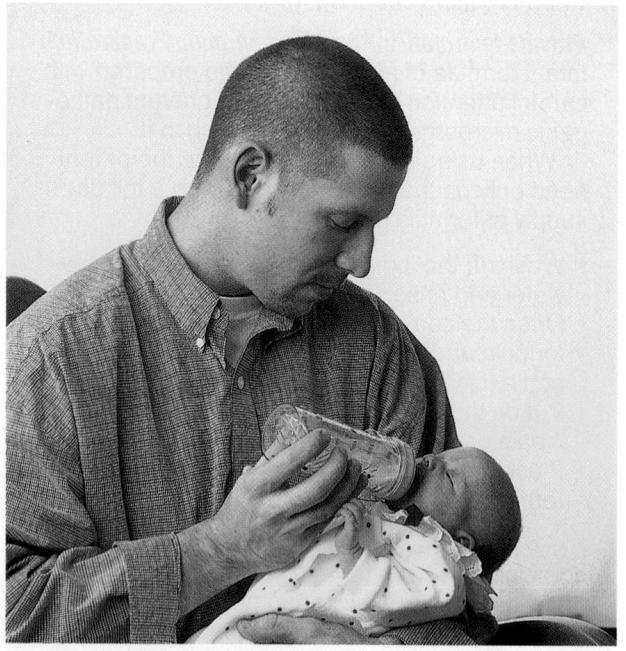

FIGURE 25.9 A newborn receives a bottle feeding from her father. Notice the en face position.

TABLE 25.6

Common Problems in Formula-Feeding

Problem	Possible Causes	Nursing Interventions
Infant sucks for a few minutes, then stops and cries	Either nipple is blocked and infant is unable to get milk or flow is too fast and baby has choking sensation.	Show parent how to test flow of milk from the nipple (hold bottle upside down); milk should flow from nipple at rate of about 1 drop/sec.
Infant does not bubble well after feeding	Some infants swallow little air with feeding. Parent may be handling infant too tentatively or not burping effectively.	Observe baby feeding and parent's technique of handling; rubbing newborn's back may be more effective than patting it.
Parent reports constipation	Bowel movements from formula-fed infants are not as loose as those from breast-fed infants, so parents may be concerned.	Examine stools; assure parent and explain normal stool pattern and that straining to pass stool is normal.

Key Points

Breast-feeding is the preferred feeding method for newborns, because it supplies antibodies as well as nutrients. Urge all women at least to try breast-feeding unless they are taking a drug that would be a contraindication or there is a potential for spreading a microorganism through the breast milk.

Linoleic acid is an essential fatty acid that is necessary for growth and skin integrity and cannot be manufactured by the body. It is supplied by both infant formula and human milk but not by nonfat milk.

Both breast milk and commercial formulas contain 20 kcal/oz. A term newborn requires 120 kcal/kg/day and 150 to 200 mL/kg of fluid.

Encourage mothers who are breast-feeding to drink fluoridated water and bottle-feeding mothers to prepare formula using fluoridated water to help build strong teeth. If a newborn will not have exposure to sunlight, the breast-feeding mother may need to take a supplement of vitamin D.

Almost all drugs pass into breast milk. A breast-feeding mother must be certain not to take any medication without contacting her primary care provider to be sure it is compatible with breast-feeding.

If a baby will be bottle-fed, be certain the parents understand the potential danger of warming bottles in a microwave oven (the inner core of milk may grow very hot).

Caution parents not to prop bottles, because it increases the risk for aspiration and otitis media. It also deprives infants of the pleasure of being held for feedings.

To avoid nursing-bottle syndrome (cavities of the lower teeth), infants should not be put to bed with a bottle.

Critical Thinking Exercises

1. Palaka Satir is the new mother you met at the beginning of the chapter. She is unsure whether she wants to breast-feed, especially because she does not know how she will manage breast-feeding when she returns to work. How would you advise her?
2. Palaka worries that her 1-day-old newborn is not receiving enough milk. How could you assure her that her baby is receiving enough milk?
3. Palaka's grandmother tells you that she always changed her babies to fat-free milk at 3 months to keep them from gaining too much weight. Would you support this practice?
4. Examine the National Health Goals related to newborn nutrition. Most government-sponsored money for nursing research is allotted based on these goals. What would be a possible research topic to explore pertinent to these goals that would be applicable to the Satir family and also advance evidence-based practice?

References

American Academy of Pediatrics Committee on Drugs. (2002). Transfer of drugs and other chemicals into human milk. *Pediatrics, 108*(3), 776–789.

American Academy of Pediatrics Committee on Nutrition. (2000). Iron fortification of infant formulas. *Pediatrics, 104*(1), 119–123.

American Academy of Pediatrics Committee on Nutrition. (2001). The use and misuse of fruit juice in pediatrics. *Pediatrics, 107*(5), 1210–1213.

Boyd, S. (2004). Treatment of physiological and pathological neonatal jaundice. *Nursing Times, 100*(13), 40–43.

Charchut, S. W., Allred, E. N., & Needleman, H. L. (2003). The effects of infant feeding patterns on the occlusion of the primary dentition. *Journal of Dentistry for Children, 70*(3), 197–203.

Department of Agriculture. (2005). *2005 dietary guidelines for Americans.* Washington, D.C.: DOA.

Department of Health and Human Services (2000). *Healthy people 2010.* Washington, D.C.: DHHS.

Geraghty, S. R., et al. (2004). Breast milk feeding rates of mothers of multiples compared to mothers of singletons. *Ambulatory Pediatrics, 4*(3), 226-231.

Jensen, D., Wallace, S., & Kelsey, P. (1994). LATCH: A breast-feeding charting system and documentation tool. *Journal of Obstetric, Gynecologic, and Neonatal Nursing, 23*(1), 27-32.

Johnson, M., Maas, M., & Moorhead, S. (2000). *Nursing outcomes classification* (2nd ed.). St. Louis: Mosby.

Katz, V. L. (2003). Prenatal care. In Scott, J. R., et al. (Eds.) *Danforth's obstetrics and gynecology* (9th ed.). Philadelphia: Lippincott Williams & Wilkins.

Kleinmann, R. E. (Ed.). (2004). *Pediatric nutrition handbook* (5th ed.). Elk Grove Village, Ill.: American Academy of Pediatrics.

La Leche League International. (1997). *The womanly art of breastfeeding* (6th ed.). Schaumberg, Ill.: La Leche League.

McCloskey, J. & Bulechek, G. (2000). *Nursing interventions classification* (3rd ed.). St. Louis: Mosby.

Riordan, J., et al. (2001). Predicting breastfeeding duration using the LATCH breastfeeding assessment tool. *Journal of Human Lactation, 17*(1), 20-23.

Schilling-McCann, J. A. (2004). *Maternal-neonatal nursing made incredibly easy.* Philadelphia: Lippincott Williams & Wilkins.

Spear, H. J. (2004). Nurses' attitudes, knowledge, and beliefs related to the promotion of breastfeeding among women who bear children during adolescence. *Journal of Pediatric Nursing, 19*(3), 176-183.

Ullah, S., & Griffiths, P. (2003). Does the use of pacifiers shorten breastfeeding duration in infants? *British Journal of Community Nursing, 8*(10), 458-463.

Van der Wijden, C., Kleijnen, J., & Van den Berk, T. (2005). Lactational amenorrhea for family planning. *The Cochrane Library (Oxford) (4)* (CD001329).

Suggested Readings

Berlin, C. M., & Briggs, G. G. (2005). Drugs and chemicals in human milk. *Seminars in Fetal and Neonatal Medicine, 10*(2), 149-159.

Dodgson, J. E., Chee, Y., & Yap, T. S. (2004). Workplace breastfeeding support for hospital employees. *Journal of Advanced Nursing, 47*(1), 91-100.

Gonzalez, K. A., et al. (2003). Evaluation of a lactation support service in a children's hospital neonatal intensive care unit. *Journal of Human Lactation, 19*(3), 286-292.

Hellings, P., & Howe, C. (2004). Breastfeeding knowledge and practice of pediatric nurse practitioners. *Journal of Pediatric Health Care, 18*(1), 8-14.

Hill, P. D., et al. (2004). Breast augmentation and lactation outcome: A case report. *MCN: American Journal of Maternal Child Nursing, 29*(4), 238-242.

Karl, D. J. (2004). Using principles of newborn behavioral state organization to facilitate breastfeeding. *MCN: The American Journal of Maternal/Child Nursing, 29*(5), 292-298.

Marks, J. M., & Spatz, D. L. (2003). Medications and lactation: What PNPs need to know. *Journal of Pediatric Health Care, 17*(6), 311-317.

Morin, K. H. (2004). Current thoughts on healthy term infant nutrition: The first twelve months. *MCN: The American Journal of Maternal/Child Nursing, 29*(5), 312-319.

Wills, S. A., & Willis, S. A. (2003). The pediatric nurse practitioner as lactation consultant. *Journal of Pediatric Health Care, 17*(6), 335-337.

Wolfberg, A. J., et al. (2004). Dads as breastfeeding advocates: Results from a randomized controlled trial of an educational intervention. *American Journal of Obstetrics and Gynecology, 191*(3), 708-712.

CHAPTER 26

Nursing Care of the High-Risk Newborn and Family

Key Terms

apnea
apparent life-
    threatening
    event
appropriate for
    gestational age
    (AGA)
brown fat
caudal regression
    syndrome
cephalopelvic
    disproportion
developmental care
dysmature
extracorporeal
    membrane
    oxygenation
    (ECMO)
fetal alcohol
    syndrome
    or exposure
gestational age
hemorrhagic
    disease of the
    newborn

hydrops fetalis
hyperbilirubinemia
intrauterine growth
    restriction
large for gestational
    age (LGA)
low-birthweight
    infant
macrosomia
ophthalmia
    neonatorum
periodic res-
    pirations
periventricular
    leukomalacia
postterm
    syndrome
preterm infants
retinopathy of
    prematurity
shoulder dystocia
small for
    gestational age
    (SGA)
term infants

Objectives

After mastering the contents of this chapter, you should be able to:

1. Define the following terms—small-for-gestational-age infant, term infant, large-for-gestational-age infant, preterm infant, and postterm infant—and describe common illnesses that occur in these and other high-risk newborns.
2. Assess a high-risk newborn to determine whether safe transition to extrauterine life has occurred.
3. List nursing diagnoses related to a high-risk newborn.
4. Identify appropriate expected outcomes for a high-risk newborn and family.
5. Plan novice-level nursing care focusing on priorities to stabilize a high-risk newborn's body systems.
6. Implement novice-level nursing care for a high-risk newborn.
7. Evaluate expected outcomes to determine achievement and effectiveness of care.
8. Identify National Health Goals related to high-risk newborns nurses could be instrumental in helping the nation achieve.
9. Identify areas related to the care of high-risk newborns that could benefit from additional nursing research or application of evidence-based practice.
10. Use critical thinking to analyze the special crisis imposed on families when alterations of newborn development or neonatal illness occur to make nursing family-centered.
11. Integrate knowledge of the needs of a high-risk infant with nursing process to achieve quality maternal and child health nursing care.

*M*r. and Mrs. Atkins are the parents of a 34-week-old, 2-lb baby boy born last night after a short, 4-hour labor. The baby took a few gasping respirations at birth but then stopped breathing. He was resuscitated by the neonatal nurse practitioner and respiratory therapist and then transported to the intensive care nursery. Mr. Atkins was not present for the birth because he was out of town on business. You notice Mrs. Atkins has not visited the intensive care nursery to see her son. She also refused to sign the birth certificate because she could not decide on a name. She said, "I don't want to give him our favorite name because he might die." Mr. Atkins telephoned early this morning and acted more upset the baby was born than relieved the baby was receiving intensive care. You hear him ask his wife, "What did you do to cause this?"

Previous chapters described caring for a newborn who is well at birth. This chapter adds information about how to care for a newborn who is ill or has a significant variation in gestational age or weight. This is important information because learning to recognize these infants at birth and organizing care for them can be instrumental in helping protect both their present and future health.

What type of help do the Atkinses need to better accept what has happened to them?

After you've studied this chapter, access the accompanying website. Read the patient scenario and answer the questions to further sharpen your skills, grow more familiar with RN-CLEX types of questions, and reward yourself with how much you have learned.

During pregnancy, screening women for risk factors that could lead to illness in a newborn such as younger or older than average maternal age, concurrent disease conditions (e.g., diabetes or HIV infection), pregnancy complications (e.g., placenta previa), or an unhealthy maternal lifestyle (e.g., drug abuse) is essential to identify infants who need greater than usual care at birth. In addition, an infant who is born **dysmature** (before term or post-term, or who is under- or overweight for gestational age) is also at risk for complications at birth and in the first few days of life. Unfortunately, not all instances of high risk can be predicted. Even the newborn from a "perfect" pregnancy may require specialized care or develop a problem over the first few days of life necessitating special interventions. With shorter hospital lengths of stay for newborns, parents need thorough education about their baby's health because these problems may require rehospitalization or additional follow-up at home. National Health Goals related to the high-risk newborn are shown in Box 26.1.

Being able to predict an infant is at high risk allows for advanced preparation so that specialized, skilled health care personnel can be present at the child's birth to perform necessary interventions, such as resuscitating a newborn who has difficulty establishing respirations. Immediate, skilled handling of any problems that occur may help to save the newborn's life and also prevent future problems, such as neurologic disorders.

Nursing Process Overview

For the Family of a High-Risk Newborn

● *Assessment*

All infants should be assessed at birth for obvious congenital anomalies and **gestational age** (number of weeks they remained in utero). Both determinations can be done by the nurse who first examines an infant. Be certain these assessments are made with an infant under a prewarmed radiant heat warmer to guard against heat loss.

Continuing assessment of high-risk infants involves the use of instrumentation such as cardiac, apnea, and blood pressure monitoring. However, no matter how many monitors are used, they never replace the role of frequent, close, common-sense observation. Carefully evaluate comments from fellow nurses that an infant "isn't himself" or "breathes oddly." These comments, although not scientific, are the same observations that a parent who knows his or her baby well reports at health visits. A nurse who knows an infant well from having cared for him or her consistently over time often senses changes before a monitor or other equipment begins to put a quantitative measurement on the factor.

● *Nursing Diagnosis*

To establish nursing diagnoses for high-risk infants, it is important to be aware of the normal assessment parameters of this population. Nursing diagnoses generally center on the eight priority areas of care for any newborn:

- Ineffective airway clearance related to presence of mucus or amniotic fluid in airway
- Ineffective cardiovascular tissue perfusion related to breathing difficulty
- Risk for deficient fluid volume related to insensible water loss
- Ineffective thermoregulation related to newborn status and stress from birthweight variation
- Risk for imbalanced nutrition, less than body requirements related to lack of energy for sucking
- Risk for infection related to lowered immune response in newborn
- Risk for impaired parenting related to illness in newborn at birth
- Deficient diversional activity (lack of stimulation) related to illness at birth

● *Outcome Identification and Planning*

Be certain when establishing expected outcomes that they are consistent with the newborn's potential. A goal that implies complete recovery from a major illness may be unrealistic for one newborn but completely appropriate for another. Plan care that is

BOX 26.1 FOCUS ON . . .

NATIONAL HEALTH GOALS

Preterm birth has the potential for leading to so many complications in newborns that National Health Goals were written specifically concerning preterm birth:

- Reduce low birthweight (LBW) to an incidence of no more than 5% of live births and very low birthweight (VLBW) to an incidence of no more than 0.9% of live births, from baselines of 7.6% and 1.4%, respectively.
- Reduce the rate of fetal and infant deaths during the perinatal period (28 weeks of gestation to 7 days or more after birth) to 4.5/1,000 live births, from a baseline of 7.5/1,000 live births.
- Reduce the rate of neonatal deaths within the first 28 days of life to 2.9/1,000 live births, from a baseline of 4.8/1,000 live births.
- Reduce the rate of deaths from sudden infant death syndrome (SIDS) to 0.25/1,000 live births, from a baseline of 0.72/1,000 live births (DHHS, 2000).

Nurses can help the nation achieve these goals by teaching women the symptoms of preterm labor so that, ideally, birth can be delayed until infants reach term. They also need to be prepared for resuscitation at birth of preterm infants and to plan developmental care that can help prevent conditions such as apnea, intraventricular hemorrhage, and periventricular leukomalacia.

Further research is needed as to how best to position infants to promote development and prevent fatigue, what measures can best prevent conditions such as intraventricular hemorrhage, and what measures can make parents feel most comfortable and allow them to best interact with their infants in neonatal intensive care units.

individualized considering a newborn's developmental as well as physiologic strengths, weaknesses, and needs. This helps to ensure that parents as well as the health care team understand the newborn's particular care priorities and potential.

● *Implementation*

Interventions for any high-risk newborn are best carried out by a consistent caregiver and should focus on conserving the baby's energy and providing a thermoneutral environment to prevent exhaustion and chilling. Painful procedures should be kept to a minimum to help an infant achieve a sense of comfort and balance. Assisting parents with participation in care such as bathing or feeding their infant may help make the child real to them for the first time and start the bonding process.

Many families of high-risk newborns will need continued support to care for their infants at home. They may need referral to a home health care or other agency. Organizations that may be helpful include:

- American Sudden Infant Death Syndrome Institute (*www.sids.org*)
- American Association of Premature Infants (*www.aapi-online.com*)
- Newborn Individualized Developmental Care and Assistance Program (www.nidcap.org)

● *Outcome Evaluation*

High-risk newborns need long-term follow-up so any consequences of their birth status, such as minimal neurologic injury, can be identified and arrangements for special schooling or counseling can be made. Examples of expected outcomes include the following:

- Infant maintains a patent airway.
- Infant tolerates all procedures without accompanying apnea.
- Infant demonstrates growth and development appropriate for gestational age, birthweight, and condition.
- Infant maintains body temperature at 98.6°F (37.0°C) in open crib with one added blanket.
- Parents visit at least once and make three telephone calls to neonatal nursery weekly.
- Parents demonstrate positive coping skills and behaviors in response to newborn's condition.

NEWBORN PRIORITIES IN FIRST DAYS OF LIFE

All newborns have eight priority needs in the first few days of life:

1. Initiation and maintenance of respirations
2. Establishment of extrauterine circulation
3. Control of body temperature
4. Intake of adequate nourishment
5. Establishment of waste elimination
6. Prevention of infection
7. Establishment of an infant–parent relationship
8. Developmental care, or care that balances physiologic needs and stimulation for best development

These are also the priority needs of high-risk newborns. Because of small size or immaturity or illness, fulfilling these needs, however, may require special equipment or care measures. Not all newborns will be able to achieve full wellness because of extreme insults to their health at birth or difficulty adjusting to extrauterine life. Indications that a newborn is having difficulty making the transition from intrauterine to extrauterine life may be apparent during the intrapartum period, at birth, or at initial assessment because of a low Apgar score (see Chapter 24).

Initiating and Maintaining Respirations

Ultimately, the prognosis of a high-risk newborn depends primarily on how the first moments of life are managed. Most deaths occurring during the first 48 hours after birth result from the newborn's inability to establish or maintain adequate respirations (NCHS, 2005). An infant who has difficulty accomplishing effective respiratory action in the first hours of life and yet survives may experience residual neurologic dysfunction because of cerebral hypoxia. Prompt, thorough care is necessary for effective intervention.

Most infants are born with some degree of respiratory acidosis. However, this is rapidly corrected by the spontaneous onset of respirations. If respiratory activity does not begin immediately, however, respiratory acidosis will increase. The blood pH and bicarbonate buffer system will fail. Newborn defense mechanisms are inadequate to reverse the process. Therefore, the effort to establish respirations must be started immediately after birth. By 2 minutes, the development of severe acidosis is already well under way (Thilo & Rosenberg, 2003).

Any infant who sustains some degree of asphyxia in utero, such as from cord compression, maternal anesthesia, placenta previa, or preterm separation of the placenta, may already be experiencing acidosis at birth and may have difficulty before the first 2 minutes after birth.

Resuscitation

Factors that commonly predispose infants to respiratory difficulty and so may require resuscitation are shown in Box 26.2. If breathing is ineffective, circulatory shunts, particularly the ductus arteriosus, may fail to close. Because left-side heart pressure is stronger than right-side pressure, blood circulates through a patent ductus arteriosus left to right or from the aorta to the pulmonary artery, creating ineffective pump action in the heart. Struggling to breathe and circulate blood, an infant uses available serum glucose quickly and may become hypoglycemic, compounding the initial problem.

For all these reasons, resuscitation becomes important for an infant who fails to take a first breath or has difficulty maintaining adequate respiratory movements on his or her own.

Resuscitation follows an organized process: (1) establish and maintain an airway, (2) expand the lungs, and (3) initiate and maintain effective ventilation. If respiratory depression becomes severe, a newborn's heart will

BOX 26.2

Factors Predisposing Infants To Respiratory Difficulty In The First Few Days Of Life

Low birthweight
Maternal history of diabetes
Premature rupture of membranes
Maternal use of barbiturates or narcotics close to birth
Meconium staining
Irregularities detected by fetal heart monitor during labor
Cord prolapse
Lowered Apgar score (under 7) at 1 or 5 minutes
Postmaturity
Small for gestational age
Breech birth
Multiple birth
Chest, heart, or respiratory tract anomalies

fail. Resuscitation then must also include cardiac massage (AHA, 2005). Box 26.3 highlights appropriate outcomes and interventions using the terminology identified by the Nursing Outcomes Classification (NOC) and Nursing Interventions Classification (NIC) for neonatal resuscitation.

Airway

For a well term newborn, usually bulb syringe suction, which removes mucus and prevents aspiration of any mucus and amniotic fluid present in the mouth or nose with the first breath, is all that is necessary to help establish a clear airway (see Chapter 24).

If a newborn does not draw in a first breath spontaneously, suction the infant's mouth and nose with a bulb syringe again and rub the back to see if skin stimulation initiates respirations. Be certain an infant is dry, including the hair and head, to prevent chilling. If a newborn has to attempt to raise body temperature, this will increase the need for oxygen, which the baby cannot supply because breathing has not yet been initiated. Warmed, blow-by oxygen by face mask or positive-pressure mask may be administered.

If a newborn's amniotic fluid was meconium-stained, do not stimulate an infant to breathe by rubbing the back or administering air or oxygen under pressure. Doing so could push meconium down into an infant's airway, further compromising respirations. Give oxygen by mask without pressure. Wait for a laryngoscope to be passed and the trachea to be deep suctioned before giving oxygen under pressure.

If deeper suctioning than by a bulb syringe is required, place an infant on the back and slide a folded towel or pad

BOX 26.3

Nursing Outcomes Classification (NOC) and Nursing Interventions Classification (NIC)

Neonatal Resuscitation

NOC: Respiratory Status, Gas Exchange
Respiratory status, gas exchange is defined as the alveolar exchange of carbon dioxide or oxygen to maintain arterial blood gas concentrations (Johnson, Maas, & Moorehead, 2000). Some specific indicators suggesting that this outcome has been achieved include the following:

- Uncompromised ease of breathing
- Absence of restlessness, cyanosis, and dyspnea
- Arterial blood gas values, including Po_2, Pco_2, pH, and oxygen saturation, within normal limits
- Chest x-ray findings within expected parameters

NIC: Resuscitation, Neonate
Resuscitation, neonate, is defined as the administration of emergency measures to support newborn adaptation to extrauterine life (McCloskey & Bulechek, 2000). Some important activities involved when implementing this intervention include:

- Setting up necessary equipment before birth, including testing resuscitation bag, suction, and oxygen flow to ensure proper function
- Drying with a prewarmed blanket and placing neonate under radiant warmer on back with neck slightly extended, using a rolled blanket under the shoulders to assist with correct positioning

- Suctioning nose and mouth with a bulb syringe
- Using tactile stimulation
- Inserting laryngoscope to visualize trachea and intubating to remove meconium from lower trachea if appropriate; repeating procedure until return is clear
- Monitoring heart rate and respirations
- Initiating positive-pressure ventilation for apnea or gasping
- Ventilating with properly fitting, tightly sealed resuscitation bag filled with 100% oxygen at a rate of 40 to 60 breaths per minute using 20 to 40 cm of water (for initial breaths) and 15 to 20 cm of water for subsequent pressures, continuing ventilations until adequate spontaneous respirations begin and color becomes pink
- Administering chest compressions for heart rate of less than 60 bpm or less than 80 bpm with no increase in conjunction with ongoing assessment until heart rate is greater than 80 bpm
- Auscultating breath sounds
- Inserting endotracheal tube for prolonged ventilation or poor response to bag and mask ventilation followed by auscultation of breath sounds to confirm placement
- Securing the airway
- Administering medications as ordered

under the shoulders to raise them slightly so the head is in a neutral position. Slide a catheter (8F to 12F) over the infant's tongue to the back of the throat (Fig. 26.1). Do not suction for longer than 10 seconds at a time (count seconds as you suction) to avoid removing excessive air from an infant's lungs. Use a gentle touch. Bradycardia or cardiac arrhythmias can occur because of vagus stimulation (at the posterior oropharynx) from vigorous suctioning. In most newborns, this degree of resuscitation will initiate responsive respirations and a strong heartbeat. Color, muscle response, and reflexes will improve.

An infant who still makes no effort at spontaneous respirations requires immediate laryngoscopy to open the airway. Once a laryngoscope has been inserted, deep tracheal suctioning may be performed. After deep suctioning, an endotracheal tube can be inserted and oxygen administered by a positive-pressure bag and mask with 100% oxygen at 40 to 60 breaths per minute.

In the first few seconds of life, a newborn this severely depressed may take several weak gasps of air and then almost immediately stop breathing; the heart rate begins to fall. This period of halted respirations is termed primary apnea. After 1 or 2 minutes of apnea, an infant again tries to initiate respirations with a few strong gasps. However, the child cannot maintain this effort longer than 4 or 5 minutes. After this, the respiratory effort will become weaker again and the heart rate will fall further until an infant stops the gasping effort altogether. An infant then enters a period of secondary apnea. Although usually a phenomenon that occurs after birth, both types of apnea may occur in utero.

During the period of the first gasps, resuscitation attempts are generally successful. Once a newborn is allowed to enter the secondary apnea period, however, resuscitation measures become difficult and may be ineffective. Because it is impossible to distinguish between the two periods simply by observation, resuscitation must always be started as if secondary apnea were occurring.

An obstetrician, pediatrician, neonatologist, anesthesiologist, or neonatal nurse practitioner skilled in laryngoscope and endotracheal tube insertion should be present at the birth of all infants identified as high-risk so a laryngoscope can be quickly passed. Laryngoscope insertion is easy in theory; in practice, the wide variation in size of infants' posterior pharynx and trachea and the emergency conditions always present make it very difficult (Fig. 26.2).

Laryngoscopes are equipped with different-size blades. Size 0 or 1 is used with newborns. The endotracheal tube fits inside the laryngoscope. Infants under 1,000 g need a 2.5-mm endotracheal tube; those over 3,000 g need a 4.0-mm tube. Because preterm infants are prone to hemorrhage because of capillary fragility, gentle care during insertion is crucial.

Lung Expansion

Once an airway has been established, a newborn's lungs need to be expanded. A well newborn inflates his or her lungs adequately with the first breath. The sound of a baby crying is proof that lung expansion is good because the vocal sounds are produced by a free flow of air over the vocal cords.

An infant who breathes spontaneously but then cannot sustain effective respirations may need oxygen by bag and mask to aid lung expansion. The mask should cover both the mouth and the nose to be effective. It should not cover the eyes, because it can cause eye injury mechanically from the mask or drying of the cornea from oxygen administration. Administer 100% oxygen by face mask and pressure bag at a rate of 40 to 60 compressions per minute. To prevent cooling, oxygen should be administered both warmed (between 89.6° and 93.2°F, or 32° and 34°C) and humidified (60% to 80%).

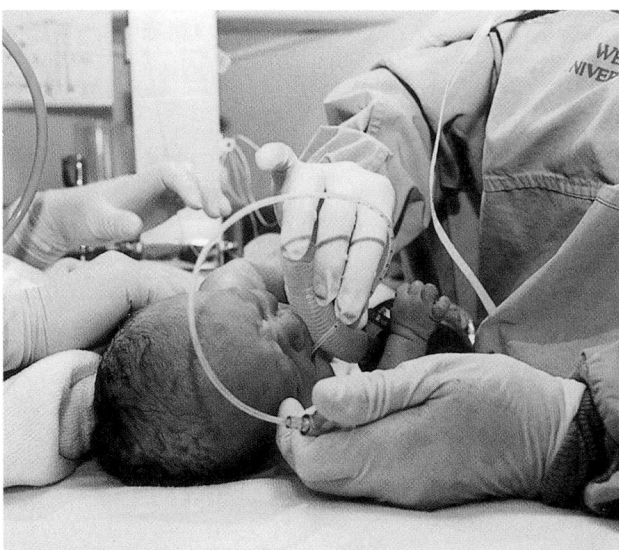

FIGURE 26.1 Suctioning a newborn with mechanical suction controlled by a finger valve. Suction is applied as the catheter is withdrawn. If the catheter is rotated as it is withdrawn, the risk of traumatizing membrane is reduced.

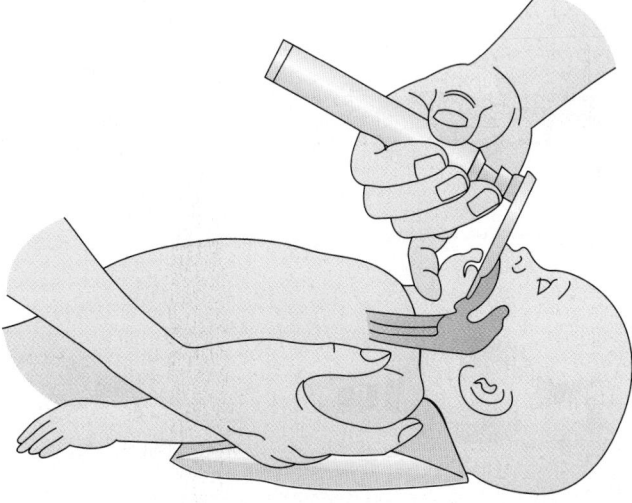

FIGURE 26.2 Intubation. Place the head in a neutral position with a towel under the shoulders. The blade of the laryngoscope is inserted to reveal the vocal cords. An endotracheal tube for ventilation is then passed into the trachea, past the laryngoscope.

The pressure needed to open lung alveoli for the first time is approximately 40 cm H_2O. After that, pressures of 15 to 20 cm H_2O are generally adequate to continue inflating alveoli (Thilo & Rosenberg, 2003). The pressure from anesthesia bags is controlled solely by the pressure of a hand against the bag. Other types of bags such as the Ambu-bag can be set with a blow-off valve that limits the pressure in the apparatus (Fig. 26.3).

It is important not to let oxygen levels in the newborn fluctuate, as fluctuation can cause bleeding from immature cranial vessels. In addition, no pressure above what is necessary should be used because excessive force can rupture lung alveoli. On the other hand, if adequate insufflation is not achieved, a newborn stands little chance of survival. To be certain oxygen is reaching the lungs with resuscitation, monitor the newborn's oxygen level with pulse oximetry. Auscultate the chest for the sound of breathing.

Be sure to listen to both lungs to be certain both sides are being aerated. If air can be heard on only one side or sounds are not symmetric, the endotracheal tube is probably at the bifurcation of the trachea and blocking one of the mainstem bronchi. Drawing it back half a centimeter will usually free it and allow oxygen to flow to both lungs.

When oxygen is given under pressure to a newborn this way, the stomach also quickly fills with oxygen. If the resuscitation continues for over 2 minutes, inserting an orogastric tube and leaving the distal end open will help deflate the stomach and decrease the possibility that vomiting and aspiration of stomach contents will occur.

Drug Therapy

Stimulants have little place in newborn resuscitation unless an infant's respiratory depression appears to be related to the administration of a narcotic such as morphine or meperidine (Demerol) to the mother during labor. In these instances, a narcotic antagonist such as naloxone (Narcan) injected into an umbilical vessel or intramuscularly into a

BOX 26.4 FOCUS ON . . .

PHARMACOLOGY

Naloxone (Narcan)

Classification: Naloxone is a pure narcotic antagonist.

Action: Administered parenterally to reverse the effects, such as respiratory depression, that may occur with opioid narcotic agents (Karch, 2004).

Pregnancy risk category: B

Dosage: Initially 0.01 mg/kg IV. Dosage may be repeated at 2- to 3-minute intervals.

Possible adverse effects: Hypertension, irritability, tachycardia

Nursing Implications
- Assess respiratory status carefully, including rate, depth, and character of respirations.
- Anticipate the need for repeat doses.
- Maintain a patent airway at all times.
- Have emergency resuscitation equipment readily available and prepare to resuscitate if necessary.

thigh will relieve the depression (Box 26.4). The dose of naloxone is determined by institutional policy but is usually 0.01 to 0.1 mg/kg body weight (Karch, 2004). If there is suspicion of maternal drug abuse, naloxone is used cautiously because it might cause acute withdrawal in the neonate. In addition to naloxone, other drug therapies also may be used (Boxes 26.5 and 26.6).

Ventilation Maintenance

To allow a newborn to adjust to and maintain cardiovascular changes, effective ventilation (continued respirations)

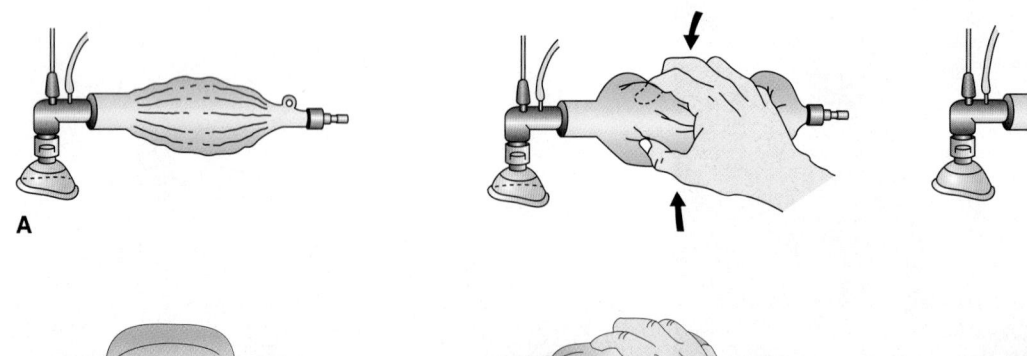

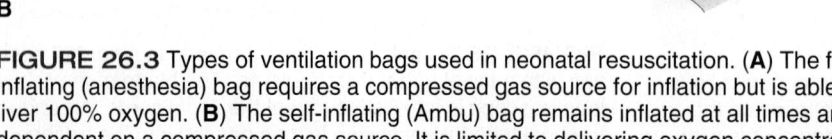

A

B

FIGURE 26.3 Types of ventilation bags used in neonatal resuscitation. **(A)** The flow-inflating (anesthesia) bag requires a compressed gas source for inflation but is able to deliver 100% oxygen. **(B)** The self-inflating (Ambu) bag remains inflated at all times and is not dependent on a compressed gas source. It is limited to delivering oxygen concentration of 40%, which may be inadequate for resuscitation at birth.

BOX 26.5 FOCUS ON . . .

PHARMACOLOGY

Drugs used in resuscitation

Drugs commonly used in newborn resuscitation include:

Atropine: Reduces bronchial secretions, keeping the airway clear during resuscitation. Reduces vagus nerve effects, relieving bradycardia.

Calcium chloride: Increases heart contractility.

Dopamine: Increases systemic blood perfusion by increasing blood pressure through beta-agonist action.

Epinephrine: Strengthens or initiates cardiac contractions; increases heart rate and blood pressure.

Lidocaine: Counteracts ventricular arrhythmias by decreasing automaticity of ventricular cells.

Sodium bicarbonate (NaHCO₃) or tromethamine: Corrects metabolic acidosis. Caution: Do not give these agents unless ventilation is adequate or acidosis can be increased by retained CO_2.

Many preterm infants have such respiratory distress at birth that they need continued therapy, including:

Surfactant: All preterm infants weighing under 1,500 g receive surfactant administered by endotracheal tube at birth (see Box 26.6). Some newborns need administration of additional surfactant to prevent symptoms of respiratory distress syndrome.

Nitric oxide: Nitric oxide is a potent vascular dilator. Because it dilates the capillaries next to alveoli, it reduces the pulmonary resistance and therefore increases oxygenation.

Liquid ventilation: Liquid ventilation is the instillation of liquid fluorocarbon (Perflubron) into the lungs. It fills and clings to alveoli. Perflubron is not absorbed by the body but instead leaves the lungs by evaporation. It acts as an anti-inflammatory and can reduce oxygen toxicity and perhaps infection because bacteria cannot live in the medium. Adverse effects may be pneumothorax and mucus plugging.

BOX 26.6 FOCUS ON . . .

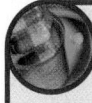

PHARMACOLOGY

Surfactant (Survanta)

Action: Surfactant restores naturally occurring lung surfactant to improve lung compliance.

Pregnancy risk category: X

Dosage: 4 mL/kg intratracheally; four doses in first 48 hours of life

Possible adverse effects: Transient bradycardia, rales

Nursing Implications
* Suction infant before administration.
* Assess infant's respiratory rate, rhythm, arterial blood gases, and color before administration.
* Ensure proper ET tube placement before dosing.
* Change infant's position during administration to encourage drug to flow to both lungs.
* Assess infant's respiratory rate, color, and arterial blood gases after administration.
* Do not suction ET tube for 1 hour after administration, to avoid removing drug.

ing the infant warm is important to prevent acidosis. Positioning an infant on the back with the head of the mattress elevated approximately 15 degrees allows the abdominal contents to fall away from the diaphragm, offering additional breathing space.

If secretions are accumulating in the respiratory tract, they must be suctioned. If the newborn has an endotracheal tube in place, perform tracheal suctioning. "Bagging" an infant for a minute before suctioning can improve an infant's oxygen level and prevent it from dropping to dangerous levels during suctioning. Use pulse oximetry or transcutaneous oxygen monitoring to monitor oxygen level if available (see Chapter 40). The cause of the respiratory distress must be determined and appropriate interventions undertaken to correct the difficulty (see Chapter 40).

Establishing Extrauterine Circulation

Although establishing respirations is the usual priority at a high-risk infant's birth, lack of cardiac function may be present concurrently or may develop if respiratory function cannot be quickly initiated and maintained. If an infant has no audible heartbeat, or if the cardiac rate is below 80 bpm, closed-chest massage should be started. Hold an infant with fingers supporting the back and depress the sternum with two fingers (see Chapter 41). Depress the sternum approximately one third of its depth (1 or 2 cm) at a rate of 100 times per minute (AHA, 2005). Lung ventilation at a rate of 30 times per minute should be continued and interspersed with the cardiac massage at a ratio of 1:5.

Continue to monitor transcutaneous oxygen or pulse oximetry to evaluate respiratory function and cardiac efficiency. If the pressure and the rate of massage are adequate, it should be possible, in addition, to palpate a femoral pulse.

must be maintained. A healthy newborn accomplishes this task on his or her own. All infants, especially those who had difficulty establishing respirations at birth, should be carefully observed in the next few hours to be certain respirations are maintained.

An increasing respiratory rate in the newborn is often the first sign of obstruction or respiratory compromise. If the respiratory rate is increased, undress the baby's chest and look for retractions (inward sucking of the anterior chest wall on inspiration). Retractions reflect the difficulty the newborn is having in drawing in air (tugging so hard to inflate the lungs that the anterior chest muscles are drawn in).

A newborn who is having difficulty with maintaining respirations should be placed under an infant warmer and have the weight of clothing removed from the chest. Keep-

If heart sounds are not resumed above 80 bpm after 30 seconds of combined positive-pressure ventilation and cardiac compressions, 0.1 to 0.3 mL/kg of epinephrine (1:10,000) may be sprayed into the endotracheal tube to stimulate cardiac function (AHA, 2005). Newborns who still have difficulty initiating cardiac function need to be transferred to a transitional or high-risk nursery for continuous cardiac surveillance.

Maintaining Fluid and Electrolyte Balance

After an initial resuscitation attempt, hypoglycemia (decreased blood glucose) may result from the effort the newborn expended to begin breathing. Dehydration may result from increased insensible water loss from rapid respirations. Fluids such as Ringer's lactate or 5% dextrose in water are commonly used to maintain fluid and electrolyte levels. Electrolytes (particularly sodium and potassium) and glucose are added as necessary, depending on electrolyte analysis.

The rate of fluid administration must be carefully maintained because a high fluid intake can lead to patent ductus arteriosus or heart failure. When using a radiant warmer, there is an increase in water loss from convection and radiation. The newborn on a warmer, therefore, will require more fluid than if he or she were placed in a double-walled incubator.

Urine output and urine specific gravity must also be carefully monitored. An output less than 2 mL/kg/h or a specific gravity greater than 1.015 to 1.020 suggests dehydration. Elevated specific gravity may also be caused by inappropriate antidiuretic hormone secretion or kidney failure due to a primary illness.

If an infant has hypotension without hypovolemia, a vasopressor such as dopamine may be given to increase blood pressure and improve cell perfusion. If hypovolemia is present, the cause is usually fetal blood loss from a condition such as placenta previa (see Chapter 15) or twin-to-twin transfusion. With hypovolemia, typically tachypnea, pallor, tachycardia, decreased arterial blood pressure, decreased central venous pressure, and decreased tissue perfusion of peripheral tissue, with a progressively developing metabolic acidosis, will be present. The hematocrit may be normal for some time after acute blood loss because blood cells present are in proportion to plasma. Normal saline or Ringer's lactate may be administered to increase blood volume. Control the rate carefully to prevent heart failure, patent ductus arteriosus, or intracranial hemorrhage from fluid pressure overload.

Checkpoint Question 1

Baby Atkins was given a drug at birth to reverse the effects of a narcotic given to his mother in labor. What drug is commonly used for this?

a. Sodium chloride
b. Morphine sulfate
c. Penicillin G
d. Naloxone (Narcan)

Regulating Temperature

Any high-risk infant may have difficulty maintaining a normal temperature. In addition to stress from an illness or immaturity, an infant's body is often exposed during procedures such as resuscitation and blood drawing.

It is important to keep newborns in a neutral-temperature environment, one that is neither too hot nor too cold, as doing so places less demand on infants to maintain a minimal metabolic rate necessary for effective body functioning. If the environment is too hot, they must decrease metabolism to cool their body. If it is too cold, they must increase metabolism to warm body cells. If an infant should become chilled, the increased metabolism required calls for increased oxygen; without this oxygen available, body cells become hypoxic. To save oxygen for essential body functions, vasoconstriction of blood vessels occurs. If this process continues for too long, pulmonary vessels become affected and pulmonary perfusion becomes decreased. An infant's PO_2 level falls and PCO_2 increases. The decreased PO_2 level may open fetal right-to-left shunts again. Surfactant production may halt, which may further interfere with lung function. To supply glucose to maintain increased metabolism, an infant begins anaerobic glycolysis, which pours acid into the bloodstream. An infant becomes acidotic, and with acidosis comes the increased risk of kernicterus (invasion of brain cells with unconjugated bilirubin) as more bilirubin-binding sites are lost and more bilirubin is free to pass out of the bloodstream into brain cells. In short, because of becoming chilled, heart action, breathing, and electrolytic balance are all affected.

To prevent a newborn from becoming chilled after birth, wipe the infant dry, cover the head with a cap, and place him or her immediately under a prewarmed radiant warmer or in a warmed incubator (Fig. 26.4) or skin-to-skin against the mother. Air, incubator, or radiant warmer temperatures should be kept regulated to maintain an infant's axillary temperature at 97.8°F (36.5°C). Be certain that during procedures an infant is not placed directly on cool x-ray tables, scales, or an unheated radiant warmer to prevent heat loss.

Radiant Heat Sources

Radiant heat warmers are open beds that have an overhead radiant heat source. Such units have Servocontrol probes, which when placed on an infant's skin continually monitor his or her temperature. Abdominal skin temperature, when measured this way, should be 95.9° to 97.7°F (35.5° to 36.5°C). If the temperature falls below this level, an alarm will sound. Tape the probe or disk in place onto the infant's abdomen between the umbilicus and the xiphoid process. Do not tape it under an infant or it will register a falsely high reading. Be sure it is not over the rib cage, where the thin subcutaneous tissue will not allow an accurate reading. Also do not place it over the liver, because increased metabolism may lead to falsely high readings. A plastic bridge or shield placed over the child will better preserve heat by reducing convection and radiation losses; plastic wrap placed over an infant will produce this same effect. When performing care or leaning over an infant, be careful your head doesn't block

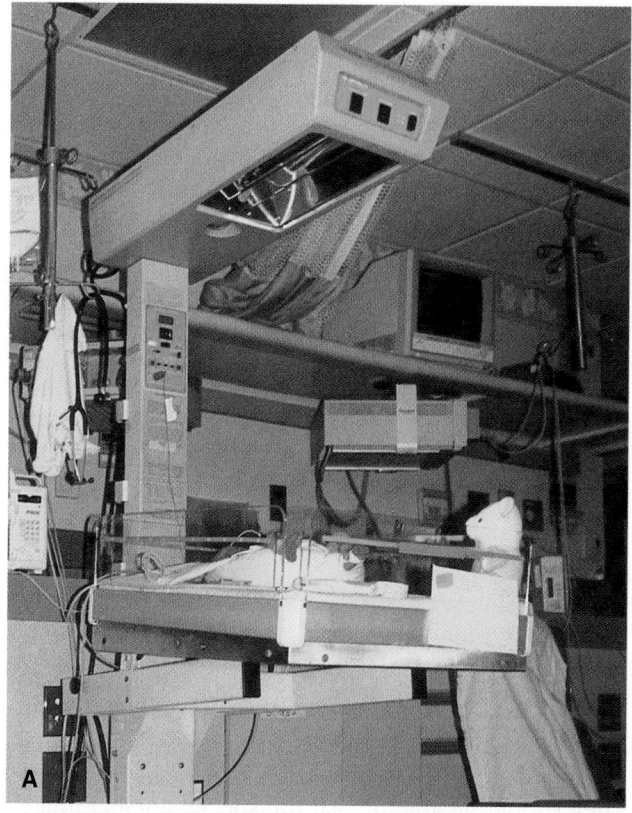
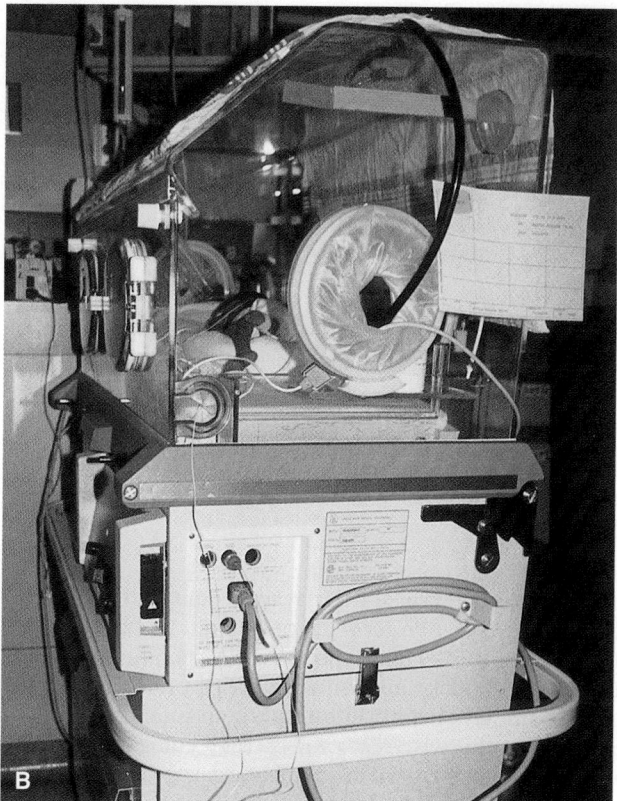

FIGURE 26.4 Neutral thermal environment. **(A)** The neonate in the intensive care bed with overhead radiant warmer can be examined periodically with ease. **(B)** Use of an incubator allows maintenance of a neutral thermal environment for neonates not requiring minute-to-minute intervention.

the heat from an overhead source and keep it from reaching the baby. An additional warming pad placed under an infant may be necessary for very preterm infants or for lengthy procedures to maintain body heat.

Incubators

After an initial resuscitation attempt, newborns may be cared for in incubators. The temperature of incubators varies with the amount of time portholes remain open and the temperature of the area in which the incubator is placed. Placing it in direct sunlight or near a warm radiator can increase the internal temperature markedly. For this reason, a newborn's temperature must be checked at frequent intervals to be certain the temperature level designated is being maintained. Use of an additional acrylic shield inside the incubator helps prevent radiation and convection heat loss when portholes are opened for care.

Similar to radiant warmers, some incubators have Servocontrol mechanism units that monitor an infant's temperature and automatically change the temperature of the incubator as needed. Portholes must remain closed to keep the Servocontrol operating efficiently.

As an infant's condition improves, weaning from an incubator may be necessary. Dress an infant as if he or she were going to be in a bassinet, then set the incubator about 2°F (1.2°C) below the infant's temperature. After a half-hour, assess whether the infant is able to maintain body temperature. If so, lower the incubator temperature another 2°F and continue until room temperature is reached. If an infant cannot maintain adequate temperature as the incubator temperature level is lowered, he or she is not yet ready for room-temperature air, and the weaning process needs to be slowed or stopped until the baby is more mature or better able to self-regulate temperature.

Kangaroo Care

Kangaroo care is the use of skin-to-skin contact to maintain body heat. An infant is undressed except for a diaper and perhaps a cap. The parent sits in a chair and holds the infant snugly against his or her chest, skin to skin (Anderson et al., 2005). Typically, an infant and parent are placed in a quiet corner with lights dimmed. A blanket is placed over them to provide privacy. This method of care not only supplies heat but also encourages parent–child interaction.

Establishing Adequate Nutritional Intake

Infants who experienced severe asphyxia at birth usually receive intravenous fluids so they do not become exhausted from sucking or until necrotizing enterocolitis (NEC) has been ruled out, as this could result from the temporary reduction in oxygen to the bowel (see Chapter 45 for a discussion of NEC). If an infant's respiratory rate remains rapid

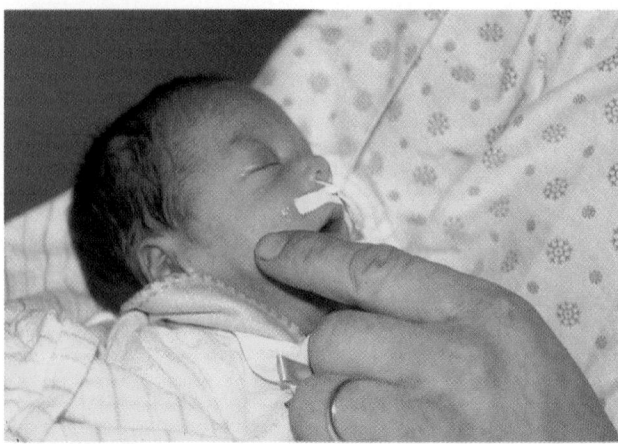

FIGURE 26.5 Infants who are ill at birth often need supplemental feedings by nasogastric or gastrostomy tube.

and NEC has been ruled out, gavage feeding may be introduced (Fig. 26.5). Preterm infants should be breast-fed if possible. If breast-feeding is not possible, a mother can manually express breast milk or use a breast pump to initiate and continue her milk supply until an infant is mature enough or otherwise ready for breast-feeding. Expressed breast milk may be used in an infant's gavage feeding. Preterm infants reveal hunger by the same signs as term infants, such as rooting and crying and sucking motions. All babies who are gavage-fed need oral stimulation from nonnutritive sucking and should be supplied with a pacifier at feeding times. Exceptions are infants too immature to have a sucking reflex and infants who must not swallow air, such as those with a tracheoesophageal fistula awaiting surgery. The techniques of gavage feeding, intravenous feeding, and gastrostomy feeding are all discussed in Chapter 36.

Establishing Waste Elimination

Although most immature infants void within 24 hours of birth, they may void later than term newborns because due to all the procedures that may be necessary for resuscitation, their blood pressure may not be adequate to optimally supply their kidneys. Carefully document any voidings that occur during resuscitation. This is proof that hypotension is improving and the kidneys are being perfused. Immature infants also may pass stool later than the term infant because meconium has not yet reached the end of the intestine by birth.

Preventing Infection

Contracting an infection could drastically complicate a high-risk newborn's ability to adjust to extrauterine life. Infection, like chilling, increases metabolic oxygen demands, which the stressed newborn may not be able to meet. In addition, infection stresses the immature immune system and already stressed defense mechanisms of a high-risk newborn. Infections may have prenatal, perinatal, or postnatal causes. In some instances, such as preterm rupture of the membranes, it is the infection (e.g., pneumonia or skin lesions) that places an infant in a high-risk category.

Common viruses that affect infants in utero are the cytomegalovirus and toxoplasmosis viruses. An infant with either of these infections may be born with congenital anomalies from the virus invasion (see Chapter 11). The most prevalent perinatal infections are those contracted from the vagina during birth, such as group B streptococcal septicemia, thrush from *Candida* infection, and herpes infections. Postnatal infection is probably most commonly spread to a newborn from health care personnel. Skin care is important to prevent skin breakdown and open portals of entry. All persons coming in contact with or caring for infants must observe good handwashing technique and standard precautions to reduce the risk of infection transmission. Health care personnel with infections have a professional and moral obligation to refrain from caring for newborns.

Establishing Parent–Infant Bonding

Women diagnosed as having a high-risk pregnancy should be offered a tour of a neonatal intensive care unit (NICU) during pregnancy so if their infant should be admitted to an NICU, they will be more comfortable in the high-tech environment.

Be sure parents of a high-risk newborn are kept informed of what is happening during resuscitation at birth. They should be able to visit the special nursing unit to which the child is admitted as often as they choose, to wash and gown and hold and touch their child. This helps to make the child's birth more real to them. Should the child not survive the illness, these interactions can help make the death more real. Only when both birth and death seem real can parents begin to work through their feelings and accept these events.

All parents handle newborn babies tentatively until they have "claimed" them or have become better acquainted. It may be months before the parents of a child who has been ill since birth can handle their baby comfortably and confidently. Urge parents to spend time with an infant in the intensive care nursery as the infant improves. Be sure they have access to health care personnel after discharge to help them care confidently for the child at home.

If an infant dies despite newborn resuscitation attempts, the parents need to see the infant without being covered by a myriad of equipment. This is a time for parents to reassure themselves their newborn was a perfect baby in every other way except lung function or whatever the infant's fatal disorder was. Thinking this way can give them confidence to plan for other children or simply to continue their lives after such a stressful experience.

Developmental Needs

Most high-risk infants enjoy "catch-up" growth once they stabilize from the trauma of birth or whatever caused them to be classified as high risk. They quickly move to playing with age-appropriate toys. Some parents may need support before and after their infants are discharged home to begin to view them as well and capable of doing all the things they are now capable of doing. Anticipatory guidance helps them to be ready for the next developmental step.

Follow-Up of High-Risk Infants at Home

Each time parents visit a high-risk nursery, assess their level of knowledge about their child's condition and development. Thorough education and referral to a home care agency may be necessary to help parents continue with the level of care that is required when their infant is discharged home (see Chapter 35). Before discharge, the safety of their home for the care of such a small infant needs to be evaluated. Transporting a preterm infant in a car requires special care, including a blanket or commercial head support, because a very small infant does not fit securely in a standard infant car seat (AAP, 2005).

High-Risk Infants and Child Abuse

When a child is ill or born preterm, the expected reaction of the parents would be to protect the child even more than the average child so no further harm can result. In reality, particularly in reference to preterm children, the opposite may occur. Preterm children are at high risk for abuse (Sirotnak & Krugman, 2003). This is probably due to the separation of the child from the family at birth, which interferes with bonding. Child abuse is discussed in Chapter 55.

What if... Mrs. Atkins is about to visit her preterm newborn for the first time. She states, "I'm so scared. He's so tiny and frail. How can I even hold him?" How should you respond to this new mother to make her visit easier?

THE NEWBORN AT RISK BECAUSE OF ALTERED GESTATIONAL AGE OR BIRTHWEIGHT

Infants are evaluated as soon as possible after birth to determine their weight and gestational age. Classification by growth charts and gestational history is important to determine the immediate health care needs of a newborn and in anticipating possible problems. Birthweight is normally plotted on a growth chart such as the Colorado (Lubchenco) Intrauterine Growth Chart (see Appendix E). Infants born after the beginning of week 38 and before week 42 of pregnancy (calculated from the first day of the last menstrual period) are classified as **term infants.** Approximately 90% of all live births are term. Infants born before term (less than the full 37th week of pregnancy) account for approximately 7% to 19% of all births and are classified as **preterm infants,** regardless of their birthweight. Infants born after the onset of week 43 of pregnancy are classified as postterm infants (Moore & Martin, 2003).

Normally, birthweight varies for each gestational week of age. Infants who fall between the 10th and 90th percentiles of weight for their age regardless of gestational age are considered **appropriate for gestational age (AGA).** Infants who fall below the 10th percentile of weight for their age are considered **small for gestational age (SGA).** Those who fall above the 90th percentile in weight are considered **large for gestational age (LGA).** Infants weighing under 2,500 g are **low-birthweight infants.** Those weighing 1,000 to 1,500 g are very-low-birthweight infants. Those born weighing 500 to 1,000 g are considered extremely-very-low-birthweight infants. Preterm infants may be AGA, SGA, LGA, low birthweight, or very low or extremely very low birthweight.

Infants who are found to be preterm, postterm, SGA, LGA, low birthweight, or very low birthweight have immediate needs that are different from or more pronounced than the needs of the usual term newborn (Box 26.7). Each of these categories carries its own set of problems and potential risks.

The Small-for-Gestational-Age Infant

An infant is SGA if the birth weight is below the 10th percentile on an intrauterine growth curve for that age. SGA infants may be born preterm (before week 38 of gestation), term (between weeks 38 and 42), or postterm (past 42 weeks). SGA infants are small for their age because they have experienced **intrauterine growth restriction (IUGR)** or failed to grow at the expected rate in utero (Garite, Clark & Thorp, 2004). This characteristic makes them distinctly different from infants whose weight is low but who are average for gestational age.

Causes

The mother's nutrition during pregnancy plays a major role in fetal growth, so lack of adequate nutrition may be a major contributor to IUGR. Pregnant adolescents have a high incidence of SGA infants: an adolescent has her own nutritional and growth needs, and these, when coupled with the increased nutritional needs of pregnancy, can affect a growing fetus. However, the most common cause of IUGR is a placental anomaly: either the placenta did not obtain sufficient nutrients from the uterine arteries or it

---

BOX 26.7 FOCUS ON . . .

DIVERSITY OF CARE

The weight of infants at birth is at least partially culturally determined. In the United States, for example, low-birthweight infants are most apt to be born to African-American women and girls under 15 years of age (DHHS, 2000). This statistic points to a need to be aware that some women are at higher risk for giving birth to low-birthweight infants than others. A number of factors may contribute to this, including lack of knowledge about the importance of prenatal care, lack of transportation to prenatal appointments, and poor nutritional status. Assessing the particular needs of these mothers is important in preventing the problems that low-birthweight infants experience at birth.

was inefficient at transporting nutrients to the fetus. Placental damage, such as partial placental separation with bleeding, limits placental function because the area of placenta that separated becomes infarcted and fibrosed, reducing the placental surface available for exchange. A developmental defect in the placenta can also prevent it from functioning properly. Women with systemic diseases that decrease blood flow to the placenta, such as severe diabetes mellitus or pregnancy-induced hypertension (both diseases where blood vessel lumens are narrowed), are at higher risk for delivering SGA babies than others. Mothers who smoke heavily or use narcotics also tend to have SGA infants (Rahimian & Varner, 2003).

In other instances, the placental supply of nutrients is adequate but an infant cannot use them because the infant has contracted an intrauterine infection such as rubella or toxoplasmosis or has a chromosomal abnormality.

Assessment

Prenatal Assessment. The SGA infant may be detected in utero when fundal height during pregnancy becomes progressively less than expected. However, if a woman is unsure of the date of her last menstrual period, this discrepancy can be hard to substantiate. A sonogram can then demonstrate the decreased size. A biophysical profile including a nonstress test, placental grading, amniotic fluid amount, and ultrasound examination can provide additional information on placental function. If poor placental function is apparent from such determinations, it can be predicted an infant will do poorly during labor because of periods of relative hypoxia during contractions. Cesarean birth is the birth method of choice in such circumstances.

Appearance. Generally, an infant who suffers nutritional deprivation early in pregnancy, when fetal growth consists primarily of an increase in the number of body cells, is below average in weight, length, and head circumference. An infant who suffers deprivation late in pregnancy, when growth consists primarily of an increase in cell size, may have only a reduction in weight. Regardless of when deprivation occurs, an infant has an overall wasted appearance. The child may have a small liver, which may cause difficulty regulating glucose, protein, and bilirubin levels after birth. An infant also may have poor skin turgor and generally appear to have a large head because the rest of the body is so small. Skull sutures may be widely separated from lack of normal bone growth. Hair is dull and lusterless. The abdomen may be sunken. The cord often appears dry and may be stained yellow.

In contrast, because an infant's age is more advanced than the weight implies, the child may have better-developed neurologic responses, sole creases, and ear cartilage than expected for a baby of that weight. The skull may be firmer, and the infant may seem unusually alert and active for that weight. The SGA infant needs careful assessment for possible congenital anomalies occurring as a result of the poor nutritional intrauterine environment.

Laboratory Findings. Blood studies at birth usually show a high hematocrit level (less than normal amounts of plasma in proportion to red blood cells are present due to lack of fluid in utero) and an increase in the total number of red blood cells (polycythemia). The increase in red blood cells is probably due to a state of anoxia during intrauterine life. The polycythemia causes increased blood viscosity, a condition that puts extra work on the infant's heart because it is more difficult to effectively circulate this thick blood. As a consequence, acrocyanosis (blueness of the hands and feet) may be prolonged and persistently more marked than usual. If the polycythemia is extreme, vessels may actually become blocked and thrombus formation can result. If the hematocrit level is more than 65% to 70%, an exchange transfusion to dilute the blood may be necessary.

Because SGA infants have decreased glycogen stores, one of the most common problems is hypoglycemia (decreased blood glucose, or a level below 40 mg/dL). Such infants may need intravenous glucose to sustain blood sugar until they are able to suck vigorously enough to take sufficient oral feedings.

NURSING DIAGNOSES AND RELATED INTERVENTIONS

●

Nursing Diagnosis: Ineffective breathing pattern related to underdeveloped body systems at birth

Outcome Evaluation: Newborn maintains respirations at a rate of 30 to 60 breaths per minute after resuscitation at birth.

Birth asphyxia is a common problem for SGA infants, both because they have underdeveloped chest muscles and because they are at risk for developing meconium aspiration syndrome due to anoxia during labor. Fetal hypoxia causes a reflex relaxation of the anal sphincter and increased intestinal movement. When gasping for breath in utero, the fetus draws meconium discharged into the amniotic fluid into the tracheobronchial tree. Acting as a foreign substance, it blocks airflow into the alveoli, leading to hypoxemia, acidosis, and hypercapnia. For this reason, many SGA infants require resuscitation at birth. Closely observe both respiratory rate and character in the first few hours of life. Underdeveloped chest muscles can make them unable to sustain the rapid respiratory rate of a normal newborn.

Nursing Diagnosis: Risk for ineffective thermoregulation related to lack of subcutaneous fat

Outcome Evaluation: Infant's temperature is maintained at 36.5°C (97.8°F) axillary.

SGA infants are less able to control body temperature than normal newborns because they lack subcutaneous fat. A carefully controlled environment is essential to keep an infant's body temperature in a neutral zone (see Chapter 24).

Nursing Diagnosis: Risk for impaired parenting related to child's high-risk status and possible cognitive or neurologic impairment from lack of nutrients in utero

Outcome Evaluation: Parents express interest in infant and ask questions about what the child's care needs will be at home.

Although SGA infants may gain weight and appear to thrive in the first few days of life, their cognitive development may have been impaired because of lack of oxygen and nourishment in utero. Babies who were growing normally in utero but whose gestation was interrupted preterm (true preterm babies) usually gain weight and height so rapidly that by the end of the first year of life they are near the 50th percentile on growth charts. SGA infants, however, may always be below normal on standard growth charts. This inability to reach normal levels of growth and development may interfere with bonding because the child does not meet the parents' expectations. Eventually, it can interfere with the child's self-esteem if the child is never able to meet parental expectations.

One way to promote early parental bonding with the child is to discuss ways parents can promote an infant's development once they are at home. An SGA infant needs adequate stimulation during the infant period to reach normal growth and developmental milestones. Encourage parents to provide toys suitable for their child's chronologic age, not physical size. Because an infant tires easily in the first few weeks of life, play periods must be spaced with rest periods or hypoglycemia or apnea can occur.

Checkpoint Question 2

Why are small-for-gestational-age newborns at risk for difficulty maintaining body temperature?

a. They are preterm so are born relatively small in size.
b. They are more active than usual so throw off covers.
c. They do not have as many fat stores as other infants.
d. Their skin is more susceptible to conduction of cold.

The Large-for-Gestational-Age Infant

An infant is LGA (also termed **macrosomia**) if the birthweight is above the 90th percentile on an intrauterine growth chart for that gestational age. Such a baby appears deceptively healthy at birth because of the weight, but a gestational age examination will reveal immature development. It is important that an LGA infant be identified immediately so that an infant is given special care appropriate to his or her gestational age rather than being treated as a term newborn (Ehrenberg, Mercer & Catalano, 2004).

Causes

Infants who are LGA have been subjected to an overproduction of growth hormone in utero. This happens most often to infants of mothers with diabetes mellitus and women who are obese (Surkan et al., 2004). Extreme macrosomia may occur in fetuses of diabetic mothers whose symptoms are poorly controlled, because these fetuses are exposed to high glucose levels. Multiparous women are also prone to deliver large babies because with each succeeding pregnancy, babies tend to grow larger. Other conditions associated with LGA infants include transposition of the great vessels, Beckwith syndrome (a rare condition characterized by overgrowth), and congenital anomalies such as omphalocele.

Assessment

A fetus is suspected of being LGA when a woman's uterus is unusually large for the date of pregnancy. Size can be deceptive, however. Because a fetus lies in a flexed fetal position, he or she does not occupy significantly more space at 10 lb than at 7 lb. If a fetus does seem to be growing at an abnormally rapid rate, a sonogram can confirm the suspicion. A nonstress test to assess the placenta's ability to sustain the large fetus during labor may also be performed. To see if an LGA fetus is mature, lung maturity may be assessed by amniocentesis.

If an infant's large size was not detected during pregnancy, it may be first recognized during labor when the baby cannot descend through the pelvic rim. Cesarean birth may be necessary because of **cephalopelvic disproportion** (the biparietal diameter is closer to 10 cm than the usual 9 cm) or **shoulder dystocia** (the wide shoulders cannot pass through the outlet of the pelvis).

Appearance. At birth, the LGA infant may show immature reflexes and low scores on gestational age examinations in relation to his or her size. A baby may have extensive bruising or a birth injury such as a broken clavicle or Erb-Duchenne paralysis from trauma to the cervical nerves if he or she was born vaginally (see Chapter 51). Because the head is large, it may have been exposed to more than the usual amount of pressure during birth, causing a prominent caput succedaneum, cephalhematoma, or molding.

The LGA newborn requires the same cautious care necessary for a preterm infant. Specific criteria for initial or continuing assessment are shown in Table 26.1.

Cardiovascular Dysfunction. Observe LGA infants closely for signs of hyperbilirubinemia (increased serum bilirubin level), which may result from absorption of blood from bruising and polycythemia. Polycythemia has been caused by an infant's system attempting to fully oxygenate all body tissues. This effort puts extra stress on the heart, so the heart rate of LGA infants should be carefully observed. If cyanosis is present, it may be a sign of transposition of the great vessels, a serious heart anomaly (see Chapter 41).

Hypoglycemia. An LGA infant also needs to be carefully assessed for hypoglycemia in the early hours of life because the infant uses up nutritional stores readily to sustain his or

TABLE 26.1

Important Assessment Criteria for a Large-for-Gestational-Age Infant

Assessment	Rationale
Skin color for ecchymosis, jaundice, and erythema	Bruising occurs with vaginal birth; jaundice may occur from breakdown of ecchymotic collections of blood; polycythemia causes ruddiness of skin.
Motion of extremities on spontaneous movement and in response to a Moro's reflex to detect clavicle fracture (crepitus or swelling may then be palpated at the fracture site) or Erb's palsy due to edema of the cervical nerve plexus	Clavicle or cervical nerve injuries may occur due to problem of birth of wider-than-normal shoulders.
Asymmetry of the anterior chest or unilateral lack of movement to detect diaphragmatic paralysis from edema of the phrenic nerve	This cervical nerve may be stretched by birth of wide shoulders.
Eyes for evidence of unresponsive or dilated pupils; vomiting, bulging fontanelles, and a high-pitched cry suggestive of increased intracranial pressure	Compression of 3rd, 4th, and 6th cranial nerves by increased pressure limits eye response; other signs of increased intracranial pressure may occur.
Activities such as jitteriness, lethargy, and uncoordinated eye movements that suggest seizure activity	Seizures may be caused by increased intracranial pressure; hypoglycemia seizures in newborns often produce only vague symptoms.

her weight. If the mother has diabetes that is poorly controlled, an infant will have an increased blood glucose level in utero, which causes the infant to produce elevated levels of insulin. After birth, these increased insulin levels will continue for up to 24 hours of life, possibly causing rebound hypoglycemia.

NURSING DIAGNOSES AND RELATED INTERVENTIONS

Nursing Diagnosis: Ineffective breathing pattern related to possible birth trauma in large-for-gestational-age newborn

Outcome Evaluation: Newborn initiates breathing at birth; maintains normal newborn respiratory rate of 30 to 60 breaths per minute.

Some LGA infants have difficulty establishing respirations at birth because of birth trauma. Increased intracranial pressure from birth of the larger-than-usual head may lead to pressure on the respiratory center. This, in turn, can cause a decrease in respiratory function. A diaphragmatic paralysis may occur due to cervical nerve trauma as the head is bent sideways to allow for birth of the large shoulders. This prevents active lung motion on the affected side. If an infant was born by cesarean birth, transient fluid can remain in the lungs and interfere with effective gas exchange. Careful observation will detect these conditions.

Care of an infant with transient lung fluid is discussed later in this chapter.

Nursing Diagnosis: Risk for imbalanced nutrition, less than body requirements related to additional nutrients needed to maintain weight and prevent hypoglycemia

Outcome Evaluation: Infant's weight follows percentile growth curve; skin turgor is good; specific gravity of urine is 1.003 to 1.030; serum glucose is above 40 mg/dL.

As a rule, the LGA infant needs to be breast-fed immediately to prevent hypoglycemia. An infant may need supplemental formula feedings after breast-feeding to supply enough fluid and glucose for the larger-than-normal size for the first few days. Newborns who are offered bottles often have more difficulty than others learning to breast-feed. Offer the mother and baby support to overcome this hurdle.

Do not overestimate this infant's ability to suck effectively at birth. An infant may seem as if he or she should do well with breast-feeding because the baby is already the size of a 2-month-old infant. However, an infant is an inexperienced newborn, so sucking may not be effective enough for the infant to obtain the larger-than-usual amount of milk needed.

Nursing Diagnosis: Risk for impaired parenting related to high-risk status of large-for-gestational-age infant

Outcome Evaluation: Parents hold infant; speak of the child in positive terms; state accurately why their infant needs to be closely observed in postnatal period.

Parents may underestimate this infant's needs because of the child's large size. He or she seems so big and healthy; parents may be confused about why their infant needs careful watching. They may read more into the child's condition than is present (he or she must be sick in some way they are not being told about), and so bonding does not happen as instinctively as it might. If the woman sustained a cervical or perineal tear or required a cesarean birth, she needs some time to air any resentment she may feel toward the infant for causing her extra pain. Otherwise, her perception that her infant is the cause of her additional distress may interfere with her ability to bond with the child.

An LGA infant needs the same developmental care all other infants need. Singing or talking to the baby, stroking the child's back, and rocking the baby are all important for the large infant's development. Encourage parents to treat their baby as a fragile newborn who needs warm nurturing, not as a tough big infant who has grown past that stage. Also remind parents an infant's birthweight is not a correlation of the child's projected adult size. Otherwise, parents may fear their infant may grow to be a larger-than-usual adult.

A Preterm Infant

A preterm infant is usually defined as a live-born infant born before the end of week 37 of gestation; another criterion used is a weight of less than 2,500 g (5 lb 8 oz) at birth. About 7% of all pregnancies end in preterm birth, and all such infants need neonatal intensive care from the moment of birth to give them their best chance of survival without neurologic after-effects (Petrou, 2003). A lack of lung surfactant makes them extremely vulnerable to respiratory distress syndrome (Rodriguez, 2003).

The maturity of a newborn is determined by physical findings such as sole creases, skull firmness, ear cartilage, and neurologic findings that reveal gestational age, as well as the mother's report of the date of her last menstrual period and sonographic estimations of gestational age.

Preterm babies, regardless of their weight, need to be differentiated at birth from SGA babies (who also may have a low birthweight). The two conditions result from different situations and therefore will cause different problems involving adjustment to extrauterine life. A preterm infant is immature and small but well proportioned for age. Unlike the SGA infant, this baby appears to have been doing well in utero. For an unexplained reason, the trigger that initiates labor was activated too early and birth has resulted, even though the baby is immature. Preterm infants are invariably low-birthweight infants. Characteristics of SGA and preterm infants are compared in Table 26.2.

Incidence

Preterm birth occurs in approximately 7% of live births of white infants. In African-American infants, the rate is doubled to approximately 14% (Thilo & Rosenberg, 2003).

When a preterm infant is recognized by a gestational age assessment, watch for the specific problems of prematurity, such as respiratory distress syndrome, hypoglycemia, and intracranial hemorrhage.

Causes

Preterm infant deaths account for 80% to 90% of infant mortality in the first year of life (NCHS, 2005). Infant

---

TABLE 26.2

Differences Between Small-for-Gestational-Age and Preterm Infants

Characteristic	Small-for-Gestational-Age Infant	Preterm Infant
Gestational age	24–44 wk	Younger than 37 wk
Birthweight	Under 10th percentile	Normal for age
Congenital malformations	Strong possibility	Possibility
Pulmonary problems	Meconium aspiration, pulmonary hemorrhage, pneumothorax	Respiratory distress syndrome
Hyperbilirubinemia	Possibility	Very strong possibility
Hypoglycemia	Very strong possibility	Possibility
Intracranial hemorrhage	Strong possibility	Possibility
Apnea episodes	Possibility	Very strong possibility
Feeding problems	Most likely due to accompanying problem such as hypoglycemia	Small stomach capacity; immature sucking reflex
Weight gain in nursery	Rapid	Slow
Future restricted growth	Possibly always be under 10th percentile due to poor organ development	Not likely to be restricted in growth as "catch-up" growth occurs

mortality could be reduced dramatically if the causes of preterm birth could be discovered and corrected and all pregnancies brought to term. However, the exact cause of premature labor and early birth is rarely known.

There is a high correlation between low socioeconomic level and early termination of pregnancy. In women from middle and upper socioeconomic groups, only 4% to 8% of pregnancies are terminated early. However, in women from low socioeconomic levels, as many as 10% to 20% end before term. The major influencing factor in these instances appears to be inadequate nutrition before and during pregnancy, as a result of either lack of money for or lack of knowledge about good nutrition. Additional factors that seem to be related to preterm birth are shown in Box 26.8. Iatrogenic causes, such as elective cesarean birth and inducing labor according to dates rather than fetal maturity, also result in preterm births. Testing fetal maturity by amniocentesis or ultrasound is used to avoid inducing labor prematurely.

Assessment

History. Although a detailed pregnancy history may sometimes reveal the reason for a preterm birth, the pregnancy history is often normal up to the beginning of labor.

When interviewing the parents of a preterm infant, be careful not to convey disapproval of reported pregnancy behaviors such as cigarette smoking or working a 12-hour shift that may have contributed to preterm birth. Once an infant is born, a new mother needs a high level of self-esteem and all of her inner resources to sustain her through the crisis. Being overburdened by guilt may be detrimen-

tal to her attempts to bond with her infant. A good answer to her direct inquiries about causes is, "No one really knows what causes prematurity."

In many instances, preterm labor might have been halted had a woman been able to recognize she was in true labor and not having Braxton-Hicks contractions. In a first labor, this can easily occur because a woman does not know what true labor feels like. Television often depicts women in labor as having agonizingly painful contractions or the opposite, simply announcing, "This is it," and then proceeding to give birth within the 30-minute show. In reality, the first-time mother does not realize that labor usually begins with subtle signs and mild contractions, not with a dramatic announcement. With preterm labor, often a woman reports that she was having intestinal cramps. Because each labor proceeds differently, even a multipara may miss the signs of early labor until it is too far advanced to be reversed. Reassure a woman it is understandable she did not realize what was happening until cervical dilatation had occurred and labor could not be reversed.

Appearance. On gross inspection, a preterm infant appears small and underdeveloped (Fig. 26.6). The head is disproportionately large (3 cm or more greater than chest size). The skin is generally unusually ruddy because the infant has little subcutaneous fat beneath it; veins are easily noticeable, and a high degree of acrocyanosis may be present. The preterm neonate, 24 to 36 weeks, typically is covered with vernix caseosa. However, in very preterm newborns (less than 25 weeks' gestation), vernix is absent because it is not formed this early in pregnancy. Lanugo is usually extensive, covering the back, forearms, forehead, and sides of the face, because this amount is present until late in pregnancy. Both anterior and posterior fontanelles are small. There are few or no creases on the soles of the feet.

Physical findings and reflex testing are used to differentiate between term and preterm newborns (Fig. 26.7). The eyes of most preterm infants appear small. Although difficult to elicit, pupillary reaction is present. Ophthalmoscopic examination is extremely difficult and often uninformative because the vitreous humor may be hazy. A preterm infant has varying degrees of myopia (nearsightedness) because of lack of eye globe depth.

The cartilage of the ear is immature and allows the pinna to fall forward. The ears appear large in relation to the head.

BOX 26.8

Factors Associated With Preterm Birth

Low socioeconomic level
Poor nutritional status
Lack of prenatal care
Multiple pregnancy
Previous early birth
Race (nonwhites have a higher incidence of prematurity than whites)
Cigarette smoking
Age of the mother (highest incidence is in mothers younger than age 20)
Order of birth (early termination is highest in first pregnancies and in those beyond the fourth pregnancy)
Closely spaced pregnancies
Abnormalities of the mother's reproductive system, such as intrauterine septum
Infections (especially urinary tract infection)
Obstetric complications, such as premature rupture of membranes or premature separation of the placenta
Early induction of labor
Elective cesarean birth

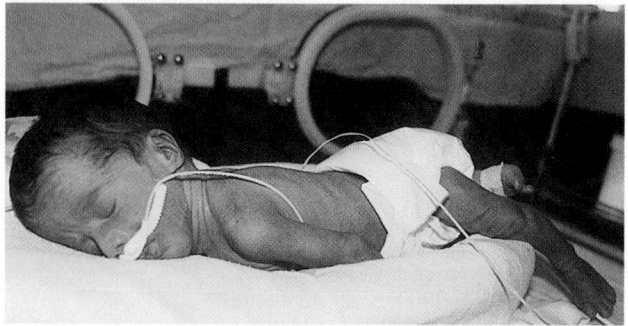

FIGURE 26.6 An immature infant. Notice the lax position of limbs due to immature muscle development.

A

Premature Infant

Full-term Infant

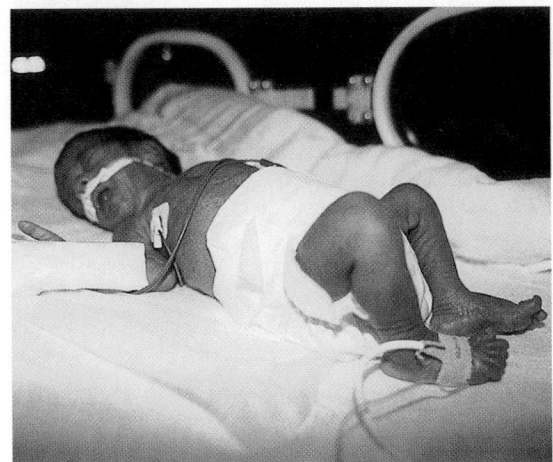
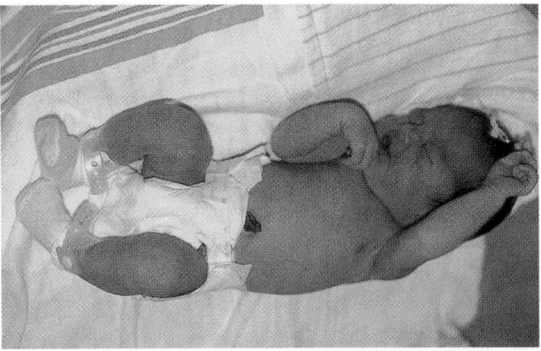

RESTING POSTURE *The premature infant is characterized by very little, if any, flexion in the upper extremities and only partial flexion of the lower extremities. The full-term infant exhibits flexion in all four extremities.*

B

Premature Infant, 28–32 Weeks

Full-term Infant

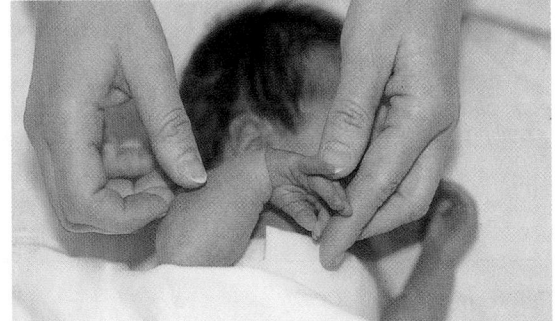
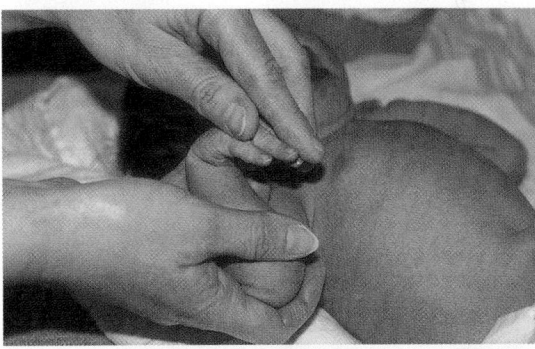

WRIST FLEXION *The wrist is flexed, applying enough pressure to get the hand as close to the forearm as possible. The angle between the hypothenar eminence and the ventral aspect of the forearm is measured. (Care must be taken not to rotate an infant's wrist.) The premature infant at 28–32 weeks' gestation will exhibit a 90° angle. With the full-term infant it is possible to flex the hand onto the arm.*

FIGURE 26.7 Examples of physical examination findings and reflex tests used to judge gestational age. (**A**) Resting posture. (**B**) Wrist flexion. *(continued)*

The level of the ears should be carefully inspected to rule out chromosomal abnormalities (see Chapter 7).

Neurologic function in the preterm infant is often difficult to evaluate as the neurologic system is still so immature. The observation of spontaneous or provoked movements may yield findings as important as reflex testing. If tested, reflexes such as sucking and swallowing will be absent if an infant's age is below 33 weeks; deep tendon reflexes such as the Achilles tendon reflex are also markedly diminished. During an examination, a preterm infant is much less active than a mature infant and rarely cries. If the infant does cry, the cry is weak and high-pitched.

Laboratory Findings. Laboratory values for a preterm infant are compared with those of the term infant in Appendix F.

Potential Complications

Because of immaturity, preterm infants are prone to a number of specific conditions.

Anemia of Prematurity. Many preterm infants develop a normochromic, normocytic anemia (normal cells, just few in number). The reticulocyte count is low because the bone marrow does not increase its production until approximately 32 weeks. An infant will appear pale and may be lethargic and anorectic. The fault appears to be immaturity of the hematopoietic system combined with destruction of red blood cells due to low levels of vitamin E, which normally protects red blood cells against oxidation. Excessive blood drawing for electrolyte or blood gas *(text continues on page 767)*

C

Premature Infant

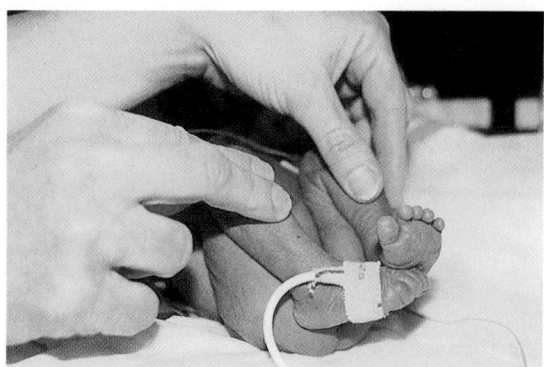

Full-term Infant

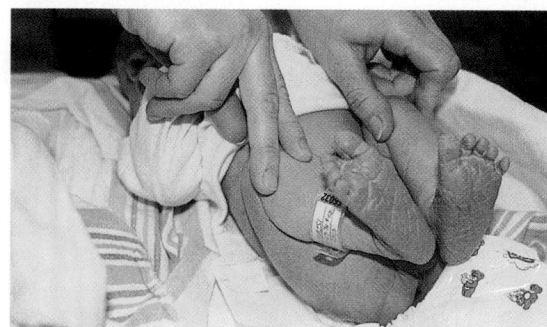

Response in Premature Infant

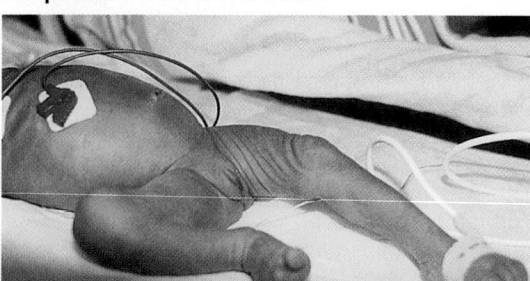

Response in Full-term Infant

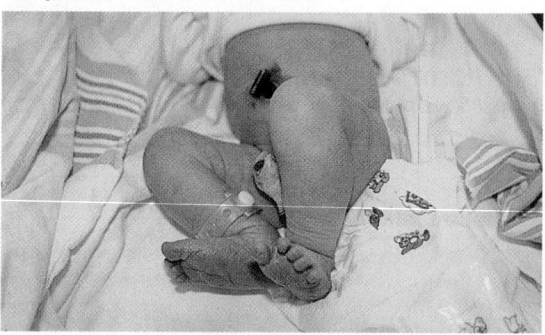

RECOIL OF EXTREMITIES   *Place an infant supine. To test recoil of the legs (1) flex the legs and knees fully and hold for 5 seconds (shown in top photos), (2) extend the legs fully by pulling on the feet, (3) release. To test the arms, flex forearms and follow same procedure. In the premature infant response is minimal or absent (bottom left); in the full-term infant extremities return briskly to full flexion (bottom right).*

D

Premature Infant

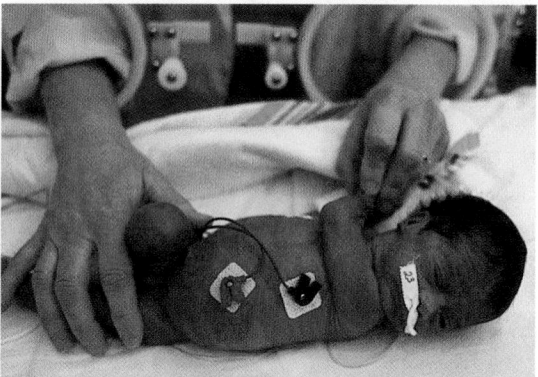

Full-term Infant

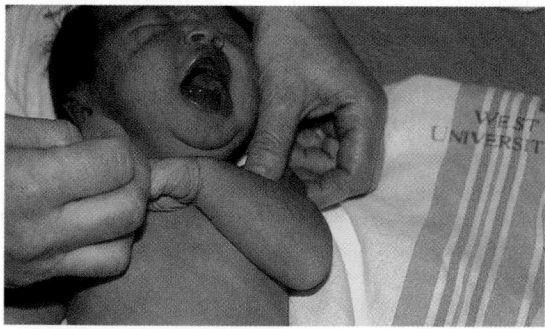

SCARF SIGN   *Hold the baby supine, take the hand, and try to place it around the neck and above the opposite shoulder as far posteriorly as possible. Assist this maneuver by lifting the elbow across the body. See how far across the chest the elbow will go. In the premature infant the elbow will reach near or across the midline. In the full-term infant the elbow will not reach the midline.*

FIGURE 26.7 (continued) (C) Recoil of extremities (legs). **(D)** Scarf sign.

Premature Infant   **Full-term Infant**

E

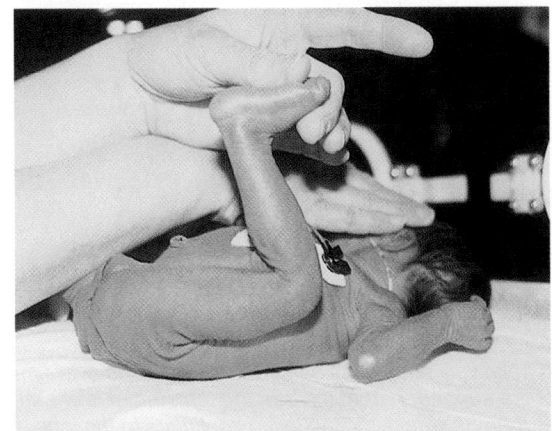
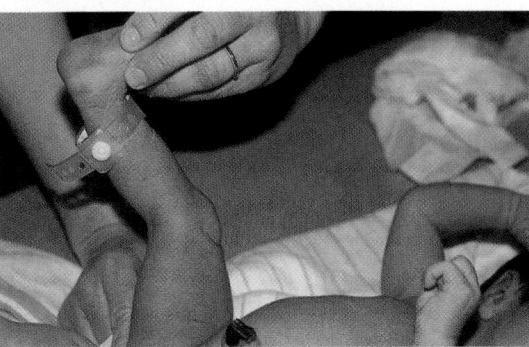

HEEL TO EAR   *With the baby supine and the hips positioned flat on the bed, draw the baby's foot as near to the ear as it will go without forcing it. Observe the distance between the foot and head as well as the degree of extension at the knee. In the premature infant very little resistance will be met. In the full-term infant there will be marked resistance; it will be impossible to draw the baby's foot to the ear.*

Premature Infant   **Full-term Infant**

F

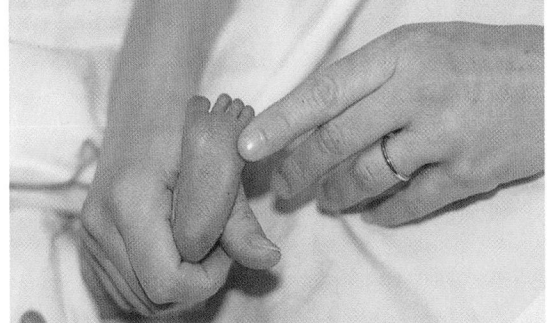
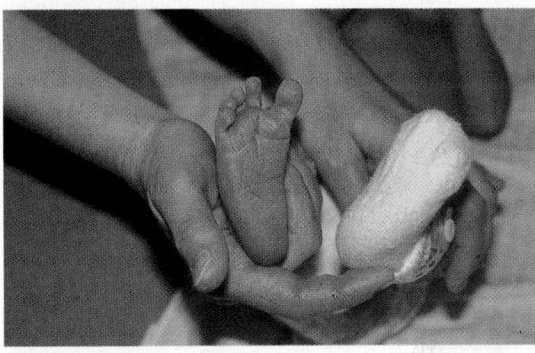

SOLE (PLANTAR) CREASES   *The sole of the premature infant has very few or no creases. With the increasing gestation age, the number and depth of sole creases multiply, so that the full-term baby has creases involving the heel. (Wrinkles that occur after 24 hours of age can sometimes be confused with true creases.)*

Premature Infant   **Full-term Infant**

G

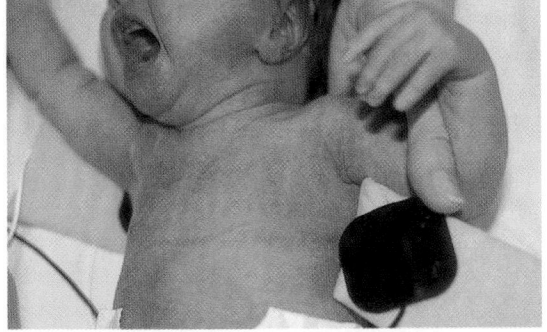
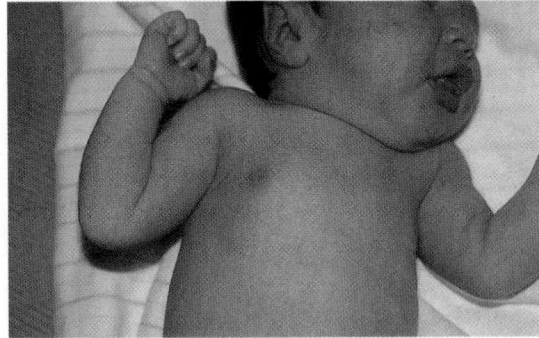

BREAST TISSUE   *In infants younger than 34 weeks' gestation the areola and nipple are barely visible. After 34 weeks the areola becomes raised. Also, an infant of less than 36 weeks' gestation has no breast tissue. Breast tissue arises with increasing gestational age due to maternal hormonal stimulation. Thus, an infant of 39 to 40 weeks will have 5 to 6 mm of breast tissue, and this amount will increase with age.*

FIGURE 26.7 (continued) (**E**) Heel to ear. (**F**) Plantar creases. (**G**) Breast tissue. *(continued)*

H

Premature Infant, 34–36 Weeks

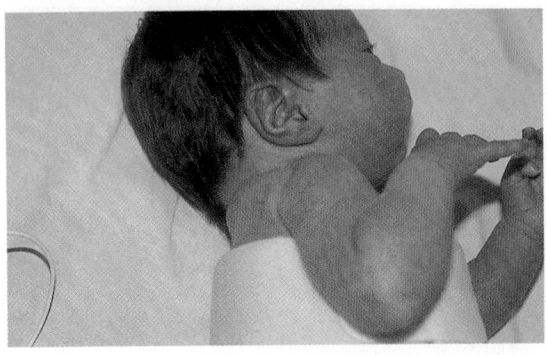

Full-term Infant

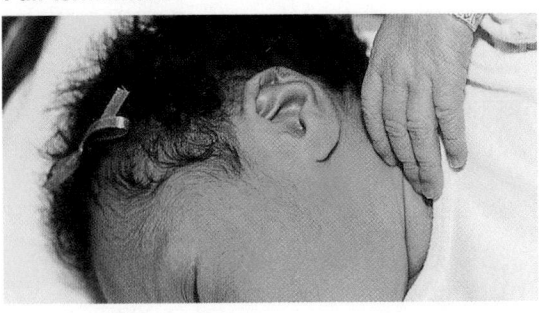

EARS   At fewer than 34 weeks' gestation infants have very flat, relatively shapeless ears. Shape develops over time so that an infant between 34 and 36 weeks has a slight incurving of the superior part of the ear; the term infant is characterized by incurving of two thirds of the pinna; and in an infant older than 39 weeks the incurving continues to the lobe. If the extremely premature infant's ear is folded over, it will stay folded. Cartilage begins to appear at approximately 32 weeks so that the ear returns slowly to its original position. In an infant of more than 40 weeks' gestation, there is enough ear cartilage so that the ear stands erect away from the head and returns quickly when folded. (When folding the ear over during examination be certain that the surrounding area is wiped clean or the ear may adhere to the vernix.)

I

Premature Male

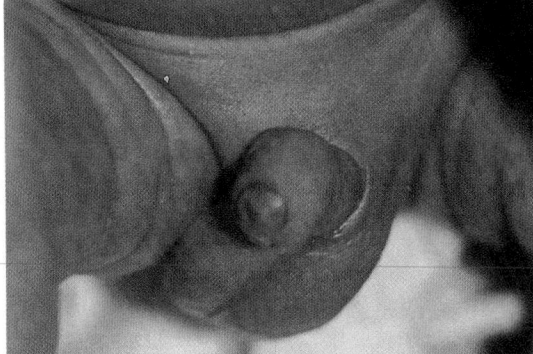

Full-term Male

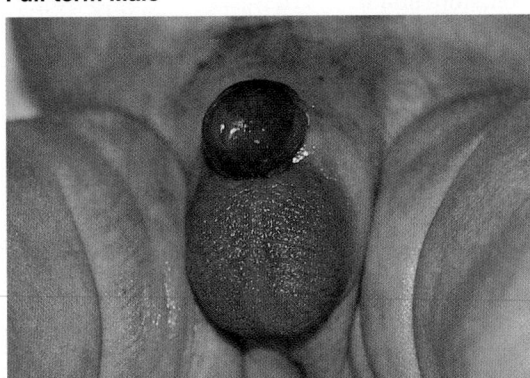

MALE GENITALIA   In the premature male the testes are very high in the inguinal canal and there are very few rugae on the scrotum. The full-term infant's testes are lower in the scrotum and many rugae have developed.

J

Premature Female

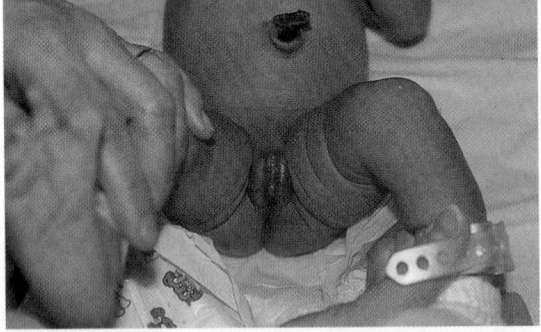

Full-term Female

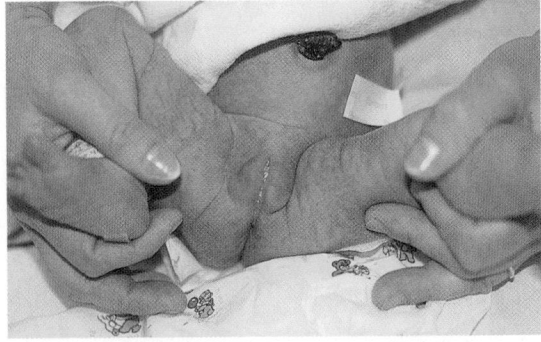

FEMALE GENITALIA   When the premature female is positioned on her back with hips abducted, the clitoris is very prominent and the labia majora are very small and widely separated. The labia minora and the clitoris are covered by the labia majora in the full-term infant.

FIGURE 26.7 (continued) **(H)** Ears. **(I)** Male genitalia. **(J)** Female genitalia. (© Caroline Brown, RNC, MS, DEd.)

trolytes such as sodium, potassium, and chloride may be necessary, depending on the newborn's blood studies. As with a term neonate, vitamin K should be administered at birth. However, the amount administered is more often 0.5 mL instead of 1 mL because of an infant's small size. Vitamin A is important in improving healing and possibly reducing the incidence of lung disease. Vitamin E seems to be important in preventing hemolytic anemia in preterm infants.

Breast Milk. There is increasing evidence that although preterm infants grow well on the increased caloric distribution of commercial formulas, the best milk for them, the same as term infants, is breast milk (Lindemann, Foshaugen & Lindemann, 2004). The immunologic properties of breast milk apparently play a major role in preventing neonatal necrotizing enterocolitis, a destructive intestinal disorder that often occurs in preterm babies.

The mother who wants to breast-feed can manually express breast milk for her infant's gavage feedings. If she cannot bring this in daily, the expressed breast milk can be frozen for safe transport and storage. The sodium content of breast milk in a mother whose infant has been born preterm is higher than that of milk at term. Therefore, it is better for an infant to receive his or her own mother's breast milk rather than banked milk. This high level of sodium is necessary for fluid retention in a preterm infant.

Nursing Diagnosis: Ineffective thermoregulation related to immaturity

Outcome Evaluation: Infant's temperature is 97.6°F (36.5°C) axillary.

A preterm newborn has a great deal of difficulty maintaining body temperature because he or she has a relatively large surface area per kilogram of body weight. In addition, because an infant does not flex the body well but remains in an extended position, rapid cooling from evaporation is more likely to occur.

A preterm infant has little subcutaneous fat for insulation, and poor muscular development does not allow a child to move as actively as an older infant to produce body heat. A preterm infant also has a limited amount of **brown fat,** the special tissue present in newborns to maintain body temperature. A preterm infant cannot shiver, a useful mechanism to increase body temperature; at the same time, he or she cannot sweat and thereby reduce body temperature because of an immature central nervous system and hypothalamic control. This makes a preterm infant depend on the environmental temperature provided to keep warm. In a birthing room, typically kept at 62° to 68°F (16.6° to 20°C), preterm infants must be kept under radiant heat warmers or warmed by skin-to-skin contact. A 1,500-g infant exposed to this low a temperature loses 1°C of body heat every 3 minutes if left unprotected.

Unless there are obvious abnormalities noted when the child is born, physical assessment of a preterm infant, even weighing, should be delayed until the infant can be placed in the warmth of an incubator or under a radiant warmer with a Servocontrol.

If an infant is going to be transported to a department within the hospital, such as the x-ray department, or to a regional center for specialized care, keeping the newborn warm during transport is crucial. Remember infants lose heat by radiation as well as conduction. If a warmed incubator is placed near a cold window or air conditioner or in a cold transport ambulance, an infant will lose heat to the distant source. An additional heat shield or plastic wrap may be placed over an infant on a radiant warmer to help conserve heat during transport.

Nursing Diagnosis: Risk for infection related to immature immune defenses in preterm infant

Outcome Evaluation: Temperature is maintained at 97.6°F (36.5°C) axillary; further signs and symptoms of infection such as poor growth or a reduced temperature are absent.

The skin of a preterm baby is easily traumatized and therefore offers less resistance to infection than the skin and mucous membranes of a mature baby. In addition, preterm infants have a lowered resistance to infection. They have difficulty producing phagocytes to localize infection and have a deficiency of IgM antibodies because of insufficient production. To help prevent infection, linen and equipment used with preterm infants must not be shared with other infants. Staff members must be free of infection, and handwashing and gowning regulations must be strictly enforced.

Nursing Diagnosis: Risk for impaired parenting related to interference with parent–infant attachment resulting from hospitalization of infant at birth

Outcome Evaluation: Parents visit frequently and hold infant; speak of him or her in positive terms.

In a preterm infant, the first and second periods of reactivity normally observed in newborns at 1 hour and 4 hours of life (see Chapter 24) may be delayed. In some infants, no period of increased activity or tachycardia may appear until 12 to 18 hours of age. If the purpose of a period of reactivity is to stimulate respiratory function, this places a preterm infant at an even greater threat of respiratory failure, because respiratory efforts may not be stimulated. A second consequence of a delayed period of reactivity is the loss of an opportunity for interaction between parents and the newborn in the early postpartum period.

At one time, a preterm infant was handled as little as possible by hospital staff to conserve the infant's energy. Parents were strictly isolated from the nursery to prevent the introduction of infection. When the child reached a "magic" weight of 4.5 or 5.5 lb, the parents were called and told their child was ready to be discharged. Some nursery personnel offered to allow the mother to feed her infant once under supervision before the day of discharge. In other nurseries, the mother was simply handed the smallest infant she had ever seen and told to take the child home and "mother" this stranger.

Although it is extremely important to conserve a preterm infant's strength by reducing sensory stimulation as much as possible and handling an infant gently, it is now recognized that a preterm infant needs as much loving attention as a term newborn. Rocking an infant, singing and talking to him or her, and gentle holding are measures to help an infant develop a sense of trust in people, which will enable the child to relate satisfactorily to them in the future. Holding the baby using kangaroo care (holding an infant with skin-to-skin contact) is yet another way to increase bonding. Encourage parents to begin interacting with their infant in as normal a manner as possible as soon as possible to strengthen bonding (Box 26.11). Box 26.12 highlights appropriate outcomes and interventions related to bonding using the terminology identified by the Nursing Outcomes Classification (NOC) and Nursing Interventions Classification (NIC).

Before effective bonding can be established, parents may need time to come to terms with their feelings of disappointment and guilt. A nurse can be instrumental in helping them air these feelings and develop a more positive attitude toward their preterm infant.

If an infant cannot be removed from an incubator or radiant heat warmer, he or she can still be han-

dled and stroked in the incubator or warmer. Because parents may not be psychologically ready for birth when a preterm baby is born, it may be more difficult for them to believe they have a child than if the baby were born at term. Encourage the mother to express breast milk for her infant if the child is too young to nurse. If a woman decides not to breast-feed, she should be encouraged to come to the hospital and hold the baby before and after gavage feedings or to give bottle feedings. By feeding her baby or expressing milk for the feedings, she is directly participating in the care and taking on responsibility for the infant's welfare.

If the baby is transferred to a regional center, make sure the parents have an opportunity to see the baby before the transfer. A photograph of the baby for them to keep is helpful in making the birth more real. Encourage them to visit the distant site as often as possible. Notes to convey messages from the baby to them can be taped to the incubator or warmer.

On the days they cannot visit, parents can still stay in touch by telephone or nursery e-mail. By the time a baby is ready for discharge, the parents should be able to feel they are taking home "their" baby, one whom they know and are ready to love.

Parents visiting a high-risk nursery often need a great deal of attention and support from nursing personnel. Remember that although radiant warmers, incubators, ventilators, and monitors are familiar equipment to nurses, they are unusual and frightening to parents. A parent may want very much to touch an infant but be so afraid touching

---

BOX 26.11 FOCUS ON . . .

 FAMILY TEACHING

Guidelines for Parents of a Newborn in Intensive Care

Q. Mrs. Atkins tells you, "I'm always afraid I'll touch the wrong thing when I visit our son in the neonatal intensive care unit. What can I do to feel more comfortable there?"

A. Here are some guidelines that should be helpful:

- Learn the name of your child's primary nurse or care manager and physician. Make a point of talking to them when you visit, so the information you receive is consistent, and these people can get to know you.
- Discuss with your child's care manager or primary nurse the time you will usually visit, so she or he can reserve this time for you. It also helps them to schedule the baby's procedures and rest times so there is time during your visits for you to hold your child and interact with him.
- Ask for explanations of any equipment or medications being used with your child, so you understand the plan of care. Insist on being included in care decisions.
- If you cannot visit on any day, telephone the nursery and ask to talk to your child's primary care nurse or

physician. Such telephone calls are not viewed as a bother but are welcomed as the mark of a concerned parent.

- If you planned to breast-feed, ask if you can supply expressed breast milk for your infant as soon as feedings are started. This contribution may help to give you a feeling of having a greater part in your baby's care.
- Supply a tape recording of your voice, so your baby can learn to recognize it, and a small toy for your baby's bed. These actions not only supply auditory and visual stimulation for your child but also help to give you a more "normal" feeling toward infant care.
- Use your baby's name when you talk about him (not "the baby") to help you gain a firm feeling that this is your baby, not the nursery's.
- If your child is hospitalized a distance from home, ask if transfer to a local hospital in a less technical environment will be possible at a later date.

BOX 26.12

Nursing Outcomes Classification (NOC) and Nursing Interventions Classification (NIC)

Bonding

NOC: Parent–Infant Attachment

Parent–infant attachment is defined as the behaviors that demonstrate an enduring affectionate bond between a parent and infant (Johnson, Maas, & Moorhead, 2000). Some specific indicators suggesting that this outcome has been achieved include the demonstration of the following by the parents:

- Assigning specific attributes to the infant
- Verbalizing positive feelings toward the infant
- Holding the infant close, touching, stroking, patting, kissing, and talking to the infant
- Using eye contact, smiling, and vocalizing with the infant in the en face position
- Responding to infant's cues

Indicators suggesting achievement of this outcome include the demonstration of the following by the infant:

- Responding to cues
- Seeking proximity with the parents
- Exploring the environment

NIC: Attachment Promotion

Attachment promotion is defined as the facilitation of the development of the parent–infant relationship (McCloskey & Bulechek, 2000). Some important activities to address when implementing this intervention include:

- Encouraging the parents to visit the infant frequently, touching and holding the infant, especially if infant is being transferred to another facility
- Encouraging parents to hold the infant close to the body
- Sharing information gained from the initial assessment of the newborn
- Reinforcing eye contact with the infant
- Explaining equipment used to monitor the infant
- Taking a Polaroid photo of the infant to leave with the parents before infant is transported
- Informing parents of care being given to the infant and of the behavioral characteristics that the infant exhibits while being cared for in the other facility

- Pointing out infant state changes and cues indicating responsiveness
- Reinforcing the normal aspects of infant

NIC: Kangaroo Care

Kangaroo care is defined as the promotion of closeness between parents and a physiologically stable preterm infant by preparing the parent and providing the environment for skin-to-skin contact (Johnson, Maas, & Moorhead, 2000). Some important activities to address when implementing this intervention include:

- Discussing the parents' reaction to the preterm infant and the image that they have of the infant
- Encouraging the parent to initiate infant care
- Determining if infant physiologically meets the guidelines for kangaroo care
- Preparing a quiet, draft-free environment, with parent sitting in rocking chair, wearing comfortable, open-front clothing
- Instructing how to move infant from incubator, warmer bed, or bassinet and how to manage equipment
- Positioning diaper-clad infant prone and upright on parent's chest
- Encouraging the parents to focus on infant, gently stroking and rocking as appropriate
- Encouraging use of auditory stimulation
- Supporting parents in nurturing and providing hands-on care
- Instructing parents to decrease activity when infant shows signs of overstimulation, distress, or avoidance
- Encouraging parent to let infant sleep, or breastfeed during care
- Urging parent to provide kangaroo care from 20 minutes to 3 hours at a time consistently
- Monitoring the infant's physiologic status, discontinuing kangaroo care if infant becomes compromised or agitated

---

might set off an alarm that he or she stands back with arms folded instead (Fig. 26.9).

Because preterm infants are hospitalized for long periods, parents can be baffled by receiving information from a parade of different health care professionals or a different person every time they visit. Primary nursing or case management with one nurse as the consistent caregiver helps to reduce the number of people who contact the parents and who communicate the baby's nursing needs to the rest of the staff.

Making parents and the baby's siblings welcome in a high-risk nursery is yet another major role for the nurse of high-risk infants (Box 26.13). Siblings should not visit if they have a cold or fever. Their immunizations should be up to date and they should not have been recently exposed to a communicable disease, such as chickenpox.

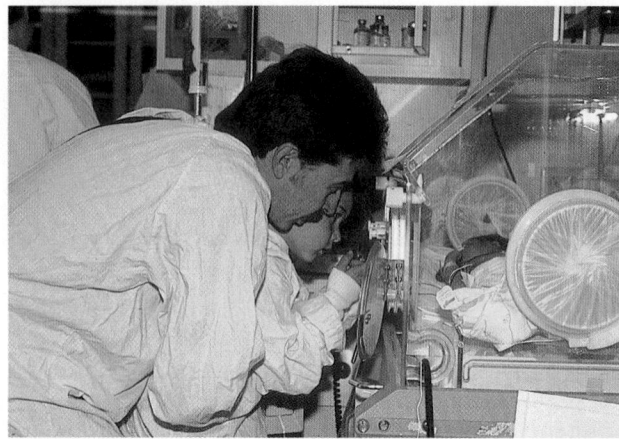

FIGURE 26.9 Encourage families to visit with immature infants to establish bonding. (© Caroline Brown, RNC, MS, DEd.)

Nursing Diagnosis: Deficient diversional activity (lack of stimulation) related to preterm infant's rest needs

Outcome Evaluation: Infant demonstrates interaction with caregivers by attuning to faces or voices.

Preterm infants need rest to conserve energy for growth and respiratory function, to combat hypoglycemia and infection, to stabilize temperature, and to develop inner balance and attentiveness. To allow for this, procedures should be organized to maximize the amount of rest available to an infant.

If this is not a coordinated effort, an infant may be awakened constantly for procedures. Preterm infants may have more difficulty blocking out stimuli than term infants do because their nervous systems are immature. They may react negatively by such behaviors as gagging, crying, splaying fingers and toes, or going limp when exposed to bright lights, noise, or overly strenuous handling. Because these infants have little strength to move away from an unwanted stimulus, it is a caregiver's responsibility to be sensitive to these cues and move the object or noise away from the infant. Until ready to take in stimuli, the newborn may need to be shielded from noise and light as much as possible. Pain should be kept to a minimum.

At the same time as a preterm infant needs rest, he or she needs planned periods of pleasing sensory stimulation. Like all newborns, preterm infants respond best to stimulation that appeals to their senses—sight, sound, and touch. A passive face, picture, or decal may be appealing for only short periods.

The view from inside an incubator can be distorted by the acrylic dome. Most people view an infant in an incubator from the side. This means an infant's face is rarely in the same line of vision as the adult's (an en face position). It is important to look directly at an infant in the straightforward position so the infant is provided with the stimulation of a human face. As an infant matures, he or she should have a mobile (perhaps black and white) or a bright object placed in view. As an infant's posi-

---

BOX 26.13 FOCUS ON . . .

COMMUNICATION

Mrs. Atkins gave birth to a 2-lb boy at 34 weeks of pregnancy, 2 days ago. The infant has been classified as a small-for-gestational-age preterm infant. Although you have told Mrs. Atkins twice that she is welcome to visit the neonatal intensive care unit (NICU), you notice that her chart indicates that she has not yet done so.

Less Effective Communication

Nurse: Mrs. Atkins, I've noticed you haven't been to the nursery to see your son yet.
Mrs. Atkins: I'm waiting for my husband to come in.
Nurse: Will that be today?
Mrs. Atkins: Tomorrow. He's out of town on business.
Nurse: Have you telephoned the nursery to ask about your son?
Mrs. Atkins: No. I'm waiting for my husband. We'll do it together.
Nurse: Okay. Let me know if there is anything else you need.

More Effective Communication

Nurse: Mrs. Atkins, I've noticed you haven't been to the nursery to see your son yet.

Mrs. Atkins: I'm waiting for my husband to come in.
Nurse: Will that be today?
Mrs. Atkins: Tomorrow. He's out of town on business.
Nurse: Have you telephoned the nursery to ask about your son?
Mrs. Atkins: No. I'm waiting for my husband. We'll do it together.
Nurse: Often it's intimidating to visit or telephone a high-risk nursery. I know it is important to you to go as a family, but I hate to see you miss these first few days with your son. What if I go with you?
Mrs. Atkins: Could you? I don't want to go alone.

Visiting a NICU is intimidating for parents, not only because of the high-tech equipment that surrounds their baby but also because their baby often appears much smaller or sicker than they imagined. In the first scenario, the nurse assumed that waiting for the husband to come to the hospital was what was important to the mother. In the second scenario, the nurse asked enough questions to realize that having another person accompany her to the nursery was the mother's need, a need the nurse could meet.

tion is changed from side to stomach to opposite side, the object should be moved to be in line with the child's vision.

An infant in a closed incubator may be able to hear nothing but the sound of the incubator motor. An infant may see people looking or nodding at him or her and may see their mouths moving, but he or she cannot benefit from the sound of their voices because this is obscured by the continuous hum of the motor. Provide some "talk time"—words spoken softly but clearly to an infant's ear—during each nursing shift to offer normal contact.

Even an infant who cannot be removed from an incubator should not suffer from lack of touch. Gently stroking an infant's back or smoothing the back of the head should not be tiring. Transcutaneous oxygen determinations allow you to recognize when an infant is comforted by handling (oxygen saturation remains steady or increases) and when the child is growing tired (oxygen saturation falls). There should be time during every nursing shift for this interaction, particularly if clinical interventions with an infant include uncomfortable procedures such as suctioning or blood drawing. As soon as an infant can be out of an incubator or removed from a warmer, he or she needs special time just to be rocked and held.

Nursing Diagnosis: Risk for disorganized infant behavior related to prematurity and environmental overstimulation

Outcome Evaluation: Newborn's vital signs remain within normal limits; infant demonstrates increasing ability to adapt to stimuli; demonstrates decreasing levels of irritability, crying, respiratory pauses, tachypnea, and color changes.

The amount of rest and stimulation required by preterm infants for healthy development is best individualized. **Developmental care** (care designed to meet the specific needs of each infant) can lead to increased weight gain and decreased crying and apnea spells in preterm infants (Box 26.14). Box 26.15 highlights appropriate outcomes and interventions for developmental care using the terminology identified by the Nursing Outcomes Classification (NOC) and Nursing Interventions Classification (NIC).

Because preterm infants have immature central nervous systems, their reactions or adjustments to stimuli may be different from those of term infants. The environment of an intensive care unit is totally different from what an infant would have experienced if he or she had remained in utero until term. Based on these two premises, nursing care must be geared toward making the environment of an infant as atraumatic as possible while helping the infant adjust to new experiences with his or her limited ability.

The usual sound level of nurseries has been documented to be about 40 to 50 dB; a radio playing raises this to 60 to 65 dB. The closing of port-

BOX 26.14 FOCUS ON . . .

EVIDENCE-BASED PRACTICE

Does Developmental Care Make a Measurable Difference in Preterm Infants' Outcome?

For this study, 92 preterm infants, weighing less than 1,250 g and with ages less than 28 weeks, were divided into two care groups. An experimental group received individualized developmental care; the control group received routine nursery care. The results of the study were dramatic. The infants who received developmental care had shorter durations of parenteral feeding, briefer transitions to full oral feeding, and shorter intensive care nursery and hospital stays. They had better weight, length, and head circumferences than routine-care infants; they also had enhanced autonomic, motor, state, attention, and self-regulatory functioning, and a lower incidence of necrotizing enterocolitis. Their families were rated as having less family stress and more appreciation of their infants than families in the routine-care group.

This is an important study for nurses, because nurses are the health care professionals who not only set the tone for care in a neonatal intensive care nursery but are also most influential in making developmental care both a reality and a success. Appreciating how important developmental care can be for preterm infants should provide motivation to make the necessary changes to institute such care in a nursery setting.

Source: Als, H., et al. (2004). A three-center, randomized, controlled trial of individualized developmental care for very-low-birthweight preterm infants: Medical, neurodevelopmental, parenting, and caregiving effects. *Journal of Developmental & Behavioral Pediatrics, 24*(6), 399–408.

holes or tapping on the sides of incubators raises the sound level inside them to 80 dB or more. Other abnormal stimuli are bright lights for 24 hours a day, frequent handling, and painful procedures.

When a preterm infant is stressed, behaviors such as respiratory pauses, tachypnea, color changes, tremors, sighing, flaccidity, finger splaying, and gaze averting occur. Such behaviors are alerts that the environment has become too stimulating and needs to be modified. Activities such as dimming the lights or covering an incubator, turning an infant to the side and containing his body with rolled towels, offering nonnutritive sucking, and maintaining a "quiet hour" to reduce sound are all ways to reduce stimuli.

Nursing Diagnosis: Parental health-seeking behaviors related to preterm infant's needs for health maintenance

Outcome Evaluation: Parents describe schedule for basic immunizations and health assessments and state who will provide ongoing health care.

BOX 26.15

Nursing Outcomes Classification (NOC) and Nursing Interventions Classification (NIC)

Developmental Care

NOC: Child Development (various age determinations)

Child development is defined as the milestones of physical, cognitive, and psychosocial progression by specific age determinations, such as 2 months, 4 months, 6 months, 12 months, 2 years, and so on (Johnson, Maas, & Moorhead, 2000). Some specific indicators suggesting that this outcome has been achieved for the child at 2 months of age include the following:

- Closed posterior fontanelle
- Ability to lift head, neck, and upper chest with support on forearms when prone
- Frequently open hands
- Fading of grasp reflex
- Demonstration of interest in auditory and visual stimuli
- Smiling
- Evidence of pleasure in interactions, especially with primary caregivers

NIC: Developmental Care

Developmental care is defined as structuring the environment to provide care in response to the behavioral cues and states of the preterm infant (McCloskey & Bulechek, 2000). Some important activities associated with implementing this intervention include:

- Providing space on the unit and at the bedside for the parents
- Supplying accurate, factual information about the infant's condition, treatment, and needs

- Informing parents about developmental concerns and issues
- Assisting parents to become acquainted with their infant
- Teaching parents to recognize cues and states
- Demonstrating infant capabilities and how to elicit infant's visual and auditory attention
- Pointing out infant's self-regulatory activities
- Providing time-out when infant exhibits signs of stress
- Providing boundaries to maintain flexion of extremities while still allowing room for extension and supports to maintain positioning
- Monitoring stimuli, decreasing environmental ambient light and environmental noise
- Positioning incubator away from noise sources
- Timing infant care and feeding around sleep/wake cycle
- Clustering care to promote longest possible sleep interval and energy conservation
- Using slow, gentle movements when handling, feeding, or caring for the newborn
- Promoting parent participation in feeding, including use of nonnutritive sucking
- Establishing consistency and predictable routines
- Providing stimulation using tape-recorded instrumental music, mobiles, massage, rocking, and touch as appropriate

---

Discharge from an NICU is a major transition for parents as well as the infant. Before discharge, the parents of a preterm infant need to learn and practice any special methods of care necessary for their infant and interventions to help maximize their child's development. Some parents tend to overprotect preterm infants, such as not allowing visitors or not taking an infant outside. Let parents know their concern is normal, but overprotection is not necessary.

Ongoing health maintenance of a preterm infant follows the usual pattern of well-child care. Basic immunizations are given according to the chronologic age of an infant. In many communities, NICUs maintain their own well-child conferences for infants who were hospitalized there. This allows for long-term follow-up studies on the effect of oxygen or drug therapy and continuity of care. Many parents prefer bringing their infant back to such a facility rather than establishing a new network of health care because they have already established trust and confidence in that health care team. This often

also increases their self-esteem because they hear the staff's delight in the progress made by their child. However, preterm infants can be followed by any health care provider for well-child care.

When plotting the height and weight of preterm infants at well-child visits, remember to account for early birth on the growth chart by double charting—that is, plotting the child's weight and height according to the chronologic age (a pattern that probably in the early months places the child below the 10th percentile). Then, in another color, plot the height and weight according to an infant's "setback" or adjusted age, or the age an infant would be if he or she had been born at term. A preterm baby typically gains "catch-up" weight in the first 6 months of life, so by 1 year of age a baby plots over the 10th percentile on a growth chart without accounting for a setback age.

Evaluate growth and development of a preterm infant by the same manner. A preterm infant can be expected to meet first-year milestones not at the chronologic age but at the setback age.

To evaluate the parents' transition to having so small an infant at home, ask at health promotion visits if the parents are:

- Beginning to feel more comfortable with their infant
- Able to allow the child to stay with a baby-sitter or another family member
- Beginning to incorporate their infant normally into their family life
- Making plans for the infant beyond the immediate newborn period

The Postterm Infant

A postterm infant is one born after the 42nd week of a pregnancy (Moore & Martin, 2003). Most nurse-midwives and obstetricians recommend inducing labor at 2 weeks postterm to avoid postmature births. However, when gestational age has been miscalculated or if for some other reason labor is not induced until week 43 of pregnancy or after, the pregnancy may result in a postterm infant.

An infant who stays in utero past week 42 of pregnancy is at special risk because a placenta appears to function effectively for only 40 weeks. After that time, it seems to lose its ability to carry nutrients effectively to the fetus. The fetus who remains in utero with a failing placenta may die or develop **postterm syndrome.** Infants with this syndrome have many of the characteristics of the SGA infant: dry, cracked, almost leather-like skin from lack of fluid, and absence of vernix. They may be lightweight from a recent weight loss that occurred because of the poor placental function. The amount of amniotic fluid may be less at birth than normal, and it may be meconium-stained. Fingernails will have grown well beyond the end of the fingertips. Such infants may demonstrate an alertness much more like a 2-week-old baby than a newborn.

When a pregnancy becomes postterm, a sonogram may be obtained to measure the biparietal diameter of the fetus. A nonstress test or complete biophysical profile (see Chapter 8) may be done to establish whether the placenta is still functioning adequately. Cesarean birth may be indicated if a nonstress test reveals that compromised placental functioning may occur during labor.

At birth, the postterm baby is likely to have difficulty establishing respirations, especially if meconium aspiration occurred. In the first hours of life, hypoglycemia may develop because the fetus had to use stores of glycogen for nourishment in the last weeks of intrauterine life. Subcutaneous fat levels may also be low, having been used in utero. This can make temperature regulation difficult, making it important to prevent a postterm infant from becoming chilled at birth or during transport. Polycythemia may have developed from decreased oxygenation in the final weeks. The hematocrit may be elevated because of the polycythemia and dehydration, which lowers the circulating plasma level.

Any woman is anxious when she does not have her baby on her due date. She becomes extremely anxious and perhaps angry when it is determined her baby is postterm or should have been born earlier. It may seem that if a baby stayed so long in utero, he or she should be extra healthy and strong. Why, then, she asks, is her baby being transferred for special care? A mother may also feel guilty for not providing well for her infant in the last few weeks of pregnancy.

Make sure a mother spends enough time with her newborn to assure herself that although birth did not occur at the predicted time, the baby should do well with appropriate interventions to control possible hypoglycemia or meconium aspiration. All postterm infants need follow-up care until at least school age to track their developmental abilities. The lack of nutrients and oxygen in utero may have left them with neurologic symptoms that will not become apparent until they attempt fine-motor tasks.

ILLNESS IN THE NEWBORN

A number of illnesses occur specifically in newborns. These automatically cause the infant to become high risk.

Respiratory Distress Syndrome

Respiratory distress syndrome (RDS) of the newborn, formerly termed *hyaline membrane disease,* most often occurs in preterm infants, infants of diabetic mothers, infants born by cesarean birth, or those who for any reason have decreased blood perfusion of the lungs, such as occurs with meconium aspiration (Rodriguez, 2003). The pathologic feature of RDS is a hyaline-like (fibrous) membrane formed from an exudate of an infant's blood that begins to line the terminal bronchioles, alveolar ducts, and alveoli. This membrane prevents exchange of oxygen and carbon dioxide at the alveolar–capillary membrane. The cause of RDS is a low level or absence of surfactant, the phospholipid that normally lines the alveoli and reduces surface tension on expiration to keep the alveoli from collapsing on expiration.

Because surfactant does not form until the 34th week of gestation, as many as 30% of low-birthweight infants and as many as 50% of very-low-birthweight infants are susceptible to this complication.

Pathophysiology

High pressure is required to fill the lungs with air for the first time and overcome the pressure of lung fluid. For example, it takes a pressure between 40 and 70 cm H_2O to inspire a first breath but only 15 to 20 cm H_2O to maintain quiet, continued breathing. If alveoli collapse with each expiration, as happens when surfactant is deficient, forceful inspirations are still required to inflate them.

Even very immature infants release a bolus of surfactant at birth into their lungs from the stress of birth. However, with deficient surfactant, areas of hypoinflation begin to occur and pulmonary resistance increases. Blood then shunts through the foramen ovale and the ductus arteriosus as it did during fetal life. The lungs are poorly perfused, affecting gas exchange. As a result, the production of surfactant decreases even further.

The poor oxygen exchange leads to tissue hypoxia, which causes the release of lactic acid. This, combined with the increasing carbon dioxide level resulting from the formation of the hyaline membrane on the alveolar surface, leads to severe acidosis. Acidosis causes vasoconstriction, and decreased pulmonary perfusion from vasoconstriction further limits surfactant production. With decreased surfactant production, the ability to stop alveoli from collapsing with each expiration becomes impaired. This vicious cycle continues until the oxygen–carbon dioxide exchange in the alveoli is no longer adequate to sustain life without ventilator support.

Assessment

Most infants who develop RDS had difficulty initiating respirations at birth. After resuscitation, they appear to have a period of hours or a day when they are free of symptoms because of an initial release of surfactant. During this time, subtle signs may appear:

- Low body temperature
- Nasal flaring
- Sternal and subcostal retractions
- Tachypnea (more than 60 respirations per minute)
- Cyanotic mucous membranes

Within several hours, expiratory grunting, caused by closure of the glottis that creates a prolonged expiratory time, can be heard. A partially closed glottis is helpful as it increases the pressure in the alveoli on expiration, helps to keep the alveoli from collapsing, and makes oxygen exchange more complete. Even with this attempt at better oxygen exchange, however, as the disease progresses, infants become cyanotic and their PO_2 and oxygen saturation levels fall in room air. On auscultation, there may be fine rales and diminished breath sounds because of poor air entry. As distress increases, an infant may exhibit:

- Seesaw respirations (on inspiration, the anterior chest wall retracts and the abdomen protrudes; on expiration, the sternum rises)
- Heart failure, evidenced by decreased urine output and edema of the extremities
- Pale gray skin
- Periods of apnea
- Bradycardia
- Pneumothorax

The diagnosis of RDS is made on the clinical signs of grunting, cyanosis in room air, tachypnea, nasal flaring, retractions, and shock. A chest x-ray will reveal a diffuse pattern of radiopaque areas that look like ground glass (haziness). Blood gas studies (taken from an umbilical vessel catheter) will reveal respiratory acidosis. A betahemolytic, group B streptococcal infection may mimic RDS, as this infection is so severe in newborns that the insult to the lungs is enough to stop surfactant production. Cultures of blood, cerebrospinal fluid, and skin may be obtained to rule out this condition. An antibiotic (penicillin or ampicillin) and an aminoglycoside (gentamicin or kanamycin) may be started while culture reports are pending.

Therapeutic Management

RDS can be largely prevented by the administration of surfactant through an endotracheal tube at birth for an infant at risk because of low gestational age (Bevilacqua & Parmigiani, 2003).

Surfactant Replacement. As a preventive measure, synthetic surfactant is sprayed into the lungs by a syringe or catheter by an endotracheal tube at birth while an infant is first positioned with the head held upright and then tilted downward. It is important an infant's airway not be suctioned for as long a period as possible after administration of surfactant to avoid suctioning the drug away. Although there are almost no unfavorable reactions to surfactant administration, some, such as mucus plugging from the solution, do occur. An infant who is receiving surfactant and then is placed on a ventilator needs close observation because lung expansion can improve rapidly. Anticipate the need to adjust ventilator settings to prevent excessive lung pressure.

Oxygen Administration. Administration of oxygen is necessary to maintain correct PO_2 and pH levels. Continuous positive airway pressure (CPAP) or assisted ventilation with positive end-expiratory pressure (PEEP) will exert pressure on the alveoli at the end of expiration and keep the alveoli from collapsing (De Paoli, Morley & Davis, 2003). This greatly improves oxygen exchange. A possible complication of oxygen therapy in the very immature or very ill infant is retinopathy of prematurity (see discussion later in chapter) or bronchopulmonary dysplasia (see Chapter 40).

Ventilation. Normally, on a ventilator, inspiration is shorter than expiration, or there is an inspiratory/expiratory ratio (I/E ratio) of 1 : 2. It is difficult to deliver enough oxygen to stiff, noncompliant lungs in this usual ratio without forcing the air into the lungs at such a high pressure and rapid rate that a pneumothorax becomes a constant fear. Infant ventilators are therefore available with a reversed I/E ratio (2 : 1). These are pressure-cycled to control the force with which air is delivered. High-frequency, oscillatory, and jet ventilation are other methods of introducing oxygen to infants with noncompliant lungs. These systems maintain airway pressure and then intermittently "jet" or oscillate at a rapid rate (400 to 600 times a minute) an additional amount of air to inflate alveoli.

Complications of any type of ventilation are possible, such as pneumothorax and impaired cardiac output because of decreased blood flow through the pulmonary artery from lung pressure. There is also a possible risk of increased intracranial and arterial pressure and hemorrhage from changing blood pressure. Limiting fluid intake may help to decrease pulmonary artery pressure.

Indomethacin or ibuprofen may be used to cause closure of a patent ductus arteriosus, making ventilation more efficient (Shah & Ohlsson, 2005). Indomethacin has been associated with adverse effects such as decreased renal function, decreased platelet count, and gastric irritation. Carefully monitor urine output and observe for bleeding, especially at puncture sites.

Additional Therapy. Yet another method of increasing pulmonary blood flow is by using muscle relaxants. Pancuronium (Pavulon) can be administered intravenously to the point of abolishing spontaneous respiratory action. Doing so allows mechanical ventilation to be accomplished at lower pressures because there is no normal muscle resistance to overcome. The possibility of pneumothorax is reduced while P_{O_2} is increased. Obviously an infant who has no spontaneous respiratory function because of drug administration needs critical observation and frequent ABG analysis because he or she totally depends on caregivers at this point (Cools & Offringa, 2005).

The effect of pancuronium decreases as the life of the drug expires; its effect can be interrupted by the administration of atropine or injectable neostigmine methylsulfate (Prostigmin Methylsulfate Injectable). For this reason, when pancuronium is being administered, both atropine and Prostigmin should be immediately available. An infant's plan of care should be specially marked to show that pancuronium therapy is being used so in the event of a power failure, manual ventilatory assistance can be begun immediately.

Some infants are maintained on **extracorporeal membrane oxygenation** (ECMO) to ensure adequate oxygenation (Elbourne, Field & Mugford, 2005). Other therapies include liquid ventilation or administration of perfluorocarbons and inhalation of nitric oxide (Schreiber et al., 2003).

Extracorporeal Membrane Oxygenation. ECMO was first developed as a means of oxygenating blood during cardiac surgery. Its current use has expanded to the management of chronic severe hypoxemia in newborns with illnesses such as meconium aspiration, RDS, pneumonia, and diaphragmatic hernia. It is used also for near-drowning victims or infants with severe lung infection. With ECMO, blood is removed from the baby by gravity using a venous catheter advanced into the right atrium of the heart. The blood circulates from the catheter to the ECMO machine, where it is oxygenated and rewarmed. It is then returned to an infant's aortic arch by a catheter advanced through the carotid artery. ECMO is typically used for 4 to 7 days. It has many potential complications, chief of which is intracranial hemorrhage, possibly from the anticoagulation therapy necessary to prevent thromboembolism. Constant nursing care is required for a child receiving ECMO to ensure that the child's blood volume remains adequate, bleeding does not occur, and adequate oxygen is being supplied to body tissues.

Liquid Ventilation. Liquid ventilation involves the use of perfluorocarbons, substances used in industry to assess for leakage in pipes. When oxygen is bubbled through it, perfluorocarbons pick up and carry the oxygen with them. When perfluorocarbons are introduced into lungs that inflate poorly because they are deficient in surfactant, or in lungs damaged by trauma or disease, the weight of the fluid, which is heavy compared with air, helps to distend the lungs. As the liquid moves into a lung, oxygen is carried along with it; as the liquid spreads over all lung surfaces, an exchange of oxygen occurs (Hancock et al., 2004). The administration of liquid ventilation can also be used to deliver surfactant to a newborn's lungs.

Nitric Oxide. An additional measure that can help to oxygenate a newborn's lungs is the administration of nitric oxide. This causes pulmonary vasodilation, which can be helpful to increase blood flow to the alveoli when persistent pulmonary hypertension is present (Schreiber et al., 2003).

What if... while you were caring for Baby Atkins, who is ventilator-dependent and receiving pancuronium, a power failure occurred? What would be your first actions?

Supportive Care. An infant with RDS must be kept warm because cooling increases acidosis in all newborns, and for the newborn with RDS it may increase to lethal levels. Keeping an infant warm also reduces the metabolic oxygen demand. Provide hydration and nutrition with intravenous fluids, glucose, or gavage feeding because the respiratory effort makes an infant too exhausted to suck (Box 26.16).

Prevention

RDS rarely occurs in mature infants. Dating a pregnancy by sonogram and by documenting that the level of lecithin in surfactant obtained from amniotic fluid exceeds that of sphingomyelin by 2:1 are important ways to be certain an infant born by cesarean birth or has labor induced is mature enough that RDS is not likely to occur.

Using tocolytic agents such as magnesium sulfate or terbutaline can help to prevent preterm birth for a few days. Because steroids appear to quicken the formation of lecithin, it may be possible to prevent RDS in infants by administering two injections of a glucocorticosteroid, such as betamethasone, to the mother at 12 and 24 hours during this time. This is most effective when given between weeks 24 and 34 of pregnancy. Unfortunately, there is often no warning that preterm birth is imminent until hours before birth. Because the steroid does not take effect before 24 to 48 hours, some labors and births will progress too rapidly for this preventive measure to be effective.

✓ Checkpoint Question 3

Baby Atkins has surfactant administered at birth. The purpose of surfactant is to:

a. Help raise lung secretions by relaxing the airway
b. Prevent alveoli from collapsing on expiration
c. Paralyze respiratory muscles to synchronize breathing
d. Reduce gastric secretions by action on the pancreas

Transient Tachypnea of the Newborn

At birth, a newborn may have a rapid rate of respirations, up to 80 breaths per minute when crying. Within 1 hour, however, this rapid rate slows to between 30 and 60 breaths per minute. In about 10 in 1,000 live births, the respiratory rate remains at a high level, between 80 and 120 breaths per minute (Takayama, 2003). The infant does not appear to be in a great deal of distress, aside from the tiring effort of breathing so rapidly. He or she may have mild retractions but not marked cyanosis. Mild hypoxia and hypercapnia may be present. Feeding is difficult because

(text continues on page 782)

B O X 2 6 . 1 6 : **Focus on Nursing Care Planning**

A Multidisciplinary Care Map for
A Newborn with Respiratory Distress Syndrome

•

Mr. and Mrs. Atkins are the parents of a 34-week-old, 2-lb baby boy, born last night after a short, 4-hour labor.

Family Assessment

Family consists of two parents. Mr. Atkins works as a consulting engineer; Mrs. Atkins worked before pregnancy as a home decorator. Mr. Atkins was out of town on business so was not present for the infant's birth. Mrs. Atkins has not visited the intensive care nursery. She refused to sign the birth certificate because she could not decide on a name. She said, "I don't want to give him our favorite name because he might die." Mr. Atkins telephoned early this morning and acted more upset the baby was born than relieved the baby was receiving intensive care. He asked his wife, "What did you do to cause this?"

Client Assessment

Newborn, 5 hours old, delivered vaginally. Difficulty establishing respirations at birth. Resuscitated by the neonatal nurse practitioner and respiratory therapist and then transported to the intensive care nursery. Temperature 97.2°F (36.2°C). Bradycardic and tachypneic with grunting respirations. Sternal and subcostal retractions present. Skin pale and somewhat cyanotic. Chest x-ray with ground-glass appearance. Arterial blood gases (ABGs) reveal respiratory acidosis. Endotracheal (ET) intubation, mechanical ventilation, supplemental oxygen, and intravenous fluid therapy initiated.

Nursing Diagnosis

Impaired gas exchange related to immaturity of newborn's lungs and lack of surfactant

Outcome Criteria

Vital signs within acceptable parameters. Temperature maintained at 97.7°F (36.5°C). Absence of cyanosis; diminished retractions; ABG values within acceptable parameters; no sound of grunting respirations.

Team Member Responsible	Assessment	Intervention	Rationale	Expected Outcome
Activities of Daily Living				
Nurse/ neonatal nurse practitioner	Assess respiratory rate, depth, and rhythm; auscultate lung sounds; evaluate ABG results and skin color.	Maintain respiratory program as prescribed, such as oxygen by ET tube or ventilator.	Signs of increasing respiratory distress may denote lessening air exchange.	Infant maintains a stable respiratory rate and depth with assistive respiratory aids in place.
Nurse	Assess infant's axillary temperature every hour.	Maintain a neutral thermal environment so infant's temperature remains stable.	Neutral thermal environment minimizes the risk of cold stress, which increases metabolic demands for oxygen.	Infant's temperature is maintained at 36.5°C (97.8°F) axillary.
Consultations				
Nurse	Determine what developmental care resources will be available for infant care.	Consult with developmental care coordinator as to specific developmental care measures for infant.	Developmental care or trying to reduce infant stress can improve infant's outcome.	Developmental care coordinator establishes an individualized program for infant care.

(continued)

Team Member Responsible	Assessment	Intervention	Rationale	Expected Outcome
Procedures/Medications				
Nurse/ neonatal nurse practitioner; physician	Assess infant's response to respiratory support. Assess oxygen saturation levels via pulse oximetry.	Maintain ET tube, mechanical ventilation, and supplemental warm humidified oxygen. Anticipate the need for CPAP or PEEP.	The ET tube protects a patent airway. Mechanical ventilation assists with delivering necessary air to the lungs. Using warm, humidified oxygen prevents cold stress and drying of mucous membranes. Oxygen saturation levels provide information about tissue oxygenation. CPAP and PEEP exert pressure on alveoli at end-expiration, preventing alveolar collapse.	Respiratory support measures are in place, and infant's respiratory rate remains within designated parameters.
Physician/ nurse	Assess availability of surfactant for administration.	Administer surfactant via ET tube as per protocol. Refrain from suctioning for 1 hour if possible.	Surfactant restores the naturally occurring lung surfactant to improve lung compliance. Suctioning would remove the drug from its intended site.	Surfactant is administered.
Nutrition				
Nurse/ nutritionist/ physician	Assess infant's need for nourishment based on gestational age and exhaustion from rapid breathing.	Administer nutrition via enteral feedings: breast milk supplemented with high-calorie formula. Anticipate the need for total parenteral nutrition if weight gain is not sufficient.	Additional nutrients are necessary because stress of RDS requires increased caloric expenditure. Total parenteral nutrition may be necessary to meet these additional needs.	Infant tolerates enteral feedings without difficulty. Mother supplies breast milk for feedings.
Nurse	Assess blood glucose levels every 4 hours by heel stick.	Report hypoglycemia (blood glucose level below 40 mg/dL).	Glucose is a source of energy. Monitoring glucose levels helps to determine if sufficient energy is available to meet the newborn's metabolic needs.	Infant maintains a glucose level over 40 mg/dL.
Patient/Family Education				
Nurse	Assess what parents know about the cause of preterm labor.	Teach parents that the cause of preterm birth often can't be identified.	Parents will need to work together to arrange for best care for preterm infant.	Parents state they are adjusting to shock of preterm birth based on better knowledge of cause.
Psychosocial/Spiritual/Emotional Needs				
Nurse	Assess what activities parents think their very small infant can accomplish.	Invite parents to see, touch, and spend as much time as possible with newborn. Guide them in activities such as skin-to-skin contact and basic care giving.	Seeing, touching, and caring promote attachment. Guidance in activities helps to alleviate anxiety.	Parents visit in nursery or telephone at least every other day; touch and talk to newborn.

(continued)

Team Member Responsible	Assessment	Intervention	Rationale	Expected Outcome
Psychosocial/Spiritual/Emotional Needs				
Nurse	Assess if parents have worked through shock of preterm birth.	Suggest parents bring in a mobile or toy to keep near newborn.	A mobile or toy provides visual stimulation and promotes feelings of participation in the newborn's care.	Parents state they know preterm birth is no one's fault; express interest in parenting.
Discharge Planning				
Nurse	Assess what community organizations will be available to family for continued support.	Refer parents to websites helpful for preterm information; suggest they join local Parents of Preemies organization.	Parents may need continued support after they return home with a small infant.	Parents give examples of how they are making active plans for infant's discharge and care.

the child cannot suck and breathe this rapidly at the same time. A chest x-ray reveals some fluid in the central lung, but aeration is, overall, adequate.

Transient tachypnea appears to result from slow absorption of lung fluid. It may reflect a slight decrease in production of phosphatidyl glycerol or mature surfactant. These factors limit the amount of alveolar surface area available to an infant for oxygen exchange. This limitation requires an infant to increase the respiratory rate and depth to better use the surface available. Transient tachypnea occurs more often in infants who are born by cesarean birth, in infants whose mothers received extensive fluid administration during labor, and in preterm infants. Infants born by cesarean birth are probably more prone to develop this form of respiratory distress because the thoracic cavity is not compressed by the force of vaginal birth, so less lung fluid is expelled than normally.

Close observation of the newborn is a priority. Watch carefully to be certain the increased effort is not tiring. Also watch for beginning signs of a more serious disorder, because a rapid respiratory rate is often the first sign of respiratory obstruction. Oxygen administration may be necessary. Transient tachypnea of the newborn peaks in intensity at approximately 36 hours of life and then begins to fade. Typically, by 72 hours of life, it spontaneously fades as the lung fluid is absorbed and respiratory activity becomes effective.

Meconium Aspiration Syndrome

Meconium is present in the fetal bowel as early as 10 weeks' gestation. An infant with hypoxia in utero experiences a vagal reflex relaxation of the rectal sphincter, which releases meconium into the amniotic fluid. Babies born breech may expel meconium into the amniotic fluid from pressure on the buttocks. In both instances, the appearance of the fluid at birth is green to greenish black from the staining. Meconium staining occurs in approximately 10% to 12% of all pregnancies (Gelfand, Fanaroff & Walsh, 2004). It does not tend to occur in extremely-low-birthweight infants because the substance has not passed far enough in the bowel for it to be at the rectum in these infants.

An infant may aspirate meconium either in utero or with the first breath after birth. Meconium can cause severe respiratory distress in three ways: it causes inflammation of bronchioles because it is a foreign substance; it can block small bronchioles by mechanical plugging; and it can cause a decrease in surfactant production through lung cell trauma. Hypoxemia, carbon dioxide retention, and intrapulmonary and extrapulmonary shunting occur. A secondary infection of injured tissue may lead to pneumonia.

Assessment

Infants with meconium-stained amniotic fluid can have difficulty establishing respirations at birth (those who were not born breech have had a hypoxic episode in utero to cause the meconium to be in the amniotic fluid). The Apgar score is apt to be low. Almost immediately, tachypnea, retractions, and cyanosis occur.

With meconium-stained amniotic fluid, an infant should be suctioned with a bulb syringe or catheter while at the perineum, before the birth of the shoulders, to avoid meconium aspiration. Although there is some dispute as to whether all infants with meconium staining need intubation, those with severe staining are intubated and meconium is suctioned from their trachea and bronchi. Do not administer oxygen under pressure (bag and mask) until an infant has been intubated and suctioned, so that the pressure of the oxygen does not drive small plugs of meconium farther down into the lungs, worsening the irritation and obstruction.

After the initiation of respirations, an infant's respiratory rate may remain elevated (tachypnea) and coarse bronchial sounds may be heard on auscultation. An infant may continue to have retractions because the inflammation of bronchi tends to trap air in the alveoli, limiting the entrance of oxygen. This air trapping may also cause enlargement of the anteroposterior diameter of the chest (barrel chest). Blood gases will reveal a poor gas exchange, evidenced by a decreased P_{O_2} and an increased P_{CO_2}. A chest x-ray will show bilateral coarse infiltrates in the lungs, with spaces of hyperaeration (a peculiar honeycomb effect). The diaphragm will be pushed downward by the overexpanded lungs.

Therapeutic Management

Amniotransfusion can be used to dilute the amount of meconium in amniotic fluid and reduce the risk of aspiration. Some infants are delivered by cesarean birth after deeply meconium-stained amniotic fluid becomes evident during labor. After birth and tracheal suction, infants may need to be treated with oxygen administration and assisted ventilation. Antibiotic therapy may be used to forestall the development of pneumonia as a secondary problem. Lung tissue is fairly noncompliant after meconium aspiration, which may necessitate high inspiratory pressure. This can cause pneumothorax or pneumomediastinum. Infants must be observed closely for signs of trapping air in the alveoli, because the alveoli can expand only so far and then will rupture, sending air into the pleural space (pneumothorax).

Because of increased pulmonary resistance, the ductus arteriosus may remain open, causing blood to shunt from the pulmonary artery into the aorta, compromising cardiac efficiency and increasing hypoxia. Observe an infant closely for signs of heart failure (e.g., increased heart rate or respiratory distress). Maintain a temperature-neutral environment to prevent increasing the metabolic oxygen demands. Chest physiotherapy with clapping and vibration may be helpful to encourage removal of remnants of meconium from the lungs (see Chapter 40). Some infants will be maintained on ECMO to ensure adequate oxygenation.

Although meconium aspiration is a serious insult to a newborn, with therapeutic interventions, the symptoms of this will begin to fade by a week's time.

Apnea

Apnea is a pause in respirations longer than 20 seconds with accompanying bradycardia. Beginning cyanosis also may be present. Many preterm infants have periods of apnea as a result of fatigue or the immaturity of their respiratory mechanisms. Babies with secondary stresses, such as infection, hyperbilirubinemia, hypoglycemia, or hypothermia, tend to have a high incidence of apnea (Thilo & Rosenberg, 2003).

Gently shaking an infant or flicking the sole of the foot often stimulates the baby to breathe again, almost as if the child needed to be reminded to maintain this function. If an infant does not respond to these simple measures, resuscitation is necessary.

Closely observe all newborns, but especially preterm ones, to detect these apneic episodes. Apnea monitors that record respiratory movements are invaluable tools to detect failing respiration and sound a warning an infant needs attention. An infant with frequent or difficult-to-correct episodes may be placed on a ventilator to provide respiratory coordination until he or she is more mature.

To help prevent episodes of apnea, maintain a neutral thermal environment and use gentle handling to avoid excessive fatigue. Always suction gently to minimize nasopharyngeal irritation, which can cause bradycardia due to vagal stimulation. Using indwelling nasogastric tubes rather than intermittent ones can also reduce the amount of vagal stimulation. After feeding, observe an infant carefully because the full stomach can put pressure on the diaphragm. Careful burping also helps to reduce this effect.

Never take rectal temperatures in infants prone to apnea; the resulting vagal stimulation can reduce the heart rate (bradycardia), which can lead to apnea. Theophylline or caffeine sodium benzoate may be administered to stimulate respirations. The mechanism by which these drugs reduce the incidence of apneic episodes is unclear, but they appear to increase an infant's sensitivity to carbon dioxide, ensuring better respiratory function. Infants who have had an apneic episode severe enough to require resuscitation are at a high risk for sudden infant death syndrome (SIDS). Such infants may be discharged home with a monitoring device to be used for 2 to 6 months.

Sudden Infant Death Syndrome

SIDS is a sudden unexplained death in infancy (Livesey, 2005). It tends to occur at a higher-than-usual rate in infants of adolescent mothers, infants of closely spaced pregnancies, and underweight and preterm infants. Also prone to SIDS are infants with bronchopulmonary dysplasia, twins, Native American infants, Alaskan native infants, economically disadvantaged black infants, and infants of narcotic-dependent mothers. The peak age of incidence is 2 to 4 months of age.

Although the cause of SIDS is unknown, a number of theories about its cause have been postulated. In addition to prolonged but unexplained apnea, other possible contributing factors may include:

- Viral respiratory or botulism infection
- Pulmonary edema
- Brain stem abnormalities
- Neurotransmitter deficiencies
- Heart rate abnormalities
- Distorted familial breathing patterns
- Decreased arousal responses
- Possible lack of surfactant in alveoli
- Sleeping prone (respiratory muscles are restricted)

Typically, affected infants are well nourished. Parents report an infant may have had a slight head cold. After being put to bed at night or for a nap, the infant is found dead a few hours later. Infants who die this way do not appear to make any sound as they die, which indicates they die with laryngospasm. Although many infants are found with blood-flecked sputum or vomitus in their mouths or on the bedclothes, this seems to occur as the result of death, not as its cause. An autopsy often reveals petechiae in the lungs and mild inflammation and congestion in the respiratory tract. However, these symptoms are not severe enough to cause sudden death. It is clear these children do not suffocate from bedclothes or choke from overfeeding, underfeeding, or crying. Since the American Academy of Pediatrics made its recommendation to put newborns to sleep on their back or side, the incidence of SIDS has declined almost 50% (Li et al., 2003).

Parents have a difficult time accepting the death of a child, especially when it happens so suddenly. In discussing the child, they often use both the past and present tense as if they are not yet aware of the death. Many parents experience a period of somatic symptoms that occur with acute grief, such as nausea, stomach pain, or vertigo. Parents should be counseled by a nurse or someone else trained in counseling at the time of the infant's death; it helps if they can talk to this same person periodically for however long it takes to resolve their grief. Some supportive organizations are listed at the beginning of the chapter to help with counseling.

Autopsy reports should be given to parents as soon as they are available (if toxicology tests are included in the autopsy, results will not be available for weeks). Reading that their child's death was unexplained can help to reassure parents the death was not their fault. They need this assurance if they are to plan for other children. If there are older children in the family, they also need assurance that SIDS is a disease of infants and that the strange phenomenon that invaded their home and killed a younger brother or sister will not also kill them. If they wished the infant dead, as all children wish siblings were dead on some days, they need reassurance that their wishes did not cause the baby's death.

When another child is born, parents can be expected to become extremely frightened at any sign of illness in their child. They need support to see them through the first few months of the second child's life, particularly past the point at which the first child died. Some parents may need support to view a second child as an individual child and not as a replacement for the one who died.

Often a new baby born to a family in which a SIDS infant died is screened using a sleep study as a precaution within the first 2 weeks of life. Depending on the parents' level of anxiety, the new baby may receive this screening before hospital discharge. The baby may then be placed on continuous apnea monitoring pending the results of the sleep study.

Apparent Life-Threatening Event

Some infants have been discovered cyanotic and limp in their beds but have survived after mouth-to-mouth resuscitation by parents. An episode of this kind is called an **apparent life-threatening event** (Stratton et al., 2004). For these children as well as for preterm infants with a tendency toward apnea or new babies born to a family whose child died from SIDS, apnea monitoring is available. With apnea monitoring in place, an alarm sounds when the neonate experiences a period of apnea of 20 seconds or more or a decreased heart rate below 80 bpm (Fig. 26.10). If parents are going to use an apnea monitor at home, make certain they will be able to hear it in all parts of the house or apartment. Usually the alarm is not loud enough to be heard in the basement from an upstairs bedroom. Caution them about household noises such as a loud television, radio, vacuum cleaner, or hair dryer that may interfere with hearing the alarm. Be sure they know how to apply and reposition the apnea leads and they are comfortable enough with the monitor to see past it to the child. In addition, parents should be taught cardiopulmonary resuscitation before their infant is discharged from the hospital (Fig. 26.11).

Caring for a child at home on an apnea monitor may be extremely stressful for the parents and their relationship. They often have difficulty finding a competent baby-sitter. These parents can benefit from a community or home care referral so they have a second opinion as to how well they

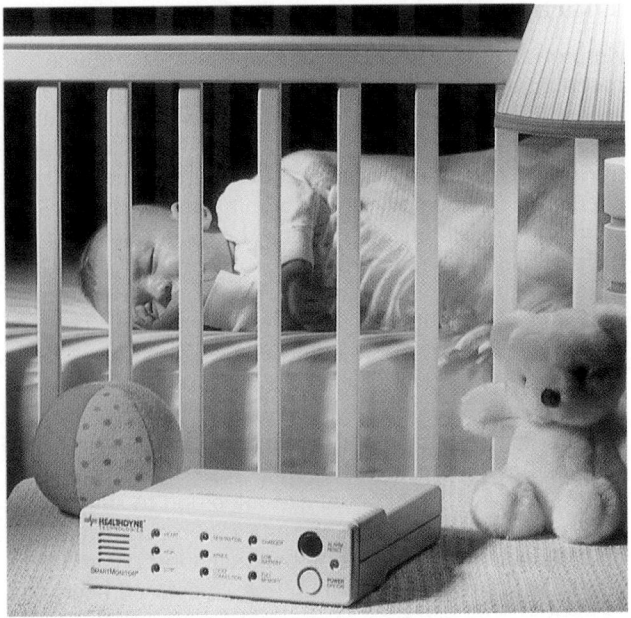

FIGURE 26.10 An apnea monitor for home monitoring. (Photo courtesy of Respironics/Healthdyne Technologies, Marietta, GA.)

are managing, as well as a listening ear to discuss the strain of having to be constantly alert for a sound that means their infant has stopped breathing. Having someone periodically review with them what steps to take should the alarm sound (jiggle the baby, begin mouth-to-mouth resuscitation, call the emergency squad) can be very comforting. Because SIDS is a baffling disease, these parents will live in fear of SIDS until their child reaches at least 1 year of age.

Periventricular Leukomalacia

Periventricular leukomalacia (PVL) is abnormal formation of the white matter of the brain (Counsell et al., 2003). It is caused by an ischemic episode that interferes with circulation to a portion of the brain. Phagocytes and macro-

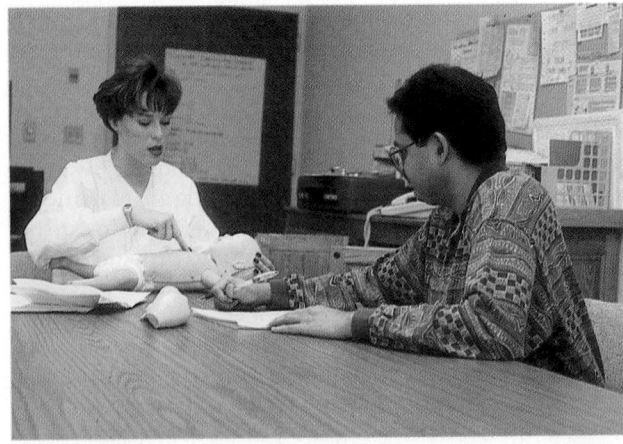

FIGURE 26.11 Parents of infants with respiratory disorders need to learn resuscitation before their infant is discharged from the hospital. Here a nurse teaches the technique using a doll.

crusted. Although facial herpes simplex lesions are probably caused by herpesvirus type 1, limiting contact does not seem excessive in light of the severity of HSV-2 disease. Urge a woman who is separated from her newborn at birth to view her infant from the nursery window and participate in planning care to aid bonding.

Human Immunodeficiency Virus Infection

Human immunodeficiency virus (HIV) infection and acquired immunodeficiency syndrome (AIDS) can be caused by placental transfer or direct contact with maternal blood during birth. The care of an infant with this infection is discussed in Chapter 42.

An Infant of a Diabetic Mother

An infant of a diabetic mother whose illness was poorly controlled during pregnancy is typically longer and weighs more than other babies (macrosomia). The baby also has a greater chance of having a congenital anomaly such as a cardiac anomaly, as if hyperglycemia were teratogenic to the rapidly growing fetus (Ehrenberg et al., 2004). **Caudal regression syndrome** (hypoplasia of the lower extremities) is a syndrome that occurs almost exclusively in such infants.

Most such babies have a cushingoid (fat and puffy) appearance. They tend to be lethargic or limp in the first days of life as a result of hyperglycemia. The macrosomia results from overstimulation of pituitary growth hormone and extra fat deposits created by high levels of insulin during pregnancy. An infant's large size is deceptive, however: such babies are often immature. RDS occurs frequently in these infants because they may be born preterm or even at term, and lecithin pathways may not mature as rapidly in them. High fetal insulin secretion during pregnancy to counteract the hyperglycemia may interfere with cortisol release. This could block the formation of lecithin and prevent lung maturity. A term frequently used for these infants is "fragile giant."

An infant of a diabetic mother loses a greater proportion of weight in the first few days of life than does the average newborn because of the loss of the extra fluid accumulated. Observe an infant closely to be certain that this large weight loss actually represents a loss of extra fluid and that dehydration is not occurring.

Complications

A macrosomic infant has a greater chance of birth injury, especially shoulder and neck injury. Cesarean birth may be necessary to avoid cephalopelvic disproportion. Immediately after birth, an infant tends to be hyperglycemic because the mother was slightly hyperglycemic during pregnancy and excess glucose transfused across the placenta. During pregnancy, the fetal pancreas responds to this high glucose level with islet cell hypertrophy, resulting in matching high insulin levels. After birth, as an infant's glucose level begins to fall because the mother's circulation is no longer supplying glucose, the overproduction of insulin will cause the development of severe hypoglycemia. Hyper-

bilirubinemia also may occur in these infants because, if immature, they cannot effectively clear bilirubin from their system. Hypocalcemia also frequently develops because parathyroid hormone levels are lower in these infants due to hypomagnesemia from excessive renal losses of magnesium (see Chapter 48).

Although infants of diabetic women are usually LGA, an infant born to a woman with extensive blood vessel involvement may be SGA because of poor placental perfusion. The problems of hypoglycemia, hypocalcemia, and hyperbilirubinemia remain the same.

Therapeutic Management

Hypoglycemia is defined as a serum glucose level of less than 40 mg/dL in a newborn. To avoid a serum glucose level from falling this low, infants of diabetic mothers are fed early with formula or administered a continuous infusion of glucose. It is important the child not be given only a bolus of glucose; otherwise, rebound hypoglycemia (accentuating the problem) may occur. Some infants of diabetic mothers have a smaller-than-usual left colon, apparently another effect of intrauterine hyperglycemia, which limits the amount of oral feedings they can take in their first days of life. Signs of an inadequate colon include vomiting or abdominal distention after the first few feedings. Careful monitoring for normal bowel movements is important.

An Infant of a Drug-Dependent Mother

Infants of drug-dependent women tend to be SGA. If the mother is dependent on a drug, an infant will show withdrawal symptoms (neonatal abstinence syndrome) shortly after birth (Box 26.18). These include such signs as:

- Irritability
- Disturbed sleep pattern
- Constant movement, possibly leading to abrasions on the elbows, knees, or nose
- Tremors
- Frequent sneezing
- Shrill, high-pitched cry
- Possible hyperreflexia and clonus (neuromuscular irritability)
- Convulsions
- Tachypnea (rapid respirations), possibly so severe that it leads to hyperventilation and alkalosis
- Vomiting and diarrhea, leading to large fluid losses and secondary dehydration

Specific neonatal abstinence scoring tools may be used to quantify and assess an infant's status. In newborns experiencing opiate withdrawal, signs usually begin 24 to 48 hours after birth, but in some infants they may not appear for up to 10 days. Generally they last approximately 2 weeks, but mild signs may appear for up to 6 months. In heroin-addicted neonates, the signs begin within the first 2 weeks of life, with an average onset of approximately 72 hours. The signs may last 8 to 16 weeks or longer. In methadone-addicted newborns, withdrawal begins later and lasts longer than heroin withdrawal. The

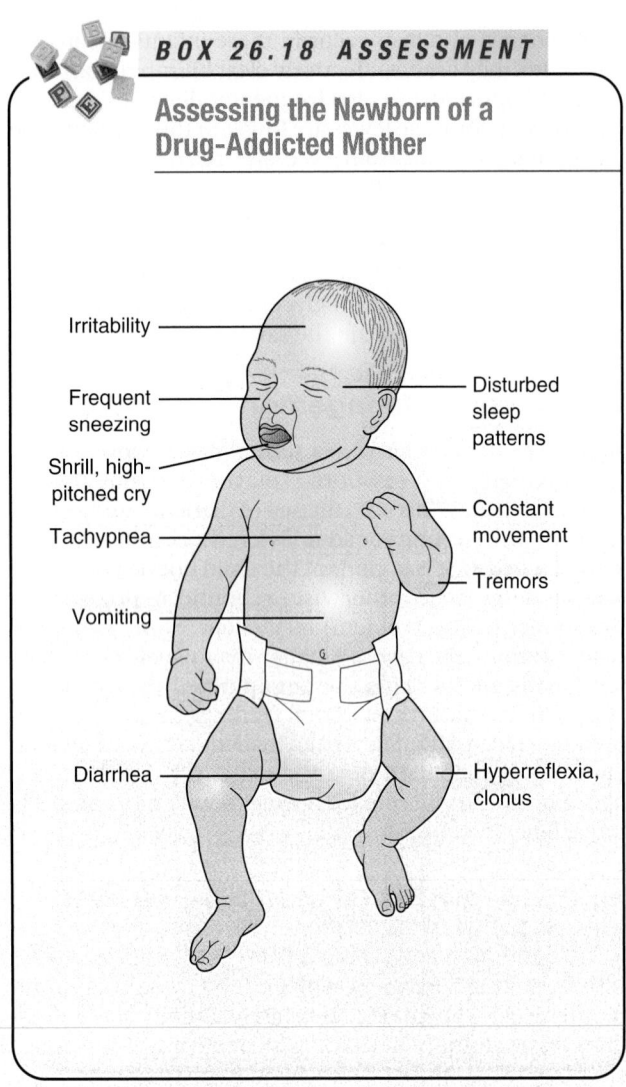

BOX 26.18 ASSESSMENT

Assessing the Newborn of a Drug-Addicted Mother

- Irritability
- Frequent sneezing
- Shrill, high-pitched cry
- Tachypnea
- Vomiting
- Diarrhea
- Disturbed sleep patterns
- Constant movement
- Tremors
- Hyperreflexia, clonus

ing ability and may have difficulty getting enough fluid intake unless gavage-fed.

Specific therapy for an infant is individualized according to the nature and severity of the signs. Maintenance of electrolyte and fluid balance is essential. If an infant has vomiting or diarrhea, intravenous administration of fluid may be indicated. The drugs used to counteract withdrawal symptoms include paregoric, phenobarbital, methadone, chlorpromazine (Thorazine), and diazepam (Valium). These are typically used if the neonatal abstinence scoring system average score is elevated on three successive occasions and nursing interventions do not reduce the score. An infant should not be breast-fed to avoid passing narcotics in breast milk to the child.

Once an infant has been identified as having been exposed to drugs in utero, the mother needs treatment for withdrawal symptoms and follow-up care as much as the infant. In addition, evaluation is necessary to determine before discharge whether an environment that allowed for drug abuse will be safe for an infant at home. Infants who are exposed to drugs in utero may have long-term neurologic problems.

Checkpoint Question 5

Why are infants of diabetic mothers fed early?

a. Their stomachs are empty at birth.
b. To help prevent hypoglycemia
c. Their mothers could not eat during labor
d. To clear mucus from their intestinal tracts

onset varies. The newborn may exhibit signs beginning at 24 to 28 hours, or these early signs may improve, then reappear at 2 to 4 weeks of age. A newborn may exhibit no signs until he or she is 2 to 3 weeks old.

There is no predictable withdrawal sequence noted for the cocaine-addicted neonate. Whether cocaine causes long-term effects varies with different studies, but factors such as maladaptive coping behaviors may be present in such newborns (Cambell, 2003).

Narcotic metabolites or quinine (heroin is often mixed with quinine) may be obtained from an infant's urine in the first hour after birth. These products are quickly cleared from the body, however, so by the time symptoms become severe, detection of narcotic substances may no longer be possible.

Infants of drug-dependent women usually seem most comfortable when firmly swaddled. Keep them in an environment free from excessive stimuli (a small isolation nursery, not a large, noisy one). Some quiet best if the room is darkened. Many infants of heroin-addicted women suck vigorously and continuously and seem to find comfort and quiet if given a pacifier. Infants of methadone- and cocaine-addicted women may have extremely poor suck-

An Infant With Fetal Alcohol Syndrome

Alcohol crosses the placenta in the same concentration as is present in the maternal bloodstream. This results in fetal alcohol exposure and **fetal alcohol syndrome** (Sharpe et al., 2004). Fetal alcohol syndrome appears in about 2 per 1,000 newborns. It is often more difficult to document than recreational drug exposure. Because it is unknown if there is a safe threshold of alcohol ingestion during pregnancy, all pregnant women are advised to avoid alcohol intake to prevent any teratogenic effects on their newborn.

The newborn with fetal alcohol syndrome has a number of possible problems at birth. Characteristics that mark the syndrome include pre- and postnatal growth restriction; central nervous system involvement such as cognitive challenge, microcephaly, and cerebral palsy; and a distinctive facial feature of a short palpebral fissure and thin upper lip. During the neonatal period, an infant may be tremulous, fidgety, and irritable and may demonstrate a weak sucking reflex. Sleep disturbances are common, with the baby tending to be either always awake or always asleep, depending on the mother's alcohol level close to birth.

The most serious long-term effect is cognitive challenge. Behavior problems such as hyperactivity may occur in school-age children. Growth deficiencies may remain throughout life. An infant needs follow-up so any future problems can be discovered. The mother needs follow-up to see if she can reduce her alcohol intake for better overall health.

Key Points

Priorities for infants born with special needs, such as preterm or postterm infants, are the same as for term infants: initiation and maintenance of respirations, establishment of extrauterine circulation, control of body temperature, intake of adequate nourishment, establishment of waste elimination, establishment of an infant–parent relationship, prevention of infection, and provision of developmental care for mental and social development.

Many high-risk infants need resuscitation at birth. Prompt action with such measures as warmth, oxygen, intubation, and suctioning are needed.

A small-for-gestational-age infant is one whose birthweight is below the 10th percentile on an intrauterine growth curve for that age infant. An infant could be preterm, term, or postterm.

Small-for-gestational-age infants have difficulty maintaining body warmth because of low fat stores and may develop hypoglycemia from low glucose stores.

A large-for-gestational-age infant is one whose birthweight is above the 90th percentile on an intrauterine growth chart for that gestational age. The infant could be born preterm, term, or postterm.

Large-for-gestational-age infants tend to be infants of diabetic mothers; they are particularly prone to hypoglycemia or birth trauma.

A preterm infant is one born before 37 weeks of gestation. Preterm infants have particular problems with respiratory function, anemia, jaundice, persistent patent ductus arteriosus, and intracranial hemorrhage. Infants who are born weighing 1,500 to 2,500 g are also termed low-birthweight infants; those born weighing 1,000 to 1,500 g are very-low-birthweight infants; those born weighing between 500 and 1,000 g are extremely very-low-birthweight infants. All such infants need intensive care from the moment of birth to give them their best chance of survival without neurologic after-effects caused by their being so close to the age of viability.

A postterm infant is one who has remained in utero past week 42 of pregnancy. Postterm infants have particular problems with establishing respirations, meconium aspiration, hypoglycemia, temperature regulation, and polycythemia.

Respiratory distress syndrome commonly occurs in preterm infants from a deficiency or lack of surfactant in the alveoli. Without surfactant, the alveoli collapse on expiration and require extreme force for re-inflation. Primary therapy is synthetic surfactant replacement at birth by endotracheal tube insufflation, followed by oxygen and ventilatory support.

Transient tachypnea of the newborn is a temporary condition caused by slow absorption of lung fluid at birth. Close observation of the infant is necessary until the fluid is absorbed and respirations slow to a normal rate.

Meconium aspiration syndrome occurs from an infant inhaling meconium-stained amniotic fluid before or during birth. Meconium is irritating to the airway and leads to both airway spasm and pneumonia. Infants need oxygen, ventilatory support, and possibly an antibiotic until the effects of the insult to the airway subside. Infants must be suctioned before oxygen administration under pressure to prevent meconium from being forced further into their lungs.

Apnea is a pause in respirations longer than 20 seconds, with accompanying bradycardia. It tends to occur in preterm infants who have secondary stresses such as infection, hyperbilirubinemia, hypoglycemia, or hypothermia. Apnea monitors are used to detect this, and infants who are at high risk for apnea may be discharged home on a home monitoring program.

Sudden infant death syndrome is the sudden, unexplained death of an infant. It is associated with infants sleeping on their stomachs (prone) and preterm birth. An important preventive measure is advising parents to position their infant on the back for sleeping.

Hyperbilirubinemia results from the destruction of red blood cells, due either to a normal physiologic response or an abnormal destruction of red blood cells. Hemolytic disease of the newborn is destruction of red blood cells from Rh or ABO incompatibility. The administration of RHIG (Rh antibodies) to Rh-negative mothers during pregnancy and after the birth of an Rh-positive infant to an Rh-negative mother has greatly reduced the incidence of the condition. Affected infants are jaundiced from release of bilirubin from injured red blood cells. Phototherapy and exchange transfusion are used to prevent kernicterus (deposition of bilirubin in brain cells, causing destruction of the cells).

Hemorrhagic disease of the newborn is a lack of clotting ability resulting from a deficiency of vitamin K at birth. This disorder is prevented by administering vitamin K to all infants at birth.

Retinopathy of prematurity is destruction of the retina caused by exposure of immature retinal capillaries to high levels of oxygen. Monitoring oxygen saturation via arterial blood gases is an important preventive measure.

Severe infections acquired at birth that may be seen in newborns include streptococcal group B pneumonia, hepatitis B infection, ophthalmia neonatorum (gonococcal and chlamydial conjunctivitis), and herpesvirus infection. Assessing newborns for symptoms of these infections is an important nursing responsibility.

Infants of diabetic women and those of drug-abusing women are at high risk at birth for further complications. Both need careful assessment for respiratory distress and hypoglycemia.

Critical Thinking Exercises

1. The Atkinses are the family you met at the beginning of the chapter. Mrs. Atkins doesn't want to visit or "waste our favorite name" on her new baby because the baby might die. How would you advise her?

2. Infants who are cared for in neonatal nurseries may need either reduced stimulation because they fatigue so easily or increased stimulation because their stay in the nursery will be so extended. What are examples of developmental care you might use with Baby Atkins?

3. Retinopathy of prematurity is an example of a disease caused by the therapy given an infant. What measures would you take to safeguard Baby Atkins against this disorder?

4. Examine the National Health Goals related to high-risk newborns. Most government-sponsored money for nursing research is allotted based on these goals. What would be a possible research topic to explore pertinent to these goals that would be applicable to the Atkins family and also advance evidence-based practice?

References

Als, H., et al. (2004). A three-center, randomized, controlled trial of individualized developmental care for very-low-birth-weight preterm infants: Medical, neurodevelopmental, parenting, and caregiving effects. *Journal of Developmental & Behavioral Pediatrics, 24*(6), 399–408.

American Academy of Pediatrics. (2005). Car safety seats: A guide for families. (*http://www.aap.org/family/carseatguide.htm*)

American Academy of Pediatrics Subcommittee on Hyperbilirubinemia. (2004). Management of hyperbilirubinemia in the newborn infant 35 or more weeks of gestation. *Pediatrics, 114*(1), 297–316.

American Heart Association. (2005). *Pediatric advanced life support.* Dallas, TX: Author.

Anderson, G. C., et al. (2005). Early skin-to-skin contact for mothers and their healthy newborn infants. *The Cochrane Library (Oxford) (4)* (CD003519).

Askie, L. M., & Henderson-Smart, D. J. (2004). Restricted versus liberal oxygen exposure for preventing morbidity and mortality in preterm or low birth weight infants. *The Cochrane Library (Oxford)(4)* (CD001077).

Bevilacqua, G., & Parmigiani, S. (2003). An observational study of surfactant treatment in infants of 23–30 weeks' gestation: Comparison of prophylaxis and early rescue. *Journal of Maternal-Fetal & Neonatal Medicine, 14*(3), 197–204.

Boyd, S. (2004). Treatment of physiological and pathological neonatal jaundice. *Nursing Times, 100*(13), 40–43.

Cambell, S. (2003). Prenatal cocaine exposure and neonatal/infant outcomes. *Neonatal Network: The Journal of Neonatal Nursing, 22*(1), 19–21.

Centers for Disease Control and Prevention. (2004). Diminishing racial disparities in early-onset neonatal group B streptococcal disease: United States, 2000–2003. *MMWR: Morbidity and Mortality Weekly Report, 53*(23), 502–505.

Cools, F., & Offringa, M. (2005). Neuromuscular paralysis for newborn infants receiving mechanical ventilation. *The Cochrane Library (Oxford) (4)* (CD002773).

Counsell, S. J., et al. (2003). Magnetic resonance imaging of preterm brain injury. *Archives of Disease in Childhood Fetal and Neonatal Edition, 88*(4), F269–274.

Department of Health and Human Services. (2000). *Healthy people 2010.* Washington, DC: DHHS.

De Paoli, A. G., Morley, C., & Davis, P. G. (2003). Nasal CPAP for neonates: What do we know in 2003? *Archives of Disease in Childhood Fetal & Neonatal Edition, 88*(3), F168–172.

Ehrenberg, H. M., Mercer, B. M., & Catalano, P. M. (2004). The influence of obesity and diabetes on the prevalence of macrosomia. *American Journal of Obstetrics and Gynecology, 191*(3), 964–968.

Elbourne, D., Field, D., & Mugford, M. (2005). Extracorporeal membrane oxygenation for severe respiratory failure in newborn infants. *The Cochrane Library (Oxford) (4)* (CD001340).

Fischbach, F. (2004). *A manual of laboratory and diagnostic tests* (6th ed.). Philadelphia: Lippincott Williams & Wilkins.

Garite, T. J., Clark, R., & Thorp, J. A. (2004). Intrauterine growth restriction increases morbidity and mortality among premature neonates. *American Journal of Obstetrics and Gynecology, 191*(2), 481–487.

Gelfand, S. L., Fanaroff, J. M., & Walsh, M. C. (2004). Meconium-stained fluid: Approach to the mother and the baby. *Pediatric Clinics of North America, 51*(3), 655–667.

Hancock, J. B., et al. (2004). Using liquid ventilation to improve lung function in patients with respiratory distress syndrome. *AANA Journal, 72*(3), 218–224.

Herrera, C., Holberton, J., & Davis, P. (2005). Prolonged versus short course of indomethacin for the treatment of patent ductus arteriosus in preterm infants. *The Cochrane Library (Oxford) (4)* (CD003480).

Johnson, M., Maas, M., & Moorhead, S. (2000). *Nursing outcomes classification* (2d ed.). St. Louis: Mosby, Inc.

Karch, A. M. (2004). *Lippincott's nursing drug guide.* Philadelphia: Lippincott Williams & Wilkins.

Li, D., et al. (2003). Infant sleeping position and the risk of sudden infant death syndrome in California, 1997–2000. *American Journal of Epidemiology, 157*(5), 446–455.

Lindemann, P. C., Foshaugen, I., & Lindemann, R. (2004). Characteristics of breast milk and serology of women donating breast milk to a milk bank. *Archives of Disease in Childhood Fetal & Neonatal Edition, 89*(5), F440–441.

Livesey, A. (2005). A multiagency protocol for responding to sudden unexpected death in infancy: Descriptive study. *British Medical Journal, 330*(7485), 227–228.

McCloskey, J., & Bulechek, G. (2000). *Nursing interventions classification* (3d ed.). St. Louis: Mosby, Inc.

Moore, L. & Martin, J. N. Jr. (2003). Prolonged pregnancy. In: J. R. Scott et al. (Eds.), *Danforth's obstetrics and gynecology.* Philadelphia: Lippincott Williams & Wilkins.

National Center for Health Statistics. (2005). *Trends in the health of Americans.* Hyattsville, MD: NCHS.

Ostlie, D. J., et al. (2003). Necrotizing enterocolitis in full-term infants. *Journal of Pediatric Surgery, 38*(7), 1039–1042.

Petrou, S. (2003). Economic consequences of preterm birth and low birthweight. *BJOG: an International Journal of Obstetrics & Gynaecology, 110*(20s), 17–23.

Puckett, R. M.,& Offringa, M. (2005). Prophylactic vitamin K for vitamin K deficiency bleeding in neonates. *The Cochrane Library (Oxford) (4)* (CD002776).

Rahimian, J., & Varner, M. W. (2003). Disproportionate fetal growth. In A. H. DeCherney & L. Nathan (Eds.), *Current obstetric & gynecologic diagnosis & treatment.* New York: McGraw-Hill.

Roberts, D., Neilson, J. P., & Weindling, A. M. (2005). Interventions for the treatment of twin-twin transfusion syndrome. *The Cochrane Library (Oxford) (4)* (CD002073).

Rodriguez, R. J. (2003). Management of respiratory distress syndrome: An update. *Respiratory Care, 48*(3), 279–286.

Schreiber, M. D., et al. (2003). Inhaled nitric oxide in premature infants with the respiratory distress syndrome. *New England Journal of Medicine, 349*(22), 2099–2107.

Shah, S. S., & Ohlsson, A. (2005). Ibuprofen for the prevention of patent ductus arteriosus in preterm and/or low birth weight infants. *The Cochrane Library (Oxford) (4)* (CD004213).

Sharpe, T. T., et al. (2004). Report from the CDC. Physician and allied health professionals' training and fetal alcohol syndrome. *Journal of Women's Health, 13*(2), 133–139.

Sirotnak, A. P., & Krugman, R. D. (2003). Child abuse and neglect. In: W. W. Hay, et al. (Eds.), *Current pediatric diagnosis & treatment* (16th ed.). New York: McGraw-Hill.

Stratton, S. J., et al. (2004). Apparent life-threatening events in infants: High risk in the out-of-hospital environment. *Annals of Emergency Medicine, 43*(6), 711–717.

Surkan, P. J., et al. (2004). Reasons for increasing trends in large for gestational age births. *Obstetrics & Gynecology, 104*(4), 720–726.

Takayama, J. I. (2003). Transient tachypnea of the newborn (TTN). In: M. W. Schwartz (Ed.), *5-Minute pediatric consult* (3rd ed.). Philadelphia: Lippincott Williams & Wilkins.

Trevett T. N. Jr., Dorman, K., Lamvu, G., & Moise, K. J. Jr. (2005). Antenatal maternal administration of phenobarbital for the prevention of exchange transfusion in neonates with hemolytic disease of the fetus and newborn. *American Journal of Obstetrics and Gynecology, 192*(2), 478–482.

Thilo, E. H., & Rosenberg, A. A. (2003). The newborn. In: W. W. Hay et al. (Eds.), *Current pediatric diagnosis & treatment* (16th ed.) New York: McGraw-Hill.

Violette, C., et al. (2003). The complex issues of herpes simplex. *Nursing Spectrum (New England Edition), 7*(1), 20–21.

Walls, M., et al. (2004). Home phototherapy: A feasible, safe and acceptable practice. *Journal of Neonatal Nursing, 10*(3), 92–94.

Wilson, H. R. (2003). Hepatitis B and you: A patient education resource for pregnant women and new mothers. *Journal of Women's Health, 12*(5), 437–441.

Suggested Readings

Altimier, L. B., et al. (2004). Developmental care: Changing the NICU physically and behaviorally to promote patient outcomes and contain costs. *Neonatal Intensive Care, 17*(2), 35–39.

Bhutani, V. K., Johnson, L. H., & Keren, R. (2003). Diagnosis and management of hyperbilirubinemia in the term neonate: For a safer first week. *Pediatric Clinics of North America, 51*(4), 843–861.

Brisch, K. H., et al. (2003). Early preventive attachment-oriented psychotherapeutic intervention program with parents of a very low birthweight premature infant: Results of attachment and neurological development. *Attachment & Human Development, 5*(2), 120–135.

Dunn, M. S., & Reilly, M. C. (2003). Approaches to the initial respiratory management of preterm neonates. *Paediatric Respiratory Reviews, 4*(1), 2–8.

Gilbert, W. M., & Danielsen, B. (2003). Pregnancy outcomes associated with intrauterine growth restriction. *American Journal of Obstetrics & Gynecology, 188*(6), 1596–1599.

Noble, L. (2003). Developments in neonatal technology continue to improve infant outcomes. *Pediatric Annals, 32*(9), 595–603.

Pollack, M. M., & Koch, M. A. (2003). Association of outcomes with organizational characteristics of neonatal intensive care units. *Critical Care Medicine, 31*(6), 1620–1629.

Toyer, R., & Fox, G. F. (2004). Patent ductus arteriosus in preterm infants: Diagnosis and treatment. *Journal of Neonatal Nursing, 10*(4), 112–115.

Tulenko, D. R. (2004). An update on ECMO. *Neonatal Network: Journal of Neonatal Nursing, 23*(4), 11–18.

White-Traut, R. C., et al. (2005). Feeding readiness in preterm infants: The relationship between preterm behavioral state and feeding readiness behaviors and efficiency during transition from gavage to oral feeding. *MCN, American Journal of Maternal Child Nursing, 30*(1), 52–59.

UNIT SIX

The Nursing Role in Health Promotion for a Childrearing Family

Team Member Responsible	Assessment	Intervention	Rationale	Expected Outcome
Nutrition				
Nurse	Employ a 24-hour recall dietary history to assess for usual calcium and vitamin D intake.	Suggest additional sources of calcium or vitamin D if needed.	Calcium is important for good bone healing and absorbed best in the presence of vitamin D.	Client states he understands calcium will help healing and is willing to ingest more as needed.
Patient/Family Education				
Nurse	Assess what parents understand about the development of trust in early life.	Suggest ways to initiate a sense of trust by demonstrating dependability and a warm, loving relationship.	A sense of trust can be reinstated at a later developmental stage if it has been lost.	Parents state they are willing to begin more active steps toward improving relationship with son.
Psychosocial/Spiritual/Emotional Needs				
Nurse	Assess what type of child parents expected to adopt.	Suggest measures that could bring parents and child closer together such as a "game night," always eating meals together, quiet "talk times" before bed.	Identifying differences between expectations and reality can help people understand dissatisfactions.	Client and parents state they are willing to begin active program of shared activities.
Discharge Planning				
Nurse	Assess if client or parents have any further needs they would like to discuss.	Discuss with client and parents adjustments client will have to make to attend school with a cast in place.	Small needs not met can grow into major needs before a return appointment and interfere further with a sense of trust.	Client and parents state they understand adjustments that need to be made and will work them out together.

a child may receive inadequate nutrition because of the family's low socioeconomic status; a parent may lack skills or not give a child enough attention; or a child could have a chronic illness. Many illnesses lower children's appetite; others, such as certain endocrine disorders, directly alter their growth rate.

Environmental influences, however, are not always detrimental. For example, children with phenylketonuria, an inherited metabolic disease, can achieve normal growth and development despite their genetic makeup if their diet (a part of the environment) is properly regulated. The following environmental influences are those most likely to affect growth and development.

Socioeconomic Level

Because health care and good nutrition both cost money, children born into families of low socioeconomic means may not receive adequate health supervision or good nutrition. Poor health supervision can leave them without immunization against measles or other childhood illnesses and therefore vulnerable to diseases that could cause permanent neurologic damage if complications occur. Poor nutrition can also leave them vulnerable to disease as anti-

body formation depends on a good protein intake (Seguin et al., 2005).

Parent–Child Relationship

Cultural norms within a family play a role in determining when a child is expected to achieve particular developmental milestones (Box 27.6). Children who are loved thrive better than those who are not. Either parent or a nonparent caregiver may serve as the primary caregiver or form a primary parent–child love relationship. It is the quality of time spent with children, not the amount of time, that is important. Loss of love from a primary caregiver, as might occur with the death of a parent, or interruption of parental contact through hospitalization, imprisonment, divorce, or inadequate parental love, can interfere with a child's desire to eat, improve, and advance.

Ordinal Position in the Family

The position of a child in the family (first-born child, middle child, youngest child, only child) and the size of the family have some bearing on a child's growth and development. An only child or the oldest child in a family, for

BOX 27.5

Categories of Temperament

The Easy Child

Children are rated as "easy to care for" if they have a predictable rhythmicity, approach and adapt to new situations readily, have a mild to moderate intensity of reaction, and have an overall positive mood quality. Most children, 40% to 50%, are rated by their parents as being in this category.

The Difficult Child

Children are "difficult" if they are irregular in habits, have a negative mood quality, and withdraw rather than approach new situations. Only about 10% of children fall into this category.

Slow-to-Warm-Up Child

Children fall into this category if they are overall fairly inactive; respond only mildly and adapt slowly to new situations, and have a general negative mood. About 15% of children display this pattern. When discussing this temperament with parents, try to use positive terms such as "ways to find a healthy fit for your child" rather than stressing ways the child is hard to manage.

BOX 27.6 FOCUS ON . . .

DIVERSITY OF CARE

Not all nations foster the growth and development of children in the same manner, in part because of cultural variations. In some countries, the predominant theory of childrearing is protective nurturing. Children are not rushed into new experiences like toilet training or beginning school. In others, it is customary to treat children in a harsh, strict manner, using shame or corporal punishment for discipline. Praising children for learning a new skill may be viewed as unnecessary or actually harmful, because this could result in a child being subject to evil forces. In some Asian cultures, an infant's personality is thought to depend not so much on genetic or environmental influences but on the year and time of birth.

Childhood in the United States covers a relatively long time period. In other countries, childhood is short because girls are asked to assume domestic responsibilities early in life and outside or farm work is required early for boys.

What foods children receive depends very much on culture also. Vegetables such as jicama and chayote, for example, may not even be recognized by children in the northeast United States but are popular with those in the Southwest.

Asking a parent questions such as, "What do you do when your baby cries?" "What kind of things do you think a 2-year-old should be able to do?" "What do you do when your 4-year-old misbehaves?" can help you to isolate and better understand cultural differences.

Recognizing cultural variations this way helps to plan care that is specific to a particular child and family.

example, generally excels in language development because conversations are mainly with adults. Children learn by watching other children, however, so a firstborn or only child, who has no example to watch, may not excel in other skills, such as toilet training at an early age.

Health

Diseases that come from environmental sources can have as strong an influence on growth and development as genetically inherited diseases. Infants cared for in neonatal intensive care units may develop some decrease in hearing because of the overstimulation of sound, an example of health being directly influenced by the environment. Children who have residual heart impairment as a result of rheumatic fever might be limited in their ability to play an active sport. The eventual degree of disability will depend not only on the damage caused by the actual disease, however, but also on the attitudes of the people around the child—how disabled they believe the child to be. Treating a child as if he or she were sick or vulnerable to sickness is referred to as "vulnerable child syndrome" (Green & Solnit, 1964). These attitudes about sick children are an influence of environment on development. Fortunately, if an illness does not last long, most children achieve "catch-up" growth afterward.

Nutrition

In the past 20 years, nutrition has become a major focus of health promotion and disease prevention in the United States because the quality of a child's nutrition during the growing years (including prenatally) has a major influence on his or her health and stature (Dudek, 2005). Poor maternal nutrition may limit the growth and intelligence potential of a child from the moment of birth. Children whose diets lack essential nutrients show inadequate physical growth. A lack of energy and stamina prevents children from learning at their best intellectual level. As many as 50% of American children are obese today (Berger, 2004). Children who eat too many carbohydrates and become obese may develop motor skills more slowly than other children because physical movement is more tiring for them. Obese children are sometimes taunted by their playmates and may become loners or have difficulty relating to their peers because of behavior problems or depression about their weight (Lumeng et al., 2003).

Nutrition also plays a vital role in the body's susceptibility to disease because poor nutrition limits the body's ability to resist infection. Lack of calcium could leave a child prone to rickets, a disease that affects growth by causing shortening or bowing of long bones. Lack of vitamins can lead to visual impairments and poor healing (Poustie et al., 2005).

Poor nutrition also plays a major role in the development of chronic illness. Of the eight leading causes of death in adults, six have been linked to dietary excesses: heart disease, cancer, cerebrovascular disease, diabetes mellitus, cirrhosis, and arteriosclerosis. It is clear, too, dietary habits have a cumulative effect; for instance, although heart disease is not one of the top causes of death in children, the arterial changes that cause it begin in childhood. Increased consumption of food and alcohol, decreased levels of exercise, and smoking all lead to a greater incidence of these diet-related diseases in adult life. Establishing healthy eating patterns early in life, therefore, can contribute to better health in the adult years.

Food Guide Pyramid Guidelines for a Healthy Diet

Basic guidelines for a healthy diet have been outlined by a variety of governmental groups, including the U.S. Department of Agriculture (USDA) and the U.S. Department of Health and Human Services. In 1992, a food guide pyramid was developed by the USDA to illustrate these guidelines. It was updated in 2005 to emphasize variety, moderation, and balance and suggest a range of daily servings from each major food group (USDA, 2005). Table 27.1 lists recommended servings for children from the five pyramid food groups. In addition, good nutrition in children should follow a number of "healthy eating" guidelines:

Eat a Variety of Foods. Choices from all food pyramid groups—dairy, meat and poultry, fruits, vegetables, cereals and grains—should be included in what children eat every day. It is also important to vary choices within each food group, as not all foods within a group are nutritionally equivalent.

Balance the Food You Eat With Physical Activity— Maintain or Improve Your Weight. Although the tendency for obesity may be inherited, being overweight in early life also plays a role. Urge parents to be certain their children receive all the nutrients they need for the substantial growth they are undergoing (including a percentage of fat, because this is important for myelination of nerves); at the same time, it is important that children not be overfed, as childhood obesity is associated with development of heart disease and type 2 diabetes in later life (Forrest & Riley, 2004). Balancing a lifestyle of physical activity with sound nutrition, such as omitting sugar-heavy soft drinks, helps to do this (Pontin, 2004).

Choose a Diet With Plenty of Grain Products, Vegetables, and Fruits. Foods with starch and fiber are more beneficial for gastrointestinal function than more processed foods. Fiber, in particular, has been linked to the lowered incidence of a variety of illnesses such as constipation and perhaps colon cancer in later life. Fiber can be included as early as during preschool years in the form of whole-grain cereals and raw fruits such as apples.

Choose a Diet Low in Fat, Saturated Fat, and Cholesterol. The American diet has changed substantially over the past 10 years to reflect this important goal. Many adults now consume low-fat diets, substituting nonfat milk for whole milk, decreasing their consumption of eggs and other high-cholesterol sources, and reducing their

TABLE 27.1

Servings of the Five Pyramid Food Groups for Children

Group	Foods	Recommended Daily Amounts		Major Nutrients Provided
		Children 2–6 yrs	*Older Children*	
Bread, cereals, rice, pasta	Whole-grain and enriched	6 servings	6–11 servings	Thiamin, niacin, riboflavin (if enriched); iron (if enriched); incomplete protein, carbohydrates
Vegetable	Vegetables (yellow and green)	3 servings	3–5 servings	Vitamin A, iron, calcium, carbohydrates (include vitamin A source at least every other day)
Fruit	Fruit	2 servings	2–4 servings	Vitamin C (include vitamin C daily); carbohydrates
Milk, yogurt, cheese	Whole milk and other milk products except butter	2 servings	2–3 servings	Calcium, phosphorus, complete protein, riboflavin, niacin, vitamin D (if vitamin D–fortified milk used), fats
Meat, poultry, fish	Muscle meats (veal, beef, pork) dry beans, eggs; fish; poultry	2 servings	2–3 servings	Complete protein, iron, thiamin, riboflavin, niacin, vitamin B_{12}, fats
Fats, oils, sweets	Candy, cake, fried foods	Use sparingly	Use sparingly	Essential fatty acids, carbohydrates

Data from Department of Agriculture. (2005). *Dietary guidelines for Americans.* Washington, DC: USDA.

consumption of red meat. For children, fat intake does not need to be restricted for the first 2 years of life. Thereafter, fat intake can be tailored to meet the guidelines of 30% total intake for both children and adults. Some foods now contain Olestra, a synthetic fat. Don't recommend this for children (or urge parents to offer this sparingly) until further study is completed because of the danger of fat-soluble vitamins being excreted and lost with the product.

Choose a Diet Moderate in Sugars. Too much sugar in a diet can contribute to both dental caries and obesity. In addition, refined sugar such as that used in soft drinks, prepared foods, candy, and chocolate represents "empty" calories: it is high in calories yet provides no essential nutrients. Although children need adequate carbohydrates for energy, parents can give their children a good start by preventing excessive sugar intake.

Choose a Diet Moderate in Salt and Sodium. The taste for salt is acquired. If unsalted or only lightly salted solid food is offered to infants, they do not develop a desire for heavily salted foods. It is helpful to assess the diet of school-age children and check whether they are eating a diet heavier in salt than necessary because of many salty after-school snacks.

If You Drink Alcoholic Beverages, Do So in Moderation. Adolescents are at increased risk for establishing unhealthy patterns of alcohol use, particularly binge drinking. Educating them about the long-term consequences of alcohol use is as important as educating them on the importance of healthy nutrition for growth (see Chapter 32).

Components of a Healthy Diet

Eating a variety of foods from all five pyramid food groups in moderation is a way of guaranteeing the intake of a balanced diet of proteins, carbohydrates, fats, vitamins, and minerals (Fig. 27.3).

Protein. Protein is the major component of bones, skin, hair, and muscle and is responsible for a wide variety of essential functions in the body. Because it is essential for growth, protein intake is crucial for children. Complete proteins contain all amino acids; incomplete proteins do not. Mixing these two types of protein (pasta and beans, for example) create common dietary staples, which then combine to furnish complete protein.

Carbohydrate. Carbohydrates are the main and preferred fuel of the body to supply energy, so they are essential to the functioning of most body systems, the neurologic system in particular. This is why carbohydrates are so important to infants and toddlers, whose brain cells are actively growing. Sugar supplies an immediate but short-term source of energy; starches, as a rule, supply sustained energy.

Fat. Dietary fat is also a source of energy to the body. It can be an immediate energy source or can be stored if not used, then released when energy is required. Some fat deposits also serve as insulating material for subcutaneous tissues; in infants, fats are necessary to ensure myelination of nerve fibers.

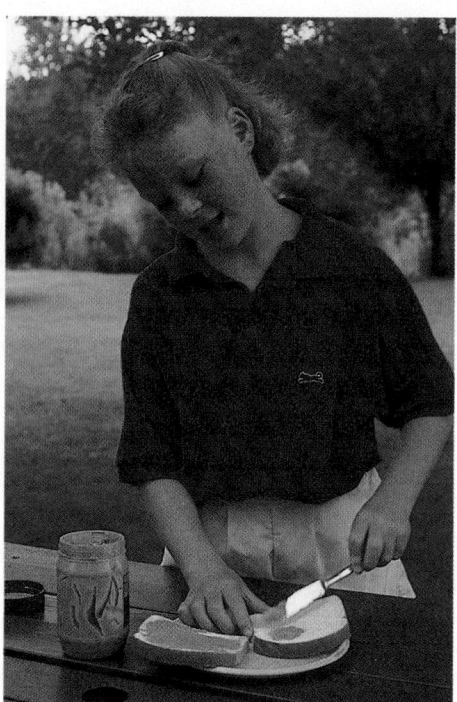

FIGURE 27.3 Good nutritional habits developed early in life provide a child with a health advantage.

Vitamins. Vitamins are organic compounds that are essential for specific metabolic actions in cells. They do not produce energy but are needed by cells to do so. For children, fat-soluble vitamins (A, D, K, and E) are mainly supplied by fortified dairy products, fortified cereals, and plant oils or fish oils. Such vitamins can leave the gastrointestinal tract and be used by the body only by being absorbed along with fat molecules. Once absorbed, they are used by the cells for growth and function or are stored in the liver and fat cells for later use. Because fat-soluble vitamins can be stored by the body, an infant or child can ingest too many of them, although overdosing usually occurs from supplements rather than dietary sources. Water-soluble vitamins (B complex and C) do not need fat for absorption but are not stored well in the body, so they must be taken daily to maintain effective levels in the body. Sources and functions of essential vitamins and results of their deficiencies are summarized in Table 27.2.

Minerals. Minerals are necessary to build new cells and regulate body processes (e.g., fluid and electrolyte balance, nerve transmission, muscle contraction), so they are vital to the health of a growing infant or child. Deficiency in a mineral such as calcium can lead to poor bone development and childhood growth. Minerals are classified according to the amounts needed daily or their importance for body functioning. If more than 100 mg is needed daily, a mineral is a **macronutrient,** or major mineral. If the amount needed is less than 100 mg, it is a **micronutrient,** or minor mineral. Trace minerals refer to those needed in only extremely small amounts. Sources and functions of

TABLE 27.2

Vitamins Essential for Health

Vitamin	Selected Dietary Sources	Function in Body	Results of Deficiency
Fat-Soluble*			
A (retinol)	Liver, carrots, spinach	Important for night vision and corneal integrity and growth	Keratinization of the eye (xerophthalmia) and blindness
D	Egg yolk, margarine, salmon, fortified milk, fortified cereals	Regulates absorption of calcium and phosphorus for bone growth	Rickets (bone deformity) in growing children
E	Margarine, corn oil, peanuts	An antioxidant that protects red blood cells from destruction by oxygen	In immature infants, severe anemia from destruction of red blood cells
K	Cabbage, spinach, pork. Best source: Green leafy vegetables	Aids blood clotting (synthesis of prothrombin)	Bleeding from lack of sufficient clotting action
Water-Soluble			
B complex:			
Thiamin	Wheat germ, yeast, pork	Important for use of glucose in cells	Beriberi, a disease that causes nerve paralysis
Riboflavin	Beef, chicken, liver, avocados, milk	Breaks down fatty acids and amino acids for energy	Red swollen tongue, inflamed eyes, fissures of lips
Niacin	Peanuts, rice bran, liver	Converts glucose to energy, involved in carbohydrate, protein, and fat metabolism	Pellagra (diarrhea, mental confusion, dermatitis, death)
B₆ (pyridoxine)	Liver, herring, salmon, chicken, fish, pork, eggs	Metabolizes amino acids and glucose	Neuritis, depression, nausea, vomiting
B₁₂ (cobalamin)	Lamb, beef kidney, egg yolk, animal products	Blood formation; DNA and RNA synthesis; myelin formation; carbohydrate, protein, and fat metabolism	Macrocytic, megaloblastic anemia (large, nonfunctioning red blood cells)
Folic acid (folacin)	Liver, asparagus, bran	Red and white blood cell structure	Poor red cell formation
C (ascorbic acid)	Broccoli, collards, citrus fruit	Collagen structure, antioxidant	Scurvy (weakness, easy bleeding, joint pain)

*All fat-soluble vitamins can be absorbed only in the presence of lipids and can be transported only in the presence of protein.

various minerals and results of their deficiencies are listed in Table 27.3.

Promoting Adequate Nutritional Intake in Vegetarian Diets

Families may select vegetarian diets for many reasons:

- Economic: Vegetables and grains are less expensive than animal food.
- Ecologic: If everyone ate lower on the food chain, world hunger could be reduced.
- Medical or health-related: Avoiding animal foods stops the ingestion of hormones and chemicals used in meat and poultry production and lowers serum cholesterol, thereby reducing the frequency of atherosclerosis and obesity; avoiding red meat may reduce the likelihood of developing colon cancer as well. Because of the association between saturated fat and bowel cancer and atherosclerosis, the number of families avoiding red meat will probably increase in the future.
- Philosophical: A belief that killing animals for food is unnecessary.
- Religious: Religions such as Hindu and Seventh-Day Adventist promote a vegetarian lifestyle.

Increasing numbers of adults of childrearing age are vegetarians; therefore, many children will eat such diets during their years of most rapid growth (Haddad & Tanzman, 2003). Although a balanced vegetarian diet can be sufficient during childhood, careful assessment and family education are necessary to ensure that it is adequate for growth. Urge parents to become knowledgeable about good nutrition so they are aware of ways to include essential nutrients for

TABLE 27.3

Minerals Essential for Health

Mineral	Selected Dietary Sources	Function in Body	Results of Deficiency or Excess
Macronutrients			
Calcium	Milk, hard cheese	Formation of bone and teeth; muscle contractility	Improper bone growth and maintenance shown by diseases such as rickets in children
Phosphorus	Milk, meats	Formation of bone and teeth; used in cell structure; aids use of glucose	Deficiency unlikely as long as calcium and protein needs are met
Sodium	Table salt	Regulates fluid volume and pH	Deficiency rare but excess leads to hypertension in genetically determined individuals
Chloride	Table salt	Formation of hydrochloric acid; regulates body fluid with sodium	Deficiency rare except with vomiting, which causes loss of hydrochloric acid
Potassium	Meats, dried fruits	Major cation of cells; essential for electrical conduction in muscle and therefore in heart action	Deficiency leading to muscle weakness and heart irritability; occurs in people taking diuretics, because potassium is excreted with urine
Sulfur	Milk, meat, eggs	Essential for protein formation and cell growth	Deficiency rare as long as protein intake is adequate
Magnesium	Cocoa, nuts, green leafy vegetables	Relaxation of muscles after contraction	Deficiency leads to muscle contraction
Micronutrients			
Iodine	Seafood, dairy, iodized salt	Formation of thyroxine and regulation of metabolic rate	Reduced basal metabolic rate and goiter (enlarged thyroid gland)
Iron	Meats, fish, dried fruits, nuts, fortified cereals	Formation of hemoglobin; transport of oxygen to body cells	Deficiency leads to microcytic (small) and hypochromic (pale) red blood cells (iron-deficiency anemia); excess leads to infiltration of tissue (hemosiderosis)
Copper	Nuts, raisins, legumes	Formation of collagen and nerve fiber	Anemia, neutropenia, and severe bone demineralization
Fluoride	Fluoridated water	Reduces dental caries and demineralization from bone	Dental caries
Zinc	Meat, eggs, seafood	Formation of eyes, male reproductive organs, insulin, and taste sensation	Diabetes-like symptoms due to decreased insulin production; poor taste sensation leading to poor food intake
Manganese	Nuts, grains, legumes	Formation of enzymes	Deficiency unlikely
Molybdenum	Organ meats, grains	Mobilizes iron in body	Deficiency apparently unknown
Cobalt	Many sources	Formation of red blood cells in bone marrow	Deficiency rare as long as animal food sources are ingested
Selenium	Seafood, kidney, liver	Immunoglobin formation and prevention of oxidation of cells	Deficiency unknown
Chromium	Meat, cheese, grains	Glucose metabolism	Deficiency seen only in severe malnutrition
Silicon	Many sources	Aids growth of connective tissue and bone	Retarded growth and bone deformity
Nickel	Many sources	Duplication of growth of cells	Has not been determined to be essential for health in humans
Vanadium	Many sources	Lipid metabolism	Has not been determined to be essential for health in humans
Tin	Many sources	Blood formation	Has not been determined to be essential for health in humans

growing children in vegetarian diets, particularly if their children participate in active sports (Barr & Rideout, 2004).

Four main types of vegetarian diets are usually seen:

- A lacto-ovo-vegetarian diet includes dairy products ("lacto"), eggs ("ovo"), and plants (vegetables, fruits, and grains).
- An ovovegetarian diet includes eggs but excludes dairy products.
- A lactovegetarian diet includes dairy products but excludes eggs.
- A vegan diet excludes all animal products and consists of only vegetables, fruits, and grains.

The vegan diet is most restrictive, so it is usually recommended that parents consult with a dietitian or nutritionist to ensure their children receive adequate nutrients on this diet. A fifth type of vegetarian diet is a macrobiotic diet, which falls between vegetarian and vegan diets. Its main sources of protein are grains, seeds, and nuts, but small quantities of egg, fish, and wild game can be added. Macrobiotic diets have different levels of restrictions. In the 1960s, a popular Far Eastern version consisted only of cereal and restricted fluid; it was so restricted it caused death from starvation and nutrient inadequacy (and created a bad reputation for macrobiotic diets). This strict level is rarely seen currently; more lenient macrobiotic diets are adequate for children. All families who eat vegetarian diets need to ensure that their children receive adequate amounts of several specific nutrients.

Protein. Lacto-ovo-vegetarian, ovovegetarian, and lactovegetarian diets provide all of the essential amino acids for growth (both eggs and dairy products provide complete proteins). Vegan diets can also supply essential amino acids by combining cereal and legume combinations such as peanut butter and wheat bread, corn and lima beans, pasta and beans, corn tortillas and beans, or chickpeas and sesame seeds. Complementary proteins do not have to be eaten at the same time to be effective, as long as varied plant proteins are consumed over the course of a day.

Calcium. Dairy products such as milk and cheese supply calcium as well as protein. When these are not eaten, calcium must be obtained from other sources, such as green leafy vegetables (e.g., broccoli or spinach) or grain products such as calcium-fortified tofu or soy flour.

Iron. Meats are the best sources of iron. With meat omitted from a diet, iron must be included from foods such as legumes, whole grains, fortified cereals, dark-green leafy vegetables, or dried fruits. Vitamin C enhances the duodenal absorption of iron found in plants, so eating fruits and vegetables rich in vitamin C (e.g., oranges or broccoli) aids iron absorption.

Vitamins. Vitamin B_{12} is unique among vitamins because it is present only in animal products (Stabler & Allen, 2004). This includes eggs and milk. Children who totally omit animal sources, therefore, need to supplement this vitamin daily. Reliable supplements of B_{12} include vitamin B_{12} tablets or fortified foods such as commercial breakfast cereals, soy beverages, and some brands of nutritional yeast.

Riboflavin is normally supplied by fortified milk. However, it may be supplied by soy milk, vegetables, or brewer's yeast, all of which contain all the B vitamins except B_{12}, so riboflavin is usually adequate in a vegetarian diet daily without additional supplementation. Good sources of riboflavin in vegan diets are whole and enriched grains and cereals, nuts, and dark-green leafy vegetables.

Vitamin D is necessary for calcium and phosphorus metabolism and is normally supplied in fortified milk. It is not present in plant foods and therefore must be supplemented in a vegan or ovovegetarian diet by vitamin D drops or tablets. Exposure to sunshine is generally an inadequate source (Dudek, 2005).

Minerals. Zinc is present primarily in animal foods but is also present in brewer's yeast, nuts, and wheat germ. Iodine is supplied normally by seafood. In a vegan or vegetarian diet, it can be supplied by seaweed and iodized table salt. Many families add a small amount of powdered kelp (a seaweed) to food two or three times a week to ensure an adequate iodine intake.

Total Calories. Plant foods have fewer total calories than meats. Therefore, one serving of nuts and one serving of legumes are recommended in place of two meat servings. All other recommended serving sizes for various caloric level patterns are the same as those presented in the usual food guide pyramid (see Appendix K).

Working with a family to help them adjust a vegetarian lifestyle to meet their growing children's needs is an important role for nurses.

What if... John's mother tells you she cannot afford to buy meat, explaining she can get more food for the family if she purchases mostly pasta and cereals? How would you help her plan meals that are low in cost but high in nutritional value?

THEORIES OF DEVELOPMENT

A **theory** is a systematic statement of principles that provides a framework for explaining some phenomenon. Developmental theories provide road maps for explaining human development.

A **developmental task** is a skill or a growth responsibility arising at a particular time in an individual's life, the achievement of which will provide a foundation for the accomplishment of future tasks. It is not so much chronologic age as the completion of developmental tasks that defines whether a child has passed from one developmental stage of childhood to another. For example, children are not toddlers just because they are 1 year plus 1 day old; they become toddlers when they have passed through the developmental stage of infancy. For reference, however, childhood is generally divided into the age periods shown in Table 27.4.

A number of theories have been proposed to describe how children grow emotionally, psychologically, and

TABLE 27.4

Basic Divisions of Childhood

Stage	Age Period
Neonate	First 28 days of life
Infant	1 mo–1 yr
Toddler	1–3 yr
Preschooler	3–5 yr
School-age child	6–12 yr
Adolescent	13–20 yr

intellectually as they pass through these different periods. Sociocultural theories stress the importance of environment on growth and development. Learning theory proposes children are like blank pages that can be shaped by learning (Horowitz, 1994). Epigenetic theories stress that genes are the true basis for growth and development. Previously discounted as too simplistic, epigenetic theories are being revised and given new credence based on new knowledge about genes now available through the National Genome Project or the mapping of all the body's genes (Clayton, 2003). Still other theories deal mainly with negative aspects of childrearing that can cause mental illness in children, either immediately or later, when a child reaches adulthood (Freud). Erikson discusses positive aspects necessary for normal growth and for development of a mentally healthy and productive adult.

Freud's Psychoanalytic Theory

Sigmund Freud (1856–1939), an Austrian neurologist and the founder of psychoanalysis, offered the first real theory of personality development (Berger, 2004). Freud based his theory on his observations of mentally disturbed adults. He described adult behavior as being the result of instinctual drives that have a primarily sexual nature (**libido**) from within the person and the conflicts that develop between these instincts (represented in the individual as the id), reality (the ego), and society (the superego). He described child development as being a series of psychosexual stages in which a child's sexual gratification becomes focused on a particular body part. Freud's stages of childhood are summarized in Table 27.5.

Infant

Freud termed the infant period the "oral phase" because infants are so interested in oral stimulation or pleasure during this time (Berger, 2004). According to this theory, infants suck for enjoyment or relief of tension, as well as for nourishment.

Toddler

Freud described the toddler period as the "anal phase" because during this time, children's interests focus on the anal region as they begin toilet training. Elimination takes

on new importance for them. Children find pleasure in both the retention of feces and defecation. This anal interest is part of toddlers' self-discovery, a way of exerting independence, and probably accounts for some of the difficulties parents may experience in toilet-training children of this age.

Preschooler

During the preschool period, children's pleasure zone appears to shift from the anal to the genital area. Freud called this period the "phallic phase." Masturbation is common during this phase. Children may also show exhibitionism, suggesting they hope this will lead to increased knowledge of the two sexes.

School-Age Child

Freud saw the school-age period as a "latent phase," a time in which children's libido appears to be diverted into concrete thinking. He saw no developments as obvious as those in earlier periods appearing during this time.

Adolescent

Freud termed the adolescent period the "genital phase." Freudian theory considers the main events of this period to be the establishment of new sexual aims and the finding of new love objects.

Criticisms of Freud's Theory

To construct his theory, Freud relied on his knowledge of people with mental illness or looked at circumstances that led to mental illness. This "looking at illness" rather than "looking at wellness" perspective limits the applicability of the theory as a health promotion measure, although the behaviors he discussed are as observable as ever.

Erikson's Theory of Psychosocial Development

Erik Erikson (1902–1996) was trained in psychoanalytic theory but later developed his own theory of psychosocial development, a theory that stresses the importance of culture and society in development of the personality (Erikson, 1993). One of the main tenets of his theory, that a person's social view of himself or herself is more important than instinctual drives in determining behavior, allows for a more optimistic view of the possibilities for human growth. While Freud looked at ways mental illness develops, Erikson looked at actions that lead to mental health. Erikson describes eight developmental stages covering the entire life span. At each stage, there is a conflict between two opposing forces. The resolution of each conflict, or accomplishment of the developmental task of that stage, allows the individual to go on to the next phase of development. Table 27.5 shows Erikson's developmental stages through adolescence compared to Freud's. Erikson's additional stages of young adulthood, middle and older age, stages important in childbearing and childrearing, are discussed below.

TABLE 27.5

Summary of Freud's and Erikson's Theories of Personality Development

	Freud's Stages of Childhood		Erikson's Stages of Childhood	
	Psychosexual Stage	*Nursing Implications*	*Developmental Task*	*Nursing Implications*
Infant	Oral stage: Child explores the world by using mouth, especially the tongue.	Provide oral stimulation by giving pacifiers; do not discourage thumb-sucking. Breastfeeding may provide more stimulation than formula feeding because it requires the infant to expend more energy.	Developmental task is to form a sense of trust versus mistrust. Child learns to love and be loved.	Provide a primary caregiver. Provide experiences that add to security, such as soft sounds and touch. Provide visual stimulation for active child involvement.
Toddler	Anal stage: Child learns to control urination and defecation.	Help children achieve bowel and bladder control without undue emphasis on its importance. If at all possible, continue bowel and bladder training while child is hospitalized.	Developmental task is to form a sense of autonomy versus shame. Child learns to be independent and make decisions for self.	Provide opportunities for decision making, such as offering choices of clothes to wear or toys to play with. Praise for ability to make decisions rather than judging correctness of any one decision.
Preschooler	Phallic stage: Child learns sexual identity through awareness of genital area.	Accept child's sexual interest, such as fondling his or her own genitals, as a normal area of exploration. Help parents answer child's questions about birth or sexual differences.	Developmental task is to form a sense of initiative versus guilt. Child learns how to do things (basic problem solving) and that doing things is desirable.	Provide opportunities for exploring new places or activities. Allow play to include activities involving water, clay (for modeling), or finger paint.
School-age child	Latent stage: Child's personality development appears to be nonactive or dormant.	Help a child have positive experiences so his or her self-esteem continues to grow and the child prepares for the conflicts of adolescence.	Developmental task is to form a sense of industry versus inferiority. Child learns how to do things well.	Provide opportunities such as allowing child to assemble and complete a short project so that child feels rewarded for accomplishment.
Adolescent	Genital stage: Adolescent develops sexual maturity and learns to establish satisfactory relationships with the opposite sex.	Provide appropriate opportunities for the child to relate with opposite sex; allow child to verbalize feelings about new relationships.	Developmental task is to form a sense of identity versus role confusion. Adolescents learn who they are and what kind of person they will be by adjusting to a new body image, seeking emancipation from parents, choosing a vocation, and determining a value system.	Provide opportunities for an adolescent to discuss feelings about events important to him or her. Offer support and praise for decision making.

Adapted from Erikson, E. H. (1993). *Childhood & society. New York:* W. W. Norton; and Freud, S. (1962). *Three essays on the theory of sexuality.* New York: Hearst Corporation, with permission.

The Infant

According to Erikson, the developmental task for infants is learning **trust versus mistrust** (other terms are learning confidence or learning to love). Infants whose needs are met when those needs arise, whose discomforts are quickly removed, who are cuddled, played with, and talked to, come to view the world as a safe place and people as helpful and dependable. However, when their care is inconsistent, inadequate, or rejecting, it fosters a basic mistrust: infants become fearful and suspicious of the world and of people. Like a burned child who avoids fire, emotionally burned children may shun the potential pain of further emotional involvement and carry this attitude through later stages of development. Such children can be "stuck" emotionally at this stage, although they continue to grow and develop in other ways.

Fortunately, because not all children achieve developmental tasks readily, each task need not be resolved once and for all the first time it arises. The problem of trust versus mistrust, for example, is not resolved forever during the first year of life but arises again at each successive stage of development. Children who enter school with a sense of mistrust may come to trust a teacher with whom they form a close relationship; given this second chance, children may overcome early mistrust. On the other hand, children who come through infancy with a vital sense of trust intact may still have a sense of mistrust activated at a later stage if their parents are divorced or separate under unpleasant circumstances.

The Toddler

Erikson defines the developmental task of the toddler age as learning **autonomy versus shame** or doubt. Autonomy (self-government or independence) builds on children's new motor and mental abilities. Children take pride in new accomplishments and want to do everything independently, whether it is pulling the wrapper off a piece of candy, selecting a vitamin tablet out of the bottle, flushing the toilet, or replying, "No!" If parents recognize toddlers need to do what they are capable of doing, at their own pace and in their own time, then children develop a sense of being able to control their muscles and impulses during this time. When caregivers are impatient and do everything for them, this enforces a sense of shame and doubt. If children are never allowed to do things they want to do, they will eventually doubt their ability to do them; they will stop trying and cannot do them. If children leave this stage with less autonomy than shame or doubt, they can be disabled in their attempts to achieve independence and may lack confidence in their abilities to achieve well into adolescence and adulthood (Fig. 27.4).

The Preschooler

Erikson defines the developmental task of the preschool period as learning **initiative versus guilt.** Learning initiative is learning how to do things. Children can initiate motor activities of various sorts on their own and no longer merely respond to or imitate the actions of other children or of their parents. The same is true for language and fantasy activities.

Whether children leave this stage with a sense of initiative outweighing a sense of guilt depends largely on how parents respond to self-initiated activities. When children are given much freedom and opportunity to initiate motor play such as running, bike riding, sliding, and wrestling or are exposed to such play materials as finger paints, sand, water, and modeling clay, their sense of initiative is reinforced. Initiative is also encouraged when parents answer a child's questions (intellectual initiative) and do not inhibit fantasy or play activity. If children are made to feel their motor activity is bad (perhaps in a small apartment or a hospital), their questions are a nuisance, or their play is silly and stupid, they may develop a sense of guilt over

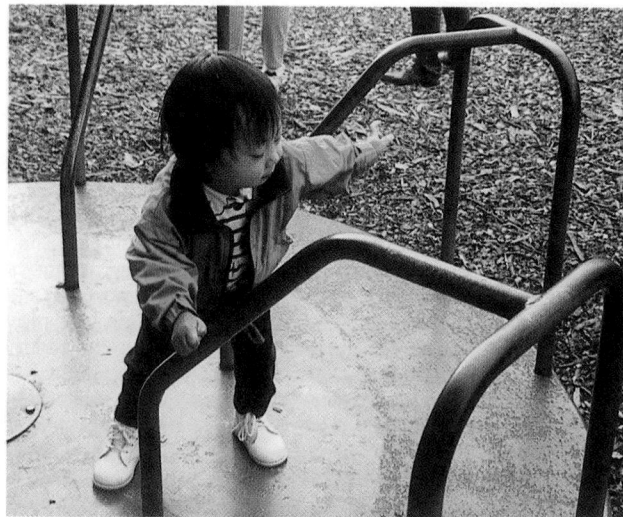

FIGURE 27.4 A toddler enjoys active, independent exploration as part of building a sense of autonomy.

self-initiated activities that will persist in later life. Those who do not develop initiative may later have limited brainstorming and problem-solving skills; they wait for clues or guidance from others before acting.

What if... John's father does not allow his preschool twins to play freely because he demands an orderly household? They begin to show signs of poor initiative. How would you counsel this parent?

The School-Age Child

Erikson viewed the developmental task of the school-age period as developing **industry versus inferiority,** or accomplishment rather than inferiority. During the preschool period, children learned initiative—how to do something. During school age, children learn how to do things well. When they are absorbed in a project, children ask, "Am I doing a good job? Am I doing this right?" When they are encouraged in their efforts to do practical tasks or make practical things and are praised and rewarded for the finished results, their sense of industry grows (Fig. 27.5). Parents who see their children's efforts at making and doing things as merely "busy work" or who don't show appreciation for their children's efforts may cause them to develop a sense of inferiority rather than pride and accomplishment.

During the elementary school years, a child's world grows to include the school and community environment, and success or failure in those settings can have a lasting impact. Children with an intelligence quotient of 80 or 90 (slightly below normal), for example, may have a particularly traumatic school experience, even when their sense of industry is rewarded and encouraged at home. Their learning style may be so different from the average child's they have difficulty competing with children of average

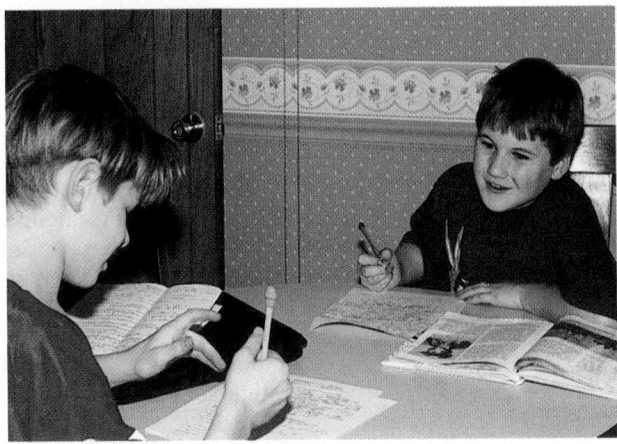

FIGURE 27.5 School-age children develop a sense of industry by working on projects that result in a feeling of accomplishment.

ability; this causes repeated failures in their efforts to learn, reinforcing their sense of inferiority. On the other hand, children whose sense of industry has not been supported at home may have it revitalized at school through the efforts of a committed teacher. A nurse during a hospitalization could also fulfill this role.

The Adolescent

Erikson believed the new interpersonal dimension that emerges during adolescence is a sense of **identity versus role confusion.** To achieve this, adolescents must bring together everything they have learned about themselves as a son or daughter, an athlete, a friend, a fast-food cook, a student, a scout, and so on, and integrate these different images into a whole that makes sense. If adolescents cannot do so, they are left with role confusion; that is, they are left unsure of what kind of person they are and are uncertain what they can do or what kind of person they can become. Some adolescents seek a negative identity: being identified as a drug abuser or runaway may be preferable to having no identity at all.

The Young Adult

The developmental crisis of the young adult is achieving a sense of intimacy versus isolation. Intimacy is the ability to relate well with other people, not only with members of the opposite sex but also with one's own sex to form long-lasting friendships.

A sense of intimacy grows out of earlier developmental tasks, because people need a strong sense of identity before they can reach out fully and offer deep friendship or love. Because there is always the risk of being rejected or hurt when offering love or friendship, individuals cannot offer it if they do not have confidence they can cope with rejection or if they did not develop a sense of trust as an infant. Parents without a sense of intimacy may have more difficulty than others accepting a pregnancy and beginning to love a newborn child.

The Middle-Aged Adult

The developmental task of middle age is to establish a sense of generativity versus stagnation. People extend their concern from just themselves and their families to the community and the world. They may become politically active, work to solve environmental problems, or participate in far-reaching community or world-based decisions.

People with a sense of generativity are self-confident and better able to juggle their various lives (mother, soccer coach, church member, teacher, political party chairperson, gourmet cook). People without this sense become stagnated or self-absorbed. Those who have devoted themselves to only one role are more likely to find themselves at the end of middle age with a narrow perspective and lack of ability to cope with change. Women without a sense of generativity may have more difficulty than others accepting a late-in-life pregnancy and a new role of childbearing and childrearing.

The Older Adult

Older adults play a role in childrearing today because many of them give childcare to young children while parents work. The developmental task of older adults is **integrity versus despair.** An older adult with integrity feels good about the life choices he or she has made; one with a feeling of despair wishes life would begin over again so that things could turn out differently. A sense of integrity is helpful in a grandparent who does childcare, as it helps children develop a sense of trust and learn initiative.

Criticism of Erikson's Theory

Erikson's main contribution to human development was the creation of stages so that development can be broken down into separate phases for study. A criticism of his theory is that life does not occur in easily divided stages, and trying to divide it that way can create superficial divisions.

 Checkpoint Question 2

John, 6 years old, is a school-age child. What must he learn, according to Erikson, to complete the developmental task of this period?

a. How to be creative
b. How to think abstractly
c. How to trust others
d. How to do things well

Piaget's Theory of Cognitive Development

Jean Piaget (1896–1980), a Swiss psychologist, introduced concepts of **cognitive development** or the way children learn and think that have roots similar to those of both Freud and Erikson and yet separate from each. Piaget defined four stages of cognitive development; within each stage are finer units or **schemas.** Each period is an advance over the previous one. To progress from one period to the next, a child reorganizes his or her thinking processes to bring them closer to adult thinking (Piaget, 1952). These stages of cognitive development are summarized in Table 27.6.

The Infant

Piaget referred to the infant stage as the **sensorimotor stage.** Sensorimotor intelligence is practical intelligence, because words and symbols for thinking and problem solving are not yet available at this early age. At the beginning of infancy, babies relate to the world through their senses, using only reflex behavior. As infants progress through this stage (which includes the schemas of primary and secondary circular reactions and coordination of secondary reactions, as defined in Table 27.6), they learn the basic concept that people are entities separate from objects. Piaget used the term "primary" to refer to activities related to a child's own body and the term "circulatory reaction" to show that repetition of behavior occurs (the infant accidentally brings his or her thumb to the mouth, enjoys the sensation of sucking, and so repeats it).

The term "secondary" refers to activities that are separate from a child's body. An example of secondary schema learning is when a baby hits a mobile, notices that this makes it move, and so hits it again. During this secondary schema, infants also learn that objects in the environment—bottle, blocks, bed, or even a parent—are permanent and continue to exist even though they are out of sight or changed in some way. For example:

- Infants will search for a block hidden by a blanket, knowing the block still exists.
- Infants can recognize that a parent remains the same person whether dressed in a robe and slippers or pants and a T-shirt.
- Infants play peek-a-boo because they realize the person playing with them exists behind his or her hands.
- Infants learn they are a separate entity from objects. They learn where their body stops and their bed, playthings, or parent begins.

A great deal of the mouthing and handling of objects by infants and the delight of watching a caregiver appear is part of primary and secondary schemas and discovering **permanence.** The world begins to make sense and the developmental task of achieving trust falls into place when the concept of permanence has been learned (infants know their parents exist and will return to them). Gaining a concept of permanence also contributes to "eighth-month anxiety," a stage in which infants continue to cry for their parents because they know their parents still exist even when out of sight.

During the final phase of the infant year (coordination of secondary reactions), infants begin to demonstrate goal-directed behavior. After noticing that hitting a mobile makes it move, infants then reach for and hit a music box nearby, in this way actively seeking new experiences. It is important for infants to have stimulating objects around for exploring in this way so that experimenting and learning can proceed.

The Toddler

The toddler period is one of transition as children complete the final stages of the sensorimotor period (defined in Table 27.6 as tertiary circular reaction and invention of new means) and begin to develop some cognitive skills of the preoperative period, such as symbolic thought and egocentric thinking. In the tertiary circular reaction schema, children use trial and error to discover new characteristics of objects and events. A toddler sitting in a high chair who keeps dropping objects over the edge of the tray is exploring both permanence and the different actions of toys. During the schema of "invention of new means," children become able to think through actions or mentally project the solution to a problem. If given a box, a toddler will investigate how the top of the box can be removed; if given a second box, even one that varies in shape, the child can foresee how the top can be removed. Toddlers following a ball that has rolled under a coffee table no longer have to follow the ball's path to retrieve it but can project where it will have rolled and walk around the coffee table to find it again.

During the period of **preoperational thought,** children relearn on a conceptual level some of the lessons they mastered as infants at the sensorimotor level, before having language. Now, children are able to use symbols to represent objects. They may have difficulty viewing one object as being different from another, however. On a walk through a department store decorated with teddy bears, for example, children are not sure whether they are seeing a succession of bears or if the same bear keeps reappearing as if it is following them, asking to be taken home.

Toddlers draw conclusions only from obvious facts they see: Daddy is shaving; therefore he must be going to work, because he went to work after he shaved yesterday. This type of faulty reasoning (prelogical reasoning) leads children to wrong conclusions and faulty judgment.

How children think has many implications for nursing. If you made John's bed yesterday and then he went to surgery, he may cry at the sight of you approaching with clean sheets today, thinking he will have to go to surgery again.

The Preschooler

Piaget saw preschool children as moving on to a substage of preoperational thought termed **intuitive thought.** During this time, children tend to look at an object and see only one of its characteristics (referred to as **centering**). For example, they see that a banana is yellow but do not notice it is also long. Centering is noticeable when children are learning about medicine (they observe it tastes bitter, but cannot understand it is also good for them).

Centering contributes to the preschooler's lack of **conservation** (the ability to discern truth, even though physical properties change) or **reversibility** (ability to retrace steps). For example, if preschoolers see beads being poured from one glass into another glass that is taller and thinner than the first one, they will notice only one changing characteristic. They might say that there are now more beads in the second glass (because the level has risen), or there are fewer beads (because the second glass

TABLE 27.6

Piaget's Stages of Cognitive Development

Stage of Development	Age Span	Nursing Implications
Sensorimotor Neonatal reflex	1 mo	Stimuli are assimilated into beginning mental images. Behavior entirely reflexive.
Primary circular reaction	1–4 mo	Hand–mouth and ear–eye coordination develop. Infant spends much time looking at objects and separating self from them. Beginning intention of behavior is present (the infant brings thumb to mouth for a purpose: to suck it). Enjoyable activity for this period: a rattle or tape of parent's voice.
Secondary circular reaction	4–8 mo	Infant learns to initiate, recognize, and repeat pleasurable experiences from environment. Memory traces are present; infant anticipates familiar events (a parent coming near him will pick him up). Good toy for this period: mirror; good game: peek-a-boo.
Coordination of secondary reactions	8–12 mo	Infant can plan activities to attain specific goals. Perceives that others can cause activity and that activities of own body are separate from activity of objects. Can search for and retrieve toy that disappears from view. Recognizes shapes and sizes of familiar objects. Because of increased sense of separateness, infant experiences separation anxiety when primary caregiver leaves. Good toy for this period: nesting toys (i.e., colored boxes).
Tertiary circular reaction	12–18 mo	Child is able to experiment to discover new properties of objects and events. Capable of space perception and time perception as well as permanence. Objects outside self are understood as causes of actions. Good game for this period: throw and retrieve.
Invention of new means through mental combinations	18–24 mo	Transitional phase to the preoperational thought period. Uses memory and imitation to act. Can solve basic problems, foresee maneuvers that will succeed or fail. Good toys for this period: those with several uses, such as blocks, colored plastic rings.
Preoperational Thought	2–7 yr	Thought becomes more symbolic; can arrive at answers mentally instead of through physical attempt. Comprehends simple abstractions but thinking is basically concrete and literal. Child is egocentric (unable to see the viewpoint of another). Displays static thinking (inability to remember what he or she started to talk about so that at the end of a sentence the child is talking about another topic). Concept of time is now, and concept of distance is only as far as he or she can see. Centering or focusing on a single aspect of an object causes distorted reasoning. No awareness of reversibility (for every action there is an opposite action) is present. Unable to state cause–effect relationships, categories, or abstractions. Good toy for this period: items that require imagination, such as modeling clay.
Concrete Operational Thought	7–12 yr	Concrete operations includes systematic reasoning. Uses memory to learn broad concepts (fruit) and subgroups of concepts (apples, oranges). Classifications involve sorting objects according to attributes such as color; seriation, in which objects are ordered according to increasing or decreasing measures such as weight; multiplication, in which objects are simultaneously classified and seriated using weight. Child is aware of reversibility, an opposite operation or continuation of reasoning back to a starting point (follows a route through a maze and then reverses steps). Understands conservation, sees constancy despite transformation (mass or quantity remains the same even if it changes shape or position). Good activity for this period: collecting and classifying natural objects such as native plants, sea shells, etc. Expose child to other viewpoints by asking questions such as, "How do you think you'd feel if you were a nurse and had to tell a boy to stay in bed?"
Formal Operational Thought	12 yr	Can solve hypothetical problems with scientific reasoning; understands causality and can deal with the past, present, and future. Adult or mature thought. Good activity for this period: "talk time" to sort through attitudes and opinions.

From Piaget, J. (1961). *The growth of logical thinking from childhood to adolescence.* New York: Basic Books, with permission.

is narrower), even when told that no beads have been added or removed. When the beads are poured back into the first glass, they still will not understand that the number of beads is unchanged. This immature perception leads children, as it did during the toddler period, to make faulty conclusions. It takes more years of development for children to learn that when thought processes (i.e., they know the number of beads did not change) and perceptions conflict, thought processes are more trustworthy.

Preschool thinking is also influenced by **role fantasy,** or how children would like something to turn out. Children use **assimilation** (taking in information and changing it to fit their existing ideas) as a part of this. For example, because a child wants to go outside and play, he or she says the outside is calling him or her to come and play. Children believe their wishes are as real as facts and dreams are as real as daytime happenings during this stage. They perceive animals and even inanimate objects as being capable of thought and feeling (they say a dog took their doll because the dog was feeling sad; they say a footstool meant to trip them). This is often called "magical thinking." Later, children learn **accommodation** (they change their ideas to fit reality rather than the reverse).

Egocentrism, or perceiving that one's thoughts and needs are better or more important than those of others, is also strong during this period. Preschoolers cannot believe that not everyone knows facts they know; if asked, "What is your name?" they may reply, "Don't you know my name?" As a part of this, children define objects mainly in relation to themselves, so that a spoon is "what I eat with," not just a curved metal object.

The School-Age Child

Piaget viewed school age as a period during which **concrete operational thought** begins as school-age children can discover concrete solutions to everyday problems and recognize cause-and-effect relationships. A child who understands beads do not change in number just because they are poured from one glass to another has grasped the concept of conservation. Conservation of numbers is learned as early as age 7 years, conservation of quantity at age 7 or 8 years, conservation of weight at age 9 years, and conservation of volume at age 11 years. Reasoning during school age tends to be inductive, proceeding from specific to general: school-age children tend to reason that a toy they are holding is broken, the toy is made of plastic, so all plastic toys break easily.

The Adolescent

Piaget saw adolescence as the time when cognition achieves its final form, that of **formal operational thought.** When this stage is reached, adolescents are capable of thinking in terms of possibility—what could be (**abstract thought**)—rather than being limited to thinking about what already is (concrete thought). This makes it possible for adolescents to use scientific reasoning or also understand deductive reasoning, or reasoning that proceeds from the general to the specific (plastic toys break easily, the toy they are holding is plastic; it will break easily).

Criticism of Piaget's Theory

Piaget has been criticized because he used only a small sample of subjects (his own children) to develop his theory. Because children today begin activities to learn reading much earlier than they did at the time the theory was devised, the age groups and "norms" may no longer be relevant. Learning computer use at an early age may be changing both the rate and type of children's cognitive development.

Checkpoint Question 3

Suppose John, 6 years old, tells you his broken leg wants to get better. What type of thinking is he using?

a. Magical thinking
b. Deductive reasoning
c. Concrete operational thinking
d. Sensorial thought

Kohlberg's Theory of Moral Development

Lawrence Kohlberg (1927–1987), a psychologist, studied the reasoning ability of boys and, based on Piaget's development stages, developed a theory on the way children gain knowledge of right and wrong or moral reasoning. These stages, as described by Kohlberg (1984), are summarized in Table 27.7.

Recognizing where a child is at according to these stages can help identify how a child may feel about an illness (e.g., whether a child thinks it is fair or not that he is ill). Recognizing moral reasoning also helps determine whether children can be depended on to carry out self-care activities such as administering their own medicine (i.e., whether a child has internalized standards of conduct so he or she does not "cheat" when away from external control). Moral stages closely approximate cognitive stages of development, because a child must be able to think abstractly (be able to conceptualize an idea without a concrete picture) before being able to understand how rules apply even when no one is there to enforce them.

The Infant

The infant period is a **prereligious stage.** Infants have little concept of any motivating force beyond that of their parents. Infants learn that when they do certain actions, parents give affection and approval; for other actions, parents scold and label the behavior "bad." To support this stage of development, it is important for caregivers to praise an infant for doing what he or she has been asked to do. Caregivers should also know the average infant is trying hard to please; if an infant falls short of doing this, it is probably due to immature development rather than any effort to displease.

The development of trust is important in moral development because infants who develop a sound sense of trust can better develop a spiritual orientation in future

TABLE 27.7

Kohlberg's Stages of Moral Development

Age (Year)	Stage	Description	Nursing Implications
Preconventional (Level I)			
2–3	1	Punishment/obedience orientation ("heteronomous morality"). Child does right because a parent tells him or her to and to avoid punishment.	Child needs help to determine what are right actions. Give clear instructions to avoid confusion.
4–7	2	Individualism. Instrumental purpose and exchange. Carries out actions to satisfy own needs rather than society's. Will do something for another if that person does something for the child.	Child is unable to recognize that like situations require like actions. Unable to take responsibility for self-care, because meeting own needs interferes with this.
Conventional (Level II)			
7–10	3	Orientation to interpersonal relations of mutuality. Child follows rules because of a need to be a "good" person in own eyes and eyes of others.	Child enjoys helping others because this is "nice" behavior. Allow child to help with bed making and other like activities. Praise for desired behavior such as sharing.
10–12	4	Maintenance of social order, fixed rules and authority. Child finds following rules satisfying. Follows rules of authority figures as well as parents in an effort to keep the "system" working.	Child often asks what are the rules and is something "right." May have difficulty modifying a procedure because one method may not be "right." Follows self-care measures only if someone is there to enforce them.
Postconventional (Level III)			
Older than 12	5	Social contract, utilitarian law-making perspectives. Follows standards of society for the good of all people.	An adolescent can be responsible for self-care because he or she views this as a standard of adult behavior.
	6	Universal ethical principle orientation. Follows internalized standards of conduct.	Many adults do not reach this level of moral development.

From Kohlberg, L. (1984). *The psychology of moral development.* New York: Harper & Row, with permission.

years or be bound by a moral conscience (they can trust in a spiritual being as well as humans around them).

The Toddler

Toddlers begin to formulate a sense of right and wrong, but their reason for doing right is centered most strongly in "mother or father says so" rather than in any spiritual or societal motivation. Kohlberg referred to this as a "punishment obedience orientation" (a child is good because a parent says a child must be good, not because it is "right" to be good).

Toddlers may not obey requests from people other than their parents because they do not view their authority as being at the same level as their parents' authority. This means that while providing nursing care, it might be necessary to ask a parent to reinforce instructions to be certain a toddler will follow them.

The Preschooler

Preschoolers tend to do good out of self-interest rather than out of true intent to do good or because of a strong spiritual motivation. When asked why it is wrong to steal from a neighbor, for example, a preschooler will answer, "Because my mother won't like me any more." Because of egocentrism, a preschooler may do things for others only in return for things done for him or her. This means it may be necessary to remind a child of actions taken on his or her behalf or trade off actions (e.g., "Lie still now for me while I change your dressing and I'll read you a story when I'm through").

Children at this age also imitate what they see, so if they see less-than-perfect role models, they may copy those wrong actions, assuming those actions are correct. Preschoolers have great difficulty knowing what rules apply to new situations because they cannot judge whether a previously learned principle of right or wrong can be applied to this new situation (does not recognize that stealing applies in a hospital setting the same as it did at home).

The School-Age Child

School-age children enter a stage of moral development termed **conventional development,** a level at which many adults continue to function. Young school-age children adhere to a phase of development termed the "nice girl, nice boy" stage. Children engage in actions that are "nice" or "fair" rather than necessarily right. Sharing, for example, is "nice." Taking turns is "fair." Stealing is not. Young school-age children may lie about their actions to disguise that they have been involved in an action that is not "nice." When asked why it is wrong to steal from a neighbor, the school-age child most often answers, "Because it's not nice or fair."

Later in the school-age period, as children learn about community resources, they become aware that community laws are enforced by crossing guards or police. They may have difficulty following self-care measures reliably when out of a nurse's or parent's sight during this time because they feel it is necessary to obey rules only when the rules can be clearly enforced. At this point, they might answer the question about stealing from a neighbor with, "You shouldn't steal because the police will arrest you."

The Adolescent

As adolescents become capable of abstract thought, they become capable of internalizing standards of conduct (they do what they think is right regardless of whether anyone is watching). This is termed **postconventional development** and is the mature form of moral reasoning. In this stage, if asked why it is wrong to steal from a neighbor, an adolescent would answer, "Because it deprives my neighbor of possessions he or she has earned." Adolescents can carry out self-care measures even when someone else is not present when they enter this stage because they can understand not only the importance of the measures to themselves but also the principle that certain things should be done simply because they are right. Many adolescents do not enter this phase of development, however, and as adults they continue at a school-age level, doing right things only when obvious authority or set rules are present.

Criticism of Kohlberg's Theory

Kohlberg's theory is frequently challenged as being male-oriented because his original research was conducted entirely with boys. Carol Gilligan (1982), a sociologist, has suggested that girls may not score well on Kohlberg's scale because, being more concerned with relationships than boys, they make moral decisions based on individual circumstances, a different criterion for decision making.

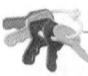

Key Points

Knowledge of growth and development is important in health promotion and illness prevention because it lays the basis for assessment and anticipatory guidance.

Genetic factors that influence growth and development are gender, race and nationality, intelligence, and health.

Environmental influences include quality of nutrition, socioeconomic level, parent–child relationship, ordinal position in the family, and environmental health.

To meet growth and development needs, children need to follow basic guidelines for a healthy diet, such as eating a variety of foods; maintaining ideal weight; avoiding too much saturated fat and cholesterol; eating foods with adequate starch and fiber; and avoiding too much sugar, the same as adults.

Temperament is a child's characteristic manner of thinking, behaving, or reacting. Helping parents understand the effect of temperament is a nursing role.

Common theories of development are Freud's psychoanalytic theory and Erikson's theory of psychosocial development. Both of these theories describe specific tasks children must complete at each stage of development in order to become a well-adapted adult.

Piaget's theory of cognitive development describes ways that children learn. Kohlberg advanced a theory of moral development, or how children use moral reasoning to solve problems they face.

Although growth and development occur in known patterns, their rate varies from child to child. Caution parents not to be concerned because two siblings are very different as long as they both fit within usual parameters.

Critical Thinking Exercises

1. John is the 6-year-old boy you met at the beginning of the chapter. He had lived in many foster homes before he was adopted. His parents state that they find him cold and unloving. What developmental task was John unable to complete because of these frequent moves at such a young age? What actions could his new parents take to try to strengthen this developmental task at this point?
2. John's mother describes her 3-year-old twins as "totally different" from each other. One is shy and quiet and agreeable; the other is aggressive and persistent. What characteristic is she describing? Which child does she probably view as easier to care for? What anticipatory guidance could you give her to help her better understand these differences in her children?
3. Children who are hospitalized for long periods may fall behind in development. What specific measures could you take to promote developmental growth and encourage a sense of autonomy if John were a hospitalized 2-year-old? To promote a sense of industry if he were hospitalized at age 10 years?
4. Examine the National Health Goals related to growth and development of children. Most government-sponsored money for nursing research is allotted based on these goals. What would be a possible research topic to explore pertinent to these goals that would be applicable to John's family and also advance evidence-based practice?

References

Anderson, J. D., et al. (2003). Temperamental characteristics of young children who stutter. *JSLHR: Journal of Speech, Language, and Hearing Research, 46*(5), 1221-1233.

Barr, S. I., & Rideout, C. A. (2004). Nutritional considerations for vegetarian athletes. *Nutrition, 20*(7/8), 696–703.

Berger, K. S. (2004). *The developing person through the life span* (6th ed.) New York: Worth Publishers.

Carey, W. B., & McDevitt, S. C. (1994). *Prevention and early intervention: Individual differences as risk factors for the mental health of children.* New York: Brunner/Mazel.

Chess, S., & Thomas, A. (1995). *Temperament in clinical practice.* New York: Guilford Publications.

Clayton, E. W. (2003). Genomic medicine: Ethical, legal, and social implications of genomic medicine. *New England Journal of Medicine, 349*(6), 562–569.

Department of Health and Human Services. (2000). *Healthy people 2010.* Washington, DC: DHHS.

Dudek, S. G. (2005). *Nutrition essentials for nursing practice.* Philadelphia: Lippincott Williams & Wilkins.

Erikson, E. H. (1993). *Childhood and society.* New York: W. W. Norton.

Eriksson, B. S., & Pehrsson, G. (2003). Relationships between the family's way of functioning and children's temperament as rated by parents of pre-term children. *Journal of Child Health Care, 7*(2), 89–100.

Forrest, C. B., & Riley, A. W. (2004). Childhood origins of adult health: A basis for life-course health policy. *Health Affairs, 23*(5), 155–164.

Gilligan, C. (1982). *In a different voice: Psychological theory and women's development.* Cambridge, MA: Harvard University Press.

Green, M., & Solnit, A. (1964). Reactions to the threatened loss of a child: A vulnerable child syndrome. *Pediatrics, 34*(8), 58–62.

Haddad, E. H., & Tanzman, J. S. (2003). What do vegetarians in the United States eat? *American Journal of Clinical Nutrition, 78*(3S), 626S–632S.

Horowitz, F. D. (1994). John B. Watson's legacy: Learning and environment. In D. Ross, et al. (Eds.), *A century of developmental psychology.* Washington, DC: American Psychological Association.

Kearney, J. A. (2003). Early reactions to frustration: Developmental trends in anger, individual response styles, and caregiving risk implications in infancy. *Journal of Child and Adolescent Psychiatric Nursing, 17*(3), 105–112.

Kohlberg, L. (1984). *The psychology of moral development.* New York: Harper & Row.

Lumeng, J. C., et al. (2003). Association between clinically meaningful behavior problems and overweight in children. *Pediatrics, 112*(5), 1138–1145.

Piaget, J. (1952). *The origins of intelligence in children.* New York: International Universities Press.

Pontin, D. (2004). A school-based program to reduce carbonated drink consumption reduced obesity in children. *Evidence-Based Nursing, 7*(4), 105–108.

Poustie, V. J., Smith, R. L., & Watling, R. M. (2005). Oral protein calorie supplementation for children with chronic disease. *The Cochrane Library (Oxford) (1)* (CD001914).

Seguin, L., et al. (2005). Understanding the dimensions of socioeconomic status that influence toddlers' health: Unique impact of lack of money for basic needs in Quebec's birth cohort. *Journal of Epidemiology and Community Health, 59*(1), 42–48.

Stabler, S. P., & Allen, R. H. (2004). Vitamin B12 deficiency as a worldwide problem. *Annual Review of Nutrition, 24,* 299–326.

U. S. Department of Agriculture. (2005). Dietary guidelines for Americans. Washington, DC: USDA.

Suggested Readings

Chen, C., Li, C., & Wang, J. (2004). Growth and development of children with congenital heart disease. *Journal of Advanced Nursing, 47*(3), 260–269.

Drummond, J., et al. (2005). Randomized controlled trial of a family problem-solving intervention. *Clinical Nursing Research, 14*(1), 299–306.

Horodynski, M. A., & Gibbons, C. (2004). Rural low-income mothers' interactions with their young children. *Pediatric Nursing, 30*(4), 299–306.

Jones, C. (2004). Genetics: Overview and issues in child health. *Paediatric Nursing, 16*(6), 37–43.

Nystrom, K., & Ohrling, K. (2004). Parenthood experiences during the child's first year: Literature review. *Journal of Advanced Nursing, 46*(3), 319–330.

Prior, M. (2003). Toddler temperament, cognition and caregiver interaction predict impulsive functioning. *Evidence-Based Mental Health, 6*(1), 20–23.

Rew, L., & Horner, S. D. (2003). Youth resilience framework for reducing health-risk behaviors in adolescents. *Journal of Pediatric Nursing: Nursing Care of Children and Families, 18*(6), 379–388.

Sankar, P., et al. (2004). Genetic research and health disparities. *JAMA, 291*(24), 2985–2989.

Squires, J., & Nickel, R. (2003). Pediatric practice: Identifying social-emotional problems in infants and toddlers. *Patient Care for the Nurse Practitioner, 1*(4), 12–15.

Thomasgard, M., & Metz, W. P. (2004). Promoting child social-emotional growth in primary care settings: Using a developmental approach. *Clinical Pediatrics, 43*(2), 119–127.

CHAPTER 28

The Family With an Infant

Key Terms

baby-bottle syndrome
binocular vision
coordination of secondary
   schema
deciduous teeth
eighth-month anxiety
extrusion reflex
fine motor development
gross motor development
hand regard
Landau reflex
natal teeth
neck-righting reflex
neonatal teeth
object permanence
parachute reaction
pincer grasp
prehensile ability
primary circular reaction
seborrhea
secondary circular reaction
social smile
thumb opposition
ventral suspension

Objectives

After mastering the contents of this chapter, you should be able to:

1. Describe normal infant growth and development and associated parental concerns.
2. Assess an infant for normal growth and development milestones.
3. Formulate nursing diagnoses related to infant growth and development and associated parental concerns.
4. Identify expected outcomes to promote optimal infant growth and development needs.
5. Plan nursing care to meet an infant's growth and development needs.
6. Implement nursing care related to normal growth and development of an infant.
7. Evaluate expected outcomes for achievement of optimal growth and development and effectiveness of care.

8. Identify National Health Goals related to infant growth and development that nurses can help the nation achieve.
9. Identify areas related to nursing care of an infant that could benefit from additional nursing research or application of evidenced-based practice.
10. Use critical thinking to analyze methods of care for an infant to be certain care is family-centered.
11. Integrate knowledge of infant growth and development with nursing process to achieve quality maternal and child health nursing care.

You meet Ms. Simpson, 19, at a pediatric clinic when she brings in her 2-month-old son, Bryan. She looks tired. She tells you she is exhausted because her baby is "awake all night, crying constantly." She stopped breast-feeding and changed him to formula to see if that would help, but it didn't. She tells you his bowel movements are normal. When you weigh Bryan, you find he has gained weight well. When you talk to him, he demonstrates a social smile.

Previous chapters described the newborn and the capabilities with which children are born. This chapter adds information about the dramatic changes, both physical and psychosocial, that occur during the first year. This is important information because it builds a base for care and health teaching for the age group.

What condition common to early infancy might Ms. Simpson be describing? Is this normal infant behavior? What factors might be playing a role? What suggestions could you make to help her enjoy caring for Bryan more?

After you've studied this chapter, access the accompanying website. Read the patient scenario and answer the questions to further sharpen your skills, grow more familiar with RN-CLEX types of questions, and reward yourself with how much you have learned.

Traditionally, infancy is designated as the period of time from 1 month to 1 year of age. In these important months, an infant undergoes such rapid development that parents sometimes believe their baby looks different and demonstrates new abilities each day. During this time, an infant triples birthweight and increases length by 50%. A baby's senses sharpen and, with the process of attachment to primary caregivers, he or she forms a first social relationship. Because of the growth and learning potential that occurs, this first year is a crucial one. Without proper nutrition, a baby will not grow and physically thrive, and without proper stimulation and nurturing care by consistent caregivers, an infant may not develop a healthy interest in life or a feeling of security essential for future development.

As a result, infant health promotion is the subject of much concern. National Health Goals addressing this important developmental stage are highlighted in Box 28.1.

Although infant health care visits are scheduled less frequently than formerly, a standard schedule is for 2-week, 2-month, 4-month, 6-month, and 12-month visits (AAP, 2005). These visits are as important for the parents as they are for the infant because they provide an opportunity for parents to ask questions about their child's growth pattern and developmental progress. They also provide opportunities for health care providers to assess for potential problems. Anticipatory guidance offered at these visits can help parents prepare for the rapid changes that mark the first year of life. When appropriate, encouraging parents to join clubs or networking groups helps to increase their knowledge base and confidence level as well.

Table 28.1 details the usual procedures at infant health maintenance visits. First-year immunizations and any risks associated with these are discussed in Chapter 33 and listed in Appendix J.

Nursing Process Overview

For Healthy Development of an Infant

● *Assessment*

Nursing assessment of an infant begins by interviewing the primary caregiver. Important areas to discuss include nutrition, growth patterns, and development. An infant's height, weight, and head circumference are important indicators of growth, so they should be measured and plotted on standard growth charts. These charts represent average growth and can determine if the baby's growth remains within the same relative percentile at each checkup. For more information about typical assessment findings, see Box 28.2.

Physical assessment of an infant must be done quickly yet thoroughly because a baby can tire or become hungry, making it difficult to judge his or her overall behavior and temperament. The primary caregiver should be present to make a child feel comfortable. Using a calm, unhurried approach helps an infant feel safe enough to accept your interventions.

● *Nursing Diagnosis*

Much of your assessment of an infant and family will focus on basic needs such as sleep, nutrition, and activity and the parents' adjustment to their new role. Examples of nursing diagnoses are:

- Ineffective breast-feeding related to maternal fatigue
- Disturbed sleep pattern (maternal) related to baby's need to nurse every 2 hours
- Deficient knowledge related to normal infant growth and development
- Imbalanced nutrition, less than body requirements, related to infant's difficulty sucking
- Health-seeking behaviors related to adjusting to parenthood
- Delayed growth and development related to lack of stimulating environment
- Risk for impaired parenting related to long hospitalization of infant
- Readiness for enhanced family coping related to increased financial support
- Social isolation (maternal) related to lack of adequate social support

BOX 28.1 FOCUS ON . . .

NATIONAL HEALTH GOALS

A number of National Health Goals focus on promotion of health during the infant year. These are:

- Increase the proportion of mothers who breast-feed until 1 year of age, from a baseline of 16% to 25%.
- Increase to at least 75% the proportion of parents and caregivers who use feeding practices that prevent baby-bottle tooth decay. Special target population: parents and caregivers with less than high school educations.
- Reduce the rate of fetal and infant deaths, from a baseline of 7.5/1,000 to 4.5/1,000.
- Increase the rate of use of child automobile restraints, from a baseline of 92% to 100%.
- Increase the percentage of healthy full-term infants who are put down to sleep on their backs, from a baseline of 35% to 70%.
- Increase to at least 90% the proportion of infants who receive all recommended immunizations for an infant at appropriate intervals (DHHS, 2000).

Nurses can help the nation achieve these goals by educating parents about the importance of not putting an infant to bed with a bottle of milk or juice, the use of infant car seats, and continuing breast-feeding for a full year. A number of areas related to these topics that could benefit from additional nursing research include effective ways mothers can comfort an infant in a car seat without removing the infant from the seat; characteristics of programs that are successful in promoting breast-feeding; and effective ways to teach about immunizations so that parents secure those required for infants.

TABLE 28.1

Health Maintenance Schedule, Infant Period

Area of Focus	Methods	Frequency
Assessment		
Developmental milestones	History, observation	Every visit
	Denver Developmental Screening Test (DDST II)	At 3 months and 1 year
Growth milestones	Height, weight, head circumference plotted on standard growth chart; physical examination	Every visit
Nutritional adequacy	History, observation	Every visit
Parent/child relationship	History, observation	Every visit
Sleep positioning counseling	Discussion of placing infants on back to sleep	Every visit up to 9 months
Injury and violence counseling	Discussion of safety measures to take with infants	Every visit
Vision and hearing screening	Observation and history	Every visit
Dental health	History, physical examination	Every visit after teeth erupt
Anemia	Hematocrit, hemoglobin	9- or 12-month visit
Lead screening	Finger stick	9- or 12-month visit
Tuberculosis screening	PPD test	12-month visit
Immunizations	Review of history and health record; teaching caregiver about any risks and side effects; administering immunization in accordance with health care agency policies	
Diphtheria, pertussis, tetanus (DPT)		2-, 4-, & 6-month visits
Haemophilus influenzae type B (HiB)		2-, 4-, 6 & 12-month visits
Varicella		12-month visit
Inactivated poliomyelitis		2-, 4-, & 6-month visits
Pneumococcal		2, 4, 6 & 12-month visits
Hepatitis B		Birth, 2-month, & 12-month visits
Influenza		Yearly at 6-month or more visit.

Centers for Disease Control & Prevention. (2005). *Recommended childhood & adolescent immunization schedule, United States, 2005*. Washington, DC: DHHS; and American Academy of Pediatrics. (2005). *Recommendations for preventive pediatric health care*. Washington, DC: AAP.

• Ineffective role performance related to new responsibilities within the family

● **Outcome Identification and Planning**
Assess that the outcomes established for infant care are realistic based on the family's circumstances. Parents of infants, especially first-time parents, must do a lot of adjusting, and this takes time. Try to suggest activities that can be easily incorporated into the family's lifestyle. If your assessment data indicate that a child needs more exposure to language and you know both parents work during the day, for example, you might suggest the parents ask their child's caretaker to talk to their infant more. Encourage parents to spend additional time each evening reading or reciting nursery rhymes to their baby. The combined interventions should increase the baby's language skills.

● **Implementation**
One of the most important interventions of an infant period is teaching new parents about normal growth and development milestones, such as the age range for rolling over or reaching for objects. Whenever possible, this information should be anticipatory so parents are prepared for changes and developments before they occur.

● **Outcome Evaluation**
Evaluate expected outcomes at each visit to detect changes in growth and development. Help parents understand that the total developmental profile, not just a single element, provides the most important description of their child. Variation is so much the rule rather than the exception that a 2-month variation from the average during the infant year is considered normal. Many 4-month-old infants, for example, have mastered

try to arrange for one person to care for their child while they are away from home or choose a day care center that will provide a consistent caregiver. Urge them to discuss their methods of childcare with alternative caregivers to prevent disrupting an infant's routine. When a child is admitted to a hospital, document and use this information.

Parents should make sure the caretaker they choose will actively interact with their child to provide a sense of trust. Passively caring for infants—not talking to them or touching or stroking them while feeding or changing them—amounts to not being with them. An increasing number of parents are installing video cameras to make sure a caretaker is actively interacting with their baby to instill a sense of trust in their child. Nursing actions designed to help an ill infant develop a sense of trust are detailed in Table 28.3.

Promoting Infant Safety

Accidents are a leading cause of death in children from 1 month through 24 years of age. They are second only to acute infections as a cause of acute morbidity and physician visits (NCHS, 2005).

Most accidents in infancy occur because parents either underestimate or overestimate a child's ability. Nursing interventions that help parents become sensitive to their infant's developmental progress not only help establish sound parent–child relationships but also provide anticipatory guidance for a child's safety (Box 28.5). Box 28.6 highlights appropriate outcomes and interventions related to infant safety using the terminology identified by the Nursing Outcomes Classification (NOC) and Nursing Interventions Classification (NIC).

Aspiration Prevention

Aspiration is a potential threat to infants throughout the first year. Round, cylindrical objects are more dangerous than square or flexible objects in this regard. A 1-inch (3.2-cm) cylinder, such as a carrot or hot dog, is particularly dangerous because it can totally obstruct an infant's airway. A deflated balloon can be sucked into the mouth, obstructing the airway in the same way. Educate parents who feed their infant formula not to prop bottles. By doing this, they are overestimating their infant's ability to push the bottle away, sit up, turn the head to the side, cough, and clear the airway if milk should flow too rapidly into the mouth and an infant begins to aspirate.

Other instances of aspiration occur because parents underestimate their infant's ability to grasp and place objects in their mouth. Even a newborn can wiggle to a new position to reach an attractive object such as a teddy bear with small button eyes. Newborns' grasp and sucking reflexes automatically cause them to grasp and pull the object into their mouth. Caution parents to be certain nothing comes within an infant's reach that would not be safe to put into the mouth. Using clothing without decorative buttons, and checking toys and rattles to ensure they have no small parts that could snap off or fall out are good steps for parents to follow. A test of whether a toy could be dangerous if an infant puts it inside the mouth is whether it fits inside a toilet paper roll. If it does, it is small enough to be aspirated. When solid foods are introduced, encourage parents to offer small pieces of hot dogs or grapes, not large chunks. Children under about 5 years should not be offered popcorn or peanuts because of this danger of aspiration.

As infants become more adept at handling toys, parents need to reassess toys for loose pieces or parts. If parents are going to offer an infant a pacifier, they should use one that has a one-piece construction with a flange large enough to keep it from completely entering the child's mouth (Fig. 28.16).

Fall Prevention

Falls are a second major cause of infant accidents. As a preventive measure, no infant, beginning with the newborn, should be left unattended on a raised surface. Normal wiggling can bring a baby to the edge of a bed, couch, or table top, resulting in a fall.

Teach parents to be prepared for their infant to roll over by 2 months of age. From that time on, they must be especially vigilant not to leave the baby unattended on a changing table or counter. If the child sleeps in a crib, the mattress should be lowered to its bottom position so the height of the side rails increases; rails should be $2\frac{3}{8}$ inches apart, narrow enough so a child cannot put his or her head between them. Two months is about the maximum length of time infants can safely sleep in a bassinet; they need the protection of a crib and high siderails before they turn over.

All of these safety precautions apply to the hospital environment as well as to the home. Be sure crib sides are raised and secure before you walk away from a crib, even for just a moment. Also ensure that the space between the mattress and headboard is small enough an infant's head could not become trapped. Make sure cords from nursing call bells or safety pins are out of an infant's reach.

Car Safety

Teaching car safety for infants (as well as for the whole family) is a vital preventive health measure. The use of car seats for newborns is discussed in Chapter 24. Car seats should continue to be used without interruption through the preschool age, or until the child reaches 40 to 60 lb. If parents are firm about keeping an infant in a car seat even when he or she gets fussy or impatient, the child will eventually become more comfortable in the seat than outside it. Infants up to 20 lb should be placed in rear-facing seats in the back seat because an inflating front-seat airbag could suffocate an infant (AAP Committee on Safety, 2005).

Safety with Siblings

As infants become more fun to play with at about 3 months, older brothers and sisters grow more interested in interacting with them. You may need to remind parents that children under 5 years of age, as a group, are not responsible enough or knowledgeable enough about infants to be left unattended with them. They might introduce an unsafe toy or engage in play that is too rough for an infant. Some

TABLE 28.3

Ways for Nurses to Help an Ill Infant Develop a Sense of Trust

Area of Care	Nursing Actions
Nutrition	Encourage mothers to breast-feed if possible; provide privacy and support as necessary.
	Hold the infant no matter what feeding method is used (gavage, total parenteral, oral, enteral). If this is not possible, hold infants for a time after or between feedings so they receive holding equal to what they would ordinarily receive.
	If infant feeding is not oral, provide a pacifier (medical condition considered) five or six times daily for sucking pleasure.
	Hold and comfort after an episode of vomiting, usually not noticeably disturbing to infants.
Dressing change	Use nonallergenic tape to avoid irritation while applied and pain when removed.
	Use a minimum of tape so the least amount has to be pulled free from sensitive skin (consider using stockinette, rolled gauze, or Kling gauze to hold a bandage in place rather than tape).
	To prevent chilling, be certain irrigation solutions are warm. Minimize exposure of the child during dressing changes to conserve warmth.
	Restrain only those body parts necessary for security.
	Talk to the infant. Hearing an explanation of what you are doing is comforting, not for the meaning of the words but for the nonthreatening tone of your voice.
Medicine administration	Flavor oral medicine to disguise disagreeable taste (being careful not to increase the amount to beyond what the child will take readily). Offer a drink of flavorful fluid afterward to counter medicinal taste.
	Never administer medicine in an infant's formula to prevent changing the formula's taste.
	Comfort the infant after injections or intravenous insertion by holding and rocking, or give immediately to a parent for this. Check intravenous sites frequently (every 30 min) for swelling to prevent infiltration and pain. Hold and play with infants despite tubing and restraints.
Rest	Encourage parents to sit and hold infants; infants sleep in a parent's arms as soundly as they do in bed.
	Rock infants to sleep if this is comforting. If contagion is not a problem, bring the crib to the nursing desk where the infant can see you until he or she falls asleep.
	Always wake infants gently, because it is frightening (for anyone) to be awakened by a stranger.
	If bed rest is necessary, check for irritated elbows, heels, and knees from the infant's skin rubbing against sheets; protect with long sleeves or pants.
Hygiene	Check the temperature of bath water for comfort and to prevent chilling.
	Change diapers frequently to reduce discomfort from irritation.
	To avoid caries and prevent pain, begin toothbrushing with first tooth.
Pain	Hold and comfort an infant in pain.
	Do not ask parents to hold a child during a painful procedure; it is difficult for them to see their child in pain. Allow them to comfort the child afterward.
	Reduce painful procedures to a minimum; combine blood drawing so only one puncture is necessary for many tests, etc.
Stimulation	Talk to infants while you care for them so they come to know you.
	Remember that infants focus longest on a human face.
	Provide a crib mirror or a mobile, because visual stimulation is satisfying to an infant.
	If no mobile is available, create one from a wire coat hanger, string, or strips of adhesive tape and objects that will suspend easily and are light enough to move from motion of the crib or an air current (colored paper, cotton balls, colored tongue blades). For safety, hang the mobile high enough for the infant to see but not reach.
	During the second half of the 1st year, remember that infants need to try to crawl. Put a pad or sheet on the floor and encourage the infant to come to you or to explore on his or her own while you stand by to offer reassurance (this is almost impossible to accomplish in a crib).

BOX 28.5 FOCUS ON . . .

FAMILY TEACHING

Accident Prevention Measures for Infants

Q. Bryan's mother is worried about keeping him safe. She asks, "How can I prevent accidents at this age?"

A. Here are some tips to help prevent specific types of accidents:

Potential Accident	Prevention Measures
General	Know the whereabouts of infants at all times.
	Be aware that the frequency of accidents is increased when parents are under stress. Take special precautions at these times.
	Choose babysitters carefully and explain and enforce all precautions when sitters are in charge.
Aspiration	Be certain any object that an infant can grasp and bring to the mouth is either safe to eat or too big to fit in the mouth. Do not feed an infant foods such as popcorn or peanuts, because these are easily aspirated. Store baby products such as powder out of infant's reach; powder is high risk for aspiration.
	Inspect toys and pacifiers for small parts that could be aspirated if broken off; don't make home-made pacifiers.
Falls	Never leave an infant on an unprotected surface, such as a bed or couch, even if the child is in an infant seat.
	Place a gate at the top and bottom of stairways; do not allow an infant to walk with a sharp object in the hands or mouth (it could pierce the throat in a fall).
	Raise crib rails and make sure they are locked before walking away from crib.
	Do not leave a child unattended in a highchair; avoid using an infant walker.
Motor vehicle	Never transport unless an infant is buckled into an infant car seat in the back seat of the car. Be aware of the proper technique for placing an infant in a car seat.
	Do not be distracted by an infant while driving.
	Do not leave an infant unattended in a parked car (can become dehydrated from excess heat, move gear shift, or be abducted).
Suffocation	Allow no plastic bags within infant's reach.
	Do not use pillows in a crib.
	Store unused appliances such as refrigerators or stoves with the doors removed.
	Buy a crib that is approved for safety (spacing of rails is not over $2\frac{3}{8}$ in [6 cm] apart).
	Remove constricting clothing such as a bib from neck at bedtime.
Drowning	Do not leave infants alone in a bathtub or unsupervised near water (even buckets of cleaning water).
Animal bites	Do not allow an infant to approach a strange dog; supervise play with family pets.
Poisoning	Never present medication as a candy.
	Buy medications in containers with safety caps; put away immediately after use.
	Never take medication in front of infants. Place all medication and poisons in locked cabinets or overhead shelves.
	Never leave medication in a pocket or handbag.
	Use no lead-based paint in any area of the home.
	Hang plants or set on high surfaces.
	Post telephone number of the poison control center by the telephone.
Burns	Test warmth of formula and food before feeding (use extra precaution with microwave warming).
	Do not smoke or drink hot liquids while holding or caring for infant.
	Buy flame-retardant clothing for infants.
	Use a sunscreen on a child over 6 months when out in direct or indirect sunlight; limit the child's sun exposure to less than 30 min at a time.
	Turn handles of pans toward back of stove.
	Use a cool-mist, not a hot-mist, vaporizer; remain in room to monitor so child cannot reach vaporizer. Keep a screen in front of a fireplace or heater.
	Monitor infants carefully near candles. Do not leave infants unsupervised near hot-water faucets.
	Do not allow infants to blow out matches (don't teach children that fire is fun).
	Keep electric wires and cords out of reach; cover electrical outlets with safety plugs.

BOX 28.6

Nursing Outcomes Classification (NOC) and Nursing Interventions Classification (NIC)

Infant Safety

NOC: **Knowledge, Child Safety**

Knowledge, child safety, is defined as the extent of understanding conveyed about safely caring for a child (Johnson, Maas, & Moorhead, 2000). Some specific indicators suggesting achievement of this outcome include the parent's ability to describe the following:

- Appropriate activities for child's developmental level
- Drowning hazards and measures to prevent drowning
- Measures to prevent electrical shock, choking, falls, and burns
- First aid techniques and CPR, including demonstration
- Proper surveillance of activities

NIC: **Teaching, Infant Safety**

Teaching, infant safety, is defined as instruction on safety during the first year of life (McCloskey & Bulechek, 2000). Some important activities involved when implementing this intervention include instructing the parent/caregiver in the following at:

0 to 3 months
- Using car seat
- Putting infant to sleep on back
- Maintaining all equipment such as swings, strollers in proper working condition

- Checking temperature of formula and bath water
- Keeping pets at a safe distance
- Never shaking, tossing, or swinging infant in air

4 to 6 months
- Avoiding use of walkers or jumpers
- Never leaving infant unattended in tub
- Using a safe highchair
- Feeding only soft or mashed foods
- Removing small objects from infant's reach

7 to 9 months
- Avoiding sources of lead poisoning
- Providing barriers to potentially dangerous areas
- Supervising infant's activity at all times

10 to 12 months
- Providing protection from glass furniture, sharp edges, and appliances
- Storing all cleaning supplies out of infant's reach
- Using childproof latches on cupboards
- Preventing infant's access to upper-story windows, balconies, and stairs
- Selecting toys according to manufacturer's age recommendations
- Ensuring barriers to pools, hot tubs, ponds, and all containers with liquid

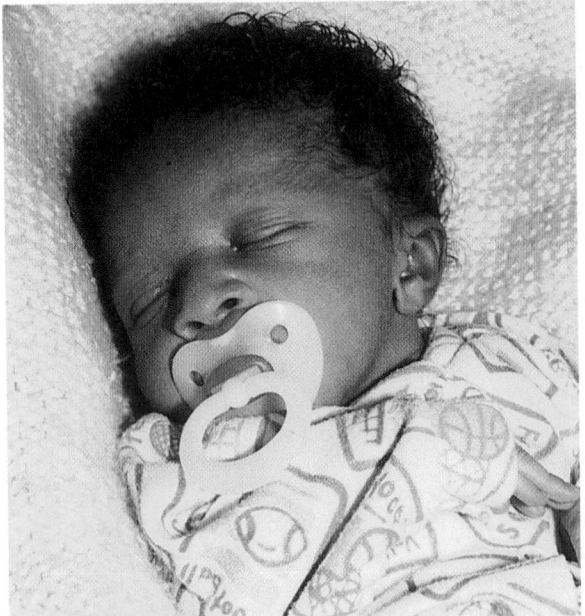

FIGURE 28.16 Many infants enjoy sucking on a pacifier to help them fall asleep.

preschoolers may be so jealous of a new baby they will physically harm an infant if left alone.

Bathing and Swimming Safety

As babies begin to develop good back support, many parents begin to bathe them in an adult tub. Caution parents never to leave an infant unattended in a tub, even when propped up out of the water or sitting in a bath ring or bath seat. Normal wiggling can easily cause the baby to slip down under the water. This applies to the hospital as well.

Many communities offer infant swim programs for babies as young as 6 months. If their child is enrolled in one of these programs, parents may become overconfident about their infant's ability to operate safely in water. Because children can dog-paddle momentarily in a swimming pool does not mean they can sustain that position for any length of time in a bathtub or pool (AAP Committee on Injury and Poison Prevention and Committee on Sports Medicine and Fitness, 2000). Being able to swim momentarily may cause children to lose their instinctive fear of water and so be in more danger when around water than children who are still naturally more cautious. Such programs may also spread microorganisms because infants this age are not yet toilet-trained (Schonberg-Norio et al., 2004).

Childproofing

When infants begin teething at 5 to 6 months, they chew on any object within reach to lessen gum-line pain. Remind parents to check for possible sources of lead paint, such as painted cribs, playpen rails, or windowsills. Paints safe for baby furniture should be marked "Safe for use on surfaces that might be chewed by children." If an infant is going to be allowed to play on the floor, parents should move furniture in front of electrical fixtures or buy protective caps for the outlets. Infants are especially fascinated by the holes and will probe them with (often wet) fingers. Parents may need to install safety gates at the top and bottom of stairways.

Urge parents to move all potentially poisonous substances from bottom cupboards and store them well out of their infant's reach. Infants of any age should not be left unattended in carriages, highchairs, grocery shopping carts, or strollers. Baby walkers are extremely dangerous because infants can maneuver them near stairways and fall the length of the stairs.

When infants begin creeping, remind parents to recheck bottom cupboards and stairways for safety. When the child begins to walk, higher areas, such as coffee tables, need to be cleared of dangerous items. In a hospital setting, assess low counter areas for dangerous objects. Do not leave possibly dangerous supplies in an infant's room.

By 10 months, achievement of a pincer grasp makes infants able to pick up very small objects. Remind parents to check play areas or areas such as table tops for pins or other sharp objects that could be swallowed. Some of an infant's toys are now also 10 months old and need to be checked to be certain they are still intact and safe.

Children who can walk may venture into the street or a swimming pool if not carefully supervised (Fig. 28.17). Although they seem very independent and able to take care of themselves, their judgment about what is dangerous is immature. In a hospital setting, a 12-month-old child can wander onto an elevator, out of the hospital, or into a laboratory area, or fall down a flight of stairs if not supervised.

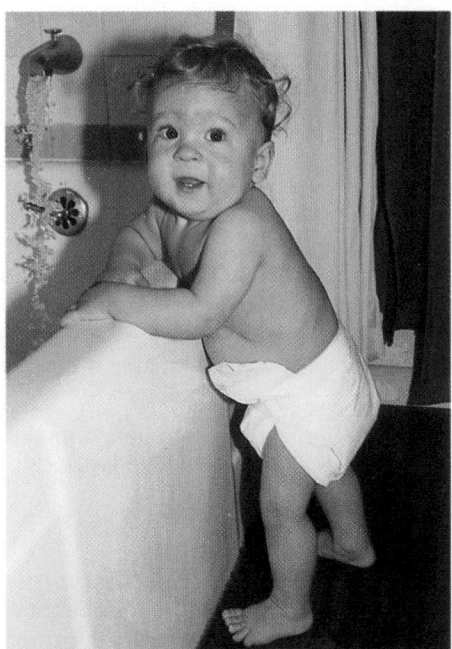

FIGURE 28.17 Once walking begins, the extended range of activities brings an infant in contact with potentially dangerous places or objects unless the house is childproofed. The bathroom is an important place to begin.

Checkpoint Question 4

You review infant safety with Bryan's mother. What are two of the most common types of accidents in infants?

a. Drowning and homicide
b. Poisoning and burns
c. Falls and auto accidents
d. Aspiration and falls

Promoting Nutritional Health of an Infant

The best food for an infant during the first 12 months of life (and the only food necessary for the first 6 months) is breast milk (see Chapter 25). With breast-feeding, as long as the mother is ingesting an adequate diet, no additional supplements such as iron or vitamins are necessary, except for fluoride if it is not included in the water supply.

If infants will not be exposed to sunshine, vitamin D may also be prescribed. How long mothers continue to breast-feed is an individual choice, although it is recommended through the entire first year (James, 2003). Prolonged breast-feeding into the preschool period is not usually recommended because it can limit nutrients and impair a child's growth.

For infants whose mothers choose not to breast-feed, a commercial iron-fortified formula may be used (see Appendix B). As with breast-feeding, supplementation is unnecessary with iron-fortified commercial formula unless the water supply does not contain fluoride. Infants who are changed to cow's milk before 1 year of age (a practice that is not recommended because the protein in cow's milk is difficult for an infant to digest) should receive a supplementary form of vitamin C and iron to make up for the deficiency of these components in cow's milk. The use of cow's milk may lead to such intestinal irritation that slight but continuous gastrointestinal bleeding occurs, resulting in anemia. Box 28.7 highlights outcomes and interventions related to infant nutrition using the terminology identified by the Nursing Outcomes Classification (NOC) and Nursing Interventions Classification (NIC).

Recommended Dietary Reference Intakes for an Infant

Because children's nutritional needs vary from infancy through adolescence, the recommended allowances of calories, protein, vitamins, and minerals also vary with each period of development.

The entire first year of life is one of extreme rapid growth, so a high-protein, high-calorie intake is needed.

BOX 28.7

Nursing Outcomes Classification (NOC) and Nursing Interventions Classification (NIC)

Infant nutrition

NOC: Knowledge, Diet

Knowledge, diet, is defined as the extent of understanding conveyed about diet (Johnson, Maas, & Moorhead, 2000). Some specific indicators suggesting achievement of this outcome include the parent's ability to:

- Describe recommendations for infant intake, including foods allowed and not allowed
- Select appropriate foods

NIC: Teaching, Infant Nutrition

Teaching, infant nutrition, is defined as instruction on nutrition and feeding practices during the first year of life (McCloskey & Bulechek, 2000). Some important activities involved when implementing this intervention include instructing the parent/caregiver in the following at:

0 to 3 months
- Feeding only breast milk or formula for first year
- Always holding infant when feeding and never propping bottle when feeding
- Limiting water intake to ½ oz to 1 oz at a time

- Avoiding use of honey or corn syrup
- Allowing non-nutritive sucking

4 to 6 months
- Introducing solid foods without added salt or sugar and iron-fortified cereal, one food at a time
- Avoiding use of juice or sweetened drinks
- Feeding from a spoon only

7 to 9 months
- Introducing finger foods and cup when infant is able to sit up
- Having infant join family at mealtimes
- Allowing self-feeding, with observation to prevent choking
- Offering fluids after solids
- Introducing limited amounts of diluted juice in a cup
- Avoiding sugary desserts and soda

10 to 12 months
- Offering 3 meals and healthy snacks
- Beginning to wean from bottle and beginning table foods
- Avoiding fruit drinks and flavored milk
- Allowing infant to feed self with spoon

Calorie allowances can be gradually reduced during the year from a level of 120 per kilogram of body weight at birth to approximately 100 per kilogram of body weight at the end of the first year to prevent babies from becoming overweight.

Although heredity plays a role, a baby who is overweight during the first year of life is more likely to become an obese adult than one whose weight is within normal limits. Breast-fed infants gain less weight than those who are formula-fed (James, 2003). Overfeeding in early life may produce large numbers of excess fat cells (adipocytes) used to store fat. Because these cells are permanent and remain filled with fat, once they are present, weight regulation can become difficult throughout life.

Introduction of Solid Food

From a nutritional standpoint, a normal full-term infant can thrive on a commercial iron-fortified formula or breast milk without the addition of any solid food until 4 to 6 months (Morin, 2004). Delaying solid food until this time helps prevent overwhelming an infant's kidneys with a heavy solute load. It also may delay the development of food allergies in susceptible infants. Most parents are eager to begin feeding their infant solid food, hoping this will help their child sleep through the night. Some parents do begin food before 6 months without apparent ill effects, possibly because much of the food is probably not processed by the gastrointestinal tract, passing through undigested due to the immaturity of the digestive system and decreased amylase and lipase secretion.

Generally speaking, infants are physiologically ready for solid food when they are taking more than 32 oz (960 mL) of formula a day and do not seem satisfied, or are nursing vigorously every 3 to 4 hours and do not seem satisfied. Infants are not ready to digest complex starches until amylase is present in saliva at approximately 2 to 3 months. Biting movements begin at approximately 3 months. Chewing movements do not begin until 7 to 9 months. Therefore, foods that require chewing should not be given until this age (Box 28.8).

Loss of Extrusion Reflex

When anything is placed on the anterior third of a newborn's tongue, it is automatically extruded or thrust out of the mouth by the tongue (extrusion reflex; Fig. 28.18). This is a life-saving reflex because it prevents infants from swallowing or aspirating foreign objects that touch the mouth. Infants extrude food when a spoonful of it is placed on the tongue in the same way. The reflex fades at 3 to 4 months. Until this time, it may be difficult to get an infant to eat solids.

Techniques for Feeding Solid Food

Table 28.4 shows the usual times and patterns for introducing solid food. Teach parents to offer new foods one

BOX 28.8 FOCUS ON . . .

FAMILY TEACHING

Tips to Help Introduce Solid Foods to Infants

Q. Bryan's mother had already started feeding him solid food. She asks, "When and how should I have begun solid foods?"

A. Infants typically are ready for solid food at 4 to 6 months of age. Use these guidelines to help when you start feeding your infant solid foods:

- Introduce one food at a time, waiting 5 to 7 days between new items.
- Introduce the food before formula or breast-feeding when an infant is hungry.
- Introduce small amounts of a new food (1 or 2 tsp) at a time.
- Respect infant food preferences; a child cannot be expected to like all new tastes equally well.
- Use only minimal to no salt and sugar on solid foods to minimize the number of additives.
- Remember that the extrusion reflex is present for the first 4 to 6 months of life, so any food placed on an infant's tongue will be pushed forward.
- To prevent aspiration, *do not* place food in bottles with formula.
- Introduce foods with a positive, "You'll like this" attitude.

at a time and allow a child to eat that item for about 1 week before introducing another new food. This system helps parents to detect possible food allergy. For example, if they start egg yolk on Monday and by Tuesday evening the child is breathing noisily or has a rash, they could suspect

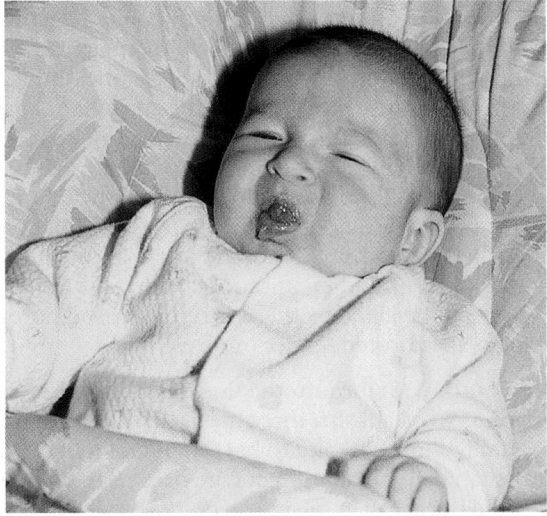

FIGURE 28.18 A 3-month-old baby demonstrates an extrusion reflex. Caution parents not to interpret this action as a food dislike but recognize it as the reflex action that it is.

the child is allergic to eggs. If two new foods had been started on Monday, it would be hard to know which one was suspect. Introducing foods one at a time also helps to establish a sense of trust in infants, because it minimizes the number of new experiences in any one day.

It is best for the first solid food feeding if an infant is held in the parent's arms as if for bottle-feeding or breast-feeding. This reduces the newness of the experience and minimizes the amount of stress associated with it. Some infants accept new experiences of this type readily, whereas other infants resist heartily. If an infant does not take readily to solid food, advise parents to wait a few days and then try again. Remind them that this is not a contest to see whose child takes cereal, vegetables, or fruit first.

Babies have distinct taste preferences even at young ages and may spit out a food because they do not like the taste. Even after the extrusion reflex has faded (at approximately 4 months), infants may appear to be spitting out food. This is because infants drink from a bottle or breast by pressing their tongue and the nipple against their hard palate. When an infant tries to eat solid food using the same technique, it appears that the child is spitting it out with the tongue. A parent who knows an infant's cues will be able to distinguish taste preferences from inadequate management of solid food. Box 28.8 lists pointers to help make the introduction of solid foods a positive experience.

Quantities and Types of Food

Infants take different quantities of food according to their preferences and needs. A newborn's stomach can hold approximately 2 tablespoons (30 mL). By 1 year, a stomach can hold no more than approximately 1 cup (240 mL). For this reason, when they begin eating solid food, infants rarely take more than 2 tablespoons (30 mL) at a time.

Cereal. The first food generally given to infants is infant cereal fortified with B vitamins and iron. These are precooked, fine dry powders to which orange juice, expressed breast milk, or infant formula is added. Orange juice is a good liquid to add because the iron in the cereal is absorbed best from an acid medium. All juices should be pasteurized for infants.

Initially, cereal should be mixed with enough fluid to make the mixture fairly liquid. As an infant adjusts to eating food from a spoon, parents can gradually thicken it. Adding sugar to cereal is unnecessary. Extra sugar in the diet can lead to diarrhea in young infants and beginning caries in older infants.

Fortified cereal costs no more than unfortified cereal, so remind parents to buy the fortified product. The first cereal introduced is usually rice cereal, because fewer children are allergic to rice products than to wheat and corn products. Usually, it is offered twice a day, morning and evening. Once the child has taken rice cereal for 1 week, parents can try another kind.

Some parents mix cereal with an infant's formula and give it to the child from a bottle. Caution parents to avoid this practice because (1) it is necessary to cut a larger hole in the bottle nipple for the cereal and milk mixture to flow freely, and there is a danger an infant may aspirate if the hole cut is too big; (2) there is a real danger of aspiration if the parent then uses that nipple for formula without

TABLE 28.4

Suggested Schedule for Introduction of Solid Foods

Age (mo)	Food to Introduce*	Rationale
5–6	Iron-fortified infant cereal mixed with breast milk, orange juice, or formula	Aids in preventing iron-deficiency anemia; the least allergenic type of food; an easily digested food
7	Vegetables	Good source of vitamin A; adds new texture and flavors to diet
8	Fruit	Best source of vitamin C, good source of vitamin A; adds new texture and flavors to diet
9	Meat	Good source of protein, iron, and B vitamins
10	Egg yolk	Good source of iron

*Wheat, tomatoes, oranges, fish, and egg whites should be omitted if there are allergies in the family, because these foods are most likely to cause allergies.

cereal added; and (3) it denies the child the opportunity of learning to eat from a spoon and experiencing different food tastes and textures.

Infant cereal is so rich in iron parents should continue feeding it at least through the first year. Ideally, children should eat infant cereal until age 3 or 4 years, as few popularly advertised products can match the nutrients of fortified infant cereal.

Vegetables and Fruit. Because their iron content is generally higher than that of fruits, vegetables are usually the second food added to the diet (at approximately 7 months of age). Parents who have a blender, strainer, or grinder can prepare their own. They simply cook a vegetable and then blend or strain it so it does not have to be chewed. Caution parents not to add butter or salt to the preparation, because infants have difficulty digesting fats until almost the end of the first year, and the added salt is unnecessary. Additional sugar is also unnecessary. By filling ice-cube trays with the blended vegetables, parents can make a 1-week supply and defrost a cube at a time. An ice cube is approximately 1 oz, or one-fourth the size of a jar of baby food.

If parents use commercial baby food, they should feed it from a dish rather than directly from the jar. This is because if the spoon carries salivary enzymes from an infant's mouth to the food, the enzymes will liquefy what remains in the jar. Also, there is danger of transferring bacteria (principally streptococci) from an infant's mouth to the jar. Then, if the parent keeps the jar for another feeding in the next 24 hours, bacteria will multiply rapidly because the contents serve as a culture medium. Baby food jars should be refrigerated once they are opened, and manufacturers recommend they be used no longer than 48 hours after they have been opened.

When vegetables are added to the diet, they are usually offered at lunch. Remind parents to offer both green and yellow vegetables. Help them to remember that their own dislike of a particular vegetable does not mean their child will feel the same way about it. If they do convey distaste for a food, the child will pick up on the feeling and will not like the vegetable either.

Fruit is usually offered 1 month after beginning vegetables (at approximately age 8 months). It can be given in addition to cereal for breakfast and dinner. Raw mashed banana is easy to prepare with just a fork; peaches are easily prepared in a blender. As with vegetables, parents should offer a selection so an infant is exposed to different tastes and textures.

Meat and Eggs. Meat is usually introduced at 9 months. Parents can grind a portion of the meat they have prepared for their own meal so it is tender, or they can use commercially prepared products. If they use commercial baby meat, urge them to use the plain meat products, not vegetable and meat dinners, because these contain mostly vegetables. Chicken has the advantage of being low in cholesterol, but this is not a priority with infants. Beef and pork have more iron than chicken, so encourage parents to offer these more frequently than chicken. When meat is added to an infant's diet, it is usually added as part of the evening meal in place of cereal.

Egg yolks are offered by 10 months of age. Egg yolks contain the bulk of the iron content of eggs; the white contains the bulk of protein. Egg yolk alone should be given at first, because the protein of the egg white can lead to allergy or can be difficult for an infant to digest. Eggs may be prepared by hard-boiling (then adding a little formula or breast milk to the mashed yolk to make it more liquid) or purchased as commercial baby food. Soft-boiling or poaching is not usually recommended, because salmonella, the chief offending microorganism that may be in eggs, may not be killed by these methods. Also, thorough cooking makes protein easier to digest.

Table Food. With the introduction of solid food, encourage parents to establish a three-meal-a-day pattern, if that is the family's lifestyle, and to have an infant join the family at the table. Generally, encourage parents to use homemade foods rather than relying on commercially prepared junior foods, although commercial foods are now prepared without excessive additives and are convenient for parents who have little preparation time. Mashed potatoes or peas and cut-up meatloaf are examples of table foods that infants older than 6 months of age like to eat and busy parents can prepare quickly. If hot dogs are offered, caution parents to cut them into small bite-size portions; otherwise, they can be aspirated. As infants begin teething, they enjoy dried bread, teething biscuits, or zwieback.

Some infants are too distracted by the activity at a family table to eat well. Parents may find these children eat more if they are fed first and then allowed to have a small amount to "feed themselves" or a cracker to chew on while just sitting at the table and being with the family.

Remind parents that highchairs are one of the most dangerous pieces of baby equipment they own. Urge them always to fasten the restraint and never leave an infant unattended in a highchair, because even a 6-month-old can squirm out of a chair with little effort. Nurses must also keep this in mind when feeding infants in a hospital setting.

Establishment of Healthy Eating Patterns

Some parents may need to be reminded there are no hard-and-fast rules for infant feeding. The rules are only guidelines based on what seems to work well with most infants. Encourage them to individualize their approach according to the cues their child is giving them for readiness.

A child who adapts to change poorly may have difficulty accepting the first solid food and may have difficulty with each new food. Parents may need support to remember a child is not conducting this struggle out of a desire for conflict but because this is a characteristic of temperament. Giving food to others is interpreted by many as giving love, so refusing food is equated with refusing love. Help parents understand this is not what is happening. Refusing a teaspoonful of carrots is refusing a teaspoonful of carrots, nothing more.

Most infants, however, eat hungrily so feeding problems tend to be reported more frequently as a second-year or toddler problem than as an infant concern. If an infant does refuse to eat, ask the parents what foods they are offering. Have them list exactly the types and amounts of foods the child ate the day before (a 24-hour dietary recall history). It may be apparent from this that enough is being eaten in a day's time and that the parents' expectations are unrealistic for the child's size and age.

If intake is inadequate and the child is, indeed, a fussy eater, ask about the parents' methods of feeding. For example, ask if they are offering a bottle first and then infant food. Infants generally accept the new experience of eating from a spoon better when they are hungry, not when their stomach is full. On the other hand, some babies, particularly those with an intense temperament, may be so hungry at mealtime they cannot tolerate the frustration of spoon-feeding until some of their hunger is relieved. They may need to drink 2 or 3 oz of formula or nurse at the breast for a few minutes before they will eat a spoonful of food.

An infant who is fatigued or overstimulated may not eat well. Providing a quiet environment away from older brothers or sisters before mealtime may solve this problem.

Encourage parents not to force infants to eat if they do not seem hungry. Healthy, happy infants will be hungry at mealtime and will eat. Those who refuse a meal may be tired, distracted, or perhaps ill. Forcing only leads to regurgitation or, if they are ill, vomiting. It also can result in feeding problems or a situation in which infants refuse to eat altogether. Infants who are eating and not thriving or not eating and therefore not thriving should be examined to determine if a cause such as a metabolic disorder or failure to thrive exists (see Chapters 48 and 55).

Weaning

Infants are capable of approximating their lips to a cup so they can drink effectively from one at about 9 months of age. The sucking reflex begins to diminish in intensity between ages 6 and 9 months, which makes this the time to consider weaning.

To wean from formula or breast milk, the mother chooses one feeding a day and then begins offering fluid by the new method at that feeding. She should choose a time of day that is not an infant's fussy period; other than that, the time is immaterial. After 3 days to 1 week, when an infant has become acclimated to the one change, the mother changes a second feeding. Should an illness such as an upper respiratory infection occur or should the child have teething discomfort, there will be setbacks, so no set number of weeks should be prescribed to complete weaning. Infants usually need more fluid during hot weather than cold weather because of increased perspiration. This may make it more difficult to begin weaning during the summer.

Self-Feeding

At approximately 6 months of age, infants become interested in handling a spoon and beginning to feed themselves. Their coordination, unfortunately, has not developed enough for them to use a spoon without a great deal of spilling, so they are much more adept at feeding themselves with their fingers (Fig. 28.19). Parents concerned with neatness can spread newspapers, a plastic tablecloth, or a towel on the floor around a highchair to catch most

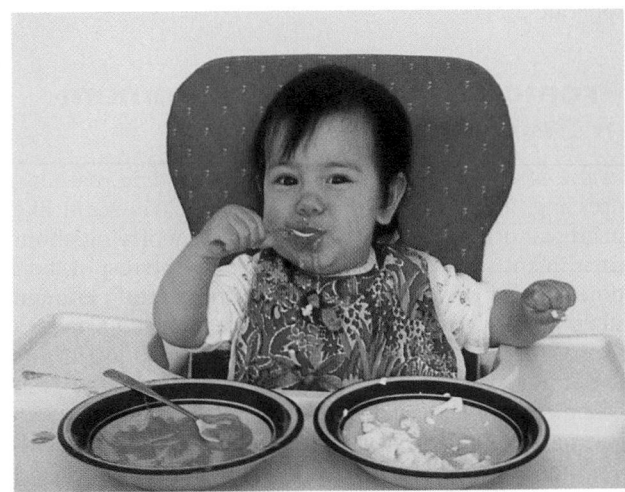

FIGURE 28.19 Self-feeding is not always a neat process for an infant.

of the dropped food, and then let the child practice. When an infant becomes fatigued or frustrated by attempts at self-feeding, a parent can then quietly help without making an issue of it. Parents who insist on continuing to spoon-feed past the time an infant wants to feed himself or herself can cause an infant to balk at eating. Often, a compromise is helpful. If a parent gives an infant a spoon, the child can poke at a cereal dish with it while the parent continues to offer him or her bites from a second spoon. In this way, the child is "in charge" of the feeding yet receptive to taking food from the parent.

When infants no longer attempt to feed themselves at a meal but merely begin to play with their food by squeezing it through their fingers or dabbing it in their hair, it is time to end the meal. This behavior indicates that they have had enough.

Adequate Intake With a Vegetarian Diet

An infant eating a vegetarian diet should continue to be breast-fed or ingest an iron-fortified, balanced, commercial formula for the entire first year. If a milk allergy is present, a soy-based formula can be used. When solid foods are added at 6 months, an assortment of foods should be provided, including vegetables such as avocados, potatoes, and broccoli; fruits such as apples, prunes (high in iron), and bananas; infant cereal; tofu; wheat germ; legumes; brewer's yeast; and synthetic vitamin D. Feeding fortified cereal throughout the first year will ensure that iron stores are built. If the diet is to include dairy products, these can be added toward the end of the first year as usual.

Because vegetarian diets are high in fiber, they may cause infants to have more frequent and looser-than-normal bowel movements. Teach parents to change diapers frequently to avoid skin irritation. Using less fibrous, more concentrated forms of protein, such as tofu and powdered nuts rather than cereal mixtures, can minimize this problem.

A sound vegetarian diet can be easily designed for the older infant who prefers finger foods, because many vegetables, fruits, and grains (e.g., pieces of oranges, peaches, tomatoes, and crackers) are easily eaten this way (Barr & Rideout, 2004).

Promoting Infant Development in Daily Activities

In the first year, caring for an infant—feeding, bathing, dressing, and so forth—occupies what may seem like nearly all of the parents' waking hours. Worrying about their infant's sleep patterns may take up the rest of their time, often because the parents are not getting enough sleep themselves. All of these basic care-related activities provide important opportunities for caregivers and infants to get to know one another and to become used to each other's personalities and patterns. Nurses can play a key role in teaching parents about these activities and stressing their importance. Box 28.9 highlights outcomes and interventions related to infant care using the terminology identified by the Nursing Outcomes Classification (NOC) and Nursing Interventions Classification (NIC).

Bathing

Except in very hot weather, an infant does not need a bath every day. If a parent is tired and would not enjoy bath time or if some days are just too rushed, a complete bath can be omitted, with only an infant's face, hands, and diaper area washed. Some infants do need their head and scalp washed frequently (every day or every other day) to prevent **seborrhea**, a scaly scalp condition often called cradle cap. If seborrhea lesions do develop, they adhere to the scalp in yellow, crusty patches. The skin beneath them may be slightly erythematous. The patches can be softened by oiling the scalp with mineral oil or petroleum jelly and leaving it on overnight. The crusts can then be removed by shampooing the hair the next morning. A soft toothbrush or fine-toothed comb can be used to help remove crusts.

Bath time should be fun for an infant and can serve many functions other than just the obvious one of cleanliness (Fig. 28.20). Especially during the second half of the first year, a child enjoys poking at soap bubbles on the surface of the water or playing with bath toys. Bath time also helps an infant learn different textures and sensations and provides an opportunity to exercise and kick, as well as a good opportunity for a parent to touch and communicate with the child. Teach parents not to leave infants alone in tubs as they could easily slip under the water.

Diaper-Area Care

The most effective means of promoting good diaper-area hygiene is to change diapers frequently, about every 2 to 4 hours. However, it is rarely good practice to interrupt the child's sleep to change diapers. If an infant develops a rash from sleeping in wet diapers, air drying or sleeping without a diaper may be a solution.

At each diaper change, the parents should wash the skin with clear water or with a commercial alcohol-free diaper wipe (and perfume-free if an infant has sensitive skin), then pat or allow to air dry. Routinely using an ointment such as Desitin or A & D ointment to keep urine and feces away from an infant's skin is good prophylaxis. Parents do not need to use baby powder. If they choose to, advise them to sprinkle the powder on their hands first, and then apply it to an infant's skin. Caution them not to shake the powder on an infant, to reduce the possibility of aspiration. They should place the container out of the infant's reach afterward, or an infant could easily spill it into his mouth and aspirate it.

Care of Teeth

It is well accepted that exposing developing teeth to fluoride is one of the most effective ways to promote healthy tooth formation and prevent tooth decay. The most important time for children to receive fluoride is between 6 months and 12 years of age. A water level of 0.6 ppm fluoride is recommended because this is the level that protects tooth enamel yet does not lead to staining of teeth. In communities where the water supply does not provide enough fluoride, the use of an oral fluoride supplement beginning at 6 months or the use of fluoride toothpaste or rinses after tooth eruption is recommended (AAP, 2001).

BOX 28.9

Nursing Outcomes Classification (NOC) and Nursing Interventions Classification (NIC)

Infant care

NOC: Knowledge, Infant

Knowledge, infant, is defined as the extent of understanding conveyed about caring for a baby up to 12 months (Johnson, Maas, & Moorhead, 2000). Some specific indicators suggesting achievement of this outcome include the parent's ability to describe the following:

- Normal infant characteristics and development
- Proper holding and positioning
- Infant safety measures
- Feeding choices and techniques
- Signs of problems such as dehydration or jaundice
- Infant bathing, diapering, cord care, temperature taking, sleep–wake patterns, communication, stimulation methods, and relaxation techniques
- Family adjustments to addition of infant
- Considerations when choosing a childcare provider
- Community resources for infant care

NIC: Parent Education, Infant

Parent education, infant, is defined as instruction on nurturing and physical care needed during the first year of life (McCloskey & Bulechek, 2000). Some important activities involved when implementing this intervention include the following:

- Determining parents' knowledge and readiness to learn, along with continued monitoring of learning needs
- Providing anticipatory guidance about developmental changes and behavioral characteristics
- Assisting with ways to integrate infant into family system
- Teaching parents skills to care for infant, including formula preparation and selection, use of pacifiers, addition of solid foods to diet, fluoride supplementation, dentition, oral hygiene, elimination patterns, and sleep patterns
- Demonstrating ways to stimulate infant's development
- Encouraging holding, cuddling, massaging, touching, talking, reading, playing, and providing pleasurable auditory and visual stimulation
- Providing examples of appropriate toys
- Assisting with interpreting infant cues
- Demonstrating infant's abilities and strengths, quieting techniques
- Monitoring parents' skill in recognizing infant's needs and reinforcing caregiver role behaviors
- Providing information about safety needs in the home and car

---

Teach parents to ask about the presence of fluoride in the drinking water in their community and help them to determine what, if any, supplementation is necessary. Breast-fed infants do not receive a great deal of fluoride from breast milk, so it may be recommended they be given fluoride drops once a day. Teach parents to begin "brushing" even before teeth erupt by rubbing a soft washcloth over the gum pads. This eliminates plaque and reduces the presence of bacteria, creating a clean environment for the arrival of the first teeth. Once teeth erupt, all surfaces should be brushed with a soft brush or washcloth once or twice a day. Children lack the coordination to brush effectively until they are school-age, so parents must be responsible for this activity well past infancy. Toothpaste is not necessary for an infant, because it is the scrubbing that removes the plaque.

The initial dental checkup should be made by 2 or 2.5 years of age; checkups should continue at 6-month intervals until adulthood.

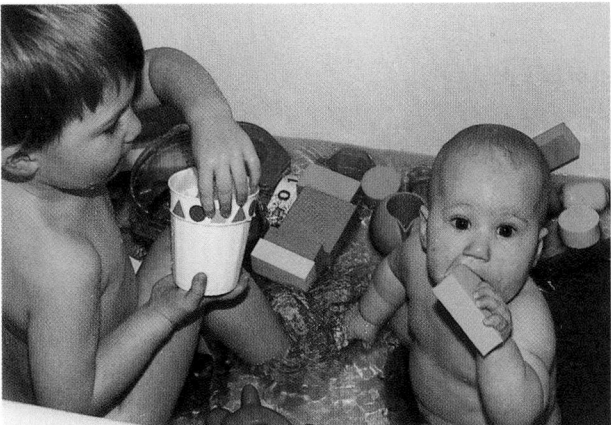

FIGURE 28.20 An 8-month-old enjoys bathtime with his big brother. Parents should always watch carefully while infants and toddlers are in the tub.

Dressing

Clothing for infants should be easy to launder and simply constructed, so dressing and undressing are not a struggle. Infants enjoy kicking and making gross body movements, so their clothing should not be binding. When they begin to creep, they need long pants to protect their knees. Until they begin to walk, they need only soft-soled shoes or merely socks or booties to keep their feet warm. Even when they begin walking, the soles of their shoes need only be firm enough to protect their feet against rough surfaces. Extremely hard soles and high ankle sides are unnecessary.

Sleep

Sleep needs and habits vary greatly among infants, but most require 10 to 12 hours of sleep at night and one or several naps during the day. Parents are usually advised to let a baby sleep in a separate space rather than in their bed so the parents do not awaken at every toss and squeak. Doing so allows infants to learn to quiet themselves and go back to sleep should they awaken briefly. This may help prevent sleep problems such as night waking in the future. Other parents prefer to have infants sleep with them in a family bed, as they believe this practice promotes a feeling of security (Mesich, 2004). Caution parents not to place pillows in an infant's bed to avoid suffocation. Always place an infant on his or her back to sleep because this position markedly reduces the incidence of sudden infant death syndrome (SIDS) (NCHS, 2005). See Chapter 26 for further discussion of SIDS.

Exercise

Infants benefit from outings in a carriage or stroller because sunlight provides a natural source of vitamin D. In hot weather, caution parents to protect an infant from sunburn by exposing the child to the sun for only very short periods, beginning with 3 to 5 minutes the first day, a little more the next day, and so on up to 15 to 20 minutes at a time. The sun is most intense between 10 AM and 3 PM, so early mornings and late afternoons are the best times for infants to be outside. These short time spans are necessary because the use of sunscreen is not recommended in children until they are at least 6 months old.

Toward the end of the first year, infants need space to crawl and then to walk, such as in an enclosed outdoor play space. In addition to providing fresh air, going for leisurely walks while pointing out the sights of the world—trees, birds, dogs, houses, neighbors—helps children develop language.

Parents can judge how much outdoor clothing to put on an infant by how much they need themselves. If an adult needs a winter coat, an infant will need a snowsuit; sweaters may be adequate for both; if an adult needs no outer clothing, an infant probably doesn't either.

It is not necessary to enroll infants in formal exercise programs for them to secure adequate exercise. Such programs may put unusual strain on muscles and tendons. Infants using infant walkers must be closely supervised, because they can be injured if they maneuver the walker too near a stairway and fall.

Promoting Healthy Family Functioning

A primary task of parents during the infant year is to learn to interpret infants' cues to decipher their needs. It is helpful if they can learn early on to perceive an infant as a separate individual with unique needs. This becomes an easier task by 2 months, when infants can indicate by their particular cry whether they are feeling cold, hungry, wet, or lonely. Parents spend a great deal of time with their infant in these first months, which gives them the opportunity to learn and recognize nonverbal cues and to become aware of their baby's needs.

Parental Concerns and Problems Related to Normal Infant Development

Some of the difficulties parents are apt to have in evaluating the health of infants are shown in Table 28.5. New parents may need reassurance and answers to questions about childcare procedures or health during an infant period because they have not yet learned their child's cues. However, the need for reassurance may be just as great in experienced parents. The unique characteristics of each child require some adjustment from parents.

Teething

Most infants have little difficulty with teething, but some appear very distressed. Generally, the gums are sore and

---

TABLE 28.5

Common Difficulties Parents Experience in Evaluating the Health of Infants

Difficulty	Suggestions for Improving Assessment
Evaluating pain	Infants manifest pain by fussiness. They can reveal arm and leg pain by immobility of the body part; ear pain by brushing or tugging at the ear; stomach pain by pulling up the legs against the abdomen.
Evaluating degree of reduced activity	Lack of interest in smiling or interaction is an important observation. Increased sleeping or lying supine with legs nonflexed (frog-legged) as if exhausted is important.
Evaluating infant temperature	All parents should learn how to take an axillary or tympanic temperature so they can report a specific degree of fever rather than a subjective finding, such as "feels hot."
Evaluating amount of vomiting or diarrhea	Knowing the number of times vomiting and/or diarrhea has occurred is important. Estimating amount in comparisons with what the child has eaten is helpful as well as estimating an amount (a cupful, etc.). Knowing whether diapers are "soaked" or "stained" with stools is important in estimating amount. Caution parents that vomiting and diarrhea are always serious in infants.

tender before a new tooth breaks the surface. As soon as the tooth is through, the tenderness passes.

Because of this pain, infants can be resistant to chewing for a day or two and be slightly cranky, possibly because they are a little hungry from not eating as much as usual. High fever, seizures, vomiting or diarrhea, and earache are never normal signs of teething. An infant with any of these symptoms has an underlying infection or disease process requiring further evaluation.

Many over-the-counter medicines are sold for teething pain. As a rule, their use should be discouraged if they contain benzocaine, a topical anesthetic, because if applied too far back in the throat, this could interfere with the gag reflex. Acetaminophen (Tylenol), 10 to 15 mg/kg every 4 hours, up to four times a day, may be used for teething discomfort. Always encourage parents to check with their infant's health care provider before giving any over-the-counter drug this way. Teething rings that can be placed in the refrigerator provide soothing coolness against the tender gums. An infant who is teething will place almost any object in the mouth, so parents must screen articles within the baby's reach to be sure they are edible or safe to chew on (Boom, 2003).

Thumb Sucking

Sucking is a surprisingly strong need: sonograms even demonstrate fetal thumb sucking in utero. Many infants begin to suck a thumb or finger at about 3 months of age and continue the habit through the first few years of life. The sucking reflex peaks at 6 to 8 months, whereas thumb sucking peaks at about 18 months.

Parents can be assured that thumb sucking is normal and does not deform the jaw line as long as it stops by school age. It does not cause "baby talk" or any of the other symptoms commonly attributed to it. The best approach is to be certain an infant has adequate sucking pleasure and then to ignore thumb sucking. Making an issue of it rarely causes a child to stop; if anything, it usually intensifies and prolongs it.

Use of Pacifiers

Whether to use pacifiers is a question parents must settle for themselves, depending on how they feel about them and their infant's needs. Infants rarely have such a need for sucking they must have a pacifier in their mouth constantly. Discussing a few pros and cons with the parents clarifies the subject.

An infant who completes a feeding and still seems restless and discontent, who actively searches for something to put into the mouth, or who sucks on hands and clothes may need a pacifier. Babies who have colic crave sucking and enjoy pacifiers because their abdomen hurts, and they interpret this as a hunger sensation. If a child is formula-fed, parents should check nipples to be certain the holes are small and the rubber is sturdy, so that an infant can suck hard enough to derive pleasure. If the nipples are satisfactory, parents could offer a pacifier after feeding for more sucking. Theoretically, a child whose sucking needs are met in infancy will not crave as much oral stimulation later in life and is less likely to become a pencil chewer, cigarette smoker, nail biter, or the like.

The use of pacifiers has been associated with an increased incidence of otitis media (Cinar, 2004). A major drawback of pacifiers is the problem of cleanliness. They tend to fall on the floor or sidewalk and are then put back into an infant's mouth. If not well constructed, they may come apart and be aspirated. Hanging a pacifier on a string around an infant's neck could cause strangulation.

Parents should attempt to wean a child from a pacifier any time after 3 months of age and certainly during the time the sucking reflex is fading at 6 to 9 months. Weaning after this age is difficult because a pacifier becomes a comfort mechanism, like a warm blanket or fuzzy toy to which a child may cling.

Head Banging

Some infants rhythmically bang their heads against the bars of a crib for a period of time before falling asleep. This is distressing behavior for parents. Besides fearing that children will hurt themselves, some parents may have heard that blind children or those with mental illness do this and worry that their child is ill in some way.

Head banging in this limited fashion—beginning during the second half of the first year of life and continuing through to the preschool period, associated with naptime or bedtime, and lasting under 15 minutes—can be considered normal. Children use this measure to relax and fall asleep. Investigating stress factors operating in the house may be helpful. If some of them can be relieved (e.g., parents' overestimation of the child's development, marital discord, illness in another family member), the head banging may decrease, or it may have already become such a strong habit that it will persist for months or even years.

Advise parents to pad the rails of cribs so infants cannot hurt themselves, and reassure them this is a normal mechanism for relief of tension in children of this age. No therapy should be necessary. Excessive head banging done to the exclusion of normal development or activity, or head banging past the preschool period, suggests a pathologic basis, and such children then need a referral for counseling and further evaluation.

Sleep Problems

Sleep problems develop in early infancy because of colic or because an otherwise healthy infant takes longer than usual to adjust to sleeping through the night. Breast-fed babies tend to wake more often than those who are formula-fed because breast milk is more easily digested, so infants become hungry sooner. In late infancy, the problem of waking at night and remaining awake for an hour or more becomes common. Although an infant may be content and not cry during this time, parents are reluctant to sleep while a child is awake, so they may become extremely fatigued. This is an increasing concern because more and more families today consist of two wage-earning parents; there is no time for parents to nap during the day to make up for sleep lost at night. Suggestions for eliminating or at least coping with night waking are (1) delay bedtime by 1 hour; (2) shorten an afternoon sleep period; (3) do not respond immediately to infants at night so they can have time to fall back to sleep on their own; and (4) provide soft toys or music to allow infants to play quietly alone during this wakeful time. Reassuring parents that infants take vary-ing lengths of time to adjust to night sleeping is helpful in assuring them their child is normal. Suggesting parents use the time they are awake at night (e.g., solve a problem at work, watch the late show, plan a shopping list) may help them view the situation as a constructive time rather than a problem.

Constipation

Breast-fed infants are rarely constipated because their stools tend to be loose. Constipation may occur in formula-fed in-fants if their diet is deficient in fluid. This can be corrected simply with the addition of more fluid.

Some parents misinterpret the normal pushing move-ments of a newborn to be constipation. When infants defe-cate, their faces do turn red, and they grimace and grunt. As long as stools are not hard and contain no evidence of fresh blood (as might occur with a rectal fissure), this is normal infant behavior.

If constipation persists beyond 5 or 6 months of age, encourage parents to check with the infant's health care provider about measures to relieve this. Adding foods with bulk, such as fruits or vegetables, and increasing fluid in-take generally relieves the problem. Apple juice (3 or 4 oz) or prune juice (0.5 to 1 oz daily) may be given as a tem-porary measure.

All infants with a history of constipation for more than 1 week should be examined for an anal fissure or tight anal sphincter. Softening stools and thereby relieving the pain of defecation often solves the problem and helps the fis-sure to heal. If an unusually tight anal sphincter exists, parents will be given instructions to manually dilate the sphincter two or three times daily until it dilates suffi-ciently. Hirschsprung's disease (aganglionic megacolon, or lack of nerve innervation to a portion of the colon) may be manifested early in life as constipation. If no stool is pres-ent in the rectum of a constipated infant on rectal exami-nation, this disease is suggested (Jamieson et al., 2004). A careful history must then be taken to assess for other symp-toms of Hirschsprung's disease: ribbonlike stools, bouts of diarrhea, and a distended abdomen (see Chapter 45).

Chronic constipation also may occur in children with congenital hypothyroidism (decreased functioning of the thyroid gland). Therefore, an infant with constipation also should be carefully observed for characteristic signs of hypothyroidism, such as lethargy, protruding tongue, and failure to meet developmental milestones (see Chapter 48). Infants with either Hirschsprung's disease or hypothyroid-ism need therapy to correct the disorder.

Loose Stools

Many new parents are unfamiliar with the consistency or color of normal newborn stools, so they mistakenly report normal stooling as diarrhea. Stools of breast-fed infants are generally softer than those of formula-fed infants. If a mother takes a laxative while breast-feeding, an infant's stools may be very loose. An infant who is formula-fed can have loose stools if the formula is not diluted properly.

Occasionally, loose stools may begin with the introduc-tion of solid food, such as fruit. Malabsorption syndrome (celiac disease), or inability to digest fat, may manifest itself first by loose stools and a distended abdomen and defi-ciency of fat-soluble vitamins (see Chapter 45).

When talking to a parent about loose stools, ask about the duration of the loose stools, the number of stools per day, their color and consistency, and whether there is any mucus or blood in them. Is there associated fever, cramp-ing, or vomiting? Does an infant continue to eat well? Appear well? Seem to be thriving? Is an infant wetting at least six diapers daily?

Infants with associated signs and symptoms such as fever, cramping, vomiting, loss of appetite, a decrease in voiding, and weight loss should be examined by their health care provider because this suggests an infectious process. Dehydration occurs rapidly in a small infant who is not eating and is losing body fluid through loose stools.

Colic

Colic is paroxysmal abdominal pain that generally occurs in infants under 3 months of age (Karp, 2004). An infant cries loudly and pulls the legs up against the abdomen. The infant's face becomes red and flushed, the fists clench, and the abdomen becomes tense. If offered a bottle, the infant will suck vigorously for a few minutes as if starved, then stop as another wave of intestinal pain occurs.

The cause of colic is unclear. It may occur in suscepti-ble infants from overfeeding or from swallowing too much air while feeding. Formula-fed babies are more likely to have colic than breast-fed babies, possibly because they swallow more air while drinking or because formula is harder to digest.

Although infants continue to thrive despite colic, the condition should not be dismissed as unimportant. It is a distressing and frightening problem for parents because an infant not only appears to be in acute pain, but the distress persists for hours, usually into the middle of the night, so no one in the family gets adequate rest. This is a difficult beginning to a parent–child relationship, which needs to be strong and binding for the parents to enjoy parenting and for an infant to thrive in their care (Box 28.10).

Take a thorough history of an infant with signs of colic because intestinal obstruction or infection may mimic an attack of colic and be misinterpreted by the casual inter-viewer. Ask parents about the duration of the problem and its frequency (it usually lasts up to 3 hours a day and occurs at least 3 days every week). Ask what happens just before the attack (e.g., if it occurs after feeding), and ask the parent to describe the attack itself and associated symp-toms. Document the number and type of bowel move-ments, because bowel movements are not abnormal with colic. Constipation; narrow, ribbonlike stools; and the presence of blood or mucus in the stool suggest other problems. A family medical history is important to obtain because allergy to milk may simulate colic.

Determine the baby's feeding pattern (breast-fed or bottle-fed). If bottle-fed, ask about the type of formula and how it is prepared. Ask parents if they are holding the baby upright so air bubbles can rise and whether they burp the infant adequately after feeding. For a breast-fed baby, a change in maternal diet (e.g., avoiding "gassy" foods) might be helpful to reduce or limit colicky periods. It may be help-

BOX 28.10 FOCUS ON . . .

EVIDENCE-BASED PRACTICE

What Is It Like to Be the Parent of an Infant?

Infants change so drastically from the time they are born until the end of the first year, parents have to also change constantly. To investigate how parents describe what this experience is like, researchers completed a literature review of 33 articles on parenthood. Results of the study showed that, overall, parents reported their first-year experience as overwhelming. Mothers reported this stemmed from worry about being satisfied and confident as a mother, the strain of being primarily responsible for a child, struggling with the limited time available for oneself, and fatigue. Fathers said that strain arose from trying to be confident as a father and partner, living up to the new demands on them, and being the protector and provider of the family. A unifying theme was "living in a new and overwhelming world."

This is an important study for nurses, because it details how important it is for nurses to ask parents of infants at health care visits how they are managing in their new role.

Source: Nystrom, K., & Ohrling, K. (2004). Parenthood experiences during the child's first year: literature review. *Journal of Advanced Nursing, 46*(3), 319–330.

ful to recommend that both breast- and formula-fed infants receive small, frequent feedings to prevent distention and discomfort. Offering a pacifier may be comforting.

Some parents try placing a hot water bottle on their infant's stomach for comfort, but this should be discouraged. A basic rule for any abdominal discomfort is to avoid heat in case appendicitis is developing. This is highly unlikely in so young an infant, but parents will remember they once used heat and may use it again when the child is older. Hot water bottles and heating pads also might burn the delicate skin of infants.

Changing formula bottles to the type with disposable bags that collapse as the baby sucks may help minimize the amount of air swallowed. Taking infants for car rides is often reported as being helpful in soothing colicky babies. Some music boxes simulate the sound of a heartbeat, which also may be helpful. Although rarely necessary, phenobarbital may be prescribed if no nonpharmacologic solutions are successful (Carey, 2003).

It is important to think of colic as a family problem or else a vicious circle may gradually begin. An infant cries and the parents become tense and unsure of themselves. An infant senses the tension and develops more colic. Help parents plan relief time from infant care to relieve their stress level and prevent this cycle.

In most infants, colic disappears almost magically at 3 months of age, probably because it becomes easier to digest food and an infant maintains a more upright position by this time, which allows less gas to form (Box 28.11).

Spitting Up

Almost all infants spit up, although formula-fed babies appear to do it more than breast-fed babies. Parents who did not handle their infant much in the health care facility where their child was born may discover spitting up only after they take the baby home. They may interpret this as vomiting or think an infant is developing an infection. Ask them to describe carefully what they mean by "spitting up." How long has the baby been doing it? How frequently? What is the appearance of the spit-up milk? Almost all milk that is spit up smells at least faintly sour, but it should not contain blood or bile.

The baby who spits up a mouthful of milk (rolling down the chin) two or three times a day (or sometimes after every meal) is experiencing normal, early-infancy spitting up. Associated signs such as diarrhea, abdominal cramps, fever, cough, cold, or loss of activity suggest illness. If an infant is spitting up so forcefully that milk is projected 3 or 4 feet away, it may be beginning pyloric stenosis (an abnormally tight valve between the stomach and duodenum), which requires surgical intervention. If the spitting up is a large amount with each feeding, parents may be describing gastroesophageal reflux, in which a lax cardiac sphincter and esophagus allow regurgitation of gastric contents into the esophagus. This also requires medical attention (see Chapter 45).

Burping the baby thoroughly after a feeding often limits spitting up. Parents may try sitting an infant in an infant chair for half an hour after feeding. Changing formulas generally is of little value. Reassure parents that spitting up decreases in amount as the baby becomes better at coordinating his or her swallowing and digestive processes (the cardiac sphincter matures). In the meantime, a bib can protect the baby's clothing and the parent. After a few months, the child will naturally stay in an upright position longer, and gravity will help to correct the problem.

Diaper Dermatitis

Some infants have such sensitive skin that diaper dermatitis (diaper rash) is a problem from the first few days of life. It occurs for a number of reasons.

When parents do not change a child's diaper frequently, feces is left in contact with skin, and irritation may result in the perianal area. Urine that is left in diapers too long breaks down into ammonia, a chemical that is extremely irritating to infant skin. Ammonia dermatitis of this type is generally a problem in the second half of the first year of life, when an infant is producing a larger quantity of urine than before. For some infants, however, it is a problem from the first week.

Frequent diaper changing, applying A & D or Desitin ointment, and exposing the diaper area to air may relieve the problem. Some infants may have to sleep without diapers at night to control the problem.

Whenever the entire diaper area is erythematous and irritated so that the outline of the diaper on the skin can be identified, one must suspect an allergy to the material in the diaper or to laundry products if a commercially washed or home-washed diaper is being used. Changing

(text continues on page 856)

A Multidisciplinary Care Map for An Infant With Colic

●

You meet Ms. Simpson, 19, at a pediatric clinic when she brings in her 2-month-old son, Bryan. She looks tired. She tells you that she is exhausted because her baby is "awake all night, crying constantly." She stopped breast-feeding and changed him to formula to see if that would help, but it didn't. She tells you his bowel movements are normal. When you weigh Bryan, you find he has gained weight well. When you talk to him, he demonstrates a social smile.

Family Assessment
Infant lives with single parent and her family (grandfather, grandmother, 26-year-old uncle, and 22-year-old aunt). Grandmother cares for infant while mother works as an exotic dancer from 12 noon to 6 PM.

Client Assessment
Well-proportioned 2-month-old boy. Height and weight at 50th percentile on growth chart. Bottle feeding with intake of approximately 4 oz of commercial formula every 4 hours. Experiencing 2 or 3 soft yellow bowel movements daily. The mother reports, "He's been crying every night lately from about 6 PM till 2 AM. His face gets red, and he pulls his legs up against his belly. I give him a bottle, he sucks for a few minutes like he's starving, and then stops, pulls up his legs, and starts to cry. He's good for my mother in the afternoon; cries from six to nine at night for me. I'm at the end of my rope." Physical examination within normal limits. Diagnosis of colic is made.

Nursing Diagnosis
Compromised family coping related to difficulty managing infant crying episodes

Outcome Criteria
Parent expresses increased confidence in caring for infant and increased feeling of control over situation within 1 week; infant sleeps for at least some of 6 PM to 2 AM period.

Team Member Responsible	Assessment	Intervention	Rationale	Expected Outcome
Activities of Daily Living				
Nurse	Assess what infant's total day is like to try and identify why crying seems confined to evenings.	Make suggestions as needed to see that different caregivers use consistency in care.	Infants with a number of daily caretakers can have difficulty adjusting to changing feeding techniques.	Parent details a day history for infant.
Consultations				
Nurse	Determine which nurse practitioner is available for consultation.	Contact nurse practitioner to do physical exam to ensure infant is healthy.	A physical exam will differentiate symptoms of colic from another more serious problem.	Nurse practitioner completes physical exam and makes recommendations.

(continued)

Team Member Responsible	Assessment	Intervention	Rationale	Expected Outcome
Procedures/Medications				
Nurse	Assess what steps parent has taken to try and relieve symptoms.	Suggest the use of a pacifier, sitting infant upright, feeding in quiet environment, riding in car, etc.	Sucking on a pacifier may increase peristalsis and promote passage of gas. An upright position may prevent distention.	Parent states she is willing to try new measures such as a pacifier.
Nutrition				
Nurse	Assess how parent prepares formula; what technique she uses for bottle-feeding and burping infant.	Review methods for formula preparation, bottle holding, and burping as needed; be certain other family members are consistent.	Proper techniques can minimize the amount of air swallowed and possible subsequent development of intestinal gas.	Parent describes formula preparation and infant feeding methods. Confirms other family members are consistent.
Patient/Family Education				
Nurse	Assess what parent knows about colic, including its incidence, usual timing, symptoms, etc.	Educate parent about common characteristics of colic, including duration, timing, and intensity of crying.	Education promotes better understanding of the problem, alleviating some of the stress and anxiety associated with it.	Parent states she understands symptoms of colic and how common it is in newborns.
Psychosocial/Spiritual/Emotional Needs				
Nurse/nurse practitioner	Assess what parent thinks is the cause of her infant crying so much in the evening.	Reassure parent she is not the cause of the child's discomfort. It's a coincidence she is giving care at the time colic occurs.	A parent can feel guilty if she is unable to soothe child. Reassurance the problem is not her fault can aid in objective problem solving.	Parent states she understands the problem is not a personal one.
Nurse	Assess parent's level of stress about constant crying.	Caution parent that crying in infants produces frustration in adults. Help parent plan respite time if possible to give relief.	Acknowledging their frustration helps to validate their feelings. A plan of action provides opportunities to regain some control over the situation. Time away can help relieve feelings of frustration and tension.	Parent states she is frustrated but also ready to work on solving problem.
Discharge Planning				
Nurse	Urge the parent to call for further suggestions if further help is needed. Explain colic generally resolves by 3 months of age.	Advise parent to contact clinic if measures are ineffective by 1 week. Anticipate the need for possible pharmacologic therapy.	Medication to reduce colic symptoms can be effective if non-pharmacologic measures are not.	Parent agrees to call in 1 week if crying has not improved.

the brand or type of diaper or washing solution usually alleviates the problem.

If a diaper area is covered with lesions that are bright red, with or without oozing, last longer than 3 days, and appear as red pinpoint lesions, suspect a fungal (monilial or candidiasis) infection. This is discussed in Chapter 43.

Miliaria

Miliaria, or prickly heat rash, occurs most often in warm weather or when babies are overdressed or sleep in over-heated rooms. Clusters of pinpoint, reddened papules with occasional vesicles and pustules surrounded by erythema usually appear on the neck first and may spread upward to around the ears and onto the face or down onto the trunk.

Bathing an infant twice a day during hot weather, particularly if a small amount of baking soda is added to the bath water, may improve the rash. Eliminating sweating by reducing the amount of clothing on an infant or lowering the room temperature should bring almost immediate improvement and prevent further eruption.

Baby-Bottle Syndrome

Putting an infant to bed with a bottle can result in aspiration or decay of all the upper teeth and the lower posterior teeth (Nainar & Mohummed, 2004); (Fig. 28.21). Decay occurs because while an infant sleeps, liquid from the propped bottle continuously soaks the upper front teeth and lower back teeth (the lower front teeth are protected by the tongue). The problem, called **baby-bottle syndrome,** is most serious when the bottle is filled with sugar water, formula, milk, or fruit juice. The carbohydrate in these solutions ferments to organic acids that demineralize the tooth enamel until it decays.

To prevent this problem, advise parents never to put their baby to bed with a bottle. If parents insist a bottle is necessary to allow a baby to fall asleep, encourage them to fill it with water and use a nipple with a smaller hole to prevent the baby from receiving a large amount of fluid.

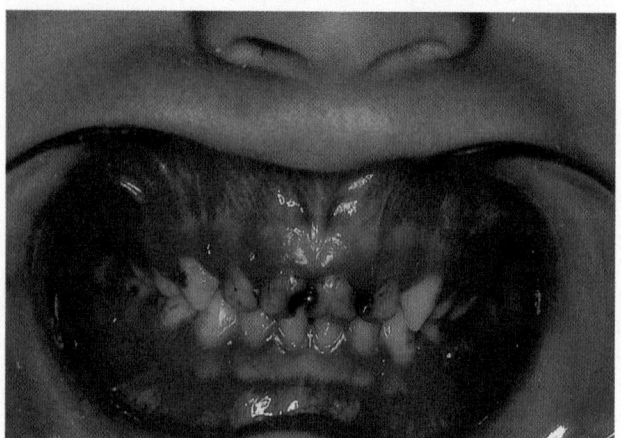

FIGURE 28.21 Baby-bottle syndrome. Notice the extensive decay in the upper teeth. (K. L. Boyd, DDS/Custom Medical Stock Photo.)

If the baby refuses to drink anything but milk, the parents might dilute the milk with water more and more each night until the bottle is down to water only.

Obesity in Infants

Obesity in infants is defined as a weight greater than the 90th to 95th percentile on a standardized height/weight chart. Obesity occurs when there is an increase in the number of fat cells due to excessive calorie intake. Preventing obesity in infants is important because the extra fat cells formed at this time are likely to remain throughout childhood and even into adulthood. If a child becomes obese because of overingesting milk, iron-deficiency anemia may also be present because of the low iron content of both breast and commercial milk. Once infant obesity begins, it is difficult to reverse, so prevention is the key (Benton, 2004).

Overfeeding in infancy often occurs because parents were taught to eat everything on their plate, and they continue to instill this concept in their children. This appears to be the case most often with formula-fed infants whose parents urge them to empty their bottle or finish a cereal serving. It can occur any time parents automatically feed an infant when the child cries, rather than investigating what the cry might really mean. As a general rule, an infant should take no more than 32 oz of formula daily. When solid food is introduced, a bottle of water can be substituted for formula at one feeding. Nonfat milk should not be given because it contains so little fat that essential fatty acid requirements may not be sufficient to ensure cell growth.

Another way to help prevent obesity is to add a source of fiber, such as whole-grain cereal and raw fruit, to an infant's diet. These prolong the stomach-emptying time, so they can help reduce food intake. Caution parents about giving obese infants foods with high amounts of refined sugars, such as pudding, cake, cookies, and candy. Encourage parents to learn more about balanced nutrition and to provide this for their entire family.

  Checkpoint Question 5

Bryan's mother is concerned about him developing baby-bottle syndrome. What would be her best action to prevent this?

a. Use plastic rather than glass bottles.
b. Boil formula to reduce the curd.
c. Don't put Bryan to bed with a bottle.
d. Check the expiration date on formula.

Concerns of the Family With a Cognitively or Physically Challenged or Chronically Ill Infant

An infant born with a cognitive or physical challenge or an illness is usually hospitalized immediately after birth for diagnosis and treatment. This can result in delayed bonding because the newborn is separated from the parents during this time. Encourage parents to visit an intensive care nursery regularly to help form a strong parent–child attachment. If parents cannot visit, urge them to telephone the hospital as frequently as they can to inquire about their child. In addition, nurses can supply Polaroid photographs of an infant for parents to take home.

Many of the developmental events of the infant year (social smile, laughing out loud, reaching for an object, uttering the first word, sitting, talking) are activities that encourage parent–child interaction because they make an infant fun to be with and naturally make a parent want to spend more time with the child. Children who are cognitively challenged may not reach these milestones. Children who are physically challenged may be unable to achieve them as well if they cannot reach up and pat their mother's face or hold out arms to be picked up by a father. If children cannot interact with parents in these ways, parents may find themselves equally unable to interact with their children. If infants leave the hospital with a cast or other equipment such as a ventilator for care, parents may be so concerned with these items that they cannot initiate normal singing and playing activities with their children.

To encourage a good parent–child relationship, point out the positive things an infant can do. Perhaps the child's facial expression says, "Pick me up," even though he doesn't reach up with his hands; perhaps his eyes follow his mother's actions even though he can't yet call to her.

Helping parents to interact more fully with their infants helps to build a sense of trust in an infant. Without a sense of trust, children have difficulty expressing themselves to others; they may not believe they are lovable or people would want to interact with them. Physically challenged individuals, no matter what their ages, need people around them to give them help at whatever point they cannot meet their own needs. It is unfortunate when a physically challenged child cannot reach out for help because he or she does not have a sense of trust.

Infants who are cognitively or physically challenged or chronically ill experience the same health and growth problems as other infants. Parents may be reluctant to bring up these concerns at health care visits because they believe such problems pale in comparison to the primary illness or condition. When taking the health histories of children with chronic or longstanding medical problems, ask parents about secondary concerns. "What about everyday things? Any problems there?" Treat these concerns seriously, so parents can feel confident about bringing them to your attention at future health care visits. Also mention they are part of normal infant development so parents can begin to view their child apart from his or her illness.

Teething pain, discomfort from diaper rash, and colic are all potential problems in infancy and may occur even more frequently in babies with other illnesses. For instance, parents may not want to "bother" an ill infant with physical care as often as they would a well child (e.g., before homes were well-heated, bathing an ill infant could cause extensive chilling, and many people still believe bathing is not appropriate for ill children). Colic may occur because parents are reluctant to tire ill infants by burping them after a feeding. Parents' attention may be so focused on the primary health problem rather than on everyday concerns, such as diaper care, that diaper dermatitis occurs. The bowel movements of physically disabled or chronically ill children may be looser than normal because of a liquid diet or medicine. Their urine may be more concentrated because of reduced intake. These conditions may also lead to diaper rash. Offering anticipatory guidance to parents can go a long way toward helping them avoid this special concern of infancy.

Nutrition and the Cognitively or Physically Challenged Infant

Nutrition is often a concern for infants who are born physically challenged or are ill at birth. Infants who have fevers because of illness have increased metabolic needs and require more calories than normal. To compound the problem, ill children may become too fatigued to take adequate feedings. If any degree of neurologic involvement exists, sucking and swallowing reflexes may not be coordinated. With gastrointestinal involvement, feeding may be impossible.

To ensure adequate calorie and protein intake, infants may need to be maintained on nasogastric tube or gastrostomy feedings, or total parenteral nutrition. These methods limit the amount of sucking that is possible. Because sucking provides pleasure as well as satisfying thirst, this is a major loss. Provide an infant with non-nutritive sucking experiences if possible to fill this need.

Infants who are ill for a long time may not eat solid foods eagerly once they are introduced because they are not hungry enough to be interested in a new eating method. Help parents to experiment with different foods to find a taste that does appeal to ill children, or teach them to limit foods to only those the child appears to like most from all five food groups.

 What if... Bryan's grandmother tells you she believes children should always finish everything on their plate, so as not to waste food? Is always cleaning a plate a good or bad habit for parents to enforce? Why or why not?

Key Points

The infant period is from 1 month to 12 months. Children typically double their birthweight at 4 to 6 months and triple it at 1 year.

Infants develop their first tooth at about 6 months; by 12 months, they have six to eight teeth.

Important gross motor milestones during the infant year are lifting the chest off a bed at 2 months, sitting at 6 to 8 months, creeping at 9 months, "cruising" at 10 to 11 months, and walking at 12 months.

Important fine motor accomplishments are the ability to pass an object from one hand to the other (7 months) and a pincer grasp (10 months).

Important milestones of language development during the first year are differentiating a cry (2 months), making simple vowel sounds (5 to 6 months), and saying two words besides "ma-ma" and "da-da" (12 months). The more infants are spoken to, the easier it is for them to acquire language.

Providing infants with proper toys for play helps development. All infant toys need to be checked to be sure they are too large to be aspirated.

Important milestones of vision development are the ability to follow a moving object past the midline (3 months) and ability to focus securely without eyes crossing (6 months).

According to Erikson, the developmental task of the infant year is the development of a sense of trust versus mistrust.

Safety is important. Infants must be protected from falls and aspiration of small objects. A skill an infant cannot accomplish one day, such as crawling, may be accomplished the next.

Solid food is generally introduced into an infant's diet at 5 to 6 months of age. Before infants can eat solid food, they must lose their extrusion reflex.

Common concerns related to infant development include teething, thumb sucking, use of pacifiers, sleep problems, constipation, colic, diaper dermatitis, baby-bottle syndrome (decayed teeth from sucking on a bottle of formula while they sleep), and obesity. Nurses play a key role in teaching parents about these problems and measures to deal with them.

Remember that parent–infant attachment is critical to mental health. Urge parents to continue to give as much care as possible to sick infants to maintain this important relationship.

Critical Thinking Exercises

1. Bryan, the 2-month-old boy you met at the beginning of the chapter, was diagnosed with colic. What are common suggestions you could make to his parents to help reduce his discomfort and crying?
2. Bryan's mother wants to "childproof" her house. What questions would you ask to assess whether the infant's house is safe for him?
3. Bryan is going to be followed in your health maintenance setting. Describe the immunization schedule you would discuss with his mother as recommended for the first year.
4. Examine the National Health Goals related to growth and development of the infant. Most government-sponsored money for nursing research is allotted based on these goals. What would be a possible re-

search topic to explore pertinent to these goals that would be applicable to Bryan's family and also advance evidence-based practice?

References

American Academy of Pediatrics. (2001). *Recommendations for using fluoride to prevent and control dental caries in the United States.* Washington, DC: AAP.

American Academy of Pediatrics Committee on Practice & Ambulatory Medicine. (2005). *Recommendations for preventive pediatric health care.* Washington, DC: AAP.

American Academy of Pediatrics. (2005). *Car safety seats: A guide for families—2005.* www.AAP.org/family/carseat guide.htm.

American Academy of Pediatrics Committee on Injury and Poison Prevention and Committee on Sports Medicine and Fitness. (2000). Swimming programs for infants and toddlers. *Pediatrics, 105*(4.1), 868–870.

Anderson, J. E. (2004). "Nothing but the tooth": dispelling myths about teething. *Contemporary Pediatrics, 21*(7), 75–80.

Barr, S. I., & Rideout, C. A. (2004). Nutritional considerations for vegetarian athletes. *Nutrition, 20*(7/8), 696–703.

Benton, D. (2004). Role of parents in the determination of the food preferences of children and the development of obesity. *International Journal of Obesity & Related Metabolic Disorders, 28*(7), 858–869.

Boom, J. (2003). Teething. In M. W. Schwartz (Ed.), *5-minute pediatric consult* (3rd ed., pp 260–261). Philadelphia: Lippincott Williams & Wilkins.

Carey, W. B. (2003). Colic. In M. W. Schwartz (Ed.), *5-minute pediatric consult* (3rd ed., pp 260–261). Philadelphia: Lippincott Williams & Wilkins.

Centers for Disease Control and Prevention. (2005). *Recommended childhood and adolescent immunization schedule, United States, 2005.* Washington, DC: DHHS.

Cinar, N. D. (2004). The advantages and disadvantages of pacifier use. *Contemporary Nurse, 17*(1–2), 109–112.

Department of Health and Human Services. (2000). *Healthy people 2010.* Washington, DC: DHHS.

Erikson, E. (1993). *Childhood and society* (3rd ed.). New York: W. W. Norton.

James, S. D. (2003). Breastfeeding. In M. W. Schwartz (Ed.), *5-minute pediatric consult* (3rd ed., pp 260–261). Philadelphia: Lippincott Williams & Wilkins.

Jamieson, D. H., et al. (2004). Does the transition zone reliably delineate aganglionic bowel in Hirschsprung's disease? *Pediatric Radiology, 34*(10), 811–815.

Johnson, M., Maas, M., & Moorhead, S. (2000). *Nursing outcomes classification* (2nd ed.). St. Louis: Mosby.

Karp, H. (2004). The "fourth trimester": a framework and strategy for understanding and resolving colic. *Contemporary Pediatrics, 21*(2), 94–99.

McCloskey, J., & Bulechek, G. (2000). *Nursing interventions classification* (3rd ed.). St. Louis: Mosby.

Morin, K. H. (2004). Current thoughts on healthy term infant nutrition: the first twelve months. *MCN: The American Journal of Maternal/Child Nursing, 29*(5), 312–319.

Mesich, H. M. (2004). Mother-infant co-sleeping: understanding the debate and maximizing infant safety. *MCN: The American Journal of Maternal/Child Nursing, 30*(1), 30–39.

Nainar, S. M., & Mohummed, S. (2004). Diet counseling during the infant oral health visit. *Pediatric Dentistry, 26*(5), 459–462.

National Center for Health Statistics. (2005). *Trends in the health of Americans.* Hyattsville, MD: NCHS.

Nystrom, K., & Ohrling, K. (2004). Parenthood experiences during the child's first year: literature review. *Journal of Advanced Nursing, 46*(3), 319-330.

Piaget, J. (1966). *The origins of intelligence in children.* New York: International University Press.

Schonberg-Norio, D., et al. (2004). Swimming and *Campylobacter* infections. *Emerging Infectious Diseases, 10*(8), 1474-1477.

ABC XYZ Suggested Readings

Ball, H. L. (2003). Breastfeeding, bed-sharing, and infant sleep. *Birth, 30*(3), 181-188.

Boyle, J., & Cropley, M. (2004). Children's sleep: problems and solutions. *Journal of Family Health Care, 14*(3), 61-63.

Elek, S. M., Hudson, D. B. & Bouffard, C. (2003). Marital and parenting satisfaction and infant care self-efficacy during the transition to parenthood: the effect of infant sex. *Issues in Comprehensive Pediatric Nursing, 26*(1), 45-57.

Gatrad, A. R., & Sheikh, A. (2004). Persistent crying in babies. *British Medical Journal, 328*(7435), 330-331.

Kramer, M. S., & Kakuma, R. (2005). Optimal duration of exclusive breastfeeding. *The Cochrane Library (Oxford) (4)* (CD003517).

Long, L. (2003). Understanding a crying baby in the first three months. *Community Practitioner, 76*(5), 175-181.

Morales, F., & Parker, S. (2003). Still not sleeping through the night: what do you try next? *Contemporary Pediatrics, 20*(10), 33-34.

Sankaran, K., et al. (2003). Sudden infant death syndrome (SIDS) and infant care practices. *Neonatal Intensive Care, 16*(3), 31-35.

Scher, A., & Dror, E. (2003). Attachment, caregiving and sleep: the tie that keeps infants and mothers awake. *Sleep and Hypnosis, 5*(1), 27-37.

Schuman, A. J. (2003). A concise history of infant formula (twists and turns included). *Contemporary Pediatrics, 20*(2), 91-98.

Secco, M. L., & Moffatt, M. E. K. (2003). Situational, maternal and infant influences on parenting stress among adolescent mothers. *Issues in Comprehensive Pediatric Nursing, 26*(2), 103-122.

Thomasgard, M., & Metz, W. P. (2004). Promoting child social-emotional growth in primary care settings: using a developmental approach. *Clinical Pediatrics, 43*(2), 119-127.

CHAPTER 29

The Family With a Toddler

Key Terms

assimilation
autonomy
deferred imitation
discipline
lordosis
parallel play
preoperational thought
punishment
tertiary circular reaction stage

Objectives

After mastering the contents of this chapter, you should be able to:

1. Describe normal growth and development of a toddler as well as common parental concerns.
2. Assess a toddler for normal growth and development milestones.
3. Formulate nursing diagnoses related to toddler growth and development or parental concerns regarding development.
4. Identify expected outcomes for nursing care of a toddler.
5. Plan nursing care to meet a toddler's growth and development needs, such as anticipatory guidance to prevent problems such as sleep disturbances, temper tantrums, or inappropriate toilet-training practices.
6. Implement nursing care to promote normal growth and development of a toddler, such as discussing toddler developmental milestones with parents.
7. Evaluate expected outcomes established for care to be certain nursing goals associated with growth and development have been achieved.
8. Identify National Health Goals related to the toddler age group that nurses can help the nation achieve.
9. Identify areas related to care of a toddler that could benefit from additional nursing research or application of evidence-based practice.
10. Use critical thinking to analyze methods of care for a toddler to be certain care is family-centered.
11. Integrate knowledge of toddler growth and development with nursing process to achieve quality maternal and child health nursing care.

*J*ason is a 2½-year-old boy you see at a pediatric clinic. His mother tells you he has changed completely in the past 6 months from an easy-to-care-for baby into a "monster" who refuses to do anything she asks. The only word he says anymore is "no." He has a temper tantrum every night at dinner over some type of food. She tells you this has changed parenting from "fun" to "a real chore."

The previous chapter discussed the growth and development of infants and the abilities infants develop in the first year. This chapter adds information about the dramatic changes, both physical and psychosocial, that occur during the toddler years. This is important information because it builds a base for care and health teaching for this age group.

What advice could you give Jason's mother to help her regain a positive relationship with her toddler?

After you've studied this chapter, access the accompanying website. Read the patient scenario and answer the questions to further sharpen your skills, grow more familiar with RN-CLEX types of questions, and reward yourself with how much you have learned.

n the toddler period, usually considered to be from age 1 to 3 years, enormous changes take place in a child and, consequently, in a family. During the toddler period, children accomplish a wide array of developmental tasks and change from largely immobile and preverbal infants who are dependent on caregivers for the fulfillment of most needs to walking, talking young children with a growing sense of **autonomy** (independence). Parents must also grow during this period. Their task is to support their child's growing independence with patience and sensitivity and to learn methods for handling the child's frustrations that arise from the quest for autonomy. This chapter provides an overview of normal growth and development of the child and family through the toddler period, covering in particular the areas to assess at routine health maintenance visits. Because healthy children and families are constantly being challenged by the process of normal development, parents often have questions about how to guide their children in different situations. This chapter also provides guidelines useful in helping parents cope with special needs and concerns relevant to this age. National Health Goals related to the toddler age group are shown in Box 29.1.

Nursing Process Overview

For Healthy Development of a Toddler

● *Assessment*

Whether a child is seen for a routine checkup or has come to a health care center because of a specific health concern, assessment begins with taking a careful health history. Asking parents about a toddler's ability to carry out activities of daily living offers assessment information not only on the child's developmental progress but also important clues about the child–parent relationship.

Careful observation is another crucial element of nursing assessment of a toddler. This is because parents may become so emotionally involved in a health concern they may not describe it with complete objectivity. On the other hand, parents see their children daily and so are the best source of information and opinion on when a child seems to be acting "out of sorts" or "different" (a typical sign a child may not be feeling well). Table 29.1 provides some guidelines to help parents evaluate illness at this age. For more information about typical assessment findings, see Box 29.2.

● *Nursing Diagnosis*

Nursing diagnoses related to normal growth and development of toddlers usually focus on the parents' eagerness to learn more about the parameters of normal growth and development or issues of safety or care. Examples are:

- Health-seeking behaviors related to normal toddler development
- Deficient knowledge related to best method of toilet training
- Risk for injury related to impulsiveness of toddler
- Interrupted family process related to need for close supervision of 2-year-old
- Readiness for enhanced family coping related to parents' ability to adjust to new needs of child
- Readiness for enhanced parenting related to increased awareness for poison prevention
- Disturbed sleep pattern related to lack of bedtime routine

● *Outcome Identification and Planning*

To help parents resolve a concern during the toddler period, focus largely on family education and anticipatory guidance. Urge them to establish realistic goals and outcomes so they can meet the rapidly changing needs of their toddler and learn to cope with typical toddler behaviors. Otherwise, parents can expect too much of a toddler and grow frustrated instead of enjoying being a parent of a child this age.

● *Implementation*

When teaching about typical toddler behavior, teach parents a good rule is to think of a toddler as a visitor from a foreign land who wants to participate in everything the family is doing, but doesn't know the customs or the language. They need to help their toddler learn these the same as they would that stranger.

Teach parents not only how to approach a current problem, but also to learn adequate methods for resolving similar situations that are sure to arise in the future. If parents do not learn methods that can be applied throughout their child's growing years, they may win battles but lose wars. For instance, parents may find that promising their child a treat when she is in the middle of a temper tantrum will stop the tantrum, but it will certainly not prevent other tantrums from occurring in the future (and, in fact, may encourage them). Health visits provide opportunities to help parents with healthy coping techniques. In addition, demonstrating good communication skills with toddlers can serve as a model for healthy communication behavior with them (Box 29.3).

BOX 29.1 FOCUS ON . . .

NATIONAL HEALTH GOALS

A number of National Health Goals relate specifically to safety during the toddler years. These are:

- Increase the rate of use of child automotive restraints in children 4 years and under, from a baseline of 92% to 100%.
- Reduce the rate of deaths caused by poisonings, from a baseline of 6.8/100,000 to 1.5/100,000 (DHHS, 2000).

Nurses can help the nation achieve these goals by continuing to educate parents about the importance of using car seats and childproofing their homes against poisoning.

Areas that could benefit from additional nursing research are methods parents can use to keep their toddlers entertained while in automobiles and specific home situations in which poisoning is apt to occur.

TABLE 29.1

Parental Difficulties in Evaluating Illness in Toddlers

Problem	Guidelines for Parents
Evaluating seriousness of illness	Toddlers typically answer "No" to almost all questions. A question such as "Does your arm hurt?" may bring a "No" response even if the arm does hurt. Observing children for indications of illness (holding an arm stiffly, rubbing abdomen, crying when they void) is more helpful. Many toddlers do not know the words to describe a feeling of nausea or a sore throat. They reveal these symptoms by not eating. If the child is normally a light eater, as many are, it is difficult for a parent to appreciate these signs.
Differentiating tiredness from illness	Toddlers tend to whine or sleep when they are either tired or ill. Reviewing the child's day and activity often helps to evaluate what is happening. If the child is not tired (it is not nap or bedtime), or there is not a break in usual routine, crying and whining or temper tantrums suggest illness.
Evaluating nutritional intake	Toddlers are normally fussy eaters compared to infants. Evaluating children as to whether they are active and growing is better than assessing any one day's food intake. Check weekly intake history.
Age-specific diseases to be aware of	The toddler period is an important age to assess speech development; children should be further evaluated if they cannot use simple sentences composed of a noun and verb ("me go") by 2 years of age.
	As children begin to walk, they should be observed for abnormal gait. Osteomyelitis (bone infection) occurs with a high frequency in toddlers; symptoms of limping, swollen joints, or arm or leg pain should be regarded as serious until ruled otherwise.
	Toddlers contract 10–12 mild upper respiratory infections a year. Otitis media (middle ear infection) may occur as a complication of these. The child with an upper respiratory infection who suddenly develops a high fever and pulls or manipulates ears should be seen by a physician.
	Children who attend day care programs have a high incidence of hepatitis A, *Giardia*, and *Shigella* infections. Teach parents to report jaundice or diarrhea promptly to a health care provider to detect these infections.

● *Outcome Evaluation*

Expected outcomes must be evaluated frequently during the toddler period because children change so much and learn so many new skills during this time that their abilities and associated parental concerns can change from day to day. Examples of expected outcomes are:

• Parents state child maintains a consistent bedtime routine within the next 2 weeks.
• Parents state they have childproofed their home by putting a lock on kitchen cupboard by next clinic visit.
• Grandmother states she has modified usual activities to conserve strength to care for toddler granddaughter by 1 week's time.

NURSING ASSESSMENT OF GROWTH AND DEVELOPMENT OF A TODDLER

Assessment of a toddler centers on the child's physical growth and skill development (Panpanich & Gardner, 2005).

Physical Growth

While toddlers are making great strides developmentally, their physical growth begins to slow.

Weight, Height, and Head Circumference

Plot weight and height on a standard growth chart at each health care visit (see Appendix E) to determine if progress is normal for each individual child. A child gains only about 5 to 6 lb (2.5 kg) and 5 in (12 cm) a year during the toddler period. As subcutaneous tissue, or baby fat, begins to disappear toward the end of the second year, the child changes from a plump baby into a leaner, more muscular little girl or boy. A toddler's appetite decreases accordingly, yet adequate intake of all nutrients is still essential to meet energy needs (Dudek, 2005).

Head circumference increases only about 2 cm during the second year compared to about 12 cm during the first year. Head circumference equals chest circumference at 6 months to 1 year of age. By 2 years, chest circumference has grown greater than that of the head.

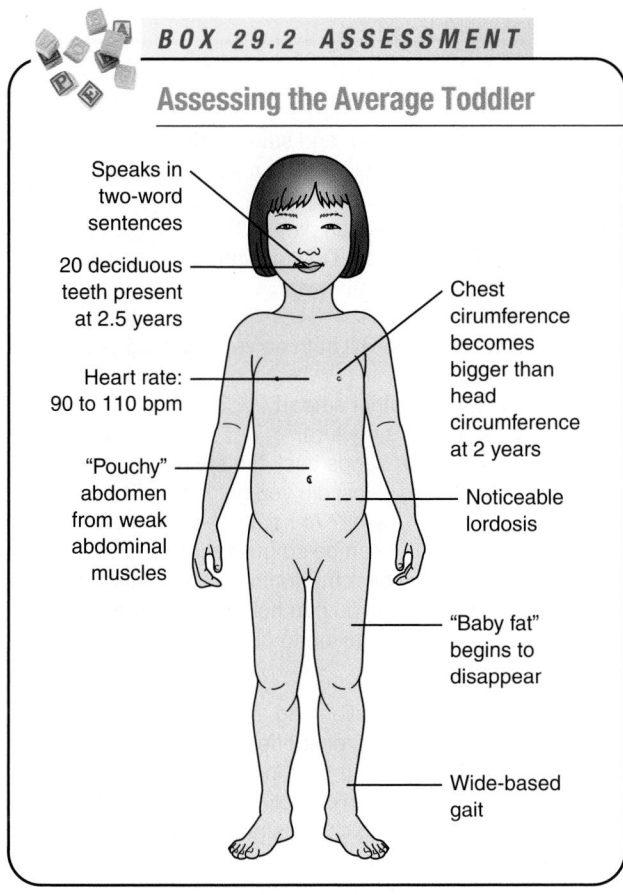

BOX 29.2 ASSESSMENT

Assessing the Average Toddler

Speaks in two-word sentences

20 deciduous teeth present at 2.5 years

Heart rate: 90 to 110 bpm

"Pouchy" abdomen from weak abdominal muscles

Chest cirumference becomes bigger than head circumference at 2 years

Noticeable lordosis

"Baby fat" begins to disappear

Wide-based gait

Body Contour

Toddlers tend to have a prominent abdomen—a pouchy belly—because although they are walking well, their abdominal muscles are not yet strong enough to support abdominal contents as well as they will later (Fig. 29.1*A*). They also have a forward curve of the spine at the sacral area (**lordosis**). As they walk longer, this will correct itself naturally. Many toddlers, in addition, waddle or walk with a wide stance (see Fig. 29.1*B*). This stance seems to increase the lordotic curve, but it keeps them on their feet.

Body Systems

Body systems continue to mature during this time:

- Respirations slow slightly but continue to be mainly abdominal.
- The heart rate slows from 110 to 90 bpm; blood pressure increases to about 99/64 mm Hg.
- The brain develops to about 90% of its adult size.
- In the respiratory system, the lumens of vessels enlarge progressively so the threat of lower respiratory infection becomes less.
- Stomach secretions become more acid; therefore, gastrointestinal infections also become less common.
- Stomach capacity increases to the point a child can eat three meals a day.
- Control of the urinary and anal sphincters becomes possible with complete myelination of the spinal cord.

- IgG and IgM antibody production becomes mature at 2 years of age. The passive immunity obtained during intrauterine life is no longer operative.

Teeth

Eight new teeth (the canines and the first molars) erupt during the second year. All 20 deciduous teeth are generally present by 2.5 to 3 years of age (Berger, 2004).

Developmental Milestones

The developmental milestones of the toddler years are less numerous but no less dramatic than those of the infant year, because this is a period of slow and steady, not sudden, growth. Toddler development is influenced to some extent by the amount of social contact and the number of opportunities children have to explore and experience new degrees of independence. It is strongly influenced by individual readiness for a new skill. Table 29.2 highlights growth and development milestones of gross and fine motor, language, and play development of the toddler years.

Language Development

Toddlerhood is a critical time for language development, although even this varies among children, because in order to master language, children need practice time. A child who is 2 years old and does not talk in two-word, noun–verb simple sentences needs a careful assessment to determine the cause. This is beyond a point of normal development.

A word that is used frequently by toddlers and that is a manifestation of their developing autonomy is "no." Toddlers may use the word to mean they are refusing a task, or they do not understand it, or they may only be practicing a sound that they have noticed has potent effects on those around them.

To learn other words, children need exposure to conversation and need to be read to often. Language develops most quickly if parents respect what toddlers have to say so children grasp the use and purpose of language.

Urge parents to encourage language development by naming objects as they play with their child (ball, block, music box, doll) or when they give their toddler something ("Here is your drink of water," "Let's put on these pajamas," and so on). This helps children grasp the fact that words are not meaningless sounds; they apply to people and objects and have uses. Always answering a child's questions is another good way to do this. Be sure answers for toddlers are simple and brief because they have such a short attention span.

Some toddlers do not develop language readily because they are not called on to use it. When they point at an object, someone hands it to them; when they climb into their highchair, someone places a meal in front of them. In other families, an older child may speak for a younger one. To assess whether parents are encouraging language development, ask them what happens when the child wants something. Do they provide opportunities for the child to ask for things before they supply them? Children should

BOX 29.3 FOCUS ON . . .

COMMUNICATION

Ms. Matthis has brought her 2-year-old son, Jason, to the clinic for a health maintenance visit. Jason is rambunctious and uncooperative. Ms. Matthis is obviously frustrated.

Less Effective Communication

Nurse: Come on, Jason, sit quietly so I can hear your heartbeat.
Jason: No!
Ms. Matthis: Jason, listen to the nurse.
Jason: No!
Nurse: If you promise to sit still, I'll let you play with the stethoscope.
Jason: Okay.
Jason plays with the stethoscope.
Ms. Matthis: Jason, now it's time to give the stethoscope back to the nurse.
Jason: No.
Nurse: There are other children waiting to see me. I really must listen to your heart now.
Ms. Matthis takes the stethoscope from Jason. Jason starts crying.
Ms. Matthis: Jason, if you stop crying and sit still, I'll take you for ice cream on our way home.
Jason: (whimpering a bit) Okay.
Ms. Matthis: Sometimes he can be so difficult.
Nurse: Oh, those terrible twos!

More Effective Communication

Nurse: Jason, I need to listen to your heart so you must be very quiet. Would you rather sit quietly on the chair or the table?
Jason: The table.
Nurse: All right, Jason, jump up.

Jason climbs onto the table and starts to fidget.
Ms. Matthis: Jason, sit still for the nurse.
Jason: No!
Nurse: If you'd like, you can play with the stethoscope for a few seconds. Do you want to listen to your mom's heart or my heart?
Jason: Mom's.
Nurse: Great, now we will both be very quiet so you can hear.
Jason listens to his mother's heart.
Nurse: Good, now it's my turn.
Jason: Okay. (Jason hands back the stethoscope.)
Ms. Matthis to Nurse: How did you get him to listen so well? At home he never listens. It can be so frustrating.
Nurse: Yes, this can be a frustrating period. By giving Jason choices, you can help him feel more in control without having to directly challenge your authority.

Toddlerhood can be a challenging and frustrating time for parents. You can teach parents effective communication skills to help toddlers assert their independence, while allowing parents to maintain discipline. It is important to show parents that offering choices rather than bribes is a far more effective and long-lasting method of modifying a toddler's behavior. In the first scenario, the nurse and mother both bribe Jason. Jason finally does what they want, but the situation is still frustrating, and his behavior change will not likely be long-lasting. In the second scenario, the nurse demonstrates how to better communicate by offering choices. The situation is much more enjoyable for everyone.

---

not be made to name an object before they can have it (because their vocabulary is so limited, the objects they could have would be restricted to 10 or fewer), but parents can reinforce language by rewording a question; for example, "You want the ball?" Reading aloud strengthens vocabulary in the same way. Reading the exact words in a book is not as important to toddlers as pointing to the pictures that accompany them. For example, Jane threw the ball ("See Jane throwing the ball?") or the dog ran away with the ball ("Look, that dog took that ball!").

The child who is very active may use fewer words than the child who is less active. The first child is too busy doing things to describe what he or she is doing; another child may be too busy obtaining objects to ask for many things. Such a child probably has a large unexpressed vocabulary; that is, the child understands more words (comprehensive vocabulary) than can be expressed (expressive vocabulary).

Because children learn language from imitating what they hear, they will speak like those around them. If they are spoken to in baby talk, their enunciation of words may be poor; if they hear examples of bad grammar, they will not use good grammar. Remind parents that pronouns are difficult for children to use correctly; many children are 3.5 or 4 years of age before they can separate the different uses of I, me, him, and her. Bilingual children interchange words from both languages.

✔ Checkpoint Question 1

What type of sentence should Jason, a 2-year-old, have mastered?

a. Red ripe tomatoes.
b. Daddy come.
c. Old MacDonald.
d. Please, please.

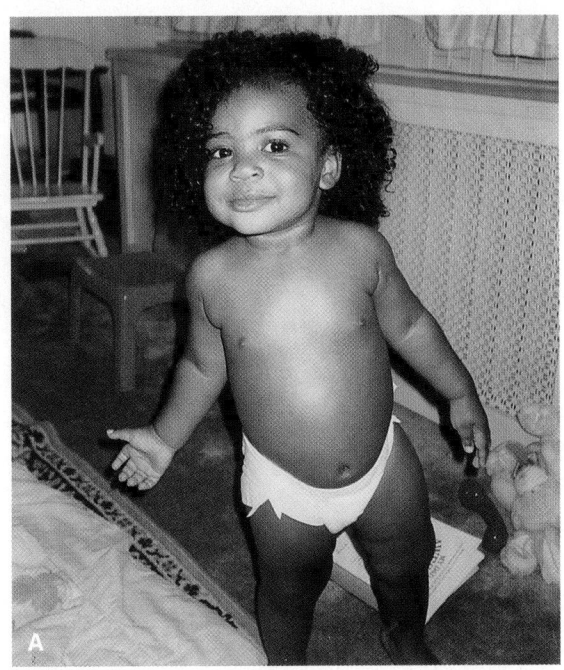
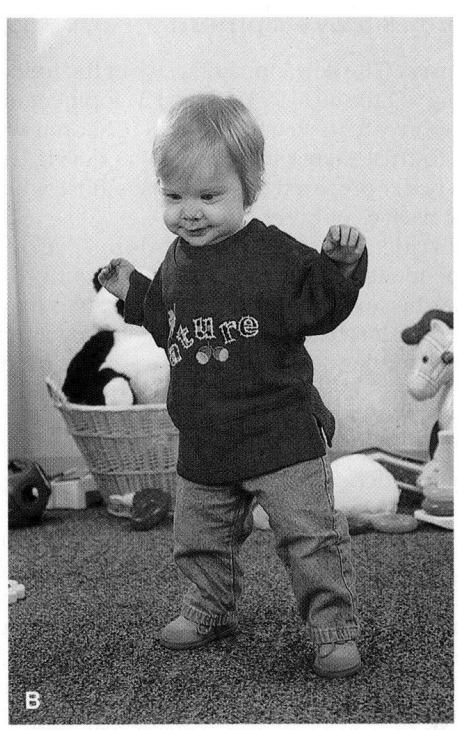

FIGURE 29.1 Physical characteristics of toddlers. (**A**) Toddlers typically have a prominent abdomen. (**B**) Toddlers typically walk with an unsteady gait for better stability.

TABLE 29.2

Milestones of Toddler Growth and Development

Age (Months)	Fine Motor	Gross Motor	Language	Play
15	Puts small pellets into small bottles. Scribbles voluntarily with a pencil or crayon. Holds a spoon well but may still turn it upside down on the way to mouth	Walks alone well; can seat self in chair; can creep upstairs	4–6 words	Can stack 2 blocks; enjoys being read to; drops toys for adult to recover (exploring sense of permanence)
18	No longer rotates a spoon to bring it to mouth	Can run and jump in place. Can walk up and down stairs holding onto a person's hand or railing. Typically places both feet on one step before advancing.	7–20 words, uses jargoning; names 1 body part	Imitates household chores, dusting, etc.; begins parallel play (playing beside not with another child)
24	Can open doors by turning doorknobs, unscrew lids	Walks up stairs alone still using both feet on same step at same time	50 words, 2-word sentences (noun-pronoun and verb), such as "Daddy go," "me come"	Parallel play evident
30	Makes simple lines or strokes for crosses with a pencil	Can jump down from chairs	Verbal language increasing steadily. Knows full name; can name one color and holds up fingers to show age	Spends time playing house, imitating parents' actions; play is "rough-housing" or active

Emotional Development

Autonomy. The developmental task of the toddler years according to Erikson (1993) is the development of a sense of autonomy versus shame or doubt. Children who have learned to trust themselves and others during the infant year are better prepared to do this than those who cannot trust themselves or others.

To develop a sense of autonomy is to develop a sense of independence. Children who are constantly told not to try things because they will hurt themselves may be left with a stronger sense of doubt than confidence at the end of the toddler period. Children who are made to feel it is wrong to be independent may leave the toddler period with a stronger sense of shame than autonomy. A healthy level of autonomy is achieved when parents are able to encourage independence while still maintaining consistently sound rules for safety.

Infants appear to have difficulty differentiating between their bodies and those of others; they think of their bodies as extensions of their parents or their primary caregivers. When infants approach toddlerhood, they begin to make the differentiation. As they recognize they are separate individuals, they realize they do not always have to do what others want them to do. From this realization comes the reputation toddlers have for being negativistic, obstinate, and difficult to manage.

This reputation is little deserved, however, and exists largely because parents misinterpret children's cues. For example, a child's refusal to accept help putting on shoes may be seen by a parent as disobedience, whereas the child may see this as insisting on performing an act he or she can do independently—a positive expression of autonomy.

Socialization. Once toddlers are walking well, they become resistant to sitting in laps and being cuddled. This is not lack of a desire for socialization but a function of being independent. Fifteen-month-old children are still enthusiastic about interacting with people, providing those people are willing to follow them where they want to go.

By 18 months, toddlers imitate the things they see a parent doing, such as "study" or "sweep," so they seek out parents to observe and initiate interactions. By 2 or more years, children become aware of gender differences and may point to other children and identify them as "boy" or "girl."

Play Behavior. All during the toddler period, children play beside the children next to them, not with them. This side-by-side play (often called **parallel play**) is not unfriendly but is a normal developmental sequence that occurs during the toddler period (Fig. 29.2). Caution parents that if two toddlers are going to play side by side, they must provide duplicate toys or an argument over one toy is likely to occur (Casby, 2003).

The toys toddlers enjoy most are those they can play with by themselves and that require action. Trucks they can make go, squeaky frogs they can squeeze, waddling ducks they can pull, rocking horses they can ride, pegs they can pound, blocks they can stack, and a toy telephone they can talk into are all favorites. These are all toys children can control, giving them a sense of power in manipulation, an expression of autonomy (Fig. 29.3).

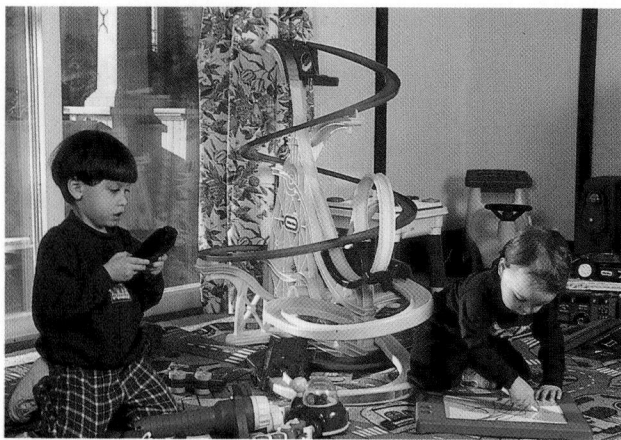

FIGURE 29.2 Toddlers play beside but not with other children (parallel play).

Some parents are not prepared for this change in play habits in their child. They wonder why a child who used to play quietly in her crib is now more interested in banging trucks together. However, they need only watch a toddler tug a pull toy, stop to see if it is following, walk again, and stop and look to see if it is still following to understand the feeling of accomplishment involved in manipulating toys.

Fifteen-month-old children are still in a put-in, take-out stage, so they continue to enjoy stacks of boxes or balls that fit inside each other. They enjoy throwing toys out of a playpen or from a highchair tray as long as someone will pick them up and return them again and again.

The 18-month-old child is walking securely enough to enjoy pull toys. Toys should be strong enough to take a great deal of abuse, because there are many things in the world toddlers do not recognize or know about. This causes them to use toys in ways other than those for which they were designed. (An infant sits and softly strokes a stuffed cat; a toddler picks it up by the tail and swings it, pounds

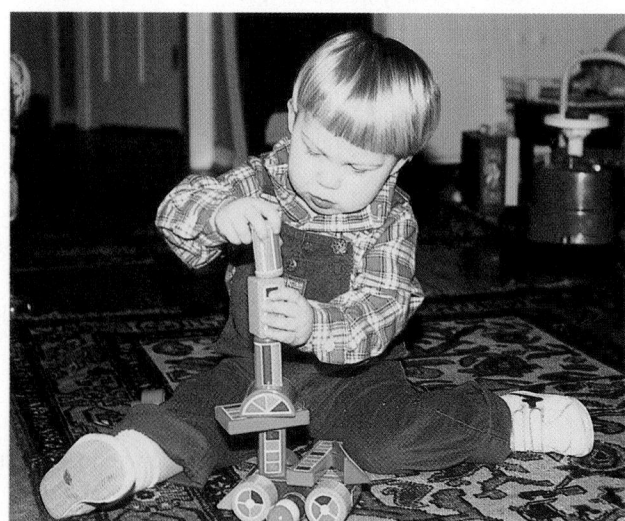

FIGURE 29.3 Toddlers enjoy toys that they can manipulate.

it, or pulls at it.) There's no need for parents to correct children about the way they are using a toy as long as it appears to give satisfaction. If toddlers find a toy frustrating because they are holding or using it incorrectly, showing them the right way will ease frustration.

By age 2, when toddlers begin to spend time imitating adult actions in their play such as wrapping a doll and putting it to bed, "setting the table," or "driving the car," they begin to use fewer toys than before. The act of imitating has become their play. By the end of the toddler period, both boys and girls begin to like rough-housing and spend at least part of every day in this very active, stimulating type of play (Fig. 29.4). Encouraging parents to schedule this type of play outdoors, where vases or other prized possessions cannot be broken, makes it more acceptable. The child who feels a need for active play is unable to sit down and eat, fall asleep, or play quiet games so may be described as "trouble." It is good to explore with parents the amount of outside or rough-housing time they allow a child each day. A trip in a stroller is not the same kind of activity as walking and running. Stroller walks are good because they provide fresh air and sunshine, but toddlers also need opportunities to engage in strenuous activity. Because of this rough activity, most toddlers have at least one black-and-blue mark on their legs at all times from tripping over their feet while trying to run too fast or jumping or bumping into a chair or doorway.

Cognitive Development

A toddler enters the fifth and sixth stages of sensorimotor thought (Table 29.3). Piaget referred to stage 5 (between 12 and 18 months) as a **tertiary circular reaction stage,** describing a toddler in this stage as "a little scientist" because of the child's interest in trying to discover new ways to handle objects or new results that different actions can achieve (Piaget, 1969). For instance, by trial and error, toddlers discover that cats do not like baths and that cookies on the center of a table can be reached by crawling up onto the table or pulling on the tablecloth. Obviously, this type of scientific investigation can lead to errors or injury.

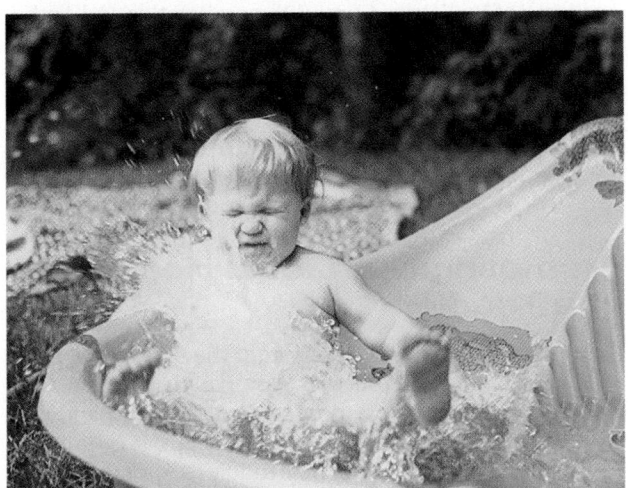

FIGURE 29.4 Toddlers usually enjoy rough and tumble play.

TABLE 29.3		
Cognitive and Psychosocial Development of the Toddler		
Age in Months	**Stage**	**Task**
Cognitive		
12–18	Sensorimotor 5	Child experiments by trial and error methods
18–24	Sensorimotor 6	Can pretend and use deferred imitation; object permanence is complete
24	Preoperational thought	Able to use assimilation or change situation to fit thoughts
Psychosocial		
24–36	Autonomy vs. shame or guilt	Learn independence and the beginning of problem solving

From Piaget, J. (1969). *The theory of stages in cognitive development.* New York: McGraw-Hill; and Erikson, E. H. (1993). *Childhood and society.* New York: W. W. Norton; with permission.

Toddlers have also advanced beyond what they could do as infants in terms of dropping objects and watching where they roll. As infants, to retrieve an article that rolled under a chair, they would crawl under the chair along the same path the object took. Many children at 15 months are able to follow a different path (walk in back of the chair) to obtain the object. This results from increased awareness that the object is permanent and, even if it follows a different direction from the one the child must take, it will be there to retrieve.

By stage 6 (between 18 and 24 months), toddlers are able to try out various actions mentally rather than having to actually perform them—the beginning of problem solving or symbolic thought. Children at this stage are also able to remember an action and imitate it later (**deferred imitation**); they can do such things as pretend to drive a car or put a baby to sleep because they have not seen this just previously but at a past time. Object permanence becomes complete.

At the end of the toddler period, children enter a second major period of cognitive development: **preoperational thought.** During this period, children deal much more constructively with symbols than they did while still in the sensorimotor period of cognition. They begin to use a process termed **assimilation.** Because they are not able to change their thoughts to fit a situation, they learn to change the situation (or how they perceive it) to fit their thoughts. This ability is what causes toddlers to use toys in the "wrong" way. For example, if they are given a toy hammer, instead of pounding with it, they might shake it to see if it rattles, using the toy in a way they had previously played (the child has changed the toy's use to fit his or her thoughts, or used assimilation).

PLANNING AND IMPLEMENTATION FOR HEALTH PROMOTION OF A TODDLER AND FAMILY

Toddlers tend to develop many upper respiratory and ear infections but otherwise come to health care facilities most often for health maintenance visits (recommended at 15, 18, and 24 months) and the immunizations important at these times. These visits allow you to focus on health promotion and provide an opportunity for early detection of any growth and development delays. Table 29.4 lists specific areas to assess during these visits.

Routine health maintenance visits also provide opportunities to support parents through the normal crises of the toddler period. Ways to encourage parents to promote the healthy development of independence in their toddler include listening carefully to their concerns, asking questions to help separate the objective circumstances surrounding a problem from the parents' possible emotional biases, and providing guidelines on how to handle specific problems.

Promoting Toddler Safety

Accidents are the major cause of death in children of all ages. Accidental ingestions (poisoning) are the type of accident that occurs most frequently in toddlers (Broderick, 2004). Although poisoning can involve medicine, it most often occurs from ingestion of cleaning products. Aspiration or ingestion of small objects such as watch or hearing aid batteries, pencil erasers, or crayons is also a major danger for children of this age. Urge parents to childproof their house by putting all poisonous products, drugs, and small objects out of reach by the time their infant is crawling, and certainly by the time their infant is walking (Box 29.4).

Other accidents that occur frequently in toddlers include motor vehicle accidents, burns, falls, and playground injuries. These occur because a toddler's motor ability jumps ahead of his or her judgment. Toddlers can walk surely and swiftly enough so that if they are left outside to play, they can very quickly travel a block away. Because they have no judgment concerning moving cars, they walk across streets with no regard for oncoming cars. To prevent serious injury, teach parents to be alert to know what their toddler is doing at all times. Until children weigh 40 to 60 lb, they need a toddler-size car seat for safety in automobiles (Fig. 29.5). They should be placed in the back seat if the car has a passenger seat airbag (AAP, 2005). They need to wear a helmet as soon as they begin riding a tricycle. Box 29.5 summarizes appropriate outcomes and interventions for toddler safety using the terminology identified by the Nursing Outcomes Classification (NOC) and Nursing Interventions Classification (NIC).

Some 15-month-old children can climb over the side rails of their cribs and enjoy exploring the house early in the morning before anyone else is awake. Parents might have to move the child to a regular bed with a side rail as early as this time to keep him or her from falling when climbing out of a crib. A safety gate on the door of the room is another way to keep a toddler contained and safe.

As the child reaches 2 years of age and begins to imitate housework or repairing a car, parents must be sure the child does not use real cleaning compounds or sharp tools. Box 29.6 summarizes accident prevention measures to encourage parents to take with their toddler.

Lead Screening

The Centers for Disease Control has set as a goal the elimination of elevated blood lead levels in children (CDC, 2005). All children between the ages of 6 months and 6 years who live in communities with buildings built before 1950 should be tested periodically for the presence of too much lead in their body (lead poisoning). Elevated lead levels are caused by eating, chewing, or sucking on objects (such as windowsills, paint chips, or furniture) that are covered with lead-based paint. Although federal law has prohibited the use of lead in the manufacture of interior and exterior paints since the mid-1970s, many older houses still contain lead paint. Additional sources of lead poisoning can include:

- Soil around the exterior of the house and potentially contaminated food grown there
- Dust or fumes created by home renovation
- Pottery made with lead glazes
- Jewelry made from lead or lead alloys
- Colored print in newspapers
- Old water pipes
- Lead-based gasoline—children who live in high-traffic areas are at high risk for contamination by lead fumes
- Lead dust brought home on the clothing of parents who work with lead products such as batteries

Because lead is toxic to body tissue, ingestion of it can lead to serious damage to the brain and nervous system, kidneys, and red blood cells. Levels as low as 10 to 15 µg/dL can cause learning and behavioral problems (Feingold & Anderson, 2004). High levels may result in seizures, cognitive challenges, coma, and even death.

Beginning symptoms of lead poisoning include irritability, headache, fatigue, and abdominal pain. Often, however, there are no symptoms before damage occurs, which is why periodic blood screening is essential. The American Academy of Pediatrics Committee on Practice and Ambulatory Medicine (2001) recommends screening for all children between the ages of 9 and 12 months and again at 24 months. A small amount of blood taken by a finger prick is analyzed. A positive result (over 10 µg/dL) must be confirmed by further testing. Therapy for lead poisoning is discussed in Chapter 52.

Promoting Nutritional Health of a Toddler

Because growth slows abruptly after the first year of life, a toddler's appetite becomes smaller than the infant's. Children who ate hungrily 2 months earlier now sit and play with their food. If feeding problems begin, it is often because parents are unaware their toddler's appetite has decreased and food consumption will be less. Because the actual amount of food eaten daily varies from one child to another, teach parents to place a small amount of food on

TABLE 29.4

Health Maintenance Schedule, Toddler Period

Area of Focus	Methods	Frequency
Developmental milestones	History, observation	Every visit
	Formal Denver Developmental Screening Test (DDST II)	18th-month visit
Growth milestones	Height, weight plotted on standard growth chart; physical examination	Every visit
Nutrition	History, observation; height/weight information	Every visit
Parent–child relationship	History, observation	Every visit
Behavior problems	History, observation	Every visit
Vision and hearing defects	History, observation	Every visit
Dental health	History, physical examination; first dental appointment	Every visit; first at 24 months
Anemia	Hematocrit/hemoglobin	24th-month visit
Lead screening	Whole blood lead level	Depending on risk level; 24-month visit
Tuberculosis	PPD test	Depending on prevalence in community
Urinalysis	Clean-catch urine	24th-month visit
Immunizations		
Measles, mumps and rubella	Check history and past records; inform caregiver about any risks and side effects.	12th- or 15th-month visit
Haemophilus influenzae type B (HiB)	Administer immunization in accordance with health care agency policies	12th- or 15th-month visit
Diphtheria, tetanus, and pertussis; inactivated poliomyelitis		15th- or 18th-month visit
Varicella vaccine		12th- or 18th-month visit
Influenza		Yearly
Anticipatory Guidance		
Toddler care	Active listening and health teaching	Every visit
Expected growth and developmental milestones before next visit	Health teaching	Every visit
Poison and accident prevention	Educate parents about toddler safety, such as using car seats and bicycle helmets, locking up poisons, and such precautions as removing drawstrings from hooded clothing to prevent strangulation.	Every visit
	Provide telephone number and location of nearest poison control center.	
Problem Solving		
Any problems expressed by caregiver during course of the visit	Active listening and health teaching regarding temper tantrums, toilet training, negativity	Every visit

From American Academy of Pediatrics. (2005). *Recommendations for preventive pediatric health care.* Washington, DC: AAP.

a plate and allow the child to eat it and ask for more rather than serve a large portion the child cannot finish. One tablespoonful of each food served is a good start. Also, cleaning a plate gives the child a feeling of independent functioning, whereas leaving food uneaten may suggest to a child that parents expected something more. It is important to

educate parents while the child is still an infant that this decline in food intake will occur so they will not be concerned when it happens.

Allowing self-feeding is a major way to strengthen independence in a toddler. Most toddlers insist on feeding themselves and generally will resist eating if a parent insists

BOX 29.4 FOCUS ON . . .

EVIDENCE-BASED PRACTICE

What Type of Accident Occurs Most Frequently Among Toddlers?

To answer this question, researchers reviewed emergency room records for toddlers. The overall annual rate was 371 accidents per 100,000 children. The leading causes of injury in young children, in descending order, were falls, poisonings, transportation accidents, ingestion or aspiration of foreign bodies, and fires/burns. Bathtub submersions remained common as a source of injury until 33 to 35 months.

This is an important study for nurses, because nurses are the people who commonly give advice on childproofing and childhood safety to parents. Knowing what injuries are most apt to occur in an age group can help organize information for health teaching.

Source: Agran, P. F., et al. (2003). Rates of pediatric injuries by 3-month intervals for children 0 to 3 years of age. *Pediatrics, 111*(6 Pt 1), 683–692.

on feeding them. An individual child may react to repeated attempts at being fed by refusing to eat at all. At the same time, toddlers may insist on the same type of food over and over because of the sense of security this offers. Offering finger foods and allowing a choice between two types of food helps promote independence while exposing children to varied foods (Briefel et al., 2004). Nutritious finger foods that toddlers enjoy include pieces of chicken, slices of banana, pieces of cheese, and crackers.

Toddlers usually do not like food that is "mixed up" such as casseroles (except maybe spaghetti); they often prefer that different foods do not touch one another on their plate. Frequently they eat all of one item before going on to another. They often prefer brightly colored foods to bland colors. Box 29.7 highlights appropriate outcomes and interventions using the terminology identified by the Nursing Outcomes Classification (NOC) and Nursing Interventions Classification (NIC) for eating habits.

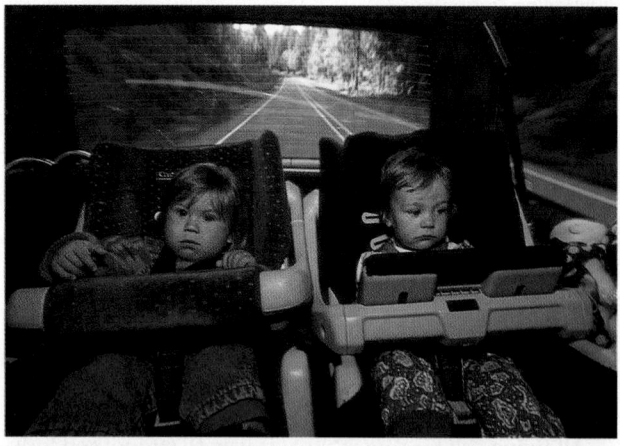

FIGURE 29.5 Toddlers should use a car seat for safety while riding in an automobile. (David J. Sams/Stock Boston.)

Toddler Nutrition

Parents may become frustrated when trying to provide adequate nutrition for their toddler because of a toddler's varying and unpredictable appetite and food preferences. Although a toddler's daily food consumption may vary greatly, energy needs are generally met when sufficient food is supplied in a positive environment. Children ages 1 to 3 years should consume 1,300 kcal daily. Protein and carbohydrate needs are often easily met during the toddler period; diets high in sugar should be avoided. Fats should generally not be restricted for children under 2 years old; however, children over 2 years old should consume no more than 30% of total daily calories from fat. Adequate calcium and phosphorus intake is important for bone mineralization. Milk should be whole milk until age 2 years, after which 2% milk can be introduced (Dudek, 2005).

Promoting Adequate Intake With a Vegetarian Diet

Vegetarian diets are adequate for toddlers if parents are well informed about needed vitamins and minerals. A vegetarian diet can be easily designed for a toddler who prefers finger foods, because many vegetables, fruits, and grains (e.g., pieces of oranges, peaches, raisins, chickpeas, tomatoes, and crackers) are easily eaten this way. The use of fortified soy milk prevents fluid, protein, B_{12}, and calcium deficiencies.

Promoting Toddler Development in Daily Activities

A toddler's new independence and developing abilities in self-care, such as dressing, eating, and to a limited extent hygiene, present special challenges for parents. Learning how to promote autonomy yet maintain a safe, healthful environment is a major goal for the family.

Dressing

By the end of the toddler period, most children can put on their own socks, underpants, and undershirt (Fig. 29.6). Some may also be able to pull on slacks, pullover shirts (the sleeves of a shirt often confuse a toddler), or simple dresses. Parents may be reluctant to encourage toddlers to dress themselves as it is often much easier and quicker to put their clothes on for them because a toddler who is dressed by parents will (usually) be wearing clothes in the correct way. When toddlers dress themselves, they invariably put shoes on the wrong feet and shirt and pants on backwards. Encourage parents to give up perfection for the benefit of the child's developing sense of autonomy. If children end up with underpants or shirt on backwards, in most instances it does not make that much difference, and toddlers are not likely to feel independent and confident if their attempts at dressing are criticized. If parents feel they must change the child's clothes, they should begin with a positive statement, such as "You did a good job," before making the switch.

During a health assessment, ask parents if their child can put on any clothing. Parents who allow this name those

BOX 29.5

Nursing Outcomes Classification (NOC) and Nursing Interventions Classification (NIC)

Toddler Safety

NOC: Knowledge, Child Safety

Knowledge, child safety, is defined as the extent of understanding conveyed about safely caring for a child (Johnson, Maas, & Moorhead, 2000). Some specific indicators suggesting achievement of this outcome include the parents' ability to describe the following:

- Appropriate activities for the child's developmental level
- Drowning hazards and preventive measures
- Use of bicycle helmets
- First aid techniques and CPR (including demonstration)
- Methods to prevent playground accidents
- Proper surveillance of outdoor activities
- Teaching about stranger awareness

NIC: Teaching, Toddler Safety

Teaching, toddler safety, is defined as instruction on safety during the second and third years of life (McCloskey & Bulechek, 2000). Some important activities involved when implementing this intervention include instructing the parent/caregiver in the following at:

13 to 18 months

- Supervising child outdoors
- Educating child about dangers of throwing, hitting, safe ways to interact with pets

- Preventing access to electrical outlets, cords, and appliances or tools
- Securing gates and doors
- Maintaining water heater temperature at 120° to 130°F

19 to 24 months

- Using car seat according to manufacturer's instructions
- Instructing child on street dangers
- Storing all chemicals, cleaners, and personal care products out of child's reach
- Ensuring multiple barriers to pools and hot tubs

25 to 36 months

- Instructing child on dangers of weapons and fires, and also how to get help when feeling scared or in danger
- Selecting toys according to manufacturer's recommendations
- Storing matches and lighters out of child's reach
- Supervising child when near swimming pool, ponds, or hot tubs
- Instructing child about stranger danger and good touch/bad touch
- Using appropriate helmet for bike riding
- Supervising child closely when in public settings

---

items the child can manage. Parents who do not allow self-dressing will probably describe the daily battle they have about dressing: "She puts up such a fuss, I don't think she will ever do it on her own." These parents may need help to understand the situation: the child may be resisting because she wants to dress herself. Don't judge how much independent exploration parents encourage by what they do in a physician's office or pediatric clinic. In these settings, they may dress a child quickly to show the child the examination is over, or they may simply be in a hurry to get home.

As soon as children are up on their feet and walking, they need shoe soles that are firm enough to provide protection from rough surfaces. However, toddlers do not need extremely firm or ankle-high shoes. Because a toddler's arches are still developing, it is better for their arches to provide foot support rather than having it provided by shoes. Sneakers are an ideal toddler shoe because the soles are hard enough for rough surfaces and arch support is limited.

Sleep

The amount of sleep children need gradually decreases as they grow older. They may begin the toddler period nap-

ping twice a day and sleeping 12 hours each night, and end it with one nap a day and only 8 hours' sleep at night. Parents who are not aware that the need for sleep declines at this time may view a child's disinterest in sleeping as a problem (Boyle & Cropley, 2004). A parent's insistence that a child get more sleep may lead to sleeping problems or refusal to sleep at all. If a child cannot fall asleep at night, maybe it is time to omit or shorten an afternoon nap. If a child is so short-tempered at dinnertime that eating is impossible, perhaps the child needs two naps a day.

Toddlers naturally fall asleep when they are tired. They may begin to resist naps, however, as well as nighttime sleep because they are aware for the first time that activities go on while they sleep, and they do not want to miss anything. Caution parents that when they say, "We'll do this after naptime," they wait until then to do it. Otherwise, a child may be reluctant to nap the next day for fear of missing another activity. Also, parents must be sure older siblings do not point out to a toddler all the exciting things a toddler missed while napping.

Other toddlers resist naptime as part of their developing negativism. Parents might minimize this by including a nap as part of lunchtime routine, not as a separate activity: the child always goes from the table directly to bed. The parent

BOX 29.6 FOCUS ON . . .

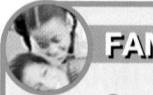

FAMILY TEACHING

Common Safety Measures to Prevent Accidents During the Toddler Years

Q. Ms. Matthis tells you, "My toddler is constantly on the go. How can I keep him safe?"

A. Accident prevention must be ongoing while your child is a toddler. Try the following precautions:

Potential Accident	Prevention Measure
Motor vehicles	Maintain child in car seat; do not be distracted from safe driving by a child in a car.
	Do not allow child to play outside unsupervised. Do not allow child to operate electronic garage doors.
	Supervise toddler who is too young to be left alone on a tricycle.
	Teach safety with pedaling toys (look before crossing driveways; do not cross streets) but do not expect that toddler will obey these rules at all times (in other words, stay close by).
Falls	Keep house windows closed or keep secure screens in place.
	Place gates at top and bottom of stairs. Supervise at playgrounds.
	Do not allow child to walk with sharp object in hand or mouth.
	Raise crib rails and check to make sure they are locked before walking away from crib.
Aspiration	Examine toys for small parts that could be aspirated; remove toys that appear dangerous.
	Do not feed toddler popcorn, peanuts, etc.; urge children not to eat while running. Do not leave toddler alone with a balloon.
Drowning	Do not leave toddler alone in a bathtub or near water (including buckets of cleaning water and washing machines).
Animal bites	Do not allow toddler to approach strange dogs.
	Supervise child's play with family pets.
Poisoning	Never present medication as candy. Buy medications with childproof caps; put away immediately after use.
	Never take medication in front of child.
	Place all medication and poisons in locked cabinets or overhead shelves where child cannot reach them.
	Never leave medication in parents' purse or pocket, where child can reach it.
	Always store food or substances in their original containers.
	Know the names of house plants and find out if they are poisonous. (Call regional poison control center for information.)
	Hang plants or set them on high surfaces beyond toddler's grasp.
	Post telephone number of nearest poison control center by the telephone.
Burns	Buy flame-retardant clothing.
	Cook on the back burners of stove if possible and turn handles of pots toward back of stove to prevent toddler from reaching up and pulling them down.
	Use cool-mist vaporizer rather than steam vaporizer or remain in room when vaporizer is operating so child is not tempted to play with it.
	Keep screen in front of fireplace or heater.
	Monitor toddlers carefully when they are near lit candles.
	Do not leave toddlers unsupervised near hot-water faucets.
	Check temperature setting for hot-water heater and turn down thermostat if it is over 125°F.
	Do not leave coffee/tea pots on a table where child can reach them.
	Never drink hot beverages when a child is sitting on your lap or playing within reach.
	Do not allow toddlers to blow out matches (teach that fire is not fun); store matches out of reach.
	Keep electric wires and cords out of toddler's reach; cover electrical outlets with safety plugs.
General	Know whereabouts of toddlers at all times. Toddlers can climb onto chairs, stools, etc., they could not manage before; can turn door knobs and go places they could not go before.
	Be aware that the frequency of accidents increases when the family is under stress and therefore less attentive to children. Special precautions must be taken at these times.
	Be aware some children are more active, curious, and impulsive and therefore more vulnerable to accidents than others.

BOX 29.7

Nursing Outcomes Classification (NOC) and Nursing Interventions Classification (NIC)

Toddler Nutrition

NOC: Knowledge, Diet

Knowledge, diet, is defined as the extent of understanding conveyed about diet (Johnson, Maas, & Moorhead, 2000). Some specific indicators suggesting achievement of this outcome include the parents' ability to:

- Describe recommendations for child intake, including foods allowed and not allowed
- Select appropriate foods
- Plan appropriate meals using diet guidelines

NIC: Teaching, Toddler Nutrition

Teaching, toddler nutrition, is defined as instruction on nutrition and feeding practices during the first years of life (McCloskey & Bulechek, 2000). Some important activities involved when implementing this intervention include instructing the parent/caregiver in the following at:

13 to 18 months
- Discontinuation of bottle feeding
- Offering of textured solids as small portions and frequent feedings

- Continued use of spoon and self-feeding
- Avoidance of force feeding
- Use of healthy snacks

19 to 24 months
- Use of drinking water for thirst
- Limitation of fluids before meals
- Inclusion of foods high in iron and protein
- Regularity of meal times

25 to 36 months
- Healthy food choices for the child, including raw and cooked vegetables, healthy snacks between meals, foods from all food groups, and iron-fortified cereals
- Use of small portions
- Creative food preparation for the picky eater
- Limitation of fat content in foods
- Avoidance of high-sugar cereals
- Child participation in food preparation
- Avoidance of food as a reward

---

can state simply, "It's naptime now," and then give a secondary choice: "Do you want to sleep with your teddy bear or your rag doll?" Toward the end of the toddler period, when children are ready to omit their afternoon naps, they may be agreeable to a "shoes-off" or quiet-play period until they begin to attend school full time.

As with any other activity of this period, a toddler loves a bedtime routine: bath, pajamas, a story, toothbrushing,

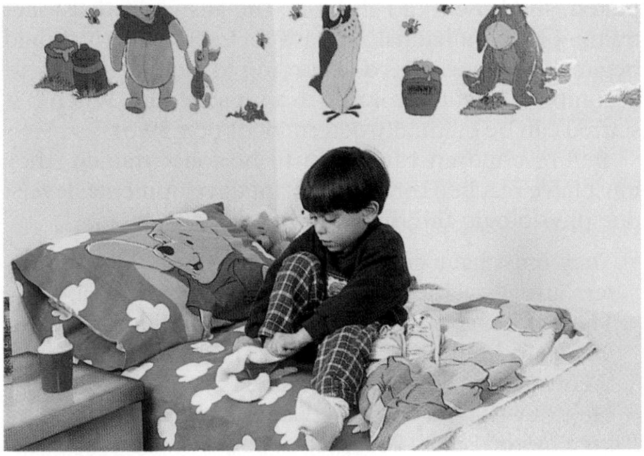

FIGURE 29.6 Getting dressed by himself is a fun morning activity for this older toddler.

being tucked into bed, having a drink of water, choosing a toy to sleep with, and turning out the lights. Parents must be careful, however, not to let a child maneuver them into such a long procedure that sleep is delayed considerably past the time initially set. Although toddlers need to be independent, they also need a feeling of security. Just as adults like to know there are guardrails along steep mountain roads, toddlers like to see parents as firm, consistent people who can be counted on to be reliable over and over.

Many toddlers are ready to be moved out of a crib into a youth bed or regular bed with protective side rails or a chair strategically placed beside it by the end of the toddler period. Moving children to a more grown-up bed is usually preferable to forcing them to sleep in a crib if they no longer feel they should be there. Either the child will not fall asleep in the crib or he or she will scale the side rail and perhaps fall.

Remind parents to stress that sleeping in a regular bed does not give children the right to get in and out of bed as they choose. Some toddlers do well if they are allowed to sleep in a regular bed and a folding gate is placed across the door to their room. This arrangement gives them a feeling of independence but still keeps them safe. When first moved to a bed without side rails, many children are found sleeping on the floor of the room in the morning. There is no harm in this unless it is cold or drafty. Dressing the child in warm pajamas or putting a blanket on the floor might be solutions to help parents accept this behavior.

Bathing

The time for a toddler's bath should depend on the parents' and the child's wishes and schedule. Some parents prefer to bathe a toddler before the evening meal because it has a quieting effect and prepares a child for eating; others prefer to give it at bedtime because it has a relaxing effect and helps the child sleep. The time, however, is not as important as the attempt to establish a sense of routine, a sense that life has order. Learning to be independent is sometimes frightening, and there is security in knowing certain events are predictable.

Toddlers usually enjoy bath time, and parents should make an effort to make it fun by providing a toy, such as a rubber duck, boat, or plastic fish. Bath time is usually so enjoyable for toddlers that parents can use it as a recreational activity or something to do on a rainy day when they can find nothing else to interest the child. Remind parents that although toddlers can sit well in a bathtub, it is still not safe to leave them alone unsupervised. They might slip and get their head under water or reach and turn on the hot-water faucet and scald themselves (Turner, 2004).

Care of Teeth

Between-meal snacks are important for growing children. Encourage parents to offer fruit (bananas, pieces of apple, orange slices) or protein foods (cheese or pieces of chicken) rather than more traditional high-carbohydrate items for snacks such as cookies not only for the nutrition involved but because they help prevent caries more than sugar snacks by limiting exposure of the child's teeth to carbohydrate. Calcium (found in large amounts in milk, cheese, and yogurt) is especially important to the development of strong teeth. In addition, children should continue to drink fluoridated water, if it is available, so that all new teeth form with cavity-resistant enamel.

Toddlers need to have a toothbrush they recognize as their own. Toward the end of the toddler period, they can begin to do the brushing themselves under supervision (almost all children need some supervision until about age 8). Remind parents it is better for a child to brush thoroughly once a day, probably at bedtime, than to do it poorly many times a day. After brushing, parents can use dental floss to clean between the child's teeth and remove plaque.

Urge parents to schedule a first visit to a dentist skilled in pediatric dental care by 2.5 years of age for assessment of dentition. Parents can prepare their child for this first and subsequent visits by reading a story about a dentist visit, maintaining a positive attitude about the visit, avoiding the use of frightening words like "drill" or "shot," and answering their child's questions honestly without going into too much detail. Because children rarely have cavities this early, the visit is usually painless (Chussid, 2003).

Promoting Healthy Family Functioning

Learning self-reliance is the primary goal of a child during the toddler period. Because of this, some parents who enjoyed caring for their child as an infant may find it difficult to have their authority challenged by a toddler. Help parents to understand their responses to these attempts at independence are crucial to the healthy development of their child. Although the child still needs firm limits to feel secure, a child must be given some room to make independent decisions in areas that the parents feel they do not need to control. An outside person, such as a nurse, can provide an important perspective on this issue.

If parents punish a child excessively at each move toward independence, he or she will not fight them indefinitely. Instead, the child will begin to feel guilty for wanting to do things independently. Adults without a sense of autonomy feel this way about independent thought. They may follow orders well, but when the job calls for a new program or function, they cannot reach into unknown areas without a great deal of consultation and help.

You may need to caution some parents not to begin to function at the same level as their toddler. An easy reaction to a toddler's refusal to allow a parent to help is, "You won't let me help you with this, so I won't do anything for you." This is a defense mechanism that prevents parents from feeling rejected. Teach parents that refusing to accept help is not refusing to accept love. Refusing to let mother put on a shoe is an instance of refusing to let mother put on a shoe, nothing more.

At bedtime, naptime, or anytime they are tired, toddlers may become much more like their old selves, wanting to sit on a parent's lap and be rocked or picked up and carried. This does not signal babyish behavior or regression in a toddler; it is a natural state between infant and preschool ages.

Parental Concerns Associated With the Toddler Period

Parental concerns of the toddler period usually arise because of a conflict over autonomy.

Toilet Training

Toilet training is one of the biggest tasks a toddler must achieve. There are so many theories concerning toilet training that understanding the procedure can become one of the biggest tasks of this period for parents. Most first-time parents ask when to start, when training should be completed, and how to go about it. The answer is that toilet training is an individualized task for each child. It should begin and be completed according to a child's ability to accomplish it, not according to a set schedule. When it is started can be culturally determined (Box 29.8).

Before children can begin to be toilet trained, they must have reached three important developmental levels, one physiologic and the other two cognitive:

- They must have control of rectal and urethral sphincters, usually achieved at the time they walk well.
- They must have a cognitive understanding of what it means to hold urine and stools until they can release them at a certain place and time.
- They must have a desire to delay immediate gratification for a more socially accepted action.

Because physiologic development is cephalocaudal, the rectal and urethral sphincters are not mature enough

BOX 29.8 FOCUS ON . . .

DIVERSITY OF CARE

In the United States, toilet training is usually introduced during the toddler period. Like so many other aspects of childrearing, though, the time when parents begin these activities is culturally determined. In other countries, toilet training may be started as soon as a child can sit, at about 6 months. Although praise is used in the United States as a common means of encouraging toddlers to learn new tasks, other cultures believe praise will bring a child harm by attracting evil spirits; strategies of shame or strict discipline are used instead. Being aware that childrearing practices are not consistent across the world is a help in understanding why parents approach childrearing problems differently and why childrearing advice must be individualized.

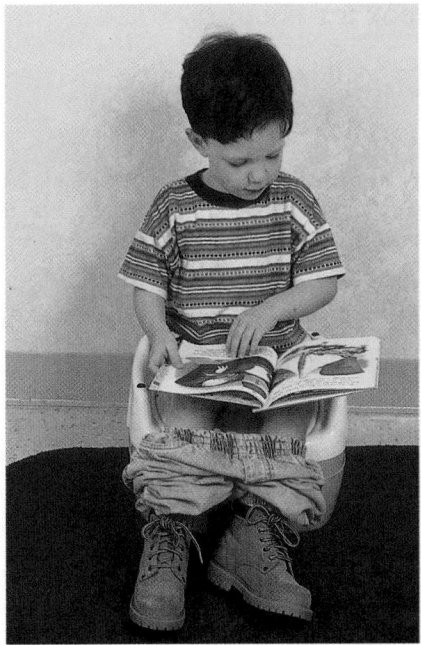

FIGURE 29.7 Toddlers are interested in toilet training as an expression of autonomy.

for control in most children until at least the end of the first year, when tracts of the spinal cord are myelinated to the anal level. A good way for a parent to know that a child's development has reached this point is to wait until the child can walk well independently.

Toilet training need not start this early, however, because cognitively and socially, many children do not understand what is being asked of them until they are 2 or even 3 years old. The markers of readiness are subtle, but as a rule children are ready for toilet training not only when they can understand what their parents want them to do but also when they begin to be uncomfortable in wet diapers. They demonstrate this by pulling or tugging at soiled diapers; they may bring a parent a clean diaper after they have soiled so they can be changed (Fig. 29.7).

Teach parents not to underestimate the difficulty of the task they are expecting their child to achieve. Infants live by a pleasure principle: they want what they want when they want it. Before they can complete toilet training, they must be able to give up an immediate pleasure—relieving themselves whenever they have the urge—to gain other pleasure later on—improved physical comfort and another step in growing up. For specific tips on how to potty train a toddler, see Box 29.9.

Some toddlers smear or play with feces, often at about the same time that toilet training is started. This occurs because they have become aware of body excretions but have no adult values toward them; stools seem little different from the modeling clay they play with. This activity can be minimized by providing toddlers with play substances of similar texture and by changing diapers immediately after defecation. Teach parents to accept this behavior for what it is: enjoyment of the body and of the self, and the discovery of a new substance. After a child is fully toilet trained, this activity rarely persists.

Ritualistic Behavior

Although toddlers spend a great deal of time every day investigating new ways to do things and doing things they have never done before, they also enjoy ritualistic patterns.

They will use only "their" spoon at mealtime, only "their" washcloth at bath time. They will not go outside unless mother or father locates their favorite cap.

The child who seems to need an excessive number of objects to cling to or an excessive number of routines, however, may be trying to say, "I need more guidelines, more rules. Don't let me be quite so independent."

What if... Jason's mother tells you he is toilet-trained, but in the hospital he refuses to use a toilet? What would you do?

Negativism

As part of establishing their identities as separate individuals, toddlers typically go through a period of extreme negativism. They do not want to do anything a parent wants them to do. Their reply to every request is a very definite "no."

It is easy for parents to believe their authority is being questioned when this happens and to worry their child is becoming so disrespectful he or she will have difficulty getting along in the world. They can be baffled by the extreme change from a happy, cooperative infant who lived to please them to this irritating, uncooperative child. They may need some help to realize this is not only a normal phenomenon of toddlerhood but also a positive stage in development. This change indicates their toddler has learned he or she is a separate individual with separate needs. It is important that toddlers do this if they are to grow up to be persons who are independent and able to take care of their own needs and desires.

BOX 29.9 FOCUS ON . . .

FAMILY TEACHING

How to Toilet Train a Toddler

Q. Ms. Matthis asks you, "How can I tell if my 2-year-old is ready for potty training? And if he is, how do I start?"

A. Try the following suggestions:

1. Children are physically ready for toilet training when they walk securely. Plan 1 or 2 weeks of psychological "readiness" activities, which will help your child realize the task of toilet training is a step toward growing up. If your child feels toilet training is something only toddlers do, he may react with extreme negativism. Readiness activities may include showing your child that other family members use the toilet; making it clear that bigger people customarily leave urine and feces in the toilet, without suggesting that these materials are dirty or distasteful; and introducing training pants and showing your child that bigger people wear underpants too.

2. Check that training pants pull down readily and that slacks are free of complicated buttons or grippers; otherwise, your child will have accidents because he cannot undress quickly enough.

3. Purchase either a potty chair that sits on the floor or an infant seat that is placed on the regular toilet. The potty chair is low and potentially less frightening to a child, but it must be emptied and cleaned after each use. If you choose an infant seat, place a footstool in front of the toilet so your child has some support for his feet.

4. Put your child on the potty chair or toilet at regular intervals (e.g., when the child wakes up in the morning, after breakfast, during midmorning, before lunch, after lunch).

5. Praise your child if he does urinate or defecate. Remind him to wash his hands.

6. Be careful not to flush the toilet while the child is sitting on it. Two-year-old children are unable to realize they will not be flushed away and may become frightened. Encourage your child to flush the toilet independently after you have helped him get redressed.

7. Do not allow a child to remain on a potty chair for much longer than 10 minutes (less than that if he is resistant). Also, do not allow your child to use the chair to eat or as a play table, so he doesn't become confused as to its purpose.

8. If your child is not ready or does not successfully use the potty on a day-to-day basis, have him return to diapers for a short period. Be careful not to make him feel as if this represents failure. Be careful not to equate "good" with being dry and "bad" with being wet. Continue with readiness activities. Reintroduce training pants and attempt toilet training again when your child seems more ready.

9. When boys have mastered defecation, it's time to include urination. Boys enjoy standing to urinate and aiming at objects in a toilet bowl, such as several pieces of breakfast cereal.

10. Some toddlers have difficulty remaining dry at night until they are 3 to 4 years old. Do not pressure your child to accomplish nighttime dryness, but assume that he is doing the best he can do. Put him into training pants for the night by explaining (not punitively) that it is hard to keep dry while he sleeps. After your child has been dry during the night for about 1 month, he has probably mastered nighttime dryness.

11. Do not wake your child during the night and carry him to the bathroom to void. This system may keep him dry during the night, but it does not help him stay dry for long periods. It may even prolong nighttime wetness, because it conditions him to void every 4 hours or so instead of retaining urine for 12 hours while he sleeps.

Parents who went away from home for the first time to college or camp might remember they behaved similarly. They may recall they rarely slept or ate sensibly; they tried, in effect, to break every rule their parents used to enforce on them. Most regained their equilibrium in time to find a midpoint between irresponsible independence and common sense. If parents can recall such circumstances, it helps them to understand this behavior in their toddler is not specific to the age but to the first feeling of independence. They can also remember they meant no vindictiveness by their behavior, so they can realize their child means none. This understanding can help to put the child's "no" into a better light.

Once it runs its course, extreme negativism passes. In the meantime, the more parents try to make children obey them, the more children are likely to resist. Some long-term parent–child interaction problems begin during this period because parents insist on being obeyed totally or are inconsistent in their approach.

A toddler's "no" can best be eliminated by limiting the number of questions asked of the child. A father does not really mean, for example, "Are you ready for dinner?" He means, "Come to the table. It's dinnertime." A mother asks, "Will you come take a bath now?" She means, "It's time for your bath." Making a statement instead of asking a question can avoid a great many negative responses.

A toddler needs experience in making choices, however. To provide the opportunity to do this, a parent might give a secondary choice. "No" is not allowed for the major task, so the parent states, "It's bath time now" but then says, "Do you want to take your duck or your toy boat into the tub with you?" Other examples are, "It's lunchtime.

Do you want to use a big or little plate?" or "It's time to go shopping. Do you want to wear your jacket or your sweater?" Although this solution is simple, it is one that parents may not arrive at by themselves because finding a solution is always more difficult for a person in the middle of a problem than for an objective observer. Once they are helped to practice this approach, however, parents usually find it helpful in smoothing out the friction caused by the negativism of the toddler period.

Checkpoint Question 2

Jason answers every request of his mother by saying, "No!" How can she minimize this?

a. Tell Jason she doesn't want him to say no anymore.
b. Answer all Jason's questions by saying, "No!"
c. Reduce the number of questions she asks Jason.
d. Explain he is not using good communication skills.

Discipline

Some parents ask during the last part of the infant year or the early toddler period when they should start to discipline their child, or when toddlers are old enough it is all right to punish them. Remind parents that "discipline" and "punishment" are not interchangeable terms. **Discipline** means setting rules or road signs so children know what is expected of them. **Punishment** is a consequence that results from a breakdown in discipline, from the child's disregard of the rules that were learned.

Parents should begin to instill some sense of discipline early in life because part of it involves setting safety limits and protecting others or property: for example, the child must stay away from the fireplace or heater; she must not go into the street; she must not hit other children. Enforcing limits, however, arises out of the day-to-day interaction with the child, out of the rhythm of childcare, not out of a set procedure such as, "Today, I'm going to teach discipline." Two general rules to follow are (1) parents need to be consistent, and (2) rules are learned best if correct behavior is praised rather than wrong behavior punished.

"Timeout" is a technique of helping children learn that actions have consequences. To use "timeout" effectively, parents first need to be certain their child understands the rule they are trying to enforce: for instance, "If you hit your brother, you'll have timeout." Parents should give one warning. If the child repeats the behavior, parents select an area that is nonstimulating, such as a corner of a room or a hallway. The child is directed to go immediately to the "timeout" space. The child then sits there for a specified period of time. If the child cries or shows any other disruptive behavior, the timeout period doesn't begin until there is quiet. When the child is quiet, the time period begins. When the specified time period has passed, the child can return to the family. A guide as to how long children should remain in their "timeout" chair is 1 minute per year of age. Using a timer, such as one for the stove that rings when time is up, lets children know when they can return to the family.

Checkpoint Question 3

Jason's mother uses "timeout" for punishment. What is a good rule for this?

a. The child should sit still for as many minutes as his age.
b. The child should sit still for as many minutes as he misbehaved.
c. Timeout activities can include quiet play or reading books.
d. Children are not ready for timeout until school age.

Separation Anxiety

As discussed in Chapter 35, fear of being separated from parents begins at about 6 months of age and persists throughout the preschool period. This universal fear of this age group is known as separation anxiety. For this reason, toddlers have difficulty accepting being separated from their primary caregiver to spend the day at a day care center or if they or their primary caregiver is hospitalized. Chapter 35 discusses nursing responsibility for care of toddlers in the hospital as well as the reactions of toddlers to the separation caused by hospitalization and the methods used to minimize these reactions.

Parents may ask what they can do about this problem. They believe they have a right to leave their child in a babysitter's or center's care, but how can they tolerate the crying at the door? Most toddlers react best to separation if a regular babysitter is employed or the day care center is one with consistent caregivers. Many are more comfortable if they are cared for in their own home. It helps if they have fair warning that they will have a babysitter. For example, they might be told, "Mommy is fixing dinner early because Mommy and Daddy are going to visit some friends tonight. Marsha is going to come and babysit for you. She'll put you to bed. When you wake up in the morning, Mommy and Daddy will be here again."

No matter how well prepared toddlers are, they may cry when the babysitter actually appears or may greet the babysitter warmly only to cry when the parents reach for their coats. It helps if parents say goodbye firmly, repeat the explanation they will be there when the child wakes in the morning, and then leave. Prolonged goodbyes only lead to more crying. Sneaking out prevents crying and may ease the parents' guilt, but it should be discouraged because it can strengthen fear of abandonment. This applies to hospital visits as well.

Temper Tantrums

Almost every toddler has a temper tantrum at one time or another. The child may kick, scream, stamp feet, shout, "No, no, no," lie on the floor, flail arms and legs, and bang the head against the floor. Children may even hold their breath until they become cyanotic and slump to the floor. When this happens, the child has a distended chest (a halt after inspiration), often air-filled cheeks, and increasing distress as the child's body registers oxygen want. This is

TABLE 29.5

Differentiating Temper Tantrums, Breath Holding, and Seizures

Assessment	Temper Tantrums	Breath Holding	Seizures
Provocation	Usually provoked—parent can state a reason for it (she asked toddler to come to dinner, but he wanted to finish an activity)	Usually provoked; child very angry; child breathes out and forgets to breathe in	Not provoked
Appearance of cyanosis	Child holds breath, becomes cyanotic, then slumps to floor	Child breathes out, becomes cyanotic, then slumps to floor	Child slumps to floor first, then becomes cyanotic

harmless breath holding; ignoring it will make it ineffective and the child will give it up. True breath holding is a neurologic problem in which a child, under stress, appears to "forget" to breathe or halts breathing after expiration, usually at the peak of anger. Breath holding can be mistaken for seizures. With some types of seizures, the cessation of breathing occurs as part of generalized seizure activity (see Chapter 49). Guidelines that are helpful in differentiating simple breath holding from neurologic disorders are shown in Table 29.5.

Temper tantrums occur as a natural consequence of toddlers' development. Toddlers are independent enough to know what they want, but they do not have the vocabulary or the wisdom to express their feelings in a more socially acceptable way. For example, temper tantrums occur most often when children are tired, just before naptime or bedtime, or during a long shopping trip or visit.

The tantrums may be a response to an unrealistic request by a parent: asking a child to comb his hair before he is coordinated enough to do so, asking her to pick up her toys before she has a feeling of family responsibility, or asking him to share before he can understand what is wanted. Also, they may occur if parents are saying "no" too frequently with regard to such things as touching the coffee table, getting dirty, using a spoon, or running and jumping so the child feels constantly thwarted. A tantrum may be a response to difficulty making choices or decisions or to pressure from activities such as toilet training. Such a child needs to express feelings in some way and does so with temper tantrums. These episodes are taxing for the parents; they are also energy-consuming for the child (Potegal, Kosorok, & Davidson, 2003).

Box 29.10 offers suggestions for managing temper tantrums. Probably the best approach is for parents to tell

BOX 29.10 FOCUS ON . . .

FAMILY TEACHING

Managing Toddler's Temper Tantrums

Q. Suppose Jason's mother tells you, "I've had it with temper tantrums. I can't stand to watch another one."

A. Here are suggestions to prevent them:
Try to determine the reason for the behavior:

- Do tantrums always occur just before bedtime? If so, you might schedule an earlier bedtime or an afternoon nap.
- Do tantrums occur every time you go shopping? If so, perhaps it would help to schedule two shorter trips each week rather than one long one.
- Do tantrums occur whenever you ask the child to do something? If so, is the child being asked to perform tasks not age-appropriate?
- Do tantrums occur in response to not being able to make a decision? If so, you may have to limit the number of choices you are asking of the child.

Next, be certain it seems like a tantrum, not something more:

- Is there a possibility you are mistaking seizure activity for temper tantrums?

- Could you be confusing neurologic breath holding with a temper tantrum?

Lastly, think through what you do when the child has a tantrum:

- Do you give either material or emotional bribes (e.g., "Come and get a cookie," or "Stop and I'll give you a kiss")? This method is rarely effective because by acceding to the child's wishes, you are encouraging your child to have more tantrums because they are so successful.
- Do you punish the child? Toddlers have a right to express opinions; they just need to be guided to learn a more controlled and mature way of doing that.
- Do you demonstrate adult behavior in managing temper tantrums? For example, if the child shouts or kicks, do you respond, "I can shout as loud as you. I can kick as hard as you"? Instead of showing the child a better way to express feelings, this reinforces the way the child is responding.

the child simply that they disapprove of the tantrum and then ignore it. They might say, "I'll be in the bedroom. When you're done kicking, you come into the bedroom, too." Children who are left alone in the kitchen will usually not continue a tantrum but will stop after 1 or 2 minutes and rejoin their parents. Parents should then accept the child warmly and proceed as if the tantrum had not occurred. This same approach works well for nurses caring for hospitalized toddlers.

NURSING DIAGNOSES AND RELATED INTERVENTIONS

Nursing Diagnosis: Risk for compromised family coping related to toddler behavior

Outcome Evaluation: Family states temper tantrums now occur less than two times daily.

Helping parents correct problems early may limit the number of tantrums they must deal with; it will not prevent them, however, because parents cannot anticipate all the circumstances that will cause this reaction. In fact, parents should not feel they must prevent all of them; they are, after all, parents, not mind readers (Box 29.11). As the child matures, increases his or her vocabulary, and is capable of better responses to stress situations, tantrums begin to fade by themselves.

What if... Jason, whom you are caring for in the hospital, has a temper tantrum in the middle of a busy hallway? Would you ignore it or move him to a quieter place?

Sibling Rivalry

Sibling rivalry, or jealousy of younger siblings, can occur during the toddler period. This is discussed in Chapter 30 with concerns of the preschool child.

Concerns of the Family With a Physically Challenged or Chronically Ill Toddler

It may be difficult for children with handicaps or disabilities to achieve a sense of autonomy or independence because they will never be totally independent. It is important for these children to develop as strong a sense of autonomy as possible, though, so they see themselves as independent and can work to become increasingly self-sufficient as they grow older. It takes courage for an adult to do such things as move a wheelchair through a busy airport or a concert crowd. Nursing actions designed to help the challenged or chronically ill child develop a sense of autonomy are outlined in Table 29.6. Most important are actions that allow a toddler to be as independent as possible. If a toddler has physical limitations, for example, he or she may be unable to explore freely or may not have the physical ability to pound and manipulate toys as the average toddler does.

A toddler with a long-term illness or who is physically challenged can be expected to exhibit normal toddler behaviors, such as temper tantrums, and to have normal outlooks, such as negativism. Parents whose child is uncoordinated or has a neurologic disease may mistake temper tantrums for seizure activity. Investigate such activity carefully, and explain to parents the difference between the two. Parents may also mistake particular toddlers' insistence on having their own way as a manifestation of illness. Remind these parents the behavior is more often an indication of age and development rather than of illness so they can respond firmly.

Toilet training is difficult for a child who is hospitalized at periodic intervals, as success usually requires a consistent caregiver; in addition, hospitalization can result in regressive behaviors. If a chronically ill child also has difficulty with ambulation, soiling accidents may occur beyond the usual age because of inability to reach a bathroom easily.

Children who survive a long-term illness are sometimes referred to as medically fragile or vulnerable children (Green & Solnit, 1964). Some parents tend to protect and shelter such a child, and you may have to remind them even though chronically ill, a toddler will demand independence and has the right to explore. A child who uses a lower-extremity prosthesis, for example, might prefer to crawl somewhere rather than wait for help to put the prosthesis in place. Although this degree of independence is good, parents may have to limit how it is expressed so the child will learn how to use the prosthesis (for example, they could make a rule the child must use the prosthesis to walk but can choose whether to use a spoon when eating).

Nutrition and the Physically Challenged or Chronically Ill Toddler

Toddlers need experience feeding themselves if at all possible. Help parents accept the accidents that occur with self-feeding, particularly if the child has difficulty with coordination; suggest finger foods if possible.

If on a special diet, children may not be allowed to eat finger foods; if they are tube fed, they receive no experience with finger foods at all. For these toddlers, parents should try to provide other, comparable experiences in independence, such as letting them choose what toy to take to bed.

BOX 29.11: Focus on Nursing Care Planning

A Multidisciplinary Care Map for A Toddler with Temper Tantrums

●

Jason is a 2½-year-old boy you see at a pediatric clinic. His mother tells you he has changed completely in the past 6 months from an easy-to-care-for baby into a "monster" who refuses to do anything she asks. The only word he says anymore is "no." He has a temper tantrum every night at dinner over some type of food. She tells you this has changed parenting from "fun" to "a real chore."

Family Assessment
Child lives with two parents in three-bedroom home. Father is a ferry boat captain; works 6 days a week. Mother is a stay-at-home mom. Finances are "Good. We've worked hard to get where we are."

Client Assessment
Well-nourished 2-year-old boy. Physical findings within normal limits. Mother reports the child is having temper tantrums "at least 20 times a day. He throws himself on the floor and pounds his head and fists." Mother unable to describe any precipitating factors for the tantrums. She states, "He seems to have them just when I start to do something. I could be playing with him one minute, and then I get up to do something, like answer the phone or start dinner, and he starts." Mother reports picking up the child immediately because she fears he will hurt himself. "I just don't know what to do anymore."

Nursing Diagnosis
Health-seeking behaviors related to measures for dealing with and reducing the number of temper tantrums.

Outcome Criteria
Mother describes measures to manage tantrums; reports tantrums have decreased to fewer than 4 a day by end of 1 week.

Team Member Responsible	Assessment	Intervention	Rationale	Expected Outcome
Activities of Daily Living				
Nurse	Ask mother to describe a typical day and to document when tantrums occur and situations that seem to provoke them.	Make suggestions to eliminate periods of stress as revealed by assessment.	Temper tantrums can increase with stress and inability of child to feel independent.	Mother reviews a typical day and identifies times when tantrums are most apt to occur.
Consultations				
Physician	Assess if child has possible neurologic symptoms.	Refer child for full neurologic workup if physical exam suggests the need.	Temper tantrums can be confused with seizures if a careful history is not taken.	Mother agrees to further neurologic testing if suggested.

(continued)

Team Member Responsible	Assessment	Intervention	Rationale	Expected Outcome
Procedures/Medications				
Nurse/ nurse practitioner	Assess what measures mother thinks would prevent temper tantrums best.	Work with the mother to develop actions (e.g., ignoring the tantrum, telling child she disapproves of behavior). Encourage mother not to pick up child unless there is actual danger of injury.	Temper tantrums are a way of expressing frustration. Rewarding the behavior prevents the child from learning more mature methods of coping with frustration.	Mother voices agreement to try suggested solutions and to telephone clinic in 5 days if there is no improvement.
Nutrition				
Nurse practitioner	Assess if child appears well nourished; assess usual dietary pattern.	As eating is a time when tantrums occur, review with mother if her actions are different at this time than others.	Eating is an area in which children can express independence.	Mother lists foods that allow child independent eating, which she will try to serve, to keep meals tantrum-free.
Patient/Family Education				
Nurse	Assess mother's knowledge of toddler behavior and temper tantrums.	Review normal toddler growth and development, explaining some temper tantrums during this period are natural occurrences.	Information about normal toddler growth and development provides a foundation for further teaching and instruction.	Mother states she understands that tantrums occur because of toddler's limited capabilities to express emotion.
Nurse	Assess why mother is so fearful child will hurt himself during a tantrum.	Inform the mother children rarely hurt themselves during tantrums.	Increased knowledge about the minimal risk of injury during tantrums should help to alleviate the mother's anxiety.	Mother states she has increased understanding about the danger of tantrums.
Psychosocial/Spiritual/Emotional Needs				
Nurse/ nurse practitioner	Assess what mother feels would be most helpful to relieve her degree of stress and frustration.	Suggest she arrange for "time out" breaks for herself by having husband or friend relieve her.	Short periods away from the child can allow her to regroup her thinking.	Mother describes a plan by which she can receive more help with child care from friend, as husband is home only 1 day a week.
Discharge Planning				
Nurse/ nurse practitioner	Review with mother the plan for added support and interventions.	Instruct the mother to keep a diary of the child's behavior and measures used during the next week. Set up an appointment for a telephone conference with the mother next week to review the diary and discuss the child's behavior.	Keeping a diary and reviewing it over the telephone aids in evaluating the child's behavior and the effectiveness of the methods used. Follow-up telephone call also provides an additional opportunity for feedback, teaching, and support.	Mother states she will follow suggestions for managing tantrums; will keep telephone and clinic appointments for follow-up care.

TABLE 29.6

Nursing Interventions to Help a Physically Challenged or Chronically Ill Child Develop a Sense of Autonomy

Area	Nursing Action
Nutrition	A special diet may limit typical finger foods. Use imagination to offer other foods not usually eaten this way as finger foods. Allow child to help pour liquid diet for a tube feeding. Toddlers are frightened by vomiting because they have no control over it. Check for possibility of nausea; toddlers have no way to express this other than by not eating.
Dressing changes	A child can hold pieces of tape or put tape in place to maintain sense of control. The child can remove an old bandage if it is not contaminated. Allow the child to view his or her incision and watch dressing changes; explaining each step of a procedure as you perform it helps the child maintain control. Restrain only those body parts necessary during a procedure to allow a child a sense of control. Remove all supplies after a procedure, or the child may "redo" the dressing.
Medication	Allow children no choice as to whether a medicine will be taken. Do allow a child to choose a "chaser," such as milk or juice, after oral medicine. Do not ask a toddler to indicate a choice of site for an injection or intravenous insertion; this is too advanced a decision for a toddler to handle.
Rest	Locate or create a ritual for bedtime (put child into bed, tuck him in, say, "Goodnight, Bobby." Tuck in bear. Say, "Goodnight, Bear"). Allow a choice of toy or cover but not a choice of bedtime or naptime hour.
Hygiene	Allow a child a choice of bathtub toy or clothing. Allow a child to wash face and hands to gain control of the situation. Allow the child to put toothpaste on a brush, but you should brush or "touch up" teeth afterward to ensure that all plaque has been removed.
Pain	Encourage a child to express pain ("Say 'ouch' when I pull off the tape"). Help channel a child's self-expression to what is acceptable (e.g., the child may shout but may not kick).
Stimulation	Provide a toddler with a toy that can be manipulated, such as boxes that fit inside one another and can be taken out again, trucks that can be pushed, and pegs that can be pounded. In a health care setting, items can usually be found that fit together (boxes from central supply or plastic vials from the pharmacy). Another action toy: buy a non-latex balloon and tie it to the crib side to be used as a punching bag; another one tied to the foot of the crib can serve as a leg exerciser.
Elimination	A child who is toilet trained needs to be encouraged to use a potty chair or toilet during an illness. Help children with ureter or bowel stomas to help with changing bags so they are as independent in bowel function as possible.

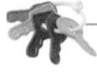

Key Points

Erikson's developmental task for the toddler period is to form a sense of autonomy or independence versus shame or doubt.

Toddlers make great strides forward in development, but their physical growth slows.

A critical milestone of toddler development is being able to form two-word sentences by 2 years of age.

Toddlers are capable of preoperational thought or are able to deal much more constructively with symbols than they could while still infants.

Important aspects of care are promoting toddler safety, including screening for lead poisoning; promoting toddler development, such as promoting daily activities; and healthy family functioning.

Toddler appetites decrease from those of the infant, so children eat proportionally less than they did as infants.

Common concerns of parents during the toddler period are toilet training, ritualistic behavior, negativism, temper tantrums, discipline, and separation anxiety.

Promoting autonomy in the child who is physically challenged or chronically ill calls for creative planning, because there may be many tasks that must be done for the child to be certain they are done safely.

aloud to a child; another is to answer questions so a child sees language as an organized system of communication. Answering a preschooler's questions can be difficult because the questions are frequently philosophical; for example, "Why is grass green?" A child may listen to an explanation of chlorophyll but then repeat the question, regardless of the clarity of the explanation, because the parent underestimated the extent of the question: a child did not want to know what makes grass green, but why, philosophically, it is not red or blue or yellow. The obvious answer to that is, "I don't know." Parents who are confident can give this answer without feeling threatened. Parents who are less sure of themselves may feel extremely uncomfortable when they realize they do not know the answers to a 4-year-old's questions (Box 30.6).

Discipline

Preschoolers have definite opinions on things such as what they want to eat, where they want to go, and what they want to wear. This may bring them into opposition with their parents. A major parental responsibility when this happens is to guide a child through these struggles without discouraging the child's right to have an opinion. "Timeout" is a good technique to correct behavior for parents throughout the preschool years (see Chapter 29). This technique allows parents to discipline without using physical punishment and allows a child to learn a new way of behavior without extreme stress.

Parental Concerns Associated With the Preschool Period

Common Health Problems of the Preschooler

The mortality of children during the preschool years is low and becoming lower every year as more infectious diseases are preventable. This results in the major cause of death being automobile accidents, followed by poisoning and falls (NCHS, 2005).

In contrast, the number of minor illnesses, such as colds, ear infections, and flu symptoms, in preschoolers is exceptionally high, more than that of any other age. Children who live in homes in which parents smoke have a higher incidence of ear (otitis media) and respiratory infections than others (DiFranza et al., 2004). Children who attend childcare or preschool programs also have an increased incidence of gastrointestinal disturbances (such as vomiting and diarrhea) from the exposure to other children (Lu et al., 2004).

Many parents find it extremely difficult to cope with the parade of constant minor colds that occur, causing stress between parent and child, an almost monthly battle of "Stay indoors until your cold is better," conflict. Children may demonstrate frequent whining or clinging behavior because they don't feel completely well. Such constant illness can cause parents to perceive a child as sickly or not able to cope with everyday life. Whereas parents encouraged independence before, they may now begin to overprotect (to shelter to too great a degree). Give reassurance that frequent minor illnesses are common in preschoolers.

BOX 30.6 FOCUS ON . . .

COMMUNICATION

Cathy's father brings her for a well-child visit. You overhear him talking to his daughter in the waiting room.

Less Effective Communication

Cathy: Why do we have to wait so long?
Mr. Edwards: It's how things work here.
Cathy: Why?
Mr. Edwards: I have no idea.
Cathy: Why is that girl here? Is she sick?
Mr. Edwards: I have no idea.
Cathy: When are we going home?
Mr. Edwards: I have no idea.
Cathy: What's that girl's name?
Mr. Edwards: I have no idea.

More Effective Communication

Cathy: Why do we have to wait so long?
Mr. Edwards: It's how things work here.
Cathy: Why?
Mr. Edwards: People have to take turns. We're waiting for our turn.
Cathy: Why is that girl here? Is she sick?
Mr. Edwards: She might be. Some children are here because they're sick and some are just in for a check-up like you.
Cathy: When are we going home?
Mr. Edwards: As soon as the nurse practitioner checks you over.
Cathy: What's that girl's name?
Mr. Edwards: I don't know. Do you want to ask her?

Preschoolers ask 300 to 400 questions a day as they explore their world. In the first scenario, the father tries to discourage questions by offering almost no answers. In the second scenario, when he tries to answer a child's questions, he is not only supplying information but is also helping a child build vocabulary. Because preschoolers ask so many questions, you may have to encourage parents to continue to answer questions this way. Otherwise, discouraging questions can become the method of interaction.

As parents become more experienced in handling these conditions, their perception of whether an illness is a problem will change.

Table 30.2 shows the usual health maintenance schedule for preschoolers. Table 30.3 lists common problems parents may have in evaluating a preschooler's illness.

Common Fears of the Preschooler

Because preschoolers' imagination is so active, this can lead to a number of fears. Fears of the dark, mutilation, and separation or abandonment are all very real to a preschooler.

TABLE 30.2

Health Maintenance Schedule, Preschool Period

Area of Focus	Methods	Frequency
Assessment		
Developmental milestones	History, observation	Every visit
	Formal Denver Developmental Screening Test (DDST II)	Before start of school
Growth milestones	Height, weight plotted on standard growth chart; physical examination	Every visit
Hypertension	Blood pressure	Every visit
Nutrition	History, observation; height/weight information	Every visit
Parent–child relationship	History, observation	Every visit
Behavior problems	History, observation	Every visit
Vision and hearing defects	History, observation	Every visit
	Formal Preschool E and audiometer testing	Before start of school
Dental health	History, physical examination	Every visit
Tuberculosis	PPD test (if there are high-risk factors)	Before start of school
Immunizations		
Diphtheria, pertussis, and tetanus	Check history and past records; inform caregiver about any risks and side effects; administer immunization in accordance with health care agency policies	Before start of school
MMR	MMR #2	Before start of school
Poliomyelitis (inactivated)	IVP #4	Before start of school
Influenza		Yearly
Anticipatory Guidance		
Preschool care	Active listening and health teaching	Every visit
Expected growth and developmental milestones before next visit	Active listening and health teaching	Every visit
Accident prevention	Counseling about street and personal safety	Every visit
Any problems expressed by caregiver during course of the visit	Active listening and health teaching regarding temper tantrums, toilet training	Every visit

American Academy of Pediatrics. (2005). *Recommendations for preventive pediatric health care.* Washington, DC: AAP.

Fear of the Dark. The tendency to fear the dark is an example of a fear heightened by a child's vivid imagination: a stuffed toy by daylight becomes a threatening monster in the dark. Children awaken screaming because of nightmares. They may be reluctant to go to bed or to go back to sleep by themselves unless a light is left on.

If parents are prepared for this fear and understand it is a phase of growth, they will be better able to cope with it. It is generally helpful if they monitor the stimuli their children are exposed to, especially around bedtime. This includes television, adult discussions, and frightening stories. Parents are sometimes reluctant to leave a child's light on at night because they do not want to cater to the fear. Burning a dim night light, however, can solve the problem and costs only pennies. Children who awake terrified and screaming need reassurance they are safe, that whatever was chasing them was a dream and is not in their room.

They may require an understanding adult to sit on their bed until they can fall back to sleep again (Fig. 30.4). Most preschoolers do not remember in the morning they had such a dream; they remember for a lifetime they received comfort when they needed it.

If parents take sensible precautions against fear of the dark or nightmares and a child continues to have this kind of disturbance every night, it may be a reaction to undue stress. In these instances, the source of the stress should be investigated. Giving sleep medication to counteract the sleep disturbance does not help solve the basic problem, so this is rarely recommended. Fear of the dark can become intensified in a hospital setting and requires careful planning to relieve.

Fear of Mutilation. Fear of mutilation is also significant during the preschool age, as revealed by the intense re-

TABLE 30.3

Parental Difficulties Evaluating Illness in the Preschool Child

Difficulty	Helpful Suggestions for Parents
Evaluating seriousness of illness or condition	Preschoolers are eager to please and tend to answer all questions such as, "Does your stomach hurt?" with a yes. Observing the child for signs of illness—refusing to eat, holding an arm stiffly, having to go to the bathroom frequently—is often more productive as an evaluation technique.
Evaluating bowel and bladder problems	Preschoolers are independent in toilet habits for the first time, so parents do not have diaper contents to evaluate. Frequent trips to the bathroom, rubbing the abdomen, and holding genitals are the usual signs of bowel or bladder dysfunction.
Evaluating nutritional intake	Preschoolers begin to eat away from home at friends' houses or at childcare, or to stay overnight with grandparents, so parents do not observe daily food intake as accurately as before. Observing whether a child is growing and active is better than monitoring any one day's food intake.
Evaluating bedwetting	Many preschoolers continue to have occasional enuresis at night until school age. If other signs are present—pain, low-grade fever, listlessness—a child should have a urine culture, as persistent bedwetting can indicate a low-grade urinary tract infection.
Evaluating activity vs. hyperactivity	Many lay magazines have articles on hyperactivity in children. Parents often wonder whether their active child is truly hyperactive. As a rule of thumb, if a child can sit through a meal (when he is hungry), watch a half-hour television show (that is his favorite), or sit still while his favorite story is read to him, he is not hyperactive.
Age-specific diseases to be aware of	Preschool age is a time for vision and hearing assessment. For the first time, a child is able to be tested by a standard chart or by audiometry.
	Urinary tract infections tend to occur with a high frequency in preschool-age girls.
	Language assessment should be done if a child is not able to make wants known by complete, articulated sentences by age 3 (exceptions are transposing *w* for *r* and broken fluency: "I want-want-want to go").

action of a preschooler to even a simple injury such as falling and scraping a knee. A child cries afterward not only from the pain but also from the sight of the injury. Part of this fear arises because preschoolers do not know which body parts are essential and which ones—like an inch of scraped skin—can be easily replaced. Boys develop a fear of castration because developmentally they are more in tune with their body parts and are starting to identify with the same-sex parent as they go through the Oedipal phase. Preschoolers can worry that if some blood is taken out of their bodies, all of their blood will leak out. They often lift a bandage to peek at an incision or cut to see if their body "stuff" is flowing out. They dislike invasive procedures, such as needlesticks, rectal temperature assessment, otoscopic examination, or having a nasogastric tube passed into their stomach, for the same reason. They need good explanations of the limits of health care procedures (e.g., a tympanic thermometer does not hurt, a finger prick heals quickly) in order to feel safe.

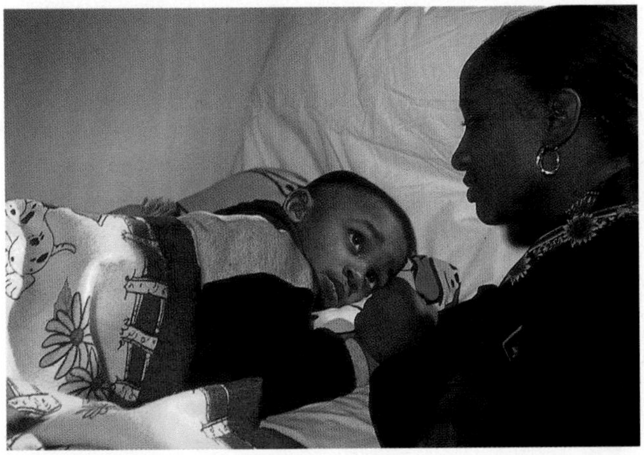

Fear of Separation or Abandonment. Fear of separation continues to be a major concern for preschoolers. For some children, it intensifies because their keen imagination allows them to believe they are being deserted when they are not. Their sense of time is still so distorted they cannot be comforted by assurances such as, "Mommy will pick you up from preschool at noon." Their sense of distance is also limited, so making a statement such as "I work only a block away" is not reassuring. Relating time and space to something a child knows, such as meals, television shows, or a friend's house, is most effective. For example, stating, "Mommy will pick you up from preschool after you have had your snack" or showing a child the work site might be more comforting (Box 30.7).

FIGURE 30.4 Having mom close by after a bad dream is a comfort to the preschooler.

BOX 30.7: Focus on Nursing Care Planning

A Multidisciplinary Care Map for A Preschooler with Fears

●

Cathy Edwards is a 3-year-old girl. Her father cares for her because her mother is hospitalized with preterm labor for a second pregnancy. Her father tells you he is concerned because Cathy talks constantly with an imaginary friend named Emma. She makes up stories about events that can't possibly be true. When corrected, Cathy stutters so badly no one can understand her. At a well-child visit, her father says he is concerned about his daughter's crying at day care.

Family Assessment
Family lives in rented apartment in inner city. Mother is hospitalized with complications of second pregnancy. Father works as city police detective. Mother is stay-at-home mom.

Client Assessment
3-year-old girl within normal limits for height, weight, and development. Child currently enrolled in all-day nursery school program while mother is hospitalized. Father picks child up after his work. Father arrived late to pick child up from nursery school last week. She states, "He forgot me." Child refuses to return to nursery school. Cries, sticks finger in mouth to make herself vomit, and complains that her stomach hurts when he tries to drop her off now.

Nursing Diagnosis
Fear related to separation and abandonment during preschool period

Outcome Criteria
Child verbalizes fear. Father demonstrates measures to minimize child's fears; reports by 2 weeks that crying episodes at school have decreased.

Team Member Responsible	Assessment	Intervention	Rationale	Expected Outcome
Activities of Daily Living				
Nurse	Ask father to detail a 24-hour day in family to gain clear picture of child's role and capabilities.	Father describes differences in family life since wife has been hospitalized, strain it causes on Cathy.	People are unable to solve a problem until the extent of the problem is clear.	Father details a typical day and expresses his wish to continue the nursery school experience.
Consultations				
Nurse	Assess if father feels referral to child guidance service is necessary to help reduce fear.	Encourage the father to talk with the nursery school staff about the problem and common methods to decrease a child's fear.	Discussion with care providers can help reinforce the measures used by the father, providing consistency and thereby helping to minimize a child's fears.	Father states he will consult with nursery school staff to help solve problem.

(continued)

social development (Burke, 2004). Children who have learned to be comfortable in a preschool group approach school comfortably and ready to learn; children who have played only infrequently in groups during the preschool age are forced into this new situation in kindergarten or first grade. They can be so busy adjusting to this new concept they are left behind in learning new skills. The terms "childcare center," "preschool," and "nursery school" are often used interchangeably, so parents cannot depend on the name of a school to define its structure. Traditionally, the main purpose of a childcare center is to provide childcare while parents work or are otherwise occupied. The preschool or nursery school is dedicated to stimulating children's sense of creativity and initiative and introducing them to new experiences and social contacts they would not ordinarily receive at home. Head Start programs and many modern childcare centers fulfill both functions.

If there are other 3- or 4-year-old children in a neighborhood with whom a child has almost daily contact, and if a parent can supervise organized play dates and projects (providing peer interaction, in which working together is the key), a preschool program may not be necessary. On the other hand, if all the neighborhood children are either older or younger or there is only one other child available to play with during the day, a preschool experience will probably be beneficial. Parents with large families point out that their child gets ample exposure to groups, that every meal is a "group session." This is not a peer group, however. Older siblings give in to the 3- or 4-year-old child, and younger siblings are not capable of peer competition. This situation does not offer the same experience as preschool does.

Be sure parents investigate preschools or childcare centers carefully before they enroll their child to be certain their child will be safe there and have an enjoyable experience. Guidelines to aid parents in this assessment are shown in Table 30.4.

To continue to evaluate their child's school experience, urge parents to make a habit of asking children what happened at school, what they learned, and the names of any new friends. For the remainder of the growing years, school will have important effects on their child's development. By taking an active role by providing input into education, parents can influence what and how their child learns.

Childcare centers are often blamed for the spread of infectious disease among the 5-and-under population because bringing together children from so many different homes to one setting each day does increase the risk of spreading contagious disease. Preschoolers may develop frequent upper respiratory infections or gastrointestinal illnesses from an early school setting. Outbreaks of cytomegalovirus and human parvovirus (fifth disease) make working in such centers a particular hazard to pregnant women. To prevent the spread of infection, children need to be taught to wash their hands frequently and cover their mouths when coughing. Childcare centers where infants as well as older children are enrolled need to take special precautions against hepatitis A or parasitic infections, as these can be spread by caregivers' not washing their hands or a changing table after changing diapers. Hepatitis may be subclinical in the preschooler, but other members of the preschooler's family may develop overt symptoms as the illness spreads through the family.

Preparing a Child for School

At the end of the preschool period, children will begin a formal school experience as they enter kindergarten. Parents may wonder whether their child is old enough for this, especially if a child's birthday is in the late summer or early fall. If this is so, urge parents to discuss their concern with school officials to determine whether their child should be registered for kindergarten or delayed for a year. As school involves a great deal of children's time and influences their future greatly, it's important for parents to take time to prepare preschoolers not only physically by being certain their immunizations are up to date (Box 30.9) but emotionally as well.

Essential to this preparation is the parents' attitude. If school is always discussed as something to look forward to, as an adventure that will be satisfying and rewarding, a child will view it from early on as a positive experience. If school is presented as a punishment ("Wait until you get into first grade—your teacher will make you sit up and behave"), there can be little delight in anticipating it.

If a child was not attending preschool, some parents may have to change their child's daily routine a few months in advance of beginning school to accustom a child to waking earlier and going to bed earlier. School has so many new components that it is wise to try to eliminate as many distractions like this as possible.

If a child is to ride a bus to school, a parent might take a child on a municipal bus as an introduction to this form of transportation. If a child is to walk, a trial walk is in order. In either instance, safety should be stressed: "Don't walk behind the bus because the driver can't see you" and "Wait for the crossing guard to help you cross streets."

If a child will be required to take a lunch to school, the parent can introduce this new experience by preparing a bagged lunch at home some noon. If a child is to purchase lunch at school, the parent can play "cafeteria" at home by serving a meal buffet-style and letting a child practice walking from one dish to another to select food.

Some kindergartens suggest children know how to tie their shoes, name basic colors, and print their name before they begin. Parents should familiarize themselves with any such suggestions from the school, but the wisdom of requiring these skills can be questioned. Identifying colors should be established by this age, but some children are not coordinated enough at 4.5 years to tie their shoes or print. A better contribution for parents to make toward their children's achievement in school is to instill in their children the concept that learning is fun and they may not always be able to do all the things other children can do, but trying to do their individual best is what is important. Trying to make children complete fine motor tasks for which they are not developmentally prepared does not instill that concept.

TABLE 30.4

Questions to Use in Evaluating Childcare Centers

Question	Finding
Management	
How long has the center been in operation?	Length of operation does not necessarily indicate quality, but it allows you to locate other parents who have used the center to ask about their experience there.
Is the center licensed, registered, approved, or inspected by the appropriate agency?	Ask in your local community what agency has the responsibility for licensing childcare centers. If not licensed, its quality is suspect.
What are the qualifications of staff members?	If staff members are teachers, more learning activities will be provided; staff should be qualified to perform cardiopulmonary resuscitation.
Is there a fast turnover rate of staff?	A fast turnover rate means little continuity of care will be provided (and probably suggests dissatisfaction with center administration).
What is the child–staff ratio?	A ratio of 3 or 4 children to one staff member provides time for quality interaction.
What is the center's policy on parental visits?	Parents should be able to drop in at any time. Be wary of facilities that restrict parental visiting in any way.
Physical Environment	
Is there adequate space in the center?	There should be opportunities for rough-and-tumble and imaginative play and naptime as well as table activities.
Does the space appear safe?	Stairways should be fenced. No paint should be peeling.
Can children get in and out of the building easily?	A first-floor plan is safest. Fire exits should be well marked. An evacuation plan should be practiced.
Is there a safe play area for children outside?	Find out how often children are taken outside: once or twice a day, or only occasionally for "outings"?
Is there a quiet place for naps?	Ask if a child can nap if tired or has to wait until a set naptime.
Can the bathroom be reached easily?	Both potty chairs and small toilet seats should be available.
If food is provided, does it meet preschool recommendations?	Food should be "preschool friendly."
Is there adequate refrigeration?	Food poisoning is a concern without refrigeration.
Staff Philosophy	
Are the workers warm and affectionate toward the children?	Watch how they greet children. They should ask questions and listen to answers.
Do caretakers spend more of their time performing janitorial tasks (cleaning) and reprimanding children, or can they devote their time to the children?	It is best if cleaning staff is separate from care staff.
Is each child assigned to a particular caregiver on a continuing basis?	Ask staff to describe their care pattern; if this is not planned, little continuity of care results.
Are the children provided stimulating toys and equipment?	Imaginative items, such as a puppet theater, finger paint, and water play, should be included.
How do the staff discipline children? Do they yell or treat the children roughly?	The method should reflect the parents' philosophy. Staff should be able to talk to children calmly without raising their voices in anger.
Is there a planned curriculum?	There should be specific individualized goals the staff hopes to accomplish.
Can the child pursue an individual interest?	Play or learning activities should be individualized.
Health Care Protocols	
How does the center care for an ill child?	There should be access to a nurse. Staff should be able to evaluate for illness.
	They should know actions to take in an emergency.
What precautions does the staff take to prevent spread of infection?	Counter where diapers are changed should be wiped with a disinfectant; tissues and handwashing facilities should be present.

TABLE 30.4

Question	Finding
Does the center follow good sanitary practices?	Be sure the center requires waterproof disposable diapers to minimize contamination of the environment and other children, and separates diaper-changing areas from other activities, especially anything related to food handling. Observe adult caregivers changing diapers. Do they wash hands after each change?
Under what conditions are children not allowed to attend the center?	A center should have a very specific policy on what illness symptoms require a child to be kept home—and they should enforce this policy strictly. For instance, a runny nose may be acceptable, but a fever is not; children with chickenpox should be kept at home until the scabs are healed over.
	Talk to parents whose children have been at the center long enough to have experienced some illnesses, and find out what the family did and how the center responded.
Children's Behavior Do the children appear happy and relaxed?	Observe for at least one morning.
Do they rush to greet any new visitors?	This could be a sign of boredom with their center's activities and a strong need for adult attention.

BOX 30.9 FOCUS ON . . .

EVIDENCE-BASED PRACTICE

Why Do Parents Decide Against Immunization?

In most communities, children cannot begin school without being fully immunized. However, some parents do not want their children immunized. To see whether parents who bring their children for immunizations share common factors with parents who neglect this area of care, researchers sent questionnaires to 129 parents of children identified as not completing recommended immunizations. Sixty-eight parents returned the questionnaires; these forms were used to obtain information. Measles, mumps, rubella (MMR) vaccine was the vaccine most frequently omitted. The reason most frequently given for children not receiving this immunization was that the vaccine was "risky" or could cause harm. Parents also perceived the information provided by health professionals about immunizations to be poor.

This is an interesting study for nurses, because it documents how important it is for parents to know what immunizations are needed at what times and to also have the latest information on the safety of vaccines. As nurses are the health care professionals who often teach this information, it should alert nurses to be certain this type of information is included in discussion of immunizations at well child visits.

Source: Smailbegovic, M. S., Laing, G. J., & Bedford, H. (2003). Why do parents decide against immunization? The effect of health beliefs and health professionals. *Child: Care, Health and Development, 29*(4), 303–311.

For children to do well in a formal school setting, they must be able to follow instructions and sit at a table and chair for a short work period. When some parents examine their child's day, they can be surprised how few instructions they give a child to follow in a day. They put on their coats, pick up their toys, and lead them to the table for dinner. Similarly, they never encourage their child to spend any time in a chair, which is something a child will have to do for at least short periods in school. Coloring at a table rather than on the floor will introduce this situation without any problem.

Finally, going to school is a form of separation and a new experience if a child has not attended childcare or preschool, so parents must make preparations for this. It might be good to arrange to have a child stay with another caregiver for part of a day. Staying at school can then be compared with that event.

These are minimum preparations parents can complete to ready their child for school. Caution both parents and children that no matter how hard they try, not everything can be anticipated; school will bring some new happenings no one predicted. If a child has been led to believe that learning is fun and new experiences are enjoyable (creating a strong sense of initiative), these unpredictable instances can be accepted as fun. The concept that new experiences are enjoyable will prepare a child not only for a first day at school but for thousands of profitable days and experiences ahead.

Broken Fluency

Developing language is such a complicated process that children from 2 to 6 years of age typically have some speech difficulty that parents may interpret as stuttering (Weir &

Bianchet, 2004). A child may begin to repeat words or syllables, saying, "I-I-I want a n-n-new spoon-spoon-spoon." This is called **broken fluency** (repetition and prolongation of sounds, syllables, and words). It is often referred to as **secondary stuttering** because a child begins to speak without this problem and then, during the preschool years, develops it. Unlike the adult who stutters, children are unaware that they are not being fluent unless it is called to their attention. It is a part of normal development and, if accepted as such, will pass. The parent who knows a persistent stutterer, however, or who was a persistent stutterer as a child may react to this normal broken fluency of the preschooler in a more emotional way than the problem deserves. If a child becomes conscious of a disrupted speech pattern, it is less likely the problem will correct itself. It is resolved most quickly if parents follow a few simple rules, listed in Box 30.10.

BOX 30.10 FOCUS ON . . .

FAMILY TEACHING

Suggestions to Reduce Stuttering in the Preschool Child

Q. Mr. Edwards says to you, "My 3-year-old daughter stutters. What can I do to stop this?"

A. What sounds like stuttering in a preschooler is often broken fluency. Helpful tips to improve fluency are:

- Do not discuss in a child's presence the difficulty she is having with speech. Do not label her a "stutterer." This makes her conscious of her speech patterns and compounds the problem. If you have to think about every word you say, it is difficult not to have trouble speaking.
- Listen with patience to what a child is saying. Do not interrupt or fill in a word for her. Do not tell her to speak more slowly or to start over. These actions make a child conscious of her speech, and her broken fluency increases.
- Talk to her in a calm, simple way. It is difficult for a child to keep up with adult speech. If adults talk slowly to her, she sees no need to rush and so speaks more clearly.
- Protect space for her to talk if there are other children in the family. Rushing to say something before a second child interrupts is the same as rushing to conform to adult speech.
- Do not force a child to speak if she does not want to. Do not ask her to recite or sing for strangers.
- Do not reward her for fluent speech or punish her for nonfluent speech. Broken fluency is a developmental stage in language formation, not an indication of regression or a chronic speech pattern.

"Bathroom Language"

Many preschoolers imitate the vocabularies of their parents or older children in the family so well during this time that they incorporate swear words into their vocabularies. Parents may have to be reminded that a child does not understand what the words mean; he or she has simply heard them, just as he or she has heard hundreds of other words and has decided to use them. Correction should be unemotional; for example, "That's not a word we like to hear you use. When you're angry, why don't you say 'fudge' (or whatever)?" The correcting is no different from that involved when a child uses poor grammar. If parents become emotional, a child realizes the value of such words and may continue using them for the attention they create.

Concerns of the Family With a Physically Challenged or Chronically Ill Preschooler

Learning how to do things when you have physical limitations can be frustrating. Being unable to understand how to do things because of physical or mental limitations can be even more so. To learn problem solving, however, is part of developing a sense of initiative. A preschooler with a disability such as cerebral palsy has a greater need for problem-solving skills than the average child, because even simple procedures such as eating or getting dressed can be difficult if a physical challenge limits the options.

Physically challenged or chronically ill preschoolers should attend a preschool program if at all possible. Many of the learning activities that preschoolers enjoy, such as playing with paint, clay, or soap bubbles, are messy. If a child must remain in bed, parents might not offer these types of experiences. A large tray of dry oatmeal or other breakfast cereal with sand shovels or cars and trucks is a good substitute activity for such a child. Although not necessarily neat, these substances (which are available even in a hospital setting) can be swept away easily at the finish of play. Table 30.5 lists nursing actions that can aid a chronically challenged child to solve problems and develop a sense of initiative.

Nutrition and the Physically Challenged or Chronically Ill Preschooler

Experiences with eating help to reinforce a sense of initiative in preschoolers. Chronically ill preschoolers who are limited in the foods they can eat (e.g., they have to maintain a diet of soft foods) or in their ability to help with food preparation may miss this reinforcement. If their appetite is diminished because of illness to the point where they take little or nothing orally, it is still important they continue to join the family at meals. In most households, this is a time for socialization, and preschoolers are ripe for the learning that goes with this type of daily interaction. Encourage parents to include the ill child in family meals and other social occasions whenever possible.

TABLE 30.5

Nursing Actions That Encourage a Sense of Initiative in the Physically Challenged or Chronically Ill Preschooler

Consideration	Nursing Actions
Nutrition	Serving toast or sandwiches cut into animal shapes with cookie cutters, cereal in the form of alphabet characters, or food arranged on a plate to make a face appeals to the imagination and may make a preschooler more interested in food.
	Respect child's food preferences.
Dressing change	Allow preschooler to measure and cut tape or draw a face on it.
	Allow child to see incision site. Explain steps of dressing change as you work to reduce unknowns and areas of fear.
	Provide extra bandages to put on a doll so child can see that bandages themselves are not to be feared.
Medicine	Allow child to choose a chaser such as juice or milk after oral medicine.
	Choosing site for injection or intravenous line is too advanced for the preschooler; do not suggest such choices.
Rest	Provide a light in the room or bring child's bed into hallway so fear of the dark is reduced and child can deal with only reality problems.
	Identify sounds the preschooler might hear in the hospital, such as an air conditioner turning on.
Hygiene	Allow child to choose bathtub toys, clothing.
	Allow child to wash own hands and face.
	Allow child to splash in water as a play activity as well as for cleanliness.
Pain	Encourage preschooler to express pain.
	Allow child to handle syringe or suction catheter, and give "shots" or suction to a doll to alleviate anger or fear.
	Encourage child to ask for analgesic if necessary.
Stimulation	Guessing games encourage a sense of initiative. Draw a dog or a house and ask child to close his or her eyes while you add one more detail to the drawing, such as an ear or a chimney; ask child to identify new item. Reverse the game and ask child what you erased from the drawing, or allow child to do own drawing.
	Provide manipulative toys, such as finger paint, soapy water, clay, or dry cereal to use as sand.
	Allow preschooler to accompany you to other departments as a way of teaching more about the hospital.
	Use "Simon Says" games not only for socialization but also to urge treatments, such as deep-breathing exercises.
	Encourage use of playroom for socialization.
	Encourage child to interact with family by drawing pictures for siblings or telephoning home.

Key Points

Although preschoolers grow only slightly and gain just a little weight, they seem much taller than when they were toddlers because their contour changes to more childlike proportions.

Erikson's developmental task for the preschool period is to gain a sense of initiative or learn how to do things. Play materials ideal for this age group are those that stimulate creativity, such as modeling clay or colored markers.

Promoting childhood safety is a major role because preschoolers' active imaginations can lead them into dangerous situations.

Appetite is not large in this age group because this is not a rapid growth time. Preschoolers can be interested in helping with food preparation.

Common parental concerns during the preschool period are broken fluency, imaginary friends, difficulty sharing, and sibling rivalry.

Preschool is often the time when a new sibling is born. Good preparation for this is necessary to prevent intense sibling rivalry.

Preschoolers have a number of universal fears, including fear of the dark, mutilation, and abandonment. All care provided for this age group must include active measures to reduce these fears as much as possible.

Preschoolers are still operating at a cognitive level that prevents them from understanding conservation (objects have not changed substance although they have changed appearance). This means they need an explanation, for example, of how they will be the same person postoperatively as they were preoperatively.

Preschoolers are self-centered (egocentric). This makes it difficult for them to share and view someone else's side of a problem. They need good explanations of how a procedure will benefit them before they can agree to it.

Many preschoolers begin preschool programs or childcare. Late in the preschool period, they may be enrolled in kindergarten. Parents often appreciate guidance on how to orient their children to these new experiences.

Preschoolers who are physically challenged or who have chronic illnesses may have difficulty achieving a sense of initiative, because they may be limited in their ability to participate in activities that stimulate initiative. They may need special playtimes set aside for stimulation and learning.

Critical Thinking Exercises

1. Cathy is the 3-year-old girl you met at the beginning of the chapter. Cathy's father is concerned because Cathy tells exaggerated stories about events at her preschool. How would you recommend her father handle this?

2. Because her family is moving, Cathy will be starting a new preschool next week. What suggestions could you make to her father about choosing a safe setting? How should he prepare Cathy for this experience?

3. Cathy's parents tell you she keeps the entire family awake at night because she is so afraid of the dark. What suggestions could you make to help relieve this problem?

4. Examine the National Health Goals related to growth and development of the preschooler. Most government-sponsored money for nursing research is allotted based on these goals. What would be a possible research topic to explore pertinent to these goals that would be applicable to Cathy's family and also advance evidence-based practice?

References

American Academy of Pediatrics Committee on Practice and Ambulatory Medicine. (2005). *Recommendations for preventive pediatric health care.* Washington, DC: AAP.

American Academy of Pediatrics. (2005). *Car safety seats: a guide for families, 2005.* (www.AAP.org/family/carseatguide.htm).

Berger, K. S. (2004). *The developing person through the life span* (6th ed.). New York: Worth Publishing.

Burke, S. (2004). Value children, value child care. *Journal of Family Health Care, 14*(4), 88-89.

Department of Health and Human Services. (2000). *Healthy people 2010.* Washington, DC: DHHS.

DiFranza, J. R., Aligne, C. A., & Weitzman, M. (2004). Prenatal and postnatal environmental tobacco smoke exposure and children's health. *Pediatrics, 113*(4S), 1007-1015.

Dudek, S. G. (2005). *Nutrition essentials for nursing practice.* Philadelphia: Lippincott Williams & Wilkins.

Erikson, E. H. (1963). *Childhood and society.* New York: W. W. Norton.

Johnson, M., Maas, M., & Moorhead, S. (2000). *Nursing outcomes classification* (2d ed.). St. Louis: Mosby, Inc.

Kohlberg, L. (1984). *The psychology of moral development.* New York: Harper & Row.

Lu, N., et al. (2004). Child day care risks of common infectious diseases revisited. *Child: Care, Health & Development, 30*(4), 361-368.

McCloskey, J., & Bulechek, G. (2000). *Nursing interventions classification* (3d ed.). St. Louis: Mosby Inc.

National Center for Health Statistics. (2005). *Trends in the health of Americans.* Hyattsville, MD: NCHS.

Piaget, J. (1969). *The theory of stages in cognitive development.* New York: McGraw-Hill.

Smailbegovic, M. S., Laing, G. J., & Bedford, H. (2003). Why do parents decide against immunization? The effect of health beliefs and health professionals. *Child: Care, Health and Development, 29*(4), 303-311.

Sothern, M. S. (2004). Obesity prevention in children: physical activity and nutrition. *Nutrition, 20*(7/8), 704-708.

Weir, E., & Bianchet, S. (2004). Developmental dysfluency: early intervention is key. *Canadian Medical Association Journal, 170*(12), 1790-1791.

Suggested Readings

Ateah, C. A., Secco, M. L., & Woodgate, R. L. (2003). The risks and alternatives to physical punishment use with children. *Journal of Pediatric Health Care, 17*(3), 126-132.

Broderick, M. (2004). Pediatric poisoning! *RN, 67*(9), 37-43.

Campbell, K., et al. (2005). Interventions for preventing obesity in children. *The Cochrane Library (Oxford) (1)* (CD001871).

Casby, M. W. (2003). The development of play in infants, toddlers, and young children. *Communication Disorders Quarterly, 24*(4), 163-174.

Friedman, J. F., et al. (2004). Child care center policies and practices for management of ill children. *Ambulatory Pediatrics, 4*(5), 455-460.

Keane, S. P., & Calkins, S. D. (2004). Predicting kindergarten peer social status from toddler and preschool problem behavior. *Journal of Abnormal Child Psychology, 32*(4), 409-423.

Loeb, S., et al. (2004). Child care in poor communities: early learning effects of type, quality, and stability. *Child Development, 75*(1), 47-65.

Spinrad, T. L., et al. (2004). The relation of children's everyday nonsocial peer play behavior to their emotionality, regulation, and social functioning. *Developmental Psychology, 40*(1), 67-80.

Timperio, A., et al. (2004). Perceptions about the local neighborhood and walking and cycling among children. *Preventive Medicine, 38*(1), 39-47.

Vaughan, E., et al. (2004). Cultural differences in young children's vulnerability to injuries: a risk and protection perspective. *Health Psychology, 23*(3), 289-298.

CHAPTER 31

The Family With a School-Age Child

Key Terms

accommodation
caries
class inclusion
conservation
decentering
inclusion
latchkey children
malocclusion
nocturnal emissions
preconventional reasoning

Objectives

After mastering the contents of this chapter, you should be able to:

1. Describe the normal growth and development pattern and common parental concerns of the school-age period.
2. Assess a school-age child for normal growth and development milestones.
3. Formulate nursing diagnoses for the family of a school-age child.
4. Identify expected outcomes based on health assessment findings.
5. Plan anticipatory guidance to prevent problems of growth and development in a school-age child (e.g., teaching about normal puberty).
6. Implement nursing care to help achieve normal growth and development of a school-age child, such as counseling parents about helping their child adjust to a new school.
7. Evaluate outcome criteria to be certain that goals of care have been achieved.
8. Identify National Health Goals related to a school-age child that nurses can help the nation achieve.
9. Identify areas related to care of school-age children that could benefit from additional nursing research or application of evidence-based practice.
10. Use critical thinking to analyze ways in which the care of a school-age child can be more family-centered.
11. Integrate knowledge of school-age growth and development with nursing process to achieve quality maternal and child health nursing care.

Shelly Lewis is a 12-year-old girl who recently started middle school. Her mother tells you that although Shelly, who is overweight, says she likes school, she has developed a lot of nervous habits such as nail biting since school started. Her mother asks you if this is normal.

The previous chapter discussed the preschooler and the abilities children develop in those years. This chapter adds information about the dramatic changes, both physical and psychosocial, that occur during the school-age years. This is important information because it builds a base for care and health teaching for this age group.

How would you advise Shelly's mother?

After you've studied this chapter, access the accompanying website. Read the patient scenario and answer the questions to further sharpen your skills, grow more familiar with RN-CLEX types of questions, and reward yourself with how much you have learned.

The term "school age" commonly refers to children between the ages of 6 and 12. Although these years represent a time of slow physical growth, cognitive growth and development continue to proceed at rapid rates. Because of this, there are many differences among children from one year to the next. For example, 7- and 10-year-old children have very different needs and outlooks, as do 11- and 12-year-old children. Because of these big differences, always assess children as individuals to understand the particular developmental needs of each child based on what developmental status he or she has achieved, not on what stage you think he or she should have reached.

Unlike the infant or toddler, whose progress is marked by obvious new abilities and skills (e.g., ability to sit up or roll over; ability to speak a full sentence), the development of a school-age child is more subtle and may be marked by mood swings; what the child enjoys on one occasion may not be acceptable on the next. For instance, a child may ask his parents for a guitar and lessons, but then after the family invests in these, he may quickly lose interest in music and prefer soccer. Children of school age may also be more influenced by the attitudes of their friends than previously. They may choose not to do something that was previously enjoyable because no friends are interested in the activity. Parents who make too much of these likes and dislikes may find themselves engaged in unnecessary conflicts with their child. The school-age period is usually the first time children begin to make truly independent judgments. As parents may not be prepared for this, this may create some very real conflicts with parents. Box 31.1 lists National Health Goals related to the school-age period.

BOX 31.1 FOCUS ON . . .

NATIONAL HEALTH GOALS

A number of National Health Goals address the health of the school-age population:

- Increase the proportion of public and private schools that require daily physical education for all students, from a baseline of 17% to a target of 25%.
- Reduce the rate of deaths caused by motor vehicle accidents to no more than 9.2 per 100,000 children, from a baseline of 15.6 per 100,000.
- Reduce the proportion of children who have dental caries (in permanent or primary teeth) to no more than 11% from a baseline of 18%.
- Increase children's rate of safety belt use in automobiles, from 69% to 92%.
- Increase the rate of helmet use by bicyclists (DHHS, 2000).

Nurses can help the nation achieve these goals by urging children to begin and maintain a consistent exercise program, brush teeth and go for dental check-ups regularly, and follow safety rules both in and around automobiles. Additional nursing research that would be helpful includes these questions: What is the ideal exercise program that is interesting enough to children that it will hold their attention for a long span of time? What are effective ways to teach street safety to children in the early school years? What strategies are most effective in helping school-age children brush teeth daily?

Nursing Process Overview

For Healthy Development of a School-Age Child

● *Assessment*

Use both history and physical examination to assess growth and development of a school-age child. Include questions about school activities and progress. School-age children are interested and able to contribute to their own health history; it is useful to interview children 10 years or older at least in part without their parents being present. During the physical examination, show your respect for the child's adult-level modesty by having him or her use a cover gown.

Parents of school-age children often mention behavioral issues or conflicts during yearly health visits. Some parents feel they are losing contact with their children during these years. This can cause them to misinterpret a normal change in behavior, especially if they are not prepared for what to expect from their child. Other parents may consider children who behave differently from their siblings as "abnormal" when children are just expressing their own personality.

When problems are discussed in the health care setting, take the history from the parent but also allow the child to express the problem. It may be necessary to obtain the opinion of school personnel (with the parents' permission) regarding the problem or even just determine whether school personnel feel a problem exists. In some instances, a counselor's opinion may be necessary. If the problem is related to a medical condition, its effect on the family should also be assessed, because the illness of a child affects the functioning of the entire family unit.

● *Nursing Diagnosis*

Common nursing diagnoses pertinent to growth and development during the school-age period are:

- Health-seeking behaviors related to normal school-age growth and development
- Readiness for enhanced parenting related to improved family living conditions
- Anxiety related to slow growth pattern of child
- Risk for injury related to deficient parental knowledge about safety precautions for a school-age child

● *Outcome Identification and Planning*

When identifying expected outcomes and planning care, keep in mind that school-age children tend to enjoy small or short-term projects rather than long, involved ones. A child with diabetes, for example, in her early school years may gain a feeling of achievement by learning to assess her own serum glucose level, but she may have difficulty continuing glucose assessment on a regular basis.

Behavior problems need to be well defined before outcomes are identified and interventions planned. Often, it is enough for parents to accept the problem as one consistent with normal growth and development.

● *Implementation*

School-age children are interested in learning about adult roles, so this means they will watch you to see your attitude as well as your actions in a given situation. When giving care, keep in mind children this age feel more comfortable if they know the "hows" and "whys" of actions. They may not cooperate with a procedure until they are given a satisfactory explanation of why it must be done.

● *Outcome Evaluation*

Yearly health visits covering both physical and psychosocial development are important at this age. It may be useful for parents to look back on problems identified at the last visit and discuss if and how they were resolved. Often, some problems and conflicts fade away without anyone really noticing. As some problems recede, however, others may emerge. At times, the same concerns of parents and the child may appear to be unresolved at each visit. Make sure no underlying problem exists that prevents resolution. Examples of expected outcomes are:

• Parent states he allows child to make own decisions about how to spend allowance.
• Child lists books his parents have read to him in past 2 weeks.
• Child states he understands his growth is normal, even though he is the shortest boy in his eighth-grade class.
• Child does not sustain injury from sports activities during the summer recess.

NURSING ASSESSMENT OF GROWTH AND DEVELOPMENT OF A SCHOOL-AGE CHILD

As school age is a relatively long time span, even though growth is slow but steady, children grow and develop extensively during this period.

Physical Growth

School-age children's annual average weight gain is approximately 3 to 5 lb (1.3 to 2.2 kg); the increase in height is 1 to 2 inches (2.5 to 5 cm). Children who did not lose the lordosis and knock-kneed appearance of toddlers during the preschool period lose these now. Posture becomes more erect.

By 10 years of age, brain growth is complete, so fine motor coordination becomes refined. As the eye globe reaches its final shape at about this same time, an adult vision level is achieved. If the eruption of permanent teeth

and growth of the jaw do not correlate with final head growth, malocclusion with teeth malalignment may be present.

The immunoglobulins IgG and IgA reach adult levels, and lymphatic tissue continues to grow up until about age 9. The resulting abundance of tonsillar and adenoid tissue in the early school years is often mistaken for disease during respiratory illness as the tonsils seem so enlarged in the back of the throat. Enlarged tonsils may also result in temporary conduction deafness from eustachian tube obstruction until this tissue recedes normally. The appendix is also lined with lymphatic tissue, so swelling of this tissue in the narrow tube can lead to trapped fecal material and inflammation (appendicitis) in the early school-age child. Frontal sinuses develop at about 6 years, so sinus headache becomes a possibility (before then, headache in children is rarely caused by a sinus infection).

The left ventricle of the heart enlarges to be strong enough to pump blood to the growing body. Innocent heart murmurs may become apparent due to the extra blood crossing heart valves. The pulse rate decreases to 70 to 80 bpm; blood pressure rises to about 112/60 mm Hg. Maturation of the respiratory system leads to increased oxygen–carbon dioxide exchange, which increases exertion ability and stamina (Berger, 2004). Scoliosis may become apparent for the first time in late childhood. All school-age children over 8 should be screened for this at all health appraisals (see Chapter 51).

Sexual Maturation

At a set point in brain maturity, the hypothalamus transmits an enzyme to the anterior pituitary gland to begin production of gonadotropic hormones, which activate changes in testes and ovaries and produce puberty. Hormone changes that occur with puberty are discussed in Chapter 4. Table 31.1 describes the usual order for secondary sex characteristics to develop.

Timing of the onset of puberty varies widely, between 10 and 14 years of age. The length of time it takes to pass through puberty until sexual maturity is complete also varies. Sexual maturation in girls occurs between 12 and 18 years; in boys, between 14 and 20. Puberty is occurring increasingly earlier, however, and, in a class of 10-year-old sixth graders, it is not unusual to discover that more than half of the girls are already menstruating. This means that for sex education to be effective, parents must introduce this material when their children are in grade school, not in middle school or high school.

Sexual and Physical Concerns

The changes in physical appearance that come with puberty can lead to problems and worries for both children and their parents. School age is a time for parents to discuss with children the physical changes that will occur and the sexual responsibility these changes require. This is also a time to reinforce previous teaching with children that their body is their own, to be used only in the way they choose. Specific measures for children to help prevent sexual abuse are discussed later in this chapter. School nurses can play a major role in this type of education as well.

TABLE 31.1

Chronologic Development of Secondary Sex Characteristics

Age (yr)	Boys	Girls
9–11	Prepubertal weight gain occurs.	Breasts: elevation of papilla with breast bud formation; areolar diameter enlarges.
11–12	Sparse growth of straight, downy, slightly pigmented hair at base of penis.	Straight hair along the labia. Vaginal epithelium becomes cornified.
	Scrotum becoming textured; growth of penis and testes begins.	pH of vaginal secretions acid; slight mucous vaginal discharge present.
	Sebaceous gland secretion increases.	Sebaceous gland secretion increases.
	Perspiration increases.	Perspiration increases.
		Dramatic growth spurt.
12–13	Pubic hair present across pubis.	Pubic hair grows darker; spreads over entire pubis.
	Penis lengthens.	Breasts enlarge, still no protrusion of nipples.
	Dramatic linear growth spurt.	Axillary hair present.
	Breast enlargement occurs.	Menarche occurs.

In both sexes, puberty brings changes in the sebaceous glands. Under the influence of androgen, glands become more active, setting the stage for acne (see Chapter 32). Vasomotor instability commonly leads to blushing; perspiration increases (Kaplan & Love-Osborne, 2003).

Concerns of Girls. Prepubertal girls are usually taller, by about 2 inches (5 cm) or more, than preadolescent boys because their typical growth spurt begins earlier. In a culture in which boys are expected to be taller than girls, this can cause concern. Sometimes a girl notices the change in her pelvic contour when she tries on a skirt or dress from the year before and realizes her hips are becoming broader. She may misinterpret this finding as a gain in weight and attempt a crash diet. She can be reassured that broad bone structure of the hips is part of an adult female profile.

Girls are usually conscious of breast development. A girl who develops ahead of her peers may tend to slouch or wear loose clothing to hide her breast development. Another girl studies herself in a mirror and wonders whether her breasts are going to develop enough. Breast development is not always symmetrical, so it is not unusual for a girl to have breasts of slightly different sizes. After the condition has been checked during a physical examination, she can be reassured that this development is normal—that one breast is not filled with a tumor to make it bigger or the other diseased in some way to make it smaller. Supernumerary (additional) nipples may darken or increase in size at puberty. Be sure girls understand that a supernumerary nipple is affected by the hormones in her body in the same way as other breast tissue, so she understands these changes are normal.

Early preparation for menstruation is important preparation for future childbearing and for the girl's concept of herself as a woman (Box 31.2). A girl who is told that menstruation is a normal function that occurs every month in all healthy women has a different attitude toward her body than a girl who wakes up one morning to find blood on her pajamas and is told bluntly, "You'd better get used to that. You'll have to put up with it for the rest of your life." In the first instance, the girl can trust her body: it is doing what every woman's body does. In the second instance, she feels her body is beyond her control. How can she accept and enjoy growing up if it involves something so unpredictable? In addition to an explanation of the reason for menstrual flow, girls need an explanation of good hygiene and reassurance they can bathe, shower, and swim during their periods. They can use either sanitary napkins or tampons; if they use tampons, they must take precautions to avoid toxic shock syndrome (see Chapter 47).

Girls also need to know that vaginal secretions will begin to be present. If this is not explained, a girl may fear needlessly that she has contracted an infection. Explain that any secretions that cause vulvar irritation should be evaluated at a health care facility, because this does suggest infection.

Most girls have some menstrual irregularity during the first year or two after menarche (the start of menstruation). This occurs primarily because a girl's cycles are anovulatory at first. With maturity and the onset of ovulation, cycles become more regular.

Girls need to know when their periods will occur so they can get used to this new phenomenon and learn to trust their bodies. A girl in college can explain matter-of-factly that she prefers not to go to the beach today because she has her period and does not want to use tampons, but for a preadolescent, this topic is too sophisticated and too emotionally charged to discuss openly. She wants to be able to plan activities to avoid having to make such explanations.

This means menstrual irregularity can be a significant concern for preadolescents. A girl may fear that irregular periods indicate a hormone imbalance. She may worry about her future ability to conceive, or she may be ill informed

BOX 31.2 FOCUS ON . . .

COMMUNICATION

Shelly is a 12-year-old girl who comes to the nurse's office at her school.

Less Effective Communication

Nurse: Hello, Shelly. What can I do for you?
Shelly: I'm having cramps.
Nurse: Are you having your period?
Shelly: No. I haven't started them yet.
Nurse: Describe your cramps to me.
Shelly: Both my sisters started their periods when they were 10.
Nurse: Are you sick to your stomach?
Shelly: I'm the only girl in my gym class who doesn't have her period yet.
Nurse: Let's talk about the cramps. What do you think is causing those?
Shelly: They're not really bad. I'll go back to class.

More Effective Communication

Nurse: Hello, Shelly. What can I do for you?
Shelly: I'm having cramps.
Nurse: Are you having your period?
Shelly: No. I haven't started them yet.
Nurse: Describe your cramps to me.
Shelly: Both my sisters started their periods when they were 10.
Nurse: Are you sick to your stomach?
Shelly: I'm the only girl in my gym class who doesn't have her period yet.
Nurse: You sound as if you're more worried about that than what you came in for.
Shelly: I need to know if I'm all right.
Nurse: Let's talk about that.

In the past, when topics such as menstruation were discussed only in whispers and neither television nor magazines advertised sanitary pads or medicine for menstrual discomfort, most 12-year-old children had little idea about what to expect at puberty. Today, with this information readily available to the public, it is easy to forget that preadolescents, because they may not read magazines or watch adult television shows, still may not know much about what to expect at puberty. Be aware that almost all prepubescent girls are concerned about puberty changes. Through effective communication and listening, you can help them talk about their problems and concerns.

about how conception occurs and fear that irregularity of her periods means she is pregnant. Malnourishment and obesity can add to the problem. Emotions can also affect menstruation. If irregularity continues beyond the first year, a careful history of the girl's school, social, and home adjustment should be taken. (Dysmenorrhea, or painful menstruation, is discussed in Chapter 47.)

For a nominal charge, manufacturers of sanitary napkins or tampons will mail an introductory kit of their products, together with well-illustrated, factual booklets, to introduce girls to menstruation. Such kits are useful if they supplement a parent's or a nurse's discussion, but they should not take the place of individual attention.

Concerns of Boys. Boys who are not prepared for the physical changes of puberty worry about them in the same way as girls. Just as girls are keenly aware of breast development, boys are aware of increasing genital size. If they do not know testicular development precedes penis growth, they can worry that their growth is inadequate. Men tend to measure their manliness by penis size, so a boy who develops late may feel inferior.

Hypertrophy of breast tissue (gynecomastia) can occur in prepuberty, most often in stocky or heavy boys. A youth with this condition may be concerned a breast tumor is present or be embarrassed about growing breasts. He can be assured this is a transitory phenomenon and, although it makes him self-conscious, will fade as soon as his male hormones become more mature and active.

Some boys also become concerned because, although they have pubic hair, they cannot yet grow a beard or do not have chest hair—outward, easily recognized signs of maturity. You can assure them that pubic hair normally appears first and that chest and facial hair may not grow until several years later.

As seminal fluid is produced, boys begin to notice ejaculation during sleep, termed **nocturnal emissions.** Preadolescent boys may believe an old myth that loss of seminal fluid is debilitating; also, boys may have heard the term "premature ejaculation" and worry this is a forewarning of a problem in years to come. Both are fallacies.

Teeth

Deciduous teeth are lost and permanent teeth erupt during the school-age period (Fig. 31.1). The average child gains 28 teeth between 6 and 12 years of age: the central and lateral incisors; first, second, and third cuspids; and first and second molars (Fig. 31.2).

Developmental Milestones

You can measure school-age children's progress by whether they meet typical developmental milestones.

Gross Motor Development

School-age development is summarized in Table 31.2. At the beginning of the school-age period (age 6), children endlessly jump, tumble, skip, and hop. They have enough coordination to walk a straight line. Many can ride a bicycle. They can skip rope with practice. A 7-year-old appears quiet compared with a rough-and-tumble 6-year-old. Gender differences usually begin to manifest in play: there are "girl games," such as dressing dolls, and "boy games," such as pretending to be pirates.

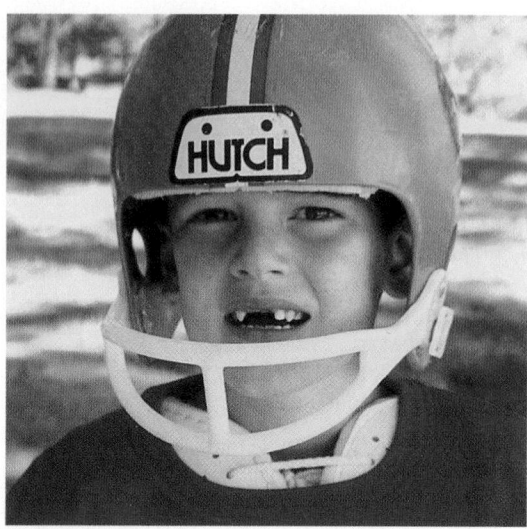

FIGURE 31.1 Early-school-age children typically have a missing upper incisor as deciduous teeth are replaced by permanent teeth.

The movements of 8-year-olds are more graceful than those of younger children, although as their arms and legs grow, they may stumble on furniture or spill milk and food. They ride a bicycle well and enjoy sports such as gymnastics, soccer, and hockey.

Nine-year-olds are on the go constantly, as if they always have a deadline to meet. They have enough eye–hand coordination to enjoy baseball, basketball, and volleyball. By 10 years of age, they are more interested in perfecting their athletic skills than they were previously.

At age 11, many children feel awkward because of their growth spurt and drop out of sports activities rather than look ungainly in their attempts. They may channel their energy into constant motion instead: constantly drumming fingers and tapping pencils or feet. This fall in sports participation may bother parents who see sports as the key to popularity or self-esteem.

Twelve-year-olds plunge into activities with intensity and concentration. They often enjoy participating in sports events for charities (e.g., walk-a-thons). They may be refreshingly cooperative around the house, able to handle a great deal of responsibility and complete given tasks.

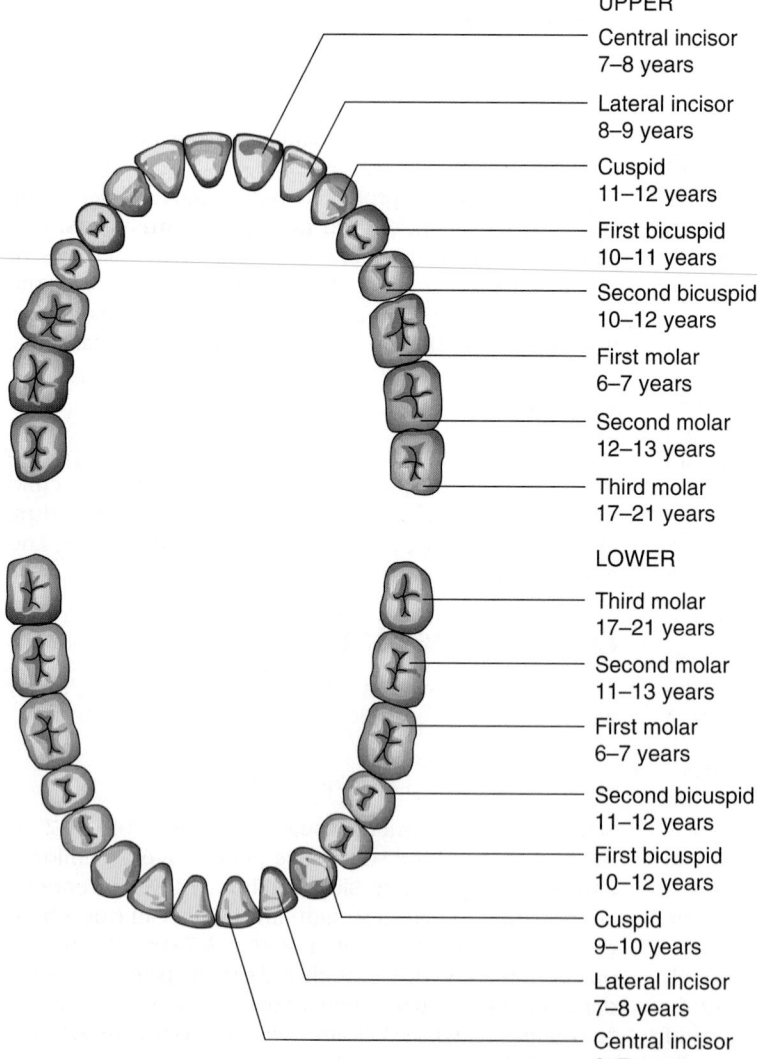

UPPER

Central incisor
7–8 years

Lateral incisor
8–9 years

Cuspid
11–12 years

First bicuspid
10–11 years

Second bicuspid
10–12 years

First molar
6–7 years

Second molar
12–13 years

Third molar
17–21 years

LOWER

Third molar
17–21 years

Second molar
11–13 years

First molar
6–7 years

Second bicuspid
11–12 years

First bicuspid
10–12 years

Cuspid
9–10 years

Lateral incisor
7–8 years

Central incisor
6–7 years

FIGURE 31.2 Eruption pattern of permanent teeth.

TABLE 31.2

Summary of School-Age Development

Age (yr)	Physical Development	Psychosocial and Cognitive Development
6	A year of constant motion; skipping is a new skill; first molars erupt.	First-grade teacher becomes authority figure; adjustment to all-day school may be difficult and lead to nervous manifestations of fingernail biting, etc. Defines words by their use: a key is to unlock a door, not a metal object.
7	Central incisors erupt; difference between sexes becomes apparent in play (video games vs. dolls); spends time in quiet play.	A quiet year; striving for perfection leads to this year being called an eraser year. Conservation (water poured from tall container to a wide, flat one is the same amount of water) is learned; can tell time; can make simple change.
8	Coordination definitely improved; playing with gang becomes important; eyes become fully developed.	"Best friends" develop; whispering and giggling begin; can write as well as print; understands concepts of past, present, and future.
9	All activities done with gang.	Gang age; a 9-year-old club is formed to spite someone, has secret codes, is all boy or all girl; gangs disband and reform quickly.
10	Coordination improves.	Ready for camp away from home; collecting age; likes rules; ready for competitive games.
11	Active, but awkward and ungainly.	Insecure with members of opposite sex; repeats off-color jokes.
12	Coordination improves.	A sense of humor is present; is social and cooperative.

Fine Motor Development

Six-year-olds can easily tie their shoelaces. They can cut and paste well and draw a person with good detail. They can print, although they may routinely reverse letters. Seven-year-olds concentrate on fine motor skills more than previously. This has been called the "eraser year" because children are never quite content with what they have done. They set too high a standard for themselves and then have difficulty performing at that level.

By 8 years of age, children's eyes are developed enough so they can read regular-size type. This makes reading a greater pleasure and school more enjoyable (Fig. 31.3).

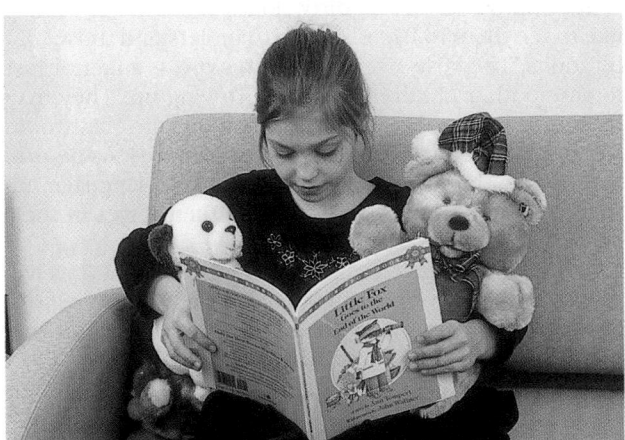

FIGURE 31.3 One of the biggest discoveries of childhood is that reading and writing are fun. Reading and writing are activities that can help a child pass the hours of illness.

Eight-year-olds learn to write script rather than print. They enjoy showing off this new skill in cards, letters, or projects. By age 9, their writing begins to look mature and less awkward.

Older school-age children begin to evaluate their teachers' ability and may perform at varying levels, depending on each teacher's expectations. The middle school curriculum involves more challenging science and mathematics courses than previously and includes good literature. This may be a child's first exposure to reading as a fulfilling and worthwhile experience rather than just as an assignment and may be the time a child is "turned on" to reading.

Play

Play continues to be rough at age 6 years; however, when children discover reading as an enjoyable activity that opens doors to other worlds, they can begin to spend quiet time with books. Many children spend hours playing increasingly challenging video games, an activity that can either foster a healthy sense of competition or create isolation from others.

By 7 years of age, children require more props for play than when they were younger. To be a police officer, a 7-year-old needs a badge and gun, whereas before a pointed finger sufficed. This is the start of a decline in imaginative play, which will continue unless a child receives adequate encouragement to use imagination. By age 7, girls begin to prefer teenage dolls if they didn't previously, and their coordination is good enough they can button the miniature dresses and pull on the tiny boots.

Around 7 years of age, children also develop an interest in collecting items such as baseball cards, dolls, rocks, or marbles. The type of item is not as important as the quantity. These collections become structured as a child reaches 8 years of age; time is spent sorting and cataloging. Most girls and boys of this age also enjoy helping in the kitchen with jobs such as making cookies and salads or frosting cakes. They start to be more involved in simple science projects and experiments.

Eight-year-olds like table games but hate to lose, so they tend to avoid competitive games. They may change the rules in the middle of the game to keep from losing.

Many children of 8 or 9 enter a phase of reading comic books. These can be read quickly, so they complement a sense of industry, the developmental task of the school-age years. If parents forbid comic-book reading, the child may read comics under the covers at night or at other children's houses. Parents would do better to set good reading examples and patiently wait out the child's acute interest in comic books. Their child is reading and will eventually seek other types of books as well.

Nine-year-olds play hard. They wake in the morning, squeeze in some activity before school, and plan something the moment they arrive home again. They may have difficulty going to bed at night because they want to play just one more game. Play is rough; children are not as interested in perfecting their skills as they will be in another year. Some parents or coaches expect children of this age to be more interested in perfecting their skills, so conflict often arises.

Many schools begin music lessons for children at about 9 years of age. Children do well if others in their group are taking similar lessons. Talent for music or art becomes evident, and children respond with new interest in school or wherever they are exposed to these arts. Nine years is also a time when children discover the Internet and how other children out there are waiting to talk to them in chat rooms. Not yet wise enough to recognize the dangers talking to strangers can create, this is an activity parents need to supervise.

Many 10-year-olds spend most of their time playing hand-held or television remote-control games. Boys and girls play separately at age 10, although interest in the opposite sex is apparent. Boys show off as girls pass their group; girls talk loudly or giggle at the sight of a familiar boy. Girls become more interested in the way they look and dress. They may feel old enough for stockings and lipstick. Slumber parties and camp-outs become increasingly popular. Children talk, giggle, and rough-house into the middle of the night.

In the 10th year, children are interested in rules and fairness. Before this time, they gave younger children breaks in games, allowing extra turns or hints. Now they strictly enforce rules (Fig. 31.4). Club activities become structured, with a president, a secretary, and rules of order.

Eleven- and 12-year-old children enjoy dancing to popular music and playing table games and are accommodating enough to be able to play with younger siblings who need the rules modified to their advantage. Time with friends is often spent just talking. If older school-age children use their bedroom as a place to meet with friends, they become more interested in seeing that it is picked up. Twelve-year-olds typically like to do jobs such as raking leaves or babysitting for money. Both boys and girls

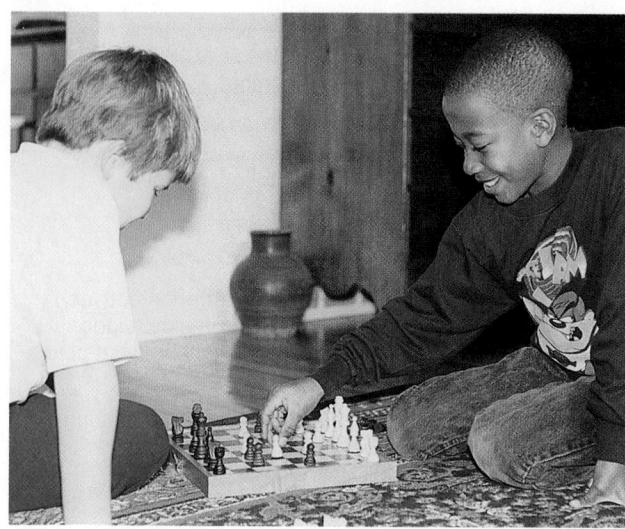

FIGURE 31.4 By 10 years of age children are ready for competition. These two children enjoy a game of chess.

seem to feel they are on the verge of something great and anxiously wait to turn 13 and become a teenager.

Language Development

Six-year-olds talk in full sentences, using language easily and with meaning. They no longer sound as though talking is an experiment but appear to have incorporated language permanently. They still define objects by their use: a key is to unlock a door; a fork is to eat with.

Most 7-year-olds can tell the time in hours, but they may have trouble with concepts such as "half past" and "quarter to," especially with the prevalence of digital clocks and watches. They know the months of the year and can name the months in which holidays fall. They can add and subtract and make simple change (if they have had experience), so they can go to the store and make simple purchases. Much of a child's talk is concerned with these concepts as he or she practices them and shows them off for family or friends.

As children discover "dirty" jokes at about age 9, they like to tell them to friends or try to understand those told by adults. They use swear words to express anger or just to show other children they are growing up. They may have a short period of intense fascination with "bathroom language," as they did during preschool years. As before, parents should make it clear they find such language unacceptable and refrain from using it themselves in their child's presence.

By 12 years of age, a sense of humor is apparent. Twelve-year-olds can carry on an adult conversation, although stories are limited because of their lack of experience.

Emotional Development

Ideally, children enter the school-age period with the ability to trust others and with a sense of respect for their own worth. They can accomplish small tasks independently because they have gained a sense of autonomy. They should have practiced or mimicked adult roles and had the opportunity to explore at preschool or other social environments. They should have learned to share, to have discovered that learning is fun and an adventure, and have learned that doing things is more important and more rewarding than watching things being done (a sense of initiative).

Developmental Task: Industry Versus Inferiority

During the early school years, children attempt to master yet another developmental step: learning a sense of industry or accomplishment (Erikson, 1993). If gaining a sense of initiative can be defined as learning how to do things, then gaining a sense of industry is learning how to do things well.

If children are prevented from achieving a sense of industry or do not receive rewards for accomplishment, they can develop a feeling of inferiority or become convinced they cannot do things they actually can do. These children will have difficulty tackling new situations later in life (new job, new school, new responsibility) because they cannot envision how they could be successful in handling them. This can result in frustration in school or work activities.

The questions a preschool child asks reflect curiosity, such as "how," "why," and "what." During the early school years, children concentrate their questions on the "how" of tasks: "Is this the right way to do this?" "Am I making this right?" "Is this good?" Often a school-age child will comment, "I can't do anything right" because his or her craft project does not look perfect or falls short of expectations. School-age children need reassurance they are doing things correctly. This reassurance is best if it comes frequently rather than infrequently after long waits.

The best type of book for school-age children has many short chapters; children feel a sense of accomplishment when they finish each chapter, rather than having to wait until the end of the book. Small chores that can be completed quickly also give this type of reward. Children can survey their finished work and see that they have done a good job. A child may dislike vacuuming, for instance, because the rug may not look very different when the task is complete. Picking up the scattered contents of a toy box, however, is a more obvious task that clearly makes a difference in the appearance of the room.

Hobbies and projects also are enjoyed best if they are small and can be finished within a short time. Most school-age children, for example, prefer putting together two or three fairly simple model-car kits to assembling one extremely complicated kit. The three kits offer three rewards; the involved one delays the reward so long the child may become bored and never complete it. With adolescence will come more respect for quality. Children will realize if they want the better model, they will have to spend the extra energy and attention—quality products involve quality work (Fig. 31.5).

Home as a Setting to Learn Industry. Parents of a school-age child need to take a step forward in development along with their child. For the first time, they realize their child looks to other role models than themselves. Parents who enjoyed fostering imagination in a preschooler

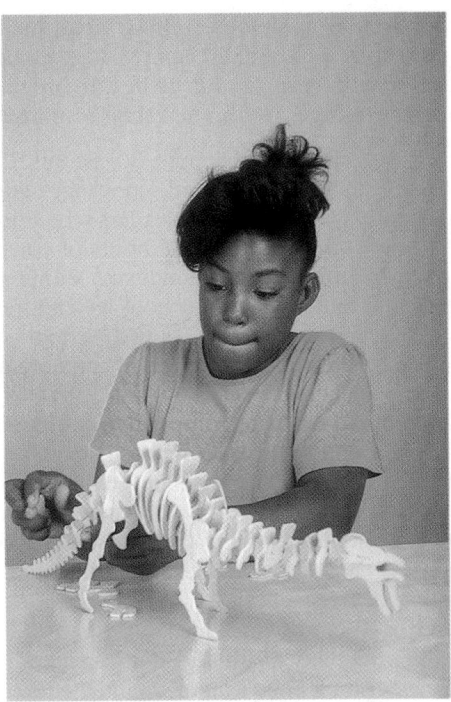

FIGURE 31.5 Assembling this simple model in a short time helps a school-age child gain a sense of industry. (© Stephen Frisch/Stock Boston.)

may feel frustrated when a school-age child begins to conform to rules and insists on the "right way" to do things. They may feel they have failed to encourage the child's creativity, but conformity is vital to children at this age. It is how they learn more about their world's rules.

Eight- or 9-year-olds begin to spend more and more time with their peers and less time with their family. They forget to do household chores they once enjoyed, such as setting the table or cleaning the garage, or they may do the work sloppily so they have more time with their friends. Although this may seem like a regression in behavior, it is actually a step of independence away from the parents and into the larger world, a developmental task that will help them become emotionally mature. This is an example of a new role the child is trying out, one of many he or she will try in the process of reaching maturity, when he will eventually find a "right-fit" role.

School as a Setting to Learn Industry. Adjusting to and achieving in school are two of the major tasks for this age group. Ideally, a child's teacher will think of learning as fun and will encourage a child to plunge into new experiences. Unfortunately, parents must monitor teachers and school activities to make sure their children are being led this way while not being pushed too hard.

Schools are increasingly assuming responsibility for education about sex, safety, avoidance of substances of abuse, and preparation for family living. These discussions are generally superficial, however, and if the classes are large, they may raise more questions than they answer. Although learning these skills with peers helps children learn other people's opinions in these areas, such classes should not replace parental teaching. If given adequate encouragement and preparation by health care providers, most parents are eager to maintain such responsibility.

Structured Activities. Girl Scouts, Boy Scouts, Campfire Girls, and 4-H clubs are respected school-age activities. If the local chapters are well run by leaders who understand children's needs, they can provide hours of constructive activity and strengthen a sense of industry. Merit badge systems are geared to the needs of school-age children, offering small but frequent rewards. As with school activities, parents should determine the worth of each organization for their individual child.

Urge parents to evaluate competitive sports programs as well. Before children can compete successfully, they must be able to lose a game without feeling devastated—in other words, to be able to say, "I lost because I played badly," not "I lost because I am a bad person." Children do not usually develop sufficient ego strength to do this until they are about 10 years old.

Another problem to consider with organized contact sports is the possibility of athletic injuries. Encourage parents to consider their child's maturity and the risk of injury (see Chapter 51) before they decide whether team competition is right for their child. Box 31.3 highlights appropriate outcomes and interventions using the terminology identified by the Nursing Outcomes Classification (NOC) and Nursing Interventions Classification (NIC) regarding school-age sports participation.

Problem Solving. An important part of developing a sense of industry is learning how to solve problems. Parents and teachers can help children develop this skill by encouraging practice. When the child asks, "Is this the right way to do this?" the parent can say, "Let's talk about possible ways of doing it."

The world depends on machinery, so mishaps and breakdowns (and therefore sudden changes) do occur. The child who can create an indoor playhouse with a card table and blanket when it is too wet or cold to use an outdoor playhouse will be able, as an adult, to find another solution to a data distribution problem when a computer malfunctions. This attitude of optimism rather than pessimism produces adults who rarely say, "It can't be done." Just as important, it leaves these adults with confidence and a sense of pride, feeling good about themselves because they have control of their environment and abilities.

Learning to Live With Others. School-age children are sometimes so interested in tasks and in accomplishing physical projects that they forget they must work with

---

BOX 31.3

Nursing Outcomes Classification (NOC) and Nursing Interventions Classification (NIC)

Sports Injuries

NOC: Safety Behavior, Personal
Safety behavior, personal, is defined as individual or caregiver efforts to control behaviors that might cause physical injury (Johnson, Maas, & Moorhead, 2000). Some specific indicators suggesting achievement of this outcome include the child's demonstration of the following:

- Balanced periods of sleep and rest with activity
- Appropriate use of helmets, seat or safety belts, and clothing for activity
- Correct use of protective devices
- Avoidance of recreational drugs, including tobacco, and high-risk behaviors

NIC: Sports-Injury Prevention, Youth
Sports-injury prevention, youth, is defined as reducing the risk of sports-related injury in young athletes (McCloskey & Bulechek, 2000). Some important activities involved when implementing this intervention include:

- Encouraging general fitness, modification of game rules based on age and ability of participants, and appropriate matching of competitors by age, weight, and stage of physical maturation

- Monitoring adherence to recommended training guidelines, compliance with safety rules, field of play for safety conditions, and proper use and condition of safety equipment
- Assisting child in selection of sport that is a good fit with interests and abilities that will promote life-long fitness behaviors
- Assisting parents and coaches in setting realistic goals for participation
- Monitoring sports physicals and return of athletes to participation following injury
- Encouraging the use of warm-up and cool-down exercises and relaxation and coping strategies
- Teaching child and family about measures to prevent injuries and signs and symptoms of overuse injuries, dehydration, heat exhaustion, use of performance-enhancing drugs, eating disorders, and stress
- Arranging for coaches and personnel to obtain annual CPR and first aid training
- Encouraging parents to be involved in child's sports programs
- Advocating for the health of young athletes

people to achieve these goals. A good time to urge children to learn compassion and thoughtfulness toward others is during the early school years, when children are first exposed to large groups of other youngsters. Writing thank-you letters and shoveling an older neighbor's sidewalk are examples of activities that can help children develop empathy toward others.

Learning to give a present without receiving one in return or doing a favor without expecting a reward is also a part of this process, and this can be taught by example. Children should see their parents doing such things with an attitude not of "What will I get?" but "What can I contribute?"

Children may show empathy toward others as early as 20 months, but cognitively they cannot relate others' experiences to their own until about 6 years of age. Therefore, it is usually ineffective to lecture a child by saying, "That was cruel to call Mary names." The child may feel she had every right to do so. A better technique is to ask a child to put herself in Mary's place for a minute and imagine how she would feel if she were Mary. A school-age child will generally be able to do this and understand why name-calling hurts and makes children feel rejected. Following this, a simple statement such as, "It doesn't feel good to be called names, does it?" may suffice.

Socialization

Six-year-old children play in groups, but when they are tired or under added stress, they prefer one-to-one contact. In a first-grade classroom, students compete actively for a few minutes of special time with the teacher. At the end of a day, they enjoy time spent individually with parents. You may have to remind parents this is not babyish behavior but that of a typical 6-year-old.

Seven-year-olds are increasingly aware of family roles and responsibility. Promises must be kept, because 7-year-olds view them as definite, firm commitments. These children tattle because they have a strong sense of justice. This tattling may dissolve play groups quickly.

Eight-year-olds actively seek the company of other children. Most 8-year-old girls have a close girlfriend; boys have a close boyfriend. Girls begin to whisper among themselves, annoying both parents and teachers.

Nine-year-olds take the values of their peer group very seriously. They are much more interested in how other children dress than in what their parents want them to wear. This is typically the gang age because children form clubs, usually "spite clubs." This means if there are four girls on the block, three form a club and exclude the fourth. The reason for exclusion is often unclear; it might be that the fourth child has a chronic disease, that she has more or less money than the others, that she was at the dentist's the day the club was formed, or simply that the club cannot exist unless there is someone to exclude. Such clubs typically have a secret password and secret meeting place. Membership is generally all girls or all boys. If an excluded child does not react badly to being shut out, the club will probably disband after a few days because its purpose is lost. The next day, the excluded member may meet with two others and snub a different child. Parents have to be careful not to intervene with this type of play,

because loyalties shift quickly: the child they defend today may be the excluded one tomorrow.

Nine-year-olds are ready for activities away from home, such as a week at camp. They can take care of their own needs and are mature enough to be separated from their parents for this length of time. Going to camp before this age usually results in homesickness and can be a negative introduction to being away from home.

Although 10-year-olds enjoy groups, they also enjoy privacy. They like having their own bedroom or at least their own dresser, where they can store a collection and know it is free from parents' or siblings' eyes. One of the best gifts for a 10-year-old is a box that locks.

Girls become increasingly interested in boys and vice versa by 11 years of age. Favorite activities are mixed-sex rather than single-sex ones. Children of this age are particularly insecure, however, and girls tend to dance with girls while boys talk together in corners. Better socialization patterns need not be rushed. Just as infants crawl before they walk, so 11-year-olds must attempt many awkward and uncomfortable social experiences before they become comfortable forming relationships with the opposite sex.

Twelve-year-olds feel more comfortable in social situations than they did the year before. Boys experience erections on small provocation so may feel uncomfortable being pushed into boy–girl situations until they know how to control their bodies better. As some children develop faster than others, every group has some members who are almost adolescent and some who are still children, making social interests sometimes difficult.

Checkpoint Question 1

Shelly has belonged to a series of clubs for 9-year-olds. A usual characteristic of clubs for this age child is:

a. The club has formal rules and regulations.
b. It is designed to help shy children socialize.
c. It is designed to spite or exclude another child.
d. Clubs include both boys and girls.

Cognitive Development

The period from 5 to 7 years of age is a transitional stage where children undergo a shift from the preoperational thought they used as preschoolers to concrete operational thought or the ability to reason through any problem they can actually visualize (Piaget, 1969; Fig. 31.6).

Children can use concrete operational thought because they learn several new concepts, such as:

- **Decentering,** the ability to project one's self into other people's situations and see the world from their viewpoint rather than focusing only on their own view
- **Accommodation,** the ability to adapt thought processes to fit what is perceived (i.e., understanding that there can be more than one reason for other people's actions). The preschooler might expect to see the same nurse in the morning that he or she had in the evening; a school-age child can understand that different nurses work different shifts.

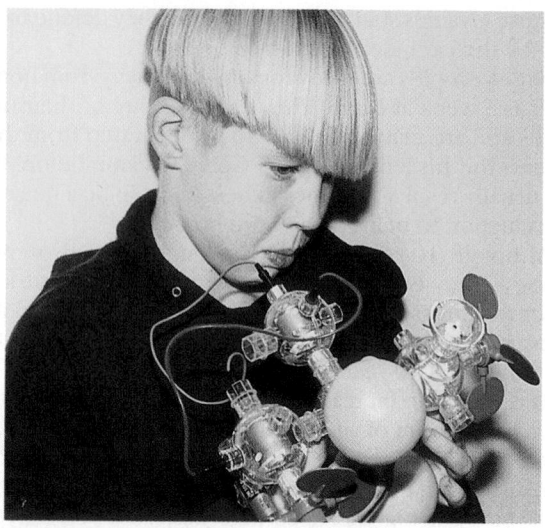

FIGURE 31.6 School-age children learn concrete operational thought or concentrate on phenomena they can actually see occurring.

- **Conservation,** the ability to appreciate that a change in shape does not necessarily mean a change in size. If you pour 30 mL of cough medicine from a thin glass to a wide one, the preschooler will say that one glass holds more than the other; a school-age child will say both glasses hold an equal amount.
- **Class inclusion,** the ability to understand that objects can belong to more than one classification. The preschooler can categorize items in only one way (e.g., stones and shells are found at the beach); a school-age child can categorize them in many ways (e.g., stones and shells are both found at the beach but are made of different materials, are different in sizes, etc.).

These cognitive developments lead to some of the typical changes and characteristics of the school-age period. Decentering enables a school-age child to feel compassion for others, which was not possible in younger years. Because he or she understands conservation, a school-age child is not fooled by perceptions as often as before; sibling arguments over food (your piece of pie is bigger than mine, his glass of cola is bigger than mine) decrease during the school-age years. The ability to classify objects leads to the collecting activities of the school-age period. Class inclusion is also necessary for learning mathematics and reading, systems that categorize numbers and words.

What if... You make a child's hospital bed one day and then give him an injection. What if the next day the child starts to cry while you're making the bed? The lack of what cognitive process led him to believe your action would be the same the second day?

Moral and Spiritual Development

School-age children begin to mature in terms of moral development as they enter a stage of **preconventional reasoning,** sometimes as early as 5 years of age (Kohlberg, 1984). During this stage, if asked, "Why is it wrong to steal from your neighbor?" school-age children will answer, "The police say it's wrong," or "Because if you do, you'll go to jail." They concentrate on "niceness" or "fairness" and cannot see yet that stealing hurts their neighbor, the highest level of moral reasoning.

School-age children begin to learn about the rituals and meaning behind their religious practices, so the distinction between right and wrong becomes more important to them than it was when they were preschoolers. Parent role modeling is also important. Remember that school-age children are rule-oriented; when they pray, they may expect their God to follow rules also (if you are good and pray for something, you should receive it). This makes children of this age confused if a prayer is not immediately answered. Because they are still limited in their ability to understand others' views, they may interpret something as being right because it is good for them, not because it is right for humanity as a whole.

What if... Shelly understands stealing from a neighbor is wrong? Will she also understand that stealing from a large department store or taking things from a health clinic is wrong?

PLANNING AND IMPLEMENTATION FOR HEALTH PROMOTION OF A SCHOOL-AGE CHILD AND FAMILY

Promoting School-Age Safety

School-age children are ready for time on their own without direct adult supervision. Many children as young as 8 or 9 stay by themselves after school (see the section on latchkey children later in this chapter). A child is generally ready for this type of experience if he or she can reliably follow instructions (don't use the fireplace; don't open the door) and can occupy himself or herself for an hour's time. Be certain school-age children know to use seatbelts in cars and bicycle safety around cars (AAP, 2005). As with adults, accidents tend to occur when children are under stress. Box 31.4 lists common measures helpful in preventing accidents in this age group.

School age is not too early for parents to look at the effect of carrying heavy backpacks on children's posture. A backpack that weighs more than 10% of the child's body weight is enough to cause a child to have to lean forward chronically to bear the weight (Hong et al., 2003).

Sexual abuse is an unfortunate and all-too-common hazard for children. Teaching points to help children avoid sexual abuse are summarized in Box 31.5 (see also Chapter 55).

BOX 31.4 FOCUS ON . . .

FAMILY TEACHING

Common Safety Measures to Prevent Accidents During the School Years

Q. Shelly's mother tells you, "My school-ager is constantly on the go. How can I keep her free from accidents when I'm not always with her?"

A. Putting preventive steps in place is the key.

Accident	Preventive Measure
Motor vehicle accidents	Encourage children to use seat belts in a car; role model their use.
	Teach street-crossing safety; stress that streets are no place for rough-housing, pushing, or shoving.
	Teach bicycle safety, including advice not to take "passengers" on a bicycle and to use a helmet.
	Teach parking lot and school bus safety (do not walk in back of parked cars, wait for crossing guard, etc.).
Community	Avoid unsafe areas, such as train yards, grain silos, back alleys.
	Do not go with strangers (parents can establish a code word with child; child does not leave school with anyone who does not know the word).
	Children should say "no" to anyone who touches them if they do not wish it, including family members (most sexual abuse is by a family member, not a stranger).
	For late school-age, teach rules of safer sex (use of condoms; inspecting partner, etc.).
Burns	Teach safety with candles, matches, campfires—fire is not fun. Teach safety with beginning cooking skills (remember to include microwave oven safety, such as closing firmly before turning on oven; not using metal containers). Teach safety with sun exposure—use sun block.
	Do not climb electric poles.
Falls	Teach that rough-housing on fences, climbing on roofs, etc., is hazardous.
	Teach skateboard, scooter, and skating safety.
Sports injuries	Teach that wearing appropriate equipment for sports (face masks for hockey; mouthpiece and cup for football; helmet for bicycle riding, skateboarding, or in-line skating; batting helmets for baseball) is not babyish but smart.
	Stress not to play to a point of exhaustion or in a sport beyond physical capability (no pitching baseball or toe ballet for an early grade-school child).
	Use trampolines only with adult supervision to avoid serious neck injury.
Drowning	Teach how to swim; dares and rough-housing when diving or swimming are not appropriate. Do not swim beyond limits of capabilities.
Drugs	Help your child avoid all recreational drugs and take prescription medicine only as directed. Avoid tobacco and alcohol.
Firearms	Teach safe firearm use. Keep firearms in locked cabinets with bullets separate from gun.
General	School-age children should keep adults informed as to where they are and what they are doing.
	Be aware that the frequency of accidents increases when parents are under stress and therefore less attentive. Special precautions must be taken at these times.
	Some children are more active, curious, and impulsive and therefore more vulnerable to accidents than others.

Promoting Nutritional Health of a School-Age Child

Most school-age children have good appetites, although any meal is influenced by the day's activity. If a child had a full day of activities, he or she may come to the dinner table ready to eat anything. If the day was full of frustration—the child received a poor mark in school, had an argument with a friend, or has a big game to think about—he or she may pick and poke at food. This is no different from the way adults feel at times, so should be respected.

Establishing Healthy Eating Patterns

School-age children need breakfast to provide enough energy to get them through active mornings at school. They eat best if parents get up in the morning and eat some themselves. Children react badly to the instruction, "Do as I say, not as I do."

Many children qualify for a free or reduced-price school lunch and breakfast. A government-regulated school lunch (type A) provides milk (8 oz), protein (2 oz), one starch serving, vegetable (¾ cup), and fruit (¾ cup). Serving sizes

BOX 31.5 FOCUS ON . . .

FAMILY TEACHING

Teaching Points to Help Children Avoid Sexual Abuse

Q. Shelly's mother wants to protect her daughter from sexual abuse. She asks you, "What are good rules to teach children without scaring them?"

A. A number of common rules are:

1. Your body is your property and you can decide who looks at it or touches it.
2. Secrets are fun things to keep. If a person asks you not to tell about something that was done to you that you didn't like, it's not a secret. It's all right to tell about it.
3. Don't go anywhere with a stranger (a stranger is someone you do not know, not someone "strange"). Don't be fooled by people asking you to give them directions or to go with them because your mother is sick or hurt or they have lost a pet.
4. Being touched by someone you like is a good feeling. You don't have to allow anyone to touch you in a way you don't like. Don't allow yourself to be left alone with a person you are uncomfortable with because he or she touches you in a way you don't like.
5. A "private part" is the part of you a bathing suit touches. If anyone asks you to show them a private part or touches a private part, tell them to stop, and tell someone else.
6. If the person you tell doesn't believe you, keep telling people until someone does believe you.

If children take a packed lunch to school, urge parents to allow them some say in the meal, because packed lunches become tedious for everyone after a while. Whether they take lunch or buy it at school, school-age children should know some elementary facts of nutrition so they do not trade a sandwich for cake or choose only desserts from the cafeteria. Ideally, children should receive guidance from school personnel, but this often is impossible in a busy lunchroom. Health care personnel, therefore, should play an active role in nutrition education at health maintenance visits.

Most children are hungry after school and enjoy a snack when they arrive home. Because sugary foods may dull a child's appetite for dinner, urge parents to make the snack nutritious: fruit, cheese, or milk, rather than cookies and a soft drink.

Teach parents to make every attempt to make mealtime a happy and enjoyable part of the day for everyone. Some school-age children learn to eat as quickly as possible (and so incompletely) to escape from the table before something unpleasant happens, such as an argument they can sense is brewing.

Fostering Industry

As a part of fostering industry, school-age children usually enjoy helping to plan meals. They can prepare foods such as instant pudding, Jell-O, salads, scrambled eggs, and sandwiches. They may eat meals they have planned or prepared more willingly than ones that are just set in front of them.

Most parents would like children to develop better table manners. Because they are in a hurry to finish eating, school-age children tend to gulp their food. Many meals are interrupted by spilled milk. As children become teenagers and are more aware of the impression they make on others, manners often improve dramatically. It is often comforting for parents to know that children typically display better table manners in other people's homes than in their own.

Recommended Dietary Reference Intakes

Although parents may have less to say about what a school-age child eats, it is important that the increasing energy requirements that come with this age (often in spurts) are met daily with foods of high nutritional value.

During the late school years, the recommended dietary intakes begin to be separated into categories for girls and boys because boys require more calories and other nutrients at this time. Because school-age children typically dislike vegetables, their intake may be deficient in fiber. Both girls and boys require more iron in prepuberty than they did between the ages of 7 and 10. Adequate calcium and fluoride intake remains important to ensure good teeth and bone growth.

Promoting Nutritional Health With a Vegetarian Diet

School-age children who are raised in vegetarian homes need to learn aspects of vegetarian nutrition if they are going to eat in a school cafeteria. Unfortunately, many

vary according to age to provide one third of a child's nutrition requirements for a day (Fig. 31.7). Check that children are actually eating school lunches, not trading items they do not want, so they receive the full benefit of the program.

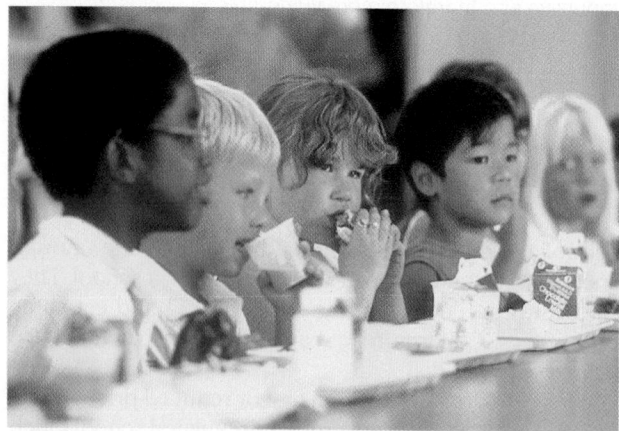

FIGURE 31.7 School lunch programs provide nutritious meals to help school-age children meet nutrition requirements.

school lunch programs offer mainly milk and meat or cheese foods, such as sloppy joe sandwiches, macaroni and cheese, or pizza. This forces children who are vegetarians to carry packed lunches with foods such as cucumber, tomato, or peanut butter sandwiches on whole-grain bread; hot soups; salads; vegetable sticks; and fruit. When eating at a friend's house, they need to learn to notify the host they eat a special diet or to choose correctly from foods they are served.

A potential problem to assess with vegetarian school-age children is whether they are obtaining enough protein and calcium to be prepared for the rapid growth spurt of puberty. Foods high in calcium are green, leafy vegetables (e.g., spinach and turnip greens), prunes, nuts, enriched bread, and cereals. Soybeans, legumes, nuts, grains, and immature seeds (e.g., green beans, lima beans, and corn) are relatively high in protein. As with any individual on a vegetarian diet, children may need a vitamin B_{12} supplement. Encourage outside activities for sun exposure to increase vitamin D. Iron may need to be supplemented, especially in girls with heavy menstrual flows (Dudek, 2005).

Promoting Development of a School-Age Child in Daily Activities

With life centered on school activities and friends, a school-age child still needs parental guidance for most daily activities, because the habits and lifestyle patterns gained during this period will form the basis for the patterns of living later in life. Figure 31.8 shows a day in the life of a family with school-age children. Along with nutritional needs, areas of concern for a school-age child and family include dressing, sleep needs, exercise, hygiene, and dental care.

Dress

Although school-age children can fully dress themselves, they are not good at taking care of their clothes until later in the school-age years. This is the right age, however (if not started already), to teach children the importance of caring for their own belongings. School-age children have definite opinions about clothing styles, often based on the likes of their friends or a popular sports or rock star rather than the preferences of their parents. Help parents be aware that a child who wears different clothing than others may become the object of exclusion from a school club or group. In schools with a gang culture, children may not be able to wear a certain color or style lest they be mistaken for a gang member. Many schools have begun requiring school uniforms to avoid this problem.

Sleep

Sleep needs vary among individual children. Younger school-age children typically require 10 to 12 hours of sleep each night, and older ones require about 8 to 10 hours. Most 6-year-olds are too old for naps but do require a quiet time after school to get them through the remainder of the day. Nighttime terrors may continue during the early school years and may actually increase during the first-grade year as a child reacts to the stress of beginning school.

During early school years, many children enjoy a quiet talk or a reading time at bedtime. At about age 9, when friends become more important, children generally are ready to give up pre-bedtime talks with parents. Some parents react strongly to this change and feel rejected. They may need some help to take at face value their child's statement, "I'm tired. I'd rather go to sleep."

Exercise

School-age children need daily exercise. Although they go to school all day, they do not automatically receive much exercise because school is basically a sit-down activity. Children who are bussed or driven by a parent to school may therefore return home without having spent much time in active exercise.

Exercise need not involve organized sports. It can come from neighborhood games, walking with parents, or bicycle riding. As children enter preadolescence, those with poor coordination may become reluctant to exercise. Urge them to participate in some daily exercise, or else obesity, or osteoporosis later in life, can result (Box 31.6).

Hygiene

Children of 6 or 7 years of age still need help in regulating the bath water temperature and in cleaning their ears and fingernails. By age 8, children are generally capable of bathing themselves but may not do it well because they are too busy to take the time or because they do not find bathing as important as their parents do.

Both boys and girls become interested in showering as they approach their teens. This can be encouraged as perspiration increases with puberty, along with sebaceous gland activity. When girls begin to menstruate, they may be afraid to take baths or wash their hair during their period if they have heard this is not safe. They need information on the importance and safety of good hygiene during their menses. Boys who are uncircumcised may develop inflammation under the foreskin from increased secretions if they do not wash regularly.

Care of Teeth

With proper dental care, the average child today can expect to grow up cavity-free. To ensure this happens, school-age children should visit a dentist at least twice yearly for a checkup, cleaning, and possibly a fluoride treatment to strengthen and harden the tooth enamel (Fig. 31.9). Some children develop a fear of dentists and, if the dentist hurts them, want to avoid going at all. The advantage of frequent visits is that if cavities are filled when they are small, the drilling required is minimal and little pain is involved. If cavities are not treated promptly in this way but are allowed to grow large, the drilling hurts, causing these children to refuse to go back to the dentist. More large cavities then grow, and a vicious circle develops. Pedodontists specialize in caring for children's teeth and understand the developmental level of their patients. Children who tend to

(text continues on page 926)

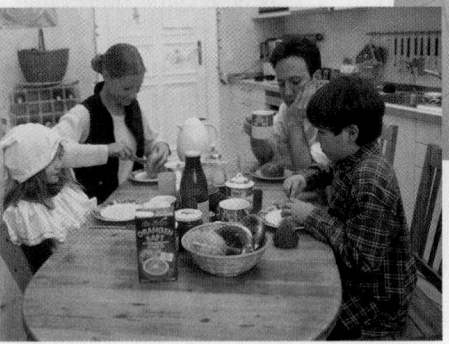

7:00 AM: The family sits down to a healthy breakfast. Claudia helps Laura with the butter.

7:30 AM: John walks Marc to school, emphasizing safety when crossing the street.

10:00 AM: Claudia and Laura bake a cake for the night's dessert. Four-year-old Laura enjoys practicing adult roles.

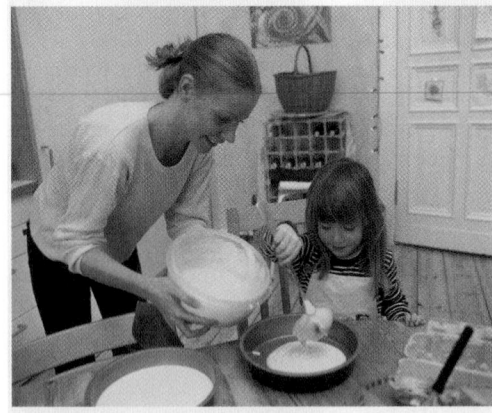

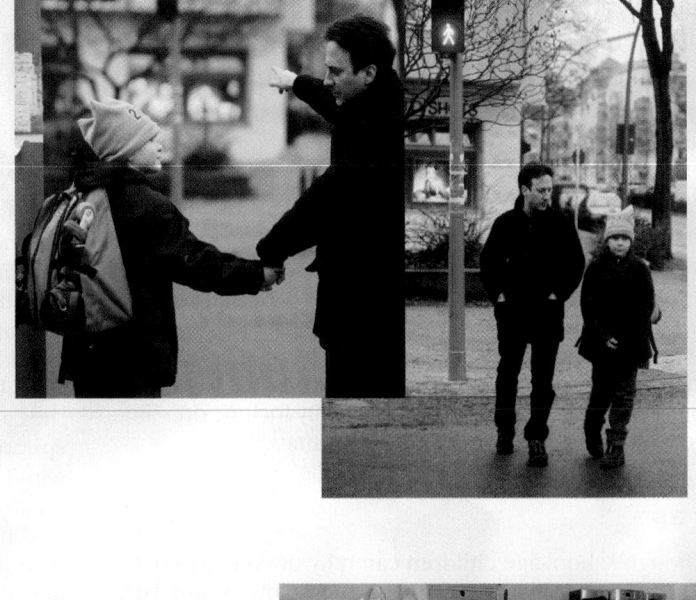

3:00 PM: Marc and Laura play together after Marc gets home from school. Their cooperative play is punctuated by an occasional argument.

FIGURE 31.8 A day in the life of a family with young children.

shoplifts more than once may need counseling; it reflects more than simple confusion about property rights.

As an overall principle, parents must set good examples if they expect their child to be honest. If one parent takes money from the other without permission, neither should be surprised to find their child attempting to do the same. If a parent changes price tags or unwraps items and eats them without paying for them in the supermarket, he or she cannot expect the child to do otherwise.

Violence or Terrorism

Children basically view their world as safe, so it is a shock when violence such as a school shooting or reports of international terrorists enter their lives. A number of organizations have proposed guidelines on how to help children deal with terrorism (NACCT, 2004). Common recommendations for parents include:

- Assure children they are safe; the violence is isolated to another part of the world and they are out of danger.
- Assure children their parents are actively involved in keeping them safe.
- Observe for signs of stress such as sleep disturbances, fatigue, lack of pleasure in activities, or signs of beginning substance abuse.
- Not allow children or adolescents to view footage of traumatic events over and over, as this decreases the ability to feel safe.
- Watch news programs with their children so they can explain that the situation portrayed is not near them and that their child is safe.
- Explain there are bad people in the world, and bad people do bad things, but help children appreciate not all people in a particular group or who look a particular way are bad. Lashing out at people who resemble them only causes more harm.
- Prepare a family disaster plan, including such things as bottled water, blankets, toiletries, pet supplies, appropriate clothing, and flashlights and information such as what immunizations their children have had (particularly tetanus) and, if a child is ill, a history of medical needs or care so that in an emergency, these items are ready.
- Designate a "rally point" where the family will meet if ever separated by a disaster or evacuation.

Some parents may be reluctant to talk to their children about a disaster plan for the family, believing that these preparations will frighten children unnecessarily, but such preparations should have the major effect of increasing a feeling of safety, not decreasing it. Fear of the unknown is always more intense than fear of something tangible.

Bullying

A frequent reason school-age children cite for feeling so unhappy that they turn guns on classmates is that they were ridiculed or bullied to the point they could no longer take such abuse (Seals & Young, 2003). Why do some children become bullies and some become victims? Traits commonly associated with school-age bullies are:

- Advanced physical size and strength for their age
- Aggressive temperament (both male and female)
- Parents who are indifferent
- Parents who are permissive with an aggressive child
- Parents who typically resort to physical punishment
- Presence of a child who is a "natural victim" (underweight, small, anxious, insecure, cautious, or sensitive, with low self-esteem)

Suggestions for school personnel to deal with bullies are:

- Supervise recreation periods closely.
- Intervene immediately to stop bullying.
- Insist that if such behavior does not stop, both school and parents will become involved.
- Therapy may be needed to correct bullying behavior if it is ingrained.
- Advise parents to discuss bullying with their school-age child and tell them how it should be reported, so that adults can intervene.

Recreational Drug Use

Once considered a college or high school problem, illegal drugs are now available to children as early as elementary school and certainly by the time they reach the seventh and eighth grades (Ellickson et al., 2003). Because alcohol is available in so many homes and often can be purchased in small stores without proof of age, this has become a commonly abused drug of this age group (Donovan et al., 2004). Cocaine and amphetamines are also becoming increasingly easy for children to obtain.

The use of hard drugs and alcohol and ways to encourage children to avoid their use are discussed in Chapter 32. Inhalants that are easily available to school-age children, and so may be abused by them, are airplane glue (toluene) and aerosolized cooking oil. Children do not become physically addicted to glue but do become psychologically dependent on it. To achieve the desired effect, they drop quantities of the glue into a paper bag, then sniff the fumes and experience a feeling of exhilaration or giddiness. This may seem a harmless procedure, but in high concentrations glue fumes can cause extensive liver damage or pulmonary edema that can be fatal. Inhalants such as cooking spray or computer keyboard cleaner give this same effect. Because these products contain Freon, they can cause severe respiratory and cardiac irregularity.

Parents should suspect glue sniffing or some other form of recreational drug use if their child regularly appears irritable, inattentive, or drowsy. School health personnel should be aware of the increase in this practice among students and look for warning signs.

Abuse of steroids to improve muscle mass can be found in children as young as sixth grade. Counsel children against this because abuse of steroids leads to cardiovascular irregularities, uncontrollable aggressiveness, and possible cancer in later life (AAP Committee on Sports Medicine and Fitness, 2005).

Cigarette smoking also begins in school-age children. With the sure knowledge that cigarette smoking plays a large part in the development of lung cancer and other serious respiratory illnesses, many parents assume their children will know not to start. Smoking is considered by children to be an adult activity, however, so adopting the habit can be considered a giant step on the road to adulthood. Although the amount of cigarette advertising targeting young people as consumers has decreased, school-age children should be taught to recognize advertising manipulation aimed at them. Caution children against experimenting with smokeless tobacco as well as this can lead to mouth and throat cancer. Children may try this after seeing professional athletes using it.

To discourage use of tobacco by school-age children, health care professionals and parents need to be role models of excellent health behaviors in hopes children will follow their good examples.

Children of Alcoholic Parents

As many as one in five children live with an alcoholic parent (Schuckit, 2005). Such children are at greater risk for having emotional problems than others because of the frequent disruption in their lives. Alcoholism may have a genetic cause, so children of alcoholics are more likely to become alcoholics. They also can learn poor coping behavior (Sims & Iphofen, 2003). Immediate problems that can occur with children of alcoholics are:

- A feeling of guilt that the child is the cause of the parent's drinking
- Constant worry that the alcoholic parent will become sick or die, leaving the child; at the same time, fear of violence from the alcoholic parent and a wish the parent would leave
- A feeling of shame that prevents the child from inviting friends home or asking for help
- Decreased ability to trust adults because the parent has been unreliable so many times
- Concern because the alcoholic parent's behavior is so erratic that no regular schedule of bedtime and meals exists
- Anger at the alcoholic parent for drinking and at the nonalcoholic parent for not doing more to correct things
- Helplessness to change the situation

Such fears may be revealed by failing marks in school, withdrawal from friends or social activities, and delinquent behavior such as stealing. With adolescence may come depression, suicidal thoughts, or abuse of drugs or alcohol. School nurses are in an excellent position to identify such children, monitor their school progress, and refer them to organizations such as Al-Anon or Alateen (*www.al-anon-alateen.org*) for support.

Checkpoint Question 3

School-agers can begin drug abuse. What is a common household product frequently abused by school-agers?

a. Grated orange peel
b. Laundry bleach
c. Aerosol cooking oil
d. Shredded cabbage

Obesity

As many as 50% of school-age children are obese by body-mass index guidelines for ideal weight. Some of these children have been overweight since infancy; their pre-pubertal natural weight gain makes them obese. Children with an endomorphic build (a natural tendency to accumulate body fat) are more likely to be obese at any time of life than those with a mesomorphic (normal) or ectomorphic (slender) build. Many families rely on fast-food meals several times a week, and such foods tend to be high in calories and fat and can lead to obesity. Soft drink machines in grade schools add to the problem (Pontin, 2004). Children of obese parents are also inclined to obesity; perhaps genetic influences have some bearing. If parents ingest a diet full of excessive calories, the child is encouraged to eat similarly; this makes environmental factors also play a role.

Obese children begin to develop many of the same health problems as obese adults, such as hypertension, type 2 diabetes, and an elevated total cholesterol level, with possible atherosclerosis. They also may be ridiculed for their size and be unable to participate on sports teams. This is strong evidence for the need for active measures to help preteens regulate their weight.

Those who become so obese that friends leave them out of activities or who cannot play sports because they tire quickly may develop such a poor self-image they have little motivation for self-improvement. A weight-reduction program for school-age children that emphasizes long-term lifestyle changes is best. Such programs should contain three aspects:

1. Intake of about 1,200 calories (no more than 30% as fat), with lifestyle changes such as a structured family meal, eliminating eating or snacking in front of the television, decreased portion sizes, and elimination of sugar-rich drinks
2. An active exercise program, including such things as monitoring and limiting time spent in physical inactivity (watching television, playing computer and video games, surfing the Internet, and talking on the telephone)
3. A counseling program to discuss aspects such as self-image and motivation to reduce weight (Stettler, 2003)

Total caloric intake cannot be reduced too drastically because children need calories to form new body tissue for continued growth. If carbohydrate intake is restricted too greatly, protein is broken down for body energy and a negative nitrogen balance is produced. Caution children not to try faddish high-protein diets (as most adults should not), because such diets do not supply enough carbohydrates and may produce a heavy renal solute load (the breakdown product of proteins) for the kidneys. It helps if children aim to lose 5 lb over a short time rather than 50 lb over a year. This short-term goal coincides better with the task of developing industry.

Surgical techniques such as an intestinal bypass are obviously extreme measures and inappropriate for children. Obese children might request one, however, in an attempt to avoid the not insignificant difficulty of long-term weight loss.

NURSING DIAGNOSES AND RELATED INTERVENTIONS

————————●————————

Nursing Diagnosis: Altered family dynamics related to lack of motivation to reduce weight

Outcome Evaluation: Child states reasonable weight loss and exercise goals; discusses feelings with nurse about being overweight and reactions from schoolmates; expresses positive feelings about self-worth.

Motivating preteens to lose weight can be difficult because they often have little regard for what will happen to them in the future. They are not upset when told obese people do not live as long as slimmer persons and have more heart attacks, because this will happen far in the future. They do, however, have a great respect for adults who are sympathetic to their problems. They are also aware slim children are usually the most popular, and they wish they could look that way. They follow better dietary regimens, therefore, if they are asked to do so by a respected adult, such as a nurse, or if they fear being left out of social interactions.

Overweight school-age children often do well if a dieters' club is formed. They are not too young to participate in formal weight-control organizations. Having tangible support from other group members helps them follow tedious and monotonous nutrition patterns. Behavior modification can also be useful in teaching children how to eat in a healthier manner.

As a way of increasing daily activity, preadolescents do well with formal exercise classes because they enjoy the support from other children. In addition, encourage them to increase informal exercise, such as walking to and from school. Encourage coaches of childhood sports to accept obese children as part of a team, not because they will necessarily benefit the team, but because the exercise will benefit the children. Exercise burns up calories, and if children's daylight hours are filled with activities and friends, they have less time to eat.

Lifestyle change is the ultimate goal for the entire family, because obesity is usually a family problem. Rather than preparing special meals for just the obese child, the entire family probably needs to eat in a healthier manner. Because preadolescents do not generally prepare their own food, the person in the home who prepares meals requires as much information on the planned weight loss as the child. The old concepts that used to hold ("A clean plate is good; how can you leave food when people in other countries are starving?") may have to be changed so children and other family members reduce their

intake appropriately. The importance of exercise should also be reflected in the home. Family members should not only encourage the obese child to exercise but also should partake in some form of daily activity themselves.

There is some danger in pointing out to preadolescents they are terribly overweight because some children become so obsessed with losing weight that they become bulimic or anorexic (Marcus & Kalarchian, 2003) (see Chapter 32). Stressing that children "become healthier" or "improve stamina" may be better advice than talking about dieting.

Concerns of the Physically Challenged or Chronically Ill School-Age Child

One of the biggest problems facing a school-age child with a long-term illness or physical challenge is time lost from school. This threatens not only academic achievement but also the child's relationships with his or her peers. It may make him or her the "odd person out" with respect to making friends or joining gangs. Whether children are confined to the home or hospitalized, helping them to keep in contact with friends by telephone, e-mail, or letters can help foster the socialization that is important for continued development. Encourage parents (or school friends) to obtain schoolwork and help these children with their homework so they can progress with learning at a usual pace and continue to build self-esteem.

Most children with physical or cognitive challenges attend regular schools and classes (**inclusion**) because federal law (PL 99-457) stipulates all children must receive equal education in the least restrictive situation possible. Placement in classrooms is determined by a committee in each school system. You may need to advocate for a child with such a committee to demonstrate, for example, that although a child uses a wheelchair or needs continuous oxygen, he or she can participate in a regular classroom setting; or that a child would benefit from a period each day with a special resource teacher. It may be necessary to meet with a school nurse, teacher, or the child's classmates (with the parents' permission) to increase their understanding and acceptance of the child's illness.

Urge parents of children with physical or cognitive challenges to assign them household chores just like other children their age and to allow them to participate in activities, such as Girl or Boy Scouts, in which accomplishment is encouraged. It is important for such children to develop a sense of industry or accomplishment so they can persevere in measures that will help them to be as independent as possible (Fig. 31.10).

When you are caring for a school-age child who is chronically ill or physically challenged, choose short-term activities that can be completed independently, as with all school-age children. Conversely, be careful not to insult a child with tasks that are obviously not age-appropriate. Table 31.5 describes some nursing actions to help

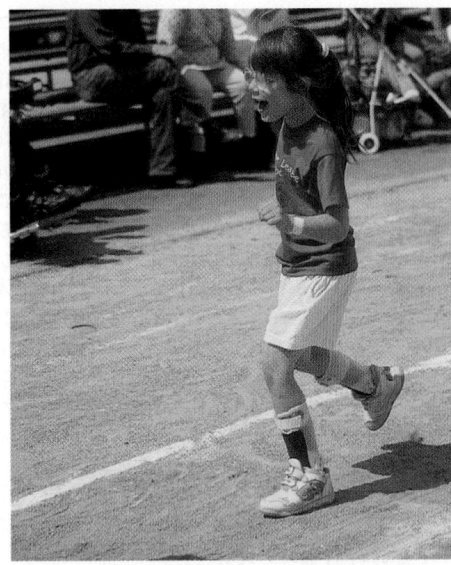

FIGURE 31.10 A school-age child who is physically challenged is elated at a finish line. This accomplishment can go far toward her developing a sense of industry. (© Jose Carillo/Stock Boston.)

foster a sense of industry in children who are physically challenged or chronically ill.

Nutrition and the Challenged School-Age Child

Food preparation and dishwashing are times for socializing in most households. A school-age child who cannot be involved in these activities because of a physical challenge needs extra time during the day to make up for these lost socializing experiences, such as a specific hour set aside for talking or sharing a project that can be accomplished in one sitting.

When eating in cafeterias or at a friend's home, a child who must eat a special diet is usually tempted to select the same food as everyone else rather than limit what he or she chooses. A child may decline invitations rather than admit to requiring a special diet or needing help with eating. Ask at health care visits if any of these problems are present. Help children with special diets to plan ways they could be comfortable in social food-based settings (e.g., bringing a party snack that is easily eaten and appropriate for the child, or politely declining particular foods). Help children who are hospitalized to select a diet that is enjoyable as well as nutritious.

TABLE 31.5

Nursing Actions That Encourage a Sense of Industry in the Physically Challenged or Chronically Ill School-Age Child

Category	Actions
Nutrition	Allow choices of food and respect food preferences.
	Provide small food servings that child can finish, encouraging sense of accomplishment.
Dressing	Allow child to make out requisitions for supplies.
	Ask for suggestions as to how bulky the child wants dressing, where to apply tape.
Medicine	Teach child name and action of medicine.
	Encourage child to keep track of medication times by clock or record.
	Child may feel more in control of injections or intravenous insertions if allowed to choose the site from among options offered.
	Allow child to choose oral medicine form (capsules or liquid) if possible.
Rest	Establish clear rules for rest periods (reading or watching television is all right; playing a game is not, etc.).
Hygiene	Respect modesty of school-age child at an adult level.
	Allow as much choice as possible (e.g., own clothing, timing of self-care).
Pain	Encourage child to express and rate pain.
	Encourage child to use distraction techniques, such as counting backward from 100 or imagery, during episodes of pain.
	Explain source and cause of pain to give child sense of mastery.
Stimulation	Encourage school work.
	Encourage activity that ends in a product (putting together a picture puzzle rather than listening to a CD).
	Encourage paper-and-pencil games, such as connect the dots, tic tac toe.
	Card games provide social interaction and also encourage simple addition skills (make a deck from paper if one is not available).
	Don't suggest competitive games for children less than age 10 yr.
	Encourage using playroom for socialization.
	Encourage child to keep in contact with school friends by telephoning or writing notes to them.

Key Points

School-age children mature slowly but steadily. Their average annual weight gain is 3 to 5 lb; their increase in height is 1 to 2 inches.

At about age 10, children begin to develop secondary sex characteristics. Preparation for this helps them accept these changes positively.

Deciduous teeth are lost and permanent teeth erupt during the school-age period.

Erikson's developmental task for the school-age period is to gain a sense of industry, or how to do things well.

Common health problems during the school-age period include minor respiratory and gastrointestinal infections as well as dental caries and malocclusion.

Common parental concerns about a school-age child are language development, fears and anxieties, and behavior problems such as stealing and using recreational drugs.

As many as 90% of parents of school-age children are dual-earner families. This means many school-age children return home before their parents. Counseling families on ways to turn this independent time alone into a positive experience is a nursing responsibility.

Children in a concrete stage of operational thought are limited to understanding concepts they can actually see. When health teaching, use concrete examples (actually let them hold a syringe, don't just talk about it) to increase their understanding.

School-age children thrive on rules. It is confusing for them when rules are changed (medicine will now be taken four rather than three times a day) unless they have a clear explanation of why the change is occurring.

School-age children are looking for good adult role models; it is hard for them to feel confidence in an adult who isn't honest with them or who fails to live up to their expectations by not following through on promises.

School-age children with a family tendency toward obesity may become overweight. Helping the family learn a healthier lifestyle is important.

Critical Thinking Exercises

1. Shelly is the 12-year-old you met at the beginning of the chapter. Her mother told you that she has developed many nervous habits since she started middle school. She asks you if this is normal. How would you answer? What suggestions would you make to her mother regarding this?

2. Shelly has become obese in the last year. School-age children develop obesity because of excessive nutritional intake, lack of exercise, and inheritance or family factors. What are suggestions you could make to help prevent Shelly from gaining more weight? What is a possible consequence of telling school-age children they are overweight?

3. Shelly's best friend is a 12-year-old boy who is confined to a wheelchair because of muscular dystrophy. Why might developing a sense of industry be particularly difficult for him? What suggestions could you make to encourage this?

4. Examine the National Health Goals related to school-age children. Most government-sponsored money for nursing research is allotted based on these goals. What would be a possible research topic to explore pertinent to these goals that would be applicable to the Lewis family and also advance evidence-based practice?

References

American Academy of Pediatrics. (2005). *Car safety seats: a guide for families, 2005.* (www.AAP.org/family/carseatguide.htm).

American Academy of Pediatrics, Committee on Sports Medicine and Fitness. (2005). Use of performance-enhancing substances. *Pediatrics, 115*(4), 1103–1016.

Berger, K. S. (2004). *The developing person through the life span* (6th ed.). New York: Worth Publishing.

Centers for Disease Control and Prevention. (2005). *Recommended childhood and adolescent immunization schedule, United States, 2005.* Washington, DC: DHHS.

Department of Health and Human Services. (2000). *Healthy people 2010.* Washington, DC: DHHS.

Donovan, J. E., et al. (2004). Really underage drinkers: alcohol use among elementary students. *Alcoholism: Clinical and Experimental Research, 28*(2), 341–349.

Dudek, S. G. (2005). *Nutrition essentials for nursing practice.* Philadelphia: Lippincott Williams & Wilkins.

Ellickson, P. L., et al. (2003). Adolescent health. New inroads in preventing adolescent drug use: results from a large-scale trial of Project ALERT in middle schools. *American Journal of Public Health, 93*(11), 1830–1836.

Erikson, E. H. (1993). *Childhood and society.* New York: W. W. Norton.

Freud, S. (1962). *Three essays on the theory of sexuality.* New York: Hearst Corporation.

Hong, Y., Lau, T. C., & Li, J. X. (2003). Effects of loads and carrying methods of school bags on movement kinematics of children during stair walking. *Research in Sports Medicine, 11*(1), 33–49.

Johnson, M., Maas, M., & Moorhead, S. (2000). *Nursing outcomes classification* (2d ed.). St. Louis: Mosby, Inc.

Kaplan, D. W., & Love-Osborne, K. (2003). Adolescence. In: W. W. Hay et al. (Eds.), *Current Pediatric Diagnosis and Treatment* (16th ed.) New York: McGraw-Hill.

Kohlberg, L. (1984). *The psychology of moral development.* New York: Harper & Row.

Marcus, M. D., & Kalarchian, M. A. (2003). Binge eating in children and adolescents. *International Journal of Eating Disorders, 34*(Suppl), S47-57.

Martin, J. T., et al. (2004). Female adolescents' knowledge of bone health promotion behaviors and osteoporosis risk factors. *Orthopaedic Nursing, 23*(4), 235–244.

McCloskey, J., & Bulechek, G. (2000). *Nursing interventions classification* (3d ed.). St. Louis: Mosby, Inc.

McDermott, I. E. (2003). Web resources for home-schooling. *Searcher: The Magazine for Database Professionals, 11*(8), 27–31.

National Advisory Committee on Children and Terrorism. (2004). Schools and terrorism: a supplement to the report of the National Advisory Committee on Children and Terrorism. *Journal of School Health, 74*(2), 39–51.

National Center for Health Statistics. (2005). *Trends in the health of Americans.* Hyattsville, MD: NCHS.

Piaget, J. (1969). *The theory of stages in cognitive development.* New York: McGraw-Hill.

Pontin, D. (2004). A school based programme to reduce carbonated drink consumption reduced obesity in children. *Evidence-Based Nursing, 7*(4), 105–106.

Salemi, A. T., & Brown, K. M. (2003). School phobia: implications for school health educators. *American Journal of Health Education, 34*(4), 199–205.

Schuckit, M. A. (2005). Alcohol related disorders. In: B. J. Sadock & V. A. Sadock (Eds.), *Kaplan and Sadock's comprehensive textbook of psychiatry* (8th ed.). Philadelphia: Lippincott Williams & Wilkins.

Seals, D., & Young, J. (2003). Bullying and victimization: prevalence and relationship to gender, grade level, ethnicity, self-esteem, and depression. *Adolescence, 38*(152), 735–747.

Sims, J., & Iphofen, R. (2003). Parental substance misuse and its effect on children. *Drug and Alcohol Professional, 3*(3), 33–40.

Stettler, N. (2003). Obesity. In M. W. Schwartz (Ed.), *5-minute pediatric consult* (3rd ed.). Philadelphia: Lippincott Williams & Wilkins.

Wahl, N. (2005). Orthodontics in 3 millennia. Chapter 1: Antiquity to the mid-19th century. *American Journal of Orthodontics & Dentofacial Orthopedics, 127*(2), 255–259.

Suggested Readings

Campbell, K., et al. (2005). Interventions for preventing obesity in children. *The Cochrane Library (Oxford) (1):* (ID #CD001871).

Clark, A. (2004). The role of the school nurse in tackling childhood obesity. *Nursing Times, 100*(23), 28–29.

Decaluwe, V., Braet, C., & Fairburn, C. G. (2003). Binge eating in obese children and adolescents. *International Journal of Eating Disorders, 33*(1), 78–84.

Jones, S. E., Brener, N. D., & McManus, T. (2003). Prevalence of school policies, programs, and facilities that promote a healthy physical school environment. *American Journal of Public Health, 93*(9), 1570–1575.

Kien, C. L., & Chiodo, A. R. (2003). Physical activity in middle school–aged children participating in a school-based recreation program. *Archives of Pediatrics & Adolescent Medicine, 157*(8), 811–815.

Marinho, V. C. C., et al. (2005). Fluoride mouth rinses for preventing dental caries in children and adolescents. *The Cochrane Library (Oxford) (1)* (CD002284).

Morris, R. I., & Strong, L. (2004). The impact of homelessness on the health of families. *Journal of School Nursing, 20*(4), 221–227.

Ramirez, M., Peek-Asa, C., & Kraus, J. F. (2004). Disability and risk of school related injury. *Injury Prevention, 10*(1), 21–26.

Venning, H. B., Blampied, N. M., & France, K. G. (2003). Effectiveness of a standard parenting-skills program in reducing stealing and lying in two boys. *Child & Family Behavior Therapy, 25*(2), 31–44.

Xiang, P., Bruene, A., & McBride, R. E. (2004). Using achievement goal theory to assess an elementary physical education running program. *Journal of School Health, 74*(6), 220–225.

The Family With an Adolescent

Key Terms

adolescence
comedones
formal operational thought
glycogen loading
identity
puberty
role confusion
stalking
substance abuse

Objectives

After mastering the contents of this chapter, you should be able to:

1. Describe normal growth and development and common parental concerns of the adolescent period.
2. Assess adolescents for normal growth and development milestones.
3. Formulate nursing diagnoses for the family of an adolescent.
4. Identify expected outcomes based on health assessment findings.
5. Plan nursing care related to growth and development concerns of an adolescent, such as planning health teaching necessary to accept pubertal changes.
6. Implement nursing care related to growth and development or special needs of an adolescent, such as organizing a discussion group on ways to prevent drug abuse.
7. Evaluate expected outcomes to be certain that goals of care have been achieved.
8. Identify National Health Goals related to adolescents that nurses could help the nation achieve.
9. Identify areas related to care of adolescents that could benefit from additional nursing research or application of evidence-based practice.
10. Use critical thinking to analyze ways in which care of an adolescent could be more family-centered.
11. Integrate knowledge of adolescent growth and development with nursing process to achieve quality maternal and child health nursing care.

Raul is a 15-year-old boy you see at an adolescent clinic. His chief concern is a head cold. He has numerous acne lesions on his forehead and cheeks. His parents tell you Raul seemed depressed for a long time after his girlfriend broke up with him but now seems happy again. They are pleased to see him maturing so much he recently gave away his collection of baseball cards to a young neighbor. You mention to Raul that a decongestant would probably make him feel better. He asks you how many pills it would take to kill someone, then jokes he was kidding. His parents tell you Raul has been joking about killing himself a lot lately. The physician in the clinic prescribes a decongestant and suggests Raul return in 6 months.

The previous chapter discussed school-age children and the capabilities children develop during that time period. This chapter adds information about the changes, both physical and psychosocial, that occur during adolescence. This is important information because it builds a base for care and health teaching for this age group.

Did Raul have some needs that were not met by his clinic visit?

After you've studied this chapter, access the accompanying website. Read the patient scenario and answer the questions to further sharpen your skills, grow more familiar with RN-CLEX types of questions, and reward yourself with how much you have learned.

Adolescence is the period between 13 and 18 to 20 years, a time that serves as a transition between childhood and adulthood. It can be divided into an early period (13 to 14 years), a middle period (15 to 16 years), and a late period (17 to 20 years). During all periods, adolescence is defined not so much by chronologic age as by physiologic, psychological, and sociologic factors. The drastic change in physical appearance and the change in expectations of others (especially parents) that occur during the period may lead to both emotional and physical health problems.

Adolescents invariably feel a sense of pressure throughout this period because they are mature in some respects but still young in others. For example, an adolescent's sexual interests are awakening, yet personal or parental pressures discourage sexual exploration. This duality causes a major dilemma for an adolescent, leading to many of the growth and developmental concerns of the age.

There is such a strong adolescent subculture today parents may feel from the minute their child enters the teenage years that all communication stops. Parents may expect difficulty guiding a child or understanding teenage values, as though entering this period locks an adolescent into a shell or pulls down a curtain between child and parents. This can become a self-fulfilling prophecy, whereby the parents actually cause the communication breakdown. At other times, communication problems can begin when a teenager refuses to respect parents' opinions or stops asking for them. Many of the problems adolescents bring to health care personnel arise from this communication impasse, no matter how it started. They often come to health care facilities with many misconceptions, seeking adult help and guidance. National Health Goals related to adolescence are shown in Box 32.1.

Nursing Process Overview

For Healthy Development of an Adolescent

● *Assessment*

Parents rarely bring adolescents for health maintenance visits, and adolescents generally don't come to health care facilities on their own unless they are ill. Unless adolescents need a physical examination for athletic clearance, therefore, they are usually not seen for health assessments as often as they were when younger. When adolescents are accompanied by their parents at health visits, it is best to obtain a health history separately from parents to promote independence and responsibility for self-care. When performing physical examinations on adolescents, be aware they may be very self-conscious. They also need health assurance and appreciate comments such as "Your hair has a nice, healthy feel," or "This is an accessory nipple. Have you ever wondered about it?" so they can learn more about their rapidly changing bodies (Box 32.2).

● *Nursing Diagnosis*

Frequently used nursing diagnoses related to adolescents and their families are:

BOX 32.1 FOCUS ON . . .

NATIONAL HEALTH GOALS

Health teaching in the adolescent years is important, because healthy habits begun at this time can influence health over a lifetime. For this reason, a number of National Health Goals relate to adolescent health:

- Reduce the number of adolescents who are overweight or obese to a prevalence of no more than 5%, from a baseline of 11%.
- Reduce tobacco use by adolescents to a rate of 16%, from a baseline of 35%.
- Reduce the rate of smokeless tobacco use by adolescents to no more than 1%, from a baseline of 8%.
- Reduce the rate of deaths caused by alcohol-related motor vehicle accidents among people ages 15 to 24 to no more than 18%, from a baseline of 21.5%.
- Reduce the rate of suicide attempts by adolescents to no more than 1%, from a baseline of 2.6%.
- Increase to 35% the proportion of adolescents who exercise regularly, from a baseline of 22% (DHHS, 2000).

Nurses can help the nation achieve these goals by educating adolescents against the use of cigarettes, smokeless tobacco, alcohol, drug abuse, and acts of violence, and by acting as support people for adolescents during times of crisis to help prevent suicide. Areas that could benefit from additional nursing research are identifying effective programs that reduce the use of smokeless tobacco or cigarette smoking, documenting the best actions for nurses to take in emergency rooms when adolescents are admitted after suicide attempts, and constructing rapid surveys to identify adolescents who are abusing drugs.

BOX 32.2 FOCUS ON . . .

DIVERSITY OF CARE

In the United States, as in most developed countries, adolescence covers a long time span. In developing countries, in contrast, adolescence tends to be much shorter because children must take full-time jobs early in life to help support their families. Socioeconomic factors definitely influence the length of adolescence across all cultures. Recognizing that adolescents may have differing responsibilities and life experiences based on cultural expectations can be useful when making an assessment. In a family in which an adolescent is expected to begin working full-time or to marry at an early age, you may need to include factors such as occupational hazards or the effects of job, family, and financial stress on an adolescent. Readiness for childbearing is also important.

These activities fulfill an adolescent's need for satisfying interaction with others and are indications of maturity and willingness to accept adult roles.

Emotional Development

Developmental Task: Identity Versus Role Confusion

According to Erikson (1993), the developmental task in early and mid-adolescence is to form a sense of **identity** or decide who they are and what kind of person they will be. In late adolescence, the task is to form a sense of intimacy or form close relationships with persons of the opposite as well as the same sex. It is the concentration on these two tasks that leads to typical adolescent behavior. The four main areas in which adolescents must make gains to achieve a sense of identity are:

1. Accepting their changed body image
2. Establishing a value system or what kind of person they want to be
3. Making a career decision
4. Becoming emancipated from their parents

If young people do not achieve a sense of identity, they develop a sense of **role confusion** or can have little idea what kind of person they are (Erikson, 1993). This can lead to their having difficulty functioning effectively as adults, because they are unable, for example, to decide what stand to take on a particular issue or how to approach new challenges or situations. Some adolescents may become delinquent or exhibit acting-out (attention-getting) behavior because they believe it is better to have a negative image than to be nobody at all. Those who do not develop a sense of intimacy at the end of adolescence can have difficulty forming long-term relationships.

Body Image. Adolescents who developed a strong sense of industry during their school-age years have learned to solve problems and are best equipped to adjust to their new body image. Nurses who care for adolescents can do much to educate them about their bodies and help them to accept the changes that mark maturity. Some adolescents, for example, are disappointed with their final height; they had hoped to be 6 ft tall and are only 5 ft 6 inches tall. In other instances, they have seen themselves as "ugly ducklings" and dreamt they would emerge as beautiful swans. They are depressed to find, at the end of adolescence, they still look much like ducks.

Adolescents are usually their own worst critics, never pleased with any aspect of their bodies. Those with low self-esteem may need parental or health care provider support to understand that a person's worth is based on more than physical appearance. They may need help to realize the characteristics that make someone creative, compassionate, and fun to be with are the qualities on which lasting relationships are built.

Help parents understand how important it is for adolescents to have immediate successes such as making the high school basketball team or having a date for the senior prom. Parental comments, such as "When you're older, these things won't be so important," are not likely to erase the hurt that comes from being 16 years old and not being

included in such major events. Compassionate understanding ("It's hard to be left out") is a better communication technique.

Self-Esteem. Like body image, self-esteem may undergo major changes during the adolescent years and can be challenged by *all* the changes that occur during adolescence, including:

- Changes in one's body and physiologic functioning
- Changes in feelings and emotional focus
- Changes in social relationships (including relationships with both family and friends)
- Changes in family and school expectations

All of these factors can have an effect on an adolescent's feelings about himself or herself, sometimes resulting in crisis.

In recent years, a number of researchers have looked at the differences in the way boys and girls handle these emotional crises of adolescence. Several researchers have proposed that adolescence is a period of particular crisis for girls who are trying to find a place in a male-dominated society. The sociologist Carol Gilligan and her colleagues interviewed more than 500 girls between the ages of 7 and 16 over a 5-year period and found many girls who, at age 11, were feisty, confident, and eager to speak their minds became, by early adolescence, hesitant to voice their opinions aloud, having pushed their earlier resistance "underground" (Gilligan, 1982). Gilligan tied this change to a growing realization among girls during adolescence that their forthrightness may not be appealing to boys; they begin to self-censor, hoping to become more popular. At the same time, girls are expected to grow up and to value independent and academic (or athletic) success over close relationships, a situation that conflicts with a girl's need to maintain personal connections. This scenario presents a double-edged sword for the developing adolescent whose concern with relationships is not valued by others and who can no longer necessarily rely on her former outspokenness to get across her concerns and opinions.

Although the turmoil of adolescence can be just as confusing to boys as it is to girls, Gilligan hypothesized there may be less pressure on boys, who may have already learned to be competitive, independent, and separated from feelings. Gilligan describes the rearing of boys as including separation from emotions and feelings at an earlier age, whereas girls are encouraged to maintain their concern for people throughout their childhood. This makes girls at risk for more conflicting feelings throughout adolescence.

Parents can help their adolescent girls deal with these conflicts by encouraging them to maintain their honesty and forthrightness. According to Gilligan, however, this option puts adolescents at risk for criticism from other adults. The cost of going underground, by repressing one's views and feelings, may, however, be higher. Long-term psychological problems, notably eating disorders, which by some statistics are said to affect as many as one in five women in the United States, may be one unfortunate result of such repression.

Value System. Adolescents develop values through talking to peers. They also need an attentive adult ear, someone who will listen to their fears, hopes, dreams, and the pressure they feel to be somebody, the pressure of wanting to do something and yet not knowing what or how.

In early adolescence, girls tend to band together with girls and boys with boys. They dress identically with other members of their group: jeans and sweatshirts, special jackets, or whatever the fashion may be. On the surface, this makes adolescents appear to be losing their identities rather than finding them (Fig. 32.3). Adolescents who are different for whatever reason (e.g., overweight or from a different socioeconomic, racial, or cultural background) often are excluded from groups in the same way they were from clubs as 9-year-olds. This behavior may seem immature, but, like banding together, it is a necessary way for adolescents to establish a sense of identity. They know they are like the rest of the group because they dress, talk, and think the same way and go to the same places. They know they are not like the excluded member. Knowing who they are *not* is one step in discovering who they are. Helping adolescents to appreciate that it is not fair to exclude others on the basis of superficial characteristics helps them move more quickly through this stage.

Some parents may be concerned about an early adolescent's lack of interest in the opposite sex. Occasionally, they worry about an intensely close girl–girl or boy–boy relationship. You can assure parents that adolescents must feel secure and pleased with their own sex before they can relate comfortably to the opposite sex.

Career Decisions. Part of the feeling of knowing what kind of person you are is knowing what kind of job you can do. Because of the thousands of opportunities available today, making a career decision becomes more and more difficult.

Many adolescents are encouraged to wait until they have been in college for 2 years before choosing a major. This delay may be an advantage because of the wide range of available options. It delays settling on a concrete goal

until about 20 years of age, however, and therefore puts off a choice that strengthens an adolescent's sense of identity. Some school-age children do poorly in school during preadolescence but, as adolescents, show increased interest in learning as they select a job field and come to see education as relevant to their future.

Emancipation From Parents. Emancipation from parents can become a major issue during the middle and late adolescent years for two reasons. Some parents may not yet be ready for their child to be totally independent, and some adolescents may not yet be sure they want to be on their own. They may fight bitterly for a right—for example, to stay out until midnight or later on a weekend—then never use the privilege once they have gained it. Winning the battle was more important than exercising the newly won right.

In some instances, the closer the tie adolescents feel with their parents, the more severe can be their struggle. Because they love and feel loved, severing bonds is difficult. As long as parents are reasonable in their restrictions, the amount of noise being made may be proof the ties are strong and separation or emancipation is not easy.

Encourage parents to give adolescents more freedom (e.g., allowing them to buy their own clothes, use their own judgment about allotting time for studying, choose their friends, join clubs, or choose after-school activities); at the same time, help parents continue to place some restrictions on adolescent behavior (e.g., "You must drive the car safely or you can't use it," "You must continue to take responsibility for household chores," "We must know where you go after school"). These are not unreasonable rules and actually help adolescents accept the responsibility that must come with independence.

Help parents also make emancipation a gradual reeling-out process. Some parents err on one side or the other, either by neglecting to let out the line at all until adolescents, feeling trapped, have no other choice but to break free and swim away; or letting it all out at once, leaving adolescents to flounder because they cannot yet swim effectively on their own.

In some instances, friction and misunderstandings arise because parents had such traumatic experiences as adolescents themselves that they fear seeing their children reach this stage. Their own experiences may cause them to react so strongly that they are unable to discuss anything with their children. This makes adolescents feel they have offended their parents in some way. They do not understand that the parental attitudes are based not on anything they may have done, but on old, unresolved conflicts being brought to the surface. In other instances, parents may view adolescent growth as threatening. Seeing their adolescent grow up may make them feel old or, if a marriage is not strong, fear that once their child becomes independent they will no longer need to stay together. They may strive to keep their child immature (producing conflict) in an effort to keep these thoughts from entering the corners of their minds.

Both parents and adolescents may need help to understand that emancipation does not mean severance but a change in a relationship. People who are independent of one another can have even better relationships than those who are dependent on one another. This step is actually

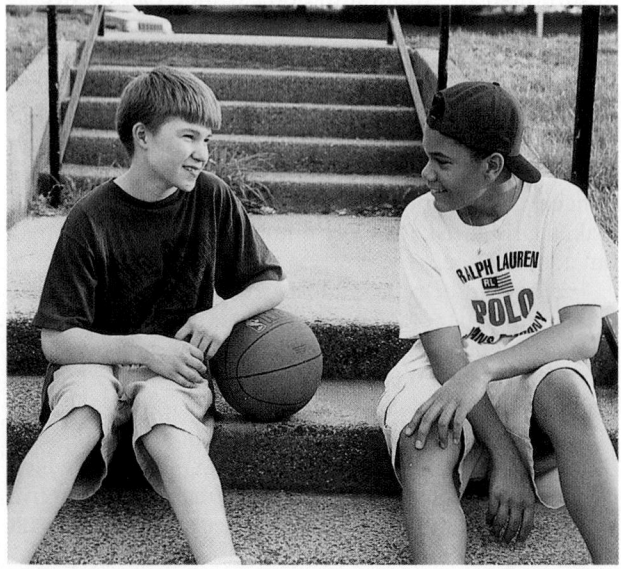

FIGURE 32.3 Adolescents have a need to interact with peers to learn more about themselves and others.

no different from the one children accomplished when they grew from infants to toddlers, when they changed from wanting to be held and rocked to wanting to run. If parents can think of it in this light, they will gain a better perspective and may begin to see they will continue to like their children as independent adults.

By the time children are 18 years of age, they have survived leaving high school. They are in college or have found a beginning job and have begun to manage their own lives, perhaps even their own apartment. They are like swimmers who have discovered the water is not as cold as they thought it would be.

Many 18-year-olds so enjoy their new independence they find it difficult to understand why adulthood is thought to be challenging. A little more maturity will help them realize that initial success as an independent young adult does not necessarily guarantee additional success, that beginning adult life may be far easier than continuing it in the years ahead.

Sense of Intimacy. Once adolescents have achieved a sense of identity in early or mid-adolescence, they are ready to work on a second developmental task, that of achieving a sense of intimacy (Erikson, 1993). The ability to form intimate relationships is strongly correlated with the sense of trust, the first developmental task in infancy. Infants who are unable to form a sense of trust may be unable to relate to others on a deep enough level to form lasting and close relationships as adults. Conversely, adults unable to gain a sense of intimacy may be unable to foster a sense of trust in an infant.

Some adolescents require help from parents or other adults to differentiate between sound relationships and those that are based only on sexual attraction. Never do adolescents need an adult to listen to them more than when they are struggling with the heart-rending feelings of young love or wondering whether a particular love relationship is temporary or lasting. It helps to put this into perspective if parents or health care personnel who counsel adolescents remember that first love is such an intense emotion, it physically hurts.

Some parents may not be able simply to listen without interjecting their own opinions, because they worry that love between adolescents will lead to a sexual relationship. Parents should feel an obligation to inform their children of their feelings about adolescent sexual relationships. They also should be realistically aware some adolescents will not follow their advice. Rates of teenage pregnancy and sexually transmitted diseases, including human immunodeficiency virus (HIV), are high and still rising. If parents suspect their adolescent is sexually active, counsel them to be sure their child is knowledgeable about safer sex practices (see Chapter 4, Box 4.5, for guidelines regarding safer sex; see Chapter 17 for a discussion of adolescent pregnancy).

Some adolescents may believe that intense sexual yearnings or peer pressure can be alleviated only by a sexual act. They can be reassured they are pleasant people to be with because of the many fine qualities they possess and that sexual intercourse can be delayed until two persons have come to know these qualities in each other and have made a mutual commitment based on a deeper level than simply physical passion.

Intimacy involves this deeper level of relationships or developing a sense of compassion or concern for people of both sexes. It means being able to discern when words will hurt, when a companion is unhappy and needs encouragement, or when a friend is floundering and needs support.

In our busy modern society in which adolescents can engage in such a variety of activities, they may need help learning how to project themselves into another person's situation and to ask themselves how the world looks from that position. This ability, *empathy,* is feeling for another or a developed sense of intimacy in its finest form.

Socialization

Early teenagers may feel more self-doubt than self-confidence. They want to look grown up, but they still look like children. The voices of most boys have not yet dependably deepened; this makes them unable to trust their voices to carry the serious tone they wish to convey. Most girls' bodies have not yet fully developed; they may look at themselves in a mirror and compare their profiles with those of girls in popular magazines and feel inadequate.

Both male and female 13-year-olds tend to be loud and boisterous, particularly when peers of the opposite sex whose attention they would like to attract are nearby. They are impulsive and very much like 2-year-old children in that they want what they want immediately, not when it is convenient for others.

Many 13-year-olds fall "in love." At this age, however, they may spend more time longing for someone than they do instituting an in-depth and rewarding relationship. They have too little experience with life, too limited a frame of reference yet to know how to offer a deep commitment to another or accept one from that person.

Fourteen-year-olds are often quieter and more introspective than they were the year before. They are becoming used to their changing bodies, have more confidence in themselves, and feel more self-esteem.

Adolescents watch adults carefully during this period, searching for good role models with whom they can identify. They usually have a hero—a film star, writer, scientist, doctor, or athlete—whom they want to grow up to be like. Fourteen-year-olds often form a friendship with an older adolescent of the same sex, trying to imitate that person in everything from thoughts to clothing. If the older adolescent has dropped out of school or plays a particular sport, the younger person may express a wish to drop out or train for that sport too.

Idolization of famous people or older adolescents fades as adolescents become more interested in forming reciprocal friendships. Attachments to older adolescents are often severed abruptly and painfully as the older teenager makes it clear he or she is more interested in being with people his or her own age. Rejection by an older member of a pair this way forces the younger member to turn to own-age friends and ends the intense hero worship so typical of early adolescence.

Most 15-year-olds fall in love five or six times a year. However, many of these relationships are based on attraction because of physical appearance, not because of inner qualities or characteristics that are necessarily compatible

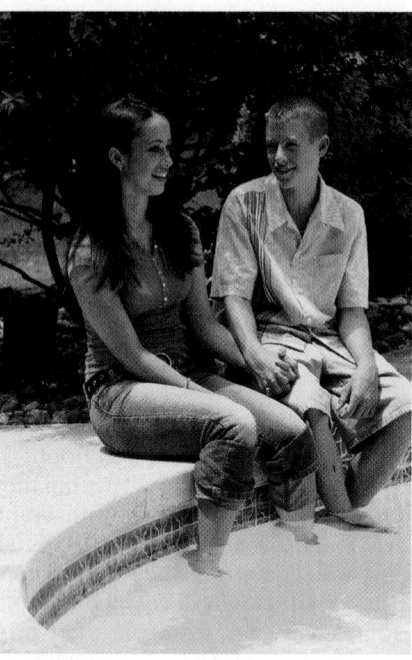

FIGURE 32.4 Although love can be fleeting, adolescents may feel intensely for another.

with their own. Because infatuation is fleeting, it can lead to extremely intense but brief attachments that fade once the two young people discover they really have little in common. Falling in love this often, however, does not mean their feelings are any less strong or they feel any less pain when the relationship ends (Fig. 32.4).

By age 16, boys are becoming sexually mature (although they continue to grow taller until about 18 years of age). Both sexes are better able to trust their bodies than they were the year before. By age 17, they tend to be quieter and thoughtful about interactions. They have left behind the childish behaviors they used in early adolescence—shoving and punching—to get the attention of the opposite sex.

Cognitive Development

The final stage of cognitive development, the stage of **formal operational thought,** begins at age 12 or 13 years and grows in depth over the adolescent years (Piaget, 1969). This step involves the ability to think in abstract terms and use the scientific method to arrive at conclusions. The problems that adolescents are asked to solve in school depend on this type of thought (e.g., a boy rowing upstream at 5 miles per hour against a current of 2 miles per hour will go how far in 1 hour?). Problem solving in any situation depends on the ability to think abstractly and logically.

With the ability to use scientific reasoning, adolescents can plan their future. They can create a hypothesis (What if I go to college? What if I don't go to college?) and think through the probable consequences. Thinking abstractly is what allows adolescents to project themselves into the minds of others and imagine how others view them or their actions (display compassion).

Moral and Spiritual Development

Because adolescents enlarge their thought processes to include formal reasoning, they are able to respond to the question, "Why is it wrong to steal from your neighbor's house?" with "It would hurt my neighbor by requiring him to spend money to replace what I stole," rather than with the immature response of the school-age child, "The police will punish me." Some adolescents, however, may have difficulty envisioning a department store or a large corporation as capable of suffering economic loss from stealing, a concept that may contribute to the frequent practice of petty shoplifting at this age.

Almost all adolescents question the existence of God and any religious practices they have been taught (Kohlberg, 1984). This questioning is a natural part of forming a sense of identity and establishing a value system at a time in life when they draw away from their families.

Checkpoint Question 2

Raul is entering the final stage of cognitive development. This stage is termed:

a. Formal operational thought.
b. Cognitive attainment.
c. Concrete operational thought.
d. Scientific formulating.

PLANNING AND IMPLEMENTATION FOR HEALTH PROMOTION OF AN ADOLESCENT AND FAMILY

Promoting Adolescent Safety

Accidents, most commonly those involving motor vehicles, are the leading cause of death among adolescents. Although teenagers are at the peak of physical and sensorimotor functioning, their need to rebel against authority or to gain attention leads them to take foolish chances while driving, such as speeding or driving while intoxicated.

In the interest of an adolescent's safety and that of others, parents need to have the courage to insist on emotional maturity rather than age as the qualification for obtaining a driver's license. Encourage adolescents to take driver education courses to learn not only the techniques of driving but also a sense of responsibility toward others. The use of seat belts should be mandatory. Some adolescents dismiss seat belts as childish, and they need convincing that it is only sensible to use every safety precaution available when in a motor vehicle.

Equally dangerous for adolescents are motorcycles, motorbikes, and motor scooters, which are appealing because of their low cost and convenience in parking. Both drivers and riders should wear safety helmets to prevent head injury; long pants to prevent leg burns from exhaust pipes; and full body covering to prevent abrasions in case of an accident. Advise adolescents who choose these forms of transportation to be as familiar with safety rules as automobile drivers. They need to wait to drive motorcycles or scooters until they are emotionally mature enough to use sound driving judgment.

Drowning is another chief accident of adolescence, even though it is largely preventable. Teaching all children to swim is not the only preventive measure, because some drownings occur when good swimmers go beyond their capabilities on dares or in hopes of impressing friends. Teaching water safety, such as not swimming alone or when tired, is as important as teaching the mechanics of swimming.

Other common causes of death in adolescents are homicide and suicide, related to the easy accessibility of guns to teenagers. Gang violence and the desire to protect themselves from this can add to this problem. Accidental gunshot injuries increase in early adolescence, often for the same reason that drowning increases: youngsters want to impress friends. Some teenagers play gunshot Russian roulette to prove to friends they are courageous. It's important that both water and firearm safety be taught creatively to adolescents by encouraging problem solving rather than lecturing, because they tend to rebel against such lectures or claim that they have heard it all before.

Athletic injuries tend to increase in number during adolescence because of the vigorous level of competition that occurs. In early adolescence, overuse injuries result from poor conditioning. Types of athletic injuries are discussed in Chapter 51. Health teaching measures to prevent accidents and athletic injuries are summarized in Box 32.3.

Promoting Nutritional Health for an Adolescent

Adolescents are experiencing so much growth they may always feel hungry (Fig. 32.5). If adolescents' eating habits are unsupervised, they tend to eat faddish or quick snack foods rather than more nutritionally sound ones because of both hunger and peer pressure. Some adolescents turn away from the five pyramid food groups to eat such great quantities of sweets, soft drinks, or empty-calorie snacks they are left poorly nourished despite their large intake. One form of rebellion is to refuse to eat foods parents stress are good for them. Parents who stock their kitchens with more nutritious foods, always keeping plenty of milk and healthy snacks such as fruit and vegetables on hand, and who are willing to meet their adolescents halfway in terms of food preferences (e.g., serving pizza once a week) can be more certain their child is eating nutritious foods during the day. Giving an adolescent some responsibility for food planning or meals (e.g., making dinner every Wednesday night) can teach some important lessons about nutrition without conflict.

Adolescents who are slightly obese because of prepubertal changes may begin low-calorie or starvation diets to lose excess weight. Some develop eating disorders such as bulimia or anorexia nervosa (see Chapter 54). A weight-loss diet may be appropriate during adolescence, but it must be supervised to ensure that an adolescent consumes sufficient calories and nutrients for growth. For example, many adolescents omit breads and cereals entirely to lose weight rather than just reducing the amounts they con-

sume. Diets such as these may be deficient in thiamine and riboflavin.

BOX 32.3 FOCUS ON . . .

FAMILY TEACHING

Measures to Prevent Accidents in Adolescents

Q. Raul's mother tells you, "My son doesn't always use mature judgment. How can I keep him safe from accidents?"

A. Teach the following points:

Accident	Health Teaching Measure
Motor vehicle	Use a seat belt whether as a driver or passenger.
	Do not drink alcohol while driving, and refuse to ride with anyone who has been drinking.
	Wear helmet and long trousers as driver or passenger on a motorcycle.
	Accepting dares has no place in safe driving.
	Take a driver education course to learn safe driving habits for both two-wheel and four-wheel vehicles.
Firearms	Always consider all guns loaded and potentially lethal.
	Learn safe gun handling before attempting to clean a gun or hunt.
Drowning	Learn how to swim. Follow safe water rules, such as never swimming alone, no diving into shallow end of swimming pools, no hyperventilating before swimming under water, no swimming beyond own limit.
	Taking dares has no place in water safety.
Sports	Use protective equipment, such as face masks for hockey, pads for football.
	Do not attempt participation beyond physical limits.
	Careful preparation for sports through training is essential to safety.
	Recognize and set own limit for sports participation.

Recommended Dietary Reference Intakes

An adolescent needs an increased number of calories to support the rapid body growth that occurs. As shown in Appendix E, males grow more than females during this period. One of the most important things adolescents can learn is that just filling their stomachs will not provide adequate nutrition. Foods that supply the necessary carbohydrates, vitamins, protein, and minerals are essential.

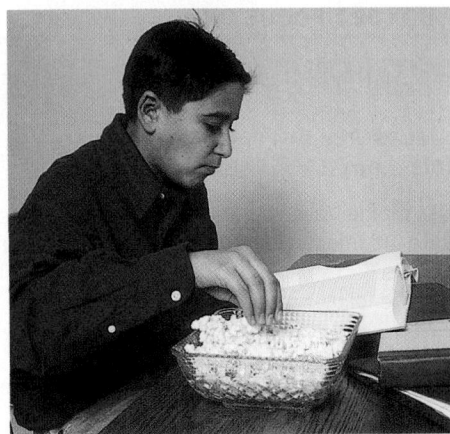

FIGURE 32.5 Adolescents experience rapid physical growth, so typically, they are always hungry. (© Billy Barnes/Stock Boston.)

The nutrients that are most apt to be deficient in both male and female adolescent diets are iron, calcium, and zinc. Large amounts of iron are necessary to meet expanding blood volume requirements. Females require a high iron intake not only because of increasing blood volume but also because iron begins to be lost with menstruation. Girls with a heavy menstrual flow (menorrhagia) may need to take an additional iron supplement to prevent iron-deficiency anemia (see Chapter 44). Increased calcium is necessary for rapid skeletal growth as well as to "stockpile" calcium to prevent osteoporosis later in life (Dudek, 2005). Zinc is necessary for sexual maturation and final body growth. Good sources of iron are meat and green vegetables; calcium is abundant in milk and milk products; meat and milk are also high in zinc.

Promoting Nutritional Health With a Varied Diet

Vegetarian Diets. Because vegetables generally contain fewer calories than meat, adolescents need to consume large amounts of them to achieve an adequate caloric intake with a vegetarian diet. Textured vegetable protein can be purchased and added to meals to increase the amount of protein supplied and help meet adolescent growth needs. Some adolescents may find it difficult to follow a vegetarian diet because it makes them different from their peers and limits the foods they can eat at parties or at school, such as pizza, meat tortillas, or hot dogs. Whether to continue to follow this type of diet is a decision an adolescent must make as part of achieving a sense of identity. Well-balanced vegetarian diets can supply enough energy for an active athlete (Barr & Rideout, 2004). Be certain all adolescent vegetarians are following a diet and not only eating fruits and vegetables as a way to lose weight (Krepcio et al., 2003).

Glycogen Loading. Athletes need more carbohydrate or energy than do people who do not engage in strenuous activity, and the source of carbohydrate that best sustains athletes comes from the breakdown of glycogen because this supplies a slow steady release of glucose. **Glycogen loading** is a procedure used to ensure there is adequate glycogen to sustain energy through an athletic event. Several days before a sports event, athletes lower their carbohydrate intake and exercise heavily to deplete muscle glycogen stores. They then switch to a diet high in carbohydrate. With the renewed carbohydrate intake, muscle glycogen is stored at approximately twice the usual level, ready to supply twice the glucose for sustained energy. The effects of frequent glycogen loading are unknown, however, so the practice is not recommended for adolescents. As a rule, the goals of nutrition that are best for everyone, such as eating a well-balanced diet, are also the best rules for athletes, rather than diets that interfere with carbohydrate, fluid, or fat intake.

Promoting Development of an Adolescent in Daily Activities

Maintaining adequate nutrition to support rapid adolescent growth is essential to continued healthy development, as discussed above. Adequate sleep, hygiene, and exercise are also important and should become an adolescent's responsibility rather than the parents'. Parents can, however, encourage adolescents to engage in healthy patterns of living—primarily through role modeling.

Dress and Hygiene

Adolescents are capable of total self-care and, because of their body awareness, may even be overly conscientious about personal hygiene and appearance. They often wash their hair every day, but then grow dissatisfied because their hair has lost so much natural oil it is dull and stringy. Both sexes try many types of shampoo, deodorant, breath fresheners, and toothpaste. They may take seriously (without admitting it) the content of ads showing toothpastes or deodorants helping win an attractive person or gaining instant success. Remember this when caring for hospitalized adolescents. Providing time for self-care, such as shampooing hair, is important to include in an adolescent's nursing care plan.

Adolescents are acutely aware of what their peers are wearing. When adolescents cannot trust or are disappointed in their bodies, it is very reassuring to be dressed exactly like everyone else. When they first begin to work, many adolescents spend their first paychecks entirely on clothing. This seems inappropriate to many parents; they want their child to learn to spend money on more lasting items or to show an interest in saving. Adolescents may have to mature fully, however, before they discover their real person shows through their clothing.

Remembering how important clothing is for adolescents also helps you plan care for them during a hospitalization. Most teenagers seem to improve markedly when allowed to wear their own clothing rather than a hospital gown.

Care of Teeth

Adolescents are generally very conscientious about toothbrushing because of a fear of developing bad breath. They should continue to use a fluoride paste rather than a brand

of having one's needs met. Loss of a parent, loss of a girl-friend or boyfriend, loss of a community, and loss of self-esteem are all significant and can trigger a suicide. Because some adolescents may be unable to believe that a parent was at fault in the case of divorce or that the death of a parent could not have been prevented, they may believe, in-stead, they somehow caused the parent to leave or to die. The loss of a girlfriend or boyfriend is particularly signifi-cant because it involves two types of loss: friendship and self-esteem. Rejection from a peer group, sports team, or school club may cause a similar loss of self-esteem.

Assessment

Adolescents need to have thorough physical examinations at health maintenance visits to assure them they are in good physical health. Assess for signs of depression such as anorexia, insomnia, excessive fatigue, or weight loss. In younger adolescents, depression may be manifested by be-havior problems such as disobedience, temper tantrums, truancy, and running away from home. Self-destructive behavior or accident proneness may be noted. Difficulties in school; acting out with chemicals, alcohol, or sexual promiscuity; or trouble with legal authorities may be fur-ther clues. Occasionally, depressed adolescents find it so hard to be alone they seek constant activity as a means of escape. In contrast, others may withdraw from contact with other persons and become completely isolated. Either behavior may be detected through assessment of activity and interaction levels.

Adolescents who attempt suicide fall into no one cate-gory, although many tend to be loners or to have difficulty expressing their feelings to others and, therefore, do not receive emotional support from friends. Others are "per-fect" students. The stress of trying to achieve continually at this level, however, is the trigger that provokes suicide. Gay and lesbian youths appear to have higher levels of suicide than others. Assess for these lifestyles as well.

If another member of a family or a close friend has com-mitted suicide, the chance that an adolescent will do so is greater than usual, as adolescents then see suicide as a method of coping and use it. The anniversary of a family member's suicide is an emotional time and may be espe-cially difficult for an adolescent; wishing to join the dead family member appears attractive. When one adolescent in a high school commits suicide, there is a good chance another will take similar action soon afterward. Adolescent suicide rates may actually reach epidemic proportions after a popular student's suicide. Students who have Internet contacts may arrange a group suicide as a method of mak-ing a statement or gaining support for the act.

Because suicide usually reflects a problem in family in-teraction, family assessment is helpful. A thorough family history may reveal conflict with one or both parents. Many adolescents express a desire to get even with someone. "They'll be sorry when I'm dead" is a frequent comment. School friends may often be aware an adolescent is con-templating suicide before the parents. Caution parents not to discount reports from their child's friends who tell them they are concerned about their child. Close to the chosen time of suicide, some adolescents may demon-strate characteristic behaviors that show they are making

preparations to end their life. Teach family and friends the typical danger signs (Box 32.13).

After a suicide attempt, ask enough questions on a health history so you know whether an adolescent made a detailed suicide plan. For example, a young person who took four aspirins and left the empty aspirin container con-spicuously on the kitchen counter just before the mother was due to arrive home from work is more likely to be only crying for help; the one who took 100 aspirins and hid the container under the bed just after the mother left for 8 hours of work is making a serious attempt. You may be the first person in a health care facility to realize that an adolescent talking about suicide is not "just talking" (it is a fallacy that people who talk about suicide do not attempt it) but has a definite, well-thought-out plan to accomplish it. An adolescent who has been admitted to a hospital unit after a serious suicide attempt may formulate a new plan that will be successful the next time unless some ac-tion is taken and the adolescent's life can be changed in some way.

BOX 32.13 FOCUS ON . . .

FAMILY TEACHING

Suicide Warning Signs

Q. Raul's father says to you, "Our neighbor's son recently committed suicide. What are warning signs of this to look for in our son?"

A. The following are commonly seen clues:

- Giving away prized possessions
- Organ donation questions, such as "How do you leave your body to a medical school?"
- Sudden, unexplained elevation of mood. Mood elevation may indicate that the individual has reached a decision about the suicide and feels relief.
- Accident proneness, carelessness, and death wishes
- A statement such as, "This is the last time you will see me."
- Decrease in verbal communication
- Withdrawal from peer activities or previously enjoyed events
- Previous attempt (80% of all completed suicides have been preceded by a failed attempt)
- Preference for art, music, and literature with themes of death
- Recent increase in interpersonal conflict with significant others
- Running away from home
- Recent experience of a friend or famous person committing suicide
- Inquiring about the hereafter
- Asking for information (supposedly for a friend) about suicide prevention and intervention
- Almost any sustained deviation from the normal pattern of behavior

NURSING DIAGNOSES AND RELATED INTERVENTIONS

---•---

Nursing Diagnosis: Risk for violence, self-directed, related to symptoms of depression or expressed desire to hurt oneself

Outcome Evaluation: Client expresses feelings of depression to health care providers or other adults; states she will contact support person should the desire to commit suicide become overwhelming.

Crisis intervention for adolescents who are contemplating suicide includes trying to alleviate their pain and depression and counseling them in an effort to help them change their perspective on the value of life. Be aware that establishing expected outcomes with adolescents who are contemplating suicide or who have made an attempt will be difficult because they are often too depressed to come up with an alternative solution to their problems (their goal is to kill themselves, not solve problems).

Try to find out the things in the child's life that are still viewed as important; build a plan that will help him or her see life is worth living enough to work through problems. Show them no one can change everything, but everyone can make one or two changes that can make a difference. After these small changes are made, a domino effect can be created to change more and more of one's circumstances.

Because adolescents resort to suicide as a method of solving problems, helping them in this area is a prime intervention strategy. Ask them "what would happen if" questions such as "Suppose you did fail a course; what would happen?" "Are there ways you can reverse the finality of the problem?" (Talk to a teacher about make-up assignments? Ask a friend for help in reviewing material? Buy a review book to help in studying?) Do not count on everyone being willing to help. A high school teacher may feel that to be asked to do outside tutoring is an imposition, and for you to advise adolescents to seek this kind of help will only add to their depression if the teacher refuses. You may have to make these contacts yourself (with an adolescent's permission) because, generally, persons who are depressed have difficulty initiating this type of action because they do not believe anyone cares enough about them to help.

A general measure is to help adolescents speak honestly about thoughts of suicide and the problems that have led them to think that death is a solution. Most problems begin to seem manageable if they can be put into words in this way. It is important not to underestimate an adolescent's determination to end his or her life. In most instances, an adolescent needs referral to a consultant well versed in suicide prevention to improve self-image and offer alternative solutions to problems.

For an adolescent's safety, a period of observation in a hospital setting is desirable after a suicide attempt to prevent the individual from inflicting personal injury and to allow him or her to be evaluated in a neutral setting, away from the stress that precipitated the attempt. This can take place in an adolescent service rather than a psychiatric service.

Antidepressant medicine alone, a therapy used with depressed adults, may be of little value in treating depressed adolescents. Some antidepressants have been associated with elevating the mood of depressed children enough to allow them to formulate a plan and commit suicide after taking them (Hampton, 2004).

Continuing evaluation by both history taking and physical examination is necessary, because the young person who has attempted suicide may attempt it again if support people and better problem-solving ability are not available at another time.

What if... Raul seems unusually happy at a clinic visit, when usually he is sad? Would you worry that this change in mood is a warning sign that he might be contemplating suicide?

Concerns Regarding Runaways

A *runaway* is commonly defined as an adolescent between the ages of 10 and 17 years who has been absent from home at least overnight without permission of a parent or guardian. The frequency of running away for adolescents may be as high as one in eight. Fortunately, most do not go far or stay away long (under 1 week); about 1 in 20 adolescent runaways stays away as long as 1 year; some never return home. Runaway adolescents are most likely to be from low- or high-income families. Unemployment, alcoholism, sexual abuse, attempted suicide, and poverty are frequent characteristics. They are slightly more likely to be male than female.

Assessment

Running away is usually preceded by an argument with parents that is often the last straw after a number of long-term disagreements. Other reasons may be personal concerns such as loneliness, pregnancy, and problems with friends, school, or the police. Incest can also be a precipitating cause, as can other parental abuse. A school history often reveals frequent truancy, failing grades, possible drug use, and runaway behavior by friends. It is a sad fact that some adolescents are "throwaways" or cannot remain at home because they have been rejected by their families.

Common health reasons for which runaway adolescents are seen at health care facilities are sexually transmitted diseases, including HIV/AIDS, rape, pregnancy, substance abuse, hepatitis, and vaginitis. They also have a high incidence of suicide attempts. When caring for adolescents with these concerns, be certain to secure a thorough history so the fact they are no longer living at home will not be missed. Be sure to be nonjudgmental in questioning. Revealing you are shocked by a report an adolescent has been sleeping on a park bench for 2 months, has been robbed, or steals to obtain money could prevent you from learning even greater concerns, such as having a sexually transmitted disease, being pregnant, or using drugs. Ask if the adolescent wants to return home. Even though a homeless state is high stress, and many adolescent runaways want to take the first step back toward their parents, they may not know how to begin the process (Rew, 2003).

NURSING DIAGNOSES AND RELATED INTERVENTIONS

Nursing Diagnosis: Ineffective individual coping related to stress of adolescent period and inadequate family resources

Outcome Evaluation: Adolescent states stress level at home is manageable; is able to describe how he can use family and community resources to help solve problems and aid in a crisis.

Adolescents may run away because they cannot solve a problem in any other way; therefore, setting goals with them may be difficult. A short-term goal to stay home through a holiday rather than a long-term one of finishing high school may be all you can achieve.

Because adolescent runaways lack references for jobs and do not necessarily qualify for public assistance programs, they generally have no secure source of income. Both males and females may resort to prostitution to support themselves, or they may resort to stealing. Police consider them to be juvenile delinquents and are required to return them to their homes if discovered. If they leave home again, they may be sentenced to an institution for care; unfortunately, these facilities are often crowded and may not have the means to meet adolescent needs other than food and clothing.

Try to imagine yourself in adolescent runaways' circumstances to determine whether your health instructions are sensible for their lifestyle. Giving them instructions to eat a high-protein diet or iron-rich foods, for example, may be ludicrous. If they do not have a source of running water, soaking a lesion or changing a dressing may be difficult. They may have no way to pay for health care, making it impossible to obtain a prescription medication, so giving them a sample of a drug is often more practical. If they don't have a means of transportation, they may be unable to return to the health care fa-

cility for frequent follow-up visits. Try to meet as many of the runaway's needs as possible, therefore, at one visit. Remember that many runaways have associated school failure so may be poor readers; discuss the information with them when giving them a pamphlet.

Be certain runaway adolescents are familiar with the national Youth Crisis Hotline, which they can telephone day or night when they want to return home. The phone number is 1-800-448-4663 (1-800-HIT HOME). Remember also they are runaways because, for some reason, their home was intolerable. Although they agree to return home, they may not remain there unless circumstances can be changed.

Nursing Diagnosis: Impaired parenting related to inability of family to adjust to adolescent needs

Outcome Evaluation: Parents list definite changes they have made in family life to better accommodate an adolescent, such as providing increased privacy or using "contracting" with adolescent.

In some instances, it is impossible for a family to reestablish itself after a child has run away because the family is dysfunctional (incest or abuse has occurred). In other instances, family life can be modified to welcome the runaway adolescent back home.

So that parents and an adolescent can learn to communicate better, it is helpful to urge them to establish ground rules for communication (shouting or threats are not allowed; no subject is too difficult to be discussed calmly; no emotion or feeling is to be called "foolish"). Once ground rules are laid, parents and the adolescent should meet to discuss how difficult it is to be an adolescent and how equally difficult it is to be the parent of an adolescent; in the past, they became so engaged in arguing that they did not appreciate the other side of the controversy.

Helping parents and adolescents establish a contract for behavior can be effective (for the right to have her own private room, an adolescent can't do drugs; for the right to stay overnight at a friend's house on Friday, she must eat with the family all other nights, for example). Contracting is effective with adolescents, but it does carry the responsibility for parents to be certain they are abiding by their half of the contract (not invading the private room) and of being prepared to enforce the contract. Some families benefit by calling on a mediator (a relative, a close friend, a minister or rabbi) to listen to both sides of an issue and make a ruling.

What if... after a fair trial of trying to make adjustments, an adolescent's parents are still unable to maintain a functional home life for him? What other arrangements would you help them make for safe care of their adolescent?

Unique Concerns of the Family With a Physically Challenged or Chronically Ill Adolescent

Achieving a sense of identity may be difficult for adolescents who have spent much of their life with an illness or other challenge. It is vital, however, for such individuals to learn to look past their particular condition to their real selves. For example, a 16-year-old girl in a wheelchair must learn to perceive herself as a teenager who is normal intellectually, is a good conversationalist, has a good sense of humor, enjoys watching football, and only incidentally uses a wheelchair to ambulate.

Some of the biggest problems of chronically ill adolescents are likely to be difficulties in being as independent as they would like to be, achieving in school, and establishing intimate relationships. Those who cannot learn to drive when their friends are learning to do so, who are not invited to dances and parties, or who are too hesitant to ask someone to go with them, may feel acute losses of self-esteem. Moreover, the loss of many hours of school due to illness or frequent hospitalization may result in the inability to pursue a desired career, at least without a delay.

Adolescence may be the first time these children realize that certain occupations or opportunities, such as a military career, may be closed to them. As they prepare to leave the security of a familiar school system, it may be the first time they examine just how they will be able to function on their own. Some may come to realize they will never be able to do so with complete independence.

Chronic hospitalization or the realization they will never be free of symptoms can cause depression in adolescents, placing them at high risk for substance abuse or suicide. Helping these adolescents realize that even completely well people must compromise life decisions for other reasons (e.g., lack of money, lack of ability or qualifications, extra personal responsibilities) helps them feel they are not so different from others. This type of guidance can be time-consuming, but sometimes the fact that an adult was willing to make this time commitment with them is enough to give these adolescents the self-esteem they need to alter aspirations and plans and find a future role consistent with their capabilities. Nursing actions that encourage a sense of identity in an adolescent with a long-term illness or who is physically challenged are summarized in Table 32.5.

TABLE 32.5

Nursing Actions That Encourage a Sense of Identity in the Physically Challenged or Chronically Ill Adolescent

Category	Actions
Nutrition	If adolescent is on special diet, discuss role of his or her food preferences with dietitian (hot dogs, pizza, etc.).
	Respect food preferences.
Dressing change	Allow adolescent to order supplies.
	Ask for suggestions as to final appearance of dressing.
	If soaks are included, have adolescent time the treatment.
	Allow adolescent to choose time for dressing change.
Medicine	Offering the adolescent a choice of site for injection or intravenous insertion encourages a sense of control.
	Teach name, action, and possible side effects of medicine.
Rest	Contract with adolescent for time and length of rest periods.
Hygiene	Respect modesty of the adolescent as being at adult level.
	Contract with adolescent for extent of self-care (will give own bath and make bed, not medicate self).
Pain	Encourage adolescent to express pain; teach distraction technique for sharp pain, such as deep breathing, counting backward from 100.
	Encourage adolescent to ask for analgesics as needed.
Stimulation	Provide tapes of favorite music with earphones.
	Provide a radio for adolescent to listen to talk show to foster active involvement.
	Encourage school work, crossword puzzles (you may need to help adolescents divide school assignments so they do not become overly fatigued and frustrated).
	Provide cards for games to increase socialization (make or have the adolescent make a card deck from pieces of paper if one is not available).
	Encourage adolescents to network with one another.
	Encourage adolescents to keep in contact with friends through telephoning, e-mail, or writing notes.

Nutrition and the Chronically Ill Adolescent

Adolescents who are not fully mobile must be aware of their total calorie intake, or as growth needs decline at the end of adolescence they can become obese. They should also be knowledgeable about good nutrition, so they can participate in meal planning, an action that helps them feel a sense of control over this area of their life. Assess how often they have a chance to eat at fast-food restaurants; although this is not a source of excellent nutrition, eating there occasionally provides an important social experience and a chance to be like their peers.

Key Points

The major milestones of development in the adolescent period are the onset of puberty and the cessation of body growth. Between these milestones, physical growth is rapid, although the development of adult coordination and thought processes is slow.

The development of secondary sex characteristics is completed during adolescence. These are rated according to Tanner stages.

The developmental task of an adolescent according to Erikson is to establish independence from parents by gaining a sense of identity versus role confusion. Adolescents, therefore, usually respond best to health care personnel who respect their attempts at independence and allow them as many choices as possible in care.

Adolescents reach a point of cognitive development termed *formal operational thought*. With this gained, they are able to think in abstract terms and use the scientific method to arrive at conclusions.

Adolescents need to consume adequate calories and especially protein, iron, calcium, and zinc to meet their increased growth needs.

To appear older than they are, some adolescents present an assured, "I know that" attitude. To be effective, health teaching may have to be introduced with "I know you know this, so I'll just review it" approach that allows an adolescent to maintain a mature front, while gaining additional information.

Being an adolescent is difficult in today's world. Be aware that, to reduce stress, some adolescents begin to use substances of abuse. Asking about an adolescent's drug experiences, if any, during a health assessment is not intruding on privacy; it is conducting safe health interviewing.

Promoting adolescent safety is an important nursing role. Motor vehicle accidents, homicide, and suicide are leading causes of death in this age group.

Common health problems in an adolescent are sometimes minor and include poor posture, fatigue, or acne; they can also be serious, such as beginning

hypertension, substance abuse, and suicide. Identifying these problems and referring an adolescent for help are important nursing actions.

Critical Thinking Exercises

1. Raul is the 15-year-old boy you met at the beginning of the chapter. His parents tell you he was depressed after the loss of a girlfriend but now is suddenly happy. He has been collecting baseball cards since he was 8. Recently, he gave his collection away to a neighborhood boy because "I won't need them where I'm going." Why might you be concerned about him? What additional questions might you ask him? If you learned he is about to leave to be an exchange student in England, how would this affect your assessment of the situation?

2. Suppose Raul tells you during history taking he does not smoke, but you smell cigarette smoke on his clothing. Although he says he doesn't use drugs, a number of blue-and-white capsules fall out of his shirt pocket when he unbuttons his shirt. What questions would you ask to determine if he is smoking cigarettes or using drugs? Describe your next action if he does admit he is not only heavily into drugs but does not intend to stop using them.

3. A shy, quiet, 14-year-old girl you care for in a hospital setting tells you she is concerned because she has not menstruated yet. This is making her feel "left out" at school. How would you counsel her? What if she were 16 and had the same concern?

4. Examine the National Health Goals related to growth and development of adolescents. Most government-sponsored money for nursing research is allotted based on these goals. What would be a possible research topic to explore pertinent to these goals that would be applicable to Raul's family and also advance evidence-based practice?

References

American Academy of Pediatrics. (2005). *Recommendations for preventive pediatric health care.* Washington, DC: AAP

American Academy of Pediatrics, Committee on Sports Medicine and Fitness. (2005). Use of performance-enhancing substances. *Pediatrics, 115*(4), 1003–1016.

Barr, S. I., & Rideout, C. A. (2004). Nutritional considerations for vegetarian athletes. *Nutrition, 20*(7/8), 696–703.

Berger, K. S. (2004). *The developing person through the life span* (6th ed.). New York: Worth Publishing.

Bonifazi, W. L. (2003). Quest for big muscles yields big problems. *Nursing Spectrum, 16*(19), 32–33.

Boyle, J., & Cropley, M. (2004). Children's sleep: problems and solutions. *Journal of Family Health Care, 14*(3), 61–63.

Campo, S., Poulos, G., & Sipple, J. W. (2005). Prevalence and profiling: hazing among college students and points of intervention. *American Journal of Health Behaviors, 29*(2), 137–149.

Comer, V. G., & Annitto, W. J. (2004). Buprenorphine: a safe method for detoxifying pregnant heroin addicts and their unborn. *American Journal on Addictions, 13*(3), 317–318.

Copperman, N., & Jacobson, M. S. (2003). Medical nutrition therapy of overweight adolescents. *Adolescent Medicine: State of the Art Reviews, 14*(1), 11-21.

Dent, C. W., Grube, J. W., & Biglan, A. (2005). Community-level alcohol availability and enforcement of possession laws as predictors of youth drinking. *Preventive Medicine, 40*(3), 355-362.

Department of Health and Human Services. (2000). *Healthy people 2010.* Washington, DC: DHHS.

Dudek, S. G. (2005). *Nutrition essentials for nursing practice.* Philadelphia: Lippincott Williams & Wilkins.

Erikson, E. H. (1993). *Childhood and society.* New York: W. W. Norton.

Fernandez, H. J., at al. (2003). Evaluation of what parents know about their children's drug use and how they perceive the most common family risk factors. *Journal of Drug Education, 33*(3), 337-353.

Ford, V. E. (2003). Coming out as lesbian or gay: a potential precipitant of crisis in adolescence. *Journal of Human Behavior in the Social Environment, 8*(2/3), 93-110.

Gilligan, C., et al. (1982). *In a different voice: psychological theory and women's development.* Cambridge, MA: Harvard University Press.

Hampton, T. (2004). Suicide caution stamped on antidepressants. *JAMA: Journal of the American Medical Association, 291*(17), 2060-2061.

Irwin, C. E, Jr. (2004). Tobacco use during adolescence and young adulthood: the battle is not over. *Journal of Adolescent Health, 35*(3), 169-171.

Johnson, M., Maas, M., & Moorhead, S. (2000). *Nursing outcomes classification* (2nd ed.). St. Louis: Mosby.

Karch, A. M. (2004). *Lippincott's nursing drug guide.* Philadelphia: Lippincott Williams & Wilkins.

Kohlberg, L. (1984). *The psychology of moral development.* New York: Harper & Row.

Krepcio, D., et al. (2003). The vegetarian teen. *Nursing Spectrum (West), 4*(8), 20-24.

Laskowski, C. (2003). Theoretical and clinical perspectives of client stalking behavior. *Clinical Nurse Specialist, 17*(6), 298-304.

Lovato, C., et al. (2005). Impact of tobacco advertising and promotion on increasing adolescent smoking behaviours. *The Cochrane Library (Oxford) (4)* (CD003439).

Lynskey, M. T. (2003). Screening for inhalant abuse in children and adolescents. *American Family Physician, 68*(5), 811-812.

McCloskey, J., & Bulechek, G. (2000). *Nursing interventions classification* (3rd ed.). St. Louis: Mosby.

Murphy-Hoefer, R., et al. (2005). A review of interventions to reduce tobacco use in colleges and universities. *American Journal of Preventive Medicine, 28*(2), 188-200.

National Center for Health Statistics. (2005). *Trends in the health of Americans.* Hyattsville, MD: NCHS.

Patel, M. M., et al. (2004). Shedding new light on the "safe" club drug: methylenedioxymethamphetamine (Ecstasy)-related fatalities. *Academic Emergency Medicine, 11*(2), 208-210.

Piaget, J. (1969). *The theory of stages in cognitive development.* New York: McGraw-Hill.

Rew, L. (2003). A theory of taking care of oneself grounded in experiences of homeless youth. *Nursing Research, 52*(4), 234-241.

Schiffman, R. F. (2004). Drug & substance use in adolescents. *MCN: The American Journal of Maternal/Child Nursing, 29*(1), 21-29.

Shaffer, D. (2005). Depressive disorders and suicide in children and adolescents. In: B. J. Sadock & V. A. Sadock (Eds.), *Kaplan and Sadock's comprehensive textbook of psychiatry* (8th ed.). Philadelphia: Lippincott Williams & Wilkins.

Shalita, A. R., & Terezakis, N. (2004). Achieving optimal results with today's acne treatment options. *Patient Care for the Nurse Practitioner, 1*(1), 12-14.

Simkin, D. R. (2005). Adolescent substance abuse. In: B. J. Sadock & V. A. Sadock (Eds.), *Kaplan and Sadock's comprehensive textbook of psychiatry* (8th ed.). Philadelphia: Lippincott Williams & Wilkins.

Tanner, J. M. (1962). *Growth at adolescence* (2nd ed.). Oxford: Blackwell.

A B C X Y Z Suggested Readings

Brajac, I., et al. (2004). Acne vulgaris: myths and misconceptions among patients and family physicians. *Patient Education and Counseling, 54*(1), 21-25.

Brewster, M. P. (2003). Power and control dynamics in prestalking and stalking situations. *Journal of Family Violence, 18*(4), 207-217.

Broderick, M. (2003). Spotting drug use. *RN, 66*(9), 48-53.

Ozer, E. M., et al. (2005). Increasing the screening and counseling of adolescents for risky health behaviors: a primary care intervention. *Pediatrics, 115*(4), 960-968.

Petrie, H. J., Stover, E. A., & Horswill, C. A. (2004). Nutritional concerns for the child and adolescent competitor. *Nutrition, 20*(7/8), 620-631.

Santana, Y. et al. (2003). Young adolescents, tobacco advertising, and smoking. *Journal of Drug Education, 33*(4), 427-444.

Schettler, A. E., & Gustafson, E. M. (2004). Osteoporosis prevention starts in adolescence. *Journal of the American Academy of Nurse Practitioners, 16*(7), 274-282.

Shenassa, E. D., et al. (2004). Safer storage of firearms at home and risk of suicide: a study of protective factors in a nationally representative sample. *Journal of Epidemiology and Community Health, 58*(10), 841-848.

Smith, J., & McSherry, W. (2004). Spirituality and child development: a concept analysis. *Journal of Advanced Nursing, 45*(3), 307-315.

Vigil, G. J., & Clements, P. T. (2003). Child and adolescent homicide survivors: complicated grief and altered worldviews. *Journal of Psychosocial Nursing and Mental Health Services, 41*(1), 30-41.

CHAPTER 33

Child Health Assessment

Key Terms

antitoxins
audiogram
auscultation
bruit
chief concern
conjunctivitis
deep tendon
    reflexes
diaphragmatic
    excursion
epispadias
esotropia
exotropia
gamma
    globulin
geographic
    tongue
hordeolum
hydrocele
hypospadias
inspection
intelligence

intercostal
    spaces
kwashiorkor
palpation
percussion
physiologic
    splitting
point of
    maximum
    impulse
ptosis
retractions
review of
    systems
sinus
    arrhythmia
strabismus
temperament
toxoid
turgor
varicocele

Objectives

After mastering the contents of this chapter, you should be able to:

1. State the purposes of health assessment in children of all ages.
2. Assess a child and family by health interview, physical examination, and development screening.
3. Formulate nursing diagnoses based on health assessment findings.
4. Identify expected outcomes based on health assessment findings.
5. Plan nursing care based on health assessment findings such as informing parents of health deviations.
6. Implement nursing care such as conducting an age-appropriate health interview or physical examination by modifying techniques based on the child's age.
7. Evaluate expected outcomes for achievement and effectiveness of care.
8. Identify National Health Goals related to health assessment of children nurses can help the nation achieve.
9. Identify areas related to health assessment of children that could benefit from additional nursing research or application of evidence-based practice.
10. Use critical thinking to analyze ways health assessment skills can be incorporated into nursing care procedures to maintain family-centered care.
11. Integrate nursing process with knowledge of health assessment to achieve quality maternal and child health nursing care.

*K*eoto Wiser is a 13-year-old you meet in an ambulatory clinic. Her father has brought both her and her 2-year-old sister, Candy, for health assessments before Keoto begins seventh grade. Her father is worried Keoto doesn't see well because she always sits close to the television set. Keoto's mother didn't want to bring her for a pre-middle school assessment because she's worried that if glasses are prescribed, her daughter won't be able to play on a school soccer team.

Previous chapters described the normal growth and development of children. This chapter adds information about techniques for assessing the health of children, including history taking, physical examination, related screening procedures for hearing, vision, and development, and immunizations. This is important information because it builds a base for care and health teaching for differing age groups.

What questions would you want to ask Keoto? What screening tests for vision would be best for this 13-year-old child? What could you do to help her adjust to wearing glasses, if they are prescribed?

After you've studied this chapter, access the accompanying website. Read the patient scenario and answer the questions to further sharpen your skills, grow more familiar with RN-CLEX types of questions, and reward yourself with how much you have learned.

ursing assessment is not only the first step in the nursing process, but also the fundamental means by which a nurse establishes and maintains contact with a child and family. Child health assessment is especially important as an opportunity to provide families with information about health promotion, signs of health and illness, and expected developmental progress in their children. This anticipatory guidance can have a long-lasting positive impact on the health of a child and family.

Effective assessment for the maternal–child population first requires you to be familiar with health maintenance standards and usual findings, because this knowledge is essential to the ability to recognize illness. Most health screening procedures are performed in ambulatory settings (e.g., well-child conferences, physicians' offices, health maintenance organizations, community clinics, and schools), but they can be used to evaluate children in all settings.

Sometimes it is necessary to complete just a partial history or a partial physical examination, such as when a child is referred for vision examination. This chapter, however, covers all aspects of physical examination so that, when necessary, a complete examination can be performed (Box 33.1). Procedures specific to particular illnesses appear in later chapters with the illness they detect. Box 33.2 lists National Health Goals related to health assessment in children.

Nursing Process Overview

For Health Assessment of the Child and Family

● *Assessment*

Health assessment of children can be a positive, educational experience for the child and family if time is taken to listen carefully to a family's concerns and responses to questions. Never rush either an interview or a physical examination. Be sure a child has time to familiarize himself or herself with the environment and equipment that will be used.

Obtaining health histories and performing physical examinations can be done independently or as part of a total preventive health care program for a child. The recommendations for standard preventive pediatric health care for the United States are shown in Table 33.1.

● *Nursing Diagnosis*

Health assessment provides the data used to identify potential problems and serves as the basis for the establishment of nursing diagnoses. Be certain not to overlook diagnoses that accentuate the healthy functioning of a child and family, even when diagnoses that address specific problems have been identified. These wellness diagnoses are crucial components of the entire assessment picture and often provide an avenue for addressing identified problems. For instance, the nursing diagnosis of "Impaired social interaction related to lack of self-esteem secondary to disability" would be appropriate for a 4-year-old child who ambulates by wheelchair who, according to the parents,

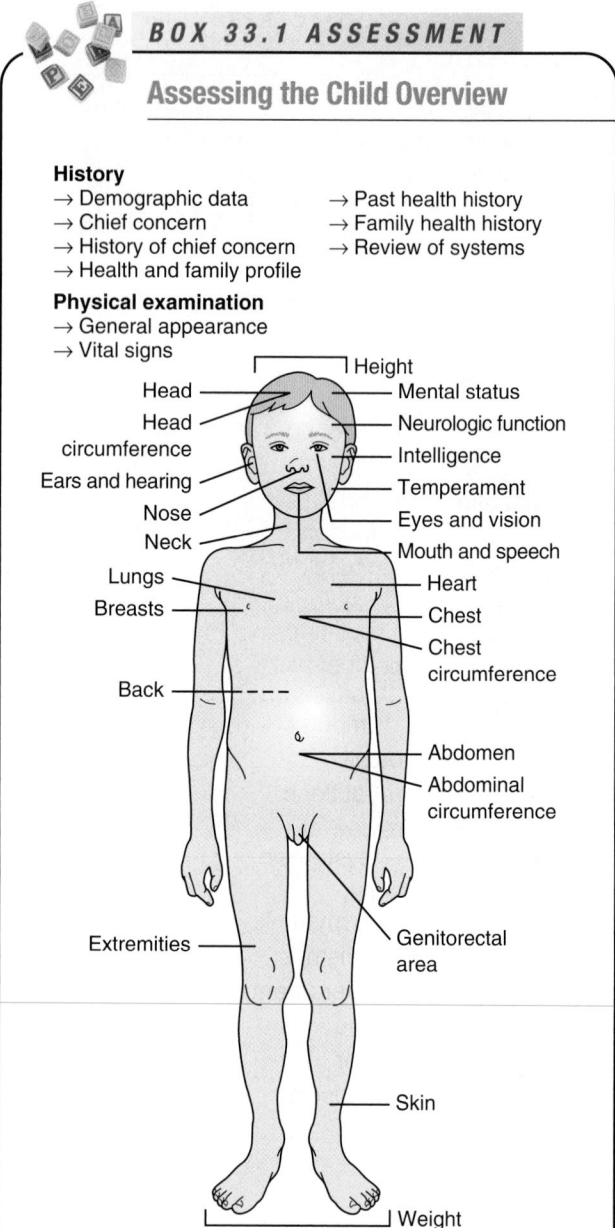

BOX 33.1 ASSESSMENT

Assessing the Child Overview

History
→ Demographic data
→ Chief concern
→ History of chief concern
→ Health and family profile
→ Past health history
→ Family health history
→ Review of systems

Physical examination
→ General appearance
→ Vital signs

Height
Head — Mental status
Head circumference — Neurologic function
Ears and hearing — Intelligence
Nose — Temperament
Neck — Eyes and vision
— Mouth and speech
Lungs — Heart
Breasts — Chest
— Chest circumference
Back — — —
— Abdomen
— Abdominal circumference
Extremities — Genitorectal area
— Skin
Weight

feels uncomfortable around other children. If the parents have difficulty adapting to their child's disability but are eager to accept advice from health care experts on how to provide the most stimulating environment for their child, the diagnosis "Readiness for enhanced family coping" would also be appropriate. Using both these diagnoses allows the development of a plan of care that takes the best advantage of this family's strengths.

● *Outcome Identification and Planning*

Nursing diagnoses serve as the basis for identifying expected outcomes. Health promotion and illness prevention are vital parts of this process. Help parents plan for their child's next developmental stage; keep them aware of important safety measures and other ways to keep children well. Remind them about immu-

BOX 33.2 FOCUS ON . . .

NATIONAL HEALTH GOALS

A number of National Health Goals relate directly to health assessment of children. These are:

- Increase the proportion of territories and states that have service systems for children with special health care needs from a baseline of 15% to a target of 100%.
- Increase the proportion of children and youth, 17 years of age and younger, who have a specific source of on-going care from a baseline of 93% to a target of 97%.
- Achieve and maintain effective vaccination coverage levels for universally recommended vaccines among young children from baselines of 84% (DTaP); 87% (hepatitis B); 91% (polio); 43% (varicella); and 92% (MMR) to a target level of 90% (DHHS, 2000).

Nurses can help the nation achieve these goals by participating actively in health assessment and conscientiously screening for and administering vaccines. Nursing research that might add more information in this area would include techniques that can be used to orient preschoolers quickly to a health care setting, effective techniques for eliciting health interview information from adolescents, and methods to help parents better record or remember what immunizations their children have received.

nizations needed in the future and be certain they know when to schedule the next health visit.

● *Implementation*
Health interviewing and physical examination both require a great deal of skill, skill that can be perfected only through practice. To perfect skills and judgment with children of different ages, take advantage of every opportunity to practice interviewing and physical examination techniques.

● *Outcome Evaluation*
Health assessment of children is an ongoing process that does not end when the first database is obtained. Data must be added at all future interactions so the database remains current and meaningful. Examples suggesting that expected outcomes have been achieved would include:

- Parents state immediately after health examination that they are satisfied with child's motor development.
- Child states after Snellen test that she is aware her vision needs correction.
- Parents state they will continue to assess child's growth by weighing child weekly.

HEALTH HISTORY: ESTABLISHING A DATABASE

The assessment of a young child begins with an interview of the child's parents. An adolescent or preadolescent may choose to be interviewed without the parents present, although many preadolescents and adolescents still prefer to have a parent with them for support.

The purpose of a health interview is to gather information that will direct physical or laboratory examinations to complete a thorough health evaluation. An extensive interview elicits facts such as parental problems in childrearing or detection of future health problems. It lays a foundation for health education and health promotion. Important principles of child health interviewing include the interview setting, the types of questions asked, and the type of information collected.

Interview Setting

An interview is best conducted in a private room with all parties seated comfortably (Fig. 33.1); if not seated, a health care provider appears rushed and can't interact at eye level. During the interview, call the parents by their names. This lets them know their input and opinions about how their child is developing are valued. A question such as, "Does Candy speak in sentences yet, Mr. Wiser?" is far more personal and a better form than, "Does baby sit up yet?" As children grow they are able to speak and answer questions directly.

Types of Questions Asked

The phrasing of questions varies depending on the type of answer desired. Closed-ended and open-ended questions are two types of effective questions; compound, expansive, and leading questions, on the other hand, are three types of questions to avoid.

Closed-Ended Question

This simplest form of question asks directly for a fact: "Does Candy walk yet?" "Did you take Candy's temperature?" This is an effective type of question if a particular point is being sought. It is limited in scope, however, because the response usually will be only a yes or no, with no further elaboration.

Open-Ended Question

An open-ended question allows a parent to elaborate. In contrast to a closed-ended question like "Did you take Candy's temperature?" the question "What did you do for Candy?" is open-ended. The parent answers with a listing of all the things he or she did: took Candy's temperature, had her lie on the couch, gave her extra fluid, and so on. It is important to ask open-ended questions with school-age children and adolescents so they are encouraged to describe a problem fully.

Compound Question

Compound questions are confusing and should be avoided because the information they elicit is often inaccurate and must be followed by a clarifying question. An example is, "Did Candy have nausea and vomiting?" The parent answers

(text continues on page 981)

TABLE 33.1

Recommendations for Preventive Pediatric Health Care

Each child and family is unique; therefore, these Recommendations for Preventive Pediatric Health Care are designed for the care of children who are receiving competent parenting, have no manifestations of any important health problems, and are growing and developing in satisfactory fashion. Additional visits may become necessary if circumstances suggest variations from normal. These guidelines represent a consensus by the Committee on Practice and Ambulatory Medicine in consultation with national committees and sections of the American Academy of Pediatrics. The Committee emphasizes the great importance of continuity of care in comprehensive health supervision and the need to avoid fragmentation of care.

Age[5]	Prenatal[1]	Newborn[2]	2–4d[3]	By 1mo	2mo	4mo	6mo	9mo	12mo	15mo	18mo	24mo	3y	4y
				Infancy[4]									**Early Childhood[4]**	
History														
Initial/Interval	•	•	•	•	•	•	•	•	•	•	•	•	•	•
Measurements														
Height and Weight		•	•	•	•	•	•	•	•	•	•	•	•	•
Head Circumference		•	•	•	•	•	•	•	•	•	•	•		
Blood Pressure													•	•
Sensory Screening														
Vision		S	S	S	S	S	S	S	S	S	S	S	O6	O
Hearing		O7	S	S	S	S	S	S	S	S	S	S	S7	O
Developmental/Behavioral														
Assessment[8]		•	•	•	•	•	•	•	•	•	•	•	•	•
Physical Examination[9]		•	•	•	•	•	•	•	•	•	•	•	•	•
Procedures General[10]														
Hereditary/Metabolic Screening[11]			•	←See separate schedule→										
Immunization[12]														
Hematocrit or Hemoglobin[13]								↑*		*		*	*	*
Urinalysis														
Procedures—Patients at Risk														
Lead Screening[16]								↑*	*			*	*	
Tuberculin Test[17]										*	*	*	*	*
Cholesterol Screening[18]														*
STI Screening[19]														
Pelvic Exam[20]														
Anticipatory Guidance[21]	•	•	•	•	•	•	•	•	•	•	•	•	•	•
Injury Prevention[22]	•	•	•	•	•	•	•	•	•	•	•	•	•	•
Violence Prevention[23]	•	•	•	•	•	•	•	•	•	•	•	•	•	•
Sleep Positioning Counseling[24]	•	•	•	•	•	•	•	•	•	•	•	•	•	•
Nutrition Counseling[25]	•	•	•	•	•	•	•	•	•	•	•	•	•	•
Dental Referral[26]													•	→

		Middle Childhood[4]				Adolescence[4]										
Age[5]	5y	6y	8y	10y	11y	12y	13y	14y	15y	16y	17y	18y	19y	20y	21y
History															
Initial/Interval	•	•	•	•	•	•	•	•	•	•	•	•	•	•	•
Measurements															
Height and Weight	•	•	•	•	•	•	•	•	•	•	•	•	•	•	•
Head Circumference															
Blood Pressure	•	•	•	•	•	•	•	•	•	•	•	•	•	•	•
Sensory Screening															
Vision	O	O	O	O	S	O	S	S	O	S	S	O	S	S	S
Hearing	O	O	O	O	S	O	S	S	O	S	S	O	S	S	S
Developmental/Behavioral															
Assessment[8]	•	•	•	•	•	•	•	•	•	•	•	•	•	•	•
Physical Examination[9]	•	•	•	•	•	•	•	•	•	•	•	•	•	•	•
Procedures-General															
Hereditary/Metabolic Screening[11]															
Immunization[12]	See separate schedule														
Hematocrit or Hemoglobin[13]	*				←———————— 14 ————————→										
Urinalysis	•				←———————— 15 ————————→										
Procedures-Patients at Risk															
Lead Screening[16]		*	*	*	*	*	*	*	*	*	*	*	*	*	*
Tuberculin Test[17]	*	*	*	*	*	*	*	*	*	*	*	*	*	*	*
Cholesterol Screening[18]	*	*	*	*	*	*	*	*	*	*	*	*	*	*	*
STI Screening[19]					*	*	*	*	*	*	*	*	*	*	*
Pelvic Exam[20]					*	*	*	*	*	*	*	* ←—— 20 ——→	*	*	*
Anticipatory Guidance[21]	•	•	•	•	•	•	•	•	•	•	•	•	•	•	•
Injury Prevention[22]	•	•	•	•	•	•	•	•	•	•	•	•	•	•	•
Violence Prevention[23]	•	•	•	•	•	•	•	•	•	•	•	•	•	•	•
Sleep Positioning Counseling[24]															
Nutrition Counseling[25]	•	•	•	•	•	•	•	•	•	•	•	•	•	•	•
Dental Referral[26]															

Key: • = to be performed

* = to be performed for patients at risk

S = subjective, by history

O = objective, by a standard testing method

↔ = the range during which a service may be provided, with the dot indicating the preferred age.

From American Academy of Pediatrics (2000). *Policy statement recommendations for preventive health care* (RE9939), *105*[03], March, p. 645, with permission.

1. A prenatal visit is recommended for parents who are at high risk, for first-time parents, and for those who request a conference. The prenatal visit should include anticipatory guidance, pertinent medical history, and a discussion of benefits of breastfeeding and planned method of feeding per AAP statement "The Prenatal Visit" (1996).

(continued)

TABLE 33.1

Recommendations for Preventive Pediatric Health Care (continued)

2. Every infant should have a newborn evaluation after birth. Breastfeeding should be encouraged and instruction and support offered. Every breastfeeding infant should have an evaluation 48–72 hours after discharge from the hospital to include weight, formal breastfeeding evaluation, encouragement, and instruction as recommended in the AAP statement "Breastfeeding and the Use of Human Milk" (1997).

3. For newborns discharged in less than 48 hours after delivery per AAP statement "Hospital Stay for Healthy Term Newborns" (1995).

4. Developmental, psychosocial and chronic disease issues for children and adolescents may require frequent counseling and treatment visits separate from preventive care visits.

5. If a child comes under care for the first time at any point on the schedule, or if any items are not accomplished at the suggested age, the schedule should be brought up to date at the earliest possible time.

6. If the patient is uncooperative, rescreen within 6 months.

7. All newborns should be screened per the AAP Task Force on Newborn and Infant Hearing statement, "Newborn and Infant Hearing Loss: Detection and Intervention" (1999).

8. By history and appropriate physical examination; if suspicious, by specific objective developmental testing. Parenting skills should be fostered at every visit.

9. At each visit, a complete physical examination is essential, with infant totally unclothed, older child undressed and suitably draped.

10. These may be modified, depending upon entry point into schedule and individual need.

11. Metabolic screening (eg, thyroid, hemoglobinopathies, PKU, galactosemia) should be done according to state law.

12. Schedule(s) per the Committee on Infectious Diseases, published annually in the January edition of *Pediatrics*. Every visit should be an opportunity to update and complete a child's immunizations.

13. See AAP *Pediatric Nutrition Handbook* (1998) for a discussion of universal and selective screening options. Consider earlier screening for high-risk infants (eg premature infants and low birth weight infants). See also "Recommendations to Prevent and Control Iron Deficiency in the United States" [1998]. *MMWR, 47* (RR-3), 1–29.

14. All menstruating adolescents should be screened annually.

15. Conduct dipstick urinalysis for leukocytes annually for sexually active male and female adolescents.

16. For children at risk of lead exposure consult the AAP statement "Screening for Elevated Blood Levels" (1998). Additionally, screening should be done in accordance with state law where applicable.

17. TB testing per recommendations of the Committee on Infectious Diseases, published in the current edition of *Red Book: Report of the Committee on Infectious Diseases*. Testing should be done upon recognition of high-risk factors.

18. Cholesterol screening for high-risk patients per AAP statement "Cholesterol in Childhood" (1998). If family history cannot be ascertained and other risk factors are present, screening should be at the discretion of the physician.

19. All sexually active patients should be screened for sexually transmitted infections (STIs).

20. All sexually active females should have a pelvic examination. A pelvic examination and routine pap smear should be offered as part of preventive health maintenance between the ages of 18 and 21 years.

21. Age-appropriate discussion and counseling should be an integral part of each visit for care per the AAP *Guidelines for Health Supervision III* (1998).

22. From birth to age 12, refer to the AAP injury prevention program (TIPP—MS 534) as described in *A Guide to Safety Counseling in Office Practice* (1994).

23. Violence prevention and management for all patients per AAP Statement "The Role of the Pediatrician in Youth Violence Prevention in Clinical Practice and at the Community Level" (1999).

24. Parents and caregivers should be advised to place healthy infants on their backs when putting them to sleep. Side positioning is a reasonable alternative but carries a slightly higher risk of SIDS. Consult the AAP statement "Changing Concepts of Sudden Infant Death Syndrome: Implications for Infant Sleeping Environment and Sleep Position" (2000).

25. Age-appropriate nutrition counseling should be an integral part of each visit per the AAP *Handbook of Nutrition* (1998).

26. Earlier initial dental examinations may be appropriate for some children. Subsequent examinations as prescribed by dentist.

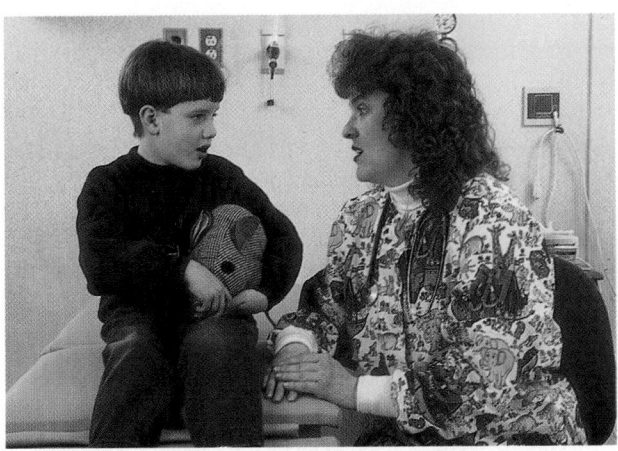

FIGURE 33.1 Maintaining good eye contact and allowing children to be as active a part as possible in the assessment process are important for good health interviewing.

yes, but it still is not known whether Candy had vomiting and nausea, just vomiting, or just nausea.

Expansive Question

This is an open-ended question gone wrong because it is too broad to answer. "What can you tell me about Candy?" leaves a parent wondering where to start. "How has Candy been since her last visit?" limits the question and makes it answerable.

Leading Question

A leading question supplies its own answer so also should be avoided. "Candy has had all her immunizations, hasn't she?" implies that Candy should have had them and perhaps the parent is a poor caregiver if he or she answers that question any way but yes. The penalty for such an exchange could be a child left vulnerable to disease.

Health Interview

Data gathering for an initial health assessment can be divided into nine sections:

1. Introduction and explanation
2. Demographic data
3. Chief concern
4. History of chief concern
5. Health and family profile
6. Day history
7. Past health history, including pregnancy history
8. Family health history
9. Review of systems

At return visits, the categories used generally include only introduction and explanation, chief concern, health and family profile, interval history, and day history.

While conducting a health interview, be certain to make a transition statement before shifting from one section of

an interview to another. Without a transition, a parent could be left wondering what importance the questions have, possibly misinterpreting their significance. For instance, if a parent has been providing information on the family's hospital insurance policy and, without a transition statement, is asked whether the child has been vomiting, a parent may think the interviewer believes the child needs hospitalization when that is not the intent at all. A statement such as, "Before we talk about Candy's current symptoms, let me ask you some general questions about your family as a whole," is an example of a good transition statement.

Introduction and Explanation

As a matter of courtesy, parents and the child should be told to whom they are talking and what topics they will be discussing. "Hello, Ms. Wiser, I'm Janet Dickson, a nurse here in the One-Day Surgery Department. I'd like to talk to you about Candy this morning" is an example of a suitable introduction. Because some families have never had the benefit of in-depth health care, it is also helpful to include a statement about the subjects that will be discussed during the interview. For example, "So that I can get a picture of Candy's overall health, I'd like to ask you questions about why you've brought her here today, your pregnancy with her, concerns you've had in the past, and questions about your typical day with Candy," would be appropriate. The parent begins to concentrate on those areas because he or she realizes health care providers in this setting are interested not just in Candy's health this particular day, but in her total health (Box 33.3).

Demographic Data

To begin collecting demographic data, identify the client. Information such as a client's name, address, gender, and the person who provided information should be included. To provide culturally competent care and make provisions for special needs, a child's culture, ethnicity, place of birth, religious or spiritual practices, and primary and secondary language should also be identified. Ask if older children have a Social Security number.

Be certain to identify the child's primary caregiver. If the parents are divorced or deceased, it is especially important to identify who has custody of the child and who has the right to sign the consent for health care treatment.

Chief Concern

After gathering demographic data, begin data collection with the reason the parents have brought the child to the health care agency: the **chief concern.** This is what parents are most anxious to discuss, so it is important they get this immediate concern off their mind early in the interview. An effective way to elicit this information is to ask an open-ended question such as, "Why did you bring Candy to the clinic today, Ms. Wiser?" Such an opening allows the parent freedom to answer in a number of areas of concern: physical, emotional, nutritional, and developmental.

BOX 33.3 FOCUS ON . . .

DIVERSITY OF CARE

Health assessment of children is a skill that is learned with practice. Successful interviewing depends on respecting cultural variations. Whether people establish eye contact with an interviewer, for example, is a characteristic that is culturally determined.

Findings and techniques in children also differ depending on racial and ethnic characteristics. Assessing for cyanosis, for example, is more difficult in dark-skinned than in fair-skinned children (mucous membrane is the best place to detect this). Because height and weight charts are standardized on middle-class white children, measurements of children who do not fit this description may not plot well on these charts. In Vietnam, touching the head of a child during physical assessment is thought to be harmful because the head is considered to be the seat of the soul.

Recognizing that people hold differing cultural expectations and characteristics can help in establishing

rapport with children and their families and help make health assessment more meaningful.

Some cultures are much more aware of the role of communicable disease in childhood illnesses than others and so advocate for all children to be immunized against these disorders. Even if awareness about the danger of disease spread exists, however, it doesn't mean all people in a community will be conscientious about having their children immunized. Other factors such as cost and convenience and ethical beliefs are also important.

Some religious groups, such as the Amish, do not encourage immunizations. In these communities, the prevalence of illnesses such as measles can rise to high numbers. Being aware that immunization rates are not consistent from place to place aids in understanding the importance of planning health education and health surveillance based on individual community needs.

If asked, "How is Candy feeling today?" or "Is Candy ill?" the parent is left to think about only physical aspects and may not voice his or her biggest concern: Candy's teething difficulty or frequent temper tantrums. For more details on eliciting information about children's chief concern, see Box 33.4.

History of Chief Concern

Once a parent has voiced a chief concern, ask him or her to describe at least six aspects of the problem:

1. Duration
2. Intensity

BOX 33.4 FOCUS ON . . .

COMMUNICATION

You see Keoto at another time at an ambulatory clinic because she has frequency and burning on urination. Her mother accompanies her for the visit.

Less Effective Communication

Nurse: Hello, Keoto. What's the reason you've come into the clinic today?
Mrs. Wiser: It hurts when she urinates.
Nurse: How long ago did that start, Keoto?
Mrs. Wiser: She started complaining about it yesterday.
Nurse: Has she had any blood in her urine?
Mrs. Wiser: She hasn't said anything about that. The important thing is the pain.
Nurse: Okay. I'm sure we need a urine specimen for culture. Let's get that to get started here.

More Effective Communication

Nurse: Hello, Keoto. What's the reason you've come into the clinic today?
Mrs. Wiser: It hurts when she urinates.
Nurse: Let's let Keoto answer for herself, Mrs. Wiser. Tell me what you think is the problem, Keoto.
Keoto: It hurts when I go to the bathroom.
Nurse: How long ago did that start, Keoto?
Mrs. Wiser: She started complaining about it yesterday.

Nurse: Keoto, when do *you* think it started?
Keoto: About an hour after I came in from my date last night.
Nurse: Have you had any blood in your urine?
Mrs. Wiser: She hasn't said anything about that.
Nurse: Keoto, have you noticed your urine is red or dark brown?
Keoto: I had bright blood last night.
Nurse: Let me take you down to the lavatory and explain about a urine specimen. While we're there, I'd like to ask you some more questions about last night.

At about 10 years of age, children are able to supply much of a health history by themselves. As children become teenagers, it is increasingly important for them to do this because they may not have shared a total history with a parent. In the above scenario, for example, when the child is asked directly for information, she supplied more than when her history was given by the mother. Some urinary tract infections occur in girls after their first sexual relations. It would be important to ask Keoto if she is sexually active (what her date last night included), not only to document the probable cause of the urinary tract infection, but also to be certain she is knowledgeable about pregnancy prevention and safer sex practices.

3. Frequency
4. Description
5. Associated symptoms
6. Actions taken

In discussing duration, determine when a child was last well to determine when he or she became ill. For example, on Saturday morning, Candy began having long crying periods. On Monday night, she developed a fever. On Tuesday afternoon, her mother brought her into the clinic for a checkup. The parent states Candy vomited three times Monday morning and thinks this was caused by teething. Unless the parent is asked when Candy was last well, she may pinpoint Monday as the beginning of the illness (the vomiting) when actually it was Saturday (the crying).

In this example, the intensity of the illness refers to the kind of vomiting the child is having. Is it drooling, spitting up, or actual vomiting? The description is the amount (a cupful? a mouthful?) and color (whether it contains blood, bile, or mucus). Associated symptoms might include fever, abdominal pain, difficulty eating, or signs of respiratory illness. A good question to use to obtain this information is, "Is Candy ill in any other way?"

Knowing the parent's actions can be important for a number of reasons. First, it helps to know whether anything a parent has been doing has been making the illness worse (e.g., offering a great deal of fluid to replace that vomited and by doing so causing more vomiting; using a home remedy or alternative therapy that actually induces vomiting). The parent's actions also reveal what the parent has previously tried but found ineffective. Telling a parent to give a child two tablets of acetaminophen (Tylenol) every 4 hours for fever if the parent has already done that and the fever has not improved would be unproductive. This information also reveals the parent's response to caring for an ill child. A parent who says, "I tucked her into bed and gave her a little tea to drink" is different from one who replies, "Nothing. I fall apart when my child is ill." If the child is going to return home under the parent's care, the second parent in the example will need more instructions and support before he or she leaves the health care setting than the first parent.

Obtaining information about the chief concern puts the parent's observations in proper perspective. In the previous example, the parent is probably not describing teething difficulty (teething does not cause vomiting); more likely, the child has a viral gastroenteritis. Unless the problem is investigated, it is easy to accept the parent's statement at face value as a teething problem without appreciating its full significance.

During this phase of the interview, it is also important to gather information about related or other health concerns. After the chief concern is documented, ask another open-ended question to elicit additional information: "Is there anything else that worries you about Candy?" Now the parent might want to talk about Candy's temper tantrums. Unless asked about a second problem, a parent can go home with the first problem cared for but the second one still not addressed. When the parent arrives home and Candy begins stomping her feet in the car, unwilling to go into the house, she can feel that the health care Candy received was less than adequate because she did not receive help with this concern.

Do not assume parents will always reveal their worst fears in the initial minute of an interview: it can be frightening to put these fears into words. As long as a concern is hanging as a nebulous thought in the mind, it is easy to tell oneself it may not be true. Only when a parent voices the thought ("Do you think Candy is retarded?" "Do you think this is leukemia?" "Could this be inherited?") does the fear become real. Before parents dare to speak openly this way, they must trust health care providers not to treat their statement lightly. For this reason, it is helpful to repeat the question about a second concern once more at the very end of the interview.

Health and Family Profile

Before pursuing the past history or development of a child, document the circumstances in which the child lives. A good introduction to a health and family profile is a sentence such as, "Before we talk about any past illnesses or happenings with Candy, let me ask you some questions about her health and your family as a whole."

Important information concerning the child's current health status includes:

- Who is the child's primary health care provider?
- How often is the child seen for routine health examinations?
- Are the child's immunizations up to date?
- What is the child's general state of health? How does it compare to the child's health 1 and 5 years ago (if appropriate)?
- Does the child have any known allergies?
- Does the child have a chronic illness or disability?
- Is the child taking any prescription medications? Over-the-counter medications? Home or folk remedies, such as herbal remedies?
- Is the child undergoing any treatments?

Important information concerning the family includes:

- Is the parent married, single, or divorced?
- Is the family nuclear or extended?
- How many children are in the family?
- What are the family's current living arrangements?
- What are the parents' occupations? (This helps establish the family's socioeconomic level and means of family support.)
- If both parents work, how do they manage child care?

Obtaining a health and family profile is sometimes delayed by medical interviewers until the end of the interview, when, theoretically, a parent or child is more comfortable and will answer these personal questions more readily. However, by following a nursing model and obtaining the information earlier in the interview, the health care practitioner can better assess the child and evaluate data.

Day History

The child's current skills, sleep patterns, hygiene practices, eating habits, and interactions with the family can all be elicited by asking a parent to describe a typical day. Day histories are fun to obtain because most parents are eager to describe their day with their child and information gained this way is surprisingly rich and pertinent, much more so than if parents are just asked how their child sleeps, eats, or plays.

Begin by asking, "Was yesterday a fairly typical day for Candy?" (The parent says yes, it was.) "Would you describe for me everything Candy did yesterday, beginning with when she first woke up?" Some parents offer this information in great detail; with others, it is necessary to backtrack for particular details: "What did she eat for breakfast? Does she use a fork and spoon? Does she sit in a high chair or on your lap?"

Play. Play, the work of children, reveals a great deal about the child's development and overall well-being. Important questions to ask about play include:

- Is Candy kept in a playpen or given room to run?
- What is Candy's favorite toy?
- Does she play active, chasing games or engage in quiet, pretending types of activities?
- Do you (the parent) spend time reading to the child?
- Do you (the parent) play with her or let her play by herself? (This allows for an estimation of the quality of interaction during the day.)

Sleep. Every child needs adequate rest for healthy growth and development. Poor sleep patterns can often reveal a psychosocial or physical health problem. Important questions regarding sleep include:

- When the child sleeps, how long does she sleep?
- Is falling asleep a problem?
- Where does she sleep? Does she have night terrors?
- Does she sleepwalk?
- Does she wet her bed (depending on whether the child is toilet-trained)?

Hygiene. Good hygiene practices promote healthy teeth, gums, and skin, prevent infections, and improve self-esteem. Poor hygiene may reflect neglect, depression, drug abuse, or low socioeconomic status. Important questions regarding hygiene include:

- How much self-care does the child do?
- Does the child take baths or showers?
- Does the child brush her teeth? How often? Does she floss regularly? (Responses depend on the age of the child.)
- Does the child wash her hands before snacks and meals?
- Has there been a recent change in hygiene practices?

Nutrition. Nutritional assessment is an important portion of a health assessment because it influences health so strongly (Dudek, 2005). Characteristics of a nutritionally healthy child that can be revealed by assessment are summarized in Table 33.2. Food and nutrient intake risk factors are summarized in Box 33.5.

Taking a history of a child's food intake can help determine whether there are any foods missing in a typical meal plan or whether any quantities seem inadequate or excessive. Be certain to assess not only the quantity of food taken but the quality as well (e.g., for the infant, cereal should be iron-fortified).

To do this, ask parents to describe a typical day (24-hour recall), listing what the child ate for each meal and between meals as well. With an older child, the 24-hour recall can be a joint parent–child venture. Providing this history can be difficult when the child consumes some meals at home and others at day care or school. It may be necessary to ask for a weekend history to get a complete picture.

When assessing the adolescent, take a 24-hour recall nutritional history without a parent present, if possible. In front of a parent, adolescents may add nutritional foods to a food intake history or leave out foods they have eaten

---

TABLE 33.2

Physical Signs of Adequate Nutrition

Assessment	Finding
Overall impression	Alert, with good energy level; positive mood
Hair	Shiny, strong, with good body
Eyes	Good eyesight, particularly at night; conjunctiva moist and pink
Mouth	No cavities in teeth; no swollen or inflamed gingivae; no cracks or fissures at corners of mouth; mucous membrane moist and pink; tongue smooth and nontender
Neck	Normal contour of thyroid gland
Skin	Smooth; normal color and turgor; no ecchymotic or petechial areas present
Extremities	Normal muscle mass and circumference; normal strength and mobility; no edema present; no tender joints; normal reflexes; legs not bowed
Gastrointestinal	No diarrhea or constipation present
Finger and toenails	Smooth, pink; not cracked or broken
Height and weight	Within normal limits on growth chart
Blood pressure	Normal for age

BOX 33.5

Food and Nutrient Intake Risk Factors

History or evidence of any of the following may pose a potential nutritional risk:

- Intake less or greater than standard for age, calories, protein, or activity
- Intake less or greater than standard for nutrients (i.e., vitamins and minerals)
- Unusual food habits, such as pica, faddism, and meal skipping
- Inappropriate use of supplements (vitamins, minerals, fortified food products)
- A physician's order for NPO or a clear liquid diet for more than 3 days without enteral or parenteral nutrition
- Inadequate transitional feeding, enteral support, or parenteral support
- Minimal or no intake from a major food group
- Fluid intake less than output
- Eating disorders such as bulimia or feeding disorders
- Food allergies
- Restricted diet

(e.g., milkshakes, potato chips, or pizza) to avoid a lecture later; on the other hand, they may leave out healthy items or add less desirable ones because they may enjoy the obvious parental disapproval, indicative of their rebellion against adult authority.

After taking a history of the child's food intake, determine whether the child is receiving foods that comply with the recommendations of the food guide pyramid (see Appendix K). If whole food groups are absent or grossly inadequate, the follow-up evaluation should include a food frequency record as a double-check to see if the 24-hour recall was truly representative of a usual day. Remember that children do not have to eat food from all groups at every meal, as long as they eat from them every day. If parents think in terms of days rather than meals, they may exert less pressure on a child at each meal.

Be sure to consider the role of food preferences and cultural, lifestyle, and financial variations when assessing food intake. The number of meals eaten at home versus outside the home, the form and content of traditional meals cooked at home, and the pattern of meals should all be considered. Any religious dietary restrictions should also be determined. Do not appear critical of a child's diet. If you convey dismay at erratic eating habits, parents or older children (especially adolescents) may begin to fabricate the food history to make it seem more acceptable.

Past Health History

For a past health history, ask whether a child has ever had any serious illnesses. Parents do not generally think of childhood diseases such as measles, chickenpox, and mumps as serious illnesses; inquire about these separately. Also inquire about the child's immunization history and whether the immunizations are up to date for the child's age. (See the discussion of immunizations later in this chapter.) Has a child had any accidents (unintentional injuries)? Any surgery? Parents may not think of a tonsillectomy as surgery because there were no stitches; ask about that separately. Did a child ever ingest anything that was inedible or harmful? Has a child been hospitalized for any reason? How many times has a child been seen in an emergency room? These last questions provide information about the degree of adult supervision, and possibly clues to abuse (Horner, 2005).

Information about the outcome of past illnesses is as important to obtain as information about the illnesses themselves. If the child had otitis media (middle ear infection) at age 2 years and received an antibiotic and recovered without complications, the parent has every reason to be confident that the child will get better from a present illness also; the parent has confidence in health care personnel. If the child had an allergic reaction to the antibiotic or was left with a hearing difficulty from the previous illness, a parent may distrust the care being given to the child now; he or she may not follow instructions well, thinking nothing works anyway. Or the parents may need extra support to follow instructions. This is important information for planning care.

When parents report a past health concern or illness, be sure to ask for details of the illness. This can help to minimize inaccurate data and ensure that the present and future care of the child is appropriate. For example, some parents believe their child is allergic to an antibiotic because while the child was taking the drug he or she developed diarrhea. There is a strong possibility the diarrhea was associated with the reason for taking the antibiotic, not with the drug itself. In this example, you would want to ask about specific symptoms and record what the parent says about allergies so the person who prescribes medication for the child can decide whether a true allergy exists.

The health of children is affected by their mother's health during pregnancy. For children under age 5 years, therefore, a pregnancy history is usually obtained. Document which pregnancy this was for the mother. Were there complications in any past pregnancies? Abortions or miscarriages? Stillbirths? Children born prematurely? A history of the pregnancy of the child being assessed can begin with a question such as, "How was your pregnancy with Candy?" This allows the mother to answer in both physical and emotional areas. After exploring details mentioned by the mother, ask about specific events that are known to occur with pregnancy, such as:

- Did the mother have any complications such as bleeding, falls, swelling of hands and feet, high blood pressure, or unusual weight gain?
- Did she take any medication?
- Were any x-ray films taken?
- Did she smoke cigarettes, drink alcohol, or use recreational drugs?
- Did the pregnancy end early or late?

Because life contingencies such as loss of finances or illness in the family during a pregnancy may affect a parent's ability to form a bond with a child, the emotional experiences of a woman during pregnancy are also important to obtain. Ask if the parents planned the pregnancy. A question such as, "A lot of pregnancies come as a sort of surprise. Is that how it was with Candy?" or "Some unmarried women want to have children and some don't. How was it with you?" lets parents know you will nonjudgmentally accept any answer they give.

Next, review labor and birth. Questions to ask may include:

- How long was labor? Was it what you expected it to be?
- Were there any complications? Was the birth vaginal or cesarean?
- Was anesthesia used for birth?
- Was the baby born vertex (head-first) or breech?

Ask about the health of the child at birth as well. Questions to ask may include:

- Did the baby cry right away?
- Did the infant room in or need care in a special nursery?
- Did the infant need special procedures or equipment at birth?
- Was there cyanosis or jaundice?
- Was the infant discharged from the birth setting with the mother?
- How did the parents feel about having a boy or girl?
- How did it feel for them to be new parents?

Family Health History

Because some diseases are inherited or familial, it is important to know which ones occur in a family. Ask if any family member has heart disease (childhood or adult type), kidney disease, a congenital anomaly, seizures, diabetes (type 1 or 2), tuberculosis, a sexually transmitted infection, or allergies or is cognitively challenged.

Review of Systems

The last step in a health interview is a summary of body symptoms or a **review of systems.** Once more, make certain to introduce this part of the history with a transition statement. Otherwise a parent may think that the local problem (vomiting) he or she has been describing suggests other problems. For example, a statement, such as, "I'd like to ask about different parts of Candy's body, from her head down to her toes, just to be certain I don't miss anything" provides a transition.

Although the important items to be covered in a review of systems differ according to the age of the child, a basic list is shown in Box 33.6.

A review of systems covers a lot of ground, but it generally takes no more than 5 minutes. However, do not rush through the questions so quickly that a parent does

---

BOX 33.6

Review of Systems

The following questions provide a guide when completing a review of systems:

Neuropsychiatric symptoms: Has the child ever had seizures? Head injury? Attention problems? Depression? Aggressive behavior? Has the parent ever had such difficulty rousing the child that the parent believed the child was unconscious? Have there been any problems with suspected substance abuse?

Eyes: Has the child had difficulty with eyes not focusing? Eye infection? Does the parent have any reason to believe that the child does not see well? Does the child wear eyeglasses? Contacts?

Ears: Ear infections? Drainage from the ears? Ear aches? Tubes in ears? Any infection from piercing? Reason to believe the child does not hear well?

Nose: Frequent drainage or cold symptoms? Difficulty breathing? Nosebleeds?

Mouth: Difficulty with teeth or teething? Mouth infections? Has the child seen a dentist (if older than age 2 years)? Does the child chew tobacco?

Throat: Throat infections? Difficulty swallowing?

Neck: Masses or swelling? Stiffness? Does the child hold his or her head straight? (Torticollis or wry neck will make the child hold the head crookedly; children with poor vision also may cock their heads to the side to try to see better.)

Chest: Is breast development in girls appropriate for age? For adolescent girls over 14 years and Tanner stage V, ask about yearly breast examination.

Lungs: Breathing problems? Infections? Pneumonia? Asthma? Does the child smoke any substance?

Heart: Has a physician ever said there was difficulty? What exactly was said?

Gastrointestinal system: Has there been an eating problem? Frequent nausea? Vomiting? (Ask separately from nausea; children with pyloric stenosis [obstruction of the pyloric opening of the stomach] have vomiting but no nausea; children with a brain tumor may also have vomiting but no nausea; pregnant teenagers may have nausea but not vomiting.) Diarrhea? Any constipation? Is the child toilet-trained? Any difficulty with this?

Genitourinary system: Pain or burning on urination? Blood in urine? Does the child have a good urine stream? If a girl is age 10 years or older, has she started menstruation? Any problems with menstruation? If an adolescent male, has he begun testicular self-examination? If an adolescent, is the child sexually active? Using contraception? Want more information on contraception? Ever had an STI? (To protect privacy, it is essential to ask the adolescent, not the parents, questions regarding sexuality.)

Extremities: Painful or swollen joints? Broken bones? Muscle sprains? Is the parent pleased with the child's coordination?

Skin: Rashes? Lesions such as warts?

Immunizations: What immunizations has the child received to date?

BOX 33.9 FOCUS ON . . .

FAMILY TEACHING

Breast Self-Examination

Q. Keoto is interested in beginning breast self exams. She asks you, "What is the best way to do it?"

A. Follow these steps each month on the day after your menstrual period ends:

Step 1. Inspect
(A) In front of a mirror, look for any change in the size or shape of the breast, puckering or dimpling of the skin, or changes in the nipple.

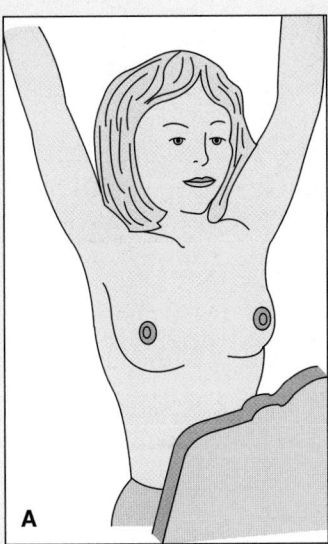

A

(B) Inspect in three positions: (1) with arms relaxed at sides, (2) with arms held overhead, and (3) with hands on hips, pressing in to contract the chest muscles. Turn from side to side to view all areas.

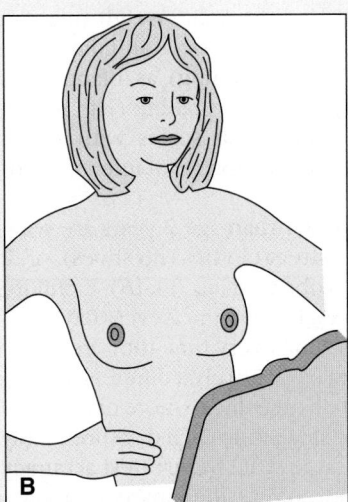

B

(C) Nipple examination: Gently squeeze the nipple of each breast between thumb and index finger to check for discharge.

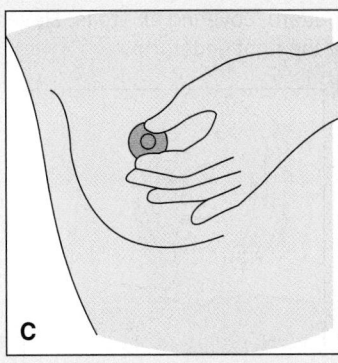

C

Step 2. Palpate or feel
(D) In shower or bath, fingers will glide over wet, soapy skin, making it easier to feel changes in the breast. Check the breast for a lump, knot, tenderness, or change in the consistency of normal tissue. To examine your right breast, put your right hand behind your head. With the pads of your fingers of your left hand held flat and together, gently press on the breast tissue using small circular motions. Imagine the breast as the face of a clock. Beginning at the top (12 o'clock position), make a circle around the outer area of the breast. Move in one fingerwidth; continue in smaller and smaller circles until you have reached the nipple. Cover all areas including the breast tissue leading to the axilla. Repeat the procedure for the left breast. At the lower border of each breast, a ridge of firm tissue may be felt. This is normal.

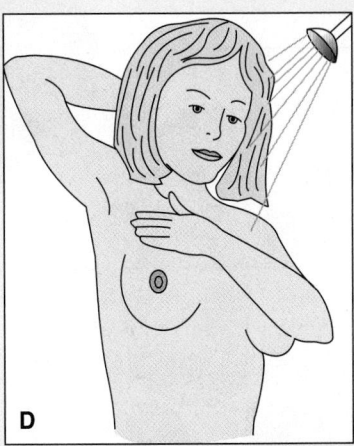

D

(continued)

BOX 33.9 FOCUS ON . . .

FAMILY TEACHING

Breast Self-Examination (continued)

(E) Underarm examination. Examine the left underarm area with your arm held loosely at your side. Cup the fingers of the opposite hand and insert them high into the underarm area. Draw fingers down slowly, pressing in a circular pattern, covering all areas. Reverse the procedure for the right underarm.

(F) Lying down. While lying flat, place a small pillow or folded towel under the right shoulder. Examine the right breast using the same circular motion as was used in the shower. Cover all areas. Repeat this procedure for the left breast. Press firmly but gently while examining your breast, rolling the tissue between your fingers and the chest wall.

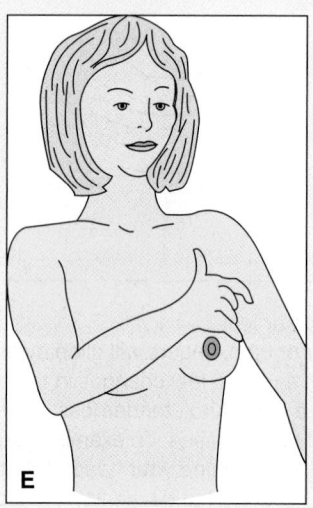

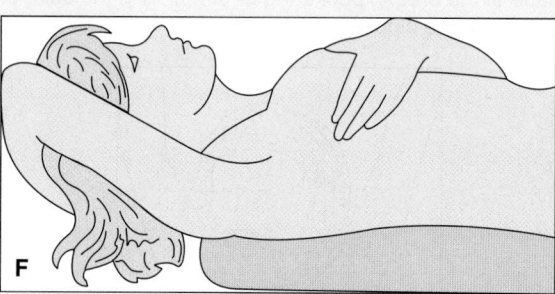

(Courtesy of the American Cancer Society, New York State Division, Inc. East Syracuse, New York.)

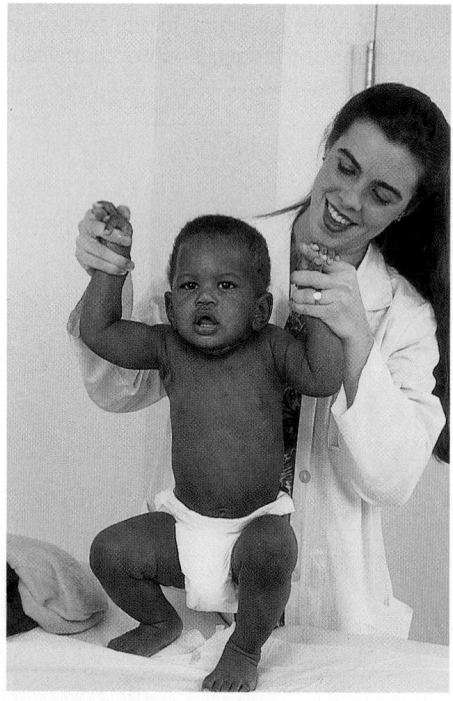

FIGURE 33.3 General appearance assessment reveals that this child is well proportioned and active.

Weight

Until they can stand well, infants are weighed on a sitting or infant scale. Because diapers can be heavy in proportion to total body weight, weigh infants nude. Always keep a protective hand over an infant on an infant scale (hovering but not touching), as infants squirm readily and there is danger of them falling (Fig. 33.4A). Cover both infant scales and adult scales with scale paper before weighing to prevent spread of infection from one child to another.

Children older than age 2 years are weighed on standing scales, in street clothes (no shoes), or, if in a hospital, in a gown or robe (see Fig. 33.4B). If children are going to have serial weights (weighed every day), be sure they wear the same clothing every time they are weighed so any discrepancy in weight is truly a difference in body weight and not a weight change due to more or less clothing. Take the weight at the same time each day (preferably before breakfast) on the same scale for greatest accuracy.

Most children and their parents want to know their weight. To convert from kilograms to pounds, multiply the kilogram amount by 2.2 (50 kg × 2.2 = 110 lb).

To assess whether weight is average for height, compare the child's weight with a standardized height/weight graph (Appendix E). In the standardized scale for children, all weights between the 10th and 90th percentiles are con-

TABLE 33.4

Significant Body Odors

Source of Odor	Possible Cause
Breath	
Alcohol	Possible recent ingestion (important if coma or neurologic symptoms are present as cause of abnormal functioning)
Camphor	Mothball ingestion
Halitosis (bad breath)	Poor dental hygiene, lung infection; foreign body in respiratory tract
Burnt rope	Marijuana use
Sweet	Acidosis (seen in a child in diabetic coma)
Body	
Stale urine	Incontinence; poor kidney functioning leading to uremia; infrequently changed diapers; neglect
Sweat	May imply that child is too fatigued or stressed to maintain hygiene
"Spoiled fruit"	Wound infection
Sweet	*Pseudomonas* infection
Urine	
Maple syrup	Protein metabolic condition
Musty or mousy	Phenylketonuria or a protein metabolism disorder
Ammonia	Urinary tract infection or poor hydration leading to concentrated urine
Stool	
Putrid	Fat in stool from inadequate absorption

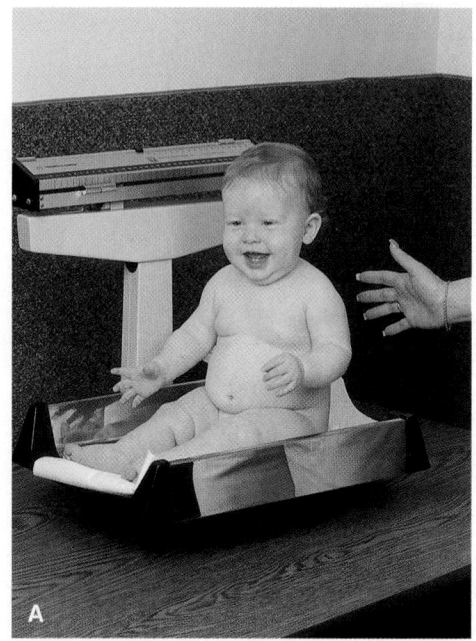

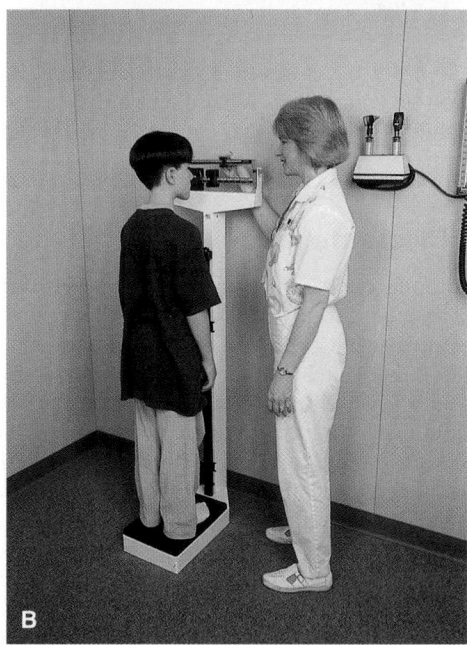

FIGURE 33.4 (**A**) Weighing an infant. Note the protective hand to ensure the infant's safety. (**B**) Weighing an older child.

sidered normal (statistically, a range of weights that includes two standard deviations from the mean or the 50th percentile). As important as the fact that a child's weight falls between the 10th and 90th percentile on a growth chart is that over time the weight follows one of the percentile curves—in other words, the child is not at the 80th percentile the first time he or she is weighed and a month later at the 40th percentile. Although both readings are within the normal range, they reflect a weight loss that would need investigation. Gaining weight in the same way could be equally serious. A child is defined as having a "failure to thrive" syndrome (medical diagnosis) if height or weight drops below the third percentile on a standardized growth chart. Any height or weight in this category definitely needs to be reported so its cause can be investigated.

Another method to determine whether a child's weight is consistent with height is to compute the body mass index (BMI). Table 33.5 describes the formula used to calculate BMI and the implications of the values obtained (see also Appendix E).

Height

In children, height is as good a determinant of health and normal nutrition as is weight. To accurately measure the height of infants and older children, see Box 33.10.

Plot height measurements for children on a standard graph, the same as for weight. Height and weight should follow the same percentiles. Remember that height/weight charts have been standardized for middle-class white American children, so there will be variations among children from different cultural backgrounds. The important thing to

TABLE 33.5

Body Mass Index Findings

To calculate the body mass index (BMI), divide the child's weight in kilograms by the square of the child's height in meters:

$$\frac{\text{Body weight in kg}}{(\text{Height in meters})^2} = \text{BMI}$$

BMI	Implication
Below 18.5	Underweight
18.5 to 24.9	Normal
25.0 to 29.9	Overweight
Over 30	Obese

look for is consistency of measurements over time (always at the same percentile).

What If... Keoto, 13 years old, weighs 93 lb? Would you be concerned? What if 6 months earlier she had weighed 110 lb and a year earlier she had weighed 105 lb?

Head Circumference

Head circumference is measured at birth and routinely on physical assessment until 1 year of age (some health care agencies measure it routinely until 2 years of age). Head growth occurs because the brain is growing, so head circumference reflects brain growth and potential neurologic function. The measurement is made by placing a tape measure around an infant's head just above the eyebrows and around the most prominent portion of the back of the head, the occipital prominence (Fig. 33.5). Babies generally push any object away from their head, so it may be difficult to carry out this otherwise simple procedure. Plot measurements on a standardized graph (see Appendix E). Head circumference should correlate with the child's length (e.g., if length is in the 40th percentile, head circumference also should be). If measurements of head circumference plot at different percentiles over time, this should be reported because it implies that brain or skull growth is in some way abnormal and needs investigation.

Chest and Abdominal Circumference

Measurements of chest and abdominal circumference are not done routinely, but only when specific pathology warrants. Chest circumference is measured at the nipple line, abdominal circumference at the level of the umbilicus.

Skin

Skin is assessed in conjunction with the examination of each body region. Assess the following:

- Temperature
- Color
- Texture
- **Turgor** (amount of fluid in body tissue; Fig. 33.6)
- Presence of any lesions

Table 33.6 summarizes various findings that may be detected. Be certain to examine a child's total skin surface at some time during an examination. As necessary, remove and replace adhesive bandages and other dressings that could hide important findings. Be certain there is adequate lighting, especially when assessing dark-skinned children.

Newborn and Infant

Newborns may appear ruddy because their layer of subcutaneous fat is thin and the intense redness of their blood circulation is visible. Erythema toxicum (newborn rash) may be present. Birthmarks (hemangiomas, mongolian spots, or nevi) may be present. After the first few days of life, a diaper rash may be present.

Toddler, Preschooler, and School-Age Child

Many children this age have minor lesions from mosquito bites or from flea bites if they own a pet. They also typically have a number of ecchymotic spots on their lower extremities from bumping into objects during active play. Ecchymotic spots on upper extremities are less common and may suggest a blood coagulation problem. In evaluating ecchymotic spots on children of all ages, though, consider the possibility of child abuse (Mulryan, Cathers, & Fagin, 2004).

Adolescent

At least a few acne lesions on the face or back are usually present in the adolescent. Lesions or rashes caused by allergies to cosmetics also may be seen. If a child has a tattoo or body piercing, assess the site for inflammation to reveal beginning infection.

Head

To examine a child's head, slide a hand over the skull, assessing for irregular configurations or tenderness. Most children have a prominent occipital outgrowth; do not mistake this natural head contour for an abnormality. Assess the texture and cleanliness of the child's hair. Children who are well nourished usually have hair of good texture; poorly nourished children tend to have dry, brittle, or limp hair. If hair is exceptionally oily, it may suggest a lack of adequate hygiene, possibly from fatigue due to an unidentified illness. If a serious protein deficiency such as **kwashiorkor** is present, the hair becomes striped with dark and light color; dark hair forms during periods of good protein intake and the light color forms during periods of protein deficit. Patches of hair loss (alopecia) suggest a fungal infection (tinea capitis), child abuse, or a possible drug reaction (chemotherapy will cause total hair loss, not patches).

BOX 33.10 NURSING PROCEDURE

Measuring a Child's Height

Purpose
To assess for optimal growth.

PROCEDURE	PRINCIPLE
Infant	
1. Until they can stand securely (at approximately age 2 years), measure infants lying down on a measuring frame or an examining table.	1. Promotes accuracy.
2. Align the infant's head snugly against the top bar of the frame and ask an assistant to secure it there. Parents can help you restrain infants for height measurements because it is a painless procedure.	2. Provides a starting point for measurement.
3. Straighten the infant's body (Figure *A*).	3. Straightens knees to ensure accuracy. Knees are difficult to straighten in infants because they always keep them flexed.

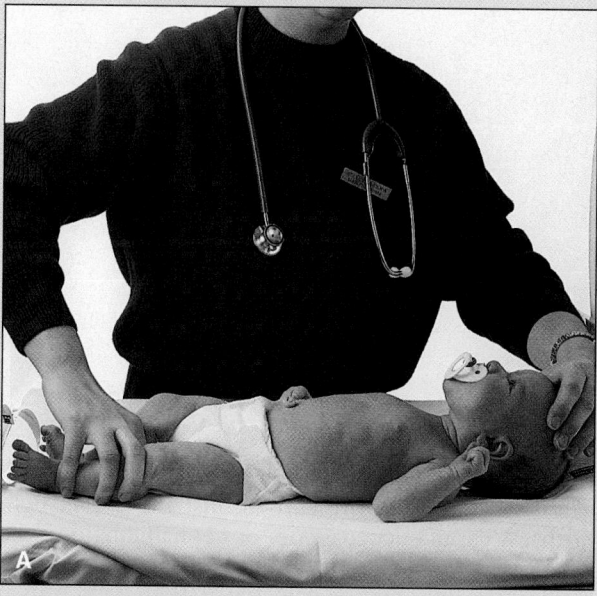

Photo by Keith Cotton

4. Hold the infant's feet in a vertical position. Bring the foot board up snugly against the bottom of the foot.	4. Completes measurement.
5. If an examining table is used, mark the spots at the top of the child's head and bottom of feet and then measure between the marks.	5. Provides for an alternative approach.
6. Plot height measurements on a standard graph.	6. Allows for interpretation of findings.
Older Child	
1. Have the child remove his or her shoes.	1. Promotes accuracy.
2. Have the child stand straight with his or her head held level.	2. Puts the child in the proper position for accurate measurement.
3. Align the measuring bar of a standing scale with the top of the head.	3. Determines the measurement.
4. If a scale with a measuring bar is not available, place a flat object such as a clipboard on the child's head in a horizontal position and read the height at the point at	4. Provides for an alternative approach.

(continued)

PROCEDURE	PRINCIPLE
which the object touches a measuring tape on the back of the scale or a flat wall surface (Figure B).	

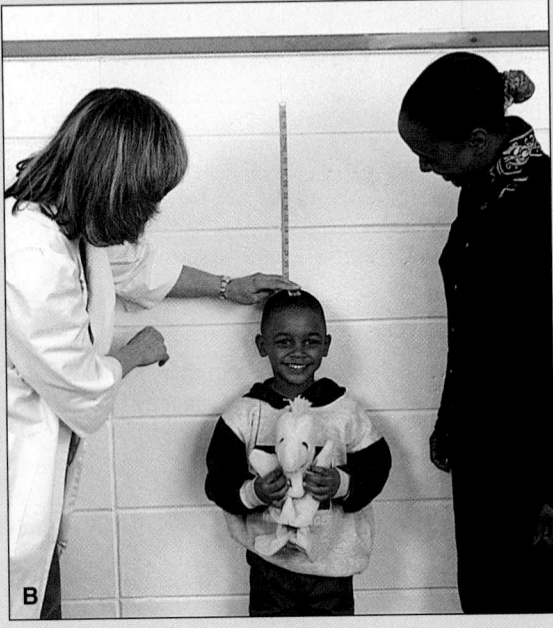

© Barbara Proud.

5. Plot height measurements on a standard graph.	**5.** Allows for interpretation of findings.

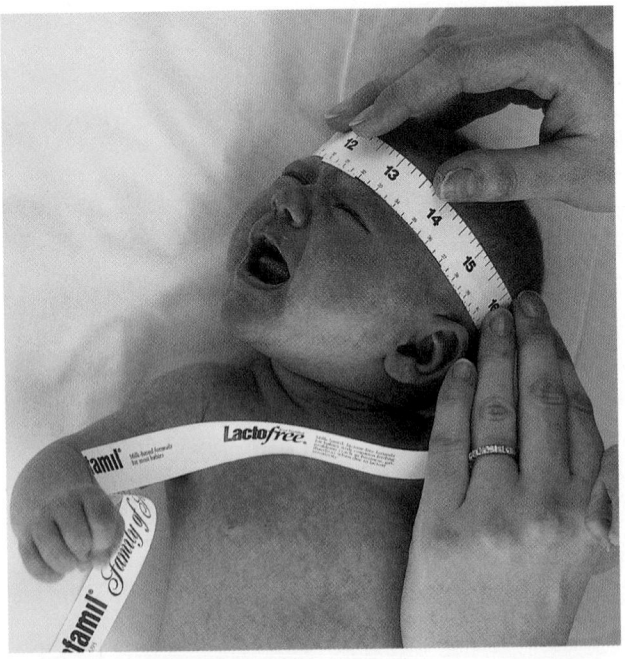

FIGURE 33.5 Measuring head circumference. The measuring tape passes just above the eyebrows and around the prominent posterior aspect of the head.

Newborn and Infant

In a newborn, the head usually shows molding (an elongated shape due to pressure against the cervix before birth). A caput succedaneum or cephalhematoma from the pressure of birth may be present (see Chapter 24). Skull suture lines may be palpable. In both newborns and infants, sit the child upright and palpate the skull for the presence of fontanelles (the places where the skull bones fuse). The anterior fontanelle is at the junction of the two parietal bones and the two fused frontal bones. It is diamond-shaped and measures 2 to 3 cm (0.8 to 1.2 in) in width and 3 to 4 cm (1.2 to 1.6 in) in length. The posterior fontanelle is at the junction of the parietal bones and the occipital bone. It is triangular and measures approximately 1 cm (0.5 in) in length (see Fig. 18.2).

With the infant sitting, fontanelles should be felt as soft spots but should not appear indented (a sign of dehydration) or bulging (a sign of increased intracranial pressure). When an infant cries, cerebral pressure increases; thus, with crying, the fontanelles may feel tense, and sometimes even the fluctuation of a pulse can be observed. The anterior fontanelle normally closes at 12 to 18 months and the posterior fontanelle by the end of 2 months. They should not be palpable after these times. The closing of fontanelles too early or too late may indicate decreased or increased brain or ventricle growth.

A scalp problem commonly encountered in infants is seborrhea (scaling, greasy-appearing, salmon-colored patches), or "cradle cap." Increasing the frequency of hair washing to once a day and applying baby oil to the scalp typically reduces this problem.

Toddler, Preschooler, and School-Age Child

Examine the hair of children who attend school or day care carefully for small white-yellow, sand-sized particles attached to hair strands—the eggs (nits) of pediculi (head lice). Nits cling and cannot be readily removed from hair by running fingers the length of the hair. The child may have recent scratch marks on the scalp and generally states that the scalp feels itchy. Pediculi spread easily in school-age children due to the sharing of combs and towels in school.

Also examine the scalp carefully for round circular areas (perhaps weeping in the center, crusting and scaling on the edges) that would suggest tinea capitis (ringworm, a fungal infection). Like pediculi, fungal infections can spread readily among school-age children; a prescription medication is necessary to best cure both conditions (see Chapter 43).

Adolescent

Adolescents may streak their hair with dye or arrange it in a way that requires gel, hair extensions, or use of a curling iron. Inspect to see that their scalp and hair are healthy underneath the styling.

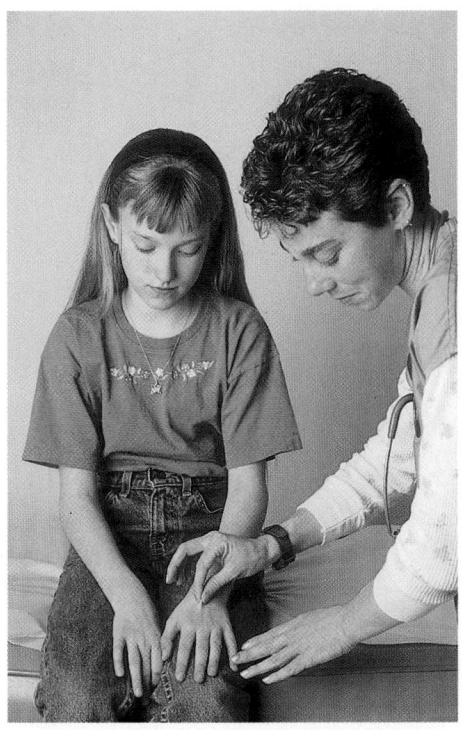

FIGURE 33.6 Assessing skin turgor. If the ridge of tissue does not immediately return to place, this suggests that the child is poorly hydrated.

TABLE 33.6

Skin Findings in Children That Suggest Illness

Finding	Indication
Central bluish color	Cyanosis from decreased respiratory function or cyanotic heart disease. Acrocyanosis (blue hands and feet) is normal in newborn for first 48 hours.
White color	Edema (accumulated subcutaneous fluid is stretching the skin)
Pale color	Anemia or decreased circulation to a body part
Reddened area	Local inflammation or increased systemic temperature
Linear abrasion	Scratch marks from local irritation from an insect bite, or allergic reaction
Ecchymoses (black and blue marks)	Recent injury to skin
Petechiae (pinpoint blood marks)	Blood dyscrasia (poor clotting ability)
Yellow color	Jaundice from increased bilirubin in subcutaneous tissue; carotenemia (excess carotene in skin)
Moistness	Excess perspiration from elevated temperature
Localized cold temperature	Decreased circulation to particular body part
Warm temperature	Local irritation or elevated systemic temperature
Poor turgor	Dehydration
Rash	Infectious childhood illness, excessive heat, allergy

Eyes

Observe eyes for symmetry and signs of frequent blinking, crusting, squinting, or rubbing. Observe lids and lashes for redness (erythema), which suggests infection. Common infections include **conjunctivitis** ("pink eye," an infection of the thin conjunctiva that covers the eye) or a **hordeolum** or stye (an infection of the gland that lubricates an eyelash). Both conditions require an antibiotic for therapy (see Chapter 50).

Assess the location of eyes in relation to the nose (not unusually wide- or narrow-spaced) and the relationship of the globe to the socket (neither sunken nor protruding from the socket [exophthalmos]). Abnormalities in these areas occur in chromosomal or metabolic illnesses such as hyperthyroidism. Inspect the sclera of the eye for spots of hemorrhage (called subconjunctival hemorrhage) or yellowing. African-American children often have a slight yellowing of the sclera and small black spots on the sclera; do not mistake these for abnormal findings. Assess that no sclera shows above the pupil (if it does, this is termed a sunset sign, an indication of increased intracranial pressure).

Palpate each eye globe with the eyelid closed to assess for tenseness, a finding suggesting glaucoma (rare in children). Determine whether the eyelids completely close (edema or neurologic illnesses may make eyelids too short to do this) when the child shuts the eyes. Also determine whether the lids retract far enough so they do not obscure vision when the child opens the eyes. When a lid obscures vision, a condition termed **ptosis,** it generally denotes neurologic involvement. The difference in Western and Eastern eye creases is shown in Figure 33.7.

Examine the inner lining of the lower eyelid (the conjunctiva) by pulling the lid down slightly with a fingertip. Here, the mucous membrane should appear pink and moist. In children with anemia, it often appears pale; with allergy or infection, it may appear unusually red and irritated. Do not initiate a blink reflex by touching the cornea with a wisp of cotton, as can be done in adults; this is momentarily painful and frightening to children.

In addition, observe whether the eyes appear to be in good alignment. **Strabismus** refers to eyes that are not evenly aligned. If an eye is always turning in, the condition is called **esotropia;** if it always turns out, **exotropia.** Two screening procedures for straight eye alignment include a Hirschberg's test and a cover test. During a Hirschberg's test, the light of an otoscope should reflect evenly off both pupils if they are in equal alignment (Fig. 33.8).

To perform a cover test (Fig. 33.9), follow these steps:

- Have the child fix his or her vision on an attractive object approximately 4 ft in front of the child.
- Hold a 3 × 5-inch card over the left eye for a count of 5. If any degree of strabismus is present, the eye will wander to its misaligned position while covered.
- Remove the card and observe the eye for movement.
- As the child again fixes his or her vision on the specified object in front, the eye will move back into line, revealing the misalignment.
- Repeat the process with the right eye. Movement after being uncovered suggests malalignment.

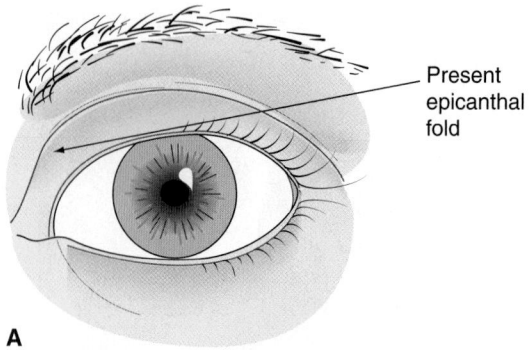

A

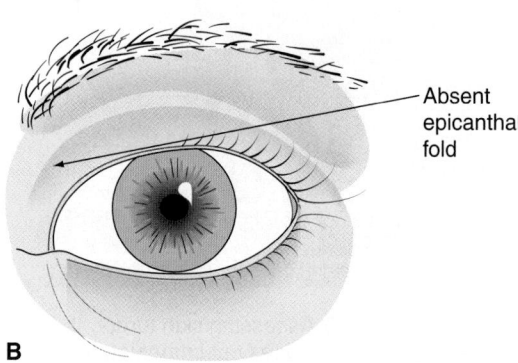

B

FIGURE 33.7 Differences in eye formation. (**A**) Western. (**B**) Eastern. The extra inner fold of tissue is an epicanthal fold.

Some children, particularly preschoolers who have wide epicanthic folds, may appear, at a quick glance, to show misalignment. A cover test is helpful in these children. There will be no eye movement after removal of the card because there is no misalignment present, only the temporary appearance of misalignment. Reasons for true misalignment are discussed in Chapter 50.

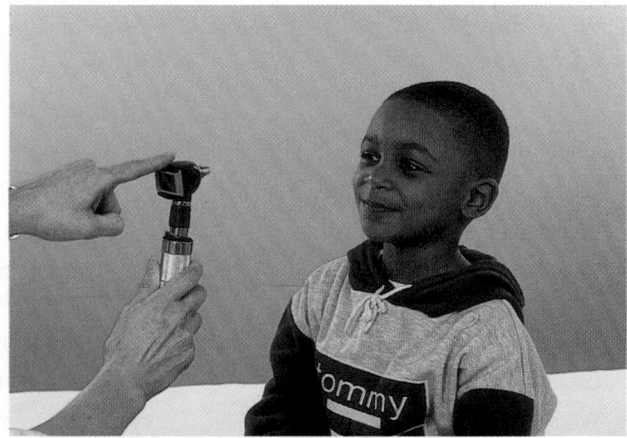

FIGURE 33.8 Testing good eye alignment by Hirschberg's test. The child is asked to look directly at the light of the otoscope. The light reflex on the pupils of both eyes will be equal if the eyes are in straight alignment.

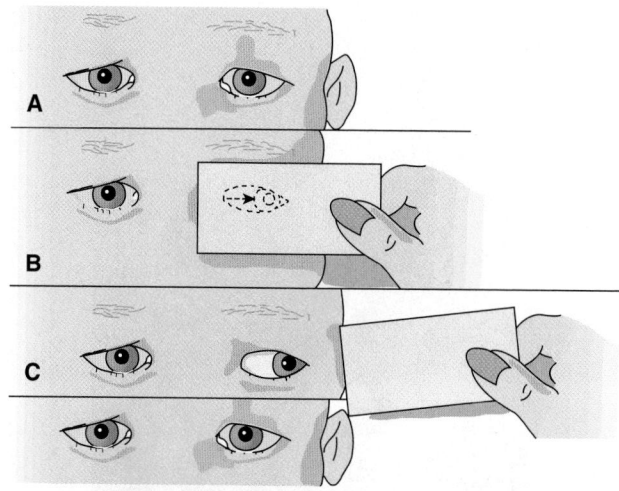

FIGURE 33.9 Cover test. **(A)** The child's eyes appear to be in good alignment. **(B)** The left eye is covered for 5 seconds. **(C)** When the card is removed, the left eye is seen to move perceptibly back to good alignment. This movement indicates that it "drifted" into a deviant position while covered, that is, that an exophoria (misalignment) is present.

Test the eyes for their ability to focus in all fields of vision by following these steps:

- Ask the child to follow a moving light (or catch the attention of an infant with a moving light) while holding the child's chin stationary.
- Move the light out to the side, then up, then down.
- Cross to the opposite side and move it up and down.
- Bring the light back to the midline and observe whether the child's eyes converge (follow the light to the nose) as the light moves in toward the nose. Infants under age 3 months cannot follow past the midline; the eyes of children under school age do not converge well.

Observe if the pupil constricts (reduces in size) in response to a light, an indication the third cranial nerve is intact. It is best to approach the child's eye from the forehead so the light suddenly appears on the pupil rather than advancing toward the child slowly. This makes the pupil constrict more dramatically. This should occur in response to a light shining directly on a pupil (direct constriction); when one pupil constricts, this will also occur in the opposite eye (consensual constriction). Record that pupils are equal in size and react to light as "PERL" (pupils equivalent, react to light). If the pupil converges (moves to follow a light in toward the nose), this is charted as "PEARL" or "PERLA" (pupils equal, react to light, accommodate).

For a final step, shine a flashlight or ophthalmoscope light into the pupil. A red reflex or the red pupil that occurs with a flash photo should appear. This is evidence that the retina is intact and the lens and cornea are clear (no tumor, cataract, scarring, or infection is present).

Newborn and Infant

Newborns often have a small, bright-red spot on the sclera (a subconjunctival hemorrhage) because the pressure of birth has ruptured a small conjunctival blood vessel. This is normal and will fade in 7 to 10 days as the blood is absorbed.

Infants can easily be tested for a red reflex, but until they are about 3 months, they cannot follow an object or light across the midline or follow a light into all six positions of gaze. Even a newborn, however, can follow a bright light to the midline. Assessing for a red reflex is important in newborns because a congenital cataract can lead to loss of central vision if not discovered early.

Toddler and Preschooler

Most young children are reluctant to let someone look into their eyes. Explaining what will happen during an eye examination is effective in reducing the child's anxiety about this part of the assessment.

School-Age Child and Adolescent

Many older children wear contact lenses (a red reflex is visible with a contact lens in place); some may be nervous about having their eyes examined because they know they should be wearing prescribed eyeglasses but are not wearing them because they do not like their appearance. Observe carefully for pupillary appearance and ability to constrict in adolescents to rule out drug abuse. Many adolescent girls are anemic and so have pale conjunctiva.

Nose

Observe the nose for flaring of the nostrils (a sign of need for oxygen). Using an otoscope light, observe the mucous membrane of the nose for color (it should be pink; pale suggests allergies, redness suggests infection). Note and describe any discharge. Document the septum is in the midline (displaced septa such as those that occur after facial injuries can interfere with respiration and make nasal intubation in emergencies difficult). Gently press one nostril closed and ask the child to inhale; repeat on the opposite side to ensure that both sides of the nose are patent (i.e., there is no choanal atresia or membrane obstructing the posterior nares). Sinuses do not fully develop until about 6 years. For children 6 or older, palpate the areas over the frontal and maxillary sinuses for tenderness, a symptom of sinus infection. Assess the sense of smell in school-age children and adolescents by asking them to identify a familiar odor such as chocolate or an orange.

Newborn and Infant

Infants are obligate nose breathers. They cannot coordinate mouth breathing, so they become disturbed when the nose is temporarily blocked to check for patency; do this only momentarily to avoid discomfort. Most newborns have milia (small white papules) on the surface of the nose.

Older Children

Many children, preschool age and older, have upper respiratory infections that cause reddened nasal mucous membranes and a purulent discharge. In contrast, allergies cause a clear discharge and pale mucous membranes. Children who have dry mucosa due to dry air (which leads to cracking and nosebleed) may be reluctant to allow inspection of their nose. Adolescents who sniff cocaine lose nasal hair and may have excoriations or abscesses in the mucous membrane. If the child has a nose piercing, inspect the site for redness or drainage.

Ears

Observe ears for proper alignment. In the average child, a line drawn from the inner canthus of the eye to the outer canthus and then to the ear will touch the top of the pinna of the ear (Fig. 33.10). Ears set lower than this are associated with chromosomal disorders such as trisomy 13. Observe the opening to the ear canal for any discharge. Touch the pinna and watch for evidence of pain (a sign of external canal infections). Observe the area immediately in front of the ear for a dermal sinus or a skin tag (a finding that is usually innocent but may be associated with kidney abnormalities). Observe the ear lobes for redness or drainage from infected piercing sites.

To examine the ear canal, follow these steps:

- Straighten the ear canal by pulling the pinna gently down and back in the child under 2 years of age and up and back in the older child.
- Select an otoscope tip. Otoscope tip sizes vary; use the smallest size possible that still gives adequate visibility.
- With the ear canal held straight, insert an otoscope tip into the external canal.
- Rest the instrument on a hand, not on the child's head (Fig. 33.11). In this position, the otoscope will move with a child, avoiding the danger that the plastic tip will scratch the canal if a child should move his or her head suddenly.
- Inspect the sides of the ear canal and locate landmarks on the surface of the tympanic membrane.

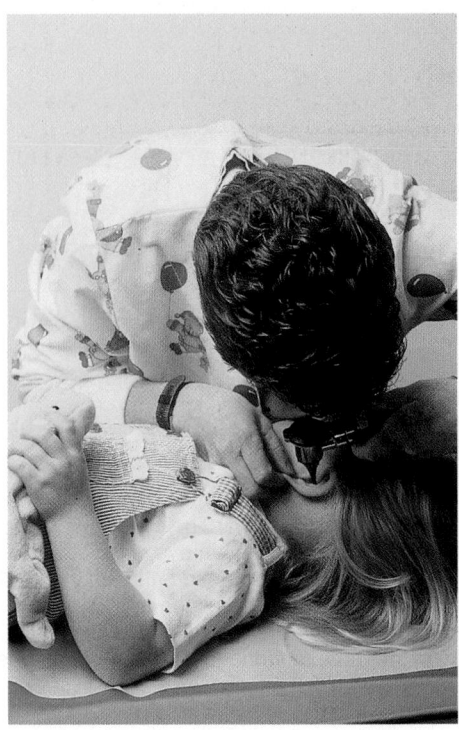

FIGURE 33.11 Otoscopic examination. Note how the nurse's hand rests between the otoscope and the child's head. Should the child move suddenly, no injury to the tympanic membrane will be sustained with this technique because the otoscope will move along with the child's head.

The outline of the malleus of the inner ear through the translucent membrane is a key landmark to visualize (Figure 33.12). The color of the membrane is pinkish gray; if the tension of the membrane is normal, a cone of light (the light reflex) should be present in one of the lower corners (at either the 5 o'clock or 7 o'clock position).

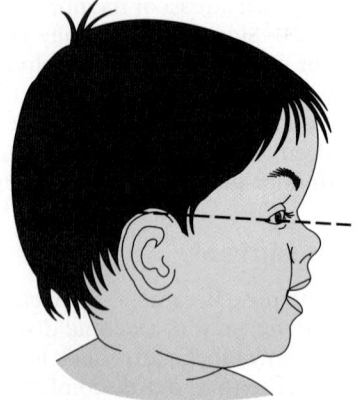

FIGURE 33.10 Normal ear alignment. When a line is drawn from the inner canthus through the outer canthus to the ear, the top of the ear pinna should meet the line. Abnormal ear alignment is associated with certain chromosomal abnormalities.

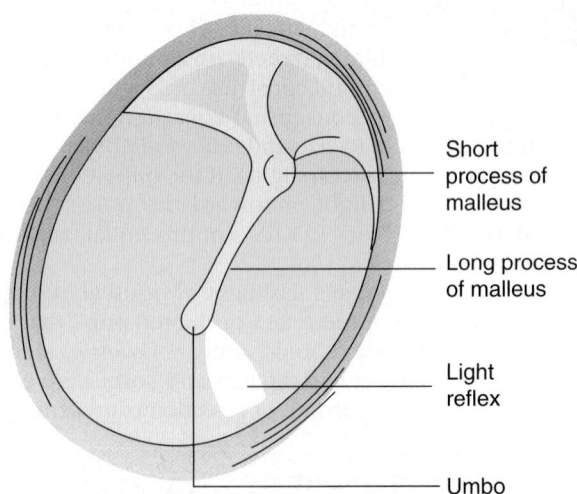

Short process of malleus

Long process of malleus

Light reflex

Umbo

FIGURE 33.12 A tympanic membrane as viewed with an otoscope.

Although many children have wax (cerumen) in their ear canals, appearing as a dark-brown, glistening substance, viewing the tympanic membrane past the wax is almost always possible.

If an ear infection is present, the tympanic membrane appears reddened and often bulges forward so the malleus is no longer discernible and the cone of light is absent. If there is fluid in the middle ear, it may be possible to see bubbles of air through the membrane. With chronic middle ear disease (serous otitis media), the tympanic membrane may be retracted, the malleus is extremely prominent, and the cone of light is again missing. If the membrane has been torn from trauma or rupture, the jagged edge and opening to the middle ear are discernible. Inspect also for any ulcerated areas that could be a cholesteatoma or an ingrowing tumor (see Chapter 50).

The mobility of the eardrum can be tested by injecting a column of air into the ear canal against the drum by a pneumatic attachment on an otoscope that looks like the bulb of a blood pressure cuff (Fig. 33.13). A normal drum is freely mobile and can be seen to move with pressure on the bulb; one with fluid behind it has decreased mobility. Before introducing air, warn the child that this "tickles."

Finally, appraise hearing. Appraisal can be done grossly in older children by assessing their response to questions. Distract an infant with a toy; then make a sound behind the infant's back, out of peripheral vision, and watch for the response. Hearing infants will show some noticeable reaction, although they have difficulty looking directly toward or locating the sound until about 4 months of age.

Newborn and Infant

Many newborns still have amniotic fluid or vernix caseosa in their ear canal, so inspecting the ear canal is ineffective.

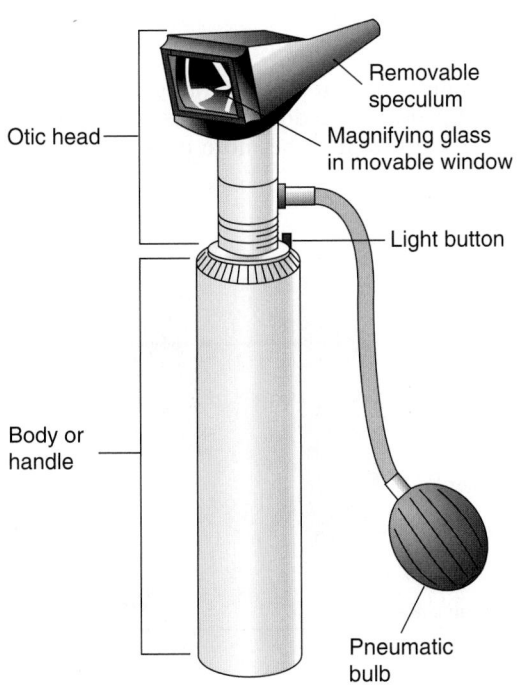

FIGURE 33.13 Otoscope with pneumatic attachment.

Be certain to assess for ear level and normal pinna contour. Assess gross hearing ability—for example, by watching the infant startle to a sudden sound or quiet to the calming effect of quiet talking.

Older Children

Middle ear infection (otitis media) is a common childhood illness. This causes the ear to be painful when examined. An external ear infection (often called swimmer's ear) causes any movement of the pinna to be painful. For these reasons and because children are told many times never to put anything into their ears, they usually resist ear examinations. Explaining what is happening helps to allay any fears. Beginning with preschool age, children may have myringotomy tubes (small circular plastic tubes placed into the tympanic membrane) to relieve chronic fluid collected in the middle ear. Inspect that the area surrounding the tube is not inflamed and the tube is not merely lying in the external canal and no longer inserted into the membrane (see Chapter 50).

Mouth

Assess the external appearance of the lips, looking for symmetry and color. Ask a child to smile and frown to evaluate the mobility of facial muscles. Count the number of teeth present and assess their condition (number missing or cavities present). Inspect the gum line (gingivae) for redness, tenderness, and edema, symptoms of periodontal disease. Inspect the buccal membrane and palate for color (pink) and the presence of any lesions. Ask a child to stick out the tongue and assess for midline position and no fasciculations (trembling). Inspect the area under the tongue for lesions in school-age children and adolescents who smoke or chew tobacco because this is the most common first site for oral cancer.

A child's tongue is normally smooth and moist. With dehydration present, it often appears roughened and dry. **Geographic tongue** is a term for the rough-appearing tongue surface that often accompanies general symptoms of illness such as fever; it may also occur normally. If a child has had the tongue pierced, inspect for redness at the site. Assess that the object is secure so there is little chance of aspiration or that it is not striking tooth enamel and wearing this away.

Inspect the uvula to be certain it is in the midline. Use a tongue blade to press down and forward on the back of the tongue (Fig. 33.14). The epiglottis can usually be observed with the tongue depressed. Observe for abnormal enlargement, palatine redness, or drainage of tonsils. Although tonsillar tissue differs greatly in size, it should not be reddened or have pus in the crypts (indentations). After initiating the gag reflex in an infant to view the back of the throat, always turn the infant's head to the side so he or she does not choke on any saliva that accumulated in the mouth during the throat examination. Infants are less able to manage this than are adults.

Do not depress the tongue of any child who is suspected to have epiglottitis or whose glottis is inflamed. Symptoms of this condition are a sore throat, drooling, fever, difficulty with respiration, dysphagia, and a barking

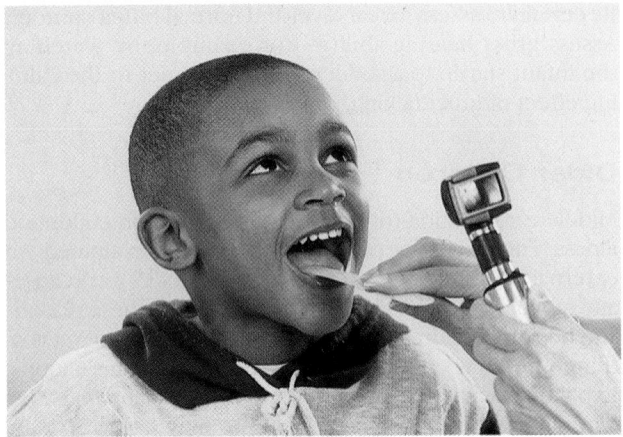

FIGURE 33.14 Inspecting the pharynx in a schoolager.

cough. If a swollen, inflamed epiglottis rises with the pressure of a tongue blade, it can obstruct the respiratory tract so completely the child is immediately unable to breathe.

Newborn and Infant

Many newborns have considerable mucus in their mouths because they are less able to handle swallowing due to immature muscle coordination. If a newborn has teeth, evaluate them for stability; if loose, they may need to be removed to prevent aspiration. Assess for white patches that do not scrape away from the buccal membrane or tongue (thrush), a common but abnormal finding in infants that needs antifungal therapy.

Older Children

Tonsillar tissue in children reaches its maximum growth at early school age, making many preschool children appear to be "all tonsils." As long as the tissue does not appear reddened or tender, it can be assumed to be normal for the age. Many children have irregular, pale-pink, elevated projections on the posterior pharynx as a normal finding. A stream of mucopurulent discharge in the posterior pharynx is not unusual if an upper respiratory infection and a "postnasal" flow of secretions are present. For a child with orthodontic appliances such as braces, assess carefully for pinpoint ulcers to be certain the wires are not causing undue discomfort or infection. Cavities appear as dark-brown areas on the tooth enamel. Many school-age children or adolescents have at least one present.

 Checkpoint Question 3

You typically gag children to inspect the back of their throat. When is it important *not* to elicit a gag reflex?

a. When children are under 5 years of age
b. When a child has symptoms of epiglottitis
c. When a boy has a possible inguinal hernia
d. When a girl has a geographic tongue

Neck

Assess the neck for symmetry (the trachea should be in the midline; any deviation suggests lung pathology). Observe the outline of the thyroid gland (barely noticeable before puberty because it is obscured by the sternocleidomastoid muscle) on the anterior neck. Palpate the area in front of the ear (location of the parotid gland) and smooth a hand over the location of lymph nodes at the sides of the neck and under the chin to palpate for swelling. Figure 33.15 shows the location of lymph node chains of the head and neck. Because children have so many upper respiratory infections, a few nodes that are freely movable, about the size of peas, are often present. Commonly, preauricular and postauricular nodes are palpable after ear infections, and postoccipital nodes are palpable after a scalp infection. Submental nodes generally denote a tooth abscess. Palpable submaxillary, anterior, and posterior cervical nodes follow throat infections.

Ask the child to move the head (or move it for the child) through flexion (touch chin to chest) and extension (raise chin as high as possible), and turn it right and left (rotation) to see that a child does this easily. Pain on forward flexion is an important sign of neurologic (meningeal) irritation.

Newborn and Infant

With infants, always assess the ability to control the head by laying the infant supine and pulling the child to a sitting position. Babies younger than 4 months of age will let their heads lag backward as they are pulled up this way; they right their heads only as they reach a sitting position. After 4 months, infants should bring their head up with them (no head lag) if their neuromuscular coordination is adequate for their age. This simple but important test yields information about overall neuromuscular control.

Adolescent

In adolescents, palpate the thyroid gland for symmetry and possible nodes. To do this, press on the right side of the gland, causing it to be more prominent on the left

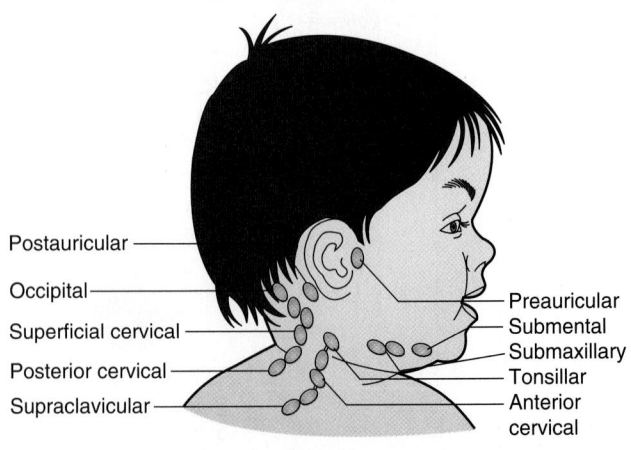

FIGURE 33.15 Location of lymph node chains in the head and neck.

side. Then palpate the left half to discern any irregularities (areas of hardness). Repeat on the right side. A finding of a thyroid node needs to be investigated. It may be only an innocent transient cyst, or it may be the first indication of thyroid malignancy. Many adolescents have some increase in the size of the thyroid at puberty; this hypertrophy should not be accompanied by any nodes.

Chest

For ease in specifying the location of chest pathology, the chest is divided into sections by imaginary lines drawn through the mid-clavicle, mid-mammary, and midsternum points on the front; the mid-axilla on the side; and the mid-scapula on the back. Pathology is described in terms of these lines (e.g., abnormal lung sound heard at left mid-axillary line). Other helpful means of locating pathology is by the suprasternal notch, the ribs, and the spaces between them (**intercostal spaces**). Intercostal spaces are numbered according to the ribs immediately above them (Fig. 33.16). Inspect both front and back surfaces of the chest for symmetry of appearance and motion. An infant with a diaphragmatic hernia (intestine herniated into the chest cavity) may have a chest enlarged on that side. An infant with atelectasis (collapsed lung) may have a chest that is smaller on the affected side. If a child has an enlarged heart, the left side of the chest may appear larger. Inspect for **retractions** or indentation of intercostal spaces or the suprasternal and substernal areas that reflect difficult respirations. Assess the proportion of anteroposterior to lateral diameter (normally 1:2). Children with chronic lung disease develop a broad (barrel) chest or one more rounded than normal (Bezyack, 2004). This and other chest abnormalities are shown in Figure 33.17.

Breasts

The degree of breast assessment depends on the child's age and development. As part of a normal breast assessment, inspect and palpate the breasts of all children to detect any abnormalities.

Newborn

Both male and female newborns may have breast edema from the influence of maternal hormones. A few drops of clear fluid may even be present from the nipples. This is normal. Document if a supernumerary nipple is present for baseline data.

School-Age Child and Adolescent

Do a breast examination on all girls past puberty. If a girl younger than 8 years is beginning breast development, precocious puberty (see Chapter 48) should be suspected. Many preadolescent boys develop hypertrophy of breast tissue due to increased hormonal influences (gynecomastia); they are generally concerned and need reassurance this is normal for their age and will fade as soon as androgen becomes their dominant hormone. Adolescent girls may be concerned their breast tissue is inadequate or that breast growth is uneven. They can be assured that not all women have completely symmetric breasts.

Inspection of breast tissue is easiest if a child sits on the examining table, arms at the sides, with both breasts exposed. Inspect for symmetry. As mentioned, it is normal and not unusual for a girl to have breasts of slightly unequal size.

Inspect breasts for edema, erythema, wrinkling, retraction, or dimpling of the skin; all suggest that a tumor is growing in deeper layers of the tissue. Erythema occurs from inflammation due to abnormal, rapidly growing tissue; edema results from the blockage of lymph channels due to tumor pressure. Breast edema makes the skin appear not only swollen but also pitted (an orange-peel effect). Note any nipple discharge or "pulled" nipple placement as another way to detect edema.

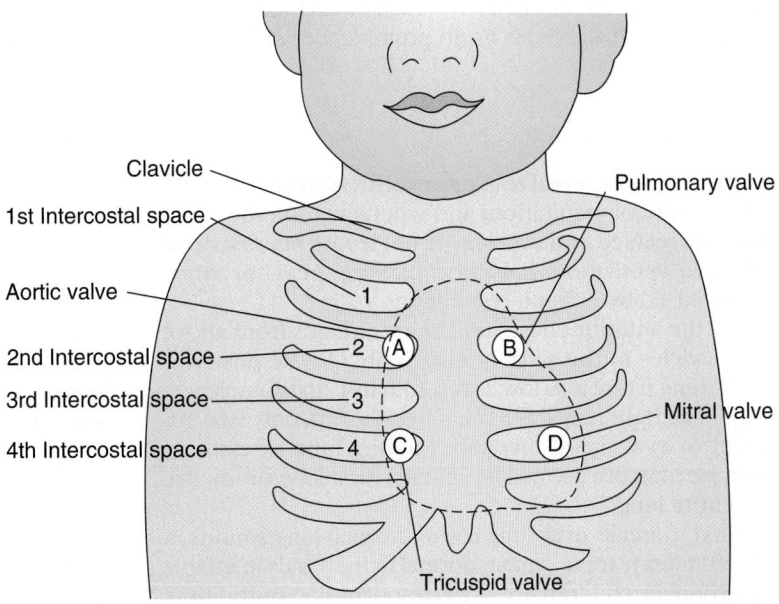

FIGURE 33.16 Intercostal (between rib) spaces are numbered according to the ribs immediately above them. The points (**A, B, C,** and **D**) to which the sounds of the heart valves radiate or where the sounds can be heard best are the listening posts of the heart.

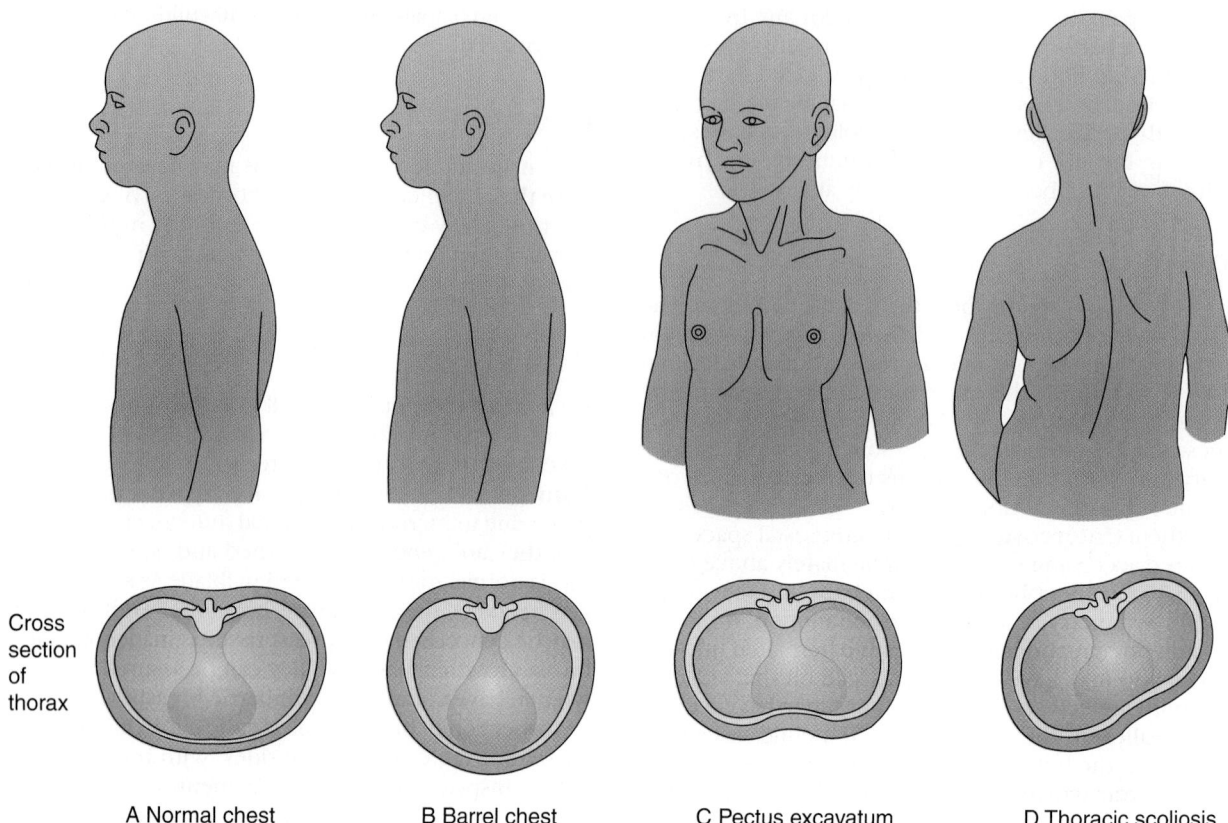

Cross
section
of
thorax

A Normal chest   B Barrel chest   C Pectus excavatum   D Thoracic scoliosis

FIGURE 33.17 Chest contours that can be assessed by inspection. (**A**) Normal chest.
(**B**) Barrel chest. (**C**) Funnel chest (pectus excavatum). (**D**) Thoracic kyphoscoliosis.

With the girl's arms at her sides to take pressure off breast tissue, palpate well into each axilla (because breast tissue extends that far), and also palpate to assess axillary lymph nodes. Normally, no nodes should be felt. Ask the girl to lie down; place a folded towel under her near shoulder. Palpate the near breast with her lying down with her arm raised and placed under her head because this spreads out breast tissue; begin at the nipple and palpate outward in a circular motion. The lower edge of each breast feels hard; do not mistake this or rib prominences underneath for a tumor.

Lungs

Various findings reveal respiratory distress in children. Assess the rate of respirations and whether respirations are easy and relaxed or if accessory muscles are necessary for effective ventilation. Palpate over lung areas for vibrations caused by difficult respirations.

On the anterior chest, lung tissue extends from above the clavicles to the sixth or eighth rib. On the posterior chest, lung tissue is as low as the 10th to 12th thoracic vertebra. The right lung has three lobes; the left, only two. Attempt to evaluate all five lobes during lung assessment because lung disease can be specific for a lobe or involve the entire lung.

Next, percuss over lung tissue. Normal lung sounds in older children are resonant; normal lung sounds in infants and younger children are hyperresonant due to the thin-

ness of the chest wall; overexpanded lungs sound hyperresonant in older children; and lungs filled with fluid sound dull in older children and less resonant in younger children. The lower anterior lobe of the right lung will sound dull because the liver covers it on the anterior surface below the fourth or fifth intercostal space. The space over the heart will also sound dull.

Diaphragmatic excursion (the distance the diaphragm descends with inhalation) is an estimation of lung volume. To establish this:

• Ask the child to take in a deep breath and hold it.
• Percuss downward to locate the bottom of the lungs (the percussion note changes from resonant to flat at that point).
• Ask the child to expire fully and momentarily hold that position.
• Percuss upward to locate the expired or empty lung position (the percussion note changes from flat to resonant).

The difference between these two points is the diaphragmatic excursion. Children who have overexpanded lungs from obstructive disease will have less diaphragmatic excursion than others.

Auscultate breath sounds by listening with the diaphragm of a stethoscope over each lung lobe while a child inhales and exhales (preferably with his or her mouth open). Listen both anteriorly and posteriorly; compare the left side with the right side for equal findings. Normal breath sounds are slightly longer on inspiration than ex-

TABLE 33.7

Breath Sounds Heard on Auscultation

Sound	Characteristics
Vesicular	Soft, low-pitched, heard over periphery of lungs, inspiration longer than expiration. Normal.
Bronchovesicular	Soft, medium-pitched, heard over major bronchi; inspiration equals expiration. Normal.
Bronchial	Loud, high-pitched, heard over trachea; expiration longer than inspiration. Normal.
Rhonchi	Snoring sound made by air moving through mucus in bronchi. Normal.
Rales (also called crackles)	Crackling or crinkling sound (like cellophane) made by air moving through fluid in alveoli. Abnormal.
Wheezing	Whistling on expiration made by air being pushed through narrowed bronchi. Abnormal; seen in children with asthma or foreign body obstruction.
Stridor	Crowing or rooster-like sound made by air being pulled through a constricted larynx. Abnormal; seen in children with upper respiratory obstruction.

piration. Consider whether there are any abnormal sounds. Table 33.7 describes normal breath sounds and transmitted airway sounds as well as adventitious sounds that, if heard, might reflect illness.

Newborn and Infant

Infants cannot breathe in and out on request. Try to listen to breath sounds early in an examination, because breath sounds are difficult to hear clearly over the sound of crying.

Heart

Heart assessment begins with visual inspection to see if there is a point on the chest where the heartbeat can be observed. This point represents the location of the left ventricle or the point where the apical heartbeat can be heard best. In children younger than 7 years of age, this point is generally lateral to the nipple line and at the fourth intercostal space. In children older than 4 years, it is at the nipple line or just medial to it and at the fifth intercostal space. This point is termed the **point of maximum impulse** (PMI) and is observable in approximately 50% of children.

Percuss the left side of the chest to discern the left side of the heart. Percussing in from the axilla, the sound will become dull as the heart is identified. A heart located further to the left than usual suggests enlargement. Normally, the percussion note changes from resonant (percussing over lung) to flat (percussing over heart) midway between the mid-axillary and mid-mammary line.

Heart Sounds

To hear heart sounds, auscultate at four main points. Although these are not the anatomic locations of heart valves, they are the listening points to which the sounds of the valves radiate and can be heard best in children (see Fig. 33.16).

- The mitral valve is heard best at the fourth or fifth left intercostal space at the nipple line.

- The tricuspid valve is heard best near the base of the sternum (fourth or fifth right intercostal space).
- The pulmonary valve is heard best at the second left intercostal space.
- The aortic valve is heard best at the second right intercostal space.

Table 33.8 describes normal and abnormal heart sounds that may be heard on auscultation. Abnormal sounds are heard best if the diaphragm of the stethoscope is used first, followed by the bell of the stethoscope.

To understand heart sounds, recall heart physiology. The first sound heard (S_1) is that of the mitral and tricuspid valves closing and the ventricles contracting (described as a "lub" sound). The second sound (described as a "dub"; S_2) is made by the closure of the aortic and pulmonary valves and atrial contraction. The first sound is generally longer and lower-pitched than the second sound. It is louder than the second sound over the heart ventricles; otherwise, it is slightly quieter.

Note the rhythm of the heart sounds. This should be regular. **Sinus arrhythmia** is a phenomenon that most

TABLE 33.8

Heart Sounds Heard on Auscultation

Sound	Cause
S_1 (first heart sound)	Closure of tricuspid and mitral valves with beginning of ventricular contraction (systole)
S_2 (second heart sound)	Closure of pulmonary and aortic valves with beginning of atrial contraction (diastole)
S_3 (third heart sound)	Rapid ventricular filling
S_4 (fourth heart sound)	Abnormal filling of ventricles

school-age and adolescent children demonstrate. With sinus arrhythmia, a marked heart rate increase occurs as a child inspires and a marked decrease in heart rate is noted as the child expires. This is a normal finding. Ask the child to hold his or her breath, and the rhythm of the heart remains the same.

With inspiration and the normal resulting increase of pressure in the lungs, the pulmonary valve tends to close slightly later than the aortic valve. This is termed **physiologic splitting** and is heard as "lub d-dub." As long as this is associated with inspiration, it is a normal finding. Fixed splitting implies there is always difficulty with the pulmonary valve closing and suggests pathology.

At times, a distinct third heart sound (S_3) may be heard due to rapid filling of the ventricles. Although this is not necessarily a serious finding, further investigation is warranted. The presence of a fourth heart sound (S_4) generally signifies heart pathology because this sound (a gallop rhythm) is caused by abnormal filling of the ventricles.

Listen to the heart in all areas; assess rate and compare this to the child's age to determine if it is a normal rate (Fig. 33.18). A heart murmur is caused by the sound of blood flowing with difficulty or in a different pathway within the heart (sounds like a swishing sound) and can be either innocent (functional) or pathogenic (organic). If a heart is pumping with abnormal force, there may be a palpable vibration termed a thrill on the chest wall. Palpate the precordium (area over the heart) for evidence of this (feels like a cat purring) or a heave (a definite outward chest movement), which also denotes a struggling heart. On hearing or palpating any accessory heart sounds or movements, try to describe them with reference to Table 33.9.

All unusual heart sounds need further identification and investigation of their cause. The skills of listening to and identifying normal and abnormal heart sounds require considerable practice. Determining the cause of an abnormal heart sound requires a cardiac specialist. Determining that an abnormal sound exists, however, and securing proper referral is an important nursing role.

Newborn, Infant, and Toddler

Listen to heart sounds in young children early in an examination, before a child begins to cry, because it is almost impossible to evaluate heart sounds over the sound of crying. Allowing a parent to hold a child while listening to the heart helps reduce fear.

School-Age Child and Adolescent

Listen carefully for sounds of murmurs in children of school age and older. Be particularly conscientious with student athletes; it seems paradoxical that they could have heart disease, yet heart disease can be fatal to them during athletic events (Trusty, Beinborn, & Jahangir, 2004). Refer them to a physician for further evaluation if any abnormalities are detected. Parents are always frightened by an unusual heart sound, but unless the child has other symptoms, they can be assured that most murmurs are innocent (functional) and caused only by the normal flow of blood across valves.

Checkpoint Question 4

Keoto has a sinus arrhythmia. This refers to:

a. A wide spaced rib cage
b. Faint, barely audible heart sounds
c. Increased heart rate on inspiration
d. An abnormal heart rate in a child

Abdomen

The abdomen is divided anatomically into four quadrants. The quadrants and the organs that lie within them are shown in Figure 33.19. To assess an abdomen, first inspect the surface for symmetry and contour. It will be slightly protuberant in infants and scaphoid in older children. Note any skin lesions or scars.

Auscultate the abdomen for bowel sounds before palpating, because palpating may alter bowel movement (peristalsis) and therefore disturb bowel sounds. Bowel sounds can normally be heard in all quadrants of the abdomen. They are high "pinging" sounds that occur normally at intervals of approximately 5 to 10 seconds. Since these sounds are high-pitched sounds, they may be heard best with the bell of a stethoscope. If the bowel is distended, the sounds occur more frequently; if the bowel is blocked so that there is no movement of contents, the sounds will be absent below the obstruction. Listen for 3 to 5 minutes before concluding that no bowel sounds are present to be certain they are not just widely spaced.

Listen along the middle of the abdomen over the aorta for irregular sounds. A **bruit** is a swishing or blowing sound that occurs if there is an outpouching of the aorta (an aneurysm), a condition that can be congenital, although it usually occurs with aging.

Palpate the abdomen in a systematic manner to include all four quadrants. First palpate lightly, then deeply. Ascertain whether any area is tender by watching the child's face while palpating; observe for guarding or the child tensing the abdominal muscles to keep you from pressing deeply at that point. If a child indicates any portion of the

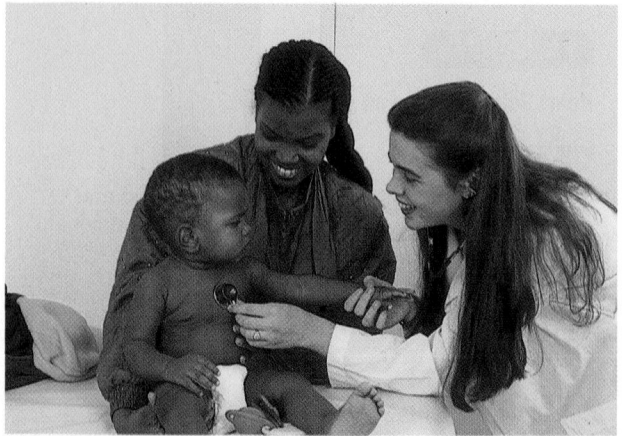

FIGURE 33.18 Auscultating heart sounds.

TABLE 33.9

Description of Accessory Heart Sounds

Assessment	Information to be Gathered
Location	At which listening post is the sound most distinct?
Quality	Can sound be described as blowing, rubbing, rasping, musical?
Intensity	*Murmurs* are graded according to the following criteria:
	Grade 6: So loud it can be heard with stethoscope not touching the chest wall; has a thrill (palpable vibration).
	Grade 5: Very loud but must touch stethoscope to chest to hear; has a thrill.
	Grade 4: Loud; may or may not have a thrill.
	Grade 3: Moderately loud; no thrill.
	Grade 2: Quiet but easily discernible.
	Grade 1: Very quiet; difficult to hear.
Timing	When in relation to S_1 and S_2 did you hear it? A sound superimposed between S_1 and S_2 is a *systolic murmur*; one between S_2 and the next S_1 is a *diastolic murmur*. Innocent murmurs (functional, denoting no pathology) are usually systolic, although there are exceptions to this; pathologic murmurs are more likely to be diastolic.
Pitch	Can the sound be described as high- or low-pitched?
Radiation and thrills	Is there an accompanying thrill? Does sound radiate so it can be heard at another location, such as back of chest?

abdomen is tender, begin assessment at the farthest point and work toward the tender area. If no tenderness is present, the order of palpation is unimportant as long as it is thorough. Note any hard areas or masses. If a tender area is detected, attempt to elicit rebound tenderness to determine its cause. To do this, press in on the abdomen, then lift your hand suddenly. This causes internal organs to vibrate. More pain with the vibration than with the original pressure is diagnostic of appendicitis.

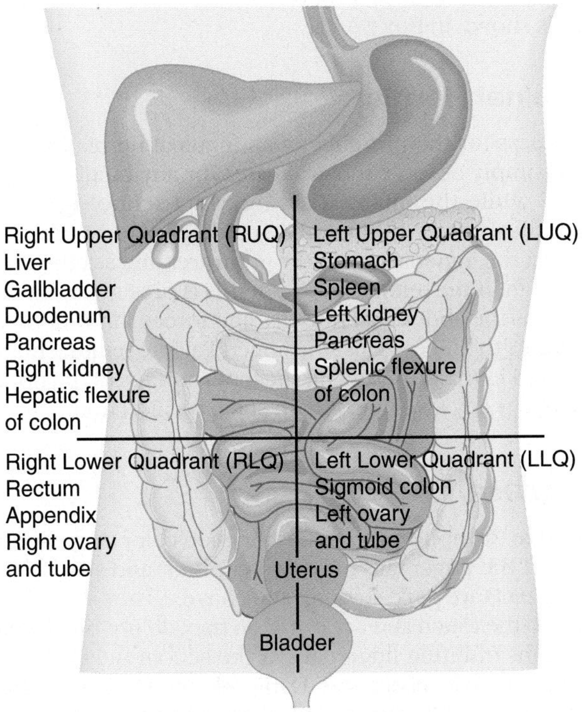

By palpating from the right lower quadrant to the right upper quadrant, the hand will bump against the lower edge of the liver 1 to 2 cm below the right ribs. On the left side, the lower edge of the spleen may be discernible in the same way. A liver or spleen larger than this is suggestive of disease. Palpate the umbilicus to try to identify the presence of an umbilical hernia. A fascial ring at the umbilicus of more than 2 cm in diameter in an infant denotes a ring of fascia larger than will normally close spontaneously; when this is present, the child will generally need surgery to prevent an umbilical hernia. Liver, spleen, and bladder size can all be documented further by percussion.

Newborn and Infant

Kidneys may be located by deep abdominal palpation in newborns and infants. The right kidney is slightly lower than the left and so is easier to locate. The optimal time to palpate the kidney of a newborn is during the first few hours of life, before the bowels begin to fill with air and obscure palpation. To palpate the kidneys:

- Place a hand under an infant's back just below the 12th rib.
- Press upward.
- Place the other hand on that side of the abdomen just below the umbilicus.
- Press deeply.
- Locate the kidney, which can be felt as a firm mass approximately the size of a walnut between the hands.

Right Upper Quadrant (RUQ)
Liver
Gallbladder
Duodenum
Pancreas
Right kidney
Hepatic flexure
of colon

Left Upper Quadrant (LUQ)
Stomach
Spleen
Left kidney
Pancreas
Splenic flexure
of colon

Right Lower Quadrant (RLQ)
Rectum
Appendix
Right ovary
and tube

Left Lower Quadrant (LLQ)
Sigmoid colon
Left ovary
and tube

Uterus

Bladder

FIGURE 33.19 Quadrants of the abdomen and underlying structures.

Preschooler and School-Age Child

Children's abdomens at this age are often "ticklish," and children may tense or guard their abdominal muscles when touched, making it difficult to palpate. Distract a child by asking a question about home or school, or let a child put his or her hand under the examiner's to help relax (Fig. 33.20).

Genitorectal Area

In both sexes, the rectum should be inspected for any protruding hemorrhoidal tissue (rare in children) or fissures. Fissures may signify chronic constipation, intra-abdominal pressure, or sexual abuse.

Female Genitalia

Inspection of external female genitalia and assessment of femoral nodes are included in every complete health assessment. An external examination consists of inspecting for Tanner stage of hair growth and configuration (an inverted triangle) and inspection of external genitalia (i.e., clitoris, labia majora, and labia minora) for normal contours. Look for signs of discharge or irritation. A vaginal discharge or fourchette tear in a young child may be an indication of sexual abuse, in an adolescent of rape (Jones et al., 2003). A pelvic examination is usually scheduled at the time the girl becomes sexually active or at age 18 (AAP, 2005). The technique for an internal pelvic examination is discussed in Chapter 10.

Male Genitalia

Inspection of male genitalia consists of observing:

- The distribution and Tanner stage of hair, which has a diamond shape
- The penis, for lesions that might suggest a sexually transmitted infection
- Appearance and placement of the urethral opening, which should be slitlike and centered at the penis tip. Children with repeated urinary tract infections develop

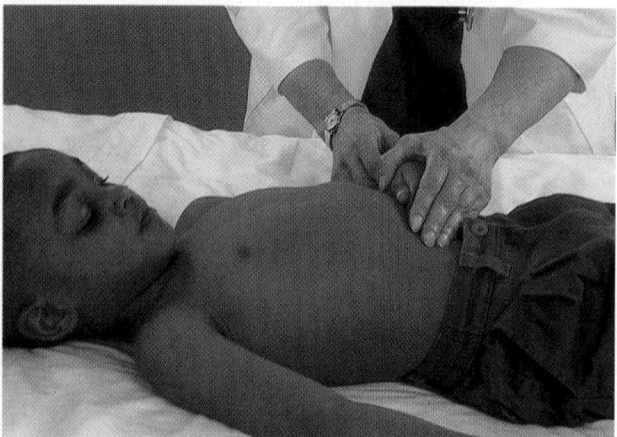

FIGURE 33.20 Decrease ticklishness during abdominal palpation by placing the child's hand under yours.

scarring of the meatal opening, making it small and round.
- The ability to retract the foreskin, if a boy is uncircumcised. Phimosis exists when the foreskin of a child older than 6 to 12 months is too tight to retract.

Hypospadias is a term for a urethral opening located on the inferior or ventral (under) surface of the penis; **epispadias** denotes a urethral opening on the superior or dorsal (upper) surface. Both these conditions need to be identified. If more than a slight deviation is present, repair is usually initiated before school age because such a urethral placement may interfere with self-image if not corrected. With adulthood, it can interfere with fertility.

Inspect the scrotum for size and the presence of testes. In most boys, the left testicle is slightly lower than the right, so the scrotum does not appear truly symmetric. Palpate to check that both testes are present by placing one hand over the top of the scrotum at the inguinal ring and then palpating the testis on that side (see Fig. 24.17). This hand position prevents the testis from slipping up into the inguinal ring and appearing to be absent on palpation. Any swelling or mass in the scrotum needs to be identified. The most likely cause of such a condition is a **hydrocele,** or a fluid-filled sac, but it could represent a serious finding such as testicular cancer in adolescents. Hydroceles can be transilluminated: when a flashlight is held in back of the scrotum, the fluid-filled cyst glows. A **varicocele** (enlarged veins of the epididymis) may be palpated. These are not important findings in young boys, but they may interfere with fertility in later life.

Assess the urethral meatus for any discharge that could reveal a sexually transmitted infection such as gonorrhea or any lesions that would suggest herpes 2 infection or syphilis (see Chapter 47). Beginning at puberty, teach boys to do testicular palpation every month. The technique for this is shown in Box 33.11.

Inguinal Hernia

To assess for the presence of an inguinal hernia in an infant, simply observe the groin area for any bulging (especially while the infant is crying). In a school-age child or adolescent, with the child standing, place a fingertip against the inguinal ring in the groin area and ask the child to cough. If the tendency for a hernia is present, coughing tightens the abdominal muscles and forces the abdominal contents to bulge against the finger. Palpate femoral nodes (located in the groin and on the inner surface of the upper thigh) for any swelling, which suggests infection.

Extremities

Observe the upper extremities for good color and warmth. Inspect the fingernails for color, contour, and shape. Normally, nails are pink, smooth, and convex. They should feel hard to the touch and not brittle so they do not break readily. Signs of bitten fingernails in the school-age child may reflect a high level of stress. Darker-skinned children's nails are more deeply pigmented. A blue or purple tinge denotes cyanosis; a yellow tinge is jaundice. Children who have decreased respiratory function or heart disease de-

BOX 33.11 FOCUS ON . . .

FAMILY TEACHING

Testicular Self-Examination

Q. Keoto's father asks you, "What is the best technique for testicular self-examination?"

A. Starting in your adolescent years, all males need to perform testicular self-examination. Follow these guidelines:

- Select a certain day each month (first day, last day, and so forth) to perform the examination.
- Perform the examination in or immediately after a shower, because that is when scrotal skin is most relaxed.
- Gently roll each testicle between your thumb and fingers, feeling for any hard lumps or nodules, change in consistency, or difference in size.
- If you notice any of these changes, call your doctor.
- Also feel for the epididymis, found at the rear of the testes. It should feel like a strong cord.
- Remember that for most males, one testicle is slightly larger than the other and hangs a little lower in the scrotal sac.

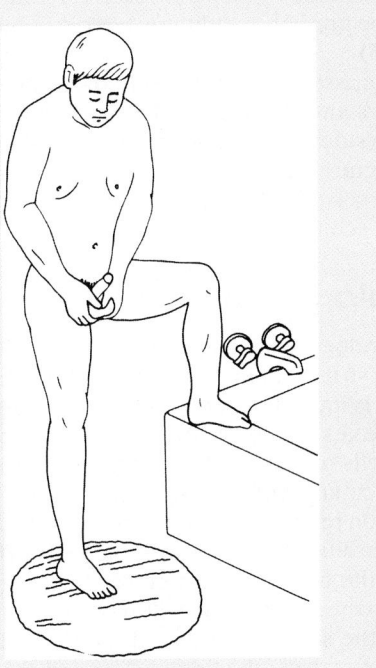

velop clubbed fingers (Fig. 33.21); children with endocarditis often have characteristic linear hemorrhages under the nails. Iron-deficiency anemia may cause extremely concave surfaces (spoon-shaped). Press against a fingernail, release the pressure, and time the refilling interval (should be under 5 seconds). Count the fingers and check for webbing between fingers. Examine for the pattern of fingerprints. Distinctive dermatoglyphics are present on fingertips from the third month of intrauterine life; these are unique to every person and show patterns of circular grooves. Abnormal fingerprints may occur with chromosomal anomalies.

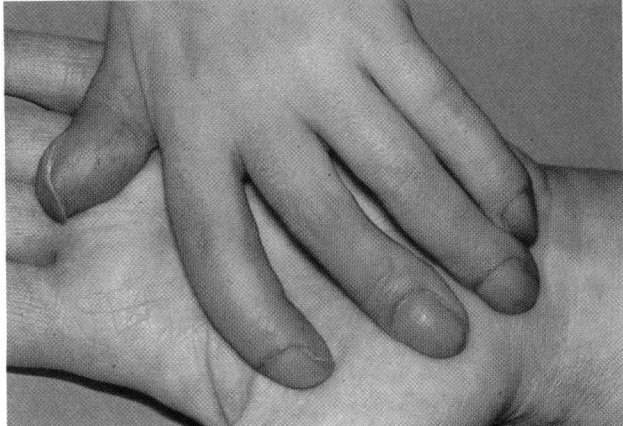

FIGURE 33.21 Clubbed fingers are a sign of cyanosis from heart or respiratory disease. (NMSB/Custom Medical Stock Photo.)

Check for normal palmar creases. Children with chromosomal abnormalities may have only one central palm crease (a simian line) on each hand rather than the normal three. Check the wrist, elbow, and shoulder joints for movement and normal range of motion; palpate joints for swelling or warmth. Palpate to be certain no lymph nodes are present in the antecubital space; palpate to check the radial pulse is present.

Inspect the lower extremities for color and warmth. Count the toes and check for webbing between toes. Check the ankle, knee, and hip joints for normal range of motion. Check for developmental hip dysplasia in infants by attempting to abduct the hip fully (see Fig. 24.18). Palpate to ensure no enlarged lymph nodes are present in the groin or popliteal areas and that femoral pulses are present and equal bilaterally. Ask the older child to walk, and observe for ease of gait, limping, or any foot displacement such as toeing in or out. Toddlers typically walk with a wide-based gait; they walk best if allowed to walk toward their parent (a safe action) rather than away. Many adolescents are self-conscious and slouch or amble rather than presenting their true, natural gait. Children who limp need further evaluation. The limp can be due to something as simple as a blister on the foot from wearing new shoes to a serious hip or bone condition (Mandracchia et al., 2004).

Back

Inspect the back for symmetry and the spinal column for any deviation. Inspect the base of the spine for a dermal sinus (a pinpoint opening) or for a tuft of hair or a hemangioma that might reveal a spina bifida occulta (a defect of the bony structure of the canal). Inspect also for any dimpling that might denote a dermal cyst (pilonidal cyst). This is an innocent finding unless it becomes infected or connects to deeper tissue layers. Assess for tenderness along the spinal column by palpating each vertebra. Lower back pain can be present as early as school age (Jones & McFarlane, 2005).

Routine assessment of the school-age child beginning at 12 years and through adolescence should include a scoliosis (sideways curvature of the spine) screening (LaMontagne et al., 2004). Box 33.12 details the steps to follow for a scoliosis screen. (See Chapter 51 for more details on scoliosis.)

Neurologic Function

A full neurologic examination takes at least 20 minutes to complete, so it is not included in a routine physical examination. It is important, however, to assess for **deep tendon reflexes** (such as triceps, biceps, patellar, and Achilles reflexes) to test for motor and sensory function and balance and coordination. Techniques for eliciting deep tendon reflexes are shown in Figure 33.22. Grade reflexes according to the scale in Table 33.10. The biceps reflex tests the fifth and sixth cervical nerves; the triceps reflex tests the seventh and eighth cervical; the patellar reflex tests the second, third, and fourth lumbar; and the Achilles reflex tests the first and second sacral. Test the sole of the foot for a Babinski reflex (see Fig. 24.8). Fanning of the toes will occur in an infant younger than 3 months; a downward reflex of the toes will occur beyond 3 months. (Some normal infants demonstrate a flaring Babinski response until they are 2; in the absence of other neurologic findings, this is not significant.)

Test for superficial reflexes: abdominal reflexes in both sexes, cremasteric reflex in boys. An abdominal reflex is elicited by lightly stroking each quadrant of the abdomen. Normally, the umbilicus moves perceptibly toward the stroke. Presence of the reflex indicates integrity of the 10th thoracic nerve and the first lumbar nerve of the spinal cord. A cremasteric reflex is elicited by stroking the medial aspect of the thigh in boys. The testes move perceptibly upward. The presence of this reflex indicates integrity of the first and second lumbar nerves.

Motor and Sensory Function

Test general facial nerve function by asking a child to make a face. The child's ability to grasp with the hands and push against a surface with the feet establishes general motor ability. Recall whether gait was adequate when the child was observed walking to assess for balance and coordination.

To test sensory function, ask a child to close the eyes and identify the location where he or she is touched at six points (at least) on different body parts.

VISION ASSESSMENT

Assessing vision is an important part of physical assessment because good vision is so important to childhood development. The extent of testing depends on the age of the child.

Any child with congenital anomalies, low birthweight, or fetal alcohol syndrome is at risk for eye abnormalities, as is a child who received oxygen at birth. During an assessment, if you notice an unreported injury or infection or signs of neglected vision, make a special note. Because the average parent is careful of a child's eyes, these findings may be indicative of child neglect.

Vision Screening

Routine vision screening is usually begun at 3 years of age. Common vision screening indicators and techniques for children of different ages are summarized in Table 33.11. Parents can provide important clues to possible problems: listen carefully any time a parent expresses concern about or questions a child's ability to see well.

Newborn and Infant

A parent's description of a child's activity can give clues to vision problems. Ask the parents if an infant's eyes follow them as they move around the room. Does an infant who is older than 6 weeks return their smile? Do the parents have any reason to think their child has difficulty seeing?

Newborns should be able to focus on a moving object such as a finger and follow it to the midline. Infants see black and white objects better than they do colored objects. They seem to see objects that are closest to them (a distance of about 19 cm [8 to 10 in]) best.

Toddler and Preschooler

Ask the parents of an older infant, toddler, or preschooler if their child does any of the following:

- Rubs his or her eyes, blinks frequently, squints, or frowns
- Covers one eye to look at objects
- Tilts the head to see things better
- Stumbles over objects in his or her path
- Holds books and toys extremely close or extremely far away to look at them

Asking whether children sit close to a television set is meaningless because almost all children do that if allowed.

School-Age Child and Adolescent

Ask the parents if their child does any of the following:

- Reports frequent headaches
- Does poorly with classwork
- Avoids sports that require long-distance vision, such as baseball or softball
- Avoids watching movies
- Skips over words when reading aloud
- Reports blurriness or double vision
- Has reddened conjunctivae or drainage from the eyes
- Blinks at bright light

BOX 33.12 NURSING PROCEDURE

Scoliosis Screening

Purpose
To assess for scoliosis (sideways curvature of the spine).

PROCEDURE	PRINCIPLE
1. Have the child remove clothing, except for undergarments. Ask the child to stand up straight, with his or her feet together and arms at sides. Observe the child from a posterior view.	1. Promotes optimal view of back.
2. Inspect for unequal shoulder or hip level, prominence of one scapula, or a curved spinal column (Figure *A*).	2. Denotes signs of spinal curvature.

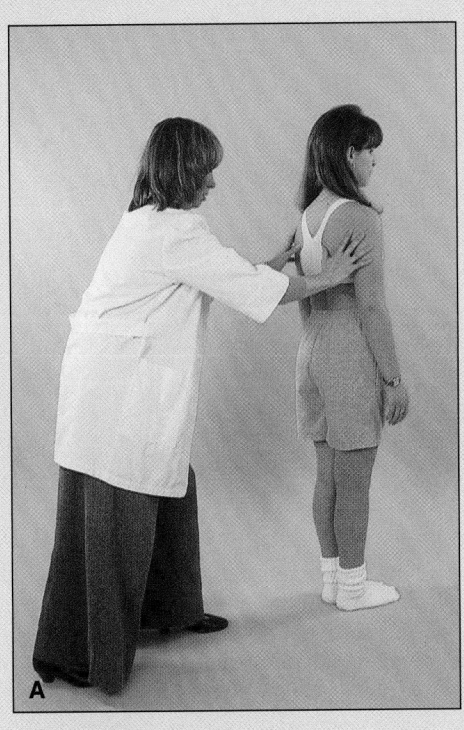

A

Ask yourself the following questions:
- Is one shoulder higher than the other?
- Is one shoulder blade more prominent than the other?
- Does one hip seem higher or more prominent than the other?
- Does the child seem to lean to one side?
- Does the spinal column appear curved?

3. Compare the level of the elbows in relation to the iliac crests. Be sure the arms are hanging down at the sides. Ask yourself the following questions:
   - Is the distance between one arm and body greater than on the other side?
   - Are the elbows uneven?
   - Do the elbows fall at the level of the crest or closer to the crest on the one side? (Normally the elbows fall above the iliac crest.)

3. Helps to determine uneven posture because it will affect level of elbows.

(continued)

PROCEDURE	PRINCIPLE
4. Ask the child to bend over and touch his or her toes while you continue to observe the back (Figure *B*).	4. Provides evidence of spinal rotation. As the child bends, the rotation of the spine accompanying scoliosis becomes more prominent.

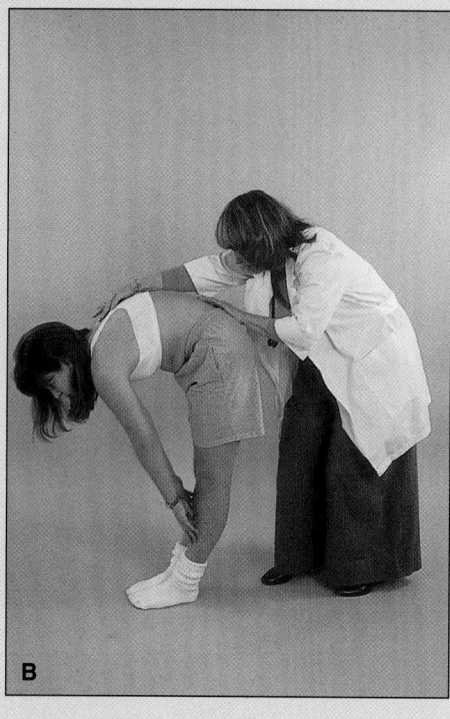

B

Ask yourself the following questions:
- Is there a hump in the back?
- Does the spinal column appear to curve?
- Is one shoulder blade more prominent than the other?

5. Refer the child to a physician for further examination if the answer to any of the above questions is yes.	5. Provides for proper referral.
6. Educate the child to inform parents or health care providers if signs of scoliosis, such as a skirt hanging unevenly, or bra straps that need to be adjusted, begin to develop.	6. Encourages health promotion.

Techniques of Vision Testing

Vision is tested by asking a child to read an eye chart. All children need good orientation to such testing so they can appreciate this is not a test in the usual sense of the word; otherwise, they may be unusually anxious or try to pass it by cheating. Vision testing needs to be started in the preschool period so children with amblyopia (lazy eye; see Chapter 50), a potentially serious vision disorder, can be identified while the condition is still correctable (Gold, 2004). In addition to usual testing, a Polaroid photo can be used to help identify strabismus (uneven gaze).

Snellen Chart

As soon as children can identify letters of the alphabet (early school age), their vision can be tested at a health checkup by using a Snellen eye chart. This chart is standardized, so set procedures must be followed when using it to test vision (Box 33.13).

Preschool E Chart

Between 3 years of age and the age they can read the alphabet, children can have their vision tested by using a preschool E chart (Fig. 33.23). This chart is also helpful in testing children who are cognitively challenged or those who do not speak fluent English. The procedure is similar to that of the standard Snellen chart:

1. The child stands 20 ft from the chart. He or she should read first with the right eye, then with the left, then both eyes, as with standard testing. Young children do not understand the importance of not pressing the card

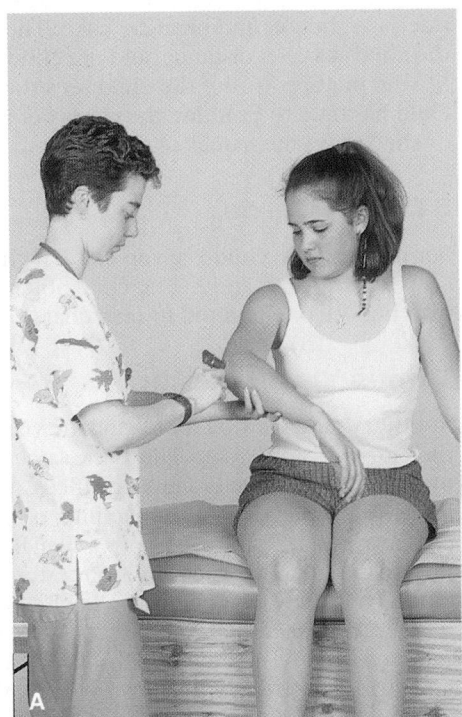
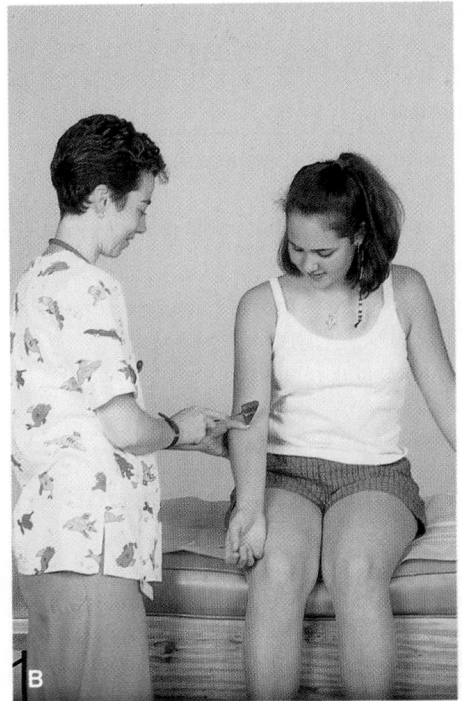
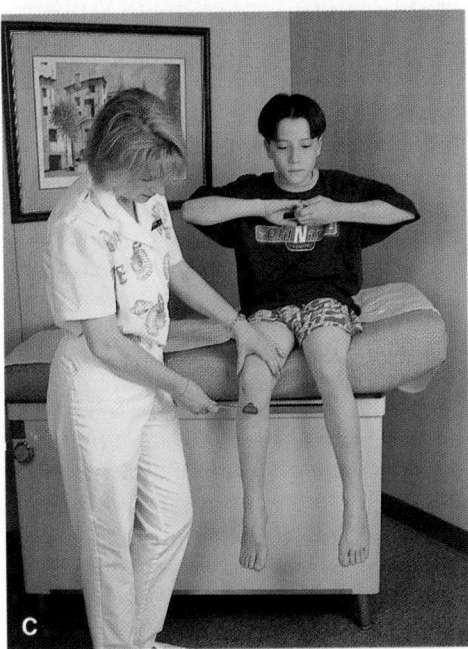
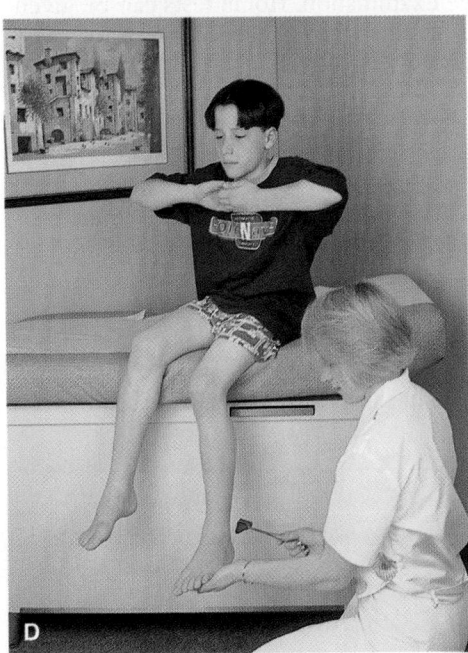

FIGURE 33.22 Deep tendon reflexes. (**A**) Triceps reflex. The triceps tendon is struck. The forearm will move perceptibly if the reflex is elicited. (**B**) Biceps reflex. The examiner's thumb is placed over the biceps tendon. The reflex hammer actually strikes the examiner's thumb. The examiner will feel the child's forearm move when the reflex is elicited. (**C**) Patellar reflex. (**D**) Achilles reflex. In both *C* and *D,* the child grasps his hands together and pulls as a means of distracting him away from what the nurse is testing. This helps to decrease muscle tension, facilitate the reflex arc, and elicit more accurate results.

against their eye or of not peeking, so a second person is often needed to hold the occluder card for children of this age.

2. It is helpful to compare the E with a table with three legs and ask the child which way the legs of the table point. By three years, children are familiar with tables,

but Es are strange symbols. Tell the child to point with the entire arm and hand in the direction the legs point so you do not confuse the hand motion.

3. Begin at the 40-ft line, as with the standard Snellen chart, and work downward until the child passes all lines or cannot read the majority of symbols on a line.

TABLE 33.10

Grading of Deep Tendon Reflexes

Grade	Interpretation
4+	Hyperactive; extremely marked reaction; abnormal
3+	Stronger than average but within normal range
2+	Average response
1+	Less than average response but within normal range
0	No response; abnormal

National Association for the Prevention of Blindness Home Test

A home eye test is available from the National Association for the Prevention of Blindness for parents to use to test children ages 3 to 6 at home. It is similar to the preschool E chart except it is smaller and the child stands only 10 ft away. The test can help alert parents that a child needs a professional eye examination. Home tests can be given or suggested to parents whose child is tired or for some other reason has not tested well in a health care facility (PBA, 2005).

Allen Cards

Preschool children may be tested with Allen cards, which consist of pictures of common objects such as a horse and rider, car, house, and birthday cake. These are shown to the child at a 15-ft distance, and the child is asked to identify the pictures (proof the child sees them). Be certain a child has time to examine the cards before the test so he or she knows the names of the objects.

STYCAR Cards

For this test, the child is given cards with nine letters: H, C, O, L, U, T, X, V, and A. The child holds up the card that matches the one pointed to on a chart.

Titmus Vision Tester

Another useful method for testing the vision of children is the Titmus Vision Tester. This is the same instrument used by many motor vehicle licensing offices. As the child looks into the eyepieces of the machine, alphabet letters or preschool Es are projected onto a well-lighted screen for the child to identify. Closed vision testers such as the Titmus have an advantage over wall charts in that a child is less easily distracted during testing. Also, because a child cannot see the vision chart beforehand, he or she cannot memorize the letters while waiting to be tested.

Color Vision Discrimination Testing

The inability to discern colors is a sex-linked recessive characteristic that tends to occur in males rather than in females, although females carry the gene for the disorder. All male children should be screened once for the disorder during their early school years.

To test a child for color awareness, ask the child to identify the colored stripes at the top of a Snellen eye chart or show the child a series of colored diagrams (Ishihara's plates). With the latter, a person with color vision can see hidden figures such as butterflies, but people with red-green or yellow-blue color vision deficits cannot. Detecting color vision deficit in children is important because many educational materials and some occupations depend on the ability to identify color. Even such a simple childhood pleasure as riding a bicycle safely on city streets depends on being able to distinguish colors, such as red from green on a traffic light.

Vision Referrals

Screen children twice before referring them to a physician for corrective eye care, as some children do not perform well on eye tests because they are easily distracted or do not know their alphabet as well as they pretend. For example, they may say they do not see a letter when they really mean they do not know or remember its name. Testing twice helps eliminate or identify this type of misleading result.

After a second screening, the following children generally require a vision referral:

- Preschool children (3 to 5 years of age) who have 20/50 vision in one or both eyes
- Children 6 years of age or older who have 20/40 vision or worse in one or both eyes
- Any child with a two-line difference between the eyes, which might be the beginning of amblyopia

TABLE 33.11

Common Vision Screening Indicators and Procedures

Age	Common Test
Newborn	General appearance*
	Ability to follow moving object to midline; focus steadily on an object at 10–12 in
Infant and toddler	General appearance*
	Ability to follow light past midline
3 yr–school age	General appearance*
	Random dot E for stereopsis (depth perception)
	Allen cards or preschool E chart for visual acuity
	Ishihara's plates for color awareness
School age–adult	General appearance*
	Snellen's test for visual acuity

* Note redness, blinking, squinting, crusting, and so forth.

BOX 33.13 NURSING PROCEDURE

Snellen Eye Chart Assessment

Purpose
To assess vision.

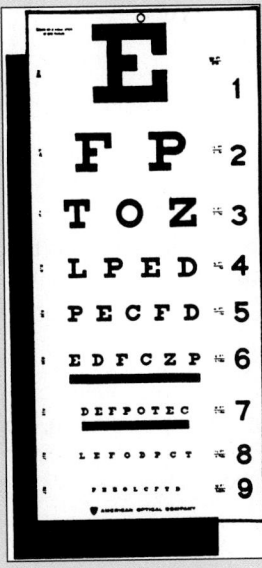

PROCEDURE

1. Hang the chart so the 20-ft line is at the child's eye level.

2. Provide a good light for the chart and place it so there is no glare. A light intensity of 20 foot-candles is recommended.

3. Measure a distance of 20 ft from the chart. Mark the floor at this point with a piece of masking tape or other similar mark. For younger children, it is helpful to cut out paper footprints and paste them to the floor with the heels of the footprints touching the 20-ft line. If the child sits in a chair, the back legs of the chair should touch the 20-ft line.

4. Provide an individual 3 × 5-in card (to cover the eye not being tested) for each child who is examined.

5. If the child wears glasses, screen while he or she is wearing the glasses. If a child has forgotten to bring glasses, defer the screening until the child can bring the glasses. Do not screen the child first without glasses and then with them, because this forces the child to strain to read the chart.

6. To begin testing, tell the child to stand with his or her shoes on the footprints (heels against the line); keep both eyes open; and cover the left eye with the occluding card. Be certain the child does not press the card against the eye (instead, the edge of the card should rest across the child's nose).

PRINCIPLE

1. The child who has to look up or down must look farther than the child who is looking straight across at the chart. A possible solution to avoid moving the chart is to have smaller children stand and taller children sit. To accommodate children in wheelchairs, the chart needs to be lowered (or else have all children sit for the test).

2. Appropriate lighting provides for optimal test conditions.

3. Twenty feet is the optimal distance from the chart for testing.

4. Covering the other eye allows for one eye to be tested at a time.

5. Testing with corrective lenses screens for corrected eyesight. After squinting, a child may have difficulty readjusting to reading with glasses, and this makes the prescription appear too weak or too strong.

6. Covering the eye not being tested provides optimal test conditions. Pressure will cause blurred vision when the child removes the card to test that eye.

(continued)

PROCEDURE	PRINCIPLE
7. Begin at the 40-ft line of the chart and, using a pointer or pencil, point to each symbol on the line from left to right (the order in which children are taught to read). If the child reads a majority of symbols in a line, he or she sees the line satisfactorily.	7. Starting at the 40-ft line is the standardized testing procedure.
8. If the child "passes" the 40-ft line, have the child read the 30- and 20-ft lines or the last line the child can read. Record the last line read. If the child fails to read the 40-ft line satisfactorily, then begin at the top of the chart and move downward to identify the last line the child can read. Record this reading. Because the 200-ft, 100-ft, and 70-ft lines have so few symbols, the child must read all the symbols on them to have read satisfactorily.	8. Moving to the 30-ft line or less reflects use of standardized testing procedure.
9. Visual acuity is always stated as a fraction. The top number is the distance in feet the child stands from the chart (always 20). The bottom of the fraction represents the last line the child read correctly. The adult with good (average) vision can read the 20-ft line from 20 ft away and thus is said to have 20/20 vision.	9. Using a fraction for visual acuity is the standardized reporting procedure.
10. It is important to test the eyes separately, then together. For example, Tony reads all the symbols on the 40-ft line with his right eye; he misses three out of four on the 30-ft line. His visual acuity for his right eye is 20 (the distance from the chart) over 40 (the last line he read correctly). With his left eye, Tony reads the 40-ft, 30-ft, and 20-ft lines correctly. His vision in that eye is 20/20. With both eyes, Tony reads the 40-ft, 30-ft, and 20-ft lines correctly. His visual acuity for both eyes is 20/20.	10. If only this last reading were taken, the right eye weakness (a symptom of amblyopia or "lazy eye") would be missed.
11. Observe the child for straining or squinting as he or she reads the chart.	11. By squinting and changing the shape of the eyeball, a child can improve his or her vision and will score higher. The child will appear to see better than he or she actually does in everyday situations.

- Any child who states or shows symptoms of visual disturbance (PBA, 2005)

HEARING ASSESSMENT

A thorough health assessment should also include an evaluation of hearing, including both history and observation, because good hearing is necessary for the development of age-appropriate skills. When taking an auditory history, be certain to ask the accompanying adult or parent an overall question such as, "Do you have any reason to believe your child doesn't hear as well as she should?" Parents and grandparents are usually attuned to hearing difficulty in children and may be suspicious of it in advance of its official detection.

Auditory Screening

Routine screening for adequate hearing levels is usually begun at 3 years of age. Testing requires knowledge of the technique and use of an audiometer. It requires a quiet, undistracted setting.

Newborn and Infant

Certain infants who are at risk should be screened at birth. This includes infants with any of the following conditions:

- History of childhood hearing impairment in the family
- Perinatal infection, such as cytomegalovirus, rubella, herpes, toxoplasmosis, or syphilis
- Anatomic malformations involving the head or neck
- Birthweight less than 1,500 g
- Hyperbilirubinemia at a level exceeding indication for exchange transfusion
- Bacterial meningitis, especially when caused by *Haemophilus influenzae*
- Severe birth asphyxia: infants with an Apgar score of 0 to 3, those who failed to breathe spontaneously within 10 minutes of birth, or those with hypotonia persisting to 2 hours of age

If a newborn's hearing is assessed, it usually is done through simple response testing—observing whether an infant stirs or responds to a sound made or delivered to the child with a commercial device (Gracey & Lankford, 2003).

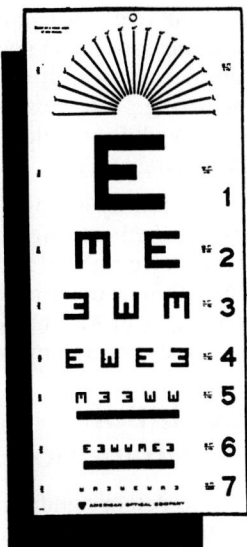

FIGURE 33.23 Astigmatic and preschool E chart. (From the American Optical Corporation, with permission.)

It can also be done by brain stem auditory-evoked response (BAER) testing. For this method, an earphone is placed on the infant and an electrode is attached to the scalp. When sound is transmitted to the child's ear through the earphone, the electrical potential created as the sound is processed by the brain stem is read by the scalp electrode, processed by a microcomputer, and plotted on a graph. This type of testing may be used at any age and is successful even in children who are comatose or anesthetized. Smaller units using transient evoked otoacoustic emissions (TEOAE) are also available. With these, a click stimulus delivered to a normal ear produces an echo from the cochlea. This can be detected by a miniature microphone to reveal even minor hearing loss. Although newborn hearing screening can lead to false-positive results because many infants of this age are still sleepy from birth analgesia and may have fluid- or vernix-filled ear canals, repeating the test usually decreases the incidence of false-positive results.

Older Children

Older children who are at risk for hearing loss are those who have been exposed to loud noises such as an explosion or loud music, were of low birthweight, have congenital anomalies, have a repaired cleft palate, or have had repeated ear infections. During history taking, ask children if they ever worry if they have difficulty hearing. Ask them how they are doing in school. Some children with a minimal hearing impairment are considered to have behavioral problems in school because they do not follow directions or appear not to be following the teacher's discussion when in fact they may be unable to hear what is being said. Be certain not to confuse difficulty hearing with shyness or recalcitrance in answering. Children with an ear infection (otitis media) or allergies should be tested after the fluids in their ears clear because their hearing may be temporarily

affected by these conditions. Cerumen in the ear canal has not been documented to substantially decrease hearing.

Principles of Audiometric Assessment

Frequency

Sound is the result of vibration; frequency is the number of vibrations a sound creates per second. When frequency is increased, the pitch of the sound increases. For audiometric testing, frequency is measured in Hertz units. Normal speech sounds fall into a narrow range, 500 to 2,000 Hz. To function adequately and speak effectively, a child must be able to hear in this range. Children are tested for a wider frequency range than this, from 500 to 6,000 Hz, on a routine screening assessment.

Loudness

Decibels are an expression of the intensity of loudness of a sound (or vigor of the vibrations). A decibel level of 0 dB is the softest sound that can be heard. Normal conversation is approximately 50 to 60 dB. The sound level at which inner ear damage can occur is about 90 dB. Sound levels of 140 dB are so intense they actually cause pain. Screening audiometry is done at 25 dB.

Hearing Loss

Table 33.12 lists levels of hearing loss. The inability of a child to hear sounds softer than 30 dB indicates the child will have some difficulty hearing normal instructions and questions. If a child cannot hear sounds softer than 50 dB, the child misses most normal conversation and will have difficulty achieving in a regular classroom environment. The hearing loss is so severe that the child will be speech-challenged because he or she does not hear normal speech sounds.

If a child can hear all frequencies at the 25-dB level, he or she has passed an audiometric screening check. If a child fails to hear two or more frequencies at 25 dB, in either or both ears, the child has failed a screening audiometry test and should be referred to a physician or an otologist. An **audiogram** is a record of audiometric testing. Figure 33.24 shows an audiogram of a child with normal hearing in the right ear (the child heard all frequencies at the 20-dB level) but an inability to hear sounds softer than 45 dB in the left ear at frequencies of 1,000, 2,000, and 4,000 Hz.

Acoustic Impedance Testing

Acoustic impedance testing is based on the principle that sound entering the ear canal meets resistance at the tympanic membrane. If the middle ear is functioning normally, there will be a symmetric pattern of resistance on a tympanogram printout. If the middle ear is functioning abnormally, the level of resistance will be greater or less than normal, so the pattern will be abnormal.

Acoustic impedance testing is performed by audiologists. For the assessment, the ear to be tested is plugged

TABLE 33.12

Levels of Hearing Loss

Hearing Loss (DB Level)	Hearing Level Present
Slight (less than 30)	Inability to hear whispered words or faint speech
	No speech challenge present
	Possible lack of awareness of hearing difficulty
	Achievement in school and home is attained by leaning forward, speaking loudly
Mild (30–50)	Beginning speech challenge possibly present
	Difficulty hearing if not facing speaker; some difficulty with normal conversation
Moderate (55–70)	Speech challenge present, possibly requiring speech therapy
	Difficulty with normal conversation
Severe (70–90)	Difficulty with any but nearby loud voice
	Vowels easier to hear than consonants
	Speech therapy required for clear speech. Possible ability to still hear loud sounds such as jets or whistle of train.
Profound (more than 90)	Almost no sound heard

with a rubber disc. Sound is then administered to the ear through the center of the disc. The resistance met at the eardrum is registered and recorded as a graph. Tympanograms are inaccurate in children younger than 7 months of age because the tympanic membrane is too compliant under that age to register normal impedance.

Conduction Loss Testing

Although not very accurate, both the Rinne and the Weber tests can be used to help determine the cause of hearing loss in older children (Box 33.14).

SPEECH ASSESSMENT

Speech problems are directly related to hearing problems: an infant who does not hear will make preliminary babbling sounds but then will not develop intelligible speech because he or she cannot hear and repeat sounds. Speech difficulties may also be related to:

- Motor development (e.g., the child cannot control tongue and facial muscles well enough to form proper words)

- Cognitive development (e.g., the cognitively challenged child cannot grasp the concept of speech or word use until later than normal, or possibly not at all)
- Cultural influences (e.g., the parents speak two languages, making it difficult for a child to accurately learn and articulate either language)

Speech screening begins by asking a child a few simple questions to determine his or her language pattern. Also ask parents if they have noticed any difficulties with their child's pronunciation or comprehension. Standardized tests, such as the Denver Articulation Screening Examination (DASE), may also be administered.

Denver Articulation Screening Examination

The DASE is designed to detect significant developmental delays and normal variations in the acquisition of speech sounds. Because it is a standardized test, its directions must be followed carefully. The test is useful only with English-speaking children.

Administration

Before the test, explain that the child will need to repeat some words he or she hears. Give enough examples so the child will understand what he or she is to do: "When I say 'boat,' then you say 'boat.'" When you are certain the child understands the directions, say each of the 22 words shown on the DASE form (Fig. 33.25A). Convey the impression that there are no right or wrong answers. Give the child approval for responding and following directions correctly, no matter how inaccurately the child repeats the word.

Scoring

The DASE is designed for use with children between ages 2.5 and 6 years. In scoring, consider the child's age to be the closest previous age shown on the percentile rank chart (see Fig. 33.25B). Score the child's pronunciation of the underlined sounds or blends in each word on the test form. A perfect raw score is 30 correctly articulated sounds. Match this raw score on the percentile rank chart with the column representing the child's age. The number at which the raw score line and the age column meet is the percentile rank of the child (how the child compares with other children of that age). Percentiles shown above the heavy line are abnormal; those below the line are normal. For example, a 3-year-old who says only 12 sounds correctly ranks in the 9th percentile (abnormal ranking); the 3-year-old who scores 20 sounds correctly ranks in the 58th percentile (normal ranking).

In addition to determining the percentile ranking, rate the child's spontaneous speech in terms of intelligibility as 1, easy to understand; 2, understandable half the time; 3, not understandable; or 4, cannot evaluate (e.g., the child does not speak in sentences or phrases during your contact with the child). Score intelligibility according to the chart in Figure 33.25B. For a final score, rate the child's total test result (normal or abnormal on the DASE or intelligibility).

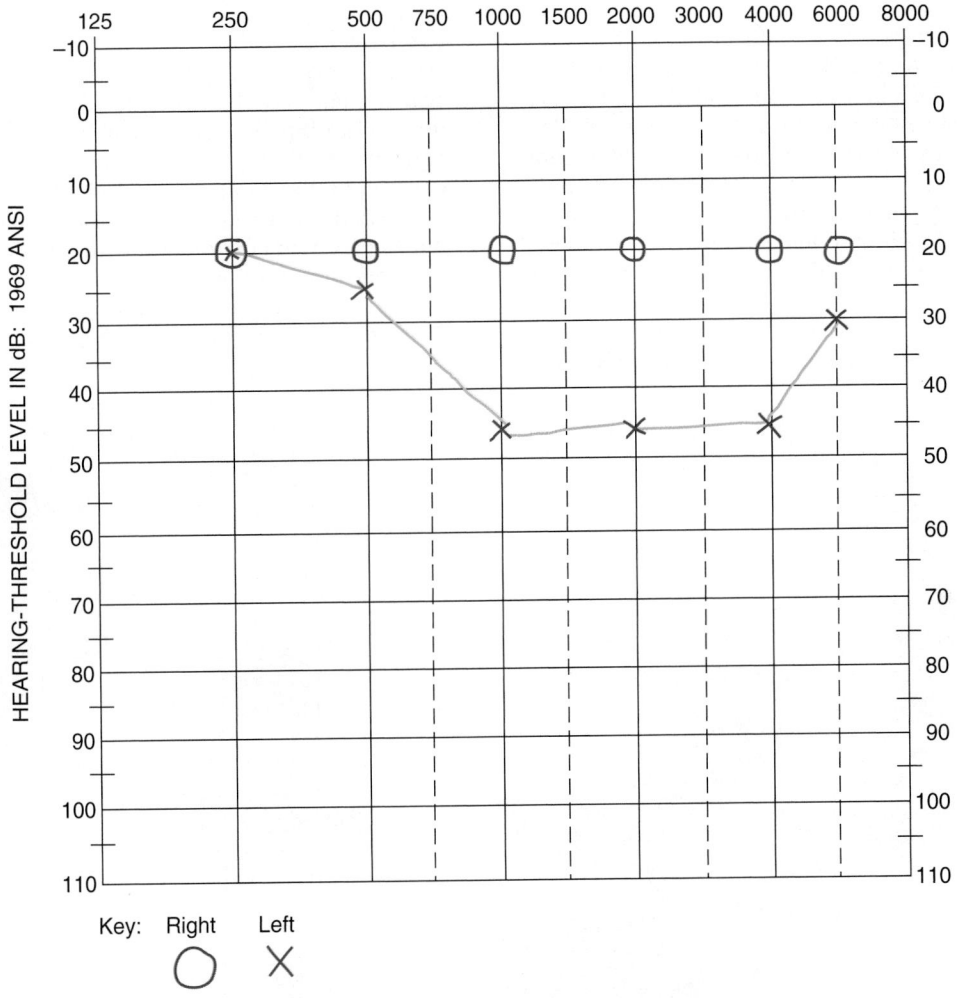

FIGURE 33.24 An audiogram done as a screening procedure. Notice that hearing is normal in the right ear (all frequencies are heard at the 20-dB level). In the left ear there is hearing loss (the frequencies 1000, 2000, and 4000 Hz are heard only at the 45-dB level). (Courtesy of Dr. H. Schill, Speech Pathology and Audiology Department, Boston University.)

Children who score abnormally on this screening test should be retested in 2 weeks. If they still score abnormally, they should be referred for complete speech evaluation.

DEVELOPMENTAL APPRAISAL

It would be ideal if children demonstrated all the developmental skills of which they are capable every time they are asked to demonstrate them. Rarely, however, do they accomplish this. Infants become hungry, sleepy, or upset during testing. Older children may become shy. A portion of developmental information on almost all health assessments, therefore, must be elicited by history taking. All previous developmental milestones must be obtained this way.

Developmental History

Many parents keep careful records of their first child's development, a less careful record of their second, a scanty record of the third, and so on. Most of this information must, therefore, be obtained by recall.

Parents may not be able to recall the month during which a skill was first demonstrated. It is often helpful to ask them to try to remember in terms of holidays or seasons. For example, they may not know at which month their infant first used a pincer grasp (grasped cleanly with index finger and thumb) but do recall the way the child pinched the ear of the family dog at a summer picnic.

If parents seem to have no recall at all of developmental milestones that are important for the child's present evaluation, suggest they ask other family members or look through family photographs to jog their memories and then call with as much information as they can gather.

In addition to getting the parents' description of the skills a child has mastered, it is helpful to watch the child perform skills and rate him or her according to standard criteria.

BOX 33.14

Rinne and Weber Tests

Rinne Test

Strike a 500-Hz tuning fork and hold the stem of it against the child's mastoid bone. Ask the child to say when he or she no longer hears the tuning fork ringing. When the child says it is no longer audible, move the fork forward so it is at the auditory meatus. Because air conduction is normally better than bone conduction, the child should hear it when it is held in front of the meatus, although he or she no longer heard it when it was held against the bone. If the child does not hear it when it is brought forward, then the child's air conduction is probably reduced.

Weber Test

Strike a 500-Hz tuning fork and hold the stem of it against the top of the child's head. The child with normal hearing in both ears will hear the sound equally well with both ears. If the child has an air conduction loss in one ear, the child will hear the sound better in that ear than in the good ear. The test must be used in conjunction with other evaluation tools because if the sound is intensified in one ear, it may mean that there is no hearing perception (there is nerve loss) in the opposite ear.

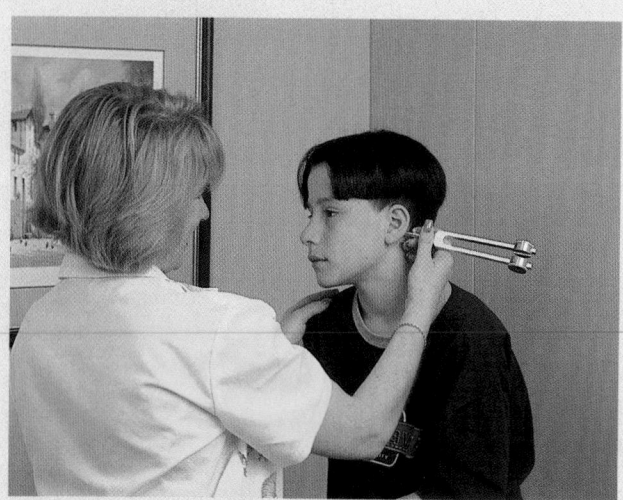

Photo by John Gallagher, with permission of Wyncote Family Medicine, Wyncote, PA.

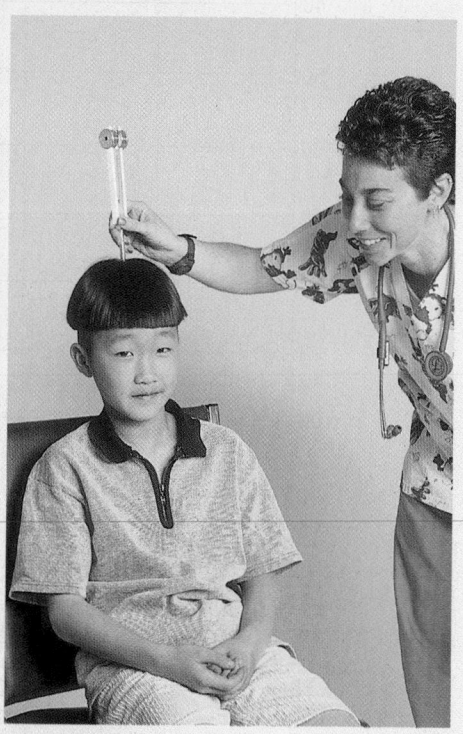

© Lesha Photography.

Denver II Developmental Screening Test

The Denver II Developmental Screening Test (see Appendix H) is the most widely used tool to assess childhood development (Frankenburg, 1994). The test can detect delays during infancy and the preschool years. Four main categories of development are rated:

1. Personal-social
2. Fine motor-adaptive
3. Language
4. Gross motor skills

Administration

The Denver II ideally should be completed when a child is approximately 3 or 4 months of age, again at 10 months, and again at 3 years. It is a supplement to the developmental evaluation by history that should be a part of every well-child assessment.

The materials to administer the test must be purchased as a kit. They include a skein of red wool, a box of raisins, a small bottle, a bell, a rattle with a narrow handle, a tennis ball, ten 1-inch brightly colored blocks, a small plastic doll, a toy baby bottle, a plastic cup, and a pencil.

Although administration of the Denver II is not difficult, it should not be attempted except by health care providers trained specifically in its procedures and interpretation. This precaution is necessary to ensure the validity of its developmental norms. Periodic retraining and proficiency testing are recommended to sustain a high degree of accuracy in administration.

A parent should be cautioned before administration that this is not a test of intelligence but of the child's level

```
┌─────────────────────────────────────────────────┬──────────────────────┐
│   DENVER ARTICULATION SCREENING EXAM             │ NAME                 │
│   for children 2 1/2 to 6 years of age           │                      │
│                                                  │ HOSP. NO.            │
│ Instructions:  Have child repeat each word after │                      │
│ you.  Circle the underlined sounds that he pro-  │ ADDRESS _____│
│ nounces correctly.  Total correct sounds is the  │                      │
│ Raw Score.  Use charts on reverse side to score  │                      │
│ results.                                         │                      │
└─────────────────────────────────────────────────┴──────────────────────┘
```

Date: _____ Child's Age:_____ Examiner: _____ Raw Score:_____
Percentile:_____ Intelligibility:_____ Result:_____

1. table	6. zipper	11. sock	16. wagon	21. leaf
2. shirt	7. grapes	12. vacuum	17. gum	22. carrot
3. door	8. flag	13. yarn	18. house	
4. trunk	9. thumb	14. mother	19. pencil	
5. jumping	10. toothbrush	15. twinkle	20. fish	

Intelligibility: (circle one) 1. Easy to understand   3. Not understandable
                               2. Understandable 1/2   4. Can't evaluate
                                   the time.

Comments:

Date: _____ Child's Age:_____ Examiner:_____ Raw Score _____
Percentile:_____ Intelligibility:_____ Result:_____

1. table	6. zipper	11. sock	16. wagon	21. leaf
2. shirt	7. grapes	12. vacuum	17. gum	22. carrot
3. door	8. flag	13. yarn	18. house	
4. trunk	9. thumb	14. mother	19. pencil	
5. jumping	10. toothbrush	15. twinkle	20. fish	

Intelligibility: (circle one) 1. Easy to understand   3. Not understandable
                               2. Understandable 1/2   4. Can't evaluate
                                   the time.

Comments:

Date: _____ Child's Age: _____ Examiner:_____ Raw Score_____
Percentile: _____ Intelligibility:_____ Result:_____

1. table	6. zipper	11. sock	16. wagon	21. leaf
2. shirt	7. grapes	12. vacuum	17. gum	22. carrot
3. door	8. flag	13. yarn	18. house	
4. trunk	9. thumb	14. mother	19. pencil	
5. jumping	10. toothbrush	15. twinkle	20. fish	

Intelligibility: (circle one) 1. Easy to understand   3. Not understandable
                                2. Understandable 1/2   4. Can't evaluate
                                    the time.

Comments:

FIGURE 33.25 Denver Articulation Screening Exam (DASE). (**A**) Test form.

of development. The child's inability to perform a task that most children of the same age can accomplish indicates a delay in that area. Further evaluation is then needed to determine the reason for this delay.

Scoring

The child is scored P (passed), F (failed), R (refused), or N.O. (no opportunity) on each item according to guidelines in the instruction manual. Each item is represented on the test form (see Appendix H) by a bar showing the ages by which 25%, 50%, 75%, and 90% of children normally have mastered that item. The left end of the bar is the 25% mark; the tick mark at the top of the bar, 50%; the left end of the colored (gray) area, 75%; and the right end of the bar, 90%. Looking at the form, notice, for ex-

ample, the item "plays pat-a-cake" in the area of personal-social development. With this item, 25% of children show the trait at 7 months, 50% between 9 and 10 months, 75% between 10 and 11 months, and 90% by ages 11 to 12 months. Interpretation of performance is detailed in the manual.

Prescreening Test

A Denver Prescreening Developmental Questionnaire (R-PDQII) is available in addition to the Denver II. The PDQII is designed to identify children who require further testing with a full Denver II. It is a questionnaire completed by the parents addressing 10 developmental items. A child who scores 8 out of 10 or fewer should be retested in approximately 2 weeks. If the initial score is

To score DASE words: Note Raw Score for child's performance. Match raw score line (extreme left of chart) with column representing child's age (to the closest previous age group). Where raw score line and age column meet number in that square denotes percentile rank of child's performance when compared to other children that age. Percentiles above heavy line are ABNORMAL percentiles, below heavy line are NORMAL.

PERCENTILE RANK

Raw Score	2.5 yr.	3.0	3.5	4.0	4.5	5.0	5.5	6 years
2	1							
3	2							
4	5							
5	9							
6	16							
7	23							
8	31	2						
9	37	4	1					
10	42	6	2					
11	48	7	4					
12	54	9	6	1	1			
13	58	12	9	2	3	1	1	
14	62	17	11	5	4	2	2	
15	68	23	15	9	5	3	2	
16	75	31	19	12	5	4	3	
17	79	38	25	15	6	6	4	
18	83	46	31	19	8	7	4	
19	86	51	38	24	10	9	5	1
20	89	58	45	30	12	11	7	3
21	92	65	52	36	15	15	9	4
22	94	72	58	43	18	19	12	5
23	96	77	63	50	22	24	15	7
24	97	82	70	58	29	29	20	15
25	99	87	78	66	36	34	26	17
26	99	91	84	75	46	43	34	24
27		94	89	82	57	54	44	34
28		96	94	88	70	68	59	47
29		98	98	94	84	84	77	68
30		100	100	100	100	100	100	100

To Score intelligibility:	NORMAL	ABNORMAL
2 1/2 years	Understandable 1/2 the time, or, "easy"	Not Understandable
3 years and older	Easy to understand	Understandable 1/2 time Not understandable

Test Result: 1. NORMAL on Dase and Intelligibility = NORMAL

 2. ABNORMAL on Dase and/or Intelligibility = ABNORMAL

* If abnormal on initial screening rescreen within 2 weeks. If abnormal again child should be referred for complete speech evaluation.

FIGURE 33.25 (continued) (B) Percentile rank form. (Reprinted by permission. Copyright 1971 by Amelia F. Drumwright, University of Colorado Medical Center, Denver, CO.)

under 6 or the retest score is 8 or below, the child should have a full Denver II.

INTELLIGENCE

Children must learn many important concepts or ideas such as near, far, here, there, number sequences, how to judge time intervals, how to reason and solve problems, and how to judge weight before they can function effectively in the world.

This type of learning—gaining concepts—is cognitive learning and is measured by intelligence tests. **Intelligence** can be defined as an ability to think abstractly, to adjust to new situations, and to profit from experience. Almost everyone has had his or her intelligence quotient (IQ) rated at some point in a school career. Although intelligence tests are not part of routine health appraisals, it is helpful to be familiar with those that are used for childhood measurements because these findings are helpful in predicting children's school success.

The IQ is the ratio of mental age as measured by an intelligence test to chronologic age. The formula for IQ is (mental age/chronologic age) multiplied by 100. A child aged 9 years old (chronologic age) who passes all the items on an intelligence test that an average 9-year-old child passes would be (9 [mental age]/9 [chronologic age]) times 100 = 100 (child's IQ). If a child passes no more items than the average 5-year-old child would, the IQ would be (5 [mental age]/9 [chronologic age]) times 100 = 55. If a child passed all the items that a 12-year-old child normally passes, the IQ would be (12 [mental age]/9 [chronologic age]) times 100 = 133.

Team Member Responsible	Assessment	Intervention	Rationale	Expected Outcome
Consultations				
Physician	Determine which school physician determines eligibility for sports teams.	Consult with school physician to determine eligibility for sports.	Schools may have restrictions on children who do not have both pairs of duplicate organs like lungs.	Qualifications for sports participation are outlined for parents and child.
Procedures/Medications				
Nurse practitioner	Obtain health history, particularly in regard to stamina, nutrition, and past ability to participate in structured activities.	Perform complete physical examination focusing on heart, lung, muscle, and nutrition status.	Physical examination can reveal additional findings regarding lung capacity and stamina.	Physical examination determines child's overall health.
Nurse	Assess whether child is familiar with Snellen vision testing.	Test child's eyesight using a Snellen eye chart.	A Snellen eye chart is a standardized test for vision appraisal.	Child completes eye exam and is told results.
Nutrition				
Nurse/ Nutritionist	Assess what parent and child know about carbohydrate loading.	Counsel regarding disadvantages of carbohydrate loading and sports participation for children.	Children and parents who are well informed can make informed choices on the benefit of nutrition practices.	Parent and child state they understand carbohydrate loading is not recommended for children.
Patient/Family Education				
Nurse	Assess past health history and recommended immunizations.	Review with parent and child the child's current immunization status and any immunizations needed.	Parents are often unfamiliar with required immunizations so need to be reminded of recommended schedules.	Parent and child agree to any immunization necessary before child returns to school.
Psychosocial/Spiritual/Emotional Needs				
Nurse	Assess what will be child's reaction if she cannot participate in school sports program.	If child is unable to participate in school sports, review with child other options: join a club; petition school sports committee.	Planning ahead can help child adjust to less-than-desired results from health assessment.	Child lists alternate ways to participate with other children at school, if sports are not an option, or describes sensible plan for petitioning for exception to rules.
Discharge Planning				
Nurse	Assess if parent or child has had questions answered by health assessment.	Answer remaining questions; schedule a return visit as needed.	If questions remain unanswered at a health assessment, needs aren't fully met.	Parent and child state they have no further questions; describe plans for next action.

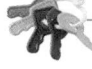

Key Points

Health assessment always causes some degree of apprehension for both parents and children because of worry some illness will be detected. Giving reassurance of wellness during examinations helps to alleviate this worry.

A health history is an important part of a health assessment. The purpose is to gather information that will supplement physical or laboratory examinations to provide a more thorough health evaluation.

The parts of a complete health history are introduction, chief concern, present health, family profile, history of past illnesses, day history, family health history, and review of systems.

Physical examination involves four techniques: inspection, palpation, percussion, and auscultation. Techniques and approaches must be varied according to the child's age.

Be certain to use examining instruments safely (e.g., supporting an otoscope base so that if a child moves, the otoscope moves with the child). Be certain young children are not left unsupervised on an examining table so they don't fall.

The components of a physical examination are vital sign assessment; general appearance; mental status assessment; body measurements; and assessment of head, eyes, nose, ears, mouth, neck, chest, breasts, lungs, heart, abdomen, rectogenital area, extremities, back, and neurologic function.

Adolescent girls can be taught breast self-examination and boys testicular self-examination at the time of a health appraisal.

Vision assessment consists of asking children to read a standardized chart such as a Snellen or Preschool E Chart, cover testing, or color discrimination assessment.

Hearing assessment consists of such assessments as audiometric testing and a Rinne and Weber test.

Development is an important part of total assessment. The Denver II Developmental Screening Test and the Denver Articulation Screening Examination are specific development tests.

The Goodenough-Harris Drawing Test correlates well with IQ and is an easy test to administer to children between the ages of 3 and 10 years to assess intelligence.

Temperament refers to a child's innate behavioral characteristics, such as activity level, rhythmicity, and tendency to approach or withdraw and adapt to situations. Assessing this can help parents better understand behavior in their child.

Assessment of immunization status is included as part of a health assessment. Childhood immunizations are a major safeguard for children against common illnesses.

Critical Thinking Exercises

1. Keoto is the 13-year-old girl you met at the beginning of the chapter. Her father has brought her to your ambulatory clinic for a middle school checkup because he is worried she needs glasses (she sits so close to the television set). Her mother was reluctant to bring her because she doesn't want her to be prescribed glasses. What questions on history would be important to ask the father or Keoto? What type of eye chart would you use with Keoto to assess her vision?

2. Keoto's 2-year-old sister, Candy, is very resistant to being examined. What techniques would you use to help the toddler adjust better to a physical examination?

3. Children should be completely undressed for physical examinations and all body surfaces inspected. What would be your response if Candy's father said he did not want to undress his child? What if he did not want to remove a Band-Aid from Candy's back?

4. Examine the National Health Goals related to health assessment of children. Most government-sponsored money for nursing research is allotted based on these goals. What would be a possible research topic to explore pertinent to these goals that would be applicable to Keoto's family and also advance evidence-based practice?

References

American Academy of Pediatrics Committee on Practice and Ambulatory Medicine. (2005). *Recommendations for preventive pediatric health care.* Washington, DC: AAP.

Bezyack, M. E. (2004). Respiratory distress: making the diagnosis in kids. *Nursing Spectrum, 17*(2), 30–31.

Carey, W. B., & McDevitt, S. C. (1978). Revision of the infant temperament questionnaire. *Pediatrics, 61*(4), 735–739.

Centers for Disease Control. (2005). *Recommended childhood and adolescent immunization schedule, United States, 2005.* Washington, DC: DHHS.

Department of Health and Human Services. (2000). *Healthy people 2010.* Washington, DC: DHHS.

Dudek, S. G. (2005). *Nutrition essentials for nursing practice.* Philadelphia: Lippincott Williams & Wilkins.

Frankenburg, W. K. (1994). Preventing developmental delays: is developmental screening sufficient? *Pediatrics, 93*(4), 586–589.

Gold, R. S. (2004). Amblyopia is a hot topic in pediatric ophthalmology. *Ocular Surgery News, 22*(18), 4–5.

Goodenough, F. L. (1926). *Measurement of intelligence by drawings.* New York: World Book Company.

Gracey, K., & Lankford, R. (2003). A parent's guide to newborn hearing screening. *Advances in Neonatal Care, 3*(6), 318–319.

Horner, G. (2005). Physical abuse: recognition and reporting. *Journal of Pediatric Health Care, 19*(1), 4–11.

Jack, S. (2004). Review: existing epidemiological evidence does not show an association between mumps, measles, and rubella vaccination and autism. *Evidence-Based Nursing, 7*(1), 25.

Jones, G. T., & McFarlane, G. J. (2005). Epidemiology of low back pain in children and adolescents. *Archives of Disease in Childhood, 90*(3), 312–316.

Jones, J. S., et al. (2003). Anogenital injuries in adolescents after consensual sexual intercourse. *Academic Emergency Medicine, 10*(12), 1378-1383.

LaMontagne, L. L., et al. (2004). Adolescent scoliosis: effects of corrective surgery, cognitive-behavioral interventions, and age on activity outcomes. *Applied Nursing Research, 17*(3), 168-177.

Mandracchia, V. J., et al. (2004). Management of osteomyelitis. *Clinics in Podiatric Medicine and Surgery, 21*(3), 335-351.

Mulryan, K., Cathers, P., & Fagin, A. (2004). How to recognize and respond to child abuse. *Nursing, 34*(10), 52-57.

Muntner, P., et al. (2004). Trends in blood pressure among children and adolescents. *JAMA: Journal of the American Medical Association, 29*(17), 2107-2113.

National Center for Health Statistics. (2005). *Trends in the health of Americans.* Hyattsville, MD: NCHS.

Peterson, C. (2004). Smallpox vaccination update. *American Journal of Nursing, 104*(7), 104-105.

Prevent Blindness America. (2005). *Test your child's eyes.* (Prevent blindness.org.)

Thomas, A., & Chess, S. (1977). *Temperament and development.* New York: Brunner/Mazel.

Thomas, M., Kohli, V., & King, D. (2004). Barriers to childhood immunization: findings from a needs assessment study. *Home Health Care Services Quarterly, 23*(2), 19-39.

Trusty, J. M., Beinborn, D. S., & Jahangir, A. (2004). Dysrhythmias and the athlete. *AACN Clinical Issues: Advanced Practice in Acute and Critical Care, 15*(3), 432-448.

Whitehill, J., Raucci, J., & Sandritter, T. (2004). Pediatric pharmacology. Childhood immunizations. *Journal of Pediatric Health Care, 18*(4), 192-199.

Suggested Readings

Bortot, A. T., Risser, W. L., & Cromwell, P. F. (2004). Coping with pelvic inflammatory disease in the adolescent. *Contemporary Pediatrics, 21*(4), 33-38.

Brennan, R. A. (2004). A nurse-managed universal newborn hearing screen program. *MCN: The American Journal of Maternal/Child Nursing, 29*(5), 320-325.

Chen, C., Li, C., & Wang, J. (2004). Growth and development of children with congenital heart disease. *Journal of Advanced Nursing, 47*(3), 260-269.

Deatrick, J. A., et al. (2003). Correlates of children's competence to make healthcare decisions. *Journal of Clinical Ethics, 14*(3), 152-163.

Duncan, M. K. W., & Sanger, M. (2004). Coping with the pediatric anogenital exam. *Journal of Child and Adolescent Psychiatric Nursing, 17*(3), 126-136.

Hay, A. D., Schroeder, K., & Fahey, T. (2004). 10-minute consultation: acute cough in children. *British Medical Journal, 328*(7447), 1062-1063.

Plunkett, A., & Beattie, R. M. (2005). Recurrent abdominal pain in childhood. *Journal of the Royal Society of Medicine, 98*(3), 101-106.

Rhoades, R. L. (2004). NIH updates guidelines for high BP in children. *Clinical Advisor, 7*(7), 52-54.

Short, M. A. (2004). Guide to a systematic physical assessment in the infant with suspected infection and/or sepsis. *Advances in Neonatal Care, 4*(3), 141-157.

Toole, K., & Perry, C. S. (2004). Increasing immunization compliance. *Journal of School Nursing, 20*(4), 203-208.

Weston, C. G. (2004). Attention-deficit/hyperactivity disorder in children: assessment, management, and outcome. *Journal of Clinical Outcomes Management, 11*(4), 241-253.

CHAPTER 34

Communication and Teaching With Children and Families

Key Terms

affective learning
behavior modification
clarifying
cognitive learning
communication
demonstration
empathy
feedback
focusing
nontherapeutic communication
paraphrasing
perception checking
positive reinforcement
psychomotor learning
redemonstration
reflecting
teaching plan
therapeutic communication

Objectives

After mastering the contents of this chapter, you should be able to:

1. Describe principles of effective communication and teaching and learning as they relate to health teaching with children.
2. Assess children for their ability to communicate and readiness to learn.
3. State nursing diagnoses related to communication and health teaching with children.
4. Identify expected outcomes for a specific child based on the child's age, developmental maturity, emotional needs, and communication or learning style.
5. Plan nursing care based on the use of communication and health teaching priorities.
6. Implement health teaching (e.g., devising a puppet show) using principles of effective communication and teaching–learning.
7. Evaluate outcome criteria to be certain outcomes established for care have been achieved.
8. Identify National Health Goals related to communication and teaching with children that nurses could help the nation achieve.
9. Identify areas of care related to effective communication or health teaching of children that could benefit from additional nursing research or application of evidence-based practice.
10. Use critical thinking to analyze ways therapeutic communication and health teaching can be further incorporated into the nursing care of children and families to make it more family-centered.
11. Integrate knowledge of effective communication and teaching–learning with the nursing process to achieve quality maternal and child health nursing care.

---

*Y*ou meet two patients of very different ages in an outpatient clinic. Wolf Whitefeather is a 3-year-old boy who is scheduled for repair of syndactyly (webbed fingers) next week. One of his favorite activities is coloring. His mother tells you she is concerned Wolf will be hard to entertain after surgery because the large pressure bandage he will have afterward will prevent him from coloring with that hand. "I don't even want to begin to talk to him about surgery," she tells you. What would be a good strategy for teaching about this type of surgery to a 3-year-old child?

Previous chapters discussed normal growth and development and how children's understanding increases with age. This chapter adds information about techniques for effective communication and health teaching with children. This is important information because it builds a base for disease prevention and health promotion for the age group.

Barry Sandoz is a 15-year-old with a recurring peptic ulcer. His mother tells you health teaching with Barry will be ineffective because he never listens to a thing adults say. Would you try to teach Barry more about his condition, or not? How would your communication with these children vary because of their age difference?

After you've studied this chapter, access the accompanying website. Read the patient scenario and answer the questions to further sharpen your skills, grow more familiar with RN-CLEX types of questions, and reward yourself with how much you have learned.

ommunication and health teaching are independent
nursing actions that accompany all nursing care. They
are probably the most frequently used interventions
for nurses working with childbearing and childrearing families because health promotion is such a priority for this
population. Education is a prime method for empowering
families to assume responsibility for their own health. It is
as important as any intervention for families experiencing
some type of illness or injury; it is especially important
when preparing a child for surgery or some other health
care procedure. New areas that require teaching are constantly arising as the health care environment continues to
grow more technical.

Communication with children can be either formal or informal. Health teaching may be offered to an individual or
to a group of children with similar learning needs. It can
also be both formal (e.g., teaching a group of preschoolers
about hospitalization) or informal (e.g., assuring a parent
his or her child is getting enough nutrition, even though the
child snacks rather than sits down to regular meals). The
same principles of effective teaching and learning apply no
matter which technique is used or whether it is offered to
an individual or to a group. National Health Goals regarding
health teaching and children are shown in Box 34.1.

Nursing Process Overview

For Health Teaching With Children

● *Assessment*
Neither communication nor health teaching can be effectively accomplished unless they are placed within
the context of the nursing process. Learner needs and
characteristics, teacher characteristics, available support people, and level of content are all factors that will
affect learning or whether communication is received,
so they must be assessed so that nursing diagnoses
that clearly state the specific health needs can be
formulated (Box 34.2).

● *Nursing Diagnosis*
Common examples of nursing diagnoses related to
communication or health teaching are:

- Impaired verbal communication related to use of
Russian as primary language
- Deficient knowledge related to importance of taking
medicine daily
- Health-seeking behaviors related to ways to improve
the child's nutritional intake
- Impaired verbal communication related to placement
of endotracheal tube
- Anxiety related to perceived amount of material
needed to be learned for home care of child

● *Outcome Identification and Planning*
After formulation of a nursing diagnosis, an individualized plan for communication or teaching needs to be
constructed. A plan should detail not only what is to be
communicated or learned but also methods as to how
this will be accomplished and evaluated. The most

BOX 34.1 FOCUS ON . . .

NATIONAL HEALTH GOALS

A number of National Health Goals address
good communication or health teaching, because it is
such an important mechanism of preventive health
care. These goals include:

- Increase the proportion of middle, junior high, and senior high schools that provide school health education
to prevent unintentional injuries, violence, suicide, tobacco use and addiction, alcohol and other drug use,
unintended pregnancy, HIV infection, AIDS, and other
STIs, unhealthy dietary patterns, inadequate physical
activity, and environmental health problems, from a
baseline of 28% to 70%.
- Increase the proportion of the nation's elementary,
middle, junior high, and senior high schools that
have a nurse-to-student ratio of at least 1:750,
from 28% to 50%.
- Increase the proportion of local health departments
that have established culturally appropriate and linguistically competent community health-promotion
and disease-prevention programs, from 35% to 50%
(DHHS, 2000).

Nurses can help the nation achieve these goals by consulting with schools and health care organizations to
develop health teaching programs and by teaching such
programs. Areas that could benefit from nursing research include ways in which busy health care providers
can better incorporate health teaching into care; what
special techniques are needed to be certain that underserved populations are addressed; and whether
material with immediate application and material for
long-term care require different teaching techniques.

effective way to ensure that expected outcomes are
achieved is to ask the child or family to join in planning. Be certain outcomes are concrete and measurable (not "Child will discuss general aspects of his
disease," but "Child will list three steps to prevent
disease").

● *Implementation*
The step of implementation involves the actual communication or teaching carried out. Teaching children
is not always easy and requires practice and knowledge of each child's particular developmental level.

● *Outcome Evaluation*
As a final step of communication or teaching, what was
communicated or learned must be evaluated. A new
plan may need to be developed to continue teaching
if communication or learning was less than optimal.
Examples of outcome criteria are:

- Child demonstrates self-injection of insulin.
- Child demonstrates anger by language rather than
punching wall.

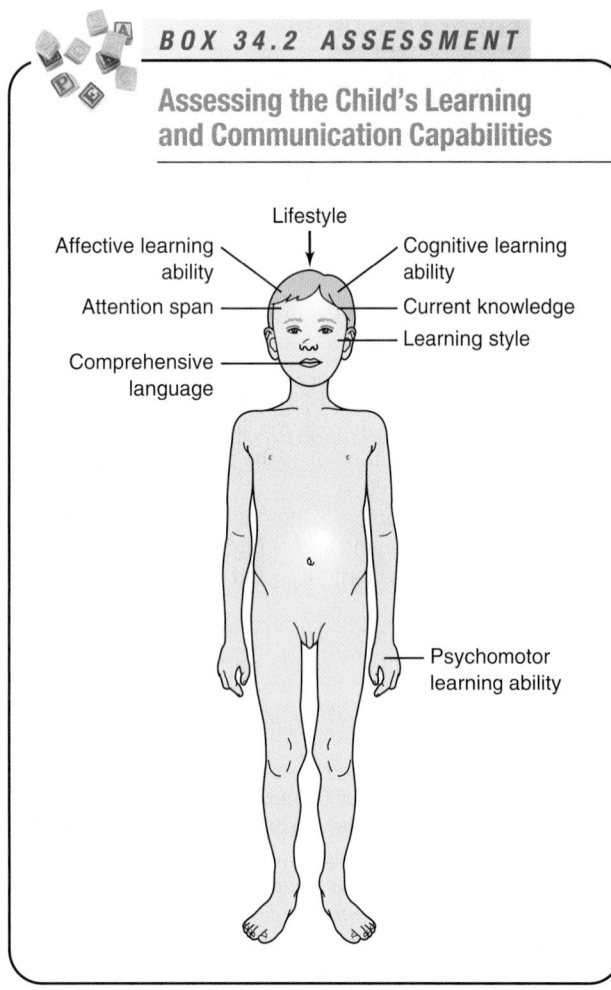

BOX 34.2 ASSESSMENT

Assessing the Child's Learning and Communication Capabilities

- Child lists foods to include in a high-protein diet.
- Family demonstrates improved family communication techniques by next clinic visit.
- Parents demonstrate effective cardiopulmonary resuscitation technique at home visit.

COMMUNICATION

Communication is the exchange of ideas between two or more persons. It can be verbal, using words, or nonverbal, using actions such as touch or eye contact or even a remote system such as mail or e-mail. It is an important process in the care of children because it can make or break an effective relationship. Communication, as a process, can be divided into two major categories: nontherapeutic (casual, everyday conversation) and therapeutic (helpful and constructive interchanges).

Nontherapeutic Communication

Nontherapeutic communication is identified by its lack of structure or planning (i.e., it lacks deliberate purpose other than socializing). Dinner conversation is an example of nontherapeutic communication.

Therapeutic Communication

Therapeutic communication is an interaction between two people that is planned (you deliberately intend to determine the true way a child feels), has structure (you use specific wording techniques that will encourage the response you expect to elicit), and is helpful and constructive (at the end of the exchange you will know much more about the child than you did at the beginning, and the child, ideally, also knows more about himself or herself).

In some instances, there is no cure for a child you care for—no surgery, no medication, no pain relief. If you practice therapeutic communication, however, you still have something to offer this child: support by your words or nonverbal communication such as touch. This is often the most valued, most appreciated, and most helpful aspect of all the care you offer.

Components of Good Communication

Communication can be broken down and diagrammed according to its essential components: the encoder, the code, the decoder, and response or feedback (Fig. 34.1).

The Encoder

The encoder is the person who originates a message. Such a person desires to share a thought or feeling with someone else. He or she molds this thought into a form suitable for transferring to another person (a code). Communication can be ineffective if the person omits cognitive processing or speaks without thinking, chooses the wrong words for the message, or accompanies the spoken words with a facial expression, tone of voice, or gesture inappropriate for the message.

The Code

The code is the message that is conveyed, as well as the medium or system used to convey it. Although this usually involves a simple spoken system, messages can also be

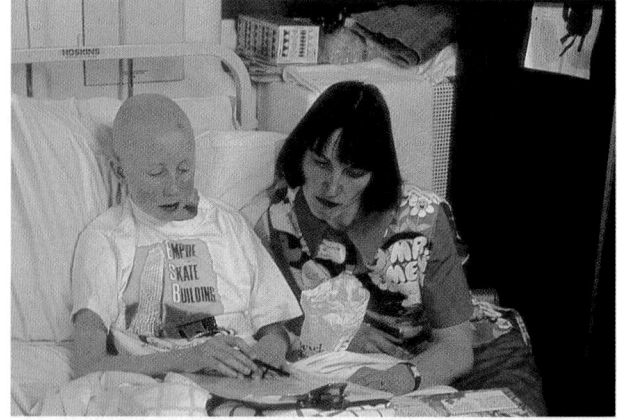

FIGURE 34.1 Health teaching is an interactive process, in which both a teacher and a learner share in the learning experience. (SPL/Custom Medical Stock Photo.)

conveyed by such methods as a painting, poem, novel, Morse code, Braille, computer, television, radio, audio or videotape, DVD, movie projector, or telephone. Communication is often ineffective because a person chooses the wrong medium for a message (e.g., delivering a lecture with many technical words when a drawing with carefully labeled parts would have made the message much clearer, or e-mailing when confronting a person directly would have been more effective).

The Decoder

The receiver (decoder) of the message not only receives it (hears it, reads it, views it) but interprets or decodes its meaning (cognitive processing). Messages are interpreted in light of the receiver's previous knowledge. They may be misinterpreted if a receiver's store of knowledge is too different from that of the sender. Messages may also be misinterpreted if the receiver misses part of the transmission, such as the wink accompanying the spoken words that would have let the receiver know the sender was joking. Under stress, children tend to narrow their ability to receive information to a small area of concern (they center). When you are dealing with children who are extremely anxious, you may find, although you gave excellent instructions (both sender and message components of communication were adequate), they did not "hear" you (did not receive or could not interpret the message because of anxiety).

Feedback or Response

Feedback is the reply the decoder returns to the sender to acknowledge the message has been received and interpreted. This could be a spoken statement, a nod of the head, a facial grimace, or the sudden slamming of a telephone receiver. With feedback, the roles of sender and receiver become reversed and another communication cycle is begun. Communication can be ineffective if children do not offer feedback (the message was either not received or understood) or offer feedback before the message is fully interpreted (acting before thinking). When you are caring for children with sensory challenges such as vision or hearing, you may have to change your usual feedback mechanisms in order to be understood, because a nod of the head or quiet response may not be received.

The Development of Language

Development of language involves not only physically being able to form and voice words but also comprehension of what they mean and how they are used. One of the first responses an infant makes at birth is to communicate. A first cry is important because it signals the infant is breathing well. It also announces to the parents the birth is real and stimulates the beginning of parent–child interaction. Early in life, when infants cry, they kick their legs and thrash their arms or react with their whole body. Some new parents comment that their newborns have bad tempers because the infant seems very angry. They are actually commenting on the way newborns respond with their total body to stimuli. Infants discontinue gesturing wildly with every need as soon as they learn a more refined communication system.

By age 2, children have mastered language well enough to be able to put two-word sentences (a noun and a verb) together. By preschool age, they not only have a vocabulary of about 900 words, but also can code them into simple jokes or stories.

School-age children enlarge their ability to communicate from close oral exchanges to use of e-mail or the telephone. They can write poetry and, by the end of the period, show an adult sense of humor by the jokes they create. Adolescents progress to a new phase in which they originate new words for objects or feelings ("cool" and so forth). This form of communication helps them separate their world from adults and keep their adolescent culture separate.

Levels of Communication

Not every conversation you engage in has the same depth level, nor should it. Throughout a day, a person may use as many as five levels, from clichés to peak communication.

First-Level: Cliché Conversation

Cliché conversation is pleasant chatting (comments such as, "Have a nice day") between people who do not intend their relationship to extend beyond a superficial level. It is important when meeting a child for the first time that you introduce yourself not only with your name but also your position and function (a student nurse who is going to take care of you; a nurse who will be visiting you in your home). This information leads the family to move the conversation from the cliché level to a more meaningful one.

Second Level: Fact Reporting

Fact reporting is simply stating facts about oneself ("I'm 12; I'm in sixth grade"). Fact reporting is necessary for you to understand children, but it does not tell you anything about their feelings or needs. Children can move from this level to a higher level of communication only when they feel they can trust you with more information.

Third Level: Shared Personal Ideas and Judgments

When children know you well, they are able to share ideas ("I always wanted to be an astronaut") and judgments ("This is too hard for me; I need to learn a different way"). This level of communication exposes them to loss of self-esteem if their views are not respected. It is the level that is the beginning of therapeutic interactions.

Fourth Level: Shared Feelings

It is difficult to share feelings until you truly trust one another, because feelings are tenuous, fragile concepts, easily destroyed and crushed by inept or uncaring comments. Listen carefully for an expression of feeling from children ("It's terrible to be always sick"). These admissions are telling you much more than how a child experiences the world; they represent trust in you and the depth of the relationship the child has established with you.

Fifth Level: Peak Communication

The fifth level of communication is a sense of oneness, or being able to know what the other person is experiencing without it actually being voiced. It sometimes occurs spontaneously in high-intensity situations but generally arises out of long-term relationships. For example, you notice that a parent sits soundlessly beside her daughter's bedside for hours at a time. When she leaves, the daughter says, "She makes me feel so much better when she's here." It would be easy to view this mother as nonsupportive (she says almost nothing during the time she's there), but by using fifth-level communication, she has given her daughter more comfort than other visitors who talk the entire time they visit.

Nonverbal Communication

What children communicate nonverbally is at least as important as the words they actually voice. Nonverbal communication can be especially important in areas such as intensive care units when the child may be unable to speak because of endotracheal tubes and ventilators. Nonverbal communication can be expressed in a variety of ways.

Distance

Although it is affected by cultural and personal variables, the distance at which you position yourself from the person you are talking to may indicate your feelings toward him or her or the type of conversation you want to have. People generally consider the space directly surrounding them (up to 18 inches) as *intimate* space, to be crossed only by people who know them well or with whom they are comfortable having close body contact. Sometimes you will notice in a heated discussion that one person moves aggressively into this space and the other automatically steps back to protect it. People in elevators separate themselves from others by this much space if the car is not full.

Whenever you touch a child, you violate this space, so always ask permission to touch ("Okay if I change your bandage now?") or with small children, announce what you are going to do ("It's time to change your bandage now"). If children agree to let you enter this space, it means they see you as safe, protective, and helpful.

The space between 18 inches to 4 feet is sensed by most people as *personal* space. This is the distance people usually stand apart from each other for casual conversation. It is a comfortable hand-shaking distance. When you stand by the side of a crib or bed or sit next to a person at home, you are within this space. It is a concerned, I-care-about-you distance but does not invade intimate space.

The distance between 4 feet and 12 feet is *social* space, the distance used to conduct business or teach a class. Conversation spoken at this distance is readily heard by others. Do not use social space to ask a personal question. If you ask a child, "How are you feeling?" as you pass in a hallway, for example, he or she will probably answer, "Fine, thank you," a programmed reply almost everyone is taught in early childhood. In contrast, if you ask that same question from a personal or intimate distance, providing privacy, the answer might be, "I'm scared I'm never going home again."

Distance beyond 12 feet is *public* space. To communicate from this distance, you need to shout; privacy is not respected at all. Waving to a friend in a hallway or across a parking lot is an example of public space communication. Most people perceive speaking on the telephone or using the mail or e-mail as either social or personal space. The tone of voice or the words used help to differentiate which area they consider it to be. A message such as, "Have I got news for you!" suggests social space. "Can you keep a secret?" brings it into intimate space.

Genuineness

Genuineness is a quality of projecting sincerity or being yourself. Children will have difficulty trusting you and therefore will be unable to move to a deep relationship with you if you change your behavior from one day to the next (e.g., from maximum patience to short-tempered), because they have to spend energy every day testing to see who you are that day. The way to achieve a feeling of genuineness is not to try to be what you are not. The insecurity that comes from pretending manifests itself as negative feelings such as aggressiveness or a bored attitude.

Warmth

Warmth is an innate quality, and some people manifest it more spontaneously than others. Basic ways in which warmth is demonstrated are direct eye contact, use of a gentle tone of voice, listening attentively, approaching a child within a comfortable space of 1 to 4 feet (closer may be threatening; farther away may be distancing), and using touch appropriately. Warmth is a quality that you display best when you know another person well. Any action that helps you to know a person better (taking a health history, talking about school or family or how a child feels about the present situation) not only lets you plan care but also allows you to become increasingly comfortable with the child and deepen the warmth of your relationship.

Empathy

Empathy is the ability to put yourself in another person's place and experience a feeling the same as that person is experiencing it. People who are capable of empathy are the best support people because they can anticipate a child's reactions or fears. At first, it seems empathy would require you to have experienced all the situations that children experience. This is not necessarily true, however, because you understand the common emotion of all situations in other ways. If you have hoped for something very strongly and then not attained it, loved someone and not had that emotion returned, lost someone or something that was so important to you that you felt actual pain, you can feel empathy for children who have received a disappointing diagnosis or who are unhappy for other reasons you have never experienced. Feeling empathy is emotionally draining because, when you assume another person's emotions, you experience them at the same depth. Nurses who are capable of empathy need to surround themselves with good support people so they have refueling resources when they need them.

Gestures

Children vary a great deal in the gestures they use to accompany their spoken words. Although this is culturally influenced, it is also an individual trait. Be careful not to assess emotion only by a child's gestures; some children wave their arms wildly describing an everyday occurrence; others would use that degree of expression only when in extreme distress. Be aware also that your own gestures are always being read by children. A statement that you approve of something is contradicted by placing your arms across your chest in a disapproving, stern manner.

Body Posture and Gait

Children who feel good about themselves usually assume an upright body posture and walk rapidly and surely; those who are depressed or insecure tend to slouch and move more slowly and timidly; those who are threatened tend to either draw back or act aggressively. Children who are in agreement with you usually maintain eye contact with you as you speak to them. Very depressed or insecure children do not do that (they feel too inferior), nor do children who are very angry. Children from some cultures do not meet your gaze because it is not culturally appropriate.

Facial expression is an important accompanying gesture. Clenched teeth, frowns, and smiles are easily interpreted by everyone. The degree of pain a child is experiencing may be more evident by facial expression than words.

General Appearance

Children who have good self-esteem tend to maintain good body hygiene and care about their appearance. Those who are depressed may not feel the effort involved in grooming is worthwhile. Personal hygiene varies, however, and it is difficult to assess it on your first contact with a child. What you see as ill-kempt may be neat and trim for that particular child; what you think of as well groomed may be comparatively sloppy for that child.

Be aware that your impression of how children dress registers very strongly on your subconscious. Do not let an unconscious dislike for a mode of dress of some child (body piercing or a turban) cause you to draw back. Preparing to give nursing care is not the same kind of activity as evaluating whether you wish to invite someone to dinner.

Touch

Touch is the most intimate and meaningful of nonverbal techniques. When words are inadequate, touch rarely is. Learn to use touch such as clapping a child's shoulder or squeezing a hand to accompany reassuring words or in place of words as a strong support signal (I'm here; I understand; it's all right to be afraid). On the other hand, be aware that some children enjoy being touched more than others. Due to individual preferences or cultural variations, some children do not like you to use this nonverbal signal with them. Assess individually for the appropriateness of using touch.

Use of Humor

Some people have a natural knack for finding humor in any situation; others do not instinctively have this quality and must cultivate it. Those who can laugh at their own mistakes are usually enjoyable people to have around, because their laughter at themselves suggests that, when you make a mistake, they will be able to accept it the same way (or at least not be angry about it).

Be careful of the use of humor with children because they are school-age before they appreciate most adult jokes. If they are fatigued or ill, they may be looking for a firm support person to be with them more than one who is amusing. You can often measure a child's progress by noting the first time after a procedure the child responds to you with a humorous statement. Remember, though, that laughter and joking can also be signs of increasing anxiety. Evaluate the use of humor to be certain a child really finds a situation amusing.

Use of Drawings

A useful nonverbal technique to learn how children feel about a frightening experience is to ask them to draw a picture of what happened or a picture of themselves. A child hospitalized for heart surgery might draw her heart prominently; surely she realizes that she cannot survive if something happens to such an important body part.

A child's use of color may be a clue as to mood (happy children tend to use bright colors; depressed children use black or dark colors). A child with good self-esteem usually fills the full page with a drawing; one with less crowds a drawing into a corner. These observations are quite variable, however; a child may have had only a black crayon with which to color or may be saving the rest of the paper for a second drawing.

Use of Music

The type of music to which children prefer to listen often also conveys their mood. The better they feel about themselves, the more likely they are to choose lively music; if they are sad, they often choose a quieter, more comforting type. Children enjoy repetition, however, and so may play the same music over and over, independent of their mood.

Techniques That Encourage Therapeutic Communication

Several techniques are effective in deepening communication patterns and relationships. These techniques can be learned if they are not a spontaneous part of your present communication pattern (Box 34.3).

Attentive Listening

Making it clear you are concentrating on what another is saying by such a motion as nodding indicates you value

BOX 34.3 FOCUS ON . . .

EVIDENCE-BASED PRACTICE

Are Fathers as Supportive as Mothers Following Their Child's Surgery?

To investigate this question, nurse researchers video-taped the behavior of parents of 142 children (78 fathers and 131 mothers) during the first hour following the child's return from surgery. Two nurses then scored the parents' behavior according to the Parental Behavior Inventory scale. The results showed that fathers and mothers demonstrated similar types of behaviors such as showing affection and giving physical care. Fathers, however, spent less time at their children's bedsides than mothers did and, overall, demonstrated fewer helping behaviors.

This is an interesting study for nurses because it demonstrates that although fathers are often the parent with children postoperatively, they may need more support than mothers to be maximally helpful to their children in a postsurgical setting. As more and more children are raised by single fathers today, this type of support becomes more and more important.

Source: Tourigny, J., Ward, V., & Lepage, T. (2004). Fathers' behavior during their child's ambulatory surgery. *Issues in Comprehensive Pediatric Nursing, 27*(2), 69–81.

BOX 34.4 FOCUS ON . . .

FAMILY TEACHING

Listening to Children

Q. Barry's mother says to you, "My son always tells me I don't listen to him. How can I be a better listener?"
A. Try the following tips:

1. Stop talking. You cannot listen if you are talking.
2. Look and act interested. Don't read or write while he talks. Listen to understand rather than to reply.
3. Remove distractions. Do not doodle, tap, or shuffle papers. Would it be quieter if you turned off the television?
4. Empathize. Try to put yourself in your child's place so you can see his point of view.
5. Be patient. Allow plenty of time. Do not interrupt. Do not edge toward the door or walk away.
6. Hold your temper. An angry person gets the wrong meaning from words.
7. Hold argument or criticism, which puts children on the defensive. They may stop talking or get angry.
8. Ask questions. This is proof that you have been listening.
9. Stop talking. This is the first and last suggestion, because all others depend on it.

what a child is saying. Children who feel valued are much more likely to confide feelings and concerns than those who sense you consider them not important (Box 34.4).

No one likes to talk to someone who does not appear to be listening or responding. Good listening, therefore, like speaking, is not passive but active. Be aware that your posture reveals to a great extent whether you are listening (sitting, not standing, to convey that you are not on the run; leaning forward, not backward; stooping to meet a child's level). Nodding, maintaining eye contact, and stopping all other activities are strong indicators you are attuned to what is being said. In some instances, it is necessary to repeat a part of what the child said, interject an appropriate "uh-huh" or "m-m-m," or make a direct statement ("I'm listening. Go on") to indicate you are listening. Be certain that when you are listening to the 20th child on any given day, you do not exhibit "end-of-the day" behavior. To be therapeutic, you have to give everyone's concerns the same alert attention.

Open-Ended Questions

A pointed or direct question used in discussing asks for a specific task; it implies all you are interested in hearing about is that one fact. An example of a direct question is, "Do you take Tylenol when you have a headache?" An open-ended question is not limited to a simple answer but invites a wide variety of responses because it is so comprehensive (e.g., "Tell me what you do when you have a headache"). A child might answer this question by describing not only the amount of analgesic she takes but also using a cold towel, staying home from school, and

closing her eyes to stop the pain. Three or four times more information has been elicited.

Open-ended questions are not effective if the topic is difficult for a child to describe (a preschooler has difficulty responding even yes or no; a paragraph of material would be impossible) or if the child is naturally shy or defensive about the subject (he knows he has not been doing the things you told him to do and would rather not admit it).

Most communication is a combination of direct and open-ended questions. Listen carefully the next time you ask someone to explain something to see if you make use of mostly direct (information-limiting) questions or open-ended (information-expanding) ones.

Reflecting

Reflecting is another technique, like attentive listening, that is so simple that its importance is easy to discount. **Reflecting** is restating the last word or phrase a child has said when there is a pause in the communication. A child says, "I'm worried," and then stops. You repeat the last word. "Worried?" The child, assured you are listening and interested, will generally enlarge on the first statement: "I'm worried I won't make the football team this year." Older school-age children may not respond well to reflection; they may interpret it as imitating them, not seeking information.

Clarifying

Clarifying consists of repeating statements others have made so you and they can be certain you understood them. This is particularly helpful if a child has been describing a set of symptoms or series of actions. You would clarify such a statement by saying, "Let me see if I understand this. You said you always get the pain first in your stomach. Then it spreads to your chest." If you are not quoting correctly, the child will interrupt and restate the problem: "No, the chest pain comes first."

Paraphrasing

Paraphrasing is restating what children have said not only to assure them you have heard correctly (as in clarifying) but to help them explain what they have been trying to say in other words. In clarifying, you repeat a child's exact words; in paraphrasing, you retain the meaning of the words but repeat them in a clearer or more condensed form. The child says, for example, "I don't talk about my problems with my parents." A paraphrasing statement might be, "You're telling me you and your parents haven't discussed home care. Is that right?" When paraphrasing, ask for confirmation that your interpretation is correct; otherwise, you may find yourself putting words in children's mouths.

When the topic is embarrassing or emotionally charged (an adolescent discussing sexual orientation), the child might use such vague terms that the explanation becomes difficult to follow. Paraphrasing using basic terms would let him know not only that you understand him but that, if he can describe the problem better with such words than with medical terminology, it is acceptable to you.

Perception Checking

Perception checking documents a feeling or emotion reported to you. This makes it a step deeper than paraphrasing. In paraphrasing, you document a statement or fact; in perception checking, you document a feeling or emotion. The child says, "I'm not at all worried about surgery. I know a lot of kids have the same thing done every day. I mean, what could happen?" You say, "You're telling me you're not worried, but the number of times you've said it makes me wonder if you really are worried. Are you?"

Always ask for validation that your perception is correct so you do not put ideas into a child's mind. Perception checking is helpful because as a rule, children are not ready to deal with emotions until they can admit they are experiencing them. When you bring an emotion out on the table this way, it allows them to confront it and deal with it for the first time. They may lose their reluctance to admit other worries because you have implied that worrying is acceptable.

Focusing

Focusing helps children to center on a subject you suspect is causing them anxiety because they comment about it indirectly or else completely avoid it. It is done by repeating something they said ("You mentioned you feel tired all the time") or by mentioning the avoided topic ("You haven't said a word about how you feel about this surgery. Is that a problem?"). Once a subject is brought up for discussion, most children respond to it. As long as it can be avoided, however, they do not have to face the problem and begin to solve it.

Supportive Statements

Supportive statements let children know you accept their behavior or at least appreciate they have dealt well with unfortunate circumstances. For example, an adolescent says, "My girlfriend dumped me while I've been here in the hospital." Such a statement deserves a supportive reply such as, "That must not feel good." The adolescent will take this response to mean you want to discuss the topic and, encouraged by your empathy, may elaborate on it as it still affects him.

Silence

If you ask a question and a child does not respond immediately, it is natural to ask another question or perhaps change the subject, assuming the child is not interested in the topic. This is a social custom that allows you to back off so you do not put someone into the awkward position of having to discuss a sensitive topic. Silence, however, is an effective therapeutic technique. If you ask an emotion-laden question ("Are you worried?") and the child does not answer immediately, allow a period of silence to pass. Because you do not hurry to fill in the silence, the child is likely to respond by hurrying an answer (to fill in the silence): when this happens, the answer is usually spontaneous and often open and uninhibited. In other instances, a child may answer the question deliberately and cautiously and, because you have provided a period of time to answer, offer additional information.

Do not overdo silence, however, either by the number of times you use it or the length of time you allow it to extend. In this era of constant noise, many individuals are extremely uncomfortable with silence. Too much silence can indicate to a child you are not interested enough to keep the conversation going.

Checkpoint Question 1

Barry tells you he hates school. Which response would be the best example of paraphrasing?

a. "Tell me again what you said."
b. "School?"
c. "You're telling me you're unhappy with school?"
d. "Hate is a strong emotion for a teenager to feel."

Factors That Can Interfere With Effective Communication With Children

Because so much of nursing care is influenced by verbal communication, it is important to avoid miscalculations in communication and to recognize common situations in which meanings can easily be distorted.

Age and Developmental Level

Age and developmental levels are important to communication ability because they influence vocabulary so greatly

(Berger, 2004). A 3-year-old child may not have the vocabulary to explain the way her knee feels (she has heard the word "ache" but only in connection with headache; she does not know that knees can ache as well). Early school-age children have difficulty describing the blurring they experience as they focus on a blackboard with less-than-perfect eyesight, because this is the way they have always seen. The ability to describe inner feelings such as anger, sadness, and fear comes only with adolescence.

Intellectual Level

Intellectual level, like age, affects vocabulary and ability both to encode and decode messages. It influences the number of languages a child speaks, reading ability, and the depth of explanation a child is capable of understanding.

Physical Factors

Physical factors such as speech impairments and hearing or vision challenges interfere with the transmission and reception of messages. When children are distracted by such sensations as fatigue or pain, they also may have a reduced ability to transmit or receive messages correctly.

Technical Terminology

Adults have heard common medical words and so usually have little difficulty understanding an explanation of one. Children, in contrast, have not heard many medical words. Listen to the explanations you give them to be certain you would have understood your explanation at their age.

Showing Disapproval

Parents and children do not come for health care to be criticized; they come to learn more about how to stay well or recover from illness. If you criticize them, they may not reveal any further information to you because they do not want you to react in the same way you did to their preliminary statements.

Suppose an adolescent says, "I never drink milk. That's for babies." Knowing milk is an important source of calcium, you respond, "That's not right. You should drink at least two glasses a day." This discourages the adolescent from telling you any more about her eating habits (she doesn't eat much protein either, but you will miss this information because she will not expose herself to your criticism again).

Be aware that nonverbal disapproval (frowning, sighing) can be just as detrimental as spoken disapproval. On the other hand, this does not mean you should show approval of wrong actions. Merely listen to them with no action or comment and make a mental note. At the end of your interaction, introduce the change in behavior you'd like to see ("Let's plan some ways you can include more calcium with your meals without drinking milk").

Not Showing Approval When Warranted

Every student has had the experience of completing a difficult assignment and receiving only criticism from a teacher—no comment that, aside from the part that was not satisfactory, the rest of the assignment was done well. This happens because the instructor assumed the student would do a good job; no reward was given for meeting minimum criteria. From the other side of the desk, however, it would have been satisfying—and offered motivation to continue to do well—to have heard the words "good job."

When discussing health care problems with children, it is easy to forget that what you accept as standard behavior may take a great deal of effort for an ill child to accomplish (coughing and deep breathing after surgery seems simple but is actually very difficult to do because it is so painful). Giving children praise for what they do well encourages them to tell you more about themselves and to try other things. If a topic is difficult for them to talk about, saying that you realize it is a sensitive topic helps them continue to discuss it.

Being Defensive

In the same way that children who request health care do not enjoy being criticized, neither does the average health care provider. If a child makes a critical remark, therefore, it is easy to respond with a defensive or protective comment rather than a therapeutic one. An adolescent might say, "We have to wait so long here; this is a really dumb clinic." It is easy to reply, "Don't say that. This is a good clinic." This type of response implies that any complaint is out of line. Try to respond instead with a supportive comment such as, "I know it makes a long day for you." No health care agency is so good that there is nothing to criticize.

Cliché Advice

Cliché advice (advice given from a formula, not individualized to the situation) is meaningless because it is too general to be helpful. Statements such as "Rome wasn't built in a day" and "You have to walk before you can run" are examples of this kind of advice. Each child considers his or her problem unique and resents being given advice that could apply to everyone.

Topping Off

"Topping off" is minimizing a child's views by telling a better story. A child tells you, for example, he has a headache; you say, "You should feel the one I have." A child says she has a problem; you say, "You want to know what problems really are? Come and work here." This implies to children their problems are inconsequential, at least in respect to yours. They will not be likely to tell you any more about themselves after such responses.

Communication Situations That Require Special Skills

Some communication situations require special skills in addition to the usual therapeutic communication techniques to promote understanding.

The Shy Child

The amount of verbal communication children use varies culturally and individually. Some children talk excessively when they are nervous; those who are shy may stop talking completely. Children who are verbal reach out to secure the help they need from others by talking; shy individuals are more likely to have their needs go unrecognized. It is difficult to assess how shy children feel when they are reluctant to communicate about such things as whether they are psychologically ready for surgery or if they understand the long-term effect a disease is going to have. If they do not give you much verbal feedback, the tendency is to believe they do not have a concern. That leaves them without support people when they most need them.

Fortunately, in most instances, once children realize they know and can trust you, shyness fades. A therapeutic response, therefore, would be not to leave them alone but to maintain an active relationship despite the lack of feedback. This does not necessarily involve talking to children but may involve checking on them frequently, remaining in the room while a physician completes an examination, helping with the adhesive strip after a technician draws a blood sample, or sitting with them for a few minutes while a medication takes effect.

The Angry Child

It is difficult to work with angry children because you feel yourself being pulled into their anger. The typical response at hearing an angry outburst is to imitate it (a child is radiating anger as tight-lipped silence, and you say nothing; he or she shouts at you, and you shout back). This is not therapeutic, however. Make a point of not allowing yourself to be drawn into children's anger that way, while at the same time acknowledging it is all right to be angry. Help them to focus their anger if at all possible so they can better understand it and begin to deal with it.

To encourage focusing, ask a child to detail what it is he or she is angry about. An adolescent who feels angry at the entire health care delivery system is highly frustrated because he cannot begin to handle the whole bureaucracy; establishing that what he is really angry about is one nurse's action builds a base for resolving the problem. If a child uses silence as a method of maintaining anger, suggesting possible reasons for the anger may be helpful ("I know Dr. Smith was just talking to you. Are you angry about something she said?" or, "I know you were asking about crutch walking before. Does it have something to do with that?"). Once the subject is out in the open, few children can resist describing the extent of or reason for their anger. Be aware, too, that when you ask someone to explain he or she is angry, you ask for the emotion and the distress that go with it to be expressed as well. Even if you are the object of the anger, you are committed to listening to the child's views.

Helping children focus anger this way moves them toward a constructive solution (focusing anger at the physical therapy department because that's where the offense occurred seems justified, but swearing at you, not eating dinner, or shouting at a parent does not). If necessary, censor the way the anger is expressed, not the right to be angry. Keep anger from affecting you by reacting to the explanation, not the tone or force of it. Keep any response on your part a tone gentler and quieter than that used toward you.

The Demanding Child

Nursing has few equals in job satisfaction (provided salary and other working conditions are adequate) because the majority of people you care for are grateful for everything you do for them. It can be upsetting, then, to discover a particular child who is not grateful for or even satisfied with anything you do. This type of child is also easy to back away from or avoid.

Demanding behavior generally stems from insecurity or fear (so afraid that something will happen to them while you are out of the room they constantly find more for you to do to keep you in the room, or so afraid of unplanned events that they structure things so that nothing unexpected can happen). Give more of yourself, not less, to counteract this response. When you have proven you are dependably there for them, children do not feel so insecure, and the need to be demanding usually fades. Withdrawing may increase the child's insecurity and the demanding behavior. Ask instead, "Is there anything else I can do for you?" not, "Haven't I already done enough?"

The Sexually Aggressive Adolescent

Sexually aggressive behavior stems from the same cause as every other aggressive and demanding behavior: insecurity. It is manifested as telling unwelcome jokes or inappropriate physical touching. This may be pronounced in adolescents who worry that illness or surgery will interfere with sexual function. Adolescents with this degree of insecurity may benefit from counseling to help them channel coping responses into more socially acceptable behaviors. Be sure they have factual information as to the extent or effect of their illness. Set limits, as necessary, to make giving care acceptable to you. Always censor the action, not the adolescent. Be aware that sexually aggressive behavior occurs in both males and females.

The Child Who Is Not Proficient in English

It is not unusual in any nursing care setting to encounter children who have a different primary language from yours; in other instances, a child's speech may be limited or difficult to understand because of an accent, dialect, or speech impairment; some children may speak your language but their use of words is so different from yours that the words have different meanings (Craig & Washington, 2004).

Most children who speak another language have a support person who can serve as an interpreter. Anticipate the instructions you will need to give the child (cough, deep breathe, save urine, and so forth) and ask the interpreter to write them out in the child's language for times the interpreter may not be present. Post them conspicuously in the room or the child's care plan so everyone giving care can be familiar with them.

Most health care facilities have a list of people who serve as translators as needed; many times, you can contact such a person by telephone to ask for a specific word you want to know. If you have to give instructions and no translator is present, do not be self-conscious about using hand gestures or drawing a picture to express the action you want (a child lying in bed), an arrow pointing to a chair, and a child sitting in a chair for, "I'm going to help you get out of bed." Allow children ample paper to draw pictures to show what they want to tell you. Supply pictures for preschool children so they can select the one they want.

Everyone has a tendency to shout at children who speak a different language as if loudness will increase understanding. Avoid doing this. When using an interpreter, be certain to speak slowly and use common words that can be translated literally. "I need to stick Mary's arm for blood" could be interpreted literally to mean putting a stick in the child's arm.

The Unconscious Child

Hearing is the last sense lost with unconsciousness and the first sense regained with consciousness. This means you always need to be aware that children who do not respond to you may be able to hear and interpret anything you say. Never say anything to unconscious children or within their hearing, therefore, that you would not say if they were fully alert. Continue to use nonverbal communication such as touch to help convey your message.

The Hearing-Challenged Child

When communicating with hearing-challenged children, check whether they use a hearing aid; if so, be certain it is turned on. Face them when you speak so they can follow your lip movements. Use hand gestures as necessary to convey your message, or write out instructions. If you have difficulty understanding what they are trying to say, ask them to write it down if they're old enough. Use common sense about how loud to raise your voice to facilitate communication. As a rule, at the point that privacy is lost, it is time to resort to written words or sign language. Children who use sign language to communicate have a right to have an interpreter present to facilitate communication, the same as children who do not use English as their primary language.

The Vision-Challenged Child

When speaking to a child who is challenged visually, be careful not to rely on nonverbal communication techniques such as hand gestures, as these cannot be seen. A statement such as, "Take a piece of gauze about this long" is meaningless. Never touch children who cannot see you without speaking to them first so you do not startle them.

Process Recording

Process recording is a method to examine how effective you are at therapeutic communication. After your next interaction with a child, take a few minutes and write down in the left column of a sheet of paper a statement the child made to you. In the middle column, write what you thought on hearing the statement. In a third column, write your response. Try to record both statements and responses verbatim or as close to the actual words used as possible. The average person can accurately recall about 3 minutes of communication this way.

Next, examine your responses to each statement: Did I encourage the child to tell me more by my response, or did I block communication? Were my responses supportive or critical or trite? Did I use open-ended questions or closed, direct ones? Did I check perceptions or did I just assume that I understood correctly what was told to me? See Box 34.5 for an example of a process recording with an adolescent patient.

HEALTH TEACHING IN A CHANGING HEALTH CARE ENVIRONMENT

In the past, when children were admitted to hospitals well in advance of surgery and remained in the hospital after surgery or therapy until they were almost totally well, there was a wide window of time for health teaching. Today, when surgery is often a 1-day experience and patients are discharged early, the window for teaching has greatly narrowed. This means nurses must use more creative approaches to achieve the same health education results in these short time spans. Discharge instructions should include both verbal and written approaches (Johnson, Sandford, & Tyndall, 2005).

Children's sophistication about learning techniques has also changed. Children today are exposed to such a diet of clever animation on TV or in movies that a simple lecture on good nutrition can seem dull and uninteresting. Children who are adept at arcade or computer games where dexterity is the requirement may no longer find handling a syringe or a feeding tube a challenging feat. Before beginning, assess each child to find out what he or she expects to learn, to identify his or her individual learning style, and to determine what teaching techniques would suit him or her best.

THE ART OF TEACHING

Teaching is more than presenting information; it is presenting information to increase someone's knowledge or insight. Before teaching can be considered effective, learning has to have occurred. Conversely, before learning occurs, teaching must have occurred in some form. Common principles of teaching are summarized in Table 34.1.

The Teacher–Learner Relationship

Effective teaching and learning depend a great deal on the teacher–learner relationship, because, as a teacher, you can only influence an individual to learn; you cannot force learning. An equal partnership encourages learning more readily than a relationship in which a teacher maintains ultimate control and authority. A teacher–learner relationship based on mutual sharing empowers and motivates an individual to learn. To foster mutual sharing in the learning process, first negotiate with the learner to establish

BOX 34.5

Process Recording

The following is a record of an interaction between a nursing student and Barry Sandoz, a 15-year-old boy who is hospitalized. Barry has been diagnosed as having a peptic ulcer.

What Client Said and Did	What I Thought and Felt	What I Said and Did
	I felt anxious meeting a new patient, although I thought he'd be friendly because he was so close to my age.	I walked into his room and said, "Good morning."
He was sitting up in bed holding his hands on his abdomen. He said, "Get me something for this pain," without even looking at me.	I felt attacked. As if he thought I should have done something sooner, but I had just arrived.	I asked, "What kind of pain are you having?"
He said, "I need a student nurse like a hole in the head. Isn't there anyone else around?"	Now, I really felt attacked.	I said, "I can get you something for pain. I just need to know what kind of pain you have."
He said, "Hydrochloric acid is carving a hole into my stomach. Is that enough explanation for you to get me something?"	I felt angry that he insisted on putting me down so.	I said, "It certainly is. And I appreciate that if I had pain like that I would not want to answer questions either."
		I left to find my instructor and get him something for pain. I returned in 15 minutes and said, "I have an injection for you."
He asked, "Did you have to take so long to do that?"	I was getting really angry.	I said nothing. I just checked his ID band and gave him the injection.
He asked, "Now could you get me my purple pill?"	I was angry at his demanding tone and threatened because I didn't even know what he meant by his "purple pill."	I said, "I'll have to check your medication sheet."
He said, "Any chance you could do that in a hurry?"	Even more angry.	I said, "Are you always so demanding?"
He turned on his side so his back was to me, clenched his teeth, and pushed his hands into his abdomen again.	I realized that my criticism was unfair because he was in pain. But it was too late to take it back.	I said, "I'm sorry. I know you're uncomfortable."
He shouted, "I am not uncomfortable! I am having my stomach ripped out! Could you help me out in any decent way with that?"	I realized I was in over my head. I thought I'd limit any further interaction so he couldn't make me angry again.	I said nothing. I just left to check on whether he could have any other medicine.
		I returned (quickly as I could) with Prilosec (his purple pill).
He asked, "Do you know if Dr. M. is still in surgery?"	Threatened again; I didn't even know how to find that out.	I said, "I can find out for you."
He said, "Hand me that book on the chair over there, before you go, will you?"	Trying to concentrate on not being angry at his demanding tone, yet I had medicine I had to give safely.	I said, "Let me see your ID band again first."
He turned his wrist over so I couldn't read his ID.	I thought: I am tired of him demanding things and getting the book was not as important as what I was doing.	I said nothing.
He said, "If I don't get to that book today, I might as well cash it in."	Getting angry again, but also "hearing" what he had said for the first time.	I said, "Cash it in?"
He said, "Don't you think I ought to? I can't go back to school with pain like this. Wouldn't dying be better than failing out?"		I was surprised how one quick response on my part had brought out so much emotion. I also knew I was in over my head again (but in a nice way).

(continued)

BOX 34.5

Process Recording (continued)

Evaluation

My overall interaction with Barry would have been better if I hadn't been caught so off guard in the beginning by assuming that he was going to be someone who had a lot in common with me (student–student, close age group). His initial response to me seemed so much more intense because I had stereotyped him that way.

My responses to him were adequate up to the point that I became angry. I should have answered his comment, "Do you always take so long to do something?" with a supportive one such as, "I know it's hard to be in pain." (I heard a nurse answer that question for a client with, "Believe it or not, sometimes I take longer," and all of us laughed. I think the client felt good about being able to appreciate something funny, but I'm glad I didn't try humor here. Silence was inadequate but at least not irritating.)

If I had been more sensitive to what Barry was saying (and less angry), I would have noticed that after I gave the injection he became nicer to me (asking if I could get him his Prilosec, not just demanding it). I was too angry to notice his change in behavior though, so I cut off his preliminary attempt to interact with me by criticizing him ("Are you always so demanding?") My supportive statement ("I'm sorry; I know you're uncomfortable") was ineffective after the criticism.

In the final interaction, I was so concerned with my own needs (get my work done) that I completely missed what he said about why the book was important to him. Fortunately, at the last minute, I got my mind off my problem and onto his and was able to produce a therapeutic response for him. He shouldn't have had to describe something with the impact of driving a truck over me before he caught my attention, though. Better listening (and thinking while I'm listening) would make me hear better and be more helpful sooner in this type of interaction.

---

learning needs and goals. Allow this negotiation to continue throughout the entire learning process as needs and goals change. Next, focus on the whole person by considering the learner's cognitive and developmental abilities, values, beliefs, feelings, experiences, and learning style. Finally, the teacher–learner relationship should be interactive. The teacher and learner should both actively participate in the process and modify the teaching plan as they learn from one another.

THE ART OF LEARNING

Learning is a two-step process involving both the acquisition of knowledge and a change in behavior based on the new knowledge. Learning has not really occurred unless the change in behavior is measurable. For example, a parent teaching a child about the need to brush teeth daily must not only elicit the child's statement that daily brushing is important but also see that the child is, in fact, brushing her teeth every day. If the topic is abstract, such as helping a child change a concept about a chronic illness, change can still be measured (the child not only talks about the illness but also begins to take actions to prevent complications). Principles of learning are summarized in Table 34.2.

Types of Learning

There are many types of learning. Learning the mathematical formula necessary to change pounds to kilograms, for example, is different from learning how to fill a syringe. Learning to be kind to a brother with a chronic illness is yet another type. Before you begin teaching, for best results, analyze the type of learning you want to see take place. This helps in setting goals and designing teaching strategies.

Cognitive Learning

Cognitive learning involves a change in the individual's level of understanding or knowledge. Learning the principle behind why a particular medicine must be injected into a muscle, as opposed to subcutaneous tissue, is cognitive learning. Cognitive learning requires adequate development, intelligence, and attention span. It can be gained through exposure to any teaching technique but is usually learned through lecture, reading, and audiovisual aids. Techniques for teaching when cognitive learning is the goal must be based on the learner's cognitive ability (Cottingham, 2004). During the school-age years, learning capability is concrete (children have difficulty picturing body parts functioning unless they actually see them doing this); during the adolescent years, it becomes possible to learn abstract concepts, and children at that point can accept that liver enzymes are released with liver damage even though they never see that occur (Piaget, 1969).

Psychomotor Learning

Psychomotor learning requires a change in a person's ability to perform a skill. Learning to hold a syringe, draw up medicine, and inject it into muscle is an example of psychomotor learning. Acquiring psychomotor skills depends on muscle and neurologic coordination. It is mastered best through demonstration and redemonstration.

Affective Learning

Affective learning involves a change in a person's attitude and is the most difficult area in which to bring about change. To teach a child the reason for and the skill of giv-

TABLE 34.1

Principles of Teaching

Principle	Rationale
Know the subject.	To effectively teach children, you must be able not only to present material but also to answer questions about it. Children's questions can be as probing as an adult's and they can often be more frequent, because children are used to asking questions of a teacher or a parent.
Know the audience.	Children vary a great deal in cognitive development depending on their age group. To teach preschoolers about health, you might choose to teach how to brush teeth using puppets as a teaching aid. The same clever puppet and tooth-brushing presentation likely would not be well received among adolescents.
Know yourself.	Analyze which teaching techniques (lecture, role playing, small group discussion, audiovisual aids) fit your teaching style. Using techniques that are comfortable allows teaching to be most effective.
Assess individual learning styles.	Most children respond well to visual images (seeing a demonstration or drawing) to complement learning. Assessing individual learning styles helps to meet each child's best way of learning.
Define expected outcomes.	Expected outcomes serve as guidelines to help you select from all you know about a subject that part which is most pertinent to an individual child. They should be realistic, measurable, and mutually established. Instruction on how to walk using crutches for an early school-age child would include how to carry school books while using crutches; for an adolescent, instruction would include how to board a city bus so he or she could get to and from a part-time job.
Provide an environment conducive for learning.	Children are easily distracted from learning because of so many new experiences in their world. Divide material into segments to keep teaching sessions short; avoid competing factors such as television or mealtime.
Be consistent.	Nothing is more confusing to a person learning something for the first time than to be told two different ways to do it. Choose one method that should work best for a child and then consistently stress that method. After a child has learned the one method, then suggest alternative methods if the child is interested.
Be honest.	Abstract concepts such as "little white lies" cannot be understood by children younger than adolescents.
Recognize that actions teach as much as or sometimes more than verbal statements.	Children watch facial expressions and nonverbal gestures as much as they listen. Be certain that a nonverbal statement is not contradicting a verbal one.
Teach from the simple to the complex.	Fundamentals must be grasped before extensive learning can proceed. Many children have little idea of body anatomy. Often you need to begin with the basics; when these are mastered, you can proceed to teach about a disease condition.
Teach principles.	Teaching children the principle behind why they are doing something gives them reason to do it. It expands learning in that it allows children to modify and change to an alternative method as long as the principle is fulfilled.
Emphasize what the child should do; mention, but do not emphasize what the child should not do.	Teaching from a positive standpoint makes learning more enjoyable. Because health care information should last a lifetime, thinking of it in a positive way makes it applicable to lifetime use. However, children need to know both the do's and don'ts regarding health issues.
Include evaluation as a final step.	The only way to determine the effectiveness of teaching is to test or evaluate if learning has occurred. Structure the time and method of evaluation when first establishing a teaching plan.

ing a self-injection, for example, may be easy; teaching the child to *like* giving a self-injection may never be possible. The goal could be that the child will *value* the procedure because it will prevent him from developing hyperglycemia. Affective learning is gained best though role modeling, role playing, or shared-experience discussion.

Influence of Age and Stage on Ability to Learn

Learning ability varies a great deal depending on a child's stage of development and the past experiences he or she has had in the specific area of learning.

TABLE 34.2

Principles of Learning

Principle	Rationale
Learning occurs best when child is ready to learn.	Interferences with learning may be physical (eg, pain or hunger) or psychological (eg, fear or anxiety). The first time a child is told that he or she must inject insulin daily, for example, the child may be too anxious to learn about it.
Learning occurs most quickly if a child can see how the new information will benefit him or her.	Sixteen-year-old children learn how to drive a car quickly because they grasp readily that being able to drive will immediately enlarge their world. Children are not ready to learn insulin injections until they can see an advantage of giving them. Make a habit of including the benefit of learning in the introduction of learning.
Learning occurs best if rewards, not penalties, are offered.	Notice the amount of shoulder patting and back slapping that high school coaches engage in (rewarding by praise). Giving positive reinforcement immediately like this makes it more effective than if such reinforcement is delayed. If you must criticize the way a task was done, first compliment children on some aspect they did well and then explain the part that needs improvement. This increases self-esteem and allows children to feel good enough about themselves so that they can accept the criticism. Never be reluctant to praise in public; always criticize in private.
Children learn best by actively participating in learning.	Active participation requires involvement in learning. Ask questions to involve participation; allow children to touch and handle equipment to increase participation.
Learning occurs best in a non-stressful and accepting environment.	No one wants to take a chance redemonstrating a procedure or asking a question if they believe that actions or opinions will not be respected. People do learn from "top sergeants," but the learning experience has so many unpleasant memories attached to it that they may not retain the learning. Health teaching is too important to be presented in a way that will lead to its being quickly discarded.
Children learn best those things that hold a particular interest for them.	Everyone is more interested in something than others. A child with diabetes mellitus who enjoys dancing might be most interested in learning regulation of insulin for exercise; a child anxious to leave for college might be most interested in selecting a diabetic diet from a cafeteria.
Learning ability plateaus.	Children learn to the point of saturation; learning and interest in learning halt at that point and do not continue until the material learned is thoroughly digested and understood. Wait until information is processed, and, at that point, the child will be interested once more.

The Infant

An infant learns by exploring the environment with his or her senses (psychomotor learning). He or she learns best from a primary caregiver because that is whom the infant most wants to please. Few health care points are actually taught at this age. Any that are taught must be presented not as a structured activity but as a game or an amusing or attractive activity. You could teach an infant to exercise a leg by showing the child how to kick a balloon tied to a crib rail or rolling a ball and encouraging the child to move and creep after it, for example.

The Toddler

Toddlers are developing a sense of autonomy (i.e., learning to be independent; Erikson, 1993). Trying to teach a 2-year-old a new activity such as eating a new food or brushing his or her teeth may be met with a sharp "No!" as the child exerts this new independence. This retort does not mean the activity is unappealing to the child, only that the child is aware he does not have to do everything he is told to do. Toddlers also sometimes resist a change in routine because they need rituals to feel secure. If an activity

will allow a child to increase a level of independent functioning, he or she will usually learn it rapidly. Teaching activities such as exercise or deep breathing by having a child imitate the action is an effective teaching method because it presents the activity as a game (so there is nothing to be resisted). Parents can be instrumental in maintaining a new skill the child has learned by incorporating it into a daily routine or a ritual.

The Preschooler

Preschool children are interested in learning, because developing a sense of initiative is the main developmental task of the period. Provided that instructions are geared to their small vocabularies, they "soak up" new methods of doing things. Because they are so imaginative and uninhibited, they have few reservations about the "right" way to do things. They will experiment with trial-and-error methods. They will both watch eagerly and freely redemonstrate a skill. They ask many questions about equipment and procedures. Keep explanations short and words simple; a preschooler's attention span rarely exceeds 5 minutes.

In terms of cognitive development, preschool children "center" or can learn only one characteristic of an object.

This can limit their ability to learn all aspects of care or more than one method of doing something on any one day (Piaget, 1969).

Preschoolers tend to be frightened of intrusive procedures (eg, rectal temperature taking, bladder catheterization, or nasopharyngeal suction). They typically remove adhesive bandages minutes after application to check on the condition of their skin underneath (that it has not disappeared); they worry that any blood removed may be the last they have. Teaching this type of procedure or explaining to a child why it is necessary calls for clear explanations and praise for learning. Use dolls or puppets to help the child visualize details whenever possible, because pointing to a place on a puppet's body is not as intrusive as pointing to the child's own body (Fig. 34.2).

Parents are often most aware of the technique that will be best to motivate their preschooler. Often, this begins with reading or telling a story about the problem.

The School-Age Child

School-age children enjoy short projects that offer an immediate reward. Therefore, they learn best if a procedure is broken down into different stages and presented as separate short procedures rather than one long one. They enjoy games, so playing "Simon Says" may be an effective way to have a child learn deep breathing, for example.

School-age children are used to learning things and accept learning a new procedure or new information as just another experience in a busy day. The "staying power" of school-age children is notoriously short, however; the ability to continue to perform at the level taught tends to decrease sharply if learning is not reinforced. Be certain, therefore, that a backup person in the home knows the health care information as well as the child so that person can reinforce it or carry out a procedure if necessary.

Toward the end of the school-age period, children become interested in doing only those things their friends are also doing. The child may interpret as unreasonable a request to do something after school (come home and take a medication) that is different from what all his or her friends are doing (e.g., stopping at the playground). Modify a teaching plan as necessary to help a child fit what he or she must learn into a school and social schedule, or else the teaching may be very short-lived (Veuglers & Fitzgerald, 2005).

As part of moral development, school-age children thrive on rules or the "right way" to do things (Kohlberg, 1984). This means if two or more people are going to be involved in teaching, they must be consistent in their approach. It is frustrating for a school-age child to be shown two ways or not have a "right way" to do something.

Parents who have been supervising their child's school learning through checking homework easily assume a role in supervising health learning also. Parents who haven't been monitoring learning previously may need support to fulfill this role.

The Adolescent

Adolescents, struggling for identity, like to learn things separately from their parents. They can be responsible for their own self-care as a rule; if they understand how the new actions they have been taught will directly benefit them, unlike school-age children, they will continue to carry those actions out conscientiously. Adolescents have a strong need to be exactly like their friends, however; they rarely continue any action that makes them different or conspicuous in front of their peers. They focus best on things they can do rather than on things they cannot.

Remember that adolescents are present-oriented; they learn procedures and new information best if they can see how it will immediately benefit them. They learn poorly if the only benefit of new information presented to them is something that will affect them at some future date. Rotating insulin injection sites, for example, prevents "pockmark" formations (*lipoatrophy*) in the skin when the person reaches approximately 30 years of age. Given this information, an adolescent tends not to rotate injection sites because the benefit is not relevant to him or her at the moment. An explanation such as, "Rotating injection sites will ensure insulin absorption and allow you to play basketball this semester" (an equally true statement) is a better adolescent motivator.

For the first time, adolescents are able to think abstractly or use scientific reasoning. This means they can create hypotheses ("what if" questions) and think through what will be the consequences from an action (Piaget, 1969). This allows them to understand the principle of what they are being taught and enforces the reason for the learning. Parents may find they are not as effective with teaching their child as they were when the child was younger. They may need to "step aside" and let you introduce the subject until the phase of adolescent rebellion passes.

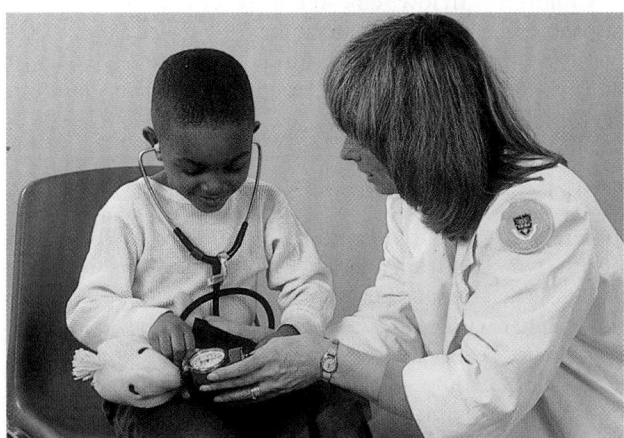

FIGURE 34.2 Teaching with dolls or toys can help to make an intrusive procedure seem less frightening for a preschooler.

 Checkpoint Question 2

You want Barry to increase his cognitive understanding of his condition. Which statement from him would best show he has increased cognitive knowledge?

a. "I feel so much better now about the care I need."
b. "I understand I have to take two types of medicine."
c. "I've finally learned how to swallow big capsules."
d. "I hate having to take medicine but will take it."

DEVELOPING AND IMPLEMENTING A TEACHING PLAN

A **teaching plan** is a design of the content to be taught and the teaching–learning techniques to be used. The first step in developing a teaching plan consists of assessing a child's current level of knowledge, ability, and motivation to learn new knowledge.

Areas of Assessment

Important areas for assessment include a child's current level of understanding; cognitive, physical, psychosocial aspects; and how the new knowledge will meld with the child's and family's lifestyle.

Language Level

Assessing language development includes assessing both the child's spoken vocabulary (how well the child speaks) and comprehensive vocabulary (how many words the child understands). Most children have a comprehensive vocabulary well above their speaking one or can understand about three times the words they actually use. Assess also "family vocabulary" or specific words the family uses. Be aware that if English is not a child's primary language, comprehensive vocabulary may not be greater than spoken vocabulary in English. Additional pictures, drawings, or diagrams may be necessary to convey meaning.

Child's Current Knowledge

Assessing how much a child currently knows about the health area in question helps to establish the needs and goals for the teaching plan. Current knowledge is in part developmentally based and in part experience based. Parents can tell you if a young child has had experience with the subject area. Some school-age children have had excellent anatomy and health classes as part of their science curriculum and are well aware of body organs. Other children may have lived with a family member with an illness and may already know what home care problems occur with that particular illness; on the other hand, what they know about the illness may be accompanied by so many misconceptions that they need a great deal of teaching to prevent being hampered by half-truths or unnecessary restraints. A helpful method of assessment, which promotes mutual sharing in the learning process, is asking children to list what they know about the health area on one side of a piece of paper and what they want to know more about on the opposite side. To reveal this type of information, young children can be asked to draw pictures of themselves, of someone with their illness, or of a good thing to do to keep well.

Child's Intellectual Capability

In many instances, intellectual capability can be inferred from developmental milestones (e.g., a child spoke in two-word sentences at 2 years) or from educational level (i.e., attends the age-appropriate class in school). However, most children regress at least slightly with illness; what one would normally expect from a 10-year-old, therefore, may be impossible for an *ill* 10-year-old. Children with chronic illnesses may not have met developmental milestones because of their lack of experiences, not because they do not have the cognitive ability to learn.

Child's Physical Capabilities

If a procedure that requires a certain level of psychomotor skill, such as medicine injection, will be necessary for care, assess the child's physical ability to perform the procedure. If you omit this step, the procedure will be frustrating because you will be asking a child to perform a skill above his or her capabilities. Assess vision and hearing ability and right- or left-hand dominance as well; these are important considerations for determining not only whether a child can accomplish procedures but also how the material will be presented.

Child's Psychological or Emotional Capabilities

To learn best, children need some motivation to learn or at least appreciate how their life will be improved through learning this new skill. It may be difficult for a young child to grasp how the new skill will make him or her feel better. Some children are too ill or too exhausted or have too much pain to be ready for learning until these factors can be alleviated. With early hospital discharge, a great deal of health education may have to be delayed until a child has returned home and feels better.

Children, like adults, may have difficulty learning about an aspect of their care they find distasteful. A child who uses food as comfort, for example, may have trouble learning about a restrictive diet because it conflicts with the way the child views food. Children with urinary or bowel disorders may have difficulty learning about these body parts if they view them as "dirty" or distasteful. School-age and adolescent children may have difficulty discussing and asking questions about a reproductive tract illness not only because they lack knowledge of the subject but also because they sense sexual functioning is not an "open" topic in their family.

Children with low self-esteem are less capable of learning self-care than others because they do not feel as capable as others. For some children, it may be necessary to plan ways to increase self-esteem first before planning active teaching.

Child's Sociocultural Values

Different cultures have different values related to good health. If a child from a family that values sports develops an illness that impairs her ability to run, for example, the family might consider the disability overwhelming. If the family believes that being able to write and read well are the keys to succeeding in life, the same leg impairment might be viewed as merely a minor complication. Study each family individually to determine which aspect of health will be most important to emphasize when teaching (Box 34.6).

An important aspect of culture is whether children are raised in an environment where they are urged to be active

BOX 34.6 FOCUS ON . . .

DIVERSITY OF CARE

Cultural differences between a teacher and a learner can complicate techniques of health teaching and evaluation of its effectiveness. Even when language is not a barrier, the way children show that they are listening or comprehending may vary from culture to culture. Looking directly at a speaker, for example, is considered disrespectful in some Asian countries. The "OK" sign traditional in the United States is interpreted as vulgar, not positive, in Spain. In South Africa or some Middle Eastern countries, a "thumbs up" sign is insulting. In India, the way people move their head to express yes and no can be opposite to those used in the United States.

Being aware of these cultural differences is important when planning health teaching for diverse cultural groups so that neither teaching nor reactions to teaching are misinterpreted.

participants in learning (allowed a lot of "hands-on" experimentation) or whether they are encouraged to be "watchers." Male/female roles also are culturally determined. This means a girl from a female-passive culture might not be enthusiastic about learning a self-care procedure because self-care is not expected of her. How long children are expected to be children (carefree, no responsibility) also varies culture to culture. In a family where children are expected to be out working and contributing to the family income by age 15, a child might have a very different attitude toward learning a self-care activity than the same-age child in a family where children are expected to remain noncontributing family members until after college (at least 21 years of age).

Child's Attention Span

The attention span of children and the capability to comprehend concepts and perform psychomotor skills differ a great deal depending on individuality and age. In general, the younger the child, the shorter the attention span (under school age, 5 minutes of attention is all that can be expected). This means you must use more "attention-getting" teaching to hold attention in younger children. Think about the clever puppet shows or animation children are exposed to today. Teaching that is not accompanied by these same attention-holding techniques needs to be very short to be effective.

Child's Lifestyle

Lifestyle refers to the common pattern of a child's life. For example, a child who attends school daily and returns home every day at 3 PM has a fairly consistent lifestyle. A busy adolescent who works part time, participates in several clubs after school, and socializes on weekends may have a varied pattern of activity every day.

Knowing family patterns helps to plan the timing of such activities as medication administration or exercise or meal times. If both parents work during the day and do not return home until 6 PM, medication may have to be administered after this time; exercises may have to be supervised in the evening, not the morning. A family that goes camping every weekend will need to plan ways to carry out a health routine at remote camp sites.

Child's Learning Style

Some children learn well from oral descriptions. Others have to see a statement in print before they can fully comprehend it. Still others are so visually oriented that they need to see a picture or a diagram before they can grasp the explanation. These different learning styles vary from child to child; few children are aware of their own learning style, so they cannot explain what it is. After caring for them for a time, it becomes easier to detect the way children learn best. Tailor a teaching plan to a learning style for the most effective learning situation.

Formulating the Plan

Formulating a teaching plan begins with establishing expected outcomes and techniques of teaching. It may need to include communication strategies for parents as well as children.

Identifying Personal Strengths and Limitations

When formulating a teaching plan, be honest about your capabilities. If you feel uncomfortable teaching a child about surgery with clever puppets dressed in scrub suits, it might be better to avoid this approach; in the wrong hands, such a method can sound so flat or complicated a child is left feeling more frightened by the presentation than comforted. The use of humor can be effective in teaching health care. Consider whether this is a teaching strength for you, however. Attempting to use a teaching method that is uncomfortable can cause children to interpret your insecurity as evidence there is something wrong with them, not with the method.

Some health teaching involves giving instructions in areas of care that may be personally embarrassing (instructing a member of the opposite sex how to obtain a clean-catch urine specimen, for example). Proceeding blindly may not result in effective teaching, because the child may be so embarrassed by your discomfort he or she cannot concentrate on the instructions. In doing this type of teaching, nothing serves you as well (as in any client contact) as honesty. Admit to the child or adolescent that you are not used to giving this type of instruction. This approach will probably evoke a response from the adolescent that he or she is not used to having anyone talk about it either. Once you have found common ground (this is not the most comfortable discussion for either of you), there is a basis for effective health teaching. Honesty also allows a child to know that your discomfort is not from lack of knowledge on the subject (the child can trust what is being said) and not the child's fault (the subject, not the child, is the disturbing factor).

Preparing Expected Outcomes

Planning outcomes is most effective when they are planned collaboratively with the child and family. They should reflect the type of learning desired: cognitive, psychomotor, or affective. They should help to establish both content and time guidelines. They should be consistent with both the child's cognitive ability to learn and the time frame it will take to learn. It is unnecessary (and often overwhelming) for a child to learn everything about his or her illness in the first day or week after a diagnosis. Likewise, information on how to stay well does not need to be presented in one setting. In many instances, it is effective to teach only part of the information needed; another nurse in another setting such as an ambulatory clinic or in the child's home can teach the remainder. For best results, state outcomes as behavioral objectives or as the activity the child is expected to demonstrate when the child has learned the new knowledge—not "Tim understands the importance of deep-breathing exercises daily" but "Tim does deep-breathing exercises daily."

Identifying Teaching Formats

Teaching techniques vary with the content to be covered, teacher–learner characteristics, and the environment for teaching.

Formal Versus Informal Teaching. Both formal and informal teaching formats are used in health education. Careful assessment is necessary to determine which format would be the best technique for a given situation. An example of formal teaching would be conducting a class on healthy eating as part of a health education course. An example of informal teaching would be explaining to a child who refuses to eat that he needs to at least drink something because his body needs more fluids to get better. Sometimes informal teaching occurs so spontaneously that it is easy to be unaware of it. It may occur, for example, in response to a question such as, "How long will I have to take this medicine?" If you answer, "For 2 weeks," that is just answering a question. If you answer, "For 2 weeks because . . . ," that is teaching.

Be careful not to equate informal teaching with disorganized, or unnecessary, teaching. It is just as important as formal teaching; it is just communicated in a less structured way. Informal teaching requires that teaching and learning principles (i.e., know the subject, recognize individual learning styles, provide an effective environment, limit time span, and so forth) are followed, just as with more formal teaching. Table 34.3 lists suggestions for incorporating informal teaching into care.

Group Versus Individual Teaching. Although most health teaching is done on an individual basis, teaching

---

TABLE 34.3

Ways to Incorporate Informal Teaching Into Care

Activity	Type of Teaching
Medication administration	Children as young as early school age should know the type and action and any expected side effects of all medication they are taking. Present medicine not by saying, "Here is your pill" but "Here is your [name of medication], medicine to help your temperature come back to normal. After you take this, you might feel yourself start to sweat. That means it's working."
Vital sign measurement	When taking vital signs such as blood pressure, temperature, and pulse, tell children what normal levels are: "Your blood pressure is 100/70. That's normal." If the child is in a high-risk category for hypertension, add some prevention measures to teaching.
Any procedure	Always tell children the purpose and principle of procedures, not "You need to drink a lot of fluid," but "You need to drink a lot of fluid because . . ."
Dressing changes	Dressing changes provide an opportunity to teach the danger of introducing infection into an open wound. The parents or child may not change this dressing, but they will apply bandages to small cuts in the future and so will benefit from teaching.
Mealtime	Provide information about nutrition: "I know you're not hungry enough to eat the entire sandwich, but could you try the meat? Meat is high in protein and that's important for healing."
Hygiene	Emphasize the necessity of good perineal hygiene to decrease the possibility of urinary tract infection.
Physical assessment	Explain aspects of self-testicular examination and describe "normal" findings as both education and reassurance.
Positioning	Teach the hazards of immobility and how change of position and ambulation increase circulation and respiratory function.
Sleep	Teach that sleep is a healing therapy and should not be considered a waste of time.
Bowel elimination	Teach children that elimination patterns vary; occasional variations in their elimination patterns are normal.

groups of children is common in some situations. Individual instruction more directly addresses the child's unique needs; group teaching can meet individual needs while adding depth to learning as children discuss information within the group. For many children, hearing that they are not the only person with their problem is comforting. Hearing another child discuss how to solve a problem may be more meaningful than hearing the same information from an adult. Peer learning not only improves knowledge but may also improve attitude and motivation to learn (Grady & Bloom, 2004).

Consider the following important guidelines when group teaching:

1. Assess for common interests and goals so that the information will appeal to as many in the group as possible.
2. Be certain that all members of the group can see and hear all others.
3. Encourage all members of the group to participate in discussions by calling on them if necessary.
4. Limit any one person from dominating the group by a statement such as, "That's a good point, Reneé. Has anyone else had a similar experience?"
5. Avoid competition in the group. No one is always right; no one is always wrong.
6. Ask group members to evaluate the experience afterward to be certain it met the group's needs.

Home Versus Institutional Teaching. Health teaching is just as important in the home as it is in a health care agency, school, or community setting. Teaching in the health care agency usually focuses on immediate acute care concerns. Teaching in the school may focus on topics such as basic health promotion and hygiene, reproductive and sex education, and drug prevention. Teaching in the home may focus on medication regimens, dressing changes, or measures to prevent complications of a particular illness. It may also involve helping a child and parents adapt a procedure to the home setting, such as accommodating a wheelchair at home. Be certain parents have obtained the supplies they will need to learn and perform the procedure.

Teaching in the home offers the advantage of being able to assess a child's environment, interactions with other family members, and overall family functioning. This may yield data that prove useful to further planning and implementation of care. It may also provide an opportunity to include other family members—siblings, grandparents, and so forth—in the teaching plan, which could strengthen the impact of teaching and ensure that all family members understand the procedures in the same way.

Always include evaluation as a step of teaching in all settings so you can feel confident that learning has occurred.

What if... Barry, who is overweight, needs to begin a lower-calorie nutrition pattern as well as a lower-cholesterol one? Would you need to teach him; his mother, who prepares his food; or his father, who does the family grocery shopping?

Determining Teaching Strategies

Because children's knowledge base, capabilities, learning styles, and attention spans vary, teaching strategies are most effective when they are intermixed and when they are selected in response to the individual situation and child to be taught. The more interactive the method, the better.

Lecture.   Lecture (or directly explaining information) is the most efficient and time-saving method of offering information to both individual children and to groups. A lecture, however, does not allow for much participation, and it is effective only in short, well-structured periods. It is rarely effective for children who are not yet school age.

Demonstration.   **Demonstration** is actually performing a procedure such as a dressing change or instillation of eye drops so the child can see clearly how the procedure should be done. Do not demonstrate a procedure unless you have all the necessary equipment to do it. If you stop in the middle of a demonstration to say, "Be sure to use a sterile syringe, not what I'm using," the poor technique demonstrated may be the lesson learned, not the good technique. The purpose of demonstration is to show how the procedure actually is done; having to imagine steps is little different than reading about it. School-age children, because of their stage of cognitive development (concrete operations), learn best by demonstration.

Redemonstration.   To determine whether a child has truly grasped a demonstration, ask the child to perform a **redemonstration,** or exact imitation of the procedure (Fig. 34.3). Redemonstration is best if it immediately follows demonstration. Praise the effort to redemonstrate even if the redemonstration is not of the quality desired. No one likes to be put on the spot, and children may be

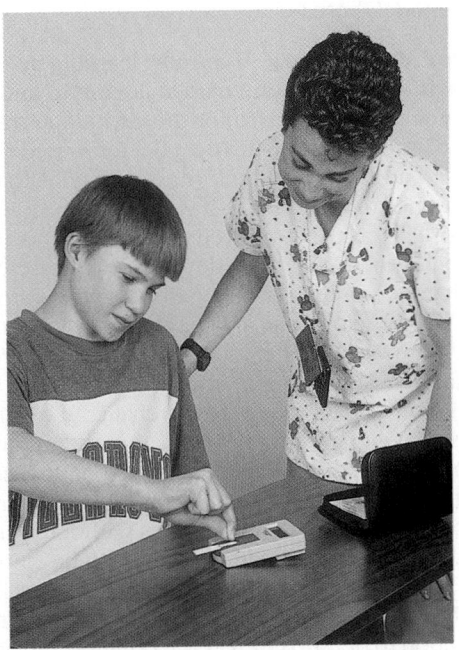

FIGURE 34.3 An adolescent redemonstrates blood glucose monitoring.

unwilling to expose themselves again by a second demonstration if criticized. Be aware that there are many different ways to do almost everything. Children do not have to follow your motions exactly, as long as their technique accomplishes the same goal. An effective way to correct a wrong action is to say, "That's one way of doing that; most children, however, find it easier to. . . ." This type of criticism is nonthreatening because it acknowledges the child's effort in a positive way before offering a correction.

Discussion. Discussion is a shared learning experience in which children ask questions about particular concerns and these are answered based on their individual circumstances, or children are asked questions about some problem, such as how they anticipate managing some aspect of care, and together the problem is solved. At the beginning of health education, children tend to ask few questions because they do not know enough about an illness or health issue to anticipate concerns. As their knowledge increases, so does their ability to project and modify information to fit their own lifestyle. Remember that children tend to think in the present: a problem that will arise once tomorrow is usually more important to a child than one that can be predicted to arise repeatedly in years to come. School-age and adolescent children enjoy discussion.

Role Modeling. Role modeling is demonstrating a certain attitude or behavior you want a child to learn. Be certain when health teaching not only to present facts but also to radiate a positive attitude. Showing frustration at getting a bubble out of medicine in a syringe demonstrates, for example, that giving injections is frustrating; showing a bored attitude toward nutrition instructions implies that nutrition information is boring. The child picks up the role modeling cues as readily as the spoken message. Role modeling is an important technique used to teach new parents newborn care; as they watch a nurse hold, comfort, and talk to their newborn, they quickly learn to model these behaviors.

Behavior Modification. Typically, learning occurs best with **positive reinforcement** (a child tries to understand a new procedure, is praised for the effort, and tries even harder). **Behavior modification** is a term used for a system aimed at *erasing* some form of behavior that interferes with health functioning. It was originally designed to help people who are cognitively challenged erase socially unacceptable behavior. Currently it has many uses, including such concerns as controlling disruptive classroom behavior. The basic premise of behavior modification is that a child is rewarded for healthful behavior, whereas unhealthful behavior is ignored or unrewarded (Jason & Fries, 2004). For example, a cognitively challenged child may have a socially unacceptable habit of constantly rocking back and forth. The child is not scolded or criticized for rocking, but the action is ignored. On the other hand, preferred behavior (sitting for 5 minutes without rocking) is praised. As another example, a child might be ignored for being a picky eater, then praised for the few bites he does eat well. Children respond best to behavior modification if, in addition to praise, they receive a tangible reward such as a star on a chart or an extra privilege of some sort for good behavior.

A behavior modification program must be discussed with the child before it is begun, because no behavior can be modified, just as no new behavior can be learned, until the child truly wants a change to occur. It might be necessary to ask older children to sign a learning contract to be certain that both teacher and learner agree on the method to be used. Many older children are able to use self-rewards to reinforce a behavior modification program (e.g., rewarding themselves by playing a video game or going to a movie after an afternoon of efficient studying or an hour of doing breathing exercises).

Behavior modification is a technique that must be used with common sense and concern so that children are not being manipulated more than they are being helped to achieve a more healthful lifestyle. It is a legitimate device to use in helping a child with attention deficit hyperactivity disorder sit still long enough to eat a meal or learn in school. It can be helpful in encouraging children to do as much self-care as possible.

Trying to modify beliefs or values by behavior modification is unethical and is one reason why behavior modification is often criticized as a learning technique. However, some behavior changes also require a change in values to be effective and long term. For example, a child's behavior of talking back to parents can be extinguished by ignoring or not responding to the behavior, and praising polite communication. At the same time, this method teaches the child to value improved communication and parental approval in order to meet his or her needs.

Selecting Teaching Tools

Teaching tools are the mechanical devices used to present content. They vary based on content, teacher–learner characteristics, and environment.

Visual Aids. "A picture is worth a thousand words" is not an idle quotation but a realistic one. Because small children know little about their bodies or where body organs are located, using visual aids such as drawings or photographs of anatomy can be very helpful. Figure 34.4 shows abdominal contents as an example of such a drawing. You could use such an illustration to show a preschooler how food moves through the body. Figure 34.5 is an example of a good tool to use while naming body parts. Pointing to a figure drawing and saying, "This is the part of your tummy the doctor will fix," is less threatening than actually pointing to the child's abdomen. Clarifying body parts this way is important because young children may have no clear understanding of where a body part such as a hand ends and an arm begins.

Do not be afraid to draw a picture of a heart, a kidney, a bladder, or any other organ to make a point about anatomic structure. Children are more interested in understanding procedures or the reason for a health maintenance measure than criticizing your artwork (they likely do not know anatomy well enough to be able to tell if a drawing is distorted).

Pamphlets. Pamphlets are helpful teaching aids with school-age children and adolescents because they usually contain brief, easily understood information and are often cleverly illustrated with cartoon characters to make them

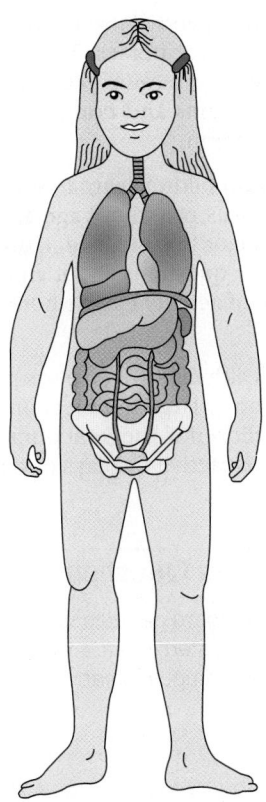

FIGURE 34.4 Anatomic drawings are helpful to illustrate basic health education topics as well as health care procedures.

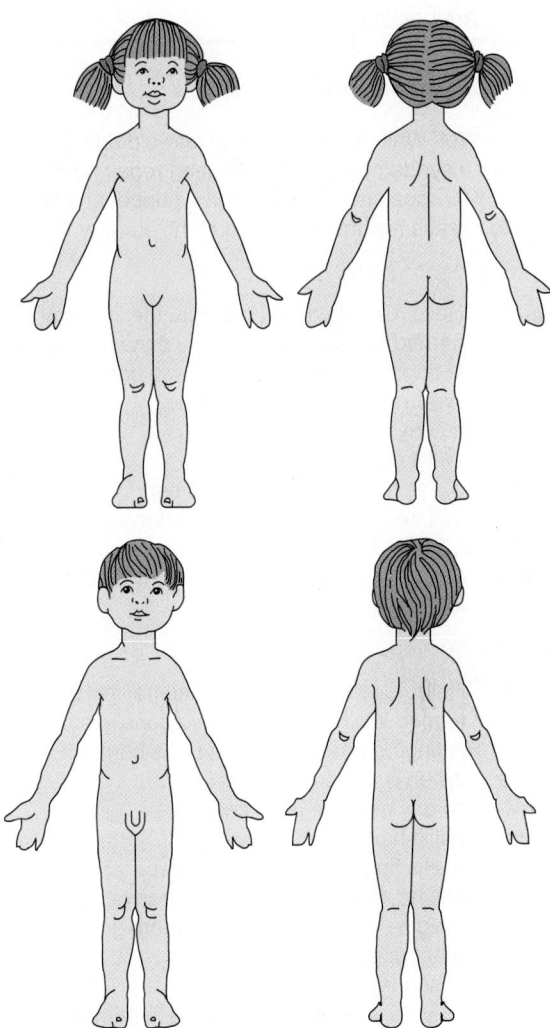

FIGURE 34.5 Simple line drawings such as these can be used to explain to a child exactly what part of his or her body will be "fixed" in surgery. For many children, having this pointed out on a drawing seems much less intrusive than having it pointed to on their own bodies.

enjoyable. Be certain to read any pamphlet before offering it to a child to be certain the information included in it is accurate. Medical advances are made so quickly that a 1-year-old pamphlet may contain a gross inaccuracy in the light of subsequent knowledge.

If a pamphlet contains some statements that are inaccurate or that do not apply to a child, do not simply cross out the information that would be contradictory before offering it (most children deliberately read what they have been told not to read); take the time to explain why it doesn't apply. Also, do not be misled into believing that because someone is given a clever pamphlet, he or she will necessarily read it and learn from it. Sit with a school-age child and read the pamphlet together; talk with an adolescent about the pamphlet's contents later to ensure it has been read.

Learning Games. For memorizing certain kinds of information, such as what foods are high or low in potassium or sodium, flash cards are a helpful learning tool. Many children enjoy playing trivia-type board games. Instead of the usual categories of information, make up new cards with questions such as "Where is insulin produced in your body?" If the child can answer the question correctly, he or she advances a designated number of spaces on the board. Children learn information quickly this way because the reward for learning is so immediate. Having parents play the game with their child educates the parents at the same time.

Word scrambles are easy games to develop. Crossword puzzles are fairly easy to design; one might be developed

to address the activities that are important for a child to do after surgery such as deep breathe, exercise legs, and not eat immediately.

Videotapes, Slides, and Films. Many health care agencies, homes, schools and community centers have videotape or DVD playback equipment or projectors that can be used to show a short tape or slide presentation as part of a health education program. Most households have VCRs or DVD players, so tapes or disks can be sent home for families to view. As with pamphlets, view the material first before showing it; be certain to check that the vocabulary used is appropriate for an individual child or family.

Puppets and Dolls. Many children are shy about talking with strangers; this shyness, in addition to their concern about what will happen to them, may make it difficult for them to discuss or explain what they know about their health, illness, or intended surgery. However, they may be able to open up to an uncritical puppet or doll (Box 34.7).

BOX 34.7 FOCUS ON . . .

COMMUNICATION

Wolf Whitefeather is the 3-year-old boy scheduled for a syndactyly (webbed fingers) repair next week. You speak with him through a puppet at a clinic visit to assess his understanding of the surgery.

Less Effective Communication

Nurse: Hello. Could you tell me what the little boy named Wolf is going to have done in surgery?
Wolf: His fingers got sick when he was born.
Nurse: When is he having them fixed?
Wolf: The day after we go to church.
Nurse: Will it hurt?
Wolf: No. His fingers are going to sleep.
Nurse: Will he have a big bandage afterward?
Wolf: So big he can't see how his fingers got cut.
Nurse: Okay. Thank you for talking to me. I'll see you Monday.

More Effective Communication

Nurse: Hello. Could you tell me what the little boy named Wolf is going to have done in surgery?
Wolf: His fingers got sick when he was born.
Nurse: When is he having them fixed?
Wolf: The day after we go to church.
Nurse: Will it hurt?
Wolf: No. His fingers are going to sleep.
Nurse: Will he have a big bandage afterward?
Wolf: So big he can't see how his fingers got cut.
Nurse: What does that mean? Cut?
Wolf: Cut so they're not there any more.
Nurse: Why do you think that's going to happen?
Wolf: I think he's been bad.

The two scenarios above are good examples of what asking children about what they expect to happen in surgery can reveal. When asked what he means by "cut," it becomes obvious that Wolf needs additional teaching, probably using a drawing to illustrate what will be done. After surgery, when his fingers are covered by a pressure dressing so he can't see them, he will need additional reassurance that his fingers are still intact underneath the gauze.

Preschool children are particularly receptive to puppets and dolls because they can believe the puppet or doll is actually talking to them.

Teaching preschool children about what to expect from a hospital experience is often taught by using a series of puppets to represent different hospital personnel such as a surgeon, a nurse, and a nurse's assistant. Children can practice giving the doll "shots" or submitting it to the procedures they will experience (see Chapter 35 for a discussion of therapeutic play).

Mass Media. Television and radio are examples of effective mass media that teach many children topics about self-help or self-care. Consulting on the topics to present or helping develop the material used in health messages can be an important role for nurses. Messages originated for these media must be attention-getting and brief to compete with the programs and commercial messages that precede or follow them.

Computers. Many children learn to solve problems using computers as early as preschool age and are exposed to computers at home or in child care. Using a computer application to answer questions about an illness is effective because this type of activity can be both entertaining and informative.

Health Fairs. Health fairs are displays presenting health-related information to large numbers of people. They are effective with children if they encourage active participation through interactive displays or computer games.

✔ **Checkpoint Question 3**

You want to use a board game to teach Barry more about his hypercholesterolemia. At what age are children first ready for competition and so enjoy board games?

a. 3 years
b. 6 years
c. 10 years
d. 14 years

Preparing Teaching Supplies

To avoid having to reorganize equipment or instructions each time a procedure is taught, put together a basket or box containing all the information and equipment needed to teach a particular task. This helps ensure that teaching is organized and is economical in that everyone on a hospital unit is not opening new equipment for demonstrations. It also helps to ensure that everyone is teaching the same information. Nothing is more confusing to anyone learning a new skill than to be taught two different principles for doing it or two different techniques.

Implementing the Plan

Health teaching can begin immediately and flow easily if goals have been developed well and strategies for teaching have been designed carefully.

Resource People

Many health care agencies, including home care agencies, have specific people who are available for health teaching about specific subjects (e.g., diabetes, stomal care, or respiratory exercises in the hospital or home setting; drug prevention in a community setting). Using such people is helpful because they know all the "tricks of the trade" for teaching that particular subject.

Some children do not learn as well from such designated teachers, because they see them infrequently, as they do from a primary nurse whom they see daily. Some parents react badly to the thought that it takes an expert to tell them about the care needed (if care is so complicated, how can they possibly learn it?). They also find it inconvenient to be told that their questions cannot be answered until the following day when the designated teacher is available to answer them. Be sure that if a designated teacher does teach a subject, you coordinate your teaching with him or her. Make a point of introducing the person to a child so the child does not view him or her as a suspicious stranger.

Parent Education

With very young children, parents as well as children need teaching. It is good practice with all children to be certain that at least one adult in the household has the necessary information or can perform the required skill as well as the child. Let the child choose this person. The individual who everyone assumes is a child's chief support person may not be the person the child perceives as the most reliable choice and, therefore, not the one the child wants as a health care backup. This person, when identified, needs as much information as the child does about why the health measure is important.

What if... Wolf, 3 years old, refuses to tell you whether he has pain or not because you are a "stranger" and he doesn't talk to strangers? What would you do?

Evaluating the Effectiveness of Teaching

Evaluation, or assessing whether teaching has been effective, is the final step in teaching. Evaluation occurs not only after the teaching plan has been implemented but throughout the entire learning process. This ongoing evaluation helps the teacher and learner modify the teaching plan to better meet changing needs.

There is some advantage in asking children questions before and after teaching to prove that teaching was effective and the child has safely learned a new health care measure. Demonstration of a change of behavior or attitude, however, is the real proof that learning has occurred.

HEALTH TEACHING FOR A SURGICAL EXPERIENCE

Teaching to prepare a child for surgery is an example of teaching that requires planning for several stages of learning (Box 34.8). The child and the child's parents often feel anxious about surgery and its results, so teaching must first address this anxiety. Do not downplay a family's fears, but allow the child and family caregivers opportunities to express their concerns as part of the teaching–learning process (Mitchell, Johnston, & Keppell, 2004).

Assessing Current Level of Knowledge

Many children's surgeries are done on an ambulatory or 1-day basis. Before admission, discuss with parents the preparation they have made for this experience and what specifically they have told a child about what will happen. It is good to ask also whether a child's concerns about the experience seem more or less than the parents had anticipated. Ask if there has been an unpleasant surgery or hospitalization in the family that a child might have heard discussed. Has the child seen anything recently on a medical show on TV that might have been upsetting?

Formulating and Implementing the Plan

It is best to prepare a child for surgery or hospitalization in stages because it is difficult for a child to absorb everything at once. However, contact before surgery may be limited to only one office or clinic visit, so time constraints can force information to be more compacted.

Be certain to discuss preparations for surgery such as coming for blood work and not eating the morning of surgery. If the child will have general anesthesia, it is important to emphasize that anesthetized sleep is "special" sleep. Otherwise, toddlers or preschoolers may be reluctant to fall asleep after surgery for fear people will come and do strange things to them. Do not say a child will be "put to sleep." Dogs and cats who are "put to sleep" are not seen again. To help prepare a young child for surgery, a doll could be used: its abdomen washed, an injection given to make it sleepy, and a hospital gown put on. It could be carried to a cart made from a cardboard box. After saying goodbye to its parents, the doll could be wheeled to surgery by a puppet nurse.

The surgery procedure should be discussed but minimized. "After you're asleep, the doctor will fix your tummy. You won't feel anything because of the special sleep. When you wake up, you'll be in a room called a recovery room where you'll stay until you're wide awake." Be honest concerning pain: "Your tummy will feel sore afterward, but I'll give you something to make it feel better" is a fair statement.

It is important to alert children that nurses and doctors in surgery wear surgical masks. Assure toddlers and preschoolers that the persons behind the masks are doctors and nurses, some of whom the child has probably already met, not superheros or bandits.

It is good to mention recovery rooms in preparation, because this is often an area parents neglect to mention. In fact, parents may not be aware that, in some institutions, they will not be allowed in the recovery room and may have promised the child, "As soon as you wake up, I'll be there." Clarify the parents' misconceptions about recovery rooms, and reiterate that the child will get to see his parents back in his own room once he is fully awake. This both makes the parents' preparation correct and saves the child from feeling deceived.

Explain postsurgery items, such as the use of oxygen, monitors, bedpans, bandages, or intravenous equipment. Furnishing a doll with such equipment is especially helpful in preparing younger children (Fig. 34.6). This prevents preschoolers from feeling overwhelmed by being taken to an intensive care unit and shown actual monitors and respirators. After surgery, be certain to evaluate whether a child's preparation was adequate, both to

BOX 34.8: Focus on Nursing Care Planning

A Multidisciplinary Care Map for
A Preschooler Undergoing Surgery

●

Wolf Whitefeather is a 3-year-old boy who is scheduled for repair of syndactyly (webbed fingers) next week.

Family Assessment
Client lives with mother in two-bedroom mobile home. Parents separated. Mother works at hospital in Medical Billing. Grandmother does childcare 4 hours a day; child attends Head Start program in afternoon. Mother describes finances as "I'm making it." Father will visit after surgery; mother has custodial authority.

Client Assessment
Favorite activity: coloring. His mother tells you she is concerned Wolf will be hard to entertain after surgery because the large pressure bandage he will have afterward will prevent him from coloring with that hand. "I don't even want to begin to talk to him about surgery," she tells you. When nervous or frightened, child has a habit of biting his hand; he has done this constantly since admission.

Nursing Diagnosis
Deficient knowledge related to what to expect in surgery

Outcome Criteria
Child describes expected outcomes of surgery. Demonstrates a minimum of nervous behaviors such as biting hand, can play "Simon Says" for hand exercises postsurgery, and describes how pain will be relieved by "special button" (patient-controlled analgesia).

Teaching Points
Child is shy with strangers; mother states that he learns best by "hands-on" experiences; "cocks head" when puzzled. Also learns better from his mother than from his father (father tends to be authoritarian).

Cognitive Learning to Be Taught
Why surgery is necessary

Psychomotor Skills to Be Taught
To keep hand in elevated position after surgery

Affective Aspects to Be Taught
Accepts surgery as a growth experience

Team Member Responsible	Assessment	Intervention	Rationale	Expected Outcome
Activities of Daily Living				
Nurse	Assess what child and parent understand about care necessary postoperatively.	Introduce postoperative hand exercises child will need to do by playing "Simon Says."	Games are an appealing way to keep the preschooler interested and motivated in doing exercises.	Child demonstrates opening and closing hand to help prevent contractions post-procedure.
Consultations				
Surgeon	Assess which anesthesiologist or nurse anesthetist is available for consult.	Request anesthesia/analgesia consult.	Child is too young to be cooperative during surgery; needs pain relief afterward.	Anesthesia service meets with child and parent and determines best form of anesthesia & pain management.

(continued)

Team Member Responsible	Assessment	Intervention	Rationale	Expected Outcome
Procedures/Medications				
Nurse practitioner/ resident physician	Assess health history.	Complete physical exam.	Health assessment helps ensure readiness for surgery.	Child cooperates with history and exam.
Nurse	Assess Wolf's and parent's knowledge of surgery and postoperative procedures.	Introduce dressing and show how child's hand will be suspended postoperatively by letting Wolf dress and suspend puppet's hand.	Therapeutic play provides an excellent medium for teaching and learning with toddlers and preschoolers.	Child demonstrates he understands how hand will be positioned by showing position with puppet.
Nutrition				
Nurse	Assess if child and parent know child will be NPO for general anesthesia for surgery.	Teach parent importance of NPO preoperatively and immediately postoperatively.	Maintaining NPO status helps prevent aspiration with anesthesia.	Child and parent state they understand necessity for NPO status and will adhere to requirement.
Patient/Family Education				
Nurse	Assess child's cognitive level and ability to learn.	Using puppets, teach that child's hand must be washed with antiseptic wash solution before surgery.	Reducing skin bacteria prior to surgery can help prevent osteomyelitis.	Child cooperates with preprocedure washes.
Nurse	Reassess who is child's main support person.	Ask mother, as support person, to reinforce preparation.	Wolf learns best from mother; reinforcement from her could help Wolf go into the operation viewing it as a growth experience.	Mother reinforces necessity for surgery and accompanying pre- and postoperative procedures.
Psychosocial/Spiritual/Emotional Needs				
Nurse/pain management team member	Assess what past experiences, if any, child has had with pain.	Teach that child will have pain after surgery but that it can be relieved by a "special button" on his intravenous line.	Preparing a child for postoperative procedures and explaining how pain will be relieved before surgery (when the child still feels well) can help reduce the amount of learning the child needs to accomplish after surgery, when he doesn't feel well.	Child and parent state they know there will be pain and understand method to be used for control.
Discharge Planning				
Nurse	Assess if child and parent feel equipped to change bandages, carry out hand exercises at home.	Review with parent a schedule of care based on Head Start and grandmother involvement.	Helping a parent walk through how postprocedure activities can be managed helps ensure adherence.	Mother states she has a plan for how to consistently arrange care given by three caregivers.
Nurse/ physician	Assess when return visit is needed and is convenient for parent.	Schedule return visit for postsurgery evaluation.	Follow-up care is necessary to evaluate success of surgery.	Parent states she understands importance of follow-up visit and will keep appointment.

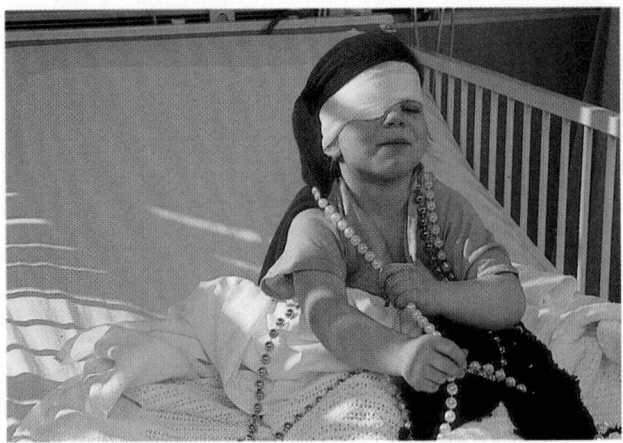

FIGURE 34.6 Pretending to be a pirate helps this young child prepare for having to wear an eye patch after surgery.

document that the experience was as trauma-free as it could be and to evaluate your expertise in teaching children (Cote, 2003).

Key Points

Communication is the exchange of ideas between two or more persons. It can be verbal or nonverbal.

Therapeutic communication is a planned interaction, has structure, and is constructive. Nontherapeutic communication lacks deliberate purpose other than socializing.

Successful communication requires an encoder, a code, a decoder, and feedback or response.

Levels of communication are (1) cliché, (2) fact reporting, (3) shared ideas, (4) shared feelings, and (5) a sense of knowing what another wants without it needing to be voiced.

Typical methods of nonverbal communication are using distance, gestures, body posture and gait, touch, use of drawings, and empathy.

Techniques that encourage therapeutic communication are attentive listening, open-ended questions, reflecting, clarifying, paraphrasing, perception checking, focusing, supportive statements, and silence.

Some situations require special communication techniques such as interacting with demanding or shy children, children who are visually or hearing challenged, or children who are not proficient in English.

Establishing a teacher–learner relationship based on mutual input and setting expected outcomes are effective ways to meet the unique needs and goals of the child and family.

There are three types of learning: cognitive, psychomotor, and affective. For something to be learned well, all of these areas may need to be involved.

To individualize a teaching program for a child, assess the child's attention span, cognitive or intellectual capability, lifestyle, and learning style and your own teaching strengths and limitations.

In many instances, there is a great deal of material a child must learn about an illness. If possible, divide material into lessons that must be taught immediately and lessons that can be taught at spaced return health visits.

The format and strategies of teaching used with children vary depending on the child's age and developmental level. Various types to consider are formal versus informal, single or group teaching, lecture, discussion, and role playing.

Behavior modification is a special technique aimed at erasing some form of behavior that interferes with good health.

Children are learning many other things besides health information every day. This may make the retention of information not as great as you would like. You may need to schedule frequent reviews and updates to keep information current.

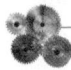

Critical Thinking Exercises

1. Wolf Whitefeather is the preschooler you met at the beginning of the chapter. He will be having surgery in a week for bilateral syndactyly (webbed fingers). His mother asks you how to prepare him for this. What suggestions would you make? The child will be left with a noticeable scar and some lack of function after surgery, so he cannot be reassured that everything will be all right. How will this affect your teaching?

2. Barry Sandoz's family has hypercholesterolemia. It is recommended that Barry begin a low-cholesterol diet. He says, "Don't tell me anything about foods I can't eat. I've heard it all." You say, "Heard it all?" He says, "Don't repeat what I said. That really bugs me." You know he needs to learn more about foods to eat so he can eat safely in the school cafeteria. What would you do?

3. Wolf has to learn how to use a peak flow meter at least once daily to monitor asthma symptoms. How would you teach this skill to so young a child? Suppose his mother says there's no reason to teach him how to read the meter because she will do it for him. Would your teaching plan be different?

4. Examine the National Health Goals related to communication and teaching with children. Most government-sponsored money for nursing research is allotted based on these goals. What would be a possible research topic to explore pertinent to these goals that would be applicable to the Whitefeather family and also advance evidence-based practice?

References

Berger, K. S. (2004). *The developing person through the life span* (6th ed.). New York: Worth Publishing.

Cote, C. J. (2003). Preoperative preparation, premedication and induction of the pediatric patient. *Current Reviews for Nurse Anesthetists, 25*(19), 215–224.

Cottingham, A. (2004). "Now wash your hands please": Teaching health concepts to very young children. *Paediatric Nursing, 16*(8), 33–35.

Craig, H. K., & Washington, J. A. (2004). Grade-related changes in the production of African-American English. *JSLHR: Journal of Speech, Language, and Hearing Research, 47*(2), 450–463.

Department of Health and Human Services. (2000). *Healthy people 2010.* Washington, DC: DHHS.

Erikson, E. H. (1993). *Childhood and society.* New York: W. W. Norton.

Grady, M. A., & Bloom, K. C. (2004). Pregnancy outcomes of adolescents enrolled in a CenteringPregnancy program. *Journal of Midwifery & Women's Health, 49*(5), 412–420.

Jason, L. A., & Fries, M. (2004). Helping parents reduce children's television viewing. *Research on Social Work Practice, 14*(2), 121–131.

Johnson, A., Sandford J., & Tyndall, J. (2005). Written and verbal information versus verbal information only for patients being discharged from acute hospital settings to home. *The Cochrane Library (Oxford)(1)* (CD003716).

Kohlberg, L. (1984). *The psychology of moral development.* New York: Harper & Row.

Mitchell, M., Johnston, L., & Keppell, M. (2004). Preparing children and their families for hospitalisation: A review of the literature. *Neonatal, Paediatric & Child Health Nursing, 7*(2), 5–15.

Piaget, J. (1969). *The origins of intelligence in children.* New York: International Universities Press.

Tourigny, J., Ward, V., & Lepage, T. (2004). Fathers' behavior during their child's ambulatory surgery. *Issues in Comprehensive Pediatric Nursing, 27*(2), 69–81.

Veuglers, P. J., & Fitzgerald, A. L. (2005). Effectiveness of school programs in preventing childhood obesity: A multilevel comparison. *American Journal of Public Health, 95*(3), 432–435.

Suggested Readings

Barlow, J., & Parsons, J. (2005). Group-based parent-training programmes for improving emotional and behavioral adjustment in 0- to 3-year-old children. *The Cochrane Library (Oxford)(1)* (CD003680).

Bishai, D., et al. (2003). Contracting with children and helmet distribution in the emergency department to improve bicycle helmet use. *Academic Emergency Medicine, 10*(12), 1371–1377.

Gillis, L. (2003). Use of an interactive game to increase food acceptance: A pilot study. *Care, Health and Development, 29*(5), 373–375.

Horner, S. D. (2004). Effect of education on school-age children's and parents' asthma management. *Journal for Specialists in Pediatric Nursing, 9*(3), 95–102.

Kreisel, K. (2004). Evaluation of a computer-based nutrition education tool. *Public Health Nutrition, 7*(2), 271–277.

Larroude, B. (2004). Multicultural-multilingual group sessions: Development of functional communication. *Topics in Language Disorders, 24*(2), 137–140.

Li, T. (2004). A bilingual web site for Chinese-speaking families and professionals. *ASHA Leader, 9*(10), 10–11.

McKlindon, D. D., & Schlucter, J. (2004). Family matters. Parent and nurse partnership model for teaching therapeutic relationships. *Pediatric Nursing, 30*(5), 418–420.

Stalker, K., & Connors, C. (2003). Communicating with disabled children. *Adoption and Fostering, 27*(1), 26–35.

Sutherland, T. (2003). Comparison of hospital and home base preparation for cardiac surgery. *Paediatric Nursing, 15*(5), 13–16.

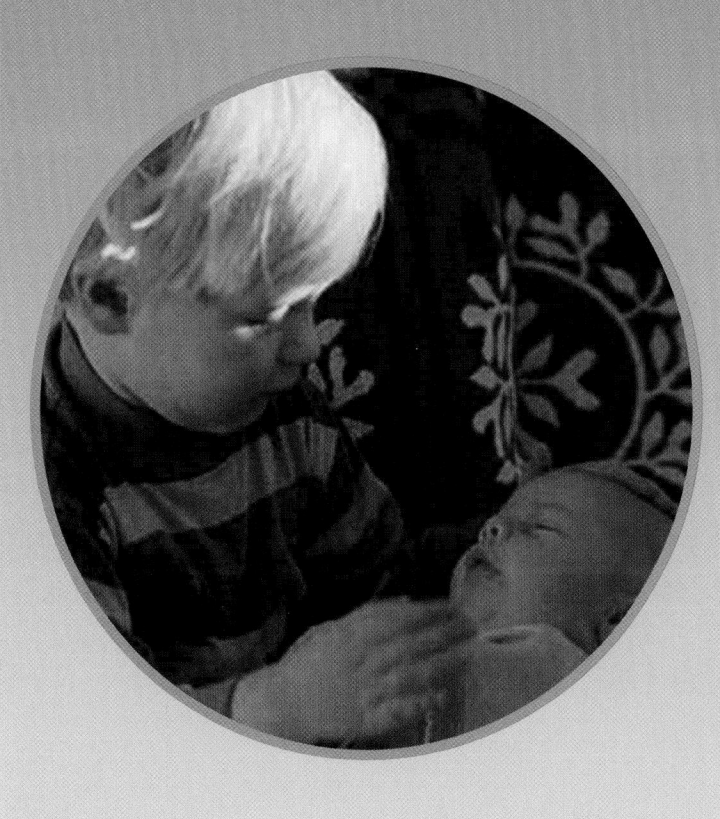

UNIT SEVEN

The Nursing Role in Supporting the Health of Ill Children and Their Families

●

CHAPTER 35

Nursing Care of the Ill Child and Family

Key Terms

calorie counting
case management nursing
direct care
home care
hospice care
indirect care
nonrapid eye movement (NREM) sleep
play therapy
primary nursing
rapid eye movement (REM) sleep
sensory deprivation
sensory overload
skilled home care
sleep deprivation
therapeutic play

Objectives

After mastering the contents of this chapter, you should be able to:

1. Describe illness and home care, ambulatory, and in-hospital experiences as they must appear to children.
2. Assess the impact of an illness, especially one requiring a hospital stay, on a child.
3. Formulate nursing diagnoses related to the stress of illness in children.
4. Establish expected outcomes for an ill child.
5. Plan nursing care to reduce the stress of illness, such as helping parents plan for hospitalization or home care.
6. Implement measures such as orientation, education, and therapeutic play to reduce the stress of illness.
7. Evaluate expected outcomes for achievement and effectiveness of care for the ill child.
8. Identify National Health Goals related to hospitalization or health care nurses can help the nation achieve.
9. Identify areas related to illness in children that could benefit from additional nursing research or application of evidence-based practice.
10. Use critical thinking to analyze ways in which illness care can be made more family-centered and less traumatic for children.
11. Integrate knowledge about a child's response to illness with the nursing process to achieve quality maternal and child health nursing care.

*B*ecky is a 7-year-old who burned her foot in a campfire accident. She is going to be admitted to the hospital for 1-day surgery to have the wound debrided. Becky's parents tell you that Becky "hasn't been herself" since the injury. She has reverted to temper tantrums and sulking, more like a 4-year-old than one of early school age. Even though she has been told eating meat is important because it provides protein for healing, she refuses to eat anything but Jell-O or soup. In the admission suite of the hospital, she picked up a doll and twisted its leg off. "What can I do with her?" her mother asks you. "How can we get our old daughter back again?"

Previous chapters described the normal growth and development of children and their special needs at each stage of development. This chapter adds information about the additional needs of children when they become ill. This is important information because it builds a base for nursing care and health teaching.

Becky is obviously showing some effects of her accident. What type of additional explanation might be helpful to her? What advice would you give her mother to help her better prepare Becky for the upcoming debridement procedure?

After you've studied this chapter, access the accompanying website. Read the patient scenario and answer the questions to further sharpen your skills, grow more familiar with RN-CLEX types of questions, and reward yourself with how much you have learned.

Illnesses that require the attention of health care professionals are outside the usual occurrences of childhood, so most children typically have little knowledge about them. Helping a child and family prepare for or adjust to such an experience is a fundamental nursing role. This role goes well beyond just providing information on what to expect throughout an illness.

Nurses can work to provide orientation programs before hospital admissions and advocate for more open parental visiting and overnight stay policies if these are not already in effect (Griffin, 2003). In addition, nurses can help families provide a therapeutic environment for the care of an ill child in the home. For individual families, nurses can perform a number of interventions that promote comfort, safety, security, and continued growth and development. Play is one of the more powerful tools available to a nurse working toward this objective. National Health Goals related to children and illness are shown in Box 35.1.

Nursing Process Overview

For an Ill Child

● *Assessment*

Assessment for an ill child begins with an interview of a child and parents to identify ways they think the illness will change their lives. This could include a wide range of situations such as increased expenses, changes in schedules to visit or stay with a hospitalized child, the need for one parent to take a leave from work to care for an ill child at home, the need to schedule frequent ambulatory visits, consultation to handle body image changes, and the need to arrange for child care for other children. Because these needs change as the course of an illness changes, assessment must be ongoing (Box 35.2).

● *Nursing Diagnosis*

Nursing diagnoses vary greatly depending on the extent of a child's illness, the care needed, and the age of a child. Those often used with families of children seen in ambulatory settings include:

- Health-seeking behaviors related to lack of knowledge regarding illness
- Anxiety related to pending hospital admission
- Risk for social isolation related to planned hospitalization

Nursing diagnoses established for children in the home are the same as those that would be established with the same findings in a health care facility. Often, however, because of the increased participation of the family necessary for home care, nursing diagnoses are more family-oriented. Home care can place a heavy burden on a family. The stress of being responsible for an ill child's daily health status can have a negative impact on a parent's self-esteem or a couple's marriage, or it can prevent parents from spending time with their other children. Examples of possible nursing diagnoses are:

BOX 35.1 FOCUS ON . . .

NATIONAL HEALTH GOALS

Illness can be a major stress to children and so become a major threat to mental health. Two National Health Goals address the mental health of children:

- Increase the proportion of children with mental health problems who receive treatment.
- Increase the number of states and territories that have an operational mental health plan that addresses cultural competence (DHHS, 2000).

Helping with assessment of children's stress level and reducing the stress of hospitalization or health care are ways that nurses can help the nation achieve these goals. Areas where additional nursing research or evidence-based practice could aid understanding are: What measures do parents need to make them feel most comfortable in a hospital setting; what are the deterrents to therapeutic play on hospital units and how could these be removed; and are there additional contributions nurses could make to shorten hospital stays for children?

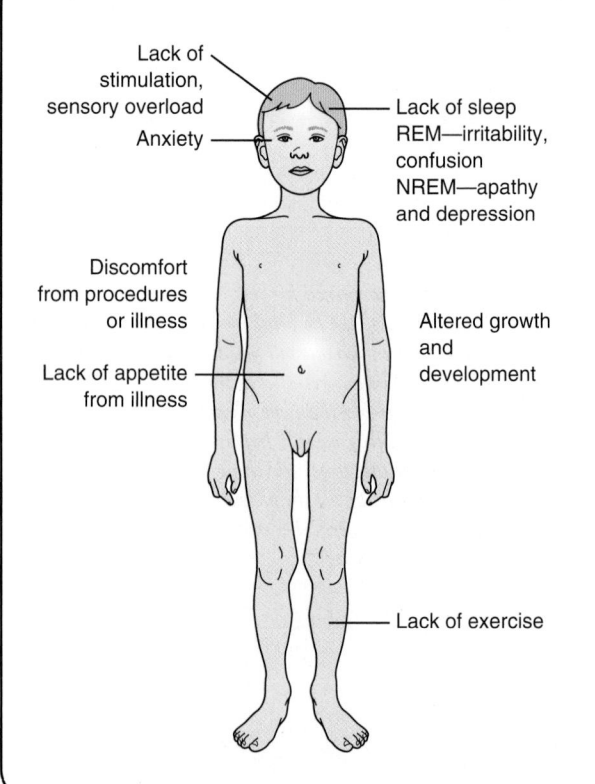

BOX 35.2 ASSESSMENT

Assessing a Child for Effects of Illness

Lack of stimulation, sensory overload

Anxiety

Lack of sleep
REM—irritability, confusion
NREM—apathy and depression

Discomfort from procedures or illness

Altered growth and development

Lack of appetite from illness

Lack of exercise

- Readiness for enhanced family coping related to increased time together because of home care
- Health-seeking behaviors related to skills needed to continue home care
- Risk for delayed growth and development related to lack of usual childhood activities
- Interrupted family processes related to dependence of ill child
- Disabled family coping related to changes in family routine brought about by home care needs of ill child

Outcome Identification and Planning

Planning for the care of an ill child requires consideration of all aspects of a child's and family's life: financial, social, and personal. When children become ill, many of their needs, such as those for nutrition, play, and family support, change. If a child will need long-term home care or hospitalization, the entire family may find their priorities changing. Unless these changing needs are examined, recognized, and met, a child may achieve physical wellness again but not mental or emotional health. A family may be left severely incapacitated. Identifying additional needs in this way and putting in place necessary services or interventions is an important nursing role.

Implementation

Five hazards that may occur with children with all illnesses are (1) experiencing harm or injury, such as physical discomfort, pain, mutilation, and death; (2) being separated from routines, parents, peers, and respected adults; (3) facing the unknown (new and strange sights and sounds and happenings); (4) facing uncertain limits (unclear definition of acceptable and expected behavior); and (5) experiencing a loss of control (loss of competence or loss of the ability to make decisions).

Being aware of these potential problems is important to guard against those that are preventable and to reduce a child's anxiety associated with those that cannot be prevented (such as facing new sights and sounds). Discussing these hazards with older children is important so that implementations to reduce their impact can be tailored to each child. Reading to a child, role playing, and puppetry are all useful techniques for easing the younger child's experience. Be certain that the techniques used are appropriate not only to the child's age but also to his or her individual learning style. Be certain that children participate in making any decision that is age-appropriate for them (Hallstrom & Elander, 2004).

Nursing interventions for home care often involve teaching family members how to give care. This may include encouraging members to voice the frustration they feel at being constantly confined at home or what they perceive to be a lack of progress in their child's condition. If the child has a terminal illness, parents may need support to express their grief. They can also grow discouraged because the work they are accomplishing is making the child comfortable but not preventing death.

Outcome Evaluation

Evaluation of expected outcomes for ill children should include specific measures such as whether discomfort was kept to a minimum during the experience. Indicators to evaluate outcomes that are long term should include whether the child was able to return to his or her usual behavior after the experience. The following are examples suggesting achievement of outcomes regarding a hospital experience:

- Parents state that their level of anxiety regarding hospitalization of their infant is now at a tolerable level.
- Parents have effectively changed work schedules to be able to stay with their child in the hospital.
- Social isolation of toddler is minimized through case manager nursing assignment.

Because a home setting is less structured than a health care facility, evaluation will show that some goals for care are more difficult to accomplish in the home; for the same reason, because there is more room for innovation at home, some goals will be more easily accomplished. Examples suggesting achievement of outcomes in the home setting might include:

- Parents state they have been able to make adjustments to accommodate care of ill child at home.
- Child states he or she enjoys respite care in hospice setting one weekend a month.
- Parents state they are actively trying to supply adequate growth experiences for siblings in light of home care of oldest child.

THE MEANING OF ILLNESS TO CHILDREN

The response of children to illness depends on their cognitive ability, past experiences, and level of knowledge. From early school age, children generally know quite a bit about the workings of their major body parts. As general guidelines, early grade-school children are usually able to name the function of the heart, lungs, and stomach. They may not be able to do that for the kidneys or bladder. This lack of information may reflect the difficulty some parents have in discussing elimination with their children.

Younger children may think the cause of illness is magical (no one knows where it comes from) or that it occurs as a consequence of breaking a rule (e.g., walking in the rain or eating candy after school). With this perspective, they can think that getting well again is possible only if they follow another set of rules, such as staying in bed and taking medicine. By fourth grade, children are generally aware of the role that germs play in illness but may be fooled by thinking that all illness is caused by germs. Because of this, they may see a passive role for themselves in getting well, because illness comes from outside influences. At about eighth grade, children are able to voice an understanding that illness can occur from several causes, such as being susceptible to chickenpox because they did not get the vaccine and playing with a child who had chickenpox. Once they accept this, they can take an active role in getting better. These concepts parallel cognitive development (see Chapter 27).

Knowing how children of each age view illness affects the planning of nursing care, influencing how explanations should be worded. For example, saying that you are going to "stick" a child for blood work could be interpreted by a young child as meaning you are actually going to put a stick in him or her. Saying a child will receive a dye for a test can be interpreted as the child will "die" during the procedure. Children who think illness comes as punishment for breaking rules can interpret nursing procedures (e.g., taking a rectal temperature or giving an injection) as punishment. They can be confused about explanations of procedures because some words sound alike or have double meanings (e.g., "drawing" as in making a picture versus drawing blood). Because of these distorted perceptions, explanations of procedures do not always relieve children's stress.

Differences in Responses of Children and Adults to Illness

Keeping in mind that children are not just small adults is important when evaluating how children react to illness, perceive an illness, or react to health care (Fig. 35.1). Their body images, as evidenced in their drawings, are different from those of adults. They can have difficulty telling which body parts are indispensable and which are not (this is why it is wise to talk to preschool and early school-age children about "fixing" body parts, such as tonsils, rather than "taking them out").

Inability to Communicate

Very young children do not have the vocabulary to describe symptoms. Headache is an example of a symptom that children younger than 5 years have a great deal of difficulty describing. Dizziness and nausea can be equally bewildering because children this age do not know the words to express these phenomena.

By the time they reach school age, most children can describe symptoms with accuracy. They may intensify their concerns, however, if they believe someone expects symptoms to be more serious. They may minimize symptoms if they are afraid illness will interfere with an activity.

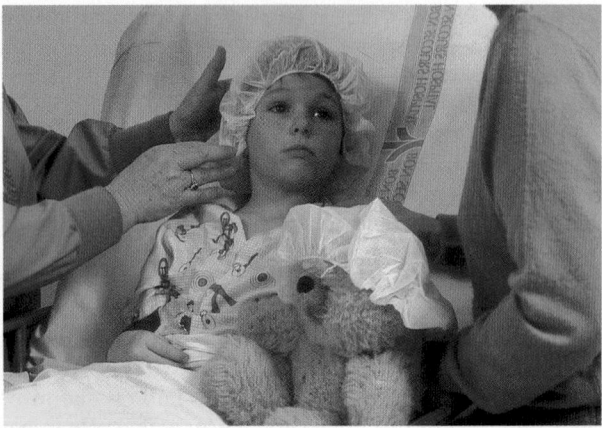

FIGURE 35.1 Illness is potentially traumatic because of the unknown and pain and discomfort that may be involved. Children need extra attention and reassurance to calm their fears.

Because of this, evaluate a child's symptoms as much by observation as by a child's report. The crying, whining preschooler who is "just not herself" probably has a symptom she cannot describe. A school-age child who guards her abdomen (keeps abdominal muscles rigid) is in pain just as clearly as a child who verbalizes a source of discomfort. This makes keen, astute observations necessary to ascertain the extent of a child's illness at any given time.

Inability to Monitor Own Care and Manage Fear

Adults who are ill often ask about medications prescribed for them or procedures they are scheduled to undergo. For example, if a hospitalized man knows he is to receive a diuretic three times a day and by 10 AM has not been given it, he usually reminds someone of the oversight. School-age and younger children cannot monitor their own care this way because they may not know which medicine or procedures they are to receive. If they do know, they may be confused about time. In addition, children have fears that adults do not have. The infant, for example, fears separation above all else; the toddler and preschooler fear such things as separation, the dark, the unknown, intrusive procedures, and mutilation of body parts. The school-age child and adolescent are concerned about the loss of body parts, loss of life, and loss of friends. Adults have fears also, but most have learned to cope with them. Children in a strange environment (such as a hospital) require proportionally more support and active intervention to cope with their stress and fears (Mitchell, Johnston, & Keppell, 2004).

Nutritional Needs

In addition to psychological differences, there are major physiologic differences in the way illness affects children compared with adults. This is because children have different physiologic needs and respond to imbalances in different ways.

Children need more nutrients (calories, protein, minerals, and vitamins) per pound of body weight than adults, for example, because their basic metabolic rate is faster, and they must take in not only enough to maintain body tissues but also enough to allow for growth. The infant requires 120 kcal per kilogram of body weight per day; the adult requires only 30 to 35. An ill child who must limit food intake because of nausea or vomiting, therefore, may require hospitalization, even though this might be unnecessary for an adult under the same circumstances.

Fluid and Electrolyte Balance

In the adult, extracellular water (that in plasma and outside body cells) represents approximately 23% of total body water; in a newborn, extracellular water is closer to 40%. This means that an infant does not have as much water stored in the cells as an adult does and so is more likely to lose a devastating amount of body water with diarrhea or vomiting. Because of this, there is no such thing as "only diarrhea" or "simple diarrhea" in a child younger than 1 year. The full implications of both vomiting and diarrhea are discussed in Chapter 45.

Systemic Response to Illness

Because their bodies are immature, young children tend to respond to disease systemically rather than locally. The child with pneumonia, for example, may be brought to an emergency room not because of a cough (although the child has one) but because of accompanying systemic symptoms such as fever, vomiting, and diarrhea. Nausea and vomiting, in fact, occur so frequently in children with any type of illness these symptoms do not have the diagnostic value they have in adults. Systemic reactions can delay diagnosis and therapy and cause increased fluid and nutrient loss, circumstances that compound an initial illness and can result in hospitalization.

Age-Specific Diseases

Because of their growth requirement and their immaturity, children are susceptible to some diseases that do not affect adults. For example, because infants are growing, a lack of vitamin D will cause rickets, but this same lack does not affect adults. Most adults have achieved immunity to common infectious diseases; children, however, are susceptible to childhood diseases such as measles, mumps, and chickenpox. Children younger than 5 years who have a high temperature may respond with generalized seizures (febrile seizures), a phenomenon that rarely occurs after this age. Children younger than 1 year of age are subject to iron-deficiency anemia because fetal red blood cells are destroyed after birth and are replaced by mature red blood cells only very slowly.

Checkpoint Question 1

Young children are more at risk for dehydration with vomiting than adults are. This is because:

a. They have a smaller stomach and intestines than adults.
b. They have proportionally more extracellular water than adults.
c. Children metabolize fluid more slowly than do most adults.
d. They maintain more fluid inside body cells than do adults.

CARE OF THE ILL CHILD AND FAMILY IN THE HOSPITAL

The parents of children admitted to intensive care units can be predicted to experience a high degree of stress during their child's hospitalization both because of the severity of their child's illness and the high-tech ICU setting (Board & Ryan-Wenger, 2003). Based on the theory that hospitalization creates a high degree of stress for children, only those who cannot be managed successfully on an ambulatory basis are now admitted to the hospital. This was not always true. For example, in the past, most children with head injuries automatically stayed overnight for observation. Currently, unless a child is unconscious or shows other signs of neurologic injury, he or she is sent home to be observed

by parents for signs of increased intracranial pressure. This policy requires that time be spent to teach parents skills such as how to take a pulse or evaluate consciousness. Teaching them requires patience because parents under stress can have difficulty comprehending instructions. However, because psychological trauma and excessive health care costs are prevented by allowing a child to return home, it is important teaching.

As another example, instead of being admitted to the hospital, many children will have procedures such as tonsillectomy done on an ambulatory or outpatient basis. This prevents the major problem of separation anxiety, but it does not necessarily reduce parents' or children's anxiety about the procedure. Some parents actually feel less confident and more anxious with ambulatory procedures than they did with in-hospital admissions because they sense their responsibility for preparation and follow-up care will be significantly greater. They often comment that modern care is not as good as when children were admitted, and that this change is a result of cost containment by insurance companies. Although it is true that short hospital stays reduce cost, it is helpful to inform parents that ambulatory or outpatient procedures are as safe as those performed with hospital admissions, and that ambulatory procedures are scheduled to prevent separation as well as contain cost.

Preparing the Ill Child and Family for Hospitalization

Many childhood illnesses such as febrile seizures, appendicitis, poisonings, and asthma attacks strike suddenly, making advance preparation for hospital admission impossible. However, when hospitalization is planned ahead of time, for orthopedic or second-stage surgeries, for example, preparation is possible (Mitchell, Johnston, & Keppell, 2004). As a rule, parents eagerly seek guidance from nurses on what and how much to tell their children about an anticipated admission. The preparation a parent makes for a child obviously varies according to the child's age and individual experience. No matter what the child's age, however, parents should be encouraged to convey a positive attitude. Statements such as, "They'll make you behave in the hospital" or "Wait until you have to stay in bed all day" should be avoided.

Children can worry unnecessarily if they are told about their approaching hospitalization too far in advance. Conversely, few things are more frightening for children than to hear conversation halt as they enter a room or to hear adults spelling out unknown words. As a rule, therefore, children between 2 and 7 years of age should be told about a scheduled ambulatory or inpatient hospitalization as many days before the procedure as the child's age in years. For example, a 2-year-old should be informed 2 days before hospitalization; a 4-year-old, 4 days before; and so forth. Children older than 7 years should be told as soon as the parents are aware of it.

On the day of admission, it is important for you to discuss the preparation the child has received to ensure that the child and family accurately understand the child's condition and upcoming procedures. Based on that, you can provide further health teaching and clear up any misunderstandings (Box 35.3).

BOX 35.3 FOCUS ON . . .

COMMUNICATION

Becky is a 7-year-old you are going to admit to your hospital unit for burn debridement. Her mother and her arrive together on the unit.

Less Effective Communication

Nurse: Hello, Becky. How are you?
Becky: Good.
Nurse: Do you know why you're coming into the hospital?
Mrs. Miller: We've talked about surgery. She knows that's why she's here.
Nurse: Did you bring a favorite toy, Becky?
Becky: I brought a book to color.
Nurse: You sound ready. Let's get you admitted.

More Effective Communication

Nurse: Hello, Becky. How are you?
Becky: Good.
Nurse: Do you know why you're coming into the hospital?
Mrs. Miller: We've talked about surgery. She knows that's why she's here.
Nurse: Tell me why you're here, Becky.
Becky: To read a book. I brought a book.
Nurse: Let's talk about everything you told her, Mrs. Miller, about surgery.
Mrs. Miller: Well, I didn't want to introduce anything scary.
Nurse: Let's take some time and talk about the whole procedure.

The above poor communication example happened because the nurse assumed that when the parent said she had prepared her daughter, she had prepared her in the same way the nurse would have prepared her. The communication improved when the nurse stopped assuming about the level of preparation and asked direct questions of the mother and child about what they knew.

NURSING DIAGNOSES AND RELATED INTERVENTIONS

●

Nursing Diagnosis: Deficient knowledge related to preparation for hospitalization

Outcome Evaluation: Parents and child both state they feel prepared for hospitalization; child has brought some personal items important to self. Child describes with accuracy and detail appropriate to age the reason for hospital stay; asks questions and expresses feelings appropriate to age about hospitalization.

Preparing Family Caregivers. Parents experience anxiety about a child's hospitalization as well as their child. Therefore, planning for hospitalization should begin as soon as the parents know that hospitalization will be necessary, not only to relieve their child's anxiety but also their own. Some parents, however, may be so concerned about the reason for hospitalization that they cannot begin this type of preparation until they are better prepared themselves. Easing parental anxiety regarding illness and hospitalization is particularly important because infants and children can keenly sense a parent's stress. No amount or type of preparation for children will be effective if they react to their parents' unspoken tension. Even though parents may say, "Don't worry, everything will be all right," a child can sense if parents really do not believe that everything will be all right, a situation that can hamper recovery.

As part of preparation, urge parents to ask questions about the hospitalization so they become as familiar as possible with what will happen. If they are well informed in this way, they will (at least theoretically) have as low an anxiety level as possible. If they arrive at a hospital unit with questions unanswered, fill in gaps immediately.

Advise parents to ask about things such as what diagnostic procedures will be necessary, how long the hospital stay will be, and what kind of dressings or other equipment will be used. If you are practicing in a doctor's office or clinic where surgery or a hospital admission is first proposed, become familiar with these facts to serve as the parents' backup informant. Many parents ask a nurse for their main information or ask to have the physician's explanation clarified to be certain they have understood it correctly. An organization that offers helpful information on hospitalization of children is the National Association of Child Care Professionals (*www.naccp.org*).

Preparing an Infant. Because an infant cannot understand explanations of surgery or treatments, preparation will be minimal. Special items such as a favorite toy, blanket, or pacifier should be packed. These objects provide a special kind of security for which there is no substitute.

A primary caregiver should plan to spend a great deal of time in the hospital with an infant. For rooming-in, he or she needs to make plans for older children or a spouse ahead of time. If a parent cannot arrange to room-in, make plans to have a consistent nurse assigned to the infant. This can both help decrease parental anxiety and minimize separation anxiety in the infant.

Preparing a Toddler or Preschooler. Three chief fears of a toddler or preschooler are fear of the unknown, fear of abandonment or separation, and fear of mutilation. These children, therefore, need preparation clearly aimed at alleviating these fears. Bringing a favorite toy or personal item such as a blanket can help. Referred to as "transitional objects," these items are symbols of the longed-for return home. Some parents buy a new toy to replace a child's favorite one because they are ashamed of a teddy bear with one ear or one eye missing. A new bear may mean nothing to the child, however, and clinging to it may not offer comfort.

When making hospital beds or changing paper on examining tables, watch for ragged blankets and threadbare stuffed animals; these can cling to sheets and can be easily discarded. Throw nothing away without first asking a child or parent if it is important. What looks like a useless alphabet block to you may mean security and home to a child.

When children are admitted to a hospital in an emergency, parents rarely have time to bring toys. In these instances, suggest a parent give a child a familiar object, such as the parent's wallet (money and papers removed) or a sweater. The child will hold these in the same way as a favorite toy. The child's outside shoes can serve this same purpose if the parents leave them with the child.

A number of helpful books about hospitalization are available for parents to read with children and also learn more about children's health care. These can be obtained from local bookstores, libraries, or Internet book sites, or by writing directly to the publishers (Box 35.4). For preschool preparation, a

parent could read one of these books to a child, adapting the story to include information specific to the child. Some books fail to orient children well to hospitalization because they are too sweet (as if the child were going to a picnic rather than a hospital). Others may omit pertinent facts, such as surgery will involve some pain (stress the child will be given medicine so the pain will go away) or that when bedrest is required, the child will have to use a bedpan. Using a bedpan is difficult for toddlers and preschoolers to accept because they have just been toilet-trained and have been told repeatedly they must use only the bathroom.

Because the imagination of preschoolers is at a peak, role playing is an effective means of preparing a child of this age for a new experience. To do this, a parent could encourage a child to act out a hospitalization experience with puppets or dolls. Or the child could change into pajamas and get into bed. The parent could then act out a physical examination, a meal in bed, a bedpan (a round cake pan simulates this), or anesthesia administration (a strainer can be used for an induction mask). At the end of the session, the parent should stress that when the child's tummy or throat is better, he or she will change back to street clothes and come home. Remind parents it is always better to use the word "fix" rather than "cut" when talking about surgery with young children, because "cut" automatically suggests pain and mutilation.

Preparing a School-Age Child or Adolescent. School-age children enjoy reading, so books about surgery and hospitalization are helpful. Be sure both school-age children and adolescents receive factual explanations of what will happen during such an experience. This should include also what will not happen: for example, surgery will require a small abdominal incision, but it will not create a scar that will show when wearing a bathing suit.

Many community hospitals sponsor hospital orientation programs for children's groups or school groups during which hospitalization is discussed. These programs are beneficial because they lay a foundation for all children about what to expect in a hospitalization; then, if they must be admitted on an emergency basis, they may not be so frightened. Programs are offered by nurses at the hospital or on visits to children's groups or schools (Fig. 35.2). Box 35.5 provides guidelines for setting up hospital tours or discussions for early school-age children.

Be certain that parents have the necessary factual information themselves so that they can provide accurate and appropriate explanations to school-age children. If they do not know the answer to a question, caution them that the best response is simply, "I don't know" rather than a guess. This prevents a child from feeling betrayed when the real answer is different. At approximately 9 years of age, when children first begin to understand the full meaning of death, parents need to be especially careful to explain that an anesthetic causes a "special sleep,"

BOX 35.4

Books on Hospitalization for Children

Bridwell, N. (1998). *Clifford visits the hospital.* New York: Scholastic Publishers. (Grades pre-K–3)

Civardi, A. (1994). *Going to the hospital.* Tulsa, OK: EDC Publications. (Infant–preschool)

Duncan, D. (1994). *When Molly was in the hospital: A book for brothers and sisters of hospitalized children* (Minimed Series Vol. 1). Windsor, CA: Rayve Productions. (Grades K–4)

Ganz, P., & Scofield, T. (1996). *Life isn't always a day at the beach: A book for all children whose lives are affected by cancer.* Lincoln, NE: High Five Publishing. (Grades K–6)

Hautzig, D. (1985). *A visit to the Sesame Street hospital.* New York: Random House. (Grades K–3)

Jennings, S., et al. (2000). *Franklin goes to the hospital.* New York: Scholastic Publishers. (Grades pre-K–3)

Krall, C. B., & Jim, J. M. (1987). *Fat Dog's first visit: A child's view of the hospital.* Atlanta: Pritchett & Hull Associates. (Preschool)

Mills, J. C., & Sebern, B. (2003). *Little Tree: A story for children with serious medical illness.* Washington, DC: Magination Press. (Early school-age)

Rey, H. A. (1976). *Curious George goes to the hospital.* Boston: Houghton Mifflin Co. (Grades 2–3)

Rogers, F. (1997). *Going to the hospital.* New York: PaperStar Publishers. (Grades K–3)

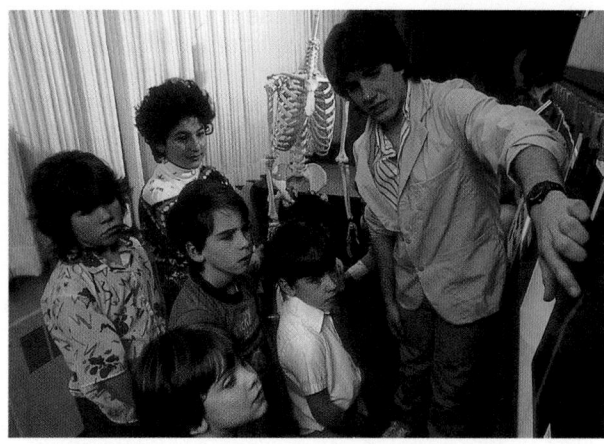

FIGURE 35.2 Children learn what to expect from hospitalization during a prehospital program.

not that a child is "put to sleep." Animals who are "put to sleep" are not seen again. Talking to another child who has undergone the same experience and come through it intact is yet another helpful way to introduce children and adolescents to hospitalization. Although parents cannot usually supply such a person in advance, on admission to the hospital, a

---

BOX 35.5

Guidelines for Conducting Hospital Tours With Early School-Age Children

1. Keep groups small (about 10 children per group) so individual reactions to the presentations can be assessed.
2. Allow or encourage parents to join the tour so their anxiety about the hospital can also be relieved.
3. Conduct the tour for only 20 to 30 minutes to meet the short attention span of children.
4. Use an indirect method to present various aspects of a hospital, such as puppets, films, or a slide show, to decrease anxiety.
5. Present the features of a hospital in a non-threatening environment, such as the hospital playroom. Avoid the emergency room, ICUs, or operating rooms while touring, because these are anxiety-producing areas for children. Talk about these areas by using slides or photographs instead.
6. Present explanations about hospitalization in concrete terms and at the child's level of understanding. Include only what the child will see, hear, and feel.
7. Avoid dwelling on unpleasant and threatening events or intrusive procedures, such as blood drawing or anesthesia, that may create anxiety.
8. Allow children opportunities to ask questions.
9. Allow children opportunities to play with dolls and hospital equipment, both to decrease anxiety and satisfy curiosity.

---

visit to a recovering patient is often possible and is a constructive way to give reassurance.

If hospitalization is to be more than 1 week long, a parent must think about continuing the child's schooling. Advise parents to ask their physician at what point their child will be able to do homework. Many school systems provide tutors; children's hospitals often have their own teachers from the local school system to carry out this service.

What if... Becky's mother brought pots and pans to the hospital as Becky's favorite play items? Would you suggest she bring an actual toy?

Preparing a Child With a Different Cultural Background. Perhaps the most important aspect to consider when preparing a child from a different culture for hospitalization is that it is your customs that seem different to the child and family. Ask enough questions and practice good listening skills to gain information about the particular needs of a child and family. When cultural differences do exist, be prepared to act as a liaison between the family and the health care team. If a different language is interfering with communication, a translator may be necessary in this preparation phase. Provide the opportunity for parents to voice their fears and ask questions at the time of hospitalization or treatment. When families speak a different language or are unfamiliar with hospital routine, allow more time and more opportunities for discussion and communication.

Preparing a Physically Challenged or Chronically Ill Child. Physically challenged or chronically ill children frequently come to ambulatory health care settings for care; they often are admitted to the hospital for care, possibly remaining in the hospital for an extended visit and continuing care at home. Think through ways in which a new hospitalization or visit will be like past ones and other ways in which it will be different to determine how best to prepare a child. Help children to maintain contact with their families and school friends during a long hospitalization or home care experience by encouraging telephone calls, e-mails, letters, and visits.

Admitting an Ill Child and Family

Whether an ambulatory or inpatient hospital unit admission, children and parents need to be admitted as a single entity to encourage parents to feel they are true partners in care. A child coming to a hospital for an elective admission generally arrives at a reception area, where significant facts are obtained, such as name, age, address, and hospital insurance coverage. The child and parents are then brought to the hospital unit. Remember that first impressions count. If parents are left standing at a counter while nurses chat, they can easily feel that no one appreciates their concern and that possibly their child will not receive optimal care. It is true that at certain times on a children's unit all nurses will be busy finishing treatments for other children before they can take the time to admit a new child. Even so, one nurse should take the time to introduce himself or herself and find a comfortable place for the family to wait until someone is available. When introducing yourself to children, stoop down so that your face is level with the child's face (Fig. 35.3). Call the child by name or ask for a nickname. Calling all children "honey" or "pumpkin" can cause children to worry they have been confused with another child.

On admission to a health care facility, all children should have an armband attached giving their name and hospital chart number. Because their hands are not much larger than their wrists and their feet are not much larger than their ankles, neonates (infants younger than 1 month of age) often need two bands in place as an extra safeguard. If a band falls off, secure it back onto the child: never tape it to the crib or bedside stand, as this is not adequate protection: if an infant is placed in the wrong crib by mistake, he or she may be given a medicine that is lethal before the mistake is realized.

Assessment on Admission

Assess each child's level of preparation for a hospitalization on admission to the facility. Be aware of not only what the child describes orally but also what facial expressions or nervous manifestations may be indicating.

Interview parents on hospital admission for a nursing history to obtain the information needed to plan nursing care (Chapter 33 describes a full child database interview history). Many hospitals have information checklists for parents to bring with them. Obtaining information in this way is highly efficient, but it may not be as satisfying to worried parents as hearing a nurse taking a few minutes to ask questions personally or specifically review the completed form. The information that is necessary to obtain about a child is shown in Table 35.1. This is then included in the child's plan of care as a vital step of assessment.

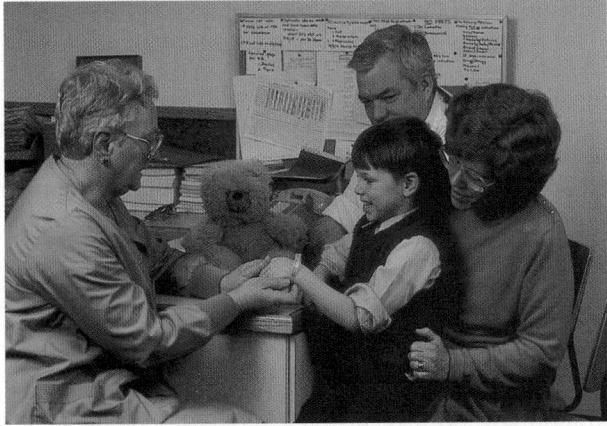

FIGURE 35.3 A child is admitted to a hospital unit. Notice how the nurse greets the child at the child's own level.

Make a note of any medication or food allergy on the child's plan of care and, if pertinent, post this information by the child's bed because unlike an adult, a child cannot call these things to the attention of health care personnel when food or medication is offered.

Take and record the child's temperature, pulse, and respirations. Measure height and weight to determine overall growth and to allow for determination of surface area, the measurement on which medication dosage is calculated. Whether blood pressure needs to be taken depends on the age (usually in children over 3 years of age) and condition of the child. Obtain a specimen for urinalysis as another routine procedure. Be sure to explain all equipment used and allow the child to touch and handle it as much as possible to help reduce anxiety.

Inspect for gross motor ability when weighing a child and measuring height. Listen for language ability (although children in strange situations may say nothing). Perform a physical examination (see Chapter 33) to gain the information necessary for nursing diagnosis and planning.

The way children deal with hospitalization is based on the same factors that determine how they deal with any crisis: perception of the event, whether support people are available, and effectiveness of past coping experiences or skills. After assessment, analyze whether a child's coping ability seems to be enough to balance the hazards of inpatient or ambulatory care hospitalization.

NURSING DIAGNOSES AND RELATED INTERVENTIONS

———◆———

Nursing Diagnosis: Parental and child anxiety related to the need for child's hospitalization

Outcome Evaluation: Parents and child state accurately the reason for child's hospital admission and therapy child will receive; state that although worried, they feel confident they can manage their anxiety.

To help reduce family anxiety regarding hospitalization, be certain the family is oriented to a hospital stay before admission by discussing the need for hospitalization and what they can expect when the hospitalization is first suggested to them in an ambulatory care setting. When children are admitted for emergency care, this type of orientation must be completed immediately, as soon as their physical needs are met. Whether children are admitted for an ambulatory care admission or are being hospitalized for a potentially longer stay, be certain that the parents and the child are oriented to the unit, the personnel who will be caring for them, and any routines.

On admission, the parents and the child both need at least basic information. If the child's diagnosis is uncertain, what steps are being taken to

TABLE 35.1

Information Necessary for the Child's Plan of Care on Admission

Area of Information	Specific Knowledge
Chief concern	Determine what the parents' understanding is of why the child is being admitted. (This view may differ widely from the physician's view regarding the reason the child is being admitted.) What has the child been told about the reason for hospitalization?
Family profile	Obtain child's name and birthday. Who lives at home (include pets)? Ask about parents' occupation and education levels. Who is the child's primary caregiver? Have there been any disruptive happenings lately in the child's life, such as a move or a divorce, that would make the child particularly insecure at this time? Will a parent be staying with the child? If parents are separated or divorced, what will arrangements be? Who has legal authority to sign medical permission?
Past experience with illness or separation	Ask about previous hospital experiences and how the child feels about them. Has there been a recent hospitalization for anyone in the family that resulted in a bad outcome? Has the child been away from the parents before? Overnight at a grandparent's? Summer camp? What is the child's past experience with taking medicine? Has the child swallowed pills before? Does the child have any known allergies to food or medications? (Document these by asking for exact symptoms and happenings.)
Daily routines	Ask about the child's regular bedtime and sleep times. Does the child nap? Does the child have a bedtime ritual? What type of bed does he or she sleep in? Does the child sleep with a favorite toy or blanket? What is his or her bathtime routine? Does the child brush his or her own teeth and hair or need help? What words does the child use for voiding and defecating? Is the child completely toilet-trained? If a preschooler, is the child accustomed to using a potty chair or toilet? Does the child have enuresis (bedwetting)? What is the child's usual meal plan? Are there foods the child does not eat? What is the child's favorite toy? Does he or she have it with him or her? What are the child's favorite games and hobbies or interests? Are there television programs the parents especially like the child to see or not see?
Developmental survey	Ascertain the child's developmental level. Does child feed self? Use a spoon, cup, bottle? Dress self? If school age, what grade in school?
Special information	Obtain any special information about the child that would make him or her more comfortable in the hospital.

confirm it? It helps if these steps are named specifically: for instance, blood work, x-ray studies, observation, recording of vital signs, or calling in a consultant. What is the tentative plan for the child? Complete bedrest or infection control procedures until the results of blood work or cultures are back? Special diet? Special procedures? If the primary care provider has written no orders as yet, be honest: "The specific plan of care isn't written yet. I'll let you know as soon as I'm sure what it will be." Although this answer does not provide a family with information, it does tell them you appreciate how difficult and bewildering it is when a child is admitted to a health care facility.

For an emergency admission, parents may have little understanding of the child's condition or the treatment plan. Conversely, someone might have taken a great deal of time to explain what was happening while the child was being cared for in the emergency room or brought to the unit. To deter-mine the parents' knowledge level, ask them if they have any questions about their child's condition or the course of treatment they want to discuss with the inpatient facility's health care team.

If parents must leave rather than remain with a child, be certain they see the child's room before they go. This is important to convince a child the parents will know where they can find him or her when they return. If there are other children in the room, introduce a new child to them. Let children wear their own clothes if possible rather than change into hospital gowns.

Promoting a Positive Hospital Stay

Promoting a positive hospital stay is important to the health of both children and their families. Several nursing actions are important to make the difference between a successful and an unsuccessful hospital experience.

Minimizing Length of Hospital Stay

Hospitalization should be limited to the shortest time possible. At one time, all children having tonsillectomies and herniorrhaphies, for example, were admitted at least overnight. Currently, these types of surgeries are performed early in the morning, and after a short recovery period a child returns home.

Be certain diagnostic procedures are scheduled for a child's, not the hospital's, convenience so that no child stays in a hospital longer than is necessary. Pressure from concerned nurses who insist on having a voice in policies can make a big difference in a department's willingness to cooperate with scheduling.

Providing Continuity of Care

To ensure that children are exposed to as few substitute care people as possible and to maintain the consistency and quality of care, nursing assignments should be made so one nurse gives as much care to the same child as possible (either **primary nursing** or **case management nursing**; Fig. 35.4). These staffing patterns allow the same nurse to admit the child, take the nursing history, establish nursing diagnoses, set goals for care in cooperation with the parents and the child, and evaluate progress toward achieving goals. It allows children to have one main nurse to whom they can relate. It allows parents to establish meaningful contact with hospital staff and maintains continuity of care, planning, and implementation.

Decreasing Separation Anxiety

It is difficult to explain the meaning that a primary caregiver has for a child, but the intensity of the relationship

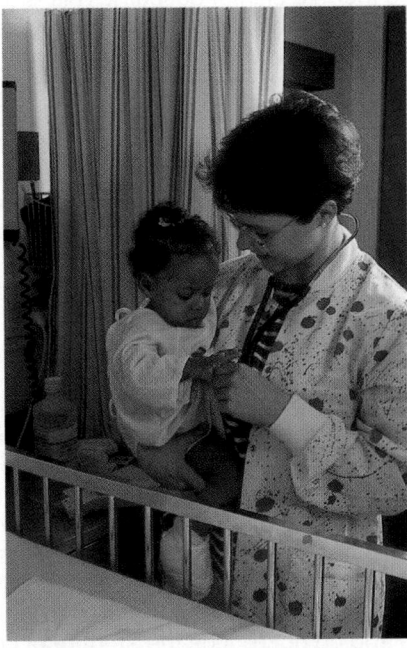

FIGURE 35.4 Each hospitalized child should have one nurse who is "hers" to minimize the effect of separation from parents (primary care nursing). (Susan Leavines/Photo Researchers, Inc.)

can be demonstrated. As early as 4 months of age, the infant registers disapproval if his or her primary caregiver walks away. As early as 5 months of age, the infant registers anxiety when strangers are present or when a person other than the usual caregiver gives care. The infant fixes his or her eyes on the stranger, becomes restless, perhaps thrashes arms or legs, and begins to cry. This activity peaks at approximately 8 months of age, so it is commonly called "8-month anxiety." It is a developmental milestone that shows an infant is able to distinguish a primary caregiver from other persons. It also means a child has reached a stage in emotional development at which he or she reacts poorly to separation or to the threat of it.

Toddlers and preschoolers can be as affected by separation as infants. In some instances, they express their feelings better, louder, and longer than infants. Although many toddlers and preschoolers attend day care and have had prior experiences with separation, others may have had only limited experiences. Being hospitalized may be the first time they are away from parents in a strange setting or away from home overnight. If this is so, many preschoolers may wonder whether they will ever live with their parents again. Problems of separation are especially intense in younger children because they do not understand time. Statements such as, "Mom will visit again tomorrow" or "Dad will be here by 6 o'clock" are meaningless to children younger than 5 years because they do not know what either "tomorrow" or "6 o'clock" means.

School-age children and adolescents react better than younger children to the separation imposed by hospitalization because they have experiences they can use for comparison. They have been to school for whole days; perhaps they have stayed with a grandparent or a friend overnight; they may have been to camp. This can make hospitalization a time for developing self-esteem and confidence in their ability to be independent. Even in light of this, ill school-age children and adolescents may still feel anxious about being separated from their parents. They appreciate their parents' presence and need reassurance that their parents support and love them.

Remember that parents may have an equally difficult time being separated from children. You may need to spend time with them assuring them that their child will receive good care at all times, even when they are absent.

To appreciate why preventing separation is so important, it is helpful to review the research that provided the foundation for this method of care. Spitz (1945) was one of the first researchers who documented the effects of separation on children. He observed children in a penal nursery and in a foundling home who were separated from their mothers for both short and long periods. From this observation, he was able to document how poorly children responded to separation from their parents. Bowlby conducted additional studies after World War II (Bowlby, 1966). Building on Spitz's and Bowlby's work, Robertson (1958) studied the effect of hospitalization on children and supplied labels for separation effects (Table 35.2). Although defined 50 years ago, these findings are still applicable to children today.

Effects of hospitalization can be so severe that they can be compared to posttraumatic stress disorder, the development of characteristic symptoms following exposure

TABLE 35.2

Stages of Separation Anxiety

Stage	Manifestations
Protest	The child cries loudly and demandingly; rejects any attempts to be comforted by nurse or substitute primary caregivers.
Despair	The child becomes less active and cries monotonously or wails in a state of mourning; may turn away from parent's approach; often lies on abdomen, facial expression flat; may lose weight and develop insomnia; loses developmental skills; prone to minor ailments such as upper respiratory infections; IQ will measure lower than previous measurement.
Denial	The child is silent, face expressionless; represses feelings for absent caregiver to protect self; deterioration in developmental milestones is apparent; may respond quickly but superficially to all caregivers; may have difficulty forming close relationships later in life.

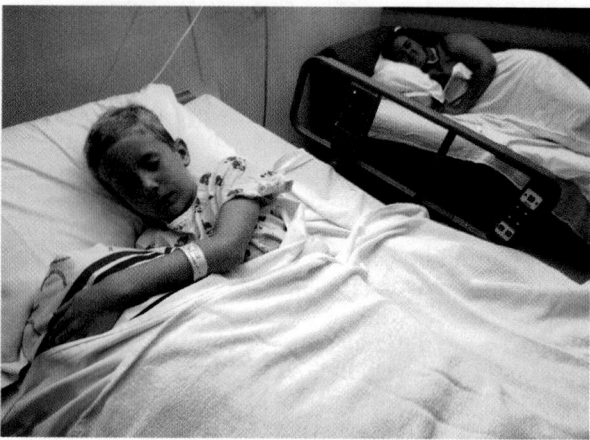

FIGURE 35.5 Rooming-in helps alleviate separation anxiety for both the child and the caregiver.

to an extremely traumatic situation (Cohen, 2005). Children who develop this condition demonstrate persistent symptoms of anxiety such as difficulty falling asleep, irritability, outbursts of anger, difficulty concentrating or completing tasks, or stomachaches and headaches. They re-experience the traumatic event through dreams or flashbacks (Pine & McClure, 2005).

Reducing the ill effects of separation and hospitalization to the extent possible should be a high priority for health care providers. Nurses play a major role in this on both direct care and management levels. Unfortunately, despite the best preparation by parents or nurses, not all of these effects of hospitalization can be prevented.

NURSING DIAGNOSES AND RELATED INTERVENTIONS

Nursing Diagnosis: Anxiety of child related to separation during hospitalization

Outcome Evaluation: Child actively relates to hospital personnel and hospital routine in ways appropriate to child's age and stage of development; manifests a minimum of nervous symptoms.

Promoting Open Parent Visiting. When possible, children younger than 5 years should have their primary caregiver room-in with them when they are in a hospital (Fig. 35.5). Children younger than 10

to 12 years continue to enjoy the feeling of security this provides. This policy is expensive for a hospital because a bed or cot must be provided for this person as well as for the child, and despite the presence of this person, no reduction in nursing staff is possible. In many instances, because so much parental education is needed, requirements for health care personnel actually increase. However, such policies greatly reduce symptoms of separation anxiety.

Not all parents can stay in the hospital continuously. Mothers and fathers who cannot stay may need help in smoothing the transition of their coming or going. For example, when a toddler first sees his parents after being separated, his reaction might be to ignore them (a sign of despair). This is a defense mechanism: "I won't show them I love them until they show me they love me; that way I won't be hurt again." The parents' reaction to being treated this way may be anger. If this makes the parents go and play with a child in the next bed—a "well, be that way then" reaction—the toddler's worst fears are fulfilled: his parents do not love him any more. However, if you urge the parents to speak to the child for a few minutes or try to interest him in a toy, a child will generally reach out to be comforted and act relieved the parents are there.

Parents often need help in saying goodbye when it is time to leave a child to go eat a meal or go home for the night (if the parent is not sleeping in). Assure parents that although someone will not be in their child's room every minute while they are gone, the child will be well cared for. When the parents of an infant are leaving, go into the room a few minutes before they leave and hold or play with the infant. Help a parent to say once, "I have to go now," and then go. Prolonged departures only delay the process and do not reduce the amount of crying that may occur. After parents leave, infants may cry until they fall asleep from exhaustion. Hold and rock them, letting them know that they are safe.

If the parents of a toddler or preschooler have to leave, urge them first to give a warning they will soon have to go: "I have to leave now to fix dinner." When the time to go has come, a parent should say firmly he or she must go and then explain when he or she will return. Time for a preschooler is best measured in terms of events rather than clock hours. "I'll be back after you've eaten supper," "after you wake up tomorrow," or "after nap time" gives the child a concrete event by which to measure time. Like infants, toddlers need someone with them when their parents leave; they like to be held or played with so they know they are not alone.

When parents leave a school-age child or adolescent, urge them to provide definite times when they will return and to leave suggestions for activities a child could do to occupy the time ("Why don't you finish your book? Start your homework and I'll check it when I come back"). Remind them it is more comforting to say specifically, "I will be back around 9 tomorrow morning" rather than, "I will be back sometime tomorrow."

Providing Opportunities for Parents to Participate in Child's Care. Participating in their child's care can make parents feel more in control, thereby reducing anxiety. Therefore, encourage parents to give as much care as possible during a hospital stay, such as bathing or feeding their child, giving oral medicine, helping with procedures such as warm soaks, or checking their child is awake from anesthesia. Most parents are eager to help and do these things spontaneously. Be certain they receive proper instruction on the tasks they will be able to do. Be sure parents who change diapers or feed children know whether the number of diaper changes or the amount of food intake should be recorded; ask them to report when they do these things or write them down on a flow sheet attached to the child's door or crib.

Occasionally parents may be reluctant to give care for fear of being judged inadequate. You can assure them they are the persons from whom their child would most like to receive care. A parent may point out that he or she is paying for nursing care and so wants the nurses to give care. This type of parent will usually soften if approached professionally and assured that nurses are willing to help but for the best interests of the child, the parent is the better caregiver.

Children may be apprehensive about undergoing a procedure without a parent present. There is rarely any reason a parent cannot accompany a child into a treatment room to help with undressing, measuring weight and height, and taking a temperature or accompanying a child to another department for a sonogram or blood work. Most importantly, the mother or father can comfort the child in these strange surroundings.

Although helping with procedures can strengthen the parent–child relationship, remind parents their most important role is being parents. Sitting and rocking or reading to their child and just being there will be their best role to minimize the adverse effects of hospitalization. When a child is to have surgery, it may be especially difficult for parents to separate from their child so the child can leave for the operating room. Helping them do this is an important part of preoperative nursing care.

Supporting Sibling and Grandparent Visitations. Sibling visitation refers to allowing the brothers and sisters of hospitalized children to visit. Allowing this alleviates loneliness on both sides and helps prevent other children at home from imagining the ill child is sicker than is true. It helps the ill child continue to feel part of the family and allows grandparents to offer much-needed support. Siblings who visit need to be free of communicable disease. Nurses may need to help parents divide their time between the ill child and siblings during a visit (short, frequent visits may be better for young children than long ones). Before a visit, ensure that the ill child's room is safe for younger children's visits (e.g., no poisonous substances or electric wires within reach).

Checkpoint Question 2

Suppose Becky shows signs of separation anxiety. The first stage of separation anxiety is marked by:

a. Loud, demanding crying.
b. Silent, sullen protest.
c. Quiet introspective thought.
d. Inability to respond verbally.

Minimizing Negative Effects of Procedures. Ill children often undergo numerous diagnostic and therapeutic procedures that have the potential to cause pain, fear, and anxiety. Details related to specific procedures are discussed in Chapter 36. General guidelines to make any procedure less painful or frightening are discussed in the following sections.

NURSING DIAGNOSES AND RELATED INTERVENTIONS

Nursing Diagnosis: Fear or anxiety related to diagnostic or therapeutic procedures

Outcome Evaluation: Child voices satisfaction with comfort measures; describes how he or she participated in a procedure.

Reducing or Eliminating Pain. Some pain and discomfort is unavoidable in association with health care. Limit this whenever possible, however, by such measures as advocating for the use of intermittent infusion devices such as heparin locks (see Chapter 37) to eliminate multiple punctures for intravenous medication or blood sampling, administering ample analgesia, including alternative therapy techniques such as distraction or imagery, providing traditional comforts such as a change of clothing or position, reading to a child, and planning a special project. Children do not always express discomfort as freely as adults; therefore, closer assessment may be necessary to reveal how they feel. Because pain increases with anxiety, reducing a child's anxiety with good preparation and encouraging a sense of control can also help to eliminate discomfort (see Chapter 38).

Maintaining the Child's Bed as a Safe Area. To assure children that their bed is an area that is safe, all painful procedures should be done in a treatment room, away from the child's bed. Be sure this rule is not broken, because only one painful experience at the bedside can be enough to significantly increase a child's anxiety. This rule should include finger sticks for blood work; although done quickly, they cause pain and stress. In addition, dressing changes, although not necessarily painful, can cause worry and so should be done in a treatment room, not at a child's bedside.

Helping Children to Maintain Control. Events are always more frightening if they appear to be beyond our control. Explaining to children what will happen (i.e., what they will feel or what they will see) and helping them to make choices whenever possible limit this type of fear because these actions offer a sense of control (Fig. 35.6). In almost any procedure, there is some choice a child can make (use a straw to drink or not, decide what size of tape to use on a bandage, or walk one way in the hall or the other). Letting a child participate in signing a consent form can be an additional way to help the child maintain control.

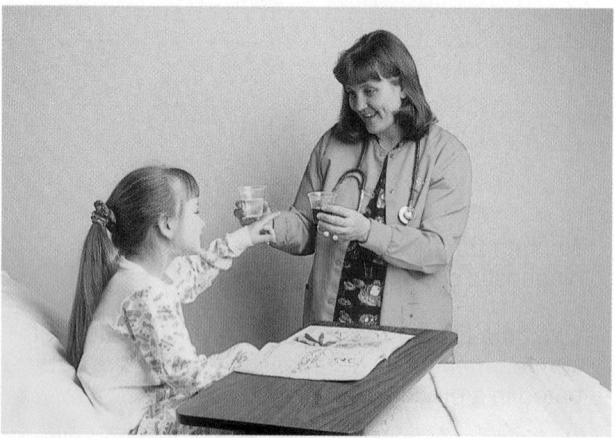

FIGURE 35.6 Include children in procedures whenever possible to offer them a feeling of control. Here a nurse gives a child a choice of fluids to drink with her medication.

Providing Adequate Play Facilities

Play is the medium through which children learn. To continue development during hospitalization, children need to be able to play as normally as possible, no matter how long their stay. Children's hospital units should be equipped with a playroom or play space in which children can feel secure and in which they know they will not be hurt. No medical procedures, not even painless ones, should be performed in this area. Children who are on bedrest need toys or crafts supplied for them also.

Because hospitalization is a traumatic experience, children need the opportunity to express their feelings through therapeutic play before painful procedures (LeRoy et al., 2003). The uses of play and guidelines for providing therapeutic play are discussed later in this chapter.

Setting Limits on Behavior

Setting limits on behavior can help promote a positive hospital stay because it can help to provide a sense of security and safety for the child. The average child is motivated to follow instructions and rules and demonstrate good behavior during a hospital stay because he or she wants to get well again and return home as soon as possible. The occasional child who misbehaves in a hospital setting usually does so because he or she lacks a clear understanding of what is expected or is demonstrating that his or her personal needs have not been recognized and met.

A child who needs frequent reminders to stop running in the hallway, for example, is probably bored with staying in a room. Providing more activities (playing a game with the child) or allowing more structured exercise (letting the child accompany a nursing aide to take a blood specimen to a laboratory) can prevent further unsafe activity.

Children who refuse to cooperate for procedures generally do so out of fear of the unknown rather than deliberate misbehavior. The better prepared a child is for such a procedure, therefore, the better the child is apt to accept it. For potentially painful procedures such as a bone marrow aspiration, lumbar puncture, blood sampling, or cast removal, any behavior short of hysterical screaming can be considered "good" behavior.

If limit setting is necessary, such as with a child who hits or bites other children, confer with the child's parents about the need for limit setting and what measures they would suggest. Gain their cooperation and approval so that what you do is consistent with their care (Regalado et al., 2004). Using "time out" periods or removing the child to a nonstimulating area for a short time is an effective measure. Be certain the child understands the rules (if the child bites or hits, he or she will have to sit alone for a designated period). The next time the child misbehaves, give one warning that the behavior is against the rules; if the behavior does not improve, take the child to the "time out" spot. If the child is disruptive, begin timing the period from when the child quiets down. When the child has been quiet for the specified duration (usually 1 minute per year of age), he or she can leave the "time out" place and rejoin activities.

Discharge Planning

Discharge planning is an important link between hospital and home.

NURSING DIAGNOSES AND RELATED INTERVENTIONS

Nursing Diagnosis: Parental health-seeking behaviors related to care for child at home after hospital discharge

Outcome Evaluation: Parents state accurately the care their child will need at home; describe and demonstrate any procedures they will need to perform with child.

Many children, particularly those having surgery, are hospitalized for only a few hours; as soon as they are able to take and retain fluid and have voided once, they are discharged. This represents such a short time that preparation for discharge must start even before they are admitted to the hospital (Barber-Parker, 2004).

If a child has been admitted on an inpatient basis, preparation for discharge should begin on the day of admission. If some procedures will need to be continued at home, allow parents to perform them in the hospital at least once so that they can become comfortable with the necessary technique and discover any problems while help is still available. Urge parents to think through problems they might have with a procedure at home. Suppose a parent will be doing warm sterile soaks for an open lesion at home. How will he or she sterilize water? Where can the parent buy dressings? Can the parent afford them? What can he or she use to keep the soaks warm for 20 minutes? What suggestions would be helpful to give the parent for keeping the child quiet and content for 20 minutes, so that the child does not move a great deal and knock off the dressing? These are real problems that must be worked out before a parent can perform the procedure at home. Do not leave this kind of instruction until the last day, because then there will not be time left to solve such problems.

Discharge planners can be indispensable in helping ready parents for home care. In a general hospital setting, however, if a discharge planner is unfamiliar with specific procedures (or children), he or she may not be as helpful on a practical level as anticipated. Some parents require follow-up help in their homes that will be provided by a community or home health care nurse. Do not leave the full responsibility for teaching to these home care nurses, however. Teach the parents what they must do on the first day they are at home before further help arrives. Be certain they know the person to contact if plans do not work out as anticipated and that they have a definite return appointment for follow-up care.

Many preschool children manifest behavior problems such as thumb-sucking, bed wetting, temper tantrums, and nightmares after returning home from a hospital stay; school-age children may manifest these behaviors to a lesser extent. You can assure parents these behaviors are part of a child's normal response to hospitalization. These behaviors do not happen because the child has been "spoiled" by the hospital staff or by the parents during the illness but because the experience was too intense for the child to handle, even with all the precautions taken to prevent stress. As children realize they are safely back home and the experience is over, these behavior reactions become less frequent and eventually disappear.

CARE OF THE ILL CHILD AND FAMILY IN THE HOME

Home care is care of children in their own home, provided by or supervised through a certified home health care or community health care agency.

In recent years, as hospital stays have decreased in length, the need for rehabilitation periods at home has grown substantially. Acute care or postsurgical clients need follow-up home visits. Children with chronic conditions such as bronchial pulmonary dysphasia, cystic fibrosis, and childhood cancer are totally cared for at home rather than in hospital settings when at all possible. Many children in terminal stages of disease are also cared for at home (**hospice care**).

Several factors have contributed to the success of the home as a health care setting. Technological advances have made it possible for potentially complicated procedures, such as the administration of total parenteral nutrition and ventilation therapy, to be performed safely at home. There is also a strong economic incentive to provide care in the home (it is less costly for health care plans). Perhaps the greatest benefit of home care for children is the opportunity it brings to include the entire family in health care planning and the ability to focus not only on a specific health problem but also on promoting healthy behaviors for the entire family.

Several types of agencies and services help to meet the growing demands for home health care. Home care agencies, which may be free-standing or allied with a health care facility, provide services by a wide variety of disciplines such as nurses, therapists, and physicians. Specialized services such as providing supplies for total parenteral nutrition, oxygen therapy, or laboratory analysis may be furnished by special service companies. Voluntary agencies often provide services such as transportation, vans to carry children to and from health care agency assessments, or respite care so parents can have a break from continual care.

Be certain that parents whose child is admitted to a home care program know what their responsibilities will be, when home care personnel will visit, any modifications of their home that need to be made, and the dates and times of return visits to a health care facility. Be certain the parents have a telephone number they can call if they have questions about care or their child's condition.

Advantages of Home Care

Although home care of children is not without drawbacks, it has two clear advantages: reduced cost and increased comfort and support.

Reduced Cost

As with adults, in most instances it is less costly to the health care delivery system to care for a child at home than in a hospital setting. Cost containment, however, must be weighed against the safety and quality of care. Because not all home settings are safe for care and not all parents have the commitment necessary for home care, it is not an alternative for all families. In addition, although home care is cost-effective for health care agencies, it may not be cost-effective for the family. Costs that health insurance would have paid for, such as dressings and medications, had the child been hospitalized may no longer be covered once the child is transferred to home care.

Comfort and Support

Unlike a child who is separated from family and friends in a hospital facility, a child being taken care of at home has important support people nearby. For children who are acutely but not terminally ill, this extra emotional support may not be as immediately important as physical care. For those who are chronically ill or dying, being close to their family and friends may be the most important aspect of their care. For these children, home care is ideal.

Disadvantages of Home Care

There are some disadvantages to home care that make it a poor option for some families. Sometimes the physical care required (for example, tracheal suctioning or a complicated medication regimen) can be overwhelming for family caregivers. The financial strain of at least one parent being needed at home full-time and, therefore, not earning an income, the social isolation this creates for the caregiver, and the disruption of normal family life are other major disadvantages that can outweigh the benefits of home care.

Assessing an Ill Child at Home

Nursing assessment of a child at home is similar to assessment of a child in a hospital or other health care facility. Being in the home may actually make it easier to obtain data on the family and family functioning. If an in-depth history or physical examination is necessary, be sure to provide the same level of privacy for a child that he or she would be provided in a clinic or hospital. To do this, it may be necessary to find a room or space that is quiet and free from the distractions of other family activities.

Often, nursing responsibility includes determining whether a child should be cared for at home. This type of assessment begins with investigation to determine whether the child's condition is compatible with home care as well as whether the family is capable of handling the stress of home care. Ongoing assessment of the suitability of the home environment and overall family functioning is necessary for continued home care. Even though health care providers have initially established that the family is able to provide home care for the child, the situation may change: the child's condition may require more monitoring than originally believed, the demands may be too great for the family to bear, or family composition may change, making a responsible caregiver no longer available. Important aspects to be included in an assessment are described in the following sections.

Identifying the Primary Care Provider

Begin assessment by identifying a child's primary caregiver. Although traditionally this is the mother, in today's families, if a father works more flexible hours, he may be the parent best able to give the bulk of care. In some homes, a grandparent or an older sibling will be the person primarily responsible for care. Arrange to include this person in planning and problem solving because this person knows best what strategy of care will be most effective with the child, as well as what strategy will be most appropriate in light of the physical layout of the home and the family's financial ability and lifestyle.

Determining Knowledge Level of Family

Before a child can be cared for at home, teaching will be required so the family understands the child's illness and principles of care. A teaching plan for the family should include the things to be learned immediately and additional care measures that will need to be taught as the child's condition changes.

Identifying Available Resources

The term "resources" refers not only to material objects (e.g., hospital bed, portable oxygen, or glucometer) but also to whether family members are able to deal with the chronic stress of fatiguing, around-the-clock nursing care. Assess physical surroundings, such as: Is there adequate floor space for a hospital bed, oxygen equipment, and so forth? Is a fire company nearby, able to respond in case cardiopulmonary resuscitation (CPR) is needed? Is a backup resource available to power needed equipment if a blackout should occur? Does the family have a telephone? Could the child be evacuated easily in case of a fire? Does the family have transportation to a health care facility for follow-up care? Table 35.3 lists additional important assessments to make, depending on the age of the child.

Determining Current Level of Family Functioning

A family that is supportive of all family members and provides an environment conducive to each member's continued growth and development is more likely to be able to manage home care than a family with a history of ineffective or destructive coping strategies—that is, a family in which parents have unrealistic expectations of family members, one with a history of abusive relationships, or one that is coping ineffectively with other stressors in

TABLE 35.3

Assessment Criteria for Home Care by Age Group

Age	Points to Assess
All age groups	Are there adequate three-pronged plugs for the care equipment needed? If oxygen will be used, is there a sign to omit smoking in the room? Is the oxygen away from a fireplace, gas space heater, or stove? Does the family know not to light candles near oxygen in a power failure or for a birthday? Is there adequate space for supplies? If a special diet is necessary, does the person who will cook have adequate knowledge of food preparation? Do caregivers know the emergency call system procedure in their community? How to reorder supplies? Has the power company been notified if an electrical appliance is necessary for life support? What would be the caregiver's actions in a power failure? What emergency steps should the caregiver take if the child is suddenly worse? Is there a smoke detector in the child's room?
Infant	Is there a suitable sleeping place? Do side rails of a crib lock securely? Can the infant be heard from the parents' room at night? Is there a functioning refrigerator if formula will be used? Is there protection from mosquitoes? Is the home free of rodents that might attack a small infant?
Toddler and preschooler	Is there a safe area for play free from stairs and poisoning possibilities? Are there screens or locks on windows to prevent child from crawling onto a ledge? Is there provision for stimulation and learning activities?
School-age child and adolescent	What is the provision for schooling (possibly an intercom with a regular classroom or home tutor)? Is peer interaction possible? If adolescent is self-medicating, will reminder sheets or some other reminder system be necessary?

their lives. Even a family that appears to be functioning well, however, may be so adversely affected by the stress of home care that its members' ability to be successful with home care can be limited. For example, the loss of employment income, resentment over missed promotions, or cramped living space could put the family at risk for ineffective coping. Consider not only the family's current status but also how it will be affected in the future when determining the advisability of home care. Remember that every family operates differently and handles stress in different ways. Events that may seem overwhelming for a visiting health care provider may actually be easy for the family to handle. Conversely, problems that seem minor could be disruptive enough to affect the family's ability to provide adequate care for their child at home (Box 35.6).

Planning and Implementing Care

Nursing in the community requires a great deal of independent judgment because neither a nursing supervisor nor an attending physician is on the premises to offer advice. It also calls for creativity in adjusting procedures to the confines of a home and the lifestyle of a family. In addition, it requires nurses to be assertive enough to help a family secure adequate funding and resources for home care.

Care at home may include **direct care,** in which a nurse remains in continual attendance or visits frequently and actually administers care, or **indirect care,** in which a nurse plans and supervises care given by others, such as home

BOX 35.6 FOCUS ON . . .

DIVERSITY OF CARE

Whether home care is successful or not can be influenced by male–female roles. In a family in which men and women share responsibility, for example, care tasks as well as time away from the stress of home care can be distributed equally. In contrast, in cultures in which the male is dominant and child care is strictly delegated to the woman, women can become exhausted from trying to keep house, prepare meals, care for other children, and give total care to a medically fragile child at the same time.

Evaluating families individually is important to see what the family's usual childrearing practices are as well as how care is given during illness.

Although play is a universal activity of children, not all parents realize how important it is to children. Children's play activities vary greatly depending on cultural and socioeconomic circumstances. When a child is not proficient in English and that is the language of health care providers, games such as stacking blocks or building with Tinkertoys can be played despite communication difficulty. Playing tapes or records of well-loved children's songs can also be effective, because the child doesn't need to be able to understand the words to enjoy the music or clap with the rhythm.

health care aides or the parents. Nursing care is considered **skilled home care** if it includes physician-prescribed procedures such as dressing changes, administration of drugs, health teaching, and observation of the client's progress or status through such measures as monitoring vital signs or measuring fluid intake and output. In many instances, classifying nursing care as skilled or not determines whether it will be paid for by third-party reimbursement.

Although home care interventions vary depending on the child's physical condition and stage of illness, nursing interventions such as teaching family members how to give care and encouraging them when they become frustrated remain a priority.

NURSING DIAGNOSES AND RELATED INTERVENTIONS

———●———

Nursing Diagnosis: Interrupted family process related to stress of caring for ill child at home

Outcome Evaluation: Parents state they feel able to manage home care; family meets weekly to discuss problems and share accomplishments.

Providing a Therapeutic Environment. For home care to be successful, a home must be one that is able to accommodate and adapt to the health care needs of the child. Modifications may be necessary.

Children cared for at home often require a room similar to that provided in a health care agency. Be sure the house is properly equipped or that medical equipment brought into the home can be accommodated (Fig. 35.7). Hospital beds can be rented from medical supply companies. If a family cannot afford one, they can elevate a house bed on wooden or

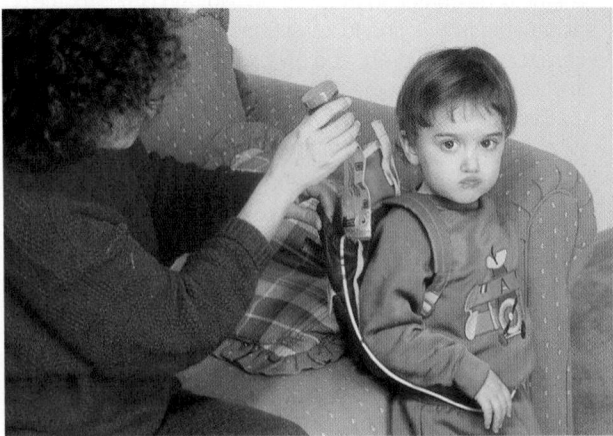

FIGURE 35.7 Procedures at home need to be modified to adjust to the setting. Here a young boy uses a backpack to carry an ambulatory bag for his gastrostomy tube feeding. (John Meyer/Custom Medical Stock Photo.)

concrete blocks. Many home mattresses are not firm; a piece of plywood slid under the mattress improves firmness. A cardboard box or additional pillows can be placed under the mattress to elevate the head of a regular bed to a gatch position. Bed trays can be purchased at any department store or made from a heavy cardboard box.

If a child uses a wheelchair to ambulate, parents need to consider what adaptations of their home will be necessary. A local carpenter can build a ramp across the house steps to allow wheelchair access. Unless the child will be using a motorized wheelchair, the ramp should have a railing for the child to grasp to pull the chair upward or to stop the wheelchair from moving down too fast; the child then can enter and leave the house independently. Wheelchair lifts or elevators can be purchased and mounted alongside house steps, but they are usually more expensive.

Because it is difficult to move a wheelchair across a high-pile carpet, covering the carpet with plastic is helpful. Throw rugs usually have to be removed because they become tangled in wheelchair wheels. Placing furniture along the walls allows increased safe turning space for a wheelchair.

It is impossible to reach high shelves from a wheelchair. To encourage a child to help with meal preparation in the kitchen, urge parents to move supplies the child will use often, such as boxes of cereal, to a lower cabinet. A pair of tongs can help a child reach supplies in upper cupboards. If the counter is too high to prepare foods, placing a board across the wheelchair arms provides a workspace. If a stove has controls at the back, it is difficult for a person in a wheelchair to use. Caution parents that if a child attempts to reach across a hot burner to reach the controls, he or she could be badly burned. A microwave oven placed on a low table can be a solution that allows a child to warm up meals and prepare snacks independently.

Installing a safety rail by the toilet in the bathroom helps the child to transfer from wheelchair to toilet. A chair placed in the bathtub alongside safety rails allows a child to transfer to the bathtub.

Federal law mandates that all public buildings provide easy access for people in wheelchairs or using walkers. In some towns, buildings may not be equipped this way because no one has ever asked for the service before. Urge parents to contact their city council if a problem exists. Advocate for children if the parents' approach is met with less-than-prompt action so that the child (and other people who use wheelchairs) will have access to facilities such as the public library, zoo, museums, and shopping malls.

Promoting Healthy Family Functioning. Although many families are good candidates for home care, they continue to need advice to adapt constructively to the crisis of illness and home management, as the stress and problems that can occur from being responsible for an ill child can lower parents' self-esteem. The time involved can harm their marital relationship or prevent parents from spending time with other children. Physical care requirements can disrupt the normal family routines and shift the focus of attention onto the ill child and away from other children in the family (Fig. 35.8). The needs of the parents may also be neglected (Box 35.7).

Help these families by promoting communication and encouraging family members to identify and share their feelings about the new situation at home. Encourage members to voice the frustration they feel at being constantly confined at home or what they perceive to be a lack of progress in their child's condition. If a child has a terminal illness, support parents to express their grief and not grow discouraged, because the work they are accomplishing is making the child comfortable before death. Continued successful coping will require the family to acknowledge and take seriously the impact of home care on each family member and work together to solve identified problems. They may need to renegotiate roles and responsibilities within the family or seek outside help.

When a family is not functioning well at the beginning of home care or does not adjust to a child's illness, nursing measures to support family functioning become even more important. A family whose coping strategies are maladaptive and ineffective may not be able to care for a sick family member at home for long.

NURSING RESPONSIBILITIES FOR CARE OF AN ILL CHILD AND FAMILY

Nursing responsibilities will vary, naturally, with the type, extent, and seriousness of a child's illness, age, care setting, and individual circumstances. A number of responsibilities, however, such as promotion of normal growth and development, sleep, stimulation, and play, cross all ages and phases of care. Chapter 36 discusses specific responsibilities related to diagnostic tests or interventions. Chapter 38 discusses the important role of promoting comfort in an ill child.

Promoting Growth and Development of an Ill Child

It is easy for children to fall behind in growth and development because of an illness unless health care providers monitor for this.

NURSING DIAGNOSES AND RELATED INTERVENTIONS

Nursing Diagnosis: Risk for delayed growth and development related to effects of illness

Outcome Evaluation: Child demonstrates only limited signs of regression to previous stage; is able to continue doing the things he or she most recently accomplished.

Illness represents a crisis event. In a crisis state, children, like adults, are susceptible to change and growth with only the slightest intervention. Without intervention, they are likely to be overwhelmed.

Promoting Growth and Development of an Ill Infant. To promote optimal growth and development, try to change an infant's normal routine as little as possible. Sameness provides security to a child and encourages the development of trust. When admitting an infant to a hospital, ask parents what type of bed the child normally sleeps in. A child who is used to sleeping in a bassinet may feel loose and insecure in a large crib. You'd need to swaddle such a child in a receiving blanket in a large crib to offer the same close, bound feeling of a smaller sleeping area.

Also, attempt to change the infant's diet as little as possible. Unless a child is diagnosed with failure to thrive or is obviously underweight, illness is not an ideal period in which to introduce new foods or formula. Unless their physical condition warrants a change, infants who breast-feed should continue to do so for as many feedings as possible. Expressed breast milk can be given by bottle to the child when the mother is not available. Overall, because infants cannot begin to understand the strange feelings accompanying illness, they need increased swaddling and comforting. As their condition improves, they need to be provided with stimulation and play opportunities.

Promoting Growth and Development of an Ill Toddler or Preschooler. Because illness can limit autonomy and prevent children from learning how to do new things, try to find opportunities to promote both

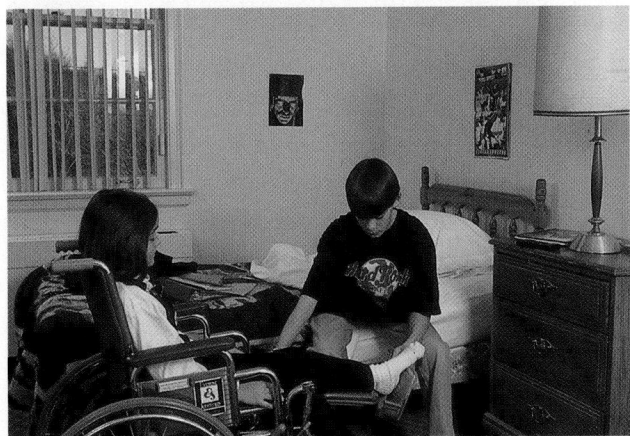

FIGURE 35.8 Home care of a child is family care. Here a brother helps his sister settle into her wheelchair.

A Multidisciplinary Care Map for A Child Undergoing 1-Day Surgery

•

Becky is a 7-year-old who burned her foot in a campfire accident. She is going to be admitted to the hospital for 1-day surgery to have the wound debrided.

Family Assessment

Child lives with parents and two older brothers (10 and 14 years) in a three-bedroom sub-urban home. Father works as sound technician at a recording studio; mother was a grade-school teacher, now is stay-at-home mom; home schools all three children. Father rates finances as, "All right. We have everything we need."

Client Assessment

Client burned left foot on a campfire while on a family weekend camping trip. Was play-ing hide and seek with brothers and ran into fire. Treated at local hospital for third-degree burn; transferred to burn center for follow-up care. Becky's parents tell you that Becky "hasn't been herself" since the injury. She has reverted to temper tantrums and sulking, more like a 4-year-old than one of early school age. Even though she has been told eating meat is important because it provides protein for healing, she refuses to eat anything but Jell-O or soup. In the admission suite of the hospital, she picked up a doll and twisted its leg off. "What can I do with her?" her mother asks you. "How can we get our old daughter back again?"

Nursing Diagnosis

Anxiety related to hospital admission and burn debridement

Outcome Criteria

Child accurately describes what debridement will entail; cooperates with procedures with age-appropriate responses. Describes measures she will need to take after returning home to aid burn healing.

Team Member Responsible	Assessment	Intervention	Rationale	Expected Outcome
Activities of Daily Living				
Nurse	Assess the degree of self-care child usually carries out.	Allow child maximum inclusion in procedures.	Ability to carry out self-care helps "normalize" hospital procedures.	Child participates in self-care to extent possible with post-procedure bandage.
Consultations				
Nurse	Consult with Child Life service on what type of therapeutic play would be most beneficial.	Conduct therapeutic play with child before and after debridement procedure.	Therapeutic play can be helpful to children to re-lieve their anxiety about a hurtful procedure.	Child participates in ther-apeutic play; demon-strates less anxious behaviors following debridement.

(continued)

Team Member Responsible	Assessment	Intervention	Rationale	Expected Outcome
Procedures/Medications				
Nurse	Assess what is child's greatest concern about debridement procedure.	Prepare child for surgery, stressing anesthesia will be used to relieve pain during procedure; analgesia will be available after procedure.	A clear understanding of what is to happen helps to relieve anxiety; knowing pain relief is available is invaluable to well-being.	Child and parent state they understand what procedure will entail; child cooperates in age-appropriate ways.
Nutrition				
Nurse/ nutritionist	Assess what are child's favorite foods.	Suggest ways mother could incorporate protein into soup (meat soups) to increase protein in child's diet.	Jell-O is a protein source; adding meat to what child eats will provide protein yet respect child's choice of food.	Mother details ways she can increase child's protein intake without opposing child's food preferences.
Patient/Family Education				
Nurse/nurse practitioner	Assess what child and parent understand about debridement procedure.	Educate family about procedure and pre- and postoperative care.	Well-prepared child and family can better cooperate with care to make experience a positive one for child.	Child and parents ask questions about procedure; state they understand what it will entail.
Psychosocial/Spiritual/Emotional Needs				
Nurse/nurse practitioner	Take history about burn accident.	Review with mother what she believes has caused the change in child's attitude. Does she think child or parent feels guilt about accident?	Children can believe they are being punished by procedures if they believe an accident was their fault; guilt can also influence parent's relationship with child.	Child and parent state they both should have been more diligent to avoid accident, but accidents happen even in the best circumstances.
Discharge Planning				
Nurse	Assess what will be a typical day for child after return home.	Plan with parent what measures child will need to carry out to keep bandage clean, exercise foot, return to home schooling.	Prospective planning can help avoid problems in home care.	Child and parent review a typical day and decide on actions that will promote healing.
Nurse/ physician	Assess when follow-up visit will be necessary.	Schedule follow-up visit as determined by surgeon.	A follow-up visit will help ensure burn is healing without further complications.	Child and parent state they understand importance of follow-up visit and will keep appointment.

autonomy in toddlers and initiative in preschoolers. Urge parents to encourage children to make choices about their care whenever possible. For example, coloring in a medication schedule is the kind of task that helps to encourage initiative in a preschooler.

If admitted to the hospital, toddlers and preschoolers who are not used to sleeping in cribs may resent being put in a crib unless the reason is explained to them ("All our beds here have side rails"). Watch toddlers closely to be certain they do not climb over crib rails to get out of bed. A child who does try may be safer in a bed than a crib.

As with infants, illness is a poor time to change the eating habits of toddlers and preschoolers. Because children of this age insist on self-feeding, they generally do poorly eating in bed and often do better sitting at low tables. Many child-care units in hospitals organize tables for toddlers and preschoolers to eat together. Some children do well at these tables, but others are too distracted by the activity and the noise and may need a separate low table by their bed to eat well. All children may eat better when their parents are present (Box 35.8).

Illness is also a poor time to begin toilet-training, even if it is appropriate to the child's age. If the parents have already begun toilet-training, continue it with as normal a routine as possible.

Promoting Growth and Development of an Ill School-Age Child. School-age children need to continue to work on a sense of industry while ill. This means learning more about how and why things are done. Explain about specific procedures and involve them as much as possible in planning their care to help foster a sense of industry.

Remember that children who are ill are not at their best and so may not act as mature as usual. This means a 7-year-old whose parents describe him as very mature may seem to function at the level of a 5-year-old. Children of any age should not be held to their chronologic age when they are ill. In a hospital, school-age children enjoy sharing a room with another child close in age so they can play games together. School-age children do well with competition when they are healthy but often do poorly with competition when they are ill. They may revert to playing types of games they would normally dismiss as too young for them.

School-age children and adolescents should continue schooling if they are ill for a long time, provided their condition will allow it. Because it is age-appropriate, ill children do well with school activities or working with a tutor. It is such a normal, everyday activity that it provides security in an otherwise insecure situation. It also reassures them that they are expected to get better and to return to school when this is over.

During the times a child will not be attending school, working on projects such as needlecraft, helping plan family menus, writing for brochures about the place the family plans to visit on vacation next year, or viewing videotapes on science or nature are activities that not only help pass the time but also encourage learning. School-age children also are developing moral responsibility and may find comfort in spiritual practices. Ways to assist with spiritual needs are shown in Table 35.4.

Encourage school-age children to carry out self-care and, if cared for at home, to contribute to household routines, such as helping with dishes or picking up after themselves, as much as they are able. This not only takes some burden off caregivers but also makes a child feel like an intrinsic part of the family.

Promoting Growth and Development of an Ill Adolescent. An adolescent who is struggling to develop a sense of identity may find it very difficult to be ill because the limitations imposed by an illness can make the development of a sense of identity difficult. Help adolescents to continue to participate in activities they did before becoming ill, if possible, to help them feel their world is not totally changing. Encourage them to maintain self-care activities and good hygiene practices to help preserve self-esteem.

Illness can be difficult for adolescents also because peer relationships are so important to them. They may miss acting in a school play, playing on a sports team, or competing for a scholarship. A girl-friend or boyfriend may fall in love with someone else while an adolescent is hospitalized. This makes them feel excluded and hurt. For these reasons, it is important for them to have visitors from their peer group, just as much as infants need visits from parents. Giving hospitalized adolescents prepaid telephone cards to use to contact friends is an easy way for them to maintain contact with individuals who are important to them.

Adolescents appreciate being hospitalized in a special adolescent unit or at least in a room free of childish decor. Adolescent hospital units should be organized with the same considerations for visiting parents as other children's units, though; anxiety and pain of separation are not limited to the under-13 set. Urge parents to stay overnight if they and the adolescent wish. Although adolescents enjoy having parents stay overnight because it is reassuring to know they are concerned, adolescents also enjoy being separated from their parents (assuming everything is going all right) so may not want their parent present all day and night.

Often adolescents convey a blasé attitude toward procedures: having x-rays taken is nothing; surgery is a cinch; a cast change is a snap. Listen carefully to make certain an adolescent really feels this way and is not trying to convince himself or herself a procedure is harmless. Remember ado-

---

BOX 35.8 FOCUS ON . . .

EVIDENCE-BASED PRACTICE

Do Children Eat Better in a Hospital When a Family Member is Present?

For this study, 200 hospitalized children were observed for 3 days to determine their food and fluid intake. The results showed that children did not eat a significantly higher level of protein or calories when a family member was present. Both patient and parent satisfaction was significantly higher, however, in the group who had parents present.

This is an interesting study for nurses because it emphasizes the importance of advocating for family-centered care or care that encourages parents to join their child in their hospital room for meals. It also gives assurance to nurses that children's intake does not suffer when a nurse supervises their mealtimes.

Source: Williams, R., et al. (2004). A comparison of calorie and protein intake in hospitalized pediatric oncology patients dining with a caregiver versus patients dining alone. *Journal of Pediatric Oncology Nursing, 21*(4), 223–232.

TABLE 35.4

Nursing Interventions To Meet Children's Spiritual Needs

Action	Implementation
Prayers	School-age children may be learning and saying prayers. Ask on hospital admission whether a child says grace with meals or a prayer at bedtime. Write it on the plan of care so that nurses can help with this. Remember that saying grace also applies to unconventional meals, such as a tube feeding. Bedtime prayers may be especially important by lending security in a strange environment.
Religious services	Many children of school age and older enjoy attending a religious service in a hospital chapel. Include time for this in the plan of care and be certain that transportation by wheelchair or cart is available.
Visits from clergy	Many school-age children and adolescents enjoy an active recreation or social program at a church facility when well. They enjoy a visit from clergy when they are ill, not so much for its religious importance as for support from a respected adult. Free the child's time as necessary for such visits.
Religious articles	A child's parent may wish to attach a religious article to the child's clothing or pillow or to post it over the bed. Be careful when changing linen that you do not throw away such articles. Mark their presence and importance on the plan of care.

lescents are extremely worried about their body parts. Make sure they know what is going to happen in surgery and in other departments such as x-ray. It is easy to assume from their attitude that they know more than they do.

PROMOTING NUTRITIONAL HEALTH OF AN ILL CHILD

Nursing responsibilities related to nutrition for ill children include maintaining optimal nutritional status in the face of illness or treatment that interferes with adequate intake; correcting nutritional deficiencies or otherwise aiding children and families to follow the nutritional care plan devised by the health care team; and educating the child and family regarding specific nutritional needs as well as overall sound nutritional health. Specific procedures for promoting nutrition such as measuring fluid intake and output and providing enteral feedings, gastrostomy tube feedings, and total parenteral nutrition are discussed in Chapter 36.

NURSING DIAGNOSES AND RELATED INTERVENTIONS

Nursing Diagnosis: Risk for imbalanced nutrition, less than body requirements, related to lack of appetite

Outcome Evaluation: Child maintains skin turgor and age- and size-determined weight pattern; ingests 80% of prescribed diet daily.

An acute illness in a child, such as pneumonia, is often accompanied by a loss of appetite; gastrointestinal illnesses often cause nausea and vomit-

ing. Because most acute illnesses last only a few days, there is no need for children to eat more than a small amount during this time as long as they can drink fluid. Trying to force them to eat only increases nausea and vomiting, which increases the possibility of creating an electrolyte imbalance. When an illness lasts for more than a few days, however, providing adequate nutrition becomes increasingly important because children need nutrients not only to repair ill or diseased tissue but also to maintain normal childhood growth.

Important points to address when planning nutrition for ill children are summarized in Table 35.5. Children who are hospitalized often tolerate hospital-prepared food, which can be repetitious and bland, better than adults do. Provided that it is the kind of food they like, such as hot dogs and hamburgers, these appeal to children more than the elaborate dishes with spices and sauces preferred by adults. Children who are receiving care at home need as much nursing supervision of their diet as those in health care agencies (possibly more) because they may not have a dietitian planning meals to ensure adequate nutrition. Assess not only the quantity but also the quality of food to ensure that intake is optimal. Ask whether nutrition supplements are being offered to increase intake (Ball, Kertesz, & Moyer-Mileur, 2005).

Encouraging Fluid Intake. Increasing oral fluid intake has traditionally been termed "forcing fluid." It is better to avoid this term with children, however, because they can interpret the instruction to mean that someone is going to physically force them to swallow fluid. A physician's order should state in detail the amount of fluid a child is to receive during 24 hours, because the amount differs so much for different ages. The following are some practical guidelines for encouraging fluid intake at any age:

- Offer small, full glasses frequently rather than half-full larger glasses; children are mid–school

TABLE 35.5

Areas to Consider When Planning Nutrition for Ill Children

Area	Importance
Meaning of food	Early in life, infants learn to associate eating with being held and loved; if they cannot eat for some reason (e.g., nothing by mouth for surgery), they may view the restriction as punishment or restriction of love.
Opportunity for socialization	Mealtime is often a time of the day when children socialize with other family members; they may feel lonely eating alone and consequently may have a poor appetite.
Level of stress	Children under stress may either feel a loss of appetite or experience a need to snack frequently; planning is necessary to see that children maintain adequate intake if not hungry and that their snacks are nutritious.
Custom	Custom is important: for example, many children like foods served separately and resist eating them if they are mixed into a casserole.
Culture	Most children eat best foods with which they are familiar; in many instances, parents can bring in favorite foods from home to provide culturally preferred items.
Environment	Hunger is associated with the sight and smell of food; many children are normally in the kitchen while meals are being prepared; they may not be hungry when food is served to them without their having seen and smelled it being prepared.

age before they evaluate the amount of fluid in a container rather than the size of the container.
- Determine the child's favorite fluid, and then offer it.
- Try changes of temperature in fluid offered (hot cocoa, then cold juice, then hot soup) for variety. Broth can be a nice change of liquid (many commercial types are quick to prepare, but be aware of their high sodium content).
- Keep in mind that popsicles and Jell-O are fluids (Fig. 35.9).
- Know that children can drink more of a clear fluid (ginger ale, water) than a thicker fluid (milk shakes or cream soups), because thicker fluids are absorbed from the stomach much more slowly.
- Use soothing beverages such as Kool-Aid, Snapple, or milk for children with mouth lesions. They may be unable to drink fruit juices because the acid content stings their mouths; carbonated beverages may also cause discomfort.
- Because ice melts to one half its volume, count a glass of ice chips as only a half-full glass of fluid.
- Unless contraindicated, let children drink fluids with a straw; this is a novelty to many who do not normally use these and encourages intake.
- Introduce a game, such as "Simon Says" (Simon says, "Drink") or a board game in which a child takes turns and with each turn has to take a drink.

Encouraging Food Intake. **Calorie counting,** as the name implies, involves counting the number of calories that children ingest in 1 day. To do this, record all the foods that a child eats during each 24-hour period, being certain to include snacks, candy, or gum. A dietitian then will analyze the list and determine the caloric intake. Be certain when doing this

that you describe the types of food and amounts (not "some toast," but "half a slice of whole wheat toast"). Be sure that everyone caring for the child is aware that calories are being counted so that they also record this information accurately.

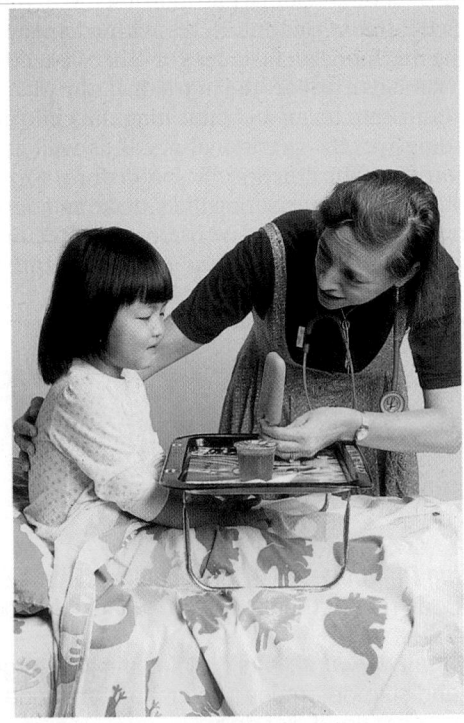

FIGURE 35.9 A nurse offers this young child a popsicle, a good source of fluid when children don't feel thirsty or hungry.

Checkpoint Question 3

You want to encourage Becky to drink a lot of water. Which action would do this best?

a. Scold her for not cooperating to make herself well again.
b. Offer her small glasses of fluid so she can drink these frequently.
c. Offer her large glasses of fluid so she doesn't have to drink so often.
d. Alert her if she doesn't drink fluid, she will have to receive an IV.

PROMOTING SAFETY FOR AN ILL CHILD

A prime consideration of nursing interventions is to keep a child safe during illness care.

NURSING DIAGNOSES AND RELATED INTERVENTIONS

Nursing Diagnosis: Risk for injury related to procedures or therapy necessary for care

Outcome Evaluation: Child remains free of injuries and accidents, such as a fall from bed or injury from medical equipment.

Promoting safety for children is a responsibility for all health care providers. Care of an ill or physically challenged child at home includes assessing the safety of the house and providing family teaching. It also includes making provisions for emergencies. For example, a family may need to install a counter-level telephone or purchase a cell phone so a child in a wheelchair can call for emergency help. They might need to make a plan for how to evacuate an ill child from the home in an emergency such as a fire.

Safety on a children's unit or clinic is the responsibility of everyone, from the administrator of the institution to part-time health care personnel. To make a child health care environment a safer place, follow these steps:

- Always be sure of the location of all children in your care.
- Ensure that doors or gates are provided near stairways or elevators.
- Ensure that back doors of health care facilities have working alarms to prevent children from going out and strangers from coming in.
- Be sure windows are covered by screens or guards so children cannot climb up on sills and fall out.

- Check that the side rails of beds and cribs are in good repair and raised appropriately.
- Always raise bedside rails after a child has received preoperative or sedative medication.
- Test a crib rail after it is raised to ensure the lock has caught so the rail will remain raised.
- Push bedside tables or stands away from cribs so a child cannot climb over the railing and use the stand as a step down.
- Be certain crib caps are provided for small children to prevent them from climbing out of bed.
- Fasten the seat belt restraint for infants in high chairs. Never leave an infant in a high chair (at home or in a hospital) without someone close enough to reach the child if he or she should fall from the chair.
- Ensure that electrical cords or appliances such as hair dryers are not used in bathrooms, where they could come in contact with water.
- Be careful of the placement of TV/call cords or Venetian blind cords so they cannot lead to strangulation.
- Never leave children younger than 5 years alone in a bathtub; they could turn on the hot water and scald themselves or slip under the water and drown.
- Never leave equipment or items that would be harmful to eat within the reach of children.
- Adhere to all fire precaution measures.
- Closely follow standard precautions to prevent the spread of infections.

Promoting Fire Safety. Fire precautions both in the home and in the hospital are essential in preserving the safety of ill or disabled children. Adults can usually take responsibility for removing themselves from a burning structure, but children depend on care providers. Ensure that there is a plan of action in case of a fire and that everyone in the home, in the clinic, or on a hospital unit knows it. To be certain a home is safe, having a smoke detector on each floor is a wise precaution. A downstairs bedroom is not only safest in case of a fire but also allows a child more self-care ability. Fire departments supply free decals for the bedroom windows of children or those who are physically challenged so they can be easily located in a fire. Encourage parents to contact their local fire department for this safety measure.

Electrical equipment such as respiratory and cardiac monitors, radiant heat warmers, special-care equipment, and electrical heating pads are often used in the care of children. Do not use equipment with frayed cords or equipment that is not properly grounded. Plugs should be three-pronged for extra safety; do not overload circuits with additional plugs. Electrical outlets should have safety caps to cover them when they are not in use so toddlers cannot poke objects into them and electrocute themselves.

Adhering to Standard Precautions. In every health care setting, closely follow standard precautions to protect the ill child, family, and staff from infections. Because of a compromised immune system, ill children may be more susceptible to repeat or secondary infections than usual. Proper handwashing technique, disposal of tissues and waste materials, and efforts to minimize exposure to other ill children or adults are all effective methods to decrease the risk of infection. For more details on infection control, see Chapter 43.

PROMOTING ADEQUATE SLEEP FOR AN ILL CHILD

Ill children need adequate rest and sleep so their body tissues can effectively use nutrients for repair and normal growth can continue. Children may not sleep well when they are ill because of discomfort, pain, administration of medications, or intensified symptoms of chronic sleep problems. They may not sleep well in a hospital because it is a strange setting; they may have to undergo so many procedures that they also do not nap or rest as much during the day as usual. Children who are recovering from trauma such as injuries from a car accident or burns may be unable to sleep because of nightmares about the accident. These nightmares can cause them to suffer sleep deprivation in the same way as a child who is frequently awakened for procedures during the night. Encourage parents to stay with these children for support and comfort.

Sleep Patterns

Sleep is influenced by anxiety level, state of health, habit, medication, and environment at the time of sleep. Stages of sleep are summarized in Table 35.6. Figure 35.10*A* shows a pattern of normal sleep. As a sleep cycle begins, a child first enters **nonrapid eye movement (NREM) sleep.** This type of sleep occurs in up to 80% of total sleep time. As a child falls deeper and deeper asleep, he or she passes from stage I to stages II, III, and IV of NREM sleep over a period of 20 to 30 minutes. **Rapid eye movement (REM) sleep** follows. In infants, most of sleep time is REM sleep, whereas young adults have the least amount of this type of sleep. The sleep pattern of a child who is awakened frequently during the night for procedures would resemble that shown in Figure 35.10*B*.

The purpose of NREM sleep, the first phase of sleep, is rest and restoration of the body; this stage keeps body cells functioning and healthy. During the periods of stage III and IV NREM sleep, the secretion of growth hormone (somatotropic hormone) from the pituitary is at its highest level. Growth hormone is necessary for protein synthesis and growth of new cells and for repair and maintenance of all cells. Corticosteroids and adrenaline from the adrenal gland, which are instrumental in the catabolism or breakdown of cells, are at their lowest levels. This balance of hormones produces the ideal combination for protein synthesis and cell growth and repair.

The purpose of REM sleep is less clear. The rapid eye movements may serve to coordinate binocular vision.

TABLE 35.6

Stages of Sleep in Children

Stage	Description	Nursing Implications
NREM		
I	A feeling of drifting or falling. Often described as twilight sleep. Temperature and heart rate decrease slightly; EEG waves show peaked, frequent waves (alpha waves).	A child can be roused easily from this early sleep by the slightest noise or even the silent presence of another person in the room. Reduce noise level in room to promote sleep.
II	Sleep deepens. Temperature and heart rate decrease slightly more.	It is more difficult to wake a child from sleep when this point has been reached
III	Sleep deepens still further. An EEG tracing reveals mixed spindle and delta (slow) waves. Temperature and heart rate decrease further. This period lasts about 10 min.	It is very difficult to wake a child from stage III sleep. Use patience to wake a child fully to offer medicine.
IV	Approximately 20 to 30 min after beginning to fall asleep, a child enters stage IV sleep. Respirations are slow and deep, temperature and heart rate slow even more, and blood pressure decreases; EEG shows delta (slow, steady) waves. A child remains at a stage IV sleep level for approximately 30 min, then progresses back through stages III and II until he or she then passes into a phase of REM sleep.	A child will be confused and unable to orient himself/herself readily if awakened from stage IV sleep. Use patience until a child is fully awake, particularly if asking a question.
REM	Eyes move in rapid, involuntary motions. Respirations are irregular; body turnings, movements, and penile erections may occur. Lasts 10 to 30 min and then a new sleep cycle with NREM sleep begins.	Dreaming occurs during REM sleep. Although a child appears to be close to waking because of the active eye movements, he or she is really very soundly asleep. A child may wake afraid and crying, disturbed by a frightening dream.

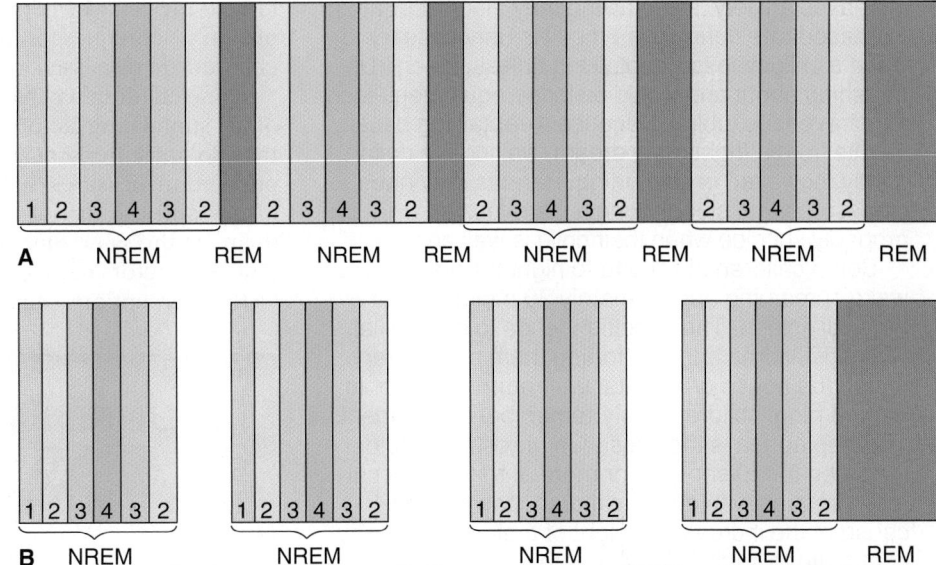

FIGURE 35.10 Sleep patterns. (**A**) Normal sleep pattern. Notice how the periods of REM sleep increase in length during the last half of the night. (**B**) The sleep pattern of a child who has been awakened frequently during the night. Notice how little REM sleep is present.

Dreams that occur during this time apparently serve as a release of tension or help to integrate new knowledge and experience with old in the brain's memory system. Vital signs may fall during NREM sleep. During REM sleep, vital signs rise to near-normal levels. These periods of REM sleep interspersed with NREM sleep, therefore, may be a fail-safe measure to prevent vital signs from falling too low during sleep.

Sleep Deprivation

Children who do not receive enough sleep can suffer **sleep deprivation** just as adults do. After approximately 4 days of poor sleep, they show difficulty in concentrating and experience episodes of disorientation and misperception.

If the sleep loss is mainly REM deprivation, children show symptoms of irritability and difficulty concentrating. Lack of stage IV NREM sleep, in contrast, tends to cause apathy, physical fatigue, and depression and can slow recovery. This is the same phenomenon that can happen in adolescents if they are studying for exams. It easily occurs in younger children during illness if they are awakened frequently for treatments.

NURSING DIAGNOSES AND RELATED INTERVENTIONS

———•———

Nursing Diagnosis: Disturbed sleep pattern related to timing of medication, discomfort, or sleep disorder

Outcome Evaluation: Child sleeps through the night without interruption (when therapeutic regimen allows); is alert and active during the day; is able to take nap during the day if that is part of usual sleep schedule.

Because sleep is so important for ill children, you need to take special steps to ensure that children are able to sleep during an illness. Be certain children are as free of pain and worry as possible. Try to let them maintain as normal a bedtime routine as possible (bath, change to nightclothes, nighttime story, prayers). Provide an atmosphere conducive to sleep (lights out, quiet surroundings, reassuring support people). Children who are bored with bedrest may catnap constantly during the day and then be wide awake at night. Providing more interesting activities for them during the day can help reduce their naps and increase nighttime sleep.

Managing Chronic Sleep Problems. Some children may have chronic sleep problems such as night terrors, nocturnal enuresis, somnambulism (sleepwalking), sleep talking, and sleep apnea. These sleep problems can intensify with illness and increase sleep deprivation in ill children.

Somnambulism is a common sleep problem in children. It apparently occurs during NREM sleep, probably during the deepest part of stage IV. It is frightening for children to wake and realize they have been sleepwalking. Sleepwalking can be potentially dangerous when a child is ill because, while getting out of bed, he or she could dislodge intravenous tubing or oxygen equipment. It is untrue that sleepwalkers should not be wakened; instead, wake them gently, help them get reoriented, and then return them to bed after reassuring them they are safe. Be certain that the side rails are raised on the bed of a child who tends to sleepwalk. In a hospital, it may be necessary to move a child's bed out into the hallway at night near the nurses' desk if a parent will not be sleeping over, so the child can be observed for sleepwalking.

Sleeptalking seems to occur during REM sleep. Dreaming of some frightening or puzzling situation, a child calls out a name or instruction such as, "Stop!" Because illness is a stressful situation that increases anxiety, sleeptalking may also occur at an increased rate during this time. It is unnecessary to wake a child who is sleeptalking unless the child is thrashing about and would dislodge equipment such as intravenous tubing. Because sleeptalking usually results from a frightening dream, waking the child gently, however, is comforting. Parents may need to be assured that sleeptalking is harmless and will probably subside when their child is well again.

Some children are prone to night terrors, or wake screaming approximately 20 minutes after they fall asleep. The condition tends to be familial. Waking children and comforting them helps everyone in the house or hospital unit return to sleep. In the morning, children rarely remember the incident.

Sleep apnea is the cessation of respirations during sleep for 20 seconds or more. It tends to occur more frequently in obese children, possibly because of the increased weight of their chest. It may contribute to sudden infant death syndrome or failure to thrive (Bonuck, 2005) (see Chapter 26). Infants who are diagnosed with this condition may be prescribed respiratory monitors to evaluate their breathing pattern and warn against any cessation of respirations.

PROMOTING ADEQUATE STIMULATION FOR AN ILL CHILD

Children are in constant interaction with both their internal environment (body) and their external environment (surroundings) by means of their five senses and the central nervous system. This makes them capable of responding to changes in environment and by so doing meet basic needs. Any illness that changes their ability to respond can cause either sensory deprivation or sensory overstimulation.

Sensory Deprivation

Sensory deprivation is the condition of being deprived of, or lacking of, adequate sensory, social, physical, or cognitive stimulation. When this happens, children tend to lose the ability to make decisions and become easily confused and depressed. Some children are more prone to sensory deprivation than others.

Ill children may have sensory deprivation because they are confined to their homes or hospital rooms and their varied activities such as school, sports, and clubs are replaced with hours of watching television or playing video games. Hospital regulations for intensive care units may limit parental interaction. When parental interaction is limited this way, children generally receive less-than-normal cognitive stimulation. Such children need cognitive stimulation from warm, reassuring health care personnel.

Children with hearing or visual deficits are more prone than others to sensory deprivation. Children with forms of sensory nerve loss or those receiving chemotherapy may lose their sense of touch, taste, or proprioception (sense of where they are in space). After losing these forms of perception, children may draw back from interacting with other people because they are self-conscious about the

loss, so they may be deprived of social and cognitive stimulation. Techniques for interacting with sensory-deprived children are discussed in Chapter 50.

Some children receive medication to lessen awareness of the stimulating factors in their environment. To ensure they do not suffer sensory deprivation, give them definite orientation measures, such as always mentioning the time of day and the day of the week in conversations with them. At the same time, they often must have overly stimulating factors reduced, such as the number of visitors, so that perceptions can be interpreted clearly.

NURSING DIAGNOSES AND RELATED INTERVENTIONS

Nursing Diagnosis: Deficient diversional activity related to lack of appropriate toys and peers

Outcome Evaluation: Child demonstrates alert and interested attitude toward self-care and play activities.

Providing Stimulation for Children on Bedrest. Children on bedrest cannot secure materials for cognitive stimulation by themselves or to participate in physical activities, except to a limited degree. A room where walls and windows offer no visual appeal and therapeutic equipment provides the only sound offers them little sensory stimulation. If no one comes into the room, they may suffer from social deprivation. When possible, encourage a child with restricted mobility to move out of bed into a wheelchair; this can provide some mobility and transportation to a place of interest, such as near a window or, in a hospital, near the nurses' desk. Watching television, a common activity for children on bedrest, provides little cognitive stimulation after the first 24 hours. Children can also be exposed to inappropriate programming if this is not carefully monitored (DiMaggio, Sharif, & Hoffman-Rosenfeld, 2003).

Occasionally, a child must remain in bed to reduce stimulation (e.g., to rest the heart or to increase kidney function), but generally bedrest is prescribed mainly to inactivate one part of the body, such as a fractured bone. When possible, other stimulation, such as a favorite toy, games, books, or simply talking with someone, must be provided for the child to maintain physical bedrest; otherwise, he or she will become bored and irritable and will thrash and turn instead of lying still (Fig. 35.11).

If a child is home on bedrest and the bedroom is away from the main home activities, encourage family members to include the ill child in as many family activities as possible—bring the television set into the child's bedroom so the entire family gathers there, or set up a card table in the room so everyone can eat there—or encourage the child to join the rest of the

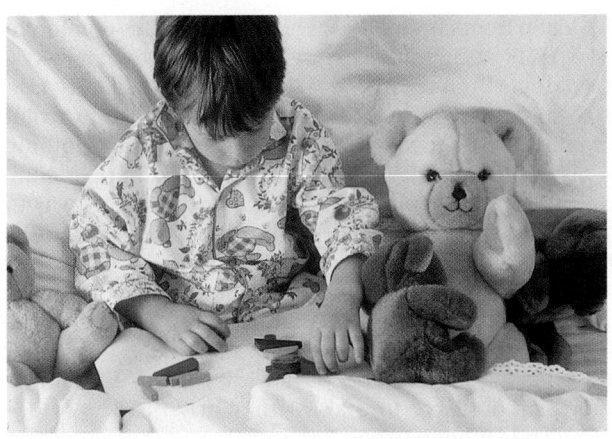

FIGURE 35.11 Children on bedrest need stimulation. Here, a young child enjoys putting together a puzzle.

family for activities by resting on the couch in the living room, a lounge chair in the backyard, or sitting in the kitchen. This principle applies to hospitalized children as well. To interact more easily, a toddler may rest in a parent's lap rather than in a bed.

Providing Stimulation for Children on Transmission-Based Precautions. Children who are placed on transmission-based precautions because of the possibility of contagious illness may experience severe sensory deprivation if everyone who enters the room must wear a gown and mask or if the number of visitors must be kept to a minimum. If gloves are part of precautions, a child can experience a significant loss of skin-to-skin contact as well. Transmission-based precautions are discussed in Chapter 43. Careful planning must be done to ensure that a child who is isolated this way is not psychologically isolated and that every possible measure is carried out to maintain sensory, social, physical, and cognitive stimulation. For example, try to visit with a child at a time in addition to those times in which you must perform procedures so you can simply talk; place the bed so the child can see out of the room; encourage him or her to telephone friends; make posters for the walls so they're no longer bare; or encourage interactive play such as electronic games. For ideas on providing stimulation to children in specific age groups, refer to Chapters 28 to 32.

Sensory Overload

Sensory overload, in contrast to deprivation, occurs when a child receives more stimulation than he or she can tolerate or process. Children with sensory overload react similarly to those with sensory deprivation (i.e., they are confused, unable to make decisions, and severely fatigued). Sometimes it is difficult to determine the cause of these symptoms (whether they are caused by sensory deprivation or overload) unless assessed carefully.

The lights in ICUs, for example, are never turned out. Although children may find this comforting, it can also result in excessive stimulation. In addition to constant light, there is excessive sound (e.g., whir of machines, buzzing of ventilators, ringing of alarms, or mix of voices in consultation). Most ICUs have no windows because the wall space is used for monitoring equipment; therefore, night and day are not easily distinguished. It is easy for a child to become confused about time and place in such a setting. For children who are cared for at home in a family room where people talk constantly, the television is always on, and activity never ceases, sensory overload may also occur. An important nursing role is reducing sensory stimulation attributed to overload. Orient children to the time of day by making frequent references to it or by providing calendars and clocks. If necessary, provide eye covers or ear plugs to reduce stimulation.

PROMOTING PLAY FOR AN ILL CHILD

Play, often described as "the work of children," is an invaluable component of child health care. Providing a space and opportunity for play can help a child feel more comfortable and allow for an important release of energy for a child who is confined to a room or bed. Play also may be used to help assess a child's level of knowledge and feelings about his or her condition so that more individualized nursing care can be planned. Depending on a child's age, play can also be a useful tool in health teaching (see Chapter 34).

Defining play is not a simple task because play activities vary greatly from child to child and among different age, cultural, and socioeconomic groups. A common definition is that play is any voluntary activity engaged in for the purpose of enjoyment. If a child views an activity as enjoyment, therefore, no matter what it is and whether it would be fun or not for an adult, it is play.

Play is clearly the means by which children develop increasing cognitive, psychomotor, and social capabilities. Touching a soft rabbit, passing colored blocks from one hand to the other, pounding with a plastic hammer, feeding a doll, and playing board games are all ways in which children are exposed to and learn about different textures and colors, experience the feeling of possessing and owning, and learn about competition, winning, and losing. A soft toy tells a child more clearly than can be described that this is what the word "soft" means. Colored blocks show him or her how parts can join to make a whole, how things stacked too high will fall (there are limits one cannot go beyond), and practice makes perfect. As a child talks with playmates during play, he or she develops both language and social skills. The repetitive acts involved in most games encourage the development of musculoskeletal skills. Play is not something a child does when he or she has nothing else to do then; it is something the child *has* to do. During illness, it provides a feeling of security because it is an activity that has continuity with everyday life.

The manner in which children play differs as they mature. Types of play and the age groups in which these types are seen most frequently are shown in Box 35.9.

Assessing Child Health Through Play

Children who are acutely ill do not play or play very little because they do not have the strength, the attention span,

BOX 35.9 FOCUS ON . . .

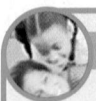

FAMILY TEACHING

Understanding Different Play Types

Q. Becky's mother tells you, "When Becky was younger, she didn't like toys as much as the boxes they came in. What's normal for children and play?"

A. Children play differently at different ages. Examples of typical play patterns include:

Type of Play/Age	Description	Example
Observation/ Infant	Child watches particular play intently, although not actively engaged in it.	Watching a mobile
Parallel/ Toddler	Two children play side by side but seldom attempt to interact with each other.	Playing separately with similar push toy
Associative/ Preschooler	Children play together in a similar activity; there is little organization of responsibilities	Engaging in typical backyard play
Cooperative/ School-age	Children play with an organized structure or compete for desired goal or outcome.	Playing organized games with rules

or the interest in activities required for play. They continue, however, to enjoy being read to, and they find comfort in holding a favorite toy even if they do not actively manipulate it. Once children are over the acute phase of an illness, interest in play returns. Whether a child is spontaneously playing, then, is a good index of health. The toys a child uses at play are a good indication of his or her growth and development level and emotional state.

The average parent knows a child's play preferences and his or her current favorite game or toy. Asking for this information at a health interview helps to assess a child's developmental level and whether it is age-appropriate. It also helps to assess the quality of parenting (if parents view play as important or are familiar with the child's activities).

Providing Play in Ambulatory Settings

Children in ambulatory departments are under a great deal of stress. They sit in a waiting room and glance fearfully at the door that leads to the examining room. They hear children crying beyond the door and wait in terror for what lies in store for them when it is their turn.

Most parents know that when their child is coming to a hospital to be admitted, they should pack the child's favorite toy. Often they do not think of an ambulatory visit as a sufficiently threatening circumstance to warrant bringing a favorite toy, however, so the child has nothing to play with. Having a parent sit beside them is so comforting they may ignore or hesitate moving 4 feet away to get the toys furnished by the health care facility unless they are urged to do so.

It's best if ambulatory departments are stocked with toys that can be played with quickly and by single children. There should be a low table and chairs so a parent can come to a table and play with a child. Examining rooms should have toys also—they may be used to distract a child while a procedure such as an ear examination is performed, and because the wait in an examining room may be as long as the wait in a waiting room. Well siblings who accompany a parent and sick child to the facility can play with toys to distract them as well so that a parent can concentrate on the ailing child. Some hospitals furnish computer games for older children for this reason. Examples of ways that play can be used in an ambulatory care setting are shown in Table 35.7.

Providing Play in the Hospital

Ideally, all hospital units in which children are cared for should have a play space big enough for most of the children on the unit to come to. There should be enough space to accommodate children who are not fully ambulatory, such as those with casts or in wheelchairs (Fig. 35.12).

TABLE 35.7

Ways to Incorporate Play Into Ambulatory Nursing Care

Nursing Care	Play Activity
Aid with physical assessment	Distract child's attention with puppet during respiratory and cardiac assessment.
	Play "Simon Says" to encourage child to take deep breaths for respiratory assessment.
	Allow child to listen to own heart with stethoscope.
	Play "Follow the Leader" to assess gait.
	Draw a face on the tongue blade used to assess throat.
	Show child how to "blow out" the otoscope light.
	Draw child's outline on the table examining paper and give it to him or her to take home to color.
Health teaching	Use puppets as teacher.
	Create word scrambles or crossword puzzles.

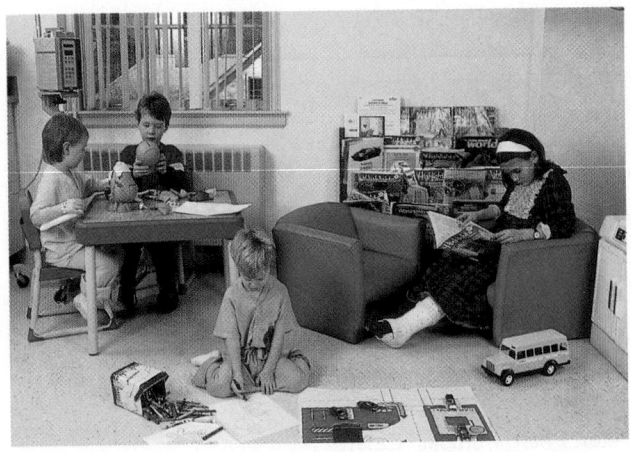

FIGURE 35.12 Children enjoying themselves in a hospital playroom, which is spacious and well equipped with age-appropriate toys and activities.

Tables for board games and play materials such as crayons and paints should be available. Children can release a great deal of anger or tension by splashing water, squeezing or pouring sand, or smearing finger paint.

School-age children can play games such as shuffleboard or tossing sand bags for tension relief and competition. Adolescents enjoy table tennis and pool tables. A great deal of "play" in older school-age children and adolescents centers on conversation with peers.

Children who are hospitalized for 1 week or more may enjoy putting on a puppet show or playing school, store, or house. A corner of a playroom should be devoted to this kind of imaginative play: a structure that will serve as a store front, puppet stage, house, or school, and dolls, cribs, empty food boxes and cans, and puppets should be provided. Large blocks (6 × 12 inches) are available for playrooms so that such structures can be built and rebuilt each day. For ill children, the blocks are best if made of cardboard, not wood, because ill children tire easily when lifting heavier wood blocks. Table 35.8 lists games that require no equipment other than that readily available on a nursing unit for children who have brought nothing of their own to play with or who have grown bored with existing games.

Providing play equipment and supervision for a recreational play program in most instances is economically feasible through donations and volunteers. Generally toys for a playroom can be secured through donations from clubs in the community. For safety reasons, children need to be supervised while they play. Because they do not feel well in a hospital or are shy in these different surroundings, they usually enjoy having a concerned adult to watch over them and suggest new activities. Such adults may be volunteers. Supervision is an excellent after-school activity for members of a future nurses' club. Ideally, child life or play specialists supervise such play.

If play supervisors are unavailable through other sources, the nursing staff must free such personnel as necessary to lead play activities. This shows that play is important—for example, that supervising finger painting is as important a duty for assistive personnel as straightening beds, or that

organizing a puppet show for long-term clients is as important as giving a bed bath. A clear sign that the nurses on a particular children's unit understand little about their young patients' needs is a locked playroom door and the explanation, "We have no one to staff it."

Providing Play for Children on Bedrest

Children who are on bedrest, at home or in a hospital, need to have play periods built into their day. The length of time for play and the toys individual children can play with depend on their age and physical and emotional states. Suggestions for play activities for children on bedrest are shown in Table 35.9.

Infants need toys in their cribs, such as mobiles, blocks, soft toys, and rattles. They also need to be out of cribs, sitting on a parent's or a nurse's lap, or sitting in strollers or swings. As soon as they are able, they need some time on the floor (with a sheet under them) to practice crawling or walking. At about 3 months, when an infant discovers the hands, those become his or her "toys." For a child learning to crawl or "cruise" or walk, that activity is his or her toy or interest for the month.

Toddlers need put-in and take-out types of toys such as blocks that can be repeatedly dropped into a bottle or that can be stacked to play with in bed. They enjoy listening to tapes of songs and nursery rhymes. Toddlers are in constant motion. They need to be out of bed as much as their physical condition allows, playing with take-apart, put-together, or pull-and-push toys. Preschoolers need creative materials such as modeling clay or sand. School-age children need quiet games such as books or crayons or markers by their bedside. While in bed, they enjoy radios, compact disk players, or tapes. Most activities for hospitalized children must be short-term projects because children are called away for treatments or procedures, and because when they are ill their attention span is shorter than usual. Short-term projects always appeal to the school-age child because they help this age child achieve a sense of industry.

Watching TV is a nonparticipant activity, so it is not the best activity for children. There is some value in watching nature programs or "after-school specials" on television that depict school-age children in real-life situations coping with problems common to the child's age group. Encouraging parents or friends to watch a game show with a school-age child and help the child guess the solution to a puzzle or watch "Sesame Street" with a preschooler can make the activity a participatory one. Watching a soap opera with an adolescent and then discussing the people and their problems can also turn television watching into active participation.

Safety With Play

Be certain to screen all toys for safety. They should be washable to prevent spreading disease, with no sharp edges and no small parts that could be swallowed or aspirated. A cylinder 1 inch in diameter, such as a rubber hot dog, is the most dangerous size for a toy because it

TABLE 35.8

Games and Activities Using Materials Available on a Nursing Unit

Age	Activity
Infant	Make a mobile from roller gauze and tongue blades to hang over a crib.
	Ask the pharmacy or central supply for different-size boxes to use for put-in, take-out toys. (Do not use round vials from pharmacy; if accidentally aspirated, these can completely occlude the airway.)
	Blow up a glove as a balloon; draw a smiling face on it with a marker. Hang it out of infant's reach.
	Play "patty cake," "so big," "peek-a-boo."
Toddler	Ask central supply for boxes to use as blocks for stacking.
	Tie roller gauze to a glove box for a pull toy.
	Sing or recite familiar nursery rhymes such as "Peter, Peter, Pumpkin Eater."
Preschool	Play "Simon says" or "Mother, may I?"
	Draw a picture of a dog; ask child to close eyes; add an additional feature to the dog; ask child to guess the added part, repeat until a full picture is drawn.
	Make a puppet from a lunch bag or draw a face on your hand with a marker.
	Cut out a picture from a newspaper or a magazine (or draw a picture); cut it into large puzzle pieces.
	Pour breakfast cereal into a basin; furnish boxes to pour and spoons to dig.
	Furnish chart paper and a magic marker for coloring.
	Make modeling clay from 1 cup salt, ½ cup flour, ½ cup water from diet kitchen.
	Play "Ring-Around-the-Rosey" or "London Bridge."
School-age	Play "I Spy" or charades.
	Make a deck of cards to play "Go Fish" or "Old Maid"; invent cards such as Nicholas Nurse, Doctor Dolittle, Irene Intern, Polly Patient.
	Play "Hangman."
	Furnish scale or table paper and a marker for a huge drawing or sign.
	Hide an object in the child's room and have the child look for it (have the child name places for you to look if the child cannot be out of bed).
Adolescent	Color squares on a chart form to make a checker board.
	Have adolescent make a deck of cards to use for "Hearts" or "Rummy."
	Compete to see how many words the adolescent can make from the letters in his or her name.
	Compete to guess whether the next person to enter the room will be a man or woman, next car to go by window will be red or black, and so forth.
	Compete to see who can name the most episodes of "Star Trek" or "The Brady Bunch."

totally occludes the trachea if it is aspirated. A toy smaller than this would cause only partial obstruction; something larger could not be inhaled into the trachea. As a rule, if a toy can fit through the center of a toilet tissue tube, it is too small for safe play.

Be certain toys offered will not lead children into danger. Tossing a ball to a toddler on bedrest is generally a safe activity. One who has a large cast in place, however, might lean over to retrieve a dropped ball and fall out of bed. Chasing a ball could lead to collisions with door frames or oxygen equipment.

If children become bored with a toy because it is not stimulating enough or they have had it for too long a time,

they may begin to use the toy in an unsafe way. After a toddler grows tired of stacking blocks, for example, he or she may begin to throw them. Children who normally play safely with modeling clay but who are on a restricted diet may eat it because they are hungry. Knowing where children are and what activity they are engaged in at all times is the best prevention against unsafe play.

For the child cared for at home, parents may need to purchase new toys. This is especially true if the bulk of the toys they furnished previously were for outside play such as balls or Rollerblades or skateboards. Because of an illness, they may now need to provide more "sit-down" toys such as markers, puzzles, or board games.

TABLE 35.9

Play Activities for Children on Bedrest

Care Measure	Play Activities
Bathing	Allow child to play in bath water with water toys.
	Play a game such as "I Spy" while giving a bed bath.
Encouraging fluid	Hold a "tea party" for a preschooler and drink "tea" with important but imaginary guests.
	Play a board game with a school-age child in which each turn starts with taking a drink.
	Draw a circle and let child color in a section each time he or she drinks until the circle is full.
	Play "Simon Says," in which Simon says, "Drink."
Deep breathing exercises	Have child blow soap bubbles in a glass of soapy water with a straw.
	Have child blow a cotton ball across the surface of a bedside table.
	Play "Simon Says," in which Simon says, "Take a deep breath."
	Allow the child to score points for reaching a high number on an incentive spirometer.
Muscle-strengthening exercises	Have child throw bean bags or large wads of paper (computer waste) at a wastebasket.
	Play "Simon Says," in which Simon says, "Raise your arms," and so forth.
	Have child throw and catch a ball.
	Have child squeeze and mold modeling clay.
	Encourage child to kick balloon suspended near foot of bed.
	Help a preschooler pretend he or she is a butterfly, airplane, and so forth.
Procedure such as blood transfusion	Save a favorite game or activity only for these times.
Health teaching	Use puppets as teacher.
	Make up board games, word scrambles, and crossword puzzles.

Child Life Programs

Child life programs are incorporated into all major children's hospitals and are an integral feature of child health care (LeRoy et al., 2003). As part of a child life program, a child life specialist offers children the opportunity to reenact and thereby master the anxiety associated with illness. Through therapeutic play, child life specialists provide programs that prepare children for hospitalization and, once hospitalized, prepare children for surgery or for procedures that could be painful. They consult with parents about good toys to choose for home care. These specialists help children air their frustration about painful or intrusive procedures, prevent social isolation of children by means of an active recreation program, and ensure that the total health care environment is conducive to children's well-being.

Such a program not only aids in promoting children's mental health but also leads to more cooperative responses of children to treatments or procedures. It is complementary to play programs initiated by nurses.

 Checkpoint Question 4

You worry about Becky aspirating a toy you give her. Which of the following items is most apt to be aspirated?

a. Pages in a coloring book
b. Clothing from a baby doll
c. Pieces of colored chalk
d. Blocks 2 inches square

Therapeutic Play

Anything almost automatically becomes less threatening when a person can talk about it. Many children cannot talk about what is happening to them during illness, however, because of fear or because their vocabulary is so limited they cannot describe their feelings.

Because play is the language of children, children who have difficulty voicing their thoughts in words can often speak clearly through play. **Play therapy** is a psychoanalytic technique used by psychiatrists to help children understand their feelings and thoughts and motivations better. In play therapy, the therapist attempts to interpret the child's verbal and nonverbal cues. Interpreting nonverbal cues and helping the child understand them this way requires the skill of a psychiatric nurse-clinician or others with specialized training. **Therapeutic play** is a play technique that can be used by nurses to better understand children's feelings and thoughts (Mitchell, Johnston, & Keppell, 2004). For therapeutic play, only the child's verbal cues are used as responses. Box 35.10 highlights appropriate outcomes and interventions for therapeutic play using the terminology identified by the Nursing Outcomes Classification (NOC) and Nursing Interventions Classifications (NIC).

Therapeutic play can be divided into three types:

1. Energy release
2. Dramatic play
3. Creative play

Energy Release

Children release energy by pounding, hitting, running, punching, or shouting. Furnishing children with materials that allow them to do these things helps them release anxiety as well. Toddlers pound pegs with a plastic hammer or pretend to cut wood with a toy saw. Other examples include giving modeling clay to a preschooler (an anxious child often pounds it flat; a relaxed child, however, will build it into shapes) or tying a balloon to an overbed trapeze for a school-age child or adolescent to punch.

Dramatic Play

Dramatic play is acting out an anxiety-producing situation. It is most effective with preschool children because they are at the peak of imagination. During illness, the situations about which children need to express feelings are illness-related, and therefore the equipment needed for therapeutic play is common health care equipment: dolls, doll beds, play stethoscopes, intravenous equipment, syringes, masks, and gowns. Puppets of doctors, nurses, mothers, fathers, and children help young children express their feelings. Anatomically correct dolls are used to help children describe their feelings about sexual abuse.

It is good to have a play session with a child near the beginning of his or her illness to see whether the child communicates any fears about this experience through play. This initial session also serves as a way of preparing the child for events that will occur during the illness (Fig. 35.13). Repeat a play session after any painful or traumatic procedure such as surgery so that the child can express new feelings. A list of procedures that fall into this category is shown in Table 35.10. If such play sessions reveal fears, a child should be scheduled for other play sessions, perhaps one daily.

Furnish children with a wide range of equipment and then let them choose those items with which they wish to play. Children invariably choose a piece of equipment that has been used with them. They poke at a doll with a syringe or enjoy giving it a "shot." They wrap the doll in bandages or put tubes into its mouth or stomach, acting out things that were done to them or that they saw done to other children on a nursing unit or at a clinic visit they fear will be done to them. Allow play to be nondirective

---

BOX 35.10

Nursing Outcomes Classification (NOC) and Nursing Interventions Classification (NIC)

Play

NOC: Play Participation

Play participation is defined as the use of activities as needed for enjoyment, entertainment, and development by children (Johnson, Maas, & Moorhead, 2000). Some specific indicators suggesting achievement of this outcome include the following behaviors by the child:

- Participating in appropriate play
- Expressing emotions and enjoyment
- Using social and physical skills and imagination
- Using role playing

NIC: Therapeutic Play

Therapeutic play is defined as the purposeful and directive use of toys or other materials to assist children in communicating their perception and knowledge of their world and to help gain mastery of their environment (McCloskey & Bulechek, 2000). Some

important activities involved when implementing this intervention include:

- Providing a quiet, interruption-free environment for a sufficient amount of time
- Communicating the purpose of the play session to the child and parents
- Providing safe, developmentally appropriate, stimulating, creative play equipment, including real or simulated hospital or medical equipment
- Encouraging manipulation of equipment and sharing of feelings, knowledge, and perceptions
- Monitoring child's reactions and anxiety level throughout session
- Identifying misconceptions or fears through comments made
- Continuing play sessions on regular basis as appropriate

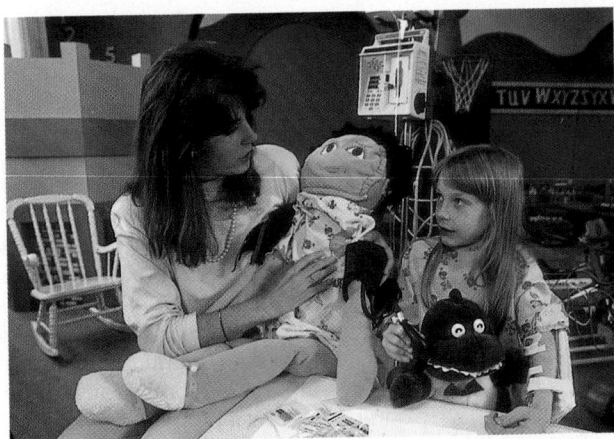

FIGURE 35.13 Therapeutic play allows children the opportunity to voice their fears of illness and procedures. (Daemmrich/Stock Boston.)

(let the child proceed at his or her own pace, choosing freely what equipment to play with and what he or she wants to do with the equipment). As a child works through an experience this way, the experience becomes less fearful and the child gains increased control over it.

Observe for children who may be using equipment in an unusual way, such as hitting dolls with stethoscopes or poking them in the eye with a thermometer (suggesting they are confused about the purpose of such equipment). Such behavior can alert you to the importance of explaining the purpose of equipment to children. Listen to what children say as they play. A comment such as, "I'm giving shots to all the bad dolls" suggests the child thinks injections are punishment. It would be important to stress the next time the child needs an injection that medicine is to make the child feel well again. A comment such as, "This doll is going to surgery, so you won't have her anymore" could suggest the child thinks she will not return from surgery (she may have heard a family member describe someone who died after surgery and is asking for reassurance that such a thing is not going to happen to her). Do not be surprised about the force with which children insert nasogastric tubes into dolls. In part, this reflects how they perceive these procedures, but it also represents energy or anxiety release, in the way that pounding or hitting releases anger.

To better understand how a child feels, repeat what the child says verbally: "You're giving the bad dolls shots?" or ask the child to tell you more about what he or she said: "Do you think that's the only kind of children who get

TABLE 35.10

Therapeutic Play Techniques for Children After Procedures

Procedure	Play Activity (Provide a doll and . . .)
Radiograph	Table and box labeled "x-ray machine"; children sometimes worry that x-rays have injured them, just as laser rays in science fiction shows do.
Blood drawing	Syringe, alcohol wipes, tourniquet, or finger lancets; remember that finger sticks are as frightening for children as are needles.
Clean-catch urine	Alcohol wipes and a collection cup; children are often more embarrassed by urine collection than adults realize.
Intravenous therapy	Intravenous tubing, as well as restraints and armboard; some children are as angry about being restrained as having the needle inserted.
Endoscopy such as bronchoscopy, cystoscopy	Catheters or a penlight to simulate a scope
Scans	Intravenous fluid and tubing, because scans usually require the intravenous injection of isotopes
Bone marrow	Alcohol wipes, syringe
EEG, EKG	Electrode leads that attach to a box; children might be afraid of these procedures because of their fear of electricity.
Surgery	An anesthesia mask and a blunt kitchen knife; watch and listen for where the child cuts and how he or she describes the experience.
Dental examination	Suction catheter, a penlight to simulate a drill, and a 4 × 4 piece of plastic to simulate a dental dam; some children are angered by the use of plastic in their mouth.
Dressing changes	Gauze and adhesive tape
Cast application or removal	Provide plaster to soak and apply; simulate a cast cutter with an electric razor or hair dryer.
Nasogastric tube insertion, enema, catheterization	Appropriate tubes
Temperature assessment	Thermometer

shots—bad children?" Don't rush to reassure ("Don't worry, that isn't going to happen to you"). Quick reassurance rather than being reassuring tells the child he or she should not ask any more questions or that the topic is not open for discussion.

Sometimes even children who seem well prepared may be taken by surprise during a procedure. For example, 7-year-old Tanya, seen in an ambulatory setting for a diagnostic workup after a urinary tract infection, showed little interest in dolls and syringes and tubing in the playroom. She had been prepared by her mother for the experience and seemed to understand what would happen during her x-ray procedure. After returning from the x-ray room, where she had a voiding cystourethrogram, however, she was obviously upset. Her nurse brought her a rag doll, a doctor and a nurse figure, a play x-ray machine, and some tubing that could simulate a urinary catheter and encouraged Tanya to play with them. Tanya picked up the girl doll and put her under the x-ray machine. She imitated the doctor doll shouting, "Pee in front of everybody!" Tanya's mother had not realized that she would have to void during a cystourethrogram and so had not prepared her for that. Tanya felt betrayed by not being really prepared for this embarrassing situation. Her play brought her emotion out in the open, where it could be talked about and handled. When Tanya was scheduled the next day for ureteral reflux surgery, her nurse was alerted to make the preparation absolutely thorough.

Children older than 9 or 10 years find playing with dolls too childish to be of benefit. They enjoy handling syringes, however, and being able to see and handle such equipment as nasogastric tubes in advance of their being placed. Active handling helps to eliminate fear because it identifies exactly what the child has to face; it meets their concrete-level learning needs.

Creative Play

Some children are too angry to be able to act out their feelings through dramatic play. However, they may be able to draw a picture that expresses their emotions or conveys the extent of their knowledge. To encourage this, give a child a blank paper and crayons or markers. If a child seems reluctant to draw something spontaneously, suggest a topic: "Why don't you draw a picture of yourself?"

Some children are so concerned with particular parts of their bodies that when asked to draw pictures of themselves, they draw only the body part about which they are worried. Such a child generally is saying he or she needs to talk about that part of the body, to be given reassurance that it is going to be all right. Figure 35.14A shows a picture drawn by Becky when she was admitted to the hospital for 1-day surgery for debridement of a campfire burn on her left foot. She stated on admission she was being admitted to have the burn on her foot "cleaned out." This sounds like a child who understands what debridement involves. Note, however, that the figure she drew has no left leg. One has to wonder whether she was concerned she was going to surgery to have more than debridement. After the word "debridement" was explained to her, she drew the picture in Figure 35.14B. The child in the drawing now has a left and a right leg, the left leg covered by

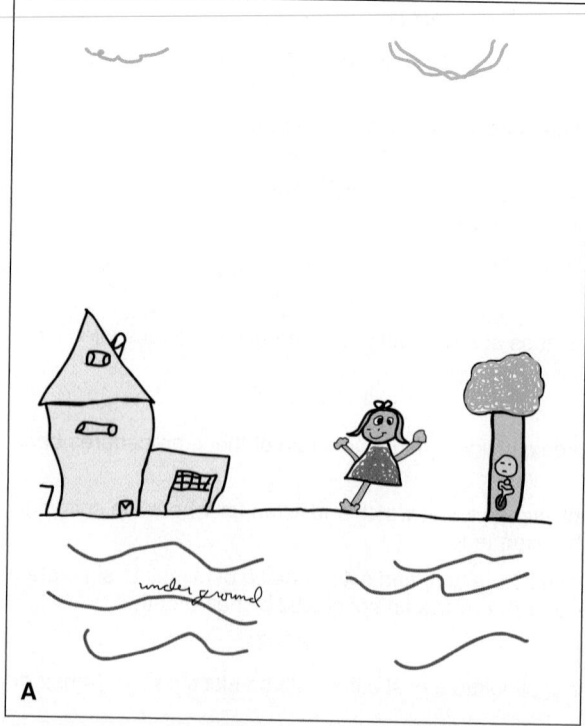

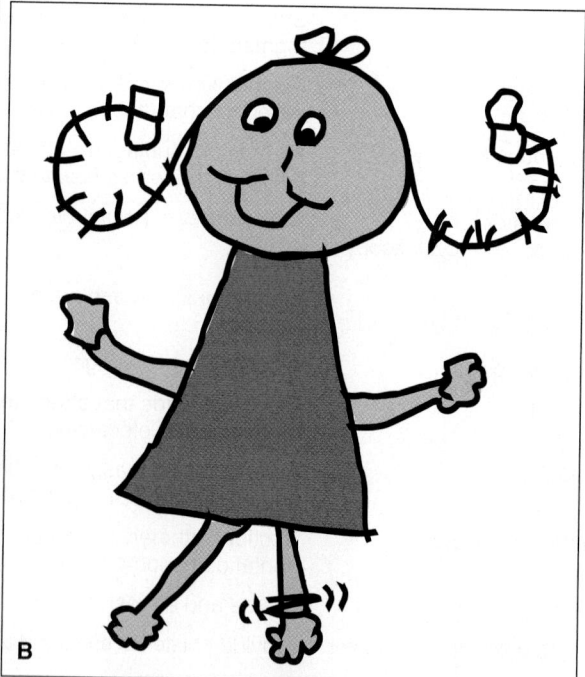

FIGURE 35.14 (A) Children who are concerned about body parts may draw pictures with that part missing or exaggerated. Note the missing left leg here. **(B)** After reassurance that her leg will be all right, the girl who did the drawing in *A* now draws a girl with two legs.

a bandage. Through a drawing, this child was able to say something she could not express without this help.

Many ill children draw pictures that reflect punitive images: a boy or girl tied to a bed or shut behind bars, or doctors and nurses frowning at them, obviously unhappy with them. Such children may need assurance that they are not being punished; they need to stay in bed or are being cared for by doctors and nurses to be made well (Fig. 35.15). Other children draw pictures that are symbolic of death: airplanes crashing, boats sinking, buildings on fire, children in graveyards. They need assurance that they will not die.

Other concerns such as fear of abandonment and loss of independence may also be manifested in drawings. For example, preschoolers may draw a child in one corner of a picture and an adult in a far corner. They may comment that the parent cannot find the child because she's gone to the hospital. They need to be reassured their parents know where they will be and will visit them each day after work.

Older school-age children and adolescents may not be interested in drawing but can be interested in making a list of procedures or experiences they like and dislike. Examine the dislike list for procedures such as "shots" or "chemo." Mark the nursing care plan for nurses to take special time to explain these procedures and to offer special support when they must be done.

What if... while you're playing with her, Becky draws a purple person with only three body parts? Would this worry you? Why or why not?

Guidelines for Conducting Therapeutic Play

Use common sense when conducting therapeutic play. Be certain not to interpret a child's black and gloomy

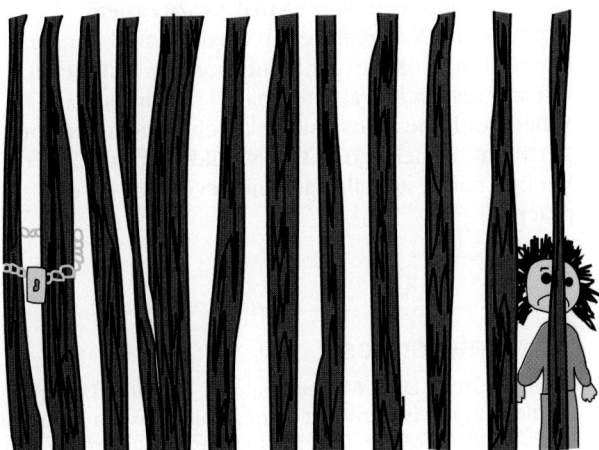

FIGURE 35.15 A picture drawn by a hospitalized child. Note the prison-like appearance of the crib. (Courtesy of Rita Crever.)

drawing as meaning the child is depressed; a black marker may have been the only one available. Many children 4 to 5 years of age draw a person lacking many body parts because that is the best human form they can draw.

Remember, too, that all children occasionally treat dolls badly. A 2-year-old pounding and banging a rag doll may not be expressing anger toward the doll image at all, but may be intent on discovering the feel of a new texture and is unaware for the moment that the object is a doll.

A conference with health care team members, including a psychologist or a psychiatric nurse specialist, may be called for if a child continues to express mutilating behavior after normal reassurance. Guidelines for conducting therapeutic play are summarized in Box 35.11.

BOX 35.11

Guidelines for Therapeutic Play

1. Allow a child to choose the articles with which he or she wants to play (something may be too frightening for a child to play with immediately; he or she needs time to work up to the activity).
2. Provide the materials specific to the child's experiences of which you, the nurse, are aware (e.g., nasogastric tube, syringe, or bandages), but do not supply only those things; a child may have misunderstandings and fears of situations you cannot know about.
3. Allow play to be unstructured; let the child use the materials however he or she wishes. If a child seems uninterested in materials, initiate play with him or her (e.g., give a doll an injection) to see if this reduces his or her anxiety enough to be able to handle items.
4. If a child cannot manipulate materials himself or herself (due to such things as a cast or traction), ask the child what he or she would like you to do with it.
5. Reflect only what the child expresses (verbal expression).
6. Do not criticize play; this inhibits further expression.
7. Use a therapeutic response—not "Don't worry, that won't happen," but "Are you worried that could happen?"
8. Ask children to describe paintings, not "That's a good picture of yourself," but "Tell me about your picture."
9. Do not be reluctant to use real equipment (e.g., real catheters and blood lancets). Handling real equipment best helps to reduce stress.
10. Supervise therapeutic play, because some equipment could cause an accident (and therapeutically responding to the child's comments is necessary).

Checkpoint Question 5

Becky will have a large bandage on her foot after surgery. Which type of therapeutic play would be best for her?

a. Letting her hold and handle a medicine syringe
b. Giving her a doll and a bandage to change
c. Helping her insert an NG tube into a puppet
d. Teaching her a rhyme about good girls

such as a smoke detector, a safe area for oxygen storage, and a safe refrigerator for food or medicine are present.

Home care can be exhausting for parents. Be certain they devise a schedule of care that allows them enough rest. Advocate for medicine or treatment schedules that allow for administering medications during the day rather than a schedule that requires medication administration at night.

Parents may need respite care to continue to be effective care providers, just as professionals need time off. Help parents to take turns giving care so that each has some free time during the week.

Key Points

Illness may be more traumatic for children than for adults because of children's inability to communicate and monitor their own care and because they have different nutrition, fluid, and electrolyte needs. The stress of hospitalization can be so acute that it can result in posttraumatic stress syndrome.

Separation from parents because of hospitalization can have permanent psychological effects on children. Methods to reduce this include keeping hospital stays as brief as possible, promoting open parent and sibling visiting, and providing primary or case management nursing.

Currently, many medical procedures can be done on an ambulatory basis. Advocating for care to be done in such settings is a nursing responsibility.

The presence of parents during health care can help reduce trauma to children. Making parents as welcome as possible makes it possible for them to room-in. Include parents in both the planning and the implementation of care. Parents reinfect children with fear if their own fear is not reduced.

Preschoolers may have the most difficult time during hospitalization because they have so many fears. Preparation and promotion of therapeutic play are essential to reduce trauma to a tolerable level.

Because hospitalizations currently are so brief, parents need good discharge instructions to continue to care for children safely at home. Providing clear instructions and danger signs for parents to watch for is a nursing responsibility.

Home care is increasing as a way of providing care to chronically ill children. It has the advantages of being cost-effective and providing meaningful comfort and support to a child. Disadvantages are that parents can become fatigued, the loss of a job for the primary caregiver can cause financial hardship, and social isolation and disruption of normal home life may occur.

Not all homes are ideal for home care. Assess that a primary care provider is present; the family is knowledgeable about the care necessary; necessary resources are available; and safety features

Critical Thinking Questions

1. Becky is the 7-year-old you met at the beginning of the chapter. Her foot was burned in a campfire accident. Since then she has refused to eat anything but Jell-O or soup. In the hospital playroom, she picked up a doll and tore off its leg. Her mother asked you why her daughter is acting this way. What suggestions would you make to her? The burn occurred because Becky was left momentarily unsupervised by a campfire. Is there a possibility her mother may not be acting her usual self because of guilt over the injury?

2. Suppose Becky's parents are called out of town on a family emergency, so Becky has no family with her for a week. What measures would you take to help make hospitalization and separation less traumatic for her?

3. Becky will be cared for at home after her surgery. Her mother is concerned that because Becky's home stay will be lengthy, she will be cut off from her friends for a long time. What suggestions could you make to help Becky maintain contact with her friends? Her mother is concerned she will become exhausted because of the need for round-the-clock care. What suggestions could you offer to make care easier?

4. Examine the National Health Goals related to care of ill children. Most government-sponsored money for nursing research is allotted based on these goals. What would be a possible research topic to explore pertinent to these goals that would be applicable to Becky's family and also advance evidence-based practice?

References

Ball, S. D., Kertesz, D., & Moyer-Mileur, L. J. (2005). Dietary supplement use is prevalent among children with a chronic illness. *Journal of the American Dietetic Association, 105*(1), 78–84.

Barber-Parker, E. D. (2004). Family matters. How to prepare families for discharge in the limited time available. *Pediatric Nursing, 30*(3), 212–214.

Board, R., & Ryan-Wenger, N. (2003). Stressors and stress symptoms of mothers with children in the PICU. *Journal of Pediatric Nursing: Nursing Care of Children and Families, 18*(3), 195-202.

Bonuck, K. A. (2005). Sleep-disordered breathing and failure to thrive: Research vs. practice. *Archives of Pediatric and Adolescent Medicine, 159*(3), 299-300.

Bowlby, J., et al. (1966). *Maternal care and mental health.* New York: Schocken Books.

Cohen, J. A. (2005). Posttraumatic stress disorder in children and adolescents. In: B. J. Sadock & V. A. Sadock (Eds.), *Kaplan and Sadock's comprehensive textbook of psychiatry* (8th ed.). Philadelphia: Lippincott Williams & Wilkins.

DiMaggio, D. M., Sharif, I., & Hoffman-Rosenfeld, J. (2003). TV guides: Exposure of hospitalized children to inappropriate programming. *Ambulatory Pediatrics, 3*(2), 98-101.

Department of Health and Human Services (2000). *Healthy people 2010.* Washington, DC: DHHS.

Griffin, T. (2003). Family matters. Facing challenges to family-centered care, I: Conflicts over visitation. *Pediatric Nursing, 29*(2), 135-137.

Hallstrom, I., & Elander, G. (2004). Decision-making during hospitalization: Parents' and children's involvement. *Journal of Clinical Nursing, 13*(3), 367-375.

Johnson, M., Maas, M., & Moorhead, S. (2000). *Nursing outcomes classification* (2nd ed.). St. Louis: Mosby, Inc.

LeRoy, S., et al. (2003). Recommendations for preparing children and adolescents for invasive cardiac procedures. *Circulation, 108*(20), 2550-2564.

McCloskey, J., & Bulechek, G. (2000). *Nursing interventions classification* (3rd ed.). St. Louis: Mosby, Inc.

Mitchell, M., Johnston, L., & Keppell, M. (2004). Preparing children and their families for hospitalisation: A review of the literature. *Neonatal, Paediatric & Child Health Nursing, 7*(2), 5-15.

Pine, D. S. & McClure, E. B. (2005). Anxiety disorders: Clinical features. In B. J. Sadock & V. A. Sadock (Eds.), *Kaplan & Sadock's comprehensive textbook of psychiatry.* Philadelphia: Lippincott Williams & Wilkins.

Regalado, M., et al. (2004). Parents' discipline of younger children: Results from the National Survey of Early Childhood Health. *Pediatrics, 113*(6 Suppl.), 1952-1958.

Robertson, J. (1958). *Young children in hospitals.* London: Tavistock.

Spitz, R. A. (1945). Hospitalism: An inquiry into the genesis of psychiatric conditions in early childhood. *Psychoanalytic Study of the Child, 1*(3), 53-59.

Williams, R., et al. (2004). A comparison of calorie and protein intake in hospitalized pediatric oncology patients dining with a caregiver versus patients dining alone. *Journal of Pediatric Oncology Nursing, 21*(4), 223-232.

Suggested Readings

Banks, J. B. (2002). Childhood discipline: Challenges for clinicians and parents. *American Family Physician, 66*(8), 1447-1452.

Battrick, C., & Glasper, E. A. (2004). Children's nursing. The views of children and their families on being in hospital. *British Journal of Nursing, 13*(6), 328-336.

Board, R. (2004). Father stress during a child's critical care hospitalization. *Journal of Pediatric Health Care, 18*(5), 244-249.

Boyd, S. (2004). Within these walls: Moderating parental stress in the NICU. *Journal of Neonatal Nursing, 10*(3), 80-84.

Darbyshire, P. (2003). Mothers' experiences of their child's recovery in hospital and at home: A qualitative investigation. *Journal of Child Health Care, 7*(4), 291-312.

Hopia, H., et al. (2005). Child in hospital: Family experiences and expectations of how nurses can promote family health. *Journal of Clinical Nursing, 14*(2), 212-222.

McKlindon, D. D., & Schlucter, J. (2004). Family matters. Parent and nurse partnership model for teaching therapeutic relationships. *Pediatric Nursing, 30*(5), 418-420.

Santacroce, S. J. (2003). Parental uncertainty and posttraumatic stress in serious childhood illness. *Journal of Nursing Scholarship, 35*(1), 45-51.

Shields, L., & Nixon, J. (2004). Hospital care of children in four countries. *Journal of Advanced Nursing, 45*(5), 475-486.

Stratton, K. M. (2004). Parents' experiences of their child's care during hospitalization. *Journal of Cultural Diversity, 11*(1), 4-11.

Tennyson, D. H. (2003). Hospital-affiliated pediatric urgent care clinics: A necessary extension for emergency departments? *Health Care Manager, 22*(3), 190-202.

Nursing Care of a Child Undergoing Diagnostic Techniques and Other Therapeutic Modalities

Key Terms

aspiration studies
barium contrast studies
bronchoscopy
clean-catch urine specimen
colonoscopy
computed tomography (CT)
electrical impulse studies
endoscopy
gavage feedings
magnetic resonance imaging (MRI)
positron emission tomography (PET)
radiopharmaceuticals
single photon emission computed tomography (SPECT)
total parenteral nutrition (TPN)
ultrasound

Objectives

After mastering the contents of this chapter, you should be able to:

1. Describe common nursing interventions used in the health care of children to aid diagnosis and therapy.
2. Assess children as to developmental stage and knowledge level before beginning diagnostic or therapeutic procedures.
3. Formulate nursing diagnoses related to common diagnostic or therapeutic procedures used with children.
4. Identify expected outcomes for a child undergoing a diagnostic or therapeutic procedure.
5. Plan nursing interventions to aid in diagnosis or therapy for children.
6. Implement nursing interventions relevant to diagnostic or therapeutic procedures.
7. Evaluate expected outcomes related to diagnostic and therapeutic procedures to see if goals were achieved.
8. Identify National Health Goals related to diagnostic and therapeutic procedures for children that nurses could help the nation achieve.
9. Identify areas related to nursing procedures with children that could benefit from additional nursing research or application of evidence-based practice.
10. Use critical thinking to analyze ways diagnostic and therapeutic procedures can be modified to be more family-centered.
11. Integrate knowledge of common diagnostic and therapeutic procedures with nursing process to achieve quality maternal and child health nursing.

T. J. Balliff is a preschooler who is scheduled to have a magnetic resonance imaging (MRI) study for a possible head injury. "How can I agree to this?" his mother asks you. "He's afraid of the dark. How can I allow him to be wheeled into a long dark machine that way?"

Previous chapters described the growth and development of well children. This chapter adds information about how to care for children who are having procedures done for therapy or to gather and document information. This is important information because it builds a base for both care and health teaching.

How would you explain MRI to T.J. to make the procedure more acceptable to him?

After you've studied this chapter, access the accompanying website. Read the patient scenario and answer the questions to further sharpen your skills, grow more familiar with RN-CLEX types of questions, and reward yourself with how much you have learned.

Illness can be particularly stressful if many diagnostic and therapeutic procedures are necessary for care. In today's health care climate, there is less time for teaching and preparation than once available, so good planning and follow-through become essential. Chapter 35 described measures to make an illness experience a more positive one. Health teaching, discussed in Chapter 34, is also a cornerstone in this process. As everything that nurses do with and for ill children can have a major influence on a child's progress toward health as well as on the child's and family's perception of professional health care and the ability to carry out healthful practices in the future, even more interventions are needed.

Many nursing actions offer an opportunity to accomplish several goals. Supporting a child and family during a diagnostic procedure, for instance, not only can aid in efficient diagnosis but also may help establish a trusting relationship between the family and health care providers that will make all future interactions more successful. This chapter describes the most common diagnostic and therapeutic techniques used in the care of ill children, including modifications needed to make these procedures safe and reduce associated stress, depending on the child's age and outlook. National Health Goals that address this area of child health practice are shown in Box 36.1.

BOX 36.1 FOCUS ON . . .

NATIONAL HEALTH GOALS

A key component of minimizing the stress of hospitalization and procedures for children, and thereby maximizing safety, is to limit the length of time children spend in the hospital. A number of National Health Goals address reducing the length of time that children spend in hospitals. One example is:

- Reduce hospitalization rates for children with pediatric asthma to 17 per 10,000, from a baseline of 23 per 10,000.

A major role of health care providers is to keep children free from disease so that they undergo a minimal number of procedures. A National Health Goal also addresses this:

- Increase the proportion of persons appropriately counseled about health behaviors (DHHS, 2000).

Nurses can help the nation achieve these goals by providing health counseling to aid in preventing children from becoming ill and subsequently requiring hospitalization.

Areas related to these goals that could benefit from additional nursing research and application of evidence-based practice include determining what teaching techniques are most effective in keeping children well; what methods are efficient at ensuring that children's hospitalizations are as short as possible; and what techniques or supplies are most satisfactory to children when procedures are performed.

Nursing Process Overview

For a Child Undergoing Diagnostic or Therapeutic Procedures

● *Assessment*

Before performing procedures such as assisting with a diagnostic test or collecting laboratory specimens, first carefully evaluate a child's age and developmental stage, as well as any special needs the child may have. Even the most common and painless procedures produce a certain amount of stress for the child and parents. During complex diagnostic procedures, this stress level is almost certain to increase even further. Unfamiliar doctors and nurses, high-tech supplies and equipment, and strange surroundings all add up to a frightening experience for most adults; imagine how frightening they can seem to children.

Assess a child's level of anxiety associated with unfamiliar equipment, circumstances, and surroundings as well as the child's knowledge concerning a technique before initiating a procedure or beginning health teaching. It may be possible to increase cooperation by acknowledging and respecting the child's past experience with similar procedures.

● *Nursing Diagnosis*

Common nursing diagnoses related to diagnostic and therapeutic procedures are as varied as the procedures themselves. Some examples are:

- Fear related to new and strange surroundings of the procedure room
- Pain related to lumbar puncture
- Deficient knowledge related to technique for 24-hour urine collection
- Deficient diversionary activity related to lack of appropriate toys and lengthy procedure
- Imbalanced nutrition, less than body requirements, related to lack of familiar foods
- Risk for injury related to a biopsy procedure

● *Outcome Identification and Planning*

Illness in itself creates anxiety in a child; unless a child is helped to feel comfortable and safe, every procedure can result in even more stress. An important nursing goal is to cause the least degree of anxiety possible while completing interventions. To achieve this goal, plan specific ways to prepare children in advance, such as the best way to explain a procedure to a particular child and also how to ensure a child is not overwhelmed by the number of diagnostic or therapeutic procedures performed in any one day. With small children, it may make more sense to stagger ambulatory diagnostic tests over a number of days to preserve a child's coping ability. Conversely, some older children (and parents) do better if they can complete all necessary tests in 1 day, so they do not have to anticipate more testing over a long period. Use nursing judgment and data from periodic assessments to help primary care providers determine the type of schedule that is in the child's and family's best interest.

● *Implementation*

Whether assisting with a procedure or performing a therapeutic intervention, it is necessary to function in several roles at the same time: performing (or assisting with) the procedure, providing active support to the child and parents, and observing and then documenting the child's reactions. Providing support is a major role, and there are many ways to do this, such as holding a child's hand or placing a hand on the parent's shoulder. Playing a distracting game with an older child can also be helpful. Important observations to be made include signs of discomfort, changes in vital signs, or other signals of distress such as pallor or dizziness. Maintain a flowsheet of observations during a procedure. After a procedure, the procedure, the child's reaction, and specimens obtained can then be documented accurately and efficiently in the child's record.

As a final follow-through step, think of therapeutic play techniques to introduce that would be helpful in relieving stress caused by the procedure.

● *Outcome Evaluation*

Evaluating expected outcomes related to diagnostic and therapeutic procedures not only helps in determining the effect of the procedure on a child but also aids in future planning, should other procedures be required. Recording that a particular child who did not appear nervous during a procedure later admitted to being "more scared than I've ever been before," for example, can help another nurse provide reassurance to this child, even when the child is masking his emotions the next time. Examples suggesting achievement of expected outcomes are:

- Child says she is able to cope with further bone marrow aspiration.
- Child lists steps to take to collect 24-hour urine at home.
- Child participates in 1 hour of active play daily.
- Child eats a minimum of 1,000 calories per day.
- Child experiences minimal loss of blood (less than 10 mL) during diagnostic procedure.
- Parent outlines plan to use alternative therapies to reduce the child's anxiety.

NURSING RESPONSIBILITIES WITH DIAGNOSTIC AND THERAPEUTIC TECHNIQUES

The most efficient way to reduce children's stress from hospitalization is to reduce the number of hospitalizations necessary (Flores, 2005). When hospitalization becomes necessary, the responsibilities of a nurse when assisting with procedures performed on children include:

- Helping obtain informed consent as needed
- Explaining the procedure to the child and his or her parents to be certain they are well informed
- Scheduling the procedure
- Preparing the child physically and psychologically

- Obtaining equipment for the procedure
- Accompanying a child to a treatment room or hospital department where the procedure will be performed
- Providing support during the procedure
- Ensuring adherence to standard precautions
- Assessing a child's response to the procedure
- Providing care to a child and specimens obtained once the procedure is completed
- Overseeing or cooperating with other health care disciplines to ensure the safety and efficacy of all procedures

Obtaining Informed Consent

Consent to perform a procedure must be obtained if a procedure carries any risk that would not be present if it were not performed. For a parent to sign a consent form, he or she must be knowledgeable about the content of the procedure and the risks of having or not having it performed. Although obtaining consent is the physician's responsibility, seeing that it is obtained is a nursing responsibility. Acting as an advocate for a family if they do not understand the consent form, the procedure, or the risks of the procedure is an important nursing role. Be certain the rights of emancipated minors are respected and that in single-parent families, the custodial parent is the one who has given the permission.

Explaining Procedures

To be able to explain procedures clearly and answer questions about them appropriately, try to observe as many procedures as possible. Asking a child after any procedure what sensations he or she experienced can help a child work through a possibly frightening situation (often called "debriefing") and can also increase your knowledge of common procedures.

As a general guide, a child needs a detailed description of the procedure, such as, "I'll clean your finger. You will feel a small pinprick," and an explanation of the following:

- Why the procedure is being performed—for example, "The doctor needs to look at your blood to see why you're so sick."
- Where the procedure will be done—for instance, the x-ray department or a treatment room
- Any unusual sensations to be expected during the procedure, such as, "Alcohol for cleaning your skin will feel cold."
- Any pain involved: "The needle will sting, although I'll put some cream on first to dull the feeling."
- Any strange equipment used, such as an x-ray machine
- The approximate length of time the procedure will take
- Any special care after the procedure—for example, "You will need to lie quietly for 15 minutes afterward."

Be certain to use age-appropriate language when explaining procedures. Be careful not to use words that might be confusing during an explanation, such as "transducer" or "electrode," without defining them. Try to associate the procedure with something with which the child is already familiar and comfortable (e.g., an x-ray machine is "a big camera"). Try not to use the word "test" in explanations because school-age children associate the word "test" with a pass/fail situation. This can make them unduly worried after a procedure about whether they have "passed" it.

If you are unfamiliar with what a procedure entails, do not guess. Nothing is more confusing to a child or parents than being told two different versions of something. Most technical personnel will take the time to describe important information a child should know about a study or procedure to you so you can relay this to the child, because having a well-informed patient makes their job easier. Be certain parents receive an explanation of the procedure as well as the child. A child has difficulty relaxing if parents are still anxious because they do not understand what is going to happen. Encourage parents to stay with a child during most procedures, because they can be extremely helpful in reducing a procedure's threatening aspects.

Scheduling

Most diagnostic procedures are scheduled on an ambulatory basis. Try to arrange for the child to have time for meals and some free play time between procedures. If food or fluid must be restricted for procedures, monitor the child's degree of discomfort and physiologic needs related to this; advocate as necessary for a time lapse between examinations or improved coordination in scheduling to decrease the time spent without food or fluid.

Preparing the Child and Family Physically and Psychologically

Physical preparation varies depending on what procedure is to be performed. In many instances, preparing a child for an examination (e.g., barium enema) involves another procedure (a saline enema), so physical preparation becomes education for the real examination. In all instances, explain both the preparative and actual procedures. Appropriate explanations aid in reducing anxiety and fear.

For many procedures, especially those that may be painful, such as a bronchoscopy, conscious sedation may be used (Ernst, Silvestri, & Johnstone, 2003). Conscious sedation refers to a depressed level of consciousness induced by the intravenous administration of a sedative such as midazolam in combination with a narcotic such as morphine sulfate and perhaps a hypnotic such as propofol. About 60 minutes before the procedure, children may be given oral chloral hydrate both to relieve apprehension and make them feel sleepy.

While under conscious sedation, children are able to maintain their ability to breathe independently and also respond appropriately to verbal commands such as to lift their head. They feel no pain, however, because of the analgesic administered. Conscious sedation is used in both ambulatory and inpatient settings. Before conscious sedation is begun, emergency equipment, including respiratory and pharmacologic measures, must be readily available. The child's level of consciousness and ability to respond, heart rate, respiratory rate, blood pressure, and oxygen saturation are monitored during the procedure. Using conscious sedation is very effective to allow children to accept a potentially painful procedure emotionally and physically. Be certain a child is prepared both for

the diagnostic procedure and the use of conscious sedation (Burton & Germann, 2004).

Accompanying the Child

If a procedure will be done at a different site from the primary care clinic or hospital unit with which a child is comfortable, ideally a nurse who the child knows should accompany the child to the other department and remain with the child for the procedure, or at least until the child has met a primary person who will be with him or her during the assessment. Having a parent accompany a child is of additional invaluable help. Older children do well without being accompanied as long as they have been introduced in advance to the new person who will give them care.

Before leaving a patient unit or clinic, have the child void for comfort unless this is contraindicated. Check for any medication or specific assessment procedures such as a blood pressure recording that should be given or done before leaving the unit for another department, in case the child is away from the primary unit for an extended time. If a child is an inpatient, check also that the identification band is securely in place and readily visible despite any intravenous equipment. If there will be a considerable wait in another department, ask the child if he or she would like to bring along an activity such as a game or book. Hallways can be cool. Provide adequate blankets for comfort, especially for infants. Always use cart straps and side rails for safety.

Providing Support

Children do well with diagnostic and evaluative procedures as long as they have adequate support from a concerned provider or parent. Provide this both verbally (explain what is going to happen; assure a child he or she is sitting still effectively) and nonverbally (a hand on the arm or a nearby presence).

Modifying Procedures According to the Child's Age and Developmental Stage

A child's age and potential understanding of procedures must be considered when planning the number and order of tests and the way they are performed.

The Infant

The number of painful or uncomfortable procedures done on infants should be kept to a minimum to avoid interfering with an infant's developing sense of trust. Parents should be allowed to accompany their infant to hospital departments and remain during procedures to offer support. Some parents may ask to hold their child during a procedure that causes pain, but do not ask parents to restrain the child during such a procedure. Their role should be a supportive and comforting one, not a policing one.

Infants need to be picked up and comforted after procedures (a child of any age likes a hug or honest compliment for cooperation). Obtaining blood specimens (which can deplete an infant's small blood stores) and x-rays (which are possibly harmful to immature bone marrow) should be kept to a minimum in infants. Help parents understand why these procedures are being limited so they do not think their infant's care is being compromised by so few diagnostic procedures.

The Toddler and Preschooler

Toddlers and preschoolers resist any diagnostic testing that involves any degree of discomfort or pain or that is unfamiliar to them. Give children of this age short explanations of what to expect, close to the time of the procedure so that little time can be spent worrying over it.

The School-Age Child and Adolescent

School-age children are interested in the theory and reason for procedures. Often they can be persuaded to cooperate for a procedure by being promised a look at their x-ray or a point-of-care meter readout afterward. Be careful to ensure that viewing the results is actually possible before promising this to children; otherwise, it can be difficult to obtain any further cooperation. Adolescents may project an air of maturity or sophistication beyond their years in order to remain in control of themselves in the face of frightening procedures. Do not be misled into thinking a child this age would not appreciate an explanation or a comforting hand on a shoulder during a procedure.

What if... T. J.'s hospital roommate, a 14-year-old adolescent who was scheduled for a series of diagnostic tests, says, "I'm not a kid, you know," and refuses to listen when you start to explain a procedure? Later, he acts angry because he has been "tricked" into having the procedure. How could you give explanations to him without offending him? What do you think is the basis for his actions?

Promoting Safety During Procedures

Safety is an important component of all patient care. Children's immaturity, which makes them unable to form mature judgments, leaves them vulnerable to harm unless their caretakers give special consideration to promoting safety.

NURSING DIAGNOSES AND RELATED INTERVENTIONS

Nursing Diagnosis: Risk for injury related to diagnostic procedures

Outcome Evaluation: Child remains free of injury from diagnostic equipment.

As a basic safety measure, before giving any food or performing any procedure, read the name on the child's identification armband. If an armband must be removed because it interferes with an intravenous infusion site, cut it away but immediately anchor it to another extremity with adhesive tape. Ask the admissions department to provide a new armband as soon as possible. Do not leave the old one off while waiting for a replacement band; this leaves the child susceptible to the danger of mistaken identity during the waiting period.

Because of their natural curiosity, children tend to fuss with equipment to see what will happen if they turn a knob or spin a dial. This means they need close monitoring while procedures are performed to ensure they do not touch any buttons or in other ways accidentally harm themselves. After a procedure, be sure to remove all equipment from a room. Children may pick up scissors or forceps left at bedsides and incur eye injuries; syringes and needles can cause puncture injuries. They may drink antiseptics such as alcohol or povidone–iodine left at bedsides and poison themselves. Young children can choke on small objects such as needle covers.

Use of Restraints

The purpose of a restraint is to keep a child safe during a procedure. Restraints must always be used with care, because if improperly applied or used, they can cause more harm than help (Tomlinson, 2004). Children can have difficulty distinguishing between restraint and punishment, so restraint should never be used more often or for any longer a time than necessary. Be certain parents receive an explanation of why their child has a restraint in place—for example, because of a particular danger of this procedure, it is safer for their child.

Check restraints every 15 minutes to see they are not occluding circulation; remove them every hour so the body part can be exercised (provided the exercise does not dislodge a device or interfere with a treatment). No part of a child's body other than that which is necessary should be restrained. When a child has a scalp vein infusion in place, such as for injection of a radioactive isotope for a nuclear medicine scan, for example, the child's arms may need to be immobilized so that he or she does not touch the infusion. The child's trunk may be immobilized so the child does not turn. The child's lower extremities may not have to be restrained, however, so he or she can still actively kick and exercise them. When a nurse or a parent is with the child, in most instances, all restraints can be removed.

Several types of restraints may be used to secure a child during a procedure or to prevent a child from touching equipment. The various types of restraints are shown in Table 36.1 and Figure 36.1.

Providing Care After Procedures

After a procedure, assess how well a child reacted to the procedure by both observation and history. Allowing children to explain what happened helps them retrace the pro-

TABLE 36.1

Safety Restraints

Type of Restraint	Purpose	Method
Wheelchairs and carts	Promote safety while transporting children to and from a procedure. Remind children to stay in a wheelchair while being transported. Prevent children from rolling off a cart while being transported.	For a wheelchair, use a vest restraint. Attach straps to the frame of the wheelchair with enough slack so the child has some mobility. For a cart, fasten a restraining belt and raise the side rails. Even with restraints in place, never leave a child unattended in hallways outside departments in a wheelchair or on a cart. Not only is this unsafe because the child may attempt to get down from the cart or wheelchair, but the anxiety of waiting in a strange department for a procedure is too acute for him or her to handle.
Clove-hitch restraints	Secure one arm or leg for a procedure, such as an intravenous infusion (see Chap. 37).	Use disposable restraints, gauze, or soft muslin tape. Soft muslin tape "gives" a little if the child exerts pressure against it so it will not pull too tight and reduce circulation or cause pain. Tie the restraint as shown in Figure 36-1A. If a child struggles against restraints, fold several layers of soft gauze around the wrist or ankle under the restraint. Secure the restraint to the underpart of the bed. Never tie restraints to side rails: when a side rail is lowered, it will jerk the child's arm or leg and possibly cause an injury. Release arm and leg restraints whenever someone can be with the child to keep the limb in the desired position.
Jacket restraints	Restrain children younger than 6 months in a supine position. (This method is not effective with older children because they are too active: they maneuver so much that they may squirm out of the jacket or put so much pressure on the trachea that they suffocate.)	Fasten the ties at the back of the jacket. Tie strips attached to the sides of the jacket under the mattress to keep the child in one position (see Fig. 36-1B).
Elbow restraints	Prevent children from touching the head or face—for example, during scalp vein infusion or after cleft lip or cleft palate repair.	Use a double-layered piece of soft muslin, which has pockets wide enough to fit tongue depressors. Place pockets vertically. Wrap the restraint around the child's arm. Secure the restraint with ties, tape, or pins (see Fig. 36-1C). It may be necessary to pin the restraint to the child's undershirt to prevent slippage. If No-No sleeves, a commercial elbow restraint, are used, slip the No-No sleeve up over the infant's arm and secure it by the Velcro strips (see Fig. 36-1D). The baby should wear a long-sleeved infant shirt under the sleeve to prevent irritation. Observe the child to be certain the sleeve is not too tight and interferes with circulation.
Mummy restraints	Temporarily immobilize young children for a procedure involving the head, neck, or throat—for example, during insertion of a nasogastric tube or drawing blood.	Use this only for the duration of the procedure because it is a total body restraint. Follow the steps shown in Figure 36-1E. If the child is exceptionally strong, a few safety pins can be used to hold the restraint even more firmly. For the infant who needs continuous observation for respiratory function, fold the mummy restraint so the chest is exposed. For newborns or infants, use a "Papoose Board," a commercial restraint used in the same way as a full or mummy restraint (see Fig. 36-1F).

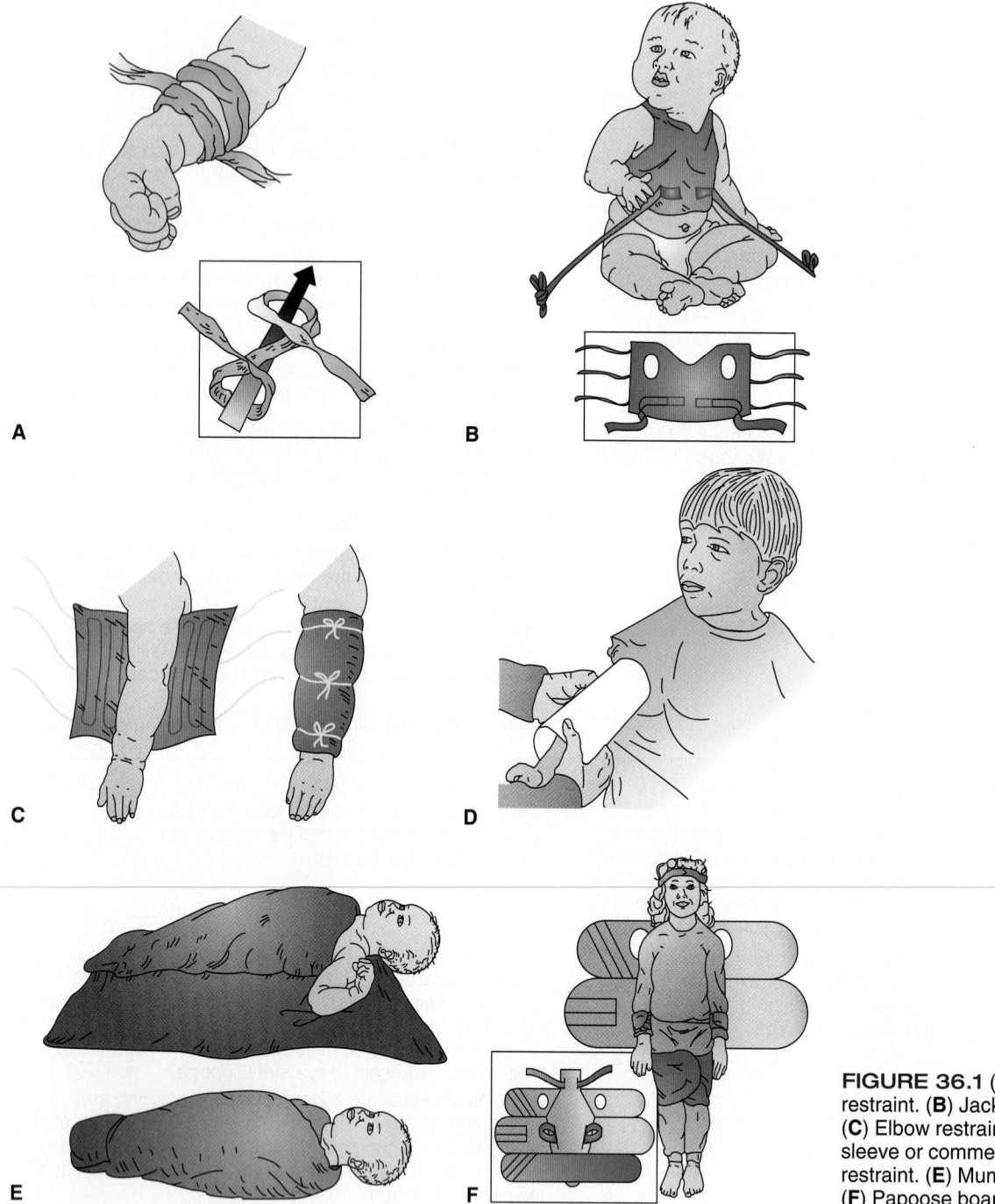

FIGURE 36.1 (**A**) Clove hitch restraint. (**B**) Jacket restraint. (**C**) Elbow restraint. (**D**) No-no sleeve or commercial elbow restraint. (**E**) Mummy restraint. (**F**) Papoose board.

cedure in their mind so they can conquer their fear of it. Fill in gaps in information as necessary to improve a child's perception of the procedure. Providing therapeutic play is another measure to reduce anxiety (see Chapter 35).

Be certain tissue samples obtained after a procedure such as bone marrow aspiration are sent to the proper department for analysis as soon as possible. Guard against specimens being dropped or improperly labeled; children do not have extra body fluids such as blood to sacrifice for additional specimen collection.

If conscious sedation was used, be sure children are awake before they are discharged home or return to an in-patient hospital unit. Using a postanesthesia score sheet (Fig. 36.2) is an effective method to rate recovery from anesthesia.

Children can be discharged as soon as 30 minutes after conscious sedation if the airway is patent and respiratory status is stable (no retraction, stridor, or wheezing); oxygen has not been needed for at least 15 minutes; oxygen saturation is 95% or greater in room air; and the child is awake and reactive, has adequate circulation and normal blood pressure, has heart and respiratory rates appropriate for age, and is reasonably free of pain (Burton & Germann, 2004).

Activity:	Description:	Score:
Activity	Able to move four extremities	2
	Able to move two extremities	1
	Able to move no extremities	0
Respiration	Regular, able to deep breathe/cough	2
	Dyspnea, limited and obstructed breathing	1
	Apneic	0
Circulation	BP within 20 mm Hg of preprocedure	2
	BP within 20–25 mm Hg of preprocedure	1
	BP 25 mm Hg above preprocedure level	0
Level of consciousness	Awake, alert	5
	Drowsy, but easily aroused	4
	Stupor, aroused by vigorous stimuli	2
	Responds to pain only	1
	No response to pain	0
Skin color	Pink, warm, dry	2
	Pale, dusky, blotchy, clammy	1
	Cyanotic, diaphoretic, cold	0
Ambulation	Ambulates with minimum help	5
	Ambulates with minimum support	4
	Unable to ambulate	2

FIGURE 36.2 Post-Anesthesia Recovery Score. A passing score is at least 10 with a level of consciousness score no lower than 4. (From Tolia, V., et al. [2000]. Sedation for pediatric endoscopic procedures. *Journal of Pediatric Gastroenterology and Nutrition, 30*[5], 477–485.)

Parents often have questions about what care their child will need after they return home. Tips for parents following conscious sedation are highlighted in Box 36.2.

Checkpoint Question 1

You are going to restrain T.J. to draw a blood sample from his hand. What type of restraint would be best?

a. Ask his mother to hold him tightly on her lap.
b. Apply a jacket restraint to confine his body.
c. Ask a fellow nurse to hold his hand firmly.
d. Use a mummy restraint so he can't be hurt.

COMMON DIAGNOSTIC PROCEDURES

Diagnostic and therapeutic procedures used with children vary widely depending on a child's condition and age. As in adults, blood, urine, and stool studies are commonly used. These are discussed under techniques of specimen collection. Respiratory illnesses require special procedures; these are discussed in Chapter 40. Biopsies (surgical procedures to remove tissue for examination) are discussed in Chapter 53. Stress testing is discussed in Chapter 41.

Electrical Impulse Studies

Electrical impulse studies are those that include electrical conduction. Children need special preparation for studies such as electrocardiograms (ECGs; Fig. 36.3) or electroencephalograms (EEGs) because they have been warned not to play with electric wires and may worry about being burned or electrocuted. They can be reassured that the electricity passes from their body to the machine, not the other way around; except for electromyelograms, children can be assured that these tests are painless. Electrodes are attached to the body by paste, which is easily removable (Gambrell, 2004). If possible, give the child a portion of the test strip afterward as a souvenir.

X-Ray Studies

A variety of x-ray studies are used to inspect internal body tissues. These range from the simple x-ray to the more complicated computed tomography (CT) scan or dye contrast study.

Flat-Plate X-Rays

X-rays are used both to diagnose illness and check the placement of apparatus such as gastrointestinal feeding tubes (Tedeschi, Altimier, & Warner, 2004). As a rule, children accept x-rays well because an x-ray machine can be compared with a camera, an instrument with which they are familiar (Fig. 36.4). Caution children that although you or a parent may be able to accompany them to the x-ray department, you will not be allowed to stay in the room while the picture is actually taken. If it is necessary for you to remain in the room to restrain a child, do not do this without lead apron and lead glove protection. Such protection is also necessary for portable x-rays taken at a child's or infant's bedside.

Dye Contrast Studies

To visualize a body cavity, some type of radiopaque dye may be swallowed or injected into the cavity and then

BOX 36.2 FOCUS ON . . .

FAMILY TEACHING

Care After Conscious Sedation

Q. T.J.'s mother asks you, "My son received conscious sedation for his MRI. What special care will he need when he comes home?"

A. Here are some tips to help you when you get your son home:

- Keep in mind that most children sleep after leaving the ambulatory care facility or hospital. Some are sleepy for the remainder of the day.
- Don't allow the child to walk alone for at least 4 hours. The child may suddenly feel dizzy and fall without warning.
- Wait until getting home to give the child something to eat or drink, to avoid car sickness. Conscious sedation may cause children to feel nauseated more easily than usual.
- For the first 12 hours after the child wakes, don't ask him to do any activity that requires alertness, coordination, or balance, such as riding a bicycle, swimming, or doing homework. The sedative can affect the child's coordination and balance.

- Remember that the child may forget things readily for the rest of the day. This forgetfulness should go away after a night's sleep.
- Keep in mind that a sedative may cause children to behave in unexpected ways, such as losing self-control or becoming very emotional. By the next day, the child's behavior should return to normal.
- Give infants clear liquids (water, apple juice, tea) after getting home. Wait approximately 30 minutes to make sure the child does not choke or vomit. Then milk, formula, or other foods may be given.
- Do not allow children to drink until they can hold a cup without help, to make sure they are awake enough to keep from choking. Wait approximately 30 minutes. If there is no vomiting or choking, the child can have the foods he or she usually eats.
- Call your primary care provider if the child has pain or recurrent vomiting, or if any of the effects above last for more than 12 hours.

examined on x-ray. **Barium contrast studies,** for example, are used to observe the outline of the gastrointestinal tract. Barium may be swallowed to outline the upper gastrointestinal tract or instilled by enema to outline the lower portion. Caution the child that barium, even if flavored,

does not taste terribly good. In studies such as an intravenous pyelogram (IVP), dye is injected intravenously; as it circulates to the kidneys, an x-ray is taken. Children must be thoroughly prepared for dye contrast procedures. Because iodine is incorporated in most of the radiopaque ma-

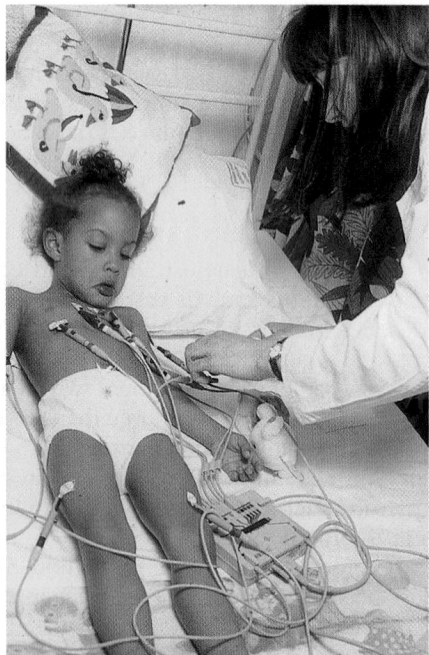

FIGURE 36.3 Administering an ECG. Children can be assured this is a painless procedure. (John Watney/Photo Researchers, Inc.)

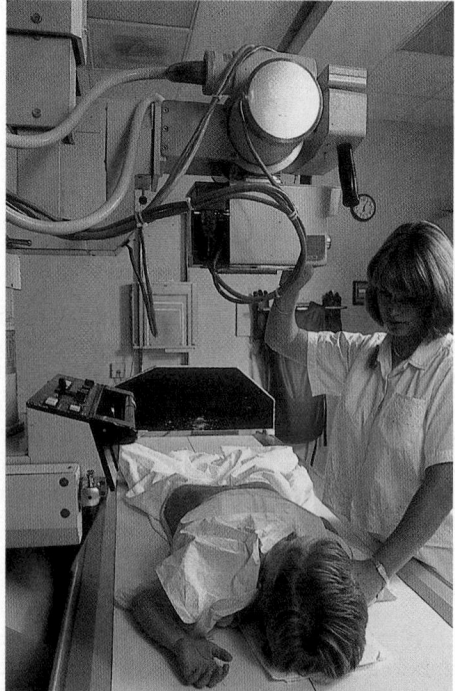

FIGURE 36.4 Positioning of a child for an x-ray. (© Bachmann/Stock Boston.)

a parent to confirm for a child that the procedure is all right, because they have been told not to let adults touch this part of their body.

To be certain that school-age children and adolescents understand the procedure, have them repeat the instructions given to them; then send them to a nearby bathroom to carry out the procedure by themselves.

Suprapubic Aspiration

Suprapubic aspiration involves the withdrawal of urine by insertion of a sterile needle into the bladder through the anterior wall of the abdomen. It is used to obtain urine for culture in infants who cannot void on command. It is usually done by physicians, although nurse practitioners or nurses in specialty units may perform it. The steps for this procedure are as follows:

1. The anterior abdominal wall is cleaned with an antiseptic.
2. The urinary meatus is blocked by gloved finger pressure, confining urine in the bladder.
3. A needle is inserted just above the pubis into the bladder.
4. Urine is aspirated through the needle into a sterile syringe.

Although suprapubic aspiration for urine appears complicated, it is not. The bladder is the most anterior of abdominal organs and, when distended with urine, is easily accessible just under the abdominal wall (Fig. 36.12). Be-

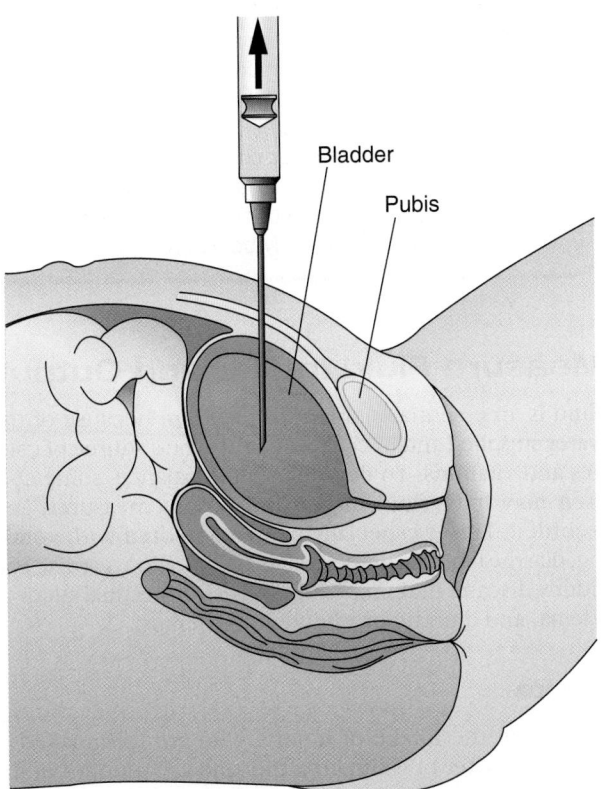

Bladder

Pubis

FIGURE 36.12 A suprapubic bladder aspiration. The full bladder is easily accessible by an abdominal puncture.

cause the needle can cause a bladder spasm, however, it can produce sharp discomfort. Parents may not have heard of this procedure and may wonder why their child had urine drawn by needle and syringe instead of by catheter. The method is used because theoretically the risk of bladder infection from needle insertion is less than that from catheter insertion (Fischbach, 2004).

Catheterization

Bladder catheterization is accomplished most easily in children up to school age if a small (#5 or #8) feeding tube is used instead of a urinary catheter. This thin tube passes readily through the meatus of even an infant. Before beginning catheterization, be certain to observe the perineum of girls to locate the urinary meatus; it is not as readily observable in infants and young children as it is in women. Cleanse the perineum or penis well before inserting the tube to reduce the risk of infection.

Catheterization is an invasive procedure, so children must be prepared in advance. Caution children that the catheter will sting for an instant as it is inserted and they will have to lie still until the urine specimen is obtained. They need both support to submit to the procedure and praise afterward for their cooperation. Preschool boys may need assurance that the procedure has no long-term consequences to reduce their fear of castration.

Obtaining Stool Specimens

Stool specimens are frequently obtained to be analyzed for blood or ova and parasites. Obtain stool specimens from children who are toilet-trained by asking them to use a potty seat or by placing a collector cap device on a toilet. For effective communication, be certain you know the word the child uses for stool. Transfer the specimen to a collection cup with tongue blades. To obtain a specimen from a child who is not toilet-trained, scrape stool from a diaper using tongue blades and place it in a stool collection cup. Some stool specimens need a preservative added to the container. If it is important to keep urine from contaminating the stool specimen, place a separate urine collector bag on an infant.

Be certain stool specimens are sent to the laboratory promptly so they do not dry and have to be collected a second time, because they can be difficult to obtain until at least 24 more hours. If the stool specimen is for ova and parasites, see that it arrives in the laboratory in less than 1 hour. Do not refrigerate ova and parasite specimens because refrigeration destroys the organisms to be analyzed.

 Checkpoint Question 2

T. J. will have a 24-hour urine specimen collected. You would time this from:

a. The time of the discard specimen.
b. The first urine voided in the morning.
c. A set time, such as 8 AM.
d. The first voiding after the discard urine.

HOT AND COLD THERAPY

Children who sustain muscle sprains or undergo procedures such as bronchoscopy or tonsillectomy may have cold applications prescribed to prevent inflammation and edema (Fig. 36.13). If inflammation or edema is already present, application of heat may be prescribed to help it resolve. It is important to implement measures to prevent both burns and boredom in the child during treatments. Guidelines for hot and cold applications are shown in Box 36.6.

NUTRITIONAL CARE

Because almost all illnesses affect children's nutritional and fluid balance, assessment of these areas sheds a great deal of light on a child's general health. Nutritional assessment begins by asking a child or parent for a 24-hour recall of all the foods eaten during that time, followed by more specific measures such as intake and output measurements. Common therapies for nutritional deficiencies include enteral feeding, gastrostomy, and total parenteral nutrition (TPN).

NURSING DIAGNOSES AND RELATED INTERVENTIONS

---●---

Nursing Diagnosis: Risk for imbalanced nutrition, less than body requirements, related to chronic illness

Outcome Evaluation: Skin turgor is good; no signs of dehydration are present; child gains a minimum of 1 pound weekly as evidence that nutritional needs are being met.

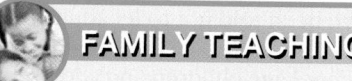

BOX 36.6 FOCUS ON . . .

FAMILY TEACHING

Guidelines for Hot and Cold Applications With Children

Q. T. J.'s mother tells you, "I need to apply cold compresses to my child's head to reduce swelling. How do I do this?"

A. When applying any type of hot or cold therapy such as cold or warm compresses, use the following guidelines:

- Apply neither heat nor cold for longer than 20 minutes unless prescribed otherwise, because after this time, the vasoconstriction caused by cold and the vasodilatation caused by heat is reversed.
- When using electrical sources of heat with toddlers and preschoolers, never make a game of plugging in and pulling out the apparatus that makes the light come on or a dial glow. Otherwise, the child may play with it after you leave.
- Supply a special activity for a child to enjoy while a hot or cold application is in place (playing a board game or reading a story to the child), so that the procedure is not viewed as a chore but as a pleasant time to look forward to.
- Put tape on the gauge of an electric appliance at the point where you want it, so that you will be able to tell if the child changes the setting.
- To be certain that solutions or heat sources are not too hot, always test them with your inner wrist or the dorsal surface of your hand before applying them to the child.
- Do not apply ice packs or ice directly to the skin. Cover the pack or ice with a towel or other cover to prevent frostbite and cell damage from cold.
- Be cautious using heat or cold applications with a child who is receiving an analgesic, because the child's perception of heat or cold may be reduced, and he or she could easily be burned.

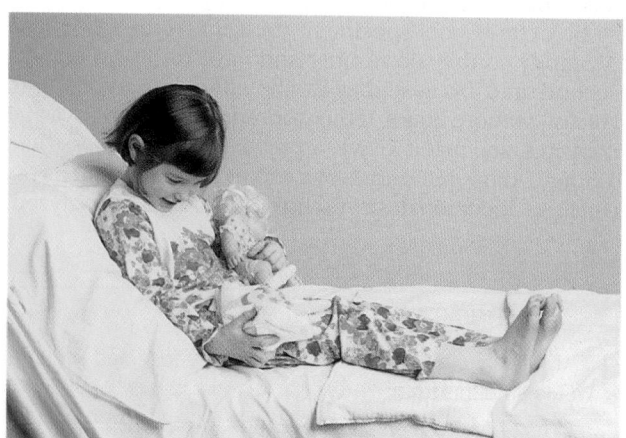

FIGURE 36.13 A rubber glove used as an ice pack. A face drawn on it helps to make it seem friendlier. Wrap gloves in washcloths to help avoid latex allergy.

Measure Fluid Intake and Output

Fluid is an essential element of nutrition because of the water supplied and because it can also be a source of calories and vitamins. To document fluid balance, some children may have fluid intake and output measured and recorded. This is especially true for children with vomiting, diarrhea, burns, hemorrhage, dehydration, cardiac and kidney disease, draining wounds, gastrointestinal suction, edema, and diuretic or intravenous therapy.

Intake

Estimating the intake of infants who are formula-fed is simply a matter of estimating the kind and amount of fluids that were swallowed. Intake in breast-fed infants is merely recorded as "breast-fed." If it is necessary to estimate the amount more closely than this, an infant can be weighed before and after a feeding. The difference in weight (in grams) is the number of milliliters of breast milk ingested. This measurement is not very accurate, however, because if the child voided or had a bowel movement, weight would be affected by these losses.

With preschool children, be certain to record fluids ingested during snacks as well as meals, because children this age usually have many during the day. At approximately 10 years of age, children can be depended on to record their own intake as long as they have a list of how many milliliters are contained in each glass or cup they use (an average cup is 150 mL; a glass, 180 mL). Remind them that soup, flavored frozen ice such as Popsicles, and sherbet are liquids and should be counted.

Output

Diapers can be readily used as a method of measuring urine output. Weigh a diaper before it is placed on an infant and record this weight conspicuously (mark it on the front of the plastic covering with a ballpoint pen). Reweigh the diaper after it is wet and subtract the difference to determine the amount of urine present. This difference will be in grams. Because 1 g = 1 mL, the amount can be recorded in milliliters. In infants who have liquid stools, it is difficult to separate stool from urine because these blend together in a diaper. Separate urine from stool by applying a urine collector; check it frequently for filling.

Girls often void along with bowel movements when they use a toilet, which means that a urine specimen is easily lost. To separate urine from bowel movements, teach older children to void first before trying to move their bowels.

Enteral Feedings

Enteral feedings, also called nasogastric tube feedings, are a common means of supplying adequate nutrition to an infant who is unable to suck or tires too easily when sucking, or to an older child who cannot eat. Enteral feedings have the advantage over parenteral nutrition because they preserve the stomach mucosa and also decrease the risk of intravenous infection. In infants, such feedings are traditionally called **gavage feedings** (Box 36.7 and Table 36.2).

Whether enteral catheters should be passed through the nares or the mouth is controversial. Orogastric insertion allows for easier breathing because the nose is not blocked. Because newborns are nose breathers, it seems reasonable that passing a catheter through the mouth in this size infant will lead to less distress than passing it through the nose. Orogastric insertion can also decrease the possibility of striking the vagal nerve and causing bradycardia. If the tube is to be left in place, however, it may be passed through a nostril. For the older child, insertion through a nostril is more comfortable.

Children are generally offered bolus or intermittent feedings rather than continuous infusions to more closely mimic a normal feeding pattern. Children with long-term neurologic disabilities may have enteral tubes left in place for continuous feedings administered by an enteric feeding pump. Give mouth care at least twice a day to children who are receiving nasogastric tube feedings; otherwise, their mouths become dry and ulcers can form.

Gastrostomy Tube Feedings

Children may have gastrostomy tubes inserted for feeding. Such feedings may be necessary for children who cannot swallow or those with esophageal atresia, severe gastroesophageal reflux, or esophageal stricture (Crawley-Coha, 2004). With the use of regional anesthesia, the tube is inserted through a puncture wound in the abdominal wall into the stomach (Fig. 36.14). The tube used in children is usually actually an indwelling urinary catheter (Foley catheter) rather than a true gastrostomy tube. This is because a Foley catheter can be removed easily and changed should it become plugged. In addition, the balloon is small enough not to obscure and fill the small stomach space.

As with nasogastric feedings, gastrostomy feedings should be at room temperature to prevent chilling. Before a feeding, elevate the child's upper trunk 30 to 40 degrees so the fluid will remain in the stomach and not flow upward into the esophagus, possibly causing aspiration. Do this by holding an infant in the lap or placing him or her in an infant seat. For an older child, use pillows or elevate the head of the bed. Use a syringe to aspirate the tube for any stomach residual. After noting the amount, replace this fluid so the child doesn't lose the electrolytes it contains. To administer the feeding, attach a syringe to the tube and allow the specified amount to flow by gravity only (to prevent reflux and possible aspiration).

After the feeding, flush the tube with a specified amount of clear water to clear it of the feeding solution. Keep the child's head elevated for at least 1 hour after a feeding to help prevent esophageal reflux.

If a child has had esophageal surgery, suspend the unclamped tube in an elevated position. Leaving the tube unclamped and elevated ensures that if the child should vomit, vomitus will be evacuated from the stomach by the tube rather than past new sutures in the esophagus. If a tube is left elevated and unclamped, cover it with a clean piece of porous gauze to prevent bacteria from entering it.

Infants who are fed by gastrostomy tube miss the pleasure of sucking. Offer a pacifier to suck on during the procedure unless contraindicated. Talk or sing to the child as if the feeding were being given orally.

The biggest problem with gastrostomy tubes is that they may not fit snugly, so formula or gastric secretions can leak around the tube onto the abdominal skin. Gastric secretions are irritating because of their high hydrochloric acid content. To protect infant skin, consult a wound, ostomy, continence nurse specialist (WOCN) for wound care. Often commercially available skin protectants can be placed around the tube to protect the skin. One method of helping to provide a snug fit for the tube is to place a soft nipple used with premature infants (enlarge the nipple opening slightly) over the catheter (nipple tip up) so the base of the nipple fits against the skin protectant. Tape the tube to the nipple at the tip, which brings the balloon of the tube up against the stomach wall and prevents leakage. Tape the nipple to the skin and skin protectant securely using nonadhesive tape. Clean the skin around the nipple daily with a product such as half-strength hydrogen

(text continues on page 1130)

BOX 36.7 NURSING PROCEDURE

Initiating an Enteral Feeding for an Infant

Purpose
To supply nutrition by an enteral tube.

PROCEDURE	PRINCIPLE
1. Loosely swaddle the infant using a mummy restraint.	1. Mummy restraints effectively contain arms and legs without causing any unwarranted pressure on the infant.
2. Measure the space from the bridge of the infant's nose to the earlobe to a point halfway between the xiphoid process and the umbilicus using a no. 8 or no. 10 feeding tube. If the infant is older than 1 year of age, measure from the bridge of the nose to the earlobe to the xiphoid process.	2. Measuring the tube ensures that it will be long enough to enter the stomach. If a tube is passed too far, it will curl and end up in the esophagus; if not passed far enough, it will also be in the esophagus. Both situations could lead to aspiration of the feeding.

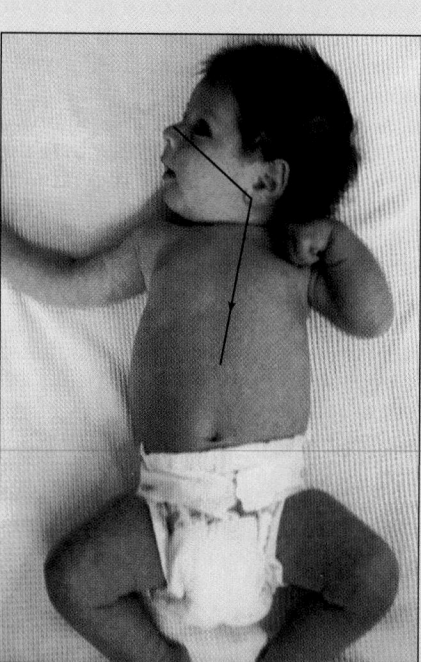

PROCEDURE	PRINCIPLE
3. Mark the tube at the measured point with a small clamp or piece of tape. Lubricate the tip of the catheter with water.	3. Lubrication helps the tube pass through the esophagus without trauma. An oil lubricant is never used because although the tube is going to be passed into the stomach, occasionally it can accidentally pass into the trachea. Oil left in the trachea could lead to lipoid pneumonia, a complication an infant already burdened with a disease may not be able to tolerate.
4. Pass the catheter with gentle pressure to the point of the clamp or tape. If the catheter is inadvertently passed into the trachea rather than the esophagus, the infant usually will cough and become dyspneic. If this happens, withdraw and replace the catheter.	4. Using gentle pressure helps to ensure comfort and safety.
5. Assess the catheter for position (confirm that it is not in the trachea) before administering a feeding (see Table 36-2).	5. Assessing for proper placement helps to ensure that the feeding will enter the stomach, not the infant's respiratory tract.

(continued)

PROCEDURE	PRINCIPLE
6. Aspirate stomach contents to assess amount. If the amount aspirated is small (a few milliliters), merely replace it at the beginning of the feeding. If large (large is determined by comparing it to the physician's order), replace it through the tubing, and reduce the amount of the feeding by that amount.	6. Assessing stomach content amount aids in determining if the previous feeding was absorbed. Replacing stomach secretions rather than discarding them helps prevent electrolyte loss.
7. After being certain that the catheter is in the stomach, attach a syringe or special feeding funnel to the tube. Elevate the infant's head and chest slightly to encourage fluid to flow downward into the stomach.	7. Elevating the infant's upper body allows the feeding to flow by gravity.
8. Add the specific kind and amount of feeding prescribed to the syringe or funnel and allow it to flow by gravity into the infant's stomach. Don't elevate the syringe end of the tube more than 12 inches above the infant's abdomen (see figure below).	8. Excessive elevation can cause the feeding to flow too quickly, filling the esophagus and increasing the risk for aspiration. Hurrying feedings by using the plunger of the syringe or a bulb attachment for more pressure also can lead to aspiration.

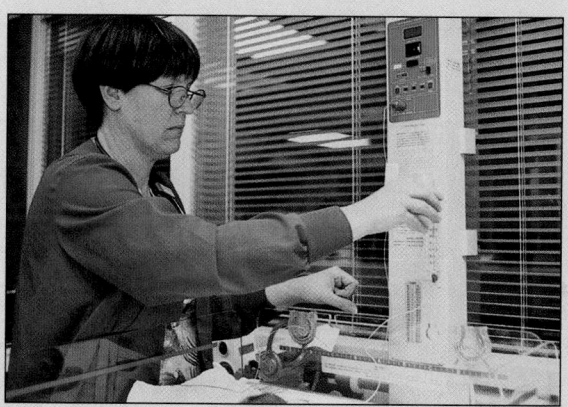

© Barbara Proud.

PROCEDURE	PRINCIPLE
9. Offer a pacifier (nonnutrient sucking) during the feeding if the infant appears to enjoy this.	9. Nonnutrient sucking can help satisfy the infant's normal need to suck, which would otherwise go unsatisfied with gavage feedings.
10. When the feeding has passed through the tube, reclamp the tube securely and gently and rapidly withdraw it.	10. Clamping the tube before it is withdrawn is important to prevent any milk remaining in the tube from flowing out as the tube is removed and thereby reduce the risk of aspiration.
11. If the tube is to remain in place, flush it with 1 to 5 mL of clear water and cap it.	11. Flushing a tube helps prevent clogging and plugging of the tube with the feeding solution. Capping a tube helps to prevent air and bacteria from entering.
12. If the tube is to be left in place, tape it below the nose and to the cheek. Do not tape it to the forehead.	12. Taping a tube to the forehead can put pressure on the anterior naris, leading to ulceration.
13. Bubble the baby after an enteral feeding as you would after a bottle or breast feeding. If a parent is present, encourage him or her to do this.	13. Bubbling helps in preventing air accumulation and regurgitation of feeding. Encouraging parental participation aids in promoting close contact, which is essential to the baby's development.
14. Unswaddle and place the infant on the right side with the head slightly elevated or hold and rock the infant in this position.	14. Placing on the right side helps the feeding solution enter the pyloric valve, promoting stomach emptying.
15. Assess that the infant appears comfortable. If a parent observed the procedure, answer any questions or concerns.	15. Assessing the infant after the feeding aids in outcome evaluation. Helping parents feel comfortable with alternative feeding methods can help increase their self-esteem and promote bonding with the infant.

TABLE 36.2

Methods to Determine Proper Gavage Tube Placement

Method	Considerations
Attach syringe to the tube and aspirate stomach contents. Test for pH (below 7 is acid).	In most instances, stomach contents aspirated this way are returned to the stomach before the feeding; in small infants, the amount of stomach contents is subtracted from the prescribed amount of feeding; because stomach contents are highly acid, discarding them at each feeding can lead to alkalosis.
Inject 5 mL air into the gavage tube and listen over the stomach with a stethoscope to the sound of injected air.	The injected air is heard as a whistling or growling sound; do not use an adult-size stethoscope on small infants to listen for it; the diaphragm of the stethoscope will be partially over lung, and where one is hearing the air injection is unknown.

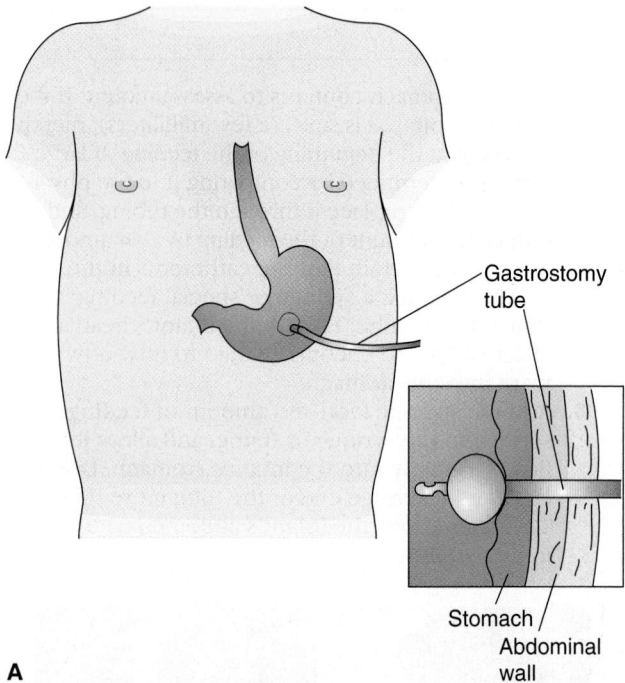

A

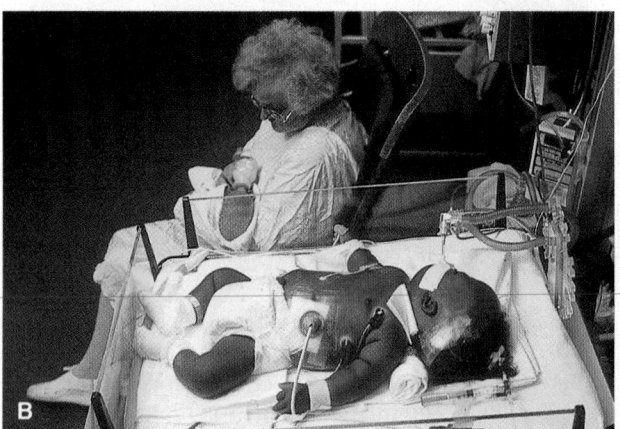

B

FIGURE 36.14 Children who are ill often need supplemental feeding by nasogastric or gastrostomy tube feedings. (**A**) Internal placement of a gastrostomy tube. (**B**) An infant with a gastrostomy tube in place. (W. McIntyre/Photo Researchers, Inc.)

peroxide; change the skin protectant as directed by the manufacturer's instructions. At the time of the change, expose the skin to air for approximately 1 hour.

A major complication associated with the use of a gastrostomy tube is that it can move into the duodenum through the pyloric sphincter and cause obstruction. Observe and report any vomiting, abdominal distention, or brown or green tube drainage (duodenal secretions that would suggest the tube has moved). Testing residual aspiration fluid to see that it is acid is a guarantee that the tube is in the stomach (stomach secretions are acid; duodenal secretions are alkaline). Putting a mark on the tube with an indelible pen just above the nipple lets you check that the tube has not migrated into the stomach but is remaining securely in place.

Tubes are replaced approximately every 6 weeks. To replace a tube, deflate the catheter balloon by withdrawing the water in it and then gently pull the tube free. Insert a clean catheter into the stomach opening approximately 1 inch beyond the balloon; inflate the balloon with 2 to 4 mL water. Attach a nipple and tape in place.

Most children receiving gastrostomy feedings will have the tube in place for an extended time. Teach the child's parents how to feed their child by this method, how to remove and to replace a tube, and the danger signs to watch for (e.g., vomiting, abdominal discomfort, or skin excoriation). Help parents to view this as an alternative way of feeding, not a totally different one. Be certain they are comfortable with the procedure before the child is discharged from the hospital, so they can effectively feed the child by this method. Reinforce with them the understanding that it does not hurt their child to have the tube replaced or to have pressure put against the tube, so that they need not worry about holding their child snugly. Many children on long-term gastrostomy feedings have gastrostomy buttons implanted for easier stomach access (Fig. 36.15). For feeding, a catheter is inserted through the device; the catheter is removed following the feeding. With this in place, only a small access device is visible, not a large bulky tube.

Percutaneous endoscopic gastrostomy (PEG) tubes are feeding tubes that are passed using endoscopy through the esophagus into the stomach and then pulled through a stab wound to the outside of the abdominal wall. The tube is then held in place by an external restraining disc. Although tubes may be passed as far as the jejunum by this same method, such tubes bypass normal stomach digestion rather than support it, so are much less used in children. The overall use of such tubes is limited because a small child's esophagus may not be wide enough to insert the tube by this route.

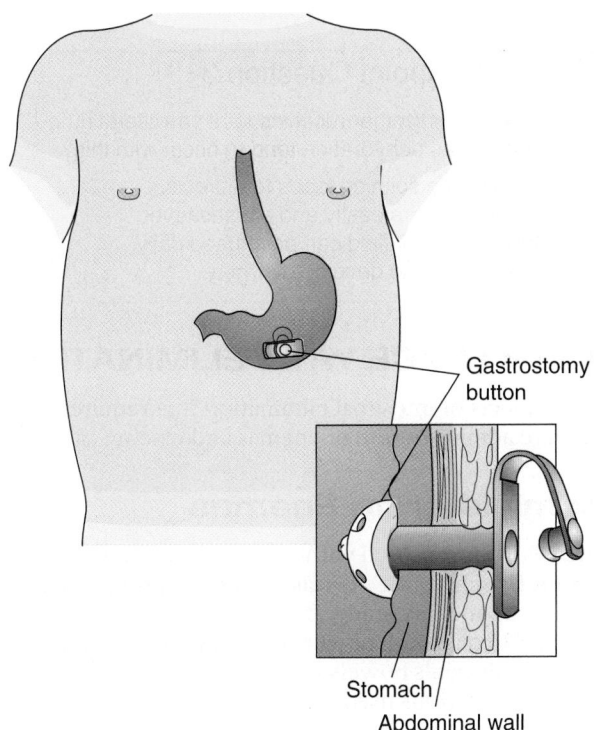

Gastrostomy button

Stomach

Abdominal wall

FIGURE 36.15 Placement of a gastrostomy button.

What if... a parent whose child has a gastrostomy tube in place tells you she's going to take the child to a restaurant so the child learns about "eating out." Would you agree with her that this is a good idea?

Total Parenteral Nutrition

NURSING DIAGNOSES AND RELATED INTERVENTIONS

Nursing Diagnosis: Imbalanced nutrition, less than body requirements, related to malabsorption of nutrients

Outcome Evaluation: Skin turgor is good; no signs of dehydration are present; child loses no weight during therapy; intestinal cramps and distention lessen.

Total parenteral nutrition (TPN) has become one of the most important therapies for children who have gastrointestinal illnesses that prevent proper absorption of basic caloric or fluid requirements or respiratory illnesses that make infants too exhausted to suck. Traditional intravenous therapy contains fluid, electrolytes, and sugars but not protein and fat, which are essential for the maintenance and growth of body tissues. With TPN, all of a child's nutritional needs can be met by a concentrated hypertonic solution of intravenous therapy containing glucose, vitamins, electrolytes, trace minerals, and protein. An intralipid solution (emulsified fat able to be administered intravenously) given once or twice per week supplies needed fatty acids. Children with chronic diarrhea or vomiting, inflammatory bowel disease, bowel obstruction, anorexia, or extreme immaturity are examples of children who benefit greatly from TPN.

TPN solutions may be administered via a central intravenous access site or via a peripherally inserted central venous catheter (PICC). If a central access site is chosen, a catheter is inserted through the right external jugular vein into the superior vena cava or directly into the subclavian vein under strict aseptic conditions (see Chapter 37). The catheter is secured at the site of insertion with sutures and covered with a sterile dressing to help reduce bacterial contamination. A major vein of this type is chosen to avoid inflammation reactions and resulting venous thrombosis from the high-caloric and high-osmotic fluid that will be infused (Ainsworth, Clerihew, & McGuire, 2005).

TPN solution is prepared in a pharmacy under sterile conditions according to prescription. A millipore filter, which removes small particles in the solution that might cause an embolus to form, is inserted into the tubing. The solution should be administered by means of a constant infusion pump so the rate can be governed. As a general rule, if the rate should fall behind, do not increase it the next hour to make up the amount of fluid, or serious cardiovascular overload could result because of the concentrated fluid being administered.

Infection is a major danger of TPN because the solution is a perfect medium for the growth of bacteria or *Candida* organisms. The dressing over the insertion site and the intravenous tubing are changed every 1 to 2 days to avoid infection; the tubing should not be used for drawing blood or for adding medications (unless a double-barreled tube is used), because either process has the potential to introduce infection. Sterile technique is required in changing bottles of solution so that the tubing is not contaminated. Some health care facilities require nurses to wear both masks and gloves while doing this to avoid airborne and direct contamination. Fewer restrictions are necessary for home care. The insertion site should be inspected at the time of the dressing change for indications of local infection, such as redness, tenderness, or discharge.

A second major problem that can occur with TPN is dehydration. A TPN solution contains approximately twice the amount of glucose normally administered in an intravenous solution to ensure that the amino acids in the solution will be used for protein synthesis, not for energy. Dehydration may occur as the kidneys recognize the amount of glucose in the bloodstream as excessive and start to reduce it by excreting it (the same phenomenon that leads to high urine output in persons with diabetes mellitus). When TPN is begun, test urine for glucose and for specific gravity with each voiding. If two or more consecutive samples indicate a 3+ or 4+ glucose level, either the rate of the infusion or the amount of glucose in the solution may need to be decreased, or insulin added to the solution, to counteract the excess glucose. Generally, decreasing the concentration of glucose and then gradually increasing it again allows the child's body to adjust to the glucose overload.

After the first few days of TPN, a rebound effect (the child's body produces increased insulin) may cause hypoglycemia. A urine sample that suddenly is negative for glucose after several serial specimens have been highly positive is therefore not necessarily an encouraging sign; rather, it may be a warning that the child's glucose level is dangerously low. TPN solution should never be discontinued abruptly but gradually tapered, or a glucose rebound effect could also occur. If a TPN catheter should be accidentally pulled out by a child, the child must be immediately assessed for hemorrhage from the insertion site and closely observed in the next few hours for signs of hypoglycemia (i.e., lethargy, incoordination, fidgeting, or seizures). Parents need to be alerted to these concerns for safe home care.

Remember that to a child, eating is more than a means of receiving nourishment; it is also a means of receiving comfort and love. Even though children are able to voice the reason they must have TPN and appear to understand they are receiving all the needed nutrients by the infusions, they still may miss eating food and the natural social interaction that comes with it. While in a hospital, they may be upset by the smell of food from a hospital unit kitchen or by the fact that playmates have to leave to eat a meal. Finding an activity for the child receiving TPN to do while other children eat (e.g., help to check supplies on the emergency cart or stamp laboratory slips) may be helpful to supply the interaction the child misses. Ask whether a child can be allowed chewing gum or occasional hard candy for chewing and taste sensations. Tooth brushing twice a day is necessary to keep the oral mucous membrane healthy because the child is not chewing. An infant needs sucking pleasure from a pacifier.

Many children on long-term TPN are cared for by parents at home. Careful coordination with the home care agency is necessary to ensure that parents are familiar with the system and know how to obtain TPN fluid so the child's care continues safely. Make sure parents arrange for special time each day with the child to make up for the time normally spent interacting at meals.

Checkpoint Question 3

T. J.'s younger brother receives total parenteral nutrition. Why does dehydration tend to occur with this?

a. The glucose solution leads to diuresis.
b. Infection occurs easily and causes fever.
c. Only 100 mL of fluid can be infused daily.
d. Children tend to develop diarrhea.

ASSISTANCE WITH ELIMINATION

Two aspects of intestinal elimination that require special care are administration of enemas and ostomy care.

Administering Enemas

Enemas are rarely used with children unless they are therapy for Hirschsprung's disease or a part of preparation for surgery or an x-ray study. If an enema is necessary, offer a careful explanation of what the child can expect. As the sizes of children's bowels vary greatly, the usual amounts of enema solutions used are:

Infant: Less than 250 mL (exact amount should be stipulated by physician's order)
Preschooler: 250–350 mL
School-age child: 300–500 mL
Adolescent: 500 mL

For an infant, use a small, soft catheter (#10 to 12 French) in place of an enema tip to prevent rectal trauma. Infants and children up to ages 3 or 4 years cannot retain enema solutions, so they must rest on a bedpan during the procedure. Pad the edge of the pan so it is not cold or sharp. Place a pillow under the infant's or young child's upper body for positioning and comfort. Lubricate the catheter generously with a water-soluble lubricant and insert it only 2 to 3 inches (5 to 7 cm) in children and only 1 inch (2.5 cm) in infants. Be certain to hold the solution container no more than 1 foot above the level of the sigmoid colon (12 to 15 inches above the bed surface) so the solution flows at a controlled rate. If a child experiences intestinal cramping, clamp the tubing to halt the flow temporarily and wait until the cramping passes before instilling any more fluid. An older child can be asked to take a deep breath to help the cramping sensation pass. The amount of solution used in infants is so small that this is not usually a problem. If the enema solution is to be retained, such as an oil solution, hold the child's buttocks together for about a count of 10 after administration.

Until late school age, children cannot retain an enema as adults can (rarely more than 5 to 10 minutes). For this reason, be certain the bathroom the child will use is available before administering the enema.

Commercial enemas, such as Fleet enemas, are not routinely administered to children younger than 2 years because of the harsh action of the sodium biphosphate and sodium phosphate they contain. Tap water is not used because it is not isotonic and causes rapid fluid shifts of water in body compartments, leading to possible water intoxication. Normal saline (0.9% sodium chloride) is, therefore, the usual solution. It can be made by parents at home by adding 1 teaspoonful of salt to 1 pint (500 mL) of water.

After enema administration, praise a child for cooperating. Allow a preschooler an opportunity for therapeutic play, because this is a frightening procedure for a child of this age.

Providing Ostomy Care

An ostomy is an opening of the bowel on the surface of the abdomen. Ostomies in newborns are created to relieve bowel obstruction caused by conditions such as ileal atresia, necrotizing enterocolitis, and imperforate anus (Rogers, 2003). In older children they are constructed for conditions such as inflammatory bowel syndrome. If an ostomy is created in the ileum (an ileostomy), the stoma is located on the right side of the abdomen and drains liquid stool, which is extremely irritating to the skin because of the digestive enzymes it contains. If an ostomy is created in the sigmoid portion of the bowel (colostomy), the stoma is on the left lower abdomen and passes normally formed stool (Fig. 36.16).

An ileostomy requires the use of a collecting ostomy appliance to contain acid stool and prevent excoriation of the abdominal skin. Older children also may use an appliance with a colostomy. For an infant colostomy, parents may choose (with support and advice) whether to use an appliance.

Two basic problems commonly arise when using an ostomy appliance with an infant: it may be difficult to locate one small enough to contain liquid drainage without leaking, and the skin under the appliance may become extremely irritated. Consulting with a wound, ostomy, continence nurse specialist (WOCN) can be helpful. Clear plastic colostomy bags without a ring can often be cut more easily to fit the size of the stoma and the contour and size of an infant's abdomen than a ring type. A commercial skin sealant is helpful to harden the skin surrounding the stoma. Apply it according to the brand directions and fan to dry. If a spray is used, protect the infant's face so that

he or she does not inhale the solution. Apply the chosen stoma collection appliance. Tuck it inside the diaper to help keep the infant from pulling it loose.

Check the appliance or bag for collecting stool at least every 4 hours. To protect the underlying skin, do not remove a self-adhering bag if it is full, but drain collected stool from the bottom of the appliance into a basin or paper cup for disposal. To reduce odor, flush the appliance bag with a warm water and soap solution, using a bulb-type syringe (an Asepto syringe), and rinse with clear water. Change the bag no more frequently than the point at which leakage occurs (perhaps as long as 1 week) to reduce skin irritation. To remove a bag that was placed with a sealant, be certain to use the designated solvent to prevent pulling or harming underlying skin. Then wash the solvent away with soap and water or it will become an irritant itself. Because most infants enjoy tub bathing, a long, soaking bath is an excellent way to loosen an appliance.

If an appliance or bag is not used, stool will be discharged onto the abdomen three or four times a day (no different than a usual newborn or infant stool pattern). Wash and dry the stoma and surrounding skin area well. Follow your agency's protocol for skin care, such as applying karaya powder, an ointment such as Desitin, or a skin protectant to protect the skin. Apply ample absorbent gauze (fluffed) and an absorbent pad. Secure in place with nonadhesive tape or a binder. Check the dressing approximately every 4 hours. Remove and replace it when soiled, washing the skin well and applying new powder or ointment as necessary. Without an appliance in place, stool is kept from touching the skin only by the protection of the ointment and frequent changing of the dressing. Turning an infant from side to side after every feeding may be helpful in keeping stool from flowing continuously to one side. Leaving the abdominal skin exposed to air for at least 1 hour per day also helps protect skin integrity.

Stress to parents that caring for an infant with an ostomy is little different from usual. All parents must change their infant's diapers frequently and clean the diaper area. Stress that the stoma has no nerves, so a parent can feel free to wash it without hurting the child and that compression

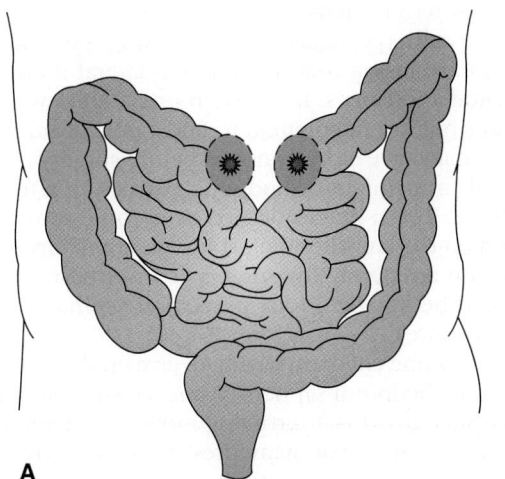
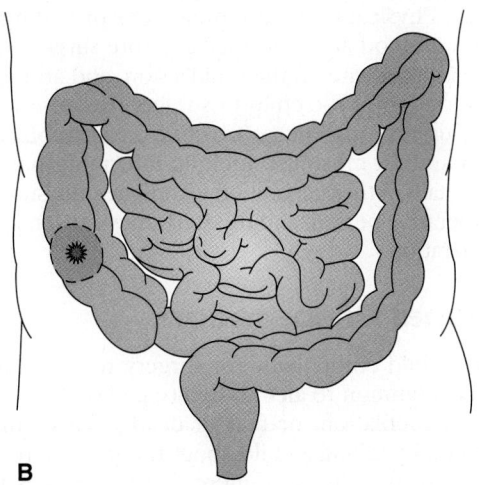

FIGURE 36.16 Different sites for ostomies. (**A**) A double-barrel colostomy. (**B**) A single-barrel colostomy.

against the stoma will not cause the child pain. These explanations can help the parents feel comfortable placing the infant on his or her abdomen or holding the infant closely against their body for comfort.

Colostomies are rarely irrigated in children. On occasion, to prepare a child for second-stage abdominal surgery, irrigation of the "blind-end" bowel (bowel between the rectum and colostomy) of a double-barreled colostomy may be ordered daily to keep it lubricated and to maintain bowel tone. The exact amount of fluid to be used should be specified by the surgeon. Typically, the amount is small, approximately 40 to 100 mL in infants. Normal saline (0.9% sodium chloride) should be used in place of tap water, which could lead to water intoxication because tap water is not isotonic.

Children who have had a colostomy since infancy adapt well to it because they have never known another method of defecation. Parents should begin toilet-training for urine control at the usual time. In contrast, school-age children often have a great deal of difficulty adjusting to a colostomy. Encourage children to perform self-care as fully and as soon as possible so they can be independent. Preschool children usually benefit from therapeutic play that helps them work through their feelings. Provide some time for older children to discuss concerns about being accepted by others and how to answer questions about a colostomy from other children. Adolescents with a colostomy may have questions regarding sexuality and need reassurance that this should not interfere with intimate relationships. They may appreciate open discussion of how they see this affecting their life.

PREPARATION OF A CHILD FOR SURGERY

Preparing a child for surgery is a major responsibility for a child health nurse because surgery is always a potentially frightening procedure. Such preparation differs according to the type of surgery being performed, but certain activities apply to all surgery and all children. Psychological preparation of both child and parents is aimed at reducing a child's fears about the procedure and consists primarily of providing health teaching and opportunities for therapeutic play. Physical preparation includes providing for restrictions on food and fluid intake before surgery, preparing the incision site on the child's skin, and arranging for transportation of the child to surgery. Because many children's surgical procedures are done on an ambulatory basis, preparation must also include informing parents about the details of the preparation techniques, the surgery, the postoperative period, and the steps they must take toward preparation.

Emotional Preparation

Preparing a child emotionally for surgery requires minimizing fears common to all children (e.g., fear of separation, fear of mutilation, or fear of death). This can be accomplished by telling a child about the procedure and describing any specific equipment and techniques that will be used, such as anesthesia, eye bandages, nasogastric tubes, sutures, or special aftercare. A teaching plan is essential for explaining all of these features of surgery to the child (see Chapter 34). Be certain all preparation is appropriate to the child's age. More children undergoing surgery receive a general anesthetic rather than a local or regional anesthetic, as might be used with adults, because this minimizes their fears of intrusive or mutilating procedures, and because children who are not yet adolescent are not mature enough to cooperate adequately during surgery.

Physical Preparation

Most children will be placed on nothing by mouth (NPO) status for surgery. The length of the time the child will remain NPO depends on the child's age. Adolescents and school-age children may be restricted from taking food or fluid from midnight until the time of surgery the following morning; however, if infants younger than 6 months were held NPO for as long a time as this, they would be taken to surgery in dehydration. Therefore, infants younger than 6 months may be kept NPO for as little as 4 hours. At the end of the 4 hours, as the infant becomes hungry, he or she will begin to cry and fuss for fluid. Parents need an explanation that infants who vomit during surgery because of recent feedings may aspirate; therefore, even though an infant is becoming hungry, he or she must be restricted from ingesting fluid. Although a hungry child will usually not suck on one for long, a pacifier can be offered.

Preparation of surgical sites varies. In most instances, shaving of the area and final cleansing are done in a holding room adjacent to the operating room after the child is anesthetized. A povidone–iodine wash may be ordered before transport to the operating room for some types of surgery. Washing a particular body part in this manner can be interpreted as an intrusive procedure by a preschooler. Give a great deal of assurance that the solution being used will not sting but is only cleaning.

Transportation

Check children's identification bands to ensure they are legible and secure before transport. If not, replace or secure them before surgery.

Immediately before transport, remove barrettes and bobby pins from the child's hair and check the mouth for loose teeth (particularly in children ages 6, 7, and 8 years, who are losing their central and lateral incisors) or for dental appliances. It is rare to find a child with full dentures but not uncommon to find a post or screw-in tooth that may have to be removed before surgery or a retainer used to maintain orthodontic correction after brace removal. Teeth braces do not need to be removed. Make certain the anesthesiologist knows about any loose teeth before an airway for surgery is inserted (a loose tooth could be knocked totally free and aspirated during the procedure).

For some children, having to give up their own pajamas or their bedroom slippers or outside shoes to change to a hospital gown is a terrifying moment. Giving up underpants is a step that many preschool and early school-age children cannot tolerate. For this reason, many children are allowed to wear their own pajamas or clothes until they are under an anesthetic.

In ambulatory settings, children may walk to surgery. If they will ride in a cart, this should have been introduced during preparation. Be sure to fasten a restraining strap for safety (presented with, "Here's your seat belt; it's just like going in a car."). Preschoolers may enjoy taking a favorite toy or blanket to surgery with them. Ideally, they should be allowed to keep this with them until they are under an anesthetic. Parents should be allowed to accompany their children to the operating suite. Some parents can accompany their child into an anesthesiologist's induction room; for others, this is inappropriate or too anxiety-producing. A nurse whom the child knows should accompany the child to the operating room and remain there until the child is under the anesthetic, if possible. Even if the child has been well prepared for the surgical experience and the change in personnel on arrival to the surgical suite, saying goodbye to parents at the door of the surgical suite and the actual sight of strange personnel can lead to high levels of anxiety and fear.

Although it may not be cost-effective to have a staff nurse wait with a child until he or she is under an anesthetic, the nurse's wait will probably not be long if the child has been called for surgery when the surgical suite is almost ready. The psychological benefit of a familiar nurse's comforting presence can make the difference between a positive and negative hospital experience.

POSTOPERATIVE WOUND CARE

Children frequently have a dressing or bandage in place to cover a surgical incision or sutured laceration. Such dressings differ from adult dressings in terms of material, size, and methods used to secure them. Keeping a dressing dry to avoid introducing infection to the wound in infants and toddlers who are not toilet-trained can be a major problem. In many instances after surgery, collodion (a clear substance similar to nail polish) or other commercially available "wound glues" are used to cover the incision. Applied to a suture line to serve as the dressing, these products keep the suture line from coming in contact with urine or feces. Since these materials are clear, they allow good visualization of the healing surface as well. Assure parents that such a covering is adequate and actually preferable if the incision is in the groin, such as a hernia repair.

If a gauze dressing is used, it can be covered with plastic and securely held in place with nonadhesive, waterproof tape. Be certain when cutting plastic to cover a dressing not to leave an extra piece behind in the crib; the child could pull it over his or her head and suffocate.

Occlusive dressings (hydrogel sheets, hydrocolloids, or polyurethane films) are dressings especially designed to provide a healing surface over a wound. These need to be applied and removed according to each product's directions.

The skin of infants and young children is usually too sensitive for adhesive tape to be used to secure dressings. Use nonadhesive tape (silk or paper) instead or secure a dressing with a nonadhering bandage (Kling) or roller gauze. Young children, as a rule, find bandages comforting and accept them as a "badge of courage," displaying them proudly. Apply adhesive bandages (Band-Aids) generously after venipuncture or finger punctures for this reason. Preschool children have little concept of how long healing takes; they are often surprised that their incision or wound has not yet healed the day after surgery. Preschoolers are often worried that a part of their body under a dressing is missing and find it reassuring to see that the body part is still there (they may pull a dressing away to do this). It is better to know what something is like than to worry about the unknown. Therefore, do not discourage children from looking at their incision during dressing changes. Even if the area looks raw and unhealed, it may look better than what the child has envisioned was under the dressing. Teach parents and children how to continue wound dressings when they return home.

REDUCING ELEVATED TEMPERATURE IN CHILDREN

Fever is such a common symptom in children that reducing temperature or giving a parent instructions on how to reduce the temperature at home becomes a common intervention with children (Box 36.8).

BOX 36.8 FOCUS ON . . .

EVIDENCE-BASED PRACTICE

Do Parents Understand What is Meant by "Fever"?

In this study, 235 parents of children attending either a hospital or neighborhood health clinic were surveyed as to their knowledge about elevated temperatures and the actions they take when this occurs in their children. Forty-five percent of the study population were Latino, 15% were African-American, and 25% were white. An interesting finding of the study was that 42% of respondents did not know what temperature would represent a fever. Eighteen percent (1 in 5) of parents did not have a thermometer to use to assess their child's temperature. Parents who had not graduated from high school had 5 times the odds of not using a thermometer to check for fever and triple the odds of not asking a health care provider for fever advice. Parents of uninsured children were 5 times less likely than others to bring their febrile child to the emergency department.

This is an important study for nurses because it points out an elementary necessity of health teaching: before discussing a health care practice with parents, be certain they have adequate resources to carry out the health care measure. For example, telling the one fifth of these parents who did not have thermometers to take their child's temperature would have been an ineffective instruction.

Source: Taveras, E. M., Durousseau, S., & Flores, G. (2004). Parents' beliefs and practices regarding childhood fever: A study of a multiethnic and socioeconomically diverse sample of parents. *Pediatric Emergency Care, 20*(9), 579–587.

NURSING DIAGNOSES AND RELATED INTERVENTIONS

──●──

Nursing Diagnosis: Risk for hyperthermia related to illness affecting temperature regulation, medications, or surgery

Outcome Evaluation: Child's temperature returns to 98.6°F (37°C) orally within 2 hours.

Because the temperature-regulating mechanism in children is immature, fever tends to be more marked in children than in adults and may even be out of proportion to the seriousness or extent of their disease. An increased temperature occurs because a child's temperature-regulating point (set point) has been elevated. The child's temperature cannot be reduced until the set point returns (or is returned) to normal.

Acetaminophen (Tylenol) is an excellent antipyretic (i.e., it acts to reduce the temperature set point), so it is the drug most often prescribed to reduce fever in children (Box 36.9). Children's ibuprofen is also effective (Box 36.10).

Parents often do not give an adequate dose of an antipyretic such as acetaminophen because they are afraid their child will have a bad reaction to it. This results in the high fever continuing. Encourage them to give a full dose of the antipyretic every 4 hours, up to five doses a day, until their child's temperature is reduced. Conversely, caution them not to give too

BOX 36.9 FOCUS ON . . .

PHARMACOLOGY

Acetaminophen (Tylenol)

Action: Used for moderate temperature elevation or pain; does not have anti-inflammatory properties (Karch, 2004)

Pregnancy risk category: B

Dosage: Oral: 10–15 mg/kg every 4–6 hours as needed; may repeat 4 or 5 times per day; do not exceed 5 doses in 24 hours

Possible adverse effects: Elevated liver enzymes, jaundice, rash

Nursing Implications
• Caution parents that drug can cause severe liver toxicity with overdose.
• Educate parents not to administer a larger dose or more frequently than prescribed.
• Encourage parents to increase the child's fluid intake to aid in reducing fever.

BOX 36.10 FOCUS ON . . .

PHARMACOLOGY

Ibuprofen (Advil, Pediaprofen)

Action: Used to reduce inflammation, fever, and mild to moderate pain

Pregnancy risk category: B; D if used in last trimester

Dosage: (for fever or pain) 5–10 mg/kg every 6–8 hours; do not exceed 40 mg in 24 hours

Possible adverse effects: Gastric upset, headache, dizziness, nausea, occult blood loss, prolonged bleeding, peptic ulceration

Nursing Implications
• Use with caution in children with gastrointestinal irritation.
• Drug can cause renal failure if child becomes dehydrated; encourage fluid intake.
• Administer with food or drink to minimize gastrointestinal irritation.

much or a severe overdose with liver or kidney toxicity can occur (Karch, 2004). An antipyretic is generally ordered for any child whose oral or tympanic temperature is more than 101°F (38.4°C) or whose rectal temperature is more than 102°F (39.0°C). Caution parents not to give acetylsalicylic acid (aspirin) to children with fever because aspirin is associated with Reye's syndrome, a severe neurologic disease (see Chapter 49).

Teach parents that fever is actually a body protection measure, and unless it is exceptionally high (more than 106°F [41.1°C]), it does no specific harm. In fact, there is some evidence that fever may be of value in helping to combat infection, because it aids in destroying microorganisms. In addition to antipyretic administration, the parents should dress children with fever in lightweight clothing, such as summer pajamas. Remove all clothing but the diaper from an infant. Many parents dress febrile children warmly in flannel nightgowns to keep them from "getting a chill." This increases the child's temperature and does not prevent the shaking, trembling reaction that comes with high fever. Placing a cool cloth (not ice) on the child's forehead feels comforting. Although sponging children to lower temperature may be effective in a small group of children (Meremikwu & Oyo-Ita, 2005), it is no longer recommended for children as a whole, because it can lead to extreme chilling and shock to an immature nervous system and has little advantage over the use of oral antipyretics.

Caution parents that common antipyretics for children's fever taste like candy. Be sure they know to lock antipyretics away or children can help themselves to more "candy" when a parent's back is turned.

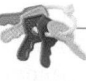

Key Points

Preparing children for procedures reduces anxiety. Prepare a child and parents by trying to relate a procedure to something with which the child is already familiar, such as comparing an x-ray machine to a camera.

Include parents in both the planning and implementation of care, as parents can reinfect children with fear if their own fear is uncontrolled. Try to give explanations on two levels: "I'm going to change the dressing on her suture line" for a parent; "I'm going to put a clean bandage on your tummy" for the child.

Minimize the number of painful procedures; for instance, combine blood sampling procedures, if possible.

Perform any procedures that will cause pain in a treatment room or away from the child's bedside so the bed remains a "safe" place.

Perform treatments without chilling or exposure. Even small children expect modesty to be respected.

Allow a child to voice anger or fear of a procedure. Provide therapeutic play after a procedure to help reduce these reactions.

Children enjoy adults who are secure in their actions. Practice as necessary the steps of a procedure before you begin so you can demonstrate confidence and skill.

Once you have announced that a procedure needs to be done, proceed to do it; waiting for something to happen is often as stressful as actually having it done.

Involve children in procedures, as this gives them a sense of control. Allow a child to examine electrodes or apply gel for electrode contact before a procedure. Give a child a portion of an ECG strip as a badge of courage after the procedure, or let the child apply his or her own adhesive bandage.

Praise children for cooperation even if none was visibly obvious. For painful procedures, any behavior short of hysterical screaming counts as cooperation.

Following the use of conscious sedation, observe children carefully until they are fully awake. Check for the return of the child's gag reflex before offering any fluids to minimize the risk of aspiration.

Help make feeding by a route such as a gastrostomy tube as close to normal as possible by talking to the child to simulate mealtime conversation and socialization.

Critical Thinking Exercises

1. T. J. is the 4-year-old you met at the beginning of the chapter who is frightened of dark places. He is scheduled to have an MRI of his head, which means he will be wheeled into a huge, dark, noisy, hollow tube. How would you prepare him for this?

2. T. J. is also scheduled for a CT scan with dye injected. His mother asks you to assure her that her son will not have a reaction to the dye. How will you answer her?

3. T. J.'s new brother had bowel surgery at birth and now has a temporary colostomy. His grandmother cares for him two mornings a week while his mother attends school. The grandmother tells you that she cannot imagine how she can care for an infant with a colostomy. What could you do to try to make her feel more comfortable with the baby's care? Will his care really be much different from that for other newborns?

4. Examine the National Health Goals related to health care of children. Most government-sponsored money for nursing research is allotted based on these goals. What would be a possible research topic to explore pertinent to these goals that would be applicable to the Balliff family and also advance evidence-based practice?

References

Ainsworth, S. B., Clerihew, L., & McGuire, W. (2005). Percutaneous central venous catheters versus peripheral cannulae for delivery of parenteral nutrition in neonates. *Cochrane Library (Oxford)(2)* (CD004219).

Bohrn, M., & Siewert, B. (2004). Acute abdominal pain: What not to miss. *Patient Care for the Nurse Practitioner, 1*(3), 1–8.

Brown, J. M., & Padman, R. (2003). Case study of a UFO (unidentified foreign object). *Pediatric Asthma, Allergy & Immunology, 16*(4), 187–192.

Burton, J. H., & Germann, C. A. (2004). Guide to procedural sedation and analgesia. *Emergency Medicine, 36*(7), 43–46.

Crawley-Coha, T. (2004). A practical guide for the management of pediatric gastrostomy tubes based on 14 years of experience. *Journal of WOCN, 31*(4), 193–200.

Department of Health and Human Services (2000). *Healthy people 2010.* Washington, DC: DHHS.

Ernst, A., Silvestri, G., & Johnstone, D. (2003). Guidelines from the American College of Chest Physicians. *Chest, 123*(5), 1693–1717.

Fischbach, F. T. (2004). *Manual of laboratory and diagnostic tests* (7th ed.). Philadelphia: Lippincott Williams & Wilkins.

Flores, G. (2005). Preventing hospitalisations for children. *Lancet, 365*(9455), 201–202.

Gambrell, M. (2004). Seizures 101. *Nursing, 34*(8), 36–42.

Karch, A. M. (2004). *Lippincott's nursing drug guide.* Philadelphia: Lippincott Williams & Wilkins.

Lafleur, K. J. (2004). Taking the fifth [vital sign]. *RN, 67*(7), 30–37.

Meremikwu, M., & Oyo-Ita, A. (2005). Physical methods for treating fever in children. *The Cochrane Library (Oxford) (4)* (CD004264).

Rogers, V. E. (2003). Ostomy care. Managing preemie stomas: More than just the pouch. *Journal of WOCN, 30*(2), 100–110.

Rohrschneider, W. K., et al. (2003). MRI to assess renal function in children. *European Radiology, 13*(5), 1033–1045.

Schwartz, M. W. (2003). Cardiology laboratory. In *5-minute pediatric consult.* Philadelphia: Lippincott Williams & Wilkins.

Shah, V., & Ohlsson, A. (2005). Venipuncture versus heel lance for blood sampling in term neonates. *The Cochrane Library (Oxford) (4)* (CD001452).

Taveras, E. M., Durousseau, S., & Flores, G. (2004). Parents' beliefs and practices regarding childhood fever: A study of a multiethnic and socioeconomically diverse sample of parents. *Pediatric Emergency Care, 20*(9), 579-587.

Tedeschi, L., Altimier, L., & Warner, B. (2004). Improving the accuracy of indwelling gastric feeding tube placement in the neonatal population. *Neonatal Intensive Care, 17*(1), 16-18.

Tomlinson, D. (2004). Physical restraint during procedures: Issues and implications for practice. *Journal of Pediatric Oncology Nursing, 21*(5), 258-263.

Willock, J., et al. (2004). Peripheral venipuncture in infants and children. *Nursing Standard, 18*(27), 43-50.

Zucker, M. L., & LaDuca, F. M. (2004). Monitoring in the NICU: The value of point-of-care testing. *Neonatal Intensive Care, 17*(2), 44-46.

Suggested Readings

Arantes, A., et al. (2004). Concise communications. Pediatric risk of mortality and hospital infection. *Infection Control and Hospital Epidemiology, 25*(9), 783-785.

Boyd, S. (2004). Within these walls: Moderating parental stress in the NICU. *Journal of Neonatal Nursing, 10*(3), 80-84.

Chandar, J., et al. (2005). Role of routine urinalysis in asymptomatic pediatric patients. *Clinical Pediatrics, 44*(1), 43-48.

LeRoy, S., et al. (2003). Recommendations for preparing children and adolescents for invasive cardiac procedures. *Circulation, 108*(20), 2550-2564.

Mitchell, M., Johnston, L., & Keppell, M. (2004). Preparing children and their families for hospitalisation: A review of the literature. *Neonatal, Paediatric & Child Health Nursing, 7*(2), 5-15.

Montagnino, B. A., & Mauricio, R. V. (2004). The child with a tracheostomy and gastrostomy: Parental stress and coping in the home: A pilot study. *Pediatric Nursing, 30*(5), 373-380.

Rutledge, D. N., Donaldson, N. E., & Pravikoff, D. S. (2003). Use of restraints: Acute nonpsychiatric care. *Online Journal of Clinical Innovations, 6*(2), 1-69.

Snyder, B. S. (2004). Preventing treatment interference: Nurses' and parents' intervention strategies. *Pediatric Nursing, 30*(1), 31-40.

Tanel, R. E. (2004). ECGs in the ED. *Pediatric Emergency Care, 20*(8), 553-554.

Ziegler, D. (2004). Is there a therapeutic value to physical restraint? *Children's Voice, 13*(4), 30-32.

Nursing Care of the Child Undergoing Medication Administration and Intravenous Therapy

Key Terms

absorption
distribution
excretion
intermittent infusion devices
Intracath
metabolism
pharmacokinetics
vascular access port

Objectives

After mastering the contents of this chapter, you should be able to:

1. Describe common methods of medication and intravenous therapy used in the health care of children.
2. Assess the developmental stage and knowledge level of children and adolescents before beginning medication or intravenous therapy.
3. Formulate nursing diagnoses related to medication or intravenous therapy with children.
4. Identify expected outcomes for children receiving medication or intravenous therapy.
5. Plan nursing interventions to aid in making medicine and intravenous therapy maximally effective.
6. Implement nursing interventions concerned with medication and intravenous therapy and children, such as introducing patient-controlled analgesia.
7. Evaluate expected outcomes related to medication and intravenous therapy with children.
8. Identify National Health Goals related to medication or intravenous therapy that nurses could help the nation achieve.
9. Identify areas related to medication or intravenous therapy with children that could benefit from additional nursing research or application of evidence-based practice.
10. Use critical thinking to analyze ways that medicine or intravenous therapy can be modified to be more family-centered.
11. Integrate knowledge of medication and intravenous therapy with nursing process to achieve quality maternal and child health nursing.

Terry, an 8-year-old with Down syndrome, comes to the ER. She is diagnosed with osteomyelitis, a bone infection. When you give her a tablet of acetaminophen (Tylenol) for pain, she spits it out. She does the same when you repeat with a second tablet. Her mother tells you Terry can't swallow pills. Her father tells you, "You'll have to give her the medicine intravenously."

Previous chapters described the difficulty children may have adjusting to illness and also diagnostic and therapeutic procedures that are frequently used with children. This chapter adds information about techniques for administering medication and intravenous (IV) therapy to children. This is important information as almost all illnesses today involve some form of medicine or IV administration.

What would you do? How would you gain Terry's cooperation?

After you've studied this chapter, access the accompanying website. Read the patient scenario and answer the questions to further sharpen your skills, grow more familiar with RN-CLEX types of questions, and reward yourself with how much you have learned.

Most adults have little difficulty understanding that taking medicine will be important to relieve whatever symptoms they are experiencing from an illness. Because children do not necessarily have this same level of understanding, they may resist taking medicine unless its importance is thoroughly explained to them and the medication is given to them by a method that best meets their preference. Many children do not have enough coordination to swallow oral medicine until they are 6 or 7 years of age. This can make taking oral medication difficult. Almost all children fear intrusive procedures. This can make them resist accepting medication given by a rectal, nasal, intramuscular, or IV route. Because children range in size from as small as 3 pounds if premature to 180 pounds by late adolescence, there is no "standard" dose of medicine. This can make it difficult to determine the correct dose. In addition, children have difficulty reporting adverse effects of medicine as accurately as adults. This can make it difficult to determine if side effects or adverse effects are occurring. All these things make medicine administration for children one of the most challenging interventions in nursing. National Health Goals that address this area of child health practice are shown in Box 37.1.

BOX 37.1 FOCUS ON . . .

NATIONAL HEALTH GOALS

When administering medicine to children or teaching children and parents how to take medicine, remember that medicines can be as dangerous in overdoses as they are helpful in the correct doses. They can be ineffective if the doses are inadequate or missed. Poisoning and drug abuse are addressed by the following national health goals:

- Reduce the incidence of childhood poisonings, from a baseline of 348/100,000 population to a target of 292/100,000 population.
- Increase the proportion of adolescents not using alcohol or any illicit drug during the past month, from a baseline of 79% to a target of 89%.
- Reduce the rate of steroid use among adolescents in the past year, from a baseline of 1.5% to 0.4% (DHHS, 2000).

Nurses can help the nation achieve these goals by educating parents about safe drug storage (locked in elevated cabinets) and teaching children and parents about effective nonpharmacologic ways to relieve stress or anxiety to help reduce drug dependence.

Areas related to these goals that could benefit from additional nursing research to strengthen evidence-based practice would include studies on the most effective ways to teach parents about safe drug storage, the phenomenon that drug poisoning increases when families are under stress, and effective ways to impart information to adolescents about the seriousness of drug abuse and its possible consequences.

Nursing Process Overview

For a Child Needing Medication/Intravenous Therapy

● *Assessment*

Because children vary so greatly in size and individual need, medication administration to children begins by assessing the child's height and weight so a correct dose of medicine or amount of IV fluid can be calculated based on the child's surface area. Also crucial to assessment is the child's developmental age. This is important because it will reveal if a child can swallow oral medicine or can use such self-medication methods as patient-controlled analgesia; in addition, it will help you determine which site would be best for an intramuscular or IV injection. Also assess the child's chronological age and cognitive level to aid in planning the level of explanation that will be needed. Include an assessment of the child's past experience with taking medicine to help predict what his or her response to medicine administration might be. Lastly, inquire about the family's cultural beliefs and attitudes toward medications, including use of herbal or folk remedies (Box 37.2). Following medicine administration, careful observation must continue to determine if the medication is having its desired effect and if any unwanted or adverse effects are occurring.

BOX 37.2 FOCUS ON . . .

DIVERSITY OF CARE

People's attitude about the worth or wisdom of medicine is not consistent across cultures. Not all families, therefore, can be expected to accept medicine administration as enthusiastically as others; some families believe an herb or home remedy actually will be preferable. Because of this, a family may accept a prescription but then not fill it or administer the medicine. In addition to prescribed medicine, some families give herbal remedies that can duplicate or counteract a medicine's effect. Keep in mind, too, that medicine is expensive and difficult for many families without health insurance to afford.

As part of health histories, always ask if a child commonly takes any type of herbal or home remedy and if he or she has been given anything specific for the present illness. When you give parents a prescription, ask them if they think they will have any difficulty with obtaining or giving it, assessing for the medicine's effect, or returning for a follow-up appointment to evaluate the medicine's effect. Such questions allow parents to say they have questions about the medicine or are uncertain whether they should give it because of a cultural belief.

● *Nursing Diagnosis*

Common nursing diagnoses related to medicine administration vary widely. Some examples are:

• Disturbed sleep pattern related to q4h timing of medication administration
• Deficient knowledge related to action and side effects of medicine
• Fear related to IV administration of medicine
• Discomfort related to rash as side effect of medicine
• Health-seeking behaviors by parent related to desire to learn more about different types of medicine available for child's illness

● *Outcome Identification and Planning*

Planning for medicine administration for children involves the same safe rules of administration as those for adults. Extra consideration is necessary at each step, however, because determining the right form and route of the medicine (e.g., liquid or capsule, oral or intramuscular) varies so widely. Establishing that a dose is accurate for that size child can involve recalculating the dose using a nomogram that shows body surface area. The schedule for administration must be not only one that is effective for the drug's action but also one that will not interfere with school activities, eating, or sleep (Weller et al., 2004).

Explain to the child the effects that can be expected from the medicine. Be certain to give this explanation at an age-appropriate level, and be sure it is consistent with any prior explanation that a parent or other health care provider has given. The American Academy of Pediatrics website (*http://www.aap.org/*) offers information on general medicine administration and tips on how to read medicine labels and is a useful site to recommend to parents.

● *Implementation*

Medicine and IV interventions with children include both administering medicine to ill children and teaching parents and children how to continue to take the medicine when at home or at school. As long as a child is uncomfortable or has definite disease symptoms, parents tend to give medicine conscientiously. However, when symptoms fade, a child returns to school, and the family returns to its busy everyday schedule, it is easy for parents to forget to give medicine. This can leave children open to a recurrence of the condition or symptoms, such as pain or recurrent infection, because the organisms causing the illness were only suppressed, not killed. Helping parents fill out administration schedules to post in a readily visible location, such as on the refrigerator or a bathroom mirror, can be as important an act as explaining the drug's action to help ensure all doses of medicine will be given.

● *Outcome Evaluation*

Expected outcomes associated with medication administration should ensure that a child received the medicine as prescribed and that the medicine had the desired effect. Specific examples suggesting outcome achievement are:

• Child states she understands she must continue to take thyroid hormone for a lifetime.
• Parents list the adverse effects of the drug and state the telephone number they will call if adverse symptoms occur.
• Adolescent describes an administration program that includes four doses daily but allows time for sports activities after school.
• Child contracts to allow IV therapy if it is inserted into nondominant hand.

MEDICATION ADMINISTRATION

Medications in children are given by a variety of routes: orally, intranasally, transdermally, topically, rectally, and via injection (e.g., subcutaneous, intramuscular, IV, intraosseous, or epidural) or by inhalation. Epidural administration is described in Chapter 38. Inhalation techniques are discussed in Chapter 40.

Safe medication administration is a priority in child health nursing because children have such a wide weight range. This wide weight range, combined with the relative immaturity of body systems in children, means there is rarely a "standard" pediatric dosage of a particular drug; therefore, each dose of a drug must be calculated individually. To administer drugs safely, it is important to have a good understanding of **pharmacokinetics** (the way a drug is absorbed, distributed throughout the body, metabolized, inactivated, and excreted). Each drug, each dose, and each child must be carefully and individually evaluated to ensure that the six rights of medicine administration—right medicine, right client, right dose, right route, right time, and right client instruction—are provided (Croskerry et al., 2004).

Pharmacokinetics in Children

The four basic processes of absorption, distribution, metabolism, and excretion determine the intensity and duration of a drug's action. The immaturity of body systems in children (and especially in newborns) plays a major role in drug action throughout each of these processes.

Absorption

Drug **absorption** (transfer of the drug from its point of entry in the body into the bloodstream) is influenced by the route of administration as well as by the concentration and acidity of the drug. Some routes of administration in children are limited and so are rarely used. For example, children younger than school age usually cannot hold tablets under their tongue for sublingual administration; they tend to swallow them instead. The small muscle size of young children limits sites for intramuscular injection. Infants pull off transdermal patches because they do not understand that this is a drug. Gastrointestinal absorption may be so immature at birth that oral absorption in newborns can be reduced. Vomiting and diarrhea, frequent symptoms of childhood illnesses, also interfere with absorption because a drug would not remain in the gastrointestinal tract long enough to be absorbed.

Distribution

Distribution refers to the movement of the drug through the bloodstream to a specific site of action. Many drugs are distributed bound to serum albumin (manufactured by the liver). This binding action limits the amount of free drug in the circulation, thereby providing protection against toxic levels of a drug. As free drug is used, the bound drug is released to maintain a therapeutic level. Newborns with immature liver function may not have enough serum albumin to transport drugs readily. This is particularly true if elevated bilirubin levels are present, because bilirubin is also carried by serum albumin. Bound to serum albumin this way, bilirubin is harmless. In free form, however, it can leave the bloodstream and enter other body tissues. If it enters the brain cells, it destroys their ability to function (kernicterus). If a newborn who has a high level of bilirubin from destruction of fetal hemoglobin receives a drug such as sulfonamide that competes for albumin binding sites, a large quantity of bilirubin may be left unbound and the infant may develop kernicterus. In addition, newborns have sluggish peripheral circulation, so distribution in children this young may not be effective. Any child with cardiovascular disease also may have limited distribution of drugs because of poor circulation.

Metabolism

Metabolism involves the conversion of the drug into an active form (biotransformation) or an inactive form (inactivation). Because a child's basic metabolic rate is faster than that of an adult, certain drugs are metabolized more rapidly in children. This means the drug must be administered more frequently to a child to maintain effective drug levels than it would be in adults. Some drugs, such as the salicylates and chloramphenicol, are metabolized directly by liver enzymes. Because liver enzymes are not fully developed in newborns, these drugs cannot be metabolized and so will reach toxic levels rapidly. Older children with liver disease who have impaired liver enzymes also have a decreased ability to inactivate or transform drugs.

Excretion

The **excretion** (elimination of raw drug or drug metabolites, a process that largely prevents properly administered drugs from becoming toxic) of drugs is potentially limited until about 12 months of age, when kidney function becomes mature. If a child has kidney disease, excretion potential is limited at any age. A few drugs are excreted in bile (e.g., digitoxin). In the newborn with sluggish bile formation, excretion of these drugs is questionable. Monitoring intake and output is important in children receiving drugs to be certain that urine excretion or an outlet for drug metabolites is adequate.

What if... Terry's mother tells you her child's school has a "no drug" policy, so the school nurse will not be able to give Terry even a prescription drug in school? How would you advise her?

Adverse Drug Effects in Children

Children respond to drugs in much the same way as adults, but they may experience unique or exaggerated side effects because of immature liver function or rapid metabolism during periods of rapid growth. The newborn may suffer adverse effects from drugs taken by the mother prenatally or from drugs taken by a breast-feeding mother.

Safe Storage of Drugs

Since young children do not appreciate that overdoses of medicine can be serious and even fatal, they may help themselves to additional medicine and poison themselves (Broderick, 2004). Adolescents can deliberately take extra doses of drugs such as steroids or pain medicine, hoping for an added effect. Oxycodone (OxyContin), for example, is an analgesic that may be prescribed for adolescents (Kokki et al., 2004); it is also frequently abused by them. Children, like adults, may hoard drugs and then use them in a suicide attempt.

When working with children, always be certain medicine is stored in a safe place. On an adult unit, for example, a medication cart can be left in the middle of a hallway or in a patient room while you answer the phone or perform another activity. On a children's unit, this would be inappropriate. A toddler walking past such a cart could easily explore it and remove a handful of pills. For the same reason, never leave medicine on a bedside table for a child to take later if he or she is playing a game or taking a shower; a nearby toddler could take the medicine first (Stucky, 2003).

When teaching parents about administering medicine at home, stress that they need to keep drugs in a safe place. In most homes, this is in a locked medicine cabinet or drawer above the height their child could reach. Remind parents that most childhood poisonings occur when a family is under stress; during these times, the family may forget usual procedures such as locking away a drug. Reinforce the need to take special precautions to lock away medications at these times. Also tell parents they should never take medicine in front of children (children can imitate this action with the parent's medication) or pour or prepare medicine in the dark. Because almost all medicine bottles dispensed from local pharmacies look and feel the same, it is easy to pour the wrong liquid, extract the wrong pills, or read the bottle instructions incorrectly without adequate light.

Safe Administration of Drugs

Administering drugs safely to children requires that you first determine that you are giving the right drug to the right child, in the right dosage and by the right route, at the right time. You also need to ensure that the parents or child have the right information about the medicine.

Right Medicine

Most medication errors are made in situations where the number of medications being given is high and speed in administration is crucial. Intensive care units and emergency

BOX 37.3 FOCUS ON . . .

EVIDENCE-BASED PRACTICE

How Many Medicine Errors with Children Occur During Hospital Admissions?

Opportunities for medication errors during children's hospital admissions are more numerous than for adults, because unlike adult doses, drug doses for children are usually calculated individually based on the child's age, weight, and clinical condition. To see what types of errors occur, researchers examined 16 recently published studies on drug errors in children. Results revealed that medication errors occur at a rate of about 2 per 100 admissions in U.S. hospitals. Wrongly prescribed doses are the most common type of medication error.

This is an important study for nurses because it points out the importance of checking pediatric medicine doses before administration to be certain that the dose has been calculated accurately and that a common error, such as placing a decimal point in the wrong place, has not occurred. It emphasizes the importance of the nurse's role in serving as a child's last-chance protector against medicine errors.

Source: Wong, I. C., et al. (2004). Incidence and nature of dosing errors in pediatric medications: A systematic review. *Drug Safety, 27*(9), 661–670.

departments, therefore, are the highest areas for risk of medication errors (Conrad & Gillis-Ring, 2003; Box 37.3). As the number of medicines available grows, so does the possibility that two drugs have similar names. The prescriber may write an order using a generic or a trade name. That makes this first step in medicine administration—identifying you have the correct drug—even more important than ever.

Right Child

Children cannot be depended on to give their correct names. Anxious to please, a preschooler will answer the question, "Are you Johnny Jones?" with "yes." He may also agree with any other name you propose. A school-age child who wants to avoid taking any medicine may deny he or she is the person whose name you call. To prevent these types of errors, never ask children their names for identification. Instead, read their identification arm bands and compare them with the medication sheet or medical record. In ambulatory care settings or homes, ask a parent to confirm the child's identity.

Right Dosage

The correct dosage of most drugs for children is based on body surface area using a nomogram (Fig. 37.1). To calculate surface area using such a chart, find the child's height in the left column (e.g., 40 cm); next, find the child's weight in the right column (e.g., 20 kg). Hold a ruler or straightedge to connect the two points. The mark at which the ruler crosses the center column is the child's body sur-

face area (0.38 m^2 in the example). Compare this to the drug manufacturer's recommended dose. Take and record height and weight measurements at health visits or on hospital admission (or as frequently as daily during an admission) to obtain this information for dose calculation.

Before administering any medication to a child, confirm that the dose ordered is correct for the child's weight or body surface. Every pediatric unit or clinic should have a drug reference, such as the *Physicians' Desk Reference*, for this purpose. However, there are always exceptions to a rule. For example, a child with a gunshot wound may receive more than the usual dose of antibiotics because the risk of infection is very high. A 3-year-old weighing only as much as a 1-year-old would receive a dose of an antibiotic consistent with that given to a 1-year-old (not the child's actual age) because of small body size. Because of such exceptions, an ordered dose that does not conform to the standard dose may still be correct; however, recheck the dose for accuracy with the prescriber before it is administered. Preventing medication errors in children is everyone's responsibility.

Although most medication on hospital units is supplied in unit doses, nurses may still need to calculate fractional dosages (Box 37.4). By verifying drug dosages, nurses serve as a child's first line of defense against dosage error (Cohen, 2005).

Right Route and Time

Possible routes of administration for medicine in children are discussed below. Each of these methods requires special techniques, as most children do not enjoy taking medicine and need strong support during administration.

Right Information

Because so many medications are advertised directly today on television or in magazines, many parents are already aware of drug names and the action of individual drugs. However, because they have been given only snatches of information (or listened to or read only that much), they also may have misconceptions about a particular drug. Be certain when giving medicine to a child or handing a prescription to a parent that you explain the drug's purpose and action, when and how it should be taken, and any side or adverse effects the parent should be aware of. People under stress do not "hear" well, so although the prescriber may have reviewed this same information with them when the prescription was written, this may be the first time they actually hear it.

Checkpoint Question 1

You are going to give acetaminophen (Tylenol) to Terry in the emergency room. She has no ID band in place as yet. What would be the best way to identify her?

a. Ask her what is her name.
b. Tell her you need to know her name.
c. Ask a parent to identify her for you.
d. Ask to see her school bus pass I.D.

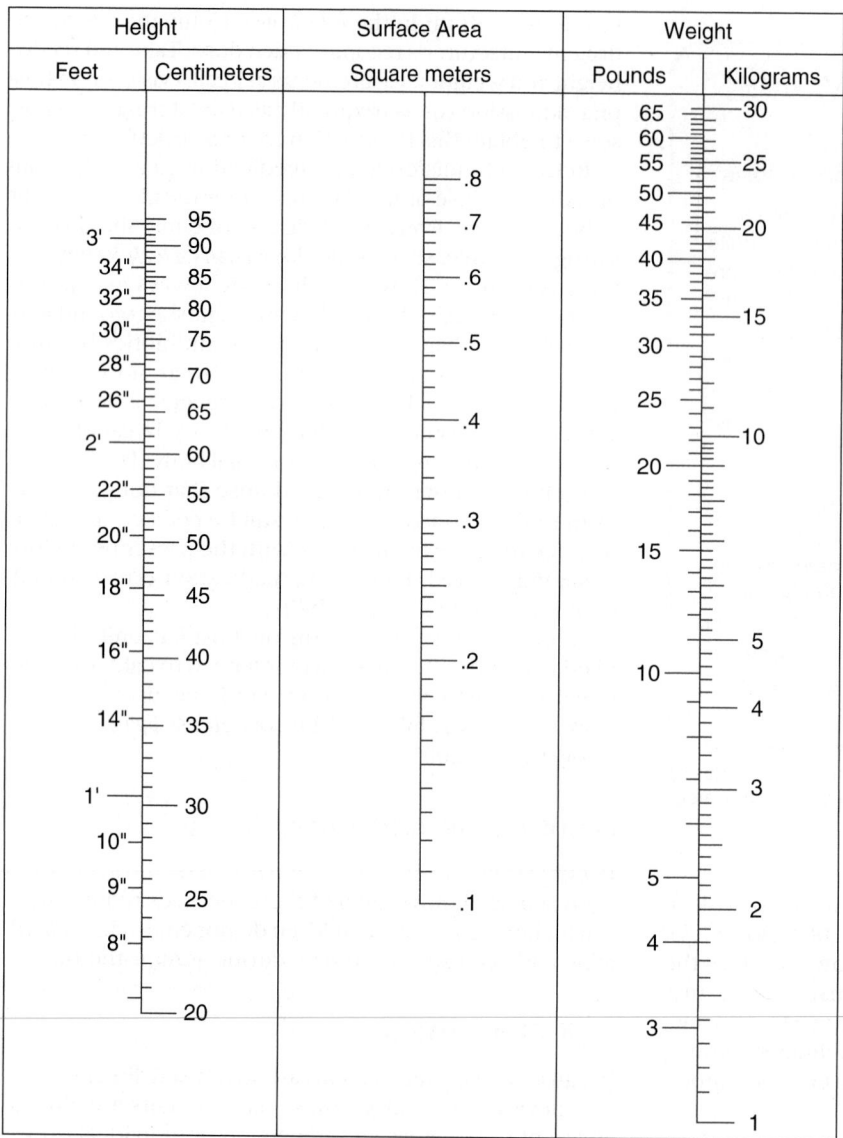

FIGURE 37.1 A nomogram to estimate body surface area. To use such a chart, draw a line from the child's height to the child's weight. The point at which it crosses the middle line is the child's surface area.

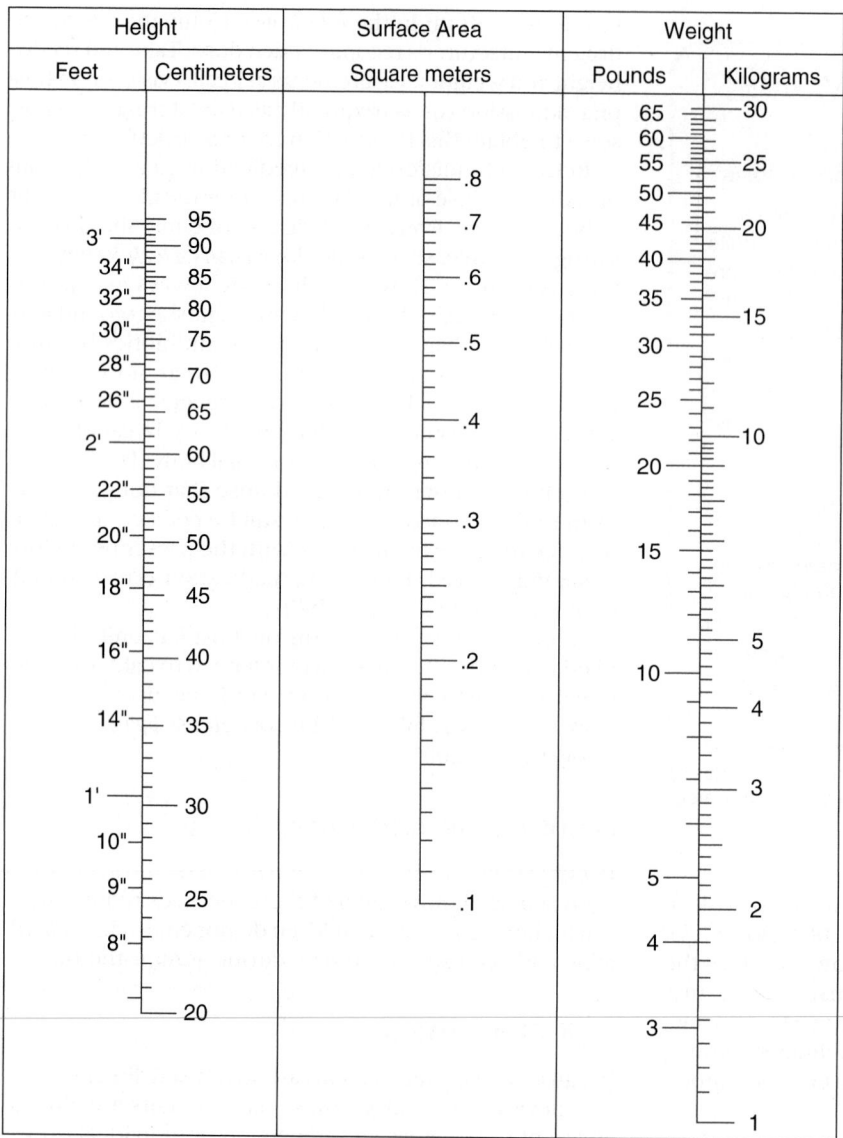

Height		Surface Area	Weight	
Feet	Centimeters	Square meters	Pounds	Kilograms

BOX 37.4

Fractional Calculation of Medication Dosages

To calculate a fractional drug dose use the formula:

$$\frac{\text{Strength Desired (D)}}{\text{Strength You Have (H)}} \times \frac{\text{Quantity Desired (QD)}}{\text{Quantity You Have (QH)}}$$

= Answer

For example, you have an order for 90 mg acetaminophen. It is supplied as 125 mg drug in 5 mL liquid. Using the formula:

$$\frac{90 \text{ mg (D)}}{125 \text{ mg (H)}} \times \frac{\text{QD (what you are asking)}}{5 \text{ mL (QH)}} = ?$$

$125 \text{ QD} = 450(5 \times 90)$

450 divided by 125 = 3.6 mL

Oral Administration

Children younger than 9 years old often have difficulty swallowing tablets. For children younger than 3 years of age, it is virtually impossible. Most oral medication for young children, therefore, is furnished in liquid form.

In infants, oral medication can be given with a medicine dropper or a unit dose syringe (without a needle). Gently restrain the child's arms and head by holding the child against your body with the head raised. Never give medicine with the child lying completely flat; otherwise, the child may choke and aspirate. A crying child is already opening his or her mouth for you; otherwise, gently open the mouth by pressing on the child's chin. Press the bulb of the medicine dropper or use the plunger of the syringe so that the fluid flows slowly into the side of the child's mouth. The end of the syringe or dropper should rest at the side of the infant's mouth to help prevent aspiration (Fig. 37.2). An infant also may be given fluid from a small glass or spoon. Allow the fluid to flow a little at a time so

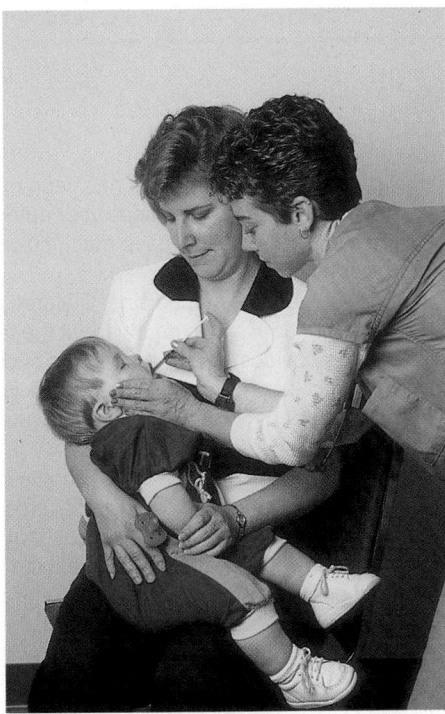

FIGURE 37.2 To administer oral medicine with a syringe, place the medicine at the side of the child's mouth.

that the child has time to swallow between small sips. As oral solutions are pleasantly flavored, most infants resist the first drop but then suck the remainder of the medicine into their mouth.

Because firm pressure was used to give the medicine to the infant, he or she may be frightened afterward. Take time to sit and comfort or let a parent do this afterward. This action is as important as checking the correct dosage of the drug because protecting a child's mental health is as important as protecting physical health.

Preschoolers and early school-age children respond well to rewards such as stickers they can paste into a book each time they take their medicine. For older children, hand them the glass of medicine as if they are expected to take it. Offer a "chaser" if necessary and not contraindicated (Box 37.5). If a child has difficulty swallowing tablets, they can be crushed and added to a teaspoonful of applesauce or a flavored syrup. If pills are not to be chewed (capsules or enteric-coated tablets), be certain the child knows not to chew them. Some children are old enough to swallow tablets but have never done it before. You can use small bits of ice for practice; they melt rapidly and do not stick in the back of the throat or esophagus. Have the child put the ice on the back of the tongue, take a sip of water, and swallow the water. Praise the child for learning this new skill.

Another useful technique to help a child swallow pills is to push them into a teaspoonful of ice cream or pudding. Children tend not to chew this type of food; rather, they swallow it along with the pill. If using this technique, push the pill into the ice cream or pudding in front of the

BOX 37.5 FOCUS ON . . .

COMMUNICATION

You want to give acetaminophen (Tylenol) to Terry, 8 years old, for her fever and sore throat.

Less Effective Communication

Nurse: I have your medicine, Terry. Swallow these for me?

Terry: No. My throat is too sore.

Nurse: If you don't swallow them, I'll put them into a shot and give it that way. And that will really hurt.

Terry: I'd rather get a shot, my throat is so sore.

Nurse: Well, I can't do that. Tylenol doesn't come that way.

Terry: Then I'm not going to take it.

More Effective Communication

Nurse: I have your medicine, Terry. Swallow these for me.

Terry: No. My throat is too sore.

Nurse: That's why I want you to swallow them. They'll take away the soreness.

Terry: I'd rather get a shot, my throat is so sore.

Nurse: This type of medicine has to be swallowed. Would you rather have orange juice or soda pop to drink after it?

Terry: Soda pop.

Nurse: Okay. Take a big swallow and it'll be gone.

The nurse in the first scenario makes some important medication administration errors: first, he *asks* the child if she will swallow the tablets rather than *telling* her to swallow them; second, he threatens the child; even worse, he threatens with a measure he cannot enforce (acetaminophen doesn't come in an injectable form). When the child refuses the request and contradicts his threat, he is left powerless. A better approach is shown in the second scenario: here, the nurse explains the advantage of taking the medicine and conveys that he expects the child to be cooperative. Allowing a secondary choice, such as a choice of beverage, offers children a sense of control but does not allow them to say no to the primary request.

child. The intent is not to hide the pill, but to help the child learn to swallow medicine.

Box 37.6 gives guidelines for administering oral medication to children or teaching parents how to give medicine at home.

What if... Terry's father tells you Terry is such a "picky eater" that she rarely eats a full meal? When should he give a medicine that should be taken with a meal?

BOX 37.6 FOCUS ON . . .

FAMILY TEACHING

Guidelines for Administering Oral Medication

Q. Terry's mother tells you, "All my children fight me any-time they need to be given medicine. How can I get them to take medicine without a battle?"

A. Use the following guidelines to help make this task a bit easier:

- Do not say, "*Can* you drink this for me?" If an adult seems unsure whether a child can do it, the child may develop grave doubts himself.
- Do not say, "*Will* you drink this for me?" This leaves the child the opportunity to say no and creates the awkward position of having to admit that the child really does not have a choice in the matter; the child *must* take the medicine.
- State firmly, "It's time for you to drink your medicine now." Give the child a secondary choice that allows a sense of control: "It is time to drink your medicine now; do you want milk or water to swallow after it?" is a suitable choice, assuming both milk and water are compatible with the medication.
- Never refer to medicine as candy. If they think it is candy, children may help themselves to fatal amounts of medicine when everyone's back is turned.
- Do not bribe children to take medicine. Bribing may work for one dose, but when a second dose is due, the child will ask for a bigger bribe; for a third dose, an even bigger one. At some point (generally reached quickly), it is impossible to supply such large bribes and therefore it is impossible to enforce the rules.
- Do not threaten. Statements such as, "Take this quickly or I'll ask the doctor to make it into a shot" cannot be followed through. The child calls the bluff (many medicines do not come in a form that can be injected intramuscularly), and once more the child is in control. A statement such as, "Take this or I'll call

your doctor" is unfair (the physician has been made the villain) and ultimately undermines your authority (it is obvious that you must not have much power, or you would not need help).

- Do not lie about the taste of medicine. Children expect honesty from adults. If in doubt about the taste, taste it (with the obvious exception of drugs such as digitoxin). Most children's medicines are artificially flavored with raspberry, orange, or cherry syrup, so they do not taste bad.
- If a medicine tastes bitter, mix it with a spoonful of strained applesauce or a teaspoonful of flavored syrup. Do not mix medicine with a full jar of baby food, because the child will then have to eat the entire jar of food to get all of the medicine. As a rule, encourage children to take medicine straight, then follow it with a pleasant-tasting drink to take away any bitter taste.
- If a medicine is supplied in tablet form, crush or dissolve it in water and mix it with syrup or apple-sauce for a better taste if appropriate. Be certain before removing the particles from a capsule that the medicine will work properly when not in capsule form: some are encapsulated to keep them from dissolving in the stomach and to bring them into the intestine, where they have their therapeutic effect. The same precaution must be followed when giving enteric-coated tablets.
- Never leave medicine by a child's bed for the child to take "in a minute" or "after your shower." The child may become involved with another activity "in a minute" and will not take it, or when he or she is not looking, a smaller child could find the medicine appealing and swallow it.

Intranasal Administration

Having someone drop medicine into the nose can be very uncomfortable. Tell the child you understand this, but that the medicine is important because it will help him or her get better. Tell the child what you are going to do: "I'm going to place two drops of medicine into your nose. Then I want you to sniff for me [demonstrate]. Then I'll put two drops into the other side of your nose and I want you to sniff again."

Place the child on his or her back. A school-age child could extend the head over the side of the bed so that it is lower than the trunk. Preschoolers generally are too frightened by this strange position and do better with a pillow under their shoulders so that their head extends over the pillow and rests downward. An infant may need to be restrained in a mummy restraint for nose drop administration (see Chapter 36 for a discussion of appropriate restraints).

Instill the appropriate number of drops into one nostril. Turn the child's head to the side—to the left after the left nostril, to the right after the right nostril—so that the medicine stays in the nose longer. If the child is a preschooler or older, ask him or her to further "sniff" the medicine. Have the child remain in the head-flat position for at least 1 minute to let the medicine come in contact with the mucous membrane of the nose. If a child gets up immediately, the medicine will flow out and will be less effective.

Give a child high praise even if he or she did not cooperate at all. Praise tells the child you understand how hard it was to stay still.

More and more medicines today are being provided as liquids to be sprayed into the nostrils. Children over about age 6 can do this independently but need to be introduced to the technique. Acknowledge that spraying a liquid into the nose is uncomfortable because it tickles or causes a sneezing sensation. Have the child sit or stand upright, hold the spray bottle upright with the tip just inside one side of

attention to the planned treatment regimen or care priorities sooner than those without close friends or relatives to whom they can turn for comfort and support. For the latter, you may need to act not only as a source of information and support but also as a sounding board and advocate until the parents can begin to develop positive coping mechanisms that will help them come to terms with this unexpected event. Referrals for support groups may be beneficial, allowing parents to learn they are not alone in this situation.

● *Implementation*

Nursing interventions for a baby born physically challenged include immediate life-sustaining measures such as providing for adequate intake of nutrients when a disorder prevents the infant from sucking. Educating the parents about pre- and posttreatment procedures and encouraging them to hold, touch, and talk with their baby are especially important to the future emotional well-being of the child and family.

Parents may suffer a loss of self-esteem with the child's birth, feeling as if the baby is proof that something in the combination of their genes or the prenatal environment they provided was inadequate (Box 39.2). They may need to hear positive comments about themselves and need to be given support until they can realize that by caring for the child they are accomplishing more, not less, than other couples.

You can expect parents to move through the same stages of grief as those whose child has died at birth. Chapter 56 describes those stages and helpful nursing interventions in more detail.

Parents are acutely aware of what people think of their child. They watch closely how nurses and other health care providers handle their baby to see if they are giving as much attention to their baby as to other babies. To encourage the parents to accept the child, be certain to treat the child in the same manner as any other—for example, rocking the baby after feeding or cooing and talking to the baby as much as with other babies. Otherwise, parents may think that if a professional finds their child distasteful, how will they dare show the child to their family and friends? If you are able to look past the anomaly to the whole child, however, they begin to do so, too. Through positive role modeling, you can set the stage for healthy parent–child interaction every time you handle an infant born with a physical or developmental challenge.

Parents may also need the assistance of support groups and community organizations. The following organizations can be helpful sources of support for parents:

- National Easter Seal Society (*www.easterseals.com*)
- Spina Bifida Association of America (*www.sbaa.org*)
- March of Dimes Birth Disorders Foundation (*www.marchofdimes.com*)
- American Cleft Palate/Craniofacial Association (*www.cleftline.org*)

● *Outcome Evaluation*

Evaluation should focus on expected outcomes established for a child's physical health and developmental needs, as well as the family's ability to cope with whatever special care and growth needs the child may have in the future. Be sure parents have numbers to call for questions, follow-up care, and support.

Evidence suggesting achievement of expected outcomes may include:

- Child is ambulatory with walker by 2 years of age.
- Parent describes positive features of child by 2 weeks.
- Parents state they understand talipes anomaly is a correctable condition by 1 month.

BOX 39.2 FOCUS ON . . .

DIVERSITY OF CARE

The cause of most congenital anomalies is unknown, although they probably arise from a combination of environmental and genetic factors. Still, many people persist in believing that infants with congenital anomalies are born to people less deserving than others or to those who have sinned or have been looked on by someone with envy during pregnancy. That eating raisins during pregnancy causes brown spots, and that strawberries cause hemangiomas, are beliefs that are still prevalent.

The way that parents carry infants may contribute to the formation of hip dysplasia. Infants who are carried straddled on their parents' hips, the way Latin American mothers carry their infants, may have less hip dysplasia than those carried with their legs consistently brought together, such as Native American infants carried on swaddling boards.

New parents need a chance to talk about why they believe their child's disorder occurred, to relieve their guilt that they were the cause and to allow them to regain sufficient self-esteem to be able to raise a child with a congenital disorder.

Ensuring that women ingest a folic acid supplement during pregnancy has decreased the incidence of ventral and dorsal nonclosure disorders. Teaching women from all cultures that taking this important supplement before and during pregnancy is a major nursing responsibility.

RESPONSIBILITIES OF THE NURSE AT THE BIRTH OF AN INFANT BORN PHYSICALLY OR DEVELOPMENTALLY CHALLENGED

Most physicians and nurse-midwives believe that relating the news of congenital physical or developmental anomalies to parents is their responsibility. However, because the physician or nurse-midwife must deliver the placenta and suture the perineum if an episiotomy was used for birth, if a neonatal specialist is not immediately available, many minutes may pass before this person is ready to make a second inspection of the baby, assess the extent of the disorder from the physical symptoms present, and tell the parents about the baby's condition and prognosis. This delay affects the parents in two ways: It leaves them believing they have just given birth to a perfect child among people who do not share their enthusiasm, or they have just given birth to a child so deformed all the professionals in the room find it too horrible to even talk to them. Because parents are aware of the atmosphere in a birthing room, the second response is by far more likely. In terms of parent–child interaction, this response is unhealthy. Parents may begin anticipatory grieving for what they believe is a severely deformed child. Even when they are told later the disorder is not extensive and is easily correctable, and that as soon as the correction is made the child will be fine, the anticipatory grief reaction may be hard to stop. They may continue to cut themselves off emotionally from their child.

For this reason, nurses need to be familiar with the most frequently encountered physical or developmental anomalies so that as the person who at that moment in the birth process is most available for patient education, they can explain the problem to parents. In other instances, nurses must be ready to serve as back-up informants to answer parents' questions after they have been told by a primary care provider their child has been born less than perfect. It is probably best to explain to parents what the disorder consists of and what the usual prognosis is before showing the baby to them. Parents may find it hard to look at an infant with a cleft lip or palate or exposed abdominal contents, for example, and also listen. Their minds are so consumed with the sight, so unlike the child they had imagined, that they cannot hear. A typical explanation would be: "Your baby's upper lip isn't completely formed. That's called a cleft lip. Your doctor will call one of the plastic surgeons here to look at your baby. This is a problem that can be repaired so well surgically you'll barely be able to tell your baby had this problem. I'll bring the baby over so you can see her. Remember when you look at her this can be repaired. She seems perfect in every other way."

These statements define and limit the problem for the parents. They also give them direction about where and how they should proceed in beginning to seek help for their child.

GASTROINTESTINAL SYSTEM PHYSICAL AND DEVELOPMENTAL DISORDERS

Many of the most common congenital anomalies involve the GI system because the GI tract forms first as a solid tube, then undergoes canalization. If this canalization does not occur, a partial or complete blockage or obstruction can occur. Other disorders of the tract, such as cleft lip and cleft palate, are the results of midline closure failure extremely early in intrauterine life. All of these disorders can interfere with an infant's ability to feed at birth. You may need to reinforce a mother's resolve to breast-feed as appropriate to aid in her success with this method of feeding.

Ankyloglossia (Tongue-Tie)

Ankyloglossia is an abnormal restriction of the tongue caused by an abnormally tight **frenulum,** the membrane attached to the lower anterior tip of the tongue (Kalu & Moss, 2004). Normally, in newborns, the frenulum appears short and is positioned near the tip of the tongue. As the anterior portion of the infant's tongue grows, the frenulum becomes located farther back. In most instances, therefore, an infant suspected of being tongue-tied has a normal tongue at birth; it just seems short to parents who are unaware of a newborn's appearance. This condition rarely causes speech difficulty or destructive pressure on gingival tissue. If it does, then surgical release can be performed, but this is rare.

Showing parents other newborns or photographs of normal tongues is helpful in convincing them a short frenulum is normal. Explore with them why they are concerned. Is there a child in the family with a speech disorder or a cleft lip and palate? Do the parents need assurance in any other way that their child is all right?

Thyroglossal Cyst

A thyroglossal cyst arises from an embryogenic fault that leaves a cyst formed at the base of the tongue, which then drains through a **fistula** (opening) to the anterior surface of the neck (Lindstrom et al., 2004). This condition may occur as a dominantly inherited trait. The cyst may involve the hyoid bone (the bone at the anterior surface of the neck at the root of the tongue) or may contain aberrant thyroid gland tissue. As the cyst fills with fluid, swelling and obstruction can lead to respiratory difficulty from pressure on the trachea. If infected, the cyst appears swollen and reddened, with drainage of mucus or pus from the anterior neck.

The cyst is surgically removed to avoid future infection of the space or, if thyroid tissue is present, the possibility of carcinoma later in life. Observe infants closely in the immediate postoperative period for respiratory distress, because the operative area will develop some edema from surgical trauma. Position infants on their sides so secretions drain freely from their mouths. Intravenous fluid therapy is given after surgery until the edema at the incision recedes somewhat and swallowing is safe once more (approximately 24 hours). If the mother is breast-feeding but the infant is NPO, encourage her to express her milk manually to preserve her milk supply. Observe infants closely the first time they take fluid orally to be certain they do not aspirate. Be certain parents feed them before they are discharged from the surgical unit so they can see that the infant is swallowing safely. This is important to help them develop confidence in themselves as parents and their ability to feed the infant at home in a relaxed and comfortable way.

Cleft Lip and Palate

The maxillary and median nasal processes normally fuse between weeks 5 and 8 of intrauterine life. In infants with **cleft lip,** the fusion fails to occur in varying degrees, causing this disorder to range from a small notch in the upper

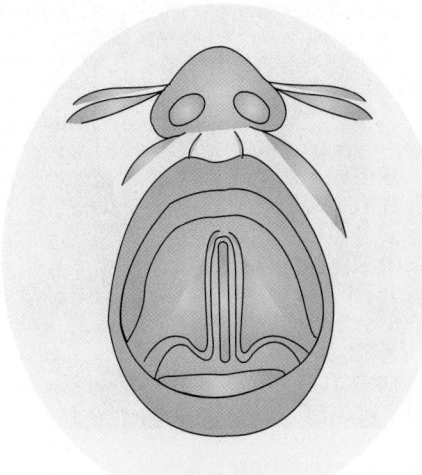

FIGURE 39.1 Appearance of a cleft palate. Both the hard and soft palate are involved.

lip to total separation of the lip and facial structure up into the floor of the nose, with even the upper teeth and gingiva absent. The deviation may be unilateral or bilateral. The nose is generally flattened because the incomplete fusion of the upper lip has allowed it to expand in a horizontal dimension (see Fig. 7.12). Cleft lip is more prevalent among boys than girls. It occurs at a rate of approximately 1 in every 700 live births (Kirschner, Carman-Dillon, & Low, 2003).

Cleft lip occurs as a familial tendency or most likely occurs from the transmission of multiple genes. It is twice as prevalent in the Japanese population and occurs rarely in African Americans. Formation may be aided by teratogenic factors present during weeks 5 to 8 of intrauterine life, such as a viral infection or possibly a deficiency of folic acid. Parents of a child with a cleft lip should be referred for genetic counseling to ensure they understand that future children are at a greater risk than usual for this problem.

The palatal process closes at approximately weeks 9 to 12 of intrauterine life. A **cleft palate,** an opening of the palate, is usually on the midline and may involve the anterior hard palate, the posterior soft palate, or both (Fig. 39.1). It may be a separate anomaly, but as a rule it occurs in conjunction with a cleft lip. As a single entity, it tends to occur more frequently in girls than boys. Like cleft lip, it appears to be the result of polygenic inheritance or environmental influences. In connection with cleft lip, the incidence is approximately 1 in every 1,000 births. As a single entity, it occurs in approximately 1 in every 2,000 births (Kirschner, Carman-Dillon & Low, 2003).

Assessment

Cleft lip may be detected by a sonogram while the infant is in utero. If not detected then, it is readily apparent on inspection at birth. Cleft palate can be determined by depressing the newborn's tongue with a tongue blade. This reveals the total palate and the extent of a cleft palate. Be sure to have good lighting to visualize the palate clearly.

Because cleft palate is a component of many syndromes, a child with a cleft palate must be assessed for other congenital anomalies.

Therapeutic Management

If a cleft lip is discovered while the infant is still in utero, fetal surgery can repair the condition, although this procedure is not usually attempted. In many children, however, the disorder is not discovered until birth. For these infants, a cleft lip is repaired surgically shortly after birth, sometimes at the time of the initial hospital stay or between 2 and 10 weeks of age. Because the deviation of the lip interferes with nutrition, infants may be a better surgical risk at birth than they are after a month or more of poor nourishment. Early repair also helps infants experience the pleasure of sucking as soon as possible. It is equally important from a psychological standpoint that these disorders be repaired early. Parents may find it extremely difficult to bond with an infant whose face is deformed in this way. This is not a sign of a "bad" parent, but it is reality and a problem that requires intervention. A revision of the original repair may be necessary when the child reaches 4 to 6 years of age.

The repair of cleft palate is usually postponed until a child is 6 to 18 months old to allow the anatomic change in the palate contour that occurs during the first year of life to take place. Repairs made before this change (the palate arch increases) may be ineffective and may have to be repeated.

Currently, the results of surgical repair of cleft lip and cleft palate are excellent (Fig. 39.2). It is helpful to show

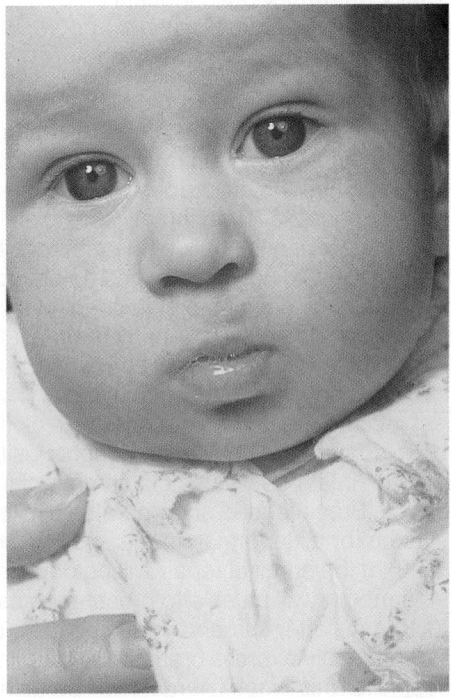

FIGURE 39.2 Infant showing surgical repair of cleft lip. Parents can be encouraged that the results of cleft lip repair are generally excellent. (Photo Researchers, Inc.)

parents photographs of babies with good repairs to assure them that their child's outcome can also be this successful. Don't use the older term for this condition, *harelip,* when talking with parents about the problem. Before modern surgical techniques were available, children were left with large lip scars, gross speech impediments, and a poor appearance after surgery. The word "harelip" tends to be associated with these negative outcomes rather than with the current positive outlook.

Some infants with a cleft lip have an accompanying deviated nasal septum, which may need to be repaired in later years for good air exchange. Because palate repair narrows the upper dental arch or because the original cleft may have involved the dental arch, there may be less space in the upper jaw for the eruption of teeth, causing poor teeth alignment. These children need follow-up treatment by a pedodontist, or a dentist skilled in children's dental problems, so that as the child grows, extractions or realignment of teeth can be done as indicated.

NURSING DIAGNOSES AND RELATED INTERVENTIONS

————————●————————

Nursing Diagnosis: Risk for imbalanced nutrition, less than body requirements, related to feeding problems caused by cleft lip or palate

Outcome Evaluation: Child ingests an adequate diet of 50 kcal/lb (110 kcal/kg) in 24 hours; weight is maintained within 10% of birthweight.

Preoperative Period. Before a cleft lip or palate is repaired, feeding the infant is a problem because the infant has difficulty maintaining suction. In addition, it is important that the child does not aspirate.

It may be possible for an infant with a cleft lip to breast-feed because the bulk of the mother's breast tends to form a seal against the incomplete upper lip. Although the baby needs the enjoyment of sucking, some surgeons do not want a baby to breast-feed or suck on a nipple before surgical correction of the disorder to avoid any local bruising of tissue. Therefore, the best feeding method for the child with cleft lip may be to support the baby in an upright position and feed the infant gently using a commercial cleft lip nipple. A Breck feeder, an apparatus similar to a bulb syringe, or a Haberman feeder may be used (Fig. 39.3). If the surgical repair will be done immediately, the mother will be able to breast-feed as early as 7 to 10 days after surgery. Teach her how to pump or manually express breast milk to maintain a milk supply for this time. If surgery will be delayed for 1 month, she will need to decide whether she wants to continue to express milk for this long a time; continuing support from the nursing staff could be important to encourage her to do this.

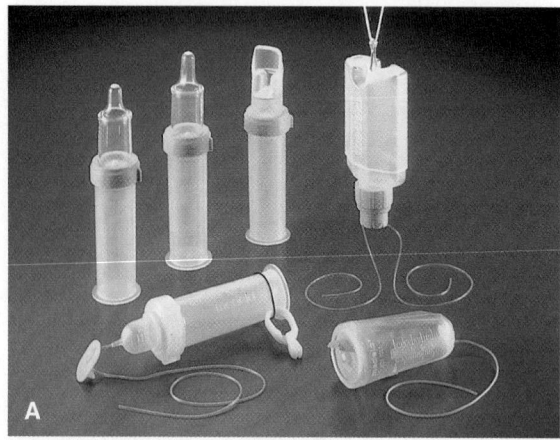

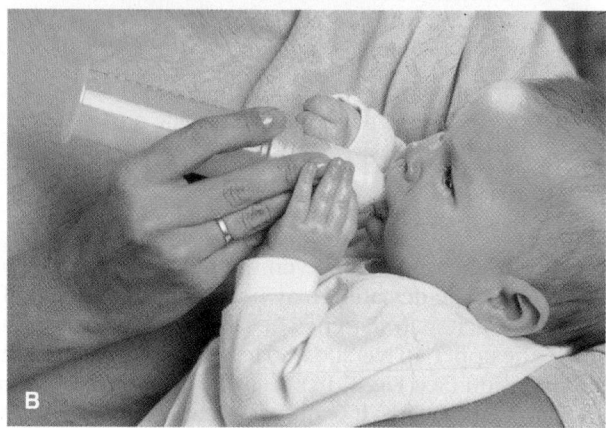

FIGURE 39.3 (A) Specialty feeding devices used for infants with cleft lip and cleft palate. **(B)** An infant uses a Haberman Feeder™.

Be certain an infant with a cleft lip is bubbled well after feeding because of a tendency to swallow air caused by the inability to grasp a nipple or syringe edge securely with the mouth. If a cleft extends to the nares, an infant will breathe through the mouth, causing the oral mucous membranes and lips to become dry. Offering small sips of fluid between feedings can help keep the mucous membranes moist and prevent cracks and fissures that could lead to infection.

Infants with cleft palate cannot suck effectively either, because pressing their tongue or a nipple against the roof of their mouth could force milk up into their pharynx, leading to aspiration. The most successful method for feeding this infant, like the child with cleft lip, is to use a commercial cleft palate nipple that has an extra flange of rubber to close the roof of the mouth. The nipple can be used with a plastic bottle that can be squeezed gently to increase the flow of the feeding to compensate for poor sucking. A Breck feeder may also be used.

If surgery is delayed beyond 6 months of age or the time solid food would be introduced, teach parents to be certain any food offered is soft.

Particles of coarse food could invade the naso-pharynx and cause aspiration. Infants whose surgery is delayed to this point can be fitted with a plastic palate guard to form a synthetic palate and help prevent this.

Postoperative Period. After surgery for cleft lip or palate, an infant is kept NPO for approximately 4 hours. The infant is then introduced to liquids (plain water). Begin the process with only a small amount to prevent vomiting.

It is important that no tension is placed on a lip suture line; avoiding tension helps keep the sutures from pulling apart and leaving a large scar. During this immediate postoperative period, the infant is usually fed using a specialized feeder because this causes less suture line tension than bottle- or breast-feeding.

After palate surgery, liquids are generally contin-ued for the first 3 or 4 days, and then a soft diet is followed until healing is complete. Ask the parents what fluids the child prefers so they will be available after surgery.

After a cleft palate repair, when the child begins eating soft food, he or she should not use a spoon, because a child will invariably put it against the roof of the mouth and possibly disrupt sutures. If being fed rather than being allowed to use a spoon himself evokes an intense reaction, it is better to leave a child on a liquid diet until the sutures are removed. Be certain milk is not included in the first fluids of-fered because milk curds tend to adhere to the su-ture line. After a feeding, offer the child clear water to rinse the suture line and keep it as clean as possible.

Nursing Diagnosis: Risk for ineffective airway clearance related to oral surgery

Outcome Evaluation: Child's respiratory rate remains between 20 to 30 respirations per minute without retractions or obvious distress.

Because of the local edema that occurs after cleft lip or palate surgery, observe children closely in the immediate postoperative period for respira-tory distress. Before surgery, the infant with a cleft lip breathed through the mouth. After surgery, the infant now has to breathe through the nose, pos-sibly adding to respiratory difficulty. Generally, however, this is not a problem because newborns normally are strict nose-breathers.

Infants may need suction to remove mucus, blood, and unswallowed saliva. When performing suctioning, be gentle and do not touch the suture line with the catheter. After cleft lip surgery, place infants on their side to allow mouth secretions to drain. Support them well so they don't turn onto their abdomen, as this could put pressure on the suture line, possibly tearing it. Placing them in an infant chair is another possibility.

Nursing Diagnosis: Impaired tissue integrity at inci-sion line related to cleft lip or cleft palate surgery

Outcome Evaluation: Incision line appears clean and intact and free of erythema or drainage during postoperative period.

After cleft lip surgery, the suture line is held in close approximation by a Logan bar (a wire bow taped to both cheeks; Fig. 39.4) or an adhesive bandage such as a Band-Aid simulating a bar that brings together the incision line but does not cover the incision. Assess the Logan bar or Band-Aid-simulated bar after each feeding or cleaning of the suture line to be certain it is secure and continues to protect the suture line from tension. Furnish ade-quate pain relief so, if possible, the infant does not cry, because crying increases tension on the sutures. To help avoid crying, try to anticipate the infant's needs. Have formula ready to feed on demand—do not wait until after the infant is awake and crying. Help the parents use whatever mea-sures, such as rocking, carrying, or holding, that are necessary to make the infant feel secure and com-fortable. The baby also will need to be bubbled well after a feeding because there is a tendency to swal-low more air than the average infant.

Nothing hard or sharp must come in contact with a recent cleft suture line. Observe infants after palate repair carefully to be certain they do not put toys with sharp edges into their mouths. They should not use a straw to drink, nor should they brush their own teeth—they will certainly brush the suture line accidentally. Keep elbow restraints in place as necessary so they do not put their fingers in their mouth and poke or pull at the sutures. Most children run their tongue over their sutures because of the odd feeling in the roof of their mouth, and most children this age do not respond to a caution not to do this. Because this often occurs when chil-dren have nothing to think about, help the parents provide diversional activities such as reading or singing to them.

If parents will be continuing to give an analgesic such as acetaminophen (Tylenol) after they return home, be certain they are aware of the correct dosage and time schedule for administration. Be

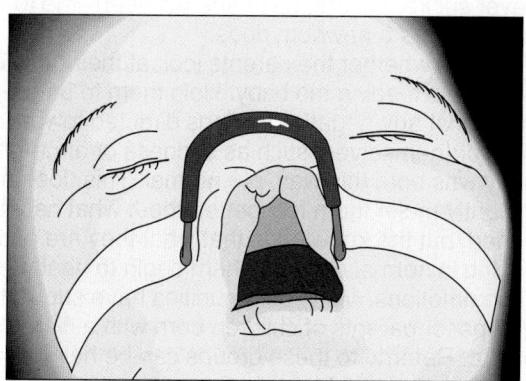

FIGURE 39.4 A Logan bar is an apparatus that may be used to protect the surgical incision for a cleft lip repair.

sure parents can demonstrate measures to protect the suture line at home until healing is complete.

Nursing Diagnosis: Risk for infection related to surgical incision

Outcome Evaluation: Infant's temperature is below 98.6°F (37°C) axillary; incision site is clean, dry, and intact without erythema or foul drainage.

Infection, and subsequent scarring, may result if crusts from serous drainage are allowed to form on a cleft lip suture line. Most surgeons prescribe cleaning the suture line with sterile water, sterile saline, or 50% hydrogen peroxide in sterile water used with sterile cotton-tipped applicators after every feeding or whenever the normal serum that forms on suture lines accumulates. Use a smooth, gentle, rolling motion to apply the solution. Do not rub, because this can loosen sutures. If hydrogen peroxide is used, it will foam as it reacts with the protein particles at the suture line. Rinse the area with sterile water afterward. Gently dry the suture line with a dry sterile cotton-tipped applicator. Remember that an infant has sutures on the inside of the lip that need the same meticulous care as those visible on the outside.

Nursing Diagnosis: Risk for impaired parenting related to the birth of an infant who is physically challenged

Outcome Evaluation: Parents state a belief in a positive outcome for child; demonstrate positive coping behaviors, evidenced by holding and helping with infant care.

To promote bonding, parents need to hold and interact with their infant during both the preoperative and postoperative periods. Caution them the incision line will appear swollen in the immediate postoperative period. Reassure them this appearance will improve over time. As soon as the child's sutures have been removed, the infant may be bottle-fed (with an ordinary bottle) or breast-fed. Caution both the breast-feeding mother (who has been maintaining her milk supply through expression) and the formula-feeding mother that because the infant has never sucked before, he or she will need time to learn, just as a newborn does.

Notice whether the parents look at their baby's face while feeding the baby. Help them to understand that any negative feelings directed toward the child or themselves, such as sadness or anger their baby was born this way, are normal. This does not instantly make them feel better about what has happened, but the knowledge that what they are experiencing is normal can help them begin to deal with such emotions. Many communities have support groups for parents of children born with a cleft lip or palate. Referral to these groups can be helpful (Pelchat et al., 2004).

Nursing Diagnosis: Risk for situational low self-esteem related to facial surgery

Outcome Evaluation: Child participates in normal childhood activities that involve contact with other people; states activities he or she enjoys at health care visits; demonstrates age-appropriate developmental milestones.

If a scar remains after cleft lip surgery, a child may need some help adjusting to it until a cosmetic repair can be completed later in life. Reinforce the child's positive attributes, stressing that the scar is only one small aspect of who he or she is. As children reach adolescence, you may need to review the familial inheritance pattern of cleft lip so adolescents are informed of the possible risk of transmission to their own children.

Nursing Diagnosis: Risk for infection (ear) related to altered slope of eustachian tube with cleft palate surgery

Outcome Evaluation: Parents state possible signs and symptoms of ear infection and state importance of early treatment; parents list signs of diminished hearing and appropriate agencies for support and guidance.

Changing the contour of the palate when it is repaired also changes the slope of the eustachian tube to the middle ear. This can lead to a high incidence of middle ear infection (otitis media) because organisms are more readily able to reach this area. Review the signs of infection (e.g., fever, pain, pulling on the ear, or discharge from the ear) with parents of children with a cleft palate. Also remind them of the importance of reporting pharyngeal infection to their primary care provider promptly so it can be treated before the infection spreads to the middle ear. Because the eustachian tube may remain partially closed because of its changed position, serous otitis media (accumulation of fluid in the middle ear) also tends to occur more frequently in these children than in others. If this happens, myringotomy tubes may be inserted to drain middle ear fluid and help protect hearing. Be certain that parents understand the need for routine screening for hearing loss during childhood, because this is a common early sign of serous otitis media.

Nursing Diagnosis: Risk for impaired verbal communication related to cleft palate

Outcome Evaluation: Family members voice satisfaction with child's speech; developmental milestone of clearly articulated two-word sentences by age 2 years is met.

Infants with a cleft palate will begin to make speech sounds at the normal time (age 2 months), although their speech may be guttural and harsh. By 9 months, when other infants begin to say meaningful words ("bye-bye," "mama," "dada"), assuming the cleft palate is still unrepaired, their sounds will be unclear. Some parents try to discourage their baby from talking, thinking if he or she does not talk until after the cleft palate repair is made, a speech impediment will not develop. Speech occurs at a specified developmental time, however, and despite the un-fused palate should be encouraged at these age-appropriate times. A child with a cleft palate can enunciate vowel sounds with the most clarity, so these are the sounds a parent should encourage the child to voice. Words such as "me," "they," "no," "mama," "home," "moon," "rain," "yell," and "row" are words consisting largely of vowel sounds and can be enunciated most clearly by the child before a cleft palate repair.

Almost all children who have had cleft palates continue to have accompanying speech problems after the repair. The soft palate must function for the child to pronounce "p" and "b" sounds. If cleft palate surgery is going to be delayed much past age 2 years (as might happen if the child has other con-genital anomalies, such as heart disease), a plastic prosthesis to cover the incomplete palate may be prescribed. This allows the child to articulate more normally.

Children do not spontaneously outgrow faulty speech patterns, so training by a speech therapist may be necessary. Commonly used exercises chil-dren are asked to perform include blowing games, such as blowing a feather or a table tennis ball (a blowing motion is what is required to pronounce "p" and "b").

Pierre Robin Syndrome

The Pierre Robin syndrome is a triad of micrognathia (small mandible), cleft palate, and glossoptosis (a tongue malpo-sitioned downward). It is an example of cleft palate occur-ring as only one part of a syndrome (Wagener et al., 2003). Children may have associated disorders of congenital glau-coma, cataracts, or cardiac disorders. They need thorough physical and genetic assessments to be certain that none of these associated disorders is present.

Observe all infants with Pierre Robin syndrome care-fully to be certain they are not developing an airway ob-struction. They may need frequent nasopharyngeal suction to remove unswallowed saliva. Beginning at birth, children with this syndrome are apt to have episodes in which they have difficulty breathing because, due to their small jaws, their tongues are too large for their mouths. This discrep-ancy causes the tongue to drop backward and obstruct the airway. Obstruction is most likely to occur when the child is in a supine position. Unlike well infants, no infant with this syndrome should be placed in a supine position to sleep; they are in grave danger of anoxia if left in this posi-tion. Use a side-lying position instead. Occasionally, infants have such extensive airway obstruction that attaching a su-ture to the anterior aspect of the tongue and pulling it for-ward is used to provide relief (Kirschner et al., 2003). The suture is attached to the mucous membrane of the lower lip, creating an artificial tongue-tied condition.

Parents need instructions to feed these infants with the same care and concern given all children with cleft palate. A gastrostomy tube or button may be inserted to relieve feeding difficulty (see Chapter 36). As the child grows older, the jaw will grow somewhat, although the mandible will always be small. Growth, coupled with a repair of the cleft palate, will decrease the respiratory problems.

Parents of the child with Pierre Robin syndrome take on a great deal of responsibility when they assume their in-fant's care. Be certain they have the name and number of a health care provider they can call when they have ques-tions. Many of these parents grow exhausted during the first few weeks of their child's life, afraid they may fall soundly asleep at night and miss their child having respira-tory difficulty. As their confidence grows in their ability to provide care, this problem lessens, but it may be months or even years before a high level of confidence is achieved.

Tracheoesophageal Atresia and Fistula

Between weeks 4 and 8 of intrauterine life, the laryngotra-cheal groove develops into the larynx, trachea, and begin-ning lung tissue. The esophageal lumen forms parallel to this. A number of anomalies may occur if the trachea and esophagus are affected by some teratogen that does not allow the two organs to separate but remain connected.

Esophageal atresia is obstruction of the esophagus. Often a fistula (opening) occurs between the closed esoph-agus and the trachea. The five usual types of esophageal atresia that occur are:

1. The esophagus ends in a blind pouch; there is a tra-cheoesophageal fistula between the distal part of the esophagus and the trachea (Fig. 39.5A).
2. The esophagus ends in a blind pouch; there is no con-nection to the trachea (see Fig. 39.5B).
3. A fistula is present between an otherwise normal esophagus and trachea (see Fig. 39.5C).
4. The esophagus ends in a blind pouch. A fistula con-nects the blind pouch of the proximal esophagus to the trachea (see Fig. 39.5D).
5. There is a blind end portion of the esophagus. Fistulas are present between both widely spaced segments of the esophagus and the trachea (see Fig. 39.5E).

These are all serious disorders because during a feed-ing, milk can fill the blind esophagus and overflow into the trachea, or a fistula can allow milk to enter the tra-chea, resulting in aspiration. The incidence of tracheo-esophageal fistula is approximately 1 in 3,000 live births (Katz & Conway, 2003).

Assessment

Tracheoesophageal atresia must be ruled out in any infant born to a woman with hydramnios (excessive amniotic fluid). Hydramnios occurs because normally a fetus swal-lows amniotic fluid during intrauterine life. A fetus with a tracheoesophageal atresia cannot swallow, however, so the amount of amniotic fluid can grow abnormally large. Many infants with tracheoesophageal fistula are born preterm because of the accompanying hydramnios, com-pounding their original problem with immaturity. The in-fant needs to be examined carefully for other congenital anomalies that could have occurred from the teratogenic

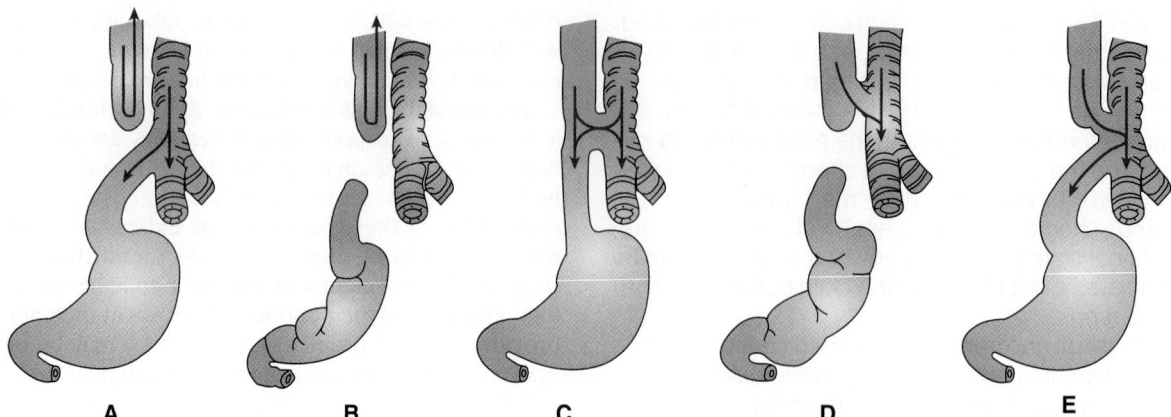

A   B   C   D   E

FIGURE 39.5 Esophageal atresia and tracheoesophageal fistula. (**A**) In the most common type of esophageal atresia, the esophagus ends in a blind pouch. The trachea communicates by a fistula with the lower esophagus and stomach (approximately 90% of infants with the defect have this type). (**B**) Both upper and lower segments end in blind pouches (5% to 8% of infants with the defect have this type). (**C**) Both upper and lower segments communicate with the trachea (2% to 3% of infants with the defect have this type). (**D**) Very rarely, the upper segment ends in a blind pouch and communicates by a fistula to the trachea, or (**E**) a fistula connects to both upper and lower segments of the esophagus.

effect at the same week in gestation, such as vertebral, anorectal, and renal disorders (VATER syndrome).

Diagnosing a tracheoesophageal fistula before an infant is first fed is important. Otherwise, the infant will cough, become cyanotic, and have obvious difficulty breathing as fluid is aspirated. A newborn who has so much mucus in the mouth that he or she appears to be blowing bubbles should be suspected of having tracheoesophageal fistula. The condition can be diagnosed with certainty if a catheter cannot be passed through the infant's esophagus to the stomach or the stomach contents cannot be aspirated. Use of a firm catheter is necessary, because a soft one will curl in a blind-end esophagus and appear to have passed. If a radiopaque catheter is used, it can be demonstrated coiled in the blind end of the esophagus on x-ray. A flat-plate x-ray of the abdomen also may reveal a stomach distended with the air that is passing from the trachea into the esophagus and stomach. Either a barium swallow or a bronchial endoscopy examination can also reveal the blind-end esophagus and fistula.

Therapeutic Management

Emergency surgery for the infant with tracheoesophageal fistula is essential to prevent the development of pneumonia from leakage of stomach secretions into the lungs or dehydration or an electrolyte imbalance from lack of oral intake. Antibiotics may be prescribed to help prevent infection. A gastrostomy may be performed (under local anesthesia) and the tube allowed to drain by gravity to keep the stomach empty of secretions and prevent reflux into the lungs. Upper right lobe pneumonia from aspiration is one of the major complications of this disorder.

Surgery consists of closing the fistula and anastomosing the esophageal segments. It may be necessary to complete the surgery in different stages and to use a portion of the colon to complete the anastomosis if the esophageal seg-

ments are far apart from each other. Observe infants closely at postoperative days 7 to 10, when sutures dissolve, because leaks occurring at anastomosis sites can occur at this time. If this occurs, fluid and air leak out into the chest cavity, and pneumothorax (collapse of the lung) can occur.

In some infants, some stenosis or stricture at the anastomosis site remains. If this occurs, esophageal dilatation at periodic intervals to keep the repaired esophagus fully patent may be necessary. Gastroesophageal reflux may also occur after a repair if the esophagus is left shorter than usual (Kovesi & Rubin, 2004). This can lead to recurrent fistula formation from the presence of stomach acid in the esophagus.

The ultimate prognosis for children with this disorder will depend on the extent of the repair necessary, the condition of the child at the time of surgery, and the presence or absence of other congenital anomalies. If the disorder is amenable to surgical correction, and surgery can be performed before pneumonia develops, the prognosis is good. However, the mortality rate for the condition remains high because of the presence of other congenital disorders and low birthweight that often accompanies the tracheal abnormality.

NURSING DIAGNOSES AND RELATED INTERVENTIONS

Outcomes established for the child with tracheoesophageal fistula must be realistic in terms of the extent of the disorder, the timing of anticipated surgery, and the stage of grief or readiness for decision making and planning the parents have reached.

Nursing Diagnosis: Risk for imbalanced nutrition, less than body requirements, related to inability to achieve oral intake

Outcome Evaluation: Child maintains weight within 10% of birthweight; maintains weight in same percentile on growth curve.

Before surgery, because oral fluid cannot be given until the esophagus is repaired, intravenous therapy or total parenteral nutrition can supply fluid and calories. This is continued for a time after surgery until the possibility of vomiting from the anesthetic is decreased. Then the infant may be fed orally, may be continued on total parenteral nutrition, or may be started on gastrostomy feedings, depending on whether the surgery could be completed in one stage or not. Early introduction of oral fluid may help to ensure patency of the esophagus because it helps to decrease adhesion formation from the anastomosis and allows the infant the enjoyment and practice of sucking. If formula is given by gastrostomy feedings, introduce it into the tube slowly and allow it to run by gravity pressure only to prevent fluid from entering the esophagus and putting pressure on the suture line. After the feeding, the end of the tube should be elevated, covered by sterile gauze, and kept in the elevated position. Don't clamp it closed. In this way, any air introduced during the feeding will bubble from the tube and not enter the esophagus and pass the fresh suture line. This also helps to ensure that if the infant should vomit the feeding, the vomitus will be projected into the gastrostomy tube and will not contaminate the fresh sutures. Most newborns enjoy sucking a pacifier during gastrostomy feedings for sucking pleasure. If a mother wishes to breast-feed, she can manually express breast milk for the gastrostomy feedings.

If the child is to return home to await a second-stage operation, the gastrostomy tube will be left in place for a month or two. Therefore, parents must learn how to do gastrostomy feedings. Be certain they know to continue usual infant care, such as holding or talking to the infant in the face of this different feeding method.

Nursing Diagnosis: Risk for infection related to aspiration or seepage of stomach secretions into lungs

Outcome Evaluation: Child's temperature remains below 98.6°F (37°C) axillary; absence of rales on auscultation.

Preoperative Care. Before surgery, position the infant upright in an infant chair or on the right side to prevent gastric juice from entering the lungs from the fistula. Because the infant cannot swallow mucus, frequent oropharyngeal suctioning is necessary. A catheter may be passed into the blind-end esophagus and attached to low continuous or intermittent suction to keep this segment of the esophagus from filling with swallowed saliva and causing aspiration from overflow. Irrigation of the catheter may be nec-

essary to keep it patent, because mucus tends to dry and plug it.

If surgery will be delayed, the infant may have a cervical esophagostomy (the distal end of the blind esophagus is brought to the surface just over the sternum so that mucus can drain). Apply a protective ointment liberally to protect skin. Use absorbent gauze around the opening to absorb moisture and prevent excoriation of the skin. A consult by a wound, ostomy, and continence therapy nurse may be needed to prevent further skin irritation.

Keeping the infant under a radiant heat warmer with a high-humidity oxygen source helps to maintain body heat and liquefy bronchial secretions while awaiting surgery. Try to keep the infant from crying; with crying, air enters the stomach from the trachea, distending the stomach and causing vomiting with aspiration into the lungs. A pacifier may help relax a baby and also satisfy a sucking need.

Postoperative Care. After surgery, the infant will have one or two chest tubes in place because the chest cavity was entered for the repair. The posterior tube drains collecting fluid; the anterior tube allows air to leave the chest space, re-expanding the lung. Care of the child with chest tubes is discussed in Chapter 41.

In the first few days after surgery, observe the infant closely for respiratory distress. Continue to suction the infant as ordered because mucus tends to accumulate in the pharynx from surgical trauma. Suctioning must be done only shallowly, however, to prevent the suction catheter from touching the suture line in the esophagus. Turn the child frequently to discourage fluid from accumulating in the lungs. Humidified oxygen helps to keep respiratory secretions moist. Keep an infant laryngoscope and endotracheal tube readily available at the bedside in case extreme edema develops, increasing the infant's risk for airway obstruction.

Nursing Diagnosis: Risk for impaired skin integrity related to gastrostomy tube insertion site

Outcome Evaluation: Skin surrounding gastrostomy tube remains clean and dry, without erythema.

Gastric secretions, which are highly acidic, may leak onto the skin from the gastrostomy site, leading to skin irritation. Protect the skin by using a cream or commercial skin protection system. Consulting with a wound, ostomy, and continence therapy nurse can be helpful to reduce the possibility of skin irritation.

Omphalocele

An **omphalocele** is a protrusion of abdominal contents through the abdominal wall at the point of the junction of the umbilical cord and abdomen (Fig. 39.6). The herniated organs are usually the intestines, but they may include stomach and liver. They are usually covered and contained

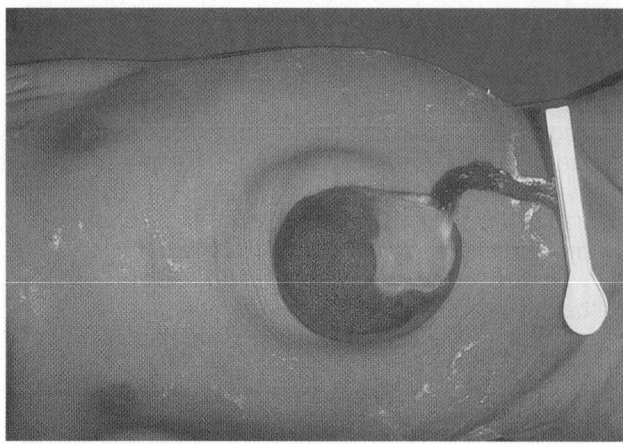

FIGURE 39.6 Omphalocele. This large example seen at birth contains intestine and liver. (Ansary/Custom Medical Stock Photo.)

by a thin transparent layer of peritoneum. This condition occurs because at approximately weeks 6 to 8 of intrauterine life, the fetal abdominal contents, growing faster than the fetal abdomen, are extruded from the abdomen into the base of the umbilical cord. At 7 to 10 weeks, when the abdomen has enlarged sufficiently, the intestine returns to the abdomen. Omphalocele occurs when the abdominal contents fail to return in the usual way.

Assessment

The incidence of omphalocele is 1 in 6,000 live births. Many omphaloceles are diagnosed by prenatal sonogram (Blazer et al., 2004). It may be revealed by an elevated MSAFP examination (see Chapter 10) during pregnancy (Ward, 2003). If not, the presence of omphalocele is obvious on inspection at birth. When an omphalocele is identified in utero, cesarean birth may be performed to protect the exposed intestine. If this is the only disorder identified, however, vaginal birth can be allowed to proceed. Be sure to document the omphalocele's general appearance and its size in centimeters at birth.

Therapeutic Management

Most infants will have immediate surgery to replace the bowel before the thin peritoneal membrane surrounding it ruptures or becomes infected. If the omphalocele is large, infants may be prescribed a topical application of a solution such as silver sulfadiazine to prevent infection of the sac, followed by delayed surgical closure. It is often difficult to replace the entire bowel because the infant's abdomen, which did not need to grow to accommodate the abdominal contents, is smaller than usual. If the total bowel were replaced into this small abdomen, respiratory distress might result from the pressure of the visceral bulk on the diaphragm and lungs. The bowel might not have room for effective peristalsis. For this reason, only a portion of the bowel is usually replaced. The remainder is contained by a Silastic pouch suspended over the infant's bed. Over the next 5 to 10 days, bowel is gradually returned to the ab-

domen. During this time, the infant can be fed by total parenteral nutrition to supply nutrients and keep the bowel from filling with air or stool.

NURSING DIAGNOSES AND RELATED INTERVENTIONS

Outcomes established for the infant with omphalocele must be realistic in terms of the extent of the disorder, the timing of anticipated surgery, and the stage of grief or readiness for decision making and planning that the parents have reached. Omphalocele is a shock to parents; it is a condition that is obviously severe and yet one that is generally unknown.

Nursing Diagnosis: Risk for infection related to exposed abdominal contents

Outcome Evaluation: Child's temperature remains below 98.6°F (37°C) axillary; skin surrounding omphalocele remains clean, dry, and intact, without erythema or foul drainage.

Before surgery, it is important that the lining of peritoneum covering the omphalocele not be ruptured or allowed to dry out and crack; if this happens, infection and malrotation of the uncontained intestine can occur, complicating the surgical repair. Exposure of intestine to air also causes a rapid loss of body heat. Therefore, immediately place the baby in a warmed incubator. Do not leave infants under a radiant heat source because this will quickly dry the exposed bowel. To keep the sac moist, cover it with either sterile saline-soaked gauze or a sterile plastic bowel bag until surgery. Because of the large amount of exposed intestinal surface, the saline used must be at body temperature to prevent lowering body temperature.

The prognosis for a final successful surgical repair is good. Except for a large abdominal scar, the child who had an omphalocele will be the child originally envisioned by his or her parents. If the size of the scar is a problem for the child in later life, cosmetic surgery can reduce its appearance.

Nursing Diagnosis: Risk for imbalanced nutrition, less than body requirements, related to exposed abdominal contents

Outcome Evaluation: Child's weight remains within 10% of birthweight; skin turgor is good; specific gravity of urine is 1.003 to 1.030.

A nasogastric tube is inserted at birth to prevent intestinal distention, which would enlarge the bowel lumen, making it even more difficult to replace. Don't feed the infant orally or allow him or her to suck on a pacifier until the bowel repair is complete, as doing so would distend the exposed bowel with food or air and also make its return to the abdomen more difficult. Some infants have an accompanying **volvulus** (a twisting of the bowel causing obstruction), which is another reason to omit oral feedings. After surgery, the infant is maintained on total parenteral nutrition. Once the final stage of bowel repair is completed, a normal infant diet can be introduced gradually. Observe infants carefully for signs of obstruction (e.g., abdominal distention, constipation or diarrhea, or vomiting) when they begin oral feedings.

Infants with omphalocele will be hospitalized or receive home care for a long time (a minimum of 1 or 2 months) waiting for a second-stage or even a third-stage operation, depending on the extent of bowel involved. If the infant is hospitalized, encourage parents to visit frequently. Be sure the infant has age-appropriate toys available for stimulation.

Parents can become distressed that their child's operation is being done in such small stages. Offer support to help them accept that this treatment method is the best way to manage this type of intestinal disorder.

Gastroschisis

Gastroschisis is a condition similar to omphalocele, except that the abdominal wall disorder is a distance from the umbilicus and abdominal organs are not contained by peritoneal membrane but rather spill freely from the abdomen (Williams, Butler, & Sundem, 2003). Also, a greater amount of intestinal content tends to herniate, increasing the potential for volvulus and obstruction. The surgical procedure is the same as that for omphalocele. Children with gastroschisis often have decreased bowel mobility, and even after surgical correction they may have difficulty with absorption of nutrients and passage of stool. Long-term follow-up may be necessary to ensure that nutrition and elimination are adequate. For unknown reasons, it seems to be increasing in incidence from about 2 in 10,000 births to 4.5 per 10,000 births (Laughon et al., 2003).

Checkpoint Question 1

What is the most important consideration in the care of the child with an omphalocele at birth?

a. Position the infant on his stomach to contain the intestine.
b. Wrap the omphalocele in cold icy gauze to prevent fever.
c. Keep the infant seated upright under a radiant warmer.
d. Contain the intestine in a sterile saline-lined bowel bag.

Intestinal Obstruction

If canalization of the intestine does not occur in utero at some point in the bowel, an **atresia** (complete closure) or **stenosis** (narrowing) of the fetal bowel can occur. The most common site is the duodenum (McCollough & Sharieff, 2003).

Obstruction may occur because the mesentery of the bowel twisted as the bowel re-entered the abdomen (after being contained in the base of the umbilical cord early in intrauterine life) or from the looseness of the intestine in the abdomen of the neonate (this continues to be a problem for the first 6 months of life). Obstruction also can occur because of thicker-than-usual meconium formation, blocking the lumen (meconium plug or meconium ileus).

Assessment

Intestinal obstruction may be anticipated if the mother had hydramnios during pregnancy (amniotic fluid could not be absorbed effectively by the fetus) or if more than 30 mL of stomach contents can be aspirated from the newborn stomach by catheter and syringe at birth (fluid is not passing freely through the tract). If the obstruction is not revealed by either of these findings, then symptoms of intestinal obstruction in the neonate are the same as at any other time in life: the infant passes no meconium or may pass one stool (meconium that formed below the obstruction) and then not pass any more; the abdomen becomes distended and tender. As the effect of the obstruction progresses, the infant will vomit. Remember that many neonates spit up feedings when burped. This rapid ejection of milk smells barely sour. True vomiting is usually sour-smelling (stomach acid has acted on it) and occurs spontaneously without coughing or back-patting.

Obstructions are rare above the ampulla of Vater, the junction of the bile duct with the duodenum, so vomitus will be bile-stained (greenish). Because meconium is black, vomitus may also be dark. Bowel sounds increase with obstruction because of the increase in peristaltic action that occurs as the intestine attempts to push stool pass the point of obstruction. Waves of peristalsis may be apparent across the abdomen. The infant may evidence pain by crying—hard, forceful, indignant crying—and by pulling the legs up against the abdomen. The child's respiratory rate will increase as the intestine fills and the diaphragm is pushed up against the lungs and lung capacity decreases. An abdominal flat-plate x-ray or sonogram will reveal no air below the level of obstruction in the intestines. A barium swallow or barium enema x-ray film may be used to reveal the position of the obstruction.

Therapeutic Management

When bowel obstruction is confirmed, an orogastric or nasogastric tube is inserted and then attached to low suction or left open to the air to prevent further gastrointestinal distention from swallowed air (see Chapter 36). Always use low intermittent suction with decompression tubes in neonates. Pressure greater than this can irritate and ulcerate their stomach lining.

Intravenous therapy is necessary to restore fluid, and immediate surgery is scheduled because bowel obstruction is an emergency that must be treated before dehydration, electrolyte imbalance, or aspiration of vomitus occurs (McCollough & Sharieff, 2003).

Repair of the obstruction (with the exception of meconium plug syndrome) is accomplished through an abdominal incision. The area of stenosis or atresia is removed, and the bowel is anastomosed. If the repair is anatomically difficult or the infant has other anomalies that interfere with overall health, a temporary colostomy may be constructed and the infant discharged to home care, with surgery rescheduled at about 3 to 6 months of age. Care of the child with a colostomy is discussed in Chapter 36. A final surgical procedure will restore the child to full health unless a large portion of the bowel had to be removed, which would have an impact on nutrient absorption (short bowel syndrome).

NURSING DIAGNOSES AND RELATED INTERVENTIONS

---●---

Nursing Diagnosis: Risk for deficient fluid volume related to vomiting

Outcome Evaluation: Child's skin turgor is good; pulse rate is 100 to 120 bpm; no further vomiting occurs; urine output is at least 30 mL/h.

Once an obstruction is suspected, keep an infant NPO to prevent the bowel from filling, and compounding the problem, and to prevent vomiting and aspiration. Vomiting in neonates is always serious, not only because aspiration may occur but also because infants lose fluid rapidly, which results in dehydration. They also lose chloride (a component of the hydrochloric acid found in the stomach contents), and this leads to metabolic alkalosis. The body attempts to compensate for the loss of chloride by excreting potassium, which can cause infants to become hypokalemic quickly. Keeping an infant NPO, restoring fluid by intravenous therapy, and monitoring laboratory values for electrolyte balance until surgery can be scheduled are crucial.

Meconium Plug Syndrome

A **meconium plug** is an extremely hard portion of meconium that has completely blocked the intestinal lumen, causing bowel obstruction (Burge & Drewett, 2004). The cause is unknown but probably reflects normal variations of meconium consistency. Meconium plugs usually form in the lower end of the bowel because this meconium formed early in intrauterine life and has the best chance to become dry and obstruct the bowel lumen. It may be associated with Hirschsprung's disease and is strongly associated with cystic fibrosis.

Assessment

Because the obstruction is low in the intestinal tract, signs of obstruction such as abdominal distention and vomiting may not occur for at least 24 hours. Typically, the infant will be identified first as an infant who has had no meconium passage and is past 24 hours of age. A gentle rectal examination may reveal the presence of hardened stool, although the plug may be too high up in the bowel to be palpated. An x-ray or sonogram may reveal distended air-filled loops of bowel up to the point of obstruction. A barium enema study not only may reveal the level of obstruction but also may be therapeutic in loosening the plug.

Therapeutic Management

The administration of saline enemas (never use tap water in newborns because it can lead to water intoxication) may cause enough peristalsis to expel the plug. Instillation of acetylcysteine (Mucomyst) with diatrizoate (Hypaque) rectally may be prescribed to dissolve the plug. Gastrografin, a highly osmotic radiographic substance, can be administered as an enema. The substance pulls fluid into the bowel because of its low osmotic pressure, allowing the stool to soften and the plug to pass.

Once the thickened portion of meconium has been passed, the infant should have no further difficulty and, over the next several hours, may pass a great amount of stool. The infant must be observed for further passage of meconium (should occur at least once daily) over the next 3 days, however, to be certain that additional plugs do not exist farther up in the bowel. If an infant is going to be discharged before this time, instruct parents on the importance of observing for meconium and also about phoning their primary care provider should the infant have no further bowel movements while at home.

Occasionally, a neonate passes a small plug of hardened meconium—hard enough it would have caused an obstruction except that it is so small—in the first 1 or 2 days of life. Be certain to record and report such a finding, because the infant will need close observation for continued defecation, the same as for the infant who actually had an obstruction, to be certain that there is not a larger and truly obstructing plug higher in the bowel.

Assess the family history of a newborn who has a meconium plug for cystic fibrosis, a recessively inherited disorder (see Chapter 40), or aganglionic megacolon (Hirschsprung's disease), a polygenic inherited disorder (see Chapter 45), as these disorders may be the cause of the hardened meconium. Hypothyroidism is yet another disorder that may present with constipation or hardened stool in newborns. Additional signs of hypothyroidism include a large protruding tongue, lethargy, and subnormal body temperature. Both hypothyroid and cystic fibrosis screening is done along with phenylketonuria screening. Be certain this blood test is obtained in any newborn with a meconium plug.

Meconium Ileus

Meconium ileus (obstruction of the intestinal lumen by hardened meconium) is a specific phenomenon that occurs almost exclusively in infants with cystic fibrosis (Burge & Drewett, 2004). With cystic fibrosis, the enzyme that moistens and makes all body fluids free-flowing is absent. All body fluids are therefore thick and tenacious. Cystic fibrosis (see Chapter 40) is most often thought of as a lung disorder, because the most severe manifestation of tenacious secretions is in the lung; tenacious lung fluid leads to stasis and infection and alveolar obstruction that reduces air exchange. Intestinal and pancreatic secretions are affected also, however, and this may be signaled at birth by hardened obstructive meconium at the ileus level from lack of pancreatic trypsin secretion (meconium ileus). This will lead to the usual symptoms of bowel obstruction: no meconium passage, abdominal distention, and vomiting of bile-stained fluid. If the obstruction is too high for enemas to reduce it, the bowel must be incised and the hardened meconium surgically removed. The infant must be further assessed for cystic fibrosis in the following months.

What if... on the second day of life you notice Baby Sparrow, who was born with meconium staining, is spitting up green mucus? Would it be safe to assume this is meconium-stained mucus? Is there a possibility the baby is vomiting bile-stained vomitus?

Diaphragmatic Hernia

A diaphragmatic hernia is a protrusion of an abdominal organ (usually the stomach or intestine) through a defect in the diaphragm into the chest cavity (Moyer et al., 2005). This usually occurs on the left side, causing cardiac displacement to the right side of the chest and collapse of the left lung. It occurs in approximately 1 in 3,000 live births. There is no difference between male and female incidence (Lovrekovic, 2003).

It occurs because early in intrauterine life, the chest and abdominal cavity are one; at approximately week 8 of growth, the diaphragm forms to divide them. If it does not form completely, the intestines can herniate through the diaphragm opening into the chest cavity (Fig. 39.7).

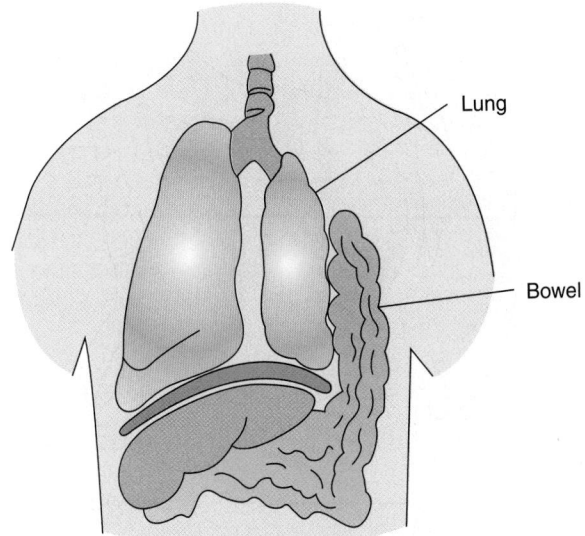

FIGURE 39.7 Diaphragmatic hernia. The bowel loop in the chest compresses the heart and lung on that side.

Assessment

Diaphragmatic hernia is occasionally detected in utero by a sonogram. If extreme, surgery to remove the bowel from the chest can be attempted by fetoscopy while the fetus is still in utero. More often, however, the condition is diagnosed at birth. Newborns with a diaphragmatic hernia will have respiratory difficulty from the moment of birth, because at least one of the lobes of their lungs cannot expand completely (and may not have formed fully). Their abdomen generally appears sunken because it is not as filled with intestine as in the normal newborn. Breath sounds will be absent on the affected side of the chest cavity. There may be cyanosis and intercostal or subcostal retractions. These infants have a potential for developing persistent pulmonary hypertension because blood cannot perfuse readily through the unexpanded lung. This leads to right-to-left shunting through the foramen ovale in the heart and also causes the ductus arteriosus to remain patent. One condition, then, has led to another, and heart involvement complicates an already complicated lung picture. The mechanics of right-to-left heart shunts are further discussed in Chapter 41.

Therapeutic Management

The mortality rate of children with diaphragmatic hernia ranges from 25% to 40%, with death often due to associated anomalies of the heart, lung, and intestine (Lovrekovic, 2003).

Treatment is emergency surgical repair of the diaphragm and replacement of the herniated intestine back into the abdomen. Such a repair usually requires a thoracic incision and the placement of chest tubes. If the disorder of the diaphragm is large, an insoluble polymer (Teflon) patch may be used in reconstruction. The repair is complicated if there is not enough room in the abdomen for the intestine to be returned. In these infants, the abdominal incision may not be closed but left open to allow the intestine to protrude abdominally. It is covered by silicone elastomer (Silastic) and left to be closed at a later date after the abdomen has grown.

Over the next week, the compressed lung (if it is normal) will gradually expand and begin to function. If it is hypoplastic from the pressure of the intestine in utero, it will not expand; it will be removed at the time of surgery.

NURSING DIAGNOSES AND RELATED INTERVENTIONS

Nursing Diagnosis: Risk for ineffective airway clearance related to displaced bowel

Outcome Evaluation: Child's respiration rate is 30 to 50 breaths per minute; Po_2 is 60 to 100 mm Hg; Pco_2 is 30 to 35 mm Hg; lungs are clear to auscultation.

The infant with a diaphragmatic hernia breathes better with the head elevated, as this allows the herniated intestine to fall back as far as possible into the abdomen, providing a maximum amount of respiratory space in the chest. Positioning the infant so the compressed lung is down also allows the unaffected lung to expand most completely. A nasogastric tube or a gastrostomy tube is inserted immediately to prevent distention of the herniated intestine, which would cause further respiratory difficulty. Be certain only low intermittent suction is used to avoid injuring the lining of the stomach. Keep the infant NPO, again, to prevent the bowel from filling and becoming distended.

After surgery, continue to maintain the infant in a semi-Fowler's position in an infant chair to keep the pressure of the replaced intestine off the repaired diaphragm. Keep the infant in a warmed humidified environment to encourage lung fluid drainage from the now uncompromised lung. Suction as necessary. Chest physiotherapy may be ordered to ensure that lung secretions do not pool and to prevent pneumonia. Positive-pressure ventilation may be ordered to increase lung expansion, although this pressure is kept to a minimum to prevent tearing the undeveloped or previously unopened lung tissue. Maintaining arterial oxygen (Po$_2$) at a high level of 100 mm Hg and the Pco$_2$ at a low level of 30 to 35 mm Hg may help to prevent arterial vasoconstriction of the hypoplastic lung, thereby improving lung function.

Infants with diaphragmatic hernia are critically ill. They may be treated with nitric oxide or maintained on extracorporeal membrane oxygenation (ECMO; a heart–lung machine) after surgery until lung tissue is able to function (Tulenko, 2004; see Chapters 26 and 41).

Nursing Diagnosis: Risk for imbalanced nutrition, less than body requirements, related to NPO status

Outcome Evaluation: Child's skin turgor remains good; weight is maintained within 10% of birthweight or between a percentile curve on growth chart.

Infants diagnosed with diaphragmatic hernia are kept NPO, because filling of the intestine with food or activating peristaltic motion will further impair lung function, and if a volvulus occurred with replacing the intestine, bowel obstruction will be present.

After surgery, to prevent pressure on the suture line in the diaphragm by a full stomach and bowel, nutrition will be supplied intravenously, such as with total parenteral nutrition. When starting oral feedings, be certain to bubble the infant well after feeding to reduce the amount of swallowed air and limit bowel pressure against the diaphragm.

Umbilical Hernia

An umbilical hernia is a protrusion of a portion of the intestine through the umbilical ring, muscle, and fascia surrounding the umbilical cord (Borkowski, 2004). This creates a bulging protrusion under the skin at the umbilicus. It is rarely noticeable at birth while the cord is still present but becomes increasingly noticeable at health care visits during the first year.

Umbilical hernias occur most frequently in African-American children and more often in girls than in boys. The structure is generally 1 to 2 cm (0.5 to 1 inch) in diameter but may be as big as an orange when children cry or strain. The size of the protruding mass is not as important as the size of the fascial ring through which the intestine protrudes. If this fascial ring is less than 2 cm, closure will usually occur spontaneously and no repair of the disorder will be necessary. If the disorder is more than 2 cm, surgery for repair will generally be indicated to prevent herniation and intestinal obstruction or bowel strangulation. This usually is done when the child is 1 to 2 years of age.

Some parents believe that holding an umbilical hernia in place by using "belly bands" or taping a silver dollar over the area will help to reduce the hernia. These actions can actually lead to bowel strangulation and should be avoided.

Surgery is generally accomplished on an ambulatory outpatient basis. The child returns from surgery with a pressure dressing, which remains in place until the sutures are well healed. Remind parents to sponge-bathe the child until they return for a postoperative visit and the dressing is removed. If the child is not yet toilet-trained, they need to keep diapers folded down below the dressing to prevent contaminating the suture line with stool.

Imperforate Anus

Imperforate anus (Fig. 39.8) is stricture of the anus. In week 7 of intrauterine life, the upper bowel elongates to pouch and combine with a pouch invaginating from the perineum. These two sections of bowel meet, the membranes between them are absorbed, and the bowel is then patent to the outside. If this motion toward each other does not occur or if the membrane between the two surfaces does not dissolve, imperforate anus occurs. The disorder can be

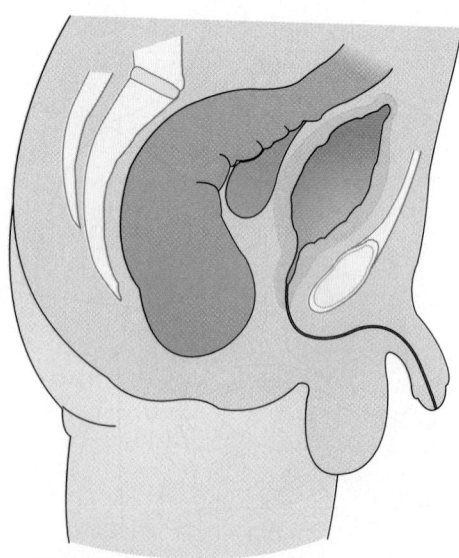

FIGURE 39.8 Imperforate anus. The lower bowel ends in a blind pouch.

relatively minor, requiring just surgical incision of the persistent membrane, or much more severe, involving sections of the bowel that are many inches apart with no anus. There may be an accompanying fistula to the bladder in boys and to the vagina in girls, further complicating a surgical repair. The problem occurs in approximately 1 in 5,000 live births, more commonly in boys than girls. Imperforate anus may occur as an additional complication of spinal cord disorders, because both the external anal canal and the spinal cord arise from the same germ tissue layer (Telega, 2003).

Assessment

Inspection of a newborn's anal region may reveal that no anus is present, although this observation may not be helpful, because the anus can appear normal and the condition can still exist far inside, so that it is missed on simple inspection. Occasionally, the condition may be revealed because a membrane filled with black meconium can be seen protruding from the anus. A "wink" reflex (touching the skin near the rectum should make it contract) will not be present if sensory nerve endings in the rectum are not intact. If these methods fail to detect the condition, it can be discovered in a newborn by the inability to insert a rubber catheter into the rectum. No stool will be passed, and abdominal distention will become evident. An x-ray or sonogram will reveal the disorder if the infant is held in a head-down position to allow swallowed air to rise to the end of the blind pouch of the bowel. This method is also helpful to estimate the distance the intestine is separated from the perineum or the extent of the correction that will be needed.

Formerly, when all newborns stayed in the hospital 3 to 4 days after birth, imperforate anus was always discovered. When infants failed to pass stools after the first 24 hours, the reason was investigated. Currently, because newborns are discharged at 2 or 3 days or even a few hours after birth, possibly no one will notice that an infant has not passed a stool in that time. For an infant born in a birthing center or at home, follow-up, therefore, must include assessment of whether the infant is defecating. Collect a urine specimen on infants with imperforate anus so it can be examined for the presence of meconium to help determine whether the child has a rectal–bladder fistula. Placing a urine collector bag over the vagina in girls may reveal a meconium-stained discharge or a rectovaginal fistula.

Therapeutic Management

The degree of difficulty in repairing an imperforate anus depends on the extent of the problem. If the rectum ends close to the perineum (below or at the level of the levator ani muscle) and the anal sphincter is formed, repair involves simple anastomosis of the separated bowel segments. The repair becomes complicated if the end of the rectum is at a distance from the perineum (above the levator ani muscle) or the anal sphincter exists only in an underdeveloped form. All repairs are complicated if a fistula to the bladder or vagina is present. If the repair will be extensive, the surgeon may create a temporary colostomy, anticipating final repair when the infant is somewhat older

(6 to 12 months). For a successful repair, it is unnecessary for an internal rectal sphincter to be present as long as the subrectal muscle is judged to be intact.

NURSING DIAGNOSES AND RELATED INTERVENTIONS

Nursing Diagnosis: Imbalanced nutrition, less than body requirements, related to bowel obstruction and inability for oral intake

Outcome Evaluation: Child's weight remains within 10% of birthweight or is maintained on a percentile curve on a growth chart; skin turgor is good.

Preoperative Care. Before surgery, keep the infant NPO to avoid further bowel distention. A nasogastric tube attached to low intermittent suction for decompression will be inserted to relieve vomiting and prevent pressure on other abdominal organs or the diaphragm from the distended intestine. Intravenous therapy or total parenteral nutrition will be started to maintain fluid and electrolyte balance.

Postoperative Care. The newborn will return from surgery with a nasogastric tube still in place. When bowel sounds are present and the nasogastric tube is removed, small oral feedings of glucose water, formula, or breast milk are begun.

Some infants, who are scheduled for repair in a second-stage operation and who have a temporary colostomy, are not permitted high-residue foods to lessen the bulk of stools. Although this is rarely a problem with infants because their diet naturally is a low-residue one, do not assume that parents know what low residue means. Examples include rice cereal and strained fruits and vegetables. They should avoid unrefined rice and grains, vegetables with fibers, or fruits with peels.

Nursing Diagnosis: Impaired tissue integrity at rectum related to surgical incision

Outcome Evaluation: Incision line remains free of erythema or drainage until it heals by about day 7 after surgery.

If a rectal repair was completed, remember there is a fresh suture line at the rectum. Take axillary or tympanic temperatures rather than rectal temperatures to avoid loosening a suture. Infants should also have no enemas, suppositories, or any other intrusive rectal procedures. It might be helpful to hang a sign above the infant's crib cautioning against any intrusive rectal procedure. Infants may be given a stool softener daily to keep the stool from becoming hard and tearing the healing suture line. Clean the suture line well after bowel movements by irrigating it with normal saline. Placing a diaper under, not on, the infant may be helpful so bowel movements can be cleansed away as soon as they occur. Do not place the infant on the abdomen because, in this position, newborns tend to pull their knees under them, causing tension in the perineal area. A side-lying position is best.

An infant may need rectal dilatation done once or twice a day for a few months after surgery to ensure proper patency of the rectal sphincter. Review this technique (gently inserting a lubricated cot-covered finger into the rectum) with the parents and document that they are able to perform this procedure before the child is discharged. Be certain they also understand the importance of the procedure. The best surgical repair could end in failure if constriction occurs because the parents do not follow up with this procedure. If infants are to be discharged with a prescription for a daily stool softener, be certain parents understand why this is also important and have a plan for remembering the correct times and dosage.

Nursing Diagnosis: Risk for impaired parenting related to difficulty in bonding with infant ill from birth

Outcome Evaluation: Parents hold and comfort infant; describe positive characteristics of infant.

An imperforate anus may be a difficult anomaly for a parent to accept because it deals with a body area that they may not feel comfortable discussing (Nisell et al., 2003). If it involves a temporary (or permanent) colostomy, learning to care for their infant may be difficult. For these reasons, parents need a great deal of support following the diagnosis. If a final surgical repair can be completed, they can be assured their child will have normal bowel function thereafter. If a final repair could not be surgically achieved, they have the even harder task of caring for a child with a permanent ostomy. They can be assured that children who always have ostomies accept these well as they grow older because they have never known any other method of defecation (see Chapter 36 for a discussion of care priorities for the child with an ostomy).

Checkpoint Question 2

What is an important nursing measure for a newborn with a diaphragmatic hernia?

a. Feed the infant immediately to decrease air in the intestine.
b. Keep the infant positioned head down so the intestine can expand.
c. Wrap the infant's abdomen tightly to better contain intestine.
d. Position the infant in an infant chair to contain intestine in abdomen.

NERVOUS SYSTEM PHYSICAL AND DEVELOPMENTAL DISORDERS

The most common developmental disorders of the nervous system at birth include abnormal accumulation of cerebrospinal fluid (hydrocephalus), which has several causes, and abnormalities associated with neural tube closure (meningocele or spinal dysraphism).

Hydrocephalus

Cerebrospinal fluid (CSF) is formed in the first and second ventricles of the brain and then passes through the aqueduct of Sylvius and the fourth ventricle to empty into the subarachnoid space of the spinal cord, where it is absorbed. **Hydrocephalus** is an excess of CSF in the ventricles or the subarachnoid space (Kestle, 2003). In the infant whose cranial sutures are not firmly knitted, this excess fluid causes enlargement of the skull. If fluid can reach the spinal cord, the disorder is called communicating hydrocephalus or extraventricular hydrocephalus. If there is a block to such passage of fluid, the disorder is an obstructive hydrocephalus or intraventricular hydrocephalus. Hydrocephalus is also classified as to whether it occurs at birth (congenital) or from an incident later in life (acquired). The cause of congenital hydrocephalus is unknown, although maternal infection such as toxoplasmosis or infant meningitis may be factors (Kang, 2003).

An excess of CSF in the newborn occurs for one of three main reasons. The first is overproduction of fluid by a choroid plexus in the first or second ventricle, as could occur from a growing tumor (rare). A second reason is obstruction of the passage of fluid in the narrow aqueduct of Sylvius (the most common cause). Other common sites of obstruction include the foramina of Magendie and Luschka, the openings that allow fluid to leave the fourth ventricle. Obstruction occurs because infections such as meningitis or encephalitis may leave adhesions behind that block fluid flow. Hemorrhage from trauma or a growing tumor also may obstruct the passage of CSF. An Arnold-Chiari disorder (elongation of the lower brain stem and displacement of the fourth ventricle into the upper cervical canal) is yet another cause.

Lastly, hydrocephalus may occur from an interference with the absorption of CSF from the subarachnoid space if a portion of the subarachnoid membrane is removed, as occurs with surgery for meningocele, or after extensive subarachnoid hemorrhage, when portions of the membrane absorption surface become obscured.

Assessment

Hydrocephalus occurs in approximately 3 to 4 per 1,000 live births (Kang, 2003). With an obstruction present, excessive fluid accumulates and dilates the system above the point of obstruction. If the atresia is in the aqueduct of Sylvius, the first, second, and third ventricles will dilate. If it is at the exit from the fourth ventricle, all ventricles will dilate. Symptoms may develop rapidly or slowly, depending on the extent of the atresia.

If hydrocephalus is present prenatally, it can sometimes be detected on a sonogram and can even be shunted in utero (von Koch et al., 2003). The condition is generally not evident during pregnancy or even at birth, however, because of the effect of intrauterine pressure. It becomes evident in the first few weeks or months of life. The infant's fontanelles widen and appear tense, the suture lines on the skull separate, and the head diameter enlarges. As the fluid accumulation continues, the scalp becomes shiny and scalp veins become prominent. The brow bulges in a typical appearance (bossing), and the eyes become "sunset eyes" (the sclera shows above the iris because of upper lid retraction). Infants show symptoms of increased intracranial pressure, such as decreased pulse and respirations, increased temperature and blood pressure, hyperactive reflexes, strabismus, and optic atrophy. They may become either irritable or lethargic, and they fail to thrive. They may have a typical shrill, high-pitched cry (Box 39.3).

Treatment is most effective when the disorder is recognized early, because once intracranial pressure becomes so acute that brain tissue is damaged and motor or mental deterioration results, even the best shunting procedure cannot replace and repair the damage to the brain cells. Assisting with detection of hydrocephalus is an important role for nurses in ambulatory child health settings. All children under age 2 years should have their head circum-ference recorded and plotted on an appropriate growth chart at health care visits, so a child whose head is growing abnormally can be detected.

Measure the head circumference of all infants within an hour of birth and again before discharge from the health care facility to establish a baseline. Older children who have suffered head trauma severe enough to be seen in a medical facility should have their head circumference noted at the time of the accident; if other symptoms of increased intracranial pressure appear, head circumference may be a meaningful part of the store of information available concerning the child's condition.

In addition to the general enlargement of the head, note any asymmetry that is occurring, because this may suggest the point of obstruction. A skull that is enlarging anteriorly with a shallow posterior fossa, for example, suggests the obstruction is in the aqueduct or third ventricle.

The infant's motor function becomes impaired as the head enlarges, because of both neurologic impairment and atrophy caused by the inability to move such a heavy head. However, as long as a child has more than 1 cm of cerebral tissue present, motor function often is not impaired. Even with an extremely enlarged head, children's intelligence may remain normal, although fine motor development may be affected.

Hydrocephalus can be demonstrated by sonography, computed tomography (CT), or magnetic resonance imaging (MRI). A skull x-ray film will reveal the separating sutures and thinning of the skull. **Transillumination** (holding a bright light such as a flashlight or a specialized light [a Chun gun] against the skull with the child in a darkened room) will reveal the skull is filled with fluid rather than solid brain (Fig. 39.9). If the hydrocephalus is a noncommunicating type, dye inserted into a ventricle through the anterior fontanelle will not appear in CSF obtained from a lumbar puncture.

Therapeutic Management

The treatment of hydrocephalus depends on its cause and extent. If it is caused by overproduction of fluid,

BOX 39.3 ASSESSMENT

Assessing an Infant With Hydrocephalus

Enlarged fontanelles

Separated suture line

Prominent scalp veins

"Bossing" of forehead

Increased head circumference

"Sunset" eyes

Lethargy or irritability

Shrill cry

Signs of increased cranial pressure
↓ pulse
↑ temperature
↓ respirations
↑ blood pressure

Hyperactive reflexes

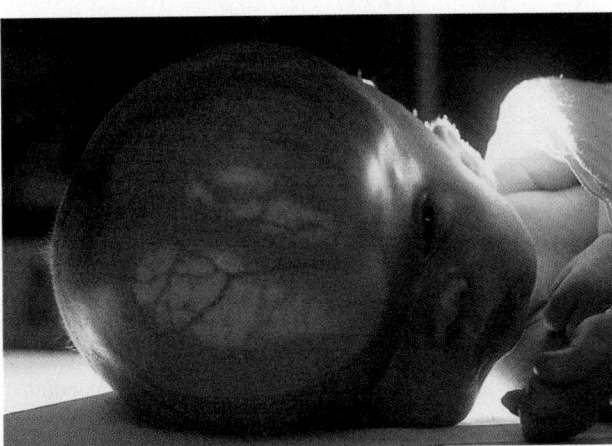

FIGURE 39.9 An infant with hydrocephalus. Transillumination reveals a fluid-filled skull. (Southern Illinois University/Photo Researchers, Inc.)

acetazolamide (Diamox) may be prescribed to promote the excretion of fluid. Destruction of a portion of the choroid plexus may be attempted by ventricular endoscopy, or if a tumor in that area is responsible for the overproduction of fluid, removal of the tumor should provide a solution. Hydrocephalus is usually caused by obstruction, however, so the treatment usually involves laser surgery to reopen the route of flow or bypassing the point of obstruction by shunting the fluid to another point of absorption.

As ventricular endoscopy is perfected and obstructions in the third or fourth ventricle can be relieved, the next generation of children with hydrocephalus may not need artificial shunting (Kang, 2003). Children today may still undergo a shunting procedure, however, and you may care for many older children or adults who have shunts in place. A shunting procedure involves threading a thin polyethylene catheter under the skin from the ventricles to the peritoneum (Fig. 39.10). Fluid drains by this route into the peritoneum and is absorbed across the peritoneal membrane into the body circulation. This type of shunt has to usually be replaced as the child grows and it becomes too short. As another complication, it may become enclosed in a fold of peritoneum and become obstructed.

The prognosis for infants with hydrocephalus is improving every day, as shunting and surgical procedures become more common and more effective (Box 39.4). The ultimate prognosis for a child depends on whether brain damage occurred before shunting and, if a shunt is in place, whether the parents can recognize when it needs to be replaced to prevent increased intracranial pressure.

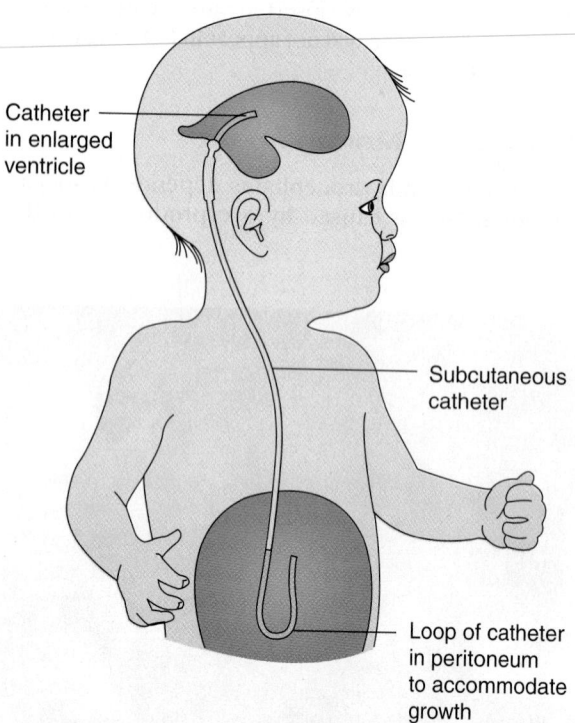

Catheter in enlarged ventricle

Subcutaneous catheter

Loop of catheter in peritoneum to accommodate growth

FIGURE 39.10 A ventriculoperitoneal shunt removes excessive cerebrospinal fluid from the ventricles and shunts it to the peritoneum. A one-way valve is present in the tubing behind the ear.

NURSING DIAGNOSES AND RELATED INTERVENTIONS

Nutrition and parent–child bonding are two major concerns for the infant with hydrocephalus. Box 39.5 illustrates these and other concerns, as do the following nursing diagnoses.

Nursing Diagnosis: Risk for ineffective cerebral tissue perfusion related to increased intracranial pressure

Outcome Evaluation: Child shows no increased temperature and blood pressure, or decreased pulse rate, decreased respiratory rate, or decreased level of consciousness; PERLA; muscle strength equal and strong bilaterally; head circumference is maintained at age-appropriate level.

After a shunt is inserted, the infant's bed is usually left flat or raised only about 30 degrees so the head remains level with the body. This is because if the child's head is raised excessively, CSF may flow too rapidly and decompression can then occur too rapidly, leading to possible tearing of cerebral arteries.

A one-way valve is inserted in the shunt that opens when CSF has accumulated to the extent that pressure has increased. It closes when enough fluid has drained to reduce the pressure. The surgeon who performed the shunting procedure will write specific orders about how often the infant is to be turned and to what side after surgery. Often infants are not turned to lie on the side with the shunt to prevent putting pressure on the valve, which might cause it to open and rapidly decompress CSF.

Assess for signs of increased intracranial pressure after surgery: tense fontanelles, increasing head circumference, irritability or lethargy, decreased level of consciousness, poor sucking, vomiting, an increase in blood pressure (difficult to measure accurately in infants unless Doppler instrumentation is used), increasing temperature, and a decrease in pulse and respiratory rates (see Chapter 49 for a neurologic assessment). Also assess for symptoms of infection (i.e., increased temperature, increased pulse rate, general malaise, and signs of meningitis such as a stiff neck and marked irritability) (Box 39.6). Be certain a child receives adequate pain management, because crying elevates CSF pressure.

Nursing Diagnosis: Risk for imbalanced nutrition, less than body requirements, related to increased intracranial pressure

Outcome Evaluation: Child's weight remains within 5th to 95th percentile on height and weight chart; no vomiting occurs.

BOX 39.4 FOCUS ON . . .

COMMUNICATION

Baby Sparrow is scheduled to have a ventriculoperitoneal shunt inserted this afternoon. You talk to his mother before surgery.

Less Effective Communication

Nurse: Is there anything I can explain to you about your son's surgery, Ms. Sparrow?

Ms. Sparrow: No. I just want to see him back here with a smaller head.

Nurse: The shunt won't actually make his head smaller. Its purpose is to keep his head from growing any larger.

Ms. Sparrow: What is the chance that he'll die in surgery?

Nurse: All surgery has a risk, certainly, but he should do well.

Ms. Sparrow: But there is a chance he'll die in surgery?

Nurse: You're worrying over nothing. Why don't you relax and go get something to drink until he gets back?

More Effective Communication

Nurse: Is there anything I can explain to you about your son's surgery, Ms. Sparrow?

Ms. Sparrow: No. I just want to see him back here with a smaller head.

Nurse: The shunt won't actually make his head smaller. Its purpose is to keep his head from growing any larger.

Ms. Sparrow: What is the chance that he'll die in surgery?

Nurse: All surgery has a risk, certainly, but he should do well.

Ms. Sparrow: But there is a chance he'll die in surgery?

Nurse: You sound more worried than I'd expect. Is there something specific you're worried about?

Ms. Sparrow: I'd like him to die in surgery. How am I going to take care of a child with such a deformed head?

Nurse: Let's sit down and talk about this some more.

Because surgical procedures are so safe today and the results of surgery for newborns are so successful, it is easy to begin to think of these disorders as more inconvenient than serious: the infant, after all, will grow up with only a few minor problems. To a parent, however, the difference between a child born with one of these conditions and the "perfect" child the parent envisioned can be great. Careful listening is necessary to appreciate the extent of a parent's understanding of the problem. Handling a problem by giving quick reassurance, as in the first scenario above, can lead to missing a parent's concern. Better listening, as in the second scenario, reveals the true problem.

Because an abdominal incision is involved to thread the catheter into the peritoneum, most children have a nasogastric tube placed during surgery. Keep them NPO until bowel sounds return and the tube can be removed. Introduce fluid gradually in small quantities after removal of the tube. Vomiting that results from the introduction of fluid too soon after any surgery causes increased intracranial pressure.

Like other infants, infants with hydrocephalus should be held when being fed if possible. Be certain to support their heads well when moving them to avoid strain on their neck from their heavier than usual head. Hold their head with the whole palm, not just the fingertips, because the skull can thin to such a degree that it can actually be punctured with a stiff, forceful touch. Urge parents to use a rocking chair with an armrest to provide support for their arm while feeding the infant. Otherwise, the infant's head can be so heavy that they cannot spend as much time holding the infant after a feeding as they might otherwise. No contraindications for breast-feeding exist. Help breast-feeding mothers to find a comfortable position for feeding so that they can be successful with this.

Note how the child sucks. Increased intracranial pressure may be noted first because of poor or in-effective sucking. Vomiting after feeding, without nausea (difficult to detect in a small infant), is also a sign of increased intracranial pressure.

Observe for constipation, because straining while passing stool causes increased intracranial pressure. This is not usually a problem of infants who are totally breast- or formula-fed. However, it can be a problem when children return for shunt replacement at an older age. Urge parents to increase fluid and roughage in the diet as a preventive measure.

Nursing Diagnosis: Risk for impaired skin integrity related to extra weight and immobility of head

Outcome Evaluation: Child's skin remains clean, dry, and intact, without signs of erythema or ulceration.

The head of the infant with hydrocephalus can become so heavy the infant cannot move it freely. As the skin of the head stretches thin, skin breakdown can occur on the pressure points. Wash the child's head daily and change the position of the head approximately every 2 hours so that no portion of the head rests against the mattress for a long period. A synthetic sheepskin pad or an air, water, or alternating air mattress may help to relieve pressure points. If a Kling or stockinette bandage is used to hold a surgical head dressing in place, place a piece

BOX 39.5: Focus on Nursing Care Planning

A Multidisciplinary Care Map for A Child with Hydrocephalus

●

At 3 months of age, Baby Sparrow develops hydrocephalus after repair of his neural tube disorder. He is scheduled for a ventriculoperitoneal shunt insertion.

Family Assessment

Child lives with 16-year-old mother and her parents and 4 siblings. Child's father works as motorcycle mechanic; visits infant frequently. Mother no longer attending school because of child care. Has not named child as yet. Mother asking many questions about the surgery. "This'll fix everything, right? I want a healthy baby."

Client Assessment

3-month-old infant whose head circumference has continued to increase since myelomeningocele surgery at birth. Head circumference at birth was 40th percentile, at 60th percentile at 6 weeks of age and now at 80th percentile. Mother noted infant had increasing irritability and lethargy over the last few weeks.

Anterior fontanelle 4 cm x 4 cm; posterior fontanelle 3 cm × cm. Sagittal suture line separated ¼ inch. Scalp veins prominent. Eyes appear sunset. Parents report two episodes of forceful vomiting yesterday. "His cry is so high-pitched and shrill, and he doesn't want anything to drink." Mother is breast-feeding. Cerebral perfusion pressure 55 mm Hg. Blood pressure 100/40; pulse 100 bpm; respirations 16. Afebrile.

Nursing Diagnosis

Risk for ineffective cerebral tissue perfusion related to increased intracranial pressure from hydrocephalus

Outcome Criteria

Infant's vital signs are within age-appropriate parameters; head circumference is maintained at current level; infant responds to auditory stimuli. Cerebral perfusion pressure remains above 50 mm Hg.

Team Member Responsible	Assessment	Intervention	Rationale	Expected Outcome
Activities of Daily Living				
Nurse	Assess if infant is able to turn because of increased head size.	Provide an environment for child that is stimulating yet not tiring (mobile, soft toys in crib). Urge parent to interact with child.	Lack of mobility can lead to pressure ulcers on head as well as insufficient 3-month development.	Child's parent plays with infant. Infant appears interested in age-appropriate toys. No irritated areas on head.
Consultations				
Nurse/ physician	Assess if neurosurgeon is available for consultation.	Arrange for consultation for mother with neurosurgeon to discuss surgery and child's prognosis.	Viewing a child as totally disabled can cause a parent to not appreciate the child's capabilities.	Neurosurgeon meets with mother to discuss that child's IQ appears normal; shunting will halt head growth.

(continued)

Team Member Responsible	Assessment	Intervention	Rationale	Expected Outcome
Procedures/Medications				
Nurse	Assess infant's neurologic status postoperatively, including response to sound, pupillary response, increasing irritability or lethargy.	Position the infant with the head of the bed elevated 15° and prevent hyperextension, flexion, or rotation of the head. Record cerebral perfusion pressure.	Elevating head of bed aids shunt functioning, helping reduce intracranial pressure. Cerebral perfusion pressure reveals extent of intracranial pressure.	Child's cerebral perfusion pressure remains greater than established parameter. Responds to sound; no increasing irritability or lethargy.
Nurse	Measure and record head circumference every 4 hours. Assess anterior fontanelle for tenseness and bulging.	Document head circumference and appearance of anterior fontanelle.	Head circumference, if increasing, or a tense, bulging fontanelle indicates accumulating CSF.	Child's head circumference does not increase in size; fontanelles no longer feel tense.
Nutrition				
Nurse/ nutritionist	Observe mother breast-feeding infant.	Encourage mother to breast-feed infant; assist mother with positioning the infant properly, supporting the head without flexion or hyperextension during feeding.	Breast milk is the optimal nutrition for an infant. Proper positioning is important to avoid neck vein compression, which could increase intracranial pressure.	Mother breast-feeds successfully following surgery.
Nurse	Monitor intake and output closely.	Administer osmotic diuretic and corticosteroids as ordered.	Adequate hydration is necessary to ensure renal function. Osmotic diuretics decrease intracranial pressure. Corticosteroids reduce inflammation.	Child's output remains over set parameter. Diuretic and corticosteroids administered as necessary.
Patient/Family Education				
Nurse/ nurse practitioner	Assess the parents' understanding of hydrocephalus and treatment measures.	Review the structure and function of the brain and explain how hydrocephalus develops. Clarify any misconceptions.	Reviewing and clarifying aid in learning and strengthen understanding.	Mother states she understands purpose of shunt to relieve excess CSF.
Psychosocial/Spiritual/Emotional Needs				
Nurse/ nurse practitioner	Assess mother's acceptance of child in light of many congenital disorders and no name for baby as yet.	Observe mother's interaction with infant; remind her that congenital disorders occur in a proportion of all births.	Young mother may have had little experience with life crises. Needs support from health care providers for this crisis.	Mother states she understands child's condition is neither her nor the child's fault; states she can handle the present crisis.
Discharge Planning				
Nurse	Assess if child's parents have questions about care he will need for future shunt care; if they understand postsurgery appointment is important.	Assist parents with caring for the child as much as possible; offer positive reinforcement frequently.	Caring for the child promotes active participation and parent–infant bonding. Positive reinforcement enhances self-esteem and aids in coping.	Mother and grandmother state they understand future care necessary for shunt; will contact neurosurgeon if any questions as to child's progress. Will keep postsurgery appointment.

(continued)

Team Member Responsible	Assessment	Intervention	Rationale	Expected Outcome
Discharge Planning				
Nurse	Assess if home care follow-up will be necessary.	Make referral for home care if needed. Refer parents to support group of other parents of children with hydrocephalus.	Support groups can decrease feelings of isolation, provide opportunities for further learning. Follow-up home care provides continuing support, guidance, and education.	Mother and grandmother state they will attend a support group at least once to evaluate benefit for them. Agree to at least one home visit for follow-up care.

BOX 39.6 FOCUS ON . . .

FAMILY TEACHING

Caring for a Child With a Ventriculoperitoneal Shunt

Q. Following ventriculoperitoneal shunt surgery, Baby Sparrow's mother asks you, "What do I need to do to care for him?"

A. Here are some helpful things to remember:

- Observe for signs of increased intracranial pressure, such as drowsiness, vomiting, headache, irritability, and anorexia.
- Observe the pump site daily for any sign of swelling or redness.
- Have your child sleep with his head slightly elevated at night to help ensure fluid flow through the tube. Do not allow your child to fall asleep with his head hanging over the side of a couch or bed.
- Do not allow your child to become constipated, because hard stool might press against and obstruct the shunt. Encourage fruit, vegetables, cereal, and a generous amount of fluid in his diet.
- Do not call attention to the pump behind your child's ear; teach him not to touch the pump when he's nervous or as an attention-getting action.
- Be certain your child wears a helmet for tricycle and bicycle riding (as should all children) to avoid injury to the shunt. Otherwise, there are no special precautions that need to be taken for normal play.
- If your child develops signs of infection such as an increased temperature, phone your primary care provider. Also remind the person that your child has a shunt in place. This is probably a simple infection of childhood but could indicate an infected shunt.
- Be certain to keep your regularly scheduled health assessment visits. As your child grows taller, the shunt will eventually need to be replaced for proper functioning.

of gauze or cotton behind the child's ear before the bandage is applied to prevent skin surfaces from touching and becoming excoriated. Make sure the bandage does not become wet from backward-draining oral secretions or shunt leakage.

Nursing Diagnosis: Deficient knowledge related to home care needs of child with hydrocephalus

Outcome Evaluation: Parents state fears regarding ability to provide care but are able to manage care; state signs of increased intracranial pressure for which to watch; demonstrate competence in shunt care.

Caring for a child with a shunt in place is an ongoing responsibility for parents. If parents do not seem to be asking many questions about the child's care after surgery, do not assume this is because they are taking the child's care in stride. They may be too frightened or not understand neuroanatomy enough to know what questions to ask. An opening such as, "Most parents are a little nervous when they think about taking a child home with a shunt in place; do you feel that way?" gives them an opportunity to admit how they feel. Talking about how nervous they feel about the responsibility will not immediately make them more comfortable with the child's care. However, it can provide them with a starting point to bring the care down to a manageable size. Assure them the health care providers caring for their child are interested in helping and supporting them.

If a valve has been inserted in the shunt, it can be palpated underneath the skin just behind the ear. Remind parents to stress to their child that this strange object is not to be felt continually. A child nervously fidgeting with a pressure pump can inadvertently evacuate CSF from the ventricles at a dangerously rapid rate.

Before an infant is discharged after surgery, be certain the parents have ample opportunity to feed and provide care so they can be comfortable and feel they "know" their infant. Because irritability, lethargy, vomiting, and a change in the baby's cry are signs of increased intracranial pressure, be certain parents know to report these immediately to their primary care provider. Before parents can report a change in the infant's disposition in this way, they must know the infant well. A referral for home care follow-up may be appropriate to offer further support.

Nursing Diagnosis: Risk for delayed growth and development related to potential neurologic challenge

Outcome Evaluation: Child demonstrates regular observable growth and achieves age-appropriate developmental milestones.

Although children may have mild learning or motor problems, the cognitive functioning of a child with hydrocephalus may remain intact despite extreme thinning of the brain cortex. Therefore, after a shunting procedure, although the head may remain larger than normal, intelligence may be normal. Like all children, children with hydrocephalus need stimulation: they need to be talked to, smiled at, and played with. If the child's head is enlarged, turning it to look at things can be difficult. It may be necessary to reposition mobiles or pictures so the child receives adequate visual stimulation. Role-model talking and singing to the child to help parents include these actions in their care.

At the time of discharge, be certain parents have the telephone number of the person they should call if they have a question or concern about their child's condition or care, and a referral for home care follow-up, if appropriate. They also need an appointment for the child's first checkup. Be sure they understand that infection of the shunt is a possibility and a severe complication because it can lead to meningitis. If this should occur, the infant will show signs of increased intracranial pressure as well as those of infection. In addition to being hospitalized, receiving the usual treatment for meningitis (see Chapter 49), and receiving intravenous antibiotics, the child may have an extraventricular shunt placed to promote drainage. This allows antibiotics to be administered directly to the CSF and ensures that infected CSF is not draining to the peritoneal cavity, where it could cause peritonitis.

As the child reaches preschool and school age, parents need to confer with the school nurse to make the nurse aware that the child has a shunt in place and that the child may need special head protection for sports activities.

✓ **Checkpoint Question 3**

Baby Sparrow may be developing increased intracranial pressure. What vital sign changes occur with this?

a. Decreased temperature; increased blood pressure
b. Increased respirations; decreased pulse rate
c. Increased temperature; decreased pulse rate
d. Decreased blood pressure; increased temperature

Neural Tube Disorders

Because the neural tube forms in utero first as a flat plate and then molds to form the brain and spinal cord, it is susceptible to malformation. The term **spina bifida** (Latin for "divided spine") is most often used as a collective term for all spinal cord disorders, but there are well-defined degrees of spina bifida involvement, and not all neural tube disorders involve the spinal cord. All of these disorders, however, occur because of lack of fusion of the posterior surface of the embryo in early intrauterine life. They can be compared with cleft palate or cleft lip—these are also closure disorders.

The incidence of neural tube disorders has fallen dramatically in recent years, from 3/1,000 to 0.6/1,000. Such disorders may occur as a polygenic inheritance pattern, but poor nutrition, especially a diet deficient in folic acid, appears to be a major contributing factor (Lumley et al., 2005). As a result, pregnant women are advised to ingest 400 micrograms of folic acid daily to help prevent these disorders (CDC, 2004). The risk of bearing a second child with a neural tube disorder once one child is born with such a disorder increases to as much as 1 in 20. Also, women who have had one child with a spinal cord disorder are advised to have a maternal serum assay or amniocentesis for alpha-fetoprotein (AFP) levels to determine if such a disorder is present in a second pregnancy (levels will be abnormally increased if there is an open spinal lesion). Serum assessment of AFP (MSAFP) is done at week 15 of pregnancy, when AFP reaches its peak concentration. AFP level testing is routine in many prenatal settings. If the result is elevated, an amniocentesis is then done to assess the level of AFP in amniotic fluid. A sonogram is also helpful to determine the presence of the disorder (see Chapter 10 for further discussion of these prenatal assessments).

Types of Disorders

Anencephaly. Anencephaly is absence of the cerebral hemispheres. It occurs when the upper end of the neural tube fails to close in early intrauterine life. It is revealed by an elevated level of AFP in the maternal serum or on amniocentesis and confirmed by a sonogram.

Infants with anencephaly may have difficulty in labor because the underdeveloped head does not engage the cervix well. Many such infants present in a breech position. On visual inspection at birth, the disorder is obvious (Fig. 39.11). Children cannot survive with this disorder because they have no cerebral function. Because the respiratory and cardiac centers are located in the intact medulla, however, they may survive for a number of days after birth.

When the condition is discovered prenatally, parents are offered the option of abortion. An ethical problem has arisen in a number of instances when parents, aware that the child cannot survive, elect to carry the infant to term so the organs can be used for transplant. Nurses need to think through their feelings about caring for such infants, because it can be difficult to give care to a child who will most likely die or who has been born only to help others live.

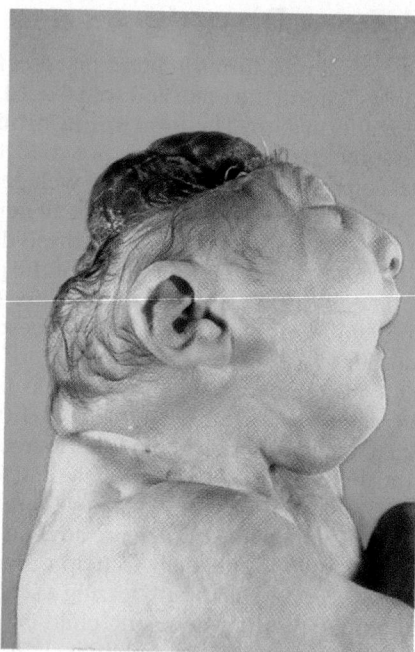

FIGURE 39.11 An infant with anencephaly. (Joseph R. Siebert, PhD/Custom Medical Stock Photo.)

Microcephaly.   Microcephaly is a disorder in which brain growth is so slow that it falls more than three standard deviations below normal on growth charts. The cause might be a disorder in brain development associated with an intrauterine infection such as rubella, cytomegalovirus, or toxoplasmosis. Microcephaly may also result from severe malnutrition or anoxia in early infancy.

The prognosis for a normal life is guarded in children with microcephaly and depends on the extent of restriction of brain growth and on the cause. Generally the infant is cognitively challenged because of the lack of functioning brain tissue. True microcephaly must be differentiated from craniosynostosis (normal brain growth but premature fusion of the cranial sutures), which also causes decreased head circumference. Infants with craniosynostosis have abnormally closed fontanelles and often show bulging (bossing of the forehead and signs of increased intracranial pressure). With surgery, craniosynostosis can be relieved and brain growth will be normal.

Spina Bifida Occulta.   Spina bifida occulta occurs when the posterior laminae of the vertebrae fail to fuse. This occurs most commonly at the fifth lumbar or first sacral level but may occur at any point along the spinal canal. The normal spinal cord is shown in Figure 39.12*A*. The disorder may be noticeable as a dimpling at the point of poor fusion; abnormal tufts of hair or discolored skin may be present (Guggisberg et al., 2004). Simple spina bifida occulta is a benign disorder; it occurs as frequently as in one of every four children (see Fig. 39.12*B*).

The term "spina bifida" is often used wrongly to denote all spinal cord anomalies. Because of this wrong usage, parents, when told that their child has a spina bifida occulta, may interpret this as meaning their child has an extremely serious disorder. Help clarify the degree of defect for them.

Meningocele.   If the meninges covering the spinal cord herniate through unformed vertebrae, a meningocele occurs. The anomaly appears as a protruding mass, usually approximately the size of an orange, at the center of the back (see Fig. 39.12*C*). It generally occurs in the lumbar region, although it might be present anywhere along the spinal canal. The protrusion may be covered by a layer of skin or only the clear dura mater.

Myelomeningocele.   In a myelomeningocele, the spinal cord and the meninges protrude through the vertebrae the same as with a meningocele. The difference is that the spinal cord ends at the point, so motor and sensory function is absent beyond this point (see Fig. 39.12*D*). Because this results in lower motor neuron damage, the child will have flaccidity and lack of sensation of the lower extremities and loss of bowel and bladder control. The infant's legs are lax, and he or she does not move them; urine and stools continually dribble because of lack of sphincter control. Children often have accompanying talipes (clubfoot)

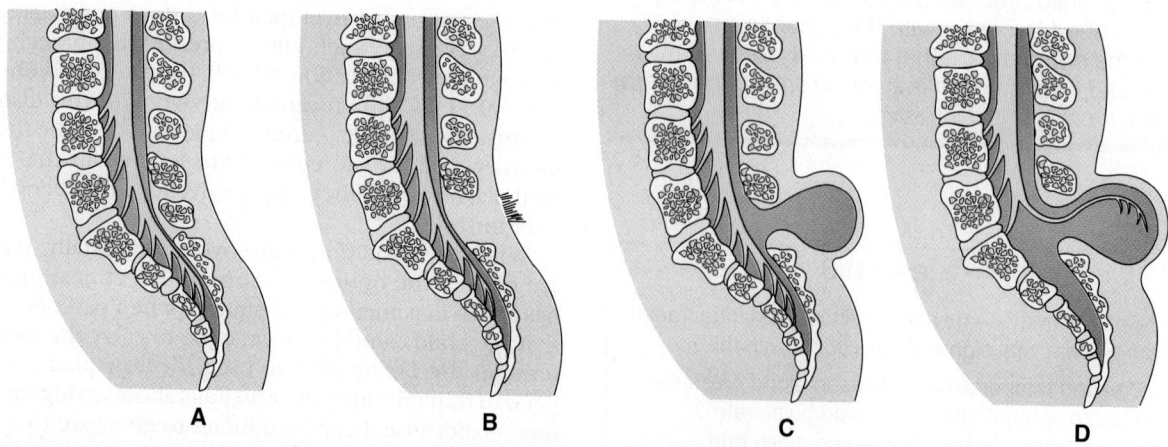

FIGURE 39.12 Degrees of spinal cord anomalies. (**A**) Normal spinal cord. (**B**) Spina bifida occulta. (**C**) Meningocele. (**D**) Myelomeningocele.

disorders and developmental hip dysplasia. Hydrocephalus accompanies myelomeningocele in as many as 80% of infants due to the lack of a subarachnoid membrane for CSF absorption; the higher the myelomeningocele occurs on the cord, the more likely it is that hydrocephalus will accompany it. It is generally difficult to tell from visual appearance whether the disorder is myelomeningocele or the simpler meningocele (Fig. 39.13). A CT or sonographic scan or MRI will reveal this.

Encephalocele. An encephalocele is a cranial meningocele or myelomeningocele. The disorder occurs most often in the occipital area of the skull but may occur as a nasal or nasopharyngeal disorder. Encephaloceles generally are covered fully by skin, but they may be open or covered only by the dura. It is difficult to tell from the size of the encephalocele if only CSF is trapped in the protruding meninges or whether brain tissue could also be involved. Transillumination of the sac will reveal solid substance or fluid in the sac. CT, MRI, or sonography will reveal the size of the skull disorder.

Assessment

Neural tube disorders may be discovered during intrauterine life by sonography, fetoscopy, amniocentesis (discovery of increased AFP in amniotic fluid), or analysis of AFP in the maternal serum. If the condition is discovered in utero, it may be possible to close the lesion by fetoscopic surgery (Tulipan, 2003). Infants may be born by cesarean birth to avoid pressure and injury to the spinal cord. Observe and record whether an infant born with a neural tube disorder has spontaneous movement of the lower extremities to assess if the child has lower motor function. Also assess the nature and pattern of voiding and defecation. A normal infant appears to be "always wet" from voiding but actually voids in amounts of approximately 30 mL and then is dry for 2 or 3 hours before voiding again. An infant without motor or sphincter control voids continually. This pattern is the same for defecation. Observing these features aids in differentiating between meningocele and myelomeningocele. Differentiation will be further established by sonography or MRI.

Therapeutic Management

Children with spina bifida occulta need no immediate surgical correction. The parents should be made aware of the defect, however, so they are not surprised when someone points it out to them in later life. Some children may eventually need surgery to prevent vertebral deterioration due to the unbalanced spinal column.

Treatment for a meningocele, myelomeningocele, or encephalocele involves surgery to replace the contents that are replaceable and to close the skin disorder to prevent infection. In the past, surgery for neural tube disorders was done only after the infant had survived the newborn period. Currently, it is done as soon after birth as possible (usually within 24 to 48 hours) so infection through the exposed meninges does not occur.

Parents need to be cautioned that the prognosis for the child depends on the extent of the disorder. Surgery is not without risk, and brain disorders accompanying an encephalocele may limit the child's cognitive potential. The loss of meninges by surgery may limit the rate of absorption of CSF. This may lead to a buildup, resulting in hydrocephalus. Parents need a great deal of support to care for a child with a myelomeningocele because their child has multiple challenges. The child with myelomeningocele will continue to have paralysis of the lower extremities and loss of bowel and bladder function after surgery because the absent lower cord cannot be replaced. Table 39.1 provides a classification of motor function ability according to the location of spinal cord disruptions.

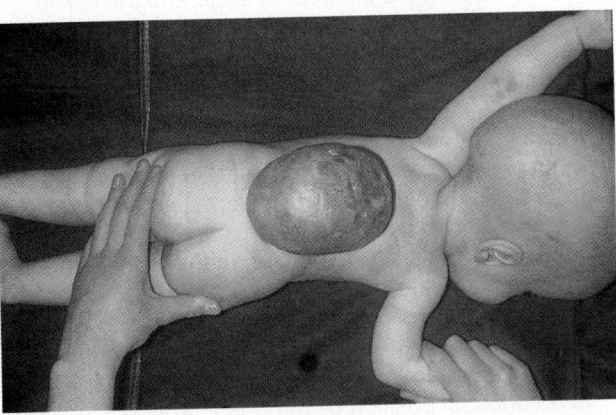

FIGURE 39.13 A myelomeningocele. The infant also has hydrocephaly and a subluxated hip. (NMSB/Custom Medical Stock Photo.)

TABLE 39.1

Motor Function Ability in Myelomeningocele

Spinal Cord Lesion	Resultant Effects
T6–12	Complete flaccid paralysis of the lower extremities; weakened abdominal and trunk musculature in higher lesions; kyphosis and scoliosis common; ambulation with maximal support
L1–2	Hip flexion present; paraplegia, ambulation with maximal support
L3–4	Hip flexion, adduction, and knee extension present; hip dislocation common; some control of hip and knee movement possible; ambulation with moderate support
L5	Hip flexion, adduction, and varying degrees of abduction; knee extension and weak knee flexion; paralysis of the lower legs and feet; ambulation with moderate support
S1–2	As above, with preservation of some foot and ankle movement; ambulation with minimal support
S3	Mild loss of intrinsic foot muscular function possible; ambulation without support

NURSING DIAGNOSES AND RELATED INTERVENTIONS: IMMEDIATE CONCERNS

Although parents of an infant with a myelomeningocele were told before surgery that their child's spinal disorder is a type that means motor and sensory function are absent in the child's lower extremities, the parents do not necessarily "hear" this information. Only after surgery do they begin to comprehend the extent of the condition. When the child is discharged from the hospital, be certain the parents understand what the next step in follow-up care will be. This prevents them from feeling deserted when they most need support—the time when they first begin to appreciate what this problem will mean to them in the coming years, and what it will mean to their child throughout life.

Nursing Diagnosis: Risk for infection related to rupture or bacterial invasion of the neural tube sac

Outcome Evaluation: Neural tube sac remains intact; axillary temperature remains below 98.6°F (37°C).

If the exposed meningeal sac is allowed to dry, it can crack, allowing CSF to drain and microorganisms to enter. Pressure on the protruding mass can rupture the sac, leading to quick decompression of the CSF (which can lead to herniation of the brain stem into the spinal cord and interference with respiratory and cardiac centers) and possibly to infection (meningitis). Such pressure may also force CSF from the sac into the spinal column, increasing intracranial pressure. Therefore, it is crucial to prevent drying of and pressure on the exposed membrane.

Preoperative Positioning. Before surgery, use sterile gloves and sterile linens when caring for the infant. Position infants carefully to prevent pressure on the exposed meninges, either in a prone position or supported on their side. When they are on their side, use a rolled blanket or diaper placed behind their upper back (above the disorder) and a separate one behind their lower back (below the disorder). This way, no pressure will be exerted on the lesion, and the infant will be protected from rolling backward onto it. Placing infants on their abdomen has the added advantage of keeping the flow of feces and urine away from the disorder as well as keeping the lesion free from pressure. A folded towel under the abdomen helps to flex the infant's hips, reduce pressure on the sac, and ensure good leg position. If an infant is on his or her side, putting a folded diaper between the legs prevents skin surfaces from touching and rubbing (and also helps to keep the hips from internally rotating). Always notice the position of the infant's legs. If they are paralyzed because of lack of motor control, the infant cannot move and straighten them to a comfortable position.

Placing a piece of plastic or sturdy plastic wrap below the meningocele on the child's back like an apron and taping it in place is another method of preventing feces from touching the open lesion. A sterile wet compress of saline, antiseptic, or antibiotic gauze over the lesion may be used to keep the sac moist. Rather than remove this to wet it again and risk rupturing the sac, merely add additional fluid.

Although no pressure should be exerted on the open lesion by a top sheet, make certain that the child is adequately warm. The presence of the sac adds to the amount of body surface area exposed, thereby increasing heat loss. The infant may need to be kept in an incubator to maintain body heat if a large area of the back cannot be covered. Use caution when placing the infant under a radiant heat source for warmth because radiant heat can dry the lesion and cause cracking. Any seepage of clear fluid from the disorder should be reported promptly, because this is probably escaping CSF. Checking any leakage for evidence of glucose will confirm the fluid is CSF (urine or mucus will not test positive for glucose).

Postoperative Care. After surgery, a child is again placed on the abdomen until the skin incision has healed (about 7 days). The same careful precautions against allowing urine or feces to touch the incision area are necessary.

Nursing Diagnosis: Risk for imbalanced nutrition, less than body requirements, related to difficulty assuming normal feeding position.

Outcome Evaluation: Child's skin turgor is good; weight is maintained within 10% of birthweight; specific gravity of urine remains between 1.003 and 1.030.

To maintain nutrition, help the parents hold the infant in as normal a feeding position as possible. Make certain that a supporting arm does not press against the lesion. Remind the parents that when bubbling the infant, they should not pat the back over the disorder. If the disorder is large and the risk in picking up the infant is too great, the infant may be fed while lying on his or her side in bed or prone on a specialized bed frame. Raise the infant's head slightly by slipping a folded diaper under it. Stroke the head, arms, or upper back while the infant sucks to give the child the same comfort and assurance at feeding time as a baby receives while being held. The infant may enjoy a pacifier after feeding, because he or she does not experience the same enjoyment of sucking while feeding that would be experienced if he could be held and cuddled. All new parents have some difficulty getting comfortable with feeding an infant. Parents who must feed their child in an unusual position or with the infant on a support frame will have even more difficulty. Role-model a warm, comforting parental role so parents begin to form a positive parent–child interaction.

Children with increased intracranial pressure tend to suck poorly. If this complication develops after surgery, breast-feeding may be difficult. Parents need a realistic explanation of the treatment planned for the child so they can decide whether to continue breast-feeding. If it is necessary to forgo breast-feeding for this child, you can assure parents that the child will thrive on commercial formula.

Nursing Diagnosis: Risk for ineffective cerebral tissue perfusion related to increased intracranial pressure.

Outcome Evaluation: Child's head circumference remains within present percentile on growth chart; signs and symptoms of increased intracranial pressure are absent.

Preoperative Care. Increasing head size from poor absorption of CSF (hydrocephalus) is a complication of neural tube disorders. To detect increased head size (development of hydrocephalus), measure head circumference once daily (or more frequently if ordered) in the preoperative period. Head circumference measurements are accurate only if the tape measure is placed on the same points of the child's head each time. Placing an indelible or ballpoint pen mark on the forehead just above the eyebrows and at the most prominent point of the occiput allows different people to measure the head during the day and yet be sure that they all measure at the same point.

Postoperative Care. Children may develop hydrocephalus after surgery, probably because of interference with subarachnoid absorption of CSF. The shortening of the meninges can create an Arnold-Chiari disorder (see below) or can cause traction of the hindbrain into the spinal cord. Observe the child frequently for signs of increased intracranial pressure such as changes in vital signs, neurologic signs such as pupillary changes, or an increase in head circumference or bulging fontanelles, as well as behavioral changes such as irritability or lethargy.

Nursing Diagnosis: Risk for impaired skin integrity related to required prone positioning.

Outcome Evaluation: Infant's skin remains intact, without erythema or ulceration.
Preserving skin integrity is a major problem before surgery because the constant prone position puts pressure on the infant's knees and elbows. Laying the infant on a synthetic sheepskin helps reduce friction; after surgery, use paper tape or stockinette for dressing changes or place protective dressings such as Stomahesive on the skin under the area where the tape will touch. Change diapers frequently to prevent excessive contact of acid urine with skin. If hydrocephalus has developed, the head will be heavy and pressure areas at the temples can occur if the head is not repositioned every 2 hours.

NURSING DIAGNOSES AND RELATED INTERVENTIONS: LONG-TERM CONCERNS

Nursing Diagnosis: Impaired physical mobility related to neural tube disorder

Outcome Evaluation: Child ambulates with the least amount of accessory equipment possible.
Help parents begin to plan stimulation activities for the infant that he or she can accomplish with limited mobility. Encourage them to take the infant to the places a child would normally accompany parents—relatives' homes, shopping, the zoo, and so forth. Encouraging the child to be independent will help him or her to lead as active a life as possible (Fig. 39.14).
Parents will need to perform passive exercises to prevent muscle atrophy and formation of contractures if a child has impaired lower extremity motor control. The child may need leg braces to help maintain good alignment and enable walking with crutches. Parents are generally anxious to do something for their child and follow routines of passive

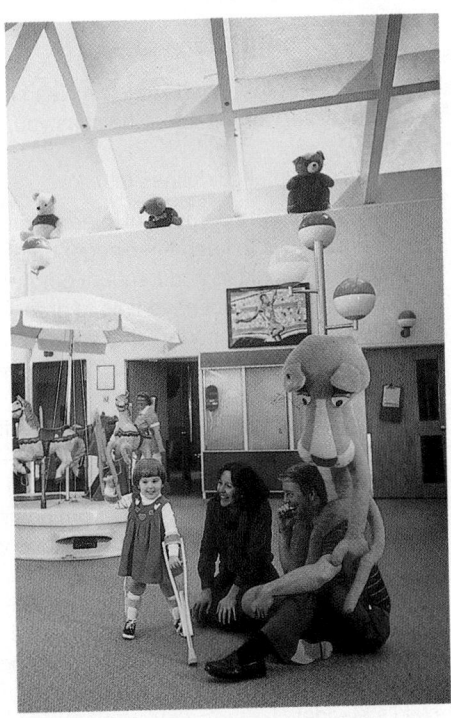

FIGURE 39.14 A child born with a neural tube disorder demonstrates her ability to walk using braces and a crutch. (Alexander Tsiara/Photo Researchers, Inc.)

exercises well if they are given sufficient support for their accomplishments at health care visits. As the child grows older, tendon transplants or osteotomy may be necessary to prevent contractures and poor bone alignment. Because children with myelomeningocele have no sensation in their lower extremities, parents must make a routine of inspecting the child's lower extremities and buttocks daily for any area of irritation or possible infection. Teach children as they grow older to do this themselves. When children are using a wheelchair, be certain they press with their arms on the armrests to raise their buttocks off the wheelchair seat at least once every hour. This will help provide adequate circulation to the lower extremities.

Nursing Diagnosis: Risk for impaired elimination related to neural tube disorder

Outcome Evaluation: Child demonstrates ability to independently manage bowel and bladder elimination by school age.

To ensure bladder emptying, an intermittent clean urinary catheterization technique is taught to parents (inserting a clean catheter through the urethra into the bladder every 4 hours to drain urine from the bladder; Box 39.7). As children reach early school age, they can learn this technique for themselves

(Campbell et al., 2004). Prescription of a drug such as oxybutynin chloride (Ditropan) may improve bladder capacity and allow a child to need less frequent catheterization (Box 39.8). It is possible to place artificial bladder sphincters in some children to help establish continence. In some children, a continent urinary reservoir or ureterosigmoidostomy (see Chapter 46) is constructed to bypass the nonfunctioning bladder. Children who are begun on intermittent clean catheterization from birth require fewer bladder augmentation procedures as they grow older.

Arnold-Chiari Disorder (Chiari II Malformation)

An Arnold-Chiari disorder is caused by overgrowth of the neural tube in weeks 16 to 20 of fetal life. The specific anomaly is a projection of the cerebellum, medulla oblongata, and fourth ventricle into the cervical canal. This causes the upper cervical spinal cord to jackknife backward, obstructing CSF flow and causing hydrocephalus. A lumbosacral myelomeningocele is also present in approximately 50% of children with this anomaly (Stevenson, 2004).

The prognosis for the child with an Arnold-Chiari malformation depends on the extent of the disorder and the

---

BOX 39.7 FOCUS ON . . .

FAMILY TEACHING

Instructions for Clean Intermittent Catheterization

Q. Baby Sparrow's mother needs to learn clean intermittent catheterization for her son. She asks you, "How do I do this?"

A. Here are some helpful guidelines to follow:

1. Remember that the purpose of intermittent catheterization is to keep the bladder empty by using clean technique and frequent emptying so microorganisms do not have time to grow in urine in the bladder. It is important that you always use clean equipment and that you catheterize at least every 4 hours to accomplish this.

2. Always carry catheterization equipment with you when away from home (a plastic bag containing a clean catheter and water-soluble lubricant). This enables you to stay longer away from home if you wish. If you will be using a public lavatory, you might want to include a presoaped washcloth rather than have to use rough paper towels.

3. To begin catheterization, wash your hands in warm, soapy water. This reduces the chance you will introduce germs from your hands into your child's bladder.

4. Next wash around your child's urinary meatus with a clean washcloth or paper towel and warm, soapy water. Rinse the washcloth and wash again with

clear water. This reduces the chance that germs on the child's skin will be pushed into the bladder.

5. Coat a clean catheter with a water-soluble lubricant. This reduces friction and makes the catheter slide into the bladder easily.

6. Quickly but gently insert the catheter into the urinary meatus approximately 6 inches. Urine should begin to flow immediately through the catheter. Let this drain into a collecting basin.

7. When urine stops flowing, gently remove the catheter. Clean the catheter with soap and water, rinse with clear water, and replace in the plastic bag with the lubricant.

8. Be certain that on special days (e.g., family celebrations or vacation) you do not forget the importance of catheterization.

9. As your child reaches school age, you can teach him how to do this himself. Be certain he will be able to have access to a school bathroom every 4 hours during the day.

10. Phone your health care provider if urine is blood-tinged, smells foul, or is cloudy rather than clear or if your child appears to have pain in his abdomen or lower back or has an elevated temperature. These may be symptoms of a urinary tract infection.

BOX 39.8 FOCUS ON . . .

PHARMACOLOGY

Oxybutynin Chloride (Ditropan)

Classification: Oxybutynin is an anticholinergic, urinary antispasmodic.

Action: Relaxes smooth muscle to relieve symptoms of bladder instability associated with neurogenic bladder (Karch, 2004).

Pregnancy risk category: C

Dosage: 5 mg orally, b.i.d.

Possible adverse effects: Drowsiness, dizziness, blurred vision, decreased sweating

Nursing Implications

- Advise the parents to give or have the child take the medication exactly as prescribed.
- Alert the parents about the need for frequent bladder examinations during treatment to document the drug's effect.
- Ask the child to report drowsiness or blurred vision. Caution the child not to attempt activities that require balance while taking the drug.
- Caution the child and parents that with decreased sweating, body temperature can rise. Encourage the parents to keep the child's environment cool and avoid high temperatures.

surgical procedure possible. Because of the upper motor neuron involvement, gagging and swallowing reflexes may be absent, increasing the risk for tracheal aspiration.

SKELETAL PHYSICAL AND DEVELOPMENTAL DISORDERS

Several steps that compromise fetal physical growth can result in skeletal disorders in the newborn.

Absent or Malformed Extremities

Congenital skeletal disorders may result from reasons such as maternal drug ingestion, virus invasion during pregnancy, or amniotic band formation in utero. Statin drugs, taken by many women 35 to 40 years of age for elevated cholesterol, may be an offender (Edison & Muenke, 2004). In most instances, however, the cause of the anomaly cannot be established. Children born without an extremity or with a malformed extremity can be fitted with a prosthesis early in life. In most instances, children will have better function if the malformed portion of an extremity is amputated before a prosthesis is fitted. This is a difficult decision for parents to make, however, because it is one that they cannot undo later. They need assurance that hands with missing fingers, for example, will not later grow to become normal. A well-fitted prosthesis that a child learns to use at an early age will provide more function and allow a more normal childhood and adult life than if the original

disorder is left unchanged (Fig. 39.15). Lower extremity prostheses are fitted as early as age 6 months (so an infant will learn to stand at the normal time). Upper extremity prostheses are fitted this early also, so an infant can handle and explore objects readily.

Introducing a prosthesis early also prevents a child from adjusting to a missing extremity, such as writing with the feet or sliding across a floor rather than walking. Children can become so proficient at these adjustments that later in life they do not see the advantage of a prosthesis and refuse to use one. Although these self-adjustments may be cute in infants, in the long run they greatly limit a child's potential.

Learning to use a hand prosthesis takes weeks to months. Help parents think of interesting activities when introducing the prosthesis so the child can see immediately how useful it will be to him or her. Gait training for use of lower extremity prostheses begins with the use of parallel bars and proceeds to independent walking and mastery of steps.

Children who are born with an absent extremity may need help in mastering not only the use of a prosthesis but also a positive body image of themselves as whole. If possible, in the newborn period, introduce parents to the rehabilitation team who will be following their child. Further steps then will be outlined for them to help them move past the helplessness they may feel to more positive action. Visiting with a child who uses a prosthesis well can be a great help in convincing parents that their child can lead a normal life. Children with a congenital extremity loss do not grieve over the lost extremity as do adults or older children, which means they are often better prepared to move quickly to rehabilitation.

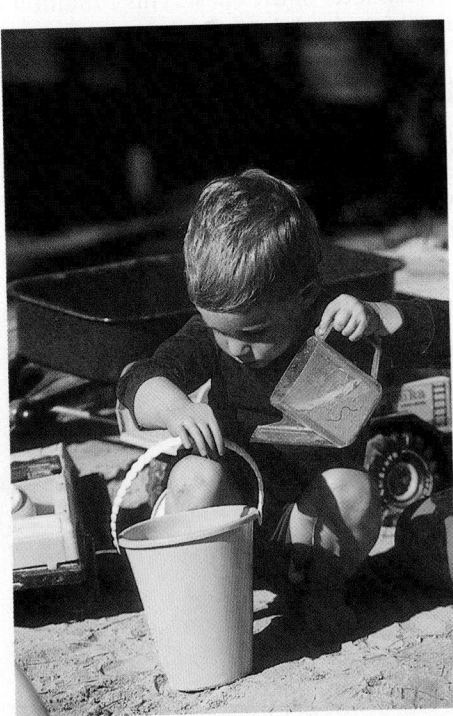

FIGURE 39.15 A young child learns to use a hand prosthesis during play. (M. Grecco/Stock Boston.)

Finger and Toe Conditions

Polydactyly is the presence of one or more additional fingers or toes (Gore & Spencer, 2004). When an entire extra finger or toe forms, the supernumerary digit is usually amputated in infancy or early childhood. These extra fingers are often just cartilage or skin tags, and removal is simple and cosmetically sound. In **syndactyly** (two fingers or toes are fused), the fusion is usually caused by a simple webbing (Fig. 39.16); separation of the digits into two sound and cosmetically appealing ones is usually successful. In other instances, the bones of the fingers or toes are also fused, and cosmetic appearance and function cannot be fully reconstructed.

These hand anomalies are always upsetting to parents (one of the first things that new parents do is count the fingers and toes of newborns). They may need time to air their feelings and concerns. They may need reassurance at health maintenance visits throughout their child's development that he or she is normal in other ways so they can accept and help the child develop self-esteem. Children need this same type of assurance so they can think of themselves as well people.

Chest Deviations

Pectus excavatum is an indentation of the lower portion of the sternum (Smith, 2004). Children usually are born with this condition, but they may also develop it after chronic obstructive lung disease or rickets. As a result, lung volume decreases and the heart is displaced to the left. This condition can be repaired, either for cosmetic reasons or to expand lung volume. With pectus carinatum, the sternum is displaced anteriorly, increasing the anterior-posterior diameter of the chest. This condition also can be repaired for physiologic or cosmetic reasons.

Torticollis (Wry Neck)

Torticollis is a term derived from *tortus* (twisted) and *collum* (neck). Torticollis (wry neck) occurs as a congenital anomaly when the sternocleidomastoid muscle is injured and bleeds during birth. This tends to occur in newborns

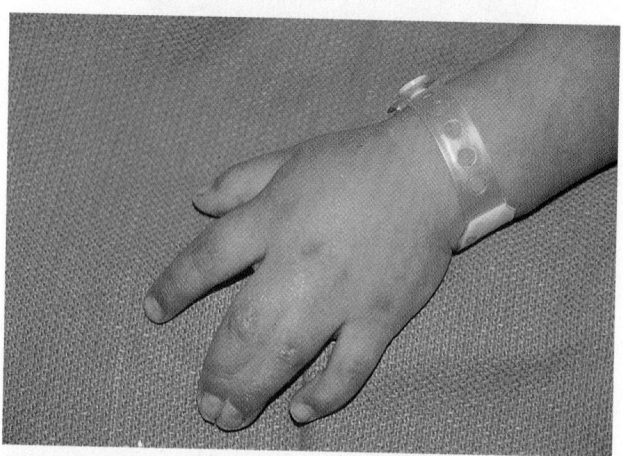

FIGURE 39.16 Syndactyly. (JPD/Custom Medical Stock Photo.)

with wide shoulders when pressure is exerted on the head to deliver the shoulder. The infant holds the head tilted to the side of the muscle involved; the chin rotates to the opposite side. The injury may not be noticeable in the newborn and may become evident only as the original hemorrhage recedes and fibrous contraction occurs at 1 to 2 months of age. A thick mass over the muscle can usually be palpated at this time.

To relieve torticollis, parents need to begin a program of passive stretching exercises and always encouraging the infant to look in the direction of the affected muscle. Parents could encourage this by holding the child to feed in such a position that the child must look in the desired direction. Placing a mobile on the child's crib to encourage the child to look toward the affected side also is helpful. The parents should speak to and hand the child objects from the affected side to make the child look that way.

If manual stretching is begun early and consistently by the parents, further treatment usually is not necessary. Help parents understand that these actions are important therapy and not just games. Otherwise, the exercises seem so simple parents may not take them seriously. In the few instances in which simple exercises are not effective and the condition still exists at 1 year of age, surgical correction followed by a neck immobilizer will be necessary. If extreme injury to the muscle occurred, torticollis can lead to the continued elevation of one shoulder. Although a rare complication, this has the potential to lead to scoliosis later in life.

Parents may ask about the use of botulism (Botox) injections, because adults who develop spastic torticollis may receive this type of treatment (Walker, 2003). This type of treatment is not recommended for infants.

Craniosynostosis

Craniosynostosis is premature closure of the sutures of the skull. This may occur in utero or early in infancy because of rickets or irregularities of calcium or phosphate metabolism; it also may occur without any known cause. It occurs more often in boys than girls.

This condition needs to be detected early because premature closure of the suture line will seal the skull closed and compromise brain growth. When the sagittal suture line closes prematurely, the child's head tends to grow anteriorly and posteriorly. If the coronal suture line fuses early, the orbits of the eyes become misshapen, and the increased intracranial pressure may lead to exophthalmos, nystagmus, papilledema, strabismus, and atrophy of the optic nerve with consequent loss of vision. Premature closure of the coronal suture line is associated with syndactyly. Therefore, closely observe all infants with syndactyly for head circumference. Conversely, assess all infants with craniosynostosis for syndactyly. Cardiac anomalies, choanal atresias, or disorders of elbows and knee joints are also associated with craniosynostosis.

Measure head circumference on all children age 2 years or younger at health maintenance visits and compare these measurements with normal head circumference charts. The posterior fontanelle normally closes at 2 months of age, the anterior fontanelle at 12 to 18 months. Children whose fontanelles close before these typical times need

The child has only streak (small and nonfunctional) ovaries, so that with the exception of pubic hair, secondary sex characteristics do not develop at puberty. Females with this disorder cannot reproduce because of limited ovarian function. The incidence of the syndrome is approximately 1 per 1,000 live births.

Although children with Turner's syndrome may be cognitively challenged, more commonly intelligence is normal. Some children may have learning disabilities.

Growth hormone can be helpful to achieve additional height (Cave, Bryant, & Milne, 2005). If treatment with estrogen is begun at approximately 13 years, secondary sex characteristics will appear. Long-term estrogen supplementation may also be important to prevent osteoporosis in these girls (Hanton et al., 2003). If girls continue taking estrogen for 3 out of every 4 weeks, they will have withdrawal bleeding that results in a menstrual flow. This flow, however, does not correct the problem of sterility. The gonadal tissue is scant and inadequate for ovulation because of the basic chromosomal aberration.

Klinefelter's Syndrome

Infants with Klinefelter's syndrome are boys with an XXY chromosome pattern (47XXY) (Hall et al., 2003). The incidence is about 1 in 1,000 live births. Characteristics of the syndrome may not be noticeable until puberty when the child does not develop secondary sex characteristics. The testes are small and produce ineffective sperm. Boys with the disorder tend to develop gynecomastia (increased breast size). The syndrome may be associated with an increased risk of developing male breast cancer.

Fragile X Syndrome

Fragile X syndrome is an X-linked pattern of inheritance in which one long arm of an X chromosome is weakened. The incidence is about 1 in 1,000 live births. It is the most common cause of cognitive challenge in boys (Kornman et al., 2005).

Before puberty, boys with fragile X syndrome typically have maladaptive behaviors such as hyperactivity and autism. They have reduced intellectual functioning, with marked deficits in speech and arithmetic. They may be identified by the presence of a large head, a long face with a high forehead, a prominent lower jaw, and large protruding ears. Hyperextensive joints and cardiac disorders may also be present. After puberty, enlarged testicles may become evident. Affected individuals are fertile and can reproduce. Carrier females may show some evidence of the physical and cognitive characteristics.

Although the intellectual function of children with the syndrome cannot be improved, both folic acid and phenothiazine administration may improve symptoms of poor concentration and impulsivity.

Down Syndrome (Trisomy 21)

Trisomy 21 (47XX21+ or 47Xy21+), the most common chromosomal abnormality, is seen as frequently as 1 in 800 live births. The syndrome occurs most frequently in the pregnancies of women who are over 35 years of age:

the incidence is as high as 1 in 100 live births for these women. Paternal age (over 55) may also contribute to the increased incidence (Chung, 2003). Because of prenatal diagnosis, the incidence of Down syndrome apparently is decreasing (Box 39.10).

The physical features of children with Down syndrome are so marked that fetal diagnosis is possible by sonography in utero. The nose is broad and flat, the eyelids have an extra fold of tissue at the inner canthus (an epicanthal fold), and the palpebral fissure (opening between the eyelids) tends to slant laterally upward. The iris of the eye may have white specks in it, called Brushfield's spots. Even in the newborn, the tongue may protrude from the mouth because the oral cavity is smaller than normal. The back of the head is flat, the neck is short, and an extra pad of fat at the base of the head causes the skin there to be so loose it can be lifted up (like a puppy's neck). The ears may be low-set. Muscle tone is poor, giving the baby a rag-doll appearance. This can be so lax that when the child lies supine, the child's toe can be touched against the nose (not possible in the average mature newborn). The fingers of many children with Down syndrome are short and thick, and the little finger is often curved inward. There may be a wide space between the first and second toes and the first and second fingers. The palm of the hand shows a peculiar crease (a simian line) or a horizontal palm crease rather than the normal three creases in the palm (see Fig. 7.15B).

Children with Down syndrome usually have some degree of cognitive challenge, but the degree can range from that of less involvement (IQ 50 to 70) to one requiring total care (IQ less than 20). The degree of cognitive challenge is not evident at birth. Those with near-average IQs may represent mosaic chromosomal patterns. The fact that the brain is not developing well is shown by a head size that is generally under the 10th to 20th percentile.

BOX 39.10 FOCUS ON . . .

EVIDENCE-BASED PRACTICE

Are Down Syndrome Births Growing in Number as More Women Have Babies Later in Life?

To answer this question, researchers used birth certificate records to survey the number of Down syndrome births occurring annually. The results of the survey showed that although an increase in Down syndrome births had been predicted because of the increasing age at which women are having their first babies, Down syndrome births are actually declining, down 15% from what was expected. In 2001, women 15 to 34 years of age had 45% fewer affected pregnancies, and women 35 to 49 years of age had 53% fewer such births.

This is an interesting study for nurses because it points out the importance of keeping abreast of trends in care; knowing trends helps with distribution of resources and improves care.

Source: Egan, J. F. X., et al. (2004). Down syndrome births in the United States from 1989 to 2001. *American Journal of Obstetrics and Gynecology, 191*(3), 1044–1048.

In addition to the above difficulties, children with Down syndrome appear to have altered immune function, making them prone to upper respiratory infections. Perhaps for this same reason, acute lymphocytic leukemia occurs approximately 20 times more frequently in children with Down syndrome than in the healthy population. Congenital heart diseases, especially atrioventricular disorders, stenosis or atresia of the duodenum, strabismus, and cataract disorders also are common. Even if children are born without an accompanying disorder such as heart disease, their lifespan generally is only 50 to 60 years, as aging seems to occur faster than in other people.

Children with Down syndrome need to be exposed to early educational and play opportunities (see Chapter 54). Because they are prone to infection, sensible precautions such as using good handwashing technique should always be taken when caring for them. In infancy, the enlarged tongue may interfere with swallowing and cause choking unless the child is fed slowly.

As with all newborns, children with Down syndrome need physical examination at birth so that the genetic disorder can be detected and counseling and support for parents and siblings can begin.

✔ Checkpoint Question 5

What is a typical description of an infant with Down syndrome?

a. Holds arms stiff and pronated.
b. Muscles are hypotonic or flaccid.
c. Head is larger than other infants.
d. Skin is ruddy and vein-streaked.

Key Points

Learning about the way a child will be physically challenged early on helps parents and child adjust to it. Advocate for parents by helping them obtain as much information as they need about their child's condition.

Parent–infant bonding is often difficult to establish when a child is hospitalized at birth. Assess family relationships at health maintenance visits to see that bonding is occurring.

Cleft lip and palate result from the failure of the maxillary process to fuse in intrauterine life. Surgical repair is possible early in life, with a good prognosis for both these conditions.

Tracheoesophageal atresia and fistula occur from failure of the trachea and esophagus to divide appropriately in intrauterine life. Surgical intervention often needs to be performed in several stages.

Omphalocele is the protrusion of abdominal contents through the abdominal wall at birth, protected only by a peritoneal membrane. When the membrane is not present, this is called gastroschisis. Although several stages of repair are often necessary, surgical correction has a good outcome.

Intestinal obstruction can result from atresia (complete closure) or stenosis (narrowing) of a part of the bowel. Correction is surgical removal of the narrowed bowel portion.

A meconium plug occurs when an extremely hard portion of meconium blocks the lumen of the intestine. Infants with meconium plug syndrome need to be observed for continuing bowel function and need to be assessed for cystic fibrosis, because a meconium plug is often a symptom of this.

Diaphragmatic hernia occurs when the abdominal organs protrude through a defect in the diaphragm into the chest cavity. This prevents the lungs from fully expanding at birth. These infants are critically ill at birth and need extensive surgical correction.

Imperforate anus is stricture of the anus, resulting in inability to pass stool. The infant may have a temporary colostomy created before a final surgical correction.

Physical developmental disorders of the nervous system include hydrocephalus (excess CSF in the ventricles) and spina bifida (incomplete closure of the spinal cord). Infants with hydrocephalus need surgery to relieve a ventricular obstruction or have a shunt implanted from their ventricles to the peritoneal cavity to remove excess CSF. Children with myelomeningocele, the most severe form of neural cord disorder, face permanent loss of lower neuron function and require continued rehabilitation.

Absent or malformed extremities may range from absence of a finger to absence of an entire limb. Children may need physical therapy and teaching on how to use a prosthesis to have full function.

Developmental hip dysplasia is the improper formation and function of the hip socket; talipes deformities are foot and ankle deformities. Children may need extensive bracing and casting to correct these disorders.

Common nondisjunction genetic disorders that cause developmental concerns include Down syndrome (trisomy 21), trisomy 13 syndrome, trisomy 18 syndrome, Turner's syndrome, and Klinefelter's syndrome. Most of the children affected by these disorders are cognitively challenged.

Critical Thinking Exercises

1. Bobby Jo Sparrow is a 16-year-old teenager whose newborn has been admitted to the neonatal intensive care unit because of a neural tube disorder and congenital hip dysplasia. Ms. Sparrow is obviously upset over the diagnosis. She says, "I'm a good person. The

only thing I did wrong during pregnancy was to take some cough medicine, so how could this have happened?" How would you answer her? What type of advice would be most helpful to her?

2. Baby Sparrow has developmental hip dysplasia and will be placed in a large cast. What suggestions could you make to his mother to help her instill a strong sense of trust in her child? A sense of autonomy?

3. You notice Baby Sparrow's mother is obviously upset at her child's appearance. She doesn't want to feed the baby and voices the thought of placing her for adoption. In contrast, the child's father, age 22, handles the baby warmly and asks questions about surgery. No grandparents visit. What interventions would you want to begin with this family?

4. Examine the National Health Goals related to children born with physical or developmental disorders. Most government-sponsored money for nursing research is allotted based on these goals. What would be a possible research topic to explore pertinent to these goals that would be applicable to the Sparrow family and also advance evidence-based practice?

References

Blazer, S., et al. (2004). Fetal omphalocele detected early in pregnancy: Associated anomalies and outcomes. *Radiology, 232*(1), 191-195.

Borkowski, S. (2004). Clinical challenge. Unsightly congenital protrusion on a toddler's abdomen: The little girl's mother expressed concern about the disfiguring appearance of the umbilical growth. *Clinical Advisor, 7*(8), 122-127.

Burge, D., & Drewett, M. (2004). Meconium plug obstruction. *Pediatric Surgery International, 20*(2), 108-110.

Campbell, J. B., et al. (2004). Complications associated with clean intermittent catheterization in children with spina bifida. *Journal of Urology, 171*(6 Pt 1), 2420-2422.

Cave, C. B., Bryant, J., & Milne, R. (2005). Recombinant growth hormone in children and adolescents with Turner syndrome. *The Cochrane Library (Oxford) (4)* (CD003887).

Centers for Disease Control. (2004). Spina bifida and anencephaly before and after folic acid mandate, United States, 1995-1996 and 1999-2000. *MMWR: Morbidity and Mortality Weekly Report, 53*(17), 362-365.

Choong, Y. F., et al. (2003). Goldenhar and cri-du-chat syndromes: A contiguous gene deletion syndrome? *Journal of AAPOS: American Association for Pediatric Ophthalmology & Strabismus, 7*(3), 226-227.

Chung, E. K. (2003). Down (trisomy 21) syndrome. In M. W. Schwartz, *5-minute pediatric consult.* Philadelphia: Lippincott Williams & Wilkins.

Davidson, R. S. (2003). Clubfoot. In M. W. Schwartz, *5-minute pediatric consult.* Philadelphia: Lippincott Williams & Wilkins.

Department of Health and Human Services. (2000). *Healthy people 2010.* Washington, DC: DHHS.

Edison, R. J., & Muenke, M. (2004). Central nervous system and limb anomalies in case reports of first-trimester statin exposure. *New England Journal of Medicine, 350*(15), 1579-1582.

Egan, J. F., et al. (2004). Down syndrome births in the United States from 1989 to 2001. *American Journal of Obstetrics and Gynecology, 191*(3), 1044-1048.

Flynn, J. M. (2003). Developmental dysplasia of the hip. In M. W. Schwartz, *5-minute pediatric consult.* Philadelphia: Lippincott Williams & Wilkins.

Glassford, B. (2003). Ethical issues. A case study in caring: Trisomy 18 syndrome. *American Journal of Nursing, 103*(7), 81-83.

Gore, A. I., & Spencer, J. P. (2004). The newborn foot. *American Family Physician, 69*(4), 865-872.

Guggisberg, D., et al. (2004). Skin markers of occult spinal dysraphism in children: A review of 54 cases. *Archives of Dermatology, 140*(9), 1109-1115.

Hall, S., et al. (2003). Providing information on Klinefelter syndrome. *British Journal of Midwifery, 11*(3), 164-168.

Hanton, L., et al. (2003). The importance of estrogen replacement in young women with Turner syndrome. *Journal of Women's Health, 12*(10), 971-977.

Kalu, P. U., & Moss, A. L. (2004). An unusual case of ankyloglossia superior. *British Journal of Plastic Surgery, 57*(6), 579-581.

Kamath, S. U., & Bennet, G. C. (2004). Does developmental dysplasia of the hip cause a delay in walking? *Journal of Pediatric Orthopedics, 24*(3), 265-266.

Kang, P. B. (2003). Hydrocephalus. In M. W. Schwartz, *5-minute pediatric consult.* Philadelphia: Lippincott Williams & Wilkins.

Karch, A. M. (2004). *Lippincott's nursing drug guide.* Philadelphia: Lippincott Williams & Wilkins.

Katz, D., & Conway, D. H. (2003). Tracheoesophageal fistula (TEF) and esophageal atresia. In M. W. Schwartz, *5-minute pediatric consult.* Philadelphia: Lippincott Willliams & Wilkins.

Kestle, J. R. W. (2003). Pediatric hydrocephalus: Current management. *Neurologic Clinics, 21*(4), 883-895.

Kirschner, R. E., et al. (2003). Surgical airway management in Pierre Robin sequence: Is there a role for tongue-lip adhesion? *Cleft Palate-Craniofacial Journal, 40*(1), 13-18.

Kirschner, R. E., Carman-Dillon, C. A., & Low, D. W. (2003). Cleft lip and palate. In M. W. Schwartz, *5-minute pediatric consult.* Philadelphia: Lippincott Willliams & Wilkins.

Kornman, L., et al. (2005). Pre-conception and antenatal screening for the fragile site on the X-chromosome. *The Cochrane Library (Oxford) (4)* (CD001806).

Kovesi, T., & Rubin, S. (2004). Long-term complications of congenital esophageal atresia and/or tracheoesophageal fistula. *Chest, 126*(3), 915-925.

Laughon, M., et al. (2003). Rising birth prevalence of gastroschisis. *Journal of Perinatology, 23*(4), 291-293.

Letourneau, N., et al. (2003). Deciding on surgery: Supporting parents of infants with craniosynostosis. *AXON, 24*(3), 24-29.

Lindstrom, D. R., et al. (2004). Anterior lingual thyroglossal cyst: Antenatal diagnosis, management, and long-term outcome. *International Journal of Pediatric Otorhinolaryngology, 67*(9), 1031-1034.

Lovrekovic, G. (2003). Diaphragmatic hernia. In M. W. Schwartz, *5-minute pediatric consult.* Philadelphia: Lippincott Willliams & Wilkins.

Lumley, J., et al. (2005). Periconceptional supplementation with folate and/or multivitamins for preventing neural tube defects. *The Cochrane Library (Oxford) (3)* (CD001056).

McCollough, M., & Sharieff, G. Q. (2003). Abdominal surgical emergencies in infants and young children. *Emergency Medicine Clinics of North America, 21*(4), 909-935.

Moyer, V., et al. (2005). Late versus early surgical correction for congenital diaphragmatic hernia in newborn infants. *The Cochrane Library (Oxford) (4)* (CD001695).

Nisell, M., et al. (2003). International pediatric nursing. How a family is affected when a child is born with anorectal malformation. *Journal of Pediatric Nursing: Nursing Care of Children and Families, 18*(6), 423–432.

Pelchat, D., et al. (2004). Parental satisfaction with an early family intervention program. *Journal of Perinatal and Neonatal Nursing, 18*(2), 128–144.

Scherl, S. A. (2004). Common lower extremity problems in children. *Pediatrics in Review, 25*(2), 52–62.

Smith, K. A. (2004). Pectus excavatum: More than meets the eye. *Orthopaedic Nursing, 23*(3),190–194.

Souchet, P., et al. (2004). Functional treatment of clubfoot: A new series of 350 idiopathic clubfeet with long-term follow-up. *Journal of Pediatric Orthopaedics, 13*(3), 189–196.

Stenchever, M. A. (2003). Mortality associated with trisomy 13 and trisomy 18. *ACOG Clinical Review, 8*(6), 5–6.

Stevenson, K. L. (2004). Chiari Type II malformation: Past, present, and future. *Neurosurgical Focus, 16*(2), E5.

Tanaka, N., et al. (2003). The comparison of the effects of short-term growth hormone treatment in patients with achondroplasia and with hypochondroplasia. *Endocrine Journal, 50*(1), 69–75.

Telega, G. (2003). Imperforate anus. In M. W. Schwartz, *5-minute pediatric consult.* Philadelphia: Lippincott Willliams & Wilkins.

Tulenko, D. R. (2004). An update on ECMO. *Neonatal Network: The Journal of Neonatal Nursing, 23*(4), 11–18.

Tulipan, N. (2003). Intrauterine myelomeningocele repair. *Clinics in Perinatology, 30*(3), 521–530.

von Koch, C. S., et al. (2003). In utero surgery for hydrocephalus. *Child's Nervous System, 19*(7–8), 574–586.

Wagener, S., et al. (2003). Management of infants with Pierre Robin sequence. *Cleft Palate-Craniofacial Journal, 40*(2), 180–185.

Walker, F. O. (2003). Botulinum toxin therapy for cervical dystonia. *Physical Medicine and Rehabilitation Clinics of North America, 14*(4), 749–766.

Ward, K. (2003). Genetics and prenatal diagnosis. In J. R. Scott, et al. *Danforth's obstetrics and gynecology* (9th ed.). Philadelphia: Lippincott Williams & Wilkins.

Williams, T., Butler, R., & Sundem, T. (2003). Management of the infant with gastroschisis: A comprehensive review of the literature. *Newborn and Infant Nursing Reviews, 3*(2), 55–63.

Suggested Readings

Baumann, S. L., Dyches, T. T., & Braddick, M. (2005). Being a sibling. *Nursing Science Quarterly, 18*(1), 51–58.

Berrocal, T., et al. (2004). Congenital anomalies of the tracheo-bronchial tree, lung, and mediastinum: Embryology, radiology, and pathology. *Radiographics, 24*(1), e17–e22.

Conway, A., & Moloney-Harmon, P. (2004). Ethical issues in the neonatal intensive care unit. *Critical Care Nursing Clinics of North America, 16*(2), 271–278.

Deurloo, J. A., et al. (2003). Gastroesophageal reflux: Prevalence in adults older than 28 years after correction of esophageal atresia. *Annals of Surgery, 238*(5), 686–689.

Johansson, B., & Ringsberg, K. C. (2004). Parents' experiences of having a child with cleft lip and palate. *Journal of Advanced Nursing, 47*(2), 165–173.

King, J., & Askin, D. F. (2003). Gastroschisis: Etiology, diagnosis, delivery options, and care. *Neonatal Network: The Journal of Neonatal Nursing, 22*(4), 7–12.

Roberts, G., Palfrey, J., & Bridgemohan, C. (2004). A rational approach to the medical evaluation of a child with developmental delay. *Patient Care for the Nurse Practitioner, 1*(5), 1–21.

Rowland, R., Wisenor, D. & Roberts, G. H. (2003). Down syndrome. *Journal of Continuing Education Topics & Issues, 5*(1), 172–177.

Sridhar, A. V. & Nichani, S. (2004). Late presenting congenital diaphragmatic hernia. *Emergency Medicine Journal, 21*(2), 261–262.

Van Riper, M. (2003). Living with illness. A change of plans: The birth of a child with Down syndrome doesn't have to be a negative experience. *Journal of Nursing, 103*(6), 71–74.

Nursing Care of a Child With a Respiratory Disorder

Key Terms

adventitious sounds
anoxia
arterial blood gases
aspiration
atelectasis
clubbing
cyanosis
expiration
hypoxemia
hypoxia
inspiration
paroxysmal coughing
percussion
pneumothorax
rales
retraction
steatorrhea
stridor
tachypnea
tracheostomy
tracheotomy
vibration
wheezing

Objectives

After mastering the contents of this chapter, you should be able to:

1. Describe common respiratory illnesses in children.
2. Assess a child with a respiratory disorder.
3. Formulate nursing diagnoses related to respiratory disorders in children.
4. Identify expected outcomes that address the priority needs of a child with a respiratory disorder.
5. Plan nursing care for a child with a respiratory disorder.
6. Implement nursing care for a child with a respiratory disorder.
7. Evaluate expected outcomes for achievement and effectiveness of care.
8. Identify National Health Goals related to children with respiratory disorders that nurses could help the nation achieve.
9. Identify areas related to care of children with respiratory disorders that could benefit from additional nursing research or application of evidence-based practice.
10. Use critical thinking to analyze ways nursing care for a child with a respiratory disorder could be more family-centered.
11. Integrate knowledge of respiratory disorders in children with nursing process to achieve quality maternal and child health nursing care.

Michael is a 4-year-old who is brought to the ER by paramedics after responding to an emergency call by his grandmother at his home. He has a sharp, barking cough and is obviously short of breath. "I can't breathe!" Michael shouts at you. "I gave him some chocolate. Is he allergic to that?" his grandmother shouts. Michael is diagnosed as having laryngotracheobronchitis (croup) and admitted to an ambulatory care unit.

Previous chapters described the growth and development of well children. This chapter adds information about the dramatic changes, both physical and psychosocial, that occur when children develop respiratory disorders. This is important information because it builds a base for care and health teaching.

What emergency care does Michael need? What about Michael's action would lead you to believe his airway is not yet completely obstructed?

After you've studied this chapter, access the accompanying website. Read the patient scenario and answer the questions to further sharpen your skills, grow more familiar with RN-CLEX types of questions, and reward yourself with how much you have learned.

Respiratory disorders are among the most common causes of illness and hospitalization in children. Overall, respiratory dysfunction in children tends to be more serious than in adults because the lumens in a child's respiratory tract are smaller and therefore more likely to become obstructed. Because respiratory disorders range from minor illnesses such as a simple upper respiratory tract infection to life-threatening lower respiratory tract diseases, such as pneumonia, and because the level of acuity can change quickly, respiratory disorders are often difficult for parents to evaluate. Both a child and parents need a great deal of nursing support when disease interferes with the function of breathing, because even very young children can panic when breathing becomes labored. Early diagnosis and treatment are essential in preventing a minor problem from turning into a more serious one.

Because respiratory disorders are such a common cause of childhood illness and hospitalization, National Health Goals have been established for children with respiratory illnesses (Box 40.1).

BOX 40.1 FOCUS ON . . .

NATIONAL HEALTH GOALS

A number of National Health Goals focus on respiratory illness in children:

- Reduce the rate of tobacco use by adolescents, from a baseline of 35% to a target of 21%.
- Reduce the incidence of invasive pneumococcal infections in children younger than 5 years, from a baseline of 76/100,000 to a target of 46/100,000.
- Reduce the incidence of tuberculosis, from a baseline of 6.8/100,000 cases yearly to a target level of 1.0/100,000.
- Reduce indoor allergen levels such as dust mites.
- Increase or maintain the number of territories or states that monitor diseases such as asthma that can be caused by exposure to environmental hazards, from a baseline of 6 to 25.
- Reduce the rate of asthma deaths in children aged 5 to 14 years, from a baseline of 3.3/million to a target level of 1.0/million.
- Reduce the rate of hospital emergency department visits for children with asthma younger than 5 years, from 150/10,000 to 80/10,000 (DHHS, 2000).

Nurses can help the nation achieve these goals by teaching children to avoid beginning cigarette smoking, teaching children with asthma to learn ways of increasing activity and what steps to take to reduce the severity of an attack, and reminding parents to come for child health maintenance visits so that children can receive pneumococcal immunization or screening for tuberculosis, as appropriate.

Additional nursing research is needed about the accuracy of parents in self-reading and interpreting tuberculosis screening tests; motivations for children to keep participating in asthma exercise programs; and information required by new parents to better manage respiratory illness in infants and young children.

Nursing Process Overview

For a Child With a Respiratory Disorder

● Assessment

Respiratory illness can begin at birth when a newborn has difficulty initiating a first breath or establishing regular respirations. Rating a newborn using an Apgar score can help to quickly identify a newborn who may be experiencing respiratory difficulty at this early stage.

As a nurse in a well-child clinic or health maintenance organization, you are often the first health care provider to talk to a parent about a child's respiratory illness. It is important to establish both the onset and duration of the problem so that its seriousness can be determined. Infants who cannot finish a bottle feeding because of exhaustion or rapid breathing or children who cannot run with other children because they do not have enough breath, for example, should be suspected of having a chronic respiratory disorder. An episode of sudden coughing is more suggestive of an acute respiratory disorder.

A child admitted to the hospital with a respiratory disorder is usually in an acute stage of the illness. The child's condition may worsen rapidly in the first few hours until a prescribed medication, such as an antibiotic or bronchodilator, begins to take effect. Nursing assessment that a child is developing tachypnea or retractions may be the first indication of a child's worsening condition.

● Nursing Diagnosis

Nursing diagnoses established for a child with a respiratory disorder focus both on the alteration in mechanisms of breathing and on the emotional distress such problems can create. "Ineffective airway clearance" is a common diagnostic category used in this area. The problem may be related to any one of a variety of factors, such as ineffective cough, fatigue, weakness, viscous secretions, pain, aspiration of a foreign body, or lack of knowledge about the importance of coughing.

The diagnostic categories "Impaired gas exchange" and "Ineffective breathing pattern" also may be used, although because a nurse does not generally prescribe definitive treatment for these problems (except when caused by hyperventilation), it may be more appropriate for a nursing diagnosis to focus on the effects of impaired gas exchange or ineffective breathing on daily activities and psychosocial health (Carpenito, 2004). Examples of possible nursing diagnoses are:

- Activity intolerance related to insufficient oxygenation
- Fatigue related to impaired gas exchange
- Fear related to inability to breathe without effort
- Impaired social interaction related to difficulty in keeping up with physical activities of peers
- Deficient knowledge related to need for continued treatment

● Outcome Identification and Planning

If a child is experiencing an acute respiratory problem, the expected outcomes and plan of care will focus on supporting the child and family through prescribed therapy and keeping parents informed about their child's health status and response to treatment. Often the treatment period for respiratory illness is prolonged, so parents of children with chronic conditions need to learn how to continue therapy at home. Helping parents to plan programs of exercise and teaching chest physiotherapy and the actions of prescribed medications are important nursing activities. Parents also need to understand that their approach to these programs must change as their child grows older. With an infant, they simply need to perform the prescribed procedures. A game might be a good way to get a toddler or preschooler to breathe deeply ("Simon says, cough. Simon says, take five deep breaths"). Parents need to plan exercise programs for school-age children around their school day. Otherwise, children may have difficulty carrying out the program or may be able to carry it out only sporadically. If parents include other family members, such as older siblings (within reason) or grandparents, in a respiratory therapy program, this can help to diffuse the burden of care and also to unite the family in working toward a common goal.

- **Implementation**

Collaborative nursing interventions in the care of a child with respiratory dysfunction include suctioning to remove respiratory secretions, administering oxygen, and providing humidification and expectorant therapy to help maintain clear airways. Some of the most important nursing interventions in this area are independent nursing functions: placing a child in an upright position to help her cough more effectively; providing an interesting game to teach a child the importance of strengthening chest muscles; supporting a child and family through the anxiety created when a child is not breathing normally; and teaching parents of a child with chronic respiratory dysfunction the basics of percussion or chest physiotherapy techniques. All of these interventions require sound nursing judgment and skill to carry out or teach effectively.

Referring parents and children to community resources and organizations for support is also a key nursing function. Some organizations to recommend as support to parents of the child with a respiratory disorder include:

- American Lung Association (*www.lungusa.org*)
- National Easter Seal Society (*www.easterseals.com*)
- National Asthma Education and Prevention Program (*www.nhlbi.nih.gov*)
- Asthma & Allergy Foundation of America (*www.aafa.org/*)
- Cystic Fibrosis Foundation (*www.cff.org*)

- **Outcome Evaluation**

An acute respiratory illness such as pneumonia is extremely frightening for parents as well as the child. After the child has recovered, talk with the parents to determine whether they have come to terms with their fear and can treat the child as a well child again. Otherwise, overprotection of a child by the parents may result in a well but dependent child. This pattern is one that nursing evaluation can help to prevent.

Expected outcomes for a child with chronic respiratory disease will change as a child grows and develops. No matter what the specific concerns are, however, evaluation should always include examination of how well a child individually and the family as a whole have adapted to managing the limitations imposed by the disorder while maintaining a lifestyle that fosters growth and development for all family members.

Examples indicating achievement of outcomes are:

- Infant maintains respiratory rate of at least 20 breaths/min.
- Child describes a reduced program of school activities he will maintain to reduce fatigue.
- Child's PO_2 is maintained at 80 to 100 mm Hg in room air.
- Child lists steps she will take if breathing becomes impaired while at school.
- Parents demonstrate correct techniques for performing respiratory therapy at home.

ANATOMY AND PHYSIOLOGY OF THE RESPIRATORY SYSTEM

The respiratory system can be separated into two divisions for discussion: the upper respiratory tract, composed of the nose, paranasal sinuses, pharynx, larynx, and epiglottis; and the lower tract, composed of the bronchi, bronchioles, and alveoli. Through inspiration, the respiratory system delivers warmed and moistened air to the alveoli; transports oxygen across the alveolar membrane to hemoglobin-laden red blood cells; and allows carbon dioxide to diffuse from red blood cells back into the alveoli. Through expiration, carbon dioxide-filled air is discharged to the outside. Levels of oxygen and carbon dioxide in the lungs, blood, and body cells are shown in Figure 40.1.

The respiratory center is located in the medulla of the brain. Peripheral receptors located in the aortic arch and carotid arteries sense diminished PO_2 levels and respond by increasing the respiratory rate. Central respiratory receptors in the medulla sense increased PCO_2 levels along with body acidity, temperature, and blood pressure as another stimulus to respiration. Depth of respiration is influenced by proprioceptors located in the lung periphery that register lung fullness. An inhibitory center in the pons halts inspiratory impulses before the lungs become overextended. Often children with chronic lung disease such as cystic fibrosis have adapted so well to a chronically high PCO_2 level that central receptor sites no longer register this as abnormal. In these instances, the main stimulus for respiration is a low oxygen level. In such children, administering high levels of oxygen can be dangerous because it alleviates oxygen want or their main respiratory stimulus.

Respiratory Tract Differences in Children

Embryologic development of the respiratory tract is discussed in Chapter 8. The ethmoidal and maxillary sinuses are present at birth; the frontal sinuses (the sinuses most

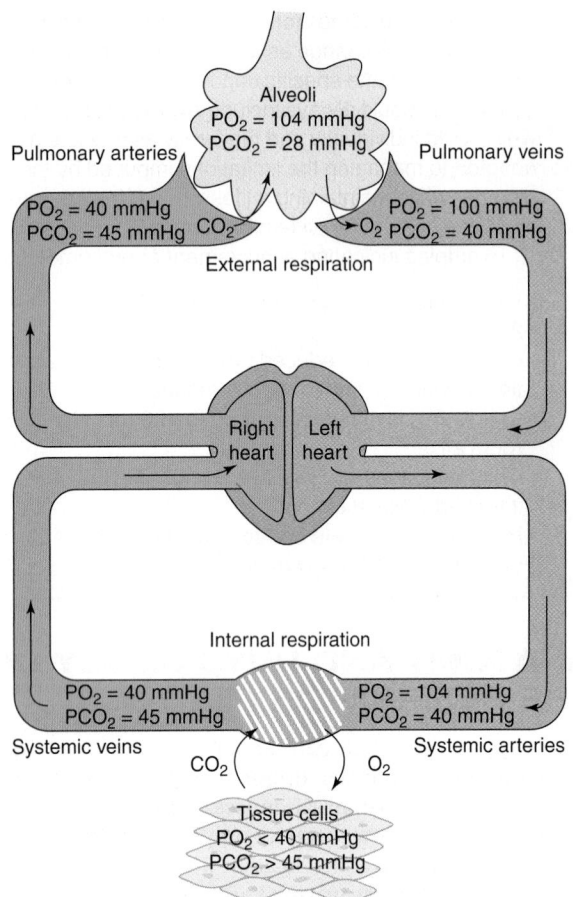

FIGURE 40.1 Partial pressure of gas (mm Hg) as measured in peripheral and systemic circulation. Because of the differences in partial pressure of the gases in the different areas, O_2 moves from alveoli to pulmonary capillaries (i.e., the gas moves from the area of greater concentration to one of a lesser concentration). When it reaches the tissue capillaries, O_2 partial pressure in cells is less, so O_2 goes into the tissues and CO_2 moves out.

frequently involved in sinus infection) and the sphenoidal sinuses do not develop until 6 to 8 years of age. Due to rapid growth of lymphoid tissue, tonsillar tissue is normally enlarged in early school-age children.

Respiratory mucus functions as a cleaning agent by moving invading organisms or other particles out of the lungs. However, newborns produce little respiratory mucus, which makes them more susceptible to respiratory infection than older children. Excessive production of mucus in children up to 2 years of age can actually lead to obstruction because the bronchial lumens are so small in a child of this age.

After 2 years of age, the right bronchus is noticeably shorter, wider, and more vertical than the left. This is the reason inhaled foreign bodies most often lodge in the right bronchus. Infants' chest muscles are not fully developed, so they use their abdominal muscles to assist in inhalation. The change to thoracic breathing begins at 2 to 3 years of age and is complete at 7 years. Because accessory muscles are used more in children than adults, weakness of these muscles from disease may more easily result in respiratory failure in children than in adults.

In infants, the walls of the airways have less cartilage than in older children and adults and so are not as strong and more likely to collapse after expiration. An advantage of immature development is that a lessened amount of smooth muscle in the airway means an infant does not develop bronchospasm as readily as an older child or adult. Therefore, **wheezing** (the sound of air being pushed through constricted bronchioles) may not be a prominent finding in infants even when the lumen of the airway is severely compromised.

ASSESSING RESPIRATORY ILLNESS IN CHILDREN

Assessment of respiratory illness in children includes an interview, physical examination, and laboratory testing. If the child is in acute distress, the interview and health history may cover only the most important details: when the child first became ill and what symptoms are present. It is important, however, to get as accurate a picture as possible, because the problem could be the result of a variety of circumstances (Box 40.2).

Symptoms of **hypoxemia** (deficient oxygenation of the blood), for example, are often insidious. Peripheral vasoconstriction (a mechanism to save the available oxygen for central life-sustaining body organs) leads to a pale appearance. Tachypnea and tachycardia (efforts to oxygenate cells better), anxiety, and confusion (caused by limited cerebral perfusion) may occur. A poor feeding pattern may be one of the first signs noted in the infant because an infant cannot suck and breathe rapidly at the same time. Cardiac arrhythmia may occur because of inadequate cardiac tissue perfusion. Always ask about home remedies that may have been used in an attempt to increase breathing space or effort (Box 40.3).

Physical Assessment

Physical assessment of a child with a respiratory disorder includes observation of presenting symptoms such as cough, cyanosis, or pallor, as well as evaluation of respirations and breath sounds. Breath sounds are best heard if an infant or child is not crying. Spending time comforting a child to prevent crying is time well spent.

Cough

A cough reflex is initiated by stimulation of the nerves of the respiratory tract mucosa by the presence of dust, chemicals, mucus, or inflammation. The sound of coughing is caused by rapid expiratory air movement past the glottis. Coughing is a useful procedure to clear excess mucus or foreign bodies from the respiratory tract. It becomes harmful and needs suppression only when there is no mucus or debris to be expelled and the amount of coughing becomes exhausting. This might occur with respiratory tract inflammation. **Paroxysmal coughing**

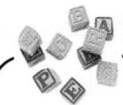

BOX 40.2 ASSESSMENT

Assessing the Child for Signs and Symptoms of Respiratory Dysfunction

History

Chief concern: Cough, rapid respirations, noisy breathing, rhinitis, reddened sore throat, lethargy, cyanosis, difficulty sucking, fever.

Past medical history: Poor weight gain, difficulty with respirations at birth, prematurity.

Family history: History of family member with asthma; other family members with respiratory infection.

Physical examination

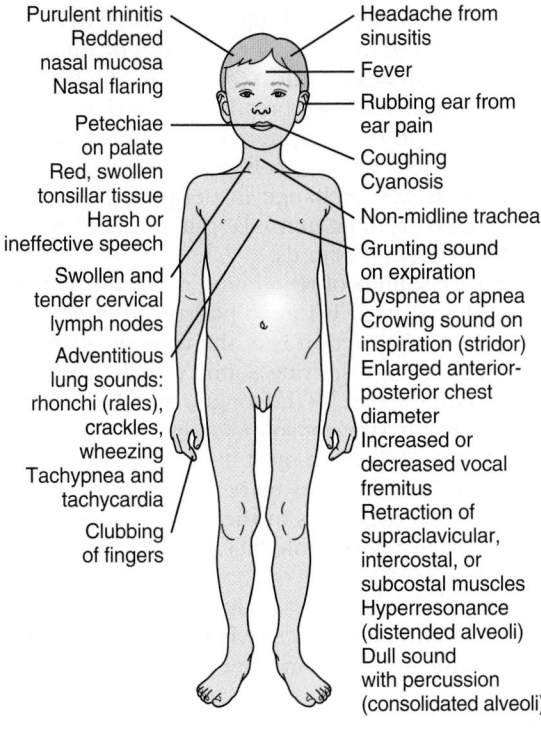

Purulent rhinitis
Reddened nasal mucosa
Nasal flaring

Petechiae on palate
Red, swollen tonsillar tissue
Harsh or ineffective speech

Swollen and tender cervical lymph nodes

Adventitious lung sounds: rhonchi (rales), crackles, wheezing
Tachypnea and tachycardia

Clubbing of fingers

Headache from sinusitis

Fever

Rubbing ear from ear pain

Coughing
Cyanosis

Non-midline trachea

Grunting sound on expiration
Dyspnea or apnea
Crowing sound on inspiration (stridor)
Enlarged anterior-posterior chest diameter
Increased or decreased vocal fremitus
Retraction of supraclavicular, intercostal, or subcostal muscles
Hyperresonance (distended alveoli)
Dull sound with percussion (consolidated alveoli)

BOX 40.3 FOCUS ON . . .

DIVERSITY OF CARE

Upper respiratory illnesses occur universally, making them a concern of parents the world over. Home remedies for such illnesses vary greatly, however. Hanging garlic around a child's neck is a frequent therapy in Mediterranean countries. "Cupping" or applying pressure to the back to "draw out" an infection (which leaves red circular ecchymotic marks on the child's back) may be used in Asian cultures. Although the therapeutic value of these remedies may not be proven, it is important to the nurse–patient and nurse–family relationships to respect family traditions.

refers to a series of expiratory coughs after a deep inspiration. Commonly, this occurs in children with pertussis (whooping cough) or those who have aspirated a foreign body or a liquid they attempted to drink.

Although helpful in removing mucus, coughing increases chest pressure and so may decrease venous return to the heart. This lowers cardiac output and can lead to fainting (syncope). Paroxysmal coughing may increase the pressure in the central venous circulation to such an extent that bleeding into the central nervous system (CNS) can result. Because young children often vomit after a series of coughs, they may be suspected initially of having a gastric disturbance even though they are coughing.

Rate and Depth of Respirations

Tachypnea (an increased respiratory rate) often is the first indicator of airway obstruction in young children. When assessing respiratory rate, particularly in infants, try to count respiratory rate before waking the infant, because crying distorts respiratory rate. Assess also the depth and quality of respiration, as these also reveal **anoxia** or lack of oxygen in body cells.

Retractions

When children must inspire more forcefully than normally to inflate their lungs because of an airway obstruction or stiff, noncompliant lungs (as in newborns with pulmonary dysplasia), intrapleural pressure is decreased to the point that the nonrigid parts of the chest (the intercostal spaces) draw inward, creating **retractions** (Fig. 40.2). Retractions occur more commonly in newborns and infants than in older children because the intercostal tissues are weaker and less developed in the younger child. Retraction of upper chest muscles (supraclavicular or suprasternal) suggests upper airway obstruction; retraction of intercostal or subcostal muscles suggests lower airway obstruction.

Restlessness

When children or infants have decreased oxygen in body cells (**hypoxia**), they become anxious and restless. In infants, restlessness coupled with tachypnea may be one of the first signs of airway obstruction. Be careful not to interpret the excessive movements of infants with respiratory distress as a sign that they are improving; anxious, restless stirring may be their only way of signaling that their respiratory obstruction is becoming acute.

Cyanosis

Cyanosis (a blue tinge to the skin) indicates hypoxia. It becomes apparent when the P_{O_2} is under 40 mm Hg or the level of unoxygenated hemoglobin increases to over 3 g/100 mL (because incompletely oxygenated red blood cells in the circulation are what give blood a dark color). If children have a low red blood cell count, cyanosis may not be apparent because there are not enough red blood cells to give the arterial blood its color. This occurs at hemoglobin levels below 5 g/100 mL. The degree of cyanosis present, therefore, is not always an accurate indication of the degree of airway difficulty. When children have accompanying

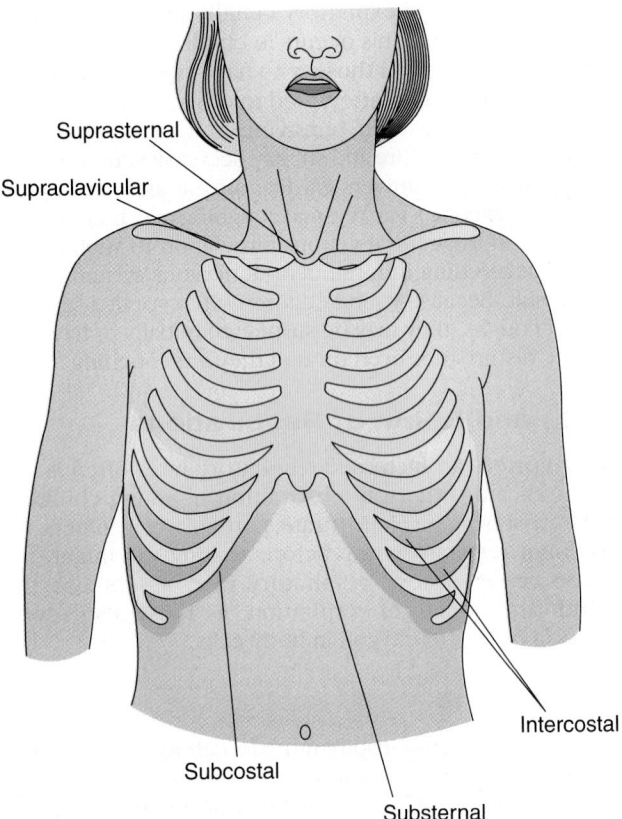

FIGURE 40.2 Sites of respiratory retraction.

peripheral vasoconstriction caused by shock, cyanosis of the extremities also may or may not be apparent.

As the P_{O_2} drops and cyanosis results, children increase their respiratory effort in an attempt to supply more oxygen to the tissues. When they do this, the difference in pressure between the intralumen of a not yet fully developed trachea and the surrounding tissue becomes so great that the trachea may collapse, compounding the obstruction problem.

Clubbing of Fingers

Children with chronic respiratory illnesses often develop **clubbing** of the fingers, a change in the angle be-

tween the fingernail and nailbed because of increased capillary growth in the fingertips (Fig. 40.3). The increased capillary growth occurs as the body attempts to supply more oxygen routes (more capillaries) to distal body cells.

Adventitious Sounds

Normal breath sounds are reviewed in Chapter 33. **Adventitious sounds** (extra or abnormal breathing sounds) are caused by pathologic conditions and can be heard on lung assessment in children with respiratory disorders. Normally, on chest auscultation, the inspiratory sound is softer and longer than the expiratory sound. This is referred to as vesicular breathing. If you listen over the trachea, this pattern in terms of the length of **inspiration** (breathing in) and **expiration** (breathing out) is reversed. This is bronchial or tubular breathing. If you hear bronchial breath sounds in the periphery of the lungs, where normally you would expect to hear a vesicular pattern, it indicates that gas exchange in peripheral alveoli is so compromised (as in pneumonia) that you are listening to transmitted tracheal sounds.

Accessory sounds of respiration result from the vibrations produced as air is forced past obstructions such as mucus. If the obstruction is in the nose or pharynx, the noise produced is a snoring sound (rhonchi). If the obstruction is at the base of the tongue or in the larynx, you will hear a harsh, strident sound on inspiration. This is laryngeal stridor. It is often most marked when a child is in a supine position and less marked when a child sits upright. If an obstruction is in the lower trachea or bronchioles, it is most noticeable on expiration. An expiratory whistle sound (wheezing) occurs. If alveoli become fluid-filled, fine crackling sounds (**rales**) are heard. Diminished or absent breath sounds occur when the alveoli are so fluid-filled that little or no air can enter them.

Chest Diameters

With chronic obstructive lung disease, children may be unable to exhale completely, allowing air to be chronically trapped in lung alveoli (hyperinflation). This produces an elongated anteroposterior diameter of the chest, sometimes termed a pigeon breast. There is an accompanying

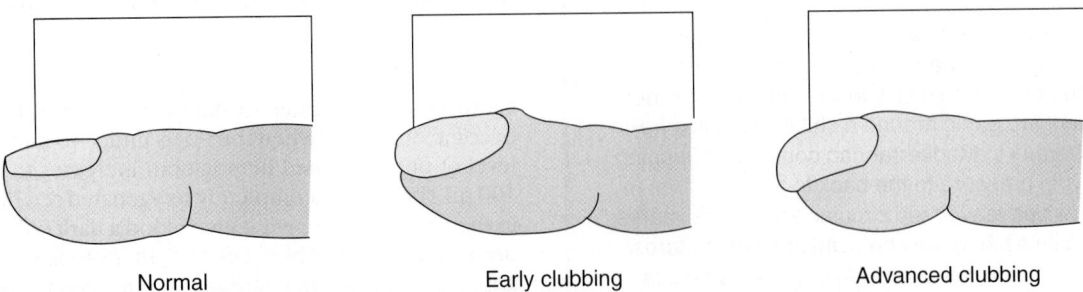

Normal   Early clubbing   Advanced clubbing

FIGURE 40.3 Clubbing of the fingers. (*Left*) The angle between the nail and digit is normally about 20 degrees in a child. (*Center*) Flattened angle represents early stage of clubbing. (*Right*) In advanced clubbing, the nail is rounded over the end of the finger. Note also that the distal phalanx is bulbous and of greater depth than the proximal portion of the finger (interphalangeal depth).

tympanic or hyperresonant (loud and hollow) sound heard on percussion over lung spaces.

Laboratory Tests

A number of laboratory tests can be used to confirm or rule out the presence of a respiratory problem and to help identify the cause and severity of the problem. These include analysis of arterial blood gases, nasopharyngeal culture, and sputum analysis.

Blood Gas Analysis

Blood gas analysis is an invasive method for determining the effectiveness of ventilation and acid–base status. The normal values of **arterial blood gases** (ABGs)—the amount of oxygen and carbon dioxide in the blood—are shown in Table 40.1.

Blood gas analysis provides important information about oxygenation of the blood, as values may indicate not only whether the arterial partial pressure of oxygen (P_{O_2}) is adequate but also whether the oxygen saturation of hemoglobin is adequate. The oxygen saturation level will fall if adequate oxygen cannot reach the bloodstream because of respiratory distress or if the hemoglobin is defective and cannot carry a full complement of oxygen (as with sickle cell anemia or thalassemia major). If a child has a severe anemia, the saturation level may be adequate (95% to 100%), but body cells may still not be receiving enough oxygen because of the limited number of red blood cells present. With increased P_{CO_2} or decreased P_{O_2}, a low pH, or decreased temperature, the ability of hemoglobin to accept oxygen diminishes so, again, cells may become hypoxic.

P_{CO_2} measures the efficiency of ventilation. In children who are hypoventilating (breathing very shallowly), P_{CO_2} will be increased because they cannot blow off CO_2; in children who are hyperventilating (breathing deeply), P_{CO_2} will be decreased because they are blowing off too much. When children cannot evacuate accumulated CO_2 because of an obstruction or hypoventilation, the partial pressure of CO_2 in the arterial blood rises and the concentration of carbonic acid (formed when carbon dioxide dissolves in plasma) also rises. This leads to acidosis (a decrease in serum pH or an increase in acidity).

If respiratory distress is incomplete, the body can compensate for developing acidity for a long time by increasing kidney tubular reabsorption of bicarbonate. When respiratory distress is relieved (by removal of an obstruction or by assisted ventilation), the amount of bicarbonate present in the bloodstream may exceed the amount of acid produced at that point, and the child's condition may change from acidosis to alkalosis. With alkalosis, the respiratory rate decreases as a means to conserve CO_2. As a result, periods of apnea may occur. Children require close observation during this time, including frequent blood gas and electrolyte determinations to ensure prompt treatment to reverse these changes when they occur. Respiratory alkalosis and respiratory acidosis are compared in Table 40.2. Box 40.4 shows steps for evaluating ABGs.

To analyze blood gases, arterial blood rather than venous blood must be used (arterial blood will reflect how well the lungs are oxygenating the blood, whereas venous blood will reflect only the oxygenation of the particular extremity from which the blood was drawn). In the young infant, the temporal artery may be used as a site for blood gasses; in newborns, an umbilical artery catheter can be used. In older children, the radial artery is the site of choice because of the collateral circulation present at the wrist. (If clotting should occur in the radial artery, the hand would still be well nourished by collateral circulation; see the Allen test in Box 40.5.)

For an ABG assessment, a specimen is withdrawn into a heparinized syringe (to prevent clotting). After any arterial puncture, always firmly compress the site. Otherwise, blood from the punctured vessel can seep into subcutaneous tissue, possibly causing a large hematoma and obscuring the site for further assessment. If frequent

---

TABLE 40.1

Arterial Blood Gas Values

Measure	Definition	Normal Value	Clinical Significance
P_{O_2}	Partial pressure of oxygen in arterial blood	80–100 mm Hg	Decreased if child cannot inspire adequately
P_{CO_2}	Partial pressure of carbon dioxide in arterial blood	35–45 mm Hg	Increased if child cannot expire adequately
O_2 saturation	The percentage of hemoglobin carrying oxygen	95%–100%	Decreased if O_2 cannot reach red blood cells, if unoxygenated cells are being mixed with oxygenated ones, or if hemoglobin is defective
pH	The hydrogen ion concentration of blood	7.35–7.45	Decreased if CO_2 is being retained as carbonic acid in blood
HCO_3	The bicarbonate concentration in blood	22–26 mEq/L	Increased in respiratory alkalosis; decreased in respiratory acidosis
Base excess	Bicarbonate available for buffering	–2.5 or +2.5 mEq/L	(+) = alkaline excess (–) = alkaline deficit

TABLE 40.2

Comparison of Respiratory Alkalosis and Respiratory Acidosis

Acid–Base Condition	Cause	Findings
Respiratory alkalosis	Hyperventilation	Rapid, deep breathing Confusion, unconsciousness Elevated plasma pH (above 7.45) Elevated urine pH (above 7) Decreased P_{CO_2} (below 40 mm Hg) Plasma bicarbonate –Initially normal –Compensated: below 20 mEq/L Base excess: 0 or a negative reading such as –4
Respiratory acidosis	Hypoventilation trapping carbon dioxide in alveoli	Shallow breathing; inability to expire freely Confusion, disorientation Decreased plasma pH (below 7.35) Decreased urine pH (below 6) Elevated P_{CO_2} (over 40 mm Hg) Plasma bicarbonate –Initially normal or elevated –Compensated: above 25 mEq/L Base excess: 0 or a positive reading such as +4

specimen collections are required, an arterial catheter, inserted either peripherally or centrally, may be used. Doing so allows frequent specimen collections without the trauma of additional punctures. Be sure to apply dressings over the area where an arterial catheter exits the skin to help prevent a young child from fussing or playing with the site. Soft restraints, such as an elbow or hand restraint, may be needed to keep a child from dislodging the catheter.

In small infants, when it is impossible to obtain arterial blood directly, heel or finger sticks may be used. If the heel or finger is warmed for about 20 minutes in warm water before the procedure, local blood flow increases so much that the blood gas levels of the capillaries approach those of arteries.

Be certain to note the use of oxygen, if any, and its liter flow on laboratory slips for ABG assessments. Also note the site where the specimen was obtained. While being transported to the laboratory, ABG specimens should be kept on ice to ensure accurate results (CO_2 levels decline in room air).

The oxygen saturation of hemoglobin can be obtained noninvasively using pulse oximetry and transcutaneous oxygen monitoring.

Pulse Oximetry. Pulse oximetry is a continuous, non-invasive technique for measuring oxygen saturation. For the measurement, a sensor and a photodetector are placed around a vascular bed, most often a finger in a child or a foot in an infant (Fig. 40.4). Infrared light is directed through the finger from the sensor to the photodetector. Because hemoglobin absorbs light waves differently when it is bound to oxygen than when it is not, the oximeter can detect the degree of oxygen saturation (SaO_2) in the hemoglobin.

Oxygen saturation is closely aligned with P_{O_2} (Fig. 40.5). When SaO_2 is 95%, the P_{O_2} is within the normal range of 80 to 100 mm Hg. When SaO_2 has fallen to 90%, the P_{O_2} is 60 mm Hg. An easy rule to remember concerning the relationship between SaO_2 and P_{O_2} is the 60 to 30, 90 to 60 rule: when SaO_2 is 60, P_{O_2} is 30; when SaO_2 is 90, P_{O_2} is 60. Any SaO_2 reading under 90, therefore, is cause for concern.

One advantage of pulse oximetry is that it is noninvasive. A second advantage is that the continuous monitoring provided by a pulse oximeter allows you to modify your care appropriately. If an oxygen level should begin to fall while you are handling an infant, for example, you could immediately stop care until the infant's P_{O_2} again returns to normal. A disadvantage is that the sensor is small and must be checked frequently to see that it remains in place. Excess light in a room may distort the reading. Therefore, the sensor may need to be covered with a blanket in a neonatal intensive care unit or brightly lit nursery for readings to be accurate. Young children also tend to remove the sensors just as they frequently remove adhesive bandages from their fingers.

Transcutaneous Oxygen Monitoring. Transcutaneous monitoring is another means of continuous, noninvasive measurement of oxygen saturation. For this determination, electrodes heated to 44°C are attached to an infant's chest. The heat causes vasodilation underneath the skin and brings the peripheral arterial blood to the surface to be read for oxygen content. This is converted to mm Hg for a monitor readout. The oxygen saturation level read by this method correlates with intra-arterial P_{O_2}, the same as with pulse oximetry. Transcutaneous monitoring has a disadvantage compared with pulse oximetry because the probe position needs to be changed every 3 to 4 hours to

BOX 40.4

Quick Assessment of Arterial Blood Gases

Use a systematic format to assess ABGs quickly:

1. Evaluate the pH: Normally, pH falls between 7.35 and 7.45. A pH below 7.35 denotes acidemia; one above 7.45 reflects alkalemia. If the patient has more than one acid–base imbalance at work, the pH identifies the process in control.
2. Evaluate P_{CO_2}: The partial pressure of arterial CO_2 (P_{CO_2}) normally ranges between 35 and 45 mm Hg. A P_{CO_2} greater than 45 mm Hg indicates ventilatory failure and respiratory acidosis from CO_2 accumulation. A P_{CO_2} less than 35 mm Hg indicates alveolar hyperventilation and respiratory alkalosis.
3. Evaluate HCO_3: A bicarbonate (HCO_3^-) less than 22 mEq/L or a base excess (BE) less than −2 mEq/L denotes metabolic acidosis. A bicarbonate level greater than 26 mEq/L or a BE greater than 2 mEq/L reflects metabolic alkalosis. If the two measurements conflict, the BE is the better indicator of metabolic status.
4. Determine which is the primary and which is the compensating disorder: Often, two acid–base imbalances coincide; one is primary, the other is the body's attempt to return the pH to normal. When both the P_{CO_2} and the HCO_3^- are abnormal, one denotes the primary acid–base disorder and the other denotes the compensating disorder.
    a. To decide which is which, check the pH. *Only a process of acidosis can make the pH acidic; only a process of alkalosis can make the pH alkaline.* For example, if steps 2 and 3 indicate that the patient has respiratory acidosis and metabolic alkalosis and the pH is 7.25, the primary disorder must be respiratory acidosis. The remaining disorder is compensating for the primary problem.
    b. When pH rises (becomes alkalotic), P_{CO_2} decreases in amount (will be below 35 mm Hg). When pH decreases (becomes acidotic), P_{CO_2} increases (will be above 45 mm Hg). When an opposite problem exists this way (pH increased; P_{CO_2} decreased), the problem is respiratory in origin.
    c. pH and HCO_3 normally move in the same direction (when pH is elevated, HCO_3 is elevated). When these two measurements correspond this way (pH decreased, HCO_3 decreased), then the cause of the problem is metabolic in origin.
    d. Three states of compensation are possible: *noncompensation,* reflected in an alteration of only P_{CO_2} or HCO_3^-; *partial compensation,* in which both P_{CO_2} and HCO_3^- are abnormal and, because compensation is incomplete, the pH is also abnormal; and *complete compensation,* in which both P_{CO_2} and HCO_3^- are abnormal but, because compensation is complete, the pH is normal. To identify the primary disorder when compensation is complete, consider a pH between 7.35 and 7.40 indicative of primary acidosis and a pH between 7.40 and 7.45 indicative of primary alkalosis.
5. Evaluate oxygenation: Normally P_{O_2} remains between 80 and 100 mm Hg. A P_{O_2} between 60 and 80 mm Hg reflects mild hypoxemia; between 40 and 60 mm Hg, moderate hypoxemia; and below 40 mm Hg, severe hypoxemia.
6. Interpret the findings: Your final analysis should include the degree of compensation, the primary disorder, and the oxygenation status; for example, "partially compensated respiratory acidosis with moderate hypoxemia."

BOX 40.5

Allen Test

Before obtaining an ABG from the radial artery, it is important to establish that the child has collateral circulation to the hand. Otherwise, the needle puncture may block the artery and block blood flow to the hand.

To prove that there is collateral circulation, compress both the radial and ulnar arteries on the inner side of the wrist and elevate the hand until color disappears. Release the pressure over the ulnar artery and observe for a color change in the hand. If the hand does not pinken (proof the blood has flowed into the hand), the radial artery on that wrist should not be used for catheter insertion.

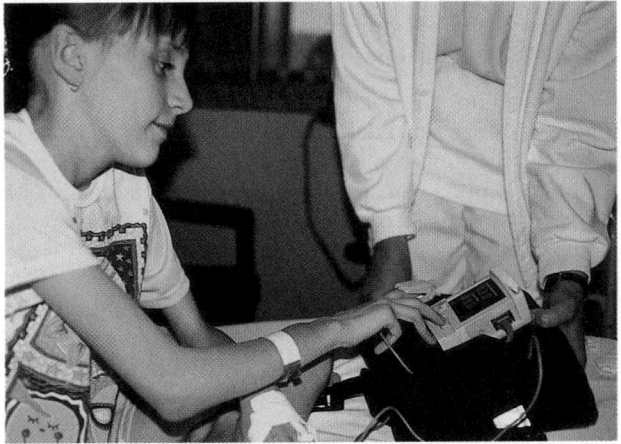

FIGURE 40.4 A school-aged child wearing a pulse oximeter checks her oxygen saturation level.

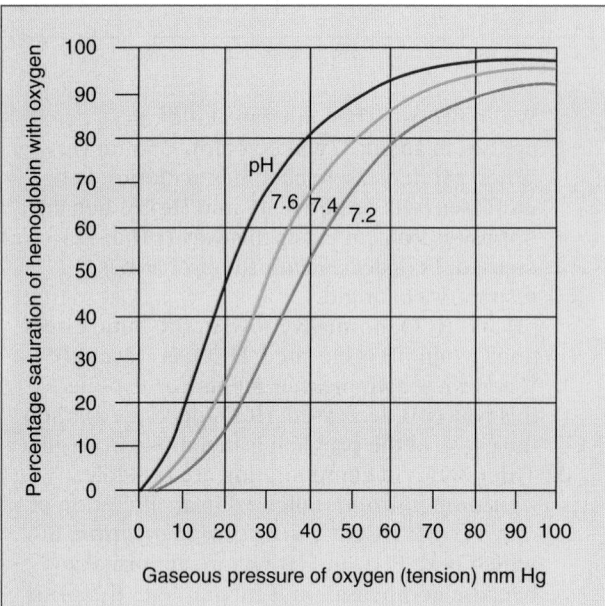

FIGURE 40.5 Oxyhemoglobin dissociation curve.

prevent a burn to the skin, and sensor recalibration is necessary with each position change.

Nasopharyngeal Culture

When done efficiently, nasopharyngeal cultures cause little discomfort and reveal a great deal of information about the microorganisms causing a disease. However, most children are terribly frightened by having something placed in their noses or throats and so may resist accordingly. Firm, calm support during the procedure while you touch a moistened swab to the mucus membrane of the nose or throat is essential. Nose and throat cultures can reveal only the organisms present in the upper respiratory tract. As a result, they may not show organisms causing a lower respiratory tract infection. A throat culture will miss pathogenic organisms if the culture tip is not touched to the infected aspect of the pharynx.

Respiratory Syncytial Virus Nasal Washings

Nasal washings are obtained to diagnose an infection by the respiratory syncytial virus (RSV). For this, a child is placed in the supine position, and 1 to 2 mL sterile normal saline is dropped with a sterile needleless syringe into one nostril. The nose is then aspirated using a small, sterile bulb syringe. The secretions removed are placed in a sterile container to be sent to the laboratory for analysis. Nasal washings are even more uncomfortable for children than nasal swabbing because of the saline that is instilled. Provide comfort to a child afterward and assure the child the specimen collection is over.

Sputum Analysis

Because they cannot raise sputum with a cough, sputum collection is rarely feasible in children younger than school age. Older children, however, are able to cough and raise sputum. Teach them exactly what you want (a specimen of what they are coughing up, not just clearing from the back of their throat). Then ask them to breathe in and out several times, cough deeply and spit mucus they have raised into a sterile specimen jar.

Diagnostic Procedures

In addition to cultures, a number of other diagnostic procedures are used to identify respiratory disorders in children. Many of these procedures are also used with adults, with modifications to account for the physical and developmental differences of children. Bronchoscopy (visualization of the bronchi through a bronchoscope) is discussed in Chapter 36. Radiologic examination (chest x-ray and bronchography) and pulmonary function testing are discussed in the following sections.

Chest X-Ray

Chest x-ray films will show areas of infiltration or consolidation in the lungs; if a foreign body is opaque, an x-ray study will show its location. Chest x-ray films are more difficult to obtain in infants than in older children, because infants cannot take a breath and hold it when instructed. It is therefore difficult to picture the lungs at their most expanded position. Computed tomography (CT) scans may be ordered for children with chronic lung disease because this technique can best mark disease progress.

Bronchography

On a chest x-ray, the air-filled larynx, trachea, and major bronchi are revealed as dark spaces. Any obstruction or distortion in the organs is apparent. For further definition of structures, a radiopaque solution may be introduced into the respiratory tract by an ultrasonic nebulizer or by a catheter inserted into the trachea before the x-ray study is performed. Children may require conscious sedation for this because nebulization can be frightening. Afterward, children may have an increase in mucus production from bronchial irritation by the procedure. Observe them carefully after such a procedure for possible respiratory obstruction from accumulating mucus.

Pulmonary Function Studies

The process of ventilation, or the work of breathing, involves three main forces: (1) an inertial force that must be overcome to change the speed and direction of air when the lungs change from exhalation to inhalation, or vice versa; (2) an elastic force to help the lungs expand with inhalation and "snap back" with exhalation; and (3) the flow resistance force or resistance to the movement of air through the bronchial tree that must be overcome. Flow resistance must be at a minimum for best ventilation. It becomes increased when the bronchioles are narrowed or plugged with mucus. Pulmonary function tests measure the forces of inertia, elasticity, and flow resistance.

The alveoli of the lungs are never completely empty at the end of expiration because the bronchioles collapse, trapping air in the alveoli. In contrast, alveoli are never completely filled on inspiration because their potential for expansion exceeds that necessary for good respiratory function. Children with obstructive lung diseases such as asthma or cystic fibrosis have some difficulty moving air into the lungs, but they have even more difficulty moving air out of the lungs. Even if they do expire the same amount of air as the average child, they expire it over a longer period. Children with restrictive ventilatory disorders, such as neuromuscular disorders, have equal difficulty with inspiration and expiration.

A number of lung capacity studies can be done to determine the degree of obstruction or restricted ventilation ability. For these studies, the child breathes into a spirometer, a device that records the force of air exchange.

Children younger than 4 years of age are usually unable to participate in pulmonary function tests because these tests require their cooperation. All children need good preparation and teaching for these tests because they must breathe forcefully through the mouth into a mouthpiece on cue. Some tests require the nose be closed by a clamp or clip or an assistant's hand while the child blows out. This can be a frightening feeling for children with respiratory disease. They may need some trial runs to assure themselves that they can breathe with the clamp in place. Without good orientation to the equipment, they may become so anxious about their performance that they develop tachypnea or fail to inhale or exhale at their full capacity, so the test results are skewed.

Common pulmonary function tests are outlined in Table 40.3. The results of pulmonary function studies help determine the nature and extent of a child's respiratory problem and the best methods for achieving more effective ventilation.

HEALTH PROMOTION AND RISK MANAGEMENT

A number of ways to promote respiratory health are available for parents and children. The common cold is the most common respiratory disorder seen in children. Children as young as toddlers can be taught to help avoid spreading colds through their family by washing their hands, properly disposing of tissues, and covering their mouth while coughing. These measures need to be stressed again with school-age children to help prevent them from contracting or spreading germs through their schoolroom. The incidence of *Haemophilus influenzae* type B, the cause of bronchiolitis, as well as influenza can be reduced by ensuring that children receive their routine immunizations against these (HIB and influenza vaccine). Children with chronic respiratory illnesses also should receive the pneumococcal vaccine. Parents of children with asthma can take major steps to reduce exacerbations by environmental control. Reducing respiratory irritation by reducing secondary smoke can help prevent asthma, upper respiratory infections, and otitis media.

THERAPEUTIC TECHNIQUES USED IN THE TREATMENT OF RESPIRATORY ILLNESS IN CHILDREN

The primary goal of nursing interventions in the care of children with respiratory disorders is to maintain or re-establish the airway to help ensure that adequate oxygen reaches the blood. Often this includes interventions aimed at liquefying and removing mucus secretions so they do not clog the bronchial pathways. Such clogging prevents adequate oxygenation and contributes to the development of bronchial and alveolar infections.

Expectorant Therapy

Any irritation of the respiratory tract causes the production of large amounts of mucus. The amount produced can become so great that the natural mechanisms for clearing it (coughing and upward cilia action) are no longer adequate. If a child is breathing rapidly because of respiratory distress, the frequent passage of air over the mucus tends to dry it and make it more viscid, compounding the removal problem. A number of measures may be used to liquefy and raise mucus.

TABLE 40.3

Pulmonary Function Tests

Test	Measurement	Clinical Implications
Vital capacity (VC)	The maximum amount of air expelled after a maximum inspiration	Decreased if bronchial lumens are narrowed or obstructed
Tidal volume (TV)	The amount of air inhaled and exhaled in a normal respiratory movement	Decreased if bronchial lumens are constricted
Residual volume	The amount of air remaining in the lungs after a maximum expiration	Increased if there is air trapping in alveoli, as in obstructive lung disease
Functional residual capacity (FRC)	The volume of air remaining in the lungs after a normal expiration	Increased if ability to breathe out is impaired
Forced expiratory volume (FEV)	The amount of air expired in 1 sec	Decreased in obstructive disease that prevents free expiration

Liquefying Agents

Pharmacologic agents (expectorants) such as guaifenesin (Robitussin), given orally, are designed to liquefy mucus in the trachea and bronchi. Instilling saline nose drops or using saline nasal sprays can be effective in moistening and loosening dried mucus in the nose (Karch, 2004).

Humidification

Humidification is the provision of moisture to the airway. Common methods of delivering moisture include vaporizers and nebulizers.

Vaporizers. Vaporizers emit a stream of air moistened by fine droplets of water into a room, providing either a cool or a warm mist to the entire room. Caution parents when using warm mist that a serious scald burn can result if children accidentally pull a vaporizer over on themselves. To avoid this type of accident, they should be certain the vaporizer is never placed within reach of the child. Although cool mist can create a clammy atmosphere in a room, this can be advantageous for a child who also has a fever, helping to cool and moisten the whole environment. Caution parents to clean vaporizers thoroughly after use to prevent the growth of *Pseudomonas* or other pathogenic organisms.

Nebulizers. Nebulizers are mechanical devices that provide a stream of moistened air directly into the respiratory tract. Most are hand-held masks that fit over the nose and mouth and are attached to an electrical pump as a power source (Fig. 40.6). Ultrasonic nebulization delivers such minuscule droplets into the respiratory tract that even the smallest bronchioles can be moistened. Nebulizers also serve as an important means for the delivery of respiratory tract medications (Fink, 2004). Drugs such as antibiotics or bronchodilators can be combined with the nebulized mist and sprayed into the lungs.

Many children find nebulizer treatments uncomfortable because the feeling of the mist in their upper respiratory tract can be frightening or irritating. Assure them that aerosol administration is the most effective route for moisture and medication to reach and cause an effect in the respiratory tract.

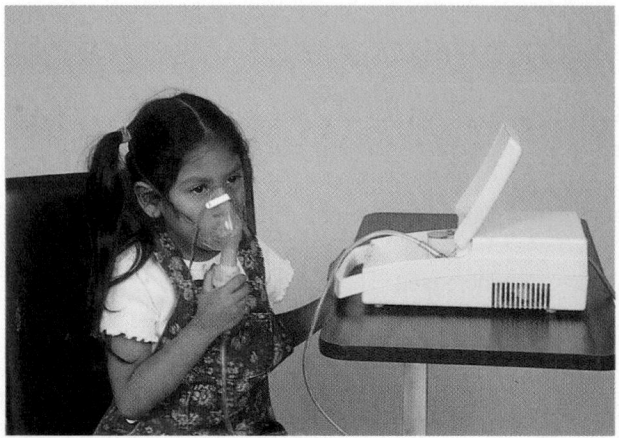

FIGURE 40.6 Child using a nebulizer.

During aerosol medication administration, watch carefully for signs of both local tracheal or bronchial effect (spasm or edema) that might result from airway irritation as well as systemic symptoms that might result from absorption of a medication by the membrane.

Coughing

As a rule, encourage coughing rather than suppressing it in children because it is an effective method of raising mucus. Changing a child's position and suggesting mild exercise and deep breathing are helpful techniques to initiate coughing. If a cough is caused by mucus dripping from the nose because of nasal congestion, a decongestant such as pseudoephedrine (Sudafed) will best halt the draining mucus and therefore the cough. Caution parents not to give adult cough syrups to children. A number of these contain codeine in doses that may be too high for the child's weight.

Chest Physiotherapy

Simply changing a child's position helps mucus to move, initiate a cough reflex, and be expelled. When a child is positioned so the chest is lower than the abdomen, gravity aids in the removal of mucus from the lower lobes and bronchi. When a child sits upright, gravity aids drainage from the upper lobes and bronchi. When lying supine, anterior bronchi drain; when prone, posterior bronchi drain. Frequent changes of position are important, therefore, to prevent mucus from pooling in certain lung areas. If a child has a localized mucus problem, lying predominantly in one position can encourage drainage of that lung segment. When the child is repositioned and the mucus drains into new bronchi, this will often cause a cough from irritation caused by this new drainage.

Three techniques are involved with chest physiotherapy (CPT) to further loosen mucus for expectoration: postural drainage, percussion, and vibration. Each technique can be used alone, but they are usually more effective at moving mucus toward the mainstem bronchus when performed together.

CPT is best scheduled before meals or at least an hour after a meal so the subsequent coughing does not cause vomiting. Techniques are described in Box 40.6 and summarized below. Limit CPT to approximately 30 minutes each time, because these techniques can be tiring. Modifications in the techniques or shortening of the time periods may be necessary, depending on a child's ability to tolerate the position changes and the techniques.

Common postural drainage positions for the infant are shown in Figure 40.7. An infant may be positioned on your lap, whereas a slant board or other surface is needed for postural drainage with an older child. Not all positions are tolerated well. Be ready to modify the positions used depending on the child's condition and tolerance.

To perform **percussion** (cupping), strike a cupped or curved palm (palm down) against the chest. This technique causes a loud, thumping noise that sounds as if it hurts, but you can assure parents it does not. In infants and some small children, a specialized device, a nipple, or

BOX 40.6 NURSING PROCEDURE

Chest Physiotherapy

Purpose

To encourage the loosening and raising of mucus from the respiratory tract through the use of postural gravity drainage and percussion (clapping) and vibrating techniques.

PROCEDURE	PRINCIPLE
1. Wash your hands; identify child; explain procedure to child.	1. Handwashing prevents spread of microorganisms. Identifying the child ensures that you are performing the procedure on the right child. Explaining the procedure beforehand promotes child's understanding and adherence and helps to minimize anxiety.
2. Assess child as to status; analyze appropriateness of procedure; modify plan as necessary.	2. Chest physiotherapy is physically exhausting; can increase intracranial pressure when head is lowered in dependent position. Wait 1 h after meals to avoid inducing vomiting with coughing.
3. Assemble supplies: pillow or slant board, disposable tissues (sputum cup if specimen for culture is desired); percussion device (if infant); nebulizer with correct fluid and medicine if prescribed.	3. Organizing care increases efficiency and helps prevent tiring child. Nebulization before postural drainage may be prescribed to promote bronchodilation, dilute mucus, and aid mobility of secretions.
4. Select a drainage position (see Fig. 40.7). Position child appropriately but comfortably. Auscultate and percuss lung area for baseline determinations.	4. Positions aid in the gravity drainage of secretions.
5. Use percussion and clapping technique (see figure) for 1–2 min and vibrate during 4 or 5 exhalations the section of chest indicated for the position. Observe child closely for respiratory distress.	5. Percussion and vibration loosen bronchial mucus and allow it to be coughed from the respiratory tract. As mucus moves, it may plug a bronchus; observe for cyanosis, tachypnea, dyspnea, and violent coughing as signs of this.

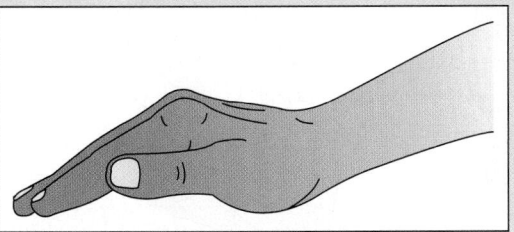

PROCEDURE	PRINCIPLE
6. Ask child to deep breathe and cough to raise secretions. Auscultate lung section to ascertain clearing of secretions.	6. Coughing also helps move secretions.
7. Reposition; percuss and vibrate the chest areas in additional drainage positions as prescribed. Continue to observe for signs of respiratory distress. Provide rest as necessary between positions.	7. Position changes allow for loosening and drainage in other lung segments. Child may grow tired after repeated percussion/vibration.
8. At finish of prescribed positions, return child to bed. Provide mouthwash if desired (and age-appropriate); discard used tissues.	8. Coughed sputum may taste unpleasant. Use standard precautions to avoid touching soiled tissues.
9. Evaluate effectiveness, cost, comfort, and safety of procedure. Plan health teaching as necessary, such as benefits of procedure.	9. Evaluation allows for determining effectiveness of the procedure and need for modifications for future treatments. Health teaching is an independent nursing action always included in nursing care.
10. Record procedure, description of sputum raised, and child's reaction to procedure. If sputum specimen is obtained, send to laboratory for analysis.	10. Documentation provides evidence of nursing care, child's status, and effectiveness of interventions.

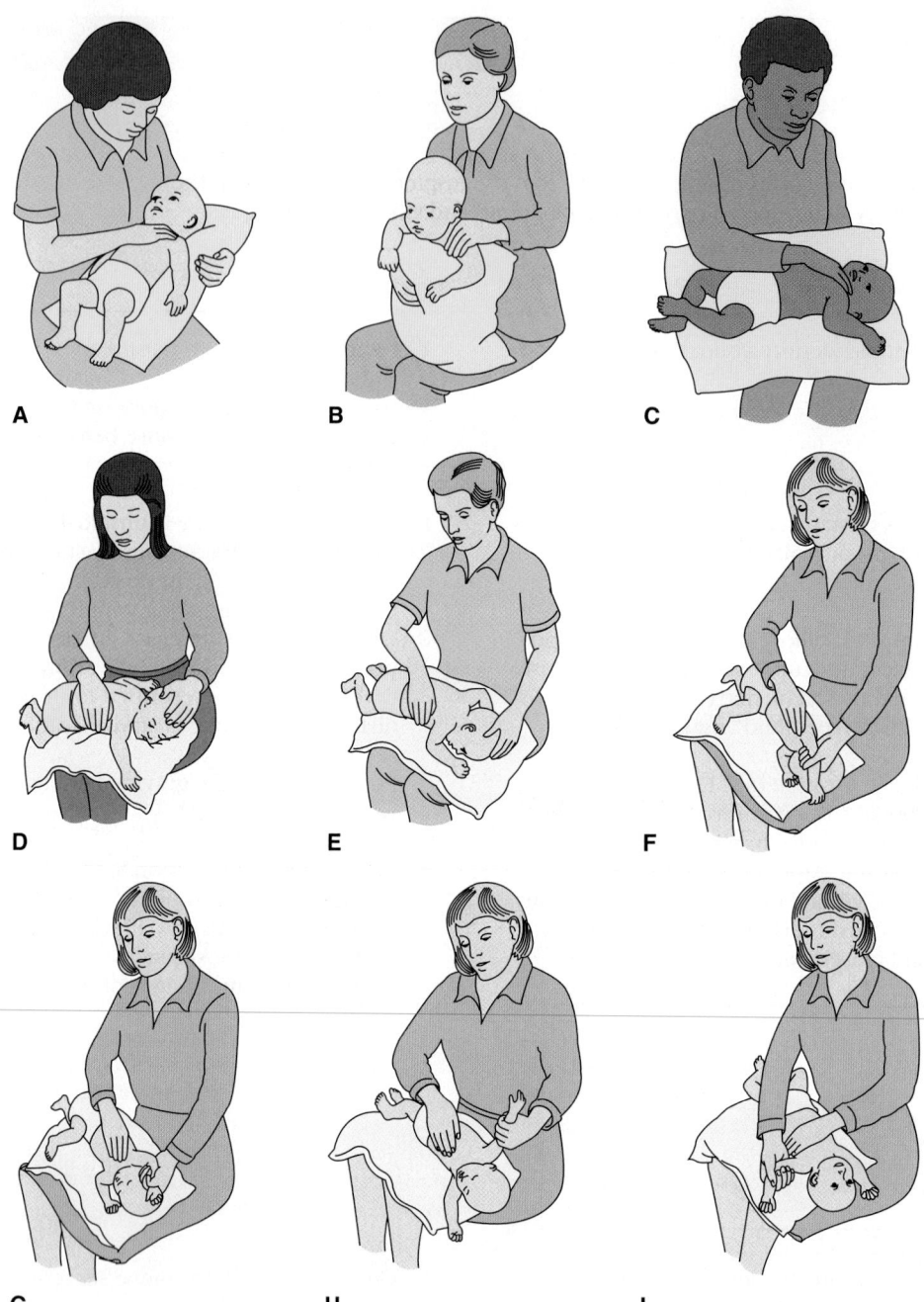

FIGURE 40.7 Positions for bronchial drainage for major segments of all lobes in infants. This procedure is most readily performed with the infant in your lap, with your hand on the chest over the area to be cupped or vibrated. (**A**) Apical segment of left upper lobe. (**B**) Posterior segment of left upper lobe. (**C**) Anterior segment of left upper lobe. (**D**) Superior segment of right lower lobe. (**E**) Posterior basal segment of right lower lobe. (**F**) Lateral basal segment of right lower lobe. (**G**) Anterior basal segment of right lower lobe. (**H**) Medial and lateral segments of right middle lobe. (**I**) Lingular segments (superior and inferior) of left upper lobe.

a small oxygen mask may be used as the palm of the hand is too big (Fig. 40.8). These devices concentrate the motion and may increase the amount of mucus removed.

Vibration is done by pressing a vibrating hand against a child's chest during exhalation. Like percussion, it mechanically loosens and helps move tenacious secretions up-

ward. Vibration also may be accomplished by a mechanical vibrator or a vibrating vest.

Position a child so the lobe of the lung to be drained is in a superior position. Because percussing or vibrating is exhausting, a child may not have all lobes drained at each session. For example, before breakfast, the upper right

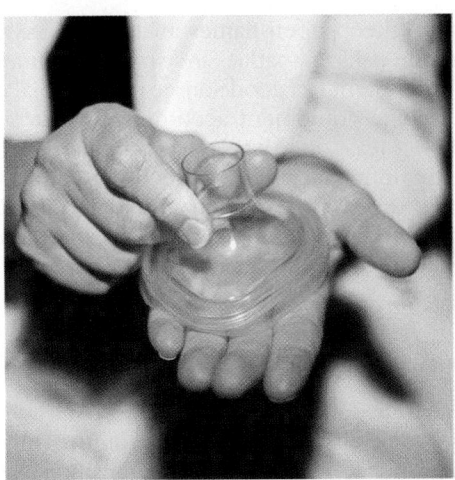

FIGURE 40.8 Alternative percussion device. To assist with percussing an infant or small child, a nipple or mask such as that from a manual resuscitation bag may be used.

and the left upper and lower lobes might be done; before lunch, the right lower lobe and right middle lobe might be done; before supper or at bedtime, the upper and lower lobe on both sides might be done.

After each position, ask the child to cough. Children cough best if you demonstrate the proper technique by taking a deep breath, blowing it out, taking a second deep breath, blowing that out, taking a third deep breath, and then coughing. The irritation of mucus in the major airway by the third breath makes a cough happen almost spontaneously.

Formerly, CPT was done in hospital settings by respiratory therapists. However, in today's health care climate of managed care, nurses are now often the health care provider who performs CPT and teaches it to parents. One or both parents may need to learn the technique before their child is discharged so that it can be continued conscientiously at home. Although not effective with all children, it is used most frequently with children with cystic fibrosis (van der Schans, Prasad, & Main, 2005).

Mucus-Clearing Devices

A mucus-clearing device (a Flutter device) can be used to aid in the removal of mucus. This device looks like a small plastic pipe. A stainless-steel ball inside the device moves when the child breathes out, causing vibrations in the lungs (Fig. 40.9). This vibration helps loosen mucus so that it can be moved up the airway and expectorated. This device is used most frequently with children who have cystic fibrosis or pneumonia to help remove mucus from the lungs.

What if... Michael needs to cough to raise bronchial mucus. What if he refuses to? How can you get him to cough?

Therapy to Improve Oxygenation

Improving oxygenation almost automatically relieves breathing distress (Frey & Shann, 2004).

Oxygen Administration

Oxygen administration elevates the arterial oxygen saturation level by supplying more oxygen to red blood cells by the respiratory tract. Oxygen may be delivered to infants by flooding an incubator or by using a plastic hood, mask or canula. Plastic oxygen hoods are tight-fitting enclosures that can keep oxygen concentration at nearly 100% (Fig. 40.10). Always check that the hood fits snugly over the infant's head, making sure it does not rub against the infant's neck, chin, or shoulders. Be sure the gas does not blow directly into the infant's face.

Although a nasal catheter or nasal prongs can be used for infants, they are usually reserved for older children. These provide a concentration of approximately 50% with an oxygen flow of 4 L/min. Most children do not like nasal prongs because they are intrusive. Assess their nostrils carefully when using these as the pressure of prongs can cause areas of necrosis, particularly on the nasal septum.

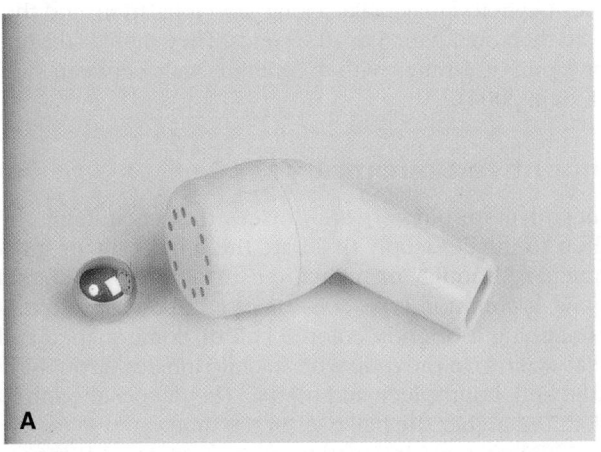

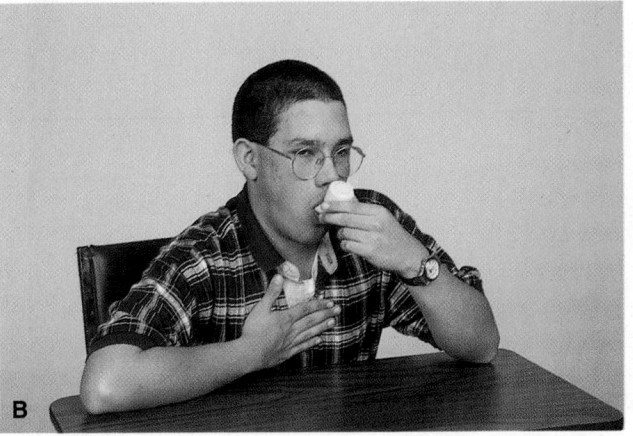

FIGURE 40.9 (**A**) Flutter device. The metal ball (shown) is enclosed in the chamber and causes the vibration. (**B**) Adolescent using flutter device.

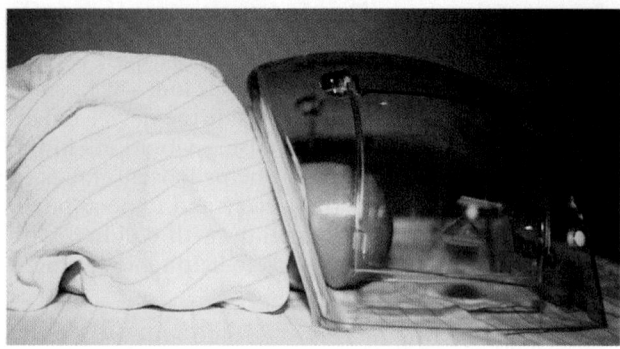

FIGURE 40.10 Oxygen hood for an infant.

A snug-fitting oxygen mask is yet another method for supplying nearly 100% oxygen and is the method frequently used in emergencies (Fig. 40.11). Masks are often not well tolerated by children because they tend to slip and obstruct their view. If necessary, let them hold a mask rather than strapping it in place to allow them more control.

Regardless of the delivery method used, oxygen must be administered warmed and moistened. Without proper humidification, oxygen dries mucous membranes and thickens secretions, thus compounding breathing difficulty. Oxygen, like any other drug, requires careful administration and follow-up assessment. If concentrations are too low, oxygen is not therapeutic; in concentrations greater than those desired, it can be toxic. If newborns are subjected to oxygen concentrations over 100 mm Hg for an extended time, retinopathy of prematurity can occur (see Chapter 26). In any child, administering oxygen concentrations of 70% to 80% for an extended period may lead to a thickening of the lung alveoli and a loss of lung pliancy (oxygen toxicity or bronchopulmonary dysplasia). For these reasons, oxygen should not be given in high concentrations for long periods unless adequate facilities for blood gas analysis are available (ATS, 2003).

When caring for a child with any form of oxygen equipment, follow good safety rules. Because oxygen supports combustion, keep open flames away from oxygen and minimize the risks of sparks. Since oxygen is humidified, oxygen equipment is a good source of microbial contaminants. Change equipment according to your agency's policy, but at least once a week to keep bacterial counts within safe limits. Monitor and record a child's oxygen saturation level via pulse oximetry or transcutaneous pulse oximetry as indicated. Obtain ABG measurements with any change in condition or oxygen flow or as otherwise ordered.

Pharmacologic Therapy

Children notice difficulty with exchange of air when their airways become obstructed because of unusual mucus production, bronchoconstriction, or inflammation. A number of drugs may be used in children to reverse these processes. Nasal sprays such as normal saline can be administered to moisten and loosen nasal secretions. Antihistamines given by this route can reduce mucus production and thereby enlarge the airway. Decongestants cause vasoconstriction, leading to shrinkage of the mucous membranes, which expands breathing space. Expectorants such as guaifenesin (Robitussin) help to raise mucus. Most of these agents also cause drowsiness, so their doses must be regulated, especially in adolescents who will be driving. Bronchodilators such as albuterol (Ventolin), terbutaline (Brethine), and levalbuterol (Xopenex) are examples of drugs used to open the lower airway. Antibiotics may be given intravenously, intramuscularly, orally, or inhaled through nebulization to reduce infection and limit purulent mucus and inflammation. Corticosteroids taken either orally or by inhalation enlarge the airway by reducing further inflammation (Karch, 2004).

Metered-Dose Inhalers. A metered-dose inhaler (MDI) is a hand-held device that provides a route for medication administration directly to the respiratory tract. The child inhales while pressing a trigger on the apparatus. Small children may need a spacer device attached to the apparatus, a plastic extension tube or chamber that helps better coordinate inhalation with the medication delivery. For successful use, children need to follow five general rules: shake the canister, exhale deeply, activate the inhaler as they begin to inhale, take a long slow inhalation, and then hold their breath for 5 to 10 seconds. They should take only one puff at a time, with a 1-minute wait between puffs (Karch, 2004).

Incentive Spirometry

Incentive spirometers are devices that encourage children to inhale deeply to aerate the lungs fully or move mucus. Although manufactured in different configurations, a common type consists of a hollow plastic tube containing a brightly colored ball or dome-shaped disk that will rise in the tube when a child inhales through the attached mouthpiece and tubing. The deeper the inhalation, the higher the ball rises in the tube.

Children need instruction on how to use this type of device, because their first impression is that they should blow out against the mouthpiece rather than inhale

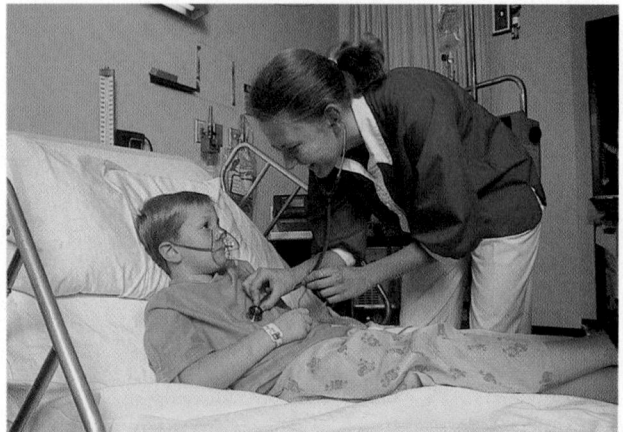

FIGURE 40.11 A nurse assesses a child's lungs while he receives oxygen therapy via a mask. (Steve Woit/Stock Boston.)

the back of the pharynx and the palatine arch. Laboratory studies will indicate an increased white blood cell count.

If the inflammation is mild, children rarely need more than an oral analgesic such as acetaminophen or ibuprofen for comfort. Warm heat applied to the external neck area using a warm towel or heating pad also can be soothing. By school age, children are capable of gargling with a solution such as warm water to help reduce the pain. Before this age, children tend to swallow the solution unless the procedure is well explained and demonstrated to them.

Because children's throats feel so sore, they often prefer liquids to solid food. Infants, especially, must be observed closely until the inflammation and tenderness diminish to be certain that they take in sufficient fluid to prevent dehydration (Bagarazzi, 2003).

Streptococcal Pharyngitis

Group A beta-hemolytic streptococcus is the organism most frequently involved in bacterial pharyngitis in children. All streptococcal infections must be taken seriously because they can lead to cardiac and kidney damage from an autoimmune process (Posner, 2003).

Assessment. Streptococcal infections are generally more severe than viral infections. The fact that symptoms are mild, however, does not rule out streptococcal infection. With a streptococcal pharyngitis, the back of the throat and palatine tonsils are usually markedly erythematous (bright red); the tonsils are enlarged and there may be a white exudate in the tonsillar crypts. Petechiae may be present on the palate. A child typically appears ill with a high fever, an extremely sore throat, difficulty swallowing, and overall lethargy. Temperature is usually elevated to as high as 104°F (40°C). The child often has a headache. Swollen abdominal lymph nodes may cause abdominal pain. A throat culture, often completed as a quick office procedure, confirms the presence of the *Streptococcus* bacteria.

Therapeutic Management. Treatment consists of a full 10-day course of an oral antibiotic such as penicillin G or clindamycin. Cephalosporins or broad-spectrum macrolides such as erythromycin may be prescribed if resistant organisms are known to be in the community. Help parents understand the importance of completing the full 10 days of therapy. The prolonged treatment is necessary to ensure the streptococci are eradicated completely. If they are not, the child may develop a hypersensitivity or autoimmune reaction to group A streptococci that results in rheumatic fever (although the chance of rheumatic fever occurring is probably as low as 1%) or glomerulonephritis.

Symptoms of acute glomerulonephritis (blood and protein in urine) appear in 1 to 2 weeks after the pharyngitis. For this reason, 2 weeks after treatment, children may be asked to return to the health care facility with a urine specimen to be examined for protein so that developing acute glomerulonephritis can be detected (Meyers, 2003).

To ensure that a child receives the full antibiotic course, help parents make a reminder sheet to place on a cabinet or refrigerator door. In addition, instruct them about measures for rest, relief of throat pain, and maintaining hydration, the same actions as for a common cold. Because it is impossible for parents to discriminate between a pharyn-

gitis caused by a virus (and needing no therapy other than comfort measures) and a streptococcal pharyngitis (needing definite therapy to prevent life-threatening illnesses), a child with pharyngitis always should be examined by health care personnel.

Checkpoint Question 2

Suppose Michael is diagnosed as having a streptococcal pharyngitis. The chief danger of such an infection is:

a. Lymph nodes will swell and obstruct the airway.
b. Infection may spread and cause a tooth abscess.
c. A small number of children develop kidney disease.
d. Four out of five children will develop lung abscesses.

Retropharyngeal Abscess

In infants, the lymph nodes that drain the nasopharynx are located behind the posterior pharynx wall. These nodes may become infected in an infant following an acute nasopharyngitis or pharyngitis. Since these nodes disappear by preschool age, the problem is usually limited to young infants (Rutstein, 2003).

Assessment. Typically, infants have an upper respiratory tract infection or sore throat for a few days. Suddenly, they refuse to eat. They develop a high fever and may drool because they cannot swallow saliva past the obstruction in the back of their throat. They "snore" with respirations as the pharynx becomes further occluded. To allow themselves more breathing space, they may hyperextend the head, a very unusual position for infants.

Physical assessment reveals enlargement of the regional lymph nodes. The mass in the posterior pharynx may not be visible if it is below the point of vision. An ultrasound or x-ray study using a swallowed contrast medium will reveal the bulging tissue in the pharynx. Laboratory studies will reveal leukocytosis.

Therapeutic Management. Because the most common cause of retropharyngeal abscess is group A beta-hemolytic streptococcus, benzathine penicillin G or penicillin V is effective. As a result of their poor swallowing, infants' mouths may need to be suctioned to remove secretions. Be careful not to touch the suction catheter to the posterior pharynx because this might rupture the abscess, possibly leading to aspiration of the abscess contents (producing respiratory obstruction or a pneumonia caused by the aspirated purulent material). Blood vessels invade some retropharyngeal abscesses, so rupture of the structure also could lead to profuse bleeding (dangerous to the child both because of the loss of blood from major arteries such as the carotid artery and because the blood could be aspirated).

Place infants in a side-lying position to allow difficult-to-swallow mouth secretions to drain forward. Limit oral intake to fluids. A hard food such as a toast crust (a food often recommended for teething) could rupture the abscess with its hard edges.

Although some postpharyngeal abscesses resolve on their own, some need to be incised by a surgeon to promote drainage. This is done with the child in a Trendelenburg position so that drainage from the abscess can be suctioned away to prevent aspiration. After surgery, maintain the child in a Trendelenburg or a side position to encourage further drainage and prevent aspiration. Monitor vital signs closely. Observe any drainage from infants' mouths to detect fresh bleeding. Frequent swallowing is also a sign of postpharyngeal bleeding. Increased respiratory rate suggests airway obstruction.

Oral fluid is introduced as soon as the infant's swallowing and gag reflexes are intact after surgery. Although the throat is undoubtedly still sore, most infants suck eagerly and need supplemental intravenous fluid administration following surgery for only a short time.

On admission to the hospital, parents may be thoroughly frightened by the extent of the child's symptoms (gurgling or snoring sound, high temperature, dyspnea). Allow parents to handle the infant and care for him or her while overnight in the hospital to help them allay their fears and regain confidence in their ability to give care.

Tonsillitis

"Tonsillitis" is the term commonly used to refer to infection and inflammation of the palatine tonsils. "Adenitis" refers to infection and inflammation of the adenoid (pharyngeal) tonsils.

Tonsillar tissue is lymphoid tissue that filters pathogenic organisms from the head and neck area. The palatine tonsils are located on both sides of the pharynx; the adenoids are in the nasopharynx. Tubal tonsils are located at the entrance to the eustachian tubes. Lingual tonsils are located at the base of the tongue. All of the tonsils, referred to collectively as Waldeyer's ring, are easily infected because of the bacteria that pass through or are screened through them with lymph (Smith & Osborne, 2003).

Assessment

Infection of the palatine tonsils presents with all of the symptoms of a severe pharyngitis. Children drool because their throat is too sore for them to swallow saliva. They may describe swallowing as so painful it feels as if they are swallowing bits of metal or glass. In addition, they usually have a high fever and are lethargic. Tonsillar tissue appears bright red and may be so enlarged the two areas of palatine tonsillar tissue meet in the midline. Pus can be detected on or expelled from the crypts of the tonsils.

In addition to fever, lethargy, pharyngeal pain, and edema, the symptoms of adenoidal tissue infection also include a nasal quality of speech, mouth breathing, difficulty hearing, and perhaps halitosis or sleep apnea. The mouth breathing, change in speech, and apnea result from the postpharyngeal obstruction by the enlarged tissue. The difficulty with hearing occurs because of eustachian tube obstruction. Long-term obstruction this way can further cause serous and acute otitis media (middle ear infection).

Tonsillitis occurs most commonly in school-age children. The responsible organism is identified by a throat culture. In children younger than 3 years of age, the cause is often viral. In school-age children, the organism is generally a group A beta-hemolytic streptococcus (Curtin-Wirt et al., 2003).

Therapeutic Management

Therapy for bacterial tonsillitis includes an antipyretic for fever, an analgesic for pain, and a full 10-day course of an antibiotic such as penicillin or amoxicillin. If the cause is viral, no therapy other than comfort or fever reduction strategies is necessary. Although the pain of the infection will subside a day or two after the antibiotic administration is begun, remind parents that children need the full 10-day course of antibiotic to eradicate streptococci completely from the back of the throat. After a tonsillar infection, tonsillar tissue may remain hypertrophied, or it may atrophy and appear smaller than it did previously.

Tonsillectomy. Tonsillectomy is removal of the palatine tonsils. Adenoidectomy is removal of the pharyngeal tonsils. In the past, tonsillectomy was a common procedure after tonsillitis, but today it is not recommended unless all other measures to prevent frequent infections prove ineffective. Tonsillar tissue is removed by ligating the tonsil or by laser surgery. Because sutures are not placed, the chance for hemorrhage after this type of surgery is higher than after surgery involving a closed incision. The danger of aspiration of blood at the time of surgery and the danger of a general anesthetic compound the risk.

Chronic tonsillitis is about the only reason for removal of palatine tonsils. Adenoids may be removed if they are so hypertrophied they cause obstruction or sleep apnea. At one time, adenoids and palatine tonsils were always removed together; today, depending on the symptoms and the extent of hypertrophy and infection, children may have a tonsillectomy, an adenoidectomy, or both.

Tonsillectomy or adenoidectomy is never done while the organs are infected, because an operation at such a time might spread pathogenic organisms into the bloodstream, causing septicemia. Parents often ask why an operation to remove tonsils must be delayed until the child is well again. They think that as long as the tonsils are sore, they should be immediately removed. Help them understand why this is not possible and why it is safer to schedule surgery for a later date. Most parents report an improvement in their child's general health and performance after tonsillectomy surgery, as this ends the chronic infections.

NURSING DIAGNOSES AND RELATED INTERVENTIONS

Nursing Diagnosis: Risk for fluid volume deficit related to blood loss from surgery

Outcome Evaluation: Child's pulse and blood pressure remain normal for age; there is absence of extensive bleeding; intake and output are within acceptable parameters.

Tonsillectomies are done as ambulatory or 1-day surgery following completion of a complete history and physical examination and laboratory tests, including bleeding and clotting times, complete blood count, and urinalysis. Teach parents to use common sense in their child's care during the week before hospital admission so that the child does not have a cold or recurrent tonsillitis at the time planned for surgery. An important aspect of immediate assessment on the day of surgery is to observe for loose teeth; if present, they could be dislodged during surgery and aspirated. If loose teeth are present, mark this on the front of the child's chart and report it to the anesthesiologist.

After surgery, observe vital signs carefully to make certain the child is not bleeding from the denuded surgical area. Place the child on the side or abdomen with a pillow under the chest so that the head is lower than the chest. This allows blood and unswallowed saliva to drain from the child's mouth rather than back to the pharynx, where it might be aspirated (Fig. 40.16).

If hemorrhage occurs after tonsillectomy, it can be acute and intense. Because children will swallow any blood that is oozing from the surgical site, a child can be bleeding heavily and yet little blood is apparent. To detect bleeding, assess for subtle signs of hemorrhage, such as an increasing pulse or respiratory rate, frequent swallowing, throat clearing, or a feeling of anxiety. A child's first line of defense against hemorrhage is a nurse who recognizes these subtle signs of bleeding before the bleeding becomes so intense that signs of shock occur.

If you find that the surgical site is bleeding, elevate the child's head and turn him or her on the side to reduce vascular pressure on the operative site. Use a good light to inspect the posterior throat. Have a dental mirror available so the surgeon can thoroughly inspect the bleeding area. If the surgical area is bleeding heavily, the child may need to be returned to surgery for a suture or two to halt bleeding.

The most dangerous periods for a child after a tonsillectomy are the first 24 hours, when the clots covering the denuded surgical area are forming, and days 5 to 7, when the clots begin to lyse or dissolve. If new granulation tissue is not yet present when the clots dissolve, hemorrhage from the denuded surface can occur.

If children have no complications from surgery, are able to swallow fluids, and have voided, they are discharged later the same day of surgery. Parents need careful instructions concerning the danger signs to watch for during the first day home (frequent swallowing, clearing the throat, increasing restlessness). They are usually advised to restrict their child's activity (no gymnastics, swimming) until after the seventh day, when firm healing should have taken place. The child needs a return appointment to a health care facility approximately 2 weeks after surgery for follow-up assessment to make sure the surgical area has healed without complication.

Nursing Diagnosis: Pain related to surgical procedure

Outcome Evaluation: Child states level of pain is tolerable.

Tonsillectomy is an uncomfortable and painful procedure for children. Be sure they receive good preparation for the procedure and for the sensations they will experience afterward. Although tonsils are removed, it is better to talk about tonsils being "fixed" rather than taken out; children may be extremely frightened to know that a body part will be removed, however small it is.

Children's throats are extremely sore following a tonsillectomy. Liquid analgesics are better tolerated than pills or tablets because they are easier to swallow. Rectal administration is a possibility for very young children. Occasionally, a child may require intravenous pain relief.

Most children are thirsty immediately after surgery, and drinking is helpful because swallowing fluid causes active pharyngeal movement, increasing the blood supply to the area and reducing edema and pain. Children commonly are promised by well-meaning people they can have all the ice cream they want after a tonsillectomy. However, because milk products form tenacious secretions that are difficult to swallow, ice cream is not a food of choice. Offer instead frequent sips of clear liquid, Popsicles, or ice chips. Avoid acid juices because these sting the denuded tissue. Carbonated beverages also can irritate the area unless they stand for a time to become

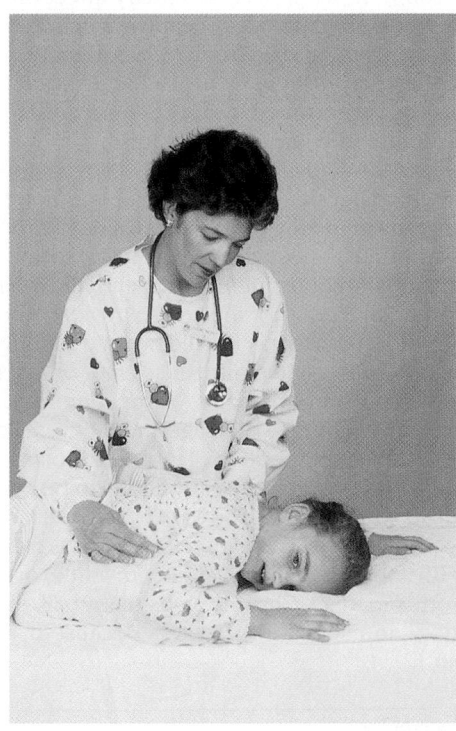

FIGURE 40.16 Positioning a child after tonsillectomy. The pillow under the chest helps secretions flow out of the mouth.

"flat." Avoid red fluid such as Kool-Aid, which if vomited can be mistaken for swallowed blood.

Children can then gradually advance after 24 to 48 hours to a diet of soft foods such as gelatin, mashed potatoes, soups, and cooked fruits. They should continue to eat only soft foods for the first week (no toast crusts or other foods that could cause pharyngeal irritation if not chewed well). Be certain parents know whom they should call (clinic, hospital, or pediatrician) if they have a question or concern about their child's condition or care. Caution parents that some children develop a mild earache after tonsillectomy for the first week, probably caused by shifting pressure on the eustachian tube.

Checkpoint Question 3

Suppose Michael's 4-year-old roommate spits up dark-red blood following her tonsillectomy. Your best action in relation to this would be:

a. Suction the back of her throat.
b. Encourage her to cough vigorously.
c. Perform a Heimlich maneuver.
d. Continue to observe her for bleeding.

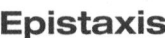

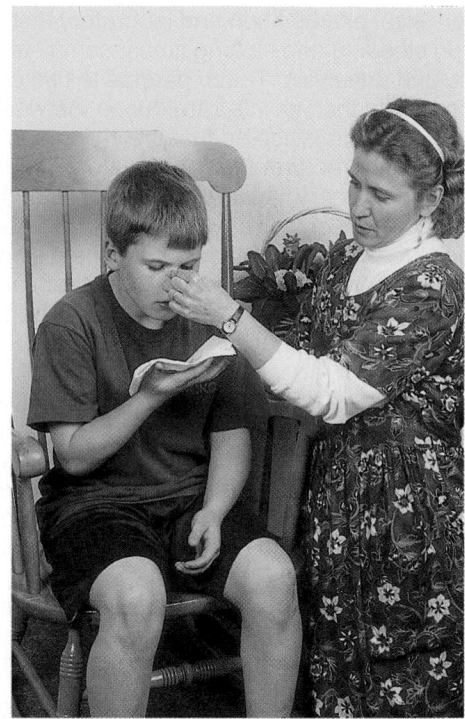

FIGURE 40.17 Emergency therapy for a nosebleed is to sit the child up and apply pressure to the sides of the nose.

Epistaxis

Epistaxis (nosebleed) is extremely common in children and usually occurs from trauma, such as picking at the nose, from falling, or from being hit on the nose by another child. In homes that lack humidification, the hot dry environment makes children's mucous membranes dry, uncomfortable, and susceptible to cracking and bleeding. In all children, epistaxis tends to occur during respiratory illnesses. It also may occur after strenuous exercise, and it is associated with a number of systemic diseases, such as rheumatic fever, scarlet fever, measles, or varicella infection (chickenpox). It can occur with nasal polyps, sinusitis, or allergic rhinitis. Some families show a familial predisposition.

Nosebleeds are always frightening because of the visible bleeding and a choking sensation if blood should run down the back of the nasopharynx. The fear is generally out of proportion to the seriousness of the bleeding.

Keep children with nosebleeds in an upright position with their head tilted slightly forward to minimize the amount of blood pressure in nasal vessels and to keep blood moving forward, not back into the nasopharynx (Osterhoudt, 2003). Apply pressure to the sides of the nose with your fingers (Fig. 40.17). Make every effort to quiet the child and to help him or her stop crying, because crying increases pressure in the blood vessels of the head and prolongs bleeding. If these simple measures do not control the bleeding, epinephrine (1:1,000) may be applied to the bleeding site to constrict blood vessels. A nasal pack may be necessary to provide continued pressure.

Teach parents that every child has occasional nosebleeds. Chronic nasal bleeding, however, should be investigated to rule out a systemic disease or blood disorder.

Sinusitis

Sinusitis is rare in children younger than 6 years of age because the frontal sinuses do not develop fully until age 6 (Chung, 2003). It occurs as a secondary infection in older children when streptococcal, staphylococcal, or *H. influenzae* organisms spread from the nasal cavity. Children develop a fever, a purulent nasal discharge, headache, and tenderness over the affected sinus. A nose and throat culture will identify the infectious organism.

Treatment for acute sinusitis consists of an antipyretic for fever, an analgesic for pain, and an antibiotic for the specific organism involved. Oxymetazoline hydrochloride (Afrin), supplied as nose drops or a nasal spray, shrinks the edematous mucous membranes and allows infected material to drain from the sinuses. To avoid a rebound effect, this type of nasal spray should be used for only 3 days at a time; otherwise, it actually causes more nasal congestion than was present originally. Warm compresses to the sinus area may encourage drainage and relieve pain. Some children need acetaminophen (Tylenol) for pain.

Sinusitis is considered by many adults to be a minor illness. It needs to be treated, however, because it can have serious complications if the infection spreads from the sinuses to invade the facial bone (osteomyelitis) or the middle ear (otitis media). Chronic sinusitis can also interfere with school and social interactions because of the constant pain.

Laryngitis

Laryngitis is inflammation of the larynx. It results in brassy, hoarse voice sounds or inability to make audible voice sounds. It may occur as a complication of pharyngitis or from excessive use of the voice, as in shouting or loud cheering. Laryngitis is as annoying for children as it is for adults. Sips of fluid (either warm or cold, whichever feels best) offer relief from the annoying tickling sensation often present. The most effective measure, however, is for the child to rest the voice for at least 24 hours, until inflammation subsides. For infants with laryngitis, attempt to meet their needs before they have to cry for things. Simply caution older children not to speak. Provide them with a paper and pencil or chalkboard for communication.

Congenital Laryngomalacia/ Tracheomalacia

Congenital laryngomalacia means that an infant's laryngeal structure is weaker than normal and collapses more than usual on inspiration. This produces laryngeal **stridor** (a high-pitched crowing sound on inspiration) present from birth, possibly intensified when the infant is in a supine position or when sucking (Carden et al., 2005).

Assessment

The infant's sternum and intercostal spaces may retract on inspiration because of the increased effort needed to pull air into the trachea past the collapsed cartilage rings. Many infants with this condition must stop sucking frequently during a feeding to maintain adequate ventilation and to rest from their respiratory effort, which is exhausting.

Therapeutic Management

When parents wake at night and listen in a quiet house to the sound of stridor, it seems unbearably loud. This makes it difficult for them to believe it is safe for them to care for the infant at home.

Most children with congenital laryngomalacia need no routine therapy other than to have parents feed them slowly, providing rest periods as needed. The condition improves as infants mature and cartilage in the larynx becomes stronger at about 1 year of age. Many parents sleep at night with the child's crib next to their bed or with one hand resting on the infant's chest so they can be assured during the night the child is continuing to breathe. At health care visits, assess whether the parents are receiving enough sleep at night and are not becoming too exhausted to be able to continue their daily activities. Showing them a weight chart that demonstrates their child is growing and thriving despite this problem can be reassuring.

Be certain parents know the importance of bringing the child for early care if signs of an upper respiratory tract infection develop. If not, laryngeal collapse will be even more intense during these times, and complete obstruction of the trachea could occur. Any time stridor becomes more intense, advise parents to have the infant seen by their primary care provider, because generally this indicates beginning obstruction and probably the beginning of an upper respiratory tract infection. As parents become more accustomed to the sound their infant makes while breathing, they will become astute reporters of change in their infant's condition; listen to them carefully when they report a change to prevent overlooking this important information.

Croup (Laryngotracheobronchitis)

Croup (inflammation of the larynx, trachea, and major bronchi) is one of the most frightening diseases of early childhood for both parents and children. In children between 6 months and 3 years of age, the cause of croup is usually a viral infection such as parainfluenza virus. In previous years, the most common cause was *H. influenzae*. However, since immunization against this organism has been included in a routine immunization series, the incidence of croup from this cause has declined by 90% (Phillips, 2003).

Assessment

With croup, children typically have only a mild upper respiratory tract infection at bedtime. Temperature is normal or only mildly elevated. During the night, they develop a barking cough (croupy cough), inspiratory stridor, and marked retractions. They wake in extreme respiratory distress. The larynx, trachea, and major bronchi are all inflamed. These severe symptoms typically last a number of hours and then, except for a rattling cough, subside by morning. Symptoms may recur the following night. Cyanosis is rarely present, but the danger of glottal obstruction from the laryngeal inflammation is very real. Pulse oximetry and transcutaneous SaO_2 monitors are helpful measures to document whether hypoxemia is occurring.

Therapeutic Management

One emergency method of relieving croup symptoms is for a parent to run the shower or hot water tap in a bathroom until the room fills with steam, then keep the child in this warm, moist environment. If this does not relieve symptoms, instruct parents to bring the child to an emergency department for further evaluation and care. When a child is seen at the emergency room, cool moist air with a corticosteroid such as dexamethasone, or racemic epinephrine, given by nebulizer, can reduce inflammation and produce effective bronchodilation to open the airway (Bjornson & Johnson, 2004). Intravenous therapy may be prescribed to keep the child well hydrated. Maintain accurate intake and output records and test urine specific gravity to ensure that hydration is adequate.

NURSING DIAGNOSES AND RELATED INTERVENTIONS

Nursing Diagnosis: Ineffective airway clearance related to edema and constriction of airway

Outcome Evaluation: Respiratory rate is below 22 breaths/min; no cyanosis is present; P_{O_2} is 80 to 100 mm Hg; $S_{a}O_2$ is over 95%.

Attach a sensor for pulse oximetry monitoring and remain constantly with a child with croup, not only to observe closely for increasing respiratory distress but also to reduce the child's anxiety. Take vital signs as often as every 15 minutes, because extreme restlessness and thrashing, increased stridor, increased heart and respiratory rates, and cyanosis are symptoms of oxygen deprivation. In some children, it is difficult to distinguish between fright from the newness of the experience (and their sense of their parents' fright) and the anxiety that comes from oxygen deprivation. Keep a continuous record of vital signs and activity as a way to demonstrate increasing respiratory rate and restlessness. ABGs may be obtained to assess for sufficient oxygenation if pulse oximetry is not being used. A tracheostomy or endotracheal intubation along with oxygen therapy may be necessary if symptoms do not diminish. (It is difficult to intubate children with croup because of the severe respiratory tract edema.)

Laryngospasm with total occlusion of the airway can occur when a child's gag reflex is elicited or when the child is crying. Therefore, do not elicit a gag reflex in any child with a croupy, barking cough, and provide comfort to prevent crying.

Croup is a frightening disease for parents because their child is suddenly ill with severe symptoms. When the severe symptoms disappear by morning, parents may feel foolish they rushed to a hospital with the child in the middle of the night. Assure them that their initial judgment was correct. When they brought the child in, he or she was seriously ill. Parents may be reluctant to see their child discharged in the morning until they are convinced that he or she is now well enough to go home (Box 40.10).

What if... Michael, who had loud stridor when he was admitted, suddenly has no stridor present? Would you be relieved (his condition must be improving) or worried (his airway may be so blocked that not enough air is entering to make the sound of stridor)? How should you respond?

Epiglottitis

Epiglottitis is inflammation of the epiglottis (the flap of tissue that covers the opening to the larynx to keep out food and fluid during swallowing). Although it is rare, inflammation of the epiglottis is an emergency because the swollen epiglottis cannot rise and allow the airway to open. It occurs most frequently in children from 2 to about 7 years of age (Cromer & Foley, 2004).

Epiglottitis can be either bacterial or viral in origin. *H. influenzae* type B has been replaced as the most common bacterial cause of the disorder by pneumococci, streptococci, or staphylococci. Echovirus and respiratory syncytial virus also can cause the disorder.

Assessment

Symptoms begin as those of a mild upper respiratory tract infection. After 1 or 2 days, as inflammation spreads to the epiglottis, the child suddenly develops severe inspiratory stridor, a high fever, hoarseness, and a very sore throat. The child may have such difficulty swallowing that he or she drools saliva. The child may protrude the tongue to increase free movement in the pharynx.

If a child's gag reflex is stimulated with a tongue blade, the swollen and inflamed epiglottis can be seen to rise in the back of the throat as a cherry-red structure. It can be so edematous, however, that the gagging procedure causes complete obstruction of the glottis and respiratory failure. Therefore, in children with symptoms of epiglottitis (dysphagia, inspiratory stridor, cough, fever, and hoarseness), *never attempt to visualize the epiglottis directly with a tongue blade or obtain a throat culture* unless a means of providing an artificial airway, such as tracheostomy or endotracheal intubation, is readily available. This is especially important for the nurse who functions in an expanded role and performs physical assessments and routinely elicits gag reflexes.

With epiglottitis, laboratory studies will show leukocytosis (20,000 to 30,000 mm^3), with the proportion of neutrophils increased. A blood culture to evaluate for septicemia and ABGs to evaluate respiratory sufficiency may be ordered. However, because excessive crying can precipitate entrapment of the epiglottis and obstruction, such tests may be delayed in preference to a lateral neck x-ray film or sonogram, which will show the enlarged epiglottis. Do not allow a child with possible epiglottitis to go to these departments accompanied only by parents or a nursing aide, in case obstruction occurs in the x-ray or sonograph room.

Therapeutic Management

Children need moist air to reduce the epiglottal inflammation. If cyanosis is present, they need oxygen. An antibiotic, such as a second-generation cephalosporin (e.g., cefuroxime), may be prescribed until a throat culture indicates a specific antibiotic drug. Because they can't swallow, children need intravenous fluid therapy to maintain hydration. They may need a prophylactic tracheostomy or endotracheal intubation to prevent total obstruction, although it is often difficult to intubate children with epiglottitis because the tube cannot be passed beyond the edematous epiglottis. After antibiotic therapy begins, the epiglottal inflammation recedes rapidly. By 12 to 24 hours, it has reduced enough that the airway may be removed. Antibiotic administration will continue for a full 7 to 10 days. Siblings of the ill child may be prescribed prophylactic antibiotic therapy to prevent them from developing the same symptoms.

Initially, the symptoms of epiglottitis are not unlike those of croup. As a result, parents may not realize the extent of the occlusion in their child, especially if the child has had croup on other occasions. They may question why a prophylactic tracheostomy was necessary this time when it was not used when the child had croup. Explain to them the difference between the two diseases (Table 40.5).

popcorn, nuts, and coins. As a rule, nuts or popcorn should not be given to children younger than school age. These objects are coated with oil, and as they swell with moisture in the respiratory tract, they cause not only obstruction but also lipid pneumonia, a persistent and difficult-to-treat type of pneumonia. Foreign bodies that are inhaled this deeply are rarely coughed up spontaneously, despite the severe coughing that ensues. Because objects such as plastic and nuts cannot be visualized well on x-ray film, an x-ray study may be inconclusive.

Therapeutic Management

Children who are seen in emergency departments after aspirating a foreign body are in distress from pain and are choking and coughing. Their parents are frightened by the degree of distress. Parents may feel bad about having offered the child (or allowed the child to reach) a food such as a peanut. Children need quick orientation to the treatment environment, as they move from the emergency department to x-ray and then possibly to surgery or a treatment room. If possible, allow the parents to go with them as appropriate. Throughout, be vigilant in observing the child for coughing up the foreign body or developing increasing respiratory distress.

A bronchoscopy may be necessary to remove the foreign body (Brown & Padman, 2004). Children are often given conscious sedation for a bronchoscopy (for details of a bronchoscopy procedure and conscious sedation, see Chapter 36). After bronchoscopy, assess the child closely for signs of bronchial edema and airway obstruction that occurs from mucus accumulation due to the bronchus manipulation. Obtain frequent vital signs (increasing pulse and respiratory rates suggest increased edema and obstruction).

Keep a child NPO for at least an hour after a bronchoscopy. Check for return of the gag reflex. Once the gag reflex is present, offer the first fluid cautiously to prevent additional aspiration. Cool fluid may feel more soothing and also helps to reduce the soreness in the throat. Breathing cool, moist air or having an ice collar applied may further reduce edema.

Obviously, parents need to be cautioned about the dangers of aspiration to keep it from happening again. Do not lecture them, however. A parent whose child has just been through this experience already recognizes the danger of aspiration and realizes he or she needs to be more careful in the future.

DISORDERS OF THE LOWER RESPIRATORY TRACT

The structures of the lower respiratory tract are subject to infection by the same pathogens that attack the upper respiratory tract. Inflammation and infection of the lungs or bronchi is particularly troublesome: it occurs in various forms and is caused by several organisms. Other illnesses that occur in the lower respiratory tract, such as asthma and cystic fibrosis, can lead to secondary pneumonia infections and chronic illness.

Influenza

Influenza involves inflammation and infection of the major airways. It is caused by the orthomyxoviruses influenza types A, B, or C. It is marked by a cough, fever, fatigue, aching pains, a sore throat, and often accompanying gastrointestinal symptoms such as vomiting or diarrhea. The disease spreads readily through a home or a classroom because children are contagious on the day before symptoms appear and for about the next 5 days.

Children usually need an antipyretic such as acetaminophen (Tylenol) to control fever. Oseltamivir (TamiFlu), a new antiviral drug that halts viral proliferation, can be taken by children over 1 year of age (Karch, 2004). Because TamiFlu only halts virus replication, it needs to be taken at the first sign of illness. Although most children recover without incident, influenza can lead to bronchitis or pneumonia. The condition can be largely prevented by yearly influenza vaccine. Because the influenza virus mutates yearly, the influenza vaccine is specific for only that year and must be readministered yearly (Goldrick, 2004).

Bronchitis

Bronchitis, or inflammation of the major bronchi and trachea, is one of the more common illnesses affecting preschool and school-age children. It is characterized by fever and cough, usually in conjunction with nasal congestion. Causative agents include the influenza viruses, adenovirus, and *Mycoplasma pneumoniae,* among others.

Assessment

A child usually has a mild upper respiratory tract infection for 1 or 2 days; he or she then develops a fever and a dry, hacking cough, which is hoarse and mildly productive in older children. The cough is serious enough to wake a child from sleep. These symptoms may last for a week, with full recovery sometimes taking as long as 2 weeks.

On auscultation, rhonchi and coarse crackles (the sound of rales) can be heard. A chest x-ray will reveal diffuse alveolar hyperinflation and some markings at the hilus of the lung.

Therapeutic Management

Therapy is aimed at relieving respiratory symptoms, reducing fever, and maintaining adequate hydration. An antibiotic is prescribed for bacterial infections. If mucus is viscid, an expectorant may be needed to help the child raise it. It is important that children with bronchitis cough to raise accumulating sputum. Cough syrups to suppress coughing, therefore, are rarely indicated.

Bronchiolitis

Bronchiolitis is inflammation of the fine bronchioles and small bronchi. It is the most common lower respiratory illness in children younger than 2 years, peaking in incidence at 6 months of age. It occurs most often in the winter and spring. Many children who develop asthma later in life have numerous instances of bronchiolitis during their first year of life. Viruses, such as adenovirus, parainfluenza virus, and respiratory syncytial virus (RSV), in particular, appear to be the pathogens most responsible for this illness (Zsolway, 2003).

Assessment

Typically, infants have 1 or 2 days of an upper respiratory tract infection, then suddenly begin to demonstrate nasal flaring, intercostal and subcostal retractions on inspiration, and an increased respiratory rate. They may have a mild fever, leukocytosis, and an increased erythrocyte sedimentation rate, indicating the amount of bronchial inflammation present. Both accumulating mucus and inflammation block the small bronchioles, so air can no longer enter or leave alveoli freely. Most infants develop alveolar hyperinflation because air enters more easily than it leaves inflamed, narrowed bronchioles. The expiratory phase of respiration is prolonged, and wheezing may be present. After initial hyperinflation, areas of atelectasis may occur as the air that cannot be expired is absorbed. Tachycardia and cyanosis develop from hypoxia. Infants soon become exhausted from rapid respirations. A chest x-ray may show pulmonary infiltrates caused by a secondary infection or collapse of alveoli (atelectasis). Pulse oximetry shows low oxygen saturation. A throat culture will identify the offending organism.

Therapeutic Management

For children with less severe symptoms, antipyretics, adequate hydration, and maintaining a watchful eye for progression to more serious illness is all that is necessary. Hospitalization is warranted for children in severe distress (e.g., if the infant is tachypneic, has marked retractions, seems listless, or has a history of poor fluid intake).

Antibiotics are not commonly used in the treatment of bronchiolitis, because bacteria are rarely a causative factor. Children with chronic pulmonary disease may receive anti-RSV immunoglobulin if RSV was identified as the causative agent (Zsolway, 2003).

If symptoms are severe, children need humidified oxygen to counteract hypoxemia and adequate hydration to keep respiratory membranes moist. Nebulized bronchodilators, epinephrine, and steroids may be used, although there is little evidence they make a major difference in reducing symptoms (King et al., 2004). Some children need ventilatory assistance to achieve adequate ventilation. All infants with bronchiolitis need to be carefully observed because if RSV is the cause, apnea may occur. In some infants, extracorporeal membrane oxygenation (the same as that used for heart surgery) is necessary to maintain adequate oxygenation.

Feeding is often a problem because infants tire easily and therefore cannot finish a feeding. Intravenous fluids may be given for the first 1 or 2 days of illness to eliminate the need for oral feeding.

NURSING DIAGNOSES AND RELATED INTERVENTIONS

Nursing Diagnosis: Parental anxiety related to respiratory distress in child

Outcome Evaluation: Parents state that their anxiety level is tolerable as signs and symptoms of disease decrease.

Be certain that parents receive a good explanation of their child's condition. Most parents are aware of bronchi but are unfamiliar with the word "bronchiole." This leaves them unsure how a simple cold has become so severe. They wonder whether they should have sought medical attention sooner. This may cause them to lose confidence in themselves as parents. Assure them that bronchiolitis begins as only a cold and that it was impossible to know that this cold would take a more serious turn.

The acute phase of bronchiolitis lasts 2 or 3 days. After this time, the child's condition improves rapidly. Although mortality from bronchiolitis is less than 1%, it is a serious disorder of infancy; without treatment, a larger number of infants certainly would die (Hernandez, 2003).

Respiratory Syncytial Virus (RSV) Bronchiolitis

RSV is a pathogenic RNA virus that is the most common cause of bronchiolitis in young children. Symptoms begin as a mild upper respiratory infection that quickly extends to include the bronchioles. The infant becomes lethargic and possibly cyanotic. Dehydration occurs as the child becomes too fatigued to suck. Respiratory distress with nasal flaring, retractions, grunting, rales, rhonchi, and expiratory wheezing noted on auscultation occur. All infants with an RSV infection must be monitored closely because the virus tends to cause apnea or periodic halting of respirations. The diagnosis is confirmed by throat or nasal culture.

Therapy is supportive (supplemental oxygen and hydration therapy), although life-threatening apnea may require ventilatory support with mechanical ventilation. Ribavirin, an antiviral agent, is effective against RSV, but ribavirin aerosol treatment is controversial as the drug is teratogenic and could be harmful to pregnant caregivers. Because RSV infection spreads readily from one child to the next, infants should be isolated for care. Nursing care should be organized so nurses do not care for infants infected with RSV and those who are not.

The disease peaks in severity between 48 to 72 hours. Recurrent apneic episodes are rare, so home monitoring for apneic episodes is usually not necessary. Two products are available for the prevention of RSV infection: Respiratory Syncytial Virus Immune Globulin Intravenous (RSV-IGIV), made from RSV antibody positive donor serum, and Palivizumab, a humanized monoclonal antibody produced by recombinant DNA technology. These may be given prophylactically to premature infants during the winter months (Zsolway, 2003).

Asthma

Asthma, an immediate hypersensitivity (type I) response (see Chapter 42), is the most common chronic illness in children, accounting for a large number of days of absenteeism from school and many hospital admissions each year. It tends to occur initially before 5 years of age, although in these early years it may be diagnosed as frequent occurrences of bronchiolitis rather than asthma (Table 40.6). The condition may be intermittent, with symptom-free periods, or chronic, with continuous symptoms. If a parent has asthma, the chance a child will also develop asthma is increased (Clayton, 2003).

Asthma tends to occur in children with atopy or those who tend to be hypersensitive to allergens. Mast cells release histamine and leukotrienes that result in diffuse obstructive and restrictive airway disease because of a triad of inflammation, bronchoconstriction, and increased mucus production. Most children with asthma can be shown to have sensitization to inhalant antigens such as pollens, molds, or house dust. Food also may be involved. Severe bronchoconstriction can occur because of exposure to cold air or irritating odors, such as turpentine or smog, as well as inhalation of a known allergen. Air pollutants such as cigarette smoke may lower the threshold for hypersensitivity reactions and worsen the condition. Although there may be a seasonal factor responsible for a particular child's symptoms, most children have multiple sensitivities and are affected all year long. Aspirin can be a trigger, so cau-

tion adolescents with asthma that if they begin to take aspirin as an adult, it may initiate an attack.

Mechanism of Disease

Asthma primarily affects the small airways and involves three separate processes: bronchospasm, inflammation of bronchial mucosa, and increased bronchial secretions (mucus). All three processes act to reduce the size of the airway lumen, leading to acute respiratory distress. Bronchial constriction occurs because of stimulation of the parasympathetic nervous system (cholinergic mediated system), which initiates smooth muscle constriction. Inflammation and mucus production occur because of mast cell activation to release leukotrienes, histamine, and prostaglandins. Once viewed as a long-term, poorly controlled disorder, newer therapy makes this a reversible or manageable disorder (Kallstrom, 2004).

Assessment

The word "asthma" is derived from the Greek word for panting, a description of the child's distress. Typically, after exposure to an allergen or trigger, an episode begins with a dry cough, often at night as bronchoconstriction begins. Because bronchioles are normally larger in lumen on inspiration than expiration even with bronchoconstriction, children may inhale normally or have little difficulty. They develop increasing difficulty exhaling, however, as it becomes more and more difficult to force air through the narrowed lumen of the inflamed bronchioles filled with mucus. This causes the typical dyspnea and wheezing (the sound caused by air being pushed forcibly through obstructed bronchioles) typically associated with this disorder. Remember that wheezing is heard primarily on expiration. However, when severe, wheezing may be heard

TABLE 40.6

Comparison of Bronchiolitis, Pneumonia, and Asthma

Assessment	Bronchiolitis	Pneumonia	Asthma
Cause	Usually respiratory syncytial virus	Possibly bacterial (pneumococcal, or *H. influenzae*), viral, or mycoplasmal; possibly secondary to aspiration	Hypersensitivity type I immune response
Age of child	Under 2 yr	All through childhood	Onset 1–5 yr
Onset pattern	Follows an upper respiratory infection	Follows an upper respiratory infection	Follows initiation by an allergen
Appearance	Fatigued, anxious, shallow respirations, increasing anteroposterior diameter of chest	Fatigued, anxious, shallow respirations	Wheezing, exhausted, frightened
Cough	Paroxysmal, dry	Productive, harsh cough	Paroxysmal, with thick mucus production
Fever	Low grade	Elevated	None
Auscultatory sounds	Barely audible breath sounds, crackles, expiratory wheezing	Decreased breath sounds, rales	Wheezing

on inspiration as well. Hearing it on inspiration means the child is having extreme breathing difficulty. If the child coughs up mucus, it is generally copious and may contain white casts bearing the shape of the bronchi from which it was dislodged.

History. Assessment should include a thorough history of the development of the child's symptoms—for example, what the child was doing at the time of the attack, and what actions were taken by the parents or child to decrease or arrest the symptoms. When an acute attack has passed, ask the parent or child to describe the home environment, including any pets, the child's bedroom, outdoor play space, classroom environment, and type of heating in the house, to see whether more environmental control could reduce future occurrences.

Physical Assessment. A physical assessment includes examining for the specific symptoms of asthma. In many children, the initial wheezing is so loud it can be heard without a stethoscope. In others, it is evident only by auscultation. Asthma affects all lobes of the lungs, so although the wheezing may be more prominent in one lobe than in another, it is generally audible in all lung fields. Audible wheezing in only one lobe suggests that only one bronchus is plugged, which suggests that a foreign body such as a peanut is more likely responsible than asthma. Cyanosis may be present. The eosinophil count is elevated.

Bronchospasm leads to CO_2 trapping and retention; therefore, arterial oxygen saturation monitored by a pulse oximeter will begin to decrease because of the child's inability to fully aerate the lungs. The child becomes frightened because of an acute feeling of suffocation. A peak flow meter shows decreased ability to exhale.

Air-filled lungs are hyperresonant to percussion (i.e., they make a louder, hollower noise on percussion than usual). In normal respiration, the inspiration phase of breathing is longer than the expiration phase. During an asthma attack, however, the child must work so hard to exhale that the expiration phase becomes longer than the inspiration phase. Time the two phases to demonstrate this. Also observe for retractions, because children use intercostal accessory muscles to achieve full breaths.

As constriction becomes acute, the sound of wheezing may decrease because so little air can leave the alveoli. Hypoxemia and possibly cyanosis will become severe. When blood gases show an increased Pco_2 level and the sound of wheezing suddenly stops, respiratory failure is imminent.

During attacks, children with asthma are generally more comfortable in a sitting or standing position rather than lying down. If seated in a chair, they lean forward and raise their shoulders to give themselves more breathing space. Do not urge children to "lie down and relax," as this can cause severe anxiety and increased difficulty in breathing. Children who do agree to lie down are either at the end of an attack and so beginning to feel less threatened by the dyspnea or are so exhausted by the paroxysms of coughing they no longer have the strength to sit upright.

Over time, as a child has many bouts of asthma, he or she develops a shield-like or barrel-shaped chest from constant overinflation of air in alveoli. Clubbing of the fingers (from the growth of excess capillaries initiated when

oxygen deprivation is sensed in distal parts) may be noticeable. If a child has been treated for a long period with steroids, he or she may develop growth restriction.

Pulmonary Function Studies

Good pulmonary function depends on good ventilation (both drawing adequate air into the lungs and expelling it again), adequate transfer of gases across the alveolar capillary membranes, and adequate volume and distribution of pulmonary capillary blood flow to transport oxygen to body cells. In children with asthma, the vital capacity (air that they are able to exhale) may be low or the capacity may be normal, but, because of narrowed bronchioles as a result of bronchospasm, the expiratory rate will be abnormally long (more than 10 seconds, rather than the normal 2 or 3 seconds). If a child has bronchial plugging, the vital capacity will be low because of air absorption behind blocked bronchi. A gross measure of vital capacity is to ask a child to blow out a match. A child with an average vital capacity should be able to do this when the match is held at 6 inches. When a vital capacity test is abnormal, it may be repeated after an inhalation treatment to show the effect of the treatment.

Peak Expiratory Flow Rate Monitoring. Children with asthma often use a home peak flow meter daily to measure gross changes in peak expiratory flow over time and help in planning an appropriate therapeutic regimen (Fig. 40.20). Children with asthma should be able to tell you their usual reading and personal best score.

To use a peak flow meter, a child places the indicator on the apparatus at the bottom of the numbered scale, and takes a deep breath. He or she places the meter in the mouth and blows out as hard and fast as possible. He or she then repeats this two more times and records the highest number achieved as the peak flow meter result. During a 2-week period when the child feels well, this should be done daily. The highest number achieved during this time is recorded as the child's personal best.

Children are assigned "zones" to rate their expiratory compliance:

- Green zone (80% to 100% of their personal best) means no asthma symptoms are present, and they should take their routine medications.
- Yellow zone (50% to 80% of personal best) signals caution. An episode of asthma may be beginning.
- Red zone (below 50% of personal best) indicates an asthma episode is beginning. A child should immediately take his or her prescribed medication such as an inhaled beta-2-agonist, then repeat the peak flow assessment. If the second reading is not in the green zone, the parent should alert the primary care provider of the impending asthma attack.

Therapeutic Management

Therapy for children with asthma involves planning for the three goals of all allergic disorders: avoidance of the allergen by environmental control; skin testing and hyposensitization to identified allergens; and relief of symptoms by pharmacologic agents.

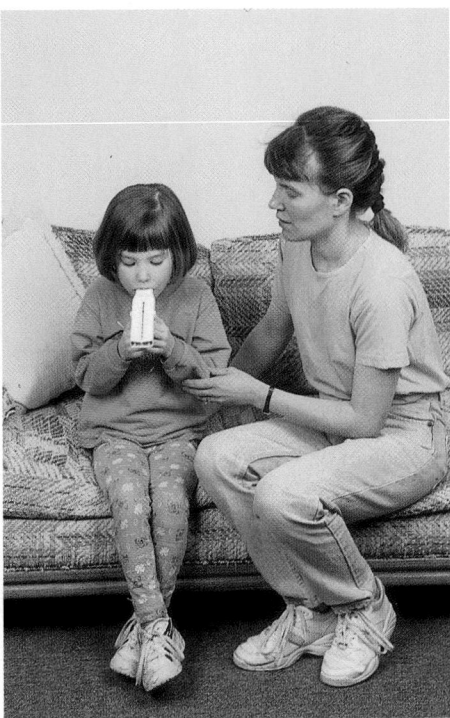

FIGURE 40.20 Children with any chronic illness require periodic evaluation and sometimes home monitoring. Here a child with asthma practices using a home peak flow meter to track her peak expiratory flow readings on a daily basis.

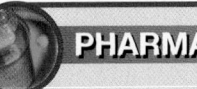

BOX 40.11 FOCUS ON . . .

PHARMACOLOGY

Albuterol Sulfate (Proventil, Ventolin)

Classification: Albuterol is a beta-2-adrenergic agonist.

Action: Acts selectively to cause bronchodilation and vasodilation for relief of bronchospasm (Karch, 2004).

Pregnancy risk category: C

Oral Dosage:
- Children older than 14 years—2 or 4 mg, 3 or 4 times daily; not to exceed 32 mg/day
- Children ages 6 to 14 years—2 mg, 3 or 4 times daily, not to exceed 24 mg/day
- Children ages 2 to 6 years—0.1 mg/kg, 3 times daily, not to exceed 2 mg/day; gradually increasing to 0.2 mg/kg, 3 times daily, not to exceed 4 mg/day

Inhaled Dosage: Children 12 years of age and older— 2 puffs every 4 to 6 hours: 2.5 mg (0.5 mL of 0.5% solution diluted with 2.5 mL of 0.9% sodium chloride) OR 3 mL of 0.083% solution, 3 or 4 times daily

Possible adverse effects: Restlessness, apprehension, anxiety, fear, nausea, cardiac arrhythmias, paradoxical airway resistance with repeated, excessive use of inhalation preparations, sweating, pallor, and flushing

Nursing Implications
- Instruct parents and child in method to administer drug. Teach child and parents about use and care of nebulized solution or metered-dose inhaler and spacer devices, if ordered.
- Caution child and parents not to exceed the number of ordered puffs, to prevent possible tolerance to drug.
- If more than one inhalation is ordered, advise child to wait 1 to 2 minutes before taking the second puff.
- If the child is also receiving an inhaled corticosteroid, advise the child and parents to have the child use the albuterol first to open the airways and then wait approximately 5 minutes before using the corticosteroid, to maximize its effectiveness.

Cough suppressants are contraindicated with asthma because, as a rule, as long as children can continue to cough up mucus, they are not in serious danger. When they stop coughing up mucus, thick plugs form that then may lead to pneumonia, atelectasis, and further acidosis.

A child with mild but persistent asthma usually is prescribed an inhaled anti-inflammatory corticosteroid such as fluticasone (Flovent) daily. Children who have moderate persistent symptoms usually are prescribed a long-acting bronchodilator at bedtime in addition to the inhaled anti-inflammatory daily corticosteroid. Children who have severe persistent asthma symptoms take a high dose of both an oral corticosteroid and an inhaled corticosteroid daily as well as a long-acting bronchodilator at bedtime. In addition, children may be prescribed a short-acting beta-2-agonist bronchodilator, such as albuterol or terbutaline, to use if an attack should begin (Box 40.11). Cromolyn sodium is a mast cell stabilizer given by a nebulizer or metered-dose inhaler that can prevent bronchoconstriction and thereby prevent the symptoms of asthma (Box 40.12). Cromolyn sodium is not effective once symptoms have begun.

Another group of drugs used in the treatment of asthma are leukotriene receptor antagonists such as montelukast (Singulair). This drug is also used for prophylaxis and chronic treatment of asthma in children over 6 years of age. It is not effective in an acute attack.

Metered-dose inhalers require that the child trigger the inhaler at the same time he or she breathes in (Fig. 40.21A).

Because it is difficult for children younger than approximately 12 years to do this, placing a spacer tube between the inhaler and the mouthpiece better coordinates inhaling and trigger release (see Fig. 40.21B). If children are to receive medication by nebulizer or inhaler, be certain they know how to use these properly. It is easy for children to take this type of medication lightly (the belief it is "not really medicine" because it is not swallowed). As a result, overdose from constant use of nebulizers or metered-dose inhalers can occur.

Dehydration occurs rapidly in children during an asthma attack because they have decreased oral intake (children stop drinking because they are coughing, or coughing makes them vomit and parents stop offering fluid) as well as increased insensible loss that occurs from tachypnea. Dehydration may contribute to increased mucus plugging

BOX 40.12 FOCUS ON . . .

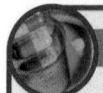

PHARMACOLOGY

Cromolyn Sodium (Intal)

Classification: Cromolyn sodium is a mast cell inhibitor.

Action: Inhibits the release of histamine, slow-releasing substance of anaphylaxis, and leukotriene, thereby decreasing the overall allergic response. In asthma, it is used prophylactically to prevent severe bronchospasms (Karch, 2004).

Pregnancy risk category: B

Dosage: Initially, 20 mg inhaled (via spinhaler inhalant or as nebulized solution) 4 times daily at regular intervals; one ampule orally 4 times daily one-half hour before meals and at bedtime (ampule is not recommended for use in children under the age of 5 years)

Possible adverse effects: Dizziness, headache, nausea, dry and irritated throat, cough, nasal congestion, epistaxis, sneezing

Nursing Implications
- Instruct parents and child that this drug is not effective in an acute attack.
- Caution child and parents to take the drug exactly as prescribed and to continue other agents, such as bronchodilators.
- Instruct child and parents in the use of metered-dose inhaler or nebulizer for administration of cromolyn sodium.
- If the oral form is prescribed, instruct parents to open the ampule and pour the contents into a glass of water and to wait for the medication to dissolve. Caution parents not to substitute the oral form for the inhalant form and vice versa.
- Instruct parents and child to watch for a possible recurrence of asthma symptoms if dosage is decreased.
- Know that this drug is only given once the acute episode is over and the child's airway is clear, to prevent a further episode.
- Caution child and parents not to exceed the number of ordered puffs via inhaler, to prevent possible tolerance to drug.
- If more than one inhalation is ordered, advise child to wait 1 to 2 minutes before taking the second puff.
- If the child is also receiving an inhaled bronchodilator, advise the child and parents to have the child use the bronchodilator first to open the airways and then wait approximately 5 minutes before using the cromolyn sodium, to maximize its effectiveness.

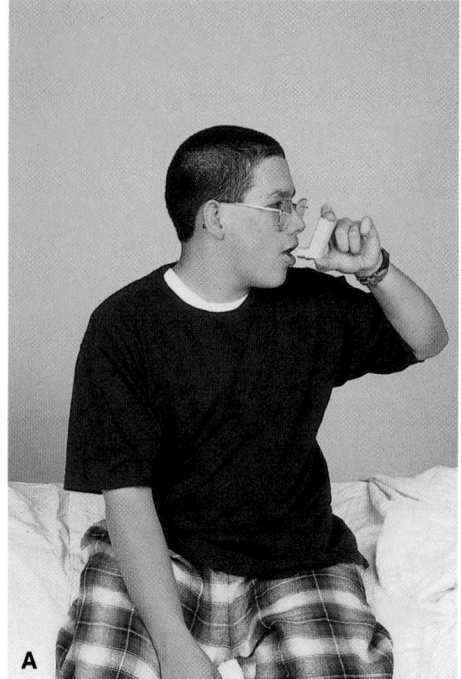

A

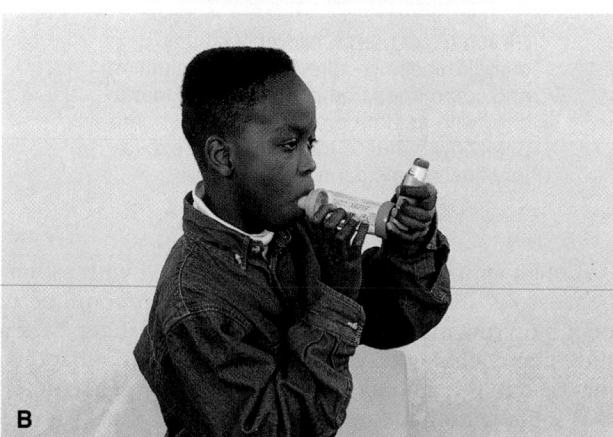

B

FIGURE 40.21 (**A**) Many children with asthma use a metered dose inhaler to administer a bronchodilator to themselves. Be certain children respect such medicine as medicine so they use sensible precautions. (**B**) Younger children need a "spacer" with inhalers so they do not need to correlate administration with inhalation.

NURSING DIAGNOSES AND RELATED INTERVENTIONS

Nursing Diagnosis: Fear related to sudden onset of asthma attack

Outcome Evaluation: Parents and child express confidence in their ability to prevent attacks and effectively manage any that occur.

and further airway obstruction. Encourage children to continue to drink fluids (ask about favorite beverages and offer small sips of them). Avoid milk or milk products because they cause thick mucus and difficulty swallowing. In an emergency setting, an intravenous line is established to supply continuous fluid therapy and also provide a route for emergency drug administration.

Asthma is a frightening disease. At the time it is diagnosed, parents may have already gone through a long period of wondering what was wrong with their child. After diagnosis, parents may be afraid to allow the child to sleep overnight away from them or leave him or her alone with a baby-sitter. Help parents find a middle ground: to allow a child enough freedom for growth and development while still being certain he or she is safe. Taking steps to slow breathing, better emptying alveoli through pursed-lip breathing, and administering medications to prevent symptoms are key measures for children to learn. Many children have long periods without attacks. When a new one occurs after a long absence, it is almost as frightening as the original attack because everything seems so new again.

Nursing Diagnosis: Health-seeking behaviors related to prevention of and treatment for asthma attacks

Outcome Evaluation: Parents and child accurately state triggers that cause an attack; child correctly demonstrates breathing exercises, use of inhaler, and peak expiratory flow meter.

Children need to learn how to avoid possible triggers through environmental control. (For more information about controlling triggers in the home, see Chapter 42.) If foods are a trigger, children need to learn to be responsible for their own diets so they can avoid these foods. Children as young as 6 years can learn what foods they cannot eat and can take responsibility for telling a friend's parent or a schoolteacher that they must not eat certain foods. They must learn to use a metered-dose inhaler or nebulizer if prescribed. At the same time, they must not become inhaler-dependent or carry the inhaler with them constantly, afraid to go anywhere without it. This will invariably result in their using the inhaler much more often than is necessary.

To prevent children with asthma from losing chest mobility and to decrease their tendency to develop a barrel chest, they may be taught a number of breathing or mobility exercises to do daily at home. Such exercises are aimed at increasing expiratory function (diaphragmatic or side expansion breathing). Recommended activities include bending side to side, bending forward and touching the left foot with the right hand, and swinging the arms rhythmically in front of the body like a windmill (jumping jacks). These exercises can be incorporated into a bedtime or after-school routine (Box 40.13). (Parents [and nurses] who do mobility exercises with children find the exercises are helpful to them as well, as they help tighten the abdominal muscles.) Using an incentive spirometer daily is another method for children to use to exercise the lungs and keep chest muscles supple.

The prognosis in children who develop asthma is good if they adhere to their treatment regimen. Children do not outgrow asthma, although most of them may become symptom-free as adults, probably be-

BOX 40.13 FOCUS ON . . .

EVIDENCE-BASED PRACTICE

Can School Nurses Have an Impact on Children's Asthma Management?

To answer this question, nurse researchers determined the asthma prevalence and absentee rates caused by asthma in a large school district over 3 years. Approximately 5% of children in this school system were diagnosed as having asthma. Students with asthma were absent between 0.5 to 1.25 days more than children without asthma. Following interventions by school nurses, such as asthma education or a home visit, students were more likely the next year to bring their asthma medication to school, to use a peak flow meter at school, and to have reduced asthma severity.

This is an interesting study for nurses because it directly demonstrates the impact nurses can have on management of a chronic childhood disease such as asthma. It also documents the common prevalence of asthma and its effect on children's education.

Source: Taras, H., et al. (2004). Impact of school nurse case management on students with asthma. *Journal of School Health, 74*(6), 213–219.

cause the lumens of major airways enlarge with adulthood.

Do not convey to parents the impression that asthma is a disease that will be simply outgrown. Although asthma may not always last into adulthood, parents need to maintain careful environmental control, conscientious administration of medication, and hyposensitization, if indicated, to keep the child free of symptoms during childhood.

Status Asthmaticus

Under ordinary circumstances, an asthma attack responds readily to the aerosol administration of a bronchodilator such as albuterol, terbutaline, or levalbuterol (Xopenex). When children fail to respond and an attack continues, they are in status asthmaticus. This is an extreme emergency because if the attack cannot be relieved, the child may die of heart failure caused by the combination of exhaustion, atelectasis, and respiratory acidosis from bronchial plugging.

Assessment

A child with status asthmaticus is in acute respiratory distress. Both heart rate and respiratory rate are elevated. Sao_2 and Po_2 are low; Pco_2 is elevated because the bronchi are so constricted the child cannot exhale, resulting in CO_2 accumulation. The rising Pco_2 rapidly leads to acidosis. In contrast to the loud wheezing initially heard in an asthma attack, children with status asthmaticus may have so little air able to pass in or out of their lungs that breath sounds are limited. Pulse oximetry will reveal the poor oxygenation.

Status asthmaticus is often initiated by pulmonary infection, which acts as the triggering mechanism for the prolonged attack. If this occurs, obtain cultures from coughed sputum, and be prepared to administer a broad-spectrum antibiotic until the culture results are available. Be certain the sputum obtained for culture was coughed from deep in the respiratory tract and not just from the back of the child's throat.

Therapeutic Management

By definition, a child in status asthmaticus has failed to respond to first-line therapy. Continuous nebulization with an inhaled beta-2-agonist and intravenous corticosteroids may be necessary to reduce symptoms. The Po_2 usually is maintained at more than 90 mm Hg with oxygen administration. This is best given by face mask or nasal prongs. These methods supply good oxygen concentrations and yet leave the child's face unobscured for easy observation. To prevent drying of pulmonary secretions, always give oxygen with humidification. Oxygen is best administered at a concentration of 30% to 40%, not 100%. If concentrations greater than 40% are needed, a Venturi mask that allows for rebreathing may be used. Some children in severe status asthmaticus have such a carbon dioxide buildup (because they cannot exhale properly) that they develop carbon dioxide narcosis with no stimulation for inhalation. The child's respiratory stimulus, therefore, is hypoxia, or lack of oxygen. If 100% oxygen were administered, the oxygen lack would disappear, and respirations would cease. The idea "if a little is good, a lot is better" does not apply here. After it has been ascertained that the child is not in acidosis (from blood gas and pH studies), oxygen levels may be increased, but for initial therapy, unless prescribed otherwise, keep the level at 40%.

During the acute stage of status asthmaticus, children need increased fluid to combat dehydration and keep airway secretions moist. Drinking tends to aggravate coughing, so an intravenous infusion such as 5% glucose in 0.45 saline is usually prescribed to supply fluid. If a child can drink, do not offer cold fluids because these tend to aggravate bronchospasm.

Monitor intake and output; measure the specific gravity of urine. Under stress, antidiuretic hormone is released, so fluid retention and overhydration may occur.

An increasing Pco_2 is a danger sign because it indicates the degree of hypoventilation. In severe attacks, endotracheal intubation and mechanical ventilation may be necessary to maintain effective respirations (Clayton, 2003).

Bronchiectasis

Bronchiectasis is chronic dilatation and plugging of the bronchi. It may follow pneumonia, aspiration of a foreign body, pertussis, or asthma. It is often associated with cystic fibrosis (Wagener & Headley, 2003).

Children develop a chronic cough with mucopurulent sputum. Young infants may have accompanying wheezing or stridor. If a large area of lung is involved, children may have cyanosis. As the disease becomes chronic, children develop symptoms of chronic lung disease, such as clubbing of the fingers and easy fatigability. Their physi-

cal growth may become restricted. Their chest may become enlarged from overinflation of alveoli caused by the air trapped behind inflamed bronchi.

Chest physiotherapy may be necessary to raise the tenacious sputum. An antibiotic will be necessary if infection is present. The cause of the bronchiectasis must be identified and relieved before the chronic process can be relieved. Surgery to remove the affected lung portion may be necessary.

Pneumonia

Pneumonia (infection and inflammation of alveoli) occurs at a rate of 2 to 4 children in 100. It may be of bacterial origin (pneumococcal, streptococcal, staphylococcal, or chlamydial) or viral in origin, such as respiratory syncytial virus (RSV). Aspiration of lipid or hydrocarbon substances also causes pneumonia. Pneumonia is commonly divided into two types: hospital acquired (pneumococcal or streptococcal pneumonia) and community acquired (chlamydia, viral pneumonias) (Thibodeau & Viera, 2004). It is the most common pulmonary cause of death in infants younger than 48 hours of age. It occurs most often in late winter and early spring. Newborns who are born more than 24 hours after rupture of the amniotic membranes and those who aspirated amniotic fluid or meconium during birth are particularly prone to developing pneumonia in their first few days of life (Greenberg, 2004). When it is known that the fetal membranes have been ruptured for more than 24 hours before birth, prophylactic broad-spectrum antibiotics may be given to prevent pneumonia. The differences between bronchiolitis, pneumonia, and asthma are summarized in Table 40.6. *Pneumocystis carinii* pneumonia, the type seen almost exclusively with HIV/AIDS infection, is discussed in Chapter 42.

Pneumococcal Pneumonia

The onset of pneumococcal pneumonia is generally abrupt and follows an upper respiratory tract infection. In infants, pneumonia tends to remain bronchopneumonia with poor consolidation (infiltration of exudate into the alveoli). In older children, pneumonia may localize in a single lobe, and consolidation may occur. With this, children may have blood-tinged sputum as exudative serum and red blood cells invade the alveoli. After 24 to 48 hours, the alveoli are no longer filled with red blood cells and serum but fibrin, leukocytes, and pneumococci. At this point, the child's cough no longer raises blood-tinged sputum but thick purulent material.

Assessment. Children develop a high fever, nasal flaring, retractions, chest pain, chills, and dyspnea. Some children report the pain as being abdominal. The fever with pneumococcal pneumonia may rise so high and fast a child has a febrile seizure (see Chapter 49).

Children with pneumococcal pneumonia appear acutely ill. Tachypnea and tachycardia develop. Because the lung space is filled with exudate, respiratory function will be diminished. Breath sounds become bronchial (sound transmitted from the trachea) because air no longer or only poorly enters fluid-filled alveoli. Crackles (rales) may be present as a result of the fluid. Dullness on percussion over a lobe indicates that total consolidation has occurred. Chest x-rays will usually show this type of lung consolidation in older children but only patchy diffusion in young children. Laboratory studies will indicate leukocytosis.

Therapeutic Management. Before antibiotic therapy was available for pneumonia, it was almost always a fatal disease, especially in infants, so parents may be more worried about a child's condition than is warranted (Box 40.14).

Therapy for pneumococcal pneumonia is antibiotics. Either ampicillin or a third-generation cephalosporin is effective against pneumococci. Amoxicillin-clavulanate (Augmentin) also may be prescribed for penicillin-resistant organisms. Children need rest to prevent exhaustion. Plan nursing care carefully to conserve the child's strength. At the same time, turn and reposition a child frequently to avoid pooling of secretions. Intravenous therapy may be necessary to supply fluid, especially in infants, because infants tire so readily with sucking they may not be able to achieve a good oral intake. They may need an antipyretic such as acetaminophen to reduce fever.

Humidified oxygen may be necessary to alleviate labored breathing and prevent hypoxemia. Assess oxygen saturation levels frequently via pulse oximetry. Chest physiotherapy encourages the movement of mucus and prevents obstruction. Older children may need to be encouraged to cough so that secretions do not pool and become further infected.

Following pneumonia, children usually have a period of at least a week when they tire easily and need frequent, small feedings. Parents need to be cautioned that this degree of fatigue is an expected outcome and not a complication in itself. Children with chronic illness, those who have had a splenectomy, or those who are immunocompromised should receive a pneumococcal vaccine to prevent pneumococcal pneumonia.

Chlamydial Pneumonia

Chlamydia trachomatis pneumonia is most often seen in newborns up to 12 weeks of age because the chlamydial organism is contracted from the mother's vagina during birth. Symptoms usually begin gradually with nasal congestion and a sharp cough; infants fail to gain back their birthweight. Symptoms progress to tachypnea, with wheezing and rales audible on auscultation. Laboratory assessment will show an elevated level of immunoglobulin IgG and IgM antibodies, peripheral eosinophilia, and a specific antibody to *C. trachomatis*. Such an infection is treated with a macrolide antibiotic such as erythromycin with good results (Bhargava, 2003).

Viral Pneumonia

Viral pneumonia is generally caused by the viruses of upper respiratory tract infection: the RSVs, myxoviruses, or adenoviruses. Symptoms begin as an upper respiratory tract infection. After a day or two, additional symptoms such as a low-grade fever, nonproductive cough, and tachypnea begin. There may be diminished breath sounds and fine rales on chest auscultation. RSV may cause apnea. Chest x-rays will show diffuse infiltrated areas.

Because this is a viral infection, antibiotic therapy usually is not effective. The child needs rest and, possibly, an antipyretic for the fever; intravenous fluid may be necessary if a child becomes exhausted or is dehydrated and refusing fluids. After recovery from the acute phase of illness, a child will have a week or two of lethargy or lack of energy, the same as occurs with bacterial pneumonia. Parents may be confused because their child is not receiving an antibiotic, despite the diagnosis of pneumonia. Explain the difference between viral and bacterial infections so they can better understand their child's therapy and plan of care.

BOX 40.14 FOCUS ON . . .

COMMUNICATION

B. J. Silver is a 2-year-old who has been admitted to your hospital unit with pneumonia. His mother called home to tell the grandmother about the diagnosis. Since she returned from the telephone, Mrs. Silver seems tearful and visibly upset.

Less Effective Communication

Nurse: Is something wrong, Mrs. Silver? You seem upset.

Mrs. Silver I am. I didn't realize pneumonia was so serious until I talked to my mother.

Nurse Because it's serious is the reason that B.J.'s been admitted to the hospital.

Mrs. Silver She told me my brother had pneumonia when he was a baby. Is this oxygen? My mother said to check B.J.'s getting oxygen.

Nurse It sure is. He's also going to get an antibiotic. Why don't you stay with him while I get the equipment for that?

More Effective Communication

Nurse Is something wrong, Mrs. Silver? You seem upset.

Mrs. Silver I am. I didn't realize pneumonia was so serious until I talked to my mother.

Nurse Because it's serious is the reason that B.J.'s been admitted to the hospital.

Mrs. Silver She told me my brother had pneumonia when he was a baby. Is this oxygen? My mother said to check B.J.'s getting oxygen.

Nurse Let's talk about everything your mother told you about pneumonia. Because the treatment has changed so much, what happened years ago isn't the same as what happens now.

Before the advent of antibiotics, a diagnosis of pneumonia in a young child was almost automatically a fatal diagnosis. Ask enough questions to be certain parents understand that pneumonia, although serious, is not the fatal diagnosis of years ago.

Mycoplasmal Pneumonia

The mycoplasma organisms are similar to yet larger than viruses. Mycoplasmal pneumonia occurs more frequently in older children (over 5 years) and more often during the winter.

The symptoms of mycoplasmal pneumonia make it difficult to differentiate from other pneumonias. The child has a fever and a cough and feels ill. Cervical lymph nodes are enlarged. The child may have a persistent rhinitis.

Mycoplasmal organisms generally are sensitive to erythromycin or tetracycline. Erythromycin is the preferred drug for children younger than 8 years of age, because tetracycline tends to stain teeth brown and possibly stunt long bone growth (Karch, 2004).

Lipid Pneumonia

Lipid pneumonia is caused by the aspiration of an oily or lipid substance. It is much less common than it once was because children are not given oil-based tonics, such as castor oil or cod liver oil anymore, as they were in the past. Today it is most often caused by aspirated oily foreign bodies such as peanuts or popcorn. A proliferative inflammatory response occurs when lung lipases act on the aspirated oil. This is then followed by diffuse fibrosis of the bronchi or alveoli. The area then becomes secondarily infected.

A child may have an initial coughing spell at the time of aspiration. A period follows during which the child is symptomless; then a chronic cough, dyspnea, and general respiratory distress occur. A chest x-ray shows densities at the affected site.

Antibiotic therapy is ineffective unless a secondary bacterial infection has occurred. Surgical resection of a lung portion may be necessary to remove a lung segment if the pneumonitis does not heal by itself.

Hydrocarbon Pneumonia

A number of common household products such as furniture polish, cleaning fluids, turpentine, kerosene, gasoline, lighter fluid, and insect sprays have hydrocarbon bases. These products are a common cause of childhood poisonings and result in hydrocarbon pneumonia.

Assessment. Children who swallow a hydrocarbon-based product usually exhibit gastrointestinal symptoms such as nausea and vomiting. Next, they become drowsy and develop a cough from inhalation as vapors from the stomach rise and are inhaled. As bronchial edema occurs from irritation and inflammation, respirations become increased and dyspneic.

Physical assessment shows an increased percussion sound caused by the presence of air trapped in the alveoli beyond the point of inflammation. Rales may be heard as air passes through collecting mucus. Because air cannot reach and inflate the alveoli fully, breath sounds may be diminished.

Therapeutic Management. Irritation from fumes of hydrocarbon ingestion may occur when children initially swallow the fluid. If they are given an emetic to induce vomiting, it can cause them to aspirate vomitus or cause additional irritation. Parents should telephone a poison control center to ask for advice if their child has swallowed any poison, rather than inducing vomiting. In the emergency room, gastric lavage may be done by health care personnel with great care to remove the substance from the stomach and help prevent inhalation.

The child is usually admitted to a hospital observation unit for a short time. Obtain vital signs and observe the child's general appearance carefully for evidence of increased respiratory tract obstruction or increasing drowsiness or other symptoms of CNS involvement from CNS intoxication. Cool, moist air administered by a nebulizer with supplemental oxygen may be prescribed to decrease lung inflammation. If febrile, a child needs an antipyretic. Frequent changes of position will prevent pooling of secretions, which could lead to a secondary infection. Chest physiotherapy will help to move secretions and reduce areas of stasis.

The initial inflammation reaction from hydrocarbon aspiration may lead to such occlusion that emphysema (pocketing of air in alveoli) occurs, causing rupture of the alveoli into the pleural space, with consequent pneumothorax and atelectasis.

Often, children who swallow a household cleaner or other substance are aware they should not have been handling substances kept under the sink. As a result, they cannot help but interpret the hospitalization, blood drawing, and other uncomfortable procedures as punishments for their action. They may benefit from therapeutic play with puppets or dolls that will help alleviate their guilt and anger at being "punished" so severely.

Hydrocarbon pneumonia is slow to resolve, so the child will be ill for some time. After the illness, reinforce with parents the need to keep poisons in a safe place. Offer a listening ear so they can explain they were unaware of the extreme danger of these everyday household products.

Atelectasis

Atelectasis is the collapse of lung alveoli. It may occur in children as a primary or secondary condition.

Primary Atelectasis

Primary atelectasis occurs in newborns who do not breathe with enough respiratory strength at birth to inflate lung tissue or whose alveoli are so immature or so lacking in surfactant that they cannot expand. This is seen most commonly in immature infants or in infants with CNS damage. It may occur if infants have mucus or meconium plugs in the trachea.

When atelectasis occurs, the newborn's respirations become irregular, with nasal flaring and apnea. After a few minutes, a respiratory grunt and cyanosis may occur. The sound of a respiratory grunt is caused by the newborn's glottis closing on expiration. At first, this is a helpful action because it increases pressure in the respiratory tract, keeps alveoli from collapsing, and allows for better alveoli exchange surfaces. This action is also tiring, however, and as the infant tires, hypoxemia will increase, and the infant will become hypotonic and flaccid. The Apgar score will invariably be low.

As infants cry or are administered oxygen, more alveoli become aerated and cyanosis may decrease. The cause of the atelectasis must be established so that therapy directed to the specific cause can be initiated.

Secondary Atelectasis

Secondary atelectasis occurs in children when they have a respiratory tract obstruction that prevents air from entering a portion of the alveoli. As the residual air in the alveoli is absorbed, the alveoli collapse. The causes of obstruction in children include mucus plugs that may occur with chronic respiratory disease or aspiration of foreign objects. In some children, atelectasis occurs because of pressure on lung tissue from outside forces, such as compression from a diaphragmatic hernia, scoliosis, or enlarged thoracic lymph nodes (Fig. 40.22).

The signs of secondary atelectasis depend on the degree of collapse. Asymmetry of the chest may be noticed. Breath sounds on the affected side are decreased. If the process is extensive, tachypnea and cyanosis will be present. A chest x-ray will show the collapsed alveoli (a "whiteout").

Children with atelectasis are prone to secondary infection because mucus, which provides a good medium for bacteria, becomes stagnant without air exchange.

Therapeutic Management

Atelectasis caused by inspiration of a foreign object will not be relieved until the object is removed by bronchoscopy. Atelectasis caused by a mucus plug will resolve when the plug resolves or is moved or expectorated. Children may need assisted ventilation to maintain adequate respiratory function until this time.

Make certain the chest of a child with atelectasis is kept free from pressure so that lung expansion is as full as possible (to allow as much breathing space as possible). If restraints are being used to keep an infant positioned, make certain that body restraints are not crossing the chest area and interfering with chest expansion. Check clothing to be certain it is loose and nonbinding. Make certain the child's arms are not positioned across the chest, where their weight could interfere with deep inspiration.

A semi-Fowler's position generally allows for the best lung expansion because it lowers abdominal contents and increases chest space. Increase the humidity of the child's environment to prevent further bronchial plugging; suction and chest physiotherapy may be necessary to keep the respiratory tract clear and free of mucus. Observe closely for increased respirations or cyanosis, as these indicate failing oxygenation. Atelectasis is a serious disorder that must be considered as a possibility in all children with respiratory distress.

Pneumothorax

Pneumothorax is the presence of atmospheric air in the pleural space; its presence causes the alveoli to collapse (Fig. 40.23). Pneumothorax in children usually occurs when air seeps from ruptured alveoli and collects in the pleural cavity. It also can occur when external puncture wounds allow air to enter the chest (Kravitz, 2003).

Pneumothorax occurs in approximately 1% of newborns, probably due to rupture of the alveoli from the extreme intrathoracic pressure needed to initiate a first inspiration. The infant develops tachypnea, grunting respirations, flaring of the nares, and cyanosis. Auscultation reveals absent or decreased breath sounds on the affected side. Percussion may not be revealing, despite the hollow air space; as so much air is present, this may be hyperresonant. A more revealing sign may be the shift of the apical pulse (mediastinal shift) away from the site of the pneumothorax and the resulting atelectasis. A chest film will show the darkened area of the air-filled pleural space.

The child needs oxygen therapy to relieve respiratory distress. A thoracotomy catheter or needle may be placed in the pleural space and atmospheric air aspirated or low-pressure suction with water-seal drainage applied to remove accumulated air. In most children with pneumothorax, symptoms are relieved within 24 hours after suction is begun. The use of water-seal drainage with children is discussed in Chapter 41.

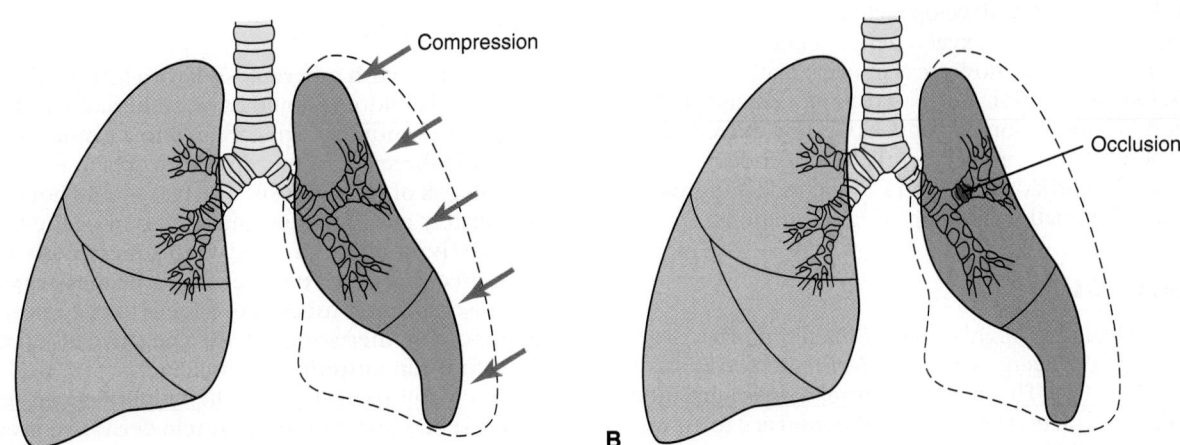

FIGURE 40.22 (A) Atelectasis caused by compression of lung tissue. **(B)** Atelectasis caused by obstruction.

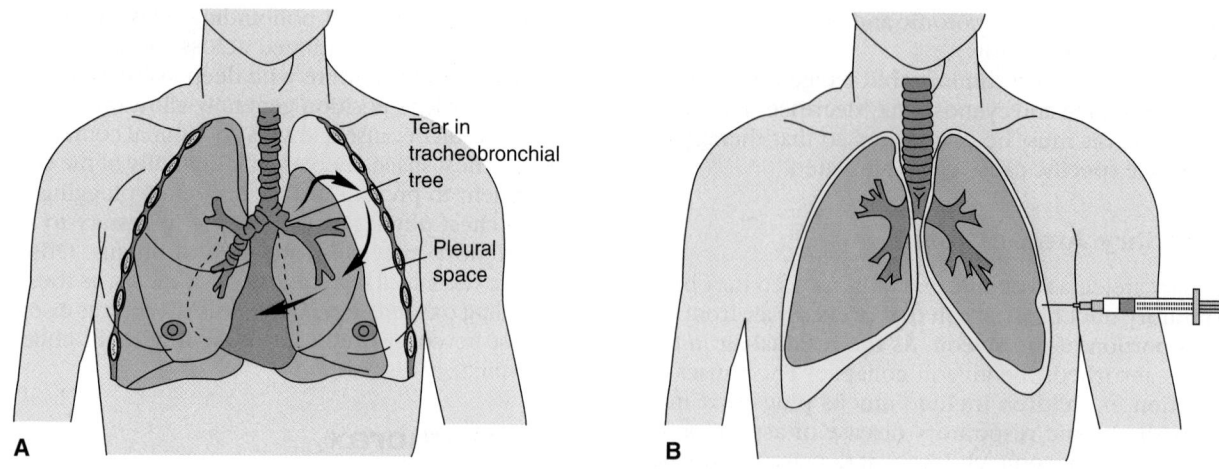

FIGURE 40.23 (**A**) Pneumothorax. A tear in the tracheobronchial tree has caused air to move into the pleural space; the lung collapses and the mediastinum shifts to the unaffected side. (**B**) Aspiration of air from the pleural space allows lung to reexpand after a pneumothorax.

If the air in the pleural space is from a puncture wound such as a stab wound, cover the chest wound immediately with an impervious material, such as petrolatum gauze, to prevent further air from entering. In an emergency, an impervious object can be your gloved hand.

Pneumothorax is always a potentially serious respiratory problem. The extent of the symptoms and the outcome will depend on the cause of entry of air into the pleural space and whether it can be removed.

Bronchopulmonary Dysplasia

Bronchopulmonary dysplasia (BPD) is chronic pulmonary involvement that occurs in 10% to 40% of infants who are treated for acute respiratory distress in the first days of life. The condition is thought to occur from a combination of surfactant deficiency (decreased from lung trauma), barotrauma (lung damage from ventilator pressure), oxygen toxicity (from high levels needed to counteract the original respiratory distress), and continuing inflammation. The condition most often occurs in infants who received mechanical ventilation for respiratory distress syndrome at birth (Good, 2003).

Infants with BPD develop tachypnea, retractions, nasal flaring, tachycardia, oxygen dependence, and abnormal x-ray findings that show areas of overinflation and atelectasis. On auscultation, decreased air movement can be detected. Although some infants have such decreased lung function that they are left ventilator-dependent, administration of a corticosteroid and a bronchodilator greatly reduces inflammation and improves respirations.

Tuberculosis

Tuberculosis is a highly contagious pulmonary disease. The causative agent is *Mycobacterium tuberculosis* (tubercle bacillus). The mode of transmission is inhalation of infected droplets. The incubation period is 2 to 10 weeks (Watson, 2003).

Children generally contract this disease from someone in the immediate family. When any member of a family contracts tuberculosis, all family members must be tested (a Mantoux skin test) to screen for the disease. In some children, the contact is not known, and the disease is first detected when symptoms appear. Children who are homeless or severely impoverished or who have chronic illness or malnutrition tend to be more susceptible than other children because of their overall susceptibility to infection.

When *M. tuberculosis* invades a child's lung, there is primary inflammation. The child develops a slight cough. As the disease progresses, anorexia, weight loss, night sweats, and a low-grade fever occur.

Leukocytes and lymphocytes invade the lung area, effectively walling off the primary infection. The wall surrounding the bacteria then calcifies and confines the organism permanently. This development of a primary focus is the most usual form of tuberculosis in children. If a child is in poor health or does not have adequate calcium intake for the body to confine the infection, tuberculosis may spread to other lung areas or to other parts of the body (miliary tuberculosis). Other body sites that may be affected are bones and joints, lymph nodes, kidneys, and the subarachnoid space (tuberculous meningitis).

Assessment

Most children with tuberculosis have a history of a recent contact. All children should have a tuberculin test as part of basic preventive health care at 9 to 12 months of age, and yearly thereafter if they live in an area in which there is a high risk of tuberculosis. The test should not be done immediately after measles immunization or the test will read falsely negative (a child with tuberculosis will be considered free of the disease). Also, the measles vaccine can cause a primary tuberculosis focus to become miliary; it is important, therefore, to have a negative tuberculin result before administering this vaccine.

For a Mantoux test, also called a purified protein derivative (PPD) test, 5 units of protein derivative vaccine is injected intradermally, usually on the left lower arm. A health care professional inspects the area in 72 hours and notes the reaction. A positive reaction (the formation of

5 to 15 mm of reddened induration) indicates the child has been exposed to tuberculosis or has developed antibodies to the foreign products of the tuberculosis organism (Fischbach, 2005). Children with positive reactions need follow-up with a chest x-ray to ascertain the importance of the reaction; that is, whether a current infection exists. Skin testing should not be done on children who are known to have had tuberculosis. Such a child will have such an intense reaction that the skin at the site of the test may slough and necrose.

To confirm a diagnosis of active disease, sputum may be analyzed. Make certain the child understands that you want him or her to expectorate mucus raised from the lungs, not just from the back of the throat. Have the child demonstrate a deep cough to you so you can be sure you are both talking about the same thing. Infants and children younger than 5 years do not raise sputum but swallow it. In young children, therefore, gastric lavage may be necessary to obtain the sputum specimen (because tuberculosis bacteria are acid-fast, they are not destroyed by gastric secretions). Schedule this test early in the morning before the child eats. This prevents vomiting and also allows for the collection of large numbers of organisms because the child has been coughing sputum and swallowing it all night. To collect the specimen, a nasogastric tube is passed either nasally or orally. The stomach contents are then aspirated and placed in a sterile container for laboratory processing. Analysis is generally done for 3 consecutive days because individual specimens may not contain organisms.

Having a large tube passed into the stomach is uncomfortable, and the concept itself is frightening. Offer support during the procedure. Encourage children to express their feelings about the procedure afterward. They may enjoy playing with a plastic catheter and a doll into which a tube can be inserted after the procedure (therapeutic play). It is revealing to see the force and the anger they use to insert the tube into the doll. This helps you to understand how they envision the procedure being done to them.

In the early course of tuberculosis, because the initial focus of the tuberculosis is so small, it may not be evident on a chest x-ray. As local inflammation occurs, however, cloudiness in the inflamed area will be noticeable on the film, as will calcification as it occurs.

Children who have primary tuberculosis are not infectious because they have a minimal pulmonary lesion and little or no cough. They need not be isolated. As soon as drug therapy has been started, they can return to regular activities, including school.

Before drug therapy was available, a diagnosis of tuberculosis meant a hospital stay of approximately a year. Parents who believe that tuberculosis is still treated this way will need assurance that it is all right for their child to return home and attend regular school as soon as he or she starts taking medication.

Therapeutic Management

A number of medications are effective against tuberculosis. Isoniazid (INH) is the drug of choice. INH may produce peripheral neurologic symptoms if pyridoxine (vitamin B) is not administered concurrently. Rifampin is often used in combination with INH. Para-aminosalicylic acid (PAS) is bacteriostatic to *M. tuberculosis* and for a long time served as the mainstay of therapy. However, PAS administration may lead to such gastrointestinal disturbances in children that it is not used as much as in the past. If it is prescribed, it should be administered after meals, never on an empty stomach.

Ethambutol is used with older children. It must be used with caution with infants because one side effect is optic neuritis; the inability to do adequate eye examinations in children under school age to discover this side effect can make ethambutol unsafe for long-term use.

In addition to drug therapy, children should receive a diet high in protein, calcium, and pyridoxine, especially if INH is being used, to wall off organisms in lung tissue.

Because tuberculosis therapy can last up to 18 months, a major concern during treatment is that the tuberculosis organism will become resistant to commonly used drugs. Children should have periodic chest x-rays for the rest of their life to make certain their disease does not become active again later in life. A woman who had tuberculosis as a child should tell her primary care provider about this when she becomes pregnant; lung changes that occur in pregnancy as a result of the pressure of the growing uterus against the lungs can break down calcifications and reactivate tuberculosis. Children who develop another chronic disease that interferes with appetite, and therefore with calcium intake, also have a high risk of reactivation of calcium-contained tuberculosis.

Because children will be taking medicine for a long time, they need periodic health care visits to evaluate the extent of drug adherence. Assess that they receive regular childhood immunizations so they do not contract a second disease until they have fully recovered from tuberculosis. It is most important to prevent pertussis (whooping cough) because the paroxysmal cough caused by this illness could easily reactivate tuberculosis lesions.

The bacille Calmette-Guerin (BCG) vaccine is available against tuberculosis, but it is not used routinely in the United States. A skin test will be strongly positive after effective BCG vaccination. For this reason, most people advocate placing children on prophylactic INH when there is known tuberculosis in the home rather than vaccinating them against tuberculosis. With this method, as long as a repeat PPD test remains negative, you know that they are disease-free. After BCG vaccine is administered, the value of skin testing would be lost.

Cystic Fibrosis

Children with cystic fibrosis (CF) have a generalized dysfunction of the exocrine glands. Mucus secretions of the body, particularly in the pancreas and the lungs, are so tenacious that they have difficulty flowing through gland ducts. There is also a marked electrolyte change in the secretions of the sweat glands (chloride concentration of sweat is two to five times above normal). The cause of the disorder is an abnormality of the long arm of chromosome 7. This results in the inability to transport small molecules across cell membranes; this leads to dehydration of epithelial cells in the airway and pancreas and dried secretions.

The disorder is inherited as an autosomal recessive trait. It occurs in approximately 1 in 2,500 live births. It occurs most commonly in whites, rarely in blacks and Asians. Although the disease can be fatal in early life, as many as 50% of children now live to be more than 30 years of age. With the availability of lung transplants, full life expectancy is possible. Because the gene that causes the disorder can be isolated, chorionic villi sampling or amniocentesis can be done early in pregnancy to detect fetuses who have the disease. All newborns can be screened at birth by a simple heel puncture blood sample for the disorder (Merelle et al., 2005). In the future, it is expected that gene therapy will be available to reverse the effect of the involved gene.

Boys with CF may not be able to reproduce because they have persistent plugging and blocking of the vas deferens from tenacious seminal fluid. Girls may have such thick cervical secretions that sperm penetration is limited. Artificial insemination or in vitro fertilization can be accomplished if they desire to become pregnant.

Pancreas Involvement

The acinar cells of the pancreas normally produce lipase, trypsin, and amylase, enzymes that flow into the duodenum to digest fat, protein, and carbohydrate. With CF, these enzyme secretions become so thickened that they plug the ducts; eventually, there is such back-pressure on the acinar cells that they become atrophied and then are no longer capable of producing the enzymes. The islets of Langerhans and insulin production are little influenced by this process until late in the disease because they have endocrine (ductless) activity.

Without pancreatic enzymes in the duodenum, children cannot digest fat, protein, and some sugars. The child's stools become large, bulky, and greasy (**steatorrhea**). The intestinal flora increases because of the undigested food; this, when combined with the fat in the stool, gives the stool an extremely foul odor, often compared to that of a cat's stool. The bulk of feces in the intestine leads to a protuberant abdomen. Because children are benefiting from only about 50% of the food they ingest, they show signs of malnutrition—emaciated extremities and loose, flabby folds of skin on their buttocks. The fat-soluble vitamins, particularly A, D, and E, cannot be absorbed because fat is not absorbed, so children develop symptoms of low levels of these vitamins. These four symptoms—malnutrition, protuberant abdomen, steatorrhea, and fat-soluble vitamin deficiencies—are the same four symptoms that are part of celiac disease (malabsorption syndrome), so they are referred to as the celiac syndrome (see Chapter 45).

Meconium in a newborn is normally thick and tenacious. In approximately 10% of children with CF, it may be so thick, because pancreatic enzymes are lacking, that it obstructs the intestine (meconium ileus). The newborn develops abdominal distention with no passage of stool. Meconium ileus should be suspected in any infant who does not pass a stool by 24 hours of life (McCollough & Sharieff, 2003). Rectal prolapse from straining to evacuate hard stool is another common finding in infants with CF.

Lung Involvement

Pockets of infection begin in pooled thick secretions of the bronchioles. The organisms most frequently cultured from lung secretions in children with CF are *Staphylococcus aureus, Pseudomonas aeruginosa,* and *H. influenzae.* Secondary emphysema (overinflated alveoli) occurs because the air cannot be pushed past the thick mucus on expiration, when all bronchi are narrower than they are on inspiration. Bronchiectasis and pneumonia occur. Atelectasis occurs as a result of complete absorption of air from alveoli behind blocked bronchioles. The child's fingers become clubbed because of the inadequate peripheral tissue perfusion. The anterior-posterior diameter of the chest becomes enlarged. Respiratory acidosis may develop because obstruction interferes with the ability to exhale carbon dioxide.

Sweat Gland Involvement

Although the sweat glands themselves do not appear to be changed in structure, the electrolyte composition of perspiration is changed. In children with CF, the level of chloride to sodium is increased two to five times above normal. Some parents report they knew their newborn had the disease before they had laboratory tests done because when they kissed their child, they could taste such strong salt in the perspiration.

Assessment

If CF is not diagnosed by a screening blood sample at birth, it is diagnosed by documenting the chromosomal abnormality, and the history and the combination of the abnormal concentration of chloride in sweat, the absence of pancreatic enzymes in the duodenum, the presence of immunoreactive trypsinogen in the blood, and pulmonary involvement.

CF may be suspected in a newborn when he or she loses the normal amount of weight at birth (5% to 10% of birthweight), but then, because the infant cannot make use of the fat in milk, does not gain it back at the usual time of 7 to 10 days and perhaps not until 4 to 6 weeks of age. Nurses are the individuals who often weigh babies and may be the first to detect this lack of weight gain. Nurses may also be the first health care provider to suspect CF because meconium is so tenacious the infant is unable to pass stool. All babies with meconium ileus are tested for CF. This can be done by a chromosome analysis or analysis of serum immunoreactive trypsin (IRT) in the stool, which is elevated because obstruction in the pancreas occurs as early as during fetal life.

Children who are not diagnosed at birth may be seen in a health care setting at about 1 month of age because of a feeding problem. Using only about 50% of their intake because of their poor digestive function, they are always hungry. This causes them to eat so ravenously they tend to swallow air. This is manifested as colic or abdominal distention and vomiting. The appearance of typical CF stools (large and greasy) is an important finding because children with simple colic do not show these changes in stool consistency.

Respiratory infections begin to occur at 4 to 6 months of age. Even at this early stage of the disease, wheezing and rhonchi may be heard on chest auscultation.

By the time a child with CF is a preschooler, a cough is a prominent finding. On percussion, the chest is hyperresonant, reflecting the emphysema present. Rales and rhonchi are heard. Clubbing of the fingers may already be apparent. It is rare for a child to go undiagnosed beyond this time because the symptoms of the illness have become so persistent and evident.

Sweat Testing. Sweat testing is a time-honored method for detecting the abnormal concentrations in sweat in children with CF. Sweat is collected and analyzed for sodium chloride content. With chromosomal determination available, sweat tests are no longer necessary, but parents may ask about the procedure if they hear about it from friends. A normal concentration of chloride in sweat is 20 mEq/L. A level of more than 60 mEq/L chloride in children is diagnostic of CF.

Duodenal Analysis. Analysis of duodenal secretions for detection of pancreatic enzymes may be done to show the extent of the pancreatic involvement by passing a nasogastric tube into the duodenum and then aspirating secretions for analysis. This test may take a considerable amount of time because the tube is allowed to pass through the pylorus and into the duodenum by natural peristaltic action. You can tell that a tube has passed from the stomach into the duodenum by aspirating secretions from the tube and testing them for pH. Stomach secretions are acid (pH less than 7.0); duodenal secretions are alkaline (pH more than 7.0). The initial insertion of the tube typically is frightening to children because they may choke and gag as it passes the pharynx. Children, however, are generally surprised that once the initial insertion is done, the tube is not uncomfortable. They need a great deal of support during the procedure, however, because it is so unusual for them and initially so uncomfortable. Duodenal analysis may also be done by endoscopy; for this, children usually receive conscious sedation (Burton & Germann, 2004).

The secretions removed from the duodenum are sent to the laboratory for analysis of trypsin content, the easiest pancreatic enzyme to assay. Keep the secretions cold during transport. They should be analyzed immediately for accurate results.

Stool Analysis. Stool may be collected and analyzed for fat content, although description of the large greasy appearance may be all that is necessary.

Pulmonary Testing. A chest x-ray generally confirms the extent of the pulmonary involvement (pockets of emphysema and perhaps beginning pneumonia infiltration are present). Pulmonary function tests may be done to determine if atelectasis and emphysema are present.

Therapeutic Management

Therapy for children with CF consists of measures to reduce the involvement of the pancreas, lungs, and sweat glands.

NURSING DIAGNOSES AND RELATED INTERVENTIONS

Nursing Diagnosis: Imbalanced nutrition, less than body requirements, related to inability to digest fat

Outcome Evaluation: Child's height and weight follow percentile growth curves; quantity of stool decreases; signs and symptoms of vitamin deficiency are absent.

Children with CF are placed on a high-calorie, high-protein, moderate-fat diet. Water-miscible forms of vitamins A, D, and E are supplemented. During the hot months of the year, extra salt may be added to food to replace that lost though perspiration. Medium-chain triglycerides are used with the diet because these are more readily digested than other oils.

Generally, infants with CF cannot be totally breast-fed because there is not enough protein in breast milk for them (they need large amounts because they cannot make use of all the protein they ingest). Breast-feeding with supplementary formula is required. Some of these children, unfortunately, are initially diagnosed as having a milk allergy and are treated by being placed on a soybean formula. This does not contain enough protein either, and their malnutrition increases greatly while they are taking this formula. A high-protein formula, such as Probana, is generally recommended.

Children with CF have a ravenous appetite and eat well. Before each meal or snack, they need to take a synthetic pancreatic enzyme, pancreatic lipase (Cotazym or Pancrease), to replace the enzyme they cannot produce (Box 40.15). These synthetic enzymes are supplied in large capsules that must be opened for young children because they cannot swallow such a big capsule; infants, in particular, may not have enough gastric acids to dissolve the capsule. The powder from the capsule is then added to a small amount (no more than a teaspoonful) of food. It should not be added to hot food, or a large portion of enzyme activity will be destroyed. Also, it must not be added to the infant's bottle of formula, because the infant may not drink the entire bottle and therefore will not receive the total benefit of the enzyme. When children are taking a synthetic source of pancreatic enzyme this way, the size of stools and the accompanying foul odor decreases. Children begin to gain weight. In adolescence, children may have a great deal of difficulty eating enough to maintain weight, even with enzyme therapy, because their growth spurt requires so many additional calories.

BOX 40.15 FOCUS ON . . .

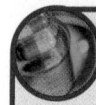

PHARMACOLOGY

Pancrelipase (Cotazym)

Classification: Pancrelipase is an enzyme replacement.

Action: Used to aid digestion in children with cystic fibrosis.

Pregnancy risk category: C

Dosage:
- Children 6 months to 1 year of age: 2,000 U orally per meal
- Children 1 to 6 years of age: 4,000 to 8,000 U orally with each meal and 4,000 U with snacks
- Children 7 to 12 years of age: 4,000 to 12,000 U orally with each meal and with snacks

Possible adverse effects: Nausea, abdominal cramps, diarrhea, hypersensitivity

Nursing Implications
- Administer the drug before or with meals and snacks. Instruct parents and child to do the same.
- Caution child and parents to avoid inhaling powder or spilling it on the hands, because it may irritate the skin or mucous membranes.
- Do not crush or let the child chew the enteric form of the drug.
- Instruct the child and parents about possible adverse effects and encourage them to contact their health care provider should any become severe.

If children with CF become overheated, they begin to lose excessive sodium and chloride through perspiration and become dehydrated. Caution parents to keep their house temperature at 72°F or below and to offer water frequently. They also need to supervise outside play to guard against overexertion or heat exposure.

Nursing Diagnosis: Ineffective airway clearance related to inability to clear mucus from the respiratory tract

Outcome Evaluation: Child's temperature is below 100.4°F (38.0°C); Po_2 is 80 to 90 mm Hg; Pco_2 is less than 40 mm Hg.

Unfortunately, the pulmonary effects of CF progress despite supplementation with pancreatic enzyme; infection from plugged airways is always a possibility. Therefore, it is important to try to keep bronchial secretions as moist and freely flowing as possible so they can drain from the bronchial tree. This is done by frequent nebulization or aerosol therapy followed by chest physiotherapy.

Humidified Oxygen. Oxygen is supplied to children by mask, prongs, ventilators, or nebulizers. Mist can be supplied by an ultrasonic compressor and delivered through a nebulizer mask, which makes the droplet size so small the mist reaches the smallest bronchial spaces.

Aerosol Therapy. Three or four times a day, children may be given aerosol therapy by means of a nebulizer to provide antibiotics or bronchodilators. Antibiotics are specifically determined by culture. A mucolytic, such as acetylcysteine (Mucomyst), can be added to the mist to aid in diluting and liquefying secretions. A child's cough will become loose and productive after using aerosol therapy. Provide a box of tissues so the child can cough up these loose secretions. Observe the child to ensure that he or she can cough and keep the airway clear. Never give cough syrups to suppress a cough, because getting secretions out is essential for air exchange and to prevent infection. Likewise, question an order for codeine as an analgesic, because codeine suppresses the cough reflex.

Chest Physiotherapy. Because the bronchial secretions with CF are so tenacious, even with liquefaction by mist or aerosol therapy, children may be unable to raise them. To aid drainage of secretions, children need chest physiotherapy frequently, approximately three or four times a day.

Activity. Children with CF need to maintain their usual activities as much as possible. When in bed, they need frequent position changes so that, at various times of the day, all lobes of their lungs will be encouraged to drain by being in a superior position. Be certain they sit up part of each day to drain the upper lobes. This change in position also helps to prevent skin breakdown over bony prominences.

Frequent Observation. Observe children with CF frequently because their condition can change rapidly. If a portion of a lung becomes obstructed from a plug of mucus, a child can quickly experience respiratory difficulty. The right side of the heart tends to enlarge in children with chronic respiratory disease because the congestion in the lungs increases pressure in the pulmonary artery and the right ventricle. After a period of stress or exercise, children may begin to show signs of cardiac failure because their already enlarged heart cannot compensate any further.

Respiratory Hygiene. The sputum that a child coughs up may have a disagreeable taste or odor. Offer frequent mouth care, toothbrushing, and a good-tasting mouthwash to make the child's mouth feel fresh.

Adequate Rest and Comfort. Any child who has compromised lung function has a degree of dyspnea that leads to exhaustion. To counteract this, provide periods of rest during the day, but do not group too many activities or procedures together all at once, as this could exhaust the child. Plan a rest period before meals so that the child is not too tired to eat. Also plan for a long rest period before chest physiotherapy so that the child will be able to tolerate it better. Achieving a balance between allowing periods of rest and yet not doing all procedures at once is not an easy task.

Growth and Development. Children need to be exposed to as many normal life experiences as possible. This may be difficult because it is important not to tire the child out or expose him or her to crowds of people (possibly increasing the risk for infection). Assist the parents with planning age-appropriate activities with the child.

Nursing Diagnosis: Risk for impaired skin integrity related to acid stools

Outcome Evaluation: Child's skin does not exhibit areas of erythema or ulceration; rectal prolapse is not present.

Until children are regulated on pancreatic enzymes, the stool is particularly irritating because of its high fat content. Children who are not toilet-trained need to have their diapers changed immediately after they wet or pass stool so that they do not develop skin irritation and breakdown in the diaper area.

After a bowel movement, check the rectum for rectal prolapse. Because of weak musculature of the rectal area, this is a common complication. A prolapse of rectal mucosa appears as a bright-red mass protruding from the anal sphincter. This mucosa must be replaced promptly before its blood supply is compromised. Place the child on the slant board used for chest physiotherapy with the head lower than the buttocks; then, with a lubricated, gloved hand, gently replace the prolapsed rectal mass. Afterward, compress the buttocks together to maintain gentle pressure on the anus for a few minutes. This is much less of a problem in children who are receiving pancreatic enzymes than in those who are not, because the incidence of rectal prolapse decreases with better nutrition.

Nursing Diagnosis: Risk for compromised family coping related to chronic illness in a child

Outcome Evaluation: Family members state they have adequate resources to cope with current circumstances.

The parents of children with CF are asked to assume a great deal of responsibility for care of their child. Begin discharge planning when a child is first admitted to a hospital in terms of what changes need to be made to accommodate the child at home and to familiarize parents with the necessary care measures. For example, many children with this disorder sleep with oxygen by cannula at night when they are at home. Parents need to be taught the functions of oxygen and how to regulate the flow. This type of learning is most effective if a little is taught every day (for example, "Could you turn the oxygen on for me, Mrs. Smith? I'm ready to tuck Brian in to sleep" rather than a sit-down, let-me-tell-you-how-oxygen-works lecture given close to the day of discharge). Teach parents how to do chest physiotherapy the same way.

The family will have to think through how the care of this child will affect their home life. They are going to be spending a great deal of time caring for the child, so they will need to balance work, care of the child, and care of the rest of the family. Many parents become fatigued after the first week of having the child at home; they may believe that if they fall soundly asleep at night, they may not hear the child call if he or she should be in distress. As they grow more confident in their ability to evaluate the child's condition before bedtime, their apprehension will lessen, but real confidence may not come for months, even years. This may always be a problem for some parents.

Be sure that the parents have the telephone number of the health care provider they should call if they feel overwhelmed. Encourage parents to join a support group, so that there are other people available to understand and to whom they can voice their concerns. At these times, one of the most important needs they have is to verbalize to someone what it feels like to be the parent of a child with CF, including feelings of guilt they may be experiencing because the disease is inherited.

Children should attend regular school if at all possible so they are provided with socialization experiences with other children. If this is not possible, a home tutor can be arranged for them. Urge children to participate to the extent they can in physical fitness activities in school or with friends. Use a reminder sheet as necessary so they can remember to take pancreatic enzyme with them if they are going to be eating lunch in the school cafeteria or outside the home.

Ensure that children with CF receive periodic health assessments and routine childhood immunizations. It is not unusual for children with a chronic disease to fall behind in routine check-ups and immunizations if they are hospitalized at the times these are routinely done. It is particularly important that children with CF receive the pertussis and measles vaccines, because these two infections cause severe respiratory complications. Children also should receive influenza, meningococcal, and pneumococcal vaccines.

As children with CF reach adolescence, they are candidates for lung transplants. Some of these are done as lower lobe transplants from a living donor. People who donate a single lobe in this manner report that they feel little loss of lung capacity afterward. A lung transplant is advantageous for children with CF because the new lung does not possess the defective gene that caused mucus to be so thick. Lifespan can greatly improve.

Checkpoint Question 5

Children with cystic fibrosis take the pancreatic enzyme pancrelipase before each meal. You would prepare this by:

a. Opening the capsule and adding it to warm tea.
b. Adding it to at least 8 ounces of milk to drink.
c. Sprinkling it on a small amount of applesauce.
d. Teaching the child how to swallow large capsules.

Key Points

Respiratory tract disorders tend to occur more frequently in children than adults, because the lumens of bronchi are narrow and obstruction and infection can occur more easily.

Infants with respiratory illness need extremely close observation because they cannot describe oxygen deprivation. Young children do not comprehend the fact that oxygen supports combustion. Observe them more frequently than adults to be certain that no flames, such as birthday candles, are brought within 10 feet of an oxygen source.

Acute nasopharyngitis (common cold) is the most common infectious disease in children. There is no specific therapy for a common cold other than comfort measures.

Tonsillitis is infection and inflammation of the palatine tonsils. Adenitis is infection and inflammation of the adenoid tonsils. Children with recurring infections may have their tonsils surgically removed.

Laryngotracheobronchitis (croup) is inflammation of the larynx, trachea, and major bronchi. Epiglottitis is inflammation of the epiglottis. Both of these conditions can cause severe impairment of the airway. Children with epiglottitis should never be assessed for a gag reflex with a tongue blade because the elevated epiglottis can completely occlude the airway.

Bronchitis is inflammation of the major bronchi and trachea. Bronchiolitis is inflammation of the fine bronchioles. Both conditions are caused by bacterial or viral invasion.

Respiratory syncytial virus infection is an infection that accounts for the majority of lower respiratory infections in young children. Infants with RSV infections must be observed closely because they are prone to apnea.

Asthma, a type I hypersensitivity reaction, is a diffuse and obstructive airway disease with wheezing as the most common symptom. Newer drugs such as leukotriene receptor antagonists and careful environmental control have aided in the management of this disorder.

Pneumonia may occur from a variety of organisms (viral, pneumococcal, chlamydial, mycoplasmal, lipid, and hydrocarbon). Except for viral pneumonia, children need specific antibiotics, depending on the organism present.

Tuberculosis is a lung infection that is growing in incidence, with some strains becoming very resistant to the usual therapy. The entire family needs drug therapy if one member develops a primary lesion.

Cystic fibrosis is a disease in which there is generalized dysfunction of the exocrine glands. This results in malabsorption and tenacious pulmonary secretions, leading to infection and pneumonia. Lung transplantation can be used to replace the diseased lung tissue and increase the child's lifespan.

Critical Thinking Exercises

1. Michael is the 4-year-old you met at the beginning of the chapter. His grandmother brought him to the emergency room because his respirations were rapid and he had a sharp, barking cough. He is diagnosed as having laryngotracheobronchitis (croup). Both he and his grandmother shouted information at you. What about Michael's actions would lead you to believe his airway is not yet extremely constricted? Would you encourage him to lie down and rest? What emergency care does Michael need?
2. One of Michael's ambulatory roommates has a permanent tracheostomy tube in place from pulmonary dysplasia as an infant. Her parents are going to enroll her in kindergarten starting next month. What precautions would you want to review with her parents to keep this experience safe?
3. When the 4-year-old in the ambulatory bed next to Michael returns from tonsillectomy surgery, what observations would be most important to make? Why is the 7th day after tonsillectomy surgery a particularly important day for close observation?
5. Examine the National Health Goals related to respiratory disorders in children. Most government-sponsored money for nursing research is allotted based on these goals. What would be a possible research topic to explore pertinent to these goals that would be applicable to Michael's family and also advance evidence-based practice?

References

American Heart Association. (2005). *Pediatric advanced life support.* Dallas, TX: Author.
American Thoracic Society. (2003). Statement on the care of the child with chronic lung disease of infancy and childhood. *American Journal of Respiratory and Critical Care Medicine, 168*(3), 356–396.

Bagarazzi, M. L. (2003). Pharyngitis. In M. W. Schwartz (Ed.), *5-minute pediatric consult* (3rd ed.). Philadelphia: Lippincott Williams & Wilkins.

Bhargava, S. (2003). Chlamydial infections. In M. W. Schwartz (Ed.), *5-minute pediatric consul.* (3rd ed.). Philadelphia: Lippincott Williams & Wilkins.

Bjornson, C. L., & Johnson, D. W. (2004). Pediatric practice. That characteristic cough: When to treat croup and what to use. *Patient Care for the Nurse Practitioner, 1*(1), 1–12.

Bonafos, G., et al. (2004). Choanal atresia and rare craniofacial clefts. *Cleft Palate-Craniofacial Journal, 41*(1), 78–83.

Brown, J. M., & Padman, R. (2004). Case study of a UFO (unidentified foreign object). *Pediatric Asthma, Allergy & Immunology, 16*(4), 187–192.

Burton, J. H., & Germann, C. A. (2004). Guide to procedural sedation and analgesia. *Emergency Medicine, 36*(7), 43–46.

Carden, K. A., et al. (2005). Tracheomalacia and tracheobronchomalacia in children and adults: An in-depth review. *Chest, 127*(3), 984–1005.

Carpenito, L. (2004). *Nursing diagnosis: Application to clinical practice* (9th ed.). Philadelphia: Lippincott Williams & Wilkins.

Chung, E. K. (2003). Sinusitis. In M. W. Schwartz (Ed.), *5-minute pediatric consult* (3rd ed.). Philadelphia: Lippincott Williams & Wilkins.

Clayton, R. G, Jr. (2003). Asthma. In M. W. Schwartz (Ed.), *5-minute pediatric consult* (3rd ed.). Philadelphia: Lippincott Williams & Wilkins.

Cromer, M., & Foley, K. (2004). How to recognize a supraglottic infection. *Emergency Medicine, 36*(4), 13–16.

Curtin-Wirt, C., et al. (2003). Efficacy of penicillin vs. amoxicillin in children with group A beta-hemolytic streptococcal tonsillopharyngitis. *Clinical Pediatrics, 42*(3), 219–225.

Department of Health and Human Services. (2000). *Healthy people 2010*. Washington, DC: DHHS.

Dougherty, J. M., et al. (2003). Pediatric tracheostomy and ventilator care. *Nursing Spectrum (Midwest), 4*(6), 24–29.

Fink, J. B. (2004). Aerosol delivery to ventilated infants and pediatric patients. *Respiratory Care, 49*(6), 653–665.

Fischbach, F. (2005). *A manual of laboratory and diagnostic tests* (6th ed.). Philadelphia: Lippincott Williams & Wilkins.

Fiske, E. (2004). Tracheostomy home care guide. *Advances in Neonatal Care, 4*(1), 54–55.

Frey, B., & Shann, F. (2004). Oxygen administration in infants. *Archives of Disease in Childhood Fetal and Neonatal Edition, 88*(2), F84–88.

Good, J. M. (2003). Bronchopulmonary dysplasia. In M. W. Schwartz (Ed.), *5-minute pediatric consult* (3rd ed.). Philadelphia: Lippincott Williams & Wilkins.

Goldrick, B. A. (2004). Emerging infections. Influenza 2004–2005: What's new with the flu? *American Journal of Nursing, 104*(10), 34–36.

Graessle, W. R. (2003). Otitis media. In M. W. Schwartz (Ed.), *5-minute pediatric consult* (3rd ed.). Philadelphia: Lippincott Williams & Wilkins.

Graham, S. (2004). Continuous positive airway pressure: The story of change in a neonatal intensive care unit. *Journal of Neonatal Nursing, 10*(4), 130–134.

Greenberg, M. (2004). Resuscitation of the neonate: Principles and practice. *Current Reviews for Nurse Anesthetists, 26*(20), 239–249.

Hernandez, M. E. (2003). Bronchiolitis. In M. W. Schwartz (Ed.), *5-minute pediatric consult* (3rd ed.). Philadelphia: Lippincott Williams & Wilkins.

Kallstrom, T. J. (2004). Evidence-based asthma management. *Respiratory Care, 49*(7), 783–792.

Karch, A. M. (2004). *Lippincott's nursing drug guide.* Philadelphia: Lippincott Williams & Wilkins.

King, V. J., et al. (2004). Pharmacologic treatment of bronchiolitis in infants and children: A systematic review. *Archives of Pediatrics & Adolescent Medicine, 158*(2), 127–137.

Kravitz, R. M. (2003). Pneumothorax. In M. W. Schwartz (Ed.), *5-minute pediatric consult* (3rd ed.). Philadelphia: Lippincott Williams & Wilkins.

McCollough, M., & Sharieff, G. Q. (2003). Abdominal surgical emergencies in infants and young children. *Emergency Medicine Clinics of North America, 21*(4), 909–935.

Merelle, M. E., et al. (2005). Newborn screening for cystic fibrosis. *The Cochrane Library (Oxford) (4)* (CD001402).

Meyers, K. E. C. (2003). Glomerulonephritis. In M. W. Schwartz (Ed.), *5-minute pediatric consult* (3rd ed.). Philadelphia: Lippincott Williams & Wilkins.

Osterhoudt, K. C. (2003). Nosebleeds (epistaxis). In M. W. Schwartz (Ed.), *5-minute pediatric consult* (3rd ed.). Philadelphia: Lippincott Williams & Wilkins.

Phillips, S. C. (2003). Croup (laryngotracheobronchitis). In M. W. Schwartz (Ed.), *5-minute pediatric consult* (3rd ed.). Philadelphia: Lippincott Williams & Wilkins.

Posner, J. C. (2003). Strep infection—invasive group A beta-hemolytic streptococcus. In M. W. Schwartz (Ed.), *5-minute pediatric consult* (3rd ed.). Philadelphia: Lippincott Williams & Wilkins.

Pritchard, M., Flenady, V., & Woodgate, P. (2005). Preoxygenation for tracheal suctioning in intubated, ventilated newborn infants. *The Cochrane Library (Oxford) (4)* (CD000427).

Rutstein, R. M. (2003). Retropharyngeal abscess. In M. W. Schwartz (Ed.), *5-minute pediatric consult* (3rd ed.). Philadelphia: Lippincott Williams & Wilkins.

Smith, L. M., & Osborne, R. F. (2003). Infections of the head and neck. *Topics in Emergency Medicine, 25*(2), 106–116.

Spence, K., & Barr, P. (2005). Nasal versus oral intubation for mechanical ventilation of newborn infants. *The Cochrane Library (Oxford) (4)* (CD000948).

Taras, H., et al. (2004). Impact of school nurse case management on students with asthma. *Journal of School Health, 74*(6), 213–219.

Teets, J. M., & Borisuk, M. J. (2004). Pediatric thoracic organ transplants: Challenges in primary care. *Pediatric Nursing, 30*(1), 23–30.

Thibodeau, K. P., & Viera, A. J. (2004). Atypical pathogens and challenges in community-acquired pneumonia. *American Family Physician, 69*(7), 1699–1706.

van der Schans, C., Prasad, A., & Main, E. (2005). Chest physiotherapy compared to no chest physiotherapy for cystic fibrosis. *The Cochrane Library (Oxford) (4)* (CD001401).

Wagener, J. S., & Headley, A. A. (2003). Cystic fibrosis: Current trends in respiratory care. *Respiratory Care, 48*(3), 234–247.

Watson, B. (2003). Tuberculosis. In M. W. Schwartz (Ed.), *5-minute pediatric consult* (3rd ed.). Philadelphia: Lippincott Williams & Wilkins.

Zsolway, K. W. (2003). Respiratory syncytial virus (RSV). In M. W. Schwartz (Ed.), *5-minute pediatric consult* (3rd ed.). Philadelphia: Lippincott Williams & Wilkins.

Suggested Readings

Bezyack, M. E. (2004). Respiratory distress: Making the diagnosis in kids. *Nursing Spectrum, 17*(2), 30–31.

Buysse, C. M., de Jongste, J. C., & de Hoog, M. (2005). Life-threatening asthma in children: Treatment with sodium bicarbonate reduces PcO_2. *Chest, 127*(3), 866–870.

Clayton, S. (2005). Paediatric asthma: Overcoming barriers to an improved quality of life. *British Journal of Nursing, 14*(2), 80-85.

Farber, H. J., & Oliveria, L. (2004). Trial of an asthma education program in an inner-city pediatric emergency department. *Pediatric Asthma, Allergy & Immunology, 17*(2), 107-115.

Hay, A. D., Schroeder, K., & Fahey, T. (2004). 10-minute consultation: Acute cough in children. *British Medical Journal, 328*(7447), 1062.

Horner, S. D. (2004). Effect of education on school-age children's and parents' asthma management. *Journal for Specialists in Pediatric Nursing, 9*(3), 95-102.

Lessard, M. J. (2004). Pediatric asthma: An epidemic to be controlled. *Nursing Spectrum, 8*(1), 20-21.

Low, D. E., Pichichero, M. E., & Schaad, U. B. (2004). Optimizing antibacterial therapy for community-acquired respiratory tract infections in children in an era of bacterial resistance. *Clinical Pediatrics, 43*(2), 135-151.

Naim, M. Y., Smith, R., & Schears, G. (2004). Severe respiratory distress. *Clinical Pediatrics, 43*(4), 403-405.

Salyer, J. W. (2004). Respiratory care of bronchiolitis patients: A proving ground for process improvement. *Respiratory Care, 49*(6), 581-583.

CHAPTER 41

Nursing Care of the Child With a Cardiovascular Disorder

Key Terms

acyanotic heart disease
afterload
balloon angioplasty
cardiac catheterization
congestive heart failure
contractility
cyanosis
cyanotic heart disease
diastole
echocardiography
electrocardiogram
fluoroscopy
innocent heart murmur
left-to-right shunt
organic heart murmur
phonocardiogram
polycythemia
postcardiac surgery syndrome
postperfusion syndrome
preload
right-to-left shunt
systole
vasculitis

Objectives

After mastering the contents of this chapter, you should be able to:

1. Describe the common cardiovascular disorders of childhood.
2. Assess a child with a cardiovascular dysfunction.
3. Formulate nursing diagnoses for a child with a cardiovascular disorder.
4. Establish appropriate outcomes based on the priority needs of a child with a cardiovascular disorder.
5. Plan nursing care for a child with a cardiovascular disorder.
6. Implement nursing care for a child with a cardiovascular disorder.
7. Evaluate expected outcomes for achievement and effectiveness of nursing care.
8. Identify National Health Goals related to cardiovascular disorders and children nurses could help the nation achieve.
9. Identify areas related to the care of children with cardiovascular problems that could benefit from additional nursing research or application of evidence-based practice.
10. Use critical thinking to analyze ways that nursing care of children with cardiovascular disorders could be more family-centered.
11. Integrate knowledge of cardiovascular disorders with nursing process to achieve quality maternal and child health nursing care.

---

*M*egan is a newborn who was born with tetralogy of Fallot. By 1 hour of age, she developed rapid respirations, tachycardia, and cyanosis. An echocardiogram revealed the typical four structural defects of the syndrome. Megan's parents will be taking her home for a month to await cardiac surgery. They tell you their doctor instructed them to "watch her carefully" during that time. "What does that mean?" they ask you. Will they be able to take her outside in a stroller? Should she sleep in their bedroom? Exactly what should they watch for?

Previous chapters described the growth and development of well children. This chapter adds information about the child who is ill with heart disease and the stress that such a serious diagnosis places on a family. This is important information because it builds a base for care and health teaching for children with these disorders.

What advice would you give Megan's parents?

After you've studied this chapter, access the accompanying website. Read the patient scenario and answer the questions to further sharpen your skills, grow more familiar with RN-CLEX types of questions, and reward yourself with how much you have learned.

The cardiovascular system, the body system on which all other systems depend, consists of the heart, which acts as a pump; the blood, which provides the fluid and cells for transport of oxygen and nutrients; and the blood vessels, which provide the means and routes for transport throughout the body. The regular pumping of the heart propels oxygen and needed nutrients through the bloodstream to cells and allows waste products to be removed from cells and transported to the lungs or kidneys for excretion. The cardiovascular system also transports regulatory materials such as hormones, enzymes, and antibodies to the body systems. It can adapt to changing body needs by adjusting the rate and force of heart pumping, modifying the size of the blood vessels, and altering the volume and composition of the blood.

Most cardiovascular disorders in children occur as a result of a congenital anomaly; either the heart has developed inadequately in utero, or the heart cannot adapt to extrauterine life for some reason. Open-heart surgery often is the only treatment that will correct the primary congenital problem. Children also may experience acquired cardiovascular disorders, such as rheumatic fever or Kawasaki disease. All these disorders can lead to heart failure or infection or inadequate heart function.

Cardiovascular disorders are frightening for both children and their parents, as even small children realize the importance of their hearts in sustaining life, and they recognize the seriousness of any illness that undermines the heart's activity. For the families of children with a cardiovascular disease, understanding the functioning of the heart and circulation is an important first step toward coping with the illness. Cardiac disorders are a major focus of health promotion and disease prevention measures in both adults and children. National Health Goals related to cardiovascular illness and children are shown in Box 41.1.

Nursing Process Overview

For Care of the Child With a Cardiovascular Disorder

● Assessment

Assessment of the child with a cardiovascular disorder includes both careful history taking and physical examination, because many of the signs and symptoms of heart disease in children are subtle. A variety of diagnostic studies such as echocardiography or electrocardiography or cardiac catheterization may be used to confirm the diagnosis and prepare for surgery. Teaching about these tests and providing psychological support to children and their families are two major responsibilities of nurses throughout the assessment process.

● Nursing Diagnosis

Nursing diagnoses associated with heart disease in children usually speak to the effect of poor circulation on body tissues or the effect a serious disorder can create on the child or parents. Examples are:

- Decreased cardiac output related to congenital structural disorder
- Ineffective tissue perfusion related to inadequate cardiac output
- Deficient knowledge related to care of the child pre- and postoperatively
- Fear related to lack of knowledge about child's disease
- Interrupted family processes related to stresses of the diagnosis and care responsibilities
- Ineffective coping related to lack of adequate support people

BOX 41.1 FOCUS ON . . .

NATIONAL HEALTH GOALS

Cardiovascular illness is a major health problem in adults. However, the illness and its effects can be prevented or at least minimized by instituting measures early in childhood. A number of National Health Goals address ways that children should modify nutrition or exercise to achieve better cardiovascular health:

- Increase the proportion of children and adolescents ages 5 through 17 who engage in vigorous physical activity that promotes cardiorespiratory fitness 3 or more days per week, for 20 or more minutes per occasion, from a baseline of 65% to at least 85%.
- Increase the proportion of persons aged 2 years and older who consume less than 10% of calories from saturated fat, from a baseline of 36% to a target level of 75%.
- Reduce the proportion of children and adolescents who are overweight or obese, from a baseline of 11% to a target level of 5% (DHHS, 2000).

Nurses can help the nation achieve these goals by educating parents and children about the importance of reducing obesity and planning exercise and nutrition programs for sound cardiovascular health. It is equally important for nurses to caution parents not to start their children on reduced-fat diets until they are 2 years old, to allow for myelination of nerve cells.

Nursing research is needed to determine what weight loss programs are the most effective for children, what reduced-fat foods make the best finger foods for preschoolers, what snacks schools could provide in snack machines that would have a reduced fat content and would also be eaten by children, and what are effective ways to increase physical activity in adolescents who do not participate in any type of organized sport or exercise program.

• Impaired parenting related to inability to bond with critically ill newborn

If the concerns in the latter three diagnoses are not identified when a child is ill, they may continue long after a child is treated and returns home.

If a child will be undergoing surgery or cardiac catheterization, nursing diagnoses will focus on the psychological needs of the child and family for preparation and postprocedure care in addition to physical concerns after the procedure (e.g., hypothermia related to cooling during surgery; powerlessness related to conscious sedation during cardiac catheterization).

● *Outcome Identification and Planning*

Nursing planning is essential to help parents and children understand heart anatomy. A sound knowledge base will help them understand the need for diagnostic testing. Additional teaching is necessary to prepare parents and children for procedures or surgery and recovery at home. Teaching parents to conscientiously administer cardiac medications is another area where planning plays an important role. Part of this planning includes establishing appropriate outcomes to help a child and parents adjust to a serious diagnosis, now and in the future (e.g., coping with their present fears and caring for the child at home).

● *Implementation*

Nursing interventions in the care of the child with a cardiovascular disorder include teaching, providing an opportunity for children and their families to express fears about a child's illness and treatment plan, providing physiologic and psychological support such as comfort measures after surgery, and caring for a child in cardiac failure. An equally important role is teaching prevention of heart disease. Measures such as promoting nonsmoking and exercise, maintaining appropriate weight, and eating a low-fat diet are discussed in Chapter 31. For additional help, parents may wish to contact the American Heart Association (*www.americanheart. org*) for educational materials and family support groups in their area.

● *Outcome Evaluation*

Outcome evaluation should be both long term and short term for the child and family. It is important for families to receive adequate immediate support during procedures and treatment. If long-term care is necessary, evaluating the family's ability to think of their child not in terms of illness but in terms of wellness is also key. Provide opportunities for parents to express their concerns about their child at follow-up visits to help address any misconceptions about their child's future.

Examples suggesting achievement of outcomes are:

• Child's heart rate remains within accepted parameters for age.
• Child demonstrates age-appropriate coping skills related to diagnosis and possible surgery.
• Parents demonstrate competence with procedures required for care of their child.

• Parents exhibit positive coping skills related to their child's diagnosis and required care to foster optimal growth and development in their child.
• Parents verbalize positive aspects about their child.

THE CARDIOVASCULAR SYSTEM

Embryologic development of the heart is described in Chapter 8. Cardiac adaptations at birth are described in Chapter 24. After these adaptations, the heart can be thought of as consisting of two pumps: the right side pumps blood to the lungs, where it is oxygenated before returning to the left side of the heart; the left side pumps the oxygenated blood to the peripheral tissues through systemic arteries. After supplying nutrients and collecting wastes, the blood returns through the veins to the right side of the heart, where the cycle begins again. Contraction of the chambers is termed **systole;** relaxation is termed **diastole.** Normal heart anatomy is shown in Figure 41.1.

Most heart disease in children occurs because embryonic structures necessary for fetal life did not close at birth or the heart originally formed inappropriately. For example, a septal defect between the right and left sides of the heart may remain open. Because pressure and volume on the left side of the heart are greater than on the right side, blood will flow through the connecting opening left to right, or from the area of stronger heart action to the area of weaker heart action, compromising right-sided function.

Cardiac output (CO) is the volume of blood pumped by the ventricles each minute. It is calculated by multiplying stroke volume (the volume of blood a ventricle ejects during systole) by the heart rate (beats per minute). CO is affected by three main factors: preload, contractility, and afterload. **Preload** is the volume of blood in the ventricles at the end of diastole (the point just before contraction). **Afterload** refers to the resistance against which the ventricles must pump. **Contractility,** the ability of the ventricles to stretch, refers to the force of contraction generated by the myocardial muscle. The Frank-Starling law predicts that the stroke volume can be increased by increasing the stretch of the fibers. Excessive stretch, however, results in a decrease in cardiac output as the heart tires. Much of the therapy of heart disease is aimed at reducing preload and afterload and increasing contractility to promote better cardiac output.

ASSESSMENT OF HEART DISORDERS IN CHILDREN

The assessment of heart disease in children begins with a thorough history and a physical assessment. More specific diagnostic studies, such as electrocardiography or echocardiography, are ordered as indicated. Because all children with heart disorders have an increased risk of poor tissue perfusion, which may affect growth and development, developmental testing also is incorporated into the assessment.

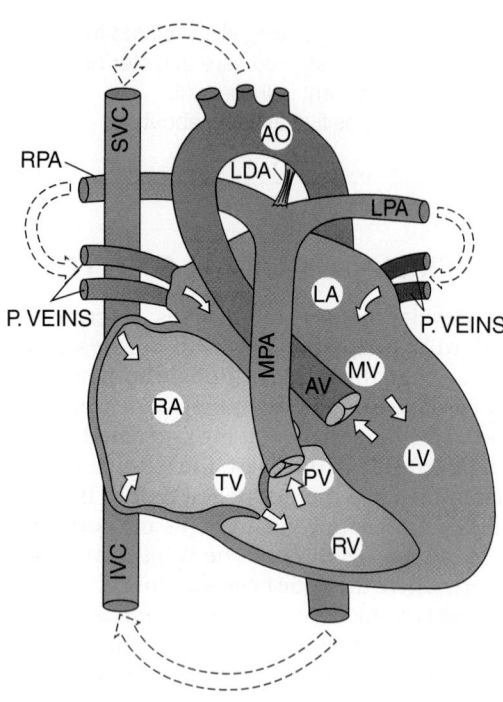

AO–Aorta
AV–Aortic valve
IVC–Inferior vena cava
LA–Left atrium
LPA–Left pulmonary artery
LV–Left ventricle
MPA–Main pulmonary artery
MV–Mitral valve
LDA–Ligamentum ductus arteriosus
PV–Pulmonary valve
P. Vein–Pulmonary vein
RA–Right atrium
RPA–Right pulmonary artery
RV–Right ventricle
SVC–Superior vena cava
TV–Tricuspid valve

FIGURE 41.1 Anatomy of the normal heart.

History

Some congenital heart disorders, such as atrial septal defects, may have a polygenic inheritance pattern. Because the heart arises from the same embryonic origin as the kidney, heart disorders often occur in conjunction with renal disease. Heart disorders also occur as an anomaly in chromosomal disorders (Ward, 2003).

As a result of technological advances in prenatal health care, such as prenatal ultrasound, which can show poor heart action or a distended heart, heart disease may be recognized as early as fetal life. However, even with these advances, heart disease may not be detected before birth. In the newborn period, because the newborn heart rate is so rapid that extra sounds of abnormal circulation may not be heard, heart disease still may not be detected. Because of relatively high pulmonary resistance, defects of the septum may not be readily apparent at birth. Infants with heart disease generally have tachycardia and tachypnea. The infant who is breathing rapidly has to stop sucking on a bottle or breast frequently to breathe. The infant who is easily fatigued because of ineffective heart action has to stop sucking to rest before finishing a feeding. Heart disease may be first discovered, therefore, when an infant is brought to a primary care setting at 1 or 2 weeks of age because the child is having difficulty drinking enough fluid.

A history should include a thorough pregnancy history to try to determine whether an intrauterine insult could have led to poor fetal formation. Cardiac anomalies can occur as a result of intrauterine infections such as toxoplasmosis, cytomegalovirus, or rubella. Also ask whether the mother took any medication during pregnancy, whether nutrition was adequate, or whether she was exposed to any radiation, because these may also contribute to congenital heart disorders.

A mark of older children with heart disease is that they become easily fatigued. When obtaining the history, ask how much activity it takes before a child becomes tired: an hour of strenuous play? A short walk? Be sure parents are not confusing sedentary activities (the child who prefers to sit and read) with activities that are the result of fatigue (e.g., coming home from school and falling asleep day after day).

Ask about a child's usual position when resting. Some infants with congenital heart disease prefer a knee–chest position, whereas older children often voluntarily squat. These positions are unusual in children but trap blood in the lower extremities because of the sharp bend at the knee and hip, allowing the child to oxygenate the blood remaining in the upper body more fully and easily. Also ask about frequency of infections, because children with heart disease have a higher incidence of lower respiratory tract infections than do other children, probably due to less than usual pulmonary circulation. Children with left-to-right shunts tend to perspire excessively because of sympathetic nerve stimulation. Ask if there is an indication of this. Urine is produced only when cardiac function is adequate to perfuse the kidneys. Ask if an infant is wetting diapers or if an older child is voiding normally to discover this. Edema from retained fluid is a late sign of heart disease in children. If it does occur, periorbital edema generally occurs first. **Cyanosis** (a blue tinge to the skin) may occur if a shunt allows deoxygenated blood to enter the arterial system. Such infants generally fail to thrive and are below normal height and weight on a standard growth chart. Children with coarctation of the aorta, discussed below, who have high blood pressure in the head and upper extremities have a history of nosebleeds and headaches. Because of corresponding low blood pressure in the lower extremities, such children may have pain in the legs on running (reported as "growing pains").

Physical Assessment

Physical assessment of a child with a suspected heart disorder begins with measuring height and weight and comparing these findings against standard growth charts. A thorough physical examination should then be done, with particular emphasis on certain body parts or systems (Box 41.2).

Because a major part of the physical assessment will include inspection, palpation, and auscultation of the chest for heart function, it is best if a child is relaxed and not crying. Provide age-appropriate toys that can distract a child readily. Provide a bottle of glucose water in case an infant grows hungry. Play with a child if possible before an examination so he or she is acquainted with you.

General Appearance

Inspect toes and fingers (particularly the thumbs) for clubbing and color. If you press on a fingernail, it will blanch white and then quickly return to pink in a child with good circulation and oxygenation. In a child with poor tissue perfusion, the pink color returns slowly (more than 5 seconds).

The mucous membranes of the mouth are the most likely place for cyanosis to be visible, so always assess the buccal membrane and lips for a blue color. Any time hemoglobin is reduced below 4 to 6 g/100 mL, cyanosis may not be evident because the severe anemia masks it. Cyanosis persisting for over 20 minutes after birth (except for acrocyanosis) suggests serious cardiopulmonary dysfunction. If the cyanosis increases with crying, cardiac dysfunction is suggested, as this implies the infant cannot meet the increased circulatory demands of extrauterine life. If the cyanosis decreases with crying, pulmonary dysfunction is suggested because crying deepens respirations and aerates more lung tissue.

A ruddy complexion may be present in some children with heart disease because the body overproduces red blood cells (**polycythemia**) in an attempt to better oxygenate body cells. Also observe for lethargy and rapid respirations, symptoms that the heart is an ineffective pump.

Inspection of the chest may reveal a prominence of the left side and obvious heart movement (the apex beat, or point of maximum impulse). If a chest is extremely flat, loud innocent murmurs, accentuated heart sounds, and palpable cardiac activity may be very noticeable because of the proximity of the heart to the chest wall.

Pulse, Blood Pressure, and Respirations

The techniques for assessing pulse and blood pressure are described in Chapter 36. Normal findings for children of different ages are shown in Appendix G. Abnormal pulse patterns that tend to occur in children with heart disorders are shown in Table 41.1. Tachycardia is a pulse rate more than 160 bpm in an infant and more than 100 bpm at 3 years of age or older. An increase in pulse rate over these standards needs further investigation. Tachycardia

---

BOX 41.2 ASSESSMENT

Assessing the Child With a Cardiovascular Disorder

History
Chief concern: Fatigue, cyanosis, frequent upper respiratory infections, feeding difficulty, poor weight gain, growth failure.
Past medical history: Infection during pregnancy, difficulty with resuscitation at birth.
Family history: Other members with heart disorders.

Physical examination
Decreased height and weight
Easily fatigued

- Frequent nose bleeds
- Cyanosis of mucous membrane or polycythemia (redness)
- Tachypnea or tachycardia
- Displaced apex beat
- Heart murmur
- Enlarged liver
- Absent femoral pulses
- Faint peripheral pulses
- Clubbing of fingers
- Pain in legs

TABLE 41.1

Abnormal Pulse Patterns

Pulse Pattern	Description
Water hammer	Very forceful and bounding pulse (Corrigan's pulse); capillary pulsations possibly apparent even in the fingernails; suggestive of cardiac insufficiency, as in patent ductus arteriosus
Pulsus alternans	A pulse of one strong beat and one weak beat; suggestive of myocardial weakness
Dicrotic	A double radial pulse for every apical beat; symptomatic of aortic stenosis
Thready	Weak and usually rapid pulse; suggestive of ineffective heart action

is particularly significant if it persists during sleep, when the possibility of excitement and activity is removed.

Murmurs of no significance are termed functional, insignificant, or innocent murmurs. In discussing such murmurs with parents, the term **innocent heart murmur** is best to use because it most clearly describes that the sound heard is not important or is nothing to worry about. Such murmurs probably reflect a normal variation of vibration in the heart or pulmonary artery.

Although innocent murmurs are of no consequence, parents need to be told when their child has one because this finding will undoubtedly be discovered again at a future health assessment. Teach parents that although an innocent murmur is present, it is not a sign of any heart disease. Activities need not be restricted, and the child will require no more frequent health appraisals than other children. Also teach parents that innocent murmurs do not turn into serious murmurs; otherwise, some parents can view them as a prelude to heart disease. They may become more pronounced during febrile illness, anxiety, or pregnancy. This is why they may be audible for the first time at a hospital admission or at a sick-child visit. At future health assessments, parents may need to be reassured again that a murmur is innocent.

If a murmur occurs as the result of heart disease or a congenital defect, it is termed an **organic heart murmur.** The characteristics of innocent and organic murmurs are compared in Table 41.2.

Describe any murmur that you hear according to the following criteria:

- Its position in the cardiac cycle (e.g., early systolic, midsystolic, late diastolic)
- Duration (how long the sound lasts)
- Quality (blowing, rasping, rumbling)
- Pitch (high- or low-sounding noise)
- Intensity (loudness)
- Location (where it is heard best or the point of maximum intensity)
- Presence of a thrill (a palpable purring sensation)
- The response of the murmur to exercise or change of position.

TABLE 41.2

Comparison of Innocent and Organic Murmurs

Characteristic	Innocent	Organic
Timing	Systolic	Systolic or diastolic
Duration	Short	Longer
Quality	Soft, musical	Harsh, blowing
Intensity	Soft	Loud
Position in which heard	Usually supine positions	Heard in all positions
Affected by exercise	Yes	No

The intensity, or loudness, of the murmur is graded according to the standard criteria shown in Table 33.9.

Diagnostic Tests

The diagnostic studies performed on a child with suspected heart disease vary with the specific lesion suspected.

Electrocardiogram

An **electrocardiogram** (ECG) is a written record of the electrical voltages generated by the contracting heart. It provides information about heart rate, rhythm, state of the myocardium, presence or absence of hypertrophy (thickening of the heart walls), ischemia or necrosis due to inadequate cardiac circulation, and abnormalities of conduction. It also can provide information about the presence or effect of various drugs and electrolyte imbalances.

On an ECG waveform tracing, an upward pattern indicates a positive voltage, whereas a downward pattern indicates a negative voltage. The heartbeat is initiated by the sinoatrial (SA) node in the right atrial wall near the entrance of the superior vena cava. From the SA node, the electrical impulse spreads over the atria, reaching the atrioventricular (AV) node in the lower right atrium. From there, it spreads through the AV bundle (bundle of His) and the Purkinje fibers to the walls and septum of the ventricles. At the point that the ventricles have filled, the electrical flow has reached a peak, causing the ventricles to contract.

A normal ECG consists of an atrial wave (the P wave, denoting atrial depolarization), a brief hesitation before the AV node is activated, then the prominent ventricular peak (the QRS spike), another brief hesitation, and then a large slow wave caused by ventricular recovery (the T wave, denoting repolarization), and often an incompletely understood additional slow wave (the U wave; Fig. 41.2). A longer-than-normal P wave suggests that the atria are hypertrophied and it is taking longer than usual for the electrical conduction to spread over the atria. A lengthened P-R interval suggests that there is difficulty in coordination between the SA and AV nodes (first-degree heart block). A heightened R wave indicates that ventricular hypertrophy is present. An R wave that is decreased in height means that the ventricles cannot contract fully, as happens if they are surrounded by fluid (pericarditis). Elongation of the T wave occurs in hyperkalemia; depression of the T wave is associated with anoxia; depression of the ST segment is associated with abnormal calcium levels.

Checkpoint Question 1

Megan has a heart murmur from tetralogy of Fallot, a congenital heart disorder. This type of murmur is termed:

a. Innocent
b. Functional
c. Organic
d. Symmetrical

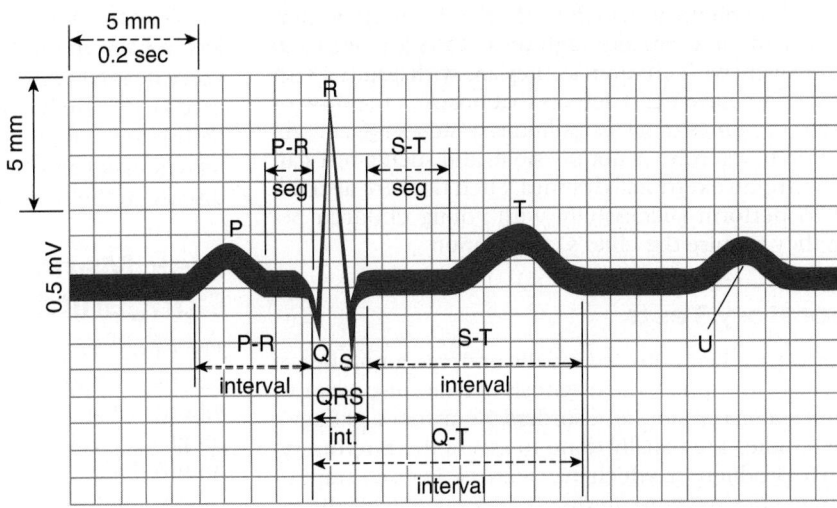

FIGURE 41.2 A normal ECG configuration.

X-ray

X-ray examination can furnish an accurate picture of the heart size and the contour and size of the heart chambers. It can reveal fluid collecting in the lungs or pulmonary artery from cardiac failure. It also can be used to confirm the placement of pacemaker leads. In a posteroanterior view (in children over 1 year of age), if the cardiac width is more than half the chest width, it indicates that the heart is unusually enlarged. In infants, because of the more horizontal position of the heart, this ratio must be increased to more than half.

In addition to a chest x-ray, an upper gastrointestinal (UGI) series may be done. This is because the esophagus is located so close to cardiac chambers that when it is visualized with barium, it can help define cardiovascular structures. Even with this technique, interpretation of atrial or ventricular hypertrophy in infants and children by x-ray is difficult. X-ray findings are therefore usually complemented by ECG, a more sensitive and accurate measure of ventricular enlargement.

Fluoroscopy, a form of radiography, provides a permanent motion-picture record of important information about the size and configuration of the heart and great vessels, lungs, thoracic cage, and diaphragm. Because prolonged observation is necessary to record this information, special precautions must be taken to protect the child and health care personnel from radiation during an assessment.

In radioangiocardiography, a radioactive substance such as technetium is injected intravenously into the bloodstream. As the substance circulates through the heart, it may be traced and recorded on videotape. The procedure involves a low dose of radiation and may be used to demonstrate, in particular, septal shunts.

Generalized angiography, or instillation of dye followed by x-rays, has little value in demonstrating pediatric heart defects. Selective angiocardiography, however, performed as part of a cardiac catheterization, allows identification of specific heart abnormalities if followed by serial x-ray films. After a contrast medium has been introduced into a specific heart chamber, closed-circuit video equipment records fluoroscopy pictures. Angiocardiography is not without hazard: deaths have been reported from sensitiv-

ity to the dye used, cardiac arrhythmias, and pulmonary edema.

Echocardiography

Echocardiography, or ultrasound cardiography, has become the primary diagnostic test for heart disease (Lambert, Fox, & Chhiv, 2004). High-frequency sound waves, directed toward the heart, are used to locate and study the movement and dimensions of cardiac structures, such as the size of chambers, thickness of walls, relationship of major vessels to chambers, and the thickness, motion, and pressure gradients of valves. This technique is referred to as M-mode, a single beam that reveals chamber contractility; two-dimensional, a technique used to reveal chamber and vessel size; and Doppler technique, which reveals the velocity of blood flow. Remind parents that echocardiography does not use x-rays so it can be repeated at frequent intervals without exposing children to the possible risk of radiation. It may be done using a transesophageal probe to better reveal heart chambers. Fetal echocardiography can reveal heart anomalies as early as 18 weeks into a pregnancy. This can alert staff to be prepared with immediate resuscitation or other needed equipment at the baby's birth (Simpson, 2004).

Phonocardiography and Magnetic Resonance Imaging

A **phonocardiogram** is a diagram of heart sounds translated into electrical energy by a microphone placed on the child's chest and then recorded as a diagrammatic representation of heart sounds. The technique can measure the timing of heart sounds that occur too quickly or at too high or too low a sound frequency for the human ear to detect by direct auscultation. Magnetic resonance imaging (MRI) may also be used to evaluate heart structure or size or blood flow (Reddy & Higgins, 2003).

Exercise Testing

Exercise tests using treadmill walking to demonstrate that the pulmonary circulation can increase to meet the increased respiratory demands of exercise may be performed with children, although these tests are not used as extensively with children as they are with adults. With children who have heart defects that obstruct the flow of blood to the lungs (such as pulmonary stenosis), accommodation to exercise is not possible, and such a test can cause extreme exertional dyspnea. Such tests are also difficult to perform successfully with young children because they require the child's cooperation.

Laboratory Tests

Children with heart disease usually undergo a number of blood tests to support the diagnosis of heart disease or to rule out anemia or clotting disorders. Hematocrit or hemoglobin studies are usually done to assess the rate of erythrocyte production, which may increase in an attempt to produce more oxygen-carrying red blood cells. If the increase in the number of red blood cells is extreme (polycythemia), there will be a corresponding increase in blood volume and possibly an increase in blood viscosity. Newborns are normally slightly polycythemic. In a newborn, polycythemia is defined as a hemoglobin level over 25 g/100 mL or a hematocrit level over 70%. In an older child, polycythemia is defined as a hemoglobin level over 16 g/100 mL or a hematocrit level over 55%. An elevated erythrocyte sedimentation rate (ESR) denotes inflammation and is useful in documenting that an inflammatory process, such as occurs with rheumatic fever, Kawasaki disease, or myocarditis, is present (Fischbach, 2005).

Blood gas levels also are determined. To test for this, a child is given 100% oxygen for 15 minutes. If the child still has a Po_2 less than 150 mm Hg after this time, a shunt directing deoxygenated blood into oxygenated blood can be suspected. Oxygen saturation levels also are assessed; children with a deoxygenated to oxygenated shunt will have a lower-than-normal oxygen saturation level in arterial blood. Normally, arterial blood oxygen saturation is 95% to 100%; oxygen saturation is usually less than 92% when venous arterial shunts are present.

Before cardiac catheterization or surgery, blood clotting must be assessed. Expect prothrombin and partial thromboplastin times and platelet count studies to be completed before the procedure. Some children with polycythemia from heart disease have an associated reduced platelet count (thrombocytopenia). Because platelet formation is necessary for blood coagulation, the platelet count must be corrected before cardiac surgery.

In children with heart failure, a serum sodium level may be obtained to ensure that an increased sodium level is not causing edema. All children receiving diuretics should have serum potassium levels determined because diuretics tend to deplete the body of potassium. Low serum potassium levels potentiate or increase the effect of cardiac glycosides, such as digoxin. For this reason, serum potassium levels are also usually obtained in children receiving these medications.

HEALTH PROMOTION AND RISK MANAGEMENT

Cardiac disease prevention in adults has received extensive attention in health literature. Because the risk factors that lead to adult heart disease, such as obesity, high cholesterol serum levels, and lack of consistent exercise, involve health habits that begin in childhood, prevention of cardiac disease has shifted from an adult to a child focus. Early interventions to reduce risk factors in early life should have a major impact on reducing the incidence of heart disease in the next generation.

Risk Management for Congenital Heart Disease

The cause of congenital heart disease often cannot be documented, although it is associated with familial patterns of inheritance and possibly triggers such as infection during pregnancy. All women of childbearing age should be immunized against rubella (German measles) and varicella (chickenpox) because these viruses are known to cause heart damage to a fetus if the mother contracts them during pregnancy. Because some types of congenital heart disorders have a familial incidence, parents who have a family member born with a heart defect need to alert their primary care provider so that other children can be carefully screened prenatally and at birth for a similar disorder.

Risk Management for Acquired Heart Disease

Acquired heart diseases in children that have identified risk factors include rheumatic fever, hypertension, and hyperlipidemia. Rheumatic fever is an autoimmune response that follows a group A beta-hemolytic streptococcal infection. Ensuring that all parents know that children with streptococcal infections from otitis media, streptococcal pharyngitis, and impetigo should receive adequate antibiotic therapy is essential for disease prevention (Hoffman, 2003).

Although hypertension (elevated blood pressure) occurs mainly because of a genetic predisposition, a high intake of sodium (such as table salt), lack of exercise, and obesity increase the chances that a susceptible child will develop the disorder by late childhood (Schulman, 2003). If infants are never introduced to high-sodium foods, perhaps by the time they are selecting their own meals they will continue to eat a low-sodium diet, helping to prevent the development of hypertension in later life. For this reason, baby food manufacturers have stopped adding salt and monosodium glutamate to infant food. Urging school-age children and adolescents to reduce their intake of canned soups, cheese, lunch meats, and hot dogs, all foods with high sodium content, can reduce salt intake in these age groups. School nurses can play an important role in this effort by monitoring the foods served daily in school cafeterias and advocating for more nutritious menus. Beginning when a child is 3 years of age, blood pressure should be included as part of routine assessment to detect hypertension as early as possible (NCHS, 2005).

Although the tendency toward hyperlipidemia is inherited, a diet high in saturated fat has been implicated in the development of the syndrome. It is important that fat intake not be restricted in infants because they need fat and the calories it provides for brain growth. School-age children and adolescents, however, should reduce their fat intake to 30% of total calories (the same recommendation as for adults). The use of vegetable oils in place of saturated fat should begin when children begin solid food. Children from high-risk families (a family member has had an early myocardial infarction or hyperlipidemia) should be regularly screened for elevated cholesterol and triglyceride levels beginning at about 3 years of age. Children with total cholesterol values above 170 mg/dL should receive nutritional counseling and instruction about a regular exercise program to enhance their health (Liacouras, 2003).

NURSING CARE OF THE CHILD WITH A CARDIAC DISORDER

Most parents have many questions about how to care for a child with heart disease. Encourage them to learn as much as possible about their child's disorder. Encourage them to handle and feed their newborn in the hospital so they can feel secure in caring for him or her at home. Be certain they recognize that not all children with heart disease have the same disease or need the same degree of restriction. If this is not made clear to parents, they may unnecessarily limit their child's activity, assuming that because another child was told not to do some activity, their child should not do it either.

NURSING DIAGNOSES AND RELATED INTERVENTIONS

———◆———

Nursing Diagnosis: Parental health-seeking behaviors related to desire to be informed about child's disorder

Outcome Evaluation: Parents accurately state the nature of their child's illness and unique needs of the child; can name primary care providers who will follow child's progress; state they will telephone or e-mail if they have any questions.

Provide Information About Care. Parents generally ask whether it is safe to let a baby with heart disease cry. If the infant has a cardiac disorder such as tetralogy of Fallot in which cyanotic spells tend to develop, the baby should not be allowed to cry for long periods of time (no baby should). However, crying for a few minutes while a parent warms formula or fully awakens at night will, as a rule, not harm the baby.

Another common question is, "Does our child need special nutrition?" As with all newborns, breast-feeding is the preferred method of feeding, and the average infant with heart disease can be successful at this (Barbas & Kelleher, 2004). Salt is rarely restricted during early life because infants need sodium to regulate water balance. Because

anemia stresses the heart, infants are generally given an iron supplement, either with formula or separately, to prevent iron deficiency anemia during the first year. Like all infants, they should receive supplemental vitamins with formula or when breast-feeding is stopped. Because some infants with congenital heart disease tire readily, frequent small feedings during the day may be necessary. If a child is an extremely poor eater, a high-calorie formula or enteral or gastrostomy feedings may be necessary to supply enough calories for growth.

"How much activity can we allow the baby?" This answer depends on the type and extent of the heart disorder. As a rule, infants or young children naturally limit their own activity. Parents may need guidance, however, in setting limits on activity. Roughhousing with infants, such as tossing them up in the air and watching them squeal and laugh, or playing games such as chasing a ball may not be advisable. Encourage parents to observe their infant carefully to recognize the first signs of respiratory distress and the point at which a child's activity is beginning to exceed his or her tolerance. Caution parents to observe the child carefully and thoughtfully as new activities are introduced and new interests are gained, so that the child's activity is limited to what the heart can accommodate.

"What do we do if he becomes ill?" Although children with congenital heart disorders are usually seen by a cardiologist for health supervision, it is important that they are also seen by health care personnel who can ensure they are receiving normal childhood immunizations and health guidance. As a rule, infants with heart disorders need prompt treatment for minor illnesses. The fever that accompanies a cold, for instance, can increase the metabolic rate of a child who has a severe congenital heart disorder to beyond the point at which the child's heart can compensate. Dehydration must be avoided in children with polycythemia or the polycythemia may become so severe that clotting or thrombophlebitis may result. It is also important that infections be treated vigorously to avoid infectious endocarditis.

Children with congenital heart disorders or rheumatic fever need prophylactic antibiotic therapy before they have oral surgery (tooth extractions or tonsils removed). This is because the streptococcal organisms generally present in the mouth can lead to infectious endocarditis if the organisms enter the bloodstream during surgery. It is a good rule for parents to ask that their children be given prophylactic antibiotics before they visit the dentist at all, because they cannot always anticipate what procedures the dentist will do at any one visit. Oral penicillin is the preferred prophylactic antibiotic; erythromycin can be used for a child sensitive to penicillin. Some parents need reassurance that their child will not become immune to penicillin if it is taken this way over long periods. Children with congenital heart disorders should receive routine immunizations and influenza vaccines and should be considered for pneumonia vaccine.

Review Steps for Follow-Up Care and Emergencies.
Before parents leave the hospital with a newborn who has a congenital heart disorder, be certain they have the name and number of the person to call if they have a question about their infant's health (their primary care provider and an emergency telephone number as a back-up). Review with them the steps to take if their child should become cyanotic, such as placing him or her in a knee–chest position. Be certain they have an appointment for a first health assessment. This helps to reassure them that the responsibility of caring for this child will not be theirs alone but will be shared by concerned health care personnel. In many instances, parents are first-time parents. If they are unsure whether their child is in distress or ill, urge them to err on the side of caution by telephoning or bringing the child to their primary care setting. Everyone who cares for infants or children with heart disease appreciates the responsibility parents feel and the difficulty they can have in making health judgments about their child.

Most parents feel relieved to know they can have home follow-up after a hospitalization. In addition to providing opportunities for child and family assessment, home visits allow parents to discuss the frightening responsibility they feel and to obtain a second opinion about their child's health. Teach cardiopulmonary resuscitation (CPR) and how to activate the community's emergency medical system (EMS) before they leave the hospital. It may be reassuring for the parents to visit their closest EMS station so they know the staff is acquainted with their child should an emergency call be necessary.

The Child Having Cardiac Catheterization

Cardiac catheterization, a procedure in which a small radiopaque catheter is passed through a major vein in the arm, leg, or neck into the heart to secure blood samples or inject dye, helps to evaluate cardiac function (Kern et al., 2004). Diagnostic cardiac catheterization is used to help diagnose specific heart disorders in anticipation of surgery. Interventional cardiac catheterization is used to correct an abnormality, such as dilating a narrowed valve by the use of a balloon catheter or other device. With both types, the pressure of blood flow in all heart chambers and total cardiac output can be evaluated. Blood specimens can be obtained to determine oxygen saturation levels, or a contrast dye can be injected for angiography. Electrodes can be introduced to record electrical activity and diagnose arrhythmias.

This procedure may be done as ambulatory or 1-day surgery using conscious sedation. Children must have a recent chest x-ray, ECG, and electrolyte levels, and blood must be typed and cross-matched before the procedure. Take and record pedal pulses for a baseline assessment. Also measure and record height and weight. This information is used to determine catheter size and the amount

of sedation to be administered. Because the vessel site chosen for catheterization must not be infected at the time of catheterization (or obscured by a hematoma), do not draw blood specimens from the projected catheterization entry site before the procedure (generally a femoral vein). Children scheduled for the procedure are usually kept NPO for 2 to 4 hours beforehand to reduce the danger of vomiting and aspiration during the procedure.

In the cardiac catheterization room, ECG and pulse oximetry leads are attached. The site for catheterization is locally anesthetized with EMLA cream or intradermal lidocaine, and a catheter is threaded through a large-bore needle into a blood vessel. The specific vessel used differs according to the technique being planned. In neonates, an umbilical artery can be catheterized. For right-side heart catheterization, a right femoral vein or a vein in the antecubital fossa usually is used. Left-side heart catheterization can be performed using either a venous or an arterial approach. If done by the arterial route, a catheter is inserted into either the femoral or brachial artery. If a venous route is used, the catheter is inserted into the right femoral vein. Under fluoroscopy, the catheter is advanced to the right atrium and then through the foramen ovale. Once the catheter is in a selected heart chamber, radiopaque dye can be injected to outline the heart configuration (Fig. 41.3).

Cardiac catheterization has a mortality rate of under 0.1% when done as an elective procedure and approximately 2% to 5% when performed in a severely distressed child (Kern et al., 2004). Arrhythmias may occur while the catheter is being passed through the heart chambers or when contrast dye is being injected. Such arrhythmias generally are transitory or stop abruptly with withdrawal of the catheter. Inadvertent perforation of the heart may occur during passage of the catheter. Other complications include bleeding from the insertion site (secondary to heparin introduced into the catheter to reduce the possibility of clot formation) and thrombophlebitis (from platelet aggregation due to irritation by the catheter, a foreign body). Because cardiac catheterization may be necessary so that the cardiac surgeon can visualize and plan a cardiac repair, the key to making cardiac surgery safe, the benefit of the procedure outweighs the risks.

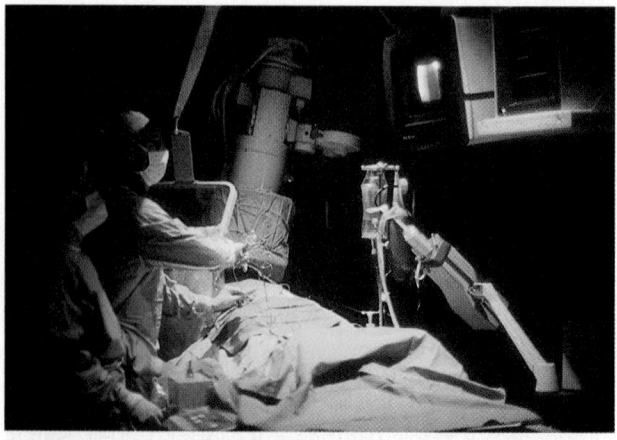

FIGURE 41.3 A child undergoing a cardiac catheterization. (© Hough/Custom Medical Stock Photo.)

NURSING DIAGNOSIS AND RELATED INTERVENTIONS: PREPROCEDURE PHASE

───●───

Nursing Diagnosis: Anxiety related to lack of knowledge about cardiac catheterization procedure

Outcome Evaluation: Parents and child (when possible) state goal of procedure and reasons for preparation and aftercare measures; state that anxiety is less after teaching.

Because most cardiac catheterizations are done with children under conscious sedation, children may need more information about what is going to happen during this procedure than they will need for cardiac surgery, when they will be fully anesthetized. Provide explanations about the procedure for the child with the parents present, if possible. This allows parents to help reinforce the information. After this explanation, provide parents with a more detailed explanation of the procedure and allow time to ask any questions they do not want to ask in the child's presence.

Parents often need a review of heart anatomy. Although the cardiologist may have already done this, many parents appreciate reinforcement and a review of this information. Show them the pathway the catheter will take during the procedure.

Be aware that consenting to a cardiac catheterization experience brings with it the realization that cardiac surgery may be necessary. As a result, parents may be so concerned with what the procedure may reveal that they cannot listen well to preprocedure explanations. Allow them to accompany their child to the catheterization room and, if possible and appropriate, to remain there for support during the procedure if they choose.

Review with the child what he or she will see in the catheterization room. Small children can become overwhelmed by seeing the actual equipment. Therefore, try building a facsimile room out of small cardboard boxes (representing the x-ray machine, the fluoroscopy screen, the ECG machine, and so forth). A puppet or small doll can serve as the patient in the miniature room. Dress the puppets in surgery suits and masks like those worn by cardiac catheterization personnel and act out what the child can expect to happen. Older children prefer a tour of the cardiac catheterization area and the opportunity to meet the personnel.

If children have never seen ECG leads or restraints before, let them touch and feel the equipment. Caution them the total procedure may be as long as 3 to 4 hours and that they will need to lie still during this time. Help them master imagery or

another stress-reduction technique to help reduce apprehension.

Do not underestimate what children know about their heart's purpose and function; even preschoolers know their heart is vital to their body. Reassure them that the doctors are only taking a look at their heart during this procedure, not cutting it or removing any part of it.

Teach children of all ages that when the catheter is inserted, it will not hurt. Caution them, however, that they may feel a momentary speeding up of their heart, a feeling that is uncomfortable. When dye is inserted, they may feel a stinging sensation. Do not use the word "dye," which young children may misinterpret as "die." Instead, say "medicine." Caution them that the lights will be turned off after the medicine is injected so a doctor can watch the medicine on a television screen (fluoroscopy) as it passes through the heart. Let children know that after the procedure, a pressure dressing will be placed over the catheter insertion site to reduce the risk of bleeding. They will need to keep that extremity flat and unbent to prevent the dressing from loosening.

NURSING DIAGNOSES AND RELATED INTERVENTIONS: POSTPROCEDURE PHASE

───●───

Nursing Diagnosis: Risk for ineffective cardiopulmonary and peripheral tissue perfusion related to cardiac catheterization

Outcome Evaluation: Child's vital signs remain within established parameters; absence of arrhythmia; absence of bleeding or hematoma formation at catheterization site; pedal pulse is present distal to catheterization site.

When a child returns from the procedure, assess the pressure dressing over the catheterization site to be certain it is snug and intact and no bleeding is present. Instruct the child not to bend the hip (if the femoral site was used) or the elbow (if the brachial site was used) to keep the pressure dressing secure and to prevent hematoma formation. This is particularly important when an artery was used for catheterization; a loose dressing on an artery will cause a large blood loss in a very short time. Palpate pulses and assess color, temperature, and circulation (blanch the toe or fingernail and watch to see that it turns pink again readily) distal to the insertion site to ensure that blood flow in the extremity is unobstructed. If there is bleeding at the insertion site, apply firm, continuous pressure and notify the physician who performed the procedure immediately.

Children often appreciate being asked to describe their experience afterward. Saying out loud how frightened they were—by the x-ray machine being pushed in over them or by the thought of a tube going all the way into their heart—helps alleviate their fear and allows better acceptance of the procedure. Praise them for their cooperation during a very stressful experience. Introduce therapeutic play if needed.

Keep the child flat in bed for 2 to 3 hours until he or she is completely awake from conscious sedation. This helps to prevent not only oozing at the insertion site but also postural hypotension, which may occur when a child rises suddenly after lying flat while under sedation for such a long period. In the immediate postcatheterization period, a child's blood pressure may be 10% to 15% lower than the precatheterization level because of the hypotensive effect of the radiopaque dye.

Cardiac arrhythmias and bradycardia may occur from the mechanical action of the catheter having touched the conduction nodes of the heart. Assess pulse, blood pressure, and respirations at frequent intervals (about every 15 minutes) for the first several hours. Monitor the pulse for a full minute to aid in recognizing abnormalities. Be alert for signs of arrhythmias. Small children cannot describe the odd feeling that accompanies an arrhythmia. Older children might describe it as the heart "fluttering" or "skipping beats." Therefore, be alert for signs of increasing anxiety in the child after a catheterization; this may be the child's way of reporting these feelings.

Infants may need intravenous (IV) fluid during the procedure and for several hours afterward to prevent dehydration, which could result from being NPO for a long period of time. If an infant is polycythemic, IV fluid helps minimize the risk of vessel thrombi. Regulate IV fluid carefully to prevent heart failure from fluid overload.

Assess temperature immediately after the procedure to determine a baseline. Some children have a transient elevation in temperature already due to physiologic dehydration as a result of having been NPO or as a reaction to the dye. Others have slightly subnormal temperature readings from lying in a cool procedure room for a lengthy period. This below-normal body temperature quickly compromises respiratory and heart action because, to raise body temperature, infants must increase their metabolic rate. This requires rapid breathing and increased heart action, which can lead to exhaustion. Infants may need to be placed under radiant heat warmers to help regain and maintain normal body temperature and also to allow accurate temperature determinations.

The adverse effects of cardiac catheterization may be spells of apnea, sternal retractions, or dyspnea. If oxygen was administered during the catheterization procedure, it may be continued for a period of time after the procedure to reduce the stress of respirations. Like arrhythmias, dyspnea, bradycardia, and blood pressure anomalies may be transient, but all should be reported so they can be evaluated.

Nursing Diagnosis: Risk for infection related to presence of cardiac catheterization incision site

Outcome Evaluation: The child's temperature remains less than 100.4°F (38.0°C) axillary; the catheter insertion site appears free of erythema or drainage.

If the dressing for a cardiac catheterization is over the femoral artery or vein, keep it clean of stool and urine. Waterproofing the dressing with plastic may be necessary. Also check the insertion site for signs of infection, because any opening in the skin is a portal of entry for bacteria. Alert parents to observe the catheter insertion site daily for redness. Most parents are advised to monitor their child's temperature daily for about 3 days and to omit tub baths and strenuous exercise for their child for 2 to 3 days to aid healing.

 Checkpoint Question 2

Megan is scheduled for a cardiac catheterization. Why might a child develop cardiac arrhythmias after this procedure?

a. The dye inserted can create inflamed heart chambers.
b. The many x-rays taken lead to a weakened heart muscle.
c. The catheter can irritate nerves in the heart septum.
d. Latex allergy can cause symptoms of unusual heart rate.

The Child Scheduled for Cardiac Surgery

There are many different types of congenital heart disorders, and many different procedures are available to correct them. Open-heart surgery, however, remains the chief cure for congenital heart disease (Bute, 2004). Open-heart surgery is made possible by the use of cardiopulmonary bypass or extracorporeal membrane oxygenation (ECMO). The venous return to the heart is diverted from the right atrium or inferior and superior vena cava to a heart–lung machine, where it is artificially oxygenated. It is returned to the body's arterial system by way of the aorta, bypassing the heart. The heart, practically bloodless, now can be opened and operated on. Blood returns to the coronary and pulmonary capillary beds under pressure from the aorta so that even though blood bypasses the heart, it still receives an adequate blood supply for self-maintenance during the bypass procedure (Tulenko,

2004). Very ill infants may be maintained on ECMO using the same technique after surgery.

During surgery, hypothermia (reducing the child's body temperature to 68° to 79°F [20° to 26°C]) is used to reduce the child's metabolic needs and slow the heart rate. If extreme hypothermia is used (59° to 68°F [15° to 20°C]), usually in an infant, the body temperature drops so low that the heart stops beating and the surgeon can work in a quiet and bloodless field. Measuring temperature to be certain the infant is rewarmed is a major responsibility (Maxton, Justin, & Gillies, 2004).

Preoperative Care

Before surgery, obtain vital signs (blood pressure, temperature, pulse, and respirations) to establish baselines. Count pulse and respiratory rates for a full minute for accuracy. Some children may need baseline pulse determinations done at several pulse points or blood pressures taken in both upper and lower extremities. Before obtaining a blood pressure, have a child rest for about 15 minutes and take the recording with the child lying down. Also record height and weight, because these parameters are necessary for the estimation of blood volume for the heart–lung machine and for medication dosages. Weighing also is helpful in estimating blood loss or edema after surgery. In children receiving digoxin, it is usually withheld 24 hours before surgery because cardiac surgery may cause arrhythmias in the presence of cardiac glycosides.

The immediate surgical preparation of children varies from one institution to another but usually includes preparing the skin incision site. The skin over the surgical incision area is scrubbed with an antiseptic solution to ensure as clean a surgical field as possible. Most children and parents are startled to learn that cardiac surgery may be performed through the sternal bone or the back, not over the left side of the chest, and may question the area being prepared for the incision. An enema also may be given to keep children from straining to pass stool in the immediate postoperative period and placing additional strain on the newly operated heart.

NURSING DIAGNOSES AND RELATED INTERVENTIONS: PREOPERATIVE PHASE

———————●———————

Nursing Diagnosis: Deficient knowledge related to cardiac surgery and its outcome

Outcome Evaluation: Parents and child accurately state the reason for surgery and expected outcome.

Bringing a child to the hospital for cardiac surgery is a large responsibility for parents. They want their child to be made well, but they are also aware there is a definite risk from this surgery. They may have been protecting and guarding their

child for months or years, and they feel no less protective the morning of surgery. For this reason, parents of children being readied for cardiac surgery may watch preoperative procedures more carefully than usual. Review with them what they already know about the surgery to correct any misconceptions and inform them what laboratory tests will be scheduled. Prepare them for the amount of equipment that will surround their child after surgery, such as cardiac monitors, oxygen and IV equipment, chest tubes, and a ventilator. Parents usually appreciate visiting the intensive care unit (ICU) where their child will go after surgery. Be certain they have an opportunity to meet the ICU staff, especially if those nurses are not the same ones who are caring for the child preoperatively.

Prepare Child for Surgery and Postoperative Care. It is best if a child is prepared for surgery with the parents present. This allows the parents the opportunity to reinforce your teaching and shows a child that his or her parents approve and feel secure with these surgery plans. Parents will then need additional time to discuss the surgical procedure with you and ask questions they might not have wished to ask in the presence of their child.

Do not underestimate how much children understand about the seriousness of this surgery (Fig. 41.4). Remember when caring for them preoperatively (or any time) not to make careless remarks. For example, statements such as, "These

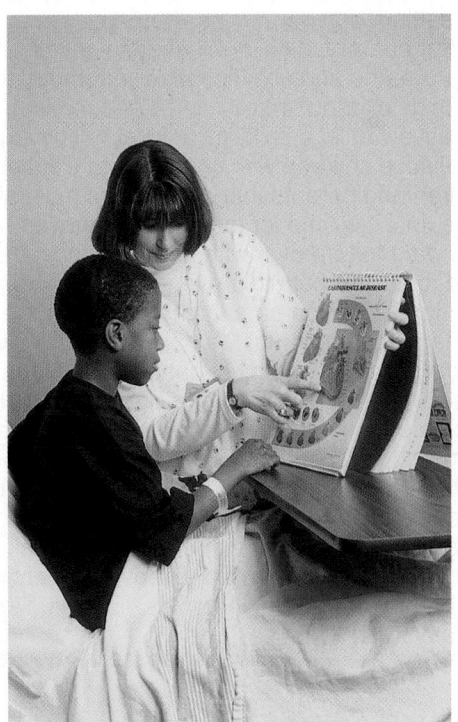

FIGURE 41.4 Orientation for cardiac surgery includes time for talking and learning more about the heart. (© Lesha Photography.)

syringes never work right" (when all you mean is you prefer another brand) or "Amy [an ICU nurse] is a real clown" (when you mean she is not only a competent nurse but has a good sense of humor besides) could be interpreted by anxious parents or children to mean a child is in less-than-competent hands. Because many children having cardiac surgery have had previous cardiac catheterizations, talking to them about their previous hospitalization experiences is helpful. Talking will reveal the things they fear the most this time. Any misconceptions they have about past experiences can then be discussed and clarified.

Both parents and children may have questions about the difference between cardiac catheterization and cardiac surgery. One important difference is that children are sedated but awake for the former but anesthetized for the latter. For some children, knowing they will be fully asleep is more reassuring; for others, it is more frightening. When they were awake, they knew that they were all right; asleep, how can they know? Encourage them to express these feelings so they can receive reassurance that anesthetized sleep is a special sleep from which they will have no difficulty waking. Meeting the anesthesiologist and receiving reassurance directly from him or her that they will be watched over while they are asleep is often helpful.

As with cardiac catheterization, it may help to make models of the equipment that will surround the child postoperatively. Parents and older children can be taken to the ICU where they will return after surgery and be shown the actual equipment and setting.

After surgery, a child will need to cough and deep-breathe and use incentive spirometry to help the lungs expand. Introduce these exercises preoperatively to let a child know what will be expected. Familiarize children with chest tubes. Caution both children and parents that chest tubes must stay in place until it is time for them to be removed. If children want to turn over with tubes in place, they need to ask for help to prevent the tubes from being dislodged. Caution parents that a chest-tube drainage reservoir must remain below the level of the child's chest and must not be raised for any reason. If children are not familiar with ECG leads, introduce these as part of preoperative preparation. Comparing these tubes or leads to being "hooked up" like an astronaut is often appealing to children. In addition, introduce children to the form of oxygen therapy they will receive after surgery (mask, cannula, or ventilator) to avoid surprises. Orienting children to oxygen equipment is discussed in Chapter 40.

Postoperative Care

After surgery and before leaving the operating room, an x-ray film is taken and the child is weighed. Future estimates of lung expansion and weight, to reveal whether edema is accumulating from poor heart function, will be checked against these two measurements.

NURSING DIAGNOSES AND RELATED INTERVENTIONS: POSTOPERATIVE PHASE

Nursing Diagnosis: Risk for ineffective cardiopulmonary tissue perfusion related to cardiac surgery

Outcome Evaluation: Vital signs are within normal limits; central venous pressure (CVP) or pulmonary artery wedge pressure is within established parameters.

Taking accurate vital signs, as often as every 15 minutes, is essential in the immediate postoperative period following cardiac surgery. Continuous cardiac monitoring and assisted ventilation with endotracheal intubation also are usually necessary. Blood pressure will probably be monitored directly by means of an intra-arterial catheter or indirectly with an automated blood pressure recording device. Hemodynamic monitoring by way of a pulmonary artery or central venous catheter will reveal information on chamber pressures and oxygen saturation (Fig. 41.5).

Adequate voiding after surgery indicates that the kidneys are receiving an adequate blood flow or the

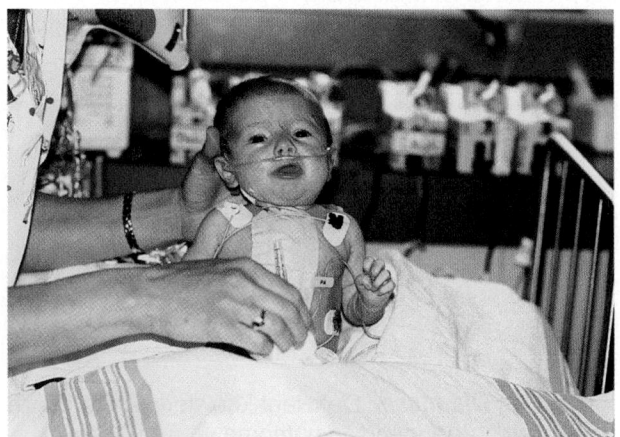

FIGURE 41.5 Because children after cardiac surgery typically have a myriad of wires and tubes attached to monitors, pumps, and equipment, parents need to be prepared for how their child will look. As the child's condition improves, use of the equipment is discontinued. Here, an infant is 2 days post-cardiac surgery. Note his level of alertness and the use of only a few monitoring devices and equipment. (© Caroline Brown, RNC, MS, DEd.)

heart is working effectively. An indwelling urinary (Foley) catheter is usually inserted at the time of surgery so urine output can be carefully recorded postoperatively (it should be 1 mL/kg/hour). Be certain to mark the amount of urine drainage present when children first return from surgery so that lack of or diminished urinary output will not be missed or misinterpreted. Individual samples may be tested for specific gravity and pH. A specific gravity below 1.010 implies that the kidneys are not concentrating urine well, perhaps because of the stress of surgery. The pH should remain slightly acid; however, extreme acidity may indicate respiratory acidosis from poor pulmonary perfusion.

Carefully record all IV fluid administered to the child after heart surgery. Fluid overload can pose a severe threat to the heart during the immediate postoperative period. Use an infusion control device to regulate the amount and rate of infusion.

Laboratory tests such as arterial blood gases (Po_2 and Pco_2), hemoglobin, hematocrit, clotting time, and electrolytes (particularly sodium and potassium) will be monitored closely to assess cardiac and pulmonary function postoperatively. Oxygen saturation levels may be monitored by pulse oximetry or transcutaneous oxygen monitoring. A drug such as dopamine may be administered to improve cardiac output.

Central Venous Pressure Monitoring. CVP may be recorded by inserting a catheter into a brachial, jugular, or subclavian vein, and ultimately into the right atrium (Fig. 41.6). CVP is an excellent way to evaluate a child's fluid volume status. CVP will rise with heart failure, indicating that the heart cannot handle the blood arriving at the atria.

Pulmonary Artery Pressure Monitoring. To assess pressure in the left side of the heart parallel to CVP

measurement, a multilumen pulmonary artery catheter, such as a Swan-Ganz catheter, can be threaded through the venous circulation through the right side of the heart and into the pulmonary artery. The pressure, registered there as a waveform on a cardiac monitor, reflects both the resistance of the lungs to the passage of blood (pulmonary artery resistance) and the ability of the left side of the heart to handle the circulating fluid volume. Such catheters must be kept from clotting with frequent irrigations or with a constant infusion system. When withdrawing blood specimen samples from the catheter, make sure no air is allowed to enter, because this would immediately flow into the left side of the heart and possibly to a cerebral artery as an embolus.

Nursing Diagnosis: Impaired gas exchange related to unexpanded lung space and collection of lung excretions

Outcome Evaluation: Child's respiratory rate remains within age-appropriate parameters; absence of rales or other adventitious breath sounds; chest tubes function normally.

Measures to Prevent Pooling of Secretions in Lungs. Suction as necessary while a child is receiving ventilatory assistance to prevent pooling of secretions in the respiratory tract. As soon as the endotracheal tube and ventilator are removed, encourage the child to cough and deep-breathe or use an incentive spirometer at hourly intervals to help mobilize secretions. Although a child may have practiced such procedures preoperatively, he or she may have difficulty carrying them out now because coughing or deep-breathing can be very painful, especially without continuous pain relief. To minimize the pain, administer the prescribed analgesia or alert the child to use the patient-controlled

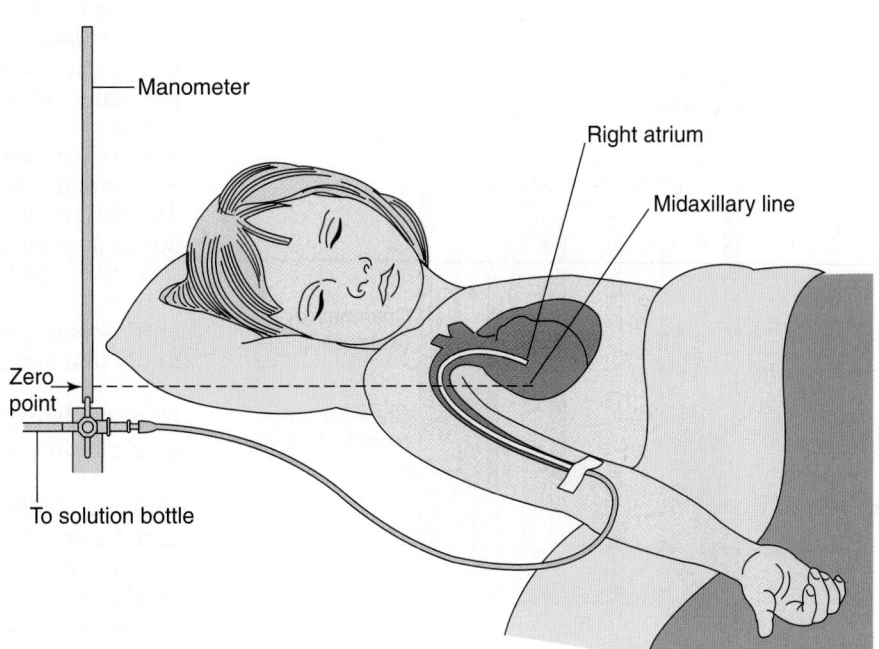

FIGURE 41.6 A CVP catheter may be inserted after cardiac surgery to monitor fluid volume. The zero point on the scale is at the level of the right atrium.

analgesia (PCA) pump 10 to 15 minutes before it is time to deep-breathe. For optimal effectiveness, demonstrating coughing again, sometimes deep-breathing with the child, may be necessary. Chest physiotherapy with percussion and vibration may be prescribed to keep lung secretions mobile. Be certain parents understand that games such as blowing cotton balls or blowing up a balloon are not really games but important exercises to help achieve lung expansion. Otherwise, they may interpret these exercises as too tiring for the child and discourage them.

Most children have two thoracotomy chest tubes inserted following surgery. The upper tube drains air to aid lung re-expansion and the lower one drains fluid to encourage lung expansion and decrease the possibility of infection. These tubes are connected to a water-seal drainage apparatus (a Pleur-Evac; Fig. 41.7).

Pleur-Evacs consist of three chambers: one to collect drainage, one to furnish a water seal, and one that can be attached to suction. A thoracotomy tube connects to the first drainage compartment. Because of the water seal, atmospheric air cannot enter the tube and flow back into the pleural space. Note how much drainage is occurring and if the level of fluid fluctuates (proof that the apparatus is airtight). On the third or fourth postoperative day, the fluctuation will cease, indicating that the lungs are fully expanded. Then it is time for the tubes to be removed.

Maintain children with chest tubes in place in a semi-Fowler's position because thoracotomy tubes drain best in this position; often there is less dyspnea as well, because the chest is elevated and the abdominal contents do not press on the lungs. Always keep thoracotomy chest tube drainage systems below the level of the child's chest so that fluid does not flow back into the pleural space.

Check that tube connections are secure and that the Pleur-Evac is not cracked or broken. Otherwise, air can enter the chest cavity and collapse the lungs (pneumothorax).

Mark the fluid level in the collecting chamber immediately after surgery. Continue to mark the level of fluid in the drainage chamber every hour so the hourly amount of drainage can be evaluated (approximately 5 mL/kg/hour is typical). Also note the color and the presence of any clots in the drainage. Drainage fluid may be blood-tinged but should not contain fresh blood. If it does, this suggests active bleeding.

A chest x-ray taken on the third or fourth postoperative day will confirm that full lung expansion has returned. The tubes are then removed by a physician or nurse practitioner while an impervious dressing is simultaneously applied to the puncture wound. Provide emotional support during thoracotomy tube removal. Children know these tubes are important for their well-being. Aside from worrying about the momentary pain of removal, they may believe that something bad will happen after the tubes are removed. Do not change any dressings over former thoracotomy tube sites, because lifting them to change them could allow air to enter.

Occasionally, despite being cautioned not to, a child may turn so suddenly after surgery that he or she pulls a thoracotomy tube out accidentally. This creates an emergency situation because air rushing into the child's chest can cause a pneumothorax with sudden dyspnea, tachycardia, cyanosis, and perhaps sharp chest pain. If a tube is only loosened or air is leaking slowly through a connection, the symptoms may be less dramatic but include restlessness and apprehension accompanying gradually increasing dyspnea. If the air entering the chest is the result of air leaking into the tubing, clamp the tube close to the child's chest with a large clamp to prevent further air from entering the chest. If the tube actually has been pulled out, immediately close the puncture wound to the chest by covering it with petrolatum gauze, a type of dressing that is impervious to air. If such gauze is not immediately available, place your gloved hand over the puncture wound and hold it snugly in place until help arrives. The child may need emergency oxygen administration to counteract the decreased amount of air exchange space he or she is experiencing as a result of partial lung collapse. Remaining calm will help a child remain calm, which will avoid increasing respiratory rate and oxygen demand.

Nursing Diagnosis: Risk for infection related to surgical incision and tube sites

Outcome Evaluation: Child's temperature remains at or below 100.4°F (38.0°C) axillary; incision site is clean, dry, and without evidence of erythema or foul drainage.

Some children are begun on a prophylactic course of a broad-spectrum antibiotic before

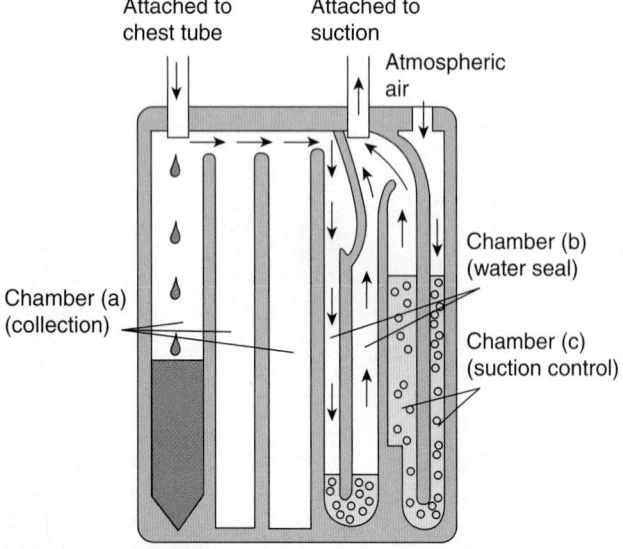

FIGURE 41.7 Pleur-Evac system for chest tube drainage.

surgery. If so, this will be continued for 24 to 48 hours postoperatively. Frequently monitor temperature postoperatively to assess for infection. Frequently assess the dressing over the surgical incision and the points of insertion of the thoracotomy tubes for drainage and erythema. Use strict aseptic technique when changing the incisional dressing to avoid introducing pathogens.

Nursing Diagnosis: Hypothermia related to cooling during surgery

Outcome Evaluation: Child's temperature is above 96.8°F (36.0°C) axillary. Capillary refill is less than 5 seconds.

If hypothermia was induced for surgery, the child's temperature will be low postoperatively and a hyperthermia blanket, warm blankets, or radiant heat may be necessary to elevate the temperature to normal. Alternatively, a child's temperature may be above normal because of an inflammatory response to hypothermia. Unless infection is developing, these temperature readings will gradually return to normal in a few days.

Nursing Diagnosis: Risk for excess or deficient fluid volume related to fluid shifts accompanying cardiac surgery

Outcome Evaluation: Child maintains weight; skin turgor is good; central venous pressure or pulmonary artery pressure is within established parameters.

Children tend to develop hypervolemia after cardiac surgery because of increased production of aldosterone by the adrenal glands and an increase in antidiuretic hormone secretion by the pituitary gland in response to stress. Also, if cardiopulmonary bypass was used, some fluid may have been shifted from the intravascular system to the interstitial spaces during surgery. After surgery, this fluid returns by osmosis to the vessels, increasing hypervolemia. On the other hand, an individual child may have experienced excessive bleeding because of the heparin used during surgery and may subsequently develop hypovolemia.

Monitor central venous or pulmonary artery pressure to evaluate a child's hemodynamic status. Monitor IV fluid administration carefully to prevent fluid overload. Typically, oral fluid intake is withheld for at least the first 24 hours after surgery. Once bowel sounds have returned, oral fluids can be introduced gradually.

Nursing Diagnosis: Parental anxiety related to lack of knowledge of postoperative routine and exercises

Outcome Evaluation: Family members accurately state plans for child's postoperative recovery; relate less anxiety after teaching and support.

Most children recover quickly from heart surgery. Passive range-of-motion exercises may be pre-scribed the day of surgery. By 24 hours, children are out of bed and ambulating. Encourage parents to do whatever they want to for their child's care during this period. It is difficult for them to accept the fact the surgery is over and their child is now a well child (or will be at the end of the recovery period).

Offering the child sips of water or helping him or her take a bath (under supervision) helps parents see that their child is returning to usual activities and doing well. Be certain that in the midst of the postoperative excitement, the child receives adequate rest the first postoperative days. You may need to monitor and regulate visits by staff and outside visitors to make sure a child is undisturbed for sustained rest periods. Urge parents to read to children or play music for them as a way to provide quiet rest periods. Caution parents not to pick up an infant under the arms, because this pulls on the chest incision. Show them how to lift an infant by placing their hands under the shoulders and buttocks instead.

Once the immediate postoperative period has passed, the child will be moved from the ICU to a routine patient unit. This may be a difficult move for both the child and the parents because they have developed confidence in the ICU staff and are reluctant to entrust the child to new personnel (even if the patient unit is the one to which the child was initially admitted before surgery). It helps the transition if the regular nursing staff visits the child daily in the ICU. Generally, place children returning from the ICU in a room near the nursing station, and place the bed so it can be easily seen from the hallway. Although you are not providing the constant attendance that the child received in the ICU, you can show that you are very observant and aware of individual needs. Stopping to look in every time you pass the room reassures the family that you are always close by. Allow parents an opportunity to voice their concern over the change in personnel and surroundings. Accepting this change can help prepare them for the day of hospital discharge, when they will be observing and caring for their child on their own.

At hospital discharge, parents need clear explanations of the activities in which the child will and will not be able to participate. Be sure they have an appointment for a checkup for the child and the telephone number they should call if they have any questions regarding their child's care. The protectiveness they felt for the child before surgery does not diminish instantly, even though surgery has been completed. They may find themselves saying, "Don't run" for months after the child has been allowed full activity. They may appreciate a listening ear for their concerns, which may include feeling they are not as important to their child as they were when the child was ill. Emphasize that well children also need continued parental supervision and guidance (Box 41.3).

BOX 41.3 FOCUS ON . . .

COMMUNICATION

Megan is a 3-month-old infant who is being discharged after cardiac surgery. You stop at her hospital room to give discharge instructions to her mother.

Less Effective Communication

Nurse: Good morning, Mrs. Carver. Let me review a few instructions with you.

Mrs. Carver: The most important thing you can tell me is how to keep a baby on bed rest.

Nurse: Most infants are so exhausted from surgery, they automatically reduce their activity, so that's not a problem. You can let her return to her usual activities at as near normal a level as possible.

Mrs. Carver: She likes to kick a mobile. It'll be hard to keep her from doing that.

Nurse: Her appetite should be back to normal in a few days. Check back with the clinic if it doesn't improve.

Mrs. Carver: I don't understand how she'll eat well if she has to be in bed all the time.

Nurse: Megan will need to continue to take digoxin until she returns for her checkup in 1 week. Do you have any questions about the dose?

Mrs. Carver: No. It'll be hard to get her to cooperate, though, when she's unhappy about having to stay in bed all the time.

Nurse: You'll need to check the incision daily and report any redness or increasing pain.

Mrs. Carver: I can do that. The thing I'll have trouble with is keeping her on bed rest.

Nurse: Infants generally limit their own activity, so that shouldn't be a problem. Wait here, now, until I call transportation to take you downstairs.

More Effective Communication

Nurse: Good morning, Mrs. Carver. Let me review a few instructions with you.

Mrs. Carver: The most important thing you can tell me is how to keep a baby on bed rest.

Nurse: Most infants are so exhausted from surgery, they automatically reduce their activity, so that's not a problem. You can let her return to her usual activities at as near normal a level as possible.

Mrs. Carver: She likes to kick a mobile in bed. It'll be hard to keep her from doing that.

Nurse: You'll need to check the incision daily and report any redness or increasing pain.

Mrs. Carver: I can do that. The thing I'll have trouble with is keeping her on bed rest.

Nurse: You've mentioned bed rest several times. Megan doesn't have to stay on bed rest. Let's talk about what activities she can do.

Because cardiac surgery is such serious surgery, most parents assume that it will take their child a very long time to recover from it. In the above scenarios, the mother has overestimated the time it will take her child to return to normal activities. Only when really listening to what the mother is saying, rather than just continuing to review discharge instructions, does the nurse recognize that the mother has not heard the first instruction—let the child return to activities at as near normal a level as possible.

Complications

A number of complications can arise after cardiac surgery because of the use of cardiopulmonary bypass and the extent of the surgery. The first of these is hemorrhage, because heparin is used to prevent blood coagulation during the cardiopulmonary bypass. Although protamine sulfate (the antidote for heparin) is administered IV immediately after surgery, some heparin is still present in the child's system. Monitor the coagulation time and vital signs and observe thoracotomy tube drainage to identify early signs of bleeding.

Shock, another possible complication, is revealed by hypotension, oliguria, acidosis, and cyanosis. It may result from hypovolemia or cardiac tamponade (bleeding into the heart muscle or pericardium, interfering with the heart's ability to contract forcibly), or it may be a reaction to prolonged extracorporeal perfusion. It is treated according to individual needs, including plasma volume expanders, continued mechanical ventilation, and perhaps a return to surgery to stop the bleeding. Heart block or arrhythmias may occur as the result of edema or trauma compromising the effectiveness of the bundle of His. An artificial pacemaker may be inserted to correct these problems. If the child had congestive heart disease before surgery, this may persist for a week or more after surgery. If it occurs as a new entity, it suggests that the surgery has caused a stricture to circulation at some point, causing either the right or left side of the heart to become overwhelmed. Measures for treating postoperative congestive heart failure are the same as those in children who have this syndrome from any cause. Neurologic symptoms, also a possible complication, may occur if the child experienced hypoxia during surgery.

A **postcardiac surgery syndrome** may develop at the end of the first postoperative week. This is a febrile illness with pericarditis and pleurisy (fluid collecting in the pleural space) that appears to be a benign inflammatory response to the surgical procedure. Anti-inflammatory therapy and bed rest reduce the symptoms. The symptoms may recur months after surgery.

Postperfusion syndrome may occur 3 to 12 weeks after surgery. The child develops a fever, splenomegaly, general malaise, and a maculopapular rash. Hepatomegaly also may be present. The white blood count reveals a leukocytosis, with lymphocytes as the predominant cell type. Such a reaction is usually caused by a cytomegalovirus infection contracted from the donor blood used in the cardiopulmonary bypass machine. The illness runs a short course, with no permanent effect.

Checkpoint Question 3

Megan will be scheduled for open-heart surgery. What type of fluid imbalance is apt to occur after cardiac surgery?

a. Hypervolemia from aldosterone production
b. Hypercalcemia from calcium release from bones
c. Hypernatremia from excess sodium retention
d. Hypokalemia from excess urine diuresis

The Child with an Artificial Valve Replacement

A number of congenital heart anomalies, such as aortic stenosis, and diseases such as rheumatic fever or Kawasaki disease can require artificial heart valve replacement (Wiegand, 2003). Valve replacement is technically more complicated in children than adults because children's hearts are smaller. Because children have a longer life expectancy than adults, valve durability also is a prime consideration. In addition, the advantage of the long-term anticoagulation therapy necessary to prevent clots from forming at the valve site must be weighed against the problem of extensive bleeding from normal childhood accidents.

Artificial valves were first obtained from pigs (porcine) or cows (bovine), but synthetic material (prosthetic) or human donors (homografts) are most often used today because synthetic materials or a child's own tissue provide the best long-term replacement. After surgery to place an artificial valve, a child is given either anticoagulation or antiplatelet therapy to prevent thrombi from forming at the valve implantation site. The drugs prescribed most commonly for anticoagulation therapy are heparin or warfarin sodium (Coumadin). Antiplatelet therapy also may be used, most often acetylsalicylic acid (aspirin) and dipyridamole (Persantine). Aspirin decreases platelet aggregation; dipyridamole decreases platelet adhesiveness. The dosage for these drugs must be periodically monitored by blood analysis to ensure they remain adequate as the child grows.

If a child should develop a bacterial infection with an artificial valve in place, organisms tend to cluster and colonize at the valve site. For this reason, a child generally is prescribed prophylactic antibiotic therapy to prevent this from becoming endocarditis. Additional therapy will be prescribed if a child is scheduled for dental work or any other invasive procedure.

Adolescent girls need counseling about avoiding pregnancy until they become adults because the artificial valve may be unable to accommodate the increased blood volume associated with pregnancy and support the adolescent's growth as well. In addition, because warfarin is teratogenic, any girl contemplating pregnancy needs to be changed to a heparin regimen before conception. Girls with artificial valves in place should not use an estrogen-based birth control pill, because this can increase blood coagulation and possibly lead to thrombi. They also should not use an intrauterine device (IUD) because an IUD may cause an increased rate of pelvic inflammatory disease, which could spread to the valve site.

Hemolytic anemia may occur as a complication of artificial valve replacement. The extreme turbulence of blood through the prosthetic valve apparently results in breakage of red blood cells. Blood replacement may be necessary if the hemolytic process persists.

The Child Undergoing Cardiac Transplantation

Children who have a hypoplastic left ventricle or extensive cardiomyopathy from any cause are candidates for heart transplantation. The procedure has become so successful that over 60,000 transplants have been performed worldwide (Burch & Aurora, 2004).

Children who will be having heart transplants may be at home or in the hospital when their family is notified that a donor heart is available. After removal from the donor, the transplant heart is perfused with a balanced electrolyte solution and chilled immediately. It can be maintained this way for 2 to 3 hours before being transplanted using cardiopulmonary bypass technique. For the procedure, the aorta of the child who will be receiving the heart is cross-clamped, and the original heart is removed except for the upper portion of the right atrium, which contains the SA node (Bahruth, 2004). Once the new heart is transplanted and the major cardiac vessels are reattached, intrathoracic hemodynamic monitoring lines and ventricle pacing wires are implanted. Transplanted hearts beat normally except for autonomic nervous system control. This means the transplanted heart varies its rate in response to the amount of blood arriving at it and the response to catecholamines rather than by nervous system control. An ECG will show two P waves (one from the residual original heart and one from the donor heart) because both SA nodes are intact.

Postoperative care is similar to that for any child undergoing cardiac surgery. The child has the same potential problems: decreased cardiac output, impaired gas exchange, risk for infection, imbalanced nutrition, and ineffective family coping. Children are prone to arrhythmias because of possible injury to the SA node during transport or transplant.

Although a long-term consequence of cardiac transplantation is severe atherosclerosis, apparently as a result of inflammation, rejection of the transplant is the number-one cause of death in cardiac transplant patients. An antithymocyte antibody preparation and drugs such as cyclosporine A, prednisone, and azathioprine are commonly used for immunosuppression in an attempt to reduce the risk of rejection. However, rejection still can occur in hyperacute, acute, or chronic forms. Hyperacute rejection occurs immediately and is manifested by coronary thrombosis. Acute rejection occurs in about 7 days and is manifested by low-grade fever, tachycardia, edema, and ECG changes. Cardiac catheterization is usually performed a week after transplant to obtain a biopsy sample from the heart muscle to evaluate for signs of acute rejection (tissue necrosis will have started to occur). This may be repeated every 2 or 4 weeks for the first year. Long-term or chronic rejection may begin as early as 6 months. At any point that rejection is beginning, additional antithymocyte globulin (ATG) or monoclonal antibodies to CD3T-lymphocytes (OKT-3) may be infused to help stop the process.

Once past the rejection period, most children adjust well to cardiac transplant. They can participate in normal growth and development activities after the procedure. Depending on the specific protocol, they return to the transplant center about once yearly for a repeat cardiac catheterization and evaluation of progress.

The Child with a Pacemaker

A child whose heart has ineffective SA node function or has difficulty in transmitting impulses from the SA node to the ventricles may have an artificial pacemaker inserted to control the heartbeat by stimulating the ventricles electronically (Woods, Schutte, & McCulloch, 2003). The pacing system consists of two components: a pulse generator that contains the battery and programmed instructions, and wire leads that connect to the heart. Most leads placed in children are an epicardial type and are attached to the epicardium (the outside wall of the heart) by suture. The generator is placed under the skin in the subxiphoid or mid- or lower abdomen. Heart disorders that will need pacing can be detected during intrauterine life by fetal monitoring. In these children, pacemakers can be implanted as soon as they are born.

Commonly, the type of pacemaker and its functions are denoted by either a three- or five-letter code. With the three-letter system, the first letter identifies the chamber paced, the second the chamber sensed, and the third the pacemaker's response to the intrinsic activity of the heart. If a fourth letter is used, it denotes whether rate modulation is possible; a fifth letter denotes whether antitachyarrhythmia function, such as the ability to produce a shock to defibrillate, is possible (Alexander et al., 2004). For example, a pacemaker that is set to pace the ventricle, sense the ventricle, and be inhibited (cannot modify the rate and does not respond as long as the heart initiates a normal beat) is a VVI pacemaker.

Teach the parents of the child with a pacemaker how to take the child's pulse accurately. They will need to do this daily at home and report any alterations in the pulse rate to their primary care provider until it is certain that the paced rate is appropriate. They also may need to telephone the health care center periodically and transmit a recording of the child's heart action to the center by means of a telephone attachment to ensure that the paced rate remains accurate.

Some parents stay awake at night worrying that the pacemaker batteries will suddenly stop operating and their child will die. Because of this fear, they may be afraid to take vacations or allow the child to go away to camp. How long a pacemaker battery lasts depends on the percentage of time pacing is needed (continuous or intermittent), the battery energy output in amplitude (the amount of battery voltage needed to create each pacing impulse), and the pulse width (the length of time the impulse is being delivered). With usual pacemaker parameters, such as an intermittent pattern, low amplitude, and narrow pulse width, a battery can last up to 15 years. In all instances, parents can be reassured that pacemaker batteries lose power slowly, not abruptly. They will have ample time to recognize weakening batteries through signs in their child such as dizziness, fatigue, fainting, or a slow pulse rate and arrange to have the pacemaker replaced before the child's heart would fail.

Occasionally, pacemaker leads in the right ventricle of infants lie in such close proximity to the diaphragm that they stimulate the diaphragm to contract with each ventricular contraction. This causes constant hiccupping. If this occurs, the leads may need a position adjustment. Another problem with infants is that there is not room to implant the generator deeply, so it can trigger airport security systems.

Help parents learn to evaluate whether toys are safe. As a rule, magnets should be avoided. Toys that emit an electrical current can interfere with a pacemaker's operation and so are not recommended. Also question the use of MRI (which involves the use of magnets) or electrocautery (which involves the use of electricity) with these children.

CONGENITAL HEART DISORDERS

About 8% of term newborns are born with a congenital cardiovascular abnormality (Fulton & Freed, 2004). This rate is even higher in preterm infants. Overall, these disorders affect equal numbers of male and female infants, but specific defects show a tendency toward sex differences. Patent ductus arteriosus and atrial septal defect, for example, are found more commonly in girls. Conditions such as valvular aortic stenosis, coarctation of the aorta, tetralogy of Fallot, and transposition of the great vessels occur more often in boys.

The usual cause of congenital heart disorders is failure of a heart structure to progress beyond an early stage of embryonic development. Maternal rubella is an example of an infection known to lead to disorders such as patent ductus arteriosus, pulmonary or aortic stenosis, atrial or ventricular septal defects, or pulmonary stenosis. Atrial and ventricular septal defects can also be familial. If a parent has an aortic stenosis, atrial septal defect, ventricular septal defect, or pulmonic stenosis, the incidence of this occurring also in the child is about 10% to 15% (Fulton & Freed, 2004).

Classification

Formerly, congenital heart disorders were classified based on the physical sign of cyanosis, or these disorders were classified as either cyanotic or acyanotic disorders.

Acyanotic heart disease involves heart or circulatory anomalies that involve either a stricture to the flow of blood or a shunt that moves blood from the arterial to the venous system (oxygenated to unoxygenated blood, or **left-to-right shunts**). These disorders cause the heart to function as an ineffective pump and make the child prone to heart failure. **Cyanotic heart disease** occurs when blood is shunted from the venous to the arterial system as a result of abnormal communication between the two systems (deoxygenated blood to oxygenated blood, or **right-to-left shunts**). Although helpful, this classification system led to difficulties because children with acyanotic heart disease can develop cyanosis, and children with cyanotic disease may not exhibit cyanosis until they are seriously ill.

To solve this problem, a second classification system has been established that addresses the hemodynamic and blood flow patterns of the disorders rather than their effect, allowing a more uniform and predictable set of signs and symptoms. As identified by this system, the four classifications include disorders with:

- Increased pulmonary blood flow
- Obstruction to blood flow leaving the heart
- Mixed blood flow (oxygenated and deoxygenated blood mixing in the heart or great vessels)
- Decreased pulmonary blood flow

Disorders With Increased Pulmonary Blood Flow

Congenital heart disorders associated with increased pulmonary blood flow involve blood flow from the left side of the heart, which is under greater pressure, to the right side of the heart, which is under less pressure, through some abnormal opening or connection between the two systems or the great arteries. Disorders of this type include ventricular septal defect (VSD), atrial septal defect (ASD), atrioventricular canal (AVC) defect, and patent ductus arteriosus (PDA).

Ventricular Septal Defect

VSD, the most common type of congenital cardiac disorder seen, accounts for about 30% of all instances of congenital heart disease, or about 3 in every 1,000 live births (Hirshfeld, 2003). With this defect, an opening is present in the septum between the two ventricles. Because pressure in the left ventricle is greater than that in the right ventricle, blood shunts from left to right across the septum (an acyanotic disorder). This impairs the effort of the heart because blood that should go into the aorta and out to the body is shunted back into the pulmonary circulation, resulting in right ventricular hypertrophy and increased pressure in the pulmonary artery (Fig. 41.8).

Assessment. A VSD may not be evident at birth. With incomplete opening of the alveoli, there is still high pulmonary artery resistance, so little blood is shunted through the defect. At about 4 to 8 weeks of age, as shunting begins, the infant demonstrates easy fatigue, and a loud, harsh pansystolic murmur becomes evident along the left sternal border at the third or fourth interspace. This typical murmur is generally widely transmitted. A thrill (vibration) also may be palpable. The diagnosis of VSD is based on examination by echocardiography with color flow Doppler or MRI, which reveals right ventricular hypertrophy and possibly pulmonary artery dilatation from the

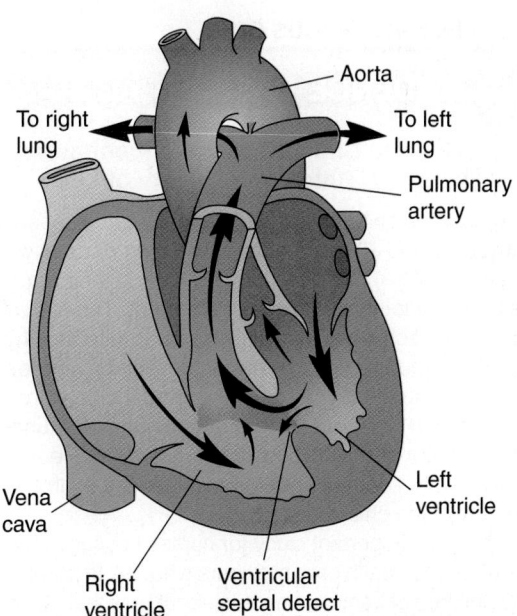

FIGURE 41.8 A ventricular septal defect.

increased blood flow. An ECG will also reveal right ventricular hypertrophy.

Therapeutic Management. Up to 85% of VSDs are so small they close spontaneously (Woods, Schutte & McCulloch, 2003). Those that are moderate in size may be closed by interventional cardiac catheterization. Larger ones (over 3 mm) require open-heart surgery. This is usually scheduled before 2 years of age to prevent pulmonary artery hypertension. Closure is important because if the defect is left open, cardiac failure from the artery hypertension can result. The heart can become infected (endocarditis) because of the recirculating blood flow.

Surgery requires the use of extracorporeal circulation and a quiet heart. In surgery, after cardiopulmonary bypass, the edges of the septal opening are approximated and sutured. If the defect is exceptionally large, a Silastic or Dacron patch can be sutured into place to occlude the space. With time, septal tissue will grow across the synthetic patch and knit it firmly into place. Postoperatively, be alert for arrhythmias because edema in the septum can interfere with ventricular conduction. Children may receive prophylactic antibiotics to prevent bacterial endocarditis for 6 months afterward. If there are no complications, children can expect a normal quality of life after the repair (Box 41.4).

Checkpoint Question 4

Suppose Megan has a simple ventricular septal defect. With this condition, in which direction would blood shunt?

a. From the left to the right ventricle
b. From the right ventricle to the aorta
c. From the right to the left ventricle
d. From the left ventricle to the left atria

BOX 41.4 FOCUS ON . . .

EVIDENCE-BASED PRACTICE

How Do Children with Congenital Heart Disease (CHD) Rate Their Quality of Life?

One hundred children with congenital heart disease, between 8 and 18 years of age, and their parents were given a quality of life questionnaire during their regular visit to a pediatric cardiology department. The results showed that children with CHD, compared to healthy children, reported reduced motor functioning and fewer feelings of autonomy. Parents reported their children had reduced quality of life in the areas of motor functioning, autonomy, and cognitive functioning. Reduced quality of life appeared not to be influenced by the severity of the child's disease.

This is an important study for nurses because nurses are often the health care providers who talk to parents and children at health care visits about how their school and home lives are going. Knowing that these children rate their quality of life lower than that of healthy children is an alert that children with CHD need extra time to discuss how they feel and support for trying activities that would make them feel better about themselves.

Source: Krol, Y., et al. (2003). Health-related quality of life in children with congenital heart disease. *Psychology and Health, 18*(2), 251–260.

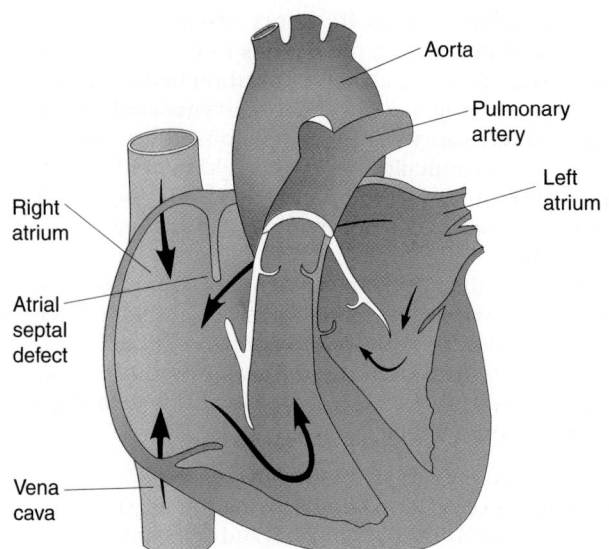

FIGURE 41.9 Atrial septal defect.

Atrial Septal Defect

An ASD is an abnormal communication between the two atria, allowing blood to shift from the left to the right atrium (an acyanotic defect). It is more common in girls than boys (Fleenor, 2003). Blood flow is from left to right (oxygenated to deoxygenated) because of the stronger contraction of the left side of the heart. This causes an increase in the volume in the right side of the heart and generally results in ventricular hypertrophy and increased pulmonary artery blood flow, the same as with a VSD (Fig. 41.9). There are two types of ASDs: ostium primum (ASD1), where the opening is at the lower end of the septum, and ostium secundum (ASD2), where the opening is near the center of the septum. ASD2 defects may be asymptomatic and not discovered until infection from recirculating blood occurs.

Assessment. A harsh systolic murmur is heard over the second or third interspace (the pulmonic area) because of the extra amount of shunted blood that crosses the pulmonic valve. As the volume of blood crossing it causes the pulmonic valve to close consistently later than the aortic valve, the second heart sound will be auscultated as split (fixed splitting). Such a sound is almost always diagnostic of ASD.

Echocardiography with color flow Doppler will generally reveal the enlarged right side of the heart and the increased pulmonary circulation. Cardiac catheterization, although rarely needed for diagnosis, would reveal the separation in the atrial septum and the increased oxygen saturation in the right atrium.

Therapeutic Management. Surgery to close the defect is done electively between 1 and 3 years of age. Closure is important because without it, a child is at risk for infectious endocarditis and eventual heart failure. It is particularly important that ASDs be repaired in girls, because they can cause emboli during pregnancy. Management is by open-heart surgery or interventional cardiac catheterization. For surgery, after a cardiopulmonary bypass, the edges of the opening are approximated and sutured. As with VSDs, if the defect is large, a Silastic or Dacron patch may be sutured into place to occlude the space. Postoperatively, carefully observe the child for arrhythmias because edema of the right atrium could interfere with SA node function. With uncomplicated surgery, children can expect a normal quality and length of life.

Atrioventricular Canal Defect

AVC, also called an endocardial cushion defect, results from incomplete fusion of the endocardial cushion, which is the septum of the heart at the junction of the atria and the ventricles (Fig. 41.10). Usually there is a low ASD continuous with a high VSD and distortion of the mitral and tricuspid valves. Although blood flow is generally left to right, blood may flow between all four heart chambers with this defect. Although rare in the general population, as many as 50% of children with trisomy 21 (Down syndrome) who have heart disease have this type of congenital cardiac defect (Chung, 2003). It leads to the same symptoms as other ASDs (i.e., right ventricular hypertrophy, increased pulmonary blood flow, and fixed S2 splitting). An ECG often will reveal first-degree heart block as impulse conduction is halted before the AV node. Echocardiography will confirm the diagnosis. Pulmonary artery banding may be done palliatively in selected infants. This increases pressure in the pulmonary artery and right side of the heart, reducing the amount of shunting. Surgery, however, is always necessary for a final repair because these defects are too large to close spontaneously. Because

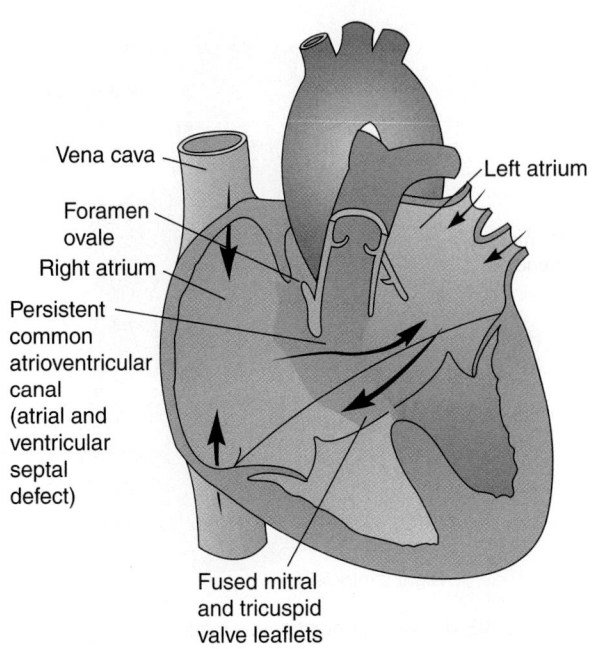

FIGURE 41.10 Atrioventricular canal defect.

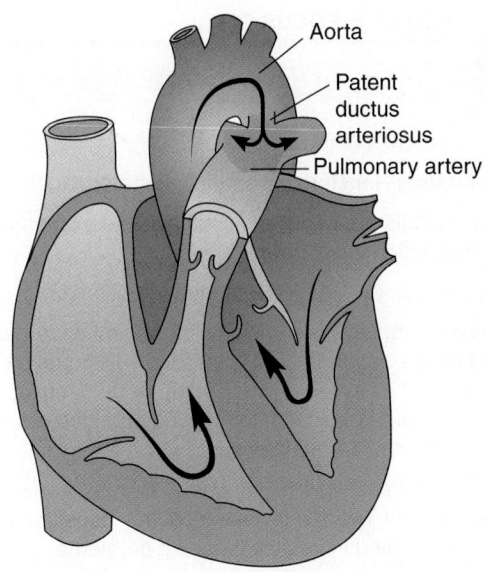

FIGURE 41.11 Patent ductus arteriosus.

surgery may involve a valve repair as well as a septal repair, mitral and tricuspid insufficiency from poor valve function may occur at a later date. Postoperatively, closely observe children for jaundice resulting from red blood cell destruction as red cells are destroyed by the newly constructed valves. Both prophylactic anticoagulation and antibiotic therapy may be necessary postoperatively, but with these drugs, the quality of life will be good.

Patent Ductus Arteriosus

The ductus arteriosus is an accessory fetal structure that connects the pulmonary artery to the aorta. If it fails to close at birth (closure should begin with the first breath, but complete closure may not occur until 3 months of age), blood will shunt from the aorta (oxygenated blood) to the pulmonary artery (deoxygenated blood) because of the increased pressure in the aorta. The shunted blood returns to the left atrium of the heart, passes to the left ventricle, out to the aorta, and shunts back to the pulmonary artery (Fig. 41.11). This causes an increased pressure in the pulmonary circulation from the extra shunted blood; this leads to right ventricle hypertrophy. The disorder accounts for about 10% of all instances of congenital heart disease (Toyer & Fox, 2004).

Assessment. PDAs are twice as common in girls as boys and occur at a higher incidence at higher altitudes. In preterm infants, the incidence may be as high as 20% to 60% (Mulreany, 2003). On physical examination, the child usually has a wide pulse pressure (the difference between systolic and diastolic blood pressures). The diastolic pressure, a measure of peripheral resistance, is low because of the shunt or runoff of blood, which reduces resistance. A typical continuous (systolic and diastolic) "machinery" murmur can be heard at the upper left sternal border or under the left clavicle in older children. In newborns, the murmur may not be quite so characteristic, perhaps a short grade II or III harsh systolic sound. An ECG is generally normal, although it may show ventricle enlargement if the shunt is large. Echocardiography provides good visualization of the patent ductus. Cardiac catheterization is generally not necessary for diagnosis but may be performed to rule out associated defects.

Therapeutic Management. One reason that the ductus arteriosus remains open in fetal life is stimulation by prostaglandins, particularly PGE, from the placenta and the low oxygen level of fetal blood. After birth, when the PGE level falls and the oxygen level increases, the ductus arteriosus is stimulated to close. If it does not close spontaneously, an infant may be prescribed IV indomethacin or ibuprofen, prostaglandin inhibitors. These lower the PGE level and encourage ductus closure. If indomethacin is given, assess for possible side effects, including reduced glomerular filtration, impaired platelet aggregation, and diminished gastrointestinal and cerebral blood flow (Box 41.5). Because it has much fewer side effects, ibuprofen is becoming the drug of choice; it can even be used as prophylaxis in preterm infants (Van Overmeire, 2003).

If medical management fails to bring about closure of the ductus arteriosus, the disorder can be closed by insertion of Dacron-coated stainless-steel coils by interventional cardiac catheterization when the child is 6 months to 1 year of age. Exceptionally large defects can be closed surgically by ductal ligation. This involves major surgery because opening the chest (thoracotomy) and manipulating the great vessels is necessary. However, it is not open-heart surgery and so does not involve the use of extracorporeal circulation; rather, it may be performed using only three small thoracotomy incisions on the chest. If surgery is not done by one of these techniques, the child is at risk for heart failure from the increased amount of blood pouring back into the pulmonary artery and infectious endocarditis developing from the recirculating blood and potential stasis in the pulmonary artery.

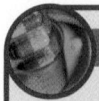

BOX 41.5 FOCUS ON . . .

PHARMACOLOGY

Indomethacin (Indocin)

Classification: Nonsteroidal anti-inflammatory agent

Action: Inhibits prostaglandin synthesis. Its exact mechanism of action is unknown.

Pregnancy risk category: B (D in third trimester)

Dosage: 0.2 mg/kg intravenously for the first dose, followed by 0.1 mg/kg (if child is less than 48 hours old), 0.2 mg/kg (if child is 2 to 7 days old), or 0.25 mg/kg (if child is over 7 days old) for second and third doses, given at 12- to 24-hour intervals.

Possible adverse effects: Headache, dizziness, somnolence, nausea, gastrointestinal bleeding, constipation, rash, apnea, and increased bleeding problems

Nursing Implications

• Administer reconstituted solution intravenously over 5 to 10 seconds.
• Space doses at specified intervals.
• Educate the parents about the rationale for using the drug.
• Observe the child closely for adverse effects. Check the infusion site carefully for signs of oozing or bleeding indicative of impaired clotting. Also assess vomitus or urine for bleeding.

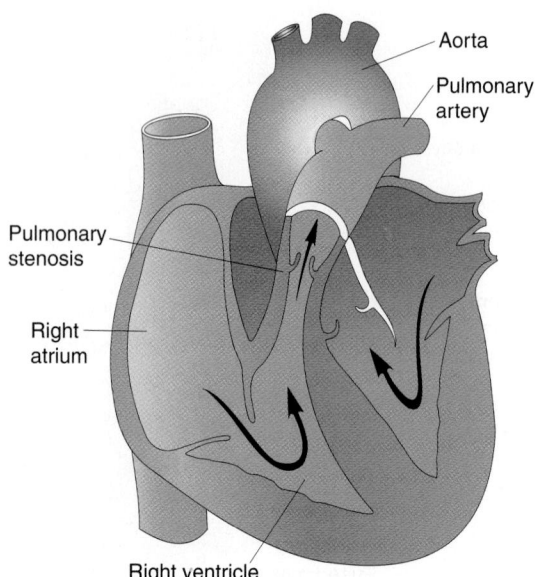

FIGURE 41.12 Pulmonary stenosis.

Disorders With Obstruction to Blood Flow

A number of congenital anomalies cause the blood flow leaving the heart to be obstructed because a vessel or a valve is narrower than usual. Pressure from blood flow increases before the narrowing and decreases after the narrowing. These are problematic defects in that they prohibit enough blood from reaching its intended site, the lungs or the rest of the body; they threaten to overwhelm the heart because of back-pressure. Obstructive defects of this category include pulmonary stenosis, aortic stenosis, and coarctation of the aorta.

Pulmonary Stenosis

Pulmonary stenosis is narrowing of the pulmonary valve or the pulmonary artery just distal to the valve (Fig. 41.12). It accounts for about 10% of congenital heart anomalies (Fulton & Freed, 2004). Inability of the right ventricle to evacuate blood by way of the pulmonary artery because of the obstruction leads to right ventricular hypertrophy.

Assessment. Infants with pulmonary artery stenosis may be asymptomatic or have signs of mild (right-sided) heart failure. If the narrowing is severe, cyanosis may be present from inability of adequate blood to reach the lungs for oxygenation or right-to-left shunting across the foramen ovale because of the increased right-sided heart pressure. A typical systolic ejection murmur, grade IV or V crescendo–

decrescendo in quality, can be heard, usually loudest at the upper left sternal border. It may radiate to the suprasternal notch. A thrill may be present in the upper left sternal area or at the suprasternal notch. The second heart sound may be widely split because of late closure of the pulmonary valve. An ECG or echocardiography will reveal right ventricular hypertrophy. Cardiac catheterization is rarely necessary for diagnosis but is used for interventional enlargement of the stenosed valve (Fulton & Freed, 2004).

Therapeutic Management. Management of the defect depends on the severity of the stenosis and the child's age. **Balloon angioplasty** by way of cardiac catheterization is the procedure of choice. With this procedure, a catheter with an uninflated balloon at its tip is inserted and passed through the heart into the stenosed valve. As the balloon is inflated, it breaks valve adhesions and relieves the stenosis. Following the procedure, although children may always have a residual heart murmur, they can expect a normal lifespan and quality of life.

Aortic Stenosis

Stenosis, or stricture, of the aortic valve prevents blood from passing freely from the left ventricle of the heart into the aorta. Because the heart cannot force blood through the strictured valve, increased pressure and hypertrophy of the left ventricle occur (Fig. 41.13). If the left ventricular pressure becomes acute, pressure in the left atrium also increases, resulting in back-pressure in pulmonary veins and possibly pulmonary edema. Aortic stenosis accounts for about 7% of congenital cardiac abnormalities (Fulton & Freed, 2004).

Assessment. Most children with aortic stenosis are asymptomatic, but physical assessment generally reveals a typical murmur, a rough systolic sound heard loudest in the second right interspace (the aortic space). The murmur may be transmitted to the right shoulder, clavicle, and up

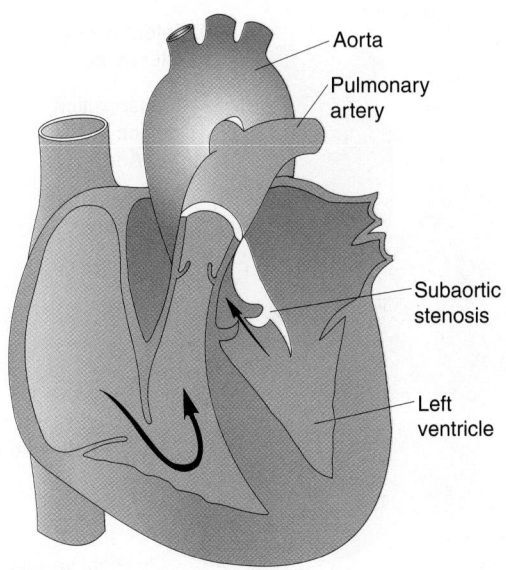

FIGURE 41.13 Aortic stenosis.

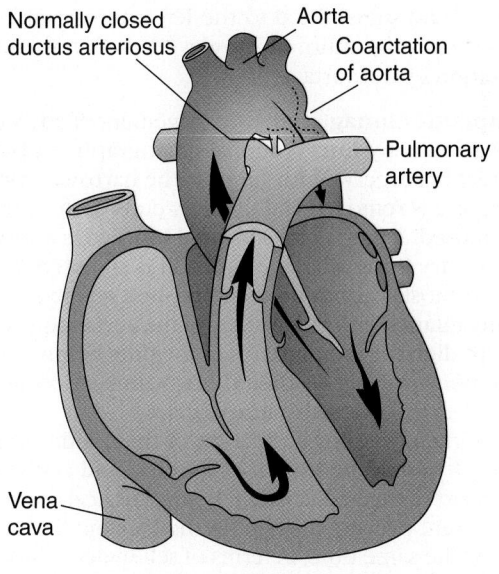

FIGURE 41.14 Coarctation of the aorta.

the vessels of the neck; it may also be transmitted to the heart's apex. A thrill may be present, particularly at the suprasternal notch. If severe, decreased cardiac output evidenced by faint pulses, hypotension, tachycardia, and inability to suck for long periods may be present. When the child is active, he or she may develop chest pain similar to angina, because the coronary arteries receive inadequate blood. Sudden death can occur when the amount of oxygen needed by the heart muscle on exertion far exceeds what is available because of the aortic stenosis.

ECG or echocardiography will reveal left ventricular hypertrophy. Cardiac catheterization is rarely necessary unless interventional therapy by this route is planned.

Therapeutic Management. Stabilization with a beta-blocker or a calcium channel blocker may be necessary to reduce cardiac hypertrophy before the defect is corrected. Balloon valvuloplasty is the surgical treatment of choice. Surgery that involves dividing the stenotic valve or dilating an accompanying constrictive aortic ring can be used for severe defects. Such a repair may lead to aortic valve insufficiency in later life, at which time further surgery may be needed. Some children will need artificial valve replacement for correction. If a prosthetic valve is used, children generally continue to receive anticoagulation or antiplatelet therapy and antibiotic prophylaxis against endocarditis. In addition, children need exercise testing before participating in competitive sports.

Coarctation of the Aorta

Coarctation of the aorta, a narrowing of the lumen of the aorta due to a constricting band (Fig. 41.14), accounts for about 6% of instances of congenital heart disease (Bird, 2003). It occurs more frequently in boys than in girls and is the leading cause of congestive heart failure in the first few months of life. There are two locations in which this commonly occurs. In the first, termed "preductal," the constriction exists between the subclavian artery and the ductus arteriosus. In the second, postductal, the constriction is distal to the ductus arteriosus.

Because it is difficult for blood to pass through the narrowed lumen of the aorta, blood pressure increases proximal to the coarctation and decreases distal to it. This results in increased blood pressure in the heart and upper portions of the body as pressure in the subclavian artery increases. Elevated upper-body blood pressure produces headache and vertigo. Because a child under 3 years of age has difficulty describing these sensations, exceptional irritability may be the main clue that these symptoms are present. Epistaxis (nosebleed) and cerebrovascular accident, an event not generally associated with children, can occur from this dangerously elevated blood pressure.

Assessment. If the coarctation is slight, absence of palpable femoral pulses may be the only symptom. Children who have an obstruction proximal to the left subclavian artery may have absent brachial pulses as well. For this reason, always include evaluation of femoral pulses in all initial newborn assessments and admission inspections to newborn nurseries. As children with coarctation of the aorta grow older, they may experience leg pain on exertion because of the diminished blood supply to their lower extremities. Because collateral circulation is necessary to allow blood to flow around the constriction, collateral arteries enlarge and may be seen on the ribs as obvious nodules as the child grows older.

The diagnosis of coarctation of the aorta may be made on the grounds of the history and physical assessment. On examination, the blood pressure in the arms will be at least 20 mm Hg higher than in the legs, a reversal of the normal pattern. Echocardiography, ECG, MRI, or x-ray examination of older children will reveal left-sided heart enlargement from back-pressure and also notching of the ribs from the enlarged collateral vessels. Occasionally, a murmur is present, but this is variable in position, intensity, and character. The most frequent type is a soft or moderately loud systolic murmur, especially prominent at the base of the heart and transmitted to the left interscapular area. The absence of a murmur, however, does not rule out coarctation of the aorta.

Therapeutic Management. Management of coarctation of the aorta is by interventional angiography (a balloon catheter) or surgery. With surgery, the narrowed portion of the aorta is removed and the new ends of the aorta are anastomosed. A graft of transplanted subclavian artery may be necessary if the narrowed section is so extensive that an anastomosis cannot be accomplished readily.

Many infants with coarctation of the aorta require therapy with digoxin and diuretics in the time before surgery can be performed. This drug therapy aims to reduce the severity of the congestive heart failure.

Planning a time for correction of the condition is important. It would be ideal if children could achieve the greater part of their adult height before surgical correction, as this might prevent a strain on the incision line as they grow. At the same time, in terms of self-image, correction is best done before children begin to think of themselves as chronically ill or before they develop a complication, such as chronic hypertension. Girls must have the defect repaired before childbearing age, or the extra blood volume during pregnancy can cause heart failure. Surgical repair is usually scheduled by 2 years of age. If the surgery is successful, without complications, the child can expect to live a normal life. After surgery, abdominal vessels receive more blood than they did previously. This may result in abdominal pain or generalized abdominal discomfort, but this is a short-term problem. Some children continue to have elevated upper body hypertension after the repair. They need continued treatment with antihypertensive agents. Some children require repeat balloon angioplasty at adolescence to re-enlarge the aortic lumen and help reduce this upper body hypertension.

Disorders With Mixed Blood Flow

Mixed disorders are cardiac anomalies that involve mixing of blood from the pulmonary and systemic circulation in the heart chambers. This mixing results in a relative deoxygenation of systemic blood flow, although cyanosis is not always visible. Mixed defects include transposition of the great arteries, total anomalous pulmonary venous return, truncus arteriosus, and hypoplastic left heart syndrome.

Transposition of the Great Arteries

In transposition of the great arteries, the aorta arises from the right ventricle instead of the left, and the pulmonary artery arises from the left ventricle instead of the right. Blood enters the heart from the vena cava to the right atrium, then flows to the right ventricle, and goes out into the aorta to the body completely deoxygenated; it returns again by the vena cava. A secondary source of blood enters the heart from the pulmonary veins, goes to the left atrium, left ventricle, and out the pulmonary artery to the lungs to be oxygenated, and returns to the left atrium, a second closed circulatory system (Fig. 41.15). This severe a defect is incompatible with life. In most instances, atrial and ventricular septal defects occur in connection with

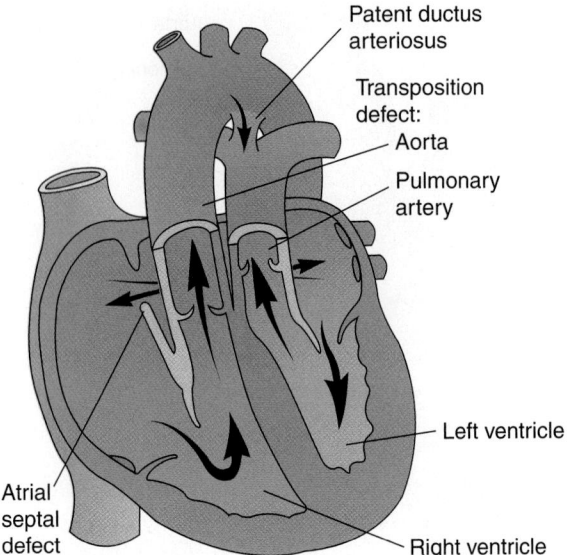

FIGURE 41.15 Transposition of the great vessels.

this transposition, making the entire heart one mixed circulatory system. It tends to occur in large newborns (9 to 10 lb) and occurs more often in boys than in girls. This disorder accounts for about 5% of congenital heart anomalies (Marino, 2003).

Assessment. Infants with this defect are usually cyanotic from birth. There may be no murmur, or there may be various murmurs, depending on the shunting of blood through atrial or ventricular defects or through the ductus arteriosus, which usually remains open. Echocardiography generally reveals an enlarged heart. An ECG may or may not reveal heart changes. Cardiac catheterization will reveal the low oxygen saturation resulting from the mixing of blood in the heart chambers.

Therapeutic Management. If no septal defect exists or if the defect is too small to allow enough mixing of blood to sustain life, PGE, a prostaglandin, will be administered to keep the ductus arteriosus patent. A balloon atrial septal pull-through operation to enlarge the septal openings may also need to be done in the infant's first few days. With this procedure, done by cardiac catheterization, a deflated balloon catheter is passed from the right atrium through the foramen ovale into the left atrium. The balloon is then inflated, and the catheter is drawn back into the right atrium. This enlarges the opening of the foramen ovale and creates an artificial ASD.

Surgical correction of transposition of the great vessels, done at 1 week to 3 months of age, involves an arterial switch procedure in which the major vessels are switched in position. The child will be transported to a major center for the surgery and care as soon as a disorder of this magnitude is diagnosed. The survival rate following surgery is as high as 95%.

Total Anomalous Pulmonary Venous Return

In this disorder, the pulmonary veins return to the right atrium or the superior vena cava instead of to the left atrium

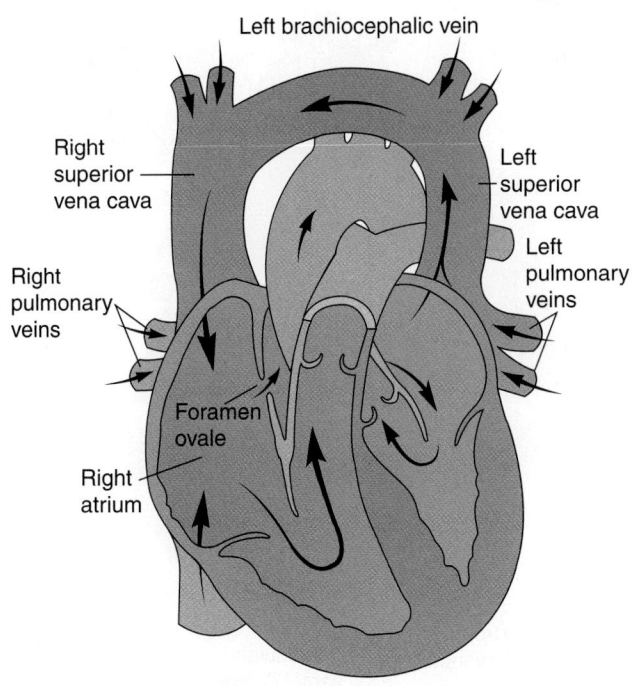

FIGURE 41.16 Total anomalous pulmonary venous return.

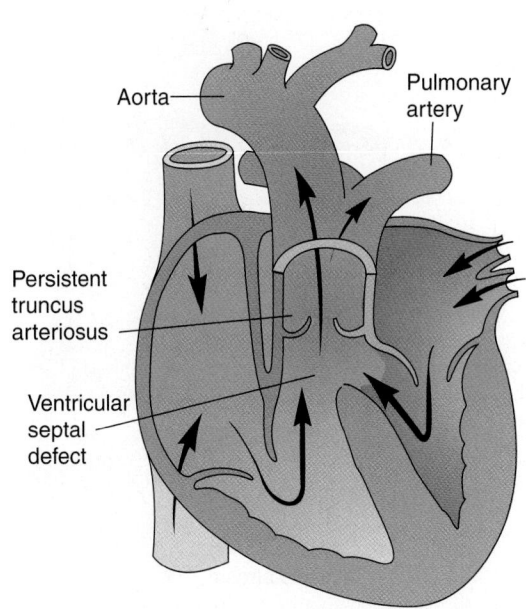

FIGURE 41.17 Truncus arteriosus.

as they normally would. For blood to reach the systemic circulation, it must shunt across a patent foramen ovale or a PDA (Fig. 41.16). This disorder accounts for only 2% of all congenital heart disorders. An absent spleen is often associated with the disorder. These infants are mildly cyanotic and tire easily. If the ductus closes or the septal defect is small, cyanosis increases in amount; right-sided heart failure develops (Dyke, Simpson, & Carter, 2004).

Surgery involves reimplanting the pulmonary veins into the left atrium. Until this can be carried out, a balloon atrial septal pull-through procedure may be necessary to enlarge a small foramen ovale. The child may be maintained on a continuous IV infusion containing PGE to help keep the ductus arteriosus open (Fulton & Freed, 2004).

Truncus Arteriosus

In truncus arteriosus, a rare defect (approximately 1% of initial cardiac lesions), one major artery or "trunk" arises from the left and right ventricles in place of separate aorta and pulmonary artery vessels (Fig. 41.17). There is usually an accompanying VSD. The child is cyanotic and may have a typical VSD murmur. Repair involves restructuring the common trunk to create separate vessels. Some children need a second surgical procedure by school age as the graft inserted to separate the aorta and pulmonary artery is outgrown.

Hypoplastic Left Heart Syndrome

In hypoplastic left heart syndrome, a rare disorder accounting for only 1% to 3% of congenital heart disease cases, the left ventricle is nonfunctional. There may be accompanying mitral or aortic valve atresia. The nonfunctioning left ventricle lacks adequate strength to pump

blood into the systemic circulation. This causes the right ventricle to hypertrophy as it tries to maintain the entire heart action (Kon, Ackerson, & Lo, 2003). Mild to moderate cyanosis develops as deoxygenated blood is shunted across the foramen ovale because of the greater pressure on the right. Echocardiography effectively diagnoses this condition. Prostaglandin therapy to maintain a PDA will be started to increase blood to the aorta. Inhaled nitrogen may be prescribed to decrease Po_2; this increases pulmonary resistance and allows the right heart to shift more blood into the left heart and aorta. Surgery has limited success in this syndrome, although a great deal of research is being done in this area and a two- or three-stage procedure (restructuring of the heart) is possible. Heart transplantation is the ultimate answer for prolonging the child's life, but the number of donor hearts available for newborns is limited (Burch & Aurora, 2004).

Disorders With Decreased Pulmonary Blood Flow

Disorders with decreased pulmonary blood flow involve some type of obstruction to pulmonary blood flow. Because of the obstruction, pressure increases in the right side of the heart. If an ASD or VSD also is present, deoxygenated blood shunts from right to left. This results in deoxygenated blood invading the systemic circulation. Common disorders include tricuspid atresia and tetralogy of Fallot.

Tricuspid Atresia

Tricuspid atresia is an extremely serious disorder because, as the name implies, the tricuspid valve is completely closed, allowing no blood to flow from the right atrium to the right ventricle. Instead, blood crosses through the patent foramen ovale into the left atrium, bypassing the lungs and the step of oxygenation. It reaches the lungs

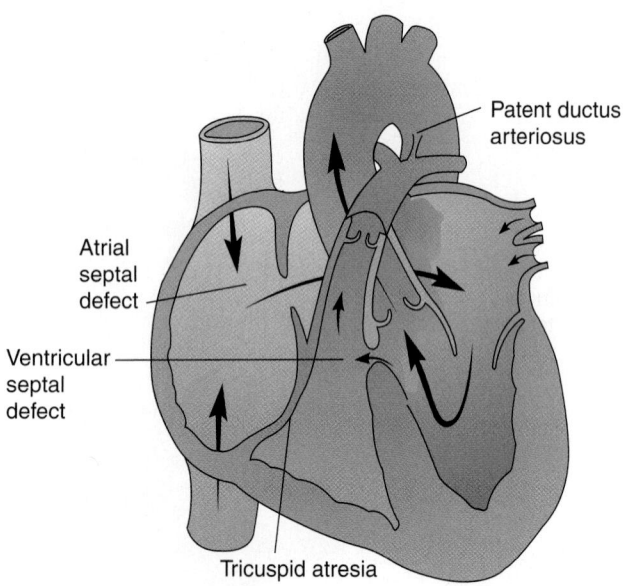

FIGURE 41.18 Tricuspid atresia.

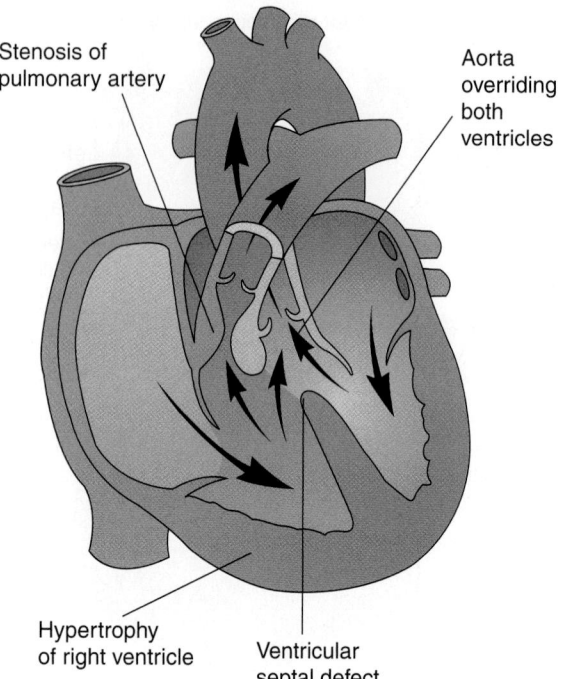

FIGURE 41.19 Tetralogy of Fallot.

for oxygenation by being shunted back through a PDA (Fig. 41.18). As long as the foramen ovale and ductus arteriosus remain open, the child can obtain adequate oxygenation. At the point they close, however, the infant will develop extreme cyanosis, tachycardia, and dyspnea. An IV infusion of PGE is started to ensure that the ductus remains open. Surgery consists of the construction of a vena cava-to-pulmonary artery shunt, which deflects more blood to the lungs, or a Fontan procedure (sometimes termed a Glenn Shunt baffle), which restructures the right side of the heart.

Tetralogy of Fallot

Tetralogy of Fallot, one of the first types of congenital heart disease described, occurs in about 10% of children with congenital cardiac disease (Ro, 2003). It is called a tetralogy because four anomalies are present: pulmonary stenosis, VSD (usually large), dextroposition (overriding) of the aorta, and hypertrophy of the right ventricle. Because of the pulmonary stenosis, pressure builds up in the right side of the heart. Blood then shunts from this area of increased pressure into the left ventricle and the overriding aorta. The extra effort involved to force blood through the stenosed pulmonary artery causes the fourth deformity, hypertrophy of the right ventricle (Fig. 41.19). As many as 15% of children with this disorder show a deletion abnormality of chromosome 22 (22q11), or the disorder can result from a documented chromosome disorder.

Assessment. Although this is an extremely serious form of heart disease, newborns may not exhibit a high degree of cyanosis immediately after birth. As they become more active, however, their skin acquires a bluish tint as cyanosis begins. Polycythemia (an increase in the number of red blood cells) occurs as the body attempts to provide enough red blood cells to supply oxygen to all body parts. This is a potential danger because the increased concentration of red blood cells causes the blood to become thick (in-

creased viscosity), and clots in blood vessels may occur, with complications such as thrombophlebitis, embolism, or cerebrovascular accident.

If the condition is not corrected, the child will generally develop severe dyspnea, growth restriction, and clubbing of the fingers. He or she tends to assume a squatting or a knee–chest position when resting. Squatting gives physiologic relief to an overstressed heart by trapping blood in the lower extremities. Unless they do this, children's hearts can be overwhelmed, leaving an insufficient amount of total circulating blood for the body to oxygenate and deliver to major body organs.

Children may develop syncope (fainting) and hypoxic episodes (sometimes called tet spells) caused by decreased blood and oxygen supply to the brain. These usually follow prolonged crying or exertion. They can be so extreme, if long term, that children develop a cognitive challenge.

Tetralogy of Fallot is diagnosed based on the history and physical symptoms, laboratory results, echocardiography, ECG, and cardiac catheterization. A loud, harsh, widely transmitted murmur or a soft, scratchy, localized systolic murmur in the left second, third, or fourth parasternal interspace may be present. It is so widely transmitted that it is often heard as well in the left clavicular area or posteriorly, in the interscapular space. Splitting of the second heart sound rarely occurs with tetralogy of Fallot because blood is forced through the shunt; the pulmonic valve does not, therefore, close later than the aortic valve.

Echocardiography and ECG both show the enlarged chamber of the right side of the heart. Echocardiography also shows the decrease in the size of the pulmonary artery and the reduced blood flow through the lungs. Cardiac catheterization and angiography will permit a definitive evaluation of the extent of the defect, particularly the pulmonary stenosis and the VSD. Laboratory findings reveal polycythemia, increased hemoglobin, hematocrit, and total red blood cell count as well as reduced oxygen saturation.

Therapeutic Management. Final management of tetralogy of Fallot is surgery to correct the heart defects, done at 1 to 2 years of age. Parents need to try to keep hypoxic episodes to a minimum during this waiting time. If a baby begins to have a hypoxic episode, administering oxygen, placing him or her in a knee–chest position (to trap blood in the lower extremities and keep the heart from being overwhelmed), and administering morphine sulfate generally reduces symptoms. If not, propranolol (Inderal, a beta-blocker) may be given orally to aid pulmonary artery dilation. A temporary or palliative surgical repair, called the Blalock-Taussig procedure, can create a shunt between the aorta and the pulmonary artery (thereby creating a ductus arteriosus). This will allow blood to leave the aorta and enter the pulmonary artery, oxygenate in the lungs, and return to the left side of the heart, the aorta, and the body. Because the subclavian artery is used in a Blalock-Taussig procedure, a child will not have a palpable pulse in the right arm after this procedure. For this reason, blood pressure and venipunctures should be avoided in the affected arm.

A full repair that relieves the pulmonary stenosis, VSD, and overriding aorta can be accomplished (a Brock procedure). Postoperatively, observe for arrhythmias, which may result from any ventricular septal repair, edema, and conduction interference.

❓ *What if...* you noticed Megan always draws her knees up tightly against her chest? Would this be a concern for you? Why or why not?

ACQUIRED HEART DISEASE

The most commonly acquired heart disease in children is **congestive heart failure** (CHF), which usually occurs as a result of a congenital heart disorder or a disease such as rheumatic fever, Kawasaki disease, or infectious endocarditis.

Congestive Heart Failure

CHF results when the myocardium of the heart cannot pump and circulate enough blood to supply oxygen and nutrients to body cells. Blood pools in the heart (excessive preload) or in the pulmonary or venous systems. This may result from a congenital disorder that lessens the effectiveness of the heart's pumping action, or it may occur after cardiac surgery or rheumatic fever, when the myocardium is weakened. Severe anemia, hypocalcemia, and myocarditis may contribute to the heart's inability to function effectively. CHF is most apt to occur in children under 1 year of age (Fulton & Freed, 2004).

The heart can compensate in several ways to move blood forward and attempt to increase cardiac output. The muscle fibers can lengthen, causing the ventricles to enlarge in an attempt to handle more blood with each heart stroke (ventricular hypertrophy). The heart can also increase the number of beats per minute. As long as these mechanisms allow for adequate cardiac output, the signs of heart failure are not apparent. However, the heart's capacity for compensation is limited, particularly in infants, an age group in which hypertrophy is restricted. Eventually, in children of all ages, the heart can no longer compensate and becomes overwhelmed by the amount of blood present, which cannot be pushed forward effectively (Lee, 2003).

Sympathetic nervous system stimulation causes the frequently seen symptoms of excessive sweating and pallor. As blood flow to the kidneys decreases, the glomerular filtration rate slows, resulting in stimulation of the renin-angiotensin system, which causes fluid and sodium retention. Aldosterone secretion by the adrenal glands further promotes sodium retention in an attempt to increase blood flow to the kidneys. Antidiuretic hormone secretion by the pituitary is also increased to help retain fluid. This additional fluid can result in dependent edema.

Assessment

One of the first signs of CHF is tachycardia as the heart attempts to beat faster to move blood forward more effectively; this is quickly followed by tachypnea or rapid breathing. When a child has primary right heart failure, increased venous pressure and hepatomegaly (enlarged liver) occur from back-pressure in the portal circulation. The child may feel irritable and restless from the abdominal pain caused by the liver distention. Lower extremity edema, usually a primary sign in adults, is often a late sign of heart failure in children (Box 41.6).

With left-sided heart failure, back-pressure causes blood to accumulate in the pulmonary system. Dyspnea is usually the dominant symptom, especially when a child lies in a supine position (this is orthopnea; it occurs due to increased pulmonary congestion). A child may have rales and may produce bloody sputum on coughing (from lung capillaries broken under increased pulmonary blood pressure). The child may appear cyanotic from interference with gas exchange in the alveoli, which begin to fill with fluid (pulmonary edema). Left-sided heart failure can ultimately lead to right-sided heart failure as extensive pressure in the pulmonary system prevents blood from leaving the right ventricle.

In an infant, heart failure is often difficult to detect because it presents with very subtle signs. The infant becomes breathless from rapid respirations, tires easily, and has difficulty feeding because of the exhaustion and dyspnea present. Often an infant becomes diaphoretic from the effort of feeding. If edema is present, it is generalized rather than dependent and often is first noticed as periorbital edema. An abrupt gain in weight may be the most obvious indication that extra fluid is accumulating. On physical examination, an infant will have an enlarged liver (a liver palpable more than 2 cm below the right costal margin) and may have ascites.

The apical heartbeat is displaced laterally and downward. As a rule of thumb, if the width of the heart is more than half the width of the chest (in a child over 1 year of age), the heart is enlarged. In addition, a galloping heart rhythm or an accentuated third heart sound may be heard

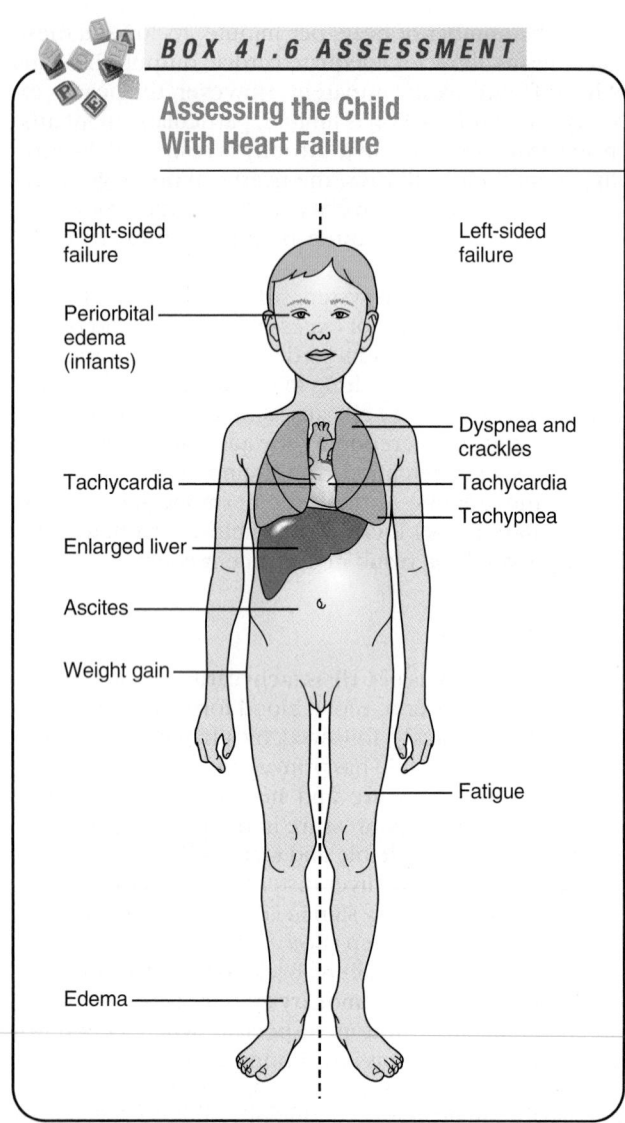

BOX 41.6 ASSESSMENT

Assessing the Child With Heart Failure

Right-sided failure

Left-sided failure

Periorbital edema (infants)

Dyspnea and crackles

Tachycardia

Tachycardia

Tachypnea

Enlarged liver

Ascites

Weight gain

Fatigue

Edema

because of the sudden distention of the ventricle during the rapid filling phase. Heart failure may be confirmed by echocardiography, which reveals the enlarged heart. Ventricular hypertrophy can be confirmed by ECG.

Therapeutic Management

Therapy for heart failure consists of reducing the workload of the heart by measures such as evacuating the accumulated fluid (reduces preload) with diuretics, slowing the heart rate and strengthening cardiac function (increases contractility) by administering an inotropic (heart-strengthening) drug, and reducing afterload with vasodilators.

Commonly used diuretics include furosemide (Lasix) and spironolactone (Aldactone). The most common drug used to increase contractility and slow tachycardia is digoxin. Drugs that decrease afterload include hydralazine, an arterial vasodilator; nifedipine, a calcium channel blocker; nitroprusside, a direct-acting vasodilator; and captopril, an angiotensin-converting enzyme (ACE) inhibitor (Karch, 2004).

NURSING DIAGNOSES AND RELATED INTERVENTIONS

Be certain that outcomes established for the care of a child with congestive heart disease are realistic in light of the child's condition as well as individualized for each child. Interventions focus on helping support heart function and helping parents deal with this crisis until the child's heart is again strong enough to maintain strong heart action (Box 41.7).

Nursing Diagnosis: Ineffective cardiopulmonary and peripheral tissue perfusion related to inadequate heart function

Outcome Evaluation: Child's pulse, blood pressure, and respiratory rate are within acceptable parameters for age group; abnormal heart sounds, edema, and ascites are absent.

Provide for Rest Periods. Rest, a major aspect of care for a child with heart failure, reduces the metabolic rate, decreasing myocardial and body oxygen demand. Most children with heart failure feel more comfortable in a semi-Fowler's position than in a supine position. This chest-elevated position lowers the abdominal contents, enlarging the thoracic cavity and allowing for easier, more comfortable lung expansion. Babies are most comfortable in an infant seat, which supports them in a semi-Fowler's position. Sedation, such as with morphine, may be necessary to encourage bed rest in some children. Most children with heart failure, however, automatically limit their activity, so the need for sedation must be considered on an individual basis.

Organize nursing care to allow periods of sustained rest. At the same time, do not attempt to perform too many procedures at once or you will exhaust the child. Be certain that both you and the child's parents understand how much rest the child is to have each day. The term "complete bed rest" is often loosely used and has different meanings to different people. Does it mean a child may eat by herself, or must she be fed? Does it mean bathroom privileges or not? Playtime or not? Unless children are exceptionally exhausted, most children need to be entertained or played with to remain on bed rest. Activities such as watching television, being read to, or listening to music can quiet a child and promote better rest than if the child is expected to rest quietly without any diversion.

Provide Oxygen as Necessary. If a child has dyspnea, hypoxemia, or cyanosis, supplemental oxygen by way of hood, mask, or nasal prongs is usually necessary. Monitor oxygen saturation levels with pulse oximetry. Assess the nostrils of the child receiving

B O X   4 1 . 7 :   F o c u s   o n   N u r s i n g   C a r e   P l a n n i n g

A Multidisciplinary Care Map for An Infant with Congestive Heart Failure

●

Megan is a newborn who was born with tetralogy of Fallot. By 1 hour of age, she developed rapid respirations, tachycardia, and cyanosis. An echocardiogram revealed the typical four structural defects of the syndrome. An hour later, Megan is in heart failure.

Family Assessment

Child's parents were divorced 1 month ago; dual custody of infant granted. Child will spend weekdays with mother, weekends with father. Father is a city bus driver; mother is a paralegal. Father to pay child support; with child support, mother rates finances as "workable."

Client Criteria

One-hour-old infant girl who appears pale to cyanotic, tachycardic, and dyspneic. Child born by vaginal birth; Apgars 9 and 6. Afebrile; pulse 150 bpm; respirations 36. Oxygen saturation via pulse oximetry 90 mm Hg. Apical heart rate displaced down and laterally. S3 heart sound noted. Lungs with harsh rhonchi and rales on auscultation. Generalized edema with hepatomegaly.

Nursing Diagnosis

Ineffective cardiopulmonary tissue perfusion related to impaired cardiac function and increased cardiac workload

Outcome Evaluation

Child's vital signs are within age-acceptable parameters; skin color pink and warm; dyspnea seems lessened. Absence of S3 heart sound; oxygen saturation more than 95 mm Hg. Lungs clear to auscultation.

Team Member Responsible	Assessment	Intervention	Rationale	Expected Outcome
Activities of Daily Living				
Nurse	Assess vital signs as prescribed. Auscultate heart and lung sounds. Monitor arterial blood gas values and oxygen saturation levels via pulse oximetry.	Place infant in infant seat to elevate head and chest 30° to 60°.	Elevating the head and chest relieves pressure on the diaphragm, enhancing lung expansion and heart function.	Child's vital signs remain within prescribed parameters. O$_2$ saturation is at 95%. Po$_2$ is 80–100 mm Hg.
Nurse	Assess actions that appear to allow the infant to be most comfortable.	Remove any constricting clothing from child's chest. Limit procedures to those that are necessary to provide adequate rest periods.	Constricting clothing interferes with chest expansion. Activity increases metabolic and myocardial oxygen demands, further impairing cardiopulmonary tissue perfusion.	Infants appears to rest comfortably in infant seat.

(continued)

Team Member Responsible	Assessment	Intervention	Rationale	Expected Outcome
Consultations				
Physician	Determine whether additional consultation will be necessary.	Consult with cardiac specialist on call as necessary.	Infants with congestive heart failure have few resources to use to compensate for failing heart action.	Cardiac specialist consults as necessary to better stabilize infant's condition.
Procedures/Medications				
Nurse	Assess apical pulse before administering digoxin. Obtain serum digoxin levels as ordered.	Administer digoxin as prescribed.	Digoxin improves myocardial contractility.	Infant receives digoxin based on adequate heart rate and serum level.
Nurse	Obtain baseline weight. Assess electrolytes for hypokalemia before administering diuretics.	Monitor weight daily at same time. Administer diuretics, such as furosemide, as ordered.	Weight is an indicator of fluid balance. Diuretics reduce edema and diminish afterload. Potassium can be removed with urine.	Infant receives diuretics as prescribed, based on weight and potassium status.
Nurse/ respiratory therapist	Assess O_2 saturation with continuous pulse oximetry.	Administer oxygen by infant hood.	Oxygen enhances tissue perfusion; Infant hoods provide oxygen without obscuring infant's face.	Infant's O_2 saturation remains at 95% or above.
Nutrition				
Nurse	Assess child's intake and output for adequacy.	Feed 1 oz commercial formula q4h as prescribed. Allow to rest halfway through feeding.	Eating requires energy expenditure, which could compromise heart function and interfere with nutrition.	Infant takes in prescribed formula without evidence of undue tiredness.
Nurse	Determine when mother will be present in hospital.	Urge mother to feed infant at least once daily.	Feeding can promote mother–child interaction.	Mother visits and feeds at least one feeding daily. States she is comfortable feeding ill infant.
Patient/Family Education				
Nurse	Assess parents' understanding of child's condition.	Educate parents as needed about congenital heart disease and congestive heart failure.	Parents need an understanding of child's illness to respect need for rest and medications.	Parents both state that they understand child's condition; necessary because both will be caregivers.
Psychosocial/Spiritual/Emotional Needs				
Nurse/ nurse practitioner	Assess whether parents feel they have enough emotional support to care for an ill infant at home.	Discuss necessity for vigilance and keeping infant free of infection.	Respiratory infection could quickly worsen child's condition.	Parents state that they understand the strain caring for an ill infant can cause. Have made arrangements for continuous care.

(continued)

Team Member Responsible	Assessment	Intervention	Rationale	Expected Outcome
Discharge Planning				
Nurse	Assess whether parents have any further questions about child's condition or needs.	Review care necessary for infant. Give parents written instructions.	Parents will be taking responsibility for a potentially ill infant.	Parents state that they feel confident in their ability to care for infant prior to corrective surgery.
Nurse	Assess whether parents are familiar with CPR techniques for infants.	Teach parents infant CPR technique using CPR mannequin.	Well-prepared parents can be the child's first line of defense.	Parents correctly demonstrate infant CPR technique on CPR mannequin.
Nurse	Assess whether parents will be able to return infant in 1 week for follow-up visit.	Schedule appointment for 1-week follow-up visit.	Weekly evaluation will help ascertain that child's condition remains stable until corrective surgery.	Parents state that they understand importance of follow-up visit and will keep appointment.

oxygen with nasal prongs every 4 hours to prevent pressure and subsequent irritation and breakdown of the interior nostrils (this is a major problem in newborns). For a child with heart failure, it is a strain to be submitted to strange, frightening equipment. Orient a child to oxygen equipment before it is brought to the bedside. Children generally experience such relief from dyspnea when they are receiving oxygen that their apprehension quickly disappears.

Administer Drugs as Prescribed to Strengthen Heart Action. Digoxin, a cardiac glycoside made from digitalis, acts directly on the heart to increase the contractility of the myocardium (and the force of contraction). It also slows the ventricular response in atrial arrhythmias. Digoxin is a potent drug, so doses must be prepared with extreme accuracy. For safest administration, digoxin should be prescribed with the dose designated in both milligrams and milliliters. When this is done, the milligram dose can be checked against the milliliter dose to be certain the decimal point of the milligram dose has not been inadvertently misplaced (i.e., 0.03 mg, not 0.3 mg). Digoxin may also be ordered in micrograms or μg (0.02 mg = 20 μg). Digoxin preparations are typically administered IV first in a large dose (the digitalizing dose). Six to 8 hours later, one fourth of the initial dose is given; another one fourth is given again in 6 to 8 more hours. An ECG and serum digoxin level are generally obtained before the second or third dose of digoxin to assess the adequacy of the dose. Following this, maintenance doses are given once daily. For children under 10 years of age, the dosage could be divided into two doses given at 12-hour intervals (Lee, 2003).

Before administering a dose of digoxin, obtain a child's apical pulse. As a rule, the pulse rate should be above 100 bpm in infants and above 70 bpm in older children. When effective, digoxin improves

the strength of the heart's contraction. Diuresis begins and relieves any edema present. Changes in the ECG (a lengthening of the P-R interval or a depression of the S-T segment) confirm that digitalization has taken place.

The "window" between effective digitalization and digoxin toxicity is very narrow. Monitor serum digoxin levels closely as prescribed. Symptoms of toxicity include anorexia, nausea and vomiting, dizziness, diarrhea, headache, and arrhythmia.

Many children are discharged on long-term administration of digoxin (Lanoxin). If parents will be administering the drug after their child's discharge from the hospital, be certain they understand the drug's correct dose and frequency of administration. Help them choose a specific time for administration to which they can adhere faithfully. Make out a reminder sheet to help them remember to give the drug. Instructions for home administration of digoxin are shown in Box 41.8.

Diuretics such as furosemide (Lasix) may be administered to decrease pulmonary edema, which will reduce afterload. This choice appears to be more effective than restricting salt and fluid in young children. Daily weights are a good way to gauge the diuretic's effectiveness. Be certain children are weighed at the same time, with the same scale, in the same clothing (or nude) every day so measurements are as accurate as possible and any weight loss can be noted easily. As large quantities of fluid can be lost through diuretics, so can potassium, which could lead to hypokalemia (low serum potassium levels). For these reasons, monitor urine output and serum electrolyte levels, including the potassium level. Normal urine output is 1 to 2 mL/kg/hour. If hypokalemia occurs, the risk for digoxin toxicity increases. Hydrochlorothiazide (HCTZ) is a typical diuretic used for long-term therapy. Because HCTZ, a thiazide diuretic, also promotes potassium excretion, a diet high in potassium and perhaps oral potassium

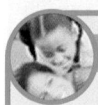

BOX 41.8 FOCUS ON . . .

FAMILY TEACHING

Giving Digoxin Safely at Home

Q. Megan's mother says to you, "The doctor has prescribed our daughter digoxin to take at home. Are there any special things we should do?"

A. Use the guidelines below to ensure safe digoxin administration at home:

- Always assess an apical pulse before administration; do not administer the drug if your child's heart rate is below 100 bpm (or as specifically instructed as she grows older).
- Always use the same measuring device (spoon or dropper) each time, so the dose given remains consistent.
- Do not change the amount or timing of the dose without specific instructions from your primary care provider.
- If you omit a single dose, give the next dose on time as prescribed.
- If you omit more than one dose, telephone your primary care provider for further instructions.
- Give digoxin 1 hour before or 2 hours after feeding, to avoid a dose being lost if the child spits up.
- If a dose is vomited, do not repeat the dose. Give the next dose at the scheduled time. If the child vomits the next dose, call your primary care provider.
- Notify your primary care provider if the child vomits more than once each day, because vomiting is a sign of digoxin overdose (toxicity).
- Notify your primary care provider if administration of the medicine or the timing of the dose is difficult for your lifestyle.

---

supplementation may be prescribed to maintain potassium levels. Liquid potassium is irritating to the gastrointestinal tract and should be given mixed with fruit juice.

Nursing Diagnosis: Risk for imbalanced nutrition, less than body requirements, related to fatigue

Outcome Evaluation: Child maintains percentile curve on growth chart; skin turgor is good.

Maintaining proper nutrition may be a problem for children with heart failure because they tire easily. Eating six to eight small meals daily is often less tiring than eating three large meals. Smaller meals also prevent the child's stomach from pressing upward on the diaphragm and compromising an enlarged heart. Sucking is hard work, so infants may need to drink smaller amounts frequently to maintain adequate fluid intake or receive a higher-calorie formula to allow for adequate calories without added fluid volume. Using soft "preemie" nipples may be helpful because they make sucking

easier. If an infant is breast-fed, the mother may need to consult a lactation consultant to coordinate a program of frequent feedings.

Nursing Diagnosis: Fear related to child's ill appearance and possible disease outcome

Outcome Evaluation: Parents and child openly discuss fears and concerns, actively question, and express confidence in treatment plan and health care team.

By school age, children with heart failure are usually aware of the seriousness of their condition. They learn this from the frequent procedures and visits to cardiologists and from the exhaustion they feel because their heart is not working well. They may lie stiffly in bed, afraid to move, afraid to burden their already overtaxed heart with even simple activities such as turning pages in a book. Offer reassurance that although their heart is a little behind in its action, the oxygen and medication they are receiving are helping. Reassure them that people are checking on them frequently and observing them closely in between as well as during procedures. Give them time to talk and use play to express their fears.

Parents of a child with heart failure need the same reassurance (provided, of course, the statements are true). They are as frightened by what the physician has told them as by their child's obviously ill appearance. It is often helpful to point out subtle signs of improvement in their child that they may not notice on their own, such as a slower heart rate or slower, less distressed respirations.

If the child will be cared for at home, review CPR techniques to be certain parents know what to do in an emergency. Be certain they have a follow-up appointment scheduled and a telephone number they can call if they have any concerns about their child's condition.

Persistent Pulmonary Hypertension

Persistent pulmonary hypertension (PPH) results when the pulmonary vascular resistance present at birth because of unopened alveoli fails to fall to normal. The disorder occurs most often in full-term infants who have experienced perinatal asphyxia from conditions such as meconium aspiration, respiratory distress syndrome, or intrauterine infection.

PPH occurs because hypoxia and acidosis from respiratory difficulty cause vasoconstriction of the pulmonary artery. The infant develops tachypnea. Pulse oximetry shows a low PO_2 from inability of blood to perfuse the lungs because of the pulmonary artery constriction. The resulting hypoxia and acidosis cause even greater vasoconstriction of the pulmonary artery. An echocardiogram slows right-to-left shunting across the patent ductus or foramen ovale.

Treatment consists of supportive therapy such as oxygen, high-frequency oscillatory ventilation, IV glucose to provide calories, antibiotics to combat infection, medications to reduce pulmonary resistance, and other drugs, such as low-dose dopamine, to elevate systemic blood pressure. Sodium bicarbonate may be necessary to relieve acidosis and to help reverse pulmonary vasoconstriction. Inhaled nitric oxide may be administered to promote pulmonary vasodilatation. Infants who do not respond to these usual measures may require ECMO to allow the lungs to rest until adequate pulmonary vasodilatation and the return of alveoli perfusion can be achieved.

PPH is a serious threat to newborns, both because of the original insult from respiratory distress that produced the syndrome and the prolonged therapy course. Because of this, a newborn may be left with neurologic damage from severe hypoxia and inadequate brain cell oxygen perfusion (Conway, 2003).

Rheumatic Fever

Rheumatic fever is an autoimmune disease that occurs as a reaction to a group A beta-hemolytic streptococcal infection (Hoffman, 2003). Inflammation from the immune response leads to fibrin deposits on the endocardium and valves, in particular the mitral valve, as well as in the major body joints. The disease often follows an attack of pharyngitis, tonsillitis, scarlet fever, "strep throat," or impetigo, because the organism common to these infections is a group A beta-hemolytic streptococcus. In 95% of children with acute rheumatic fever, an elevation of one or more antistreptococcal antibodies, an indication of a recent streptococcal infection, can be documented (Hoffman, 2003).

Although the incidence of rheumatic fever has declined greatly in recent years, the disease has not been eradicated, and in some inner cities the incidence is rising. It occurs most often in children 6 to 15 years of age, with a peak incidence at 8 years. It is seen most often in poor, crowded urban areas. Because children do not develop immunity to streptococcal infections, streptococcal infections recur; rheumatic fever also recurs.

The symptoms of the original streptococcal infection subside in a few days with or without antimicrobial therapy. Children appear well again. After 1 to 3 weeks, however, if the child was not treated with an appropriate antibiotic for the original infection, the onset of rheumatic fever symptoms can begin. Because nurses are the primary people who advise parents when to seek health care and how to adhere to medicine administration, nurses have contributed greatly to the decline of this disorder.

Assessment

The signs and symptoms of rheumatic fever are divided into major and minor symptoms according to the Jones criteria (Box 41.9). Of these, the heart involvement is the most serious. The child usually has a systolic murmur from mitral insufficiency and prolonged P-R and Q-T intervals on the ECG that reflect inflammation and slowing of impulse conduction. Chorea (sudden involuntary movement of the limbs) is a striking symptom. This loss of voluntary muscle control due to inflammation of basal ganglia occurs most often in children between 7 and 14 years of age (rarely after age 20). It occurs more frequently in girls than boys (Hoffman, 2003). Dysfunctional speech from chorea may be

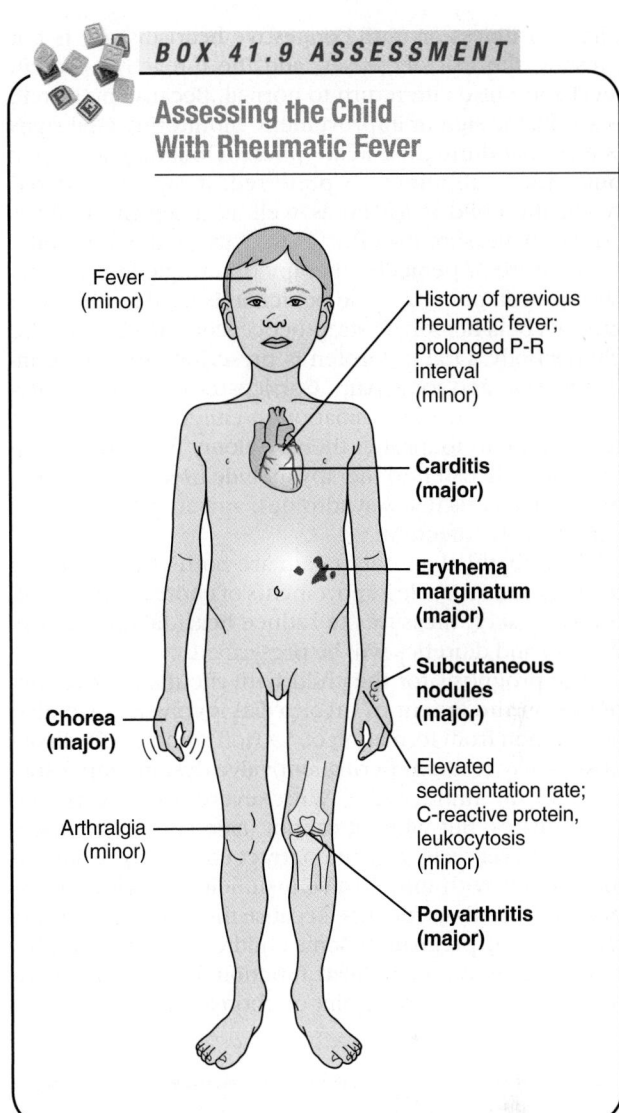

BOX 41.9 ASSESSMENT

Assessing the Child With Rheumatic Fever

- Fever (minor)
- History of previous rheumatic fever; prolonged P-R interval (minor)
- Carditis (major)
- Erythema marginatum (major)
- Subcutaneous nodules (major)
- Elevated sedimentation rate; C-reactive protein, leukocytosis (minor)
- Chorea (major)
- Arthralgia (minor)
- Polyarthritis (major)

demonstrated by asking the child to count rapidly. Children with chorea begin with clear speech, but then suddenly the sounds become garbled or they cannot speak for several seconds. If asked to protrude the tongue, children cannot keep from making undulating, jerky movements. If asked to extend their arms in front of them, they soon hyperextend their wrists and fingers. Hand grasp may be weak or may consist of spasmodic contractions and relaxation. If asked to smile, the facial expression may change rapidly from a "Cheshire cat" grin to a flat, expressionless affect or grimace. Erythema marginatum, a macular rash found predominantly on the trunk, subcutaneous nodules or painless lumps on tendon sheaths by the joints, and tender swollen large joints (polyarthritis) are additional manifestations. Important laboratory findings include the presence of an antibody anti-streptococcal titer (ASO) and an increased ESR and C-reactive protein levels (Fischbach, 2005).

Therapeutic Management

The full course of rheumatic fever is 6 to 8 weeks. Children are maintained on bed rest only during the acute phase of illness or until congestive heart disease is not present, the ESR decreases, and the C-reactive protein level and pulse rate return to normal. Because pulse rate is a valuable sign of improvement, monitoring vital signs is essential during the acute phase. Obtaining an apical pulse for a full minute is preferred. It may be ordered when the child is asleep as well as when the child is awake to measure the effect of activity on the pulse rate.

A course of penicillin therapy or a single intramuscular injection of benzathine penicillin is used to eliminate group A beta-hemolytic streptococci completely from the child's body. Oral ibuprofen is prescribed to reduce inflammation and joint pain. Corticosteroids may be prescribed to reduce inflammation in children who are not responding to ibuprofen therapy alone. Possible side effects of corticosteroid therapy include hirsutism, a round moon face (Cushing's syndrome), and an increased susceptibility to infection.

Phenobarbital and diazepam are both effective in reducing the purposeless movements of chorea. If heart failure is present, measures to reduce heart failure such as digoxin and diuretics will be prescribed.

The prognosis for the child with rheumatic fever depends on the extent of myocardial involvement. Valve destruction from formation of Aschoff's bodies (fibrin deposits) may result in permanent valve dysfunction, especially of the mitral valve. With severe myocarditis the heart dilates, but when it cannot maintain this compensation, it eventually fails to contract effectively. Children may be left with mitral valve insufficiency, which is especially hazardous for girls, because this may lead to heart failure during pregnancy. Some children need mitral valve replacement to restore heart function. Usually, there are no residual effects from joint or chorea involvement.

injection of a long-acting penicillin, such as benzathine penicillin (Bicillin), can be used with children if there is a question whether the parent will give, or the child will take, the full course of oral penicillin. Be sure to repeat prescription instructions for parents in ambulatory settings so they understand how often and how much of a drug is to be given and the need to give the drug for the full 10 to 14 days. Usually the child's symptoms will fade before then, and if the parents are not cautioned about the importance of the drug, they may give the drug for only 2 or 3 days and then discontinue it.

Prevent Recurrent Attacks. Children who have had rheumatic fever must be prevented from contracting the disease again to prevent valve damage from occurring a second time. To do this, they must take prophylactic antibiotic therapy for at least 5 years after the initial attack, or until they are 18 years of age. If some valve involvement is present, many physicians advocate maintaining the child on penicillin indefinitely. Penicillin may be prescribed as monthly injections of benzathine penicillin G or daily oral doses of aqueous penicillin (penicillin V).

Additional prophylactic measures should be instituted when dental or tonsillar surgery is planned, because most children have streptococci in their throats. With an open incision in the mouth, the risk of streptococcal invasion of the bloodstream increases.

Nursing Diagnosis: Situational low self-esteem related to chorea movements secondary to rheumatic fever

Outcome Evaluation: Child expresses frustration with inability to control movements; continues to feed and dress self with help as needed.

Children may have difficulty feeding themselves because of chorea. They may also be emotionally unstable and cry easily. Emphasize the transitory nature of the chorea; stress that it is frustrating to have to be fed and to be unable to use your hands meaningfully, but that this lack of coordination will pass without permanent effects. Provide toys and games that do not require fine coordination, because it may be frustrating to try to do something such as move checkers or chessmen on a board (a typical low-activity game). Children with chorea who are on bed rest may need to have the bedrails padded so they do not injure themselves from thrashing movements.

NURSING DIAGNOSES AND RELATED INTERVENTIONS

Nursing Diagnosis: Risk for nonadherence to drug therapy related to knowledge deficit about importance of long-term therapy

Outcome Evaluation: Child takes oral penicillin daily; absence of symptoms of throat infection; vital signs are within age-acceptable parameters.

Therapy for Initial Attack. After mild cases of streptococcal pharyngitis, rheumatic fever occurs in about 0.3% of children. After severe streptococcal infections, the attack rate may be as high as 1% to 3% (Hoffman, 2003). Either amoxicillin or penicillin is used to eliminate streptococci from the upper respiratory tract. To be effective, a drug level must be maintained for 10 to 14 days. Erythromycin is used in children sensitive to penicillin; it, too, must be continued for at least 10 days. One intramuscular

Kawasaki Disease

Kawasaki disease (mucocutaneous lymph node syndrome) is a febrile, multisystem disorder that occurs almost exclusively in children before the age of puberty. The peak incidence is in boys under 4 years of age. The incidence is higher in late winter and spring. **Vasculitis** (inflammation of blood vessels) is the principal (and life-threatening) finding because it can lead to formation of aneurysm and myocardial infarction (Callahan, 2003).

The cause of Kawasaki disease is unknown, but it apparently develops in genetically predisposed individuals after exposure to an as-yet-unidentified infectious agent. After the infection (perhaps an upper respiratory infection), altered immune function occurs. An increase in antibody production creates circulating immune (antibody-antigen) complexes that bind to the vascular endothelium and cause inflammation. The inflammation of blood vessels leads to aneurysms, platelet accumulation, and the formation of thrombi or obstruction in the heart and blood vessels.

Assessment

Kawasaki disease begins with an acute phase (stage I) of high fever (102° to 104°F [39.0° to 40.0°C]) that does not respond to antipyretics (Box 41.10). The child acts lethargic or irritable and may have reddened and swollen hands and feet. Soon the bulbar mucous membranes of the eyes become inflamed (conjunctivitis) and the child develops a "strawberry" tongue and red, cracked lips. A variety of rashes occur, often confined to the diaper area. Cervical lymph nodes become enlarged. As internal lymph nodes

> **BOX 41.11**
>
> **Criteria for Diagnosis of Kawasaki Disease**
>
> 1. Fever of 5 or more days' duration
> 2. Bilateral congestion of ocular conjunctivae
> 3. Changes of the mucous membrane of the upper respiratory tract, such as reddened pharynx; red, dry, fissured lips; or protuberance of tongue papillae ("strawberry" tongue)
> 4. Changes of the peripheral extremities, such as peripheral edema, peripheral erythema, desquamation of palms and soles
> 5. Rash, primarily truncal and polymorphous
> 6. Cervical lymph node swelling

swell, children may develop abdominal pain, anorexia, and diarrhea. Joints may swell and redden, simulating an arthritic process. White blood cell count and the ESR are both elevated.

About 10 days after the onset, a subacute phase begins. The skin desquamates, particularly on the palms and soles. The platelet count rises; this increases the possibility of clotting, which could result in necrosis of distant body cells, particularly the fingertips, if they no longer receive adequate blood. Aneurysms may form in coronary arteries, compromising heart activity. Sudden death from accumulating thrombi or rupture of an aneurysm may occur, making this the most dangerous phase.

The convalescent phase (stage II) begins at about the 25th day and lasts until 40 days. Stage III lasts from 40 days until the ESR returns to normal. To be diagnosed with Kawasaki disease, a child must manifest fever and four of the typical symptoms shown in Box 41.11, plus echocardiographic confirmation of artery disease. Children are followed by sequential echocardiograms to monitor for development of aneurysms.

Therapeutic Management

The administration of acetylsalicylic acid (aspirin) or ibuprofen decreases inflammation and blocks platelet aggregation. Abciximab is a platelet receptor inhibitor specific for Kawasaki disease (Karch, 2004). IV immune globulin can also be administered to reduce the immune response. Steroids, which may increase aneurysm formation, are contraindicated. If the child is left with coronary artery disease from stenosis of the coronary arteries, coronary artery bypass surgery may be necessary in the future.

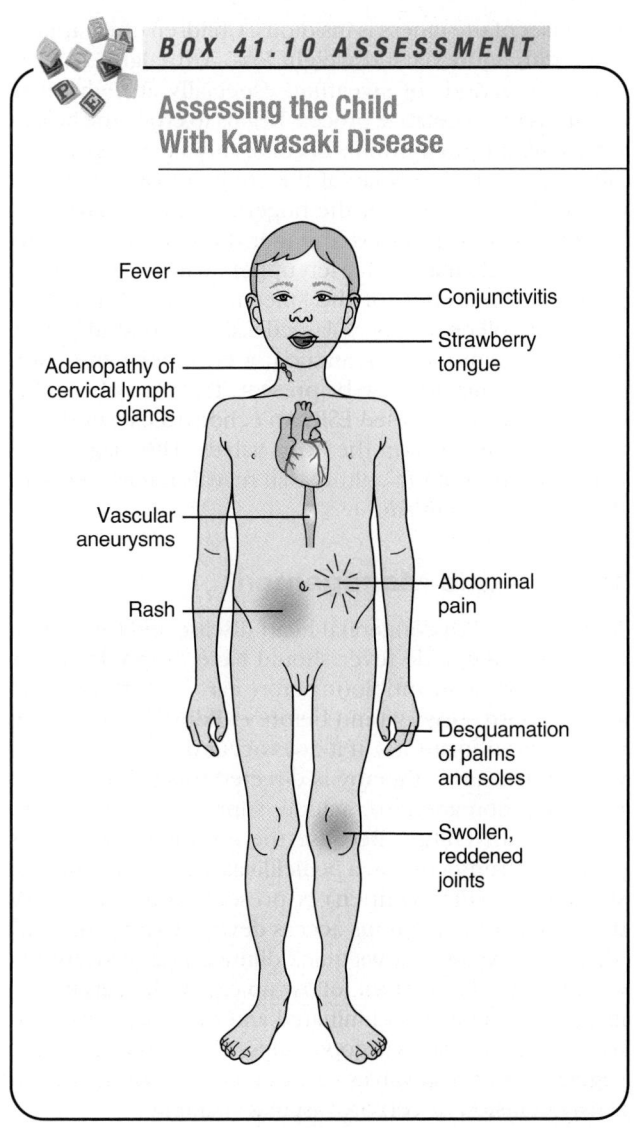

BOX 41.10 ASSESSMENT

Assessing the Child With Kawasaki Disease

- Fever
- Conjunctivitis
- Strawberry tongue
- Adenopathy of cervical lymph glands
- Vascular aneurysms
- Rash
- Abdominal pain
- Desquamation of palms and soles
- Swollen, reddened joints

NURSING DIAGNOSES AND RELATED INTERVENTIONS

Nursing Diagnosis: Risk for ineffective peripheral tissue perfusion related to inflammation of blood vessels

Outcome Evaluation: Child's pulse, blood pressure, and respiratory rate are within age-established parameters; capillary filling time is less than 5 seconds.

Observe for signs of heart failure such as tachycardia, dyspnea, rales, and edema. Inspect the extremities for color and palpate for warmth and capillary filling in toes and fingers to evaluate peripheral tissue perfusion. If a child is developing myocarditis, be alert for chest pain, arrhythmias, and ECG changes. All these are findings that need to be reported and documented.

Nursing Diagnosis: Pain related to swelling of lymph nodes and inflammation of joints

Outcome Evaluation: Child states level of pain is tolerable; rates it below 2 on a standard scale.

A child with Kawasaki disease is uncomfortable from the joint involvement, edema, pruritic rash, abdominal discomfort, and the frequent blood sampling necessary to monitor the platelet count. The high fever can lead to dry, cracked lips. Ibuprofen, administered for its anti-inflammatory action, helps reduce both the pain and itchiness (which is a low level of pain). Provide additional comfort measures such as rocking and holding. Protect edematous areas from pressure; make certain clothing is not constricting and irritating areas of rash. Applying lip balm protects lips from drying and cracking.

Because the fever remains high, offer extra fluid to help maintain hydration and reduce mouth tenderness. Keep the child free of heavy blankets or clothing and prevent overexertion. Monitor IV fluid to prevent fluid overload.

Children with Kawasaki disease lose their appetite and generally eat poorly because of the systemic illness, mouth soreness from cracks and fissures, and abdominal pressure from swollen lymph nodes. Carefully monitor and record the child's intake and output. Encourage the child to continue brushing his or her teeth (use a soft toothbrush or a padded tongue blade), even though the oral mucous membrane is tender. Soft, nonirritating foods such as gelatin (Jell-O) may be better tolerated than foods that require chewing and acidic fluids, such as orange juice, that might sting. Observe for signs of gastrointestinal obstruction, such as vomiting.

Most children with Kawasaki disease recover fully, but a few will need cardiac bypass surgery to treat aneurysms that developed in the coronary arteries.

What if... a child with Kawasaki disease has ibuprofen ordered every 4 hours but tells you she no longer has pain or fever? Should you continue to give it?

Endocarditis

Endocarditis is inflammation and infection of the endocardium or valves of the heart. It may occur in a child without heart disease but more commonly occurs as a complication of congenital heart disease such as tetralogy of Fallot, VSD, or coarctation of the aorta. The infection is generally caused by streptococci of the viridans type, although staphylococcal or fungal organisms may be at fault. The streptococcal infection tends to invade the body during oral surgery, such as with dental extractions. It also can enter from a urinary tract infection or a skin infection, such as impetigo. As the disease progresses, vegetation composed of bacteria, fibrin, and blood appears on the endocardium of the valves and heart chambers. This tends to occur more commonly on the left side of the heart, although if a heart defect is present the erosion begins at the site of the defect. Over a period of time, the invading process destroys the endocardial lining of the heart. Underlying muscle and valves are also affected (Jacobson, 2003).

Assessment

The onset of the illness is insidious. Children often appear pale, with anorexia and weight loss. Arthralgia, malaise, chills, or periods of sweating, especially at night, may occur. As the vegetative process begins to erode the heart's valves, significant murmurs become audible. Signs of heart failure appear. Petechiae of the conjunctiva or oral mucosa or hemorrhages of the fingernails or toenails (that simulate a splinter inserted under the nail) may be present. The child may notice left upper quadrant abdominal pain from infarction of the spleen; on physical assessment, the spleen may be enlarged. Laboratory studies may reveal proteinuria or hematuria; a normochromic, normocytic anemia may also be present. There may be leukocytosis and an increased ESR. An echocardiogram shows vegetative growths on the heart valves. The diagnosis is confirmed by a blood culture that reveals the presence of the invading organism.

Therapeutic Management

All children with congenital heart disease and those who have had rheumatic fever should have prophylactic administration of an antibiotic before ear, nose, throat, tonsil, or mouth surgery (and before childbirth) to prevent infectious endocarditis. If it does occur despite these preventive measures, therapy is directed toward the underlying infection and also includes supportive measures to reduce heart failure. Because the invading organism is generally streptococcus, a penicillinase-resistant penicillin such as nafcillin (Unipen) is prescribed and given IV through a central venous access device. Giving the drug into a large vessel allows quick dilution and distribution. Children need long-term follow-up care to be certain the invading organism is eliminated and the disease process has halted. Prognosis is good unless an embolus from the vegetations on the valves causes a complication such as renal occlusion or cerebrovascular accident.

Arrhythmias

Children have fewer cardiac arrhythmias than do adults, but the number of these is increasing as more and more children survive cardiac surgery for congenital heart disease but are left with a cardiac arrhythmia due to septal trauma (Stefanelli & Fischbach, 2003). Better means of monitoring cardiac rhythm patterns through the use of Holter monitors has also made detection of cardiac arrhythmia easier. Remember that most children show a normal sinus arrhythmia or a slowing of the heart rate during inspiration (increased lung size slows lung perfusion, putting enough back-pressure on the heart to slow the heartbeat), with the normal rate resuming on expiration.

Ventricular tachycardia and atrial fibrillation are syndromes that occur because of multiple or abnormal initiation of the heartbeat and can occur following surgery for congenital heart disease. These can cause episodes of syncope, palpitations, and exercise intolerance. If bradycardia occurs, it can be treated with a drug such as atropine to counteract vagal stimulation; digoxin is commonly used for decreasing and strengthening the heart rate if needed. A few children may require pacemakers implanted to maintain a steady heart rhythm (Timothy & Rodeman, 2004).

Radiofrequency ablation is a nonsurgical transvenous catheter technique that can permanently disrupt an abnormal arrhythmia focus. A technique once reserved for adults, this can now be used even for infants (Blaufox, Paul, & Saul, 2004).

Hypertension

Although primary hypertension may occur in children, hypertension in children usually occurs as a secondary manifestation of another disease such as a kidney disorder. It has a higher incidence among black children than other ethnic groups and occurs in about 1% of schoolchildren and adolescents (Box 41.12). As obesity in children is increasing, the incidence of hypertension in children is also increasing.

It is difficult to define hypertension in children because normal blood pressure varies with the age of the child. A systolic pressure reading above the 95th percentile for a given age may be used as a practical criterion (Schulman, 2003).

BOX 41.12 FOCUS ON . . .

DIVERSITY OF CARE

Hypertension, hypercholesterolemia, and congenital heart disorders occur at higher incidences in some adolescents than others because these disorders tend to be familial. Hypertension, for example, occurs at a higher rate in African Americans than in other groups. Nurses have a responsibility to educate adolescents about the importance of maintaining a sensible sodium intake and reducing saturated fat and cholesterol intake, in an attempt to minimize these familial disorders. Be knowledgeable about cultural preferences in foods when planning preventive health care.

Assessment

Beginning at 3 years of age, blood pressure should be included as a part of routine health assessment. Normal blood pressure and the technique of blood pressure recording in children are discussed in Chapter 33. To ensure accuracy, be sure a child is relaxed, after at least 1 or 2 minutes of rest, before taking a blood pressure. When children are discovered on routine physical assessments to have hypertension, the reading should be repeated at a successive visit to confirm that the abnormal reading was not a reaction to the stress of the examination or some other emotional event of that day. Only when the blood pressure is still elevated on a third occasion is hypertension diagnosed.

When a child has hypertension, a number of additional studies are performed to discover underlying disease conditions. The most common diseases associated with hypertension in children are renal and cardiac diseases such as coarctation of the aorta, Cushing's syndrome, primary hyperaldosteronism, adrenogenital syndrome, pheochromocytoma (a tumor of the adrenal gland), and brain tumor. If blood pressure is elevated, record a blood pressure in both lower extremities and upper extremities to help rule out coarctation of the aorta (which results in low pressure in the lower extremities). Obtain a urine specimen for analysis of microalbuminuria, a finding that accompanies hypertension. If red blood cells are present in urine, this suggests glomerulonephritis, a kidney disease that increases blood pressure. Children with suspected hypertension should have a funduscopic examination of their eyes to determine the presence of papilledema or spasm, or hemorrhage of the retinal arteries from the consistently elevated blood pressure. If papilledema is present, children need immediate care to prevent optic nerve damage. Further studies to rule out adrenal or renal disease may be ordered if these preliminary assessment procedures do not reveal a cause for the hypertension (Lundquist & Zimmermann, 2005).

Therapeutic Management

Therapy for hypertension depends on the underlying primary disease. Although the underlying disease conditions that lead to hypertension are serious disorders, they are also ones that can respond to therapy. Therefore, hypertension must not be dismissed lightly.

If essential hypertension (elevated blood pressure for no identifiable reason) is present and a child is obese, he or she is placed on a reducing diet and urged to increase the level of exercise to reduce weight. Salt intake is rarely limited, but it may be if intake has been excessive; girls are advised not to use oral contraceptives, which elevate blood pressure. Unfortunately, because mild hypertension produces few symptoms, often children do not adhere to nutritional suggestions or suggested exercise programs well. For these children, a single medication such as an angiotensin-converting enzyme (ACE) inhibitor (e.g., captopril [Capoten]) may be prescribed. A diuretic such as furosemide (Lasix) or vasodilators such as hydralazine (Apresoline) may also be added.

Children with hypertension need continued counseling at health care visits. Educate them and their parents about its long-term effects (increased risk of heart and blood vessel disease). Only if they understand these long-term consequences can they see the benefits of taking medication today.

Dyslipidemia

Dyslipidemia (increased lipids in blood serum) can involve cholesterol or triglycerides. Risk factors include familial hypercholesterolemia, a dominantly inherited disease occurring in 5% to 25% of children; obesity; a sedentary lifestyle; and a high-fat diet (Liacouras, 2003). For this reason, all children of parents with premature coronary artery disease (disease before the age of 55) or a family history of hypercholesterolemia (parents with blood cholesterol levels above 200 mg/dL or low-density lipoprotein [LDL] levels above 130 mg/dL) should be screened for total serum cholesterol, because there is an association between high total cholesterol and LDL and the incidence of coronary artery disease. This is particularly important if the child smokes, is obese, or has a sedentary lifestyle.

Acceptable levels of total cholesterol and LDL in children are less than 170 mg/dL and less than 110 mg/dL, respectively. Levels are borderline if they are 170 to 199 mg/dL and 110 to 129 mg/dL. They are high if over 200 mg/dL and 130 mg/dL (Liacouras, 2003).

If the total triglyceride, cholesterol, or LDL level is found to be elevated, the child's diet should be regulated in an attempt to lower these levels. Exercise also should be increased. Adolescents may be placed on the American Heart Association's step 1 diet (total fat no more than 30% of calories; cholesterol less than 300 mg/day) to attempt to bring them into adulthood with sound nutritional habits. Children rarely are placed on low-fat diets because they need calories for growth. Use of low-fat diets in infants under 2 years of age is even less common because fat is needed for myelinization of nerves.

If the child becomes an adolescent and the diet has not been effective, one of the many cholesterol-reducing agents such as cholestyramine (Questran) may be prescribed. These agents reduce the cholesterol level by binding bile acids and decreasing their reabsorption. Side effects of these drugs include large, bulky stools and possible gastrointestinal discomfort. If this therapy is ineffective, an HMG-CoA inhibitor such as atorvastatin (Lipitor) may be prescribed.

Because hypercholesterolemia has no symptoms, it is difficult to motivate children to continue a special diet and take medication. They need continued counseling at health care visits so they understand the damage that excess lipids can cause.

Cardiomyopathy

The term "cardiomyopathy" refers to a structural or functional abnormality of the ventricular myocardium that occurs following an infection such as adenovirus, cytomegalovirus, or HIV/AIDS infection and results in severe dilation of the left or both ventricles. This impairs systolic function and leads to heart failure. Idiopathic dilated cardiomyopathy (IDC) is a rare form that presents before 2 years of age, usually after a viral respiratory or gastrointestinal illness (Maron, 2004).

In the older child, symptoms appear gradually. Physical examination reveals an ill-appearing child with severe respiratory distress. Peripheral pulses are weak and blood pressure is decreased. Pulsus alternans (beat-to-beat variation) is a common finding. The liver is enlarged from backflow pressure. A chest x-ray, echocardiogram, and ECG all reveal the enlarged heart.

Therapy is directed at controlling the heart failure by bed rest, fluid restriction, and pharmacologic agents to decrease the cardiac load, improve myocardial contractility, and decrease afterload. Immune globulin may help reverse the process. If a child fails to respond to medical therapy, the prognosis is poor unless the child is eligible for cardiac transplantation.

CARDIOPULMONARY ARREST

Children with heart disease are at high risk for cardiopulmonary arrest, although this may occur in any child for reasons such as airway obstruction, trauma, anaphylactic reaction, central nervous system depression, drowning, or electrocution. Management of cardiopulmonary arrest may vary according to the cause of the arrest and the age of the patient, but the basic considerations are the same.

Many health care facilities and public buildings provide automated external defibrillators (AEDs) for use in cardiac resuscitation. Nurses who respond to emergencies need to familiarize themselves with this equipment as well as CPR technique (AHA, 2005).

Assessment

Respiratory failure is the most frequent cause of cardiac arrest because anoxia in the heart muscle quickly leads to cardiac arrest. When cardiac arrest occurs, no audible heart sounds or pulses can be obtained. No blood pressure can be recorded (don't waste time trying to obtain one). If a cardiac monitor was attached before the arrest, it will show no ECG complex. This is a helpful assessment if available, but again do not waste time attaching monitor leads if they are not already in place. The outcome for the child will depend to a great extent on the speed with which resuscitation is begun, so it is better to err on the side of unnecessary resuscitation rather than delayed resuscitation. The steps for resuscitation can be remembered as "ABCs" (airway, breathing, and circulation).

Airway

The first step in resuscitation is to shake the child and call the child's name to verify that a child is not just sound asleep. If a child does not respond to this action, call for help. Turn the child onto his or her back and open the mouth. Tip the child's head backward slightly to a neutral position or place a rolled towel or other fairly firm object under the neck to hyperextend the head slightly (a "sniffing" position). Do not overextend the neck, however, or you will occlude, not clear, the airway (AHA, 2005).

Breathing

Emergency equipment such as an Ambu-bag should be readily available in all health care settings so that mouth-to-mouth resuscitation is not necessary. If no breathing bag is available, use a protective one-way valve mask for mouth-to-mouth resuscitation to protect yourself from body secretions.

For small infants, place the bag mask over the infant's mouth and nose, creating a seal. For large infants and children, make a bag-to-mouth seal, pinching the child's nose tightly with the thumb and forefingers. Provide two slow breaths (1 to 1.5 seconds per breath). It may be necessary to adjust the head-tilt chin position to obtain optimal airway patency, although this should not be done if neck or spine trauma is suspected (AHA, 2005).

If oxygen is available, attach it to the resuscitation bag, running at a rate of about 4 L/min. However, do not wait for oxygen if it is not available. Room air's oxygen content is about 21%, so additional oxygen is helpful but not necessary for resuscitation.

Observe the child's chest with each breath you administer to see if it rises. If it does not, the airway is obstructed and air cannot reach the lungs. Perform back blows and chest thrusts for an infant or abdominal thrusts for an older child to help relieve the obstruction. Continued breaths should be given at the rate of normal respirations (20/min) in both infants and older children. When respiratory arrest has occurred and mechanical ventilation is anticipated, the child needs to be intubated to provide an open airway, as discussed in Chapter 40.

Circulation

After the two initial ventilations, feel for a carotid pulse (in an infant, the brachial pulse) or assess for other signs of circulation, such as adequate color (Fig. 41.20). It is better to use the carotid than a peripheral pulse as an indicator of cardiac function in older children, because with shock, the peripheral pulses may be absent while the heart is still beating. The carotid pulse is also the easiest to assess from your position near the child's head. In an infant, however, the neck may be too chubby for you to easily palpate the carotid pulses, so the brachial pulse is easiest to assess.

If you feel no pulse, begin chest compressions. In a newborn, enough pressure will be generated by two fingers pressed on the midsternum about a fingerbreadth below the nipple line to a depth of 0.5 to 1 inch (Fig. 41.21). Midsternal compression is used with newborns and infants to prevent excessive pressure on the ribs and the possibility of breaking either a rib or the xiphoid process (which then might puncture the heart or liver). In the older child, you need to apply the heel of your palm over the sternum (measure one or two fingerbreadths up from the sternal-costal notch and place the palm there) and compress 1 to 1.5 inches (Fig. 41.22). Compress the chest at a rate of 100 bpm in both infants and older children (AHA, 2005).

Breathing and cardiac compression must be carried out concurrently but not exactly at the same time. If there are two people available for resuscitation, one can administer breaths to the child while the other compresses the chest. If you are by yourself, you must do both. For infants, administer one breath, then compress the chest five times; administer another breath, then compress the chest five more times, and so forth. This 1:5 ratio of ventilations to compressions is necessary to effectively ventilate and circulate blood for this size child. For older children, use a 2:15 ratio as with adults. A 2:15 ratio reduces the number of times compressions must be interrupted for breaths. Be certain that you release the pressure on the chest between compressions; this allows the heart to fill more readily. Do not lift your fingers or hands off the chest, however, because doing so requires time spent to properly reposition them. Also make sure to maintain a patent airway by using the head-tilt chin lift using the hand not

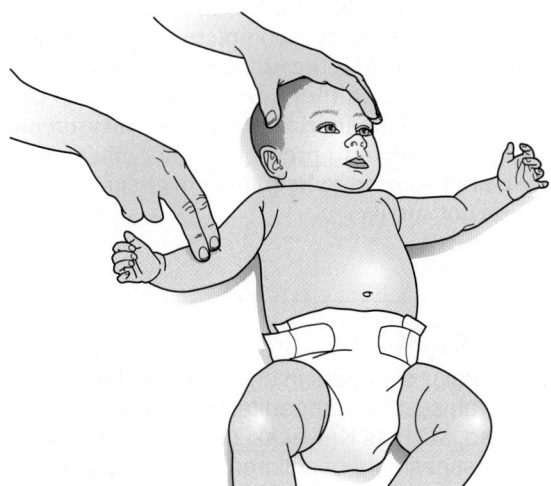

FIGURE 41.20 Assessing a brachial pulse in an infant.

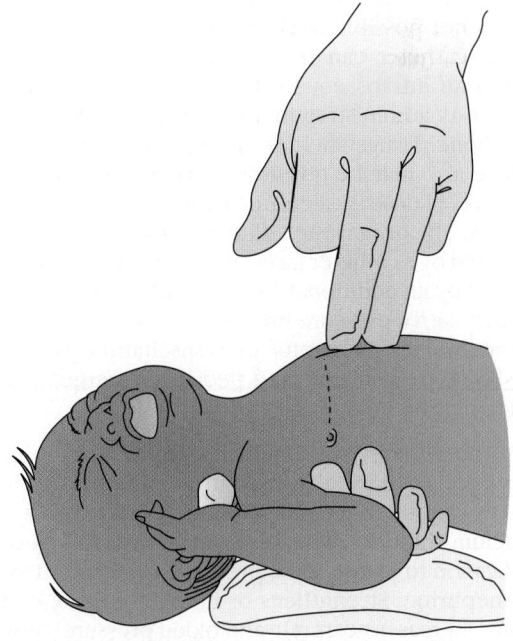

FIGURE 41.21 With cardiac resuscitation in a newborn or infant, chest compression is best done by pressing two fingers on the midsternum. Notice the slight extension of the infant's head to maintain a patent airway.

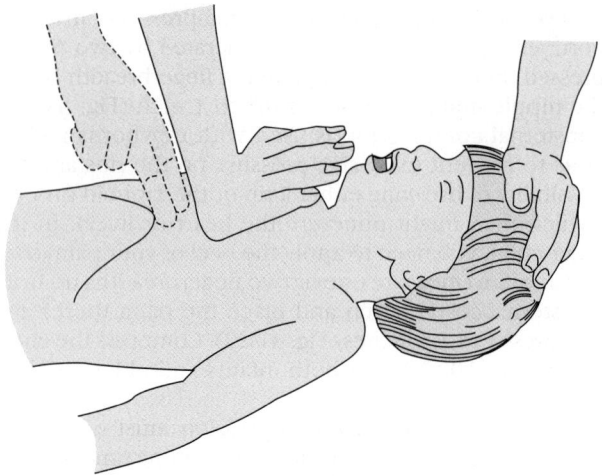

FIGURE 41.22 Locating hand position for cardiac compression in an older child.

performing the compressions. If the resuscitation attempt is successful, the child's color will improve (especially the oral mucous membrane, which is readily visible) and the carotid pulse will become palpable.

These three techniques (clearing the airway, ventilating the lungs, and circulating blood by cardiac compression) will provide adequate oxygenation to major body organs for several minutes until additional personnel arrive who can initiate further resuscitation measures. The outcome of these secondary measures depends on how well and promptly the initial measures were performed.

Secondary Measures

IV access must be accomplished for drug administration. If this is not possible in about a minute's time, an intraosseous catheter can be inserted. Drugs administered through an intraosseous route reach the circulation as rapidly as IV administration because of the rich blood supply in bone. Drugs such as epinephrine, lidocaine, and atropine also may be given by an endotracheal tube. An endotracheal dose is calculated by multiplying the IV dose by 2 or 3. The drug is then diluted with normal saline, administered by a catheter inserted deeply into the tube, and followed by an additional 1 or 2 mL of normal saline and several positive-pressure breaths.

Common drugs helpful in resuscitation procedures that should be available on a pediatric emergency resuscitation cart include:

- Atropine: Reduces bronchial secretions, keeping the airway clear during resuscitation attempts. It also reduces vagus nerve effects, relieving bradycardia.
- Calcium chloride: Increases heart contractility. A contraindication to its use is the presence of digitalis toxicity.
- Epinephrine: Strengthens or initiates cardiac contractions; increases heart rate and blood pressure; bronchodilates
- Adenosine: Relieves arrhythmias
- Lidocaine: Counteracts ventricular arrhythmias
- Bretylium tosylate: Like lidocaine, counteracts ventricular arrhythmias

- Dopamine: Increases cardiac output. It acts on alpha-receptors to cause vasoconstriction.
- Dobutamine: Acts as a direct-acting beta-agonist that increases contractility and heart rate

Checkpoint Question 5

You need to teach CPR to Megan's parents before hospital discharge. What is the ratio of ventilation to compressions used for resuscitating an infant?

a. One to five
b. One to ten
c. Two to fifteen
d. Three to fifteen

Psychological Support

A cardiopulmonary arrest is an acute emergency, and everyone who arrives at the scene should know what course of action to take. Even after heart action has been initiated, ventricular fibrillation may occur, requiring defibrillation. As soon as a child begins to respond to resuscitation, be aware that he or she begins to hear. The child is obviously frightened by the number of people and all the equipment surrounding him or her, such as cardiac monitor leads, IV tubing, and possibly an endotracheal tube. The child may have vivid memories of frightening body sensations just before going into cardiac arrest. A child may regain consciousness, therefore, struggling and fighting. Assure the child that everyone is there to help. It is extremely frightening for parents to see their child suddenly cease breathing. Although it is comforting to see emergency personnel arrive promptly and efficiently, parents are frightened to realize their child is ill enough to need such skilled personnel. Assist, inform, and comfort parents, therefore, as well as the child.

Provide specific information on the child's condition as soon as it is available, and update the parents often. Allow them to see their child as soon as possible after the resuscitation attempt is complete so they can assure themselves their child is breathing and has heart function once again. Be certain they know that follow-up procedures such as ECG monitoring or blood-gas measurements are being undertaken to prevent another emergency. In contrast, offer support to help them begin grieving if the child does not survive.

Key Points

Cardiovascular disorders in children may be either structural, such as congenital heart disease, or acquired, such as Kawasaki disease or rheumatic fever. Assessment of children with heart disease includes history and physical examination. Echocardiogram, MRI, and cardiac catheterization are procedures used frequently for diagnosis.

Children with cardiac disease may fall behind in development because they do not have the energy to play usual childhood games. Help parents to think of games that are intellectually or developmentally stimulating without being physically exhausting.

Limiting saturated fat intake and following a consistent exercise program are important strategies for children to prevent heart disease in later life.

A number of therapies are available for children with cardiac disease. For example, children born with a septal defect undergo open-heart surgical repairs; those with hypoplastic left heart syndrome may undergo cardiac transplant. Children born with ineffective SA node function may have pacemakers implanted to improve heart function.

The families of children undergoing cardiac surgery need a great deal of support from health care personnel so they can cope well enough with this major event to provide effective support to their child.

Postcardiac surgery syndrome and postperfusion syndrome are two complications that may occur after cardiac surgery. They are related to the extracorporeal circulation used during the procedure.

Congenital heart disorders are classified as those associated with increased pulmonary blood flow, decreased pulmonary blood flow, obstruction to blood flow, and mixed blood flow.

Common signs of heart failure seen in children include tachycardia, tachypnea, enlarged liver, dyspnea, and cyanosis. Signs tend to be subtle in infants and may be manifested chiefly by difficulty in feeding from exhaustion and dyspnea.

Rheumatic fever is an autoimmune disease that occurs after a group A beta-hemolytic streptococcal infection. Common signs and symptoms include fever, chorea, arthralgia, polyarthritis, erythema marginatum, subcutaneous nodules, and an elevated ESR. Taking prophylactic penicillin after the illness until age 18 helps prevent further recurrence and cardiac involvement. Some children with congenital heart disease may also need this same protective routine.

Kawasaki disease results from altered immune function. An inflammation of blood vessels leads to platelet aggregation and formation of thrombi and aneurysms.

Infectious endocarditis is an infection of the endocardium of the heart. It may be a complication of congenital heart disease.

Hypertension in children usually occurs as a result of a secondary disorder. A diet that is moderate in cholesterol content along with regular exercise and maintenance of weight proportional to height can help prevent this condition.

Children with heart disease are at high risk for cardiopulmonary arrest. Nurses and parents need to know how to perform CPR to be prepared for this emergency.

Critical Thinking Exercises

1. Megan is the newborn with tetralogy of Fallot whom you met at the beginning of the chapter. Her parents are taking her home for a month while they wait for cardiac surgery to be scheduled. They asked you what "watch her carefully" means and how much exercise they should allow her. What advice would you give them about how to care for Megan?

2. Megan is admitted to the hospital with beginning heart failure. Her most important need is to have sustained periods of rest. How would you schedule your nursing care to avoid tiring her? What advice would you give to her parents at hospital discharge about home care?

3. Megan will need to take prophylactic penicillin until she is an adolescent. She will be living with her mother during the week and visiting her father on weekends. What steps would you take to ensure adherence over this long period?

4. Examine the National Health Goals related to heart disease in children. Most government-sponsored money for nursing research is allotted based on these goals. What would be a possible research topic to explore pertinent to these goals that would be applicable to Megan's family and also advance evidence-based practice?

References

Alexander, M. E., et al. (2004). Implications of implantable cardioverter defibrillator therapy in congenital heart disease and pediatrics. *Journal of Cardiovascular Electrophysiology, 15*(1), 72–76.

American Heart Association. (2005). *Pediatric advanced life support.* Dallas, TX: Author.

Bahruth, A. J. (2004). What every patient should know . . . pretransplantation and posttransplantation. *Critical Care Nursing Quarterly, 27*(1), 31–60.

Barbas, K. H., & Kelleher, D. K. (2004). Breastfeeding success among infants with congenital heart disease. *Pediatric Nursing, 30*(4), 285–289.

Bird, G. (2003). Coarctation of aorta. In M. W. Schwartz (Ed.), *5-minute pediatric consult* (3rd ed.). Philadelphia: Lippincott Williams & Wilkins.

Blaufox, A. D., Paul, T., & Saul, J. P. (2004). Radiofrequency catheter ablation in small children: relationship of complications to application dose. *Pacing and Clinical Electrophysiology, 27*(2), 224–229.

Burch, M., & Aurora, P. (2004). Current status of paediatric heart, lung, and heart-lung transplantation. *Archives of Disease in Childhood, 89*(4), 386–389.

Bute, M. (2004). Congenital heart disease and treatment options. *Case Manager, 15*(2), 56–59.

Callahan, J. M. (2003). Kawasaki disease (mucocutaneous lymph node syndrome). In M. W. Schwartz (Ed.), *5-minute pediatric consult* (3rd ed.). Philadelphia: Lippincott Williams & Wilkins.

Chung, E. K. (2003). Down (trisomy 21) syndrome. In M. W. Schwartz (Ed.), *5-minute pediatric consult* (3rd ed.). Philadelphia: Lippincott Williams & Wilkins.

Conway, D. H. (2003). Persistent pulmonary hypertension of the newborn (PPHN). In M. W. Schwartz (Ed.), *5-minute pediatric consult* (3rd ed.). Philadelphia: Lippincott Williams & Wilkins.

Department of Health and Human Services (2000). *Healthy people 2010.* Washington, D.C.: DHHS.

Dyke, P. C. II, Simpson, S. L., & Carter, G. (2004). Anomalous systemic venous return. *Journal of Pediatrics, 144*(5), 682–683.

Fischbach, F. (2005). *A manual of laboratory and diagnostic tests* (5th ed.). Philadelphia: Lippincott Williams & Wilkins.

Fleenor, J. (2003). Atrial septal defect. In M. W. Schwartz (Ed.), *5-minute pediatric consult* (3rd ed.). Philadelphia: Lippincott Williams & Wilkins.

Fulton, D. R., & Freed, M. D. (2004). The pathology, pathophysiology, recognition, and treatment of congenital heart disease. In V. Fuster, R. W. Alexander, & R. A. O'Rourke (Eds.), *Hurst's the heart* (11th ed.). New York: McGraw-Hill.

Hirshfeld, A. B. (2003). Ventricular septal defect. In M. W. Schwartz (Ed.), *5-minute pediatric consult* (3rd ed.). Philadelphia: Lippincott Williams & Wilkins.

Hoffman, T. M. (2003). Rheumatic fever. In M. W. Schwartz (Ed.), *5-minute pediatric consult* (3rd ed.). Philadelphia: Lippincott Williams & Wilkins.

Jacobson, Z. (2003). Endocarditis. In M. W. Schwartz (Ed.), *5-minute pediatric consult* (3rd ed.). Philadelphia: Lippincott Williams & Wilkins.

Karch, A. M. (2004). *Lippincott's nursing drug guide.* Philadelphia: Lippincott Williams & Wilkins.

Kern, M. J., et al. (2004). Cardiac catheterization, cardiac angiography, and coronary blood flow and pressure measurements. In V. Fuster, R. W. Alexander, & R. A. O'Rourke (Eds.), *Hurst's the heart* (11th ed.). New York: McGraw-Hill.

Kon, A. A., Ackerson, L., & Lo, B. (2003). Choices physicians would make if they were the parents of a child with hypoplastic left heart syndrome. *American Journal of Cardiology, 91*(12), 1506–1509.

Krol, Y., et al. (2003). Health-related quality of life in children with congenital heart disease. *Psychology and Health, 18*(2), 251–260.

Lambert, M. J., Fox, J. C., & Chhiv, N. B. (2004). Cyanotic congenital heart disease: emergency department diagnosis by limited bedside echocardiography. *Topics in Emergency Medicine, 26*(3), 267–271.

Lee, H. R. (2003). Congestive heart failure. In M. W. Schwartz (Ed.), *5-minute pediatric consult* (3rd ed.). Philadelphia: Lippincott Williams & Wilkins.

Liacouras, C. A. (2003). Hyperlipidemia. In M. W. Schwartz (Ed.), *5-minute pediatric consult* (3rd ed.). Philadelphia: Lippincott Williams & Wilkins.

Lundquist, D. R., & Zimmermann, R. W. (2005). Workup for a child with high BP. *Clinical Advisor, 8*(2), 72–73.

Marino, B. S. (2003). Transposition of the great arteries. In M. W. Schwartz (Ed.), *5-minute pediatric consult* (3rd ed.). Philadelphia: Lippincott Williams & Wilkins.

Maron, B. J. (2004). Hypertrophic cardiomyopathy in childhood. *Pediatric Clinics of North America, 51*(5), 1305–1346.

Maxton, F. J. C., Justin, L., & Gillies, D. (2004). Estimating core temperature in infants and children after cardiac surgery: a comparison of six methods. *Journal of Advanced Nursing, 45*(2), 214–222.

Mulreany, M. P. (2003). Patent ductus arteriosus. In M. W. Schwartz (Ed.), *5-minute pediatric consult* (3rd ed.). Philadelphia: Lippincott Williams & Wilkins.

National Center for Health Statistics. (2005). *Trends in the health of Americans.* Hyattsville, MD: NCHS.

Reddy, G. P., & Higgins, C. B. (2003). Magnetic resonance imaging of congenital heart disease: evaluation of morphology and function. *Seminars in Roentgenology, 38*(4), 342–351.

Ro, P. S. (2003). Tetralogy of Fallot (TOF). In M. W. Schwartz (Ed.), *5-minute pediatric consult* (3rd ed.). Philadelphia: Lippincott Williams & Wilkins.

Schulman, S. L. (2003). Hypertension. In M. W. Schwartz (Ed.), *5-minute pediatric consult* (3rd ed.). Philadelphia: Lippincott Williams & Wilkins.

Simpson, J. (2004). Antenatal detection of congenital heart disease. *Hospital Medicine (London), 65*(3), 143–147.

Stefanelli, C. B., & Fischbach, P. S. (2003). Cardiac arrhythmias in children. *ACC Current Journal Review, 12*(2), 103–107.

Timothy, P. R., & Rodeman, B. J. (2004). Temporary pacemakers in critically ill patients: assessment and management strategies. *AACN Clinical Issues, 15*(3), 305–325.

Toyer, R., & Fox, G. F. (2004). Patent ductus arteriosus in preterm infants: diagnosis and treatment. *Journal of Neonatal Nursing, 10*(4), 112–115.

Tulenko, D. R. (2004). An update on ECMO. *Neonatal Network: The Journal of Neonatal Nursing, 23*(4), 11–18.

Van Overmeire, B. (2003). The use of ibuprofen in neonates in the treatment of patent ductus arteriosus. *International Journal of Clinical Practice (Supplement), 135*(4), S23–27.

Ward, K. (2003). Genetics and prenatal diagnosis. In J. R. Scott, et al. (Eds.), *Danforth's obstetrics & gynecology* (9th ed.). Philadelphia: Lippincott Williams & Wilkins.

Wiegand, D. L. (2003). Cardiovascular surgery. Advances in cardiac surgery: valve repair. *Critical Care Nurse, 23*(2), 72–76.

Woods, W. A., Schutte, D. A., & McCulloch, M. A. (2003). Care of children who have had surgery for congenital heart disease. *American Journal of Emergency Medicine, 21*(4), 318–327.

Suggested Readings

Bader, R. S., Goldberg, L., & Sahn, D. J. (2004). Risk of sudden cardiac death in young athletes: which screening strategies are appropriate? *Pediatric Clinics of North America, 51*(5), 1421–1441.

Chen, C., Li, C., & Wang, J. (2005). Self-concept: comparison between school-aged children with congenital heart disease and normal school-aged children. *Journal of Clinical Nursing, 14*(3), 394–402.

Danford, D. A. (2004). Heart murmur in a child. *Hospital Physician, 40*(6), 27–40.

Jack, P. (2004). Children born with cyanotic congenital heart disease: effects on the family. *Journal of Neonatal Nursing, 10*(6), 191–195.

LeRoy, S., et al. (2003). Recommendations for preparing children and adolescents for invasive cardiac procedures. *Circulation, 108*(20), 2550–2564.

Mennick, F. (2004). Going up? Adolescents' blood pressure levels are rising along with their weight. *American Journal of Nursing, 104*(8), 22–23.

Regan, K., & Avelar, C. (2004). Treating sudden cardiac arrest in a school setting. *School Nurse News, 21*(4), 32–36.

Rempel, G. R. (2004). Technological advances in pediatrics: challenges for parents and nurses. *Journal of Pediatric Nursing: Nursing Care of Children and Families, 19*(1), 13–24.

Tanel, R. E. (2004). ECGs in the ED. *Pediatric Emergency Care, 20*(5), 345–346.

Watt, R. H. (2004). Congenital heart disease: an overview of the condition and treatment options. *Lippincott's Case Management, 9*(4), 205–208.

CHAPTER 42

Nursing Care of the Child With an Immune Disorder

Key Terms

allergen
anaphylaxis
angioedema
antigen
autoimmunity
B lymphocyte
cell-mediated
  immunity
chemotaxis
complement
contact dermatitis
cytotoxic response
cytotoxic T cells
delayed
  hypersensitivity
environmental
  control
hapten formation
helper T cells
humoral immunity
hypersensitivity
  response
hyposensitization
immune response
immunity
immunocompetent
  cells
immunogen
immunoglobulins
lymphokines
lysis
macrophage
memory cell
phagocytosis
plasma cell
suppressor T cells
T lymphocyte
tolerance
urticaria

Objectives

After mastering the contents of this chapter, you should be able to:

1. Describe the immune process as it relates to childhood illnesses.
2. Assess a child with a disorder of the immune system.
3. Formulate nursing diagnoses for a child with a disorder of the immune system.
4. Establish outcomes for a child with a disorder of the immune system.
5. Plan nursing care pertinent to a child with an immune system disorder.
6. Implement nursing care for a child with an immune disorder such as teaching about environmental control.
7. Evaluate expected outcomes for achievement and effectiveness of care for a child with an immune disorder.
8. Identify National Health Goals related to immune disorders and children that nurses could help the nation achieve.
9. Identify areas related to care of a child with an immune disorder that could benefit from additional nursing research or application of evidence-based practice.
10. Use critical thinking to analyze ways that nursing care for a child with an immune disorder can be more family-centered.
11. Integrate knowledge of immune disorders and the nursing process to achieve quality maternal and child health nursing care.

Dexter Goodenough is a 6-year-old boy you meet in an ambulatory setting. He had atopic dermatitis (infantile eczema) as an infant. Today, his eyes look reddened and are watering; his nose is draining a clear discharge. His mother tells you he is constantly listless and other children make fun of him because of his appearance. His grades are "terrible" because the minute he gets to school, his symptoms begin. Dexter is diagnosed as having atopic rhinitis (hay fever). "Thank heavens," his mother exclaims. "I thought when I heard he had an immune system disease he had AIDS. What a relief to know it's only an allergy."

Previous chapters described normal growth and development of children. This chapter adds information about the dramatic changes, both physical and psychosocial, that occur when a child is born with or develops a disorder of the immune system. This is important information because it builds a base for care and health teaching for children with these diseases.

In light of the effect this condition is having on Dexter's life, is this "only" an allergy? What additional information would you want his mother to know about his condition? Knowing his problem is worse at school, what environmental control measures would you want to suggest for Dexter?

After you've studied this chapter, access the accompanying website. Read the patient scenario and answer the questions to further sharpen your skills, grow more familiar with RN-CLEX types of questions, and reward yourself with how much you have learned.

The immune system consists of a complex network of cells interacting to protect the body against invasion by foreign substances. The study of the immune system has grown immensely over the past several years, and almost every day brings new findings. More diseases are being attributed at least in part to a malfunctioning of the immune system, all of which makes an understanding of how the immune system works in health and disease essential for safe nursing care.

Disorders of the immune system include deficiencies of immune substances and function that affect the body's ability to ward off infection (immunodeficiency disorders); abnormal and excessive immune response to foreign substances (hypersensitivity disorders, or allergies); and abnormal and excessive immune response to self (autoimmune disorders). Immune disorders are a focus of much research and study because they may hold the key to understanding why major illnesses such as HIV/AIDS and possibly cancer occur. Immunodeficiencies and examples of allergic disorders are described in this chapter. Autoimmune disorders, which include a wide range of illnesses affecting many body systems, are addressed in the chapters that discuss the affected system (e.g., rheumatoid arthritis, which affects the joints, is discussed in Chapter 51). National Health Goals related to immune disorders and children are shown in Box 42.1.

Nursing Process Overview

For a Child With an Immune Disorder

● *Assessment*

The immune system provides protection for the body from invading organisms or antigens. A deficiency of **immunocompetent cells** (cells capable of resisting these types of foreign invaders) or alteration in their function can limit this protection. Assessment focuses on analysis of blood components, particularly the white blood cells, to determine exactly what components are altered, missing, or not functioning properly. When the immune system reacts excessively or inappropriately to the invasion of certain antigens, a thorough history and analysis of presenting symptoms are usually the best way to identify the problem and develop appropriate interventions (Box 42.2).

● *Nursing Diagnosis*

The most relevant diagnosis associated with immune dysfunction is:

• Risk for infection related to altered immune response

Nursing diagnoses for children experiencing allergic responses focus on their particular allergic symptoms. Examples of these are:

• Situational low self-esteem related to effects of contact dermatitis
• Ineffective breathing pattern related to bronchospasm of anaphylaxis
• Anxiety related to continued allergic response

BOX 42.1 FOCUS ON . . .

NATIONAL HEALTH GOALS

Of the immunologic disorders, human immunodeficiency virus (HIV) infection is the most serious, not only because it is still ultimately fatal but also because its spread has been so difficult to contain. A number of National Health Goals address this problem:

• Increase to at least 95%, from a baseline of 85%, the proportion of adolescents who abstain from sexual intercourse or use condoms if sexually active.
• Reduce occupational needlestick injuries among health care workers, from a baseline of 600,000/year to 420,000/year, a 30% improvement.
• Reduce AIDS among adolescents and adults, from a baseline of 19.5 new cases/100,000 of the population to a target level of 1.0/100,000.
• Reduce the incidence of new cases of perinatally acquired HIV infection.
• Increase the proportion of middle, junior high, and senior high schools that provide education on HIV and AIDS, from a baseline of 65% to a target level of 90% (DHHS, 2000).

Nurses can help the nation achieve these goals by initiating educational programs for children that include teaching children and adolescents about the way HIV is transmitted (sexual relations and unclean intravenous needles) and protective measures they can take to avoid contracting the disease (using safer sex practices and not using intravenous drugs).

Nursing research that could add helpful information to the area includes research that attempts to answer questions such as: How can parents of school-age children be persuaded that safer sex practices should be part of usual school-age health awareness curricula? What methods work best to educate adolescents about the danger of unprotected sex?

• Powerlessness related to difficulty determining cause of allergy
• Risk for delayed growth and development related to chronicity of HIV/AIDS

● *Outcome Identification and Planning*

Outcome identification and planning for the child with an immune disorder focuses both on present and future concerns. Relief of immediate symptoms is the first priority. This is followed by planning for long-term care and prevention of future attacks. Looking into organizations that could supply information for parents or children could be key.

● *Implementation*

A major nursing intervention in the care of children with immune disorders is client and family teaching. The family of the child with an immunodeficiency may need help in identifying ways to keep the child from contracting life-threatening infections while at the same time

BOX 42.2 ASSESSMENT

Assessing the Child With an Immune Disorder

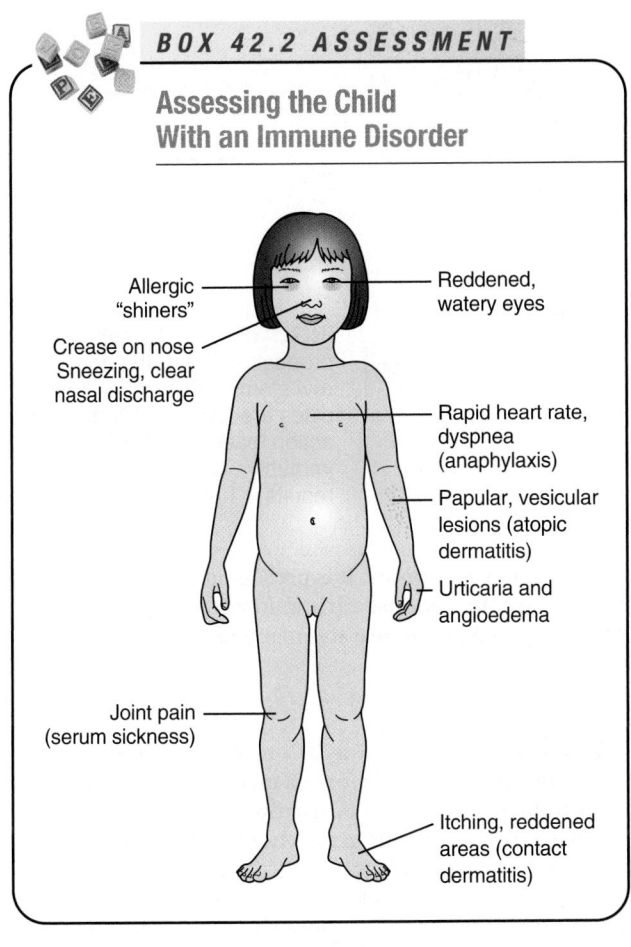

- Allergic "shiners"
- Crease on nose Sneezing, clear nasal discharge
- Reddened, watery eyes
- Rapid heart rate, dyspnea (anaphylaxis)
- Papular, vesicular lesions (atopic dermatitis)
- Urticaria and angioedema
- Joint pain (serum sickness)
- Itching, reddened areas (contact dermatitis)

- Child's respiratory rate is maintained at 20 breaths per minute with minimal wheezing.
- Child and parents state they can cope with their present level of anxiety.
- Child lists three actions she takes daily to help feel a greater sense of control.
- Child demonstrates achievement of developmental milestones within age-acceptable parameters despite chronic illness.

THE IMMUNE SYSTEM

The immune system functions to protect the body from invasion by foreign substances by several mechanisms. First, body surfaces such as the skin, cilia, and mucous membranes act as physical protective barriers. When an invading pathogen does get through this barrier, the process of **phagocytosis** (destruction of invaders) begins. **Macrophages** (mature white blood cells) engulf, ingest, and neutralize the pathogen. At the same time, an inflammatory response creates vascular and cellular changes that help to rid the body of dead tissue and the inactivated antigens. The immune system maintains cells ready to attack this way whenever necessary, directing the efforts of macrophages and supplementing the inflammatory response as necessary. It also singles out specific antigens for interactions (antibody–antigen reactions). This immune response not only furnishes immediate protection but also creates a template for how to destroy that particular antigen again in the future.

Immune Response

The **immune response** is the body's action plan devised to combat invading organisms or substances by leukocyte and antibody activity. An **antigen** is any foreign substance (molecule) capable of stimulating an immune response. Most antigens are proteins, but other large molecules such as polysaccharides may also function as antigens. Penicillin, although not antigenic by itself, may become antigenic when it combines with a higher-weight molecule, usually a protein (a process called **hapten formation**; this explains why penicillin reactions occur). If an antigen is one that can be readily destroyed by an immune response, and **immunity** (the ability to destroy like antigens) results, the antigen may be referred to as a simple **immunogen**. If, during the immune response, mediating substances are released that cause tissue injury and allergic symptoms, the antigen is termed an **allergen.** Allergens may enter the body through a variety of routes. They may be ingested (e.g., foods such as eggs or wheat), inhaled (e.g., pollen, dust, or mold spores), injected (e.g., drugs), or absorbed across the skin or mucous membranes (e.g., poison ivy).

Immune System Organs and Cells

The organs of the immune system consist of the lymph nodes, bone marrow, thymus, spleen, and tonsils. Bone marrow produces two types of lymphocytes, **B lymphocytes** and **T lymphocytes.** After being produced, lymphocytes travel throughout the lymphoid system and are

providing enough stimulation and social contact to promote normal growth and development. A similar teaching goal must be established for a child with a chronic allergic disorder. Parents need to learn ways to help their child avoid triggers or situations that provoke allergy, but they must not keep the child so isolated or fearful that the child misses out on important experiences. A referral to informational and support organizations such as these may be helpful: Asthma and Allergy Foundation of America (*www.aafa.org*), Elizabeth Glaser Pediatric AIDS Foundation (*www.pedaids.org*), Eczema Association for Science and Education (*www.nationaleczema.org*).

● *Outcome Evaluation*
Outcome evaluation with immune disorders must be ongoing because new triggers for allergies can arise at any time. New therapies for HIV/AIDS are constantly being suggested. Because the field of immunology is continually evolving, theories about immune diseases and associated treatments may change from visit to visit. Be certain parents are kept abreast of developments in the field, especially those that will affect their ability to provide an environment that is safest for their child.

Examples of outcomes suggesting achievement of goals include:

- Child voices high self-esteem even if contact dermatitis rash has not completely faded.

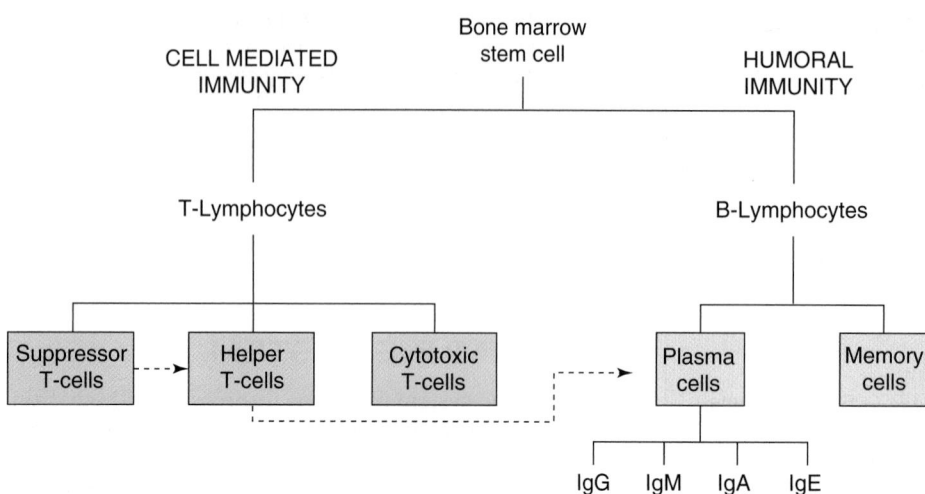

FIGURE 42.1 Lymphocyte production. From the bone marrow stem cell, T- and B-lymphocytes are formed. T-lymphocyte action leads to cell-mediated immunity. B-lymphocyte action results in humoral immunity.

stored in the lymph nodes and spleen. Both T and B lymphocytes recognize invading organisms and provide for attack of specific antigens (Fig. 42.1).

B Lymphocytes

Originating in the bone marrow (the reason for their name), the B lymphocytes develop into plasma cells and memory cells when exposed to antigens. **Plasma cells** secrete large quantities of immunoglobulins or antibodies, which bind to and destroy specific antigens (termed humoral immunity). When an antibody is formed in response to a particular antigen this way, it is specific to that antigen. An antibody against the pertussis antigen, for instance, will not have any effect on the tetanus antigen. Memory cells are responsible for retaining the formula or ability to produce specific **immunoglobulins.** Immunoglobulins are classified as IgG, IgA, IgM, IgD, and IgE. Those involved in immunity are IgG, IgA, and IgM. IgM reaches adult levels at approximately 1 year of age, IgG at 4 years, and IgA at adolescence. IgE is primarily responsible for allergic or hy-

persensitivity responses. It is present at proportions capable of extreme response early in infancy. The functions of the immunoglobulins are summarized in Table 42.1.

T Lymphocytes

T lymphocytes account for 70% to 80% of blood lymphocytes and are responsible for cell-mediated immunity. They are produced by the bone marrow but mature under the influence of the thymus gland (hence their name). When mature, T lymphocytes leave the thymus to enter specific body regions (thymus-dependent zones), mostly in the lymph nodes and spleen; there they react specifically to viruses, fungi, and parasites but have an effect on all antigens. T cells can be differentiated into three subtypes.

The first type, cytotoxic (killer) T cells, are T lymphocytes that have the specific feature of binding to the surface of antigens and directly destroying the cell membrane and therefore the cell (phagocytes). As a part of this process, cytotoxic cells secrete **lymphokines;** lymphokines contain or prevent migration of antigens and call other lympho-

TABLE 42.1

Location and Function of Immunoglobulins

Immunoglobulin	Description
IgM	Effective in agglutinating antigen as well as lysing cell walls; discovered early in the course of an infection in the bloodstream
IgG	Most frequently occurring antibody in plasma; during secondary response, it is the major immunoglobulin to be synthesized; it freely diffuses into extravascular spaces to contact antigens; in prenatal life, it diffuses across the placenta to supply passive immune protection to the fetus and until the infant can effectively produce immunoglobulins; it has the major responsibility for neutralizing bacterial toxins and in activating phagocytosis (destruction of bacteria)
IgA	Found in external body secretions such as saliva, sweat, tears, mucus, bile, and colostrum; provides defense against pathogens on exposed surfaces, especially those of the gastrointestinal tract and respiratory tract, apparently by preventing adherence of pathogens to mucosal cells
IgD	Found in plasma; may be the receptor that binds antigens to lymphocyte surfaces
IgE	Involved in immediate hypersensitivity reactions; exists bound to mast cells on tissue surfaces; when contacted by an antigen, cellular granules are released; associated with allergy and parasitic infections

cytes into the area. Interferon is an example of a lympho-kine important in preventing viral spread and helping to call leukocytes into the area (the property of **chemotaxis**).

The second type, **helper T cells** (CD4 cells), stimulate B lymphocytes to divide and mature into plasma cells and begin secreting immunoglobulins. The IgA antibody response, especially, depends on stimulation by helper T cells. Helper T cells can be identified in blood because of specific markers on their surface. Analysis of these (CD4 counts) is an important assessment of the competency of the immune system.

The third type, **suppressor T cells,** are T cells that reduce the production of immunoglobulins against a specific antigen and prevent their overproduction.

Types of Immunity

The action of B and T lymphocytes leads to two different types of immunity: humoral and cell-mediated immunity.

Humoral Immunity

Humoral immunity refers to immunity created by antibody production or B-lymphocyte involvement. The process begins when helper T cells recognize an antigen and cause activation of B lymphocytes (possibly by an intermediary macrophage). The specific B lymphocytes differentiate into plasma cells and begin creation of specific immunoglobulins that mark the antigen for destruction (Fig. 42.2). A few antigens (e.g., *Escherichia coli*) are capable of activating a B-lymphocyte response without recognition by T lymphocytes.

Primary Response. The first time a specific antigen enters the body and is identified by T lymphocytes, B-cell differentiation and growth begin. Within 6 days, IgM antibodies specific to the antigen can be measured in the bloodstream. The production of IgM antibodies peaks at 14 days and then declines until, within a few weeks, few are any longer present. At approximately day 10, IgG production begins and remains high for several weeks (Fig. 42.3).

Secondary Response. When a specific antigen enters the body a second or additional time, antibody production begins immediately because of **memory cells.** The main type of immunoglobulin produced in a secondary response is IgG (see Fig. 42.3).

Complement Activation. Complement is composed of 20 different proteins that are normally nonfunctional molecules; however, when activated by antigen–antibody contact, these molecules begin a cascade response that leads to increased vascular permeability, smooth muscle contraction, chemotaxis ("calling" leukocytes into the area), phagocytosis, and **lysis** (killing) of the foreign antigen. The affected area feels warm and looks reddened and swollen, indicating an inflammatory reaction. Although an inflammatory reaction causes some local injury to tissue around the antigen, it is helpful overall because it produces an environment harmful to the antigen. Complement reactions that persist beyond the usual time for resolution (2 to 3 days) may be responsible for many of the autoimmune disorders.

Cell-Mediated Immunity

Cell-mediated immunity is the type of immune response due to T-lymphocyte activity. **Cytotoxic T cells** attack and directly destroy invading antigens through the release of chemical compounds on the antigen membrane, injection of a toxin directly into the antigen, or secretion of lymphokines. A wheal-and-flare response occurs due to accumulation of lymphocytes around small blood vessels, resulting in minor destruction of blood vessels (see Fig. 42.2). This response is termed **delayed hypersensitivity** if the T-lymphocyte activity occurs solely without an accompanying humoral response. It is this response that causes transplant rejection.

Autoimmunity

Autoimmunity results from an inability to distinguish self from nonself, causing the immune system to carry out immune responses against normal cells and tissue. Autoimmune responses may be organ-specific (i.e., limited to one organ), as in Hashimoto's disease (see Chapter 48), or generalized and systemic (not organ-specific), as in rheumatoid arthritis and systemic lupus erythematosus (see Chapter 14). There is currently much research oriented toward the study of autoimmune responses and their possible implications in a wide variety of disorders, such as multiple sclerosis. Autoimmune disorders occur at a greater rate in some families than in others and in girls and women more than boys and men.

HEALTH PROMOTION AND RISK MANAGEMENT

As many as 15% to 30% of children today have some form of allergy (Wills-Karp & Khurana-Hershey, 2003). Preventing allergies, therefore, could have a major impact on the health of children. Early prevention can begin with encouraging women to breast-feed so that infants are not exposed to cow milk protein. Delaying the introduction of solid food until 6 months of age, once thought to reduce the development of allergies, may not be as beneficial as once thought (Zutavern et al., 2004). Delaying solid food because infants' gastrointestinal tracts are not ready for digestion, however, is still a valid reason to delay early feeding. Environmental control to reduce the number of allergens in a home can drastically reduce allergy symptoms. This should begin when parents choose furniture for a child's room, such as eliminating wool blankets, choosing toys carefully, and keeping the room free of dust. Teach parents to use a minimum of washing compounds so that children are exposed to as few chemical products as possible. Pets should not be introduced into the house. Avoiding spray products such as perfumes and air fresheners and discontinuing cigarette smoking also help (Box 42.3). These are sensible rules for parents to follow beforehand, rather than waiting for a child to develop allergic rhinitis or atopic dermatitis and then having to put more extreme measures into effect.

Health promotion is also important to prevent HIV/AIDS. Teaching children safer sex practices is an important part of this. All health care providers can help prevent

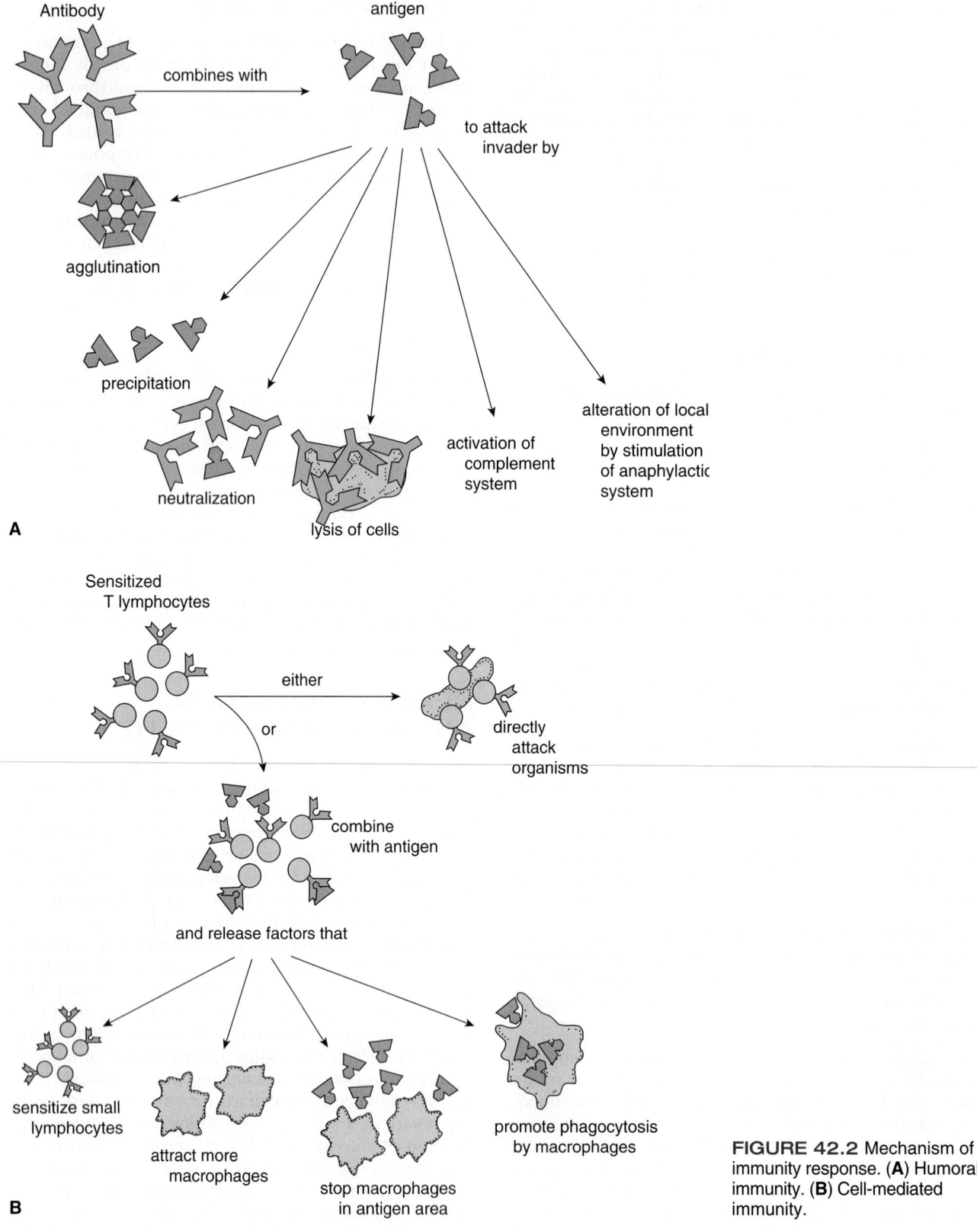

FIGURE 42.2 Mechanism of immunity response. (A) Humoral immunity. (B) Cell-mediated immunity.

the spread of HIV/AIDS by using standard precautions. The parents of children with immune deficiencies may need to be reminded periodically to take measures to keep their children free of disease, such as keeping immunizations updated and seeking help immediately for infections.

Allergies are a type of disorder that typically cause chronic rather than acute symptoms. For this reason, children who develop allergies often need to be encouraged to be vigilant in taking their medicine. For the same reason, once parents begin a child on an immunotherapy program,

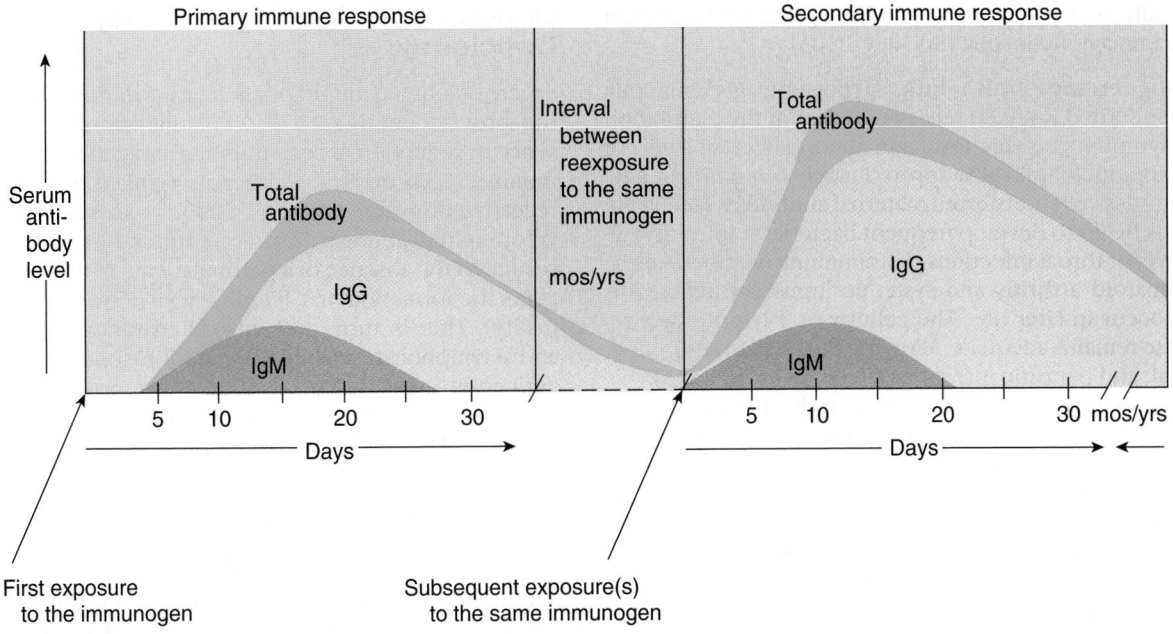

FIGURE 42.3 Primary and secondary humoral responses. IgM is the first immunoglobulin to appear in the serum.

they may need to be encouraged to continue it. It helps if children and their parents understand how allergic reactions lead to symptoms and how important it is for them to play a role in their own therapy.

Although it is probably impossible to keep children with atopic allergies free of reactions and manifestations of allergies, parents who know of familial allergy patterns can take some preventive steps in this direction. If parents are going to prepare allergy-free foods, be sure they consider the child's likes and dislikes and think through the child's weekly intake to ensure he or she receives all essential nutrients. If a child eats at school or has a meal prepared every day at a child care center, remind parents to make sure the center, babysitter, or school dietitian is aware of the child's allergies. If a child is allergic to wheat products and cannot eat bread for sandwiches, preparing

a bag lunch for school may be a difficult daily problem that only good planning can eliminate.

If a child's allergies involve pollen sensitivities, planning vacations at a time when the pollen count is lowest may make the vacation more pleasant for the family. If desensitization against a specific pollen is necessary, assist parents in planning to start desensitization so it will be effective by the time the pollen count of the offending allergen rises.

IMMUNODEFICIENCY DISORDERS

When any one portion of the immune system is not functioning adequately, an immunodeficiency results. The immunodeficiency disorder may be primary (congenital) or acquired (secondary to viral invasion or exposure to a toxic substance). Only a part or the entire system may fail in its goal of protecting the body from invading organisms.

Primary (Congenital) Immunodeficiency

Children with primary congenital immunodeficiencies are born without an essential immune substance or function or with inadequate amounts of immune substances. Usually these deficiencies become apparent relatively early in life. However, it may take a few months for B-lymphocyte deficiencies to produce symptoms, because a newborn is born with enough maternal IgG (which crossed the placenta during pregnancy) to supply protection for approximately the first 6 months of life. Help parents to understand that primary disorders are not the same as AIDS.

B-Lymphocyte Deficiencies

B-lymphocyte deficiencies create abnormally low levels of immunoglobulins either selectively (as in an IgA deficiency)

BOX 42.3 FOCUS ON . . .

DIVERSITY OF CARE

Because some families are more prone to allergies than others, some communities have a higher incidence of children with allergies than others. As a result, these communities may have more services and specialists to treat these children, a situation that develops a "community culture" of allergy acceptance and treatment. Children typically may leave school early for immunotherapy. School cafeterias commonly offer allergy-free foods. In other communities where fewer children have allergies, a child with an allergy is viewed as unique or not typical, so may need additional support.

or totally, which is referred to as hypogammaglobulinemia or agammaglobulinemia (Buckley, 2003).

Hypogammaglobulinemia. Hypogammaglobulinemia is an inherited X-linked recessive defect in the maturation of B lymphocytes that results in abnormally low levels of all immunoglobulins. At approximately 6 months of age, when passively transferred maternal antibodies fade, male infants begin to develop frequent bacterial respiratory, digestive, or throat infections. Autoimmune diseases such as rheumatoid arthritis and systemic lupus erythematosus may occur in later life. The cellular or T-lymphocyte response remains adequate, allowing the child to resist viral, fungal, and parasitic infections (Rehman et al., 2003).

This deficiency is treated with monthly intravenous immune globulin (IVIG) injections to supply immunoglobulins. Bone marrow transplantation may be successful in restoring immune competency. Parents and children, as they grow older, need to be taught the importance of recognizing infection early. Also help them set up a schedule for IVIG injections so these are not forgotten.

Common Variable Immunoglobulin Deficiencies. The most common disorder in this group is deficiency of IgA in surface secretions. The overall level of B lymphocytes is normal, but IgA production is reduced or absent, perhaps due to an increase of IgA suppressor cells or a defect in T-helper cells important for IgA synthesis. Without IgA, infection of surfaces exposed to the external environment and normally protected by mucus becomes common. Sinusitis, upper respiratory tract illness, and inflammatory bowel disease are apt to occur. There are associated atopic diseases (allergies) because without IgA on the surface mucosa, many more antigens than usual can enter the body, permitting more antigens to interact with IgE and produce allergic symptoms. Chronic irritation due to these large numbers of antigens predisposes exposed tissue to malignant transformation, so malignancy of the respiratory, gastrointestinal, and lymphoid systems occurs more readily. There is an increased risk that an antibody will cross-react with a self-antigen to cause autoimmune illness, so diseases such as systemic lupus erythematosus and rheumatoid arthritis also occur at increased rates. IgA deficiency can occur as a secondary type due to treatment with phenytoin (an anticonvulsant) and penicillamine (a copper chelating agent). IVIG contains little IgA, so therapy with IVIG does not greatly reduce symptoms. Because prevention, not treatment, is the key, parents need to be conscientious about preventing infections and perhaps administering prophylactic antibiotics to prevent respiratory infections (Perez, 2003).

T-Lymphocyte Deficiencies

T-lymphocyte immunodeficiencies involve inadequate numbers or inadequate functioning of one or more types of T lymphocytes; this affects cell-mediated immunity and also, because of helper T-lymphocyte function, possibly humoral immunity as well. DiGeorge anomaly (which includes failure of the thymus to develop) and chronic mucocutaneous candidiasis are two disorders caused by T-lymphocyte deficiency or malfunction. DiGeorge syndrome is a defect of chromosome 22 or 22q11.2 (Saitta et al., 2004).

Combined T- and B-Lymphocyte Deficiency

Severe combined immunodeficiency syndrome (SCIDS) is the most frequently seen disorder characterized by an absence or reduction of both humoral and cell-mediated immunity. SCIDS occurs as either an X-linked or autosomal recessive disorder (Andrews, 2003). It is caused by a developmental abnormality (sometimes but not always related to the absence of a particular enzyme), which prevents the formation of T lymphocytes (a stem cell abnormality). This, in turn, prevents the maturation of both T and B lymphocytes. Children cannot respond directly to antigen invasion and no antibodies are produced. Bone marrow transplantation has proven to be an effective treatment for this disorder (Perez, 2003).

Secondary (Acquired) Immunodeficiency

Secondary immunodeficiency, or loss of immune system response, can occur from factors such as severe systemic infection, cancer, renal disease, radiation therapy, severe stress, malnutrition, immunosuppressive therapy, and aging. There can be complete or partial loss of both B- and T-lymphocyte response.

Stress appears to alter the immune response by stimulating the release of corticosteroids from the adrenal gland. This suppresses the inflammatory response by inhibiting macrophage action. Immunosuppressive drugs, such as prednisone, can also suppress the inflammatory response. Radiation or chemotherapy can act to limit or destroy rapidly growing cells. Because both T and B lymphocytes are rapidly growing and dividing cells, they are killed by these drugs or radiation. Extreme infection is yet another cause for a decreased immune response because the body's continued ability to combat infection becomes exhausted.

Malnutrition can decrease immunity because rapidly growing cells need protein for synthesis; renal disease with protein loss will also deplete the amount of protein available for new lymphocyte production.

HIV Infection and AIDS

AIDS is the end stage of an acquired immunodeficiency caused by infection with the RNA human immunodeficiency retrovirus HIV (Rutstein, 2003). The virus has at least two divisions, HIV-1 and HIV-2, with a variety of further subtypes. The virus acts by attacking the lymphoreticular system, in particular CD4-bearing helper T lymphocytes. The virus enters and replicates in these lymphocytes, in the process destroying them. There is no defense against the virus, so it remains in the body for life. Infection results in loss of CD4 lymphocytes and the ability to initiate an effective B-lymphocyte response. Because B-lymphocyte or humoral immune function, which initiates the production of antibodies, is affected, antibody formation will be decreased (hypogammaglobulinemia). When monocytes and macrophages become affected as well, the person with HIV infection cannot resist normal infection and is susceptible to opportunistic ones such as fungal infections. The final result is that both the immune response and the ability to screen and remove malignant cells from the body are lost.

Transmission. HIV infection is spread by exposure to blood and other body secretions through sexual contact, sharing of contaminated needles for injection, transfusion of contaminated blood or blood products, perinatally from mother to fetus or newborn, and through breast-feeding. A few children have acquired the infection because of sexual abuse. Health care providers must maintain vigilance to guard against needle punctures, as these injuries are a source of blood transfer.

Pediatric AIDS accounts for only 1% to 2% of the total AIDS cases (CDC, 2005). Although it is decreasing in incidence, transmission of HIV from mother to child by placental spread is still the most common reason for childhood HIV infection in the United States. This transmission can occur during pregnancy, at birth, and possibly during breast-feeding. Transmission by this route has declined to less than 3% since HIV-positive women have been prescribed zidovudine during pregnancy. Nevirapine can have the same effect (Jaspan & Garry, 2003).

In the past, many children with hemophilia, because they receive so many blood product transfusions, received HIV-contaminated blood and were infected. This source of transmission now almost never occurs. The increasing rate of sexual activity and the rapidly rising incidence of sexually transmitted infections among adolescents are making this group vulnerable to growing rates of HIV infection (Thomas et al., 2003). HIV is not transmitted by animals or through usual casual contact, such as shaking hands or kissing, or in households, day care centers, or schools.

Assessment. HIV has a long incubation period of about 10 years in adults. The disorder appears to progress more rapidly in children and infants who receive the virus through placental transmission if they do not receive treatment. These individuals are usually HIV positive by 6 months and develop clinical signs by 1 to 3 years of age. Children who receive the virus from another source usually convert to HIV positivity by 2 to 6 weeks, or at least by 6 months after exposure. During this preconversion time, the child may have poor resistance to infection, such as fever, swollen lymph nodes, respiratory tract infections, and thrush.

All infants born to infected mothers test positive for antibodies to the virus at birth because of passive antibody transmission. This persists for about 18 months. The disease is diagnosed, therefore, by recovery of the HIV antigen in children under this age and antibodies to the virus in children over this age. Tests to detect the antigen are termed PCR (polymerase chain reaction) tests; those for the antibody are termed ELISA (enzyme-linked immunosorbent assay) and Western blot confirmation. CD4 counts are used to document the disease status and predict disease progression. Normal counts vary according to age because the lymphocyte count normally varies by age. Table 42.2 shows the use of Centers for Disease Control and Prevention (CDC) guidelines and CD4 counts to determine disease progress. Severe suppression indicates a condition serious enough to cause life-threatening infections (CDC, 2005).

The CDC classification of HIV infection in children has three categories:

- Category A, Mildly Symptomatic: two or more symptoms such as enlarged lymph nodes, liver, or spleen, or recurrent or persistent upper respiratory infections, sinusitis, or otitis media
- Category B, Moderately Symptomatic: more serious illnesses such as oropharyngeal candidiasis, bacterial meningitis, pneumonia, or sepsis, cardiomyopathy, cytomegalovirus infection, hepatitis, herpes simplex virus (HSV) bronchitis, pneumonitis, or esophagitis, herpes zoster (shingles), lymphoid interstitial pneumonia (LIP), pulmonary lymphoid hyperplasia complex, or toxoplasmosis
- Category C, Severely Symptomatic (AIDS): serious bacterial infections such as septicemia, pneumonia, meningitis, bone or joint infection, or abscess of an internal organ or body cavity; candidiasis (esophageal or pulmonary), encephalopathy, herpes simplex lasting over 1 month, histoplasmosis, lymphoma, tuberculosis, Mycobacterium or *Pneumocystis carinii* pneumonia. Unlike adults, children rarely develop Kaposi's sarcoma (CDC, 2005).

Therapeutic Management. Because of the success of zidovudine administration during the pregnancy of HIV-positive women, many fewer infants are born with HIV infection today (Capparelli, Rakhmanina, & Mirochnick, 2005). Those who are born with a perinatal infection, once thought to have a short life expectancy, now have an opportunity for long-term survival. To accomplish this,

---

TABLE 42.2

CD4 Cell Counts Related to Progress of Disease in Children

	Age of Child		
	Under 12 Months	*1–5 Years*	*6–12 Years*
No evidence of suppression	1,500 cells/µL	1,000 cells/µL	500 cells/µL
Evidence of moderate suppression	750–1,499 cells/µL	500–999 cells/µL	200–499 cells/µL
Severe suppression	750 cells/µL	500 cells/µL	200 cells/µL

Centers for Disease Control and Prevention. (2005). HIV/AIDS recommendations. Washington, D.C.: CDC.

therapy involves a complex regimen of nutritional supplements to prevent weight loss, vaccines to prevent infections, and highly active antiretroviral therapy (HAART) as well as antibacterial agents to combat the HIV virus and opportunistic infections (Dybul, Connors, & Fauci, 2003).

NURSING DIAGNOSES AND RELATED INTERVENTIONS

Nursing Diagnosis: Risk for infection related to decreased immune function

Outcome Evaluation: Child's temperature is within normal parameters; no cough or skin lesions are present.

Children with HIV infection and their families must maintain strict personal hygiene (e.g., frequent handwashing) and avoid close contact between the child and anyone who has a respiratory infection to try to prevent the child from contracting dangerous opportunistic infections. When infections do occur, antibiotic and antifungal treatment should be prompt and aggressive.

Combating the infection requires specific antiretroviral medications to prevent progressive deterioration of the immune system and to provide prophylactic measures against opportunistic infections. Three classes of drugs are the mainstay of therapy: nucleoside reverse transcriptase inhibitors (NRTIs), nonnucleoside reverse transcriptase inhibitors (NNRTIs), and protease inhibitors. NRTIs are designed to block production of viral DNA, limiting the ability of the virus to infect cells; zidovudine is an example (Box 42.4). NNRTIs also inhibit the DNA synthesis of viruses but act at different sites on the viral enzyme; nevirapine and efavirenz are examples. Protease inhibitors stop the ability of the virus to produce protease, limiting metastasis; amprenavir, nelfinavir, and ritonavir are examples of protease inhibitors used in children.

The CDC (2005) has recommended that children be prescribed a regimen involving multiple drugs, such as one protease inhibitor plus two NRTIs.

Many children are given prophylactic therapy for *P. carinii* pneumonia (trimethoprim/sulfamethoxazole [TMP-SMZ]) beginning at 6 months of age. Children with HIV infection are more susceptible to tuberculosis than other children, so they also must be safeguarded against contracting this. If a child develops tuberculosis, a combination of antituberculosis drugs, such as isoniazid or rifampin, is used. Preventing tuberculosis is becoming more difficult because strains of tuberculosis have become resistant to the usual drugs (Chen, 2004).

Children with HIV infection should receive routine immunizations with the killed virus vaccines, includ-

---

BOX 42.4 FOCUS ON . . .

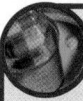

PHARMACOLOGY

Zidovudine (ZDV)

Classification: Zidovudine is a thymidine analog.

Action: Zidovudine inhibits the replication of some retroviruses, including HIV (Karch, 2004).

Pregnancy risk category: C

Dosage: 2 mg/kg every 6 hours to infants born to HIV-positive mothers, starting within 12 hours of birth to 6 wk of age. 180 mg/m^2 (720 mg/m^2/dose) orally or intravenously every 6 hours to children ages 3 mo to 12 y (dosage not to exceed 200 mg every 6 hours).

Possible adverse effects: Nausea, loss of appetite, change in taste, paresthesia, headache, fever, agranulocytopenia, and rash

Nursing Implications

- When administering the drug intravenously, infuse the drug over 60 min to avoid too rapid an infusion.
- Administer the drug around the clock for maximum effectiveness.
- Monitor blood studies frequently for changes.
- Advise child to eat frequent small meals to counteract change in taste and loss of appetite.
- If the child experiences paresthesias, institute safety precautions and instruct the child and parents in measures to prevent injury related to loss of feeling.
- Caution child and parents that ZDV does not reduce the risk of HIV transmission, except placentally. Reinforce the importance of hygiene and infection control measures.

---

ing the new pneumococcal vaccine, according to the usual schedule. Symptomatic children should not receive the varicella vaccine, and those with low CD4 counts should not receive MMR. If a child is exposed to varicella, intravenous varicella zoster immune globulin (VZIG) is prescribed in an attempt to prevent this disease. Yearly influenza vaccinations should begin at 6 months of age (Rutstein, 2003).

Nursing Diagnosis: Risk for compromised family coping related to diagnosis of HIV infection in child

Outcome Evaluation: Parents state ability to continue providing child's physical care; identify outside resources for help with care and decision making.

The diagnosis of HIV infection in an infant or child can prove devastating for a family. When the infection is transmitted maternally, this diagnosis may be the first indication of the existence of HIV infection in the mother; as such, this signals tremendous stress for the whole family. If the child contracted HIV infection from a contaminated blood transfusion or organ donation (rare with current protocols for donor screening), the family can feel so betrayed and angry that they are unwilling to cooperate with health care providers who, in their minds, are responsible for their child's illness. In any instance, the family's coping skills are sure to be compromised. Siblings may feel left out of the family circle because of the many health care appointments needed for the ill child. They may fear contracting the infection themselves. One of the first nursing priorities in the care of such a family should be to help the family re-establish their previous level of functioning so they can turn their attention to their child's emotional and physical care needs and to their own needs as well.

Physical care requirements for the child with HIV infection may be extensive, depending on the child's symptoms and disease progression. No matter what the child's physical needs, however, love and emotional support are essential to his or her well-being and psychological health. Parents or caregivers need extensive support, education, and anticipatory guidance from nurses and other members of the health care team. Encourage parents to seek medical care for their child at the first sign of illness or infection to prevent unnecessary hospitalization and pain.

Checkpoint Question 1

When Dexter's mother learned he had an immunologic disease, she was concerned that he had developed acquired immunodeficiency syndrome (HIV infection or AIDS). What is the transmission method by which most children acquire HIV infection?

a. Blood transfusion
b. Shared bath towels
c. Placental transfer
d. Sneezing and coughing

ALLERGY

Allergic diseases occur as a result of an abnormal antigen–antibody response. Allergic symptoms can be chronic and minor, such as those that occur with seasonal rhinitis, or acute and severe, as in an anaphylactic reaction. They can disrupt a child's life and development and the life of the family. When the cause of an allergic response is difficult to pinpoint, the child and parents often become frustrated. Even when the child has a known allergy, symptoms can vary from minor to acute without warning, ultimately disrupting family functioning (Box 42.5).

Hypersensitivity

The underlying cause of all allergic disorders appears to be an excessive antigen–antibody response when the invading organism is an allergen rather than a simple immunogen. This is termed a type I response or a **hypersensitivity**

BOX 42.5 FOCUS ON . . .

EVIDENCE-BASED PRACTICE

Can underlying immune system disorders contribute to the fatigue often seen in high school athletes?

To answer this question, researchers completed a health examination of 22 male and 19 female athletes who had reported persistent fatigue, recurrent infections, or both associated with intense training. Results of the health assessments revealed that 68% of athletes had some condition that was causing the fatigue. Immune disorders discovered were humoral immune deficiency (28%), allergic disease (15%), new or poorly controlled asthma (13%), and upper airway dysfunction (5%). Also discovered was nonfasting hypoglycemia (28%), sleep disorders (15%), and iron depletion (3%). One student had a thyroid disorder.

This is an interesting study for nurses because it shows the incidence of immune disorders in adolescents who were assumed (because they were athletes) to be disease-free. It also reveals the importance of immune disorders to optimal health.

Source: Reid, V. L., et al. (2004). Clinical investigation of athletes with persistent fatigue and/or recurrent infections. *British Journal of Sports Medicine, 38* (1), 42–45.

response when it happens immediately. It can also occur as a type II, III, or IV response (Table 42.3). Types I, II, and III are mediated by antibodies (humoral response), whereas type IV is mediated by the T lymphocytes (cell-mediated response).

Type I: Anaphylaxis

With a type I allergic response, IgE receptor sites attached to the surface of mast cells bind to IgE antibodies responding to the presence of an antigen. Mast cells are specialized cells found lining blood vessels and in connective tissue, the mucous membranes, and skin. The IgE immunoglobulin triggers mast cells to release intracellular granules. These contain histamine, leukotrienes, a slow-reacting substance of anaphylaxis (SRS-A), and chemotactic substances (substances to draw leukocytes into the area). Histamine and leukotrienes cause peripheral vasodilation and permeability of blood vessels. This leads to vascular congestion and edema. SRS-A causes extreme bronchial constriction and reduced vasodilation and permeability. **Anaphylaxis** is an acute reaction characterized by extreme vasodilation that leads to circulatory shock and extreme bronchoconstriction that decreases the airway lumens (Crusher, 2004).

Type II: Cytotoxic Response

In a **cytotoxic response,** cells are detected as foreign and immunoglobulins directly attack and destroy them without harming surrounding tissue. Foreign red blood

TABLE 42.3

Classification of Hypersensitivity Reactions

Type	Involved Cell	Mechanism	Effect
I Anaphylaxis	IgE	IgE attached to surface of mast cell triggers release of intracellular granules from mast cells on contact with antigens	Allergies, asthma, atopic dermatitis, anaphylaxis
II Cytotoxic	IgG or IgM	Antigen–antibody reaction leading to antigen destruction; complement is activated	Hemolytic anemia, transfusion reaction, erythroblastosis fetalis
III Immune complex disease	IgG or IgE	Antigen–antibody complexes precipitate; complement is activated, leading to inflammatory response	Rheumatoid arthritis, systemic lupus erythematosus
IV Delayed	T lymphocyte	T cells combine with antigen to induce inflammatory reactions by direct cell involvement or release of lymphokines	Contact dermatitis, transplant graft reaction

cells that are introduced to an Rh-negative woman by an Rh-positive fetus are destroyed by this process (see Chapter 26). Tumor cells may be destroyed by this process. Why this immune response fails when malignant cells begin to proliferate is not understood. Current research is attempting to devise ways to activate the natural immune response as a method of destroying malignant cells. Care of the child with a malignancy (neoplasm) is discussed in Chapter 53.

Type III: Immune Complex

A type III response is an IgG- or IgE-mediated antigen–antibody complex reaction that involves complement and initiates the inflammatory response. Complement reactions that persist beyond the usual inhibition may serve as the basis for many of the autoimmune illnesses, such as glomerulonephritis and systemic lupus erythematosus (see Chapter 46). Serum sickness also occurs as a result of a type III response.

Type IV: Cell-Mediated Hypersensitivity

In a delayed hypersensitivity response, T lymphocytes react with antigens and release lymphokines to call macrophages into the area. An inflammatory response occurs that helps to destroy the foreign tissue. A Mantoux or purified protein derivative (PPD) tuberculin test is an example of this. Redness and induration of the site do not begin initially but only after approximately 12 hours from the injection. The reaction peaks in 24 to 72 hours (a delayed response).

Contact dermatitis is another example of a delayed hypersensitivity response. Certain substances, such as cosmetics, household products, or cured leather, alter the protein of skin cells so that they become an antigen, or the foreign substance combines with the protein (hapten formation) to become an antigenic protein. Lymphocytes and macrophages infiltrate the area and attempt to destroy the offending protein. Redness and vesicles occur, and pruritus may be intense.

Assessment of Allergy in Children

History

Taking a health history of a child with an allergy can be time-consuming because many factors must be considered. A family history is important because there are familial tendencies with allergic diseases. Obtaining the exact symptoms of the allergy is important to help identify the allergen: rhinitis is probably due to an airborne antigen; urticaria (swelling and itching) is often caused by ingested antigens; and contact dermatitis (often a rash) must be from something that contacts the skin in that area. The time of the year that the allergy occurs also may give a clue to its cause. If the child's allergy exists all year, the antigen must be one that is present all year (house dust mites, pet dander, or a common food). If it occurs in the spring, it may be due to a tree pollen; in summer, a grass pollen; if it occurs just in August, ragweed is a prime suspect.

Children with allergic rhinitis (hay fever) develop common symptoms such as a horizontal crease across the nose (called a Dennie's line) from their habit of constantly wiping away nasal secretions. They also may develop dark patches under their eyes from back-pressure from nasal congestion (allergic shiners).

Many symptoms of allergy are vague, described as "colds all winter," "itching," or "runny nose." Listen carefully: even though no one symptom is acute, together such symptoms can interfere with a child's comfort, school experience, and long-term health. Having the parents and the child keep a chart of when symptoms are worse and better often helps identify a specific allergen. Children with allergic rhinitis (hay fever), for example, have more symptoms on a windy day and fewer after a rainstorm (the rain washes pollen out of the air). Children are often poor reporters of when they have symptoms because they cannot remember clearly whether they had the same rhinitis and watery eye symptoms last summer as they do this summer. A record that details when symptoms start—

for example, on arising, or only after the child reaches school—also can help identify an allergen.

Laboratory Testing

Few laboratory tests are helpful in establishing a diagnosis of allergy. A determination of IgE serum antibodies can be made. Most children with an allergy have an increased eosinophil count. Five percent or more of eosinophils on a differential count, or an eosinophil count of 250 or more cells per cubic millimeter, is significant. Another main cause of an increased eosinophil count is invasion by ova or parasites. This is why a stool specimen for ova and parasites is generally collected to rule out these problems as the cause of the increased eosinophil count. A radioallergosorbent test (RAST) may be ordered. This is an indirect radioimmunoassay in which the child's serum IgE is allowed to react with specific allergens impregnated in laboratory disks (Smith, 2003).

Skin Testing

Skin testing is done to detect the presence of IgE in the skin, or to isolate an antigen (allergen) to which the IgE is responding or to which a child is sensitive. When an allergen is introduced into the child's skin and the child is sensitive to that allergen, a wheal or flare response appears at the site of the test. This is due to the release of histamine, which leads to local vasodilation. Because this reaction appears quickly, the test should be read in 20 minutes. Systemic or aerosol administration of an antihistamine will inhibit the flare response, so the child should not receive these drugs for 8 hours before skin testing. Corticosteroid therapy does not affect immediate skin reactivity and so may be continued during skin testing.

Skin testing may be done by applying a patch or using a scratch or an intracutaneous injection technique. Patch testing has become the method of choice because it is painless and more efficient. For the child with rare allergies not typically provided by commercial patches, scratch or intracutaneous testing still may be necessary. Scratch testing is done by placing a drop of allergen solution on the skin, then scratching through the drop of liquid with a sterile needle. A relatively concentrated extract of allergen must be used for scratch testing because little allergen enters the child's skin.

Intracutaneous injections are done by injecting a small amount of a solution of allergen below the epidermis of the skin. This is usually done on the forearm so that if a sensitivity reaction does occur, a tourniquet can be applied proximal to the test site to prevent further absorption of the antigen. If the categories to be tested are extensive, the back can be used. Solutions used for intracutaneous injections are more dilute than those used for scratch testing (1:500 dilution compared with 1:5 for scratch testing). This means that the allergen extracts are not interchangeable from a group prepared for scratch testing to a group prepared for intracutaneous injections (or vice versa).

Because intracutaneous injections are given just below the epidermal layer of skin, they are almost painless. This is the same phenomenon as passing a needle or pin under the top layer of skin of a fingertip, a trick every school-age child does at least once to the horror of friends. The child needs a great deal of support for this type of skin testing, however, because it looks as if it will be painful, and the sight of a needle is frightening.

After all forms of skin testing, if the child is allergic to the test solution, a wheal and erythema (redness) will occur at the test site (Fig. 42.4). The size of the reaction is measured and graded as 1+ to 4+ or as slight, moderate, or marked. The allergens chosen for skin testing depend on the child's symptoms. Few children need more than 30 test media tried. This is because most allergies are worse at certain times of the year, and only the allergens prevalent at that time of year need to be evaluated.

Have a syringe filled with 1 mL epinephrine (Adrenalin) 1:1,000 on hand to counteract an unexpected anaphylactic reaction from skin testing. Epinephrine is given subcutaneously in doses of 0.01 mg/kg, up to 0.5 mg. Children should stay in the health care setting for at least 30 minutes after skin testing so they are there when such a reaction is most apt to occur.

Skin testing with food extracts is largely ineffective. Food allergies are best identified by eliminating a suspected food from the diet and observing whether there is an improvement in symptoms. After a time of improvement, the food is reintroduced. If it is one to which the child is allergic, symptoms will return with its reintroduction (termed "rechallenging").

Therapeutic Management

No matter what the symptoms of a child's allergy, there are three goals for therapy: reduce the child's exposure to the allergen, hyposensitize the child to produce a state of increased clinical **tolerance** (a state of not responding) to the allergen, and modify the child's response to the allergen with a pharmacologic agent.

Reducing the child's exposure to the allergen is possible when the offending allergen is a drug, food, or irritant. Reducing exposure is much more difficult when the child is found to be allergic to allergens such as molds, dust, feathers, or other substances found almost everywhere.

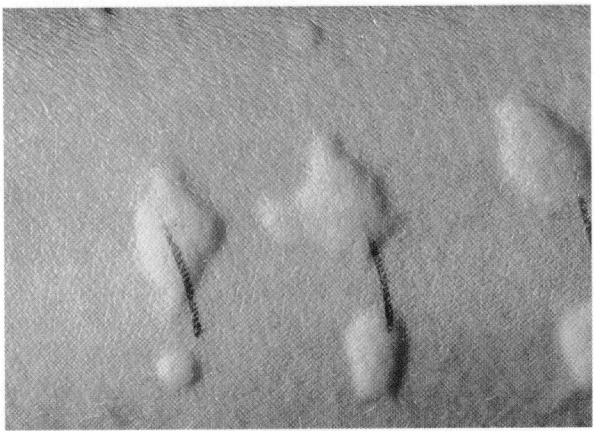

FIGURE 42.4 Allergy skin testing. Note the positive reactions. (© SPL/Custom Medical Stock Photo.)

Environmental Control

Environmental control means removal of as many common allergens as possible from the child's environment. Common measures of environmental control are shown in Table 42.4 and Box 42.6. Some parents carry out instructions to reduce potential allergens in their house without difficulty, but for others the process seems too involved to undertake. Help parents understand that environmental control can make a great deal of difference in their child's symptoms (Box 42.7). If environmental control is effective with the child, this is preferable to hyposensitization, which involves many visits to the doctor and many injections.

Hyposensitization

Hyposensitization, or immunotherapy, is done when the child's allergy symptoms cannot be controlled by avoidance of the allergen or conventional drug therapy. Because it is expensive and may not be successful, it is usually considered only after environmental control has been tried.

Hyposensitization works by increasing the plasma concentration of IgG antibodies. IgG acts to prevent or block IgE antibodies from coming in contact with the allergen. After specific allergens have been recognized with skin testing, small amounts of the allergy extract (dilute enough to be clinically subreactive) are injected into the child subcutaneously at 3- to 5-day intervals. The dose of antigen is increased in strength each time until a peak concentration is reached. The peak dose corresponds to the greatest strength that does not give clinical symptoms after injection. After hyposensitization has been achieved, the child then needs periodic injections every 3 to 4 weeks to maintain hyposensitization to this allergen. If a child is going to have an anaphylactic reaction to the injected allergen, it

TABLE 42.4

Common Measures for Environmental Control of Allergens

Area of Concern	Measures	Rationale
Child's bedroom	Encase mattress and pillow in sturdy plastic.	Reduces dust and dust mites
	Cover the zipper of plastic pillow and mattress case with adhesive tape.	Keeps dust confined
	Use blankets or quilts made of or stuffed with smooth, synthetic material; avoid wool.	Minimizes dust; wool is a good dust collector or may be an allergen itself
	Take down any ornamental items, such as a bed canopy.	Prevents dust collection
	Remove stuffed chairs and replace with wooden ones.	Removes dust collectors
	Remove venetian blinds and curtains that need to be dry-cleaned; replace with easily laundered types.	Removes dust collectors
	Remove stuffed toys unless filled with synthetic material.	Removes dust collectors and possible sources of allergens
	Remove aquariums and plants.	Removes mold spores
	Clean closet so it contains only currently used items.	Eliminates dust collectors
	Remove any fur or woolen items from child's wardrobe.	Removes possible allergens
Living room	Remove all carpets. If a rug is necessary, replace an animal hair pad with a foam rubber one.	Avoids containers for dust collection
	Provide a wooden chair for sitting.	Provides space free from allergens
	Vacuum frequently.	Minimizes dust collection
	Use linoleum or plastic laminate surface on carpet if child sits on the floor.	Provides space free from allergens
	Discourage child from lying on rug.	Reduces exposure to allergens
Bathroom	Use nonscented toilet paper, soaps, cleaners.	Minimizes exposure to potential irritants
School room	Have child sit away from blackboard, caged animals, or fish tanks.	Minimizes exposure to chalk, mold spores, and animal dander, which are allergens
	Keep locker free of collectibles	Reduces dust collection
General	Purchase a dehumidifier; add compounds to paint to decrease mold spores.	Reduces mold spores
	Use HEPA filters on furnaces, vacuums.	Filters air of possible allergens
	Do not keep a pet.	Reduces exposure to animal dander
	Dust daily with a moist cloth.	Controls dust better than dry dusting

BOX 42.6 FOCUS ON . . .

FAMILY TEACHING

Avoiding Secondary Smoke

Q. Dexter's mother says to you, "Neither my husband nor I smoke, but some of our relatives and friends do. How can we keep our child from being exposed to secondary smoke?"

A. Use the following guidelines to help avoid secondary smoke:

- Declare your home a smoke-free zone.
- If family members smoke, ask them to smoke outside.
- If at a restaurant, ask to sit in a no-smoking area, or visit only smoke-free restaurants.
- If staying at a hotel, ask for a nonsmoking room.
- Don't be reluctant to ask people around your child at a social gathering to stop smoking.
- Encourage your friends or family members who smoke to take quit-smoking courses (for their own benefit as well as yours).

generally occurs within 30 minutes after the injection. Therefore, always have the child wait in the health care setting for 30 minutes after the injection before going home.

Immunotherapy is generally continued for 2 to 3 years because the longer it is used, the longer the period of re-lief from symptoms after it is stopped. Be certain that parents know at the beginning of therapy that this therapy will not "cure" their child. It will make the child symptom-free or will decrease symptoms for a length of time, however, and it may prevent a disease such as hay fever (allergic rhinitis) from turning into asthma. Be certain children have adequate preparation for the procedure. Help them understand the importance of returning for additional injections.

A newer technique of immunotherapy is the sublingual administration of chosen allergen solutions. SLIT (sublingual immunotherapy) is administered for an equal length of time as injection therapy, but SLIT has the advantage of being painless while producing equal results.

Pharmacologic Therapy

A number of pharmacologic preparations can be used to reduce the symptoms of childhood allergies. Like hypo-sensitization procedures, these drugs do not change the sensitivity to allergens; they only relieve the symptoms.

Antihistamines block histamine release and as a result control itching, sneezing, and rhinorrhea. Diphenhydramine hydrochloride (Benadryl) is the prototype of this drug class (Box 42.8). It is effective but causes severe drowsiness. Second- and third-generation antihistamines, such as cetirizine (Zyrtec) and loratadine (Claritin), cause less drowsiness and provide a longer effect.

Decongestants, such as pseudoephedrine (Sudafed), decrease nasal edema and can help enlarge breathing space. Intranasal corticosteroids reduce inflammation, producing

BOX 42.7 FOCUS ON . . .

COMMUNICATION

The Goodenough family has been instructed on environmental control measures because Dexter has severe allergic rhinitis. Despite this, Dexter's symptoms have not improved. You meet with his parents to confirm they are carrying out these measures.

Less Effective Communication

Nurse: Have you made the changes around your house that we discussed to reduce dust?

Mrs. Goodenough: As many as we can.

Nurse: What about Dexter's bedroom? Do you have the mattress covered? Any frilly curtains down? Any stuffed animals taken out?

Mrs. Goodenough: I've done everything I can.

Nurse: In the living room, it's important he has a protected floor space, also that he doesn't sit in overstuffed chairs.

Mrs. Goodenough: I've done everything I can.

Nurse: Okay, you sound in good shape. It's puzzling, though, why, in the face of all you've done, Dexter's symptoms haven't improved.

More Effective Communication

Nurse: Have you made the changes around your house that we discussed to reduce dust?

Mrs. Goodenough: As many as we can.

Nurse: What about Dexter's bedroom? Do you have the mattress covered? Any frilly curtains down? Any stuffed animals taken out?

Mrs. Goodenough: I've done everything I can.

Nurse: It's puzzling why Dexter's symptoms haven't improved. Why don't you tell me exactly what steps you've taken?

Mrs. Goodenough: I covered the mattress. I had to leave the curtains up, though, because they match the rug. I took out a lot of the toys, but I had to leave the stuffed bears because they match the wallpaper.

Nurse: Let's review again what environmental control means and the effect it can have on reducing Dexter's symptoms.

The above scenario is an example of what can happen when nurses assume that what they mean by a term is also what a parent means by the same term. In this instance, by taking the parent's statement that she has done "everything possible" to mean she has done everything that needs to be done, the nurse makes an incorrect assumption. Following up by asking the parents to be more specific reveals better information.

BOX 42.8 FOCUS ON . . .

PHARMACOLOGY

Diphenhydramine Hydrochloride (Benadryl)

Classification: Diphenhydramine is a first-generation antihistamine.

Action: Blocks the effects of histamine at H_1 receptor sites, resulting in relief of symptoms associated with histamine release disorders such as allergic rhinitis (Karch, 2004).

Pregnancy risk category: B

Dosage: 12.5 to 25 mg t.i.d. to q.i.d. or 5 mg/kg/day or 150 mg/m²/day orally (in children weighing over 10 kg [20 lb]) up to a maximum dose of 300 mg/day

Possible adverse effects: Drowsiness, dizziness, sedation, epigastric distress, dry mouth, thickening of bronchial secretions, hypotension

Nursing Implications

- Administer drug with food if gastrointestinal upset occurs.
- Use a humidifier to keep nasal mucosa moist.
- Be alert for drowsiness, which may interfere with school or sports performance; notify the health care provider for possible change in dosage or drug.
- Encourage the child to suck on sugarless lozenges to combat dry mouth.
- Notify health care provider if child develops a lower respiratory tract disorder. Antihistamines should not be used when secretions need to be kept moist to enhance expectoration.
- Do not use this drug if the child has glucose-6-phosphate dehydrogenase deficiency. Severe hemolysis may occur.

an effect similar to decongestants. Intranasal cromolyn sodium can be used prophylactically to prevent symptoms.

COMMON IMMUNE REACTIONS

Anaphylactic Shock

Anaphylactic shock is an immediate, life-threatening, type I hypersensitivity reaction that occurs after exposure to an allergen in a previously sensitized child. Within minutes of antigen invasion (being stung by an insect or receiving an injection of a drug to which a child has been sensitized), symptoms begin (Brown, 2004).

Assessment

Initially, a child may become nauseated, with vomiting and diarrhea, because of the sudden increase in gastrointestinal secretions produced by the stimulation of histamine. This is followed by urticaria and angioedema. Bronchospasm becomes so severe the child becomes dyspneic and hypoxemic. Continued bronchospasm leads to

hypoxia. As blood vessels dilate, the blood pressure and pulse rate may fall. Seizures and death may follow as soon as 10 minutes after the allergen was introduced into the child's body (Smith, 2003).

It is sometimes difficult to distinguish anaphylactic shock from fainting (syncope). Children, as a rule, do not faint after an injection or a bee sting. Syncope rarely occurs if a person is lying prone, so if the reaction occurred while the child was lying on the treatment table, it is most likely that the reaction is anaphylactic. With syncope, although the child falls and is momentarily unconscious, the pulse and blood pressure remain normal. The child appears pale and may have intense perspiration, but he or she can be roused readily after breathing amyl nitrite (smelling salts). The child with an anaphylactic reaction cannot be roused this way.

Therapeutic Management

Preventing and recognizing anaphylaxis are as important as knowing how to respond when it occurs. Before giving drugs that are known to have a high incidence of anaphylactic reactions (e.g., penicillin, aspirin, or antitoxin serums), be certain to ask parents if the child has ever had a reaction to the drug before. If in doubt, withhold the drug until its safety can be confirmed. Check the child's chart to be certain that no prior reactions are noted. People who have hypersensitivity reactions to any injectable substance should wear a bracelet or necklace identifying the drug to which they are allergic. Some children object to this safety measure because they do not want to look conspicuous, but assure them this is important. Generally, children who have hypersensitivity reactions to insect stings are advised to undergo hyposensitization therapy because they cannot totally avoid insects.

Epinephrine is the drug of choice to treat anaphylaxis (Box 42.9). Additional emergency interventions for anaphylactic shock are summarized in Box 42.10. If anaphylaxis follows an injection or an insect sting, give the epinephrine in the opposite arm. Place a tourniquet on the extremity of the allergenic injection or sting proximal to the injection site to prevent further absorption of the allergen. Release the tourniquet every 15 minutes for a few seconds to avoid totally compromising blood flow.

If a sensitized child receives an injection or is stung by an insect while at home, parents must know the proper procedure to follow so they can give their child immediate help. In place of a tourniquet, they can apply ice to the injection or sting site to slow absorption. If a child has been prescribed an antihistamine, they should give that. Then the parents should notify an emergency squad that their child is having a severe reaction. Caution them not to attempt to give an oral medication if the child is comatose. Parents may purchase an emergency kit (e.g., Ana-Kit), an insect sting treatment kit that contains measured doses of epinephrine (often in a device called an EpiPen, which injects the epinephrine; Box 42.11) and an antihistamine.

Evaluation of the child after an anaphylactic reaction involves not only a physical examination but also evaluation to help the child avoid such a serious reaction from occurring again. This involves health teaching about the substance that caused the reaction and related substances that could have the same effect (Sheetz & McIntyre, 2005).

BOX 42.9 FOCUS ON . . .

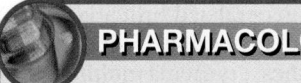

PHARMACOLOGY

Epinephrine Hydrochloride (Adrenalin)

Classification: Epinephrine is a sympathomimetic drug.

Action: Acts on both alpha- and beta-receptor sites of sympathetic receptor cells to cause increased blood pressure and heart rate. It also relaxes the smooth muscles of the bronchi. It is used to counteract the symptoms of anaphylaxis (Karch, 2004).

Pregnancy risk category: C

Dosage: 0.01 mg/kg or 0.3 mL/m^2 of a 1:1,000 solution subcutaneously every 20 min or more often if needed for 4 hours, not to exceed 0.5 mL (0.5 mg) in a single dose (for children and infants); 0.005 mL/kg (0.025 mg/kg) subcutaneously of a 1:200 suspension (in infants and children 1 mo to 1 y)

Possible adverse effects: Anxiety, restlessness, headache, nausea, arrhythmias, hypertension, palpitations, pallor

Nursing Implications
- Be sure to calculate the drug dosage and check the solution strength carefully; solution is available in different concentrations, and epinephrine is a very potent drug.
- Obtain blood pressure, pulse, and respirations and auscultate breath sounds before and immediately after administration. Assess the child for signs indicating resolution of anaphylaxis.
- Rotate injection sites to prevent necrosis.
- Have a rapidly acting alpha-adrenergic blocking agent or vasodilator readily available in case of hypertensive reaction; have a beta-adrenergic blocking agent readily available in case of arrhythmias.
- Protect the drug from light and heat. Use only solutions that are clear and colorless.

BOX 42.10

Emergency Measures For Anaphylactic Shock

Anaphylaxis is an emergency, and fast action is necessary.

- Position the child with head even with the body to counteract hypotension.
- Administer aqueous epinephrine (Adrenalin) 1;1,000 subcutaneously at a dosage of 0.01 mg per kilogram of body weight up to 0.5 mg. This relieves laryngeal edema and severe bronchospasm.
- Administer nebulized bronchodilators such as albuterol to halt wheezing.
- If hypoxia is present, administer oxygen by mask or nasal cannula.
- Notify the cardiac arrest team because both respiratory and cardiac arrest may occur.
- Anticipate use of diphenhydramine (Benadryl) IM or IV as a secondary medication, particularly if urticaria (itching and swelling) is present.
- Anticipate the need for an IV fluid line as a route for a vasopressor such as dopamine and fluid to help restore blood pressure.
- If the child is experiencing seizures, prepare to administer phenobarbital or diazepam.
- Be prepared to administer corticosteroids as second-line drugs. Corticosteroids do not act immediately but reduce inflammation, which is necessary. IV methylprednisolone is a typical drug given.
- Keep the child and family members calm; anxiety adds to bronchospasm and decreases breathing ability.

 Checkpoint Question 2

Any child can have an anaphylactic reaction to a food or drug. What is the drug of choice you would want to have available to treat anaphylactic reactions?

a. Prednisone
b. Epinephrine
c. Penicillin
d. Ibuprofen

Urticaria and Angioedema

Urticaria, or hives, refers to flat wheals surrounded by erythema arising from the chorion layer of skin; they are intensely pruritic (often described as a burning sensation). Elevations may occur so close together they tend to coalesce (blend together). Urticaria occurs from a type I or immediate hypersensitivity reaction created by the release of histamine from an antibody–antigen reaction,

similar to but of lesser intensity than anaphylaxis. In chronic urticaria, no causative allergen may be found. There is dilatation of capillaries and venules with increased permeability.

Angioedema is edema of the skin and subcutaneous tissue. This occurs most frequently on the eyelids, hands, feet, genitalia, and lips—areas where skin is loosely bound by subcutaneous tissue. Angioedema can be distinguished from other edemas because it is not dependent, is generally asymmetrically distributed, and usually occurs with urticaria. One type is inherited as an autosomal disorder on chromosome 11 (Smith, 2003). With severe angioedema, the larynx may be involved. This is serious because laryngeal edema may lead to airway obstruction and subsequently asphyxiation and death.

The allergens that most frequently cause urticaria and angioedema include drugs, foods, and insect stings. Exposure to hot or cold can also cause these reactions. The cause of the reaction should be identified so it can be avoided in the future. Although hot and cold exposure is a rare cause, children with this form must be identified because if they swim in cold water, the sudden release of histamine could cause dizziness so severe that they could drown. Therapy for urticaria or angioedema is subcutaneous epinephrine or an oral antihistamine.

BOX 42.11 FOCUS ON . . .

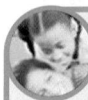

FAMILY TEACHING

Guidelines for Using an EpiPen

Q. Dexter's father says to you, "If my child is stung by a bee, I'm supposed to inject epinephrine. How do I do that?"

A. It's important you think about this in advance, because at the moment your child is stung, it will be an emergency situation.

- Purchase an EpiPen, a commercial syringe with a designated dose of epinephrine for use in emergencies.
- If necessary, purchase additional EpiPens so you have one at home, provide one for your child's school, and maybe keep one in your car to avoid having to remember to carry a single one with you.
- Store EpiPens at room temperature; don't refrigerate.
- Inspect the color of the solution in the EpiPen once a month; replace it if it is cloudy or discolored.
- If your child is stung, remove the gray safety cap from the device and wipe the outer fleshy portion of your child's thigh with an alcohol wipe.
- Place the EpiPen against the thigh until the device activates, injecting the solution into your child's thigh. If necessary, you can place the device on top of your child's clothing. The needle is long enough to pass through the clothing and into your child's skin.
- Be careful before injecting that you are holding the EpiPen with the needle toward your child. If not, you will accidentally inject your own thumb (a serious circumstance, as the dose of epinephrine could seriously injure your thumb).
- Keep in mind that the EpiPen is designed so that not all the solution in the pen will be ejected. Do not try to give the remainder of the solution.
- Remember that epinephrine will control symptoms for about 20 minutes. After administering the dose, therefore, call 911 for transportation assistance or transport your child to an emergency facility for further care.

Serum Sickness

Serum sickness is a type III hypersensitivity response of the body to a foreign serum antigen or drug. Examples of foreign sera given to children include tetanus antitoxin, diphtheria antitoxin, and rabies antiserum. These are obtained from horse serum. Children may experience a serum sickness reaction to a drug (e.g., penicillin), but this is rare.

Assessment

Symptoms of serum sickness begin 7 to 12 days after the serum injection. If the child has received the same type of foreign serum previously, symptoms may occur as early as 1 to 5 days. Children notice itching, edema, and erythema at the injection site. There is generalized urticaria (hives) with or without angioedema (generalized edema). Erythematous maculopapular rashes, erythema multiforme (a generalized macular eruption with dark red papules), or purpura (hemorrhage into the skin) may result.

There may be fever and arthralgia (joint pain). Lymphadenopathy may be present, especially of the regional nodes near the site of the injection. The child may have weight gain, nausea, vomiting, and abdominal pain. In more extreme instances, the child's nervous system may be involved and optic neuritis, stupor, and coma may occur. If edema is severe, laryngeal edema will become the paramount symptom that needs treatment.

Therapeutic Management

Serum sickness lasts days or weeks. In its usual form (i.e., urticaria, edema, arthralgia, or pruritus), the treatment is only symptomatic because the condition will improve by itself with time. However, an antihistamine such as diphenhydramine (Benadryl) or epinephrine may be helpful in relieving symptoms. A nonsteroidal anti-inflammatory drug (NSAID) such as ibuprofen (Motrin) or a corticosteroid may be necessary to relieve the fever and joint pain (Salerno, 2003).

Like anaphylactic reactions, serum sickness reactions are frightening to the child and parents. Parents need an explanation of why the reaction occurred (their child has a low threshold of sensitization to this particular substance), that it was not anyone's fault, and that it did not occur from administration of the wrong compound (assuming that proper precautions to ascertain sensitivity to the solution were taken before the incident). Because serum sickness mimics so many other diseases, parents need reassurance that it is not arthritis (the arthralgia may make them think it is) and that their child will not have long-term effects from it.

The child should not receive the foreign serum or drug that was responsible for this primary occurrence of serum sickness again. Otherwise, if administered again, the manifestation of the reaction may be anaphylaxis. The child should wear a bracelet or necklace stating the solutions to which he or she is hypersensitive. Children should have their immunizations (and records) kept current so there is never a need to give sera such as tetanus or diphtheria antitoxins.

ATOPIC DISORDERS

Individuals with atopy are prone to all allergic responses. Three disorders occur most frequently: hay fever (allergic rhinitis), eczema (atopic dermatitis), and asthma (see Chapter 40). Although these diseases show a familial tendency, different family members may have different symptoms. In one family, for example, the father may have allergic rhinitis, one child may have asthma, and another may have atopic dermatitis.

The gene responsible for an immune response is located near the human leukocyte antigen that is responsible for graft rejection. In certain children, a tendency for sensitivity to antigens or abnormality of this gene is apparently inherited. These children have a higher-than-normal production of IgE antibody that makes them more responsive to allergens than other people. However, there is also a strong environmental component to these diseases. Children whose parents smoke have a greater incidence of atopic disorders compared with children of parents who do not smoke (Smith, 2003).

Allergic Rhinitis

Allergic rhinitis is caused by a type I or immediate hypersensitivity immune response. It occurs in 10% to 15% of children (Cohet et al., 2004).

Assessment

Common symptoms of allergic rhinitis include sneezing, nasal engorgement, and a profuse watery nasal discharge. The mucous membrane of the nose is generally paler than normal. It may be edematous, adding to nasal congestion. The conjunctivae of the eyes may be pruritic, often with a distinctive pebbly appearance, and may also water. Children constantly rub their noses in an upward motion, termed an allergic salute. Over a long period, rubbing the nose this way leads to a horizontal crease across the tip of the nose, called an allergic crease. Because of congestion in the nose, there tends to be back-pressure to the blood circulation around the eye orbit, which leads to blackened areas under the eyes, termed allergic shiners (Fig. 42.5).

Children older than 6 years (when frontal sinuses develop) may report a full frontal headache. This becomes more marked with adolescence. Some children feel exhausted and lethargic and cannot function well in school. Recurrent otitis media may occur due to the swollen pharyngeal tissue (eustachian tubes are blocked to the middle ear). A smear of the nasal discharge will reveal an increased eosinophil count (more than 10% of the white cell count). RAST analysis may reveal the offending allergens.

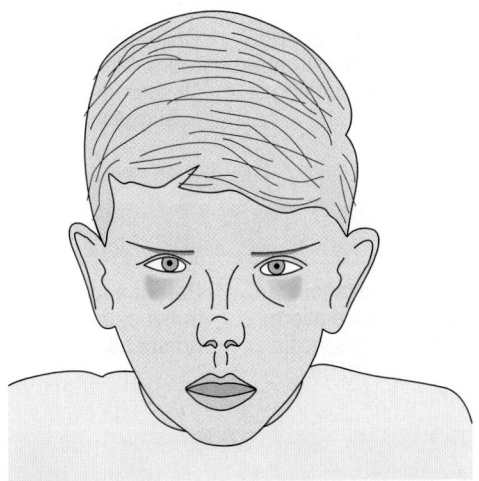

FIGURE 42.5 Back-pressure to the blood circulation around the eye orbit from allergic rhinitis may lead to dark areas under the eyes (allergic shiners). The frequent rubbing of the nose in an upward direction can lead to a peculiar horizontal crease (Dennie's line).

The allergens that cause allergic rhinitis are generally pollens or molds rather than foods or drugs. Many of these children are brought to a health care setting during peak pollen months because parents think they have a "summer cold." However, with an upper respiratory infection, the mucous membrane of the nose is more apt to be reddened than pale, and the secretions draining from the nose are apt to be thick white or yellow rather than the thin, watery secretions of allergic rhinitis. Children with an upper respiratory infection often have a fever; children with allergic rhinitis do not. With an upper respiratory infection, a sore throat and cervical adenopathy may be present, but these are rare with allergic rhinitis.

Therapeutic Management

Allergic rhinitis is managed by avoidance of allergens, use of pharmacologic agents (antihistamines, leukotriene inhibitors, or corticosteroids), or immunotherapy. Parents usually ask how sick children should be before they need to see an allergist about skin testing and definite treatment (an expensive, time-consuming, and potentially painful procedure). Individual circumstances dictate the direction of treatment. As a rule, a child whose symptoms are increasing in intensity, who has associated lower respiratory tract involvement, or whose condition interferes with activities in which he or she wants to participate needs definitive testing and treatment. Others can be managed by environmental control and medications to reduce symptoms.

Intranasal corticosteroids or antihistamines are effective in reducing symptoms in most children. Caution children and parents that antihistamines tend to cause sleepiness. Assess whether this will interfere with schoolwork. Be certain that parents understand that if nasal antihistamine sprays are given for more than 3 days, a rebound effect may occur (the nasal mucosa becomes more edematous rather than less edematous).

Avoidance of allergens may be ineffective with allergic rhinitis because a child has a sensitivity to many different pollens or grasses. If children always show symptoms at one particular time of the year, parents may be able to carry out environmental control for that period of the year. Some children with allergic rhinitis are more comfortable in air-conditioned buildings; others have strong symptoms in the presence of air conditioning, probably accounting for the high incidence of headaches that occur at school (Wills-Karp & Khurana-Hershey, 2003).

Allergic rhinitis is often considered a minor illness by parents, something that children will outgrow. However, for children who have the condition, it may not be a minor illness and it may keep them from interacting with other children during certain months because they dread going outside and initiating symptoms. Help parents understand the importance of avoiding allergens and the need for conscientious administration of intranasal corticosteroids or antihistamines to minimize symptoms (Box 42.12).

Perennial Allergic Rhinitis

Allergic rhinitis becomes perennial (year-round) when the allergen is one that is capable of affecting the child year-round, such as house dust mites or pet hair. Although

BOX 42.12: Focus on Nursing Care Planning

A Multidisciplinary Care Map for
A Child with Allergic Rhinitis
●

Dexter Goodenough is a 6-year-old boy you meet in an ambulatory set-ting. Dexter is diagnosed as having allergic rhinitis (hay fever). "Thank heavens," his mother exclaims. "I thought when I heard he had an immune system disease he had AIDS. What a relief to know it's only an allergy."

Family Assessment
Child lives with his mother and his stepfather in a beach-front cottage. Also in the family is a brother, 8 years; a stepbrother, 16 years; and a paternal grandmother. His stepfather owns a jewelry store. His mother is a stay-at-home mom. Finances are rated as "not a problem."

Client Assessment
Child's eyes are reddened and watery; his nose drains a clear discharge. His mother tells you he frequently has a headache and is constantly listless, and other children make fun of him because of his appearance. His grades are "terrible" because the minute he gets to school, his symptoms begin. Dexter is prescribed an antihistamine and environmental control.

Nursing Diagnosis
Situational low self-esteem related to feelings of inadequacy and embarrassment

Outcome Criteria
Client states he is able to function in school in spite of allergy symptoms and discomfort; is taking active measures to avoid allergens.

Team Member Responsible	Assessment	Intervention	Rationale	Expected Outcome
Activities of Daily Living				
Nurse	Assess what Dexter's classroom is like to identify potential allergens, as child's symptoms are most intense when he is at school.	Discuss potential source of allergens with mother; ask her to meet with teacher to see if modifications could be made.	Environmental control can reduce the number of allergens causing symptoms.	Child describes classroom. Mother visits classroom as necessary to suggest changes.
Consultations				
Physician	Assess if child's symptoms could be reduced with hyposensitization.	Consult with allergist about possibility of hyposensitization.	Hyposensitization can greatly reduce allergy symptoms if specific allergens can be identified.	Parent and child agree to hyposensitization if prescribed.
Procedures/Medications				
Nurse	Assess if child has had experience with taking medicine before.	Help mother set up a medicine chart that will help with antihistamine adherence.	Allergy medicine is most effective when it is taken conscientiously.	Parent states she will be conscientious about antihistamine administration.

(continued)

Team Member Responsible	Assessment	Intervention	Rationale	Expected Outcome
Nutrition				
Nurse	Assess if there are any foods child or mother feel contribute to allergy symptoms.	If foods are identified, review with mother list of foods to avoid.	Respiratory allergens are more likely involved in allergic rhinitis, but foods should be ruled out.	Mother and child describe any foods that cause discomfort for child and measures to avoid them.
Patient/Family Education				
Nurse	Assess environmental aspects at home that could be causing child's symptoms.	Discuss environmental control with parents.	Reducing allergens in the home can also aid in reducing child's symptoms.	Parents agree to any modifications necessary in their home.
Nurse	Assess if the child is exposed to secondary smoke in home.	Educate family on the damage that secondary smoke can cause.	Secondary smoke is a potent allergen and also may contribute to lung and heart disease.	Parents agree to make home smoke-free.
Psychosocial/Spiritual/Emotional Needs				
Nurse	Assess the extent of ridicule child undergoes at school.	Discuss coping measures with child. Urge mother to report bullying to school authorities.	Psychological health is as important as physical health.	Child describes experiences at school. States he is no longer bullied.
Discharge Planning				
Nurse	Assess if parent has other questions about child's allergies.	Schedule a follow-up visit for reevaluation of new medication.	Allergy control can involve a range of medicine, so it can be confusing for children or parents.	Mother states she understands the importance of follow-up visit and will keep appointment.

the child's symptoms may not result in the obvious distress associated with seasonal allergic rhinitis, the child needs treatment just as much because the symptoms occur constantly. Because the agent that causes perennial allergic rhinitis is often house dust, environmental control plays a big role in the control of the disorder. Serous otitis media may be a serious consequence of perennial allergic rhinitis (see Chapter 50).

Atopic Dermatitis (Infantile Eczema)

Atopic dermatitis is primarily a disease of infants, beginning as early as the second month of life and possibly lasting until age 2 to 3 years. It may be related to food allergy because it tends to occur more often in formula-fed infants than in breast-fed infants and more common if infants are fed solid food before 6 months. Sweating, heat, tight clothing, and contact irritants such as soap increase the pruritus. Symptoms may be more annoying in the winter, when additional irritating clothing is present, with marked improvement in the summer.

Assessment

With infantile atopic dermatitis, capillary permeability increases, causing a loss of serous fluid out into the tissues. Children develop papular and vesicular skin eruptions with surrounding erythema. The vesicles rupture and exude yellow, sticky secretions that form crusts on the skin as they dry. Because the lesions are extremely pruritic, the child scratches and further irritates the lesions, causing linear excoriations. Secondary infections of open lesions may then occur. As the infected lesions heal, the skin becomes depigmented and lichenified (shiny), and dry, flaky scales form. If secondary infection occurs, local lymph nodes will be swollen. The child may have a low-grade fever. An increased eosinophil count reveals that the condition is allergy-based.

The common sites for lesions include the scalp and forehead, the cheeks, neck, behind the ears, and the extensor surfaces of the extremities (Fig. 42.6). The palms of the hands and the soles of the feet are uninvolved. Because the lesions are uncomfortable, children with infantile atopic dermatitis may be overly fussy and irritable. They may not eat well due to this generalized discomfort.

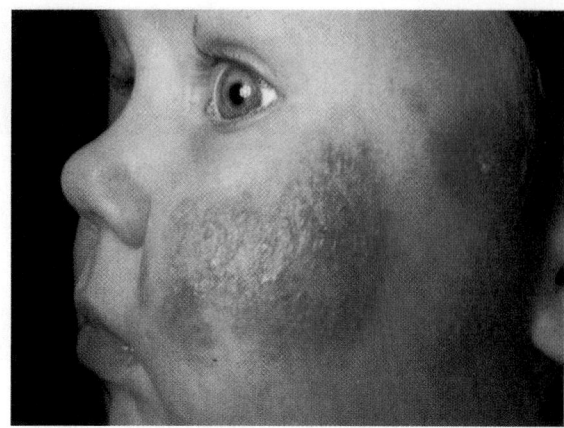

FIGURE 42.6 Infant with atopic dermatitis. (Sauer, G. C. & Hall, J. C. [1996]. *Manual of skin diseases,* [7th ed.]. Philadelphia: Lippincott-Raven Publishers.)

Although infantile atopic dermatitis is generally diagnosed while taking the family history (considering other allergic individuals in the family) and noticing the characteristic lesions and their patterns, it is sometimes difficult to distinguish from seborrheic dermatitis (cradle cap; see Chapter 28). The findings in seborrheic dermatitis and infantile atopic dermatitis are compared in Table 42.5. Seborrheic dermatitis is a fairly benign condition of infants, requiring little treatment other than frequent shampooing of the hair and soaking the lesions in mineral oil and combing them away. A child with infantile atopic dermatitis, on the other hand, will not respond to these measures but must be referred for additional treatment. Also, children with infantile atopic dermatitis should have a repeat test for phenylketonuria (PKU) done because children with PKU often have atopic dermatitis (Yan, 2003).

Skin testing is ineffective because the allergen causing infantile atopic dermatitis is often a food allergen. However, it may also be caused by pollens, dust, or mold spores. For this reason, skin testing may be attempted to isolate a causative allergen.

Therapeutic Management

The treatment of atopic dermatitis is aimed at reducing the amount of allergen exposure, if such allergens can be identified. The most likely foods to which infants are allergic are milk, eggs, wheat, chocolate, fish, tomatoes, and peanuts. The use of elimination diets to identify food allergens is discussed later in this chapter. A second major consideration in treatment is aimed at reducing pruritus so children do not irritate lesions and cause secondary infections by scratching. Hydrating the skin by bathing or applying wet dressings (wet with tap water or Burow's solution) for 15 to 20 minutes, followed by application of a hydrating emollient such as petroleum jelly (Vaseline) or even vegetable shortening (Crisco), is helpful. Do not allow infants to become chilled if a large portion of the body is to be covered with wet dressings. A stockinette dressing with holes cut out for the eyes, nose, and mouth pulled over the head will hold wet dressings in place on the face and neck. To prevent corneal irritation, be careful that such dressings do not come in contact with the eyes.

Some infants need an antihistamine to reduce itching. Topical steroids such as 1% hydrocortisone cream do a great deal to relieve the discomfort and appearance of lesions by reducing the inflammation and pruritus. If the lesions are dry, a corticosteroid ointment is most effective; if moist, a lotion may be most effective. Applying the cream or lotion and then covering the area with an occlusive dressing such as plastic wrap overnight may speed the healing process. If the lesions are secondarily infected, hydrocortisone mixed with an antibiotic (generally neomycin)

TABLE 42.5

Comparison of Seborrheic Dermatitis and Atopic Dermatitis

Finding	Seborrheic Dermatitis	Atopic Dermatitis
Age at onset	0–6 months	2–6 months
Length of disease	Rarely 1 year	2–3 years
Mood of child	Happy; parents happy	Irritable; parents tired
Location of lesions	Scalp, behind ears, near umbilicus	Cheeks, extensor surfaces, some flexor surfaces
Types of lesions	Salmon-colored erythematous lesions with greasy scales	Papulovesicular erythematous lesions with weeping and crusting
Itching	No	Severe
Depigmentation	No	Yes
Lichenification	No	Yes
White dermographism	No	Yes
Eosinophilia	No nasal mucus or blood eosinophilia	Nasal mucus or blood eosinophilia
IgE serum levels	Low	High

and a suitable base is prescribed. Caution parents not to discontinue application of cortisone cream abruptly. Although absorption with topical application is limited, some does occur. This reduces adrenal gland functioning. If the cream is discontinued abruptly, the infant's adrenal response (ability to produce epinephrine) in an emergency might be limited. Also caution the parents not to overuse the cortisone cream. More is not better and may increase the risk of systemic absorption. Because of the complications that steroid creams can create, the new immunomodulators tacrolimus (Protopic) and pimecrolimus (Elidel) may be prescribed. These represent a safer class of drugs and also alter the local immune response (Smith & Brodell, 2004).

NURSING DIAGNOSES AND RELATED INTERVENTIONS

Nursing Diagnosis: Risk for impaired parenting related to feelings of inadequacy secondary to infant's chronic atopic dermatitis

Outcome Evaluation: Parents express confidence in their ability to follow recommended therapy; express positive aspects of infant; hold infant close and smile and talk to infant.

Parents of children with infantile atopic dermatitis need a great deal of support through the course of the disease because children can be irritable from the constant pruritus. No matter how hard parents try, they cannot seem to make them happy. Parents need a listening ear so they can vent these concerns and maintain their self-esteem as parents. Support groups also can help meet this need.

Nursing Diagnosis: Impaired skin integrity related to infantile atopic dermatitis

Outcome Evaluation: Infant does not scratch lesions; parents state infant is less irritable and easier to care for. Lesions show signs of healing.

When lesions begin to heal, a skin emollient and moisturizer, such as Eucerin, or baths with a substance to lubricate the skin, such as Alpha-Keri, are prescribed to prevent excessive skin dryness. The infant should soak in the bath with the lubricant for approximately 15 minutes, then be patted, not rubbed, dry so the lesions are not aggravated. Caution parents not to use soap, because it can be drying.

Suggest that parents trim the infant's fingernails short or cover his or her hands with cotton socks to prevent scratching. Exposure to the herpes virus can cause a generalized reaction. Caution parents to screen babysitters or alert child care personnel with active herpes lesions not to care for their infants while atopic dermatitis is active.

In most infants, the lesions of infantile atopic dermatitis clear by the time the child is 3 years old. Un-

less secondary infection with scarring results, the skin surface will not be marked. Many of these children go on to develop other allergies, however, as they grow older. In the preschool years, the child's parents may report that the child has "one cold after another" (allergic rhinitis). By early school years, the child may show signs of asthma (see Chapter 40).

Atopic Dermatitis in the Older Child

Atopic dermatitis in the older child may occur at any age, but frequently it occurs at puberty or late adolescence (Yan, 2003). Atopic dermatitis that occurs at these later ages is prominent on the flexor surface of the extremities and on the dorsal surfaces of the wrists and ankles. It often occurs in the eyebrows; if the child scratches the lesions, the child may be left with scant eyebrows. Depigmentation or hyperpigmentation is usually present, and lichenification is marked. The fingernails often have a glossy sheen from the buffing action of constant rubbing and scratching. In some children, an itch–scratch cycle in response to stress may lead to an exacerbation of symptoms. For example, a child begins to feel pressured in school or upset because he or she is left out of the neighborhood group of children. The child rubs his or her skin, a nervous, comforting mannerism, and the rubbing or scratching leads to irritation of lesions. Then the lesions itch, and the child scratches vigorously because of discomfort. The more the child scratches, the worse the lesions become; the more lesions there are, the more the child scratches, and so on.

Therapeutic Management

Atopic dermatitis is a difficult disease for older children. Because they can see that the scratching leads to depigmentation or lichenification, they know they should stop scratching to keep the disorder under control. The itching is so intense, however, that they wake at night scratching and cannot stop. Adolescents are acutely aware of their appearance, so this is an especially difficult illness for them. Suggest they not use soap or use only a prescription soap to prevent skin drying. They should avoid swimming in chlorinated pools. Encourage other summer sports if possible. If children are required to swim in school, encourage them to shower well afterward to remove chlorine from the skin and apply a skin emollient and moisturizer such as Eucerin after swimming. After a period of activity in which sweating occurs, suggest that the child take a shower to remove perspiration, which is irritating to skin. Avoiding tight clothing at the flexor portions of the extremities may also help. Caution children not to use medication intended for acne cover-up on atopic dermatitis lesions because these medications are designed to dry the skin and will increase itching.

Medical treatment is basically the same as for the infant with atopic dermatitis: keeping the skin hydrated and identifying allergens and any psychological problems that are initiating an itch–scratch cycle. Application of hydrocortisone cream can make a big difference in helping lesions improve. Phototherapy with ultraviolet light may be prescribed.

Evaluation for the older child with atopic dermatitis should include evaluating how well the lesions are healing and also how well the child is adjusting to school and family. A child who enters adulthood with poor self-esteem because of a chronic allergic disorder during childhood could have difficulty achieving a high level of adult wellness.

? *What if...* Dexter's atopic dermatitis is worse every December and every June at the end of school semesters? What might you suspect as the cause of an itch–scratch cycle at this time?

DRUG AND FOOD ALLERGIES

Drug Allergies

One of the hazards of giving any medication is the risk that a child may experience a reaction to it or exhibit allergic symptoms. Because reactions to drugs differ, it is important to be familiar with the symptoms of an allergic reaction, a toxic reaction, or a known side effect to a drug.

A *toxic reaction* is one that occurs when a child has received too much of a drug. *Side effects* of drugs are those that are known to occur in addition to a therapeutic effect. When an *allergic effect* occurs, unpredictable symptoms occur. The drug itself may not be an allergen, but when the drug combines with body protein, it becomes an allergen. This is why allergic responses occur not with the initial administration of a drug but only after the protein interaction (hapten formation or sensitivity) has occurred. When drugs are applied to skin or mucous membrane, the chance of a drug allergy is highest. With the exception of acetylsalicylic acid (aspirin), allergy occurs rarely to orally administered drugs. Children with atopic diseases appear to be most prone to allergic drug reactions, although anyone can have such a reaction (Smith, 2003).

Reactions to drugs differ, but skin manifestations seen frequently include urticaria, angioedema, allergic contact dermatitis, pruritus, and purpura. Respiratory symptoms include wheezing or rhinitis. There may be thrombocytopenia and hemolytic anemia. Anaphylactic shock and serum sickness may occur. Children with a known drug allergy should wear a medical identification bracelet stating the drug to which they are sensitive.

Drugs that are frequently involved in allergic reactions are parenteral penicillin and vaccines. In most instances, discontinuing the drug or never again administering the vaccine is the only therapy needed. If urticaria or serum sickness occurs, an antihistamine (such as diphenhydramine hydrochloride [Benadryl]) is needed to relieve the symptoms. If anaphylaxis results, the treatment would be the same as for any anaphylaxis.

Food Allergies

Food allergies manifest themselves differently from one child to another, but urticaria, angioedema, pruritus, stomach pain, colic, cramps, diarrhea, respiratory symptoms, and atopic dermatitis are common symptoms (Wasserman, 2003).

A symptom such as urticaria begins to manifest itself only minutes after an offending food is eaten. Other symptoms may be delayed, making the offending food difficult to recognize. Whole protein is probably the cause of immediate reactions, whereas delayed reactions are the result of sensitivity to some protein breakdown product.

Skin testing is unreliable with food allergies because it is done with whole protein extracts. Delayed reactions, therefore, will not be detected this way. The most common foods that cause immediate allergy symptoms include egg white, fish and other seafood, berries, and nuts. Delayed food reactions are commonly caused by cereals (wheat and corn), milk, chocolate, pork, legumes, white potatoes, beef, food additives and colorings, and oranges. If children are allergic to milk, they are probably allergic to milk products as well. Children who are allergic to eggs often cannot eat any foods that contain egg, such as pudding or baked goods (Wasserman, 2003).

Assessment

Young children cannot describe why they do not enjoy eating because they do not know the word for "headache," "stomachache," or "itchiness," but they tend to avoid foods that affect them. This gives them a reputation of being "fussy eaters." This is not diagnostic of food allergies, however, because children may refuse to eat foods as a form of toddler rebellion or may be reported as fussy eaters because parents are expecting them to eat more than their small size requires.

Encouraging a child or parents to keep a food diary or a record of everything the child eats each day often is the best way to spot offending foods. They should note the presence of symptoms, if any. A food that is found on lists when symptoms were few, but not on days when the child is in distress, is not an offending food. A food that appears only on "bad days," however, can be strongly suspected as an allergen.

An elimination diet is another method that can be used to detect food allergens. For this, parents feed the child only foods that rarely cause allergy, such as rice, lamb, carrots, peas, and sweet potatoes, for about 7 days. Then they add, one by one, at 2- to 3-day intervals, foods that are suspected of causing allergy. When a food is introduced this way, the child must be encouraged to eat a lot of it that day. If symptoms occur, the food is then eliminated from the child's meals on a permanent basis. If no symptoms occur, the child can continue to eat the food.

Therapeutic Management

The treatment of food allergy is to permanently eliminate offending foods from the child's diet. This is relatively easy to do if there are only a few offending foods, but it becomes difficult when the foods are great in number or, like milk, wheat, or eggs, are found in many products. Parents must become careful shoppers, reading labels carefully to be certain the foods they are buying do not contain products to which their child is sensitive. Help school-age children learn to choose foods they can safely eat at the school cafeteria or at summer camp.

Milk Hypersensitivity

The true incidence of milk hypersensitivity is probably not as high as the number of diagnoses made. Allergy to milk is typified by failure to gain weight, diarrhea, perhaps vomiting, and abdominal pain. Because these symptoms may also occur in a gastroenteritis infection, the child may be misdiagnosed with an infection. Some infants with colic (characterized by abdominal pain, no change in stools, and no failure to gain weight) or those with lactase deficiency (they cannot ingest the lactose in milk) may also be incorrectly diagnosed as having a milk allergy. If milk allergy is suspected, children are given a casein hydrolysate formula (Ram, Ducharme, & Scarlett, 2005). When this is done, symptoms are dramatically relieved.

To establish whether the problem is truly a milk allergy, milk should be reintroduced at a later date. If the problem is a true milk allergy, signs will recur.

Peanut Hypersensitivity

A growing number of children are identified yearly as being so allergic to peanuts that even smelling peanut butter in a cafeteria or another child's lunch can provoke acute wheezing or anaphylaxis (Lack et al., 2003). School nurses need to be very aware of this danger and may need to advocate for "peanut-free" lunch rooms. Desensitization to peanuts can minimize children's response.

STINGING INSECT HYPERSENSITIVITY

Children may have severe hypersensitivity reactions to stings from bees, wasps, hornets, or yellow jackets. Although a serum sickness reaction may occur, the usual reaction to these stings is an immediate type I hypersensitivity reaction (anaphylaxis). The peak season for insect stings is summer, and more boys than girls have allergic reactions to insect stings (Posner, 2003).

Assessment

The first time a child is stung, the total reaction is probably only local edema at the site. The second time, generalized urticaria, pruritus, and edema may develop. The third time, symptoms may progress to wheezing and dyspnea. The next time, the reaction could be so severe that shock and death result. The progression of symptoms may be slower than this (involving 10 to 12 stings) if the stings occur far apart; if the stings are received close together (1 or 2 days apart, or even 3 weeks apart), the progression to fatal symptoms may occur as early as the second or third exposure.

The time interval between the fatal sting and death is extremely short, approximately 10 minutes. For this reason, these children must be identified and given medication to combat shock immediately (there is no time to transport them for emergency care).

Therapeutic Management

The best way to protect children with allergies to stinging insects is to begin hyposensitization against insect stings after the first reaction. An extract of wasp, yellow jacket, hornet, and honeybee venom accomplishes this.

The child who has not been hyposensitized must be treated immediately after the sting. This can be done by subcutaneous injection of epinephrine, which will give rapid relief (EpiPens are available for self-injection; see Box 42.11). If the child is going on a hiking or camping expedition away from parents, caution parents that the child will need to learn to administer this to himself or herself, or be certain that a responsible adult accompanying the child will be able to do it. Someone at school should be given the responsibility of administering this if a child is stung during recess or an outside gym period. If a school nurse is in attendance, this certainly is his or her job. In schools where there is no full-time nurse, another person must be designated and taught how to give the injection. If the child has antihistamine medication in addition to epinephrine, this should be given also. Ice applied to the site minimizes the amount of venom absorbed. The child should then be transported to the nearest hospital in case additional epinephrine is needed (the initial injection will be effective for only approximately 20 minutes).

Teach children who are allergic to stinging insects not to use scented preparations such as hair spray, deodorants, lotions, or perfume because these attract bees and wasps. They should not go outside barefoot because bees are often found in ground cover. They should not be assigned household chores such as mowing the lawn or weeding the garden, actions that might stir up bees. Because insects tend to cluster around garbage containers, taking out the trash is also an inappropriate chore for these children. Encourage the child to refrain from drinking from open soda cans at picnics and outside activities; bees and wasps are drawn to the sugar in the soda, and the child may be unaware that an insect has entered the open can. Caution the child to have a fast-acting insecticide handy when out of doors to use on flying insects.

 Checkpoint Question 3

Dexter is atopic or prone to allergies. In the hospital he has no toys. What would be a poor choice of a toy to make for him?

a. A paper deck of cards
b. A cloth beanbag
c. A latex glove balloon
d. A tongue-blade puppet

CONTACT DERMATITIS

Contact dermatitis is an example of a delayed or type IV hypersensitivity response; it is a reaction to skin contact with an allergen (a substance irritating to the child only with prior sensitization). The first reaction is generally erythema, followed by intensely pruritic papules and then vesicles. The allergen causing the irritation is often suggested by the part of the child's body that is affected (Kamei, 2003). For example, dermatitis from a diaper-washing compound appears in the diaper area. Allergy to cosmetics appears on the face. Oozing at the site of pierced ears suggests an allergy to the nickel used in earring posts. Poison ivy appears on the hands and arms where the child brushed against the plant (Fig. 42.7). Many children as

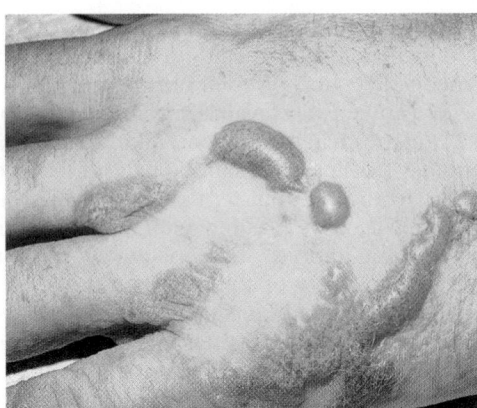

FIGURE 42.7 Poison ivy on a child's hand. (© Beckman/Custom Medical Stock Photo.)

well as health care providers are developing reactions to latex gloves (Willis-Karp & Khurana Hershey, 2003). Footwear, because of the chemicals used to tan leather, is also a frequent offender.

Assessment

Patch testing may be used to identify contact dermatitis allergens. A child should not be taking a corticosteroid at the time of patch testing because these drugs reduce delayed hypersensitivity reactions. However, the child may continue to take antihistamines or sympathomimetic drugs because these do not interfere with delayed reactions. After 48 hours, the patches used for testing are removed and the reactions are graded 1+ to 4+, the same as in regular skin testing.

Therapeutic Management

Treatment for contact dermatitis consists of removing the identified allergen from the child's environment. In children, this is generally not difficult to do. In adults, because allergens may be job-related, this is much more difficult.

Dressings moistened with water, saline, or Burow's solution relieve itching. Calamine or Caladryl lotion is also generally effective. Hydrocortisone lotions or creams reduce itching and also promote healing. Baths with baking soda or oatmeal in the water may be helpful if a large area of the body is involved. Some children need a sedative to relieve their discomfort during the period of intense pruritus.

What if... Dexter, who is allergic to leather, develops an erythematous, pruritic area on his right buttock? What would be a likely object causing the irritation?

Key Points

An antigen is a foreign substance capable of stimulating an immune response. The immune system protects the body from invasion by foreign substances.

Humoral immunity refers to immunity created by antibody production. B lymphocytes are involved in this type of reaction. Cell-mediated immunity refers to T-lymphocyte involvement.

Autoimmunity results from an inability to distinguish self from nonself, causing the immune system to carry out immune responses against normal cells.

Immunodeficiency disorders can be primary, such as B-lymphocyte and T-lymphocyte deficiencies, or secondary, such as acquired immunodeficiency syndrome (AIDS). HIV/AIDS is spread by the retrovirus HIV through blood and body secretions. Conscientious use of standard precautions is essential to prevent transmission.

Allergic disorders occur as a result of an abnormal antigen–antibody response. As many as 15% to 30% of children have some form of allergy.

Immune disorders, as a category, are long-term disorders, and children must participate in their own care to remain well (e.g., avoiding allergens, conscientiously taking an antihistamine). Involving children from the start helps them play an active role in their own care.

Anaphylactic shock is an acute type I hypersensitivity reaction characterized by extreme vasodilation and bronchoconstriction. If action is not taken immediately, the reaction can be fatal. Subcutaneous epinephrine is the drug of choice to reduce symptoms.

Environmental control refers to ways to reduce the number of allergens to which children are exposed. Hyposensitization is a method to increase the plasma concentration of IgG antibodies to prevent or block IgE antibody formation and allergic symptoms.

Atopic disorders include allergic rhinitis (hay fever), atopic dermatitis, and asthma.

Promoting breast-feeding is a prime intervention to help prevent food allergies in allergy-prone families.

Critical Thinking Exercises

1. Dexter, the 6-year-old boy you met at the beginning of the chapter, was diagnosed as having allergic rhinitis. His symptoms start when he arrives at school. Knowing this problem is worse at school, what environmental control measures would you suggest for Dexter?
2. When Dexter had atopic dermatitis (infantile eczema) as an infant, almost his entire face was covered with weeping, crusting lesions. His forehead was lined with scratch marks. His mother was exhausted because Dexter never slept due to the constant itching. What suggestions could you have made to his mother to make him more comfortable? What would you have suggested she do for herself?
3. Dexter's mother was concerned he might have AIDS. What would you want to explain to Dexter's mother about how the HIV virus is spread?

chain of infection. Nurses are instrumental in teaching parents how to prevent the spread of infection in homes and how to carry out safe practices so infection does not spread in health care facilities.

Reservoir

The **reservoir** is the container or place in which organisms grow and reproduce. The source of a human pathogen could be another human with the disease, a human carrying the disease, soil, or an animal or insect. Immunizations are helpful in limiting organisms' use of children as reservoirs for growth.

Portal of Exit

The **portal of exit** is the method by which organisms leave an infected child's body to be spread to others. This could be by upper respiratory excretions, feces, vomitus, saliva, urine, vaginal secretions, blood, or lesion secretions (Table 43.1). To break a chain of infection at this point, follow good aseptic technique and prescribed transmission-based precautions such as wearing a gown, gloves, or mask as appropriate. Teach parents good handwashing technique after the use of a bathroom or after handling diapers. Supply an adequate number of disposable tissues so droplet or airborne spread from coughing or sneezing can be limited.

Means of Transmission

The **means of transmission** of pathogens can be by direct or indirect contact, by **fomites** (i.e., inanimate objects such as soil, food, water, bedding, towels, combs, or drinking glasses) or by insects, rats, or other vermin (vectors). Direct contact implies body-to-body touching. Sexually transmitted infections (STIs) and skin disorders are spread this way. The most common means of indirect contact is the spread of mouth and nose secretions (droplet infection) through talking, sneezing, coughing, breathing, and kissing. Some droplets containing pathogenic organisms are spread immediately to another individual in this way. Some droplets fall to the ground, where the organisms dry and then are spread by dust. If small, the organisms become suspended in the air (airborne transmission) and can move with the wind to infect people at a distance. Common respiratory tract infections, for example, are spread by indirect contact.

Head lice (tinea capitis) can be spread by a fomite such as a comb if it is passed from one child to another. Insects carry and spread rickettsial diseases. Soil always contains some anaerobic organisms (those that grow without oxygen), such as tetanus bacilli. When a child receives a puncture wound, such as from stepping on a rusty nail, some dirt may be left in the closed wound, and tetanus bacilli contained in the soil can begin to multiply in the closed area. Staphylococcal gastrointestinal disorders can be spread by improperly refrigerated food.

To break a chain of infection at this point, use transmission-based precautions as appropriate and wash hands before, between, and after client care. Teach parents and children good handwashing technique and other measures as necessary.

Portal of Entry

The **portal of entry** or the opening through which a pathogen can enter a child's body can be by inhalation, ingestion,

TABLE 43.1

Methods by Which Infections Spread

Portal of Exit	Means of Transmission	Portal of Entry	Prevention Measures
Blood	Arthropod vectors	Injection into the bloodstream	Decreasing vector incidence
	Blood sampling		Careful handling of blood sampling equipment
	Transfusion		Screening of transfused blood for organisms such as human immunodeficiency virus (HIV) or hepatitis B
Respiratory secretions	Airborne droplets	Respiratory tract	Wearing mask
	Fomites		Droplet precautions
			Airborne precautions
			Handwashing
Feces	Water, food	Gastrointestinal tract	Handwashing before eating, after using bathroom or handling diapers
	Fomites		
	Vectors such as flies		
Exudate from lesions	Direct contact	Skin, mucous membranes	Contact precautions
	Contact with soiled dressings		Self-screening for sexual contacts
			Gloves

BOX 43.3 FOCUS ON . . .

EVIDENCE-BASED PRACTICE

Can the Incidence of Communicable Diseases be Reduced in School-Age Children if They Use an Alcohol Gel for Handwashing?

For this study, 253 elementary school children were given a class on how germs are spread, then randomized by classroom into an experimental group who washed their hands with an alcohol gel and a control group who followed their usual handwashing practices. Over the next 3 weeks, 69 children in the control group but only 39 children in the experimental group were absent from school because of infectious illnesses. Absenteeism attributable to infectious illness was reduced by 43% in the experimental group.

This is an interesting study for nurses because it points out how important simple handwashing can be in preventing communicable diseases and how nurses who work in facilities (such as private homes or summer camp sites) where handwashing facilities may not be readily available could also benefit from alcohol wash products.

Source: Morton, J. L., & Schultz, A. A. (2004). Healthy hands: use of alcohol gel as an adjunct to handwashing in elementary school children. *Journal of School Nursing, 20*(3), 161–167.

or breaks in the skin such as bites, abrasions, and burns. To break a chain of infection at this point, teach children to wash their hands after sneezing or coughing and before eating and after using the bathroom (Box 43.3). Teach girls to wipe their perineum from front to back after defecating or voiding to prevent organisms from spreading from the rectum to the urethra. Teach parents to wash cuts and abrasions before bandaging them.

Susceptible Host

For infection to occur, a child must be susceptible to the infection (**susceptible host**). Certain characteristics make some individuals more prone to infection than others:

- Age—infection occurs most readily in the very young and the very old
- Gender—girls, for example, have more urinary tract infections than boys
- Virulence—some organisms are stronger than others or cause disease more readily
- Body defenses present—physical, chemical, and immune responses all protect against foreign invaders. Children with immunosuppression have a reduced immune response.

Immune Response to Organisms

When a foreign organism (antigen) is identified, it can be destroyed by the phagocytic (cell-engulfing) action of white blood cells or by activation of the body's immune system. Phagocytes are unique white blood cells that are capable of cell destruction. The cells chiefly responsible for this function are neutrophils. Monocytes serve as backup cells for phagocytosis. The action of all white blood cells is summarized in Table 43.2.

The action of phagocytes on organisms produces pus (remnants of the organisms, phagocytes, and destroyed tissue). Children and parents alike may need a review of the purpose of pus because they think its presence indicates that an infection is becoming worse. More likely, it

TABLE 43.2

Types and Functions of White Blood Cells (Leukocytes)

Type	Percentage of Total Count	Origin	Function
Granular Forms			
Neutrophils	60 at birth / 33 at 2 y / 60 thereafter	Bone marrow	Active in acute bacterial infections
Eosinophils	1–4	Bone marrow	Increased in parasitic infection
Basophils	0.0–0.5	Bone marrow	Increased with inflammation
Nongranular Forms			
Lymphocytes	30 at birth / 50 at 2 y / 30 thereafter	Bone marrow / Divides into B cells and T cells	Direct reaction with antigens (T lymphocytes—centered in thymus gland); antibody production by B lymphocytes against antigens
Monocytes	5–10	Bone marrow	Backup for neutrophils in acute infection; macrophages are mature form

indicates that phagocytosis is occurring and the infection is resolving.

If bacteria escape the action of the phagocytes, they enter the blood and lymph systems and are then transported to other body locations, activating the immune system. Pathogenic organisms in the bloodstream create **septicemia,** which is always a serious development because it means the organism is being spread systemically.

With activation of the immune system, B lymphocytes (humoral immunity) and T lymphocytes (cell-mediated immunity) are produced. B lymphocytes form antibodies specific to offending antigens that either actively destroy cells or activate **complement,** a special body protein that is capable of lysing cells (see Chapter 42).

T lymphocytes (thymus-dependent) can destroy antigens by direct contact or release of lymphokines. An example of a lymphokine is **interferon,** a substance that prevents cells from being host to more than one virus at a time. This is why it is rare to see a child with two viral diseases at the same time, although it is not impossible to see a child with both a viral and a bacterial disease (e.g., scarlet fever and a common cold) at the same time. This is also why two virus vaccines are not given to a child at the same time unless they are specially designed to be given together (such as measles, mumps, and rubella). (See Chapter 42 for a more detailed discussion of the immune response and Chapter 33 for a discussion of immunizations.)

HEALTH PROMOTION AND RISK MANAGEMENT

Prevention of infectious disease begins with being certain all children are in general good health. Adequate nutrition is important to provide protein and vitamins to supply adequate white blood cells so that both phagocytic and antibody-producing B lymphocytes are available to destroy invading organisms.

A second important step is to be certain all parents are aware of the need for their children to be immunized (Box 43.4). Nurses need to ensure that immunizations are offered to children at well-child and many illness health care visits (see Chapter 33 for a discussion of immunizations).

It is important that parents also understand that although diseases such as scarlet fever, chickenpox (varicella), and mumps (infectious parotitis) are referred to as "common" childhood illnesses, they have the potential to be serious illnesses, leading to complications such as pneumonia and encephalitis. When children develop these common communicable diseases, they need to be seen by a primary health care provider to minimize the risk for these complications.

Preventing the Spread of Infections

Nosocomial or health care-associated infections (HAI) are infections that are contracted while in a hospital or other health care setting (Pellowe, Macqueen, & Coe, 2004). They represent a major threat to hospitalized children. The overall rate of nosocomial, or hospital-acquired, infection in children ranges from 0% in low-risk settings to 23% in

BOX 43.4 FOCUS ON . . .

DIVERSITY OF CARE

The responsibility expected of parents and children to help prevent the spread of communicable diseases differs from country to country and varies among cultures. In the United States, both federal and state governments have taken an active role in preventing the spread of infectious disease by requiring children to have immunizations against the most common illnesses. Parents are expected to obtain such immunizations for children by school age. Schools and school nurses, as the school system's front-line health officers, take an active role in enforcing these regulations. Community health nurses are also instrumental in administering immunizations and counseling families on how to prevent the spread of disease in their home. Nurses can also make certain that parents are aware of the latest studies available on the safety of vaccines so they do not associate common vaccines with the development of autism, for example.

War-torn countries have a great deal of difficulty maintaining this same level of disease prevention. Remember when caring for children newly arrived from another country that the child may not have the same level of immunization as usually seen. This opens an important area of health teaching, as the parents may not be aware of the importance of immunizations, which ones are required, or what community services are available to supply them.

high-risk settings such as intensive care units. Children younger than 2 years, children with a nutritional deficit, those who are immunosuppressed, those who have indwelling vascular lines or catheters, those receiving multiple antibiotic therapy, or those who remain in the hospital for longer than 72 hours are at highest risk for contracting such an infection. Children's toys may be a prime way that infection is spread (Hanrahan & Lofgren, 2004). Nurses provide a line of defense against infection by adhering to strict aseptic techniques, such as frequent and thorough handwashing, and by following protective transmission-based precautions when indicated. Nurses and other health care providers must also take precautions to protect themselves from acquiring communicable diseases, including HIV and hepatitis, by adhering to the standard precautions recommended by the Centers for Disease Control and Prevention (CDC, 2004, 2005). Box 43.5 and Appendix I summarize standard precautions and transmission-based infection control precautions.

CARING FOR THE CHILD WITH AN INFECTIOUS DISEASE

As almost all childhood infectious diseases include a fever or rash, nursing care must address relief of these symptoms.

BOX 43.5

Standard and Transmission-Based Precautions for Infection Control

To reduce the risk of disease transmission in the health care setting:

1. Wash hands immediately with soap and water before and after examining patients and after any contact with blood, body fluids, and contaminated items—whether or not you wear gloves. Use of a plain, non-antimicrobial soap is recommended.
2. Wear clean, nonsterile gloves anytime contact with blood, body fluids, mucous membrane, or broken skin is likely. Change gloves between tasks or procedures on the same patient. Before going to another patient, remove gloves promptly and wash hands immediately and then put on new gloves.
3. Wear a mask, protective eyewear, and gown during any patient care activity when splashes or sprays of body fluids are likely. Remove the soiled gown as soon as possible and wash hands.
4. Handle needles and other sharp instruments safely. Do not recap needles. Make sure contaminated nondisposable equipment is not reused with another patient until it has been cleaned, disinfected, and sterilized properly. Dispose of nonreusable needles, syringes, and other sharp patient care instruments in puncture-resistant containers.
5. Routinely clean and disinfect frequently touched surfaces including beds, bedrails, examination tables, and bedside tables.
6. Do not touch linens soiled with blood or body fluids with bare hands. Use plastic bags to transport soiled linen.
7. Place a patient whose blood or body fluids are likely to contaminate surfaces or other patients in an isolation room or area.
8. Minimize the use of invasive procedures to avoid the potential for injury and accidental exposure. Use oral rather than injectable medications whenever possible.
9. When a specific diagnosis is made, find out how the disease is transmitted. Use precautions according to the transmission risk.

Airborne Precautions

Airborne precautions reduce the risk of small-particle organisms being transmitted through the air. Micro-organisms carried by this route can be carried widely. If airborne transmission is possible:

1. Place the patient in an isolation room that is not air-conditioned or where air is not circulated to the rest of the health care facility. Make sure the room has a door that can be closed.
2. Wear a HEPA or other biosafety mask when working with the patient and in the patient's room.
3. Limit movement of the patient from the room to other areas. Place a surgical mask on the patient who must be moved.

Droplet Precautions

Droplet precautions reduce the risk of pathogens being spread through large-particle droplet contact by acts such as coughing, sneezing, and talking or through procedures such as suctioning or bronchoscopy. Large droplets do not remain suspended in the air for long periods and generally travel only short distances, so close proximity is required for spread of disease. If droplet transmission is possible:

1. Place the patient in an isolation room.
2. Wear a HEPA or other biosafety mask when working with the patient.
3. Limit movement of the patient from the room to other areas. If the patient must be moved, place a surgical mask on the patient.

Contact Precautions

Contact precautions reduce the risk of transmission of pathogens by direct contact such as skin-to-skin contact (shaking hands) or indirect contact through an intermediate object such as a comb or soiled dressing. If contact transmission is possible:

1. Place the patient in an isolation room and limit access.
2. Wear gloves during contact with patient and with infectious body fluids or contaminated items. Reinforce handwashing throughout the health facility.
3. Wear two layers of protective clothing.
4. Limit movement of the patient from the isolation room to other areas.
5. Avoid sharing equipment between patients. Designate equipment for each patient, if supplies allow. If sharing equipment is unavoidable, clean and disinfect it before use with the next patient.

Centers for Disease Control. (2004). *Recommendations for isolation precautions in hospitals.* Washington, DC: CDC.

NURSING DIAGNOSES AND RELATED INTERVENTIONS

Nursing Diagnosis: Pain related to pruritus from skin lesions

Outcome Evaluation: Child states he is more comfortable; reports less itching; is not seen scratching rash; no signs of excessive scratching or bleeding are present.

Providing comfort for the pruritus of skin lesions is important for many childhood infections. No matter what agent is causing the disease, a rash tends to be extremely itchy and uncomfortable. Fortunately, a number of simple remedies are available for reducing the discomfort. Because pruritus is a minimal form of pain, an analgesic, such as acetaminophen (Tylenol), may be helpful to reduce discomfort. An antihistamine, such as diphenhydramine hydrochloride (Benadryl), is extremely helpful. Calamine lotion is a nonprescription lotion that is cooling and soothing and often helps to relieve itching. Colloidal baths, such as baking soda or oatmeal (approximately 1 cup to 3 inches of bath water), are soothing for some children. Warn parents to take precautions to prevent clogging the drain if oatmeal is used. Caution parents to use only lukewarm water, not hot, because heat usually increases the sensation of itching. Bathing serves two purposes: it can be not only soothing but also distracting. A child, especially a preschooler, may splash for 15 to 20 minutes in a bathtub without noticing the discomfort of a rash.

Some parents bundle up children with rashes, believing that the extra clothing brings out the rash, and that if a rash does not come out, it will go in and affect a child's heart or brain. In reality, bundling up only serves to make a rash more uncomfortable and probably increases any accompanying fever. Instead, dress a child in light cotton clothing. Remove wool blankets from the bed. Cut the child's fingernails short so scratching will not open up lesions, causing secondary infection. Placing cotton gloves on the child, especially at night, may help. Comfort measures for relieving the discomfort of rashes are summarized in Box 43.6.

None of these measures is foolproof. Some may provide great relief to some children and little or none to others. Regardless of whether they offer direct relief, they do give a parent a constructive and comforting activity to carry out, providing parents with an opportunity to soothe their children and themselves.

Most infectious diseases also involve fever. Measures to combat fever in children are discussed in Chapter 36.

BOX 43.6 FOCUS ON . . .

FAMILY TEACHING

Relieving the Itchiness of a Rash

Q. Marty's mother says to you, "Our son is miserable because his rash is so itchy. What can we do to help him?"

A. Itching is a very uncomfortable sensation. Use the following to help relieve the itch of a rash:

- Dress your child in light cotton clothing so overheating and perspiration do not occur. Perspiration can make itching worse.
- Avoid wool clothing, because it can irritate skin and increase itching.
- Offer adequate fluid to maintain good hydration, because dry skin increases discomfort.
- Keep your child's fingernails short, to avoid injury to the skin from scratching.
- Teach your child to press on an itchy area rather than scratching to relieve discomfort; cold cloths applied to an area can also be helpful.
- Administer an analgesic, such as acetaminophen, as needed for comfort.
- Adding a few teaspoonfuls of baking soda to bath water can be soothing. Use lukewarm rather than hot water.
- Keep in mind that some children need an antihistamine such as diphenhydramine (Benadryl) to reduce itching. Ask your primary care provider about using it.

Nursing Diagnosis: Social isolation related to required activity restriction associated with precautions to prevent disease transmission

Outcome Evaluation: Child states reasons for restrictions; expresses interest in activities proposed by nurses or parents.

A child who is restricted from others because of infection control precautions can begin to feel lonely and depressed unless stimulation and social needs are met.

Children easily associate isolation and restriction with being punished. In a hospital setting, make as few trips as possible in and out of the room to limit the possibility of pathogen spread; on the other hand, do not make care visits seem hurried. If there is a procedure scheduled at 9:00 AM and another at 9:30 AM, stay in the room rather than leave to return again, if possible. Use the time to read a story to the child, play a card game, or talk about how strange and lonely it feels to be separated from other people.

When the child is hospitalized and requires transmission-based infection control precautions, parents must follow these precautions just as all hospital personnel do when they visit. Some parents feel so self-conscious about having to gown and wash they may stay away rather than visit. Making them feel comfortable with these procedures is a nursing responsibility. Remember that when children are admitted to a hospital, parents may not hear everything that is said to them during admission because of their anxiety. If the gowning technique was explained on admission, therefore, do not expect parents to remember the next day what was said. Explain the technique as many times as necessary.

Parents may be reluctant to give children who require transmission-based precautions their favorite toy, thinking that the hospital will insist on destroying it after the precautions are discontinued. Few pathogens exist that are not destroyed by exposure to sunlight, however, and few articles are available that cannot be further gas-sterilized to ensure that pathogens have been removed, so there is no reason to restrict toys. Check the rooms of children requiring transmission-based precautions for favorite toys, therefore, the same as in all rooms. Never leave children in a room before checking that they have a toy to play with or an activity that will keep them busy for the length of time they will be alone. See Chapter 35 for a discussion of interventions that can be used to promote adequate stimulation for a child requiring transmission-based precautions.

VIRAL INFECTIONS

Viruses are the smallest infectious agents known, so small they cannot be seen through an ordinary microscope. They are actually not true cells because they contain either ribonucleic acid (RNA) or deoxyribonucleic acid (DNA), but not both. Because they are incomplete, viruses increase in number by replication inside bacteria, plant, animal, or human cells using the biochemical products of living cells to function. Although a body cell may not be outwardly altered by a virus invasion, it could fail to function or die because of lysis of internal components or rupture. Symptoms usually do not become apparent until many cells have been interrupted in this way, so the incubation period of viral infections can be long. Some viruses are capable of invading only specific cells. The Epstein-Barr virus, for example, invades only B lymphocytes, HIV viruses invade CD4 T lymphocytes, and influenza viruses affect specific receptor sites in tracheal cells.

Viral Exanthems

The majority of childhood exanthems (rashes) are caused by viruses, and each of these diseases has specific symptoms, characteristic lesions, and a specific distribution or pattern to the rash that allows it to be identified (Figs. 43.2 and 43.3).

Exanthem Subitum (Roseola Infantum)

- Causative agent: Human herpesvirus 6 (HHV-6)
- Incubation period: Approximately 10 days
- Period of communicability: During febrile period
- Mode of transmission: Unknown
- Immunity: Contracting the disease offers lasting natural immunity; no artificial immunity is available.

Assessment. Roseola is a disease whose symptoms appear more severe than the disease actually is. It generally occurs in children between 6 months to 3 years, mainly in the spring and fall, although it can occur any time of

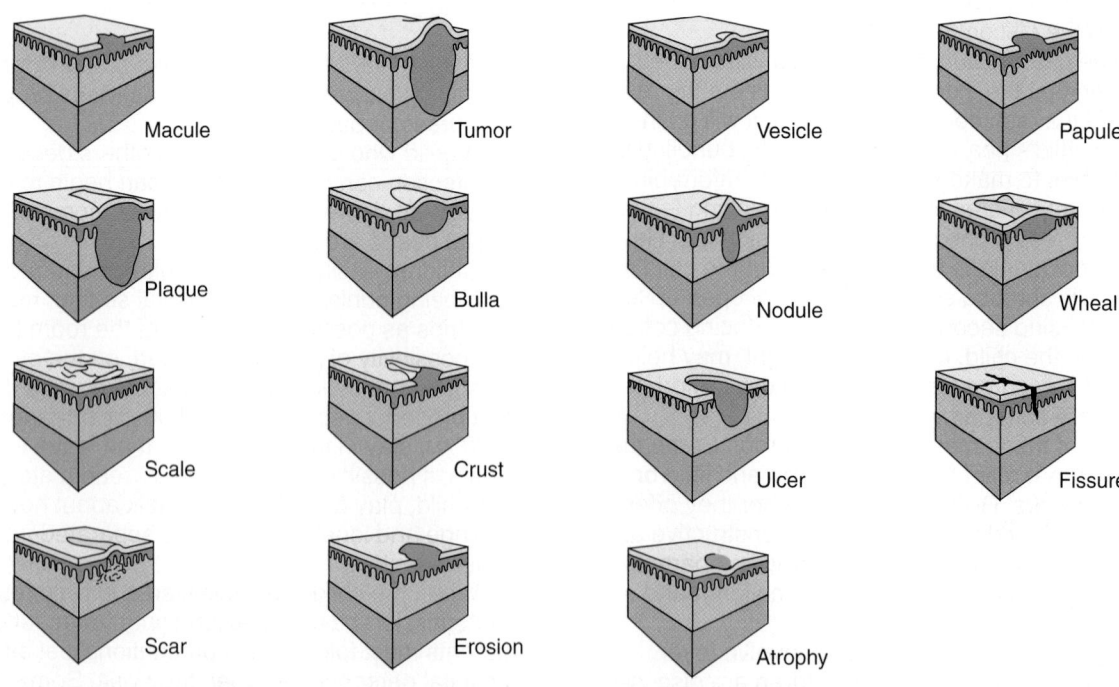

FIGURE 43.2 Primary and secondary skin lesions and their characteristics.

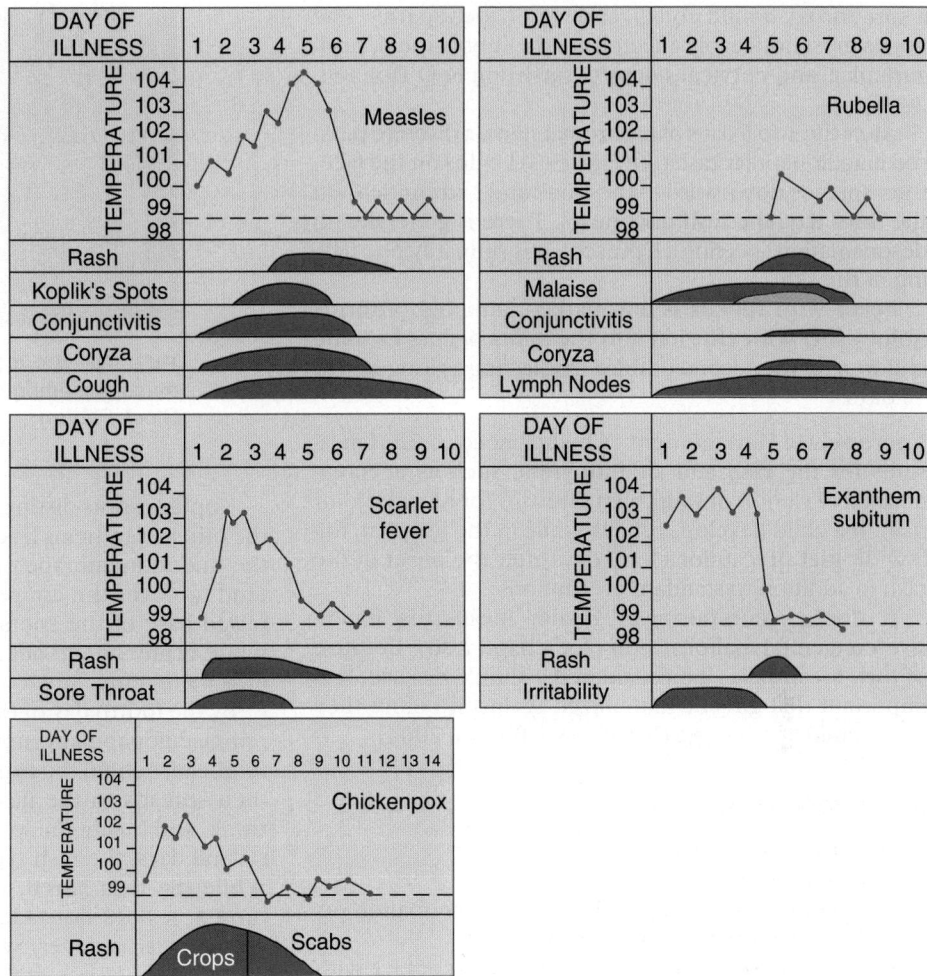

FIGURE 43.3 Differences between five acute exanthems characterized by rash.

the year. The first symptom is a high fever (104° to 105°F [40.0° to 40.6°C]). Infants may be irritable and anorexic but rarely appear as ill as this high fever suggests. They usually remain playful and alert. The pharynx may be slightly inflamed. The occipital, cervical, and postauricular lymph nodes may be enlarged. The white blood count is usually decreased, with the proportion of lymphocytes increased (Bell, 2003).

After 3 or 4 days, the fever falls abruptly and a distinctive rash appears (see Fig. 43.3). The lesions are discrete, rose-pink macules approximately 2 to 3 mm in size. They fade on pressure and occur most prominently on the trunk. The rash resembles that of rubella or measles, but it is darker, and children have no accompanying coryza (cold symptoms), conjunctivitis, or cough. Because it occurs mainly on the child's trunk, parents may report it as a heat rash. The rash lasts 1 to 2 days. The diagnosis of roseola is based on the physical signs and symptoms. The hallmark of roseola is the appearance of a rash immediately after the sharp decline in fever.

Therapeutic Management. Treatment focuses on measures to reduce the discomfort of the rash and fever. The fever will respond to acetaminophen (Tylenol) or ibuprofen (Motrin), but after 4 hours it is apt to rise again to the high level. The most frequent complication of roseola is a febrile seizure with the onset of the disease because the

temperature rises so rapidly. Management of this type of seizure is discussed in Chapter 49.

There are no long-term effects of roseola. If an infant develops this exanthem in the hospital, follow standard precautions.

Rubella (German Measles)

- Causative agent: Rubella virus
- Incubation period: 14 to 21 days
- Period of communicability: 7 days before to approximately 5 days after the rash appears
- Mode of transmission: Direct and indirect contact with droplets
- Immunity: Contracting the disease offers lasting natural immunity; a high rubella titer reveals infection has occurred.
- Active artificial immunity: Attenuated live virus vaccine
- Passive artificial immunity: Immune serum globulin is considered for pregnant women.

Assessment. Rubella is a disease rarely seen today, but when it does occur, it affects older school-age and adolescent children; it occurs most commonly during the spring. The symptoms begin with a 1- to 5-day prodromal period, during which children have a low-grade fever, headache, malaise, anorexia, mild conjunctivitis, possibly a sore throat, a mild cough, and lymphadenopathy. The nodes most noticeably affected are the suboccipital, postauricular, and cervical nodes (Armstrong & O'Donnell, 2004).

After the 1 to 5 days of prodromal signs, a discrete pink-red maculopapular rash (see Fig. 43.3) begins on the face, then spreads downward to the trunk and extremities. On the third day, the rash disappears. There is generally no desquamation (peeling); if present, it is primarily fine flaking of the skin.

Fever with rubella is not marked, although arthritis (joint pain) with effusion into the joints occurs in some children on the second or third day, lasting as long as 5 to 10 days.

Therapeutic Management. Children need comfort measures for the rash and an antipyretic such as acetaminophen (Tylenol) or ibuprofen (Motrin) for fever or joint pain. If a child develops rubella while in the hospital, follow droplet precautions for 7 days after the onset of the rash in addition to standard precautions.

If rubella occurs during pregnancy, it can cause extensive congenital malformation (see Chapter 26). Because of this, it can never be considered a simple disease. It is important that girls be immunized against it before they reach child-bearing age (Banatvala & Brown, 2004).

Measles (Rubeola)

- Causative agent: Measles virus
- Incubation period: 10 to 12 days
- Period of communicability: Fifth day of incubation period through the first few days of rash
- Mode of transmission: Direct or indirect contact with droplets
- Immunity: Contracting the disease offers lasting natural immunity.
- Active artificial immunity: Attenuated live measles vaccine
- Passive artificial immunity: Immune serum globulin

Assessment. Measles is sometimes called brown or black, regular, or 7-day measles to differentiate it from rubella (German, or 3-day, measles). Like rubella, it is rarely seen today except for periodic outbreaks that occur in newly underimmunized immigrant populations or an under-immunized college-age population. The incidence of the disease is highest in the winter and spring.

The disease has a 10- to 11-day prodromal period, during which the lymphoid tissue, particularly postauricular, cervical, and occipital lymph nodes, becomes enlarged. Children develop a high fever (103° to 104°F [39.5° to 40.0°C]) and malaise. By the second day of the prodromal period, coryza (rhinitis and a sore throat), conjunctivitis with photophobia (sensitivity to light), and a cough develop. **Koplik's spots** (small, irregular, bright-red spots with a blue-white center point) appear on the buccal membrane. Unfortunately, the coryza of measles is indistinguishable from that of a common cold (nasal congestion, a mucopurulent discharge, and a deep brassy, bronchial cough) when it begins. As a result, many children with measles are diagnosed as having a simple upper respiratory infection at this point.

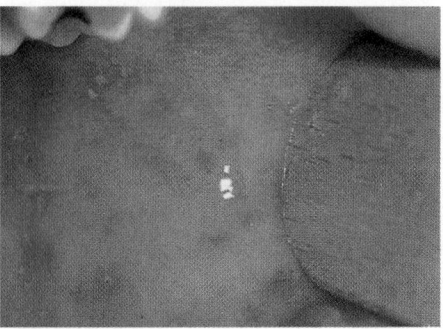

FIGURE 43.4 Koplik's spots on the oral mucous membrane. (SPL/Custom Medical Stock Photo.)

Koplik's spots distinguish the disease because none of the other exanthems has this finding. They appear first on the buccal membrane opposite the molars and then extend to cover the entire buccal surface (Fig. 43.4). The raised base of the spots may coalesce so that the blue-white centers stand out as grains of salt on the erythematous membrane.

By the fourth day of fever, the rash appears. This deep-red maculopapular eruption begins at the hairline of the forehead, behind the ears, and at the back of the neck and then spreads to the face, the neck, upper extremities, trunk, and finally the lower extremities (Fig. 43.5). After several days, the rash typically turns from red to brown. While the rash is red, it fades on pressure; when it is brown, it does not fade. This differentiates it from the rash of scarlet fever, which always fades on pressure.

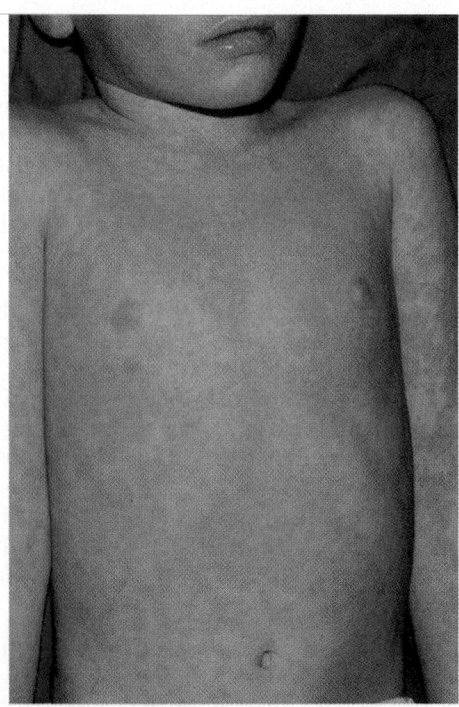

FIGURE 43.5 The typical rash of measles on a child's upper body. (© NMSB/Custom Medical Stock Photo.)

After 5 to 6 days, the rash completely fades. There is a fine desquamation after this. However, the skin of the hands and feet does not desquamate, a feature again differentiating it from scarlet fever.

Children with measles appear very ill because their cough is loud and frequent, the coryza is acute, the fever is high, and the rash is pruritic. Fortunately, on the third or fourth day of rash, when the temperature begins to fall, the other symptoms clear quickly and children feel better. Fever that lasts beyond the third or fourth day of rash or coughing that continues generally suggests that a complication of measles, such as pneumonia, has occurred.

Therapeutic Management. Children with measles need comfort measures for the rash and an antipyretic for the fever. The coryza, which does not respond to decongestants, fortunately lasts only a few days. The skin below the nose may become excoriated from the constant nasal drainage. Applying a lubricating jelly or an emollient (A and D ointment) to the area may help prevent excoriation. The child may need a cough suppressant to control the cough; otherwise, the throat can become painful from frequent irritation. Because children with measles have photophobia, it is painful for them to look at bright lights, so it may be painful for them to watch television. They are often more comfortable with the shades or curtains drawn or wearing dark glasses, so these measures should be instituted. Children need to be seen by a health care provider because the complications of measles include otitis media (middle ear infection), pneumonia, airway obstruction, and acute encephalitis (Duke & Mgone, 2003). If the child is hospitalized, follow airborne precautions for the duration of the illness in addition to standard precautions.

Chickenpox (Varicella)

- Causative agent: Varicella-zoster virus
- Incubation period: 10 to 21 days
- Period of communicability: 1 day before the rash to 5 to 6 days after its appearance, when all the vesicles have crusted
- Mode of transmission: Highly contagious; spread by direct or indirect contact of saliva or vesicles
- Immunity: Contracting the disease offers lasting natural immunity to chickenpox; because the same virus causes herpes zoster, it may be reactivated at a later time as herpes zoster.
- Active artificial immunity: Attenuated live virus vaccine
- Passive artificial immunity: There is little passive placental immunity to chickenpox. Children who are immunosuppressed, such as those with leukemia or HIV/AIDS, or those who are being treated with corticosteroids are given varicella-zoster immune globulin (VZIG). This may prevent or modify chickenpox if given within 72 hours of exposure.

Assessment. Chickenpox is another common childhood infection that is decreasing in incidence because of required immunization. The people most prone to it are those who have not been immunized, such as older children and college students. The disease is marked by a low-grade fever, malaise, and, in 24 hours, the appearance of a rash (see Fig. 43.3). The lesion begins as a macula, then

progresses rapidly within 6 to 8 hours to a papule, then a vesicle that first becomes umbilicated and then forms a crust. Each lesion is approximately 2 to 3 mm in diameter and is surrounded by an erythematous area. When the first crop of lesions appears, the child's temperature may rise markedly to 104° or 105°F (40.0° or 40.6°C).

Most of the chickenpox lesions are found on the trunk, although the face, scalp, palate, and neck also may be involved. They appear in approximately three separate series or crops, with each new lesion moving through progressive stages (Fig. 43.6). At one time, all four stages of lesions (macule, papule, vesicle, and crust) are present.

Therapeutic Management. If the scab from crusting is allowed to fall off naturally and lesions do not become secondarily infected, no scarring results. Scabs removed prematurely may leave a white, round, slightly indented scar at the site. It is important that children not scratch and remove scabs, but because the rash of chickenpox is extremely pruritic, preventing scratching becomes a difficult problem for parents. A prescribed antihistamine usually helps to reduce the itchiness to a bearable level, and an antipyretic will counteract the high fever. Acyclovir may be prescribed to reduce the number of lesions and shorten the course of the illness (Klassen et al., 2005). The development of Reye's syndrome has been associated with aspirin use during varicella and influenza virus illness (see Chapter 49), so caution parents when treating all childhood exanthems to avoid aspirin and to use acetaminophen or ibuprofen to control fever instead.

If the child is hospitalized, follow airborne and contact precautions until all lesions are crusted, in addition to standard precautions. Children may return to school as soon

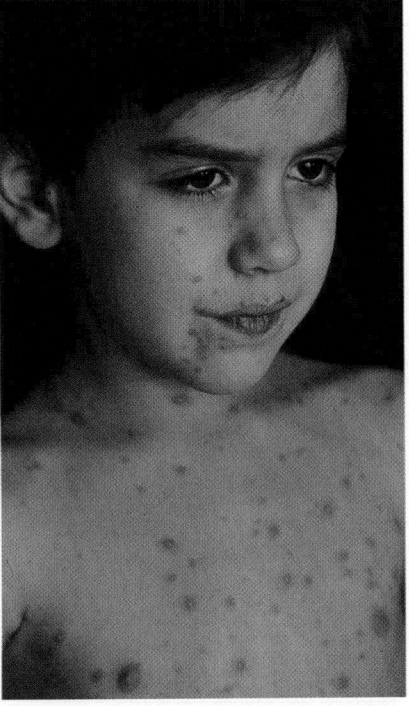

FIGURE 43.6 An older school-age boy with varicella. (© Martin/Custom Medical Stock Photo.)

as all the lesions are crusted (the crusts are not infectious). Complications include secondary infections of the lesions, pneumonia, and encephalitis.

Herpes Zoster

Herpes zoster is caused by the varicella-zoster virus, the same virus as chickenpox (Watson, 2003). Apparently, the first time children are invaded by the virus, they have symptoms of chickenpox. Thereafter, herpes zoster symptoms may appear due to reactivation of a latent virus or possibly due to a second or third exposure. Herpes zoster tends to occur in older children or young adults, although it can occur at any age.

The first manifestations are pruritus and cutaneous vesicular lesions on erythematous bases that follow the distributions of the lumbar and thoracic nerves (usually on the trunk, face, or upper back) and cause deep nagging pain (Fig. 43.7).

Treatment for herpes zoster includes measures to reduce pruritus and analgesia for pain. Acyclovir, which inhibits viral DNA synthesis, may be effective in limiting the disease. VZIG may minimize symptoms.

Smallpox (Variola)

- Causative agent: Smallpox virus
- Incubation period: 7 to 17 days
- Period of communicability: From onset of rash until all crusts have been shed
- Mode of transmission: Direct or indirect contact
- Immunity: Lasting natural immunity after contracting the disease
- Active artificial immunity: No longer recommended

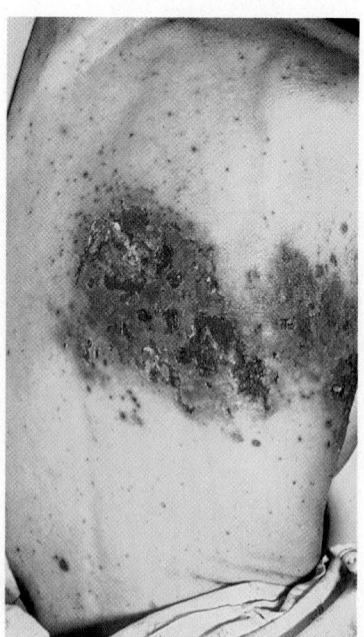

FIGURE 43.7 Herpes zoster on a child's back. (© Dr. P. Marazzi/ SPL/Science Source/Photo Researchers.)

- Passive artificial immunity: Vaccinia immune globulin (VIG)

Smallpox is a disease that has been extinct in the world since 1995. However, health care providers need to be able to recognize symptoms of it because viruses, colonies of which are stored in various laboratories throughout the world, could be used as an agent of biologic terrorism (Martin & Didion, 2003).

The disease has a 3- to 4-day prodromal period of chills, fever, headache, and vomiting. The child looks extremely ill and exhausted. On day 3 or 4, a rash and high fever appear. The lesions, most prominent on the distal extremities and face, begin as macules, then progress to papules, vesicles, and pustules, eventually crusting over a 10- to 14-day period.

Although the lesions of smallpox resemble those of chickenpox, they can be differentiated by the appearance of the pustular stage (not seen with chickenpox) and the fact that they arise as one crop of lesions and all progress at the same rate (chickenpox occurs in stages). The crusts of chickenpox are not contagious, but the crusts of smallpox are (Watson, 2003).

Smallpox is a serious illness: its mortality rate is as high as 50% and it can be spread readily from an infected person to another. Children are treated with VIG to suppress symptoms and an antibiotic to prevent secondary infection of lesions. They may need oxygen or other measures to support respiratory function and measures such as a cardiac glycoside to support cardiac function.

 Checkpoint Question 1

If a smallpox epidemic should occur, it will be important to be able to distinguish chickenpox (varicella) from smallpox. What are the stages of chickenpox lesions?

a. Macular, papular, vesicular, and crusting
b. Macular, crusting, and extensive peeling
c. Papular, vesicular, and pruritic crusting
d. Maculopapular lesions with fine flaking

Erythema Infectiosum ("Fifth Disease")

- Causative agent: Parvovirus B19
- Incubation period: 6 to 14 days
- Period of communicability: Uncertain
- Mode of transmission: Droplet
- Immunity: None

Assessment. Erythema infectiosum (the fifth important childhood exanthem) occurs most often in children 2 to 12 years of age. The first phase of the infection includes fever, headache, and malaise. A week later, a rash, which erupts in three stages, appears. It is intensely red and appears first on the face. The lesions are maculopapular and coalesce on the cheeks to form a "slapped face" appearance (Fig. 43.8). The facial lesions fade in 1 to 120 days (Vafaie & Schwartz, 2004).

A day after the facial lesions appear, a rash appears on the extensor surfaces of the extremities. One day later, it invades the flexor surfaces and the trunk. These lesions

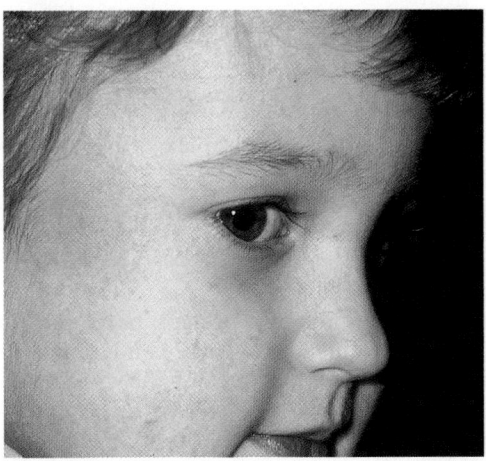

FIGURE 43.8 The rash of fifth disease.
(© Dr. P. Marazzi/SPL/Science Source/Photo
Researchers.)

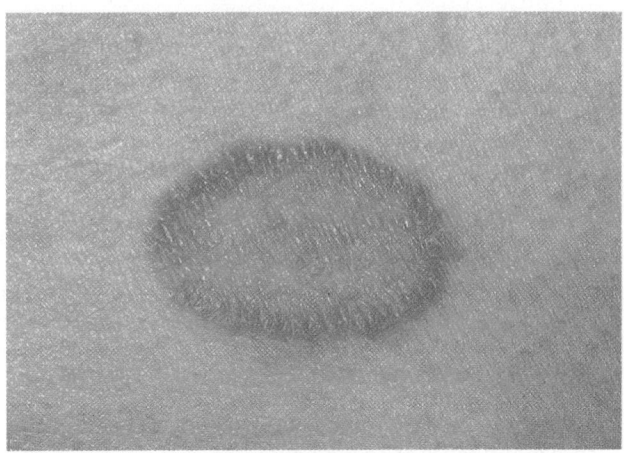

FIGURE 43.9 The "herald patch" of pityriasis rosea.
(Dr. H. C. Robinson/SPL/Science Source/Photo
Researchers.)

last for 1 week or more. When they fade, they fade from the center outward, giving the lesions a lacelike appearance. After the rash has faded, it may reappear if precipitated by skin irritation such as trauma, sunlight, hot, or cold. Some children develop a persistent arthritis.

Therapeutic Management. Treatment is typically supportive, with antipyretics and analgesics. Children also may need comfort measures for the rash (see Box 43.6). There are no known complications of fifth disease for the child; it is teratogenic for a fetus, however, so children with this disorder should avoid contact with pregnant women. Use droplet precautions in a hospital. Children can return to school as soon as the rash appears because they are no longer infectious at this point.

What if... Marty's parents tell you their doctor is ruling out fifth disease? What are the other four diseases that gave this disease its name?

Pityriasis Rosea

- Causative agent: Probably a virus
- Incubation period: Unknown
- Period of communicability: Unknown
- Mode of transmission: Unknown
- Immunity: Apparently none

Pityriasis rosea occurs in school-age and older children. Children may have a short, mild prodromal period of fever and sore throat. A herald patch, an erythematous round lesion with a scaly border, usually appearing on the trunk, is the first obvious lesion (Fig. 43.9). Approximately 1 week after the appearance of the herald patch, a generalized rash of papules, vesicles, or urticaria appears. This is generally also confined to the trunk. It follows skin lines, giving it the unique configuration of a Christmas tree (Stulberg & Wolfrey, 2004).

The rash lasts 6 to 8 weeks. It is pruritic and, because it lasts so long, is particularly worrisome to children and par-

ents. Because the lesions, particularly the herald patch, are scaly at the edges, they are often confused with tinea corporis (ringworm). Treatment is limited to oral antihistamines and other comfort measures for rash.

Pityriasis rosea appears to have no sequelae or complications; in fact, it is difficult to demonstrate in what manner it is infectious. It is a baffling rash of childhood but should be differentiated from serious (severe) exanthems.

Enteroviruses

There are three main types of enteroviruses: echoviruses (33 subdivisions), coxsackievirus A (24 subdivisions) and coxsackievirus B (6 types), and polioviruses (3 subdivisions).

Echovirus Infections

The echoviruses are responsible for a number of childhood diseases, including aseptic meningitis, diarrhea, acute respiratory illness, and maculopapular rashes. Such infections are usually benign and self-limiting. Treatment involves supportive measures. If the child is hospitalized, follow contact precautions for the duration of the illness, in addition to standard precautions.

Coxsackievirus Infections

The coxsackievirus groups are responsible, like the echovirus groups, for a variety of diseases. One of the most frequently found diseases of children caused by coxsackievirus A is herpangina. With herpangina, children have an abrupt elevation of temperature, up to 104° or 105°F (40.0° or 40.6°C) for 1 to 4 days. Anorexia, difficulty swallowing, sore throat, and vomiting may be present. Children may have headaches and abdominal pain. Small lesions, generally discrete grayish vesicles, pinpoint in size, appear on the tonsillar fauces, soft palate, and uvula (Atkinson, 2003). They may be present elsewhere in the mouth or throat as well. The lesions gradually change to shallow ulcers surrounded by a red areola.

They disappear within a few days after the temperature returns to normal. There are generally no complications.

Children need to be maintained on soft or liquid foods while their mouth and throat are sore. They may need an antipyretic for fever. If the child is hospitalized, follow contact precautions for the duration of the illness, in addition to standard precautions.

Poliovirus Infections: Poliomyelitis (Infantile Paralysis)

- Causative agent: Poliovirus
- Incubation period: 7 to 14 days
- Period of communicability: Greatest shortly before and after onset of symptoms, when virus is present in the throat and feces (1 to 6 weeks)
- Mode of transmission: Direct and indirect contact
- Immunity: Contracting the disease causes active immunity against the one strain of virus causing the illness.
- Active artificial immunity: Inactivated polio virus vaccine (IPV)
- Passive artificial immunity: None

Poliomyelitis, no longer seen in the United States, may be caused by any of the three strains of poliovirus, the rationale for immunizing children with the trivalent (three-strain) vaccine. Poliomyelitis still does occur in other parts of the world, and in war-torn or developing nations such as India and parts of Africa, the incidence is still high and rising (Alexander et al., 2004).

Assessment. The poliovirus enters the child's gastrointestinal tract, where it multiplies and produces symptoms such as fever, headache, nausea, vomiting, or abdominal pain. Moderate pain of the neck, back, and legs soon develops. The cerebrospinal fluid shows increased protein and lymphocytes.

These initial symptoms are followed by intense pain and tremors of the extremities and then paralysis, occurring either immediately or over a period of 1 to 7 days as the virus invades the central nervous system. Kernig's sign, a test for meningeal irritation, is positive. Children demonstrate a tripod sign—when sitting on the floor or on an examining table, they cannot sit without placing both the arms and hands behind them to brace themselves. Their deep tendon reflexes are hyperactive at first and then diminish as the central nervous system is fully invaded. Laryngeal paralysis makes swallowing or talking difficult, and respiratory paralysis can halt respiration.

Therapeutic Management. Treatment for poliomyelitis is bed rest with analgesia and moist hot packs to relieve pain. If the respiratory muscles are involved, long-term ventilation is necessary. Survivors tend to develop progressive muscle atrophy (postpoliomyelitis muscular atrophy syndrome) or severe arthritis in late adulthood, further reducing their ability to be self-sufficient (Nollet & de Visser, 2004).

Viral Infections of the Integumentary System

Viral infections of the skin include the herpes infections and warts (verrucae).

Herpesvirus Infections

Herpesviruses are responsible for a number of infections in children.

- Causative agent: Herpes simplex or herpes type 1 or type 2 virus
- Incubation period: 2 to 12 days
- Period of communicability: Greatest early in the course of the infection
- Mode of transmission: Direct contact
- Immunity: Immunity to a primary herpes response is gained after one incident. There is no immunity to recurrent herpes infections because the virus lies dormant in the body until it is activated by stress, sun exposure, fever, other illness, or menstruation.

When children are first invaded by a herpesvirus, they have no antibodies against the virus, so a primary form of the disease such as herpetic gingivostomatitis occurs. The virus remains latent in the neurons of local sensory ganglia, or children become permanent carriers of the herpes simplex virus (Andreae, 2004).

Acute Herpetic Gingivostomatitis. Acute herpetic gingivostomatitis is the most common form of herpes simplex invasion in children. It is an example of the primary, not the recurrent, response. It occurs in children ages 1 to 4 years. Children have a high fever (104° to 105°F [40.0° to 40.6°C]), are restless, and have anorexia and a sore mouth. Their gumline is swollen and reddened and bleeds easily. White plaques or shallow ulcers with red areolae appear on the buccal mucosa, tongue, and palate and perhaps on the tonsillar fauces. The anterior cervical lymph nodes are enlarged and tender. The disease runs its course in 5 to 7 days (Blevins, 2004).

Children need an antipyretic to reduce fever. They also need soft, acid-free foods that they can eat with minimal irritation or abrasion. Popsicles are soothing against inflamed mucous membranes. Oral acyclovir helps with healing. Use contact precautions with hospitalized children.

Children with gingivostomatitis are often very ill. The disease can become very serious, especially in infants, if their mouths become so sore that they cannot swallow readily and they become malnourished and dehydrated.

Herpes Simplex (Herpes Labialis). Herpes simplex infection, popularly known as a cold sore or fever blister, represents the recurrent form of a type 1 herpesvirus invasion that has remained dormant in the ganglia of the trigeminal or fifth cranial nerve. Herpes simplex typically appears as clusters of painful, grouped vesicles surrounded by an erythematous base on the lips or skin surrounding the mouth. After 2 or 3 days, vesicles crust, then gradually dry. Keeping lesions dry helps them to fade sooner, but keeping them lubricated with an ointment reduces pain. Topical or oral acyclovir reduces pain and increases healing. Children feel conspicuous about the appearance of herpes simplex lesions. They may need counseling to assure them that the lesions are not as obvious to others as they seem to them (Andreae, 2004).

Acute Herpetic Vulvovaginitis (Genital Herpes). Genital herpes is caused by the herpesvirus type 2, which remains dormant in the ganglia of the sacral nerves. Because this form is spread primarily by sexual contact, it is discussed in Chapter 47 with other STIs.

Eczema Herpeticum. Children with atopic dermatitis (infantile eczema) may have a generalized reaction if they contract a herpes infection (Yan, 2003). They develop a fever as high as 104° to 105°F (40.0° to 40.6°C), irritability, and crops of vesicles that erupt at the sites of eczematous skin lesions. Lesions may occur at different times during the disease course of 7 to 9 days. Generally by day 10, all lesions are crusted.

In children with severe eczema, the number of lesions that appear may be extreme. Enough body fluid can be lost through the oozing of the vesicles to cause serious fluid loss. Pain can be intense. The extent of the involvement can make children gravely ill.

Warts (Verrucae)

Warts, one of the most common dermatologic diseases in children, are caused by the papillomavirus. The virus has an incubation period of 1 to 6 months. The mode of transmission is unknown, but it is probably by direct contact (Ho, 2003).

Warts are flesh-colored, dirty-appearing papules. They generally occur on the dorsal surface of the hands, although they may occur anywhere. Plantar warts appear on the soles and are painful when children walk. They may be differentiated from calluses in that they obliterate skin lines as they grow, whereas calluses do not.

Warts on the hands or the face are generally removed if they are cosmetically unattractive to children. Plantar warts may have to be removed because of the discomfort they cause. Parents can use over-the-counter wart-removing preparations, such as Compound W, to dissolve them. Application of 40% salicylic acid may be prescribed to remove plantar warts. Carbon dioxide snow, liquid nitrogen, electrodesiccation, and curettage are also effective for removal, but these methods are painful and rarely necessary.

Children need reassurance that people do not catch warts from frogs or toads and even if left without any treatment, warts will eventually fade by themselves after about 24 months. Anogenital warts need special consideration as they can be a mark of sexual abuse (Hornor, 2004).

Viruses Causing Central Nervous System Diseases

Viruses are responsible for causing a number of central nervous system disorders such as rabies, encephalitis, and meningitis. Encephalitis and meningitis are discussed in Chapter 49.

Rabies

- Causative agent: Rabies virus
- Incubation period: 2 to 6 weeks, possibly as long as 12 months
- Period of communicability: 3 to 5 days before the onset of symptoms through the course of the disease
- Mode of transmission: The bite of rabid animals; rarely through saliva from infected animals being transferred to open lesions on a child's skin

- Immunity: Contracting the disease apparently offers active immunity, but few people have ever survived the illness to verify this.
- Active artificial immunity: Human diploid cell rabies vaccine
- Passive artificial immunity: Rabies immune globulin (RIG)

Any warm-blooded animal can contract rabies. Wild animals, such as skunks, squirrels, raccoons, and bats, constitute the most important sources of infection from rabies in the United States. However, children receive more bites and, therefore, more treatments for rabies from bites of dogs or cats. Bites of rodents are seldom found to be rabid. Bites from other children are not rabid, although therapy is required because such bites usually contain streptococci. In the animal infected with rabies, the virus can be cultured from the central nervous system, saliva, urine, lymph, and blood. When a child is bitten by an infected animal, the virus migrates from the bite area to the child's central nervous system. Cranial nerve and spinal cord nuclei become acutely damaged. Negri bodies (cytoplasmic inclusion bodies) can be isolated from nerve cells (Fishbein, 2004).

Assessment. The diagnosis of rabies is established largely from the history of an animal bite and the clinical symptoms. After the long incubation period of the virus, children begin to show prodromal signs of malaise, fever, anorexia, nausea, sore throat, drowsiness, irritability, and restlessness. They may notice numbness or hyperesthesia at the area of the bite and along the course of the involved nerves. The white blood cell count will show slight leukocytosis. The cerebrospinal fluid is usually normal, with perhaps only a slight elevation in protein and cells. As the symptoms increase, there is high fever, anxiety, and hyperexcitability. Involuntary twitching movements and generalized seizures may occur. When children try to drink, there are violent contractions of the muscles of the mouth. They may drool saliva rather than swallow it because swallowing is extremely painful. These two phenomena give the disease its popular name, hydrophobia ("water-fear").

As symptoms progress, children become comatose, with possible total body paralysis. Peripheral vascular collapse and death follow quickly in only 5 or 6 days. Postmortem examination will reveal the diagnostic Negri bodies in brain cells.

Therapeutic Management. Once the disease process begins, rabies is almost invariably fatal. The key is preventing the active process. All children who receive an animal bite should be seen by a primary care provider to evaluate the circumstances surrounding the bite and to decide whether to begin rabies prevention measures. The decision to treat must be made immediately if treatment is to be effective.

Taking a history of the incident to determine the type of animal is of primary importance. Most children are sure they know the type of animal if it was a dog; they may be unsure if it was a wild animal. Do not lead children into naming an animal just to please. If asked, "Was it a skunk? A raccoon? A squirrel?" the child may choose an animal name because he or she thinks that is the answer expected.

Instead, ask the child to describe the animal; from that description, establish the kind of animal that bit the child. It helps in rural health facilities to have a picture book of animals handy so that preschoolers in particular can identify the animal that bit them. A rabid animal usually does not act normally. It runs blindly, often staggering; it may dribble saliva rather than swallow it. It is easy to assess whether a household pet is acting this way. It is sometimes difficult to assess the actions of a wild animal because the fear it experiences at being trapped or cornered may make it run about frantically.

An unprovoked attack is highly suggestive that the animal is rabid, rather than if the bite happens during a provoked attack. Let children know that they will not be punished if they were provoking an animal so they feel free to say so. Statements such as "I was only hugging him" or "I was just feeding him" may sound innocent but may have constituted a provoked attack to the animal.

The kind of wound that a child receives also is instrumental in deciding whether to begin treatment. A bite mark is much more serious than a scratch from an animal's claws. The immunization status of the animal should be checked if available. Whether rabies exists in the community at the time of the attack will also influence the decision. An animal that has been properly immunized against rabies will rarely transmit the virus. If there have been no other reported instances in domestic animals, the chance that this dog bite is serious in terms of rabies is lower than if dogs with rabies have been reported in the area.

Inspect the wound carefully to see whether it was caused by teeth marks or scratch marks. Wash the wound well with soap and water and a suitable antiseptic. If puncture wounds are present, the wound must not be sutured and closed, because tetanus (organisms that are anaerobic and grow in deep, closed wounds, where oxygen does not reach) can develop in the wound. The animal that caused the bite should be located if possible and then confined for 5 to 10 days. If it develops any signs of rabies during this period, it will be destroyed and the brain examined for evidence of rabies. Domestic animals are not destroyed unless they show signs of rabies; if people are unaware of this, they may resist surrendering an animal for observation.

If the animal is found to be rabid, children receive both rabies vaccine and antirabies serum (RIG). This applies also if the animal escapes and its condition is unknown (it is assumed to be rabid). A portion of the RIG dose is injected into the wound site and the remainder is given intramuscularly. Antirabies vaccine is given immediately and then again on days 3, 7, 14, and 28 (Fishbein, 2004).

It may seem contradictory to give an active immunization serum (administering antigen to children) when they have received an animal bite (which administers antigen to them). This is done because the rabies virus has a long incubation period before antibody production is stimulated; administering RIG provides antibodies against the rabies virus immediately. Administering rabies vaccine allows the child to begin additional antibody formation so that by the time the rabies virus from the bite begins to have an effect (2 to 6 weeks after the bite), the child has developed sufficient antibodies to combat it and prevent the illness.

West Nile Virus Disease

Although the West Nile virus may be transmitted by contaminated blood products, it is usually spread by the bite of a mosquito after the mosquito has bitten, and acquired the infection from, a natural host such as an infected bird (Crane, 2003).

Fortunately, most children who contract the disease remain asymptomatic. A small number develop flulike symptoms such as fever, fatigue, and malaise. A few develop encephalitis, with symptoms such as mental confusion, lethargy, photophobia, headache, muscle weakness, and coma, leading to death. West Nile virus disease is diagnosed when antibodies to the virus are recovered from blood serum. There is no specific therapy for the disorder, except for supportive measures to maintain function.

Parents can help prevent the spread of West Nile disease in several important ways:

- Urge children to wear long sleeves and pants to avoid mosquito bites.
- Have children apply insect repellent with DEET if hiking near swampy areas where mosquitoes may breed.
- Urge children to avoid outside activities between dusk and dawn, when mosquitoes are most likely to bite.
- Empty potential stagnant water sources, such as bird baths, to prevent mosquitoes from breeding close to the house.

Other Viral Infections

Mumps (Epidemic Parotitis)

- Causative agent: Mumps virus
- Incubation period: 14 to 21 days
- Period of communicability: Shortly before and after onset of parotitis
- Mode of transmission: Direct or indirect contact
- Immunity: Contracting the disease gives lasting natural immunity.
- Active artificial immunity: Attenuated live mumps vaccine
- Passive artificial immunity: Mumps immune globulin

Assessment. Mumps is now a rare disease due to successful immunization programs. It is most likely to be seen in adolescents who have not been immunized. If the disease occurs, it begins with fever, headache, anorexia, and malaise. Within 24 hours, an "earache" occurs. When the child points to the site of the pain, however, he or she points not to the ear, but to the jaw line just in front of the ear lobe. Chewing movements aggravate the pain. By the next day, the parotid gland (located just in front of the ear lobe) is swollen and tender. As the parotid gland swells, it displaces the ear upward and backward. Boys also may develop testicular pain and swelling (orchitis).

It is often difficult to differentiate mumps from submaxillary adenitis (swelling of lymph nodes). The best method of differentiation is to place a hand along the child's jaw line. If the major amount of swelling is above the hand, it is probably mumps. If the largest amount of swelling is below the hand line, it is probably adenitis (Fig. 43.10).

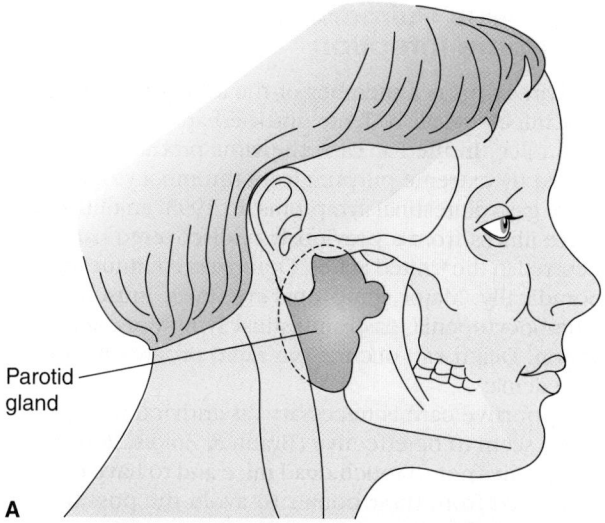

Parotid gland

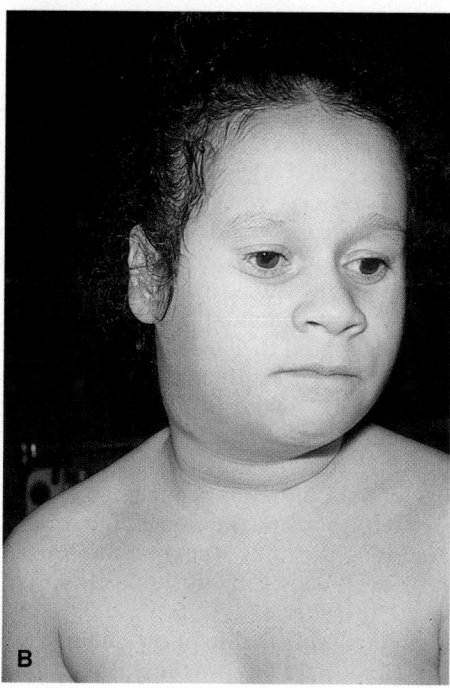

FIGURE 43.10 Infectious parotitis. (**A**) The parotid gland is located just in front of the ear. (**B**) A boy with parotitis (mumps). (© Morris Huberland/Science Source/Photo Researchers.)

Therapeutic Management. Because chewing movements are so painful, children may need soft or liquid foods until the major portion of the swelling recedes (about 6 days). It is also more difficult for them to swallow sour foods than sweet ones. They may need an analgesic for pain and an antipyretic for fever. If a child is hospitalized, follow droplet precautions in addition to standard precautions. Children should not return to school until 9 days after the onset of parotid swelling (Tsarouhas, 2003).

One attack of mumps gives lasting immunity. Some parents worry that because the child has swelling only on one side, he or she will develop mumps on the opposite side in the future. If a child does appear to have mumps

twice, the diagnosis was probably confused with cervical adenitis one of the two times.

Mumps is a potentially serious illness because a number of serious complications can arise. If mumps orchitis develops, it is generally unilateral. A single testis swells rapidly and is painful and tender. When the fever declines, testicular swelling also decreases, although the tenderness may exist for weeks. Atrophy of the testis may result. The chance that mumps orchitis will lead to complete sterility is exaggerated, however (Tsarouhas, 2003).

The complication of meningoencephalitis occurs in a few children. Severe permanent hearing impairment is a rare complication that may occur because of neuritis of the auditory nerve.

Checkpoint Question 2

Which is the best description of mumps (infectious parotitis)?

a. Cervical lymph nodes become swollen.
b. Swelling behind the child's ear occurs.
c. Swelling above the jaw line occurs.
d. The adenoid tonsils are red and swollen.

Infectious Mononucleosis

- Causative agent: Epstein-Barr virus
- Incubation period: Unknown; probably 2 to 8 weeks
- Period of communicability: Unknown; probably only during acute illness
- Mode of transmission: Direct and indirect contact
- Immunity: One episode apparently gives lasting immunity. No vaccination is available.

Infectious mononucleosis is also known as glandular fever or, because it was first discovered as a disease that is transferred readily from one person to another by kissing, the kissing disease. It occurs most commonly in adolescents and young adults, although it may occur in any age child (Osterhoudt, 2003).

Assessment. The beginning symptoms include chills, fever, headache, anorexia, and malaise. Children develop lymphadenopathy and a severe sore throat. The fever is generally high (103°F [39.5°C]) and lasts approximately 6 days.

The cervical lymph nodes, most markedly affected, are firm and tender. The tonsils feel painful and are enlarged and erythematous. A thick, white membrane may cover the tonsils (Fig. 43.11), and often petechiae appear on the palate. If the mesenteric lymph nodes enlarge, children may experience abdominal pain so sharp it simulates appendicitis. The spleen enlarges, placing the child at risk for spontaneous rupture. Hepatitis, skin manifestations (e.g., a maculopapular eruption similar to the rash of rubella), pneumonitis, and central nervous system involvement (e.g., encephalitis, meningitis, or polyneuritis) may occur.

Lymphocytosis, with lymphocytes representing more than 50% of the total white blood cell count, occurs. Of these lymphocytes, a significant number (more than 20%) are atypical; they are larger-than-normal, mature lymphocytes, and their nuclei are somewhat less dense. A serologic

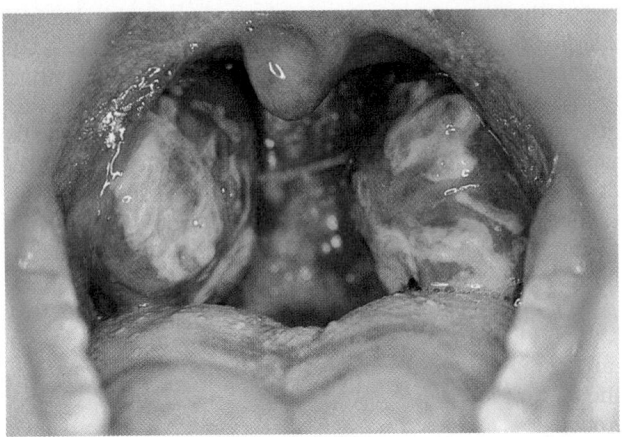

FIGURE 43.11 Appearance of the tonsils in a child with infectious mononucleosis. Note the degree of erythema, enlargement, and purulent covering. (© Dr. P. Marazzi/SPL/Science Source/Photo Researchers.)

test, known as the heterophil antibody test, is based on the fact that the antibody produced in infectious mononucleosis will agglutinate sheep red blood cells. A technique known as the Monospot test has also been developed, using horse red blood cells. This test can be performed in minutes. A positive test, along with the increased number of atypical lymphocytes apparent on a blood slide, confirms the diagnosis of infectious mononucleosis. Epstein-Barr virus antibodies can be recovered from blood serum for a final diagnosis.

Therapeutic Management. Children with infectious mononucleosis need bed rest during the acute stage of the illness (7 to 10 days) because with the splenomegaly there is a danger of spleen rupture with any trauma to that area. If a child is hospitalized, follow standard precautions. Be careful in helping children with this disease turn in bed so that no pressure is placed over the splenic area. If palpating the spleen, do so gently to avoid inadvertent rupture.

Teach children and parents the importance of maintaining a good fluid intake despite the sore throat. Cool, nonacidic fluids are often tolerated best.

Neurologic complications such as meningitis or encephalitis may occur (Orti et al., 2003). Children may notice weakness and general fatigue for up to 6 weeks after the illness. Caution them to avoid contact sports as long as the spleen is enlarged. Because infectious mononucleosis occurs primarily in young adults, it may interrupt school or career plans. Help these young adults to voice their frustration with this illness. Offer support to help them through this unexpected interruption in their life.

Checkpoint Question 3

For a child with infectious mononucleosis, why must abdominal palpation be performed gently?

a. Regional lymph nodes are painful.
b. The enlarged spleen can rupture.
c. Red cells pocket just under the skin.
d. Petechiae form easily from bruising.

Hantavirus Pulmonary Syndrome Infection

The hantavirus is a member of the arbovirus group. The virus infects small rodents and perhaps cats who have eaten mice. In the Far East, the virus produces an illness marked by extreme purpura from thrombocytopenia and severe gastrointestinal symptoms. In 1993, an outbreak of severe illness from a previously undiscovered hantavirus occurred in the United States. Outbreaks continue to occur sporadically. Major symptoms are fever, muscle aches, thrombocytopenia, gastrointestinal symptoms, and hypotension. Death can occur from rapid progressive pulmonary edema.

Supportive care is necessary, as antiviral medications do not seem to be effective (Braun & Zoidis, 2004). Caution families not to touch dead mice and to have mice exterminated from their homes to avoid the possibility of contracting this disease.

BACTERIAL INFECTIONS

Bacteria reproduce by fission, in which one cell enlarges and duplicates itself, then divides into two equal parts. They are usually single-celled organisms occurring in three main shapes: spheres (cocci), rods (bacilli), and spirals (spirochetes). Bacteria are independent, living organisms. They have a nucleus, cytoplasm, and a cell wall, and they contain both DNA and RNA.

Bacteria are most commonly observed under a microscope after being fixed to a slide by heating followed by staining. Bacteria that stain violet are gram-positive organisms; those that stain red are gram-negative organisms. Those that cannot be decolorized with acid after being stained are acid-fast. As some bacteria grow, they produce **exotoxins,** or poisons. If this happens, disease symptoms arise not from the bacteria themselves but from the effect of these toxins on the body. Tetanus, botulism, and diphtheria are diseases caused by the systemic spread of toxins produced by bacteria.

Some bacteria are capable of producing enzymes as they grow. Hemolytic streptococci, for example, produce streptokinase, which enables the bacteria to pass through blood clots. Penicillinase, an enzyme produced by certain bacteria, can destroy penicillin. Many first-generation penicillins are therefore ineffective against such organisms.

Streptococcal Diseases

Streptococci, gram-positive organisms, are found normally in the respiratory, alimentary, and female genital tracts. Most severe diseases in children result from infection with *Streptococcus pyogenes* (beta-hemolytic streptococci, group A). Beta-hemolytic, group B streptococcal infection can be contracted from vaginal secretions at birth (see Chapter 26) and so tends to occur in newborns. Streptococcal pharyngeal infection is discussed in Chapter 40 with other throat infections. Rheumatic fever and glomerulonephritis, conditions that may result as an autoimmune response to streptococci, are discussed in Chapters 41 and 46, respectively.

Scarlet Fever

- Causative agent: Beta-hemolytic streptococci, group A
- Incubation period: 2 to 5 days
- Period of communicability: Greatest during acute phase of respiratory illness; 1 to 7 days
- Mode of transmission: Direct contact and large droplets
- Immunity: One episode of disease gives lasting immunity to scarlet fever toxin. No vaccination is available, however.

Assessment. Scarlet fever occurs most commonly in the 6- to 12-year-old age group, although it may be seen in preschoolers. The incidence is highest in temperate climates, and the disease occurs usually in late winter or early spring.

The symptoms of scarlet fever begin abruptly and are those of a streptococcal pharyngitis: fever, sore throat, perhaps headache, chills, and malaise. As the beta-hemolytic, group A streptococcus grows in the child's body, it produces a number of toxins; erythrogenic toxin is the one responsible for the rash of scarlet fever. The rash appears 12 to 48 hours after the onset of the pharyngeal symptoms (see Fig. 43.3). The fever is high (103° to 104°F [39.5° to 40.0°C]) on the first day of throat symptoms and again on the day the rash appears, and then gradually returns to normal. The pulse rate may be increased out of proportion to the fever.

The rash of scarlet fever is both enanthematous and exanthematous (on both mucous membrane and skin). The tonsils are inflamed and enlarged and usually covered with white exudate. The uvula and pharynx are beefy red. The palate is usually covered with erythematous punctiform (pinpoint) lesions and perhaps scattered petechiae. The tongue, during the first 2 days of the illness, is white and appears furry. By day 3, papillae enlarge and protrude through the white coat, giving the tongue a "white strawberry" appearance. By day 4 or 5, the white coat disappears and the prominent papillae of the tongue give it a "red strawberry" appearance. A "strawberry tongue" is distinctive for scarlet fever and helps to differentiate the disease from other rashes. A throat culture reveals streptococci (Bagarazzi, 2003).

The skin rash is typically red, pinpoint lesions that blanch on pressure and feel as rough as sandpaper. Lesions are densest on the trunk and in skin folds. Few lesions appear on the face. The area around the mouth tends to be abnormally pale (circumoral pallor). There are areas of hyperpigmentation in skin folds at the joints (Pastia's sign). The rash persists for approximately 1 week. It desquamates, with large areas of skin peeling off in fine flakes.

Therapeutic Management. Children with scarlet fever usually appear ill. They need a soft or liquid diet for a few days until their throat soreness has diminished. They may need an analgesic and antipyretic, such as acetaminophen (Tylenol) or children's ibuprofen (Motrin) for pain and fever. The rash of scarlet fever tends to be pruritic, so comfort measures are necessary. Because the underlying cause of the illness is a streptococcal infection, a 10-day course of penicillin is prescribed (Bagarazzi, 2003). Caution parents to give the full amount prescribed for the full course to prevent the complications of beta-hemolytic, group A streptococcal infections (acute glomerulonephritis or rheumatic

fever). If a child is hospitalized, follow droplet precautions until 24 hours after therapy is started, in addition to standard precautions (Box 43.7).

Children who receive penicillin may not develop the typical extreme rash and obviously do not have as severe a systemic illness as those who do not receive penicillin. As a result, scarlet fever is currently popularly termed scarlatina (a small, scarlet rash). Caution parents that regardless of the name, the consequences can be grave and penicillin therapy is necessary.

Checkpoint Question 4

Marty has developed scarlet fever. What is the mark of scarlet fever lesions?

a. They appear on skin and mucous membranes.
b. The crusts that form are mildly contagious.
c. The lesions weep a clear, sticky fluid.
d. Lesions are dark brown to black.

Impetigo

- Causative agent: Beta-hemolytic streptococcus, group A (nonbullous); *Staphylococcus aureus* (bullous)
- Incubation period: 2 to 5 days
- Period of communicability: From outbreak of lesions until lesions are healed
- Mode of transmission: Direct contact with lesions
- Immunity: None

Impetigo is only mildly infectious because it seems to be transmitted only by direct contact (Foster, 2003). It is not uncommon to see several children in a family with identical lesions, however. Parents may be upset at being told their child has impetigo because at one time the lesions (dirty and crusty-appearing) were associated with poor hygiene.

Assessment. Impetigo is a superficial infection of the skin. It begins as a single papulovesicular lesion surrounded by localized erythema. As more vesicles appear, they become purulent, ooze, and form honey-colored crusts (Fig. 43.12). They are found most commonly on the face and extremities. They are often seen as secondary infections of insect bites or in children who have body piercings. If there are a number of lesions, children may have local adenopathy.

Therapeutic Management. Treatment is oral administration of penicillin or erythromycin or the application of mupirocin (Bactroban) ointment for 7 to 10 days (Box 43.8). The lesions heal most quickly if a parent or the child washes the crusts daily with soap and water.

Although rare, complications of rheumatic fever or acute glomerulonephritis may occur after impetigo, as they may after other streptococcal infections. If a child develops impetigo while in the hospital, follow contact precautions until 24 hours after initiation of therapy.

Cat-Scratch Disease

- Causative agent: *Bartonella henselae* bacteria
- Incubation period: 3 to 10 days

BOX 43.7: Focus on Nursing Care Planning

A Multidisciplinary Care Map for A Hospitalized Child with Scarlet Fever

●

Marty, a 10-year-old boy, was admitted to the hospital for appendicitis. The morning after surgery, his throat was painful and his arms were covered by a very itchy, red, macular rash. Marty was diagnosed as having scarlet fever. "How could this have happened?" his mother asks you. "He's not a bad kid. How could two bad things happen to him at once?"

Family Assessment

Child has two siblings: a 6-year-old brother and a 10-day-old newborn. Parents are migrant crop workers. Move yearly from Florida to Connecticut to follow crops. Mother rates finances as: "We have no money."

Client Assessment

Macular, pinpoint erythematous rash on abdomen, groin folds, and chest. Lesions blanch with pressure. Groin fold areas hyperpigmented. Child scratching lesions constantly. Uvula and pharynx beefy red. Tonsils inflamed and enlarged with white exudate. Temperature 103°F (39.5°C). Pinpoint lesions with two or three scattered petechiae noted on palate. Tongue white and furry. Throat culture positive for streptococcus. Other physical examination findings within normal limits for postoperative course. Child upset and crying. "I wish my Mom was here to stay with me. I'm all by myself. I can't even go to the playroom." Mother usually visits once a day in the late afternoon.

Nursing Diagnosis

Social isolation related to required restrictions associated with infection control precautions

Outcome Evaluation

Child states reason for restrictions; identifies time when restrictions will be lifted; expresses interest in activities proposed.

Team Member Responsible	Assessment	Intervention	Rationale	Expected Outcome
Activities of Daily Living				
Nurse	Assess what child understands about how communicable diseases are spread.	Explain the reasons for restrictions and infection control precautions. Institute droplet precautions.	Child may associate precautions and restrictions with feelings of being punished. Droplet precautions help reduce the spread of the disease.	Child states he understands reason for isolation. Cooperates to maintain infection precautions.
Nurse	Assess what play activity would provide stimulation.	Visit the child frequently, at least every hour, and provide him with opportunities for therapeutic play.	Frequent visits help to decrease feelings of being alone. Therapeutic play helps the child deal with resentment about condition.	Child states that although he wants to go to playroom, he has found an enjoyable activity to occupy his time in his hospital room.

(continued)

Team Member Responsible	Assessment	Intervention	Rationale	Expected Outcome
Consultations				
Physician	Determine whether hospital infection control committee is aware of contagious illness in a postoperative patient.	Consult with infection control members on the possibility surgical personnel may have been exposed to scarlet fever.	Scarlet fever is contagious for 2 to 7 days prior to outbreak of rash.	Infection control committee members state they are aware of possible spread of illness to health care personnel and institute needed precautions, such as prescribed penicillin for exposed health care personnel.
Procedures/Medications				
Nurse	Determine whether child has ever had a reaction to penicillin.	Begin antibiotic therapy (penicillin V) as prescribed.	Penicillin is effective for group A beta-hemolytic streptococcus, the causative organism of scarlet fever.	Child's parents are contacted and report child has not had a previous reaction to penicillin. Child cooperates to take oral penicillin as prescribed.
Nurse	Ask child to rate pain of sore throat and itchiness of rash on scales of 1 to 10.	Administer analgesia and antihistamine prescribed. Caution child antihistamine may make him feel sleepy.	An antihistamine such as Benadryl can greatly reduce the pruritus of a rash.	Child states the itchiness of rash and pain of sore throat have decreased to tolerable levels.
Nutrition				
Nurse/ nutritionist	Assess what fluid child would find most appealing to drink.	Provide frequent oral fluids. When soft diet is begun (child is postop appendicitis), provide soft foods.	Adequate fluid intake is important to prevent skin dryness, which increases discomfort. A soft or liquid diet is less irritating to the child's sore throat.	Child identifies favorite fluid to drink. States he is able to eat soft foods even with painful throat.
Patient/Family Education				
Nurse/ physician	Determine whether other members of family will need prophylactic antibiotic.	Explain the purpose of prophylactic penicillin for susceptible family members.	As family members were near child during prodromal period, they are susceptible to also contract the disease.	Parent identifies susceptible family members; states she will be able to fill prescription for susceptible family members and supervise them to ensure they take prescribed antibiotic.
Psychosocial/Spiritual/Emotional Needs				
Nurse	Assess whether child and parent understand the cause of scarlet fever.	Discuss the spread of infectious diseases is not related to "good or bad."	Mother voiced she was concerned because two diseases happened to her child at the same time.	Mother and child state they understand diseases are caused by infectious organisms, not moral status.

(continued)

Team Member Responsible	Assessment	Intervention	Rationale	Expected Outcome
Discharge Planning				
Nurse	Assess if parent is aware child's rash will be itchy for about a week.	Discuss possible measures parent can take to reduce pruritus (loose clothing, cool compresses) and measures to reduce pain of sore throat.	If children scratch pruritic lesions, they can cause secondary infection. Sore throats interfere with comfort and ability to eat well.	Parent states she understands common measures to reduce pruritus and will instigate them.

- Period of communicability: Unknown
- Mode of transmission: Bite or scratch from a cat or kitten
- Immunity: One episode of disease gives lasting immunity; no passive artificial immunity

Cat-scratch disease occurs most commonly in preschool children because children at that age play roughly with cats or pick them up against their will and so receive scratches. At the time the child contracts the disease, the cat does not appear ill (Batts & Demers, 2004).

The first symptom for the child is a single skin papule or pustule that lasts 1 to 3 weeks. Approximately 2 weeks after the scratch, severe local lymphadenopathy also develops. The nodes most markedly involved are those of the head, neck, and axilla. The node enlargement generally lasts 2 to 3 months. In some children, there is node suppuration (a node breaks open to the skin and drains sterile pus).

Some children have a low-grade fever and malaise. Occasionally, central nervous system involvement, such as encephalitis or meningitis, occurs. A positive reaction to a skin test of cat-scratch disease antigen is present. This, along with the history of a cat scratch and the aspiration of sterile pus from an enlarged lymph node, is diagnostic. Treatment is symptomatic, although an antibiotic may be prescribed to help shorten the course of the disease. Children may need an analgesic for painful adenopathy. Aspiration of involved nodes may be necessary to relieve pain.

Parents may ask if the cat should be destroyed. Because an attack of cat-scratch disease gives lifetime immunity and fewer than 10% of children scratched by the same cat contract cat-scratch disease, there is no need to destroy the cat for an act it may have seen as defending its safety.

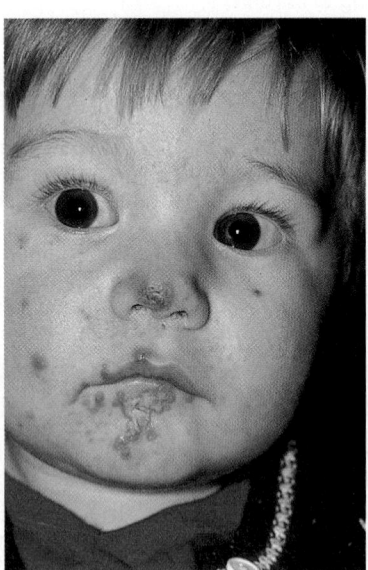

FIGURE 43.12 Impetigo in a toddler. Note the honey-colored crust appearance of some of the lesions. (© Dr. P. Marazzi/SPL/Science Source/Photo Researchers.)

BOX 43.8 FOCUS ON . . .

PHARMACOLOGY

Mupirocin (Bactroban)

Classification: Mupirocin is a topical antibiotic.

Action: Mupirocin is used to treat impetigo caused by *Staphylococcus aureus* and *Streptococcus pyogenes.*

Pregnancy risk category: B

Dosage: Small amount applied three times a day to the affected areas for 10 days

Possible adverse effects: Erythema, dry skin, pruritus, burning, stinging

Nursing Implications

- Advise parents to wash the lesions with soap and water and pat dry before applying ointment, to soften crusts for better absorption.
- Caution parents that causative organisms are infectious by direct contact. Instruct them to wash their own hands before and after applying the ointment.
- Urge parents to continue to use the ointment to ensure eradication of the causative germs. The lesions may begin to improve before 10 days have elapsed.
- Instruct the parents to use caution when applying the ointment around the eyes. Ointment is irritating to the eyes.
- Teach the parents about the signs and symptoms of secondary fungal infection that may occur and instruct them to notify a health care provider should any occur.

Staphylococcal Infections

Staphylococcal organisms are gram-positive. Colonies of staphylococci are normally found on the skin, so they are generally the organisms involved in skin infections (pyodermas). Because the organisms grow rapidly in cream foods that are not well refrigerated, such as potato salad or cream pies, they are often the organisms involved in summer food poisoning episodes. Because food poisoning produces gastrointestinal symptoms, these infections are discussed in Chapter 45.

Furunculosis (Boils)

A furuncle is a staphylococcal infection of the hair follicle. A yellow pustule forms at the site. There is localized redness, pain, and edema of the surrounding skin. Urge children not to rupture these lesions but rather to allow them to run their self-limiting course so the infection is not spread to surrounding tissue and does not become a cellulitis.

Cellulitis

Cellulitis is a staphylococcal inflammation of the deeper layers of skin. It occurs generally on the extremities or face, or surrounding wounds. The skin feels warm and is edematous and reddened. Cellulitis is treated with a systemic antibiotic. Warm soaks relieve pain and inflammation.

Scalded Skin Disease

Scalded skin disease (Ritter's disease) is a staphylococcal infection seen primarily in newborns. Children develop rough-textured skin and general erythema. Large bullae (vesicles), filled with clear fluid, form. The epidermis separates in large sheets, leaving a red, glistening, scalded-looking surface. Children need intensive intravenous antibiotic therapy to survive this extreme infection (Patel, 2004).

Other Bacterial Infections

Diphtheria

- Causative agent: *Corynebacterium diphtheriae* (Klebs-Löffler bacillus)
- Incubation period: 2 to 6 days
- Period of communicability: Rarely more than 2 weeks to 4 weeks in untreated persons; 1 to 2 days in patients treated with antibiotics
- Mode of transmission: Direct or indirect contact
- Immunity: Contracting the disease gives lasting natural immunity.
- Active artificial immunity: Diphtheria toxin given as part of DTaP vaccine
- Passive artificial immunity: Diphtheria antitoxin

Assessment. Although diphtheria is an illness that should be extinct because of available immunization, it still occurs in isolated outbreaks. When diphtheria bacilli invade and grow in the nasopharynx of children, they produce an exotoxin (a potent protein poison) that causes massive cell necrosis and inflammation. The necrosing material lends itself well to the growth of the bacilli, so the bacilli reproduce rapidly. The inflammation and necrosing cells form a characteristic gray membrane on the nasopharynx. This may extend up into the nose and down into the major bronchi, causing a purulent nasal discharge and a brassy cough. The toxin is absorbed from the membrane surface and spread systemically by the bloodstream to affect major organs, such as the heart and nervous system. If untreated, myocarditis with heart failure and conduction disturbances may occur. Central nervous system involvement can include severe neuritis with paralysis of the diaphragm and pharyngeal and laryngeal muscles. The diagnosis of diphtheria is made based on clinical appearance and on a throat culture, which reveals the presence of the bacilli (Zimmerman & Poland, 2004).

Therapeutic Management. Treatment involves intravenous administration of antitoxin in large doses. In addition, children are given penicillin or erythromycin intravenously. Complete bed rest is crucial during the acute stage of the illness. Droplet precautions must be followed until cultures are negative. Children need careful observation at all times to prevent airway obstruction. If obstruction occurs, endotracheal intubation may be necessary.

Because the diphtheria vaccine is included in routine immunizations for infants, diphtheria is almost extinct in the United States. However, isolated instances do occur, and when they do, prompt recognition and treatment are necessary.

Whooping Cough (Pertussis)

- Causative agent: *Bordetella pertussis*
- Incubation period: 5 to 21 days
- Mode of transmission: Direct or indirect contact
- Period of communicability: Greatest in catarrhal (respiratory illness) stage
- Immunity: Contracting the disease offers lasting natural immunity.
- Active artificial immunity: Pertussis vaccine given as part of DTaP vaccine
- Passive artificial immunity: Pertussis immune serum globulin

Pertussis is a serious disease of childhood. Like diphtheria, pertussis had become quite rare because of required immunizations, but it still occurs sporadically and is actually making a comeback in some locales (Schweon, 2005). Those most susceptible are children who have not been immunized because a previous vaccine had possible side effects that led parents to refuse immunization.

Assessment. Pertussis manifests itself in three stages: catarrhal, paroxysmal, and convalescent. The **catarrhal stage** begins with upper respiratory symptoms such as coryza, sneezing, lacrimation, cough, and a low-grade fever. Children are irritable and listless. In some children, a mild cough is the only symptom during this stage. It lasts from 1 to 2 weeks (Scribano, 2003).

The paroxysmal stage lasts 4 to 6 weeks. During this time, the cough changes from a mild one to a paroxysmal one, involving five to ten short, rapid coughs, followed by a rapid inspiration, which causes the "whoop," or high-pitched crowing sound, of whooping cough. Children are in obvious distress while coughing. They may become cyanotic or red-faced, and their nose may drain thick, tenacious mucus. They often vomit after a paroxysm of coughing, and they are exhausted afterward from the effort. Attacks of coughing tend to be more severe at night.

During the convalescent stage, there is a gradual cessation of the coughing and vomiting. The cough may be present for some time, but as single, not paroxysmal, coughs. During the next year, if children develop an upper respiratory infection, they may again have a return of the paroxysmal coughing with vomiting.

Pertussis is diagnosed by its striking symptoms, although in children younger than 6 months of age, the "whoop" of the cough may be absent, making it more difficult to diagnose. The *B. pertussis* bacillus may be cultured from nasopharyngeal secretions during the catarrhal and paroxysmal stages. The white cell count, particularly the lymphocyte count, increases with whooping cough: it may be as high as 20,000 to 30,000/mm³ at the end of the catarrhal stage (normal is 5,000 to 10,000/mm³).

Therapeutic Management. Children with pertussis are maintained on bed rest until the paroxysms of coughing subside. They need to be secluded from environmental factors, such as cigarette smoke, dust, and strenuous activity, that initiate coughing episodes. Nutrition may be a problem if the child is constantly coughing and vomiting. As a rule, frequent small meals are vomited less than larger meals. Infants with pertussis may be admitted to a health care facility for observation because they may have such tenacious secretions with coughing episodes that they need airway suction. Place an intercom in the infant's room so personnel can listen for paroxysms of coughing.

A full 10-day course of erythromycin or azithromycin may be prescribed (Langley et al., 2004). These drugs have the potential to shorten the period of communicability and may shorten the duration of symptoms. Droplet precautions are used until 5 days after a child starts effective therapy. Complications of pertussis include pneumonia, atelectasis, or emphysema from plugged bronchioles. Seizures from asphyxia as a result of severe paroxysms of coughing may occur. Epistaxis, subconjunctival and subarachnoid bleeding from the force of coughing, may occur. If sufficient fluid intake cannot be maintained, alkalosis and dehydration from persistent vomiting can occur.

Prevention. Little passive immunity is transferred to the newborn, so children in their early months are particularly susceptible to this disease. This is why pertussis vaccine is one of the first immunizations scheduled. Infants who have not yet been immunized or are immunocompromised and are exposed may be given pertussis immune serum globulin to protect them from contracting the disease (Scribano, 2003).

What if... an adolescent with pertussis vomits after an episode of coughing? Should you urge him to try to eat again immediately, or do you think he would be too nauseated to do so?

Anthrax

- Causative agent: *Bacillus anthracis,* a bacteria
- Incubation period: 1 to 7 days (inhalational), 1 to 12 days (cutaneous), 1 to 7 days (gastrointestinal)
- Mode of transmission: Originally contracted from contact with cow or sheep feces; not transmissible from person to person
- Immunity: Unstudied
- Active artificial immunity: A vaccine is available for people in high-risk occupations, such as veterinarians, but it is not recommended for children.
- Passive artificial immunity: Not available

Anthrax is an acute infectious disease that is contracted from exposure to the bacteria or its spores (Chang, Glynn, & Groseclose, 2003). Such bacteria live in the feces of infected cows or sheep. As the organism grows inside the human body, a toxin is produced that is the actual source of the symptoms. Children, like adults, may be affected by all three clinical forms: cutaneous, inhalational, or gastrointestinal.

Inhalational anthrax begins with a brief prodromal period of flulike symptoms, followed shortly by dyspnea, severe systemic shock, and marked evidence of mediastinal widening and pleural effusion on x-ray. The mortality for this form is over 90%.

Cutaneous anthrax is characterized by a skin lesion that begins as a papule, then passes through a vesicle stage to a painless depressed black eschar. Fever, malaise, and headache and regional lymphadenopathy may accompany the skin lesion. The mortality of cutaneous anthrax is as low as 1% with antibiotic therapy.

Gastrointestinal anthrax is contracted by eating undercooked meat infected with the organism. The child develops severe abdominal pain, fever, bloody diarrhea, and septicemia. Mortality is about 25%.

If a child is exposed to anthrax, prophylaxis with ciprofloxacin (Cipro) for those over 18 years and doxycycline for younger patients should be started. Drug therapy is continued for 60 days because of the potential persistence of spores.

Tetanus (Lockjaw)

- Causative agent: *Clostridium tetani*
- Incubation period: 3 days to 3 weeks
- Period of communicability: None
- Mode of transmission: Direct or indirect contamination of a closed wound
- Immunity: Development of the disease gives lasting natural immunity.
- Active artificial immunity: Tetanus toxoid contained in DTaP vaccine
- Passive artificial immunity: Tetanus immune globulin

Tetanus, a highly fatal disease if untreated, is caused by an anaerobic, spore-forming bacillus. The bacillus, found in soil and the excretions of animals, enters the body through a wound. If the wound is deep, such as a puncture wound, where the distal end of the wound is shut off from an oxygen source, the tetanus bacilli begin to reproduce. The organism may also enter through a burn site, which crusts, creating an anaerobic environment. As the bacilli grow, they produce exotoxins that cause the disease symptoms by affecting the motor nuclei of the central nervous system (Newcombe, 2004).

The entrance site of the bacillus does not appear infected (no pus or reddened area is present unless a secondary infection also exists). After the incubation period, the exotoxins have developed to such an extent, however, that they are capable of disrupting the nervous system.

Assessment. The first symptoms that are noticeable are stiffness of the neck and jaw (lockjaw). Within 24 to 48 hours, muscular rigidity of the trunk and extremities develops. The back becomes arched (opisthotonos), the abdominal muscles are stiff and boardlike, and the face assumes an unusual appearance, with wrinkling of the forehead and distortion of the corners of the mouth (a "sardonic grin" sign). Any stimulation, such as a sudden noise, a bright light, or a touch, causes painful, paroxysmal spasms. The sensorium is clear throughout the course of the disease, so the child is aware of the pain associated with muscle spasms. As these spasms begin to include laryngospasm, respiratory obstruction, and a collection of secretions in the respiratory tract, death by asphyxiation may occur.

Fever is an ominous sign accompanying tetanus. Children who survive the disease rarely have more than a low-grade fever.

Therapeutic Management. The child needs to be cared for in a quiet, stimulation-free room. If the wound has necrotic tissue, it may be débrided to ensure that no secondary infections arise. Enteral or total parenteral nutrition may be necessary to prevent aspiration from laryngeal spasm. Tetanus immune globulin (human) is administered to supply passive antitoxins to combat the growing organisms.

Parenteral penicillin G or erythromycin is administered to reduce the number of growing forms of the bacillus. Sedation and a muscle relaxant may be necessary to reduce the severity and pain of the muscle spasms. The child may need to be intubated and mechanical ventilation begun to maintain respiratory function.

Prevention. Tetanus is a serious disease, but it can be prevented through active immunization and suitable booster immunization. Children routinely receive tetanus immunization as part of routine DTaP immunization and a booster dose at school age; thereafter they should receive a booster dose every 10 years. At the time of a wound, the wound site should be cleaned well with soap and water and a suitable antiseptic. If the wound is deep, such as a knife stab, a nail puncture, or a dog bite, it should not be sutured but should be left open to heal by secondary intention. This reduces the possibility of an anaerobic pocket forming in the wound. If the child received basic immunization against tetanus and it has been fewer than 10 years since the last injection, no booster or antitoxin management is needed at the time of the wound.

If a child's immunization record cannot be obtained, or if it has been more than 10 years since the child received a booster injection or an initial injection for tetanus, a child will probably be treated with a booster injection and

tetanus immune globulin. A booster injection provides tetanus antigen to the child. If the child received initial immunization for this disease, the booster will cause the body to "remember" how to make tetanus antibodies, and the body will begin to produce them rapidly. By the time the invading tetanus organisms from the wound have passed their long incubation period (3 days to 3 weeks), the child will have antibodies in the system prepared to eradicate the organisms. If the initial immunizations were incomplete or are unknown, in addition to tetanus antigen the child will also receive the passive antibodies included in tetanus immune globulin (Callahan, 2003).

Lyme Disease

- Causative agent: *Borrelia burgdorferi,* a spirochete
- Incubation period: 3 to 30 days
- Period of communicability: Not communicable from one person to another
- Mode of transmission: Deer tick
- Active artificial immunity: Lyme disease vaccine

Lyme disease is caused by a spirochete, *Borrelia burgdorferi,* that is transmitted by a tick often carried on deer. The disease is the most frequently reported vector-borne infection in the United States, occurring most often in the summer and early fall. Almost immediately after the tick bite, an erythematous papule is noticeable at the site, which spreads over the next 3 to 30 days (the incubation period) to become a large, round ring with a raised swollen border (erythema chronicum migrans; Fig. 43.13). This is followed by systemic involvement that leads to cardiac, musculoskeletal, and neurologic symptoms. Cardiac involvement may be so severe that it includes heart block from atrioventricular conduction abnormalities. Neurologic symptoms commonly include stiff neck, headache, and cranial nerve palsy. Musculoskeletal symptoms occur in 50% of children and include painful swollen arthritic joints, particularly the knee (Rudd-Arieta, 2003).

Amoxicillin or penicillin V is administered at the time of the bite to young children. Doxycycline is given to those older than 8 years of age. A vaccine for the disease

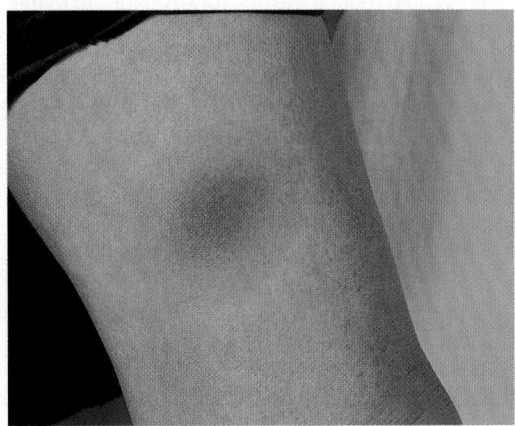

FIGURE 43.13 The rash of Lyme disease. (© Larry Mulvehill/Science Source/Photo Researchers.)

has been approved for use in adults who live or work in high-risk areas but not yet for children.

Parents should be cautioned to inspect the skin of children who have been playing in wooded areas for tick bites to help identify the disorder before debilitating symptoms occur. Other suggestions for avoiding Lyme disease are shown in Box 43.9.

OTHER INFECTIOUS PATHOGENS

Rickettsial Diseases

Rickettsiae are organisms that resemble viruses both in size and in their inability to reproduce except inside the cells of a host organism. They reproduce by fission, however, as bacteria do; like bacteria, they are complete organisms containing both RNA and DNA. They multiply inside ticks, lice, mites, or fleas (arthropods) without causing disease. They are transmitted to humans through the bite or feces of the infected arthropod. An exception is Q fever, which is spread by droplet infection. All rickettsial diseases include fever, and almost all include a rash caused by rickettsial multiplication in the endothelial cells of small blood vessels. Rickettsiae invasion triggers an immune response.

Rocky Mountain Spotted Fever

- Causative agent: *Rickettsia rickettsii*
- Incubation period: 3 to 12 days

BOX 43.9 FOCUS ON . . .

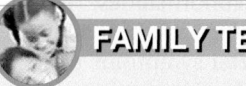

FAMILY TEACHING

Tips For Avoiding Exposure to Lyme Disease

Q. Marty's father tells you, "My children love to play in the woods, but I'm so afraid that they'll get Lyme disease. What can I do to protect them?"

A. Here are some suggestions for you and your children to help reduce the risk for exposure to Lyme disease:

- Wear protective clothing when hiking or playing in wooded areas: long sleeves, high necklines, long slacks. Tuck bottom of slacks into socks or boots.
- Wear light-colored clothing, so any tick present on clothing can be readily observed.
- Inspect skin for ticks thoroughly after hiking or playing in wooded areas. Remove any ticks found with tweezers.
- Report any area of inflammation that might be a tick bite to a health care provider for early diagnosis.
- Ask your primary care provider about the availability of Lyme disease vaccine. Currently, it is administered only to adults with high-risk occupations, but it is anticipated that the vaccine will soon be available for children living in high-risk areas.

- Period of communicability: Not communicable from one person to another
- Mode of transmission: Wood, dog, or rabbit tick
- Active artificial immunity: Rocky Mountain spotted fever vaccine

Rocky Mountain spotted fever is the most common rickettsial disease seen in the United States. It is most prevalent in the western United States and is transmitted by a tick. It is seen most often during the spring and early summer, when ticks are most commonly seen. A reddened area develops at the site of the tick bite. In 2 to 8 days, a typical rash, persistent headache, fever (as high as 104°F [40°C]), and mental confusion begin. The rash is distinctive, beginning with reddened macules, then changing to petechiae. It begins on the wrists and ankles, then spreads up the arms and legs onto the trunk. Unlike most rashes, it can cover the palms and soles (Fig. 43.14).

In untreated children, symptoms worsen to include central nervous system involvement (stiff neck and seizures) and cardiac and pulmonary symptoms such as heart failure and pneumonia. Nitrogen loss in the urine becomes extreme. An accompanying hyponatremia may also be present (Masters et al., 2003).

Therapy is with tetracycline for 7 to 10 days. Caution parents to administer the drug for the full course of therapy to ensure disease eradication and prevent the risk of complications. Rocky Mountain spotted fever was a serious childhood illness before antibiotic therapy was available, and it still has the potential to be serious if the symptoms are not reported when they first occur.

Murine Typhus

Murine typhus is seen almost exclusively in the southern United States. It is transmitted by mites and fleas that live on rats. Its symptoms are almost identical to those of Rocky Mountain spotted fever. It responds to tetracycline or a third-generation antibiotic such as ciprofloxacin (Cipro).

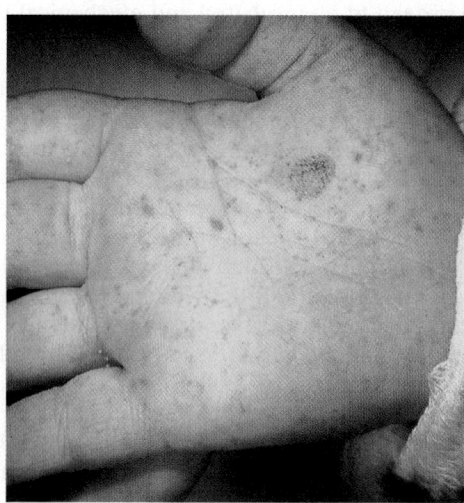

FIGURE 43.14 Typical rash of Rocky Mountain spotted fever. (Courtesy of Stuart Starr, MD, The Children's Hospital of Philadelphia.)

Chlamydial Infections

Chlamydiae are gram-negative nonmotile organisms similar to rickettsiae. Chlamydial pneumonia or vaginitis may occur in children (see Chapters 40 and 47). Psittacosis is a chlamydial infection commonly found in children.

Psittacosis

Psittacosis, caused by *Chlamydia psittaci,* is a disease transmitted to children by birds, such as parakeets, lovebirds, parrots, chickens, turkeys, and pigeons (Thom, 2004). The bird has no apparent symptoms of illness. Children develop symptoms of an upper respiratory infection, possibly accompanied by a low-grade fever, a dry cough, weakness, and anorexia out of proportion to the fever. An enlarged spleen may also be present. Children may develop patchy bronchopneumonia. The course of the disease is as long as 3 to 4 weeks. Treatment is with erythromycin for young children and tetracycline for children over the age of 8 years.

Parasitic Infections

Parasites are organisms that live on and obtain their food supply from other organisms. Frequently seen parasites in children include head lice and scabies (Table 43.3). Parents are often embarrassed when they learn that their child has lice. Reassure them that this infestation can happen to any child (Box 43.10).

Helminthic Infections

Helminths are pathogenic or parasitic worms. They may be roundworms (nematodes), flukes (trematodes), or tapeworms (cestodes). Most helminths begin life when the eggs or larvae are eliminated in the feces or urine of humans. They are then transmitted to the oral cavity by contaminated foods or hands. Because children tend to be careless about washing their hands before eating or tend to suck their thumbs, they are prone to these infections (Kucik, Martin, & Sortor, 2004).

Roundworms (Ascariasis)

The roundworm parasite lives in the intestinal tract. Eggs are excreted in the feces. Children typically ingest the eggs when they eat food with hands that are improperly washed. Larvae, which hatch from the ingested eggs, penetrate the intestinal wall and enter the circulation. From there, they may migrate to any body tissue. Children have a loss of appetite and perhaps nausea and vomiting. Intestinal obstruction may occur from a mass of roundworms in the intestinal tract. Ascariasis can be prevented by the sanitary disposal of feces to prevent contamination of the soil. A single dose of an anthelmintic such as pyrantel pamoate (Antiminth) controls the infection.

Hookworms

Hookworm eggs, like roundworm eggs, are found in human feces. They enter children's bodies through the skin and then migrate to the intestinal tract, where they attach themselves onto the intestinal villi. They suck blood from the intestinal wall to sustain themselves. If a great number of hookworms are present, severe anemia may result. Treatment is with anthelmintics to destroy the worms. Children may also need therapy for the anemia.

Pinworms

Pinworms are small, white, threadlike worms that live in the cecum. At night, the female pinworm migrates down

TABLE 43.3			
Common Parasitic Infections			
Infection	**Organism**	**Symptoms**	**Treatment**
Pediculosis capitis	Head lice	Small, white flecks on hair shaft (nits or eggs of lice)	Wash hair with shampoo such as lindane (Kwell).
		Extreme pruritus	Comb nits from hair with fine-toothed comb.
			Wash bed sheets, recently worn clothes.
			Vacuum pillows, mattresses, or other items unable to be washed.
			Teach children not to exchange combs, hair barrettes, or other personal items.
Pediculosis	Pubic lice	Same as for head lice except on pubic hair	Same as head lice
Scabies	Female mite (*Acarus scabiei*)	Black burrow filled with mite feces ½ inch long, usually between fingers and toes, on palms, or in axilla or groin	Caution adolescent that groin infestations might be spread by physical intimacy.
			Wash area with lindane (Kwell) lotion or permethrin (Elimite).

BOX 43.10 FOCUS ON . . .

COMMUNICATION

When Marty's 6-year-old brother Joshua visits him, you notice he has scratch marks on his neck and forehead. His hair shafts are covered by sand-like particles. You suspect he has pediculosis capitis or head lice.

Less Effective Communication

Nurse: Mrs. Ireland, I'm wondering if you've noticed these sand-like particles in your son's hair.

Mrs. Ireland: Well, you know boys. They don't always wash well.

Nurse: I'm concerned they may be the eggs of head lice.

Mrs. Ireland: We're not that poor. Don't insult us.

Nurse: I didn't mean to. Like you said, it's probably something else.

More Effective Communication

Nurse: Mrs. Ireland, I'm wondering if you've noticed these sand-like particles in your son's hair.

Mrs. Ireland: Well, you know boys. They don't always wash well.

Nurse: I'm concerned they may be the eggs of head lice.

Mrs. Ireland: We're not that poor. Don't insult us.

Nurse: Let's talk about head lice, and how easy it is for anyone to get them.

The above scenario is an example of what can happen if people believe one of the myths that circulate related to communicable diseases. Head lice can be spread easily in locker rooms or classrooms, so any child can contract them.

✓ Checkpoint Question 5

Marty had a pinworm infection last year. A typical symptom of this infection to assess for would be:

a. Nausea and vomiting.
b. Anal itching on awakening.
c. Loose, bloody stools.
d. Mild jaundice and itching.

Protozoan Infections

Protozoa are unicellular organisms. They absorb fluid through the cell membrane and can move from place to place by pseudopod, flagella, or cilia action. They are most pathogenic in the gastrointestinal, genitourinary, and circulatory systems. Some protozoa reproduce by simple binary fission; other forms have complex life cycles. Protozoa have the ability to form cysts or surround themselves with a membrane; this makes them resistant to destruction.

Giardiasis

Giardia lamblia is a protozoan infection that is responsible for epidemic outbreaks of diarrhea, particularly in travelers to Europe and in day care centers in the United States.

Transmission occurs when the child ingests the cysts of the organism on unclean hands. In the intestine, the cysts develop into the mature form of the organism, causing symptoms such as diarrhea, weight loss, abdominal cramps, and nausea.

Diagnosis is made by history and recognition of the mature form of the organism in the stool or on duodenal aspiration. Therapy is with metronidazole (Flagyl) for 7 days (John-Kelly, 2003).

Fungal Infections

Fungi are larger than bacteria; some are unicellular (yeasts), but generally they are multicellular (molds). Fungal infections are most often divided into groups according to the body tissue they infect. Deep mycoses invade internal organs. Transmission is by the inhalation of spores. Subcutaneous mycoses invade skin, subcutaneous tissue, and bone. Infections usually occur from introduction of the fungi into a wound. Superficial mycoses invade only the hair, skin, or nails.

Superficial Fungal Infections

Four superficial fungal infections are seen frequently in children: tinea cruris, pedis, capitis, and corporis.

Tinea Cruris. Tinea cruris (jock itch) occurs on the inner aspects of the thighs and scrotum. It is pruritic. Local application of clotrimazole (Lotrimin) or econazole (Spectazole) liquid or powder destroys the infection (Karch, 2004).

Tinea Pedis. Tinea pedis (athlete's foot) produces skin lesions between the toes and on the plantar surface of

---

the intestinal tract and out the anus to deposit eggs in the anal and perianal region. The movement of the worms causes the anal area to itch, and the child awakens at night crying and scratching. Some of the eggs are then carried from the child's fingernails to the mouth. They hatch in the child's intestinal tract, and the cycle is repeated (Silver, 2003).

The worms are large enough that they can be seen if the child's buttocks are separated when he or she is sleeping. Pressing a piece of cellophane tape against the anus and then looking at it under a microscope will generally reveal pinworm eggs.

Treatment is with a single dose of mebendazole (Vermox) or pyrantel pamoate (Antiminth). Both drugs destroy pinworms. All family members are treated for pinworm infestation because the worms are easily transmitted from person to person. Underclothing, bedding, towels, and nightclothes should be washed before reuse. Teach children to avoid nailbiting and to wash their hands before food preparation or eating to avoid transfer of pinworm eggs to the gastrointestinal tract.

the foot. Pruritic, pinpoint vesicles and fissuring, especially between the toes, may occur. It is treated with liquid preparations of an antifungal agent such as clotrimazole (Lotrimin).

Tinea Capitis. Tinea capitis (ringworm) is a fungal infection that begins as an infection of a single hair follicle but spreads rapidly in a circular pattern to produce a lesion usually approximately 1 inch in diameter (Fig. 43.15). The hairs involved in the lesion generally break off. The circle becomes filled with dirty-appearing scales. Some strains of tinea capitis may be detected because they glow green under a Wood's light. Newer strains of the organism do not do this, so the test is losing its accuracy.

Treatment is with griseofulvin given orally. Adolescents should be cautioned not to use alcohol while taking this drug; this may cause tachycardia. Safety during pregnancy is not established. Children need to avoid strong sunlight during therapy because photosensitivity may occur.

Tinea capitis is not as contagious as was once assumed. Children need not be kept home from school, although they should be cautioned not to exchange towels or combs or other potential fomites. The course of the disease may be long; it may be 3 months before all lesions have faded (Chamberlain, 2003).

Tinea Corporis. Tinea corporis is fungal infection of the epidermal layer of the skin. It presents as a scaly ring of inflammation with a clear area in the center anywhere on the body. Treatment is with a topical antifungal agent such as clotrimazole (Lotrimin).

Candidiasis

Candida albicans is the fungus responsible for candidal (monilial) infections. Candidal organisms grow in the vagina of many adult women and adolescents (candidal vaginitis) (see Chapter 47). Newborns born vaginally may develop an infection of the mucous membrane of the mouth (thrush or oral candidal infection). Thrush is characterized by white

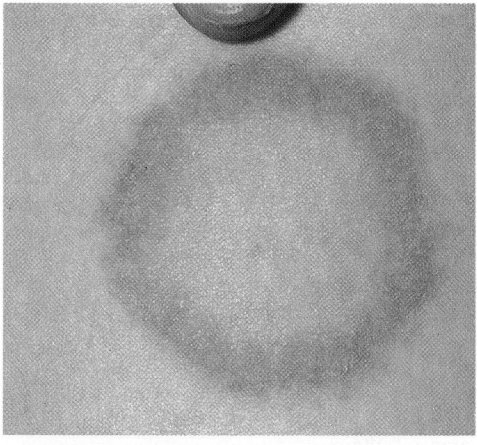

FIGURE 43.15 Ringworm. The fungus spreads rapidly, producing a circular, ringlike lesion. (© SPL/Science Source/Photo Researchers.)

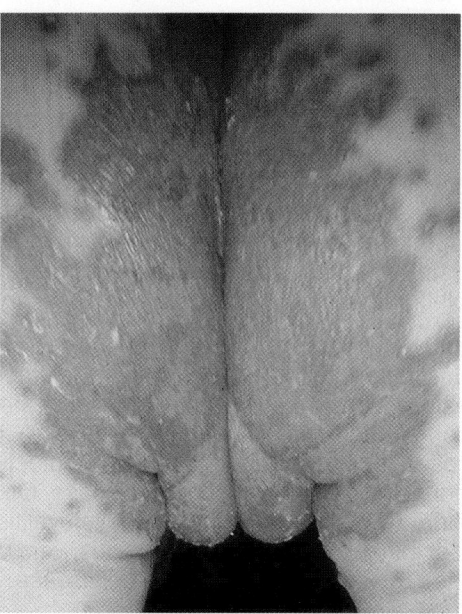

FIGURE 43.16 Monilial diaper rash. Note the intense red color of the rash. (© Custom Medical Stock Photo.)

plaques on an erythematous base on the buccal membrane and the surface of the tongue. It resembles a milk curd left from a recent milk feeding. Thrush plaques do not scrape away, however, whereas milk curds do. The mouth is painful, and the child does not eat well due to the inflammation and local pain.

C. albicans also causes a severe, bright red, sharply circumscribed diaper-area rash (Fig. 43.16). Satellite lesions also may appear. The rash is marked by its intense color, and it does not improve with the usual diaper rash measures, such as Desitin ointment, frequent changing of diapers, or exposure to air.

Nystatin is an example of an effective antifungal drug (Shah, 2003). For oral thrush, it is generally administered by mouth approximately four times a day. It should be dropped into the mouth after feedings so it will remain in contact with the lesions rather than being washed away immediately by a feeding. For diaper rash, a nystatin ointment is prescribed.

Candidiasis can become a generalized infection, especially in a newborn. There is a tendency to think of thrush as a common, almost expected disease of infants. It needs treatment, however, to prevent it from becoming more serious or systemic (Shah, 2003).

Key Points

The incubation period of an infectious disease is the time between the invasion of an organism and the onset of symptoms. The prodromal period is the time between the beginning of nonspecific symptoms and specific symptoms. Children are infectious during the prodromal period. Illness is the stage during which specific symptoms are evident. The convalescent period is the interval between the time symptoms begin to fade and the time the child returns to full wellness.

The chain of infection depends on the presence of a reservoir, a portal of exit, a means of transmission, a portal of entry, and a susceptible host. To reduce the spread of infection, use standard precautions. Transmission-based precautions—airborne, droplet, and contact—also may be necessary.

Common viral infections of childhood include exanthem subitum (roseola), rubella (German measles), measles (rubeola), chickenpox (varicella), herpes zoster, erythema infectiosum (fifth disease), pityriasis rosea, mumps (epidemic parotitis), infectious mononucleosis, and cat-scratch disease. Other important viral infections include poliomyelitis (now almost extinct), herpesvirus infections, verrucae (warts), rabies, and West Nile virus disease.

Streptococcal diseases include scarlet fever and impetigo. Staphylococcal infections include furunculosis (boils), cellulitis, and scalded skin disease. Outbreaks of diphtheria, whooping cough (pertussis), and tetanus (lockjaw) still occur.

Important tick-borne diseases are Rocky Mountain spotted fever and Lyme disease. Parasitic infections are pediculosis capitis (head lice), pediculosis pubis, and scabies. Helminthic infections are roundworms, hookworms, and pinworms. Fungal infections are tinea capitis and tinea corporis (ringworm).

Teaching parents and children about infection control measures and the need for keeping immunizations up to date is essential to reduce the risk of infectious disorders in children.

Critical Thinking Exercises

1. Marty Ireland is the 10-year-old boy you met at the beginning of the chapter. He was diagnosed as having scarlet fever the morning after surgery for appendicitis. Is it likely that Marty contracted this infection while he was hospitalized, or is it more likely that the contact occurred before hospitalization? What is the typical pattern of scarlet fever lesions? What would you recommend to his parents to help reduce the itchiness of the rash?

2. Suppose Marty's mother tells you one disease she is not worried about is Lyme disease, as her children never eat limes. How would you respond to her?

3. Suppose Marty's mother tells you she doesn't intend to have her newborn immunized because she feels the risk of developing a complication from vaccine administration is higher than letting her child contract simple childhood illnesses. How would you counsel her?

4. Examine the National Health Goals related to infectious diseases in children. Most government-sponsored

money for nursing research is allotted based on these goals. What would be a possible research topic to explore pertinent to these goals that would be applicable to the Ireland family and also advance evidence-based practice?

References

Alexander, L., et al. (2004). Ensuring preparedness for potential poliomyelitis outbreaks. *Archives of Pediatrics & Adolescent Medicine, 158*(12), 1106–1112.

Andreae, M. (2004). How to recognize and manage herpes simplex virus type 1 infections. *Contemporary Pediatrics, 21*(2), 41–42.

Armstrong, N., & O'Donnell, N. (2004). Rubella: 40 years after the epidemic. *American Journal for Nurse Practitioners, 8*(4), 51–56.

Atkinson, L. R. (2003). Stomatitis. In M. W. Schwartz (Ed.), *5-minute pediatric consult* (3rd ed.). Philadelphia: Lippincott Williams & Wilkins.

Bagarazzi, M. L. (2003). Scarlet fever. In M. W. Schwartz (Ed.), *5-minute pediatric consult* (3rd ed.). Philadelphia: Lippincott Williams & Wilkins.

Banatvala, J. E., & Brown, D. W. G. (2004). Rubella. *Lancet, 363*(9415), 1127–1137.

Batts, S., & Demers, D. M. (2004). Spectrum and treatment of cat-scratch disease. *Pediatric Infectious Disease Journal, 23*(12), 1161–1162.

Bell, L. M. (2003). Roseola: herpes 6, 7, 8. In M. W. Schwartz (Ed.), *5-minute pediatric consult* (3rd ed.). Philadelphia: Lippincott Williams & Wilkins.

Blevins, J. Y. (2004). Primary herpetic gingivostomatitis in young children. *Dermatology Nursing, 16*(4), 341–344.

Braun, P. C., & Zoidis, J. D. (2004). Viral infections of the lower respiratory tract: understanding influenza, RSV infection, hantavirus pulmonary syndrome, and SARS. *RT: The Journal for Respiratory Care Practitioners, 17*(4), 22–25.

Callahan, J. M. (2003). Tetanus. In M. W. Schwartz (Ed.), *5-minute pediatric consult* (3rd ed.). Philadelphia: Lippincott Williams & Wilkins.

Centers for Disease Control. (2004). *Recommendations for isolation precautions in hospitals.* Washington, D.C.: CDC.

Centers for Disease Control & Prevention (2005). *HIV/AIDS recommendations.* Washington, D.C.: CDC.

Chamberlain, L. (2003). Alopecia (hair loss). In M. W. Schwartz (Ed.), *5-minute pediatric consult* (3rd ed.). Philadelphia: Lippincott Williams & Wilkins.

Chang, M. H., Glynn, M. K., & Groseclose, S. L. (2003). Endemic, notifiable bioterrorism-related diseases, United States, 1992–1999. *Emerging Infectious Diseases, 9*(5), 556–564.

Crane, J. K. (2003). Here comes West Nile virus, again. *Clinical Advisor, 6*(7), 11–12.

Department of Health and Human Services (2000). *Healthy people, 2010.* Washington, D.C.: DHHS.

Duke, T., & Mgone, C. S. (2003). Measles: not just another viral exanthem. *Lancet, 361*(9359), 763–773.

Fishbein, D. B. (2004). Rabies. In M. R. Dambro (Ed.), *Griffith's 5-minute clinical consult.* Philadelphia: Lippincott Williams & Wilkins.

Foster, J. A. (2003). Impetigo. In M. W. Schwartz (Ed.), *5-minute pediatric consult* (3rd ed.). Philadelphia: Lippincott Williams & Wilkins.

Hanrahan, K. S., & Lofgren, M. (2004). Evidence-based practice: examining the risk of toys in the microenvironment of infants in the neonatal intensive care unit. *Advances in Neonatal Care, 4*(4), 184-205.

Ho, J. K. (2003). Warts. In M. W. Schwartz (Ed.), *5-minute pediatric consult* (3rd ed.). Philadelphia: Lippincott Williams & Wilkins.

Hornor, G. (2004). Ano-genital warts in children: sexual abuse or not? *Journal of Pediatric Health Care, 18*(4), 165-170.

John-Kelly, H. A. (2003). Giardiasis. In M. W. Schwartz (Ed.), *5-minute pediatric consult* (3rd ed.). Philadelphia: Lippincott Williams & Wilkins.

Karch, A. M. (2004). *Lippincott's nursing drug guide.* Philadelphia: Lippincott Williams & Wilkins.

Klassen, T. P., et al. (2005). Acyclovir for treating varicella in otherwise healthy children and adolescents. *The Cochrane Library (Oxford) (4)* (CD002980).

Kucik, C. J., Martin, G. L., & Sortor, B. V. (2004). Common intestinal parasites. *American Family Physician, 69*(5), 1161-1168.

Langley, J. M., et al. (2004). Azithromycin is as effective as and better tolerated than erythromycin estolate for the treatment of pertussis. *Pediatrics, 114*(1), 96-101.

Martin, M. E., & Didion, J. (2003). The smallpox threat: the school nurse's role. *Journal of School Nursing, 19*(5), 260-265.

Masters, E. J., et al. (2003). Rocky Mountain spotted fever: a clinician's dilemma. *Archives of Internal Medicine, 163*(7), 769-774.

Morton, J. L., & Schultz, A. A. (2004). Healthy hands: use of alcohol gel as an adjunct to handwashing in elementary school children. *Journal of School Nursing, 20*(3), 161-167.

Newcombe, P. (2004). Treating and preventing tetanus in A&E. *Emergency Nurse, 12*(6), 23-29.

Nollet, F., & de Visser, M. (2004). Postpolio syndrome. *Archives of Neurology, 61*(7), 1142-1144.

Orti, A., et al. (2003). Epstein-Barr virus mononucleosis: neurologic complications. *Clinical Pediatrics, 42*(4), 361-364.

Osterhoudt, K. C. (2003). Epstein-Barr virus (infectious mononucleosis). In M. W. Schwartz (Ed.), *5-minute pediatric consult* (3rd ed.). Philadelphia: Lippincott Williams & Wilkins.

Patel, G. K. (2004). Treatment of staphylococcal scalded skin syndrome. *Expert Review of Antiinfective Therapy, 2*(4), 575-587.

Pellowe, C. M., Macqueen, S., & Coe, L. (2004). Preventing healthcare associated infections in the neonatal unit: the use of evidence-based infection control guidelines. *Journal of Neonatal Nursing, 10*(5), 171-175.

Rudd-Arieta, M. P. (2003). Lyme disease in children: an overview. *Advance for Nurse Practitioners, 11*(6), 77-78.

Schweon, S. (2005). Whooping cough makes its return. *RN, 68*(2), 32-37.

Scribano, P. V. (2003). Pertussis. In M. W. Schwartz (Ed.), *5-minute pediatric consult* (3rd ed.). Philadelphia: Lippincott Williams & Wilkins.

Shah, S. S. (2003). Candidiasis. In M. W. Schwartz (Ed.), *5-minute pediatric consult* (3rd ed.). Philadelphia: Lippincott Williams & Wilkins.

Silver, D. L. (2003). Pinworms. In M. W. Schwartz (Ed.), *5-minute pediatric consult* (3rd ed.). Philadelphia: Lippincott Williams & Wilkins.

Stulberg, D. L., & Wolfrey, J. (2004). Pityriasis rosea. *American Family Physician, 69*(1), 87-91.

Thom, D. H. (2004). Psittacosis. In M. R. Dambro (Ed.), *Griffith's 5-minute clinical consult.* Philadelphia: Lippincott Williams & Wilkins.

Tsarouhas, N. (2003). Mumps/parotitis. In M. W. Schwartz (Ed.), *5-minute pediatric consult* (3rd ed.). Philadelphia: Lippincott Williams & Wilkins.

Vafaie, J., & Schwartz, R. A. (2004). Parvovirus B19 infections. *International Journal of Dermatology, 43*(10), 747-749.

Watson, B. (2003). Chickenpox (varicella, herpes zoster). In M. W. Schwartz (Ed.), *5-minute pediatric consult* (3rd ed.). Philadelphia: Lippincott Williams & Wilkins.

Yan, A. C. (2003). Atopic dermatitis. In M. W. Schwartz (Ed.), *5-minute pediatric consult* (3rd ed.). Philadelphia: Lippincott Williams & Wilkins.

Zimmerman, R. K., & Poland, G. A. (2004). Diphtheria. In M. R. Dambro (Ed.), *Griffith's 5-minute clinical consult.* Philadelphia: Lippincott Williams & Wilkins.

Suggested Readings

Barford, G., Rentz, A. C., & Faix, R. G. (2004). Viral infection and antiviral therapy in the neonatal intensive care unit. *Journal of Perinatal and Neonatal Nursing, 18*(3), 259-274.

Ensor, D. (2005). The significance of herpes simplex for school nurses. *Journal of School Nursing, 21*(1), 10-16.

Eppes, S. C. (2003). Diagnosis, treatment, and prevention of Lyme disease in children. *Paediatric Drugs, 5*(6), 363-372.

Goldrick, B. A. (2004). Vaccine-preventable infections in children. *American Journal of Nursing, 104*(2), 34-37.

Kaplan, D. L. (2003). Rash decisions: is this your patient's rash? *Consultant, 43*(3), 405-408.

Lott, J. W. (2004). Infectious diseases in the newborn and infant. *Newborn and Infant Nursing Reviews, 4*(1), 4-5.

Mackell, S. M. (2003). Vaccinations for the pediatric traveler. *Clinical Infectious Diseases, 37*(11), 1508-1516.

Parker, L. A., & Montrowl, S. J. (2004). Neonatal herpes infection: a review. *Newborn and Infant Nursing Reviews, 4*(1), 62-69.

Rolain, J. M., Jensenius, M., & Raoult, D. (2004). Rickettsial infections: a threat to travellers? *Current Opinion in Infectious Diseases, 17*(5), 433-437.

Swischuk, L. E. (2005). Fever in an infant. *Pediatric Emergency Care, 21*(2), 139-141.

CHAPTER 44

Nursing Care of the Child With a Hematologic Disorder

Key Terms

agranulocytes
allogeneic transplantation
aplastic anemia
autologous transplantation
blood dyscrasias
blood plasma
direct bilirubin
erythroblasts
erythrocytes
erythropoietin
granulocytes
Heinz bodies
hemochromatosis
hemoglobin
hemolysis
hemosiderosis

hypodermoclysis
leukocytes
leukopenia
megakaryocytes
normoblasts
pancytopenia
petechiae
plethora
poikilocytic
priapism
purpura
reticulocytes
sickle-cell crisis
sickle-cell trait
synergeneic transplantation
thrombocytes
thrombocytopenia

Objectives

After mastering the contents of this chapter, you should be able to:

1. Describe the major hematologic disorders of childhood.
2. Assess a child with a hematologic disorder.
3. Formulate nursing diagnoses for a child with a hematologic disorder such as sickle-cell anemia.
4. Identify expected outcomes for a child with a hematologic disorder.
5. Plan nursing care for a child with a hematologic disorder.
6. Implement nursing care related to a child with a hematologic disorder, such as reducing the possibility of infection.
7. Evaluate expected outcomes for achievement and effectiveness of care for a child with a hematologic disorder.
8. Identify National Health Goals related to children with hematologic disorders that nurses could help the nation achieve.
9. Identify areas related to care of children with hematologic disorders that could benefit from additional nursing research or application of evidence-based practice.
10. Use critical thinking to analyze ways that nursing care for a child with a hematologic disorder could be more family-centered.
11. Integrate knowledge of hematologic disorders in children with nursing process to achieve quality maternal and child health nursing care.

Lana is a 4-year-old girl diagnosed with thalassemia major. She has a prominent mandible and wide-spaced upper front teeth from overgrowth of bone marrow centers. Her skin is bronze from the number of transfusions (64) she has received in her short lifetime. Joey, a 7-year-old with sickle-cell anemia, is seen at the same clinic. His growth is only in the 5th percentile, and he's had two vaso-occlusive crises in the past year. "Why did this happen?" Lana's mother asks you. "Why were our two families so unlucky? Why didn't we have healthy children?"

Previous chapters described the growth and development of well children. This chapter adds information about the dramatic changes, both physical and psychosocial, that occur when children have a hematologic disorder. This is important information because it builds a base for care and health teaching.

What additional health teaching does Lana's mother need to help her better understand these hematologic diseases?

After you've studied this chapter, access the accompanying website. Read the patient scenario and answer the questions to further sharpen your skills, grow more familiar with RN-CLEX types of questions, and reward yourself with how much you have learned.

The blood and blood-forming tissues that make up the hematologic system play a vital role in body metabolism: transporting oxygen and nutrients to body cells, removing carbon dioxide from cells, and initiating blood coagulation when vessels are injured. As a result, any alteration in the substance or function of blood or its components can have immediate and life-threatening effects on the functioning of all body systems. For instance, an alteration in the process of coagulation can result in death from acute and uncontrollable blood loss. Inadequate red cell formation results in decreased oxygenation in tissues.

Hematologic disorders, often called **blood dyscrasias,** occur when components of the blood are formed incorrectly or either increase or decrease in amount beyond normal ranges. Most blood dyscrasias in children originate in the bone marrow, where blood cells are formed.

A common hematologic disorder in children is iron-deficiency anemia. The National Health Goals related to this disorder are shown in Box 44.1.

Nursing Process Overview

For the Child With a Hematologic Disorder

● *Assessment*

Many of the symptoms of hematologic disorders begin insidiously, with symptoms such as pallor, lethargy, and bruising (Box 44.2). These seem to be such minor symptoms that parents may not bring their child to a health care facility for some time. They are surprised to learn when they do that such subtle symptoms can signify the presence of a serious illness.

BOX 44.1 FOCUS ON . . .

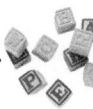

NATIONAL HEALTH GOALS

A National Health Goal that addresses iron-deficiency anemia, the most common blood disorder in children, is:

• Reduce the incidence of iron deficiency among children aged 1 to 2 years to less than 5% and among women of child-bearing age to less than 7%, from baselines of 9% and 11% (DHHS, 2000).

Nurses can help the nation achieve this goal by educating parents about the importance of women taking an iron supplement during pregnancy and adding iron-rich cereal to their infants' diets. Nursing research questions that could add important information for prevention include: what are ways of increasing adherence among pregnant women that would help ensure that all women take an iron supplement during pregnancy; and do infants maintain higher iron levels when cereal is eaten with milk or orange juice?

BOX 44.2 ASSESSMENT

Assessing a Child With a Hematologic Disorder

History
Chief concern: Fatigue, easy bruising, epistaxis.
Past medical history: Low birthweight; blood loss at birth; lack of vitamin K administration at birth.
Nutrition: "Picky eater" or presence of pica. Increasd milk intake.
Past illnesses: History of recent illness; history of recent medicine ingestion.
Family history: Inherited blood disorder; parents known to have sickle-cell trait, thalassemia minor, or hemophilia in family.

Physical examination

General appearance	*Possible significance*
Obese infant	Iron-deficiency anemia
Fatigue	Anemia
Eyes	
Retinal hemorrhage	Sickle-cell anemia
Face	
Bossing of maxillary bone	Thalassemia
Mouth	
Pale mucous membrane	Iron-deficiency anemia
Ecchymotic or bleeding gumline	Decreased coagulation ability
Heart	
Increased rate, possible murmur	Anemia
Skin	
Petechiae, ecchymosis Blood oozing from wound or injection point	Decreased coagulation ability
Jaundice	Hemolytic anemia
Pallor	Anemia
Bronze color	Frequent blood transfusion
Abdomen	
Pain on palpation	Sickle-cell anemia
Increased liver or spleen size	Hemolytic anemia
Genitourinary	
Delayed secondary sex characteristics	Sickle-cell anemia
Extremities	
Spoon nails	Iron-deficiency anemia
Joint swelling, pain	Hemophilia, sickle-cell crisis
Neurologic	
Weak muscle tone	Iron-deficiency anemia

Many hematologic disorders are inherited. When a child is diagnosed with one, parents may feel guilty or blame themselves or their partner for their child's disease. It may be difficult for parents to support a child during an illness when they need intensive support themselves because they feel the illness is their fault. Be certain both parents and children receive the support and comfort they need.

Asking at routine checkups about a child's dietary intake often reveals iron-deficiency anemia. Many babies with this problem have been drinking too much milk and not eating enough iron-containing foods. This makes them iron-deficient, but aside from paleness and irritability, they appear plump and "healthy." Their parents do not suspect their baby's appearance masks a nutritional deficiency.

● *Nursing Diagnosis*

Nursing diagnoses commonly used with children who have hematologic disorders are:

- Deficient knowledge related to the cause of child's illness
- Imbalanced nutrition, less than body requirements, related to parental lack of knowledge of need for iron-rich foods
- Anxiety related to frequent blood-sampling procedures
- Pain related to tissue ischemia
- Compromised family coping related to long-term care needs of child with a chronic hematologic disorder

● *Outcome Identification and Planning*

When helping parents plan outcomes, be certain that the outcomes are realistic for the child and family. The number of blood-sampling procedures, for example, cannot be reduced, but a child can be helped, with distraction techniques, to deal with the pain and anxiety the procedures produce.

Children with hematologic disorders often are prescribed long-term medication such as a corticosteroid. When a child appears very ill, parents are usually very conscientious about giving such medicine. When a child has a disorder with few symptoms, however, like a blood dyscrasia, it is easy for parents to forget to give the medication. In addition, a child may refuse to take the medication because it tastes bad or upsets the stomach. Planning includes helping parents devise ways to disguise the taste or remember to give the medication over the long term.

Nutritional planning is another area that needs consideration. Parents of children with iron-deficiency anemia, for example, may need to modify meal plans not only for the child but also for the entire family; this is not necessarily easy to do, because iron-rich foods are expensive. If a child is a "fussy eater," parents may need a great deal of support to insist that the child eat foods containing iron rather than giving the child what he or she wants. If the child will be restricted for long periods because the immune system is compromised as a part of the illness, planning must include ways to keep the child interested in activities that promote development. Parents may need help investigating possible resources for education and support.

● *Implementation*

Nursing interventions for children with hematologic disorders include helping to obtain specimens for testing and assisting with blood or stem cell transfusions. Remember that a finger puncture for blood is often as painful as a venipuncture (and more painful afterward because the fingertip is irritated every time the child attempts to use it). Suggesting that blood be drawn by means of an intermittent device may reduce the number of times a child is subjected to venipuncture. Applying EMLA cream before finger sticks or venipunctures also helps to reduce pain and improve cooperation with these procedures. Even so, children may need some therapeutic playtime with a syringe and a doll to express their anger about constant invasion by needles.

Because of the chronicity of some of the hematologic disorders, parents and children often need the support of outside agencies. Some organizations helpful for referral are the Aplastic Anemia Foundation of America (*www.aplastic.org*), Sickle Cell Disease Association of America (*www.sicklecelldisease.org*), American Society of Pediatric Hematology and Oncology (*www.aspho.org*), and National Hemophilia Foundation (*www.hemophilia.org*).

● *Outcome Evaluation*

Evaluation focuses on whether short-term outcomes were achieved (e.g., the moderation of pain or elimination of anxiety in the child undergoing testing or treatment) and progress is being made toward the achievement of long-term outcomes (e.g., improving the ability of the family to manage the stress of raising a child with a chronic illness or deal with frequently occurring health crises).

Examples of expected outcomes that suggest goals were achieved are:

- Parents correctly state the most frequent causes of iron-deficiency anemia.
- Child states she feels better able to cope with blood-sampling procedures through the use of imagery.
- Parents describe realistic plans to ensure adherence to long-term medication administration.
- Parents voice they understand importance of preventing dehydration in school-age child with sickle-cell anemia.

STRUCTURE AND FUNCTION OF BLOOD

Blood Formation and Components

The formation of blood cells begins in the fetal yolk sac as early as week 2 of intrauterine life. By month 2 of intrauterine life, the liver and spleen begin forming blood components. At approximately month 4, the bone marrow becomes and remains the active center for the origination of blood cells. As in extrauterine life, the spleen serves as the organ for the destruction of blood cells once their normal life span has passed.

The total volume of blood in the body is roughly proportional to body weight: 85 mL/kg at birth, 75 mL/kg at 6 months of age, and 70 mL/kg after the first year. The **blood plasma** (the liquid portion containing proteins, hormones, enzymes, and electrolytes) is in equilibrium with the fluid of the interstitial tissue spaces. Although it is important in diseases causing vomiting and diarrhea (when it may become depleted, leading to dehydration), plasma is not a major site of hematologic disease. The formed elements—the erythrocytes (red blood cells), leukocytes (white blood cells), and thrombocytes (platelets)—are the portions most affected by hematologic disorders in children.

Erythrocytes (Red Blood Cells)

Erythrocytes (red blood cells [RBCs]) function chiefly to transport oxygen to and carry carbon dioxide from body cells. RBCs are formed under the stimulation of **erythropoietin,** a hormone produced by the kidneys that is stimulated whenever a child has tissue hypoxia. Children with kidney disease often have a low number of RBCs because erythropoietin secretion is inadequate in diseased kidneys. Polycythemia, or an overproduction of RBCs, can occur in children who experience prolonged systemic hypoxia because of erythropoietin overproduction.

RBCs form first as **erythroblasts** (large, nucleated cells), then mature through **normoblast** and **reticulocyte** stages to mature, nonnucleated erythrocytes. Approximately 1% of RBCs are in the reticulocyte stage at all times. An elevated reticulocyte count indicates that rapid production of new RBCs is occurring. This is seen in children with iron-deficiency anemia once iron therapy is begun and the body is again able to produce RBCs. The absence of a nucleus in the mature red blood cell allows for increased space for oxygen transport, but it also limits the life of cells because metabolic processes are limited. At the end of their life span (about 120 days), erythrocytes are destroyed through phagocytosis by reticuloendothelial cells, found in the highest proportion in the spleen.

In infants, the long bones of the body are filled with red marrow actively producing RBCs. In early childhood, yellow marrow begins to replace this in long bones, so blood element production is then carried out mainly in the ribs, scapulae, vertebrae, and skull bones. The yellow marrow remaining in the extremities can be activated if necessary to produce additional blood products.

At birth, an infant has approximately 5 million RBCs per cubic millimeter of blood. This concentration diminishes rapidly in the first months, reaching a low of approximately 4.1 million per cubic millimeter at 3 to 4 months of age. The number then slowly increases until adolescence, when the adult value of approximately 4.9 million per cubic millimeter is reached.

Hemoglobin. The component of RBCs that allows them to carry out the transport of oxygen is **hemoglobin,** a complex protein. Hemoglobin is composed of globin, a protein (like all proteins) dependent on nitrogen metabolism for its formation, and heme, an iron-containing pigment. Deficiency of either iron stores or nitrogen, therefore, will interfere with the synthesis of hemoglobin. It is the heme portion that combines with oxygen and carbon dioxide for transport.

The hemoglobin in erythrocytes during fetal life is different from that formed after birth. Fetal hemoglobin has a special affinity for oxygen, so it can absorb oxygen at the low oxygen tension that exists in utero. It is composed of two alpha and two gamma polypeptide chains. At birth, 40% to 70% of the infant's hemoglobin is fetal hemoglobin (hemoglobin F). This is gradually replaced by adult hemoglobin (hemoglobin A) during the first 6 months of life. Hemoglobin A is composed of two alpha and two beta chains. For this reason, diseases such as sickle-cell anemia or the thalassemias, which are disorders of the beta chains, do not become apparent clinically until this hemoglobin change has occurred (at approximately 6 months of age). However, because some hemoglobin A is present even in early intrauterine life, they can be diagnosed prenatally by hemoglobin analysis or electrophoresis.

The hemoglobin amount in blood varies according to the number of RBCs present and the average amount of hemoglobin each cell contains. Hemoglobin levels are highest at birth (13.7 to 20.1 g/100 mL); they reach a low at approximately 3 months of age (9.5 to 14.5 g/100 mL), and then gradually rise again until adult values are reached at puberty (11 to 16 g/100 mL).

Bilirubin. After an RBC reaches its life span of approximately 120 days, it disintegrates and its protein component is preserved by specialized cells in the liver and spleen (reticuloendothelial cells) for further use. Iron is released for reuse by the bone marrow to construct new RBCs. As the heme portion is degraded, it is converted into protoporphyrin. Protoporphyrin is then further broken down into indirect bilirubin. Indirect bilirubin is fat-soluble and cannot be excreted by the kidneys in this state. It is therefore converted by the liver enzyme glucuronyl transferase into **direct bilirubin,** which is water-soluble. This is then excreted in bile.

In the newborn, generally liver function is so immature that the conversion to direct bilirubin cannot be made. Because of this, bilirubin remains in the indirect form. When the level of indirect bilirubin in the blood rises to more than 7 mg/100 mL, it permeates outside the circulatory system, and the infant shows signs of yellowing or jaundice. If excessive **hemolysis** (destruction) of RBCs occurs from other than natural causes, a child will also show signs of jaundice.

Leukocytes (White Blood Cells)

Leukocytes (white blood cells [WBCs]) are nucleated cells. They are few in number compared with RBCs, with approximately 1 WBC to every 500 RBCs. Their primary function is defense against antigen invasion. There are two main forms of WBCs: **granulocytes** (those with granules in the cell cytoplasm) and **agranulocytes** (those without granules in the cell cytoplasm). Granulocytes (often referred to as polymorphonuclear forms) are further differentiated as neutrophils, basophils, and eosinophils. The agranulocytic leukocytes are further differentiated as lymphocytes and monocytes.

A typical total white cell count is 5000 to 10,000 cells per cubic millimeter of blood. The WBC count in newborns is approximately 20,000 per cubic millimeter, a high level caused by the trauma of birth. In the newborn, granulocytes are the most common WBCs. By 14 to 30 days of life, the total WBC count falls to approximately 12,000 per cubic millimeter, and lymphocytes become the dominant type. By 4 years of age, the WBC count reaches an adult level (5,000 to 10,000 cells/mm^3), and granulocytes are again the dominant type. Leukocytes are produced in response to need. Their life span varies from approximately 6 hours to unknown intervals.

Thrombocytes (Platelets)

When blood is centrifuged in a test tube, plasma rises to the top as a clear yellow fluid; red cells sink to the bottom as a dark-red paste. Between these two layers a thin white strip (often termed a buffy coat) forms that consists of the WBCs and thrombocytes. **Thrombocytes** are round, nonnucleated bodies formed by the bone marrow. Their function is capillary hemostasis and primary coagulation. The normal range is 150,000 to 300,000 per cubic millimeter after the first year. Immature thrombocytes are termed **megakaryocytes.** If large numbers of these are present in serum, it indicates that rapid production of platelets is occurring.

Blood Coagulation

Effective blood coagulation depends on a complex series of events including a combination of blood and tissue factors released from the plasma (the intrinsic pathway) and from injured tissue (the extrinsic pathway). The plasma-released factors are factors VIII, IX, and XII. Factors released from injured tissues are a tissue factor (an incomplete thromboplastin or factor III), plus factors VII and X. Together, the pathways form factor V. The names for coagulation factors are given in Box 44.3.

When a vessel is injured, vasoconstriction occurs in the area proximal to the injury, narrowing the vessel lumen and reducing the amount of blood to the injured area. Platelets begin to adhere to the damaged vessel site and to one another, forming a platelet plug. This is the first stage of clotting (Fig. 44.1).

In the second stage, factors from either the intrinsic or the extrinsic system combine with platelet phospholipid to form complete thromboplastin.

In the third stage, thromboplastin converts prothrombin (factor II) to thrombin if ionized calcium is present. The production of prothrombin and factors VII, IX, and X depends on the presence of vitamin K. This stage will be incomplete if levels of any of factors VIII through XII, vitamin K, or calcium are deficient.

In the fourth stage, thrombin converts fibrinogen (factor I) to fibrin. Fibrin strands form a mesh incorporating RBCs, WBCs, and platelets to form a permanent protective seal at the site of injury. Factor XIII (fibrin stabilizing factor) acts to make the fibrin clot insoluble and permanent.

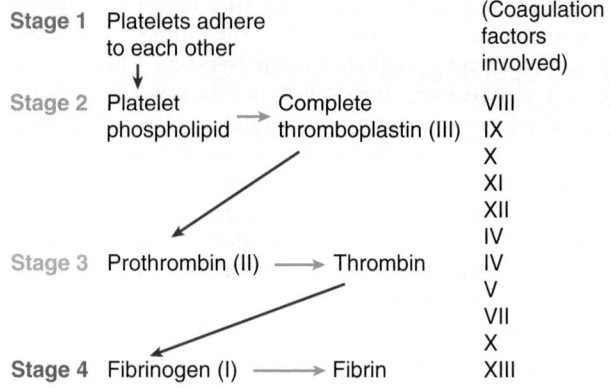

FIGURE 44.1 Steps in blood coagulation.

To prevent too much coagulation after the seal is complete, plasminogen is then converted to plasmin (a fibrinolysin) near the injury to halt the clotting sequence. Blood coagulation problems will result if any step or factor in the process is inadequate. Common tests for blood coagulation are described in Table 44.1.

ASSESSMENT OF AND THERAPEUTIC TECHNIQUES FOR HEMATOLOGIC DISORDERS

Bone Marrow Aspiration and Biopsy

Bone marrow aspiration provides samples of bone marrow so that the type and quantity of cells can be determined (Perkins, 2004). In children, the aspiration sites include the iliac crests or spines (rather than the sternum, which is commonly used in adults; Fig. 44.2) because these sites have larger marrow compartments during childhood. Also, performing the test here is usually less frightening for children. In neonates, the anterior tibia can be used.

For a bone marrow aspiration, a child lies prone on a treatment table. Use of a hard table rather than a bed is advantageous because pressure is needed to insert the needle through the surface of the bone into the marrow compartment. Conscious sedation may be used to help reduce the child's fear. Topical anesthesia helps reduce pain.

The area of the aspiration is cleaned with an antiseptic solution and draped. The overlying skin is infiltrated with a local anesthetic. After a few minutes, a large-bore needle and stylus is introduced through the overlying tissue into the bone. This involves considerable pressure. When the marrow cavity is reached, the stylus is removed, a syringe is attached to the needle, and bone marrow is aspirated (appears as thick blood in the syringe). The syringe is then removed, and marrow is expelled onto a slide and allowed to dry. After being sprayed with a preservative, it is taken to the laboratory for analysis. The aspiration needle is removed, and pressure is applied to the puncture site to prevent bleeding. After another few minutes, a pressure dressing is applied.

A child feels pain from the local anesthetic injection and hard pressure while the needle is inserted. Some report a sharp pain when the marrow is actually aspirated. If con-

---

BOX 44.3

Blood Coagulation Factors

   I: Fibrinogen
  II: Prothrombin
 III: Thromboplastin
 IV: Calcium
  V: Labile factor (platelet phospholipids)
 VII: Stable factor
VIII: Antihemophilic factor
 IX: Christmas factor; antihemophilic factor B; plasma thromboplastin component
  X: Stuart factor
 XI: Plasma thromboplastin antecedent (antihemophilic factor C)
 XII: Hageman factor
XIII: Fibrin stabilizing factor

Numbers refer to the order in which factors were discovered, not to the order of action in coagulation.

TABLE 44.1

Tests for Blood Coagulation

Test	Definition	Normal Value
Prothrombin time (PT)	Measures action of prothrombin after complete thromboplastin is added to the blood in a test tube; reveals deficiencies in prothrombin, factors V, VII, and X. International Normalized Ratio (INR) is a comparative rating of PT ratios that allows for more sensitive analysis.	11–13 sec (PT) 2.0–3.0 (INR)
Partial thromboplastin time (PTT)	Measures activity of thromboplastin after incomplete thromboplastin is added to blood in a test tube; reveals deficiencies in thromboplastin, factors VIII–XII	30–45 sec
Bleeding time	Measures the time required for bleeding at a stab wound on the earlobe to cease; reveals deficiencies in platelet formation and vasoconstrictive ability	3–10 min
Clot retraction	Measures platelet function; interval from placement of blood in a tube to the point clot shrinks and expels serum	Retraction at side of test tube in 1 h; complete in 24 h
Tourniquet	Measures capillary fragility and platelet function; response of tissue to application of tourniquet to forearm for 5–10 min	0–2 petechiae per 2-cm area
Prothrombin consumption time	Evaluates thromboplastin function; child's blood is allowed to clot and PT is then done on the serum; if clot formation used a great deal of prothrombin (as it should), serum prothrombin time will be brief; prolongation denotes defects in thromboplastin function	Approximately 20 sec
Thromboplastin generation time	Tests basic ability to form thromboplastin; difficult test to do; ordered rarely to distinguish factor VIII from factor IX defects	12 sec or less
Plasma fibrinogen	Measures stage 4 clotting process; level of fibrinogen in blood	200–400 mg/100 mL plasma
Venous clotting time (Lee-White)	Measures factor defects in stages 2 and 4; time it takes venous blood to clot in a test tube	9–12 min

scious sedation is used, monitor vital signs until the child is fully awake. Monitor pulse and blood pressure and observe the dressing every 15 minutes for the first hour after the procedure to be certain that no bleeding is occurring. Keep the child fairly quiet for the first hour by playing a quiet game or other activity. Allow young children an opportunity for therapeutic play with a doll and syringe to help them express their feelings about such a painful, invasive procedure. If the procedure was done as an ambulatory procedure, instruct parents to take the child's temperature 12 and 24 hours after the procedure to detect infection.

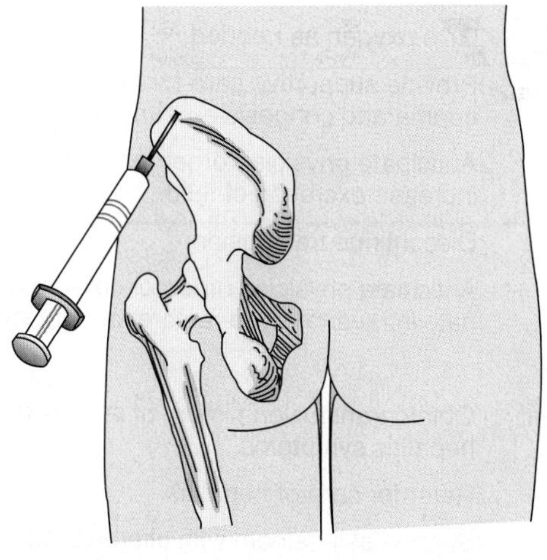

FIGURE 44.2 A common site used for bone marrow aspiration in children is the iliac crest. In neonates, the anterior tibia may be used.

Blood Transfusion

Transfusions of blood or its products is used in the treatment of many disorders, including the anemias and primary immunodeficiency disorders (see Chapter 42). A variety of forms are available, including whole blood, packed RBCs, washed RBCs (as much "foreign" matter is removed as possible to reduce the possibility of blood reaction), plasma, plasma factors, platelets, WBCs, and albumin. No matter what the blood product, it is important to be certain it has been carefully matched with the child's blood type. Blood must be infused with a solution as nearly isotonic as possible (normal saline). If blood is given with a hypertonic solution, fluid will be drawn out of the RBCs, causing them to shrink; if infused with a hypotonic solution, fluid will be drawn into the cells, and they will burst. In both instances, they will be worthless.

Packed RBCs are the most common form of transfusion in children because they help minimize the risk of fluid overload. The usual amount of blood transfused to children is 15 mL/kg body weight. The commonly accepted rate for transfusions in a child is 10 mL/kg/h unless the child has hypovolemic shock and volume equilibrium needs to be established. An infusion of packed RBCs at a proportion of 15 mL/kg can be expected to raise the hematocrit level 5 points. A transfusion of platelets will elevate the platelet count by approximately 10,000 cells. Platelets last only approximately 10 days, so transfusions of these must be repeated every 10 days.

Even if given slowly, a blood transfusion is always a strain on a child's circulation beyond that of a regular intravenous infusion, because the circulatory system must accommodate a thick, difficult-to-mobilize fluid.

Before any transfusion, ensure that a signed consent form is obtained to respect sociocultural or religious beliefs. Also obtain vital signs to establish a baseline. Monitor vital signs every 15 minutes during the first hour and approximately every half hour for the remainder of the transfusion. Give the infusion slowly for the first 15 minutes; then increase the rate to 10 mL/kg/h if no reaction occurs. Common symptoms of blood transfusion reactions are shown in Table 44.2.

Provide an enjoyable activity for a child during a transfusion. Without this, a child can become bored and may attempt to increase the infusion rate to speed up the process.

Stem Cell Transplantation

Stem cell transplantation is the intravenous infusion of hematopoietic stem cells from bone marrow obtained by

---

TABLE 44.2

Common Blood Transfusion Reaction Symptoms

Symptoms	Cause	Time of Occurrence	Nursing Interventions
Headache, chills, back pain, dyspnea, hypotension, hemoglobinuria (blood in urine)	Anaphylactic reaction to incompatible blood; agglutination of red blood cells occurs; kidney tubules may become blocked, resulting in kidney failure	Immediately after start of transfusion	Discontinue transfusion. Maintain normal saline infusion for accessible intravenous line. Administer oxygen as necessary. Anticipate physician order for diuretic to increase renal tubule flow and reduce tubule plugging and/or heparin to reduce intravascular coagulation.
Pruritus, urticaria (hives), wheezing	Allergy to protein components of transfusion	Within first hour after start of transfusion	Discontinue transfusion temporarily. Give oxygen as needed. Anticipate physician order for antihistamine to reduce symptoms.
Increased temperature	Possible contaminant in transfused blood	Approximately 1 hour after start of transfusion	Discontinue transfusion. Obtain blood culture to rule out bacterial invasion as ordered.
Increased pulse, dyspnea	Circulatory overload	During course of transfusion	Discontinue transfusion. Give oxygen as needed. Provide supportive care for pulmonary edema and congestive heart failure. Anticipate physician order for diuretic to increase excretion of fluid.
Muscle cramping, twitching of extremities, convulsion	Acid-citrate-dextrose anticoagulant in transfusion is combining with serum calcium and causing hypocalcemia	During course of transfusion	Discontinue transfusion. Anticipate physician order for calcium gluconate intravenously to restore calcium level.
Fever, jaundice, lethargy, tenderness over liver	Hepatitis from contaminated transfusion	Weeks or months after transfusion	Obtain transfusion history of any child with hepatitis symptoms. Refer for care of hepatitis.
Bronze-colored skin	Hemosiderosis or deposition of iron from transfusion in skin	After repeated transfusions	Support self-esteem with altered body image. Administer iron-chelating agent (deferoxamine) as ordered to help reduce level of accumulating iron.

marrow aspiration or from peripheral or umbilical cord blood from a donor to reestablish marrow function in a child with defective or nonfunctioning bone marrow. Donors are compatible when their human leukocyte antigen (HLA) system matches that of the recipient (Alcoser & Rodgers, 2003).

Hematologic stem cell transplantation has become a relatively common procedure for children with blood disorders such as acquired aplastic anemia, sickle-cell anemia, thalassemia, and leukemia and some forms of immune dysfunction diseases. Stem cells can be recovered from circulating peripheral blood after the stimulation of stem cell production by a cytokine or stem cell colony-stimulating factor. Stem cell transplants are most successful when the recipient has not already received multiple blood transfusions that have sensitized him or her to blood products. Success also depends on the HLA compatibility of donated stem cells to a child's blood. An identical twin is the ideal donor; a parent or sibling may be next best, although compatibility is not guaranteed. Siblings have a 25% chance of being compatible.

Allogeneic transplantation involves the transfer of stem cells from an immune-compatible (histocompatible) donor, usually a sibling, although a national registry allows compatible volunteer donors to be located. The term **synergeneic transplantation** is used when the donor and recipient are genetically identical (i.e., identical twins). In **autologous transplantation,** the child's own stem cells are used. The stem cells are aspirated from the bone marrow or obtained from circulating blood, treated to remove abnormal cells, and then reinfused.

Parents who are found to be incompatible donors may feel guilty and frustrated they could not do more for their child. If the most compatible person is a young sibling, health care personnel and parents alike may have some reservations about submitting a young child to bone marrow aspiration (Pentz et al., 2004). There is no guarantee that the graft will be accepted by the recipient, or that improvement will occur. However, with good tissue compatibility in the absence of infection, this can be effective in most children.

To prevent a child from rejecting newly transplanted donor stem cells by the T lymphocytes, a drug such as cyclophosphamide (Cytoxan) will be administered intravenously to the child before the procedure to suppress marrow and T-lymphocyte production. This may cause nausea and vomiting. Total body irradiation to destroy the child's marrow also may be done. This is a difficult time for the child because total body irradiation causes extreme nausea, vomiting, and diarrhea.

To obtain stem cells from peripheral blood, donors receive 5 days of a colony-stimulating factor to promote the release of stem cells into the peripheral blood. Blood is then collected by a plasmapheresis technique. If umbilical cord blood is used, it is drained from the placenta immediately after birth. It is then infused into the recipient by usual blood infusion technique.

If the marrow will be taken directly from the bone, on the day of the procedure, the donor is admitted to the hospital for a 1-day stay and receives epidural anesthesia or conscious sedation, as multiple bone marrow aspirations from the posterior iliac crests are necessary for retrieval.

The marrow is strained to remove fat and bone particles and any other unwanted cells. An anticoagulant is added to prevent clotting. It is then infused intravenously into the recipient's bloodstream.

Because an infused stem cell solution is fairly thick, the infusion takes 60 to 90 minutes. Do not use a filter that is normally used for the infusion of blood products, because this would filter out marrow tissue. Monitor the child's cardiac rate and rhythm during the infusion to detect circulatory overload or pulmonary emboli from unfiltered particles.

Fever and chills are common reactions to a stem cell transplant infusion. Acetaminophen (Tylenol), diazepam (Valium), or diphenhydramine hydrochloride (Benadryl) may be prescribed to reduce this reaction.

After the infusion, take the child's temperature at 1 hour and then every 4 hours to detect infection that could occur because the child's WBCs are nonfunctional from radiation or chemotherapy. Reinforce strict handwashing and limit the child's diet to cooked foods to reduce exposure to bacteria. The WBC count must be measured daily; bone marrow aspirations or venous blood samples are scheduled at regular intervals to assess the growth of the new marrow.

Almost immediately after the infusion, stem cells begin to migrate from the child's bloodstream into the marrow. If engraftment occurs (the transplant is accepted), new RBCs can be detected in the peripheral blood in approximately 3 weeks. WBCs and platelet cells may not return to normal for up to 1 year after a transplant.

? *What if...* Lana's 12-year-old sister donates stem cells to Lana, but the stem cell transplant does not "take"? How would you explain to the donor child that she did not fail?

NURSING DIAGNOSES AND RELATED INTERVENTIONS

Nursing Diagnosis: Anxiety related to lack of knowledge about procedure and expected outcome of stem cell transplant

Outcome Evaluation: Parents state the reason for the transplant; state they are agreeable to the procedure even though they know the transplant may not be successful, depending on immunologic factors that are not totally known to science.

Stem cell transplantation is an emotional experience not only for the child but also for the parents and the marrow donor (Forinder, 2004). Be certain that the child who receives the transplant and the donor understand they are not responsible for the outcome of the transplant. Its success does not depend on their behavior or what kind of person they are but on immunologic factors over which they have no control. If a sibling was the donor, he or she may become jealous of the recipient child, who is the center of attention. Be certain donors know that if bone marrow aspiration was done, the donor sites will feel tender afterward. Conscious sedation will leave them feeling exhausted for several days. Donors who have undergone bone marrow aspiration generally are asked to return to their primary care provider in 24 to 48 hours to check whether the aspiration sites are infected (local swelling, redness, intense pain, or fever).

Nursing Diagnosis: Risk for delayed growth and development related to extended restrictions and infection control precautions in hospital or at home

Outcome Evaluation: Parents express satisfaction with child's ongoing development. Objective tests of developmental stage show child within age-appropriate ranges.

Children may be restricted from interacting with other children to prevent them from contracting an infection following stem cell transplantation. At the same time, be certain they are isolated from health care providers as little as possible. Visit the room frequently; provide sterilized play materials as appropriate. Most children grow tired of a restricted diet and may crave fresh fruits and vegetables. Thick-skinned fruits such as bananas and oranges can be given soon after the procedure, but unwashed foods are avoided as they could carry bacteria.

Be certain children are well prepared for all procedures. Allow them to make as many choices as they can about their care to help them preserve a sense of control over their life. Children who receive a transplant need periods of therapeutic play incorporated into their care so they can begin to express their anger and frustration at the number of intravenous therapies or follow-up bone marrow aspirations they require. Measures to help children cope with pain, such as imagery, can help a child accept one more painful procedure. Encourage parents to spend time with their child during long periods of hospitalization for additional support.

Provisions for completing schoolwork need to be made as soon as the child has a return of RBCs in the peripheral blood (approximately 3 weeks). On the day of discharge, parents may be surprised that the child's blood replacement is not complete and that they will need to continue infection control measures and restrictions at home. Help them locate a support group in their community if possible. Be certain they feel free to call the transplant center after discharge if they have any problems. Once the danger of infection has passed and the restrictions can be discontinued, parents may still be reluctant to allow their child outside, fearing that their child may still be susceptible to infection. Frequent follow-up for the next year is necessary to ensure that a child is free of infection until the WBC count has risen to normal levels. Follow-up should also ad-

dress the parents' commitment to allowing their child to pursue age-appropriate activities and avoiding overprotection.

If children are prepared adequately for these painful or restrictive procedures and supported throughout, they should have no long-term consequences. Not all stem cell transplants are successful, however, and some children will die of the original disease that necessitated the transplant. Some children develop an infection despite all precautions and die of sepsis in the weeks immediately after the transplant.

Graft-Versus-Host Disease

Graft-versus-host disease (GVHD) is a potentially lethal immunologic response of donor T cells against the tissue of the bone marrow recipient (Alcoser & Rodgers, 2003). The symptoms range from mild to severe and include a rash and general malaise beginning 7 to 14 days after the transplant. Latent virus infections may become active. Severe symptoms include high fever and diarrhea and liver and spleen enlargement as cells are destroyed.

Because there is no known cure for GVHD, prevention is essential. Careful tissue typing; intravenous administration of methotrexate, a corticosteroid, or cyclosporine before transplant; and irradiation of blood products (which helps to inactivate mature T lymphocytes) before stem cell infusion all can help reduce the incidence of this complication. Drugs such as methotrexate and cyclosporine kill all rapidly growing cells, including WBCs and T lymphocytes, so administration of these drugs after transplantation cannot be continued because they would also slow the growth of the host's new stem cells. Depletion of mature T lymphocytes from donor bone marrow before it is infused into the child offers good results, as does the administration of corticosteroids or antithymocyte globulin (ATG), an immune serum, to children after the transplant (Bevans & Shalabi, 2004).

Checkpoint Question 1

Lana, who has thalassemia major, is scheduled for a bone marrow transplant. Which is the best instruction for her regarding this?

a. She must not move while the bone marrow is infused into her.
b. She will not be allowed to eat raw fruit following the transplant.
c. Her hip bones will feel tender from the marrow transplantation.
d. She will not need any further bone marrow aspirations after this.

Splenectomy

One of the purposes of the spleen is to remove damaged or aged blood cells. This poses a difficulty with diseases such as sickle-cell anemia and the thalassemias because the spleen recognizes the typical cells of these diseases as damaged and destroys them. This causes these children to have a continuous anemia, with hemoglobin levels as low as 5 to 9 g/mL. In some children, therefore, removal of the spleen (splenectomy) will not cure the basic defect of the blood cells but will limit the degree of anemia. Splenectomy formerly required an abdominal incision but today it can be performed by laparoscopy (Essien et al., 2003).

A second function of the spleen is to strain the plasma for invading organisms so that phagocytes and lymphocytes can destroy them. Children who have had their spleen removed appear to be very susceptible to the pneumococcal infections because this bacteria is no longer removed systematically from the body. After surgery, oral penicillin is given as a prophylactic antibiotic for a year or two to guard against infection. The child should receive pneumococcal and meningococcal vaccines as well as routine immunizations, including influenza vaccine. Teach parents about signs of infection (cough, fever, general malaise), and encourage them to report any such signs immediately.

HEALTH PROMOTION AND RISK MANAGEMENT

Many hematologic disorders such as sickle-cell anemia and hemophilia are inherited disorders. Health promotion and disease prevention, therefore, begins with ensuring that families have access to genetic counseling so they can be aware of the incidence of a disorder in their family and the potential for the disease to develop in their child.

The most frequently occurring anemia in children, iron-deficiency anemia, is preventable. This condition could be virtually eliminated in infants if all bottle-fed infants were fed iron-fortified formula for the first year and, when cereal is introduced, iron-fortified types are used. The disorder occurs again with a high incidence in adolescents because adolescent diets tend to be low in meat and green vegetables, the chief dietary sources of iron. Adolescents who begin vegetarian diets become especially prone to developing the disorder. Counseling parents of young children to maintain well-child visits and urging adolescents to ingest iron-rich foods could have a major impact on decreasing the incidence of the disorder.

Aplastic anemia, or the inability to form blood elements, can be acquired if a child is exposed to a toxic drug or chemical. Educating parents about the importance of keeping poisons out of the reach of children could help decrease the incidence of this disorder.

Nurses can also help make the therapy for these disorders much less painful and distressing than it was in the past. All hematologic disorders require obtaining blood specimens for diagnosis and continued testing for follow-up. Many therapies include blood product transfusion. The use of EMLA cream or topical lidocaine can greatly reduce the pain of venipuncture. Helping a child to use a distraction technique such as imagery can reduce apprehension or fear associated with the procedures or treatments.

DISORDERS OF THE RED BLOOD CELLS

Most RBC disorders fall into the category of the anemias, or a reduction in the number or function of erythrocytes.

BOX 44.4 FOCUS ON . . .

DIVERSITY OF CARE

Blood dyscrasias do not occur at equal rates in all countries, because many of these disorders are inherited. Sickle-cell anemia occurs mainly in African Americans; thalassemia occurs in children from Mediterranean countries. Iron-deficiency anemia, an example of a noninherited disorder, tends to occur in children from lower socioeconomic areas of many countries, because iron-rich foods often are expensive. Being aware of the differences in the incidence of blood dyscrasias can be helpful in planning care and providing health care services for an individual community. Treatment for blood disorders can be culturally influenced also. For example, Jehovah's Witnesses may refuse blood transfusions, a common therapy for blood disorders, on religious grounds.

Polycythemia, or an increase in the number of RBCs, can also occur and may be as dangerous to a child as a reduction in RBC production (Box 44.4).

Anemia occurs when the rate of RBC production falls below that of cell destruction, or when there is a loss of RBCs, causing their number, or the hemoglobin level, to fall below the normal value for a child's age. Anemias are classified according to the changes seen in RBC numbers or configuration, or according to the source of the problem. Although any reduction in the amount of circulating hemoglobin lessens the oxygen-carrying capacity, clinical symptoms of this are not apparent until the hemoglobin level reaches 7 to 8 g/100 mL. Average values for hemoglobin and RBC number are shown in Appendix F.

Normochromic, Normocytic Anemias

Normochromic, normocytic anemias are marked by impaired production of erythrocytes by the bone marrow, or by abnormal or uncompensated loss of circulating RBCs, as with acute hemorrhage. The RBCs are normal in both color and size, but there are simply too few of them.

Acute Blood-Loss Anemia

Blood loss sufficient to cause anemia might occur from trauma such as an automobile accident with internal bleeding; from acute nephritis in which blood is lost in the urine; or in the newborn from disorders such as placenta previa, premature separation of the placenta, maternal–fetal or twin-to-twin transfusion, or trauma to the cord or placenta, as might occur with cesarean birth. It can also occur from intestinal parasites (Kucik, Martin, & Sortor, 2004).

Children are in shock from acute blood loss and appear pale. As the heart attempts to push the reduced amount of blood through the body more rapidly, tachycardia will occur. Loss of RBCs needed for oxygen transport causes body cells to register an oxygen deficit, and children begin to breathe rapidly. Newborns may have gasping respirations, sternal retractions, and cyanosis. They will not respond to oxygen therapy because they lack RBCs to transport and use the oxygen. Such infants become listless and inactive.

This type of acute blood-loss anemia generally is transitory because the sudden reduction in available oxygen stimulates the release of erythropoietin from the kidney and a regeneration response in the bone marrow. The reticulocyte count becomes elevated, evidence the bone marrow is trying to increase production of erythrocytes to meet the sudden shortage.

Treatment involves control of bleeding by addressing its underlying cause. The child or infant should be placed in a supine position to provide as much circulation as possible to brain cells. Keep the child warm with blankets; place an infant in an incubator or under a radiant heat warmer. Blood transfusion may be necessary to provide an immediate increase in the number of erythrocytes. Until blood is available for transfusion, a blood expander such as plasma or intravenous fluid such as normal saline or Ringer's lactate may be given to expand blood volume and improve blood pressure.

Anemia of Acute Infection

Acute infection or inflammation, especially in infants, may lead to increased destruction of erythrocytes and therefore to decreased erythrocyte levels. Common conditions include osteomyelitis, ulcerative colitis, and advanced renal disease. Impaired production of erythrocytes due to infection may contribute to the anemia. Management involves treatment of the underlying condition. When this is reversed, the blood values will return to normal.

Anemia of Renal Disease

Renal disease causes loss of function in kidney cells, and this causes an accompanying decrease in erythropoietin production. This decreases the stimulation for RBC production in the bone marrow, and a resultant normocytic normochromic anemia occurs. Administration of recombinant human erythropoietin can increase RBC production and correct the anemia, but not the renal disease.

Anemia of Neoplastic Disease

Malignant growths such as leukemia or lymphosarcoma (common neoplasms of childhood) result in normochromic, normocytic anemias because invasion of bone marrow by proliferating neoplastic cells impairs RBC production. There may be accompanying blood loss if platelet formation also has decreased. The treatment of such an anemia involves measures designed to achieve remission of the neoplastic process and transfusion to increase the erythrocyte count.

Aplastic Anemias

Aplastic anemias result from depression of hematopoietic activity in the bone marrow. The formation and development of WBCs, platelets, and RBCs can all be affected.

Congenital aplastic anemia (Fanconi's syndrome) is inherited as an autosomal recessive trait. A child is born with a number of congenital anomalies, such as skeletal and renal abnormalities, hypogenitalism, and short stature. Between 4 and 12 years of age, a child begins to manifest symptoms of **pancytopenia,** or reduction of all blood cell components (Minturn, 2003a).

Acquired aplastic anemia is a decrease in bone marrow production that can occur if a child is exposed excessively to radiation, drugs, or chemicals known to cause bone marrow damage. Drugs that may cause this include chloramphenicol, sulfonamides, arsenic (contained in rat poison, sometimes eaten by children), hydantoin, benzene, or quinine. Exposure to insecticides also may cause severe bone marrow dysfunction. Chemotherapeutic drugs temporarily reduce bone marrow production. A serious infection such as meningococcal pneumonia might cause autoimmunologic suppression of the bone marrow.

Assessment. When symptoms begin, the child appears pale, fatigues easily, and has anorexia. These symptoms reflect the lower RBC count (anemia) and tissue hypoxia. Because of reduced platelet formation (**thrombocytopenia**), the child bruises easily or has **petechiae** (pinpoint, macular, purplish-red spots caused by intradermal or submucous hemorrhage). A child may have excessive nosebleeds or gastrointestinal bleeding. As a result of a decrease in WBCs (**leukopenia**), a child may contract an increased number of infections and respond poorly to antibiotic therapy. Observe closely for signs of cardiac decompensation (e.g., tachycardia, tachypnea, shortness of breath, or cyanosis) from the long-term increased workload on the heart (see Box 44.2 earlier in this chapter). Ask about any exposure to drugs or chemicals or recent infection.

Bone marrow samples will show a reduced number of blood elements; blood-forming spaces become infiltrated by fatty tissue.

Therapeutic Management. The ultimate therapy for both congenital and acquired aplastic anemia is stem cell transplantation. If a donor cannot be located, the disease is managed by procedures to suppress T lymphocyte-dependent autoimmune responses with antithymocyte globulin (ATG) or cyclosporine or transfusion of new blood elements (Rosenfeld et al., 2003). ATG, given intravenously, must always be administered cautiously because of the high risk for anaphylaxis. Packed RBCs and platelet transfusions are generally necessary to maintain adequate blood elements. An RBC-stimulating factor (erythropoietin) may be helpful. Colony-stimulating factors may also improve bone marrow function. Some children show improvement with a course of an oral corticosteroid (prednisone). Testosterone to stimulate RBC growth may be tried.

For children who receive a stem cell transplant, chances of complete recovery are good. For others, the course is uncertain. A decreased platelet count may persist for years after other blood elements have returned to normal. Bleeding, therefore, especially petechiae or purpura, may be a long-term problem. Any drug or chemical suspected of causing the bone marrow dysfunction must be discontinued at once and the child must never be exposed to that substance again. Children with aplastic anemia are apt to be irritable because of their fatigue and recurring symptoms. Their parents may feel responsible for causing the illness if it originated from exposure to a chemical such as an insecticide. Many parents will have less confidence in health care personnel if the illness followed treatment with a drug such as chloramphenicol. They wonder how they can trust in a drug to cure the illness if they believe that one drug caused the illness. How can they trust that their child will not be harmed further?

When discussing with parents the outcome of this disease, be conservatively optimistic. It may be easier for parents to deal with this problem if they face only one day or one blood test at a time rather than trying to predict the outcomes of all the blood tests to come. They need to feel they can discuss their frustration and bitterness about continual abnormal results with health care personnel. Establishing good communication with these parents does much to establish their trust in everyone caring for their child.

NURSING DIAGNOSES AND RELATED INTERVENTIONS

Nursing Diagnosis: Risk for infection related to dramatic decrease in number of WBCs

Outcome Evaluation: Child's temperature remains below 100°F (38.0°C) axillary; symptoms of infection such as cough, vomiting, or diarrhea are absent.

Exposure to other children must be limited as long as WBC production is inadequate to prevent infection. Remind parents of the signs and symptoms of infection and advise them to come for treatment promptly if the child shows any of these signs. In the absence of granulocytes, however, antibiotic therapy may be ineffective, and severe septicemia can result. WBCs (granulocytes) may be transfused to counteract a severe infection.

Nursing Diagnosis: Risk for disturbed body image related to changed appearance occurring as medication side effect

Outcome Evaluation: Child states he or she is a worthwhile person; does not appear to be excessively shy or reluctant to interact with peers.

Children who receive corticosteroids such as prednisone to suppress the immune response almost always experience some of the side effects, such as a cushingoid appearance, hirsutism, hypertension, and marked weight gain. Masculinizing effects, such as growth of facial and body hair, the development of acne, and deepening of the voice, may also occur as the result of long-term therapy with testosterone. Be sure both the child and the parents know that these effects are related to the medication and that they will remain for an extended period but will fade when the medication is withdrawn.

Adolescents may have an especially difficult time accepting weight gain and increased acne. They need a chance to express their feelings about their changed appearance. Reinforce and emphasize positive attributes.

Nursing Diagnosis: Risk for injury related to ineffective blood clotting mechanisms secondary to inadequate platelet formation

Outcome Evaluation: Child exhibits no ecchymotic skin areas, gingival bleeding, or epistaxis; stools are negative for occult blood.

Inadequate platelet formation interferes with blood coagulation, placing a child at risk for bleeding. Some techniques for reducing bleeding due to inadequate platelet formation include:

- Limit the number of blood-drawing procedures; combine samples whenever possible; use a blood pressure cuff instead of a tourniquet to reduce the number of petechiae.
- Apply pressure to any puncture site for a full 5 minutes before applying a bandage.
- Minimize use of adhesive tape to the skin (pulling for removal may tear the skin and cause petechiae).
- Pad side and crib rails to prevent bruising.
- Protect intravenous sites to avoid numerous reinsertions.
- Administer medication orally or by intravenous infusion to minimize the number of injection sites.
- Assess diet for foods that the child can chew without irritation (e.g., avoid toast crusts).
- Urge the child to use a soft toothbrush.
- Check toys for sharp corners, which may cause scratches. Urge the child to be careful with paper, because paper cuts can bleed out of proportion to their size.
- Assess the need for routine blood pressure determinations. Tight cuffs could lead to petechiae.
- Distract the child from rough play; suggest stimulating but quiet activities to minimize risk of injury.
- Keep a record of blood drawn; do not draw extra amounts "just in case" so children do not become more anemic.

Hypoplastic Anemias

Hypoplastic anemias also result from depression of hematopoietic activity in bone marrow; they can be either congenital or acquired. Unlike aplastic anemias, in which WBCs, RBCs, and platelets are affected, in hypoplastic anemias only RBCs are affected.

Congenital hypoplastic anemia (Blackfan-Diamond syndrome) is a rare disorder that shows symptoms as early as the first 6 to 8 months of life. It affects both sexes and is apparently caused by an inherent defect in RBC formation. No changes in the leukocytes or platelets occur. An acquired form is caused by infection with parvovirus, the infectious agent of fifth disease (Carpenter, Zimmerman, & Ware, 2004).

The onset of hypoplastic anemia is insidious, and it must be differentiated from iron-deficiency anemia. In iron-deficiency anemia, blood cells appear hypochromic and microcytic; in hypoplastic anemia, they are normochromic and normocytic but few in number.

With acquired hypoplastic anemia, the reduction of RBCs is transient, so no therapy is necessary. Children with the congenital form show increased erythropoiesis with corticosteroid therapy. Long-term transfusions of packed RBCs are needed to raise erythrocyte levels. As a result of the necessary number of transfusions, **hemosiderosis** (deposition of iron in body tissue) can occur. Therefore, an iron chelation program such as subcutaneous infusion (**hypodermoclysis**) of deferoxamine (Desferal) may be started concurrently with transfusions. Deferoxamine binds with iron and aids its excretion from the body in urine; it is given 5 or 6 days a week over an 8-hour period. This is one of the few times that an infusion is given subcutaneously. Parents can do this at home after careful instruction, often while their child is asleep at night. The parent must assess that voiding is present and specific gravity is normal (1.003 to 1.030) before drug administration.

For a subcutaneous infusion, an area beside the scapula or on the thigh is cleaned with alcohol; a short 25-gauge needle is inserted at a low angle into only the subcutaneous tissue. The medication is then allowed to infuse slowly. Periodic slit-lamp eye examinations should be scheduled to check for cataract formation, a possible adverse effect of deferoxamine.

Congenital hypoplastic anemia is a chronic condition. However, approximately one fourth of affected children undergo spontaneous permanent remission before age 13 years. If not, they are candidates for stem cell transplantation. Both the child and the parents need support from health care personnel to help them accept the many procedures and tests required.

Checkpoint Question 2

Lana has received iron chelation therapy in the past. Iron chelation therapy is:

a. A procedure to remove excess iron from the child's body.
b. A procedure to help iron move effectively into hemoglobin.
c. A therapy to increase the iron level in bone and muscle cells.
d. A therapy to convert iron into calcium to increase heart action.

Hypersplenism

Under normal conditions, blood is filtered rapidly through the spleen. If the spleen is enlarged and functioning abnormally, blood cells pass through more slowly, with more cells being destroyed in the process. This increased destruction of RBCs can cause anemia and may lead to pancytopenia (deficiency of all cell elements of blood). Virtually any underlying splenic condition can cause this syndrome.

Therapeutic management consists of treating the underlying splenic disorder, including possible splenectomy. Although the spleen's role in the body's defense mechanisms against infection is not well documented, the organ appears to be relatively important in early infancy. Its function decreases as a child grows older, and it may serve no function at all in adulthood. If the spleen is removed, there is no decrease in general immunity or in gamma globulin or antibody formation. With the removal of the spleen's filtering function, however, there seems to be an increased susceptibility to meningitis or pneumonia due to pneumococci. For this reason, a splenectomy may be delayed until after 2 years of age, when the risk of meningitis decreases. Such children should receive immunization against influenza, pneumococci, and *H. influenzae* in addition to prophylactic penicillin for 2 years after the splenectomy.

Hypochromic Anemias

When hemoglobin synthesis is inadequate, the erythrocytes appear pale (hypochromia). Hypochromia is generally accompanied by a reduction in the diameter of cells (RBCs are also microcytic).

Iron-Deficiency Anemia

Although the incidence of iron-deficiency anemia is decreasing in the United States due to improved infant nutrition, it is still the most common anemia of infancy and childhood, occurring when the intake of dietary iron is inadequate (Shusterman, 2003). Inadequate dietary iron prevents proper hemoglobin formation. Most iron in the body is incorporated in hemoglobin, but an additional amount is stored in the bone marrow to be available for hemoglobin production. With iron-deficiency anemia, RBCs are both small in size (hypocytic) and pale (hypochromic) due to the stunted hemoglobin.

Children are at high risk for iron-deficiency anemia because they need more daily iron in proportion to their body weight to maintain an adequate iron level than do adults. A daily intake of 6 to 15 mg of iron is necessary. Iron-deficiency anemia occurs most often between ages 9 months and 3 years; its frequency rises again in adolescence, when iron requirements increase for girls who are menstruating. It also is found in overweight teenagers if they ingest most of their calories from high-carbohydrate, not iron-rich, foods (Nead et al., 2004).

Causes in Infants. When an infant's diet lacks sufficient iron, he or she usually has enough in reserve to last for the first 6 months. After that, if the infant continues to be iron-deficient, he or she will have difficulty forming the RBCs needed. Infants of low birthweight have fewer iron stores than those born at term because iron stores are laid down near the end of gestation. Because low-birthweight infants grow rapidly and their need for RBCs expands accordingly, they will develop an iron-deficiency anemia before 5 to 6 months. As a preventive measure, they are given an iron supplement beginning at about 2 months of age.

Women with iron deficiency during pregnancy tend to give birth to iron-deficient babies because the babies don't receive iron stores. Low hemoglobin levels from iron-deficiency anemia lead to diffusion of plasma proteins such as albumin and gamma globulin out of the bloodstream by osmosis. The loss of transferrin, a plasma protein responsible for binding iron to protein to facilitate its transportation to bone marrow after absorption from the gastrointestinal tract, further depletes this system of iron transport.

Infants born with structural defects of the gastrointestinal system, such as gastroesophageal reflux (chalasia—an immature valve between the esophagus and stomach, resulting in regurgitation) or pyloric stenosis (narrowing between the stomach and duodenum, resulting in vomiting), are particularly prone to iron-deficiency anemia. Although their diet is adequate, they cannot make use of the iron because it is never adequately digested. Infants with chronic diarrhea are also prone to this form of anemia due to inadequate absorption. Some infants develop minimal gastrointestinal bleeding if fed cow's milk; this is why breast milk or commercial formula is recommended for the first year.

Iron-deficiency anemia can be prevented in formula-fed infants by giving them iron-fortified formula for the first year. If an infant is breast-fed, iron-fortified cereal should be introduced when solid foods are introduced in the first year. Fortunately, these cost no more than nonfortified foods. Occasionally, an infant becomes constipated while ingesting iron-rich formula, but this is the exception rather than the rule.

Causes in Older Children. In children older than 2 years, chronic blood loss is the most frequent cause of iron-deficiency anemia. This results from gastrointestinal tract lesions such as polyps, ulcerative colitis, Crohn's disease, protein-induced enteropathies, parasitic infestation, or frequent epistaxis.

Adolescent girls can become iron deficient because of frequent attempts to diet and overconsumption of snack foods low in iron. Without sufficient iron, their body cannot compensate for the iron lost with menstrual flow.

Assessment. Common symptoms of iron-deficiency anemia are shown in Box 44.5. Children with iron-deficiency anemia appear pale. Because the pallor develops slowly, however, parents may not realize how extensive it is. They may describe their child as "fair-skinned" even though the child's pallor is so extreme the skin is transparent. In dark-skinned infants, pale mucous membranes may be the most significant finding.

Infants may show poor muscle tone and reduced activity. They are generally irritable from fatigue. The heart may be enlarged, and there may be a soft systolic precordial murmur as the heart increases its action, attempting to supply body cells with more oxygen. The spleen may be slightly enlarged. Fingernails become typically spoon-shaped or depressed in contour.

A 24-hour dietary history generally reveals an abnormally high milk intake. As a rule, infants should not ingest more than 32 oz of milk a day. Infants with iron-deficiency anemia may be drinking up to 50 oz a day. One quart of milk provides only approximately 0.5 mg of iron. In contrast, 1 tablespoon of iron-fortified baby cereal supplies 2.5 to 5.0 mg of iron.

As iron-deficiency anemia develops, laboratory studies will reveal a decreased hemoglobin (a hemoglobin level less than 11 g/100 mL of blood) and reduced hematocrit level (below 33%). The RBCs are microcytic and hypochromic

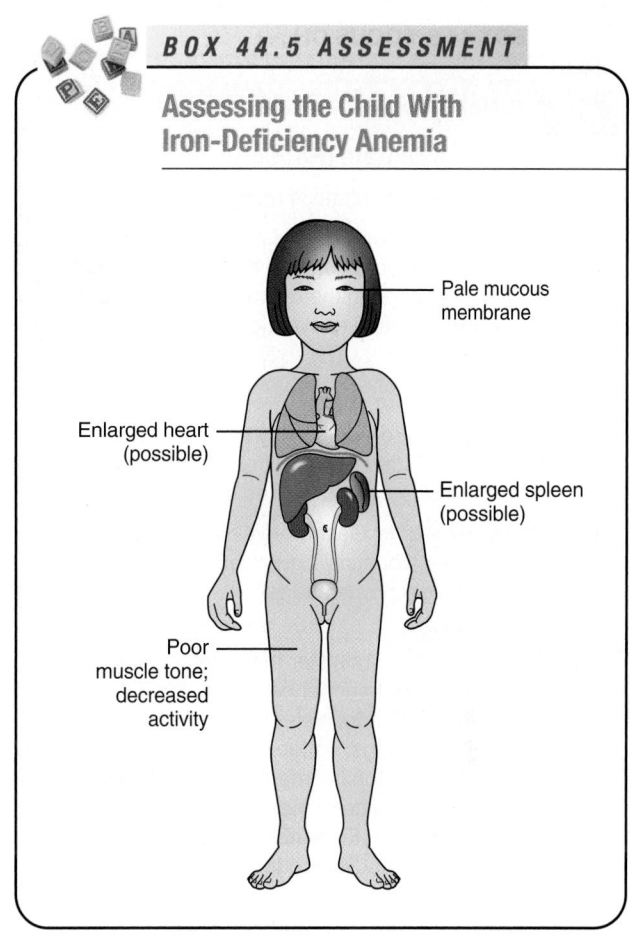

BOX 44.5 ASSESSMENT

Assessing the Child With Iron-Deficiency Anemia

- Pale mucous membrane
- Enlarged heart (possible)
- Enlarged spleen (possible)
- Poor muscle tone; decreased activity

and possibly **poikilocytic** (irregular in shape). The mean corpuscular volume is low. The mean corpuscular hemoglobin may be reduced. Serum iron levels are normally 70 µg/100 mL; with iron-deficiency anemia the level is often as low as 30 µg/100 mL, with an increased iron-binding capacity (more than 350 µg/100 mL). The level of serum ferritin reflects the extent of iron stores and is less than 10 µg/100 mL (normal is 35 µg/mL). Without iron, heme precursors cannot be used, so free erythrocyte protoporphyrins increase to more than 10 µg/g from a normal of 1.9 µg/g.

Monoamine oxidase (MAO) is an enzyme important for central nervous system maturation. Iron is incorporated into MAO, so without iron this necessary enzyme is absent and central nervous system maturation may be affected.

There may be an association in school-age children between iron-deficiency anemia and poor school achievement, probably related to chronic fatigue. Iron-deficiency anemia is also associated with pica (the eating of inedible substances such as dirt and paper). Eating ice cubes is common in adolescents. Until the anemia is corrected, parents need to supervise the child's environment to keep inedible materials out of his or her reach.

Therapeutic Management. Therapy for iron-deficiency anemia focuses on treatment of the underlying cause. Sources of gastrointestinal bleeding must be ruled out. The diet must be rich in iron and should contain extra

BOX 44.6 FOCUS ON . . .

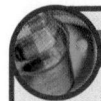

PHARMACOLOGY

Ferrous Sulfate (Feosol)

Classification: Ferrous sulfate is an iron salt.

Action: Supplies iron for red cell production. It elevates the serum iron concentration and then is converted to hemoglobin or trapped in the reticuloendothelial cells for storage and eventual conversion to a usable form of iron (Karch, 2004).

Pregnancy risk category: A

Dosage: For severe iron-deficiency anemia: 4 to 6 mg/kg/day, in three divided doses. For mild iron-deficiency anemia: 3 mg/kg/day in two divided doses.

Possible adverse effects: Gastrointestinal upset, anorexia, nausea, vomiting, constipation, dark stools, stained teeth (liquid preparations)

Nursing Implications

• Instruct parents to administer the drug on an empty stomach with water to enhance absorption. If this causes GI irritation, administer it after meals. Avoid giving it with milk, eggs, coffee, or tea.

• If the liquid preparation is ordered, advise parents to mix it with water or juice to mask the taste and prevent staining of teeth. Encourage the parents to have the child drink the medication through a straw to avoid staining of the teeth.

• Keep in mind that iron is absorbed best in the presence of vitamin C. Suggest parents give the iron with a citrus juice such as orange juice to help absorption. Some children may be prescribed vitamin C to take concurrently to increase absorption.

• Inform child and parents that iron may turn stools black.

• Encourage parents to include high-fiber foods in the child's diet to minimize the risk of constipation.

• Reinforce the need for thorough brushing of teeth to prevent staining.

• Remind parents about the need for follow-up blood studies to evaluate the effectiveness of the drug.

vitamin C, as this enhances iron absorption. An iron compound such as ferrous sulfate for 4 to 6 weeks is the drug of choice to improve RBC formation and replace iron stores (Wolf, Jimenez, & Lozoff, 2003; Box 44.6).

NURSING DIAGNOSES AND RELATED INTERVENTIONS

Nursing Diagnosis: Imbalanced nutrition, less than body requirements, related to inadequate ingestion of iron

Outcome Evaluation: Parents report child's dietary intake includes iron-rich foods; parents administer ferrous sulfate as prescribed; serum iron levels increase to normal by 6 months.

When planning care for an infant with iron-deficiency anemia, it is helpful to minimize the child's activities to prevent fatigue, particularly at mealtime, as a fatigued child will not be able to eat, let alone eat iron-rich foods.

Counsel parents on measures to improve their child's diet, such as adding iron-rich foods while decreasing milk intake to maintain iron levels and prevent recurring anemia. If the child is not fond of meat, suggest parents substitute cheese, eggs, green vegetables, or fortified cereal. Because iron-rich foods are often expensive, remind parents that these items are important and that they should not substitute less expensive, high-carbohydrate foods.

Before iron therapy is started, alert parents to possible side effects, such as stomach irritation. If oral iron is not tolerated or if there is a doubt the child will take it, an iron-dextran injection (Imferon) can be given intramuscularly. Imferon stains the skin and is extremely irritating unless it is given by deep Z-track intramuscular injection.

Of all age groups, adolescents tend to do the least well with taking medicine consistently. Help them plan a daily time for taking their iron supplement with a medication reminder chart. At first, they may reject this as childish, but assure them that everyone needs these charts. Review with them the iron-rich foods they will need to eat daily. An iron supplement is effective only if taken with iron-rich foods.

After 7 days of iron therapy, a reticulocyte count is usually done. If elevated, this means the child is now receiving adequate iron and the rapid proliferation of new erythrocytes is correcting the anemia. Iron medication must be taken for at least 4 to 6 weeks after the RBC count is normal to rebuild iron levels in the blood. In some children, maintenance therapy may continue for as long as a year.

Chronic Infection Anemia

Acute infection interferes with RBC production, producing a normochromic, normocytic anemia. When infections are chronic, anemia of a hypochromic, microcytic type occurs. This is probably caused by impaired iron metabolism as well as impaired RBC production.

The degree of anemia is rarely as severe as that occurring with iron deficiency. Administration of iron has little effect until the infection is controlled (Kang, 2003).

Macrocytic (Megaloblastic) Anemias

A macrocytic anemia is one in which the RBCs are abnormally large (Smith-Whitley, 2003). These cells are actually immature erythrocytes or megaloblasts (nucleated immature red cells). For this reason, these anemias are often referred to as megaloblastic anemias. Because these anemias are caused by nutritional deficiencies, they occur less frequently in the United States than in developing countries.

Anemia of Folic Acid Deficiency

A deficiency of folic acid combined with vitamin C deficiency produces an anemia in which the erythrocytes are abnormally large. There is accompanying neutropenia and thrombocytopenia. Mean corpuscular volume and mean corpuscular hemoglobin are increased, whereas mean corpuscular hemoglobin concentration is normal. Bone marrow will contain megaloblasts, indicating inhibition of the production of erythrocytes at an early stage. Megaloblastic arrest, or inability of RBCs to mature past an early stage, may occur in the first year of life from the continued use of infant food containing too little folic acid or from an infant drinking goat's milk, which tends to be deficient in folic acid. Treatment is daily oral administration of folic acid. Response to treatment is dramatic.

Pernicious Anemia (Vitamin B$_{12}$ Deficiency)

Vitamin B$_{12}$ is necessary for maturation of RBCs (Stabler & Allen, 2004). Pernicious anemia results from deficiency or inability to use the vitamin. Vitamin B$_{12}$, found primarily in foods of animal origin, including both cow's milk and breast milk, usually is readily available to infants. An adolescent may be deficient in vitamin B$_{12}$ if he or she is on a long-term, poorly formulated vegetarian diet.

For absorption of vitamin B$_{12}$ from the intestine, an intrinsic factor must be present in the gastric mucosa. In adults, lack of the intrinsic factor is the most frequent cause of the disorder. Symptoms of intrinsic factor deficiency can occur in the first 2 years of life (once the intrauterine stores of vitamin B$_{12}$ have been exhausted). The child appears pale, anorexic, and irritable, with chronic diarrhea. The tongue appears smooth and beefy red due to papillary atrophy. In children, neuropathologic findings such as ataxia, hyporeflexia, paresthesia, and a positive Babinski reflex are less noticeable than in adults.

Laboratory findings reveal low serum levels of vitamin B$_{12}$. The rate and efficiency of absorption of vitamin B$_{12}$ can be tested by the ingestion of the radioactively tagged vitamin. The dose absorbed in the presence and absence of a dose of intrinsic factor can be measured.

If the anemia is caused by a B$_{12}$-deficient diet, temporary injections of B$_{12}$ will reverse the symptoms. If the anemia is caused by lack of the intrinsic factor, lifelong monthly intramuscular injections of B$_{12}$ may be necessary. Parents and the child need to understand that lifelong therapy is necessary.

Hemolytic Anemias

Hemolytic anemias are those in which the number of erythrocytes decreases due to increased destruction of erythrocytes. This may be caused by fundamental abnormalities of erythrocyte structure or by extracellular destruction forces.

Congenital Spherocytosis

Congenital spherocytosis is a hemolytic anemia that is inherited as an autosomal dominant trait. It occurs most frequently in the white Northern European population (Friedman & Rodgers, 2004). The cells are small and defective, apparently due to abnormalities of the protein of the cell membrane that make them unusually permeable to sodium. The life span of erythrocytes is diminished.

The disease may be noticed shortly after birth, although symptoms may appear at any age. The hemolysis of RBCs appears to occur in the spleen, apparently from excessive absorption of sodium into the cell. The abnormal cell swells, ruptures, and is destroyed. Chronic jaundice and splenomegaly develop. The mean corpuscular hemoglobin concentration is increased because the cells are small. Gallstones may be present in the older school-age child and adolescent because of the continuous hemolysis, bilirubin release, and incorporation of bilirubin into gallstones.

Infections may precipitate a crisis or cause bone marrow failure. During such a period, the anemia increases rapidly as the hemolysis continues. Blood transfusion will be necessary to maintain a sufficient number of circulating erythrocytes until the crisis passes.

The diagnosis of the disease is based on family history, the obvious hemolysis, and the presence of the abnormal spherocytes. The treatment is generally splenectomy at approximately 5 to 6 years. This measure will increase the number of RBCs present but will not alter their abnormal structure.

Glucose-6-Phosphate Dehydrogenase Deficiency

The enzyme glucose-6-phosphate dehydrogenase (G6PD) is necessary for maintenance of RBC life. Lack of the enzyme results in premature destruction of RBCs. The disease is transmitted as a sex-linked recessive trait. It occurs most frequently in children of African-American, Asian, Sephardic Jewish, and Mediterranean descent. Approximately 15% of African-American males have the disorder (Raffini & Rheingold, 2003). Because the disease is sex-linked, males of high-risk groups should be screened in infancy.

G6PD occurs in two identifiable forms. Children with congenital nonspherocytic hemolytic anemia have hemolysis, jaundice, and splenomegaly and may have aplastic crises. Other children have a drug-induced form in which the blood patterns are normal until the child is exposed to fava beans or drugs such as antipyretics, sulfonamides, antimalarials, and naphthaquinolones (the most common drug in these groups is acetylsalicylic acid [aspirin]). Approximately 2 days after ingestion of such an oxidant drug, the child begins to show evidence of hemolysis.

A blood smear will show **Heinz bodies** (oddly shaped particles in RBCs). The degree of RBC destruction depends on the drug and the extent of exposure to it. The child may have accompanying fever and back pain. Occasionally a newborn is seen with marked hemolysis because the mother ingested an initiating drug during pregnancy.

Drug-induced hemolysis usually is self-limiting, and blood transfusions are rarely necessary. G6PD deficiency may be diagnosed by a rapid enzyme screening test or electrophoretic analysis of RBCs. Both parents and children must be told of the abnormality in the child's metabolism so they can avoid common drugs such as acetylsalicylic acid.

Sickle-Cell Anemia

Sickle-cell anemia is the presence of abnormally shaped (elongated) RBCs. It is an autosomal recessive inherited disorder on the beta chain of hemoglobin; the amino acid valine takes the place of the normally appearing glutamic acid. The erythrocytes become characteristically elongated and crescent-shaped (sickled) when they are submitted to low oxygen tension (less than 60% to 70%), a low blood pH (acidosis), or increased blood viscosity, such as occurs with dehydration or hypoxia (Wilson, Krishnamurti, & Kamat, 2003). When RBCs sickle, they do not move freely through vessels. Stasis and further sickling occur (a sickle-cell crisis). Blood flow halts and tissue distal to the blockage becomes ischemic, resulting in acute pain and cell destruction.

Because fetal hemoglobin contains a gamma, not a beta, chain, the disease usually will not result in clinical symptoms until the child's hemoglobin changes from the fetal to the adult form at approximately 6 months. However, the disease can be diagnosed prenatally by chorionic villi sampling or from cord blood during amniocentesis. It can be identified at birth by neonatal screening (Lees, Davies, & Dezateux, 2005). The abnormal form of hemoglobin in this disorder is designated hemoglobin S. A child with sickle-cell disease is said to have hemoglobin SS (homozygous involvement).

Sickle-cell disease occurs almost exclusively among African Americans. Both parents of the child with the disease will have both normal adult and hemoglobin S or be carriers (heterozygous) of the **sickle-cell trait** (have hemoglobin AS). In people with the trait, approximately 25% to 50% of hemoglobin produced is abnormal. They produce enough normal hemoglobin to compensate for the hemoglobin that is sickled and therefore show no symptoms. Sickle-cell trait occurs in approximately 1 in 12 African Americans. A child with the disease (homozygous) produces no normal hemoglobin and so shows characteristic symptoms of sickle-cell anemia. Approximately 1 in 400 African Americans has the disease (Wilson, Krishnamurti, & Kamat, 2003). A very few children have combinations of hemoglobin S and hemoglobin C or E, leading to mild anemia.

Assessment. Hemoglobin electrophoresis is used to diagnose sickle-cell anemia at birth from the few red cells that have already converted to their adult form. At approximately 6 months of age, children with sickle-cell disease begin to show initial signs of fever and anemia. Stasis of blood and infarction may occur in any body part, leading to local disease. Some infants have swelling of the hands and feet (a hand–foot syndrome) probably caused by aseptic infarction of the bones of the hands and feet. Children with sickle-cell anemia tend to have a slight build and characteristically long arms and legs. They may have a protruding abdomen because of an enlarged spleen and liver. In adolescence, the spleen size may be decreased from repeated infarction and atrophy. An atropic spleen leaves a child more susceptible to infection than normal because the spleen can no longer filter bacteria. Pneumococcal meningitis and salmonella-induced osteomyelitis become frequent illnesses; prophylactic antibiotics may be prescribed to prevent these infections (Riddington & Owusu-Ofori, 2005). A chest syndrome with symptoms similar to pneumonia may occur. The liver may become enlarged from stasis of blood flow. Eventually, cirrhosis (fibrotic degeneration) will occur from infarcts and tissue scarring. The kidneys may have subsequent scarring also, and kidney function may be decreased. The sclerae are generally icteric (yellowed) from release of bilirubin from destruction of the sickled cells; small retinal occlusions may lead to decreased vision. Regular eye examinations are necessary in children with sickle-cell disease to detect this. Cell clusters in the blood vessels of the penis may cause **priapism,** or persistent, painful erection (Friedman & Rodgers, 2004).

Sickle-Cell Crisis. **Sickle-cell crisis** is the term used to denote a sudden, severe onset of sickling. Symptoms of crisis occur from pooling of many new sickled cells in vessels and consequent tissue hypoxia beyond the blockage (a *vaso-occlusive crisis*). A sickle-cell crisis can occur when a child has an illness causing dehydration or a respiratory infection that results in lowered oxygen exchange and a lowered arterial oxygen level, or after extremely strenuous exercise (enough to lead to tissue hypoxia). Sometimes no obvious cause of a crisis can be found (Box 44.7). Symptoms are sudden, severe, and painful (Box 44.8). Aseptic necrosis of the head of the femur or humerus with increased joint pain may occur. Laboratory reports reveal a hemoglobin level of only 6 to 8 g/100 mL. A peripheral blood smear demonstrates sickled cells. The WBC count is often elevated to 12,000 to 20,000/mm³. Bilirubin and reticulocyte levels are increased.

BOX 44.7 FOCUS ON . . .

EVIDENCE-BASED PRACTICE

Does Exposure to Secondary Smoke Increase the Incidence of Sickle-Cell Crisis?

To answer this question, researchers surveyed 52 children with sickle-cell disease, aged 1 year to 18 years, and their parents as to whether anyone in their household smoked. This information was then used to compare the number of vaso-occlusive crises during the past 2 years that had been serious enough to result in hospital admission. Results of the study showed that children exposed to secondary smoke had more than twice as many sickle-cell crises during those 2 years than did unexposed patients (3.7 episodes vs. 1.7 episodes).

This is an interesting study for nurses because it adds one more reason why secondary smoke inhalation is dangerous to children. As nurses are the health care educators with whom people are most apt to talk about healthy living, nurses may be able to play a major role in reducing vaso-occlusive crises in children with sickle-cell disease.

Source: West, D. C., et al. (2003). Impact of environmental tobacco smoke on children with sickle cell disease. *Archives of Pediatrics & Adolescent Medicine, 157*(12); 1197–1201.

BOX 44.8 ASSESSMENT

Assessing a Child With Sickle-Cell Crisis

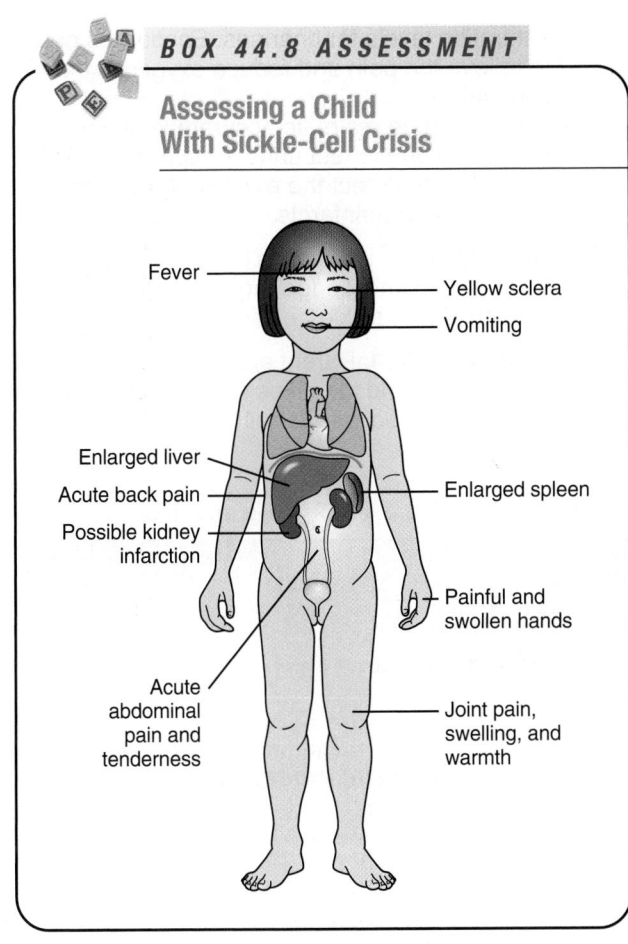

Fever

Yellow sclera

Vomiting

Enlarged liver

Acute back pain

Possible kidney infarction

Enlarged spleen

Painful and swollen hands

Acute abdominal pain and tenderness

Joint pain, swelling, and warmth

Acetaminophen (Tylenol) may be adequate pain relief for some children; for others, a narcotic analgesic such as intravenous morphine may be needed. Once the child is pain-free, he or she is able to relax, reducing the metabolic demand for oxygen and helping to end the sickling. Hydration is generally accomplished with intensive intravenous fluid replacement therapy. Tissue hypoxia leads to acidosis. The acidosis must be corrected by electrolyte replacement. Some kidney infarction may have occurred, so do not administer potassium intravenously until kidney function has been determined (the child is voiding). Otherwise, excessive potassium levels may occur, possibly leading to cardiac arrhythmias. If infection appears to be the precipitator for a sickling crisis, blood and urine cultures, a chest x-ray, and a complete blood count will be taken and the infection will be treated by antibiotics. Blood transfusion (usually packed RBCs) may be necessary to maintain the hemoglobin above 12 g/dL (termed hypertransfusion).

Hydroxyurea, an antineoplastic agent that has the potential to increase the production of hemoglobin F (fetal hemoglobin), can be used in children with sickle-cell disease to increase their overall hemoglobin level. The drug, given orally, may cause anorexia. Therefore, monitor the child's nutrition intake during this drug therapy (Wilson, Krishnamurti, & Kamat, 2003). If none of the above measures appears to be effective, children may be given an exchange transfusion to remove most of the sickled cells and replace them with normal cells. Exchange transfusion (see Chapter 26) must be done with small amounts of blood at each exchange. Otherwise, the pressure changes can cause such irregularities in blood volume that heart failure results. Stem cell transplantation is possible for the child who does not respond to usual therapies.

A cerebrovascular accident may occur from a blocked artery, causing loss of motor function, coma, seizures, or even death (Hoppe, 2005). If there is renal involvement, hematuria or flank pain may result.

Less frequent forms of crisis may occur when there is splenic sequestration of RBCs or severe anemia occurs due to pooling and increased destruction of sickled cells in the liver and spleen (a *sequestration crisis*). This leads to shock from hypovolemia. The spleen is enlarged and tender. A *hyperhemolytic crisis* can occur when there is increased destruction of RBCs. A *megaloblastic crisis* may occur if the child has folic acid or vitamin B deficiency (new RBCs cannot be fully formed due to lack of these ingredients). An *aplastic crisis* is manifested by severe anemia due to a sudden decrease in RBC production. This form usually occurs with infection.

Acute chest syndrome has become the leading cause of death in patients with sickle-cell disease. Children exhibit hypoxia, decreased hemoglobin levels, and a persistent diffuse pneumonia so severe that ventilator care may be needed. Blood transfusion is used to increase the oxygen-carrying capacity of blood, and broad-spectrum antibiotics are given to resolve the pneumonia (Friedman & Rodgers, 2004).

Therapeutic Management. The child in sickle-cell crisis has three primary needs: pain relief and adequate hydration and oxygenation to prevent further sickling and halt the crisis.

Checkpoint Question 3

Joey, who has sickle-cell anemia, has had two vaso-occlusive crises in the past year. A vaso-occlusive crisis occurs because:

a. An enlarged spleen causes blood to pool there.
b. Dehydration leads to thrombosed sickle cells.
c. Hemorrhage reduces a child's total blood volume.
d. Decreased platelet number leads to poor coagulation.

NURSING DIAGNOSES AND RELATED INTERVENTIONS

Nursing Diagnosis: Ineffective tissue perfusion related to generalized infarcts due to sickling

Outcome Evaluation: Child's respiratory rate is 16 to 20/min; cyanosis is absent; arterial blood gases within acceptable parameters including

Pco$_2$ = 40 mm Hg; Po$_2$ = 80 to 90 mm Hg; oxygen saturation of 95%; urine output greater than 1 mL/kg/h.

Oxygen may be administered by nasal cannula or mask if arterial blood gases reveal a low Po$_2$ level. Oxygen may not reach every distal body part effectively, however, if blood flowing to the part is obstructed by the sickled cells. When hemoglobin S is below 40%, there generally is adequate blood flow to body cells. High concentrations of oxygen are not used because hypoxia is a stimulant to erythrocyte production—production badly needed to replace damaged cells. Monitor the flow rate carefully and use pulse oximetry to evaluate oxy-

gen saturation levels for changes. Encourage bed rest to relieve the pain and reduce oxygen expenditure (Box 44.9).

It is important to maintain accurate intake and output records and to test urine for specific gravity and hematuria to detect the extent or presence of kidney damage from infarcts.

Nursing Diagnosis: Ineffective health maintenance related to lack of knowledge regarding long-term needs of child with sickle-cell anemia

Outcome Evaluation: Parent accurately describes disease process and identifies special precautions necessary to prevent sickle-cell crisis.

BOX 44.9: Focus on Nursing Care Planning

A Multidisciplinary Care Map for A Child with Sickle-Cell Anemia

•

Joey is a 7-year-old with sickle cell anemia. He is seen in the emergency room for a vaso-occlusive crisis.

Family Assessment

Child lives with two older brothers (10 and 12) and both parents in a 3-bedroom home. Father works as a distributor for a local water bottling company. Mother, an X-ray technician, is temporarily on duty with the National Guard in the Middle East. Father rates finances as, "Not good. Medical bills kill us."

Client Assessment

Thin, black boy whose weight is at only 5th percentile for age. Was screened and diagnosed with sickle-cell anemia at birth. Described as "picky eater"; has eaten almost no meat since mother is not at home. Father states "I don't have time to fuss" over meals. Has a history of two former vaso-occlusive crises. Missed last regularly scheduled health assessment 2 weeks ago, as father had difficulty taking off from work for visit. Was playing "tag" with older brothers on local beach this afternoon. Sclera was jaundiced and child was crying from pain by time father returned from work. Hemoglobin 6 g/100 mL; hematocrit 31%.

Nursing Diagnosis

Altered tissue perfusion related to vaso-occlusive crisis

Outcome Evaluation

Oxygen saturation level is maintained at 95% or higher; pain decreases to tolerable level; symptoms of hemolytic crisis decrease.

Team Member Responsible	Assessment	Intervention	Rationale	Expected Outcome
Activities of Daily Living				
Nurse	Assess if child understands he will need to remain in bed.	Admit child to hospital unit; restrict to bed rest.	Bed rest reduces the need for oxygen in body cells.	Child complies with bed rest; plays non-action games with parent or health care personnel.

(continued)

Team Member Responsible	Assessment	Intervention	Rationale	Expected Outcome
Consultations				
Nurse practitioner/ physician	Assess if hematology service is needed for consult.	Meet with hematology service as needed for emergency and long-range consult.	Repeated vaso-occlusive crises suggest family needs better management strategies.	Hematology service meets with physician/ nurse practitioner and parent and child as indicated.
Procedures/Medications				
Nurse/nurse practitioner	Assess degree of child's pain by use of FACES pain scale.	Administer prescribed narcotic as required.	Vaso-occlusive crises can cause sharp pain that requires strong analgesia.	Child rates pain as no higher than 2 following analgesia administration.
Nurse	Assess O_2 saturation level by pulse oximetry.	Administer oxygen by face mask to keep O_2 saturation above 95% or as prescribed.	O_2 saturation decreases as sickled cells are unable to carry a full complement of oxygen.	Child cooperates with pulse oximetry and oxygen administration. SO_2 remains above 95%.
Nurse	Determine whether child has been taking folic acid at home.	Administer folic acid as prescribed.	Folic acid is necessary to build new red cells to replace those that have been hemolyzed.	Child takes folic acid cooperatively.
Nutrition				
Nurse	Assess child's intake and output.	Begin IV therapy as prescribed.	IV therapy helps restore hydration and reduce sickle cell clotting.	Child names best hand to start infusion; cooperates with arm board restriction.
Nurse/ nutritionist	Assess child's usual dietary intake by 24-hour dietary recall history.	Demonstrate child's reduced weight to parent using height/weight chart. Plan ways to increase calorie intake.	Even "picky eaters" need to take in enough food daily to meet growth and maintenance needs.	Parent states he will try harder to serve foods child likes; child voices intent to eat at least one meat helping daily.
Patient/Family Education				
Nurse	Assess family members' understanding of the causes of sickle cell vaso-occlusive crises.	Review with family members the importance of child avoiding dehydration and oxygen deficiency.	Dehydration leads to clumping of sickled cells, cutting off circulation in distant body parts.	Family members state they are aware they must be as responsible as child for avoiding sickling circumstances.
Psychosocial/Spiritual/Emotional Needs				
Nurse	Assess the stress level of the family in light of absent mother and child with chronic illness.	Review with family ways to maintain a tight family unit (game night, common activities) to maintain family until mother returns.	When families miss a support person, they need to rally together to devise other support methods.	Father states he will try harder to meet children's needs although worrying about wife's safety is a major concern.
Discharge Planning				
Nurse	Determine whether parent has any questions about care of a child with sickle-cell anemia.	Schedule a follow-up visit in 3 days for evaluation.	Care of a chronically ill child can be a major strain on a family. Follow-up visits help share responsibility for care.	Father states he understands importance of follow-up visit and will keep appointment with child.

In many children, episodes of sickling grow less severe as a child reaches adolescence. Such children may have a normal life expectancy but still experience the stresses of chronic illness. Other children experience such devastating episodes in early childhood that the disease is fatal at an early age. Parents need support to supervise children carefully day by day when they are aware that, due to the intense episodes, the child may die despite the precautions.

Between crises, care focuses on preventing recurring crises. Although the hemoglobin level of children may remain as low as 6 to 9 g/100 mL, children adjust well to this chronic state. Children who receive frequent blood transfusions should not be given supplementary iron or iron-fortified formula or vitamins or they may receive too much iron; high levels of excess iron are deposited in body tissues (**hemochromatosis**) to a point of staining body tissue or being incorporated into body tissue with fibrotic scarring (hemosiderosis). Oral folic acid may be prescribed to help rebuild hemolyzed RBCs.

Children with sickle-cell anemia need to be followed at regular health care visits. They must receive childhood immunizations so they are not vulnerable to common childhood infections such as measles or pertussis. They are also candidates for meningococcal, pneumococcal, and influenza vaccines to prevent infection. They may be prescribed oral penicillin as prophylaxis for the first 5 years. Puberty may be delayed, and both parents and children may need counseling to accept this. Once puberty changes do occur, they are adequate, just later than normal. Parents and children with sickle-cell disease also need support and positive reinforcement to enhance the child's self-esteem and to learn how to deal with problems that occur as a result of this chronic hematologic disorder (Box 44.10).

Caution parents to bring their child to a health care facility at the first indication of infection. Some parents are reluctant to do this, afraid that they will be labeled overprotective. Assure them that health care personnel are knowledgeable about sickle-cell anemia, and they know that a child with even a minor infection could become very ill.

Parents must make decisions regarding children's activity levels. Children should attend regular school and should be allowed to participate in all school activities except contact sports (such as football), which could result in rupture of an enlarged spleen or liver. Long-distance running is also inadvisable because it can lead to dehydration. Caution parents to give the child fluids frequently, especially on long hikes and at the beach. Caution them against taking the child on board an unpressurized aircraft in which the oxygen concentration may fall during flight. During the summer, parents need to offer the child frequent drinks to prevent dehydration.

Some children who have had kidney infarcts and lessened ability to concentrate urine have chronic nocturnal enuresis (bedwetting) (Box 44.11).

BOX 44.10 FOCUS ON . . .

COMMUNICATION

Joey, who has sickle-cell disease, is seen in the emergency room with a new vaso-occlusive crisis. His right knee is discolored by a large brush burn. He's crying from pain.

Less Effective Communication

Nurse: Hello, Mr. Harrow. I need to ask some questions to see if anything triggered this new crisis.

Mr. Harrow: He better not have been doing something he's not allowed to do.

Nurse: His knee looks like he fell. Were you running, Joey? So you got dehydrated?

Mr. Harrow: He better not say he was doing that!

Nurse: Joey, how did you hurt your knee?

Joey: I don't know.

Nurse: Okay. Let's get you better and not worry about what started this.

More Effective Communication

Nurse: Hello, Mr. Harrow. I need to ask some questions to see if anything triggered this new crisis.

Mr. Harrow: He better not have been doing something he's not allowed to do.

Nurse: His knee looks like he fell. Were you running, Joey? So you got dehydrated?

Mr. Harrow: He better not say he was doing that!

Nurse: Mr. Harrow, I need to get an accurate history of what happened. I'd like Joey to tell us how he thinks the accident happened. Then later on, we can talk about what are good rules for him to be following.

Children with blood disorders have to follow a great many rules to avoid clotting or bleeding episodes, such as not playing contact sports or playing too hard in the sun. Because these forbidden activities are appealing, children occasionally break the rules. In an emergency room, it is important that children and parents both recognize that the priority at the moment is obtaining an accurate history. Until they realize this, they may be so concerned with the broken rule that they are unable to move beyond that to secure adequate therapy.

Children with sickle-cell disease are at high risk if they need surgery. The hours of being held on nothing-by-mouth status, as well as being unable to eat afterward, may lead to dehydration. Anesthesia may cause a transient hypoxia leading to sickling. Parents must be cautioned that even for such a simple operation as tooth extraction, they must alert health care personnel about their child's condition.

DIAGNOSTIC AND THERAPEUTIC TECHNIQUES

A number of typical procedures are used in the diagnosis and therapy of GI disorders. Common diagnostic procedures include fiberoptic endoscopy, colonoscopy, and barium enema. Children need good preparation for these procedures because they are potentially frightening. If children receive conscious sedation for a procedure, they need preparation for this as well as the actual procedure.

Therapy may include alternative methods of feeding such as enteral (nasogastric or gastrostomy tube feedings), total parenteral nutrition, and intravenous (IV) therapy to rest the GI tract. A colostomy or ileostomy may be created for the same reason. These tests and procedures, their meaning, their impact on children, and nursing responsibilities are discussed in Chapters 36 and 37.

HEALTH PROMOTION AND RISK MANAGEMENT

Health promotion related to GI disorders focuses on a wide area because the causes of these disorders cover a wide range. Some disorders, such as appendicitis, cannot be prevented because they occur for unpredictable causes. Some, such as celiac disease, involve genetic aspects that cannot be changed. Some, such as Crohn's disease and ulcerative colitis, are associated with an autoimmune response. Other conditions, such as vomiting and diarrhea, are often caused by foods that were refrigerated improperly or spread through improper handwashing and thus can be prevented. Hepatitis can be prevented through good handwashing (hepatitis A) and immunization (hepatitis A and B). Vitamin and protein deficiency disorders can be prevented by educating parents about the food pyramid and how to select foods that fit each of the sections.

Because any interference in nutrition pervades many aspects of children's lives, families often need help with planning care. Help families plan the necessary adaptations to their lifestyle to prevent the disease from interfering with family functioning (e.g., will day care center personnel do gastrostomy feedings? Will a nursery school accept a child with a colostomy? Can a child select a gluten-free diet at the school cafeteria?). All families should be encouraged to eat at least one meal a day together so they can have time to share experiences and "touch base" with each other. For the family with a child who has a feeding problem such as a gastrostomy feeding or total parenteral nutrition, this can be difficult. Urge such families to bring the child to the table for a social time even if the child cannot eat with the family. If watching family members eat while the child cannot is too difficult, urge the family to provide a "together" time in some other way so they do not miss out on this valuable family activity.

Some GI disorders in children, such as aganglionic megacolon, are diagnosed late because parents think the child's refusal to eat is just the sign of being a "picky eater" or a manifestation of 2-year-old autonomy. Educating parents about normal nutrition and how to distinguish things such as vomiting from illness from normal "spitting up" or severe diarrhea from a simple GI upset helps parents bring their children for care at the earliest possible time. Early intervention prevents the child from becoming dehydrated and seriously ill.

FLUID, ELECTROLYTE, AND ACID–BASE IMBALANCES

The GI system plays a major role in maintaining fluid, electrolyte, and acid–base balance. It is the main route by which substances are taken into the body and can be a major source of loss if vomiting or diarrhea occurs.

Fluid Balance

Retaining fluid is of greater importance in the body chemistry of infants than that of adults because fluid constitutes a greater fraction of the infant's total weight. In adults, body water accounts for approximately 60% of total weight. In infants, it accounts for as much as 75% to 80% of total weight; in children, it averages approximately 65% to 70%.

Fluid is distributed in three body compartments: (1) intracellular (within cells), 35% to 40% of body weight; (2) interstitial (surrounding cells and bloodstream), 20% of body weight; and (3) intravascular (blood plasma), 5% of body weight. The interstitial and the intravascular fluid together are often referred to as the *extracellular fluid* (ECF), totaling 25% of body weight. In infants, the extracellular portion is much greater, totaling up to 45% of total body weight (Fig. 45.2). In young children, this amount is 30%; in adolescents, it is 25%.

Fluid is normally obtained by the body through oral ingestion of fluid and by the water formed in the metabolic breakdown of food. Primarily, fluid is lost from the body in urine and feces. Minor losses, **insensible losses,** occur from evaporation from skin and lungs and from saliva (of little importance except in children with tracheostomies or those requiring nasopharyngeal suction). Infants do not concentrate urine as well as adults because their kidneys are immature. As a result, they have a proportionally greater loss of water in their urine. In infants, the relatively greater surface area to body mass also causes a greater insensible loss. Fluid intake is altered when a child is nauseated and unable to ingest fluid or is vomiting and losing fluid ingested. When diarrhea occurs, or when a child becomes diaphoretic because of fever, the fluid output can be markedly increased. **Dehydration** occurs when there is an excessive loss of body water (Steiner et al., 2004).

In an adult weighing 70 kg, the extracellular fluid volume is approximately 14,000 mL. Each day, the well adult ingests approximately 2,000 mL of fluid and excretes approximately 2,000 mL as urine. This means that approximately 14% of his or her total ECF (2,000 mL of 14,000 mL) is exchanged each day. In contrast to this, 7-kg infants have an ECF volume of only 1,750 mL. They ingest approximately 700 mL daily and excrete approximately 700 mL daily. Therefore, they exchange approximately 40% of their volume daily. As a result of this increased exchange rate, the infant's fluid balance may be more critically affected when he or she is ill. Adults, when they do not eat for a day because of a GI upset, and whose kidneys con-

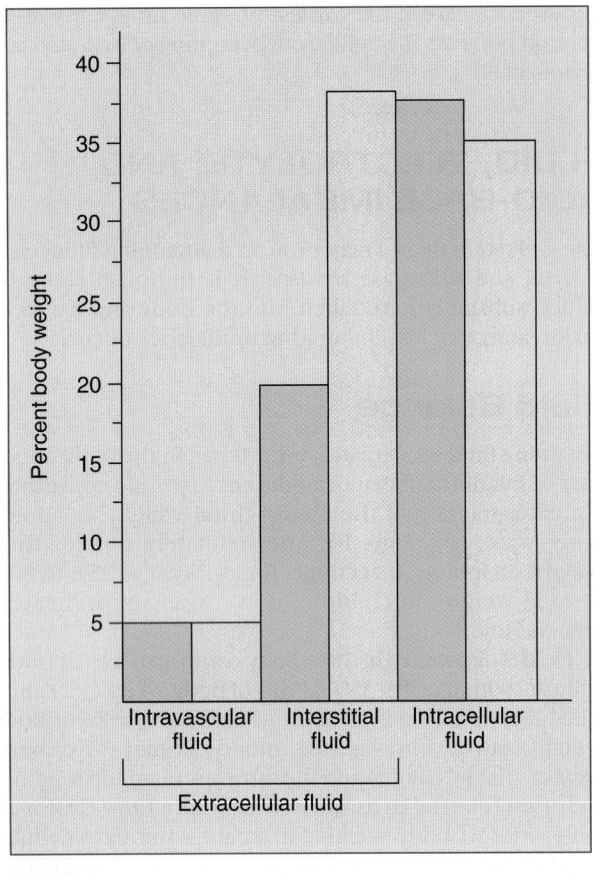

FIGURE 45.2 Distribution of fluid in body compartments.

tinue to excrete at the normal rate, will have 14% less fluid in the extracellular space by the end of the day. Infants who do not eat for a day (providing kidney function remains constant) will be 40% short of ECF by the end of the day. This is obviously a more important loss of fluid than the same loss would be in an adult; therefore, dehydration is always a more serious problem in infants than in older children and adults. Maintenance requirements of fluid for infants and children are shown in Table 45.1.

Fluid Imbalances

Under most circumstances, water and salt are lost in proportion to each other (*isotonic dehydration*). Occasionally, water is lost out of proportion to salt (i.e., water depletion or *hypertonic dehydration*). Occasionally, electrolytes are lost out of proportion to water (*hypotonic dehydration*). Each of these abnormal states produces specific symptoms.

Isotonic Dehydration

When the body loses more water than it absorbs (as with diarrhea) or absorbs less fluid than it excretes (as with nausea and vomiting), the first result will be a decrease in the volume of blood plasma. The body compensates for this fairly rapidly by shifting interstitial fluid into the blood vessels. The composition of fluid in these two spaces is similar, so the replacement by this fluid does not change plasma composition. However, this replacement phenomenon will proceed only until the interstitial fluid reserve is depleted—a danger point for the child because it is difficult for the body to replace interstitial fluid from the intracellular fluid (the fluids in these two compartments have different electrolyte contents). If an infant continues to lose fluid after this point, the volume of the plasma will continue to fall rapidly, resulting in cardiovascular collapse. Typical signs and symptoms of isotonic dehydration are summarized in Table 45.2.

Hypertonic Dehydration

Water is apt to be lost in a greater proportion than electrolytes when fluid intake decreases in conjunction with a fluid loss increase, as might occur in a child with nausea (preventing fluid intake) and fever (increased fluid loss through perspiration); profuse diarrhea, where there is a greater loss of fluid than salt; or renal disease associated with polyuria (i.e., diabetes insipidus or nephrosis with diuresis). Fluid loss is out of proportion to the loss of electrolytes, and, with such an increased loss of fluid, electrolytes concentrate in the blood. Fluid shifts from the interstitial and intracellular spaces to the bloodstream (from areas of less osmotic pressure to areas of greater pressure). Dehydration occurs in the interstitial and intracellular compartments. The red blood cell count and hematocrit will be elevated because the blood is more concentrated than usual. Levels of electrolytes (i.e., sodium, chloride,

<table>
<tr><td colspan="3">**TABLE 45.1**</td></tr>
<tr><td colspan="3">**Maintenance Requirements of Fluid Based on Caloric Expenditure**</td></tr>
<tr><td>**Body Weight (kg)**</td><td>**Caloric Expenditure**</td><td>**Daily Fluid Requirement**</td></tr>
<tr><td>3–10</td><td>100 cal/kg/d</td><td>100 mL/kg</td></tr>
<tr><td>10–20</td><td>1000 cal + 50 cal/kg for each kg of body wt more than 10 kg</td><td>1000 mL + 50 mL/kg for each kg of body wt more than 10 kg</td></tr>
<tr><td>More than 20</td><td>1500 cal + 20 cal/kg for each kg of body wt more than 20 kg</td><td>1500 mL + 20 mL/kg for each kg of body wt more than 20 kg</td></tr>
</table>

TABLE 45.2

Signs and Symptoms of Dehydration

	Isotonic	Hypotonic	Hypertonic
Thirst	Mild	Moderate	Extreme
Skin turgor	Poor	Very poor	Moderate
Skin consistency	Dry	Clammy	Moderate
Skin temperature	Cool	Cool	Warm
Urine output	Decreased	Decreased	Decreased
Activity	Irritable	Lethargic	Very lethargic
Serum sodium level	Normal	Reduced	Increased

and bicarbonate) will also likely be increased. Additional signs and symptoms are summarized in Table 45.2.

Hypotonic Dehydration

With hypotonic dehydration, there is a disproportionately high loss of electrolytes relative to fluid lost. The plasma concentration of sodium and chloride will be low. This could result from excessive GI loss by vomiting or from low intake of salt associated with extreme losses through therapeutic diuresis. It also occurs when there is extreme loss of electrolytes in diseases such as adrenocortical insufficiency or diabetic acidosis. When low levels of electrolytes occur, the osmotic pressure in extracellular spaces decreases. The kidneys begin to excrete more fluid to decrease ECF volume and bring the proportion of electrolytes and fluid back into line. This may lead to a secondary extracellular dehydration (see Table 45.2).

Overhydration

Overhydration is as serious as dehydration. It generally occurs in children who are receiving IV fluid. The excess fluid in these instances is usually extracellular. The condition is serious because the ECF overload may result in cardiovascular overload and cardiac failure.

When large quantities of salt-poor fluid (hypotonic solutions) such as tap water are ingested or are given by enema, the body transfers water from the extracellular space into the intracellular space to restore the normal osmotic relationships. This transfer results in intracellular edema manifested by headache, nausea, vomiting, dimness and blurring of vision, cramps, muscle twitching, and seizures. A situation in which intracellular edema may occur is when tap water enemas are given to a child with aganglionic disease of the intestine.

Acid–Base Imbalance

The GI system often is involved with two severe acid–base imbalances, metabolic acidosis and metabolic alkalosis. These imbalances occur with severe diarrhea or vomiting.

When dealing with acid–base balance, a key component is pH. The abbreviation "pH" refers to two French words that mean the "power of hydrogen." pH denotes whether a solution is acid or alkaline, determined by the proportion of hydrogen (H^+) ions in relation to hydroxide (OH^-) ions—the two substances that disassociate when water is broken down into its basic components ($H_2O = H^+$ and OH^-). A solution is acid (pH below 7.0) if it contains proportionately more H^+ ions than OH^- ions. It is alkaline (pH above 7.0) if the proportion of OH^- ions exceeds that of H^+ ions.

Whether body serum is becoming acidotic is determined by analyzing a sample of arterial blood for blood gases. The pH of blood is normally slightly alkaline, ranging from 7.35 to 7.45. P_{CO_2} (the amount of dissolved carbon dioxide in arterial blood) is normally 35 to 45 mm Hg. The level of bicarbonate (HCO_3) in arterial blood is normally 22 to 26 mEq/L.

Metabolic Acidosis

Metabolic acidosis may result from diarrhea. When diarrhea occurs, a great deal of sodium is lost with stool. This excessive loss of Na^+, in turn, causes the body to conserve H^+ ions in an attempt to keep the total number of positive and negative ions in serum balanced. As a result, a child becomes acidotic as the number of H^+ ions in the blood increases proportionally over the number of OH^- ions present. With metabolic acidosis, arterial blood gas analysis will reveal a decreased pH (under 7.35) and a low HCO_3 value (near or below 22 mEq/L). The lower the HCO_3 value is, presumably the more Na^+ ions that have been lost or the more extensive the diarrhea has been.

To correct this problem (a pH too low is incompatible with life), the body uses both its kidney and respiratory buffering systems. The respiratory buffering system attempts to correct the imbalance quickly. H^+ ions combine with HCO_3^- ions to form carbonic acid. This, in turn, is broken down into CO_2 and water, which is then eliminated by the lungs during expiration. This process works immediately, and, as it continues for a time, the bicarbonate level in the serum falls lower and lower as the body uses up its bicarbonate store.

In the kidneys, H^+ ions are excreted directly or combine with other substances, such as phosphate and ammonia, to form a weak acid, which is excreted. Unfortunately, this process is slow, taking up to 24 hours.

The child breathes rapidly (hyperpnea) to "blow off" CO_2 to prevent it from combining with H_2O and reforming HCO_3. Urine becomes more acid as ammonia formation in the urine is increased.

Metabolic Alkalosis

With vomiting, a great deal of hydrochloric acid is lost. When Cl^- ions are lost this way, the body has to decrease the number of H^+ ions present so the number of positive and negative charges remains balanced. This causes the child to become alkalotic as the number of H^+ ions becomes proportionally lower than the number of OH^- ions present. To further reduce the number of H^+ ions, the lungs conserve CO_2 and water by slowing respirations (hypopnea). The excessive CO_2 retained by this maneuver dissolves in the blood as carbonic acid and then is converted into excessive H^+ and HCO_3^-. With metabolic alkalosis, therefore, the serum HCO_3 invariably will be high. The higher the value, presumably the more Cl^- ions have been lost or the more extensive the vomiting has been.

The child will breathe slowly and shallowly; pH will be elevated (near or above 7.45), and HCO_3 level will be near or above 28 mEq/L.

When alkalosis occurs from vomiting, a secondary electrolyte problem often occurs. As the kidneys begin to help conserve H^+ ions, K^+ ions are exchanged for H^+ ions—that is, K^+ ions are excreted in order to retain H^+ ions. As a result of this loss of K^+ into the urine, low K^+ levels (hypokalemia) invariably accompany metabolic alkalosis.

Checkpoint Question 1

Barry has frequent bouts of vomiting. What secondary electrolyte problem often occurs when metabolic alkalosis results from vomiting?

a. Acidosis
b. Hyponatremia
c. Hypokalemia
d. Hyperchlorosis

COMMON GASTROINTESTINAL SYMPTOMS OF ILLNESS IN CHILDREN

Vomiting and diarrhea in children commonly occur as symptoms of disease of the GI tract as well as symptoms of disease in other body systems (Box 45.3). Pneumonia or otitis media, for example, may present first with vomiting or diarrhea. The danger is that either can lead to a disturbance in hydration, electrolyte, or acid–base balance. In many infants, these secondary disturbances can be more threatening to the child than the primary disease (Liacouras, 2003).

Vomiting

Many children with vomiting are suffering from a mild gastroenteritis (infection) caused by a viral or bacterial organism. The adolescent who is pregnant may also experience vomiting. The condition is always potentially serious because a metabolic alkalosis may result.

Assessment

In describing symptoms of vomiting, be certain to differentiate between the various terms that are used (Table 45.3). It is important that vomiting be described correctly because different conditions are marked by different forms of vomiting, and a correct description of the child's actions can aid greatly in diagnosis.

BOX 45.3 FOCUS ON . . .

EVIDENCE-BASED PRACTICE

What Proportion of Children Seen in Emergency Rooms Have Gastrointestinal Concerns?

For this study, the records of children seen in a major after-hour call center were analyzed to determine the most common disorders with which children presented. Of 525 children seen, 263 (50%) had lower respiratory tract concerns; 104 (20%) had gastrointestinal concerns; 84 (16%) had head, ears, eyes, nose, and throat concerns; and 74 (14%) had upper respiratory tract concerns. Thirteen percent of those with gastrointestinal symptoms, referred primarily for dehydration, required intravenous fluids. This is an important study for nurses because it documents the high incidence of gastrointestinal symptoms in children as well as how quickly small children can become dehydrated and need supplemental fluid when they have vomiting or diarrhea.

Source: Scarfone, R. J., Luberti, A. A., & Mistry, R. D. (2004). Children referred to an emergency department by an after-hours call center: complaint-specific analysis. *Pediatric Emergency Care, 20*(8), 507–513.

Therapeutic Management

The treatment for vomiting is to withhold food from the stomach for a time. If there is nothing in the stomach, vomiting cannot occur. Most parents treat vomiting in the opposite way. Every time the child vomits, they attempt to feed the child again. The child vomits again and they feed again, and so on. This prolongs the vomiting and intensifies the potential for electrolyte imbalance.

NURSING DIAGNOSES AND RELATED INTERVENTIONS

Nursing Diagnosis: Risk for deficient fluid volume related to vomiting

Outcome Evaluation: Skin turgor remains good; specific gravity of urine is 1.003 to 1.030; urine output is more than 1 mL/kg/h; episodes of vomiting decrease in frequency and amount.

To decrease vomiting, withhold food and fluid for a time (nothing by mouth [NPO]), depending on the age of the child. On the average, a period of 3 to 6 hours is usually sufficient. In the older child, after this period of fasting, offer a few ice chips, then water in small amounts—approximately 1 tbsp every 15 minutes, four times; then 2 tbsp every half-hour, four times. Popsicles can be sub-

TABLE 45.3

Differentiation Between Regurgitation and Vomiting

Characteristic	Regurgitation	Vomiting
Timing	Occurs with feeding	Timing unrelated to feeding
Forcefulness	Runs out of mouth with *little force*	Forceful; often projected 1 ft away from the infant; *projectile vomiting*—projected as much as 4 ft (most often related to increased intracranial pressure in newborns; in infants age 4–6 wk, possibly due to pyloric stenosis)
Description	Smells barely sour; only slightly curdled	Extremely sour smelling, appearing curdled, yellow, green, clear or watery, or black; perhaps fresh blood or old blood staining from swallowed maternal blood (in newborns)
Distress	Nonpainful; child does not appear to be in distress and may even smile as if sensation is enjoyable	Possible crying just before vomiting as if abdominal pain is present, and after vomiting as if the force of action is frightening
Duration	Occurs once per feeding	Continuing until stomach is empty; followed by dry retching
Amount	1–2 tsp	Full stomach contents

stituted for water. If this is retained, children can be given small sips of clear liquids, such as tea, ginger ale, or sports drinks, such as Gatorade. Children may become hungry and want whole glasses, but keeping the quantity to small sips prevents vomiting. If the child retains sips of clear liquids, he or she can be offered portions of broth, clear soup, and skim milk in addition to clear liquids. Dry crackers or toast will help assuage hunger. By the second day, children can take a soft diet; by the third day, they should be back to their regular diet.

For the infant, introduce fluid after a fasting period of approximately 3 hours in the same slow manner: 1 tbsp every 15 minutes for 2 hours, then 1 oz every 2 hours for the next 12 to 18 hours. Glucose water or a commercial electrolyte solution such as Pedialyte may be given as fluid during this time to help the infant maintain electrolyte balance. Infants progress, as do older children, gradually to clear liquids or breast milk, then a soft diet, then a regular diet. If vomiting is prolonged, infants may need IV therapy to restore hydration (Banks & Meadows, 2005).

Teach parents the importance of following these routines of gradually increasing fluid at intervals. Assure them that if children receive a small amount of fluid and do not vomit it, they will ultimately receive more fluid than if they take a large amount but, because of a gastroenteritis, vomit that amount. Parents are capable of understanding that stomach secretions are lost along with vomitus each time, and the preservation of these stomach secretions is important to keep their child well. Antiemetics are rarely necessary for children. Always ask parents if they have used an herbal remedy, to be certain that any medication prescribed will be safe with the alternative treatment (Box 45.4).

Diarrhea

Diarrhea caused by a virus is the major cause of infant gastroenteritis in developing countries (Liacouras, 2003). The most common viral pathogens that invade the GI tract include rotaviruses and adenoviruses. The most common bacterial pathogens include *Campylobacter jejuni, Salmonella, Giardia lamblia,* and *Clostridium difficile.* Diarrhea in infants is always serious because infants have such a small ECF reserve that sudden losses of water exhaust the supply quickly. The loss of extracellular sodium leads to a decrease in plasma volume (additional water is excreted) and possible circulatory collapse. Renal failure results, with irreversible acidosis and death. Breastfeeding may actively prevent diarrhea by providing more antibodies and possibly an intestinal environment less friendly to invading organisms and so should be advocated.

BOX 45.4 FOCUS ON . . .

DIVERSITY OF CARE

The incidence of gastrointestinal illnesses is not the same in all communities. Vomiting and diarrhea, for example, tend to occur because of food poisoning in communities where refrigeration is less than optimal. Celiac disease occurs most frequently in children of Northern European ancestry. Because constipation, vomiting, and diarrhea are so common, every culture has home remedies for these symptoms: cascara for constipation; psyllium for diarrhea; ginger, peppermint, licorice, or chamomile tea for nausea or vomiting. To be certain that a child seen in a health care facility does not receive two forms of the same drug (one prescribed and one given in an herb form by a parent), always ask what home remedies have been given and document these on the child's plan of care.

Diarrhea that is acute is usually associated with infection; chronic diarrhea is more likely related to a malabsorption or inflammatory cause.

Mild Diarrhea

Assessment. Normal and diarrheal stool characteristics are compared in Table 45.4. In mild diarrhea, fever of 101°F to 102°F (38.4°C to 39.0°C) may be present. Children usually are anorectic and irritable and appear unwell. The episodes of diarrhea consist of 2 to 10 loose, watery bowel movements per day.

The mucous membrane of the mouth appears dry in an infant with mild diarrhea. The pulse will be rapid and out of proportion to the low-grade fever. Skin feels warm. Skin turgor is not yet decreased. Urine output is usually normal.

Therapeutic Management. At this stage, diarrhea is not yet serious, and children can be cared for at home. As with vomiting, treatment for diarrhea must involve resting the GI tract, but this is necessary for only a short time. At the end of approximately 1 hour, parents can begin to offer an oral rehydration solution such as Pedialyte in small amounts on a regimen similar to that for vomiting (Alper, 2004). For breast-fed infants, breast-feeding should continue. Again, it may be difficult for parents to restrict fluid for a short time if they think they should overfeed children to make up for the fluid loss. Children also need measures to reduce the elevated temperature. Caution parents not to use over-the-counter drugs such as loperamide (Imodium) or kaolin and pectin (Kaopectate) to halt diarrhea. As a rule, these are too strong for young children (Karch, 2004). Also caution parents to wash their hands after changing diapers to prevent the spread of infection and to notify their health care provider if fever, pain, or diarrhea worsens.

Infants may develop a lactase deficiency after diarrhea. This leads to lactose intolerance. With lactose intolerance, the child cannot take formula or breast milk or new diarrhea will begin. Such an infant will need to be introduced to a lactose-free formula initially before being returned to the usual formula or to breast milk.

Severe Diarrhea

Assessment. Severe diarrhea may result from progressive mild diarrhea, or it may begin in a severe form. Infants with severe diarrhea are obviously ill. Rectal temperature is often as high as 103°F to 104°F (39.5°C to 40.0°C). Both pulse and respirations are weak and rapid. The skin is pale and cool. Infants may appear apprehensive, listless, and lethargic. They have obvious signs of dehydration such as a depressed fontanelle, sunken eyes, and poor skin turgor. The episodes of diarrhea usually consist of a bowel movement every few minutes. The stool is liquid green, perhaps mixed with mucus and blood, and it may be passed with explosive force. Urine output will be scanty and concentrated. Laboratory findings will show elevated hematocrit, hemoglobin, and serum protein levels due to the dehydration. Electrolyte determinations will indicate a metabolic acidosis (King et al., 2003).

It is difficult to measure the amount of fluid the child has lost, but an estimate can be derived from the loss in body weight, if known. For example, if a child weighed 10.4 kg yesterday at a health maintenance visit and today weighs 8.9 kg, he or she has lost more than 10% of body weight. Mild dehydration occurs with a loss of 2.5% to 5% of body weight. In contrast, severe diarrhea quickly causes a 5% to 15% loss. Any infant who has lost 10% or more of body weight requires immediate treatment.

Therapeutic Management. Treatment focuses on regulating electrolyte and fluid balance by oral or IV rehydration therapy, initiating rest for the GI tract, and discovering the organism responsible for the diarrhea.

All children with severe diarrhea should have a stool culture taken so definite antibiotic therapy can be prescribed. Stool cultures may be taken from the rectum or from stool in the diaper or a bedpan. Blood specimens need to be drawn for a hemoglobin level (an estimation of hydration as well as anemia); white blood cell and differential counts (to attempt to establish whether infection is present); and determinations of Pco_2, Cl^-, Na^+, K^+, and pH (to establish electrolyte needs). If a child can drink, the most effective way to replace fluid is by offering oral rehydration therapy. For a child who will not drink, an IV solution such as normal saline or 5% glucose in normal saline is started. The solution will provide replacement of fluid, sodium, and calories. Although infants usually have a potassium depletion, potassium cannot be given until it is established that they are not in renal failure. Giving potassium IV when the body has no outlet for excessive potassium can lead to excessively high potassium levels and heart block. *Before this initial IV fluid is changed to a potassium solution, therefore, be certain that the infant or child has voided—proof that the kidneys are functioning.*

Fluid must be given to replace the deficit that has occurred, for maintenance therapy, and to replace the continuing loss until the diarrhea improves. If infants have lost less than 5% of total body weight, their fluid deficit is ap-

---

TABLE 45.4

Differentiation Between Infant Normal Stool and Diarrheal Stool

Characteristic	Infant Normal Stool	Diarrheal Stool
Frequency	1–3 daily	Unlimited number
Color	Yellow	Green
Effort of expulsion	Some pushing effort	Effortless; may be explosive
pH	More than 7.0 (alkaline)	Less than 7.0 (acidic)
Odor	Odorless	Sweet or foul smelling
Occult blood	Negative	Positive; blood may be overt
Reducing substances	Negative	Positive

proximately 50 mL/kg of body weight. If infants have lost 10% of body weight, they need approximately 100 mL/kg of body weight to replace their fluid deficit. If the weight loss suggests a 12% to 15% loss of body fluid, they require 125 mL/kg of body weight to replace the fluid lost. This fluid will be given rapidly in the first 3 to 6 hours, and then it will be slowed to a maintenance rate. Once infants void, a potassium additive may be ordered to restore serum potassium.

NURSING DIAGNOSES AND RELATED INTERVENTIONS

Nursing Diagnosis: Deficient fluid volume related to loss of fluid through diarrhea

Outcome Evaluation: Skin turgor remains good; specific gravity of urine is 1.003 to 1.030; urine output is more than 1 mL/kg/h; bowel movements are formed and fewer than four per day. Stool tests negative for reducing substances and blood pH is more than 7.

Promote Hydration and Comfort. During the time infants are NPO, to minimize the risk of vomiting, which would compound the problem by adding to the dehydration, wet infants' lips with a moisturizing jelly (Vaseline) if they appear to be dry. Give them a pacifier to suck if this seems to comfort them. (They want to suck because they are very thirsty, and, if they have intestinal cramping with the diarrhea, they interpret this as hunger.)

As the infant's condition improves, oral intake is increased, changing to a soft then a regular diet. Some children become lactose intolerant after diarrhea and will need a lactose-free formula for rehydration (Liacouras, 2003). If the child with severe diarrhea also has a fever, measures to reduce the fever will be necessary (see Chapter 36). Do not obtain rectal temperatures to assess fever, because stimulating the anal sphincter could initiate more diarrhea. Assess perianal skin for irritation from liquid stools, and keep the skin clean and dry.

Record Fluid Intake and Output. Much of the nursing care of children with diarrhea focuses on careful recording of fluid intake and output. Because children have dehydration when first seen, oral rehydration or IV therapy serves as their lifeline. Be sure to maintain proper functioning of an IV infusion and site if this is used. An arm board may be necessary to prevent catheter dislodgment or interference with the infusion. Soft restraints applied to the affected and unaffected extremities may be necessary to prevent the child from pulling, playing with, or poking at the tubing or site. If soft restraints are used, be sure to release them every hour and passively exercise the child's extremities. Give parents an explanation of why the IV infusion is important so they will understand the need for the soft restraints.

In children who are not toilet trained, apply a disposable urine collection bag to help separate urine from feces. This makes it obvious that the child is voiding, confirming kidney function. Confirmation of adequate kidney function is necessary for IV K+ replacement therapy, if ordered.

Separating urine from stools also helps to judge the appearance of stools or their water content better. For each stool passed, record its color, consistency, odor, size, and the presence of any blood or mucus. Weigh soiled diapers to reveal the number of grams of stool in the diaper (1 g = 1 mL fluid). Testing the stool for acidity and for reducing substances (sugars) indicates how quickly the stool is passing through the irritated tract. A stool positive for sugar indicates that little absorption has occurred, because sugar is absorbed rapidly from ingested food. Acid stool (pH less than 7.0) shows the presence of unabsorbed sugar also (a process occurs similar to the process that causes acid to invade tooth enamel in the presence of glucose on teeth). Diarrheal stools are green from lack of time for bile to be modified in the intestine. As diarrhea improves and stool remains in the intestine for a longer period, the stool deepens in color and the acid and sugar contents fade. Testing stools for occult blood shows the extent of bowel irritation that is occurring from the acid stool. As the diarrhea improves and the irritation to the bowel lessens, occult blood disappears.

Nursing Diagnosis: Risk for impaired skin integrity related to presence of diarrheal stool on skin

Outcome Evaluation: Skin in diaper area is not erythematous or ulcerated.

Because diarrheal stool is extremely irritating to the skin, change diapers immediately after infants pass any stool. Wash the skin of the diaper area well after each stool, and cover it with an ointment such as Vaseline or A and D to protect it from further irritation. If the child is older, caution him or her to wipe away stool thoroughly.

If infants already have skin excoriation from the number of stools they have had at home, an ointment such as Desitin may help soothe the irritated skin. Exposing infants' buttocks to air is generally helpful in healing irritation. Assure older children that loss of stool by diarrhea is not "shameful" or "babyish" but to be expected because they are ill.

Nursing Diagnosis: Anxiety related to traumatic experience

Outcome Evaluation: Child interacts with parents in age-appropriate way; can be comforted after painful procedures.

All children with diarrhea are assumed to have an infectious form of gastroenteritis and therefore need contact precautions and standard precautions. Children usually are uncomfortable from the diarrhea, exhausted, and confused with these new body sensations. They need the security of someone to stay with them. When a child with severe diarrhea is admitted to the hospital, many emergency procedures must be performed, such as collecting specimens, reducing temperature, and beginning rehydration. During all of these procedures, try to remember how all of this must seem to the child in the bed. Be sure to take time during initial procedures to touch and soothe children and talk to them; once the initial admission procedures are done, sit by the bed and hold the child or gently stroke the child's head. Teach parents how to adhere to standard precautions and follow contact precautions if necessary. Encourage them to give any care possible. Children need this support to counteract the strange world into which they have suddenly been plunged.

What if... Barry's mother tells you her doctor has told her to "force fluids" for Barry whenever he has diarrhea. She asks how much she should force the child to drink. How would you answer her?

Bacterial Infectious Diseases That Cause Diarrhea and Vomiting

Salmonella

- Causative agent: One of the *Salmonella* bacteria
- Incubation period: 6 to 72 hours for intraluminal type; 7 to 14 days for extraluminal type
- Period of communicability: As long as organisms are being excreted (may be as long as 3 months)
- Mode of transmission: Ingestion of contaminated food

Salmonella is the most common type of food poisoning in the United States and a major cause of diarrhea in children. The diagnosis of the infection can be made from stool culture. Children develop diarrhea, abdominal pain, vomiting, high temperature, and headache. They are listless and drowsy. The diarrhea is severe and may contain blood and mucus (AAP, 2003). *Salmonella* infection may remain in the bowel as an intraluminal disease. When it does, it is treated, like severe diarrhea, with fluid and electrolyte replacement. It also may become systemic (extraluminal disease); in that case, it is treated with the addition of an antibiotic such as ampicillin or a third-generation cephalosporin (Sentongo & Mulberg, 2003).

Complications such as meningitis, bronchitis, and osteomyelitis may occur. Although the source of *Salmonella* generally is infected food (contaminated chicken and eggs are common sources), it may be transmitted to children by infected turtles (Box 45.5).

Shigellosis (Dysentery)

- Causative agent: Organisms of the genus *Shigella*
- Incubation period: 1 to 7 days

BOX 45.5 FOCUS ON . . .

FAMILY TEACHING

Preventing *Salmonella*-Caused Gastroenteritis

Q. Barry's mother says to you, "Our son had severe diarrhea from food poisoning. The doctor said it was *Salmonella*. How can we make sure he doesn't get that again?"

A. Anyone can get *Salmonella* food poisoning. However, it can be prevented by using the following measures:

- Wash your hands well before preparing any foods, but especially chicken and eggs.
- Remember that chicken may become contaminated with *Salmonella* at the factory where it was prepared. Wash your hands well after handling raw chicken to prevent the spread of infection to other foods being prepared.
- Clean cutting boards or food preparation surfaces with hot, soapy water and dry thoroughly after use to prevent them from becoming reservoirs of infection.
- Make a habit of preparing chicken last, after other foods are prepared.
- Cook eggs well (do not use raw eggs in milkshakes; cook soft-boiled or poached eggs at least 3 min).
- Refrigerate chicken and eggs after preparation.
- Wash hands well after playing with or feeding a pet turtle or changing the turtle's water.

- Period of communicability: Approximately 1 to 4 weeks
- Mode of transmission: Contaminated food, water, or milk products

Shigella organisms, like the *Salmonella* group, cause extremely severe diarrhea that contains blood and mucus. As the organism becomes more resistant, ampicillin or trimethoprim–sulfamethoxazole, typical drugs used for therapy in the past, are being replaced by cephalosporins. The child needs intense fluid and electrolyte replacement. *Shigella* infection can be prevented by safe food handling and cautioning families to drink only from safe water sources (AAP, 2003).

Staphylococcal Food Poisoning

- Causative agent: Staphylococcal enterotoxin produced by some strains of *Staphylococcus aureus*
- Incubation period: 1 to 7 hours
- Period of communicability: Carriers may contaminate food as long as they harbor the organism
- Mode of transmission: Ingestion of contaminated food

With staphylococcal food poisoning, a child has severe vomiting and diarrhea, abdominal cramping, excessive salivation, and nausea. Organisms are most often spread through creamed foods. It is often difficult to culture the

Lamivudine (Epivir), an antiviral agent, may be effective in reducing viral replication with hepatitis B. Interferon also may be prescribed. Of those with type B, 90% will recover completely, but 10% will develop chronic hepatitis and become hepatitis carriers. Infants who contracted the disease at birth have an increased risk for liver carcinoma later in life (Tung, 2003).

Checkpoint Question 4

Barry's family likes to eat shellfish. What form of hepatitis is most apt to be contracted by eating contaminated shellfish?

a. Hepatitis B
b. Hepatitis A
c. Hepatitis E
d. Hepatitis C

NURSING DIAGNOSES AND RELATED INTERVENTIONS

Nursing Diagnosis: Pain related to pruritus of jaundice and liver inflammation

Outcome Evaluation: Child states level of itching is tolerable; no scratch marks on skin; reports right upper quadrant pain is minimal.

Jaundice commonly causes pruritus; for some children, this results in extreme discomfort. Being certain that the child is not overheated and not perspiring reduces the itching. A cool bath is often comforting. Skin moisturizers such as Eucerin or an antihistamine may be prescribed. Teach the child distraction techniques such as putting pressure on a pruritic area or trying imagery to lessen the urge to scratch.

Chronic Hepatitis

Hepatitis is considered chronic when it persists for longer than 6 months. This is most often the result of hepatitis B, D, or C infection. Abnormal liver enzyme levels and a liver biopsy establish the diagnosis and can also predict the severity. With chronic hepatitis, fatty infiltration and bile duct damage are present. The disease may progress to cirrhosis and eventually liver failure. Therapy is supportive to compensate for decreased liver function (Tung, 2003).

Fulminant Hepatic Failure

Fulminant hepatic failure is present when acute, massive necrosis or sudden, severe impairment of liver function occurs, leading to hepatic encephalopathy. Hepatic encephalopathy is the result of ammonia intoxication caused by the inability of the liver to detoxify the ammonia being constantly produced by the intestine in the process of digestion (Gillis, 2003).

Children show mental aberrations such as confusion, drowsiness, or disorientation. Treatment involves reducing protein intake and administering lactulose to prevent absorption of ammonia in the colon or administering nonabsorbable antibiotics such as neomycin to decrease the production of ammonia by the intestinal bacteria. Liver transplantation may be necessary, but many children cannot survive the long wait for a donor organ.

Obstruction of the Bile Ducts

Obstruction of the bile ducts in children generally occurs from congenital atresia, stenosis, or absence of the duct. It also can occur from a plugging of biliary secretions, though this is rare. When the bile duct is obstructed, bile, unable to enter the intestinal tract, accumulates in the liver. Bile pigments (direct bilirubin) enter the bloodstream and jaundice occurs, increasing in intensity daily (Haber, 2003).

Assessment

Although bile duct obstruction is a congenital disorder, the chief sign (jaundice) does not develop until approximately 2 weeks of age. This delay differentiates it clinically from physiologic jaundice, which occurs in almost all newborns on the third day of life, or the jaundice of Rh or ABO isoimmunization, which typically occurs during the first 24 hours of life. Laboratory findings will also distinguish this type of jaundice from other types. Physiologic jaundice and isoimmunization jaundice occur from a rise in indirect bilirubin, whereas the jaundice of bile duct obstruction is a result of a rise in direct bilirubin. Alkaline phosphatase levels are also elevated. The AST (SGOT) level is normal in the early phase and later becomes abnormal, when prolonged obstruction and backpressure cause liver cell damage. In addition, because bile salts (necessary for fat absorption) are not reaching the intestine, absorption of fat and fat-soluble vitamins (i.e., vitamins A, D, E, and K) is poor. Calcium absorption, which depends on vitamin D absorption, also is poor. The infant's stools appear light in color from lack of bile pigments. The pressure on the liver from the obstruction becomes so acute with time that cell destruction or cirrhosis occurs. Ultimately, without liver transplantation, death from liver failure will result (Haber, 2003).

Therapeutic Management

Before treatment is begun, appropriate blood work and a liver biopsy under local anesthesia may be done to rule out hepatitis. Duodenal secretions may be collected by endoscopy to assess for bile. Radionuclide imaging may also be performed; the infant is given an IV radioactive isotope that when taken up by the liver would normally be seen flowing through the bile ducts. If a mucus plug in the duct is suspected, children may be given magnesium sulfate (installed into the duodenum to relax the bile duct) or dehydrocholic acid (Decholin) IV to stimulate the flow of bile. If atresia of the bile duct appears to be the problem, surgical correction is the treatment (a Kasai procedure). With this surgery, a loop of bowel is sutured next to the liver to create a fistula for bile flow between the liver and intestine. A double-barreled colostomy is then created (enterostomy). Bile flows out of the proximal loop into a collecting bag. It is periodically returned to the distal loop of intestine by injection. After 6 to 12 weeks, the colostomy is closed when a normal bile flow has been established. However, surgical correction is impossible in all infants with atresia because the atresia tends to occur too far back in the liver to be in an operable area. Liver transplantation is needed for children with extensive involvement.

NURSING DIAGNOSES AND RELATED INTERVENTIONS

Nursing Diagnosis: Risk for imbalanced nutrition, less than body requirements, related to inability to digest fat

Outcome Evaluation: Infant's weight remains in same percentile on standardized growth curve; absence of vitamin deficiency (e.g., cracked lips or altered bone growth); dietary record reflects intake of adequate nutrients.

Preoperative Care. Infants who are admitted for surgery for bile duct obstruction are placed on a low-fat, high-carbohydrate diet preoperatively. They are given water-soluble forms of vitamins A, D, and K to improve vitamin levels. If the vitamin K level is too low, coagulation may be affected, increasing surgical risk. Vitamin K may be administered parenterally until prothrombin levels rise to normal limits. Infants will also be well hydrated with parenteral fluids.

Postoperative Care. After surgery, infants return with a nasogastric tube in place attached to low intermittent suction. Observe carefully for abdominal distention because paralytic ileus is a frequent complication of this type of surgery. The nasogastric tube will be left in place until peristalsis has returned. Gradually, children will be introduced to oral fluids and eventually to a normal diet. If the repair is successful, the child's stools change to a yellow and then brown (normal stool) color after surgery. Description of stools is, therefore, an important postoperative observation.

If bile flow is inadequate after surgery, infants will remain on a medium-fat, high-carbohydrate diet or receive total parenteral nutrition while they await transplantation surgery.

Cirrhosis

Cirrhosis is fibrotic scarring of the liver. Cirrhosis means "yellow," or the typical color of hepatic scar tissue. It occurs rarely in children, although it may be seen as a result of congenital biliary atresia or as a complication of chronic illnesses such as protracted hepatitis, sickle-cell anemia, or cystic fibrosis.

When fibrotic infiltrates replace normal liver cells, liver function is impaired, resulting in a decreased ability to detoxify toxic substances, decreased protein synthesis, inability to produce prothrombin, decreased ability to produce bile, and, possibly, hypoglycemia. Children will have large, fatty stools resulting from the decrease in bile production; avitaminosis of fat-soluble vitamins; symptoms of hemorrhage from decreased clotting ability; and anemia.

Fibrotic infiltration interferes not only with the function of liver cells but also with the hepatic blood flow. This leads to portal hypertension from the back-pressure of blood that cannot flow readily through the scarred organ (Fig. 45.4). Children will have compromised heart action, *ascites* (an exudate of fluid into the abdomen), possibly esophageal varices (back-pressure causes them to dilate), and hypersplenism (Gillis, 2003).

Once fibrotic infiltration begins, there is no way to reverse the changes. Nursing care focuses on promoting com-

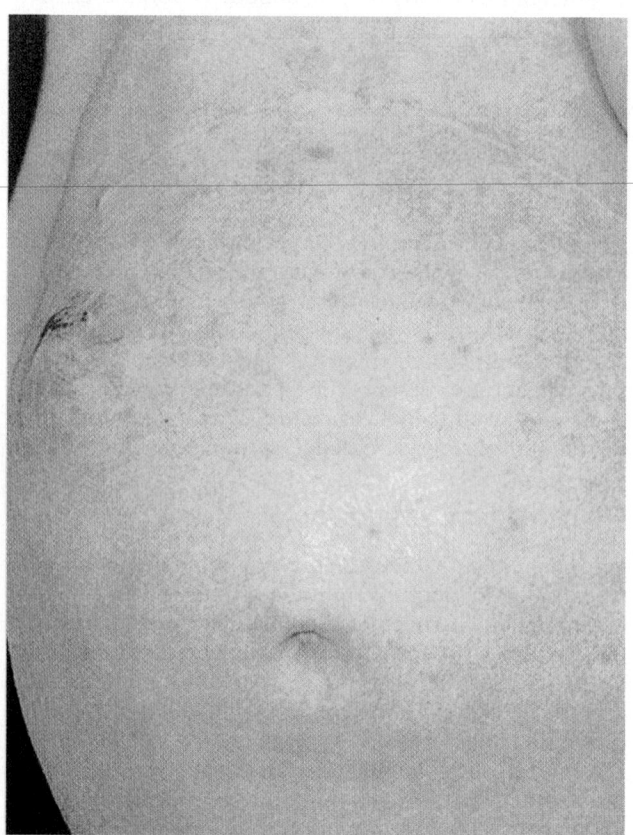

FIGURE 45.4 A child with cirrhosis of the liver. Note the abdominal distention and development of prominent, tortuous veins secondary to portal hypertension. (Zitelli, B. J. & Davis, H. W. [1997]. *Atlas of pediatric physical diagnosis* [3rd ed.]. St. Louis: Mosby-Year Book, Inc.)

fort, providing adequate nutrition by a high-carbohydrate, medium-chain-triglyceride diet, and preventing further involvement until liver transplantation can be scheduled. Cholestyramine (Questran) may be prescribed to stimulate bile flow and reduce reabsorption of bile into the circulation (this will minimize jaundice).

Esophageal Varices

Esophageal varices (distended veins) is a frequent complication of liver disorders such as cirrhosis (Gillis, 2003). They generally form at the distal end of the esophagus near the stomach secondary to back-pressure on the veins due to increased blood pressure in the portal circulation. Varices may bleed if children cough vigorously or strain to pass stool. Gastric reflux into the distal esophagus may irritate and erode the fine covering of the distended vessels, causing rupture.

Rupture of esophageal varices is an emergency because children can lose a large quantity of blood quickly from the ruptured, engorged vessels. Vasopressin or nitroglycerin may be given IV to lessen hypertension and reduce the hemorrhage. Injection of a sclerosing agent into veins may be attempted to decrease their size. Iced saline nasogastric lavage may be instituted to promote vasoconstriction. A Sengstaken-Blakemore tube or Linton-Nachlas catheter may be passed into the stomach. After insertion, balloons on the sides of the catheter are inflated to apply pressure against the bleeding vessels. As with an external tourniquet, the compression must be reduced for 5 to 10 minutes every 6 to 8 hours, or tissue necrosis can result.

Children must be monitored for future bleeding episodes. Frequent vital sign measurements and testing of stool and any vomitus for the presence of blood will indicate new GI system bleeding.

Liver Transplantation

Liver transplantation is the surgical replacement of a malfunctioning liver by a donor liver (Rand & Olthoff, 2003). Donor livers are not readily available, so the waiting time for surgery may be months. Finding an acceptable, child-sized liver may be especially difficult, so adult livers can be reduced in size for transplantation. A lobe of a liver from a living donor can be used. Often, the child is extremely ill with ascites, GI bleeding, extreme pruritus, hepatic encephalopathy, or renal dysfunction before the surgery can be performed. Nursing care after liver transplantation in a child is complex because it involves taking care of a child who has had major surgery, and also one who normally would be categorized as too ill to undergo surgery.

Despite the severity of illness and the length of surgery, children tend to recover quickly after liver transplantation. The survival rate is between 80% and 90% (Axelrod et al., 2004). Both children and parents must have thorough preoperative preparation so they understand the seriousness of the surgery and the possibility that the graft will be rejected. It helps to introduce the parents to others whose children have successfully undergone the procedure so they have support people available.

Preoperative Management

Preoperative management consists of keeping the child in the best physical condition possible so that, when a liver is available, transplantation can be performed. For many children, this includes dialysis and severe nutritional restrictions.

Surgical Procedure

Liver transplantation requires a wide subcostal incision. The vena cava is temporarily clamped during the removal of the natural liver to prevent bleeding, which means that all IV lines must be placed in the upper extremities (if placed in lower extremities, fluid could not return through the clamped venous circulation to the upper body). The total operation takes 10 to 14 hours to complete.

Postoperative Management

Rejection of a liver transplant is most often due to the function of T lymphocytes. Careful tissue matching (HLA matching) is necessary to reduce the possibility of stimulating T-cell rejection. To further reduce the action of T lymphocytes, children are given an immunosuppressive drug such as cyclosporine or tacrolimus (Prograf) before the transplantation.

Nursing care after liver transplantation surgery focuses on preventing complications that may arise from the surgery and continued immunosuppression. Children may need assisted ventilation for approximately 24 hours postoperatively to prevent pulmonary complications such as atelectasis and pneumonia because the large abdominal incision makes coughing and deep breathing difficult. In addition, ascites has placed pressure against the diaphragm, interfering with lung expansion, and preoperative pulmonary edema may be present. After discontinuation of mechanical ventilation and extubation, chest physiotherapy may be started to mobilize lung secretions.

Advocate for adequate pain control. Assess blood pressure, capillary refill, peripheral pulses, and skin color frequently to ensure adequate cardiovascular function, which is important for good tissue perfusion of the transplanted liver. The child may have a central venous pressure line or an arterial line such as a Swan-Ganz catheter inserted to assess hemodynamic status. Assess neurologic status hourly using a modified Glasgow Coma Scale (see Chapter 52).

Usually, the child is positioned flat for the first 24 hours to prevent cerebral air emboli, which may result from any air remaining in the transplanted liver. Typically, children have a nasogastric tube inserted during surgery attached to low intermittent suction postoperatively. Irrigate the tube according to agency policy to maintain patency. Assess the gastric pH by aspirating stomach contents every 4 hours; based on this assessment, administer antacids or H_2 receptor antagonists such as cimetidine or mucosal protectants as prescribed to help prevent stress ulcer. If preoperative esophageal varices are present, assess nasogastric drainage carefully for frank or occult blood.

A T-tube inserted into the bile duct for drainage allows the amount of bile being produced by the new liver to be evaluated. Once bowel sounds become active, nasogastric suction and the T-tube are usually discontinued and liquids and then solid foods are introduced gradually. If vomiting occurs and is persistent, total parenteral nutrition may be used for 3 or 4 days to rest the intestinal tract before fluid is reintroduced.

Hypoglycemia is a danger postoperatively because glucose levels are regulated by the liver, and the transplanted organ may not function efficiently at first. Assess serum glucose levels hourly by fingerstick puncture. A 10% solution of dextrose IV may be necessary to prevent hypoglycemia.

Sodium, potassium, chloride, and calcium levels are evaluated approximately every 6 to 8 hours to be certain that an electrolyte balance is maintained. Even if a low potassium level is detected, potassium is rarely added to IV solutions because of the risk that renal failure has occurred due to the stress of surgery. Plus, if the graft begins to necrose, the breakdown of cells will release potassium, elevating the level even more. Continuous cardiac monitoring is usually necessary to detect hyperkalemia (hyperkalemia causes elevation of T waves or ventricular fibrillation), hypokalemia (causes small T waves and a U wave), or other arrhythmias.

Many children develop hypertension within 72 hours after surgery. This occurs because of alterations in the renin-angiotensin system due to the not yet fully functioning transplanted liver or as a side effect of cyclosporine, tacrolimus, and steroid therapy, which is continued postoperatively to guard against transplant rejection. IV therapy with hypotensive agents such as hydralazine (Apresoline) and nitroprusside may be needed to reduce hypertension. Hypotension will occur if the transplanted liver becomes dysfunctional or if there is bleeding caused by poor blood coagulation. The child also has an increased risk for bleeding because of the number of sites for anastomosis involved with the procedure. To help detect bleeding, observe and record abdominal girth, the incision line, and drainage from any catheters or tubes placed in the incision to allow peritoneal secretions to drain.

A warming blanket may be required postoperatively to maintain normal body temperature after the long exposure of surgery. Take axillary or tympanic, not rectal, temperatures, because many children with liver damage have hemorrhoids that could rupture from the trauma of a thermometer insertion. Prevent the child from unnecessary exposure during procedures and care to help maintain normal body temperature.

NURSING DIAGNOSES AND RELATED INTERVENTIONS

Nursing Diagnosis: Risk for infection related to administration of immunosuppressive medication

Outcome Evaluation: Temperature remains within normal range; no presence of exudate or inflammation around abdominal incision.

Liver transplantation is possible because of the preoperative administration of an immunosuppressive agent that suppresses T lymphocytes, the lymphocytes responsible for rejecting transplanted organs. In addition, immunosuppressive agents are administered IV immediately postoperatively to prevent graft rejection. Because children are prone to infection while receiving immunosuppressive therapy, be sure to use strict aseptic technique, standard precautions, and careful handwashing. Clean the skin around any abdominal drains every 4 hours to avoid skin breakdown and prevent a portal of entry for microorganisms.

Serum transaminases (AST [SGOT] and ALT [SGPT]), alkaline phosphatase, serum bilirubin, and ammonia levels are assessed at least daily to detect rejection. However, children usually do not show signs of liver rejection until 5 to 7 days after surgery. In addition to changes in these laboratory values, with liver rejection the child also may develop fever and increasing abdominal girth. Also, the urine turns orange from increased urobilinogen excretion. If signs of rejection appear to be occurring, doses of cyclosporine, tacrolimus, and a corticosteroid such as methylprednisolone are increased to maximum levels.

Nursing Diagnosis: Interrupted family processes related to stress of surgery and uncertainty of transplantation outcome

Outcome Evaluation: Child and family state that although waiting is difficult, they are able to do so; identify ways they have changed their family life at home to accommodate child's illness and surgery.

Children and parents need continued support during the postoperative period while they wait to see if the graft will be rejected (LoBiondo-Wood, Williams, & McGhee, 2004). They need continued contact with health care personnel through telephone calls and clinic visits.

After successful liver transplantation, a child should be able to function normally, attending school and enjoying age-appropriate activities. Be certain by hospital discharge that parents have a return appointment for evaluation and are aware of the symptoms of graft rejection, such as jaundice, lethargy, and fever.

INTESTINAL DISORDERS

Because the intestines form a long body system, a number of either congenital or acquired disorders can occur.

Intussusception

Intussusception is the invagination of one portion of the intestine into another (Fig. 45.5). This disorder generally occurs in the second half of the first year of life (Wasserman, 2003).

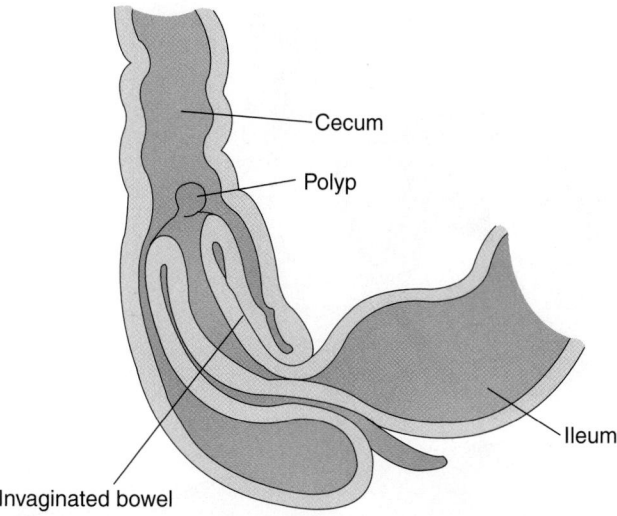

FIGURE 45.5 Intussusception. The distal ileal segment of bowel has invaginated into the cecum. A polyp serves as a lead point.

Cecum

Polyp

Ileum

Invaginated bowel

In infants younger than 1 year, intussusception generally occurs for idiopathic reasons. In infants older than 1 year, a "lead point" on the intestine likely cues the invagination. Such a point might be a Meckel's diverticulum, a polyp, hypertrophy of *Peyer's patches* (lymphatic tissue of the bowel that increases in size with viral diseases), or bowel tumors. The point of the invagination is generally the juncture of the distal ileum and proximal colon.

This condition is a surgical emergency. Reduction of the intussusception must be done promptly by either instillation of solution (or air) or surgery before necrosis of the invaginated portion of the bowel occurs.

Assessment

Children with this disorder suddenly draw up their legs and cry as if they are in severe pain; they may vomit. After the peristaltic wave that caused the discomfort passes, they are symptom-free and play happily. In approximately 15 minutes, the same phenomenon of intense abdominal pain strikes again. Vomitus will begin to contain bile because the obstruction is invariably below the ampulla of Vater, the point in the intestine where bile empties into the duodenum. After approximately 12 hours, blood appears in the stool, described as a "currant jelly" appearance. The abdomen becomes distended as the bowel above the intussusception distends (Klein, Kapoor, & Shugerman, 2004).

If necrosis has occurred, children generally have an elevated temperature, peritoneal irritation (their abdomen will feel tender; they may "guard" it by tightening their abdominal muscles), an increased white blood cell count, and often a rapid pulse.

The diagnosis is suggested by the history. Any time a parent is describing a child who is crying, be certain to ask enough questions to recognize the possibility of intussusception:

• What is the duration of the pain? (It lasts a short time, with intervals of no crying in between.)

• What is the intensity? (Severe)
• What is the frequency? (Approximately every 15 to 20 minutes)
• What is the description? (The child pulls up his or her legs with crying.)
• Is the child ill in any other way? (Yes. Vomits; refuses food; states his or her stomach feels "full.")

The presence of the intussusception is confirmed by a sonogram.

Therapeutic Management

Intussusception requires surgery to straighten the invaginated portion, or reduction by instillation of a water-soluble solution, barium enema, or air (pneumatic insufflation). If there is no lead point, just the pressure of these nonsurgical techniques may reduce the intussusception. After this type of reduction, children are observed for 24 hours because some children will have a recurrence of the intussusception within 24 hours. If this occurs, they are scheduled for an additional reduction or surgery.

NURSING DIAGNOSES AND RELATED INTERVENTIONS

Nursing Diagnosis: Pain related to abnormal abdominal peristalsis

Outcome Evaluation: Child can be comforted between spasms of pain, demonstrates interest in toys or social interactions.

Infants with intussusception are bewildered by this type of episodic pain because it is so different from any pain they have experienced before. Ordinarily, if they pinch a finger on a toy and it hurts, a parent picks them up, kisses their fingers, and the pain goes away. A parent picks them up now and the pain goes away, but it returns repeatedly. Infants need to be held and rocked and comforted in an attempt to relieve their frustration at this strange happening.

Nursing Diagnosis: Risk for deficient fluid volume related to bowel obstruction

Outcome Evaluation: Infant's skin turgor is good; pulse is 90 to 100 beats/min. Amount of diarrhea and blood loss in stool is minimal. Episodes of vomiting decrease in frequency.

Infants are kept on NPO status before surgery or nonsurgical reduction. Because they have abdominal pain, they may find comfort in sucking a pacifier. Because they have been vomiting, IV fluid therapy may be started to reestablish their electrolyte balance and to supply adequate fluid to hydrate them.

If a nonsurgical reduction is accomplished, infants are kept NPO for a few hours and then introduced gradually to regular feedings. Infants who have surgery will return with a nasogastric tube attached to low intermittent suction and an IV infusion in place. The nasogastric tube will remain in place until the suture line is healing and peristaltic function has returned. Once bowel sounds are present, oral feedings will be started gradually.

Nursing Diagnosis: Risk for impaired parenting related to infant's illness

Outcome Evaluation: Parents hold and talk to infant; express positive characteristics about infant.

Parents need to hold infants after reduction or postoperatively to promote bonding and also to comfort the infant. Provide guidance and support as they hold the infant. When oral feeding is resumed, encourage the parents to participate with this aspect of care, as it provides them with an opportunity to regain confidence in themselves as parents. Reassure them that this did not occur because of anything they did. Whenever a child's disorder begins with vomiting, many parents worry that the vomiting is somehow related to the child's method of feeding. Urge them to hold and be with the child as recovery proceeds to reassure themselves that the child is now all right again.

Volvulus

A **volvulus** is a twisting of the intestine (Fig. 45.6). The twist leads to obstruction of the passage of feces and compromise of the blood supply to the loop of intestine involved. This occurs most often because, in fetal life, a portion of the intestine first protrudes into the base of the umbilical cord at approximately age 6 weeks. At approximately age 10 weeks, it returns to the abdominal cavity. As the intestine returns to the abdominal cavity, it rotates to its permanent position. After the rotation, the mesentery becomes fixed in this position. In volvulus, this action is incomplete and the mesentery does not attach to a normal position. The bowel is left free to move and twist (Mulberg, 2003).

Usually, the symptoms are those of intestinal obstruction and occur during the first 6 months of life. Symptoms may include intense crying and pain, pulling up the legs, abdominal distention, and vomiting. The diagnosis is made based on the history and an abdominal examination, which reveals an abdominal mass. A sonogram or lower barium x-ray also will show the obstruction. Surgery is used to relieve the volvulus and reattach the bowel so it no longer is so free moving. This must be done promptly before necrosis of the intestine occurs from a lack of blood supply to the involved loop of bowel. Preoperative and postoperative care will be the same as for infants with intussusception.

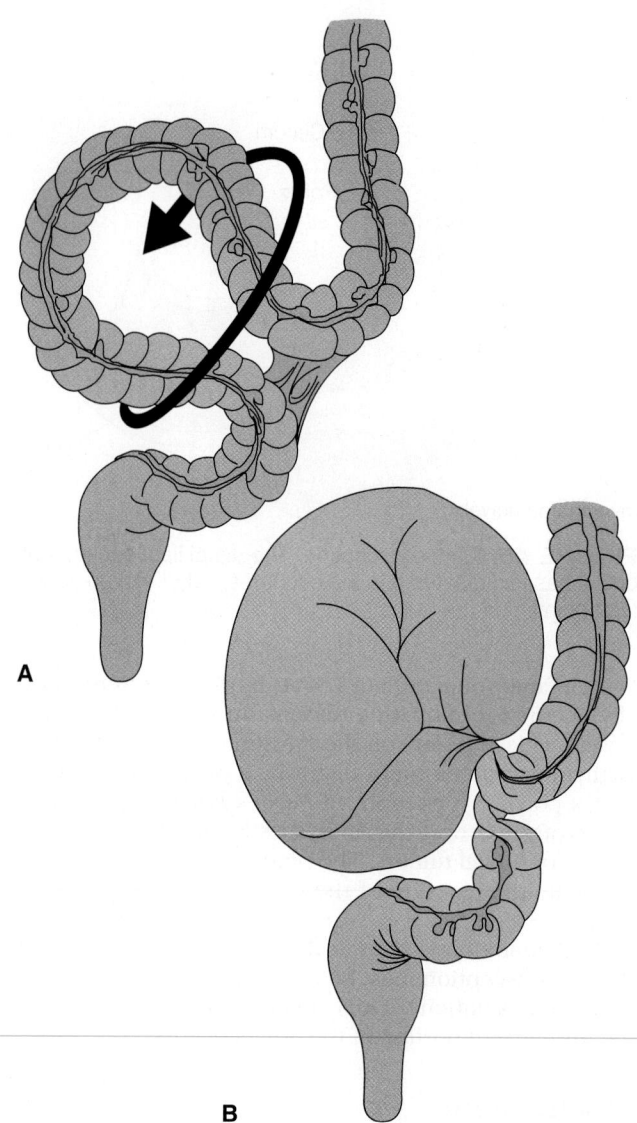

A

B

FIGURE 45.6 Volvulus of the sigmoid colon. (**A**) The unattached loop of bowel twists. (**B**) The bowel lumen is obstructed, leading to inability of stool to pass and compression of the blood supply to the looped bowel segment.

Necrotizing Enterocolitis

Necrotizing enterocolitis (NEC) is a condition that develops in approximately 5% of all infants in intensive care nurseries. The bowel develops necrotic patches, interfering with digestion and possibly leading to a paralytic ileus. Perforation and peritonitis may follow.

The necrosis appears to result from ischemia or poor perfusion of blood vessels in sections of bowel. The ischemic process may occur when, owing to shock or hypoxia, there is vasoconstriction of blood vessels to nonessential organs such as the bowel. The entire bowel may be involved, or it may be a localized phenomenon. The incidence of NEC is highest in immature infants, those who have suffered anoxia or shock, and those fed by enteral feedings. Infants with infections may develop it as a further complication of their already stressed state.

Assessment

There is a lower incidence of the condition in infants who are fed breast milk than in those who are fed formula because intestinal organisms grow more profusely with cow's milk than breast milk (cow's milk lacks antibodies). A response to the foreign protein in cow's milk may be a mechanism that starts the necrotic process. Therefore, encouraging breast-feeding may help prevent this disorder (Updegrove, 2004).

Signs of NEC usually appear in the first week of life. The infant's abdomen becomes distended and tense. The stomach does not fully empty by the next feeding time because of poor intestinal action; if the stomach contents are aspirated before a feeding, a return of undigested milk of more than 2 mL will be obtained. Stool may be positive for occult blood. Periods of apnea may begin or increase in number. Signs of blood loss due to intestinal bleeding, such as lowered blood pressure and inability to stabilize temperature, also may be present.

Abdominal x-ray films show a characteristic picture of air invading the intestinal wall; if perforation has occurred, there will be air in the abdominal cavity. Abdominal girth measurements made just above the umbilicus every 4 to 8 hours show increases.

Therapeutic Management

As soon as the condition is recognized, feedings must be discontinued, and the infant is maintained on IV or total parenteral nutrition solutions to rest the GI tract. An antibiotic may be given to limit secondary infection. Handle the abdomen gently to lessen the possibility of bowel perforation (Horton, 2005).

If bowel obstruction occurs, the infant may need a temporary colostomy performed to allow for bowel function. If the area of necrosis appears to be localized, surgery to remove that portion of the bowel may be successful. If a large portion of the bowel is removed, the infant may be prone to "short-bowel" syndrome or may have a problem with digestion of nutrients in the future. If the bowel perforates, peritoneal drainage or a laparotomy will be necessary to help remove fecal secretions from the abdomen.

NEC is a grave insult to an infant already stressed by immaturity. The prognosis is guarded until the infant can again take oral feedings without bowel complications.

Appendicitis

Appendicitis (inflammation of the appendix) is the most common cause of abdominal surgery in children. It is seen most frequently in school-age children and adolescents, although it can occur in preschoolers and even in newborns (Stern & Mulberg, 2003). The *appendix,* a blind-ended pouch attached to the cecum, may become inflamed after an upper respiratory or other body infection, but the cause of appendicitis is generally obscure. In most instances, fecal material apparently enters the appendix, hardens, and obstructs the appendiceal lumen. Inflammation and edema develop, leading to compression of blood vessels and cellular malnutrition. Necrosis and pain result. If the condition is not discovered early enough, the necrotic area will rupture and fecal material will spill into the abdomen, causing peritonitis—a potentially fatal condition.

Assessment

Most people assume that appendicitis begins with sharp pain, so they may dismiss their children's early symptoms for some time as simple gastroenteritis. Actually, pain is a late symptom in appendicitis. The history typically begins with anorexia for 12 to 24 hours. Children do not eat and do not act like their usual selves. Nausea and vomiting may then occur. The abdominal pain, when it does start, is at first diffuse. Gradually, it becomes localized to the right lower quadrant. The point of sharpest pain is often one third of the way between the anterior superior iliac crest and the umbilicus (**McBurney's point**). If the child's appendix is displaced from the usual position, the pain will not be at this typical point, so pain at any other point does not rule out appendicitis. Fever is a late symptom.

It is important in history taking to document the progress of the disease, for example:

- How was the child on Monday? (Not herself. She was not eating.)
- How was she Monday night? (She had generalized abdominal pain.)
- Tuesday morning? (She had sharp localized pain.)
- Now? (She has localized pain, vomiting, and fever.)

Until the pain becomes localized, appendicitis is difficult to distinguish from acute gastroenteritis. On abdominal examination, right lower quadrant tenderness may be elicited. Often, it is difficult to palpate children's abdomens because they guard their abdomen and make them stiff and hard by tensing their abdominal muscles. Although this interferes with abdominal examination, it is in itself an important sign that children have abdominal pain. To assist in a diagnosis of a painful abdomen, always palpate the anticipated tender area last.

Rebound tenderness is a phenomenon in which the child feels relatively mild pain when the area over his or her appendix is palpated, but, once the examiner's hand is withdrawn, the child experiences acute pain caused by the shifting of the abdominal contents. This is diagnostic for appendicitis, but it should be done with children only when necessary because it does cause acute pain. Caution children that the maneuver may cause pain. On auscultation, bowel sounds will be reduced: only one or two are heard in the same length of time that 30 are normally heard. Absence of bowel sounds on auscultation suggests peritonitis or an appendix that has already ruptured.

Laboratory findings usually indicate leukocytosis (white blood cell count between 10,000 and 18,000/mm^3), which is actually low for the extent of the infection that may be present. Ketone levels in the urine are inordinately elevated as a symptom of starvation from poor intestinal absorption.

A sonogram reveals the swollen appendix. It can also be confirmed by a CT scan. Pain in the right lower quadrant may occur as a manifestation of right lower lobe pneumonia. Therefore, children may have a chest x-ray taken to rule this out as the source of pain.

Therapeutic Management

Therapy for appendicitis is surgical removal of the appendix by laparoscopy before it ruptures (Sauerland, Lefering, & Neugebauer, 2005). Achieving surgery before rupture occurs is easier in older children, who are more capable of relating the progression of symptoms. It is more difficult in young children, whose history is not as accurate, who do not have the words to describe their symptoms, or who will not relax their abdominal muscles enough to allow for manual examination. Also, the wall of the appendix is thinner and perforates more readily in young children.

NURSING DIAGNOSES AND RELATED INTERVENTIONS

Priorities for nursing care must be established quickly because this is an emergency, and the child must be prepared immediately for surgery (Box 45.6).

Nursing Diagnosis: Pain related to inflamed appendix

Outcome Evaluation: Child states that level of pain is tolerable.

Once a diagnosis is made by a sonogram, the child needs an analgesic for pain. Cathartics and heat to the abdomen are contraindicated, because they may lead to rupture of the appendix. The abdomen will be shaved and washed with an antiseptic solution immediately before surgery. If you are assisting with the procedure, be gentle because the abdomen is tender, and compression could cause the appendix to rupture. Use lukewarm, not hot water, because heat can increase the possibility of appendix rupture by increasing edema in the appendix. Urge the child to find the best position of comfort, and assure both parents and the child that emergency steps are being carried out.

Nursing Diagnosis: Fear related to emergency nature of disorder and immediate surgery

Outcome Evaluation: Parents and child state that they understand what interventions are necessary and cooperate as necessary.

Admission for appendicitis often occurs rapidly. A parent telephones the primary care provider, who recommends the child be seen in an emergency room. Surgery is scheduled as soon as it can be arranged. A mere 30 minutes may pass from the time of the first phone call until the child is wheeled to surgery. During this time, the parent and child both need to be told exactly what is happening ("I'm going to take some blood; I'm putting your name tag on your arm") and who the people are who are caring for them ("This is Dr. Brown, the anesthesiologist. I'm Ms. Henry, a registered nurse."). Parents do not think clearly in this type of emergency, and their reactions to situations may not be their usual ones. Explain that the procedures being done for the child (e.g., blood studies or a short wait while an operating room is prepared) are necessary for safe surgery and that the danger of the appendix rupturing is not as acute a danger as they may have believed.

Remember that these children have had no preparation for hospitalization. The axiom "What they don't know won't hurt them" is not true. Lack of knowledge can make appendicitis a harrowing experience for parents as well as children. Praise them for the things they did well, such as recognizing the child was ill and bringing him or her immediately for care, to help offer a sense of control.

Nursing Diagnosis: Risk for deficient fluid volume related to NPO status

Outcome Evaluation: Child's skin fold returns flat quickly when turgor is assessed; pulse and blood pressure are within normal age limits; weight is maintained.

Preoperatively, obtain a urine sample for urinalysis and blood for a complete blood count. IV fluid therapy may be initiated to hydrate a child who has been vomiting a great deal. Postoperatively, children will be maintained on IV fluids until they can take adequate oral feedings (approximately 24 hours). With unruptured appendicitis, the postoperative course is uneventful; children are up a few hours after surgery and are discharged within a number of days. They generally return to school in another week.

Ruptured Appendix

If a child's appendix has already ruptured when the child is seen in the emergency department, the potential for peritonitis is great. When rupture occurs, children generally appear severely ill. The white blood cell count rises to more than $20,000/mm^3$. Position the child in a semi-Fowler's position so that infected drainage from the cecum drains downward into the pelvis rather than upward to the lungs. The child needs an IV fluid line inserted for hydration. Antibiotics will be begun preoperatively or when the ruptured appendix is confirmed.

During surgery, the child will have drains placed beside the surgery incision so any infectious material in the abdomen can continue to drain. Warm soaks may be ordered three or four times a day to encourage drainage. Examine the wound carefully at each dressing change. Be certain not to dislodge drains while removing soiled dressings. Report immediately any drain that is expelled; the surgeon may want to replace it to ensure a patent drainage route. Often, drains are shortened with each dressing change to encourage initially deep areas, then areas closer to the skin

A Multidisciplinary Care Map for A Child with Appendicitis

•

Barry's parents bring his older sister, 10-year-old Leann, to the emergency department because of nausea, vomiting, and abdominal pain since yesterday. Father states, "We thought it was just an upset stomach, but it isn't getting any better, and the pain is much worse now."

Family Assessment

Child lives with 2 younger siblings and both parents on a rural horse farm. Father works as a newspaper printer in town; mother cares for horses and stable. Mother reports finances as, "Good. We're enjoying this time of life."

Client Assessment

Well-nourished, 10-year-old female with a history of no major medical problems. Temperature 101.2°F; pulse 100; respirations 24. Mother reports that yesterday the child stated she was not feeling well. "She wasn't eating, and she had pains in her stomach. Last night, the pain got worse and she started vomiting." Pain now localized in right lower quadrant. Legs drawn up against abdomen. Bowel sounds sluggish. Rebound tenderness present. White blood cell count of 17,000/mm³. Ultrasound confirms appendicitis. Child is scheduled for emergency appendectomy.

Nursing Diagnosis

Pain related to presence of appendicitis

Outcome Criteria

Child states pain is not above a 2 on 1–10 pain scale.

Team Member Responsible	Assessment	Intervention	Rationale	Expected Outcome
Activities of Daily Living				
Nurse	Assess what is child's most comfortable position.	Do not palpate child's abdomen.	Palpating could rupture inflamed appendix.	Child states she knows not to put pressure on abdomen.
Consultations				
Physician	Assess what anesthetist is available for emergency surgery.	Consult with anesthetist about emergency surgery.	Emergency surgery has added risks because of lack of preparation.	Anesthesiology service consults and readies for surgery.
Procedures/Medications				
Nurse	Assess if child has ever had surgery before.	Wash abdomen and shave from nipple line to groin.	Removing abdominal hair helps prevent infection.	Abdominal preparation is completed prior to surgery.
Nurse	Assess if child's armband is in place.	Complete preoperative checklist.	Safety precautions are important to prevent misidentification during surgery.	Child's armband is in place; preoperative checklist completed and signed.

(continued)

Team Member Responsible	Assessment	Intervention	Rationale	Expected Outcome
Nutrition				
Nurse	Assess when was the last time child ate or drank. Assess skin turgor.	Keep child NPO while awaiting surgery.	Eating could evoke vomiting with aspiration during surgery.	Child cooperates to remain NPO until surgery.
Nurse	Assess if child has had prior experience with IV fluid administration.	Begin IV fluid as prescribed.	IV fluid can help prevent dehydration from previous vomiting while NPO.	Child states she understands why IV is prescribed; protects infusion site from trauma.
Patient/Family Education				
Nurse	Assess what child/parents understand about appendicitis.	Teach child and parents as needed about cause and course of appendicitis.	Better understanding of a child's condition can help child and parents accept the necessary procedures.	Child and parents state they have no questions about cause of course of appendicitis.
Psychosocial/Spiritual/Emotional Needs				
Nurse	Assess child's level of pain using a 1–10 pain scale.	Discuss surgeon's preference to not prescribe analgesic as child will soon be anesthetized in O.R.	Pain relief may be delayed until appendicitis is diagnosed.	Child states she understands her pain will be relieved as soon as anesthesia is begun.
Nurse	Assess if child has experience with nonpharmacologic pain relief measures.	Teach child a nonpharmacologic pain relief method such as imagery.	Nonpharmacologic pain relief can be very effective for abdominal pain in children.	Uses imagery as nonpharmacologic pain relief technique.
Nurse	Assess child and parents' level of apprehension about emergency situation.	Discuss positive aspects of parents' actions.	Reinforcing that parents acted with good judgment can increase self-esteem and ability to accept new developments.	Child and parents state that although their stress level is high, they are able to cope with new developments.
Discharge Planning				
Nurse	Assess if child and parents have any questions prior to leaving for operating room.	Review what will happen in O.R. and immediate postoperative course.	The better informed child and parents are of happenings, the better they will be able to cooperate.	Child and parents state they feel prepared for next step in treatment for child's condition.

to drain. IV fluid and antibiotic therapy are continued until full bowel function is restored.

Assess for signs of peritonitis with dressing changes. These signs may include a boardlike (rigid) abdomen, generally shallow respirations (because deep breathing puts pressure on the abdomen and causes pain), and increased temperature. Although the postoperative course is slower (approximately 3 weeks) after a ruptured appendix, the prognosis is still good. A local abscess or intestinal adhesions may result. Adhesion formation, a long-term effect, could interfere with fertility in girls or cause bowel obstruction in both sexes later in life.

What if... Barry's older sister had appendicitis. What if her parent tells you she "dropped everything" to rush a child to the emergency room because of appendicitis? What questions would you want to ask to see if she has thought through the situation?

Meckel's Diverticulum

In embryonic life, the intestine is attached to the umbilicus by the omphalomesenteric (vitelline) duct. This duct be-

have parents refrain from introducing new feeding methods, such as a cup or spoon, unless children are at that developmental point where they will quickly adapt to the new procedure and are, in fact, so eager to feed themselves that they will actually eat better this way.

Postoperatively, after removal of the aganglionic portion and anastomosis of the colon at the second step of the repair, infants will return with a nasogastric tube in place attached to low suction, an IV infusion, and probably an indwelling urinary (Foley) catheter. Observe the infant for abdominal distention. Assess bowel sounds and observe also for passage of flatus and stools. As soon as peristalsis has returned (approximately 24 hours after surgery), the nasogastric tube may be removed and the child may be offered small, frequent feedings of fluids, such as water or gelatin. The child is then introduced gradually to full fluids, a soft diet, a minimal-residue diet, and, finally, a normal diet for age.

Nursing Diagnosis: Risk for compromised family coping related to chronic illness in child

Outcome Evaluation: Parents state they are able to cope with the level of stress present from their child's condition.

Most parents feel tremendous relief after the second-stage surgery is complete. Caution parents that the child may still remain a "fussy eater" for a few months, because feeding problems that begin for physical reasons can continue for emotional or psychological reasons. Help parents to diminish the importance of meals gradually; to schedule periods during the day when they give their full attention to the child, such as reading a story or putting a puzzle together; and to offer praise for pleasant, not difficult, behavior. These measures will help mealtime problems gradually diminish.

Inflammatory Bowel Disease: Ulcerative Colitis and Crohn's Disease

Two conditions are categorized as inflammatory bowel disease: **ulcerative colitis** and **Crohn's disease.** Both involve the development of ulcers of the mucosa or submucosa layers of the colon and rectum. They both occur most frequently in young adults and adolescents, although, more and more frequently, symptoms first appear during school age. Both diseases occur more frequently in males than in females and show familial tendencies.

The causes of these disorders are obscure, but they probably represent an alteration in immune system response or are autoimmune processes. There is an increased number of immunoglobulins IgA and IgG present on intestinal mucosa. IgE immunoglobulins and the eosinophil count also may be elevated. Psychological factors have not been supported as a primary contributory factor to inflammatory bowel disease, but psychological problems often occur secondary to the disease, possibly intensifying symptoms.

Smoking and frequent use of antibiotics or aspirin are correlated with the occurrence of Crohn's disease (Mamula & Markowitz, 2003).

Crohn's disease is an inflammation of segments of the intestine; it may affect any part of the GI tract but most commonly involves the terminal ileum. Inflamed segments are separated by normal bowel tissue. The wall of the colon becomes thickened and the surface is inflamed, leading to a "cobblestone" appearance of mucosa. Usually, the areas of the bowel affected are higher in the intestine than in ulcerative colitis. In ulcerative colitis, typically the colon and rectum are involved, with the distal colon and rectum most severely affected, and inflammation involves continuous segments (Markowitz & Baldassano, 2003).

As inflammation becomes acute with these disorders, children develop abdominal pain from contractions of the irritated portions. These areas do not absorb nutrients or fluid well, so diarrhea and malnutrition develop. To reduce abdominal pain (which is most acute after eating, when the bowel becomes active), children begin to skip meals. They may be malnourished and have a vitamin or iron deficiency when the condition is diagnosed.

A number of complications may occur. Hemorrhage from bowel perforation during the active disease is possible. Perforation can lead to peritonitis or the formation of fistulas between bowel loops. Rectal fistula is present in as many as 20% of children. A relapse is apt to occur 6 to 12 months after therapy. With ulcerative colitis, there is an association between the disease and bowel carcinoma if the disease persists over 10 years (Markowitz & Baldassano, 2003).

Assessment

In both conditions, diarrhea and steatorrhea develop from the irritation and the unabsorbed fluid. If inflamed portions ulcerate, there will be blood in the stool. Weight loss occurs; growth failure occurs in prepubertal children. A recurring fever may be present (Table 45.6).

TABLE 45.6		
Comparison of Crohn's Disease and Ulcerative Colitis		
Comparison Factor	**Crohn's Disease**	**Ulcerative Colitis**
Part of bowel affected	Ileum	Colon and rectum
Nature of lesions	Intermittent	Continuous
Diarrhea	Moderate	Severe and bloody
Anorexia	Severe	Mild
Weight loss	Severe	Mild
Growth retardation	Marked	Mild
Anal and perianal lesions	Common	Rare
Association with carcinoma	Rare	Common

Diagnosis is established by colonoscopy and barium enema. On colonoscopy, the shallow ulcerations along the bowel can be seen; the mucosa is friable (easily irritated) and bleeds easily from inflammation. A biopsy may be performed for definite diagnosis. Observe children carefully after a bowel biopsy to detect rectal bleeding from an internal bleeding point (take blood pressure and pulse, and assess stool for occult blood).

Therapeutic Management

The child's bowel heals best if it is allowed to rest for a time. Enteral or total parenteral nutrition is usually provided for nutrition during the resting period. The child can remain home during this period as long as parents have thorough education about the child's care (see Chapter 36).

When food is reintroduced after the resting period, a high-protein, high-carbohydrate, high-vitamin diet is prescribed to replace nutrients. Children may eat cautiously at first to avoid reintroducing diarrhea; assess intake and output. An anti-inflammatory drug, such as prednisone (a corticosteroid), sulfasalazine (Azulfidine; a sulfonamide and salicylic acid), or azathioprine (Imuran; an immunosuppressive agent), generally brings about a great improvement in symptoms (Box 45.7). For ulcerative colitis, cyclosporine may be used. If medical therapy is ineffective, bowel resection to remove a portion of the bowel (colectomy) followed by an ileoanal pull-through may be necessary. In some children, such a large portion of the bowel may be removed that a colostomy or a continent ileostomy needs to be constructed (for continent ileostomy, an internal reservoir is created using a section of bowel and emptied by insertion of a catheter; Fig. 45.9).

Bowel surgery is a serious step. Because it reduces the possibility of the child's developing intestinal cancer in association with ulcerative colitis, it may be necessary in children whose disease is running a long-term, debilitating course that does not improve. Children who recover from inflammatory bowel disease should have a colonoscopy yearly for the rest of their lives.

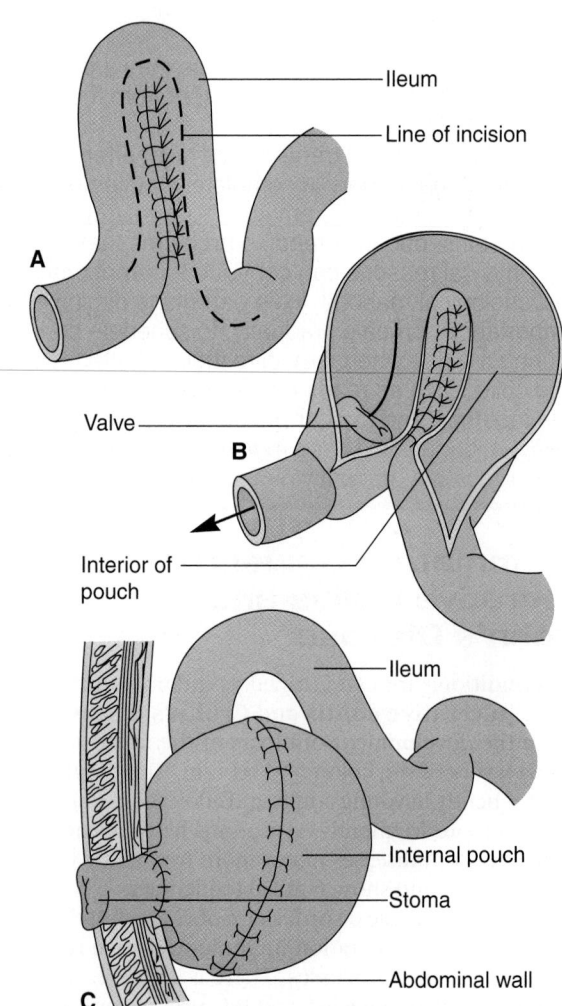

FIGURE 45.9 A continent ileostomy. **(A)** Segment of bowel is anastomosed. **(B)** Pouch for stool collection is formed. **(C)** Liquid stool is contained in pouch until drained by catheter.

BOX 45.7 FOCUS ON . . .

PHARMACOLOGY

Sulfasalazine (Azulfidine)

Classification: Sulfasalazine is a combination anti-inflammatory agent and antibiotic.

Action: Reduces the inflammation of ulcerative colitis and Crohn's disease (Karch, 2004).

Pregnancy risk category: C (D at term)

Dosage: Varied, based on severity of illness, 20 to 75 mg/kg/day. Initially, 40 to 60 mg/kg/24 h orally in four to six divided doses in children older than age 2 years. Maintenance therapy usually 20 to 30 mg/kg/day in four equally divided doses.

Possible adverse effects: Sensitivity to sunlight; dizziness; drowsiness, nausea, abdominal pains, crystalluria, and hematuria

Nursing Implications
- Caution the parents and child that the drug may turn urine orange-red and soft contact lenses yellow.
- Advise children to take with or just after meals to avoid GI irritation.
- Ensure adequate fluid intake to avoid crystallization of sulfa component in urine.
- Anticipate prescription for folic acid concurrently. Drug decreases folic acid absorption.
- Instruct the child and parents about the need to use sunscreens and protective clothing while outside.

NURSING DIAGNOSES AND RELATED INTERVENTIONS

———◆———

Nursing Diagnosis: Imbalanced nutrition related to poor absorption because of disease process

Outcome Evaluation: Child's weight follows a percentile growth curve; urine specific gravity is 1.003 to 1.030. Child states that alternative feeding method is tolerable.

Nutrition is a priority concern for children with both Crohn's disease and ulcerative colitis because malnutrition can occur from the combination of poor intestinal absorption and chronic diarrhea. Anorexia compounds the problem. Unless active steps are taken to supplement nutrition, children with inflammatory bowel disease can be left both short in stature and light in weight. Protein, vitamin, fat, and mineral deficiencies all may occur.

When nutrition is supplied by enteral or total parenteral nutrition solutions, allowing the enteral infusion to flow during the night and removing the tube during the day can make feedings more tolerable. Remember that food provides social experiences as well as nutrition. Help parents provide opportunities for mealtime stimulation in other ways.

Nursing Diagnosis: Risk for ineffective coping related to chronic illness

Outcome Evaluation: Child expresses feelings, states that she understands the disease and therapy, and suggests ways to minimize stress.

Caution children about the possible side effects, such as excessive weight gain, a round facial appearance, and facial acne, that may occur if corticosteroid therapy, such as prednisone, is used so they are not surprised by this. Assess blood pressure, intake and output, weight, and sleep patterns for any child taking steroids. Caution children that sulfasalazine (Azulfidine) turns urine an orange-yellow so they do not mistake this color change as bleeding.

Provide time to listen so children have someone outside their family to talk to about their symptoms and family or stress problems (Box 45.8). The disorder has a chronic course and can involve embarrassing episodes of diarrhea or acute abdominal pain.

Irritable Bowel Syndrome (Chronic Nonspecific Diarrhea)

Irritable bowel syndrome involves intermittent episodes of loose and normal stools or recurrent abdominal pain. It appears slightly more often in girls than in boys. It is most

---

BOX 45.8 FOCUS ON . . .

COMMUNICATION

Barry's older sister Addie has Crohn's disease. Her doctor has told her parents she won't need surgery but will need long-term therapy. You see Mrs. Abraham filling out forms by Addie's bedside.

Less Effective Communication

Nurse: Mrs. Abraham, can I help you with anything?
Mrs. Abraham: No. With Addie well again in a short time, I'm going to start back to college. I'm filling out the forms.
Nurse: Do you mean Addie doesn't need parenteral nutrition?
Mrs. Abraham: She doesn't need anything. Not even surgery.
Nurse: That's wonderful. She's very lucky.

More Effective Communication

Nurse: Mrs. Abraham, can I help you with anything?
Mrs. Abraham: No. With Addie well again in a short time, I'm going to start back to college. I'm filling out the forms.
Nurse: Do you mean Addie doesn't need parenteral nutrition?
Mrs. Abraham: She doesn't need anything. Not even surgery.
Nurse: Let's review exactly what the doctor has told you.

People under stress often do not hear instructions well. When this happens, they may need them repeated several times before they truly comprehend what was said. An easy solution when you are aware that a parent has not heard potentially bad news is to ignore the loss of information, as in the first scenario above. A better solution is to explore with the parents what they did hear and help them receive more accurate information.

---

often seen in infants 6 to 36 months of age. Most children outgrow the symptoms by 3 years of age. The cause is unknown, but it is associated with low fat intake (without fat slowing absorption, stool passes rapidly through the bowel). Excessive fluid intake also may play a role.

The symptoms are usually vague. The episodes of diarrhea may occur several times a week or as frequently as twice a day. There seems to be no relationship to meals.

Children are encouraged to eat a regular diet. Psyllium bulk agents will almost always reduce the frequency of symptoms. Probiotics or foods supplemented with lactic acid-producing bacteria may improve symptoms (Lin, 2003).

Chronic Recurrent Abdominal Pain

A number of children develop episodes of recurring abdominal pain. Although such episodes can occur for reasons such as lactose intolerance or muscle strain from sports activities, in most instances the cause is unknown (Brown, 2003). Children who experience this are commonly 6 or 7 years of age or in prepuberty (11 to 12 years of age). The pain is not accompanied by a change in bowel habits. There is no association with meals. Episodes of pain can last for only a few minutes or for hours. The intensity of the pain is mild or "annoying" rather than severe. It is generally poorly localized, although children may point to the umbilicus as the primary site. On physical examination, there is no abdominal tenderness, distention, guarding, or muscle spasm.

Symptoms of stress such as sleep disturbances, fears, or eating problems may be present. A family history may indicate problems in the family such as marital discord, financial problems, or physical illness in parents or siblings.

Although the cause of the pain cannot be identified, the pain is real. For some children, just having the opportunity to talk to an understanding person about the problem is all that is necessary to stop the attacks of pain. Other families need counseling regarding the underlying problem, such as allowing children to express their anger, reducing excessive demands on them, or giving them more attention by spending more time with them. The family may need to be referred to a family service agency for counseling.

DISORDERS CAUSED BY FOOD, VITAMIN, AND MINERAL DEFICIENCIES

There are many underfed and malnourished children in every part of the world. Although extreme diseases of food or vitamin deprivation are rare in the United States, they do exist. Such children need early identification so they can receive better nutrition before permanent damage occurs.

The average child does not develop a deficient intake of essential nutrients because, even if the child is occasionally a fussy eater, over the space of a week, he or she does ingest foods containing the necessary nutrients. Carefully assess any child who has an interference in nutrition such as a GI illness or the child receiving enteric feedings or total parenteral nutrition to make sure that nutrient deficiencies do not exist. Assess abused or neglected children closely for nutritional deficiencies, because they may not have been given adequate food.

Kwashiorkor

Kwashiorkor, a disease caused by protein deficiency, occurs most frequently in children ages 1 to 3 years, because this age group requires a high protein intake. It is a disease found almost exclusively in developing countries in Africa, Asia, and Latin America, although it does occur in the United States (Seres & Resurreccion, 2003). It tends to occur after weaning, when children change from breast milk to a diet consisting mainly of carbohydrates. Growth failure is a major symptom. Because edema is also a symptom, however, children may not appear light in weight until the edema is relieved. There is a severe wasting of muscles, but, again, this is masked by the edema.

Edema results from hypoproteinemia, which causes a shift of body fluid from the intravascular compartments to the interstitial space, causing ascites (Fig. 45.10). This

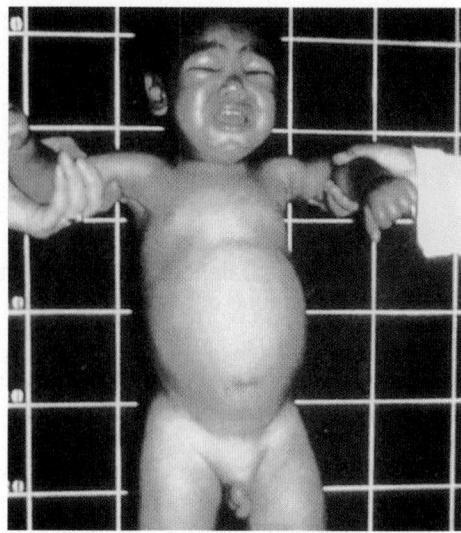

FIGURE 45.10 A child with kwashiorkor. Here the extensive generalized edema masks the severe muscle wasting. Notice the severe abdominal distention from ascites.

is the same phenomenon that causes extensive edema in children with nephrosis. The edema tends to be dependent, so it is first noted in the lower extremities. Children are generally irritable and uninterested in their surroundings. They fall behind other children of the same age in motor development.

If the child had a period of good protein intake, then poor protein intake, then good intake again, hair shafts develop a striped appearance of brown, then white, and so on—a "zebra sign." Children also have diarrhea, iron-deficiency anemia, and hepatomegaly.

Without treatment, kwashiorkor is fatal. For therapy, a diet rich in protein is essential. Even so, there is evidence to suggest that protein malnutrition early in life, even if corrected later, may result in failure of children to reach their full potential of intellectual and psychological development.

Nutritional Marasmus

Nutritional marasmus is a disease caused by deficiency of all food groups, basically a form of starvation. Although it is seen most commonly in developing countries where food supplies are short, it is seen in grossly neglected children or those with failure to thrive in the United States (see Chapter 55). These children are most commonly younger than 1 year of age. They have many of the same symptoms as children with kwashiorkor, including growth failure, muscle wasting, irritability, iron-deficiency anemia, and diarrhea. Whereas children with kwashiorkor are anorectic, children with nutritional marasmus are invariably hungry (starving) and will suck at any object offered them, such as a finger or their clothing. Treatment is a diet rich in all nutrients.

Vitamin and Mineral Deficiencies

Both vitamin and mineral deficiencies occur at a low rate in children of the United States because so many foods are

TABLE 45.7

Vitamin Deficiency Disorders

Vitamin	Cause of Deficiency	Signs and Symptoms
Vitamin A	Lack of yellow vegetables in diet	Tender tongue; cracks at corners of mouth Night blindness **Xerophthalmia** (dry and lusterless conjunctivae) **Keratomalacia** (necrosis of the cornea with perforation, loss of ocular fluid, and blindness)
Vitamin B$_1$	Most common in children who eat polished rice as dietary staple, because B$_1$ is contained in hull of rice	**Beriberi** (tingling and numbness of extremities; heart palpitations; exhaustion) Diarrhea and vomiting Aphonia (cry without sound) Anesthesia of feet
Niacin	Common in children who eat corn as dietary staple, because corn is low in niacin	**Pellagra** (dermatitis; resembles a sunburn) Diarrhea Mental confusion (dementia)
Vitamin C	Lack of fresh fruits in diet	**Scurvy** (muscle tenderness; petechiae)
Vitamin D	Lack of sunlight	Poor muscle tone; delayed tooth formation. **Rickets** (poor bone formation) Craniotabes (softening of the skull) Swelling at joints, particularly of wrists and cartilage of ribs Bowed legs Tetany

enriched (restoration of ingredients removed by processing) or fortified (additional vitamins and minerals not normally present have been added). Milk, for example, is fortified with vitamins D and A. Orange juice is fortified with calcium. White bread is enriched with B vitamins. Vitamin deficiency diseases are summarized in Table 45.7.

Iodine Deficiency

Because iodine is not supplemented in food except as iodized salt, a diet deficient in iodine may lead to hyperplasia of the thyroid gland (*goiter*) or hypothyroidism. In the United States, areas where goiter is endemic are mainly the states bordering Canada, especially the Great Lakes area, and the states between the Rocky Mountains and the Appalachians (Dudek, 2005). When the thyroid gland does not have adequate iodine to make thyroxine, its chief hormone, the gland is overstimulated by the pituitary gland, ultimately leading to the hyperplasia. Goiter tends to occur most commonly in girls at puberty and during pregnancy. An enlarged thyroid gland may lead to difficulty breathing.

Supplemental iodine or synthetic thyroxine (Synthroid) is needed. Children must also be maintained on a diet adequate in iodine, found most abundantly in seafood (Dudek, 2005).

Checkpoint Question 5

Kwashiorkor is a disorder common in developing countries. This disorder occurs because of lack of what nutrient?

a. Water-soluble vitamins
b. Fats and triglycerides
c. Quality protein
d. Vitamin K

Key Points

Children with GI disorders need to join the family for mealtime if possible. Even if they cannot eat the same foods as other family members, they benefit from the social interaction.

Some GI disorders lead to long-term therapies such as colostomy or gastrostomy feedings. Because these disorders interfere with common body functions such as eating and elimination, they are difficult for children to accept without the support of concerned health care providers.

Children lose proportionately more fluid with vomiting and diarrhea than adults do, so they need rapid assessment and interventions to avoid dehydration.

Fluid, electrolyte, and acid–base imbalances tend to occur rapidly with vomiting and diarrhea. Vomiting leads to alkalosis. Diarrhea leads to acidosis.

GI disorders almost always interfere with nutrition to some degree. This is a greater problem in children than adults because children need to ingest adequate nutrients and fluid daily for growth as well as body maintenance.

Gastroesophageal reflux (achalasia) is a neuromuscular disturbance in which the cardiac sphincter is lax, allowing for easy regurgitation of gastric contents into the esophagus. It is treated by feeding a thickened formula and keeping the infant upright after feedings.

Pyloric stenosis is hypertrophy of the valve between the stomach and duodenum. It impedes the passage of feedings, leading to vomiting.

Peptic ulcer disease may occur in children of all ages. This disease causes a shallow excavation to form in the mucosal wall of the stomach. It is treated, like adult ulcers, with antibiotics and agents to suppress gastric acidity.

Forms of hepatitis seen in children include hepatitis A and C (caused usually by eating contaminated shellfish) and hepatitis B, D, and E (caused by contaminated blood or placental spread).

Congenital obstruction of the bile ducts occurs from failure of the bile duct to recanalize in utero. This can lead to fibrotic scarring of the liver (cirrhosis). Most of these children need a liver transplant to restore liver function.

Intussusception is the invagination of one portion of the intestine into another. Volvulus is twisting of intestine. Both may lead to bowel obstruction.

Necrotizing enterocolitis is the development of necrotic patches on the intestine. It occurs almost exclusively in immature infants.

Appendicitis is inflammation of the appendix. It is always an emergency and is the most common reason for abdominal surgery in children. Laparoscopy is done to remove the appendix, ideally before it ruptures.

Celiac disease (gluten-induced enteropathy) is a change in the ability of the intestinal villi to absorb. It is apparently a dominantly inherited illness.

Inguinal and hiatal hernia can occur in children. These are surgically corrected when recognized.

Hirschsprung's disease (aganglionic megacolon) is absence of ganglionic innervation in a section of the lower bowel. Therapy may involve a temporary colostomy followed by surgery in 6 to 12 months to remove the affected bowel portion.

Inflammatory bowel disease can occur as either ulcerative colitis or Crohn's disease. Therapy is long-term. If medical therapy is unsuccessful, portions of the bowel may be surgically removed. Ulcerative colitis is associated with the development of colon cancer later in life.

Kwashiorkor (protein deficiency), nutritional marasmus (starvation), vitamins A and D (rickets), B$_1$ (beriberi), and C (scurvy) deficiencies, or iodine deficiencies occur in children when they are not provided or cannot absorb adequate nutrients. Although more common in developing countries, they can occur in a child in any community.

Critical Thinking Exercises

1. Barry is the 2-year-old boy you met at the beginning of the chapter. He was diagnosed with celiac disease. When you met him, his mother was insisting that he eat a piece of birthday cake. What health education

does his mother need to help her choose a better diet for her son? What would have been a better food, probably available at a birthday party, that he could have eaten?

2. Suppose Barry is seen in a hospital emergency department with severe diarrhea. What emergency interventions does he need to prevent an electrolyte or fluid imbalance? What measures could you take to reduce his fear of the strange hospital environment?

3. Barry's older sister, who has Crohn's disease, is being cared for at home with total parenteral nutrition. How can you help her keep pace with her friends at school? How can you help her maintain a sense of high self-esteem in light of her many hospitalizations and home care?

4. Examine the National Health Goals related to gastrointestinal disorders in children. Most government-sponsored money for nursing research is allotted based on these goals. What would be a possible research topic to explore pertinent to these goals that would be applicable to the Abraham family and also advance evidence-based practice?

References

Alper, B. S. (2004). Evidence-based medicine. Oral rehydration therapy is first-line therapy for most dehydrated children. *Clinical Advisor, 7*(6), 139–140.

American Academy of Pediatrics. (2003). Gastrointestinal infections. In L. K. Pickering (Ed.), *2003 Red book: report of the Committee on Infectious Diseases* (26th ed.). Elk Grove Village, IL: American Academy of Pediatrics.

Askin, D. F., & Diehl-Jones, W. L. (2003). The neonatal liver, part III: pathophysiology of liver dysfunction. *Neonatal Network: The Journal of Neonatal Nursing, 22*(3), 5–15.

Axelrod, D. A., et al. (2004). Association of center volume with outcome after liver and kidney transplantation. *American Journal of Transplantation, 4*(6), 920–927.

Banks, J. B., & Meadows, S. (2005). Intravenous fluids for children with gastroenteritis. *American Family Physician, 71*(1), 121–122.

Brown, K. A. (2003). Abdominal pain. In M. W. Schwartz (Ed.), *5-minute pediatric consult* (3rd ed.). Philadelphia: Lippincott Williams & Wilkins.

Chey, W. D., & Scheiman, J. M. (2003). Acid peptic disorders. In T. Yamaka, *Textbook of gastroenterology*. Philadelphia: Lippincott Williams & Wilkins.

Department of Health and Human Services. (2000). *Healthy people 2010*. Washington, DC: DHHS.

Dudek, S. G. (2005). *Nutrition essentials for nursing practice* (4th ed.). Philadelphia: Lippincott Williams & Wilkins.

Fasano, A. (2003). Celiac disease: how to handle a clinical chameleon. *New England Journal of Medicine, 348*(25), 2568–2570.

Gillis, L. A. (2003). Cirrhosis. In M. W. Schwartz (Ed.), *5-minute pediatric consult* (3rd ed.). Philadelphia: Lippincott Williams & Wilkins.

Gold, B. D. (2004). Gastroesophageal reflux disease: could intervention in childhood reduce the risk of later complications? *American Journal of Medicine, 117*(Suppl 5A), 23S–29S.

Haber, B. (2003). Biliary atresia. In M. W. Schwartz (Ed.), *5-minute pediatric consult* (3rd ed.). Philadelphia: Lippincott Williams & Wilkins.

Horton, K. K. (2005). Pathophysiology and current management of necrotizing enterocolitis. *Neonatal Network: The Journal of Neonatal Nursing, 24*(1), 37–50.

Humiston, S. G., & Marshall, G. S. (2004). Routine infant hepatitis B vaccination recommendations. *Pediatric Annals, 33*(8), 515–522.

John-Kelly, H. A., & Mulberg, A. E. (2003). Hirschsprung disease. In M. W. Schwartz (Ed.), *5-minute pediatric consult* (3rd ed.). Philadelphia: Lippincott Williams & Wilkins.

John-Kelly, H. A. (2003). Pyloric stenosis. In M. W. Schwartz (Ed.), *5-minute pediatric consult* (3rd ed.). Philadelphia: Lippincott Williams & Wilkins.

Karch, A. M. (2004). *Lippincott's nursing drug guide.* Philadelphia: Lippincott Williams & Wilkins.

King, C. K., et al. (2003). Managing acute gastroenteritis among children: oral rehydration, maintenance, and nutritional therapy. *MMWR: Morbidity and Mortality Weekly Report, 52*(RR-16), 1–16.

Klein, E. J., Kapoor, D., & Shugerman, R. P. (2004). The diagnosis of intussusception. *Clinical Pediatrics, 43*(4), 343–347.

Liacouras, C. A. (2003). Diarrhea. In M. W. Schwartz (Ed.), *5-minute pediatric consult* (3rd ed.). Philadelphia: Lippincott Williams & Wilkins.

Lin, D. C. (2003). Probiotics as functional foods. *Nutrition in Clinical Practice, 18*(6), 497–506.

LoBiondo-Wood, G., Williams, L., & McGhee, C. (2004). Liver transplantation in children: maternal and family stress, coping, and adaptation. *Journal for Specialists in Pediatric Nursing, 9*(2), 59–66.

Mamula, P., & Markowitz, J. (2003). Crohn disease. In M. W. Schwartz (Ed.), *5-minute pediatric consult* (3rd ed.). Philadelphia: Lippincott Williams & Wilkins.

Markowitz, J. E., & Baldassano, R. N. (2003). Ulcerative colitis. In M. W. Schwartz (Ed.), *5-minute pediatric consult* (3rd ed.). Philadelphia: Lippincott Williams & Wilkins.

Mascarenhas, M. R. (2003). Constipation. In M. W. Schwartz (Ed.), *5-minute pediatric consult* (3rd ed.). Philadelphia: Lippincott Williams & Wilkins.

McCollough, M., & Sharieff, G. Q. (2003). Abdominal surgical emergencies in infants and young children. *Emergency Medicine Clinics of North America, 21*(4), 909–935.

Mulberg, A. E. (2003). Volvulus. In M. W. Schwartz (Ed.), *5-minute pediatric consult* (3rd ed.). Philadelphia: Lippincott Williams & Wilkins.

Rand, E. R., & Olthoff, K. M. (2003). Pediatric liver transplantation. *Graft, 6*(2), 145–150.

Sauerland, S., Lefering, R., & Neugebauer, E. A. M. (2005). Laparoscopic versus open surgery for suspected appendicitis. *The Cochrane Library (Oxford) (4)* (CD001546).

Scarfone, R. J., Luberti, A. A., & Mistry, R. D. (2004). Children referred to an emergency department by an after-hours call center: complaint-specific analysis. *Pediatric Emergency Care, 20*(8), 507–513.

Sehgal, S., & Allen, P. L. J. (2004). Primary care approaches. Hepatitis C in children. *Pediatric Nursing, 30*(5), 409–413.

Sentongo, T. A. S., & Mulberg, A. E. (2003). Food poisoning. In M. W. Schwartz (Ed.), *5-minute pediatric consult* (3rd ed.). Philadelphia: Lippincott Williams & Wilkins.

Seres, D. S., & Resurreccion, L. B. (2003). Kwashiorkor: dysmetabolism versus malnutrition. *Nutrition in Clinical Practice, 18*(4), 297–301.

Sira, J., & Kelly, D. (2003). The impact of hepatitis B and C infection on children and their families. *AIDS & Hepatitis Digest, 1*(98), 1–3.

Sorensen, H. T., et al. (2003). Risk of infantile hypertrophic pyloric stenosis after maternal postnatal use of macrolides. *Scandinavian Journal of Infectious Diseases, 35*(2), 104–106.

Steiner, M. J., et al. (2004). Is this child dehydrated? *JAMA: Journal of the American Medical Association, 291*(22), 2746–2754.

Stem, S., & Mulberg, A. E. (2003). Appendicitis. In M. W. Schwartz (Ed.), *5-minute pediatric consult* (3rd ed.). Philadelphia: Lippincott Williams & Wilkins.

Telega, G. (2003). Inguinal hernia. In M. W. Schwartz (Ed.), *5-minute pediatric consult* (3rd ed.). Philadelphia: Lippincott Williams & Wilkins.

Tung, J. (2003). Viral hepatitis. In M. W. Schwartz (Ed.), *5-minute pediatric consult* (3rd ed.). Philadelphia: Lippincott Williams & Wilkins.

Updegrove, K. (2004). Necrotizing enterocolitis: the evidence for use of human milk in prevention and treatment. *Journal of Human Lactation, 20*(3), 335–339.

Wasserman, D. (2003). Gastroesophageal reflux. In M. W. Schwartz (Ed.), *5-minute pediatric consult* (3rd ed.). Philadelphia: Lippincott Williams & Wilkins.

Yazici, M., et al. (2003). Paraesophageal hiatal hernias in children. *Diseases of the Esophagus, 16*(3), 210–213.

Suggested Readings

Cobb, B. A., Carlo, W. A., & Ambalavanan, N. (2004). Gastric residuals and their relationship to necrotizing enterocolitis in very low birth weight infants. *Pediatrics, 113*(1 Part 1), 50–53.

Craig, W. R., et al. (2005). Metoclopramide, thickened feedings, and positioning for gastro-oesophagal reflux in children under two years. *The Cochrane Library (Oxford) (1)* (#CD003502).

Fischer, T. K., et al. (2004). Intussusception in early childhood: a cohort study of 1.7 million children. *Pediatrics, 114*(3), 782–785.

Henderson, G., Anthony, M. Y., & McGuire, W. (2005). Formula milk versus preterm human milk for feeding preterm or low birth weight infants. *The Cochrane Library (Oxford) (4)* (#CD002972).

Hoffenberg, E. J., et al. (2003). A prospective study of the incidence of childhood celiac disease. *Journal of Pediatrics, 143*(3), 308–314.

Marchetti, F., Gerarduzzi, T., & Ventura, A. (2003). Proton pump inhibitors in children: a review. *Digestive & Liver Disease, 35*(10), 738–746.

Pfeil, M., & Mathur, A. (2004). Early discharge following uncomplicated appendicectomy in children. *Paediatric Nursing, 16*(7), 15–18.

Samandari, T., Bell, B. P., & Armstrong, G. L. (2004). Quantifying the impact of hepatitis A immunization in the United States, 1995–2001. *Vaccine, 22*(31–32), 4342–4350.

Shepherd, A. J., et al. (2004). Childhood *H. pylori*: disappearing disease or chronic infection? *British Journal of Community Nursing, 9*(5), 201–205.

Zimmermann, P. G. (2003). Assessment of abdominal pain in school-age children. *Journal of School Nursing, 19*(1), 4–10.

CHAPTER 46

Nursing Care of the Child With a Renal or Urinary Tract Disorder

Key Terms

- acute transplant rejection
- Alport's syndrome
- azotemia
- Bowman's capsule
- dialysis
- enuresis
- epispadias
- exstrophy of the bladder
- glomerular filtration rate
- glomerulonephritis
- hydronephrosis
- hypospadias
- nephrosis
- patent urachus
- polycystic kidney
- postural proteinuria
- prune-belly syndrome
- vesicoureteral reflux

Objectives

After mastering the contents of this chapter, you should be able to:

1. Describe common renal and urinary disorders that occur in children.
2. Assess a child for a renal or urinary tract disorder.
3. Formulate nursing diagnoses related to renal or urinary disorders in children.
4. Establish expected outcomes related to the care of a child with a renal or urinary disorder.
5. Plan nursing care related to urinary or renal disorders in children, such as preparing a child for peritoneal dialysis.
6. Implement nursing care for a child with a renal or urinary disorder.
7. Evaluate expected outcomes for achievement and effectiveness of care for a child with a renal or urinary disorder.
8. Identify National Health Goals related to renal or urinary tract disorders in children that nurses can help the nation achieve.
9. Identify areas related to care of the child with a renal or urinary disorder that would benefit from additional nursing research or application of evidence-based practice.
10. Analyze methods for making nursing care of the child with a renal or urinary disorder more family-centered.
11. Integrate knowledge of renal and urinary tract disorders with the nursing process to achieve quality maternal and child health nursing care.

Carol Hendricks is a 4-year-old girl admitted to the hospital with nephrotic syndrome. She has marked ascites and edema. "I kept asking everyone how she could be gaining so much weight, yet she doesn't eat anything," her grandmother tells you. "My daughter said this happened because she drank part of a beer I left on the coffee table. Do you think that's what caused it? What if she needs a kidney transplant? Will I be allowed to give my kidney to her?"

Previous chapters described the growth and development of well children and the nursing care of children with disorders of other systems. This chapter adds information about the dramatic changes, both physical and psychosocial, that occur when children develop urinary tract or renal disorders. This is important information because it builds a base for care and health teaching.

How would you answer Carol's grandmother? What information does she need to better understand her grandchild's condition?

After you've studied this chapter, access the accompanying website. Read the patient scenario and answer the questions to further sharpen your skills, grow more familiar with RN-CLEX types of questions, and reward yourself with how much you have learned.

Normally, the urinary system maintains the proper balance of fluid (water) and electrolytes in the blood. When disease occurs, such as with structural abnormalities or kidney malfunction, a child may be left with excessive amounts of fluid in the body or with an imbalance of electrolytes and other substances essential to the body's functioning. Disorders involving the kidneys and urinary tract often are long term. Any urinary tract disorder can ultimately (if not originally) affect the kidneys, resulting in kidney dysfunction, with potentially fatal consequences.

Unfortunately, because symptoms may be vague, or because the child or parents do not realize the seriousness of urinary disease or are embarrassed to discuss it, children may not be evaluated at the first sign of illness. Health education to increase the awareness of the symptoms of urinary tract and kidney disorders is an important area of family health teaching. National Health Goals related to renal or urinary tract disorders and children are shown in Box 46.1.

Nursing Process Overview

For Care of a Child With a Renal or Urinary Tract Disorder

● *Assessment*

Because the symptoms of many urinary tract and renal disorders (e.g., mild abdominal pain, slowly increasing edema, or low-grade fever) are subtle, parents may not bring their child for evaluation as early in the disease as they might if symptoms were more definite.

BOX 46.1 FOCUS ON . . .

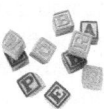

NATIONAL HEALTH GOALS

Renal disease can lead to long-term illness, so preventing it is important to improving the health of the nation. The following National Health Goals address this concern:

- Reduce the rate of new cases of end-stage renal disease, from a baseline of 289/million population to a target rate of 217/million population.
- Increase the proportion of patients with treated chronic kidney failure who receive a transplant within 3 years of registration on a waiting list, from a baseline of 41/1,000 to 51/1,000 (DHHS, 2000).

Nurses can help the nation achieve these goals by educating parents to give antibiotics conscientiously for streptococcal throat infections and being active advocates for organ transplant procedures.

Areas that would benefit from nursing research include: determining parents' or children's ability to accurately self-assess for proteinuria after streptococcal infections, identifying the specific needs of children on ambulatory peritoneal dialysis, designing ways to make low-potassium diets more appealing to children with end-stage renal disease, or designing ways that organ donation can be presented to make it more appealing to potential donors.

School nurses can play an important role in recognizing the seriousness of minor symptoms and making proper referrals for care.

Common findings from a health history and physical examination are shown in Box 46.2. The hallmark of kidney or bladder infection is pain. If children have had bladder surgery, they also may experience pain on urination or pain from bladder spasms. Be sure to assess the degree of pain, including its location and intensity, before administering an analgesic or antispasmodic. Urine specimens also provide valuable assessment information. Techniques for obtaining urine samples (i.e., clean-catch, catheterization, 24-hour collections, suprapubic aspiration, and urinalysis) are described in Chapter 36.

● *Nursing Diagnosis*

Nursing diagnoses used with children with urinary tract or renal disorders are related to the symptoms these disorders cause. Some examples are:

- Pain related to bladder irritation from urinary tract infection

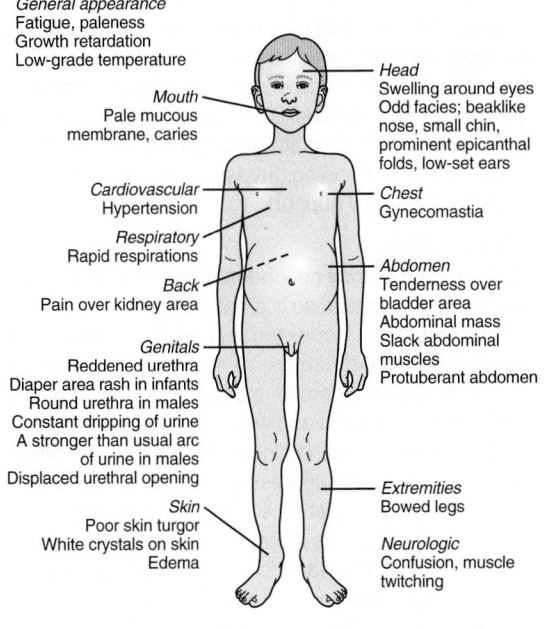

BOX 46.2 ASSESSMENT

Assessing a Child for Renal and Urinary Tract Dysfunction

History
Chief concern: Child reports burning or cries on urination; blood or "dark" urine, frequency of urination; abdominal pain, flank pain, enuresis. Parents report increase in size of abdomen, periorbital edema, poor appetite, frequent thirst, weight gain, strong odor to urine; diaper rash in infants. A school-age child may be described as a behavior problem because he or she frequently asks to use the bathroom.
Family history: History of renal disease, such as polycystic kidney, enuresis; hypertension.
Pregnancy history: Exposure to nephrotoxic drugs (antibiotics) during pregnancy. Oligohydramnios at birth.
Past illness history: Child recently had a throat or skin infection.

Physical assessment
General appearance
Fatigue, paleness
Growth retardation
Low-grade temperature

Mouth
Pale mucous
membrane, caries

Cardiovascular
Hypertension

Respiratory
Rapid respirations

Back
Pain over kidney area

Genitals
Reddened urethra
Diaper area rash in infants
Round urethra in males
Constant dripping of urine
A stronger than usual arc
of urine in males
Displaced urethral opening

Skin
Poor skin turgor
White crystals on skin
Edema

Head
Swelling around eyes
Odd facies; beaklike
nose, small chin,
prominent epicanthal
folds, low-set ears

Chest
Gynecomastia

Abdomen
Tenderness over
bladder area
Abdominal mass
Slack abdominal
muscles
Protuberant abdomen

Extremities
Bowed legs

Neurologic
Confusion, muscle
twitching

- Excess fluid volume related to decreased kidney function and fluid accumulation
- Fear related to outcome of kidney transplantation
- Imbalanced nutrition, less than body requirements, related to effects of dietary restrictions
- Social isolation related to immunosuppressant therapy
- Risk for injury related to body's inability to excrete waste products properly

Because the entire family becomes involved in long-term renal disease, other appropriate nursing diagnoses might include:

- Interrupted family processes related to the effects and stresses of the child's chronic illness
- Compromised family coping related to the chronic nature of the child's illness

● Outcome Identification and Planning

Be certain the outcomes established for care are relevant to the child's age and condition. Because renal disease may become chronic, expected outcomes need to be modified frequently to meet changing needs.

Planning for the child with a urinary tract or renal disorder often involves helping parents remember to give medicine. The child with nephrotic syndrome, for example, may take three or four different types of medicine every day at home. Be certain parents understand the types of medicine prescribed and the expected action of each. School-age children need a schedule that allows them to take medicine before they leave home in the morning or after they return in the afternoon. Some schools allow medications to be given during school hours. For these children, an order from the prescriber and the reason for the medication are required.

If a child has severe renal impairment, parents may be asked to make decisions regarding kidney removal and transplantation. Provide them with ample time for discussion. If a kidney donor is sought among relatives, the parents must help decide whether the person whose tissue matches the child's really wants to donate a kidney or is being pressured to do so. Helping parents to schedule times for hemodialysis or peritoneal dialysis or to supervise continuous ambulatory peritoneal dialysis (CAPD), to care for their other children, and to provide a life apart from their child requires nursing planning. Investigate community sources for family support.

● Implementation

Parents may or may not understand the function of the urinary system because it is not a system that receives much discussion. For example, they may confuse the words "ureter" and "urethra." The nurse can play a major role as a resource person, explaining anatomy and the tests and procedures and why they are being done.

Many children with kidney disease take a corticosteroid for immunosuppression and so develop a typical cushingoid appearance. They may have edema or ascites, which makes them appear obese. A child may be teased or criticized by some classmates because of this "different" appearance. Contacting the school nurse or making the reason for the child's appearance known to the child's teacher may be necessary to help

minimize this. Frequent contact and discussion with the child's siblings are important to help them understand the reason for so many tests and health care visits and why their sibling is receiving so much attention. It also helps open up channels of communication with all members of the family.

Referrals to support organizations such as the following may be helpful: National Kidney Foundation (*www.kidney.org*) or Kidney Dialysis Foundation (*www.kdf.org.sg/*).

If kidney damage is extensive and the child's kidneys fail or a transplant is rejected, nursing care needs to be refocused on helping the family to face the possibility of the child's death. Nursing interventions can begin to prepare the child, parents, and family for this event (see Chapter 56).

● Outcome Evaluation

Children with urinary or renal disease often need follow-up care after their acute illness. Because they are followed by a specialty renal group or clinic, parents may assume that routine health maintenance care is being given as well. Check to see that children are receiving their routine childhood immunizations (remember that children taking steroid or other immunosuppressive therapy should not receive live virus immunizations) and that parents have their questions about day-to-day childrearing concerns answered.

Children returning to health care agencies for reevaluation usually need as much preparation for procedures as those having them for the first time. Memory blurs events and sometimes confuses children. For example, they may recall that a particular test involved an injection when it did not, making them worry needlessly unless their memories are refreshed. Parents wait anxiously for the results of reevaluation studies. Ensure they are given test results as soon as a comprehensive opinion of the child's progress is available. Be sure that all involved are aware of how anxious a particular parent is to hear the results of the reevaluation.

Examples suggesting achievement of outcomes are:

- Child reports pain is at a tolerable level and decreasing in intensity after treatment.
- Family members state they are able to cope with long-term illness in child.
- Child states the value of a low-sodium diet and lists the ingredients of a low-sodium meal.
- Child states she can accept the need for kidney transplantation.
- Child states the precautions he must follow to reduce possibility of infection while on immunosuppressive therapy.
- Child remains free of any signs and symptoms of complications related to accumulated waste products.

ANATOMY AND PHYSIOLOGY OF THE KIDNEYS

Embryonic development of the urinary tract is discussed in Chapter 8. Figure 46.1 identifies the structures of the

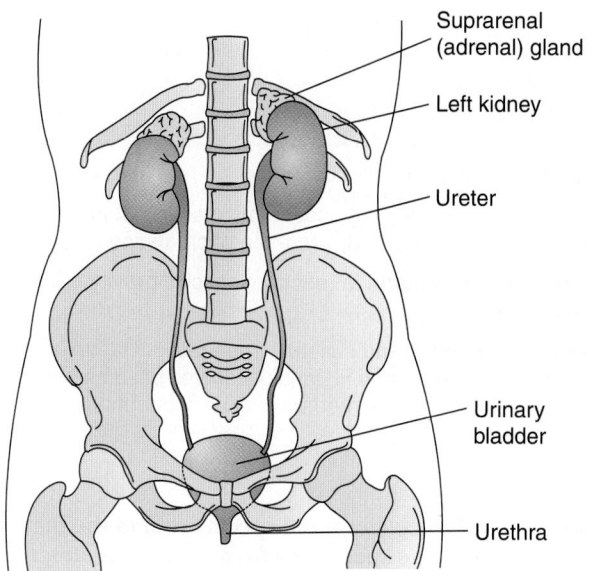

FIGURE 46.1 The urinary system.

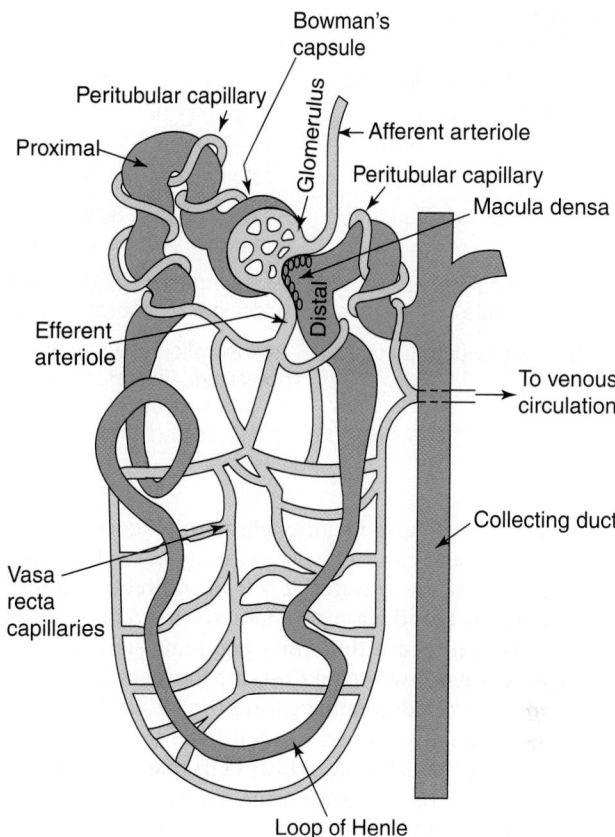

FIGURE 46.2 Basic structure of a nephron with its accompanying blood vessels.

tract. Kidneys are more susceptible to trauma in children because they are located slightly lower in relation to the ribs than in adults. They also do not have as much perinephric fat to pad them.

Nephron

A *nephron,* the functioning unit of the kidney, comprises a glomerulus (a filtrating unit) and a complex set of tubules with accompanying blood supply (Fig. 46.2). Enclosed by a double-walled chamber called a **Bowman's capsule,** the *glomerulus* is a capillary tuft supplied by a large afferent (ingoing) and a small efferent (outgoing) arteriole. It is invaginated within a tubule with a proximal and distal portion. In the glomerulus, water and solutes are filtered from the blood. This passage of water and solutes from the blood into the glomeruli is effective only as long as the blood pressure in glomerular arteries exceeds that in the tubule. The smaller efferent arteriole causes back-pressure in the glomerular arterioles, increasing the existing pressure and allowing filtration to occur readily. If blood pressure in these arterioles should fall below the tubular pressure or the tubular pressure should rise above that of the arterioles, little or no filtration will occur. For this reason, renal function must be assessed carefully in children who are hemorrhaging or are in shock with lowered blood pressure for any reason.

The solution that filtered into the tubule passes through the proximal portion, the loop of Henle, and then the distal portion. Beginning with the loop of Henle, water and electrolytes diffuse back into blood capillaries, reducing the volume of the filtrate by approximately 90%.

The glomerular filtrate enters the proximal tubule at a rate of approximately 120 mL/min. So much water is reabsorbed that the final end product (urine) left in the tubule is excreted at a rate of only approximately 1 mL/min. The proximal portion of the tubules reabsorbs most of the water, glucose, sodium chloride, phosphate (PO_4^-),

sulfate (SO_4^-), and some bicarbonate (HCO_3) ions. This is a passive process, not particularly affected by body needs. The distal portion of the tubules responds selectively to body needs. If necessary, Na^+ and HCO_3^- ions and additional water can be reabsorbed. The functions of nephron structures are summarized in Table 46.1.

Urine

The amount of urine excreted in a 24-hour period depends on fluid intake, kidney health, and age. Approximate urine output from different age groups is shown in Table 46.2. A significant decrease in urine production is termed *oliguria;* absence of urine production is *anuria.*

When renal disease occurs and glomerular or tubular function becomes impaired, nonprotein nitrogenous substances such as creatinine, urea, ammonia, and purine bodies are retained in the blood rather than being excreted. Urea is formed from the breakdown of amino acids by the liver. The amount of urea in urine is an indirect indication of kidney and liver function.

Creatinine is a product released during muscle cell metabolism. The concentration in urine remains constant, regardless of the amount of protein in the diet or body processes. Its presence or amount, therefore, can be used when comparing urine specimens. When kidney function is impaired, not only are substances retained, but also some constituents that normally are retained will be allowed to

TABLE 46.1

Functions of the Nephron

Site	Activity
Glomerulus	Secretion of water and all solutes except protein from blood
Proximal convoluted tubule	Reabsorption of 80% of glomerular filtrated water, all of glucose amino acids, vitamins, and proteins; most of sodium, chloride, and ascorbic acid; secretion of creatinine
Descending and ascending loop of Henle	Reabsorption of additional water; fluid becomes neutral in reaction; specific gravity 1.010; additional reabsorption of sodium and chloride
Distal convoluted tubule	Reabsorption of water, sodium, chloride, phosphate, and sulfate as needed; secretion of potassium, H+ ions, and ammonia (secretion of NH4+ and H+ ions conserves base because H+ ions are substituted for sodium ions; sodium is reabsorbed as sodium bicarbonate)

enter the urine. These include albumin, glucose, blood, bile pigments, and casts. Bile pigments appear in the urine when the child has elevated levels of indirect or direct bilirubin in the blood plasma (hemolysis of red blood cells or jaundice will cause this). Bile pigments stain urine a greenish yellow-brown color. Casts are formed when there is an abnormal condition that causes the kidney tubule to become lined with protein formed from red and white blood cells, epithelial cells, or fatty cells that hardens into the shape of the tubule. After urine washes the casts out, they can be detected by microscopic examination of urine. As protein deposits in this way only when fluid is slow-moving, their presence suggests slow filtration. Normal constituents of urine are shown in Table 46.3.

ASSESSMENT OF RENAL AND URINARY TRACT DYSFUNCTION

Laboratory/Diagnostic Tests

A variety of diagnostic tests may be performed, either in an ambulatory department or on an inpatient basis, to document renal or urinary tract disease (Box 46.3).

Urinalysis

One of the most revealing tests of kidney function is also one of the simplest: urinalysis. For best results, specimens collected should be fresh because urine that stands at room temperature for any length of time changes composition.

TABLE 46.2

Child's Average Urine Output in 24 Hours

Age	Amount of Urine (mL)
6 mo–2 yr	540–600
2–5 yr	500–780
5–8 yr	600–1,200
8–14 yr	1,000–1,500
Over 14 yr	1,500

Devices used to collect urine specimens and the method for obtaining urine specimens from diapers are described in Chapter 36. A chemical reagent strip can be used to detect glucose, protein, and occult blood and to measure pH. Specific gravity is best determined by use of a refractometer (requires only a single drop [see Chapter 36]).

Creatinine Clearance Rate

Glomerular filtration rate is the rate at which substances are filtered from the blood to the urine. It is measured by the amount of creatinine (the breakdown product of creatine from muscle contraction) excreted in 24 hours as determined by a 24-hour urine sample. This is known as a creatinine clearance test. A venous blood sample is taken during the 24-hour period and compared with the urine findings. A normal creatinine clearance rate is 100 mL/min. A normal urine creatinine level is 0.7 to 1.5 mg/100 mL; serum creatinine rarely exceeds 1 mg/dL (Fischbach, 2004).

Radioisotope Scanning

The administration of radioisotopes (a technetium scan) also may be used to assess glomeruli filtration ability. Radioactively tagged substances are given intravenously (IV); the rate at which these substances can be observed flowing through the kidney and excreted in urine is then determined. The level of radioisotopes used in these studies is small, and urinating removes the substance from the body immediately afterward. Children do not remain radioactive, so parents should not be afraid to stay near them or to hold them after such a study.

Urine Culture

A urinary tract infection (UTI), the presence of bacteria in urine, is diagnosed by a urine culture. Because bladder catheterization can introduce bacteria into the bladder and also is painful and intrusive, most urine specimens in children are obtained by a clean-catch procedure or sterile suprapubic aspiration (see Chapter 36). A number of instant-read commercial kits for culturing urine are available for use in ambulatory settings.

TABLE 46.3

Characteristics of Urine

Assessment	Normal Finding	Description/Implications
Color	Pale yellow	Color is influenced by urine concentration and ingredients; if fresh blood is present, urine may be red; if old blood, it may be brown or black.
Appearance	Clear	Bacteria, excessive crystals, or cells cause cloudiness; if protein content is high, it foams like beer when it is poured.
pH	4.6–8.0	Urine becomes alkaline (pH more than 7) with urinary tract infection or severe alkalosis; urine left at room temperature also becomes alkaline.
Specific gravity	1.003–1.030	Specific gravity is elevated in dehydration as kidneys try to conserve fluid, and decreased in overhydration as they try to rid the body of fluid.
Protein	0	Due to inflammation, protein molecules pass into urine; in adolescent girls, protein in urine may occur as a result of pregnancy; some children have *orthostatic proteinuria,* slight to mild proteinuria occurring only when they are standing.
Ketones	0	Ketones are released after breakdown of body protein, because of starvation.
Glucose	0	Glucose in urine occurs most frequently as a symptom of diabetes mellitus; in adolescent girls, glucosuria may occur with pregnancy.
Red blood cells	Less than 1 per high-power field Negative on dipstick	Blood may be present in urine as a result of such diseases as glomerulonephritis, urinary tract infection, or trauma; may also suggest systemic diseases such as leukemia or blood dyscrasias.
White blood cells	Less than 5 per high-power field	White blood cells are round, small configurations on a microscopic slide; they are present with bacteriuria.
Casts	0	Casts (protein configurations) are found most often in concentrated urine specimens; with cast formation, there is invariably proteinuria; casts comprise red blood cells, white blood cells, or desquamated renal epithelium; as an epithelial cast moves along the nephron, the cells begin to disintegrate, leaving a coarse granular cast; some disintegrate still further to become fine granular casts. The last stage of the process is a configuration in the shape of the tubule, termed a *waxy cast* (translucent and may be shiny and reflect light). The stage of the cast is important in indicating the flow of urine through the kidney. Hyaline casts are formations of protein appearing dull and reflecting light poorly; fatty casts are casts caused by the degeneration of tubular epithelial cells and are found in children with nephrosis. Red blood cells, white blood cells, and fatty casts are evidence of disease; other casts suggest urine stasis and probably proteinuria.
Crystals	Possibly present or not	Crystal formation is possibly indication of urine pH; uric acid, cystine, and calcium oxalate crystals are examples of crystals found in acid urine; phosphate crystals tend to be present in alkaline urine. Infection (particularly *Proteus* infection) is the most usual cause of alkaline urine. Sulfur crystals may be present if the child is receiving a sulfa drug (such as sulfamethoxazole [Gantanol]).

Blood Studies

A blood urea nitrogen (BUN) test measures the level of urea in blood and is used to assess glomerular function, or how well the kidneys can clear this from the blood-stream. However, this level may not increase until approximately 50% of glomeruli are destroyed, because the remaining glomeruli can increase in size and function to accommodate urine production. A normal value is 5 to 20 mg/100 mL.

BOX 46.3 FOCUS ON . . .

DIVERSITY OF CARE

The ease with which parents and children can discuss illnesses of the kidneys or urinary tract is culturally influenced. As a general rule, because elimination functions are typically regarded as private, this is not a body system that people discuss as comfortably as they do illnesses of other body systems. The more that modesty is stressed in a culture, the more difficult it may be for people to ask questions about kidney or urinary tract disorders. As a result, parents may wait to bring a child in to be evaluated. By being aware that this is a difficult area for parents to discuss, health care personnel can observe whether added health education is needed when caring for a child with one of these disorders.

Sonography and Magnetic Resonance Imaging

A *sonogram* or *magnetic resonance imaging* (MRI) can detect differing sizes of kidneys or ureters and can differentiate between solid or cystic kidney masses. They do not involve x-rays and so may be repeated at frequent intervals for follow-up without danger of radiation exposure.

Computed Tomography

Computed tomography (CT) scans of the kidneys are used to show the size and density of kidney structures and adequacy of urine flow. Conscious sedation may be given before a CT scan because the child must lie still for an extended time during the procedure, and the size of a CT scanner and the fact that it surrounds the child may be frightening. Be sure to prepare the child for this. A contrast medium may be injected before the procedure to better outline urine flow. If this medium is iodine based, be certain to ask about allergy to iodine before the study. Because a support person is not allowed to remain in the room during the procedure, thoroughly prepare children so they can comfortably handle the procedure by themselves.

X-Ray Studies

A plain flat-plate abdominal x-ray film can provide information about the size and contour of the kidneys. This x-ray may be referred to as a *KUB* (*k*idney, *u*reters, and *b*ladder). A small kidney shown this way is generally a hypoplastic or an underdeveloped organ. A large kidney may indicate hydronephrosis or a polycystic kidney.

Intravenous Pyelogram. An *intravenous pyelogram* (IVP) is an x-ray study of the upper urinary tract. It used to be a mainstay of diagnosis for kidney disorders but now is used less frequently (Hyde & Schwartz, 2004). A radiopaque dye is injected into a peripheral vein, circulates through the bloodstream, and is almost immediately identified as a foreign substance by the kidney and filtered out

into the urine by the glomeruli. X-ray films taken at frequent intervals show the outline of collecting systems in the kidney and of the ureters as the radiopaque dye passes through them.

In preparing children for an IVP, tell them that they will receive an injection. Say "medicine," not "dye" (or compare coloring kidneys to coloring with crayons or coloring Easter eggs), because the child may mistake "dye" for "die." Be sure children know that, after this injection, they must lie still in whatever position they are placed until all films are taken. This may be difficult for young children because x-ray tables are hard and cold and the x-ray camera overhead can be frightening. When explaining the test, compare the x-ray machine to a camera. Caution children that they may experience flushing of the face, warmth, and a salty taste in their mouth after the injection of dye. Because the dye used is iodine based, ask the parents if the child has a known allergy to iodine. This is rarely known in children because they may have had no previous studies of this kind.

Voiding Cystourethrogram. A *voiding cystourethrogram* (VCUG), a study of the lower urinary tract, reveals the structure of the urethra and bladder and the presence of reflux into the ureters (Gross, 2003). After bladder catheterization, a radiopaque dye is injected into the bladder, and the catheter is then removed. The child is asked to void into a bedpan while serial x-ray films are taken. Although the catheterization is unpleasant, being asked to void while they are observed on the x-ray table is the most stressful part of the procedure for most children because they have been taught that voiding is a private act. Children need to be told in advance that they will be asked to do this. Caution the child that a first voiding this way after catheterization may be painful. A few children have difficulty voiding a second time later in the day because they worry that the second voiding will also sting. Pouring warm water over the perineal area while sitting on the toilet or sitting in a bathtub of warm water and voiding into the water may help relieve pain. Most children, once they void this second time and realize that it is not painful, usually have no further difficulty.

A VCUG should not be done if a child has an active UTI because there is danger that the radiopaque material injected into the bladder could spread, carrying bacteria from the infection into the ureters and kidneys. Report any symptoms of UTI such as frequency, pain on voiding, or low back pain to the radiologic physician. A clean-catch urine specimen for culture may be ordered before the VCUG to rule out infection.

Checkpoint Question 1

Carol had a voiding cystourethrogram last year to help diagnose her urinary tract infection. Why is a voiding cystourethrogram a difficult test for preschool children?

a. Reading the instructions for the test is difficult.
b. Lying in an MRI machine is dark and scary.
c. They feel uncomfortable voiding in public.
d. The dye capsules may be too large to swallow.

Cystoscopy

Cystoscopy, examination of the bladder and ureter openings by direct examination with a cystoscope introduced through the urethra, is done to evaluate for possible vesicoureteral reflux or urethral stenosis. Radiopaque dye may be introduced into the bladder at the time of cystoscopy so the bladder can be visualized on x-ray (cystography). Small catheters also can be threaded into the ureters for the introduction of dye to outline them (retrograde pyelography). Because the procedure is painful and requires the child to lie still, it is usually done under conscious sedation. After the procedure, the first voiding may be painful. Once allowed, urge the child to drink plenty of fluids so he or she urinates frequently to flush out any pathogens introduced at the time of the procedure.

Renal Biopsy

Renal biopsy, which involves passing a thin biopsy needle into the kidney through the skin over the kidney, is used to diagnose the extent of renal disease and thereby predict disease outcome or progress or beginning rejection of a transplanted kidney (Filler et al., 2003). Renal biopsy may be done in the older child under only a local anesthetic, but conscious sedation may be necessary for the younger child who cannot cooperate easily. The kidney is located first by sonogram to accurately locate the place of the biopsy. The child lies prone with a sandbag under the abdomen for firmness. If the procedure is done under a local anesthetic, prepare children for the feel of a pinprick as the local anesthetic is injected; after this, they should not feel any further pain. What they may feel is pressure as the biopsy needle is inserted. Caution children that they need to lie still while the biopsy specimen is taken (if the child moved suddenly, the needle might puncture a renal artery or vein or tear vital glomeruli). Be certain children have support people to accompany them for this procedure so that they have someone to hold their hand or comfort them when they feel the pressure of the needle.

After the biopsy, press a sterile gauze square against the biopsy site for approximately 15 minutes to halt bleeding, and then apply a pressure dressing. Caution parents that a large dressing will be used and that the size of this dressing does not reflect the size of the specimen taken (the amount of tissue removed is no more than the lumen of the needle used, or approximately the size of a pencil lead).

If the procedure was done on an ambulatory basis, children can be discharged 2 to 4 hours after the procedure if vital signs are stable and they have voided. This first voiding after renal biopsy is invariably blood-tinged. Advise parents to keep children on restricted activity for 24 hours or until no more hematuria is present. Instruct parents how to keep serial urine samples, comparing each specimen with the previous one, to detect whether hematuria is becoming more or less marked. When urine no longer appears bloody, teach them to test it for occult blood to confirm that bleeding has stopped.

Measure vital signs and observe the biopsy site every 15 minutes for at least the first hour. Do not lift the dressing to assess bleeding, because doing so destroys the protective function of the pressure dressing. Encourage children to drink a considerable amount of fluid (a glass every hour while awake) during the first 24 hours to keep urine flowing freely and prevent blood from clotting in the kidney tubules and blocking urine flow. Play games with the child, if necessary, to encourage a high fluid intake (the child must take a drink each time before his or her turn at a game; play "Simon Says" and have Simon frequently say, "Drink").

A hematocrit may be ordered 24 hours after the procedure to ensure that no bleeding is continuing.

What if... Carol's grandmother telephones you after a kidney biopsy and says Carol is voiding black urine? Is there a possibility this is blood? What questions would you ask to elicit additional information? What recommendations would you make to the grandmother?

THERAPEUTIC MEASURES FOR THE MANAGEMENT OF RENAL DISEASE

When kidney function deteriorates, some method to replace kidney function must be instituted.

Peritoneal Dialysis

Dialysis is the separation and removal of solutes from body fluid by diffusion through a semipermeable membrane. *Peritoneal dialysis* uses the membrane of the peritoneal cavity to do this. Unlike hemodialysis, peritoneal dialysis does not require elaborate equipment or expense, but it does take more time than hemodialysis.

Peritoneal dialysis may be used as a temporary measure for children who experience sudden renal failure caused by trauma or shock. It is used for fairly long periods with children with chronic renal disease both in the hospital or at home to allow them to live until a kidney transplantation can be arranged (Madden et al., 2003). It is usually begun when the serum creatinine level reaches 10 mg/100 mL. Other indications are congestive heart failure, BUN of more than 100 mg/100 mL, hyperkalemia (potassium level of more than 6 mEq/L), and uremic encephalopathy (confusion or coma). *Continuous cycling peritoneal dialysis* allows the procedure to be done at home because less rigorous monitoring of the procedure is necessary.

Method for Performing Peritoneal Dialysis

Before peritoneal dialysis begins, a child's weight and vital signs are obtained to provide baseline information. Ask the child to void to reduce bladder size so that the bladder occupies as little anterior space as possible. If a child cannot void, catheterization may be necessary. The child's abdomen is cleaned just below the umbilicus with an antiseptic solution and covered with a sterile drape; a local anesthetic is injected into the abdominal wall, and a large-bore needle is inserted into the peritoneal cavity. If ascites fluid is present, a quantity of this fluid is removed and then a warmed hypertonic glucose solution (approximately 50 to 100 mL/kg of body weight) or a commercial dialysis solution is infused by gravity flow into the peritoneal cavity. This distends the abdominal wall and allows insertion of a peritoneal catheter, which is sutured in place and covered with a sterile dressing (Fig. 46.3). This catheter will remain in place for the period of dialysis.

A prescribed amount of dialysis solution is then infused into the peritoneal cavity by gravity drainage. This takes approximately 10 minutes and is recorded as inflow time. Be certain that the infusion fluid is warmed to room temperature to prevent the child from becoming chilled; warming the solution to near body temperature also appears to improve diffusion efficiency. It can be warmed in a basin of warm water or with the use of commercial warm packs at the child's bedside. Heparin is generally added at least to the first infusion to keep any blood from the abdominal puncture from plugging the tube.

Infused fluid is allowed to remain in the child's peritoneal cavity for 15 to 60 minutes (called the *equilibrium* or *dwell time*). Because the infused solution is hypertonic, fluid from extracellular spaces diffuses across the semipermeable peritoneal membrane to dilute the hypertonic solution. Urea and electrolytes diffuse with this fluid. After this designated equilibrium time, allow the fluid to drain from the peritoneal catheter into a collecting bottle (this takes approximately 10 minutes and is recorded as outflow time). More fluid generally drains from the peritoneal cavity than was infused, because excessive fluid has diffused across the peritoneum, reducing peritoneal or ascitic fluid. After a cycle of inflow, equilibrium, and outflow time, a new cycle is begun. Peritoneal dialysis may be conducted continuously for periods of 12 to 72 hours, depending on the effectiveness of the procedure in restoring the serum creatinine and BUN levels to normal.

Monitor vital signs at least every hour while children are undergoing peritoneal dialysis. During each new infusion period and while the solution is in the abdomen, carefully observe for shortness of breath, because the fluid exerts upward pressure on the diaphragm. Elevating the head of the bed helps to increase breathing space and ease respirations. If tachycardia or hypotension occurs, hypovolemia may be present. An increasing temperature (after 24 hours) may indicate peritoneal infection, a serious complication.

Frequent blood studies are necessary during periods of peritoneal dialysis to determine electrolyte concentrations. If electrolyte imbalances occur, electrolytes may be added to the infusion solution or administered IV.

The longer the peritoneal catheter remains in place, the greater the risk of peritoneal infection from the catheter insertion site. Assess the insertion site daily for signs of infection, such as redness or drainage. Obtain temperature about every 4 hours. Ask children to report any abdominal pain or diarrhea. Assess for abdominal guarding or tenderness once daily by palpating the abdomen; a rigid abdomen suggest peritonitis or infection. Follow the agency's policy for cleaning and covering the end of the peritoneal catheter (Fig. 46.4).

As for any procedure, children need to be well prepared for peritoneal dialysis. If the procedure is presented in a matter-of-fact way, children usually accept it with no more apprehension than IV therapy. Both procedures involve a needle penetration. You can assure children that they will feel the initial prick of the needle that administers the local anesthetic but will feel only pressure after that as the peritoneal needle or catheter is inserted. The procedure is intrusive, however, and frightening. Provide opportunities for therapeutic play (e.g., use a cloth doll, a dialysis tube, IV tubing, a doll's bed, or syringes and needles).

Once cycles of dialysis begin, children often grow bored lying in bed waiting for this procedure to be finished. They need planned interaction for these times—perhaps a toy or game that is allowed only during the procedure, so that it remains special. Children generally do not feel hungry while having peritoneal dialysis, because the bulk of peritoneal fluid causes pressure on the stomach and makes them feel uncomfortably full. They do well on a liquid diet or small frequent feedings during this time. So that children can feel that they have a sense of control over what is happening, let them help with the procedure by doing such things as recording the amount of solution infused and drained, and allowing them to select liquids they like for meals.

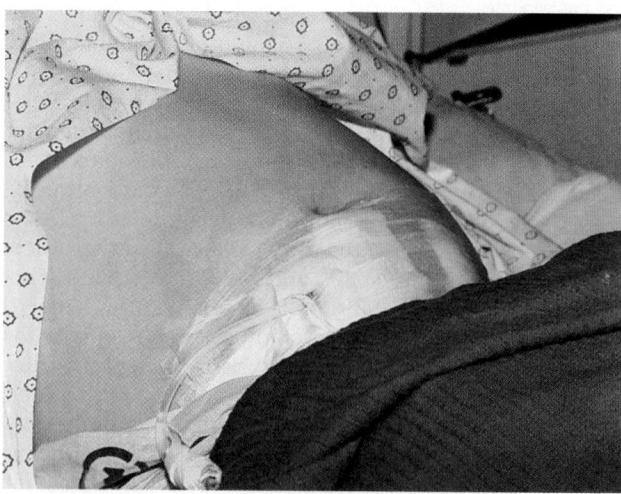

FIGURE 46.4 Peritoneal catheter inserted into a child's abdomen. A secure dressing surrounds the insertion site to prevent infection. (Courtesy of Karen M. Polise, MSN, RN, Division of Nephrology, The Children's Hospital of Philadelphia.)

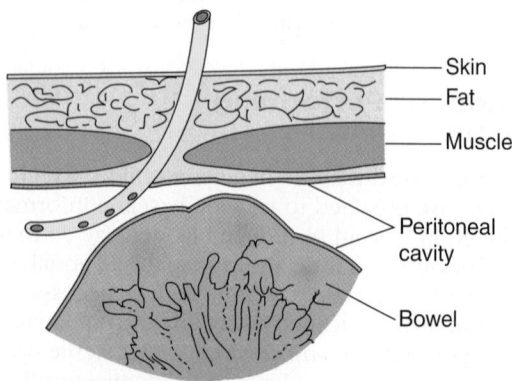

Skin
Fat
Muscle
Peritoneal cavity
Bowel

FIGURE 46.3 Insertion site for peritoneal dialysis catheter.

Peritoneal dialysis is a simple yet important concept. Help parents understand its importance so they can demonstrate a positive attitude toward it. The parents' acceptance of the procedure helps the child to accept it too.

Continuous Ambulatory Peritoneal Dialysis

Continuous ambulatory peritoneal dialysis (CAPD) allows a child to go to school or participate in other activities while receiving dialysis. With CAPD, a permanent dialysis catheter is inserted and sutured into place on the abdomen. Each day, the child or parent attaches a bag of dialysis fluid and tubing to this and infuses a prescribed dialysis solution by gravity drainage; the bag and tubing are then rolled into a compact square and carried with the child. The infused solution remains in the child for 4 to 6 hours during the day (8 hours at night); the dialysate bag is then lowered and the solution drains from the peritoneal cavity into it. The bag and fluid are then discarded and a new bag of dialysate solution is attached and raised, and new solution is infused (Munnariz, Kramer, & Carpinito, 2004).

CAPD requires careful monitoring and attention by the child or family. The parent or child must keep accurate records of infusions. Children can participate in gym programs but should not participate in contact sports or swimming. Teach parents to think ahead for holidays or family trips so they don't run short of supplies.

Because CAPD is continuous, electrolytes in the bloodstream are maintained at more constant levels than when intermittent dialysis is used. CAPD also allows greater freedom because children can return home and go back to school. There are disadvantages, however. Infection can occur because of the long-term placement of the catheter. Dehydration or hypernatremia may occur because of excess fluid removal. Because the tube remains in place at all times and the peritoneal solution constantly distends the abdomen, making the child appear obese and clothing difficult to fit, the child is frequently reminded of the illness and may have difficulty accepting this change in body image. Possible complications of CAPD are listed in Table 46.4.

Hemodialysis

Hemodialysis removes body wastes by using an external membrane as the diffusion surface. For hemodialysis, a catheter is inserted into an artery and blood is removed from the child and circulated through a dialysis coil. Urea and electrolytes in the blood diffuse into the surrounding fluid bath as the blood passes through the coil (Wright, 2004). After diffusion is complete, the blood is returned to the child's venous circulation (Fig. 46.5).

Hemodialysis can be done as a continuous process, but it is so effective that 3 hours of hemodialysis accomplishes as much as 12 hours of peritoneal dialysis. Children who have renal failure or whose kidneys have been removed can be maintained almost indefinitely by hemodialysis sessions two or three times a week or by continuous ultrafiltration or continuous arteriovenous hemofiltration. To establish a site for blood removal, children may have a double-lumen central catheter inserted into a central vein, such as the subclavian or internal jugular vein.

TABLE 46.4

Possible Complications of Continuous Ambulatory Peritoneal Dialysis

Assessment	Problem	Interventions
Redness or pain or swelling at tubing insertion	Infection	Take culture at site; administer antibiotics as prescribed; continue site care as ordered; notify physician.
Abdominal pain, increased temperature, nausea and vomiting, cloudy return in drainage solution	Peritonitis	Notify physician; administer antibiotics as prescribed; auscultate for bowel sounds.
Cramps as fluid is infused	Irritation of peritoneal cavity	Infuse solutions more slowly; warm temperature of solution to body temperature.
Difficulty with infusion or drainage of fluid	Kinked or clotted tubing; malpositioned catheter	Assess tubing for kinking; change position of child; ask child to cough to increase abdominal pressure; add prescribed amount of heparin to dialysate bag (prevents clotting).
Weight increase; moist cough, shortness of breath	Fluid overload	Decrease sodium and fluid oral intake; assess blood pressure and weight; use 4.25% exchange solution until weight is again decreased.
Weight loss, hypotension, poor skin turgor, tachycardia	Fluid loss	Increase fluid and sodium intake; assess blood pressure and weight; do not use 4.25% solution.
Blood-tinged dialysis return	Ruptured blood vessel	Assess pulse and blood pressure; observe for further bleeding in drainage; flush catheter with prescribed amount of heparin to keep clots from forming.

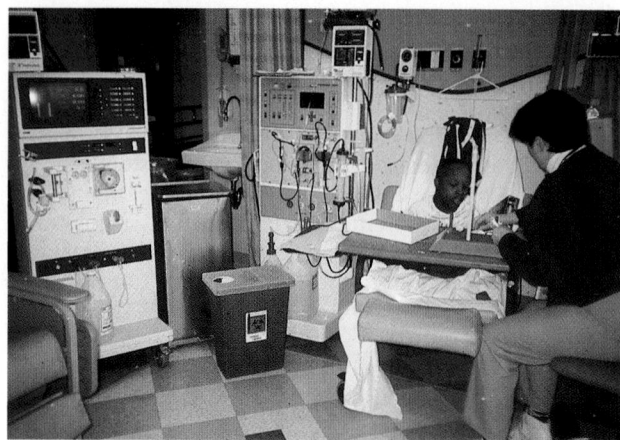

FIGURE 46.5 An adolescent receiving hemodialysis. A catheter from the child is connected to the hemodialysis equipment (in the background). Blood flows from the child through the catheter to the hemodialysis equipment for waste removal and is then returned to the child's venous circulation. (Courtesy of Karen M. Polise, MSN, RN, Division of Nephrology, The Children's Hospital of Philadelphia.)

A permanent technique is subcutaneous anastomosis of a vein and artery, creating an arteriovenous fistula (usually the brachial artery and brachiocephalic vein; Fig. 46.6*A*) or internal anastomosis of the artery and vein using a subcutaneous graft (see Fig. 46.6*B*). The possibility of infection is reduced with this method, although, unfortunately, two venipunctures, one from a low point in the shunt to remove blood and one high in the shunt to return it, are necessary for dialysis (use lidocaine or EMLA cream first to reduce pain). The ability to feel a thrill (vibration) or hear a bruit over the fistula or graft site is proof that it is open.

The risks of hemodialysis include infection introduced with venipuncture (severe because the infection automatically is septicemia) and clotting of the access site, which can lead to emboli. During hemodialysis, children may begin to show signs of confusion, vomiting, visual blurring, or hallucinations from a *dialysis disequilibrium syndrome.* This occurs because the hemodialysis is removing urea from the blood at too rapid a rate—faster than urea can be shifted from the brain to the blood. This causes fluid to shift into the brain, resulting in cerebral edema. The procedure must be temporarily halted to allow equalization to return. Muscle cramping may occur from sodium depletion. A "first use" syndrome (i.e., dizziness or muscle cramping) may occur from a reaction to the fibers in the dialysis machine coil.

Children grow bored during hemodialysis as they do during peritoneal dialysis. They need entertainment so the procedure remains acceptable. Help parents provide stimulating activities such as a play board, a ball to throw, or rings to stack for the infant. Parents may envision the infant as so ill that lying still without an activity would be best for him or her. Children need stimulation and play to avoid missing normal developmental milestones even during a long therapy such as dialysis.

When children's kidneys are removed prior to transplantation and they must remain on a continuous program of hemodialysis, they may come to resent a machine as "owning" or "controlling" them. They become aware that they cannot exist apart from it. Planning special activities to do during hemodialysis time helps to give them a feeling of control.

HEALTH PROMOTION AND RISK MANAGEMENT

A number of important interventions can help prevent urinary and renal disease in children. The first of these is the prevention of UTI in girls by educating them about perineal hygiene measures from the time they are first toilet-trained. Second is educating parents about the importance of giving the full course of antibiotics prescribed for UTI to prevent reinfection. Also important is educating parents about the importance of giving the full course of antibiotics after a streptococcal infection to prevent acute glomerulonephritis.

Teach parents to recognize the normal appearance of urine (clear and yellow) so that they can recognize abnormalities, such as red, black, or cloudy urine. Also teach parents about the signs and symptoms of UTI, such as urgency, frequency, and pain. Remind them of simple ways to prevent UTI, such as not allowing children to bathe with bubble bath.

STRUCTURAL ABNORMALITIES OF THE URINARY TRACT

Patent Urachus

When the bladder first forms in utero, it is joined to the umbilicus by a narrow tube, the *urachus.* When this fails to close properly during embryologic development, a fistula is left between the bladder and umbilicus (**patent urachus**). This occurs more commonly in males than in females. Nurses are frequently the ones to discover this condition as they notice clear fluid draining from the base

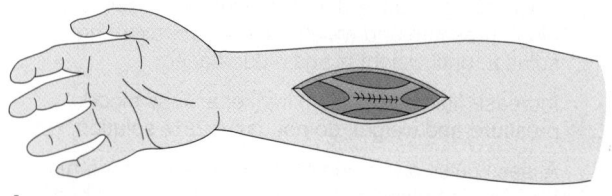

A

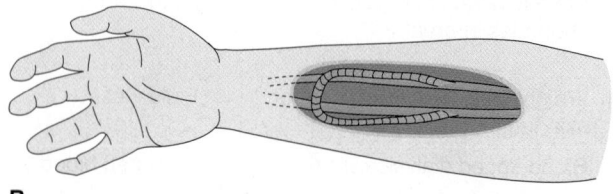

B

FIGURE 46.6 (A) An internal arteriovenous fistula. **(B)** An internal arteriovenous graft.

of the umbilical cord while changing a newborn's diaper. If the fluid is tested with Nitrazine paper for pH, its acid content will identify it as urine. A sonogram will confirm the patent connection.

A few patent urachus abnormalities heal spontaneously, but most require surgical correction to prevent pathogens from entering the fistula site and causing persistent bladder infection. This can be done in the immediate neonatal period using only a small subumbilical incision.

Exstrophy of the Bladder

Exstrophy of the bladder is a midline closure defect that occurs during the embryonic period of gestation (first 8 weeks). As a result, the bladder lies open and exposed on the abdomen. It occurs more frequently in males than females at a ratio of 2:1 (Metcalfe & Schwarz, 2004).

Assessment

Exstrophy can be revealed by fetal sonogram. There is no anterior wall of the bladder and no anterior skin covering on the lower anterior abdomen (Fig. 46.7A). The bladder appears bright red and continually drains urine from the open surface. In females, the urethra may also be abnormally formed. In males, the penis is often unformed or malformed. Pelvic bone defects, particularly nonclosure of the pubic arch, and urethral defects such as epispadias—opening of the urinary meatus on the dorsal or superior surface of the penis—may be present. The skin around the bladder quickly becomes excoriated because of constant exposure to acid urine. Untreated bladder exstrophy leads to kidney infection from ascending organisms. When children with this disorder begin to walk, they may demonstrate a "waddling" gait from the effect of the nonfused pubic arch.

Therapeutic Management

The treatment of bladder exstrophy begins with surgical closure of the bladder and, if necessary, the anterior abdominal wall with construction of a urethra (Grady & Mitchell, 2004; see Fig. 46.7B). Surgical repair may be limited if inadequate bladder tissue is present. For this reason, in some instances, the bladder is surgically removed and a ureterocecal implantation (ureters directed into the small intestine) or a *continent urinary reservoir* (an artificial bladder) is constructed (Fig. 46.8).

To construct a continent urinary reservoir, a small segment of the intestine, usually the cecum, is separated from the intestinal tract. The intestinal tract is then anastomosed so that a normal gastrointestinal (GI) tract is maintained. The separated segment is attached to the internal abdominal wall using the appendix to create an artificial urethra. The ureters are anastomosed to this segment.

Urine drains from the kidneys into the ureters, and then into the collecting bowel segment. The parent or child catheterizes the abdominal urethra three or four times daily to empty urine. The procedure is theoretically simple, but it is technically difficult to accomplish. Parents need a good review of anatomy to aid their understanding of the procedure. As the child reaches school age and begins school activities, such as showering, that exposes the condition to others, adjusting to a continent urinary reservoir can be difficult. Ensure that the child has a plan for follow-up care during the school years and in adolescence so the function of the reservoir and also the child's adjustment can continue to be assessed.

Preoperative Interventions. To minimize the possibility of infection in the bladder while the infant is waiting for surgery, keep the exposed bladder covered by a sterile plastic bowel bag. This prevents the bladder surface from adhering to bedclothes or diapers and the mucosal surface from being injured. To prevent the skin of the abdomen from excoriation due to the constant irritation of urine, protect it with a substance such as A & D Ointment, Karaya Gum, or Maalox. Consult a wound, ostomy, continence nurse for the best approach. To reduce pressure and prevent further separation of the symphysis, the orthopedic physician may ask that the infant's legs be flexed and brought together and wrapped in Ace bandages to hold them in that position. If this is done, do not separate the

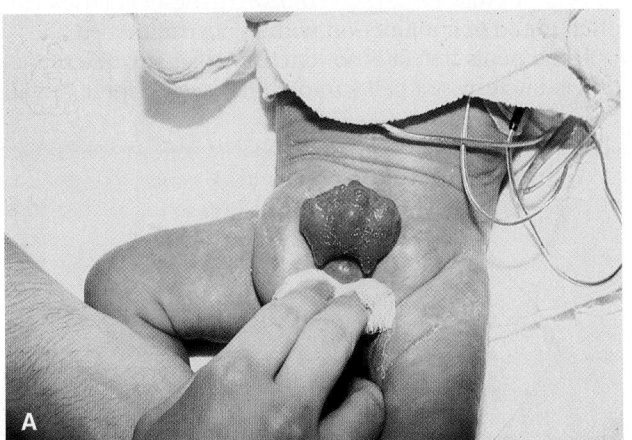
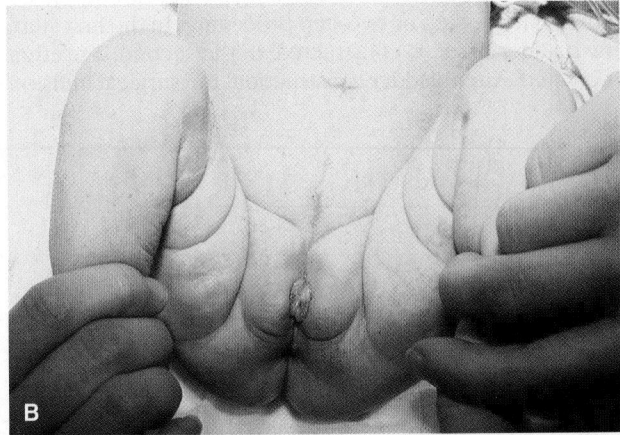

FIGURE 46.7 Bladder exstrophy. (**A**) Prior to surgical reconstruction. Note the bright-red color of the bladder. (**B**) Following surgical reconstruction. (Courtesy of Karen M. Polise, MSN, RN, Division of Nephrology, The Children's Hospital of Philadelphia.)

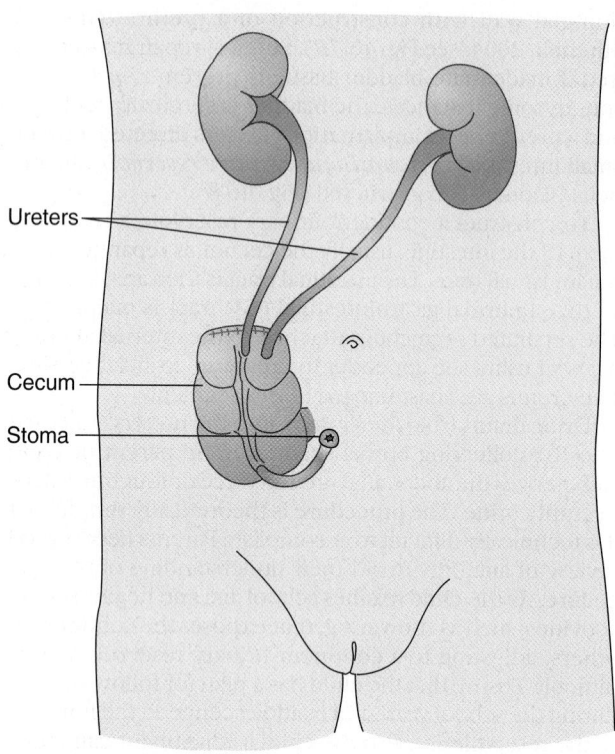

FIGURE 46.8 A continent urine reservoir. A portion of intestine is isolated; the attached ureters drain into it. The appendix creates an abdominal stoma for catheterization.

infant's legs to apply diapers; just place them under the child instead. Be certain to change diapers promptly after defecation so feces are not brought forward to the open bladder. Position the infant on his or her back, the same as for all infants, so urine drains freely. Sponge bathe rather than tub bathe the infant to prevent water from entering the ureters and becoming a source of infection.

Parents often need support to view their child as normal in all other ways but the unusual bladder formation. In some instances, the bladder repair will not be done immediately, so parents will need instructions on how to care for the child at home while waiting for surgery.

Postoperative Interventions. Surgery may be completed either as a one-step or two-step procedure. In the first step, the bladder tissue is constructed; in the second, a urethra is created. After bladder construction, the surgical incision over the bladder area must be kept free of infection. Position the infant on his or her back or in an infant chair to prevent feces from coming forward and contaminating the incision line. A suprapubic or indwelling urethral catheter for urine drainage will be inserted to allow the newly constructed bladder to rest. Immediately after surgery, urine draining from the catheter may be blood-stained, but this should clear after the first few hours. Children may notice sharp painful bladder contractions for the first few days after surgery. Analgesics and antispasmodics may be needed to keep the child comfortable. To prevent the nonfused pubic bone from separating and putting stress on the suture line, at the time of surgery, the child may be fitted with an external fixation device after an osteotomy to hold the pubic bones in approximation until they fuse.

After the second-stage urethra repair, children can be expected to experience some stress incontinence (loss of urine on physical exertion) from the constructed urethra. Kegel exercises can help strengthen the perineal muscles.

Hypospadias

Hypospadias is a urethral defect in which the urethral opening is not at the end of the penis but on the ventral (lower) aspect of the penis (Fig. 46.9A). The meatus may be near the glans, midway back, or at the base of the penis. This anomaly is fairly common, occurring in approximately 1 in 300 male newborns. It tends to be familial or may occur from a multifactorial genetic focus. **Epispadias** is a similar defect in which the opening is on the dorsal surface of the penis (Fig. 46.9B); this is corrected the same way (De, 2004).

Assessment

Be certain to inspect all male newborns at birth for hypospadias or epispadias as part of the routine physical examination. The degree of hypospadias may be minimal (on the glans but inferior in site) or maximal (at the midshaft or at the penal-scrotal junction). Many newborns with hypospadias have an accompanying short *chordee*—a fibrous band that causes the penis to curve downward (often called a cobra-head appearance; Fig. 46.9C). Also inspect carefully for *cryptorchidism* (undescended testes), often found in conjunction with hypospadias.

If the penis defect is so extensive that sex determination is unclear, sex cell karyotyping (see Chapter 7) will

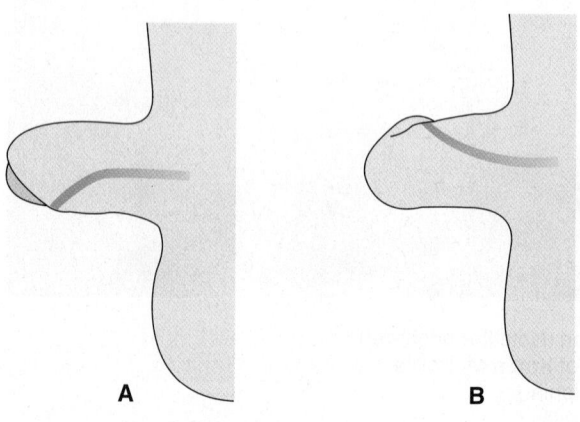

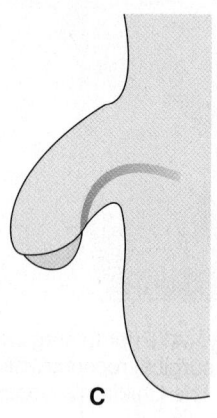

A   **B**   **C**

FIGURE 46.9 Urethral defects. (**A**) Hypospadias. (**B**) Epispadias. (**C**) Hypospadias with chordee.

be done. Hypospadias can be a difficult medical diagnosis for parents to accept because they may view it as a threat to the child's masculinity. This may cause them to have difficulty discussing this defect with relatives or health care personnel. Help parents work through these feelings by allowing them to talk about the disorder and by answering their questions honestly and openly.

Therapeutic Management

Children with hypospadias should not be circumcised because, at the time of the repair, the surgeon may wish to use a portion of the foreskin for the repair. In the newborn, a *meatotomy*—a surgical procedure in which the urethra is extended to a normal position—may initially be performed to establish better urinary function. When the child is older (age 12 to 18 months), adherent chordee may be released. If the repair will be extensive, all surgery may be delayed until the child is 3 to 4 years of age. To encourage penis growth and make the procedure easier, the child may have testosterone cream applied to the penis or receive daily injections of testosterone. It is important that hypospadias be corrected before school age so the child looks and feels normal. If left uncorrected, in later years, a meatal opening at an inferior penile site may interfere with fertility, because it does not allow sperm to be deposited close to the female cervix during coitus. Repair must be made before this time to prevent infertility.

After surgical repair, a urethral urinary drainage catheter will be inserted to allow urine output without putting tension against the urethral sutures. The child may notice painful bladder spasms as long as the catheter is in place (3 to 7 days). An analgesic such as acetaminophen (Tylenol) and an antispasmodic medication such as oxybutynin (Ditropan) may be prescribed for pain relief.

After hypospadias repair, children can be expected to be normal in both urinary and reproductive function unless accompanying anomalies of the penis were present (Stokowski, 2004).

✔ **Checkpoint Question 2**

The appearance of a child with hypospadias is:

a. The urethra opens on the underside of the penis.
b. The bladder opens on the surface of the abdomen.
c. Urine drains into the rectum and is excreted with stool.
d. The child is unable to void, as there is no urethral meatus.

INFECTIONS OF THE URINARY SYSTEM AND RELATED DISORDERS

Urinary Tract Infection

UTI occurs more often in females than in males. Pathogens appear to enter the urinary tract most often as an ascending infection from the perineum. Most urinary pathogens are gram-negative rods; *Escherichia coli* is a frequent offender. UTIs also are a common cause of nosocomial or health care-acquired infections (Shaw, 2003).

UTIs tend to occur more often in girls than in boys because the urethra is shorter in girls and because it is located close to the vagina (allowing the spread of vulvovaginitis) and close to the anus, from which *E. coli* spread. Changing diapers frequently can help reduce the risk for infection in infants. Girls should be taught early (when they are toilet-trained) to wipe themselves from front to back after voiding and defecating to avoid contaminating the urethra. There is a suggested correlation between the use of products such as bubble bath, feminine hygiene sprays, and hot tubs and UTI in girls (Bartkowski, 2003). Use of these should be discouraged. Infection also often occurs after sexual intercourse. Teach both adolescent boys and girls to void after sexual intercourse. Additional measures to prevent UTI are summarized in Box 46.4.

BOX 46.4 FOCUS ON . . .

 FAMILY TEACHING

Preventing Urinary Tract Infection (UTI) in Females

Q. Carol's grandmother tells you, "Carol had a urinary tract infection last year. How can we prevent that from happening again?"

A. Here are some important tips to help prevent UTI:

- Encourage your granddaughter to drink periodically during the day, especially in warm weather or during exercise, to keep urine flowing freely and prevent stasis of urine in ureters.
- Urge her to urinate at least every 4 hours to prevent stasis of urine in the bladder.
- Teach her not to bathe with bubble bath; this can cause vulvar and urethral irritation.
- Help your granddaughter learn to wipe from front to back after moving her bowels or urinating, to prevent moving rectal contamination forward to the urethra.
- Have your granddaughter wear cotton, not synthetic, underwear to decrease perineal irritation.
- Instruct your granddaughter to wash her vulva daily to lower the bacterial count on the perineum.
- When your granddaughter begins menstruating, encourage her to change sanitary pads at least every 4 hours to reduce the possible growth of bacteria near the urethra.
- If symptoms of UTI should occur (pain on urination, frequency, blood in urine), call your primary health care provider. If an antibiotic is prescribed, make sure that your granddaughter takes it for the full prescribed course, so all bacteria are completely eradicated. Otherwise, after a short time, bacteria will proliferate, and the infection will recur.
- When your granddaughter becomes sexually active, teach her to urinate immediately after intercourse to remove any bacteria forced into the urethra by pressure.

UTIs need vigorous treatment in childhood so they do not spread to involve the kidneys (pyelonephritis). Girls who have more than three UTIs or boys with their first UTI should be referred to a urologist to determine whether they have a congenital anomaly such as urethral stenosis or bladder–ureter reflux that causes recurrent urinary stasis. A secondary problem is more likely in boys with a UTI.

Assessment

Although it may be possible to locate a UTI precisely as urethritis, cystitis, ureteritis, or pyelonephritis, the signs and symptoms in young children often are not clear-cut. When the exact location or extent of the infection is unknown, it is referred to simply as a UTI. The typical symptoms that occur in older children or in adults—pain on urination, frequency, burning, and hematuria—may not be present. If the infection is confined to the bladder (cystitis), the child may have a low-grade fever, mild abdominal pain, and enuresis (bedwetting). If the infection is a pyelonephritis, the symptoms generally are more acute, with high fever, abdominal or flank pain, vomiting, and malaise. Any child with a fever and no demonstrable causes on physical examination should be evaluated for UTI (Bartkowski, 2003).

Urine for culture can be collected by a clean-catch technique, suprapubic aspiration, or catheterization, so that bacteria from the vulva or foreskin do not contaminate the sample. Suprapubic aspiration is generally limited to infants because the sight of the syringe is so frightening to older children; plus, the procedure can introduce infection. The use of catheterization, also frightening and a potential source of infection, is limited in children of all ages.

Urine obtained from suprapubic aspiration is generally sterile, so any growth from this source is significant. A clean-catch urine specimen is said to be positive for bacteriuria if the bacterial colony count is more than 100,000/mL. A count of less than 10,000/mL is considered a negative culture. Counts between 10,000 and 100,000/mL are repeated. Usually, the urine also is positive for proteinuria (because of the presence of bacteria). Microscopic examination may indicate the presence of red blood cells (hematuria) because of mucosal irritation. The presence of red or white blood cells and bacteria tends to make urine more alkaline, so the pH will be elevated (more than 7).

Therapeutic Management

The medical treatment for UTI is the oral administration of an antibiotic specific to the causative organism that is cultured (Shaw, 2003).

In addition to the antibiotic, the child needs to drink a large quantity of fluid to "flush" the infection out of the urinary tract. Cranberry juice is often recommended as being highly effective in acidifying urine and making it more resistant to bacterial growth. In actual practice, there is little proof of its effectiveness, so offer any fluid the child drinks readily. If the child experiences moderate to severe pain on urination that interferes with his or her ability to void, suggest that the child sit in a bathtub of warm water and void into the water. A mild analgesic, such as acetaminophen (Tylenol), may help reduce pain enough to allow voiding.

With a first UTI, treatment with antibiotics must be continued for the full prescription or the infection will return. Create a reminder sheet for parents to post in a readily visible location, such as on the refrigerator door, to help ensure adherence. A repeat clean-catch urine sample is usually obtained at 72 hours to assess the effectiveness of the antibiotic treatment.

After antibiotic therapy is stopped, at least three sterile urine specimens must be obtained to prove that bacteria are not still present. After recurrent UTIs, children may be prescribed a prophylactic antibiotic for 6 months. At periodic health checkups for the next few years, a child should void a clean-catch specimen for culture or microscopic analysis.

"Honeymoon" Cystitis

Honeymoon cystitis refers to lower UTI seen in young women shortly after they initiate a first sexual relationship. Such infections occur in connection with the local irritation and inflammation caused by initial coitus. Cystitis of this nature is occurring more and more frequently in young adolescent girls as more girls of this age group begin to engage in sexual relations. Such UTIs respond quickly to antibiotic therapy. Voiding as soon as possible after coitus may help to flush pathogenic organisms from the urethra and prevent such infections. When cystitis is seen in adolescent girls, it should alert health care providers to the possibility that a girl may be sexually active. In addition to needing counseling about personal hygiene measures to prevent UTI, the girl may need information on sexually transmitted infections, reproductive planning, and her responsibility for her maturing body.

Vesicoureteral Reflux

Normally, urine flows from the ureters into the bladder, with almost no flow reentering the ureters from the bladder. This is because the ureters enter the bladder obliquely, and a bladder skin flap or "valve" obscures the end of the ureter, preventing backflow. **Vesicoureteral reflux** refers to retrograde flow of urine from the bladder into the ureters (Wheeler et al., 2005). This reflux occurs because the valve that guards the entrance from the bladder to the ureter is defective, either from birth or because of scarring from repeated UTIs, bladder pressure that is stronger than usual, or ureters that are implanted at abnormal sites or angles. This backflow of urine happens at micturition (voiding) when the bladder contracts (Fig. 46.10).

Reflux leads to bladder infection because urine is retained in the ureters after voiding, and stasis of this urine leads to infection. It also appears that the capacity for normal bladder tissue to lyse bacteria becomes reduced due to the large residual urine volume that is always present. In addition, reflux is a potentially serious condition because it can lead to back-pressure on the kidneys, possibly leading to nephron destruction and, subsequently, hydronephrosis or dilatation of the renal pelvis. One form of reflux is inherited as a polygenic disorder (Wu, 2003).

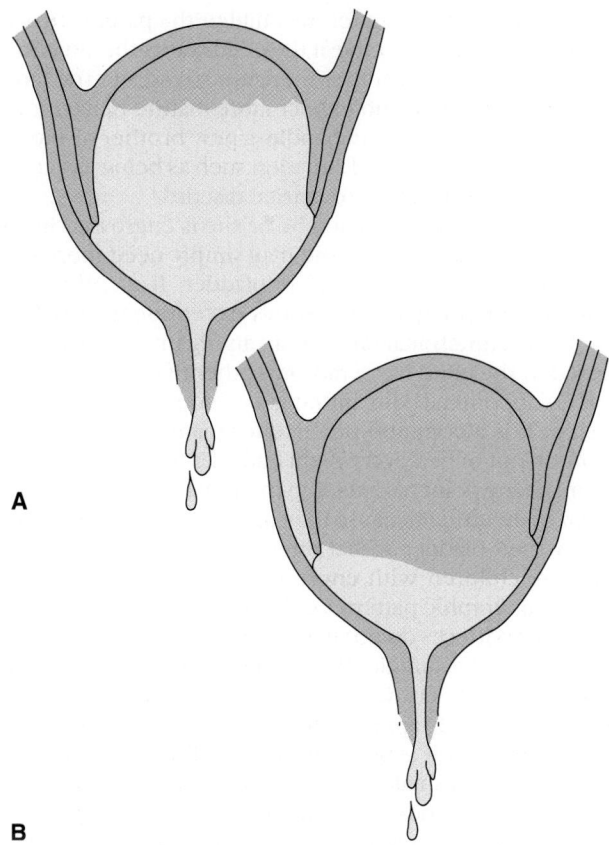

FIGURE 46.10 Vesicoureteral reflux. (**A**) Normal voiding pattern. (**B**) Reflux into ureters with voiding.

Assessment

A child with reflux is usually first seen by health care personnel because of a history of repeated UTI. A voiding cystourethrogram, CT scan, cystoscopy, or cystography with contrast material will show the ureteral reflux (Hoberman et al., 2003). Based on diagnostic studies, reflux is graded from I to V by degree of reflux, V being the most serious.

Therapeutic Management

The majority of grades of reflux resolve with maturity without a need for surgery. Until this normal growth occurs, however, reflux must be rigorously treated to decrease the possibility of glomerular scarring from infection or back-pressure. Teaching double voiding (having the child void, then in a few minutes attempt to void again) may help to empty the bladder and prevent recurrent infection from urinary stasis. Some children need to remain on prophylactic antibiotics to prevent bladder infection. Long-term maintenance with antibiotics may be as effective as surgery in reducing renal scarring in lower grades of reflux (Wheeler et al., 2005).

If continuous antibiotic therapy does not prevent recurrent UTIs, reflux can be corrected by cystoscopy. Under general anesthesia or conscious sedation, a cystoscope is passed, and polytetrafluoroethylene (Teflon) paste is injected to stabilize the ureter valves. Laparoscopic surgery

to correct the placement of ureters may be scheduled to reinsert the ureters at a more oblique angle, creating the normal valve effect.

After surgery, a suprapubic catheter remains in place to keep the bladder empty and prevent pressure against the surgical area. Two ureteral catheters (stents), threaded into the ureters to drain urine directly from the kidney pelvis, also exit at the suprapubic tube site. These are all attached as a closed drainage system to collecting bags. Sterile gauze dressings and antibiotic cream are placed around the tube insertion sites.

In preparing children for this type of surgery, be certain to prepare them for the number of tubes that will be inserted. Explain that even with the tubes in place, the child will be allowed to walk and move about soon after the operation (and should do this). Be sure that the child and parents understand the importance of keeping the urine collection bags below the level of the child's bladder to prevent urine from flowing back into the bladder. Caution them not to raise the bags above the child's bladder level when helping the child out of bed.

Observe the catheter drainage tubes closely, every hour for the first 24 hours and then at least every 4 hours. Note the color and the amount of drainage (urine), and carefully measure and record it. Initially, drainage will be bloody, but this should clear in 1 or 2 days. Assess drainage for clots (should not be over pinpoint in size). The stents should drain an equal amount, to ensure that kidney production is equal on both sides. Urine will drain primarily from the stents for approximately the first 3 days after surgery; thereafter, drainage will flow around the stents and will be mainly from the suprapubic tube.

Be sure that the ends of the catheters do not become contaminated, because then infection can spread to the surgical area or the kidneys. An antiseptic solution may be ordered placed in the drainage bags to limit the growth of bacteria in the collecting urine. Be certain any amount added is subtracted from the output amount. As soon as urine drainage from the stent catheters has decreased and blood has cleared, the stent catheters will be removed. To show that urine is clearing of blood, obtain serial urine specimens each time collecting bags are emptied and label it with the time of removal. Comparing the color of these samples will show that urine is clearing of blood. School-age children can help label the containers, which can help to improve their sense of accomplishment and control over the situation. Many children become frightened when they learn the stent catheters will be removed. Assure them that this will not be painful and can be done at an ambulatory visit without anesthesia.

Incisional pain and painful bladder spasms may occur for the first 3 days after surgery, so antispasmodics may be prescribed to reduce bladder spasm. Also, not touching or not moving the suprapubic tube helps to reduce spasms because this limits bladder irritation. The suprapubic tube is removed between 4 and 7 days after surgery (again, a nearly painless procedure). There may be slight urine leakage from the puncture site of the tube for 1 or 2 days after removal of the tube. Keep a sterile dressing in place to absorb the leaking urine. Remind the child and parents to avoid tub baths until the suprapubic tube site has closed completely.

A few children continue to have bladder reflux after ureter reimplantation. All children need follow-up care (i.e., repeated urine cultures or perhaps an IVP or sonogram at a later date) to establish that surgery was effective in halting the reflux.

Hydronephrosis

Hydronephrosis is enlargement of the pelvis of the kidney with urine as a result of back-pressure in the ureter. The back-pressure is generally caused by obstruction, either of the ureter or of the point where the ureter joins the bladder, as with vesicoureteral reflux. Although this may occur at any age, it occurs most often in the first 6 months of life. If it occurs during intrauterine life, it can be revealed by fetal sonography (Small & Copel, 2004).

Children with hydronephrosis are usually asymptomatic. They may have repeated UTIs from urinary stasis (difficult to detect in a child this age except as general irritability or crying on voiding). Elevated blood pressure caused by increasing tubular pressure (which activates the renin-angiotensin system) may be detected on a routine health assessment, although blood pressure is not taken routinely in a child of this age. With severe back-pressure, the infant experiences flank or abdominal pain. Abdominal palpation may reveal an abdominal mass (the dilated kidney pelvis). An IVP or sonogram will show the enlarged pelvis and the point of obstruction.

Hydronephrosis is a serious disorder because, if the pressure in the pelvis becomes too acute, back-pressure on the kidney will interfere with tubular function or destroy the nephrons. The treatment is surgical correction of the obstruction before glomerular or tubular destruction occurs.

DISORDERS AFFECTING NORMAL URINARY ELIMINATION

Enuresis

Enuresis is involuntary passage of urine past the age when a child should be expected to have attained bladder control (Nield & Kamat, 2004). Because this is expected at age 2 to 3 years of age for daytime and age 4 years for nighttime, enuresis is said to occur at approximately 5 to 7 years. Enuresis may be nocturnal (occurs only at night), diurnal (occurs during the day), or both. It is primary if bladder training was never achieved, acquired or secondary if control was established but has now been lost.

Most enuresis is nocturnal; daytime enuresis occurs only rarely. Functional nocturnal enuresis (that with no known cause) occurs in approximately 8% to 12% of children age 8 years or younger. It is found more frequently in boys than girls. It also tends to be familial (if it is present in a child, one of the parents probably experienced it, too).

Assessment

Children with enuresis who are older than 5 years of age need an evaluation to determine whether there is an organic cause for the disorder. During the history, ask how parents have tried to correct the problem; identify whether it is primarily a problem for the child or the parents (treatment will be most effective if the child wants the situation corrected). Assess whether there are stresses in the family, such as parents who expect more mature behavior of a child than he or she can handle, a new brother or sister, an uncomfortable school situation such as being assigned to a "shouting" teacher, or marital discord.

If a child wets only when he or she is engrossed in an interesting activity, he or she may simply need more frequent reminding to empty the bladder. If a child wets only on nights when he or she is exceptionally tired or troubled, a functional rather than an organic cause is suggested. If the child has symptoms other than bedwetting, such as abdominal pain, burning, or frequency, UTI is suggested. It is a common practice for many parents to get children out of bed every night and take them to the bathroom. At any point parents stop this practice, children may begin bedwetting because they have been conditioned to empty their bladder at that time of night.

Some children with enuresis have abnormal electroencephalographic patterns. Other children with the same abnormal patterns do not have enuresis, however, so this by itself is not a sufficiently specific finding to be helpful. In others, bedwetting seems to occur as children pass from a period of rapid eye movement sleep pattern to a type IV level, or it is primarily a sleep disorder. It may be associated with small bladder capacity (which would explain why the condition is familial).

Although usually not necessary to aid diagnosis, an IVP, VCUG, or sonogram may be done to rule out organic disease. A clean-catch urine specimen should be collected to rule out bacteriuria. Specific gravity is assessed to rule out a defect in urine concentration. Protein and glucose levels are evaluated to determine evidence of kidney disease.

Therapeutic Management

The treatment of enuresis may be complex because the cause is generally unknown. If stress factors have been identified, an attempt should be made to correct these. Some stress factors, such as birth of a new sibling, cannot be changed, but frank discussion with children regarding what causes the stress and attempts to help children cope better with their daytime activities may improve enuresis.

In many children, it helps to limit fluids after dinner. Urge parents to exercise common sense in this area. Remind them that a child may not be able to go every night without a drink from dinner until breakfast. Caution parents of children with sickle-cell anemia not to restrict fluid this way because increased sickling of cells occurs with dehydration.

Synthetic antidiuretic hormone (ADH; desmopressin [DDAVP]) administered intranasally or orally is the drug of choice to reduce urinary output (Box 46.5). Imipramine (Tofranil), an anticholinergic drug that inhibits urination, is also effective if given an hour before bedtime (Zeman, Siroky, & Babayan, 2004). Unfortunately, its side effects of insomnia, anxiety, and arrhythmias limit its use.

Alarm bells that ring when children wet at night are effective in some children. This type of system does not actually stop bedwetting. The alarm wakes the child, he or she stops voiding, and then the child gets up and uses

BOX 46.5 FOCUS ON . . .

PHARMACOLOGY

Desmopressin acetate (DDAVP)

Classification: A synthetic form of human antidiuretic hormone.

Action: Promotes resorption of water in the renal tubule or decreases bladder filling; drug of choice for enuresis (Karch, 2004)

Pregnancy Risk Category: B

Dosage: In children 6 years of age and older, 20 µg (0.2 mL) intranasally at bedtime, possibly increasing the dose up to 40 µg if necessary; or 0.2 mg orally at bedtime, titrated up to 0.6 mg to obtain the desired response

Possible Adverse Effects: Transient headache, nausea, flushing, mild abdominal cramps, fluid retention

Nursing Implications

• Instruct parents and child that child should restrict fluid after dinnertime in addition to taking medication.
• If given intranasally, advise parents to refrigerate the solution.
• Teach parents and child the proper method for intranasal administration.
• Caution child and parents that nasal administration is less effective if the child develops a cold with draining rhinitis.

the bathroom. Over time, this type of conditioning may be effective, but once the urine alarm is removed, children may relapse. Bladder-stretching exercises—drinking a large quantity of water and then refraining from voiding as long as possible—to increase the functional size of the bladder are helpful in some children. A bladder that can hold 300 to 350 mL of fluid will generally be large enough to contain urine during a night's sleep.

Enuresis is not a minor problem for either parents or for the child. Parents find it difficult to include the child on vacation trips. They may resent the daily linen washing. Children may exclude themselves from activities such as slumber parties or camping trips with friends to avoid embarrassment. As a general measure, children who wet their beds need to take baths in the morning rather than at bedtime to minimize urine odor and avoid teasing.

Enuresis may occur in hospitalized children because of the stress of their new surroundings. Preschool children may experience it because they are uncomfortable using strange bathrooms or do not understand which bathroom is theirs to use. As a rule, place as little stress or importance on enuresis as possible during an illness, and encourage parents to do the same.

Postural (Orthostatic) Proteinuria

A few children will spill albumin into the urine when they stand upright for an extended period (**postural proteinuria,** also called postural albuminuria). The amount of spilling decreases when they rest in a supine position. Children

with this condition have no apparent disease; the phenomenon is apparently attributable to the effect of gravity on glomerular function.

To determine whether postural proteinuria exists, urine is collected after the child has been recumbent during the night (a first-voided specimen) and then again after the child has been up and active for a number of hours. Make certain when collecting these urine specimens to record the child's activity accurately. If the child stood by the crib rail crying for a parent or was held in a nurse's lap for most of the night, the urine may show protein in the morning specimen because it is not truly a "resting specimen." Likewise, for the specimen to be collected after the child has been active, make certain that he or she is up and active, not lying in a supine position reading a book for most of the time. Play a game if necessary, such as follow the leader, so the child is active.

Postural proteinuria needs no therapy. However, be sure to document the condition because some of these children develop some form of kidney disorder later in life.

DISORDERS OF ALTERED KIDNEY FUNCTION

Renal disorders occur because of faulty kidney formation or illness that causes glomerular changes.

Kidney Agenesis

Agenesis means lack of growth (literally, lack of a beginning) or that no organ has formed in utero. Absence of kidneys in a newborn is suggested when the volume of amniotic fluid on sonogram or at birth is less than normal (oligohydramnios). This occurs because urine normally adds to the volume of amniotic fluid in utero. The infant with kidney agenesis often has Potter's syndrome or accompanying misshapen, low-set ears and hypoplastic (stiff, inflexible) lungs from the lack of amniotic fluid in utero. He or she will not void urine. Bilateral absence of kidneys is obviously incompatible with life unless a renal transplantation can be accomplished, but the associated condition of nonfunctioning lungs makes a successful transplantation highly unlikely.

Polycystic Kidney

Polycystic kidney means that large, fluid-filled cysts have formed in place of normal kidney tissue. The most frequent type of polycystic kidney seen in children is inherited as an autosomal recessive trait (Munson, 2004). With this, there is abnormal development of the collecting tubules. The kidneys are large and feel soft and spongy. If the disorder is bilateral, an infant will not pass urine. The mother will have had oligohydramnios during pregnancy. Children often have a typical appearance (*hypertelorism*—wide-spaced eyes, epicanthal folds, flattened nose; or *micrognathia*—small jaw), findings described as a "Potter facies." Either *transillumination* or *sonography* will show the fluid-filled cysts. In many children, the liver is filled with identical cysts. This is most evident later in life when increased portal circulation occurs (blood cannot perfuse the cystic liver structures either).

Because this kidney disease is inherited, parents, and children at adolescence, need genetic counseling to inform them that future children may also have this problem.

If the condition is unilateral, urine production will be decreased (oliguria), not absent. Because kidneys are difficult to locate in newborns, a unilateral polycystic kidney may be missed until later in life, when, with increased kidney growth, an abdominal mass can be palpated. The cystic growth offers such resistance to blood circulation that systemic hypertension often results by school age (Leonard, 2003).

The treatment for polycystic formation is surgical removal of a kidney if only one is cystic. If both kidneys are cystic, treatment is renal transplantation (difficult in the young child, because few infant kidneys are available for transplantation and because of the technical challenge presented by such small blood vessels).

Renal Hypoplasia

Hypoplasia means reduced growth. Hypoplastic kidneys contain fewer lobes than normal kidneys and are small and underdeveloped. The child with hypoplastic kidneys, in addition to having poor kidney function, may develop hypertension from stenosis of the renal arteries. If hypoplasia is bilateral, the child may need a kidney transplant in later life to maintain kidney function and prevent extreme hypertension.

Prune-Belly Syndrome

Prune-belly syndrome is severe urinary tract dilation that develops as early as intrauterine life from an unknown cause. Occurring mainly in boys, the severe dilation causes back-pressure and destruction of kidneys. The infant is born with oligohydramnios and pulmonary dysplasia because of the lack of amniotic fluid in utero (Wen, Marquez, & Cohen, 2004).

The condition is marked by the presence of three symptoms: deficiency of usual abdominal muscle tone, bilateral undescended testes, and the dilated faulty development of the bladder and upper urinary tract. The infant's abdomen appears wrinkled (like a prune) because of the poorly developed abdominal muscles (Fig. 46.11). Without surgical remodeling, the infant will develop repeated UTIs, leading to end-stage renal disease. Teach parents to protect their child's abdomen from trauma (e.g., from lap belts or baby walkers) because their child lacks abdominal support. Some children need kidney transplants because of destruction of glomeruli from back-pressure.

Acute Poststreptococcal Glomerulonephritis

Glomerulonephritis, inflammation of the glomeruli of the kidney, may occur as a separate entity but usually occurs as an immune complex disease after infection with nephritogenic streptococci (most commonly subtypes of group A beta-hemolytic streptococci). Tissue damage occurs from a complement fixation reaction in the glomeruli (*complement* is a cascade of proteins activated by antigen–antibody reactions and actually plugs or obstructs

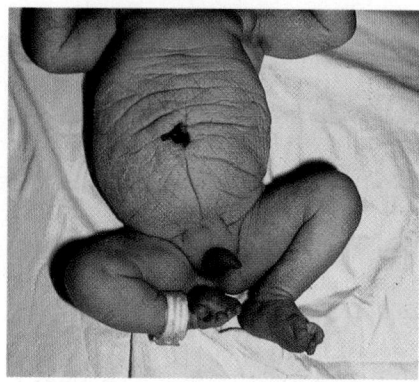

FIGURE 46.11 Prune belly syndrome. (Courtesy of Karen M. Polise, MSN, RN, Division of Nephrology, The Children's Hospital of Philadelphia.)

glomeruli). IgG antibodies against streptococci may be detected in the bloodstream of children with acute glomerulonephritis, proof that the illness follows a streptococcal infection (Schweon & Novatnack, 2003).

Intravascular coagulation occurs in the minute renal vessels. Ischemic damage leads to scarring and decreased glomerular function. This results in a reduction in the glomerular filtration rate, leading to an accumulation of sodium and water in the bloodstream. Inflammation of the glomeruli increases permeability, allowing protein molecules to escape into the filtrate.

Assessment

Acute glomerulonephritis is most common in children between the ages of 5 and 10 years, the age group most susceptible to streptococcal infections. Boys appear to develop the disease more often than girls; it occurs more often during the winter and spring, as do pharyngeal streptococcal infections. The child typically has a history of a recent respiratory infection (within 7 to 14 days) or impetigo (within 3 weeks). All children who have had a "strep" throat, tonsillitis, otitis media, or impetigo caused by streptococcal infection should have a urinalysis 2 weeks after the infection to evaluate for glomerulonephritis. Without frightening them unduly, tell parents that this is an extremely important follow-up test.

Acute glomerulonephritis is characterized by a sudden onset of hematuria and proteinuria. The protein content both of individual urine specimens and of total 24-hour urine volume is measured. Testing a single specimen will show 1^+ to 4^+ protein; a 24-hour urine specimen may contain as much as 1 g protein (normally, urine contains none).

The hematuria associated with acute glomerulonephritis is usually so gross that the child's urine appears tea-colored, reddish-brown, or smoky. Urinary sediment will contain white blood cells, epithelial cells, and hyaline, granular, and red blood cell casts. After these initial urine changes, the child develops oliguria. Specific gravity of urine is elevated. Hypertension from hypervolemia occurs. The child may have abdominal pain, a low-grade fever, edema, anorexia, vomiting, or headache. There may be cardiac involvement related to the difficulty in managing the excessive plasma fluid. Such children show signs of orthopnea, cardiac enlargement, enlarged liver, pulmonary edema, and a galloping heart rhythm. Electrocardiographic changes such as T-wave inversion and prolongation of the P-R interval may be seen. Heart failure may occur from circulatory overload.

Blood analysis will indicate a lowered blood protein level (hypoalbuminemia) caused by the massive proteinuria. Low serum complement will be present, and, as the blood volume expands, a mild anemia also will occur. As in all inflammatory diseases, the erythrocyte sedimentation rate will increase. Because the glomeruli cannot filter properly, concentrations of urea, nonprotein nitrogen (BUN), and creatinine in blood will increase. The antistreptolysin O (anti-DNase B) titer or antibody formation against streptococci is generally elevated (Meyers, 2003).

If blood pressure reaches 160/100 mm Hg as part of the acute process, encephalopathy may occur, with symptoms of headache, irritability, seizures, vomiting, coma or lethargy, and perhaps transitory paralysis. This extreme elevation in blood pressure is probably related to the expanded circulatory volume. The cerebral symptoms are caused by *cerebral ischemia* (vasoconstriction of cerebral vessels to reduce cranial pressure).

Therapeutic Management

The course of acute glomerulonephritis is 1 to 2 weeks. During this time, there is little therapy specific for the disorder. Antibiotics usually are ineffective because the disease is caused not by an active infection but by an antigen–antibody inflammatory response to a past infection. Diuretics are of little value because obstructed glomeruli bases cannot be made to function; a course of ethacrynic acid or furosemide (Lasix) may be tried. If heart failure occurs, specific measures such as placing the child in a semi-Fowler's position, digitalization, and oxygen administration may be necessary. If diastolic blood pressure rises to more than 90 mm Hg, antihypertensive therapy with a calcium channel blocker may be necessary. Phosphate binders, such as aluminum hydroxide to reduce phosphate absorption in the GI tract, or a potassium-removing resin agent, such as sodium polystyrene sulfonate (Kayexalate), may be necessary in children who have rising phosphate and potassium levels.

Bed rest is unnecessary, although children should be encouraged to participate in quiet play activities. They can attend school and engage in normal activities after 1 or 2 weeks, but competitive activity is limited until kidney function has returned to normal to avoid overstressing the kidneys.

Diet is controversial. Although limiting protein intake reduces the amount of protein lost in urine, many children who are losing large quantities of protein need high-protein diets to supplement this loss. Salt restriction may be needed to reduce severe edema. Most children do well on a normal diet for their age, however, with normal salt and protein content. Weighing the child every day and calculating intake and output are important assessments in following the course of the disease.

In most children, acute glomerulonephritis runs a limited, benign course. After most symptoms fade, proteinuria and impaired clearance of urea and creatinine may remain for as long as 2 months. Caution parents that the results of a urine protein test may remain abnormal for up to a year; if their child has this test as a routine screening procedure at a health checkup, they should not worry that this finding means reinfection or the beginning of further disease.

A few children will not completely recover from acute glomerulonephritis but will develop chronic nephritis. These children appear to suffer destruction from the initial inflammation that results in chronic renal insufficiency.

NURSING DIAGNOSES AND RELATED INTERVENTIONS

Nursing Diagnosis: Situational low self-esteem, related to feelings of responsibility for onset of serious illness

Outcome Evaluation: Child (parent) states feelings about becoming ill; discusses plans and ways to maintain health; participates in care.

Glomerulonephritis is a frightening disease for both children and their parents. Children may be frightened by the initial hematuria. They may be upset at the appearance of periorbital edema, which makes their reflection in the mirror so strange to them. Children as young as early school age are aware that kidneys are necessary for life, and this means they recognize the seriousness of kidney disease.

If children were prescribed penicillin for pharyngitis 2 weeks before the development of the nephritis but refused to take it, they may believe that they caused this disease. The parents may feel guilty because they did not force the child to take the medicine. They worry that their child will develop chronic glomerulonephritis or die during the acute phase of this attack. These parents and children need to talk about their feelings openly. Provide frequent reports of subtle positive changes in a child's condition (e.g., "His blood pressure is staying down by itself now; he does not need medicine for that any more." "He weighs 2 pounds less today than 4 days ago; that generally means his kidneys are beginning to function more efficiently again").

Be certain that parents know the date and place of a return visit for follow-up care. Because this is a perplexing disease, be sure they have a telephone number to call if they have questions about their child's care or condition.

The most frequent type of acute glomerulonephritis can be avoided by the prevention or effective early treatment of group A beta-hemolytic streptococcal infections. Acute glomerulonephritis tends not to recur with subsequent streptococcal infections, so prophylactic penicillin to prevent further streptococcal infections is unnecessary.

Checkpoint Question 3

What is typically the first symptom of acute glomerulonephritis?

a. Low blood pressure from excessive aldosterone
b. "Old blood" in urine from kidney bleeding
c. Dependent edema from protein accumulation
d. Pain on urination from urethra inflammation

Chronic Glomerulonephritis

Although chronic glomerulonephritis occasionally follows acute glomerulonephritis or nephrotic syndrome, it also occurs as a primary disease (or after acute glomerulonephritis that was clinically so mild it was undiagnosed). The child is found to have proteinuria at a routine checkup. Further investigation may indicate hypertension and the presence of red cell or white cell casts and occult blood in urine. The specific gravity of the child's urine is below normal (below 1.003). Blood studies may indicate an increased BUN or creatinine level. A renal biopsy will show permanent destruction of glomeruli membranes.

Chronic glomerulonephritis may result in either diffuse or local nephron damage. The remaining functioning nephrons increase their glomerular filtration rate to compensate for those that are damaged. At some point in this chronic disease destruction process, however, compensatory mechanisms fail, and renal insufficiency or failure will result. **Alport's syndrome** is a progressive chronic glomerulonephritis inherited as an autosomal dominant disorder (O'Connell & Siroky, 2004).

During the illness, if the child has acute symptoms of edema, hematuria, hypertension, or oliguria, bed rest may be necessary. If children have only a chronic manifestation, such as proteinuria, and if they feel well, they can maintain normal activity, including attending school. Children should not engage in competitive activities such as contact sports, however, because of the risk of kidney injury.

Therapy is nonspecific and directed at symptom relief rather than the disease process itself, because the cause of the disease is unknown. Therapy with antihypertensive drugs such as hydralazine (Apresoline) or with diuretics to increase urine output such as ethacrynic acid (Edecrin) may be necessary. Corticosteroid therapy may reduce or halt the progress of the disorder by reducing inflammation. Children have difficulty accepting long-term corticosteroid therapy because of the side effects, in particular a typical "moon face" and extra body hair (Cushing's syndrome). Talk with them about these body changes and assure them that these changes will be reversed when the drug is discontinued.

Children receiving corticosteroids are at an increased risk for infection because of the immunosuppressive activity of these drugs. They need to be shielded from other children and health care personnel with infection. Parents need to learn to take their child's temperature and recognize and report the earliest signs of infection.

Generally, the prognosis for children with chronic glomerulonephritis is poor. Although the illness may run a long-term course, eventually it leads to renal insufficiency and renal failure. Children may be maintained for long periods by peritoneal dialysis or hemodialysis. Kidney transplantation is a possibility.

Because children as young as early school age are aware of the importance of kidney function to life, most children with chronic renal disease are aware of the likely outcome of their disease. Most children are adolescents or young adults before the disease runs its ultimate course. They indicate that they appreciate having health care personnel face this outcome with them honestly if kidney transplantation cannot be performed to prolong their life.

Nephrotic Syndrome (Nephrosis)

Nephrosis, altered glomerular permeability due to fusion of the glomeruli membrane surfaces, causes abnormal loss of protein in urine. Immunologic mechanisms are involved in instigating the process. The cause may be hypersensitivity to an antigen–antibody reaction or an autoimmune process. A T-lymphocyte dysfunction may be responsible. The highest incidence is at 3 years of age, and it occurs more often in boys than in girls; it is increasing in frequency for unknown reasons (Filler et al., 2003).

Nephrotic syndrome in children occurs in three forms: (1) congenital; (2) secondary, as a progression of glomerulonephritis or in connection with systemic diseases such as sickle cell anemia or systemic lupus erythematosus (SLE); or (3) idiopathic (primary). The congenital form is rare; in children, the idiopathic form is most common (Iitaka et al., 2004).

Nephrosis can be further classified according to the amount of membrane destruction. Minimal change nephrotic syndrome (MCNS) is the type most often seen in children (80% of cases). As the name implies, little scarring of glomeruli occurs. Children with this degree of scarring respond well to therapy. Other types are focal glomerulosclerosis (FGS) and membranoproliferative glomerulonephritis (MPGN). Both of these types involve scarring of glomeruli, and these children will have a poorer response to therapy.

The four characteristic symptoms of nephrotic syndrome are proteinuria, edema, hypoalbuminemia (low serum albumin level), and hyperlipidemia (increased blood lipid level). Proteinuria occurs because increased glomerular permeability leads to protein loss in the urine and, subsequently, hypoalbuminemia. With a low level of protein in the bloodstream, osmotic pressure causes fluid to shift from the bloodstream into interstitial tissue, causing edema. As the blood volume decreases, the kidneys begin to conserve sodium and water, adding to the potential for edema. The hyperlipidemia occurs because the liver increases production of lipoproteins to try to compensate for protein loss. Lipids are too large to be lost in urine, so they rise to high levels in the blood serum. Some children have such high cholesterol levels that, when blood is drawn and placed into a test tube, a circle of white fat forms on the top of it. Figure 46.12 illustrates the process that leads to the common symptoms.

Assessment

Symptoms usually begin insidiously. Children develop edema around the eyes (periorbital edema), most noticeable when they wake in the morning from a head-

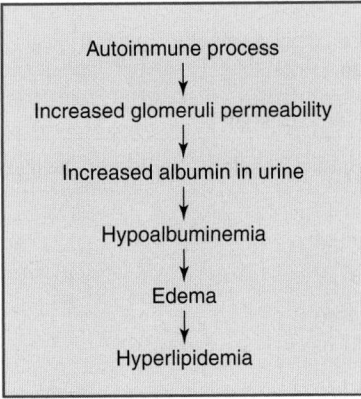

Autoimmune process

↓

Increased glomeruli permeability

↓

Increased albumin in urine

↓

Hypoalbuminemia

↓

Edema

↓

Hyperlipidemia

FIGURE 46.12 The process that results in the signs and symptoms of nephrotic syndrome.

dependent position. Parents may notice that clothing no longer fits a child around the waist, because edematous fluid is beginning to collect in the abdominal cavity (ascites). It is easy to dismiss these first symptoms as those of an upper respiratory tract infection and the normal "paunchy" belly of a toddler or preschooler. As edema progresses, the child's skin becomes pale, stretched, and taut. In boys, scrotal edema becomes extremely marked. Ascites may become so extensive that the resultant pressure on the stomach leads to anorexia or vomiting. Children may have diarrhea caused by intestinal edema and poor absorption by the edematous membrane. Because of poor nutrition, growth may stop. The child may become malnourished but yet appear deceptively obese because of the extensive edema (Fig. 46.13). When the ascites becomes even more extensive, children may have difficulty breathing as the abdominal fluid presses against the diaphragm, decreasing lung expansion. Parents report that children are irritable

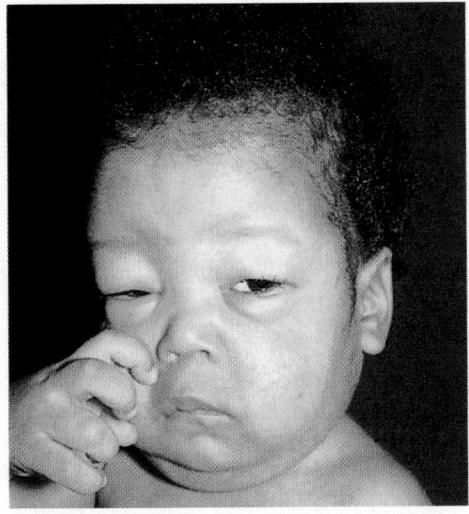

FIGURE 46.13 A 2-year-old with nephrotic syndrome. Note the extensive edema of the face and hand. (Zitelli, B. J. & Davis, H. W. [1997]. *Atlas of pediatric physical diagnosis* [3rd ed.]. St. Louis: Mosby-Year Book, Inc.)

and fussy, probably from the feeling of abdominal fullness and generalized edema. An increased risk for clotting can occur from the decreased intravascular fluid volume.

Laboratory studies will reveal marked proteinuria. A single test will show a 1^+ to 4^+ protein; a 24-hour total urine test will show up to 15 g protein (normally urine contains no protein). The protein loss with nephrotic syndrome is almost entirely albumin, differentiating it from the proteinuria of glomerulonephritis, in which protein loss tends to be nonspecific. Some children with nephrotic syndrome exhibit hematuria at the onset, but it is minimal in contrast to that seen with acute glomerulonephritis. The erythrocyte sedimentation rate (demonstrating the inflammation of the glomeruli membrane) is elevated. Features of acute glomerulonephritis and nephrotic syndrome are listed in Table 46.5. A renal biopsy may be done to determine whether there is scarring of the glomerular membrane.

Therapeutic Management

Therapy for the child with nephrotic syndrome is directed toward reducing the proteinuria and subsequently the edema with a course of corticosteroids, such as oral prednisone, and keeping the child free of infection while the immune system is suppressed. An initial dose of prednisone is given until diuresis without protein loss is accomplished; the dosage is then reduced for maintenance and continued for as long as 1 to 2 months.

Instruct parents to test the first urine specimen of the day for protein with a chemical reagent strip and keep an accurate chart showing the pattern of protein loss. Approximately once a week, they are usually asked to collect a 24-hour urine specimen so total protein loss can be measured.

After the initial 4 weeks, prednisone is generally given every other day rather than every day. Prednisone has the potential to halt growth and to suppress adrenal gland secretion. However, growth is apparently not delayed when the drug is given on alternate days and there is less alteration of adrenal steroid production (Karch, 2004). Parents may need to be assured that alternate-day therapy is best to keep them from changing the schedule to every day or giving twice the calculated dose by adding extra tablets on alternate days. To help parents remember to give medication on alternate days, have them choose either even or odd calendar days as the day of administration. Help them design a reminder chart. Prednisone tastes bitter, so parents may welcome suggestions as to how to disguise the taste, such as by mixing it with applesauce.

Be certain both the parents and the child are aware that prednisone causes a cushingoid appearance (i.e., "moon face," extra fat at the base of the neck, and increased body hair). Urge parents to plan ahead when getting refills so that the prednisone therapy is not stopped abruptly because they ran out of medication; an abrupt stop can lead to adrenal insufficiency.

Diuretics are not commonly used to reduce the edema because they tend to decrease blood volume, which is already decreased. This could lead to acute renal failure. Children who respond poorly to prednisone alone, however, may need diuretic therapy with a drug such as furosemide (Lasix). When children are taking furosemide for

TABLE 46.5

Comparison of Features of Acute Glomerulonephritis and Nephrotic Syndrome

Factor	Acute Glomerulonephritis	Nephrotic Syndrome
Cause	Immune reaction to group A beta-hemolytic streptococcal infection	Idiopathic; possibly a hypersensitivity reaction
Onset	Abrupt	Insidious
Hematuria	Profuse	Rare
Edema	Mild	Extreme
Hypertension	Marked	Mild
Hyperlipidemia	Rare or mild	Marked
Peak age frequency	5–10 yr	2–3 yr
Interventions	Limited activity; antihypertensives as needed; symptomatic therapy for congestive heart failure	Corticosteroid administration; cyclophosphamide administration; possibly a diuretic and potassium supplement
Diet	Normal for age	High-protein, low-sodium diet
Prevention	Prevention or thorough treatment of group A beta-hemolytic streptococcal infections	None known

extended periods, there is always a danger that too much potassium will be excreted, causing hypokalemia. Children on long-term diuretic therapy need frequent blood studies to determine that electrolyte levels, especially potassium, are adequate. They may need supplemental potassium and should eat foods high in potassium. IV albumin may be administered to temporarily correct hypoalbuminemia. As the serum albumin level rises, fluid shifts from subcutaneous spaces into the bloodstream. Children are then administered a rapidly acting diuretic to remove the extra fluid. It is important that the diuretic be administered after the albumin infusion or the child could develop a fluid overload and, subsequently, heart failure.

A course of cyclophosphamide (Cytoxan), because of its immunosuppressant action, may be effective in reducing symptoms or preventing further relapses of the disease in children who do not respond to corticosteroid therapy. It is important to ensure adequate fluid intake with cyclophosphamide to prevent bladder irritation and bleeding. Cyclophosphamide is also used in chemotherapy for malignancy (see Chapter 53). Be certain that parents are not misled into believing that their child has cancer because he or she is receiving a chemotherapeutic drug. Cyclosporine (Sandimmune) is another immunosuppressant that may be used.

The prognosis for children with nephrotic syndrome varies. Almost all children with MCNS respond initially to steroid therapy. Although they may have a relapse, they will then remain free of the disease. Those with FGS and MPGN types will have relapses at frequent or infrequent intervals over the next several years. Children who have frequent relapses have a relatively poor chance of ever being free of the disorder. Many develop renal failure later. Kidney transplantation may be necessary to sustain life. All children and families need emotional support while the disease runs a long-term course (Ruth et al., 2004).

 Checkpoint Question 4

What is an important nursing intervention for children with nephrotic syndrome?

a. Caution them not to eat salt, as salt irritates the bladder.
b. Encourage them to walk a mile daily for exercise.
c. Teach them to test their urine for proteinuria.
d. Teach them to take their temperature daily.

NURSING DIAGNOSES AND RELATED INTERVENTIONS

Nursing Diagnosis: Imbalanced nutrition, less than body requirements, related to poor appetite, restricted diet, and protein loss

Outcome Evaluation: Child follows normal growth curve on standard assessment scale.

Because children with nephrosis have poor appetites, maintaining them on restricted diets is difficult. A good protein intake is necessary to offset protein loss. A good potassium intake through consumption of fruits and fruit juices, particularly bananas, is necessary to maintain sufficient serum potassium levels, especially if the child is receiving a potassium-losing diuretic (Table 46.6). During acute phases of the disease, fluid or sodium may

TABLE 46.6

Foods High in Potassium

Food Group	Examples
Fruits	Bananas, peaches, prunes, raisins, oranges, and orange juice
Vegetables	Carrots, celery, lima beans, potatoes, collards, dandelion greens, spinach
Meat	Nuts, peanuts, red meat
Dairy products	Milk, whole or skim; low-sodium milk
Miscellaneous	Salt substitutes, chocolate and cocoa, bran

be temporarily restricted. If this is so, most children are happiest with many small glasses of fluid spaced throughout the day, rather than several large drinks. It helps to make a chart showing the amount of fluid the child is allowed each day. As fluid is given, color in a portion of the chart corresponding to the amount given. The child can tell from the uncolored portion how much more he or she is allowed that day. This is easier for toddlers and preschoolers (the age group usually affected by this disease) to understand rather than talking in terms of milliliters or even glassfuls.

Parents need to weigh children daily to detect fluid accumulation (use the same scale with the child in the same clothing at the same time of day), and they also must measure intake and output accurately. If the child is hospitalized, taking pulse rate and blood pressure every 4 hours will help detect hypovolemia from excessive fluid shifts to interstitial tissue.

Nursing Diagnosis: Risk for impaired skin integrity related to edema

Outcome Evaluation: Child's skin is intact, clean, and dry without erythema.

The edematous skin of children with nephrotic syndrome tends to break down easily, so they need frequent position changes while in bed. Check clothing to make certain that the elastic band at the waist of pajamas or other constricting parts is not tight. Soft gauze placed between skin surfaces, especially around the scrotum, tends to prevent skin irritation and breakdown. Edematous tissue does not heal well, so breaks in the skin easily become secondarily infected. The child who is not toilet-trained needs frequent diaper changes and thorough cleaning at each change to prevent skin breakdown in the diaper area.

Generally, children are more comfortable if they sleep with their head elevated in a semi-Fowler's position rather than the supine or prone position because this reduces periorbital edema. If children sleep in a head-flat position, edema can be so severe by morning that their eyes are swollen com-

pletely shut; their tongues are also swollen, so they cannot speak. At home, parents can provide a semi-Fowler's position by placing extra pillows on the child's bed or slipping a cardboard box under the head of the mattress to raise the end of the mattress.

Because medications are poorly absorbed from edematous skin areas, intramuscular (IM) injections should be kept to a minimum. Medication should be administered orally if possible (Box 46.6).

Nursing Diagnosis: Knowledge deficit related to chronic illness

Outcome Evaluation: Parents describe course and nature of nephrosis and their role in care of child at home.

Parents often need support to manage children at home. They need clear instructions about their responsibilities, including keeping their child free of infection, perhaps by limiting exposure to friends, and giving prednisone or oral diuretics and a potassium supplement. Review medication instructions with parents and have them repeat the instructions. Make certain they understand where and when they are to return for a follow-up visit and make certain they have a telephone number to call if they have questions or concerns about their child's care or health.

What if... you needed to give an IM injection to Carol, who has extensive dependent edema from nephrotic syndrome? Would it be best to give it in a thigh or deltoid muscle, and why?

Henoch-Schönlein Syndrome Nephritis

Henoch-Schönlein purpura is discussed in Chapter 44. Approximately one quarter of the children who develop this type of purpura develop renal disease as a secondary complication. The renal involvement becomes apparent within a few days after the manifestations of purpuric symptoms. Children may show only urinary abnormalities such as proteinuria or may have a rapidly progressing glomerulonephritis. Most children recover completely. Only a few develop chronic symptoms, but in those who do, long-term kidney disease can develop (Gusic, 2003).

Systemic Lupus Erythematosus

SLE is an autoimmune disease in which autoantibodies and antigens cause deposits of complement on the kidney glomerulus (see Chapter 14). Because of this, some children with SLE develop symptoms of acute or chronic glomerulonephritis, the ultimate cause of death in many adults with SLE (Cohen, 2003). Therapy with corticosteroids or cytotoxic agents may be effective. If kidney transplantation is required, the same damage rarely occurs in the transplanted kidney.

BOX 46.6: Focus on Nursing Care Planning

A Multidisciplinary Care Map for A Child with Nephrotic Syndrome

●

Carol is a 4-year-old girl admitted to the hospital with nephrotic syndrome. She has marked ascites and edema. "I kept asking everyone how she could be gaining so much weight, yet she doesn't eat anything," her grandmother tells you. "My daughter said this happened because Carol drank part of a beer I left on the coffee table. I didn't give her the beer; she just picked it up and drank it. Do you think that's what caused this?"

Family Assessment
Child lives with grandparents in a trailer park while mother is incarcerated on a drug charge. Grandparents are both retired. Grandfather rates finances as, "Okay. I saved some money and we both get social security."

Client Assessment
Child began "gaining weight" and becoming irritable a week ago. Yesterday, her face appeared "very puffy." Appetite has declined sharply in last two weeks. States she's "always full." Marked dependent edema (4⁺ over tibia) present. Urine tested and found to be 4⁺ for protein.

Nursing Diagnosis
Excess fluid volume related to decreased kidney function and fluid accumulation

Outcome Criteria
Child's edema decreases; urine proteinuria is less than 2⁺.

Team Member Responsible	Assessment	Intervention	Rationale	Expected Outcome
Activities of Daily Living				
Nurse	Assess whether child is able to carry out routine activities with ascites or edema.	Review with grandparents advantage of allowing child to continue usual activities.	Child's mobility may interfere with physical tasks; other children may make fun of her appearance at nursery school.	Child and grandparents state that child can continue with usual activities.
Consultations				
Physician	Assess whether grandparents have legal guardianship for child and can give permission for health care.	Contact renal service and suggest child be admitted to service for evaluation.	Nephrotic syndrome is a chronic disorder that requires conscientious, specialized health supervision.	Grandparents state they have or will obtain legal guardianship; renal service personnel meet with child and grandparents for consultation.
Procedures/Medications				
Nurse	Assess if child has experience with oral medication.	Administer oral prednisone as prescribed.	Prednisone, a corticosteroid, reduces immune response and proteinuria.	Child accepts oral prednisone and helps make out reminder sheet.

(continued)

Team Member Responsible	Assessment	Intervention	Rationale	Expected Outcome
Procedures/Medications				
Nurse	Assess if grandparents have experience with dipstick urine testing and 24-hour urine collection.	Observe grandparents' technique for dipstick urine testing and urine collection and recording results.	Testing for protein in urine will reveal extent of protein loss.	Grandparents state they feel able to test and collect urine conscientiously and record results in diary.
Nutrition				
Nurse/ nutritionist	Assess child's typical food intake for last 24 hours.	Suggest grandmother monitor child's intake to be certain it includes all food groups daily.	Ascites crowds stomach, so it can give a feeling of fullness and cause undernutrition.	Child describes yesterday's intake; grandmother voices intent to supervise child's intake to be certain it is nutritious.
Patient/Family Education				
Nurse	Assess grandparents' knowledge about kidney function and kidney disease.	Teach grandparents about kidney function and disease process as needed.	Understanding disease process can help grandparents to better carry out therapy.	Grandparents state they understand why edema has occurred and describe action of medicine to reverse this.
Psychosocial/Spiritual/Emotional Needs				
Nurse	Assess whether grandparents are having child rearing concerns.	Review natural inquisitiveness of preschool children, which can lead them into unsafe areas.	Grandparent states she didn't supervise child well so child drank beer off coffee table.	Grandparent states that although caring for a preschooler is difficult, she feels adequate to give care.
Discharge Planning				
Nurse	Assess if grandparents have transportation to return for follow-up appointment.	Schedule return appointment for 1 week at kidney clinic.	As nephrotic syndrome is a long-term disorder, child will need continued follow-up for years to come.	Grandparents state they are aware of long-term nature of disorder and will keep follow-up appointments.

Hemolytic-Uremic Syndrome

With hemolytic-uremic syndrome, the lining of glomerular arterioles becomes inflamed, swollen, and occluded with particles of platelets and fibrin. Red blood cells and platelets are damaged as they flow through the partially occluded blood vessels. As the damaged cells reach the spleen, they are destroyed by the spleen and removed from circulation. This leads to hemolytic anemia.

Ninety percent of children who develop this syndrome have recently experienced an *E. coli* GI infection. The most likely source of the *E. coli* is undercooked hamburger, because *E. coli* is found in the intestine of beef cattle. It occurs more frequently in infants who have their initial *E. coli* infection treated with an antibiotic (Brunner, Bianchetti, & Neuhaus, 2004). The syndrome occurs during the summer in children 6 months to 4 years of age.

Assessment

Children usually develop only a transient diarrhea, although this can progress to severe fluid loss and bowel wall necrosis. Fever may be so elevated that the child experiences stupor and hallucinations. Oliguria accompanied by proteinuria, hematuria, and urinary casts in urine follows. Extensive edema may occur. The oliguria will lead to increased serum creatinine and BUN. Children appear pale from the anemia; easy bruising or petechiae may be present from *thrombocytopenia* (reduced platelet level). Laboratory studies will show fibrin split products in the serum as the fibrin deposits in glomerular vessels are degraded. Thrombocytopenia is present because platelets are damaged by the irregular blood vessels. An increased reticulocyte count indicates that red blood cells are rapidly being replaced.

Therapeutic Management

The child needs supportive therapy to maintain kidney and heart function. The extreme oliguria can be treated with peritoneal dialysis; anemia can be corrected by careful transfusion of packed red cells. Peritoneal dialysis can be extremely frightening to parents and the child because it involves penetration of the child's abdomen. Be certain they understand that the actual dialysis procedure is not painful and they can hold the child during it.

Ensure that parents understand the importance of follow-up care and have an appointment for this. Help them begin to view the child as well again so they do not continue to shelter him or her unnecessarily but allow for normal growth and development.

Despite the extent of the illness, most infants with hemolytic-uremic syndrome recover completely. Some children, however, die of the acute illness or continue to have chronic renal involvement.

Acute Renal Failure

Renal failure occurs in either an acute or chronic form. The acute form most often occurs because of a sudden body insult, such as severe dehydration. The chronic form results from extensive kidney disease, such as hemolytic-uremic syndrome or glomerulonephritis (Munnariz, Kramer, & Carpinito, 2004).

Other causes of acute renal failure include prolonged anesthesia, hemorrhage, shock, severe diarrhea, or sudden traumatic injury. It also can occur in a child who is placed on cardiopulmonary bypass while undergoing heart surgery, who receives common antibiotics (aminoglycosides, penicillin, cephalosporins, and sulfonamides), who swallows a poison such as arsenic (found in rat poison), or who is exposed to industrial wastes such as mercury. The active course of acute glomerulonephritis may result in renal failure. All of these conditions appear to lead to renal ischemia, which ultimately leads to acute renal failure.

Assessment

One of the first symptoms noted with acute renal failure is *oliguria,* a urine output of less than 1 mL/kg of the child's body weight/hour. An indwelling urinary catheter may be inserted to rule out the possibility that urinary retention in the bladder rather than kidney dysfunction is causing the oliguria.

Azotemia (accumulation of nitrogen waste in the bloodstream) will occur because of the oliguria. *Uremia* (extra accumulation of nitrogen wastes in the blood, with additional toxic symptoms such as cerebral irritation) also may occur. The BUN rises progressively as renal insufficiency continues and the breakdown products of protein cannot be excreted. A level greater than 80 to 100 mg/100 mL is toxic and needs correction, usually by dialysis. Urine creatinine is another measure that can be used as an indicator of function, because it is normally excreted at a uniform rate. A rate of less than 10 mg/100 mL indicates severe renal failure. As the kidneys become unable to dilute or concentrate urine, the specific gravity of urine often becomes "fixed" at 1.010.

Hyperkalemia (elevated potassium level) may occur if potassium cannot be excreted. Hyperkalemia is manifested by a weak, irregular pulse, abdominal cramps, lowered blood pressure, and muscle weakness. Acidosis will follow shortly with acute renal failure from the inability of H^+ ions to be excreted. As total output decreases, phosphorus levels will rise in the bloodstream. A high serum phosphorus level leads to a low calcium serum level (recall that phosphorus and calcium have an inverse proportional relationship). Severe hypocalcemia can lead to muscle twitching and seizures (*tetany*); chronic hypocalcemia can lead to withdrawal of calcium from bones (*osteodystrophy*).

An IVP or radioactive uptake scan may be ordered to substantiate the lack of kidney function. Parents and children need support for this type of study, because the results may be disappointing and so different from what they hoped they would be.

Therapeutic Management

Because acute renal failure is a reaction to body stress caused by acute disease or insult, attempts to treat it focus on supporting the child's body systems while correcting the underlying condition. If the child is dehydrated (as with diarrhea or hemorrhage), IV fluid is needed to replace plasma volume. Administer such fluid slowly enough to avoid heart failure; extra fluid cannot be removed by the kidneys because they are not functioning. The fluid should not contain potassium until it is established that kidney function is adequate; buildup of potassium may otherwise cause heart block. Potassium levels greater than 6 mEq/L are corrected by the IV administration of calcium gluconate (as the glucose moves into cells, it carries potassium with it), by the oral administration of a cation exchange resin such as Kayexalate, or by dialysis. Administering sodium bicarbonate may cause a shift of potassium from the bloodstream into cells, temporarily reducing the circulating potassium level. Administration of a combination of IV glucose and insulin may also be effective (insulin helps glucose move into cells).

A diuretic such as furosemide (Lasix) may be ordered in an attempt to increase urine production. Diet should be low in protein, potassium, and sodium and high in carbohydrate to supply enough calories for metabolism yet limit urea production and control serum potassium levels. Fluid intake may be limited to prevent heart failure due to accumulating fluid that cannot be excreted. Weigh children daily (same scale, same clothing, same time of day) and maintain accurate intake and output recordings to evaluate fluid status. If children are so ill that they cannot eat, total parenteral nutrition may be used. Regulate amounts carefully to prevent fluid overload (see Chapter 36 for administration techniques).

When recovery from acute renal failure begins, children generally have a degree of diuresis as the extra fluid accumulated by the body is cleared. The increase in urine must be noted, because children may need additional fluid intake at this point to prevent hypovolemia, which could lead once more to renal failure. Parents usually remain anxious for an extended period after an episode of acute renal failure because they fear that the restoration of kidney function is only temporary. Reassure them that urine output is remaining at a normal level. This helps them to relax and interact effectively with their child.

Chronic Renal Failure

Chronic renal failure results from developmental abnormalities, when acute failure becomes long term, or when chronic kidney disease has caused extensive nephron destruction (Munnariz, Kramer, & Carpinito, 2004). The nephrons that are not destroyed by long-term disease appear to function normally; they simply are inadequate in number to sustain kidney function. Glomeruli can adjust so that kidney functions continue normally until 50% of nephrons are destroyed. After this point, kidney function diminishes by degrees until the child develops end-stage kidney disease, where the kidneys cannot maintain normal function.

Assessment

With loss of nephron function, kidneys cannot concentrate urine. This results in polyuria, possibly manifested as enuresis. The few functioning nephrons present cannot reabsorb enough sodium to maintain a functioning level of body fluid, so dehydration occurs. As additional nephrons are lost, oliguria and anuria occur. Inability to excrete H^+ ions leads to acidosis. Hypocalcemia and hyperphosphatemia occur from the kidney's inability to excrete phosphate. Osteodystrophy occurs as calcium is withdrawn from bones to compensate. Kidneys are responsible for synthesizing vitamin D to its active form. With poor kidney function, vitamin D cannot be used. Without this, calcium cannot be absorbed from the GI tract and deposited in bones. Bones become so calcium depleted that growth halts and the bones lose strength (renal rickets).

Erythropoietin, formed by the kidneys, stimulates red cell production. With decreased erythropoietin production, anemia develops. Pruritus may be present from skin irritation due to excretion of nitrogenous wastes in sweat from high levels of BUN and serum creatinine. These changes are summarized in Figure 46.14.

Therapeutic Management

Children with chronic renal failure are generally placed on a low-protein, low-phosphorus, low-potassium diet to prevent rapid urea and phosphate buildup. Children may take aluminum hydroxide gel with meals to bind phosphorus in the intestines and prevent absorption. Milk usually is not given because it is high in sodium, potassium, and phosphate—electrolytes children may have difficulty clearing. Meat is restricted and even beans are high enough in protein to be eliminated from the diet. This can be difficult for parents and children to understand because they are taught that meats are high in protein but vegetables are not. Letting children have some choice about what foods they eat each day helps to promote adjustment to this restricted diet. Whoever prepares meals needs good instructions on selecting low-protein foods. Low-electrolyte, low-protein formulas are commercially available for infants with renal failure.

Daily fluid intake may need to be restricted, although restriction should be as minimal as possible or it will present an area of tremendous conflict between the child and parents. Many children need sodium intake restricted, and others need a normal sodium intake (but no excessively salty foods such as lunch meats, potato chips, or pretzels). Other children may actually need additional salt because, due to poor tubular reabsorption, they dump sodium in urine. Low-sodium formulas such as Lonalac are recommended for children with heart failure who need a low-sodium intake. Use them cautiously in children with renal insufficiency, because their high potassium content can lead to toxic potassium blood levels. Diuretics may be ordered to help children regulate sodium and fluid levels and prevent edema.

As renal failure becomes prolonged, the child may need supplemental calcium to prevent muscle cramping, rickets, tetany, or seizures. As hypertension becomes more and more acute from the accumulating blood volume, a daily antihypertensive drug may be prescribed. A blood transfusion may be needed to correct anemia, but it must be given cautiously so volume overload does not occur. Recombinant human erythropoietin may be prescribed to stimulate red blood cell formation. Effective excretion of urea can be accomplished by dialysis or by replacing the nonfunctioning kidneys with kidney transplantation. Growth hormone may increase height in some children (Vimalachandra et al., 2005).

NURSING DIAGNOSES AND RELATED INTERVENTIONS

Nursing Diagnosis: Risk for interrupted family processes related to chronically ill family member

Outcome Evaluation: Family members express feelings about illness to each other and to nurses; participate in care of ill member.

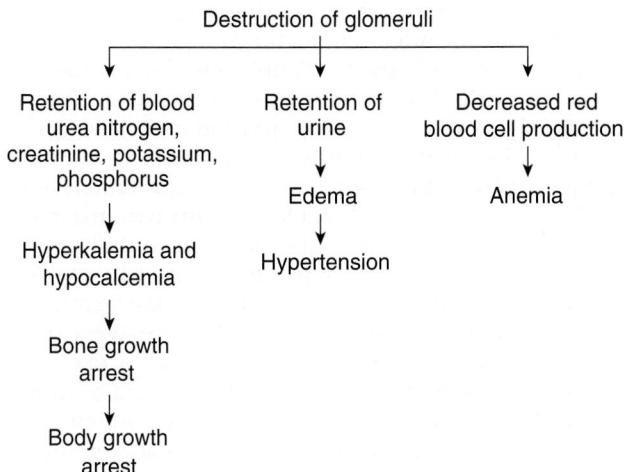

FIGURE 46.14 Pathology of chronic renal failure.

Children with renal failure grow poorly because of the alteration in calcium metabolism. Their height begins to fall below normal. It is easy for them to become depressed because of chronic fatigue and an unappetizing diet. If children are taking corticosteroids or other immunosuppressive drugs because of glomerulonephritis, they may be angry or disheartened about their change in appearance. Help them stay as active as possible by doing age-appropriate activities (Box 46.7).

Caring for a child with chronic renal disease is not only time-consuming but also financially and socially devastating for parents. Parents caring for such children at home need opportunities at periodic health assessments to voice their frustrations, fears, and anxieties. They need time to do those things important to them as individuals, whether taking a weekend trip or attending an evening show or program. Ask parents at clinic or follow-up visits, "Do you ever get out of the house or have the opportunity to do anything for yourself?" "What can we do for *you?*" Help of this kind ultimately improves children's care, because it improves the lives and mental attitudes of those around them.

KIDNEY TRANSPLANTATION

The ultimate possibility for prolonging the life of children with renal failure is kidney transplantation. With complete renal failure, children who have extensive hypertension may have their damaged kidneys removed and may be placed on hemodialysis or CAPD to await kidney transplantation. Kidney removal this way is an important step for parents and the child. Although parents realize that their child's kidneys are no longer functioning, this step removes all hope that a miracle might happen and make them function once more. Parents may ask whether it is possible to leave one of the child's kidneys, because only one kidney will be transplanted (this is not recommended, because the hypertension would continue). Parents need a thorough explanation of why hypertension is destructive (i.e., it could lead to cerebrovascular accident or coronary artery disease). They must understand that renal biopsy shows that, short of a miracle, their child's kidneys will not function again, so that removal of them is not a loss but only recognition of a loss.

Preoperative Care

Kidney transplantation is most effective (the kidney is less likely to be rejected) if the kidney is taken from a living twin or sibling. Rejection occurs at a higher incidence if a kidney comes from a cadaver or recently deceased child. If a relative's tissue-compatible kidney is used, the success rate is as high as 90% (Benfield, 2003). Most people consider that children should be of legal age to give consent to supply a kidney for transplantation, so few children have a sibling who is eligible to donate such a kidney. Tissue studies done to determine the best donor (matched for human leukocyte antigens [HLA]) may show that the person in a family most willing to donate a kidney is not the best person in terms of tissue compatibility. This can cause bitterness and hopelessness in the family, compounding an already stressed family life. Many children anticipate that the characteristics of the donor will be transmitted to them by the kidney, so they are reluctant to accept the kidney of a family member with a character trait they do not like (perhaps a bad temper). They need to be assured that transplanted organs do not carry this type of problem with them. Adult-sized kidneys may be transplanted into children, although if the child weighs less than 10 kg, this large a kidney may lead to hypertension, excessive diuresis, and abdominal complications because of the lack of space. Transplanted kidneys are placed in the abdomen, not the usual kidney space.

Tests that kidney donors can expect to have preoperatively include HLA typing, electrolyte blood analysis, complete blood count, bleeding time, urinalysis and urine culture, 24-hour urine sample for protein, a renal arteriogram, and IV pyelography. People who cannot donate a kidney include those with multiple bilateral small renal arteries, bilateral renal disease, renal infection, advanced medical illness, severe obesity, or hypertension. Although kidney removal can be done by laparoscopy, donors must understand that removal of a kidney involves major surgery. They will have urine samples collected after surgery to assess that their remaining kidney is capable of maintaining full function and they are still in good health.

Before surgery, children who are to receive a transplant may be dialyzed to clear their body of excessive potassium and fluid. If the donated kidney will be from a relative, there is adequate time for thorough preoperative preparation. If the donor kidney is from a cadaver, the announcement of surgery will be sudden and time for preoperative instruction and procedures may be limited.

BOX 46.7 FOCUS ON . . .

EVIDENCE-BASED PRACTICE

Are Young Children With Nephrotic Syndrome Able to Do Self-Care?

For this study, a nurse researcher interviewed 66 school-age children who had been hospitalized at least once for nephrotic syndrome at a local university hospital. Results showed that 83% of the 6- to 8-year-olds, 95% of 9- and 10-year-olds, and all of the 11- and 12-year-olds reported high levels of self-care. A total of 60 of the 66 children participated in their self-care at a high level.

This is an interesting study not only because it focuses on cultural influences of self-care, but also because it suggests that many children, although they have a chronic illness, do not see themselves as fulfilling a "sick role." Nursing responsibility for chronically ill children should include introducing new and challenging activities in nursing care, as children see themselves as well rather than ill.

Source: Zhimin, L. (2003). Self-care in Chinese school-age children with nephrotic syndrome. *MCN: The American Journal of Maternal/Child Nursing, 28*(2), 81–85.

Children who receive pretransplantation blood transfusions have an improved chance of transplant success. Most children, therefore, receive at least five blood transfusions while awaiting surgery. The mechanisms by which this operates are unclear, but transfusion-induced production of antibodies or immune complexes appears to mediate graft survival (Munnariz, Kramer, & Carpinito, 2004).

Human Leukocyte Antigen (HLA) Typing

The presence of antigens on erythrocytes has been documented for years. Antigens serve as the basis for blood transfusion typing and reactions. HLA is a group of antigens found on the surfaces of all cells with a nucleus, including blood components such as leukocytes and platelets. The name is derived from the fact that they were first identified on white blood cells. Such antigens are inherited from both parents and are specific for each individual. They denote tissue type or determine which tissue the immune system identifies as foreign tissue. They are carried on the short arm of chromosome 6 in each cell.

Such antigens also serve as the basis for paternity typing. They may cause reactions to blood product transfusions and bone marrow and organ transplants. When two people have like HLA antigens, they are said to be *histocompatible.* Identical twins have complete histocompatibility and family members have partial histocompatibility; any two people can have histocompatibility at least on one antigen site.

Children who are awaiting kidney transplantation are tissue typed, and this information is circulated to major medical centers. When a kidney is available for transplantation, the child's tissue type is compared with the donor kidney. For tissue typing, lymphocytes from both a donor and recipient are grown together in a culture medium and then examined for like characteristics.

Postoperative Care

After renal transplantation, children are cared for in an environment that is as sterile as possible. They are placed on immunosuppressive therapy (cyclosporine, azathioprine [Imuran], and methylprednisolone [Solu-Medrol]) to reduce the possibility of kidney rejection. Antilymphocyte globulin and antithymocyte globulin may be administered to aid immunosuppression.

Children need supportive care postoperatively. Although some transplanted kidneys begin to function immediately, hemodialysis may be continued until the implanted kidney can fully function after the insult of transplantation. Be prepared to help a child and parents through a "honeymoon" period after the transplantation.

Help children understand that acceptance or rejection of a kidney depends on a multitude of factors—the condition of renal veins and arteries, the transplanted kidney, or antigen–antibody formation—but none of these factors is related to whether the child is good or bad or deserves or does not deserve to have the transplantation work (Box 46.8).

Children with end-stage renal disease usually fail to grow despite treatment. Although the rate of growth is improved after kidney transplantation, they will probably

---

BOX 46.8 FOCUS ON . . .

COMMUNICATION

Carol's grandmother tells you Carol has "changed completely" since she became ill.

Less Effective Communication

Nurse: Mrs. Hendricks, in what way has Carol changed?

Mrs. Hendricks: She used to whine all the time, and constantly ask for things. Now she entertains herself. It's like heaven.

Nurse: That sounds wonderful. Let's review her medicine routine to be sure that's going well.

Mrs. Hendricks: That's another thing she does perfectly: never fusses a bit about anything she has to take.

More Effective Communication

Nurse: Mrs. Hendricks, in what way has Carol changed?

Mrs. Hendricks: She used to whine all the time, and constantly ask for things. Now she entertains herself. It's like heaven.

Nurse: Do you think she's acting a little too perfect?

Mrs. Hendricks: Well, it does seem a bit strange for her.

Nurse: Do you think she could be worrying that if she misbehaves, her medicine won't work?

Mrs. Hendricks: I never thought of that. I would feel better if she started to act like her old self.

What the grandmother above is describing is a "honeymoon" period that children may pass through after being told their kidneys are important for life. Parents often need help seeing this for what it is so they can begin to reassure children that behaving perfectly will not influence the outcome of their illness and because they loved them as they were, they will continue to love them regardless.

---

never reach full height. Part of this growth restriction is related to the need for corticosteroid maintenance therapy to continue immunosuppression.

Transplant Rejection

Acute transplant rejection, if it occurs, usually occurs within the first 3 months after transplantation. Children begin to develop fever, proteinuria, oliguria, weight gain, hypertension, and tenderness over the kidney. Serum creatinine and BUN levels will rise. Increasing the dose of immunosuppressants may be effective in relieving this type of rejection.

Rejection may also be *chronic,* in which the transplanted kidney gradually loses function after the first 6 months. Hypertension and anemia result. A biopsy will show vascular changes such as narrowing of arterial lumens and interstitial changes such as fibrosis and tubular atrophy. This type of rejection is difficult to halt, although it may be such a slow, steady process that it is 2 or 3 years before the kidney fails. If a kidney is rejected, it is removed and a child is returned to a program of hemodialysis. Because one kidney was rejected does not mean that a second transplant will be rejected also. Unfortunately, however, the number of kidneys available for transplantation is limited, so kidney rejection becomes an ominous sign for the child's long-term survival.

Malignant disease is more common in transplantation recipients than in the normal population, probably because of the long-term immunosuppression (Agraharkar et al., 2004). The original disease for which the child underwent transplantation may recur in the transplanted kidney. This is most apt to occur in glomerulonephritis. During adolescence, typically an age of poor adherence to medication regimens, kidney recipients need to be followed closely to be certain they are taking their immunosuppressive therapy. Parents cannot help but overprotect the child; they worry that a rough-housing session with a sibling or playing a game such as baseball may injure the transplanted kidney. The child may be afraid to engage in any activity for the same reason unless you help a family fully adjust to this major life change.

Checkpoint Question 5

How would you best explain kidney transplantation to a child?

a. A new kidney will be placed in your abdomen.
b. The new kidney will be placed in your bladder.
c. You must never eat eggs after a kidney transplant.
d. Your urine will be brown for the rest of your life.

Key Points

Many urinary tract disorders, such as polycystic kidneys, urethral obstruction, and bladder exstrophy, are evident on a fetal sonogram. Early identification allows therapy to begin in utero or immediately at birth.

Many urinary tract disorders, such as polycystic kidneys or chronic renal failure, are long-term conditions requiring years of therapy. Be certain that parents are well informed about their child's condition so they can continue to participate in planning their child's care.

Congenital structural abnormalities of the urinary tract include patent urachus, exstrophy of the bladder, hypospadias, and epispadias. Surgical correction is required for all of these.

UTI tends to occur more often in girls than boys. "Honeymoon cystitis" refers to a UTI occurring with first-time sexual intercourse.

Vesicoureteral reflux is the backflow of urine into ureters with voiding. It occurs because the valve that guards the entrance to the ureters is lax or

misplaced. Surgical correction may be necessary to prevent repeated UTI.

Renal dysfunction can occur for structural reasons such as kidney agenesis, polycystic kidney, and renal hypoplasia. Acute poststreptococcal glomerulonephritis is inflammation of the glomeruli after a streptococcal infection. It is characterized by an acute episode of hematuria and proteinuria.

Diminished kidney function leads to both fluid and electrolyte imbalances. Creative techniques are necessary to encourage children to continue to ingest a restricted-protein diet.

Nephrotic syndrome is an immunologic process that results in altered glomerular permeability. Nursing diagnoses associated with this condition may include imbalanced nutrition, risk for impaired skin integrity, and deficient knowledge.

Renal failure can be acute or chronic. Peritoneal dialysis or hemodialysis may be used to remove body wastes until kidney function can be restored.

Kidney transplantation may be an option for some children with kidney disorders. This is extensive surgery and requires the child to remain on immunosuppressive therapy to counteract transplant rejection.

Critical Thinking Exercises

1. Carol is the preschooler with nephrotic syndrome whom you met at the beginning of the chapter. Her grandmother asked you whether a sip of beer could have caused her kidney disease. What would you tell her is the cause of nephrosis? What discharge instructions can you anticipate you will need to review with Carol's grandmother?

2. Carol's grandmother is afraid Carol will need a kidney transplant. Carol tells you she hopes she has been good enough to deserve being chosen for a transplant. What would you want to teach this family about the transplantation selection process?

3. Suppose a 6-year-old girl is receiving continuous ambulatory peritoneal dialysis. She wants to go to her church camp this summer. Her parents ask you whether this would be a good experience for her. What factors would you want to know about the camp? About the child? About her procedure?

4. Examine the National Health Goals related to renal disorders and children. Most government-sponsored money for nursing research is allotted based on these goals. What would be a possible research topic to explore pertinent to these goals that would be applicable to Carol's family and also advance evidence-based practice?

References

Agraharkar, M. L., et al. (2004). Risk of malignancy with long-term immunosuppression in renal transplant recipients. *Kidney International, 66*(1), 383–389.

Bartkowski, D. P. (2003). Current diagnosis and management of urinary tract infections in infants and children. *Comprehensive Therapy, 29*(2/3), 102–107.

Benfield, M. R. (2003). Current status of kidney transplant: update 2003. *Pediatric Clinics of North America, 50*(6), 1301–1334.

Brunner, K., Bianchetti, M. G., & Neuhaus, T. J. (2004). Recovery of renal function after long-term dialysis in hemolytic uremic syndrome. *Pediatric Nephrology, 19*(2), 229–231.

Cohen, P. L. (2003). Systemic autoimmunity. In W. E. Paul, *Fundamental immunology* (5th ed.). Philadelphia: Lippincott Williams & Wilkins.

De, E. (2004). Pediatric urology. In S. B. Bauer (Ed.), *Handbook of urology: diagnosis & therapy* (3rd ed.). Philadelphia: Lippincott Williams & Wilkins.

Department of Health & Human Services. (2000). *Healthy people 2010.* Washington, DC: DHHS.

Filler, G., et al. (2003). Is there really an increase in non-minimal change nephrotic syndrome in children? *American Journal of Kidney Diseases, 42*(6), 1107–1113.

Fischbach, F. T. (2004). *Manual of laboratory and diagnostic tests* (7th ed.). Philadelphia: Lippincott Williams & Wilkins.

Grady, R. W., & Mitchell, M. E. (2004). Surgeon's corner. Complete primary repair of exstrophy. *Contemporary Urology, 16*(9), 12–17.

Gross, K. (2003). The illuminator: voiding cystourethrogram. *Images, 22*(3), 7.

Gusic, B. R. (2003). Henoch-Schönlein purpura. In M. W. Schwartz (Ed.), *5-minute pediatric consult* (3rd ed.). Philadelphia: Lippincott Williams & Wilkins.

Hoberman, A., et al. (2003). Imaging studies after a first febrile urinary tract infection in young children. *New England Journal of Medicine, 348*(3), 195–202.

Hyde, C., & Schwartz, R. K. (2004). Imaging of the genitourinary tract. In M. B. Siroky, R. D. Oates, & R. K. Babavan (Eds.), *Handbook of urology: diagnosis & therapy* (3rd ed.). Philadelphia: Lippincott Williams & Wilkins.

Iitaka, K., et al. (2004). Two cases of congenital nephrotic syndrome. *Clinical & Experimental Nephrology, 8*(2), 146–149.

Karch, A. M. (2004). *Lippincott's nursing drug guide.* Philadelphia: Lippincott Williams & Wilkins.

Leonard, M. B. (2003) Polycystic kidney disease. In M. W. Schwartz (Ed.), *5-minute pediatric consult* (3rd ed.). Philadelphia: Lippincott Williams & Wilkins.

Madden, S. J., et al. (2003). Cognitive and psychosocial outcome of infants dialysed in infancy. *Child: Care, Health and Development, 29*(1), 55–61.

Metcalfe, P. D., & Schwarz, R. D. (2004). Bladder exstrophy: neonatal care and surgical approaches. *Journal of Wound, Ostomy and Continence Nursing, 31*(5), 284–292.

Meyers, K. E. C. (2003). Glomerulonephritis. In M. W. Schwartz (Ed.), *5-minute pediatric consult* (3rd ed.). Philadelphia: Lippincott Williams & Wilkins.

Munnariz, R. M., Kramer, A., & Carpinito, G. (2004). Renal failure, dialysis, and renal transplantation. In S. B. Bauer (Ed.), *Handbook of urology: diagnosis & therapy* (3rd ed.). Philadelphia: Lippincott Williams & Wilkins.

Munson, B. L. (2004). Myths & facts about polycystic kidney disease. *Nursing, 34*(3), 75.

Nield, L. S., & Kamat, D. (2004). Enuresis: how to evaluate and treat. *Clinical Pediatrics, 43*(5), 409–415.

O'Connell, L. M., & Siroky, M. B. (2004). The abnormal urinalysis. In M. B. Siroky, R. D. Oates, & R. K. Babavan (Eds.), *Handbook of urology: diagnosis & therapy* (3rd ed.). Philadelphia: Lippincott Williams & Wilkins.

Ruth, E. M., et al. (2004). Health-related quality of life and psychosocial adjustment in steroid-sensitive nephrotic syndrome. *Journal of Pediatrics, 145*(6), 778–783.

Schweon, S., & Novatnack, E. (2003). Don't underestimate group A strep. *RN, 66*(8), 28–33.

Shaw, K. N. (2003). Urinary tract infection. In M. W. Schwartz (Ed.), *5-minute pediatric consult* (3rd ed.). Philadelphia: Lippincott Williams & Wilkins.

Small, M. J., & Copel, J. A. (2004). Ultrasound clinics. Practical guidelines for diagnosing and treating fetal hydronephrosis. *Contemporary OB/GYN, 49*(2), 59–60.

Stokowski, L. A. (2004). Hypospadias in the neonate. *Advances in Neonatal Care, 4*(4), 206–215.

Vimalachandra, D., et al. (2005). Growth hormone for children with chronic renal failure. *The Cochrane Library (Oxford) (1)* (CD003264).

Wen, C., Marquez, D. J., & Cohen, A. J. (2004). Radiological case of the month: Eagle Barrett Syndrome (also known as prune-belly syndrome ([PBS]) in an adult). *Applied Radiology, 33*(4), 34–36.

Wheeler, D. M., et al. (2005). Interventions for primary vesicoureteric reflux. *The Cochrane Library (Oxford) (1)* (CD001532).

Wu, H. Y. (2003). Vesicoureteral reflux. In M. W. Schwartz (Ed.), *5-minute pediatric consult* (3rd ed.). Philadelphia: Lippincott Williams & Wilkins.

Wright, E. (2004). Assessment and management of the child requiring chronic haemodialysis. *Paediatric Nursing, 16*(7), 37–42.

Zeman, P. A., Siroky, M. B., & Babayan, R. K. (2004). Lower urinary tract symptoms. In S. B. Bauer (Ed.), *Handbook of urology: diagnosis & therapy* (3rd ed.). Philadelphia: Lippincott Williams & Wilkins.

Zhimin, L. (2003). Self-care in Chinese school-age children with nephritic syndrome. *MCN: The American Journal of Maternal/Child Nursing, 28*(2), 81–85.

Suggested Readings

Chesney, R. (2004). The changing face of childhood nephritic syndrome. *Kidney International, 66*(3), 1294–1302.

Erickson, D. V., & Ray, L. D. (2004). Children with chronic continence problems: the challenges for families. *Journal of Wound, Ostomy and Continence Nursing, 31*(4), 215–222.

Glazener, C. M. A., & Evans, J. H. C. (2005). Simple behavioral and physical interventions for nocturnal enuresis in children. *The Cochrane Library (Oxford) (1)* (CD003637).

Landgraf, J. M., et al. (2004). Coping, commitment, and attitude: quantifying the everyday burden of enuresis on children and their families. *Pediatrics, 113*(2), 334–344.

Lux, C., & Waldrop, J. B. (2004). Advisor forum. Combating microbial resistance in pediatric UTI patients. *Clinical Advisor, 7*(9), 55–59.

Mercy, N., & Brady-Fryer, B. (2004). Bladder exstrophy: a challenge for nursing care. *Journal of Wound, Ostomy and Continence Nursing, 31*(5), 293–298.

Miller, D., et al. (2004). Challenges for nephrology nurses in the management of children with chronic kidney disease. *Nephrology Nursing Journal, 31*(3), 287–296.

Myers, P. (2003). Professional issues. Seeing visions become realities at kidney camp. *Nephrology Nursing Journal, 30*(4), 472–473.

Zamir, G., et al. (2004). Urinary tract infection: is there a need for routine renal ultrasonography? *Archives of Disease in Childhood, 89*(5), 466–468.

Zickler, C. F., & Richardson, V. (2004). Achieving continence in children with neurogenic bowel and bladder. *Journal of Pediatric Health Care, 18*(6), 276–283.

Nursing Care of the Child With a Reproductive Disorder

Key Terms

amenorrhea
anovulatory
cryptorchidism
dysmenorrhea
endometriosis
fibrocystic breast disease
gynecomastia
hermaphrodite
hydrocele
menorrhagia
metrorrhagia
mittelschmerz
orchiectomy
orchiopexy
pelvic inflammatory disease
premenstrual dysphoric
   disorder
pseudohermaphrodite
sexually transmitted infection
   (STI)
toxic shock syndrome
varicocele
vulvovaginitis

Objectives

After mastering the contents of this chapter, you should be able to:

1. Describe common reproductive disorders in children.
2. Assess a child with a reproductive disorder.
3. Formulate nursing diagnoses related to a child's reproductive illness.
4. Develop expected outcomes for a child with a reproductive disorder.
5. Plan nursing care related to reproductive disorders in children.
6. Implement nursing care for a child with a reproductive disorder, such as teaching about normal menstruation.
7. Evaluate expected outcomes for achievement and effectiveness of care.
8. Identify National Health Goals related to reproductive disorders that nurses can help the nation achieve.
9. Identify areas related to the care of children with reproductive disorders that could benefit from additional nursing research or application of evidence-based practice.
10. Analyze ways to implement more family-centered nursing care for a child with a reproductive disorder.
11. Integrate knowledge of reproductive disorders in children with the nursing process to achieve quality maternal and child health nursing care.

---

*N*avi *is a 15-year-old girl you meet in a pediatric clinic. She has been diagnosed with gonorrhea because of a purulent vaginal discharge and burning on urination. When you ask her if she is sexually active, she says no; she thinks she contracted the infection from sharing a towel in a locker room. As she leaves the clinic, you hear her tell the receptionist, "I'm glad I got this early in life. Now I won't have to worry about getting it again."*

Previous chapters described the growth and development of well children. This chapter adds information about the dramatic changes, both physical and psychosocial, that occur when children develop reproductive disorders. This is important information because it constitutes a basis for care and health teaching.

What kind of health education does Navi need?

After you've studied this chapter, access the accompanying website. Read the patient scenario and answer the questions to further sharpen your skills, grow more familiar with RN-CLEX types of questions, and reward yourself with how much you have learned.

Reproductive disorders in children range from mild infections to serious anatomic malformations that can interfere with fertility. All of these disorders require prompt and careful treatment so that children can reach adulthood in reproductive health and with a positive sense of sexuality. Reproductive infections may suggest child abuse, so they also need careful assessment to rule out this possibility (see Chapter 55).

Parents are not always as comfortable inquiring about disorders of the reproductive tract as they are about other disorders. Unless they have clear, thorough explanations of the disease process and prescribed therapy, their reluctance to pursue the subject may leave them confused or misinformed. Even young children can sense that illness affecting the genitalia or reproductive ability is viewed by some adults as different from other diseases. As they reach puberty, they need honest explanations about any effect such a condition will have on interpersonal relationships, sexual functioning, or childbearing. National Health Goals related to reproductive disorders in children are highlighted in Box 47.1.

Nursing Process Overview

For Care of a Child With a Reproductive Disorder

● *Assessment*

Assessment of reproductive health begins with the first physical examination at birth and continues at health assessments throughout childhood (Box 47.2). As with other parts of the health interview, questions regarding reproductive health and illness are generally addressed to the parents until the child is able to answer history questions reliably and independently. Once a girl has reached adolescence, a gynecologic history (Box 47.3) should be included in the health assessment. To preserve their privacy, adolescents of both

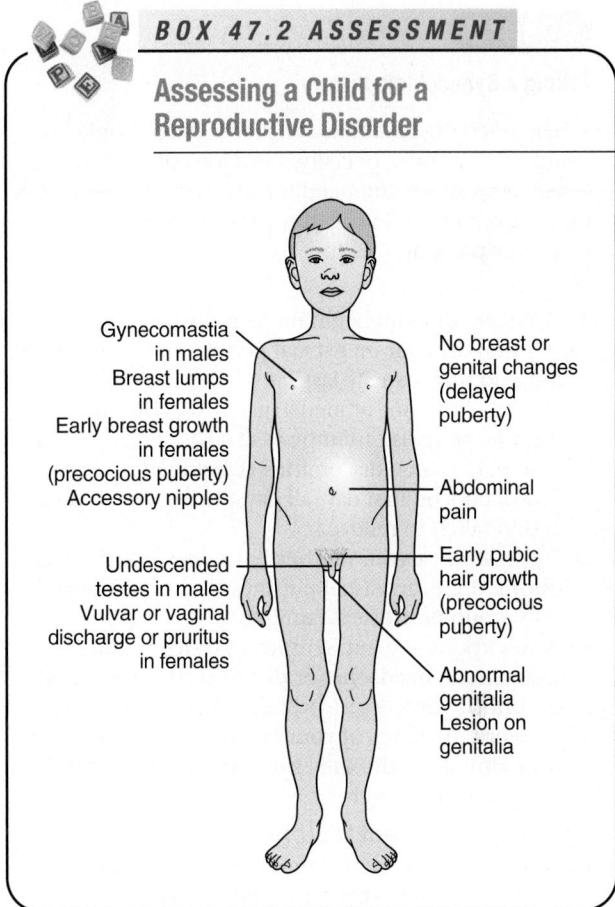

BOX 47.2 ASSESSMENT

Assessing a Child for a Reproductive Disorder

Gynecomastia in males
Breast lumps in females
Early breast growth in females (precocious puberty)
Accessory nipples

Undescended testes in males
Vulvar or vaginal discharge or pruritus in females

No breast or genital changes (delayed puberty)

Abdominal pain

Early pubic hair growth (precocious puberty)

Abnormal genitalia
Lesion on genitalia

genders may prefer not to be accompanied by a parent during a physical examination for reproductive dysfunction.

Some adolescents visit health care facilities on their own. They may be worried that they have contracted a sexually transmitted infection (STI), a disease spread

BOX 47.1 FOCUS ON . . .

NATIONAL HEALTH GOALS

Because sexually transmitted infections (STIs) not only cause short-term distress because of painful lesions but can also have long-term implications for fertility and future childbearing, a number of National Health Goals specifically address them. These goals are the following:

- Reduce the proportion of adolescents and young adults with *Chlamydia trachomatis* infections, from baselines of 12% (females) and 15% (males) to a target of 3%.
- Reduce the annual incidence of new cases of gonorrhea, from a baseline of 123 cases per 100,000 people to no more than 19 cases per 100,000 people.
- Reduce the incidence of primary and secondary syphilis, from a baseline of 3.2 per 100,000 people to no more than 0.2 cases per 100,000 people.

- Reduce the incidence of genital herpes, from a baseline of 17% to no more than 14%.
- Reduce the incidence of pelvic inflammatory disease among women aged 15 through 44 years, from a baseline of 8% to no more than 5% (DHHS, 2000).

Nurses can help the nation achieve these goals by educating adolescents about effective ways to prevent STIs and how to recognize the signs and symptoms of these illnesses. Areas that could benefit from additional nursing research and evidence-based practice in this area include the most effective ways to teach adolescents about safer sex practices, the reasons adolescents continue to believe that they cannot contract infectious diseases, and strategies that would make it easier for parents to discuss this topic with adolescents.

BOX 47.3

Taking a Gynecologic History

When assessing an adolescent for a gynecologic health history be especially conscious of the patient's sense of modesty and need for privacy. To ensure privacy, conduct the interview without the parent or caregiver present.

Menstrual History

At what age did you begin menstruating?

How often do your menstrual periods occur and how long do they usually last?

What is the amount of menstrual flow? (Document by number of pads or tampons used.)

Do you experience discomfort? (Document if discomfort occurs on first day, all days, and so forth, and action taken to relieve it.)

Do any sisters or your mother have discomfort or pain during their menstrual periods (dysmenorrhea) also (endometriosis is familial)?

Do you experience any symptoms of irritability, moodiness, headache, or diarrhea (premenstrual dysphoric disorder) 1 or 2 days before menses?

What were the dates of your last two menstrual periods? How long did they last (duration)? Was the flow light or heavy?

Reproductive Tract History

Have you had any vaginal discharge? (Document amount and whether pad is necessary—include duration, frequency, description, associated symptoms, actions taken.)

Is there vaginal itching (pruritus)?

Is there any vaginal odor?

Have you had reproductive tract surgery? Have you ever been pregnant? Have you ever had an abortion or miscarriage?

Sexual History

Have you had a sexually transmitted infection (e.g., herpes, gonorrhea, or syphilis)?

Are you currently sexually active? What is the gender of your partner?

Do you experience any discomfort during sexual activity (dyspareunia) or any spotting afterward (postcoital spotting)?

Do you have any concerns (e.g., worried about frequency, position, partner's satisfaction with coitus)? Do you experience orgasm?

Contraception History

Do you use any type of birth control? If so, what contraceptive do you use? (Document length of time used, satisfaction, any problems.)

Have you used any other type in the past?

Breast Health

Have you ever noticed any abnormality such as a lump, discharge, or pain in your breasts?

Have you ever had breast surgery?

Have you breast-fed a child?

Do you have a yearly breast examination by a health care provider?

---

by sexual relations. They may suspect that they have become pregnant or want to receive some form of contraception. Before they can admit their chief concern, however, they may "test" the health care provider by eliciting a reaction to a minor problem. Be aware that an adolescent who consults a health care provider with a seemingly minor concern may be misinterpreting symptoms and be truly worried that a minor symptom is serious; on the other hand, the adolescent actually may be seeking help for another problem. Asking the adolescent, "Is there anything else that worries you? Is there any other way we can help you today?" may help you elicit the adolescent's primary concern (Box 47.4).

A pelvic examination is unnecessary for girls who have not yet reached adolescence. However, if vaginal walls need to be inspected (because of an inflammation or infection), an otoscope and ear tip can be used in place of a speculum. Cotton-tipped applicators moistened with sterile normal saline solution can be used to take culture specimens without causing discomfort. For the adolescent girl, the pelvic examination becomes an important part of health assessment. Because the first pelvic examination can be frightening and embarrassing, spend time with the girl before the procedure to teach her about what is being assessed. A three-dimensional model of internal organs and some re-

presentative instruments may be more useful when describing the examination than a verbal description of anatomy. Let the patient look at and handle a speculum. A small speculum should be used for examining young girls. For their comfort, warm the speculum first.

Remaining beside an adolescent as a support person helps to make the examination less embarrassing. To protect her self-esteem, be sure the girl meets the person who will examine her before she is placed in a lithotomy position (Box 47.5).

A young adolescent may be uncomfortable in a lithotomy position and can be examined in a dorsal recumbent position instead (see Chapter 10 for information on assisting with a pelvic examination). Allow the adolescent to choose whether she wants a parent to remain in the room with her.

● *Nursing Diagnosis*

Nursing diagnoses formulated for reproductive illnesses in children focus not only on the result of the disease symptoms but on the anxiety this type of disorder can cause. Examples of these nursing diagnoses are the following:

• Pain related to symptoms of vaginal infection
• Disturbed body image related to fibrocystic breast disease

BOX 47.4 FOCUS ON . . .

COMMUNICATION

Navi, age 15 years, is seen at your pediatric clinic. She has mild upper respiratory tract symptoms.

Less Effective Communication

Nurse: Navi? Doctor Jensen doesn't believe you need anything for your cold. Just drink a little extra fluid and take it easy for a couple days.

Navi: Don't I need a prescription? Some penicillin or something?

Nurse: No. Colds are caused by viruses. Penicillin isn't necessary.

Navi: I want to be sure I get over this. I'd really like an antibiotic of some kind.

Nurse: One really isn't necessary.

Navi: I have a bad cough. I don't think I mentioned that.

Nurse: Doctor Jensen listened to your chest. You don't have anything serious there.

Navi: My stomach doesn't feel very good either. Can't I have something?

Nurse: Sorry. Goodbye now.

More Effective Communication

Nurse: Navi? Doctor Jensen doesn't believe you need anything for your cold. Just drink a little extra fluid and take it easy for a couple days.

Navi: Don't I need a prescription? Some penicillin or something?

Nurse: No. Colds are caused by viruses. Penicillin isn't necessary.

Navi: I want to be sure I get over this. I'd really like an antibiotic of some kind.

Nurse: One really isn't necessary.

Navi: I have a bad cough. I don't think I mentioned that.

Nurse: Doctor Jensen listened to your chest. You don't have anything serious there.

Navi: My stomach doesn't feel very good either. Can't I have something?

Nurse: It seems that you have more symptoms than you mentioned. Are you worried about something other than cold symptoms?

Navi: Well, I have this rash and . . .

Nurse: And . . . ? Go on . . .

Navi: And I'm scared I might have a sex disease.

Adolescents can have difficulty discussing reproductive tract symptoms. If they have too much difficulty, they can try to obtain an antibiotic by describing respiratory or abdominal symptoms. Being alert to this possibility helps you to recognize a "growing" history of this type.

- Anxiety related to absence or irregularity of menstrual periods in adolescent
- Fear related to surgery on genital organs

● *Outcome Identification and Planning*
Assessment of a child's knowledge about the reproductive system and ways that illness can affect reproductive and sexual functioning forms the foundation for developing appropriate outcomes. Educating the child about reproductive health may be one of the first areas to plan. When establishing expected outcomes with adolescents, remember that it will be difficult for them to meet those that require an entire change in lifestyle. It may be more effective to plan for change one step at a time.

● *Implementation*
Interventions for children with reproductive disorders should always include education about reproductive

BOX 47.5 FOCUS ON . . .

DIVERSITY OF CARE

Different cultures have different attitudes toward reproductive disorders. Adolescents in Middle Eastern countries, for example, are extremely modest, and so they are extremely uncomfortable having pelvic examinations done for reproductive disorders. Girls from these countries may be more comfortable if the examiner is a woman.

functioning and measures for maintaining reproductive and sexual health and preventing illness. Health education regarding the importance of testicular self-examination for adolescent males and breast self-examination for adolescent females (although this practice is no longer recommended as a routine assessment) should be stressed at health care visits (see Chapter 33). Guidelines for teaching about menstrual health and safer sex are covered in Chapter 4. Organizations helpful for referral for adolescents include the National Women's Health Network (*www.womenshealthnetwork.org*) and the National Adolescent Health Information Center (*http://nahic.ucsf.edu/*).

Essential nursing interventions also include supporting parents and children through difficult decisions and frightening procedures and providing close observation and empathic counseling after surgery. For example, surgery for undescended testes is a procedure that can be traumatic for a child, especially if it is performed during a developmental stage in which the child views such surgery as castrating. Being certain that the child receives good preparation for surgery and reassurance that he will not be mutilated is an essential nursing intervention.

● *Outcome Evaluation*
The responses of children to reproductive dysfunction vary both with the severity of the illness and with the specific age and fears of the child. It is safe to assume, however, that children who have experienced such an

illness are at risk for a loss of self-esteem or confusion about their body image. Therefore, outcome evaluation must include long-term evaluation of the child's coping abilities and self-image. If the child contracts an STI, evaluation should also address the child's knowledge about avoiding STIs in the future and willingness to seek help should an infection recur. An STI in a young child should be investigated to be certain that it has not resulted from sexual abuse.

The following are examples suggesting achievement of outcomes:

- Adolescent states that discomfort from vaginal infection is tolerable after beginning medication.
- Adolescent states she is able to view self as competent despite fibrocystic breast disease.
- Child states that she is able to wait 6 months without worrying about not yet having a menstrual period.
- Child states that he feels less fearful about impending surgery after talking with his health care provider.

DISORDERS CAUSED BY ALTERED REPRODUCTIVE DEVELOPMENT

Genetic sex or *biologic gender* (sex chromosomes XX or XY) is determined at conception. However, development of the reproductive system, including external genitalia, occurs over two distinct periods. Reproductive organs and genitalia begin to differentiate in utero by the 8th week, with growth and refinement occurring over the next several months. This period constitutes the first phase of reproductive development. The second phase occurs with specific endocrine changes that are triggered during puberty; this is a period of maturation of primary and secondary sexual characteristics.

Ambiguous genitalia, which is a rare condition with various causes that occur during fetal development, and precocious puberty or delayed puberty, which are second phase disorders, are examples of altered reproductive development. (For a discussion of genetic disorders, see Chapter 7.)

Ambiguous Genitalia

Understanding how reproductive organs develop in utero is important to the understanding of ambiguous genitalia. Although external sexual characteristics generally follow from the presence of the XX or XY chromosomes, under certain circumstances it is possible for structures usually considered "male" or "female" to develop in individuals of either chromosomal gender. Usually, a diagnosis of ambiguous genitalia means that external sexual organs in the child did not follow the normal course of development, so that, at birth, they are so incompletely or abnormally formed that it is impossible to clearly determine the child's gender by simple observation. For instance, a male infant with *hypospadias* (urethral opening on the underside of

the penis) and cryptorchidism (undescended testes) may appear more female than male on first inspection (see Chapter 46 for a discussion of hypospadias). A chromosomal female (XX) fetus may become "masculinized" with exposure to androgen in utero; in such cases, the clitoris may be so enlarged as to appear more like a penis, the labia may be partially fused and difficult to tell from a male perineum, or the urethra may be displaced so far forward that it is located on the clitoris. When this occurs, the newborn will appear to be a boy on initial inspection. Likewise, under certain conditions, a chromosomal male (XY) may become "feminized," with a lack of fusion of the labioscrotal folds and an incompletely formed penis (Ogilvy-Stuart & Brain, 2004).

The most common cause of in vitro virilization of females is *congenital adrenocortical syndrome.* The adrenal gland produces androgen instead of adequate cortisone, causing the clitoris to become the size of a typical newborn male's penis (see Chapter 48).

If testosterone was produced in utero but development of the müllerian duct (female) was not suppressed, a child may be intersexed (formerly termed **hermaphrodite**), with both ovaries and testes and either male or female external genitalia. Children with ambiguous genitalia are often termed pseudointersexed or **pseudohermaphrodites** because, as infants, they have some external features of both sexes, although only either ovaries or testes (or neither) are present.

Assessment

If there is any question about a child's gender, karyotyping helps to establish whether the child is genetically male or female (see Chapter 7). This involves drawing a specimen of blood, allowing the white blood cells to reach a division stage, and then examining them. *Laparoscopy* (introduction of a narrow laparoscope into the abdominal cavity through a half-inch incision under the umbilicus) or possibly exploratory surgery may be necessary to determine if ovaries or undescended testes are present. Intravenous pyelography or sonography can be used to establish whether a male has a complete urinary tract.

Therapeutic Management

Once the child's true chromosomal gender has been documented, the extent of necessary reconstructive surgery is determined in consultation with the parents. This may involve correction of a hypospadias or cryptorchidism, removal of labial adhesions, or surgical removal of an enlarged clitoris. If removal of an enlarged clitoris is involved, the parents must consider what the absence of this organ will mean to the girl in terms of later sexual enjoyment. Parents may be well advised to delay this type of surgery until the girl can decide for herself whether she wants it done (Rangecroft, 2003). Nonfunctioning ovaries or testes are generally removed to prevent malignancy later in life.

If an infant is chromosomally male but does not have an adequate penis, a decision to raise the child as a female might be made, although construction of an artificial penis is more likely.

NURSING DIAGNOSES AND RELATED INTERVENTIONS

When identifying expected outcomes, be aware that parents under stress may have difficulty making long-range plans. The birth of a child with a perplexing defect produces a particularly high level of stress, hampering parents' ability to think clearly and calmly about their situation.

Nursing Diagnosis: Anxiety related to ambiguous gender of child at birth

Outcome Evaluation: Parents voice willingness to support treatment plan, including additional necessary tests, and state they are prepared to make decisions with guidance from health care team.

If the gender of a child is unclear, the parents should be told this immediately. If told first that their child is a boy, only to be told 24 hours later that "he" is really a girl, parents can have difficulty accepting this drastic change. During this period when the baby's gender is yet to be determined, avoid calling the baby "it." Rather, say "the baby" or "your child." Explain how sexual organs form in utero and that every child has the potential to be externally female or male.

To promote bonding, help parents understand that their child is otherwise perfect (assuming this is true). As the child grows, additional counseling may be needed to help the child adjust to an abnormal appearance or function.

Precocious Puberty

Although development of breasts or pubic hair before age 8 years or menses before age 9 years may be normal, such development has traditionally been considered precocious sexual development (Midyett, et al., 2003). Often, such development is expressed as isolated breast or pubic hair growth but can proceed to complete spermatogenesis or menstrual function. Precocious puberty occurs more often in girls than in boys.

This condition is caused by the early production of gonadotropins by the pituitary gland; gonadotropins stimulate the ovaries or testes to produce sex hormones. Such stimulation can occur because of a pituitary tumor, cyst, or traumatic injury to the third ventricle next to the pituitary gland. It also can occur because of estrogen-secreting cysts or tumors of the ovary or testosterone-secreting cysts of the testes. In rare instances, it occurs because of an estrogen- or testosterone-secreting adrenal tumor. In girls, ingestion of a mother's oral contraceptive pills can also initiate menarche-like changes.

In children affected by precocious puberty, a tumor must be ruled out. If no physical cause, such as a tumor, is detected, the phenomenon appears to occur only because the *gonadostat* of the hypothalamus (the trigger that begins the development of secondary sex characteristics) was turned on several years too early. It is categorized as either central precocious puberty (gonadotropin-releasing hormone [GnRH]–dependent), in which gonadotrophic hormones are elevated, or as peripheral precocious puberty (Gn-RH–independent), which is basically elevation of sexual steroids produced by the gonads or adrenals (Kelly & Ferry, 2003).

Assessment

With precocious puberty, children have increased breast development and accelerated skeletal maturation. Girls have menstrual bleeding with little pubic or axillary hair because of still low androgen secretion. Boys have obvious genital growth. The diagnosis of early puberty is confirmed by serum analysis for estrogen or androgen; these will be at adult levels.

Therapeutic Management

A synthetic analog to GnRH is available as leuprolide acetate (Lupron) (Box 47.6). Administration of this analog desensitizes GnRH receptors, making stimulation by GnRH ineffective. The preparation is administered subcutaneously every day. After it is discontinued at age 12 or 13 years, puberty progresses normally.

BOX 47.6 FOCUS ON . . .

PHARMACOLOGY

Leuprolide acetate (Lupron)

Classification: Leuprolide is a hormonal agent, specifically a luteinizing hormone-releasing hormone (LH-RH) agonist.

Action: Occupies pituitary gonadotropin-releasing hormone (GnRH) receptors, preventing GnRH from functioning (Karch, 2004).

Pregnancy Risk Category: X

Dosage: Daily subcutaneous (SQ) or monthly intramuscular (IM) injection

Possible Adverse Effects: Nausea, vomiting, anorexia, hot flashes, headache, pain at injection site

Nursing Implications
• Administer only with the syringes supplied with the drug
• Vary injection sites to decrease local irritation
• Monitor injection sites for bruising and rash
• Instruct parents in method for proper administration
• If monthly doses are prescribed, assist parents with preparing a realistic schedule for administration. Encourage the use of a calendar for accurate timing

NURSING DIAGNOSES AND RELATED INTERVENTIONS

Nursing Diagnosis: Disturbed body image related to precocious puberty

Outcome Evaluation: Child voices an understanding of what is happening and does not evidence excessive shyness or reluctance to interact with peers.

Children who develop precociously may have difficulty interacting with peers because they appear so different from other members of their age group. Parents may worry about their children becoming sexually active, particularly about girls becoming pregnant.

Both parents and children need reassurance that, after reaching the age of normal puberty, the child will again be the same as other children; the fact that the child's sexual growth started early does not mean the genitals will be out of proportion to the rest of the body as an adult.

Parents must also understand that the child is fully fertile and able to inseminate or conceive when early puberty occurs. Oral contraceptives are not advisable for girls this young, because the increased load of estrogen hastens the closing of epiphyseal lines of long bones too early, possibly stunting the child's growth permanently.

Parents may need to be reminded that, although their child appears to be much older, the changes are only in sexual characteristics. Household tasks, responsibility, and expectations must be geared to the child's chronologic age, not to outward appearance.

Delayed Puberty

Secondary sex characteristics normally are present by age 14 years in girls and 15 years in boys. Delayed puberty, as the name implies, is the failure of pubertal changes to occur at the usual age. The family history of many children reveals a family tendency for late maturation. If so, the child needs a thorough physical examination to disclose whether some secondary sex characteristics are present or whether endocrine stimulation is beginning.

If girls have not begun to menstruate by age 17 years and pathology has been ruled out, menstrual cycles can be started by administering estrogen. Many girls worry considerably about delayed menstruation, but, once reassured that development is merely delayed, they are usually willing to wait for menarche to occur on its own. Similarly, boys who are distressed by their lack of development may receive testosterone supplements to stimulate pubic hair and genital growth (Mansbach & Gordon, 2002).

Checkpoint Question 1

Suppose a girl develops precocious puberty. What advice would you give her parents?

a. Excess estrogen causes children to be intersexed or hermaphrodites.
b. Although her sexual appearance is advanced, the girl cannot conceive.
c. To remember to treat the child appropriately for her chronologic age, not the age she appears to be.
d. To not allow the child to eat processed meats, which contain hormones.

REPRODUCTIVE DISORDERS IN MALES

Common reproductive disorders in males include structural alterations in the penis or testes such as phimosis and cryptorchidism, inflammation such as balanoposthitis, and, in adolescents, testicular cancer.

Balanitis (Balanoposthitis)

Balanoposthitis is inflammation of the glans and prepuce of the penis. It is usually caused by poor hygiene and may accompany a urethritis or a regional dermatitis.

Assessment

The prepuce and glans become red and swollen; a purulent discharge may be present. The boy may have difficulty voiding because of crusting at the meatal opening and because acidic urine touching the denuded surface of the glans causes pain (Austin & Zderic, 2003).

Therapeutic Management

Medical treatment involves local application of heat; this can be carried out with warm wet soaks or warm baths. A local antibiotic ointment may be prescribed. If *phimosis* (a tight foreskin) appears to be contributing to the condition, circumcision may be advocated after the inflammation subsides. It prevents the condition from recurring.

Although balanoposthitis is painful, a boy may tolerate the discomfort for several days because he is too embarrassed to discuss the problem. He may think it was caused by masturbation (which can contribute to the irritation) or by sexual activity and may be reluctant to seek help for fear of being criticized. He can be reassured that the problem is local and will have no long-range effect. Any discharge should be cultured to rule out an STI such as gonorrhea. On the other hand, in developing countries where balanitis can become chronic, it may be associated with the development of penile cancer (Misra et al., 2004).

Phimosis

In the normal infant, the foreskin is tight at birth and may be even held fast by adhesions. Usually, it cannot be retracted. After a few months, the adhesions dissolve and the foreskin becomes retractable; if it does not, the infant may have phimosis. With this, the foreskin remains so tight that it interferes with voiding. Balanoposthitis may develop because the foreskin cannot be retracted for cleaning. True phimosis is rare but can be corrected by circumcision (Wren, 2004). The technique of circumcision is discussed in Chapter 24.

Cryptorchidism

Cryptorchidism is failure of one or both testes to descend from the abdominal cavity to the scrotum. Normally, the testes descend into the scrotal sac during months 7 to 9 of intrauterine life. They may descend any time up to 6 weeks after birth; they rarely descend after that time.

The cause of undescended testes is unclear. Fibrous bands at the inguinal ring or inadequate length of spermatic vessels may prevent descent. Testes apparently descend because of stimulation by testosterone; hence, it is possible that a lower than normal level of testosterone production prevents descent. About 17% of premature infants and 3% to 4% of full-term infants are born with undescended testes (Wu & Kolon, 2003).

Assessment

Early detection of undescended testes is important, because the warmth of the abdominal cavity may inhibit development of the testes, ultimately affecting spermatogenesis. After puberty, sperm production deteriorates rapidly in undescended testes, and the testes may undergo a malignant change. Anchoring the testes in the scrotal sac may not prevent malignancy, but it will allow the boy to perform preventive measures such as testicular self-examination.

It is more common for the right testis to remain undescended than the left one. In approximately 20% of all cases, both testes remain undescended. Some children may be diagnosed with undescended testes when, in fact, poor examining technique caused the testes to retract. If the child is supine or the examining room is chilly, the scrotal sac may appear to be empty. Excessive palpation or stroking of the inner thigh may also stimulate the cremasteric reflex and cause retraction. In these instances, testes descend when the child is standing or after a warm bath.

An undescended testis may be at the inguinal ring (true undescended testis) or ectopic (still in the abdomen). Laparoscopy is effective in identifying undescended testes. Because testes arise from the same germ tissue as the kidneys, the kidney function of a child with ectopic testes is usually evaluated. If undescended testes and other factors (e.g., ambiguous genitals) pose questions about the child's gender, a *karyotype* may be done to determine true gender.

Therapeutic Management

Because the testes sometimes descend spontaneously during the first year of life, treatment is usually delayed for 6 to 12 months. Children may be given chorionic gonadotropin hormone to stimulate testicular descent, but this therapy is successful only in approximately 20% of cases. If necessary, surgery (**orchiopexy**) by laparoscopy by 1 year of age corrects the condition. Surgery to correct cryptorchidism is important, because undescended testes are associated with testicular cancer (Herrinton et al., 2003).

NURSING DIAGNOSES AND RELATED INTERVENTIONS

If an orchiopexy is scheduled, the focus is on parent and child teaching, preoperative preparation, and postoperative care.

Nursing Diagnosis: Deficient knowledge related to parents' and child's inexperience with surgical procedure and postoperative treatment plan

Outcome Evaluation: Parents (and child, if old enough) accurately describe what will be accomplished by surgery.

Boys who are old enough to understand need good preparation for this type of surgery. Use an anatomically correct picture to point out the exact site at which surgery will be performed. Reassure the boy that the penis itself will not be cut. The child may not voice a fear of mutilation, but you can assume that it exists, especially in preschool children.

During surgery, internal sutures may be inserted to hold the testis in place. Although the child may be discharged from the hospital on the same day, his activity will be limited until approximately the second day after surgery, to ensure that the internal suture line remains intact.

Nursing Diagnosis: Disturbed body image related to change in physical appearance

Outcome Evaluation: Child (if verbal) states that he views himself as a whole person and interacts with peers without excessive shyness or hesitancy.

Postoperative evaluation should reveal that the suture line is healing well and that both testes can be palpated in the scrotum. It should also address the boy's feelings about the surgery and the changes in his body. He may need an opportunity to express his fears about mutilation or castration by playing with puppets or dolls after surgery. Boys who have bilateral cryptorchidism may be less fertile as adults. When boys reach puberty, teach them testicular self-examination to assess any early symptoms of malignancy, such as nodules or abnormal growth (see Chapter 33).

Hydrocele

When a testis descends into the scrotum in utero, it is preceded by a fold of tissue, the *processus vaginalis.* Occasionally, fluid collects in this fold. If this occurs,

hydrocele (the fluid) can be revealed by prenatal sonography. At birth, the collection of fluid makes the scrotum of the newborn appear enlarged (Hill & Vujevich, 2004). On *transillumination* (the shining of a light through the scrotal sac), the area is illuminated by the water and shines or glows. Sonography also can reveal this fluid collection. If the hydrocele is uncomplicated, the fluid will gradually be reabsorbed into the body and no treatment is necessary. The child's parents can be assured that the hydrocele is only excess fluid and that the scrotal enlargement is not caused by an abnormal testis, tumor, or hernia.

A hydrocele may form later in life due to *inguinal hernia* (abdominal contents extruding into the scrotum through the inguinal ring, with accompanying fluid). If this happens, the hernia must be repaired for the hydrocele to be reabsorbed (see Chapter 45). Injection of a drug to decrease fluid production (*sclerotherapy*) may also be effective.

Varicocele

A **varicocele** is abnormal dilation of the veins of the spermatic cord (Fig. 47.1). It is important to identify varicoceles in adolescents, even though they are hard to document, because the increased heat and congestion in the testicles may be a cause of infertility (Raj & Wiener, 2004). No treatment is necessary unless fertility becomes a concern, at which time the varicocele can be surgically removed. The patient may report some local tenderness and edema for a few days after surgery. Edema can be minimized by applying ice for the first few hours postoperatively.

Testicular Torsion

Testicular torsion (twisting of the spermatic cord) is a surgical emergency. Although it can be present in newborns, it occurs most frequently during early adolescence (Wren, 2004). Less than normal testicular support apparently allows the spermatic cord to twist. Testicular torsion usually results from a sports activity. The boy experiences severe scrotal pain and perhaps nausea and vomiting from the severity of the pain. The testis feels tender to palpation, and edema begins to develop. If the condition is not recognized promptly (within 4 hours), irreversible change in the testis can occur from lack of circulation to the organ. Boys need to be educated about the phenomenon so that they report symptoms promptly. Laparoscopic surgery is necessary to reduce the torsion and re-establish circulation (Cole & Vogler, 2004).

Testicular Cancer

Testicular cancer is rare (only 1% of all malignancies). It usually occurs between ages 15 and 35 years, often in association with cryptorchidism (McCullagh & Lewis, 2005). Symptoms include painless testicular enlargement and a feeling of heaviness in the scrotum. The disease metastasizes rapidly, leading to abdominal and back pain due to retroperitoneal node extension, weight loss, and general weakness. **Gynecomastia** (enlargement of the breasts) may arise because of human chorionic gonadotropins (hCG) produced by the tumor. hCG and alpha-fetoprotein, tumor markers, can be detected in blood serum.

Therapy for testicular malignancy is **orchiectomy** (removal of the testis) followed by radiation or chemotherapy. After surgical removal, a gel-filled prosthesis may be inserted to provide a symmetric appearance to the scrotum. Infertility in the opposite testis results after radiation therapy. For some patients, "sperm banking," or preserving frozen sperm before the procedure, may be presented as an option for future family planning.

Teaching males to perform testicular self-examination for early cancer detection is important to help them detect symptoms at an early point (see Chapter 33).

REPRODUCTIVE DISORDERS IN FEMALES

The most frequent reproductive disorders in females involve vaginal or menstrual irregularities. Other disorders are caused by structural alterations of the reproductive organs, such as imperforate hymen, pelvic inflammatory disease (PID), or infections caused by STIs.

Menstrual Disorders

Because menstruation is an ongoing process throughout half of a woman's life, it affects her self-image significantly. An irregularity such as painful cycles can exert a major influence on daily activities. Therefore, it is a health concern requiring as much time and attention as that given to other concerns.

Menstrual disorders fall into two categories: (1) menstruation that is painful or uncomfortable and (2) infrequent or too-frequent cycles.

Mittelschmerz

Some women experience abdominal pain during ovulation from the release of accompanying prostaglandins. Pain

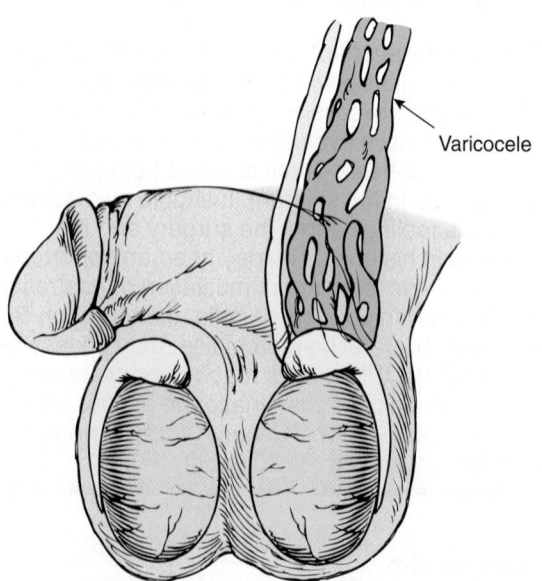

FIGURE 47.1 A varicocele. Identifying varicocele in adolescent males is important because the condition may be associated with infertility.

may also be caused by a drop or two of follicular fluid or blood that spills into the abdominal cavity. This pain, called **mittelschmerz,** can range from a few sharp cramps to several hours of discomfort. It is typically felt on one side of the abdomen (near an ovary) and may be accompanied by scant vaginal spotting.

An advantage of mittelschmerz is that it clearly marks ovulation. If pain is felt in the right lower quadrant, it can be differentiated from appendicitis by the lack of associated symptoms (i.e., nausea, vomiting, fever, abdominal guarding, and rebound tenderness) as well as by its occurrence in the menstrual cycle. Usually mittelschmerz is of limited duration and intensity and, therefore, not a great source of discomfort.

Dysmenorrhea

Dysmenorrhea is painful menstruation. For generations, it was thought to be mainly psychological, needing no treatment other than reassurance that it was a normal phenomenon and something women should endure. Today, it is known that the pain is caused by the release of prostaglandins in response to tissue destruction during the ischemic phase of the menstrual cycle (French, 2005). Prostaglandin release causes smooth muscle contraction in the uterus.

Dysmenorrhea can also be a symptom of an underlying illness such as PID, uterine myomas (tumors), or endometriosis (abnormal formation of endometrial tissue).

Assessment. Dysmenorrhea can be categorized as mild (no interference with normal activities), moderate (some interference with normal activities), or severe (interference with the majority of everyday activities). As many as 80% of adolescents have some discomfort with menstruation; in approximately 10%, the discomfort seriously interferes with daily living (Nichols, 2003). Dysmenorrhea is *primary* if it occurs in the absence of organic disease; it is *secondary* if it occurs as a result of organic disease. There may be a "bloated" feeling and light cramping 24 hours before menstrual flow. Pain is mainly noticed, however, when the flow begins. Colicky (sharp) pain is superimposed on a dull, nagging pain across the lower abdomen. Accompanying this is an "aching, pulling" sensation of the vulva and inner thighs. Some adolescents have mild diarrhea with the abdominal cramping. Mild breast tenderness, abdominal distention, nausea and vomiting, headache, and facial flushing may be present.

Therapeutic Management. Painful symptoms can usually be controlled by an analgesic such as acetylsalicylic acid (aspirin) or ibuprofen (Advil, Motrin). Acetylsalicylic acid works well as an analgesic for dysmenorrhea because it is a mild prostaglandin inhibitor. Although adolescents are usually advised not to take aspirin because of its link to Reye's syndrome, girls may take it safely at the beginning of a menstrual period as long as they do not have additional flulike symptoms. Ibuprofen is a stronger prostaglandin inhibitor and relieves more severe menstrual pain (Durain, 2004). Naproxen sodium (Aleve) is also effective. Be certain that girls know not to take these drugs on an empty stomach, because they can be extremely irritating to gastric mucosa. Low-dose oral contraceptives to prevent ovulation may also be effective if pregnancy is not desired.

One disadvantage of this therapy is the possible adverse effects of long-term estrogen administration. Adolescents may choose to be prescribed long-acting oral contraceptives so that they have menstrual periods only every 3 months (Wiegratz & Kuhl, 2004).

During the first year or two of menstruation, dysmenorrhea rarely occurs, because early menstrual cycles are usually **anovulatory** (without ovulation). As ovulation begins, typical menstrual discomfort begins.

NURSING DIAGNOSES AND RELATED INTERVENTIONS

Nursing Diagnosis: Pain related to dysmenorrhea

Outcome Evaluation: Client states that she has some control over pain through nonpharmacologic or pharmacologic methods.

Several nonpharmacologic solutions may help relieve dysmenorrhea. St. John's wort is an herb that can be used to promote general well-being. Decreasing sodium intake for a few days before an expected menstrual flow, by omitting salty foods (e.g., potato chips, pretzels, ham, other luncheon meats) and by not adding salt to foods, may help reduce "bloated" feelings. Abdominal breathing (breathing in and out slowly, allowing the abdominal wall to rise with each inhalation) may also be helpful. Applying heat to the abdomen with a heating pad or taking a hot shower or tub bath may relax muscle tension and relieve pain (Akin et al., 2004). Caution young girls not to apply heat to their abdomen for abdominal pain unless they are actually menstruating; if the pain results from an inflamed appendix, heat can cause rupture of the appendix and life-threatening peritonitis. Resting may help to relieve vulvar pain; abdominal massage (effleurage or light massage) may feel soothing. Adolescents who remain sexually active during their menses may discover that orgasm helps relieve pelvic engorgement and cramping.

Menorrhagia

Menorrhagia is an abnormally heavy menstrual flow, usually defined as greater than 80 mL per menses. It may occur in girls close to puberty and in women nearing menopause because of anovulatory cycles. Without ovulation and subsequent progesterone secretion, estrogen secretion continues and causes extreme proliferation of endometrium. It can occur because of a previously undiagnosed bleeding disorder (Braverman & Breech, 2004).

Assessment. It is difficult to determine when a menstrual flow is abnormally heavy, but one method is to ask the client how long it takes her to saturate a sanitary napkin or tampon. A sanitary napkin or tampon holds approximately

25 mL of fluid. If a pad or tampon is saturated in less than 1 hour, the flow is considered heavier than usual. There is often an unusual amount of flow in clients using intrauterine devices (IUDs). With oral contraceptives, the flow is often light; for this reason, it may seem alarmingly heavy once the pills are discontinued, but usually this is just a return of the adolescent's normal flow.

A heavy flow can indicate endometriosis (see later discussion), a systemic disease (anemia), blood dyscrasia such as a clotting defect, or a uterine abnormality such as a myoma (fibroid) tumor. It can be a symptom of infection such as PID or an indication of early pregnancy loss that is coincidentally occurring at the time of an expected menstrual period.

Determining the cause of menorrhagia is important, because it can lead to anemia from excessive iron loss. If anemia occurs, iron supplements may be necessary to achieve sufficient hemoglobin formation. The adolescent who is losing excessive blood because of anovulatory cycles may be prescribed progesterone during the luteal phase to prevent proliferative growth during this phase of the cycle; if the ability to conceive is unimportant, adolescents may be prescribed a low-dose oral contraceptive or GnRH inhibitor to decrease the flow.

Metrorrhagia

Metrorrhagia is bleeding between menstrual periods. This is normal in some adolescents who have spotting at the time of ovulation ("mittelstaining"). It may also occur in clients taking oral contraceptives (breakthrough bleeding) during the first 3 or 4 months. Additionally, vaginal irritation from infection can cause midcycle spotting. Spotting may also represent a temporarily low level of progesterone production and endometrial sloughing (dysfunctional uterine bleeding or a luteal phase defect), a condition that tends to occur near the end of the reproductive years.

If metrorrhagia occurs for more than one menstrual cycle in a teenager who is not taking oral contraceptives, she should be referred to her primary care provider for examination, because abnormal vaginal bleeding can be an early sign of uterine carcinoma or ovarian cysts.

Endometriosis

Endometriosis is the abnormal growth of extrauterine endometrial cells, often in the cul-de-sac of the peritoneal cavity or on the uterine ligaments or ovaries. This abnormal tissue results from excessive endometrial production and a reflux of blood and tissue through the fallopian tubes during menstrual flow. As many as 25% of women in the United States have endometriosis, and as many as 50% of adolescents seen for dysmenorrhea have endometriosis (Batt & Mitwally, 2003). It tends to occur most often in white nulliparous women, but there is also a familial tendency. Daughters of women with endometriosis may develop symptoms of dysmenorrhea early in life. They may want to consider having children before overgrowth of the endometrium becomes so extensive that it interferes with conception.

The excessive production of endometrial tissue may be related to a deficient immunologic response. In many women, it appears to be related to excess estrogen production or a failed luteal menstrual phase. Many women with endometriosis do not ovulate or ovulate irregularly. Therefore, endometriosis is discovered at a higher than usual rate among women undergoing infertility testing (Johnson, 2003).

In these clients, estrogen secretion continues through the cycle rather than becoming secondary to progesterone late in the cycle, as happens with normal ovulation. The resulting proliferation of tissue forces the blood back into the fallopian tubes.

Endometriosis causes dysmenorrhea when the abnormal tissue responds to estrogen and progesterone stimulation by swelling and then sloughing its layers in the same manner as the uterine lining. This causes inflammation of surrounding tissue in the abdominal cavity and an even greater release of prostaglandins. Abnormal tissue in the pelvic cul-de-sac can cause *dyspareunia* (painful coitus) because it puts pressure on the posterior vagina. Infertility may result if the fallopian tubes become immobilized and blocked by tissue implants or adhesions, preventing peristaltic motion and transport of ova (see Chapter 4).

Assessment. Pelvic examination may show that the uterus is displaced by tender, fixed, palpable nodules. Nodules in the cul-de-sac or on an ovary also may be palpable. If the endometriosis is minimal, the woman will not experience related symptoms. If the condition is moderate or extensive, she may experience dysmenorrhea or dyspareunia.

Therapeutic Management. Treatment for endometriosis can be medical or surgical, depending on the extent of the disease. Estrogen/progesterone-based oral contraceptives may stimulate implant regression as the tissue sloughs under the influence of the progesterone. Danazol (Danocrine), a synthetic androgen, can be prescribed to help shrink the abnormal tissue. Administration of a GnRH agonist, such as leuprolide acetate (Lupron), can reduce hormone stimulation (see Box 47.6). Laparotomy with excision by laser surgery is the most effective measure, but, because this is a highly invasive procedure, a course of conservative medical treatment may be tried first.

Amenorrhea

Amenorrhea, or absence of a menstrual flow, strongly suggests pregnancy but is by no means definitive, because it can also result from tension, anxiety, fatigue, chronic illness, extreme dieting, or strenuous exercise. Competitive swimmers, long-distance runners (50 to 75 miles weekly), and ballet dancers notice that intensive training causes their periods to become scant and irregular. This appears to be associated with their low ratio of body fat to body muscle, which leads to excessive secretion of prolactin. An elevation in prolactin causes a decrease in GnRH from the hypothalamus, followed by declines in follicle-stimulating hormone (FSH), follicular development, and estrogen secretion. Menstrual cycles usually return to normal within 3 months after discontinuation of strenuous training and conditioning.

Adolescents who wish to maintain a normal cycle while training for a sports event may take bromocriptine (Parlodel), which can reduce high prolactin levels by acting on the hypothalamus and initiating menstruation each month. Many adolescents, however, view the absence of menstrual periods as a benefit during sports training. If a menstrual flow is delayed and pregnancy is suspected, bromocriptine should be discontinued, because it is potentially teratogenic.

Amenorrhea also occurs among females who diet excessively, partially as a natural defense mechanism to limit ovulation and as a means of conserving body fluid. Women with *anorexia nervosa* or *bulimia* (eating disorders described in Chapter 54) often develop amenorrhea after approximately 3 months of excessive dieting or binging and dieting; as in athletes, this is caused by an increase in prolactin. Amenorrhea as a sign of pregnancy is discussed in Chapter 9.

Premenstrual Dysphoric Disorder

Premenstrual dysphoric disorder (PDD) is a condition that occurs in the luteal phase of the menstrual cycle and is relieved by the onset of menses. It has both behavioral and physiologic symptoms. Because of the variety of possible symptoms, as many as 30% of women experience some degree of PDD, a cluster of symptoms that include anxiety, fatigue, abdominal bloating, headache, appetite disturbance, irritability, and depression (McEvoy et al., 2004). For some women, these symptoms are so extreme that they are incapacitating. In some girls, premenstrual symptoms include severe migraine headaches (Granella et al., 2004).

The cause of PDD is unproven but, contrary to previous beliefs, it must be due to more than a drop in progesterone just before menses. A syndrome similar to PDD may occur in women after tubal ligation; a decrease in the blood supply to the ovary apparently results in decreased luteal function. In some women, a vitamin B–complex deficiency may lead to estrogen excess, causing an abnormal ratio of estrogen to progesterone; other related causes may be poor renal clearance leading to water retention, or hypoglycemia leading to a surge of adrenalin and low calcium levels and interference with serotonin synthesis.

Symptoms of PDD vary from cycle to cycle and throughout life. Therapy is aimed at correcting specific symptoms.

Adolescents who think they have PDD should keep a diary of when symptoms occur. If they are aware of recurring patterns that indicate PDD, they will be better able to recognize the cause. They should be certain their diet is high in vitamins and calcium and low in salt. Agents that suppress ovarian function, such as oral contraceptives or the GnRH agonist leuprolide, may be prescribed. If depression is a major symptom, an antidepressant such as buspirone (BuSpar) can be helpful. Paroxetine (Paxil) is a serotonin reuptake inhibitor that is specifically designed for PDD therapy in adults. Antidepressants are prescribed with caution in adolescents, because they may be responsible for an increase in suicidal behavior (Jick et al., 2004).

Other Reproductive Disorders in Females

Imperforate Hymen

The *hymen* is a membranous ring of tissue that partly obstructs the vaginal opening. An *imperforate hymen* to-tally occludes the vagina, preventing the escape of vaginal secretions and menstrual blood.

Before menarche, the child with an imperforate hymen usually has no symptoms. With onset of menstruation, the menstrual flow is obstructed. It builds up in the vagina, causing increased pressure in the vagina and uterus and eventually abdominal pain. Palpation of the abdomen reveals a lower abdominal mass. On vaginal examination, an intact, bulging hymen is evident.

The treatment is surgical incision or removal of the hymenal tissue. The girl may have local pain after the incision, which can be relieved by a mild analgesic and warm baths.

Careful explanation of this condition will help the girl understand that it will not interfere with sexual relations or future childbearing. Because most girls of early menstrual age have scant knowledge of anatomy, pictures of the reproductive tract help to explain that this is a local and minor problem.

Toxic Shock Syndrome

Toxic shock syndrome (TSS) is an infection that usually is caused by toxin-producing strains of *Staphylococcus aureus* organisms. Although organisms can enter the body by other means, they typically enter through vaginal walls that have been damaged by the insertion of tampons at the time of a menstrual period (Bagarazzi & Conway, 2003).

Assessment. The symptoms of TSS are described in Box 47.7. Any female who develops fever with diarrhea and vomiting during a menstrual period should suspect TSS. Remember, however, that a number of women have mild diarrhea as a normal accompaniment to dysmenorrhea.

BOX 47.7

Symptoms of Toxic Shock Syndrome*

- Temperature more than 102°F (38.9°C)
- Vomiting and diarrhea
- A macular (sunburn-like) rash that desquamates on palms and soles 1 to 2 weeks after illness
- Severe hypotension (systolic pressure less than 90 mm Hg)
- Shock, leading to poor organ perfusion
- Impaired renal function with elevated blood urea nitrogen or creatinine at least twice the upper limit of normal
- Severe muscle pain or creatine phosphokinase at least twice the upper limit of normal
- Hyperemia of mucous membrane
- Impaired liver function with increased total bilirubin and increased serum glutamate oxaloacetate transaminase (aspartate aminotransferase) at twice the upper limit of normal
- Decreased platelet count
- Central nervous system symptoms of disorientation, confusion, severe headache

---

*Three symptoms must be present for diagnosis.

Therapeutic Management. Women or adolescents with suspected TSS need a careful vaginal examination and removal of any tampon particles, as well as cervical and vaginal cultures for *S. aureus.* Iodine douches may reduce the number of organisms present vaginally. *S. aureus* is usually resistant to penicillin but not to penicillinase-resistant antibiotics (i.e., cephalosporins, oxacillins, or clindamycins). Intravenous fluid therapy to restore circulating fluid volume and increase blood pressure, or vasopressors such as dopamine (Intropin), may be necessary to increase the blood pressure. Diuretic therapy to shift fluid back to the intravascular circulation may be necessary to prevent renal and cardiac failure. Recovery occurs in 7 to 10 days; fatigue and weakness may remain for months afterward.

The rate of TSS recurrence is 28% to 64%, usually within 2 months after the first attack. Recurrence probably happens because the organism is not completely eliminated from the body. Therefore, be certain that girls complete their entire antibiotic prescription. Be sure to educate girls about menstrual hygiene (Box 47.8). All girls should use the lowest-absorbency tampon appropriate for their individual flow (Food and Drug Administration, 2004). Girls who develop TSS should avoid tampon use in the future.

Vulvovaginitis

In **vulvovaginitis,** inflammation of the vulva or vagina is accompanied by pain, odor, pruritus, and a vaginal discharge. Vaginal bleeding may be present. This condition may occur in a girl of any age, but it tends to be more frequent as girls reach puberty; the change to adult pH and the presence of vaginal secretions make the vagina more receptive to infections. Box 47.9 discusses common measures to relieve discomfort.

Preschool and School-Age Children. Vaginal discharge may occur before menarche, but bleeding is rarely seen at this age. If bleeding is present, its cause must be determined. A cystitis can cause urethral bleeding; scratching due to rectal pruritus can lead to rectal bleeding. The cause of true vaginal bleeding in this early age group is usually either irritation caused by an inserted foreign object in the vagina, infestation of pinworms, or *vaginitis* (vaginal inflammation or infection). Sexual abuse must also be investigated as a cause of any bleeding, tenderness, or infection (see Chapter 55). Precocious puberty must also be ruled out.

Treatment for pinworm is discussed in Chapter 43. If there is a foreign body in the vagina, it should be removed. Vaginal examination is necessary, first to locate the object and then to confirm that it has been fully removed. This may be difficult for girls to accept, because vaginal manipulation and stretching can be painful. Use of a small speculum helps reduce the pain. A local antibiotic ointment or warm bath may be ordered to reduce accompanying infection and inflammation afterward (Deligeoroglou et al., 2004).

Sometimes, daily bubble baths cause vulvar irritation. This can be quickly remedied by discontinuing the bubble baths; irritation from such compounds can lead not only to local discomfort but to urinary tract infection as well.

A few preschool or school-age children develop a vaginitis due to *Streptococcus* or to *Escherichia coli* introduced

BOX 47.8 FOCUS ON . . .

FAMILY TEACHING

Preventing Toxic Shock Syndrome

Q. Navi says to you, "I've heard so much about a disease called toxic shock syndrome. What is it and how can I make sure that I don't get it?"

A. Although toxic shock syndrome can occur for other reasons, it most often occurs during a menstrual flow when tampons are used. The following are measures to help prevent the syndrome:

- Use only tampons made of natural materials such as cotton, not synthetics such as cellulose or polyester, and avoid high-absorbency tampons.
- Change tampons at least every 4 hours during use.
- Alternate use of tampons with use of sanitary pads.
- Avoid handling the portion of the tampon that will be inserted vaginally.
- Do not use tampons near the end of a menstrual flow, when excessive vaginal dryness can result from scant flow.
- Do not insert more than one tampon at a time, to avoid abrasions and to keep the vaginal walls from becoming too dry.
- Avoid deodorant tampons, deodorant sanitary pads, and feminine hygiene sprays; these products can irritate the vulvar–vaginal lining.
- If fever, vomiting, or diarrhea occurs during a menstrual period, discontinue tampon use and immediately consult a health care provider, because these are symptoms of TSS.
- Anyone who has had one episode of TSS is well advised not to use tampons again, or at least not until two vaginal cultures for *Staphylococcus aureus,* the bacteria usually responsible for TSS, are negative.

from the anus by improper perineal care after voiding or bowel movements. A tight hymen then traps the microorganisms in the vagina and leads to infection. The girl needs to be reminded to wipe from front to back after voiding or bowel movements.

Adolescents. As a girl enters puberty, she may notice a slight vaginal discharge caused by increased vaginal secretions. She can be reassured that this is normal. To keep from developing vulvar irritation, girls should wear cotton underpants rather than nylon (so that moisture is absorbed better) and should dry the vulva thoroughly after bathing or swimming.

Some girls develop vulvar irritation after using personal hygiene sprays or douches. These products are unnecessary. Good hygiene can be achieved by daily washing and frequent changing of tampons or sanitary pads during menstruation. This will prevent chafing or stasis of menstrual blood and help prevent irritation and excessive odor.

BOX 47.9 FOCUS ON . . .

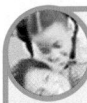

FAMILY TEACHING

Tips for Relieving the Pain of Vulvitis

Q. Navi says to you, "I have a vaginal discharge. The itching is awful. Is there anything I can do to relieve it?"

A. Here are some tips that might help:

- Wash the area twice a day with mild, non-perfumed soap and water, and pat dry. This removes secretions and decreases irritation. Wash and dry from front to back, to prevent spreading rectal contamination forward.
- Take sitz baths or apply warm, moist compresses three times a day to soothe the area and keep it free of irritating drainage.
- After drying the cleansed area, apply cornstarch for comfort and to absorb residual moisture.
- Avoid bubble baths and feminine hygiene sprays, because the ingredients may cause additional local irritation or contribute to urinary tract infections.
- Take acetaminophen (Tylenol) every 4 hours. Acetaminophen is an analgesic that relieves pain and reduces itching, a mild pain sensation.
- Avoid scratching, which may increase abrasions and introduce a secondary infection. Instead, apply a cold compress to relieve the itching sensation.
- Wear cotton underwear, which allows air to circulate and moisture to evaporate, rather than nylon or silk, which prevents air circulation and retains moisture.
- Sleep without underwear.
- Use an anesthetic spray or hydrocortisone cream only as prescribed.
- Carefully follow instructions from your health care provider about caring for a vaginal infection; only after the infection subsides will the vulvitis clear.

Pelvic Inflammatory Disease

Pelvic inflammatory disease (PID) is infection of the pelvic organs: the uterus, fallopian tubes, ovaries, and their supporting structures. The infection can extend to cause pelvic peritonitis. Although sexual transmission accounts for approximately 75% of all cases of PID (gonorrheal and chlamydial organisms are frequently responsible), infections from other causes (e.g., *E. coli, Streptococcus*) are beginning to occur more frequently and may be as severe. Adolescents have a higher incidence of PID than any other age group (Banikarim & Chacko, 2004).

PID begins with a cervical infection that spreads by surface invasion along the uterine endometrium and then out to the fallopian tubes and ovaries. It is most likely to occur at the end of a menstrual period, because menstrual blood provides an excellent growth medium for bacteria and there is loss of the normal barrier of cervical mucus during this time.

Assessment. As peritoneal tissue becomes inflamed and edematous, a purulent exudate forms. If the process is untreated, it enters a chronic phase and fibrotic scarring with stricture of the fallopian tubes results. With acute PID, the adolescent notices severe pain in the lower abdomen. She may have an accompanying heavy, purulent discharge. As the infection progresses, she will develop a fever. Leukocytosis and an elevated erythrocyte sedimentation rate will be present on laboratory testing. During a pelvic examination, any manipulation of the cervix causes severe pain. It may be difficult to palpate the ovaries because of tenderness and abdominal guarding. If the PID enters a chronic phase, the abdominal pain lessens but dyspareunia and dysmenorrhea may be extreme. If the ovaries are affected, intermenstrual spotting may occur. Diagnosis can be aided by sonography or laparoscopy.

Therapeutic Management. Therapy involves administration of analgesia for comfort plus specific broad-spectrum antibiotics such as cefoxitin (Mefoxin), doxycycline (Vibramycin), or clindamycin (Cleocin). Limiting activity also helps relieve the pain. In some women, a pelvic abscess forms and must be drained through the cul-de-sac before healing can occur.

Women who have had one episode of PID have an increased chance of a second occurrence, because the immune protection of the tubes and ovaries may be damaged. They should not have coitus with an infected partner, and they should avoid coitus during menstruation, when their protective mechanisms are lowest. Early childbearing may be recommended if they plan to have children, because extensive tubal scarring could impair fertility. It is important for adolescents to recognize the symptoms of PID and to seek early help for the best outcome.

BREAST DISORDERS

Males have few breast disorders. Gynecomastia (enlarged breast tissue) may occur temporarily in preadolescent boys in response to a rising estrogen level. Particularly noticeable in obese males, this enlargement fades with a normal increase in testosterone production (Wiesman et al., 2004). It may also occur in teens who participate in body-building sports as a result of steroid use. If this is the cause, counseling regarding drug use is crucial. Breast disorders that concern adolescent females include accessory nipples, lesions such as cysts, infection, and injury.

Accessory Nipples

As the name implies, *accessory nipples* are additional breast nipples. They occur along the mammary lines (Fig. 47.2). They usually are not as protuberant as true nipples; they also lack areolar pigmentation. Many girls are unaware that they have an accessory nipple and think it is a large mole. Accessory nipples are present at birth. Parents should be told what they are, so that they can inform their daughter later, because some growth in accessory nipples may occur at puberty or during pregnancy in response to estrogen stimulation.

In a few instances, actual breast tissue is present beneath the accessory nipple. If so, it is subject to the same

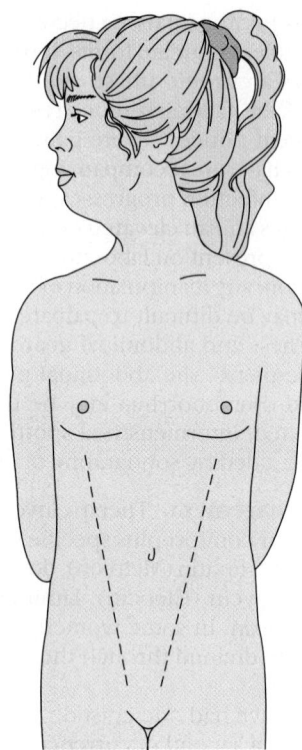

FIGURE 47.2 Nipple lines along which accessory nipples occur.

diseases as other breast tissue. If the accessory nipple or accessory breast tissue is cosmetically distressing to the adolescent, it can be removed by simple surgical excision.

What if... Navi has an accessory nipple with breast tissue underneath? Is this breast tissue susceptible to breast cancer?

Breast Hypertrophy

Breast hypertrophy is abnormal enlargement of breast tissue. In the average girl, breast development halts after puberty, as soon as progesterone levels rise to mature strength. Progesterone levels remain low until menstruation cycles are fully established. If this process is a lengthy one, breast growth may last for several years.

Breast hypertrophy can lead to both physical and emotional stress. The girl may feel pain and fatigue in the back or shoulders from attempting to maintain good posture despite the weight of heavy breast tissue. She may feel self-conscious and try to minimize her breast size by slouching, resulting in poor posture or rounded shoulders.

Adolescent girls with large breasts may find it difficult to adapt to such a new appearance. They may be treated as provocative sex objects and believe they should live up to this image. This can make it difficult for them to find their own identity. They may hear comments such as, "I wish I had your problem," rather than receiving support and understanding from parents, peers, and health care providers.

If breast hypertrophy interferes with a girl's physical and emotional well-being, surgical breast reduction is a possibility. Adolescents need to seriously consider the consequences of this procedure before undertaking it. If a large amount of glandular tissue is removed, breast-feeding may no longer be possible. The adolescent needs to be told realistically that changing her physical appearance will reduce physical discomfort, but changing her self-concept must come from within. An adolescent with large breasts must conscientiously schedule a yearly breast examination, because it is easier for a cancerous lesion to escape detection in large amounts of breast tissue than in a smaller breast. Pregnancy and lactation may be particularly difficult times, because breasts that are already large become even heavier with milk formation.

Breast Hypoplasia

Breast hypoplasia is less-than-average breast size. In most instances, this does not represent a decreased amount of glandular or functional breast tissue but a reduced amount of fatty tissue; as a rule, this will not interfere with breast-feeding in the future. If an adolescent feels that having small breasts interferes with self-esteem, she can have surgical augmentation to increase breast size.

For augmentation, an incision is made under the breast and a saline implant is inserted under the breast tissue, next to the musculus pectoralis major. It is important for the adolescent to realize that her breast tissue is not being replaced by the implant; she could still develop breast cancer in later years.

An adolescent may notice decreased nipple sensation for approximately 1 year after the implant procedure. Breasts with implants in place may feel firmer than normal on palpation due to the formation of a fibrotic band or capsule around the implant.

Breast implants do not interfere with breast-feeding. A traumatic blow to the breast, such as could occur from an automobile accident, requires examination by the augmentation surgeon to be certain that the implant did not rupture, causing its contents to leak into the breast tissue.

Breast Tenderness or Fullness

Many women notice a day or two of premenstrual breast fullness and tenderness each month. Some may find palpable granular or fine nodular lumps in their breasts during this time. This is a benign occurrence and is part of the monthly changes in hormone stimulation. If adolescents choose to do breast self-examination, it should be done after, not before, a menstrual period, because breasts tend to be tender before menstruation. If a lump or tenderness persists beyond one examination, the adolescent should consult a health care provider for additional assessment and care, because the change might signal a lesion or other problem.

Fat Necrosis

If breast tissue is struck during a fall or other traumatic injury, it can become tender, painful, inflamed or reddened, and possibly bruised. A few days later, necrosis or disintegration may occur in the fatty layer. As the area heals, fibrotic scar tissue forms. This may leave a firm, palpable lump in the breast. It is not freely movable; it can cause skin or nipple retraction or dimpling on the skin surface. Unlike malignant breast growths, post-traumatic breast lumps tend to be well delineated.

It is generally recommended that such fibrotic areas be biopsied and then excised. The surgical procedure usually leaves little scarring, and the woman no longer needs to worry about the lump in her breast. Although at one time breast trauma was thought to be a precipitating factor of breast carcinoma, no direct correlation between the two has been established. The association may exist because a woman who examines her breasts after an injury may find an already existing carcinoma.

Fibrocystic Breast Disease

Fibrocystic breast disease is the most common benign breast condition in women of all ages. It can occur as early as puberty, when estrogen rises to adult levels. More commonly, however, it affects women between the ages of 20 and 45 years. Round, fluid-filled cysts form in the connective breast tissue (Fig. 47.3). The woman is able to palpate freely movable, well-delineated breast lumps. Lumps may also be visible on the surface of the breasts (most often in the upper outer quadrant). The consistency of these lesions varies with the menstrual cycle, changing from firm and hard to soft and flexible, depending on the amount of serous fluid present. The lesions tend to shrink or even disappear during pregnancy and lactation, and they totally disappear with menopause.

Fibrocystic breasts can be painful; the breasts may feel tender and "stretched," interfering with active sports and other strenuous activity. This discomfort can be relieved with a simple analgesic, such as acetaminophen (Tylenol), or warm compresses. The formation of fibrocystic lesions may be increased in some women with the use of methylxanthines found in caffeine, theophylline, and theobromine. Advise these women to avoid coffee, cola drinks, tea, chocolate, some toffee candy, and medications such as aspirin compound or Excedrin. Discontinuing smoking can also decrease the occurrence of fibrocystic lesions. De-

creased sodium intake or short-term use of a mild diuretic just before menses can reduce fluid retention.

If these measures do not decrease the fibrocystic symptoms, cysts may be aspirated under a local anesthetic by injection of a thin sterile needle attached to a small syringe. This procedure not only reduces the size of the cyst but also provides fluid for biopsy (Lucas & Cone, 2003).

Oral contraceptives may be prescribed to reduce the symptoms. Danazol (Danocrine), a synthetic androgen, may help reduce the symptoms by suppressing estrogen formation in the ovaries.

In addition to being physically distressed, women with fibrocystic breasts may worry that each lump could be malignant. They can be reassured that the disease itself does not lead to breast carcinoma. Breast carcinoma can occur in a woman with a fibrocystic breast condition, however, and it may even metastasize before she seeks health consultation, if she assumes that all her breast lesions are benign. Therefore, these patients need more consultation than the average woman. In addition to a yearly breast examination, they need to perform monthly breast self-examinations and have an annual breast sonogram, which involves no x-ray exposure and can efficiently locate fluid-filled cysts.

Fibroadenoma

Fibroadenomas are tumors that consist of both fibrotic and glandular components and occur in response to estrogen stimulation. The tumors may increase in size during adolescence, during pregnancy and lactation, or when a woman takes an estrogen source such as an oral contraceptive.

Unlike fibrocystic lesions, fibroadenomas are round and well delineated, feeling firmer and more rubbery than fluid-filled cysts. Occasionally, they calcify and feel extremely hard. They are typically painless and freely movable and tend not to cause skin retraction. Like fibrocystic lesions, they do not become malignant.

Such tumors can be surgically excised so that the woman no longer has to worry about them. Because the incision is small, it leaves little scarring at the site.

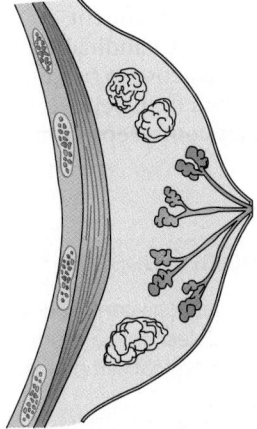

FIGURE 47.3 Round, fluid-filled cysts form in breast tissue in fibrocystic breast disease.

Checkpoint Question 2

Navi wants to have breast augmentation as soon as she's 18. What advice would you give her regarding this?

a. She will not be able to breast-feed after augmentation.
b. Breast implants cause a high degree of fibrocystic disease.
c. She cannot do breast self-examination with implants.
d. Implants do not increase the risk of breast cancer.

SEXUALLY TRANSMITTED INFECTIONS

Sexually transmitted infections (STIs) are those diseases that are spread through sexual contact. They range in severity from easily treated infections, such as trichomoniasis, to human immunodeficiency virus (HIV) infection which, despite advances in therapy, is life-threatening.

If these diseases are discovered in young children, the possibility of sexual abuse must be considered (Hornor, 2004).

Abstinence or condom use provides the best protection against STIs. Condoms should always be used, in addition to washing the genitals well with soap and water, voiding immediately after coitus, and choosing sexual partners who are at low risk for infection (avoiding persons who are intravenous drug users or those with multiple sexual partners). Educate adolescents about safer sex practices, including the need for condom use (see Chapter 4) and the importance of health screening for these disorders (Box 47.10). Also reinforce the fact that little immunity develops from STIs, which means that such diseases can be contracted repeatedly. STIs are becoming more difficult to treat because the causative organisms are becoming more and more resistant to antibiotics. The effects of STIs on pregnancy and the fetus are discussed in Chapter 14.

Candidiasis

The candidal organism is a fungus that thrives on glycogen. As many as 40% of adult females have asymptomatic candidal vaginal infections; this rate rises even higher during pregnancy, when high estrogen levels lead to glycogen levels that produce a favorable environment for fungal growth. Because oral contraceptives produce a pseudo-pregnancy state, pill users also have frequent vaginal candidal infections. When a woman is being treated with an antibiotic (which destroys normal vaginal flora and lets fungal organisms grow more readily), she is particularly susceptible to this infection. Incidence is also strongly associated with diabetes mellitus, because hyperglycemia provides a glucose-rich environment for candidal growth (Deligeoroglou et al., 2004).

Assessment

Because of the scant mucus production in the period before menses, symptoms may be most acute at this time. The adolescent notices vulvar reddening, burning and itching, and even bleeding from hairline fissures. The vagina sometimes shows white "patches" on the walls. The patches are adherent and cannot be scraped away without bleeding. A thick, cream cheese–like discharge can usually be observed at the vaginal introitus. The adolescent may notice pain on coitus or on tampon insertion. Candidal infections may also be present at other body sites, such as the oral cavity or a moist area such as the umbilicus.

Candidal infections are diagnosed by removing a sample of discharge from the vaginal wall and placing it on a glass slide; three or four drops of a 20% potassium hydroxide (KOH) solution are then added, and the mixture is protected by a coverslip. Under a microscope, typical fungal hyphae indicate the presence of *Candida* organisms (Table 47.1).

Therapeutic Management

Therapy for candidal infections includes vaginal suppositories or cream applications of antifungal preparations such as miconazole (Monistat) or clotrimazole, once a day for 3 to 7 days. Oral fluconazole (Diflucan) can be administered as a one-time oral dose (Box 47.11). Teach women to insert vaginal creams or suppositories at bedtime so that the drug does not drain from the vagina immediately afterward. During the day, a girl may want to wear a sanitary pad to avoid staining from vaginal discharge. If an adolescent is sexually active, treatment of the male partner may be necessary to break a reinfection cycle. Treatment should not be interrupted until it is complete, even during a menstrual period. Because miconazole and clotrimazole are available without prescription, adolescents need to be advised how to differentiate a candidal infection from other infections or to consult a health care provider for assistance and treatment.

If a girl has frequent candidal infections, her urine should be tested for glucose to rule out diabetes mellitus. If she is using an oral contraceptive, she might be counseled to use another contraceptive method.

BOX 47.10 FOCUS ON . . .

EVIDENCE-BASED PRACTICE

Do Adolescents Find Home Testing for Sexually Transmitted Infections (STIs) Preferable to Coming to a Clinic for Testing?

For this study, a group of ethnically diverse adolescents, 13 to 20 years old, were given opportunities to use a first-void urine sample or a self-collected vaginal swab sample as home test techniques for STIs. They were then asked which technique they preferred. Results showed that the adolescents preferred home testing to having to go to a clinic for testing. Only 22% would seek any STI screening if asymptomatic. Of the home testing methods, participants found urine collection significantly preferable to vaginal swab sampling.

This is an important study for nurses, because it documents how few adolescents understand the importance of screening for STIs. It also documents how strongly adolescents prefer to screen for disorders by themselves rather than relying on having this done at health care visits. Because nurses are the people who set the tone at health care facilities and make patients feel welcome (or not), it is an alert that any effort to make health care visits more acceptable to adolescents could be important to increase rates of health screening.

Source: Tebb, K. P., et al. (2004). Home STI testing: The adolescent female's opinion. *Journal of Adolescent Health, 35*(6), 462–467.

 Checkpoint Question 3

Candidal vaginal infections can occur as an opportunistic infection when adolescents are prescribed antibiotics. What are the typical symptoms of a candidal vaginal infection?

a. Yellow pinpoint vaginal lesions
b. Pruritic reddened vaginal walls
c. White, cheese-like vaginal discharge
d. Vaginal atrophy with final scarring

TABLE 47.1

Common Vulvovaginal Infections

Causative Agent	Symptoms	Common Therapy
Candida	Vulvar reddening and pruritus; thick, white, cheeselike vaginal discharge	Nystatin or miconazole (Monistat) suppositories or fluconazole (Diflucan) orally; bathing with dilute sodium bicarbonate solution may relieve pruritus
Trichomonas	Thin, irritating, frothy, gray-green discharge; strong, putrid odor; itching	Metronidazole (Flagyl) orally; douching with weak vinegar solution to reduce pruritus
Herpesvirus type II	Painful pinpoint vesicles on an erythematous base with a watery vaginal discharge possible; voiding may be irritating and painful	Bathing with dilute sodium bicarbonate solution, applying lubricating jelly to lesions or an oral analgesic such as aspirin may be necessary for pain relief; topically applied acyclovir (Zovirax) helps heal lesions
Gardnerella	Edema and reddening of vulva, milky gray discharge, fishlike odor	Metronidazole (Flagyl) or clindamycin
Chlamydia trachomatis	Watery, gray-white vaginal discharge, vulvar itching	Tetracycline or doxycycline; erythromycin during pregnancy
Neisseria gonorrhoeae	Possibly symptomless; may have profuse yellow-green vaginal discharge	Ceftriaxone and doxycycline; oral amoxicillin
Enterobius vermicularis (pinworm)	Rectal pruritus, especially on rising in the morning	Oral administration of an anthelmintic, such as mebendazole (Vermox)
Treponema pallidum (syphilis)	Painless ulcer on vulva or vagina	Benzathine penicillin, administered intramuscularly
Streptococcus	Vaginitis, vulvar itching; edema and reddening of vulva	Antibiotic (e.g., amoxicillin)
Foreign body	Vaginal discharge; odor	Removal of foreign body during pelvic examination

BOX 47.11 FOCUS ON . . .

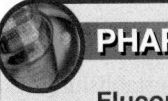

PHARMACOLOGY

Fluconazole (Diflucan)

Classification: Antifungal agent

Action: Increases fungal cell wall permeability, thereby exerting fungicidal or fungostatic action (Karch, 2004)

Pregnancy Risk Category: C

Dosage: 150 mg orally as a single dose

Possible Adverse Effects: Nausea, vomiting; diarrhea, abdominal pain, headache

Nursing Implications
- Instruct the adolescent that this drug is given as a one-time single dose.
- Teach the adolescent about safer sex measures and hygiene practices to help prevent reinfection after therapy.
- Urge the adolescent to watch for signs and symptoms of possible reinfection and report them to the primary care provider.

Trichomoniasis

Trichomonas vaginalis is a single-cell protozoan that is spread by coitus. Up to 25% of adult men and women have asymptomatic trichomoniasis. The incubation period is 4 to 20 days (Simpson & Ivey, 2004).

With a trichomonal infection, females notice vaginal irritation and a frothy white or grayish-green vaginal discharge. The frothiness of the discharge is an important typical finding. The upper vagina is reddened and may have pinpoint petechiae. Extreme vulvar itching is present. By contrast, males with the same infection rarely report any symptoms.

Assessment

The infection is diagnosed by microscopic examination of a sample of the vaginal discharge combined with lactated Ringer's or normal saline solution. Trichomonads typically appear as rounded, mobile structures. Be aware that *Trichomonas* infections cause such inflammatory changes in the cervix or vagina that a Pap test taken during this time may be misinterpreted as showing abnormal tissue.

Therapeutic Management

Oral metronidazole (Flagyl) eradicates trichomonal infections. However, a pregnancy test should be performed before Flagyl is prescribed, because this drug can be teratogenic. Treatment with Flagyl and use of condoms by sexual partners help prevent recurrence of *Trichomonas* in both parties. Because the drug interacts with alcohol to cause acute nausea and vomiting, advise the adolescent not to drink alcoholic beverages during the course of treatment.

Bacterial Vaginosis

Bacterial vaginosis is the invasion of an organism such as *Gardnerella vaginalis*. This organism thrives in the vagina, a body area with a reduced oxygen level. Vaginal discharge is milk-white to gray and has a fishlike odor. Pruritus may be intense. Microscopic examination of the discharge in normal saline solution shows gram-negative rods adhering to vaginal epithelial cells, which are termed *clue cells* (Syed & Braverman, 2004).

The treatment is oral metronidazole for 7 days; the woman's sexual partners should also be treated to prevent recurrence of the infection. Bacterial vaginosis, like other STIs, may be spread to women having sex with women as well (Bailey et al., 2004).

Chlamydia trachomatis Infection

Chlamydia trachomatis infections have become the most common bacterial cause of STI in the United States (Deligeoroglou et al., 2004). Symptoms include a heavy, grayish-white discharge and vulvar itching. The incubation period is 1 to 5 weeks. Diagnosis is made by culture of the organism. Therapy is oral doxycycline or tetracycline for 7 days. *Chlamydia* infection in a mother can cause eye infection or pneumonia in the newborn (see Chapter 14). During pregnancy, the infection is treated with erythromycin, because tetracycline is teratogenic. Because it has become so common, most public health departments require that any cases be reported.

Genital Warts (Human Papillomavirus)

Genital warts are lesions caused by the human papillomavirus (HPV). They are rapidly growing structures on the vulva, vagina, or cervix. Large growths can become cancerous and may be excised by cautery or cryotherapy. Small growths may be removed by applying podophyllin. Children (both male and female) with genital warts should be further investigated for sexual abuse (Hornor, 2004).

Herpes Genitalis

Genital herpes is caused by *herpesvirus hominis* type 2 (also called herpes simplex virus type 2, or HSV-2). This is one of four similar herpesviruses: cytomegalovirus, Epstein-Barr, varicella-zoster, and herpes types 1 and 2. Genital herpes occurs in epidemic proportions in the United States, and its incidence appears to be growing yearly (Trager, 2004). Unlike most other STIs, there is no known cure. The disease involves a lifelong process, and, although it is not a precursor to cervical cancer, women with cervical cancer have more antibodies against herpes genitalis than others do. The virus is spread by skin-to-skin contact,

entering through a break in the skin or mucous membrane. In the newborn, the virus can be systemic or even fatal (see Chapter 26).

Assessment

Herpes is diagnosed by culture of the lesion secretion from its location on the vulva, vagina, cervix, or penis or by isolation of HSV antibodies in serum. The incubation period is 3 to 14 days. On first contact, extensive primary lesions originate as a group of pinpoint vesicles on an erythematous base. Within a few days, the vesicles ulcerate and become moist, draining, open lesions. The adolescent may have accompanying flulike symptoms with an increased temperature; vaginal lesions may cause a profuse discharge. Pain is intense on contact with clothing or acidic urine.

After the primary stage that lasts approximately 1 week, lesions heal but the virus lingers in a latent form, affecting the sensory nerve ganglia. The condition will flare up and become an active infection during illness, PDD, fever, overexposure to sunlight, or stress. A secondary response usually produces only local lesions rather than systemic symptoms.

Therapeutic Management

Acyclovir (Zovirax) controls the virus by interfering with deoxyribonucleic acid reproduction and decreasing symptoms. The drug is available as a topical ointment. If applying this to a client, protect yourself with a finger cot or glove so that you do not contract the virus or absorb the drug. Sitz baths three times a day and applying a soothing substance such as cornstarch to reduce discomfort afterward may be helpful. An emollient (A & D Ointment) can also reduce discomfort, but its moisture tends to prolong the active period of the lesions. Topical imiquimod (Aldara) may be prescribed for resistant lesions.

Because of the possible association with cervical cancer, any female with genital herpes should have yearly Pap tests for the rest of her life. Condoms help prevent the spread of herpes among sexual partners.

People with herpes may have difficulty establishing sexual relationships for fear of infecting a partner. Because herpes is communicated only by direct contact, infected people need to inform their partners when they have any active lesions and avoid sexual contact or use a condom to decrease the danger of spreading the virus.

Hepatitis B and Hepatitis C

Both hepatitis B and hepatitis C can be spread by semen as well as blood and therefore are considered STIs. These are discussed in Chapter 45, with other forms of hepatitis. Because hepatitis B can be spread by sexual intercourse, adolescents need immunization against hepatitis B (see Chapter 43).

Gonorrhea

Gonorrhea is transmitted by *Neisseria gonorrhoeae*, a gram-positive diplococcus that thrives on columnar transitional epithelium of the mucous membrane. Symptoms begin after a 2- to 7-day incubation period. In males, they include *urethritis* (pain on urination and frequency of urination) and a urethral discharge. Without treatment, the infection may spread to the testes, scarring the tubules and causing permanent sterility. Untreated, the infection is easily spread among sexual partners. It often occurs concurrently with chlamydial infection (Nsuami et al., 2004).

Although symptoms of gonorrhea in females are not as visible, there may be a slight yellowish vaginal discharge. Bartholin's glands may become inflamed and painful. If left untreated, the infection may spread to pelvic organs, most notably the fallopian tubes (PID). Tubal scarring can result in permanent sterility. In both males and females, untreated gonorrhea can lead to arthritis or heart disease from systemic involvement.

An infant can contract gonorrhea in the birth canal from its mother. This leads frequently to gonorrheal ophthalmia (discussed in Chapter 14).

Assessment

A urine culture for the gonococcal bacillus, in addition to vaginal and urethral cultures, should be obtained from all children with vulvovaginitis or a urethral discharge. In males, a first voiding may reveal gonococci if a midstream urine specimen is inconclusive.

Therapeutic Management

The treatment for gonorrhea is one intramuscular injection of ceftriaxone (Rocephin) plus oral doxycycline (Vibramycin) for 7 days (Centers for Disease Control and Prevention, 2005). This treatment regimen is effective for both gonorrhea and chlamydia. Sexual partners should receive the same treatment.

Approximately 24 hours after treatment, gonorrhea is no longer infectious. Approximately 7 days after treatment, a client should return for a follow-up culture to verify that the disease has been completely eradicated (few people take this precaution). Adolescents are usually assessed for syphilis along with the gonorrheal culture, although the dose of ceftriaxone and doxycycline is also effective treatment for syphilis. Most states require that gonorrhea be reported to the health department; adolescents are asked to name sexual contacts.

NURSING DIAGNOSES AND RELATED INTERVENTIONS

●

Nursing Diagnosis: Anxiety related to having contracted a reportable STI

Outcome Evaluation: Adolescent voices confidence in his or her ability to cope with this problem and demonstrates understanding of both the illness and the treatment regimen.

People who seek treatment for an STI need to believe that they can trust health care personnel and reveal information without fear of criticism. Assure the adolescent of absolute confidentiality in naming his or her sexual contacts. Without being told who put them at risk, these people can then be notified by a health department investigator that they have been exposed to a particular STI. This vital information helps prevent further spread of the disease.

Some people are reluctant to seek treatment for gonorrhea because they have heard stories that therapy involves 10 to 15 days of intramuscular injections. Because they have no symptoms, some girls may avoid going for what they think will be extremely painful treatment. Reassure them that the treatment is simple. This is an insidious disease, and, even though no symptoms are apparent, it can have disastrous long-term effects if left untreated (Box 47.12).

Syphilis

Syphilis is a systemic disease caused by the spirochete *Treponema pallidum.* It is transmitted by sexual contact with a person who has an active spirochete-containing lesion (Trager, 2004). Like gonorrhea and chlamydia, it must be reported to public health departments.

After an incubation period of 10 to 90 days, a typical lesion appears, usually on the genitalia (penis or labia) or on the mouth, lips, or rectal area due to oral-genital or genital-anal contact. The lesion (termed a *chancre*) is a deep ulcer and is usually painless despite its size. Lymphadenopathy may be present but is unlikely to be noticed by the affected person. A lesion in the vagina may not be detected. Without treatment, a chancre lasts approximately 6 weeks and then fades.

Approximately 2 to 4 weeks after the chancre disappears, a generalized, macular, copper-colored rash appears. Unlike many other rashes, it affects the soles and the palms. A serologic test for syphilis yields a positive result at this time. There may be secondary symptoms of generalized illness, such as low-grade fever and adenopathy. With or without treatment, this stage of syphilis also fades.

The next stage is a latency period that may last from only a few years to several decades. The only indication of the disease is the serologic test, which continues to yield a positive result.

The final stage of syphilis is a destructive neurologic disease that involves major body organs such as the heart and the nervous system. Typical symptoms are blindness; paralysis; severe, crippling neurologic deformities; mental confusion; slurred speech; and lack of coordination. This third stage must be identified before the disease becomes fatal.

Assessment

Syphilis is diagnosed by recognition of the various symptoms of the three stages and by serologic serum tests, usually the Venereal Disease Research Laboratory test (VDRL),

BOX 47.12: Focus on Nursing Care Planning

A Multidisciplinary Care Map for An Adolescent With Gonorrhea

•

Navi is a 15-year-old female high school student you meet at a pediatric clinic. She describes intense vulvar irritation from a yellowish vaginal discharge.

Family Assessment

Navi lives with mother in studio apartment in inner city. Mother works at home as a freelance journalist. Mother describes finances as "good."

Client Assessment

Well-proportioned female; sexual maturity Tanner stage 3. Has not had first menstrual period as yet. Sexually active for approximately 1 year with same partner. "He doesn't use a condom any more because he's only dating me."

Vulva reddened and excoriated. Yellow-green discharge noted at vaginal introitus. Reddened areas noted on vaginal walls. One dose of intramuscular (IM) ceftriaxone (Rocephin), plus oral doxycycline (Vibramycin) for 7 days, is prescribed. She asks, "How did I get this? From my boyfriend? Does he need to be treated too?"

Nursing Diagnosis

Deficient knowledge related to cause and treatment of sexually transmitted infection (STI).

Outcome Evaluation

Adolescent states that she understands cause of STI; reports boyfriend has an appointment within 48 hours for evaluation.

Team Member Responsible	Assessment	Intervention	Rationale	Expected Outcome
Activities of Daily Living				
Nurse	Assess whether adolescent understands importance of washing hands well after using bathroom and avoiding sexual intercourse during treatment.	Discuss how disease can be spread to other body parts by unclean hands.	Gonorrhea is particularly hazardous, because it can cause eye infections with corneal scarring.	Adolescent states that she will take precautions to wash hands well; she will avoid sexual intercourse until repeat culture.
Consultations				
Nurse	Confer with STI counselor.	Meet with STI counselor regarding procedure for STI contacts.	Gonorrhea is a reportable disease.	STI counselor assumes responsibility for securing STI contacts.
Procedures/Medications				
Nurse	Assess whether adolescent has experience with taking medicine. Assess if a reminder sheet would be helpful.	Administer ceftriaxone (Rocephin) IM; give instructions for oral doxycycline (Vibramycin) for 7 days as prescribed.	The antibiotics chosen for gonorrhea treatment are also effective against Chlamydia, which is frequently associated with gonorrhea.	Adolescent accepts IM injection; states she understands importance of taking oral antibiotic for full 7 days.

(continued)

Team Member Responsible	Assessment	Intervention	Rationale	Expected Outcome
Procedures/Medications				
Nurse	Assess whether adolescent has access to a bathtub at home.	Recommend the use of sitz baths before and after school.	Sitz baths are soothing and help keep the area free of irritating discharge.	Adolescent states she will use home bathtub for sitz baths twice daily.
Nutrition				
Not applicable (NA)	Not applicable (NA)	Not applicable (NA)	Not applicable (NA)	Not applicable (NA)
Patient/Family Education				
Nurse	Assess whether adolescent is aware that STIs are spread through sexual intercourse.	Teach adolescent about the cause, means of spread, and treatment for gonorrhea.	Adolescent must be aware of STIs to prevent them in the future.	Adolescent states that she understands STIs are spread by sexual relations.
Psychosocial/Spiritual/Emotional Needs				
Nurse	Assess intensity of adolescent's pruritus or pain from vulvitis on a scale of 1 to 10.	Discuss the use of acetaminophen or ibuprofen for pain and pruritus as prescribed.	Acetaminophen and ibuprofen are effective analgesics for mild pain and itching.	Adolescent describes correct dosage of analgesics and states intention to use them.
STI counselor	Assess whether adolescent has had sexual contacts other than current boyfriend.	Ask adolescent to name any additional sexual contacts.	Sexual contacts need to be notified so they also can receive treatment.	Adolescent names any other sexual contacts; possibility of rape or abuse is ruled out.
Discharge Planning				
Nurse	Assess whether adolescent understands that she must ask boyfriend to use a condom for sexual relations.	Discuss the possibility that, because he contracted an STI, his relationship with her may not be monogamous. Explain that nonmonogamous relations make condom use even more important, not less important.	STI was spread to her by a sexual contact.	Adolescent states she will be more conscientious about insisting boyfriend use a condom.
Nurse	Assess whether child or parent has any questions about disease or therapy.	Schedule child for a return appointment in 1 week for reculture.	A repeat culture will reveal whether antibiotic therapy has been effective.	Child and parent state that they understand the importance of a repeat culture and will keep return appointment.

the automated reagin test (ART), the rapid plasma reagin test (RPR), or the fluorescent treponemal antibody absorption test (FTA-ABS).

Therapeutic Management

Benzathine penicillin G, given intramuscularly in two sites, is effective therapy. For the adolescent who is sensitive to penicillin, either oral erythromycin or tetracycline can be given for 10 to 15 days. Sexual partners are treated in the same way as the person with the active infection. Therapy effectively arrests the disease at whatever stage it has reached.

Because syphilis can be treated so easily, one would think it would be easy to eradicate. In reality, however, because the primary chancre is painless, many people are either unaware of it or choose to ignore it, thereby transmitting the disease to unsuspecting partners. Adolescents, in particular, need accurate information about syphilis to become aware of the symptoms. They should believe that they can report the disease to health care personnel and can name sexual contacts without fear of being criticized. If a woman develops syphilis during pregnancy, the disease can be spread to the fetus (see Chapter 14).

Human Immunodeficiency Virus

HIV is carried by semen as well as other body fluids, so infection with this virus is considered an STI. Invasion of the virus is discussed with other immune disorders in Chapter 42, and in relation to pregnancy in Chapter 14.

What if... Navi tells you she feels safe from contracting an STI because she knows she is up to date with her immunizations? How would you counsel her?

Key Points

Children who are born with a reproductive tract disorder frequently adjust well when young. They may need counseling at puberty or when they become aware of the impact of their disorder on sexual functioning or their ability to reproduce.

The cause of ambiguous genitalia is unknown but may be related to the level of testosterone produced in utero. The true gender of children is established by a karyotype of chromosomes.

The development of breast or pubic hair before age 8 years or menses before age 9 years is considered precocious sexual development. Children may be treated with a synthetic analog of Gn-RH to reduce development. Without effective support, such children are at high risk for disturbed body image.

Delayed puberty is the failure to develop secondary sex characteristics by the age of 17 years. Girls may be administered estrogen to promote development; boys may be administered testosterone.

Balanoposthitis (inflammation of the glans and prepuce) and phimosis (constricted foreskin) occur in boys. Phimosis can be treated with circumcision.

Cryptorchidism is failure of one or both testes to descend during intrauterine life. The condition is surgically corrected to prevent infertility and to detect testicular cancer later in life.

Testicular cancer is rare but tends to occur in young men. Boys need to be taught testicular self-examination for early detection.

Dysmenorrhea, or painful menstruation, occurs frequently in adolescent girls. Therapy is the use of a prostaglandin inhibitor such as ibuprofen.

Untreated endometriosis (the abnormal growth of extrauterine endometrial tissue) can lead to infertility

later in life. Therapy is administration of a synthetic androgen or GnRH receptor inhibitor or surgery to reduce the size of the abnormal tissue.

Vulvovaginitis (inflammation of the vulva and vagina) and PID are infections that can occur in adolescents. Therapy to prevent fallopian tube scarring and infertility later in life is essential. Girls need to be taught, in addition, ways to avoid toxic shock syndrome.

Conditions such as fibrocystic breast disease can occur in adolescents. Reducing intake of caffeine and sodium can minimize symptoms.

STIs such as candidiasis, trichomoniasis, *C. trachomatis* infection, genital warts, herpes genitalis, gonorrhea, and syphilis are increasing in incidence in the adolescent population. An important health-teaching area for adolescents is the need to follow safer sex practices.

When teaching about STIs, it is important to stress that they do not confer immunity and therefore can be contracted more than once. If an STI occurs in a young child, the potential for child abuse should be investigated.

Critical Thinking Exercises

1. Navi is the 15-year-old girl you met at the beginning of the chapter, who was diagnosed as having gonorrhea. She says she is glad she contracted the disease early in life, because now she will never get it again. She also states that she is not sexually active. What health teaching does Navi need to be better informed about her disease? What other follow-up is needed?
2. Navi has almost no breast development and also has not menstruated yet. She asks you if it is time to worry. How would you counsel her?
3. Ryan, the boy whom Navi dates, was born with undescended testes. He had surgery for this condition when he was 2 years old. He is concerned now that he is at high risk for testicular cancer. How would you counsel him?
4. Examine the National Health Goals related to reproductive disorders in children. Most government-sponsored money for nursing research is allotted based on these goals. What would be a possible research topic to explore pertinent to these goals that would be applicable to Navi's family and also advance evidence-based practice?

References

Akin, M., et al. (2004). Continuous, low-level, topical heat wrap therapy as compared to acetaminophen for primary dysmenorrhea. *Journal of Reproductive Medicine, 49*(9), 739–745.

Austin, J. C., & Zderic, S. A. (2003). Penile and foreskin problems. In Schwartz, M. W. (Ed.), *5-minute pediatric consult* (3rd ed.). Philadelphia: Lippincott Williams & Wilkins.

Bagarazzi, M. L., & Conway, D. H. (2003). Toxic shock syndrome (TSS). In Schwartz, M. W. (Ed.), *5-minute pediatric consult* (3rd ed.). Philadelphia: Lippincott Williams & Wilkins.

Bailey, J. V., Farquhar, C., & Owen, C. (2004). Bacterial vaginosis in lesbians and bisexual women. *Sexually Transmitted Diseases, 31*(11), 691-694.

Banikarim, C., & Chacko, M. R. (2004). Pelvic inflammatory disease in adolescents. *Adolescent Medicine Clinics, 15*(2), 273-285.

Batt, R. E., & Mitwally, M. F. (2003). Endometriosis from thelarche to midteens: Pathogenesis and prognosis, prevention and pedagogy. *Journal of Pediatric and Adolescent Gynecology, 16*(6), 337-347.

Braverman, P. K., & Breech, L. (2004). Management quandary. Menorrhagia in a teenager: Von Willebrand disease type 1. *Journal of Pediatric and Adolescent Gynecology, 17*(1), 61-64.

Centers for Disease Control and Infection. (2005). *STD fact sheets.* Washington, DC: DHHS.

Cole, F. L., & Vogler, R. (2004). The acute, nontraumatic scrotum: Assessment, diagnosis, and management. *Journal of the American Academy of Nurse Practitioners, 16*(2), 50-56.

Deligeoroglou, E., et al. (2004). Infections of the lower female genital tract during childhood and adolescence. *Clinical and Experimental Obstetrics and Gynecology, 31*(3), 175-178.

Department of Health and Human Services. (2000). *Healthy people 2010.* Washington, D.C.: DHHS.

Durain, D. (2004). Primary dysmenorrhea: Assessment and management update. *Journal of Midwifery and Women's Health, 49*(6), 520-528.

Food and Drug Administration, Department of Health and Human Services. (2004). Medical devices; labeling for menstrual tampons; ranges of absorbency, change from "junior" to "light." Final rule. *Federal Register, 69*(164), 52170-52171.

French, L. (2005). Dysmenorrhea. *American Family Physician, 71*(2), 285-291.

Granella, F., et al. (2004). Characteristics of menstrual and nonmenstrual attacks in women with menstrually related migraine referred to headache centres. *Cephalalgia, 24*(9), 707-716.

Herrinton, L. J., Zhao, W., & Husson, G. (2003). Management of cryptorchism and risk of testicular cancer. *American Journal of Epidemiology, 157*(7), 602-605.

Hill, M., & Vujevich, K. T. (2004). Advisor forum. Homing in on hydroceles. *Clinical Advisor, 7*(5), 46.

Hornor, G. (2004). Ano-genital warts in children: Sexual abuse or not? *Journal of Pediatric Health Care, 18*(4), 165-170.

Jick, H., Kaye, J. A., & Jick, S. S. (2004). Antidepressants and the risk of suicidal behaviors. *Journal of the American Medical Association, 292*(3), 338-343.

Johnson, J. (2003). Infertility. In Scott, J. R., et al. (Eds.), *Danforth's obstetrics and gynecology* (9th ed.). Philadelphia: Lippincott Williams & Wilkins.

Karch, A. M. (2004). *Lippincott's nursing drug guide.* Philadelphia: Lippincott Williams & Wilkins.

Kelly, A., & Ferry, R. J. Jr. (2003). Sexual precocity. In Schwartz, M. W. (Ed.), *5-minute pediatric consult* (3rd ed.). Philadelphia: Lippincott Williams & Wilkins.

Lucas, J. H., & Cone, D. L. (2003). Breast cyst aspiration. *American Family Physician, 68*(10), 1983-1986.

Mansbach, J. M., & Gordon, C. M. (2002). Demystifying delayed puberty. *Patient Care for the Nurse Practitioner, 1*(1), 1-8.

McCullagh, J., & Lewis, G. (2005). Testicular cancer: Epidemiology, assessment and management. *Nursing Standard, 19*(25), 45-55.

McEvoy, M., Chang, J., & Coupey, S. M. (2004). Common menstrual disorders in adolescence: Nursing interventions. *American Journal of Maternal Child Nursing, 29*(1), 41-49.

Midyett, L. K., Moore, W. V., & Jacobson, J. D. (2003). Are pubertal changes in girls before age 8 benign? *Pediatrics, 111*(1), 47-51.

Misra, S., Chaturvedi, A., & Misra, N. C. (2004). Penile carcinoma: A challenge for the developing world. *Lancet Oncology, 5*(4), 240-247.

Nichols, J. (2003). Dysmenorrhea. In Schwartz, M. W. (Ed.), *5-minute pediatric consult* (3rd ed.). Philadelphia: Lippincott Williams & Wilkins.

Nsuami, M., et al. (2004). Chlamydia and gonorrhea co-occurrence in a high school population. *Sexually Transmitted Diseases, 31*(7), 424-427.

Ogilvy-Stuart, A. L., & Brain, C. E. (2004). Early assessment of ambiguous genitalia. *Archives of Disease in Childhood, 89*(5), 401-407.

Raj, G. V., & Wiener, J. S. (2004). Facing the dilemma of adolescent varicoceles. *Contemporary Urology, 16*(7), 23-27.

Rangecroft, L. (2003). Surgical management of ambiguous genitalia. *Archives of Disease in Childhood, 88*(9), 799-801.

Simpson, T., & Ivey, J. (2004). Pediatric management problems: Trichomonas vaginalis. *Pediatric Nursing, 30*(3), 228-229.

Syed, T. S., & Braverman, P. K. (2004). Vaginitis in adolescents. *Adolescent Medicine Clinics, 15*(2), 235-251.

Tebb, K. P., et al. (2004). Home STI testing: The adolescent female's opinion. *Journal of Adolescent Health, 35*(6), 462-467.

Trager, J. D. (2004). Sexually transmitted diseases causing genital lesions in adolescents. *Adolescent Medicine Clinics, 15*(2), 323-352.

Wiesman, I. M., et al. (2004). Gynecomastia: An outcome analysis. *Annals of Plastic Surgery, 53*(2), 97-101.

Wiegratz, I., & Kuhl, H. (2004). Long-cycle treatment with oral contraceptives. *Drugs, 64*(21), 2447-2462.

Wren, T. (2004). Penile and testicular disorders. *Nursing Clinics of North America, 39*(2), 319-326.

Wu, H. Y., & Kolon, T. F. (2003). Cryptorchidism. In Schwartz, M. W. (Ed.), *5-minute pediatric consult* (3rd ed.). Philadelphia: Lippincott Williams & Wilkins.

Suggested Readings

Arca, M. J., & Caniano, D. A. (2004). Breast disorders in the adolescent patient. *Adolescent Medicine Clinics, 15*(3), 473-485.

Jennings, J., et al. (2004). Sex partner concurrency, geographic context, and adolescent sexually transmitted infections. *Sexually Transmitted Diseases, 31*(12), 734-739.

Jones, A. E. (2004). Managing the pain of primary and secondary dysmenorrhoea. *Nursing Times, 100*(10), 40-43.

Kaunitz, A. M. (2004). Choosing to menstruate—or not. *Patient Care for the Nurse Practitioner, 1*(1), 1-8.

Leung, A. K., & Robson, W. L. (2004). Current status of cryptorchidism. *Advances in Pediatrics, 51*(2), 351-377.

Lustyk, M. K. B., et al. (2004). Stress, quality of life and physical activity in women with varying degrees of premenstrual symptomatology. *Women and Health, 39*(3), 35-44.

Mazza, D. (2004). Dysmenorrhoea in adolescence. *Practice Nurse, 27*(10), 30-34.

Mullen, B. A. (2004). Testicular complaints and the young man. *Journal of the American Academy of Nurse Practitioners, 16*(11), 490-495.

Proctor, M. L., & Murphy, P. A. (2005). Herbal and dietary therapies for primary and secondary dysmenorrhoea. *The Cochrane Library (Oxford) (1)* (CD002124).

CHAPTER 48

Nursing Care of the Child With an Endocrine or Metabolic Disorder

Key Terms

carpal spasm
exophthalmos
glycosuria
hormones
hyperfunction
hyperglycemia
hypofunction
hypoglycemia
hypothalamus
ketoacidosis
latent tetany
manifest tetany
pedal spasm
polydipsia
polyuria
sella turcica
Somogyi phenomenon

Objectives

After mastering the contents of this chapter, you should be able to:

1. Describe the structure and function of the various endocrine glands.
2. Assess a child with a disorder of endocrine function.
3. Formulate nursing diagnoses for a child with altered endocrine or metabolic function.
4. Develop expected outcomes for a child with endocrine or metabolic dysfunction.
5. Plan nursing care such as health teaching for a child with altered endocrine or metabolic function.
6. Implement nursing care such as teaching insulin administration to a child with an endocrine or metabolic disorder.
7. Evaluate expected outcomes to be certain goals of nursing care were achieved.
8. Identify National Health Goals related to childhood endocrine or metabolic disorders nurses could help the nation achieve.
9. Identify areas related to care of children with endocrine or metabolic disorders that could benefit from additional nursing research or application of evidence-based practice.
10. Analyze ways that care of the child with altered endocrine or metabolic function can be family centered.
11. Synthesize knowledge of endocrine and metabolic dysfunctions and the nursing process to ensure quality maternal and child health nursing care.

Rob Tebecco is a 16-year-old boy with type 1 diabetes whom you meet in the emergency room, where he was taken after he became comatose while ice skating. His diabetes was diagnosed when he was 7 years old. His records indicate that his disease has generally been under good control over the past years, but in the last 6 months he has "forgotten" to take his insulin at least once a week. When you ask him about this, he tells you that ice skating practice every morning and a new girlfriend have occupied his time and interrupted what used to be a strict schedule of home-cooked meals and a rigid routine.

Previous chapters described the growth and development of well children. This chapter adds information about the dramatic changes, both physical and psychosocial, that occur when children develop an endocrine or metabolic disorder. This is important information because it builds a base for care and health teaching.

Is Rob's history unusual for an adolescent?
What health teaching do you think will most help him re-establish control?

After you've studied this chapter, access the accompanying website. Read the patient scenario and answer the questions to further sharpen your skills, grow more familiar with RN-CLEX types of questions, and reward yourself with how much you have learned.

The endocrine system is composed of a small group of ductless glands that work together with the neurologic system to regulate and coordinate all body systems (Fig. 48.1). The glands produce chemicals called **hormones,** which are secreted into surrounding tissue and picked up by the bloodstream, where they act individually and in concert to affect various organ systems. (The word *hormone* is from the Greek *hormaein,* which means "to set in motion.") Each gland of the endocrine system has specific functions that are necessary for regulating body processes; each hormone secreted acts on a specific target (or designated) organ.

Dysfunction of the glands or action of the hormones results in a variety of disorders, most of which have long-term implications. Parents—and children, as soon as they are old enough—need to understand these diseases to the best of their ability and to participate in their long-term plan of care. National Health Goals related to endocrine and metabolic disorders in children are presented in Box 48.1.

Nursing Process Overview

For Care of a Child With an Endocrine or Metabolic Disorder

● *Assessment*

Endocrine and metabolic disorders as a group commonly cause changes in normal growth or activity patterns. This is usually detected when height and weight are assessed and compared with standards for the

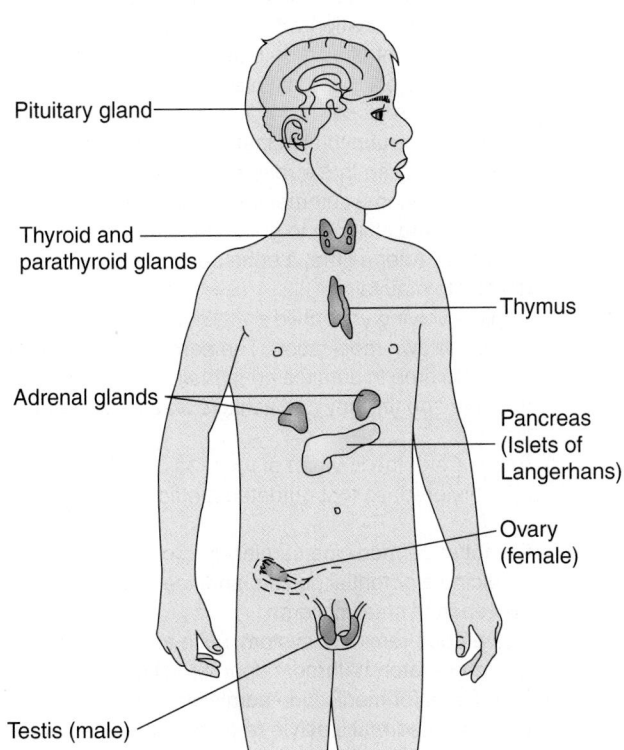

FIGURE 48.1 Location of the endocrine glands.

Pituitary gland

Thyroid and parathyroid glands

Adrenal glands

Testis (male)

Thymus

Pancreas (Islets of Langerhans)

Ovary (female)

BOX 48.1 FOCUS ON . . .

NATIONAL HEALTH GOALS

Diabetes mellitus is an endocrine disorder with serious consequences in both children and pregnant women. A number of National Health Goals address reducing the incidence of this disease:

• Reduce the annual rate of diabetes-related deaths, from a baseline of 8.8 per 1,000 to no more than 7.8 per 1,000 people.
• Increase the proportion of persons with diabetes who receive formal diabetes education, from a baseline of 45% to a target of 60%.
• Decrease the proportion of pregnant women with gestational diabetes (DHHS, 2000).

Nurses can help the nation achieve these goals by educating women about the possible effects of diabetes on pregnancy and by educating children about ways to prevent the long-term effects of the illness. Nursing research could shed additional light on these goals by asking questions such as, How should women be taught that fetal anomalies from hyperglycemia occur very early in pregnancy, so they must be certain to enter pregnancy in good glucose control? Long-term effects of diabetes are not noticeable in childhood, but how can children be educated to plan a healthy lifestyle to prevent these effects in adult life? At what age can children be expected to be responsible for glucose monitoring and insulin injection? What methods are best for encouraging children to be in charge of their own nutrition?

child's age at a health visit. Obese children may have thyroid deficiencies. Short children may have pituitary difficulties. An acute loss in weight is often the first symptom of type 1 diabetes mellitus in children. As more and more children become obese, children are developing type 2 diabetes as well.

To obtain information on activity, take a day history by asking the parent or child to describe all of the child's actions on a typical day. This type of information yields clues that are helpful in distinguishing between a normally "quiet" child and one who is experiencing inactivity and chronic fatigue as a result of decreased endocrine function. For example, the quiet child lies down after school and reads; the ill child lies down and sleeps. Taking a day history also helps to differentiate between a child who is merely active and one who is overly active because of hyperthyroidism. For example, the healthy child appears to "go constantly" but can sit through a favorite television program or a meal. The child with increased thyroid hormone production may be unable to sit quietly at all.

Also assess dietary and elimination habits. Extreme thirst or appetite may occur with an endocrine disorder such as diabetes insipidus or type 1 diabetes mellitus. Frequent voiding in children most often reflects a urinary tract infection, but it may be evidence of excessive urine excretion (**polyuria**), possibly from pituitary dysfunction or diabetes mellitus.

On physical examination, observe a child's general appearance, noting any excessive tiredness, scaling or dry skin, drooping eyelids, protrusion of the eyeballs (**exophthalmos**), or poor muscle tone (Box 48.2).

● Nursing Diagnosis

Because endocrine glands control vital body functions, nursing diagnoses relevant to children with endocrine or metabolic disorders include both physiologic functions and the child's response to those changes. Some examples of such nursing diagnoses are the following:

- Deficient fluid volume related to constant excessive loss of fluid through urination
- Risk for imbalanced nutrition, less than body requirements, related to inability to use glucose because of diabetes mellitus
- Disturbed body image related to abnormal height
- Health-seeking behaviors related to self-administration of insulin
- Deficient knowledge related to long-term treatment needs
- Fear related to potential illness outcome
- Anticipatory grieving related to presumed losses associated with diagnosis of long-term illness
- Interrupted family processes related to child's chronic illness

● Outcome Identification and Planning

Although most endocrine and metabolic disorders have long-term implications, parents and children may find it easier to work with outcomes initially that are short-term—particularly if they are having difficulty accepting the diagnosis and the long-term nature of the disorder. Because symptoms usually are not acute, children may easily forget to take medications or the parents may forget to give the medications. Helping parents create reminder charts is an effective measure to increase adherence (Box 48.3).

Evaluate the school as well as the home situation for any child with a chronic illness. You may need to instruct teachers about the child's health problem (with the parents' permission) so that they do not make excessive or inappropriate demands (e.g., insisting that

---

BOX 48.3 FOCUS ON . . .

FAMILY TEACHING

Guidelines for Successful Long-Term Medicine Administration

Q. Rob's mother says to you, "Rob keeps forgetting to take his insulin. What can we do to make sure that he continues to take it regularly for the rest of his life?"

A. Here are some helpful tips to increase the success of long-term medication therapy:

1. Teach children about the type and purpose of the medicine they will be taking. Knowing the purpose of something maintains interest and cooperation.
2. If mixing a medication with food or fluid, use only a small amount of fluid or food to avoid opposition from the child and ensure that the child takes the necessary dose.
3. Always be certain to anticipate the need to obtain prescriptions, so that a ready supply is on hand before vacations, summer camp, and holidays.
4. Avoid bribing children to get them to take their medicine. After a time, a bribe becomes too difficult to maintain.
5. Begin involving your child early in administering his or her own medication. The earlier you can involve children in administering their own medication, the sooner they can achieve an independent lifestyle.
6. Be aware of the lifespan of the medicine being administered, so that outdated medication is not used.
7. Do not store medicine carelessly. Consider all medicine a potential poison, and keep it out of the reach of small children.
8. Use a dose-reminder system, such as a chart on the refrigerator, bathroom door, or school locker.
9. Plan times for medication administration that allow for a normal lifestyle (e.g., not getting up at 2 AM or having to interrupt a school class for an injection).

BOX 48.2 ASSESSMENT

Assessing a Child With an Endocrine Disorder

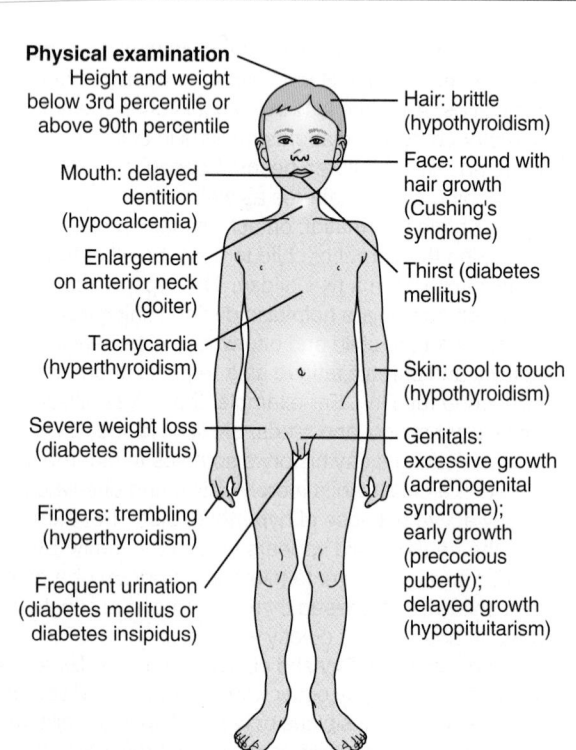

Physical examination

Height and weight below 3rd percentile or above 90th percentile

Hair: brittle (hypothyroidism)

Mouth: delayed dentition (hypocalcemia)

Face: round with hair growth (Cushing's syndrome)

Enlargement on anterior neck (goiter)

Thirst (diabetes mellitus)

Tachycardia (hyperthyroidism)

Severe weight loss (diabetes mellitus)

Skin: cool to touch (hypothyroidism)

Genitals: excessive growth (adrenogenital syndrome); early growth (precocious puberty); delayed growth (hypopituitarism)

Fingers: trembling (hyperthyroidism)

Frequent urination (diabetes mellitus or diabetes insipidus)

a child with hyperthyroidism submit neat handwriting assignments when the child cannot do so).

Selected organizations for referral include the following:

- American Diabetes Association (*www.diabetes.org*)
- Congenital Adrenal Hyperplasia Support Group (*www.cah.org.uk*)
- Little People of America (*www.lpaonline.org*)
- National Tay-Sachs and Allied Diseases Association (*www.ntsad.org*)

● *Implementation*

Interventions for children with endocrine or metabolic disorders must always be carried out with long-term aspects of care in mind. Bribing children to take a medicine, for example, is never good practice. It has no place with children who must continue to take a medication for the rest of their lives (bribery quickly becomes ineffective). As children grow older and can better understand their disorder, explanations of why they must continue to take medication need to become more detailed.

● *Outcome Evaluation*

Children with disorders of endocrine or metabolic function need to be evaluated periodically throughout childhood, because growth and changing activities necessitate changes in medication dosages or schedules. These checkups provide good opportunities for health teaching to equip children to meet new situations that arise as they mature. For example, body appearance (i.e., being like, not unlike, their peers) becomes increasingly important as children enter adolescence. Because of this, seemingly well-adjusted school-age children may develop extreme difficulty continuing to accept their illness as they get older. Adherence to a medication program may become erratic. Only by periodic reevaluation can these problems be identified so that health care plans can be modified and adapted to the child's needs, enabling the child and family to continue coping with a long-term illness.

The following examples suggest that the desired outcomes have been achieved:

- Child brings to clinic written record illustrating conscientious medicine ingestion.
- Parents list developmentally appropriate, not size appropriate, activities for their child with short stature.
- Child's blood pressure and pulse remain within normal limits for age; specific gravity of urine is between 1.003 and 1.030; skin turgor is good; child states thirst is not excessive.
- Parents demonstrate correct insulin injection technique and state they are comfortable administering an injection to their child.

THE PITUITARY GLAND

The work of the pituitary gland is directed by the **hypothalamus,** an organ located in the center of the brain that is the regulator of the autonomic nervous system. About 1 cm long, 1.0 to 1.5 cm wide, and 0.5 cm thick, the pituitary rests in the **sella turcica,** a depression of the sphenoid bone. It is covered by a tough membrane, which also joins the gland to the hypothalamus.

The pituitary gland has several distinct regions: the anterior lobe, or *adenohypophysis;* the posterior lobe, or *neurohypophysis;* and the intermediate lobe (*pars intermedia*), which lies between the anterior and posterior lobes. Each of these regions appears to have its own function and secretes specific hormones.

Pituitary Hormones

The regions of the pituitary gland store and release eight hormones. Four of these—antidiuretic hormone, thyrotropin, corticotropin, and somatotropin—are prominently involved in childhood illnesses (Table 48.1).

PITUITARY GLAND DISORDERS

Illnesses caused by pituitary dysfunction can result from a tumor growing in the pituitary or hypothalamus, interference with circulation to the gland, trauma, inflammation, structural abnormalities, erratic or nonfunctional feedback mechanisms, and, possibly, autoimmune responses.

Growth Hormone Deficiency

If production of human growth hormone (GH, or somatotropin) is deficient, children cannot grow to full size. As a result, they remain in proportion but well below the average on a standard growth chart. Deficient production of GH may result from a nonmalignant cystic tumor of embryonic origin that places pressure on the pituitary gland or from increased intracranial pressure (e.g., from trauma). In most children with hypopituitarism, the cause of the defect is unknown (Alter, 2003).

If a child with hypopituitarism is not treated, predicting exactly what height will be reached is difficult because height varies with each individual. Without treatment, however, most children will not reach more than 3 or 4 feet in height.

Assessment

The child with deficient production of GH is usually normal in size and weight at birth. Within the first few years of life, however, the child begins to fall below the third percentile of height and weight on growth charts. The face appears infantile because the mandible is recessed and immature; the nose is usually small. The child's teeth may be crowded in a small jaw (and may erupt late). The child's voice may be high pitched, and the onset of pubic, facial, and axillary hair and genital growth is delayed. History, physical findings, and a decreased level of circulating GH contribute to the diagnosis.

Evaluate the family history for traits of short stature or constitutional delay (familial late development). If at all possible, obtain estimates of the parents' height and siblings' height and weight during their periods of growth. Assess thoroughly the child's prenatal and birth history for any suggestion of intrauterine growth retardation or severe head trauma at birth, which could have injured the

TABLE 48.1

Common Pituitary Hormones and Their Purposes

Pituitary Hormone	Source and Target Organs	Actions and Effects
Antidiuretic hormone (ADH)	Secreted by the neurohypophysis *Target organ:* Kidney	• ADH helps regulate fluid volume and urine output. It decreases urinary output by increasing water reabsorption. This action increases extracellular fluid volume, resulting in a vasoconstrictor effect (increased blood pressure). When the plasma concentration increases or overall circulating vascular volume decreases, more ADH is released. • If blood pools in the body periphery, decreasing core body volume, ADH is released. • Postural changes (from a lying to a standing position) and exposure to high temperatures (blood shifts to peripheral structures to begin the cooling process) stimulate ADH release. • Trauma, pain, and anxiety increase ADH release. • When ADH levels fall, little or no water is reabsorbed, and urinary output increases. • Alcohol consumption inhibits ADH secretion; as a result, urine output increases.
Corticotropin (ACTH)	Secreted by the adenohypophysis *Target organ:* Adrenal glands	• ACTH stimulates the adrenal gland to produce glucocorticoid and mineralocorticoid hormones. Increased production of adrenal gland secretions decreases ACTH production and vice versa. • If a child receives synthetic ACTH or a corticosteroid, natural ACTH production is temporarily depressed. If these synthetic hormones are given for a long time, then stopped abruptly, the decreased amount of natural ACTH may not be enough to stimulate adrenal gland activity. The child will experience symptoms of adrenal insufficiency. • When discontinuing ACTH and high doses of long-term corticosteroids, dosage must be reduced gradually to protect adrenal function. The medication should never be stopped abruptly.
Somatotropin (growth hormone; GH)	Secreted by the adenohypophysis *Target organ:* None; acts on all body cells	• GH increases bone and cartilage growth and increases gastrointestinal absorption of calcium. If GH production is inhibited, dwarfism will occur; if GH production is excessive, gigantism or overgrowth will occur. • GH decreases catabolism of protein in cells by freeing fatty acids for energy, which, in turn, frees glucose for glycogen storage (GH is both protein and glucose sparing). • GH production increases when hypoglycemia occurs and during sleep. • GH is released from the adenohypophysis based on a release factor from both the hypothalamus and the liver. • The amount of GH secretion is influenced by exercise, sleep, nutrition, and thyroid and adrenal function.
Thyrotropin (TSH)	Secreted by the adenohypophysis *Target organ:* Thyroid gland	• TSH stimulates the thyroid gland to produce thyroid hormones (thyroxine and triiodothyronine). • Too little TSH leads to atrophy and inactivity of the thyroid gland; too much TSH causes hypertrophy (increase in size) and hyperplasia (increase in the number of cells) of the gland. • A feedback message of increased thyroid secretion lowers TSH production; decreased thyroid production increases TSH production.

pituitary gland. Assess the health history for any chronic illness, such as a heart, kidney, or intestinal disorder, that could have contributed to the decreased level of growth. Take a 24-hour nutrition history and ask carefully about urinary and bowel function. Parents often report that their child is a "picky eater," yet the 24-hour history does not reveal a poor appetite that is extensive enough to halt growth. Be certain to assess not only the child's actual height but also his or her feelings about being short.

A pituitary tumor must be ruled out as the cause of decreased GH production. Sudden halted growth suggests a tumor; gradual failure suggests an idiopathic involvement. A history of vision loss, headache, increase in head circumference, nausea, and vomiting (signs of increased intracranial pressure) also suggests a pituitary tumor. The history of a child with GH deficiency typically reveals a well child except for the abnormal lack of growth. Growth failure is so marked, however, that the parents may be suspected of child neglect (Marcus & Collins, 2004).

A physical assessment, including a funduscopic examination and neurologic testing, is necessary to detect a lesion or tumor. Blood studies for hypothyroidism, hypoadrenalism, and hypoaldosteronism are performed, because these conditions also influence growth. The wrist is examined radiographically to determine bone age. Epiphyseal closure of long bones is delayed with GH deficiency but is proportional to the height delay. A skull series, computed tomographic (CT) scanning, magnetic resonance imaging (MRI), or sonography will be performed to detect possible enlargement of the sella turcica, which would suggest a pituitary tumor. Blood is drawn for measurement of growth factor binding proteins (Alter, 2003).

Therapeutic Management

GH deficiency is treated by the administration of intramuscular (IM) recombinant human growth hormone (rhGH) two or three times a week (Box 48.4). The timing of the dose affects the hormone's effectiveness; GH is usually given at bedtime, the time of day at which GH normally peaks. Because these children have delayed epiphyseal closure, if treatment is started early, they will be able to reach a targeted height. Some may need suppression of luteinizing hormone-releasing hormone (LHRH, or gonadotropin-releasing hormone [GnRH]) to delay epiphyseal closure. Other children may need supplements of gonadotropin or other pituitary hormones if these are deficient as well.

A slight increase in the incidence of leukemia among children treated with rhGH has been noted (Alter, 2003). Parents need to be aware of this association, but should not be unduly frightened by it, because it may be due to other predisposing factors.

NURSING DIAGNOSES AND RELATED INTERVENTIONS

Nursing Diagnosis: Situational low self-esteem related to short stature

Outcome Evaluation: Child speaks positively about self; identifies friends and activities enjoyed with peers.

If a child has been consistently behind in growth since early life, parents may simply assume in early childhood that the child is going to be short as an adult. The parents then may become concerned only after the child reaches puberty and fails to develop secondary sex characteristics. If investigation reveals the child's true problem, parents may feel guilty that they did not become alarmed earlier.

BOX 48.4 FOCUS ON . . .

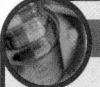

PHARMACOLOGY

Somatropin (Nutropin, Humatrope)

Classification: Somatropin is a recombinant human growth hormone (rhGH).

Action: Used for the long-term treatment of children who have growth failure from inadequate production of pituitary hormone, renal failure, or Turner's syndrome; may be used to promote healing in severe burns (Karch, 2004)

Pregnancy Risk Category: C

Dosage: Somatropin dosage is individualized. The drug is administered by injection.

Possible Adverse Effects: Injection site pain, glucose intolerance, hypothyroidism, bone problems (particularly the hip), blood abnormalities, rare intracranial hypertension in first 8 weeks of therapy

Nursing Implications
- Advise parents that radiographs of the wrist or hip are performed before therapy begins. Thereafter, parents should be alert for limping or knee or hip pain, which should be reported to their primary care provider. Slipped capital epiphysis is associated with rhGH supplementation.
- Reinforce the need for periodic thyroid function tests and funduscopic examination (to detect rare intracranial hypertension).
- Tell parents that rhGH may interact with glucocorticoid therapy (e.g., prednisone), causing a decrease in the effectiveness of the rhGH. Urge parents to inform all health care practitioners that the child is receiving rhGH.
- Keep in mind that administration of rhGH is associated with a possible increased risk of leukemia.

They may feel resentment toward health care personnel who did not alert them to the problem earlier. Encourage parents to discuss these feelings, and provide support to help them accept their child in this new light as well as participate in making the new plan of care a success (Box 48.5). You may need to remind parents to assign duties and responsibilities to children that match their chronologic age, not their physical size, in order to promote their feelings of maturity and self-esteem. Children, too, may need some help in accepting themselves at the ultimate height they achieve, especially if this is only in the 5th percentile, not the 50th (Carel et al., 2003).

Growth Hormone Excess

Overproduction of GH usually is caused by a tumor of the anterior pituitary (an adenoma). If an overproduction occurs before the epiphyseal lines of the long bones have closed, excessive growth results (Krieger et al., 2003). Weight is excessive also, but it is proportional to height. The skull circumference typically exceeds normal, and the fontanelles may close late or not at all. Such excessive growth usually becomes evident at puberty, when prepubertal growth is great. *Acromegaly* (enlargement of the bones of the head and soft parts of the hands and feet) may accompany the early excessive growth in stature, although acromegaly becomes more pronounced after the epiphyseal lines of the long bones close and linear growth is no longer possible. Acromegaly can cause the tongue to be

so enlarged and thickened that it protrudes from the mouth, giving the child a dull, apathetic appearance and difficulty in articulating words. If the condition remains untreated, a child may reach a height of more than 8 feet. Radiographs or sonograms of the skull reveal enlargement of the sella turcica.

If the cause of the increased hormone production is a tumor, laser surgery to remove the tumor or cryosurgery (freezing of tissue) is the primary treatment. If no tumor is present, irradiation or radioactive implants of the pituitary may be successful in reducing the abnormal GH production. In other children, a GH antagonist is prescribed. Because other hormones may be affected when GH secretion is halted in this way, it may be necessary for the child to receive supplemental thyroid extract, cortisol, and gonadotropin hormones in later life.

It is difficult for a child always to be bigger and taller than playmates, and the problem continues to be very real and distressing in adulthood. These children need to be identified during regular health screening to determine the cause of excessive growth and to offer treatment.

Diabetes Insipidus

Diabetes insipidus is a disease in which there is decreased release of antidiuretic hormone (ADH) by the pituitary gland (Thornton, 2003). This causes less reabsorption of fluid in the kidney tubules. Urine becomes extremely dilute, and a great deal of fluid is lost from the body. Diabetes insipidus may reflect an X-linked dominant trait, or it may be transmitted by an autosomal recessive gene. It

---

BOX 48.5 FOCUS ON . . .

COMMUNICATION

Rob, a 16-year-old with diabetes, is short in stature. While observing him and his mother, you notice that Rob is wearing clothes more suitable for a preteen than an adolescent.

Less Effective Communication

Nurse: Mrs. Tebecco, do you have any questions about Rob's care?

Mrs. Tebecco: No. I'm worried that soon he'll be wanting a driver's license. I'm lucky he's so short he can't really drive yet.

Nurse: Is he happy being so short?

Mrs. Tebecco: It's made him better at gymnastics than the taller boys. Probably because he looks so much younger than he is.

Nurse: Well, that's good. Sometimes it's hard for children with a chronic disease to be happy.

More Effective Communication

Nurse: Mrs. Tebecco, do you have any questions about Rob's care?

Mrs. Tebecco: No. I'm worried that soon he'll be wanting a driver's license. I'm lucky he's so short he can't really drive yet.

Nurse: Is he happy being so short?

Mrs. Tebecco: It's made him better at gymnastics than the taller boys. Probably because he looks so much younger than he is.

Nurse: But how does he feel about his size? How do you think he'll feel in the future?

Mrs. Tebecco: I can't even think about that. I don't want to lose my baby.

Nurse: Let's talk a little bit about how his growing up makes both of you feel before we review his insulin injection technique.

Many children with endocrine or metabolic disorders are short in stature. This characteristic causes them to be viewed as cute and petite by parents and treated as if they were younger than their true chronologic age. Parents can enjoy their child's short stature, because it makes it seem as if the child will remain a child longer, and not grow up and be independent. Exploring how parents and the child feel about this misperception can help them see that all children grow older chronologically even if they appear still young.

may result from a lesion, tumor, or injury to the posterior pituitary; or it may have an unknown cause. In a rare type of diabetes insipidus, pituitary function is adequate, but the kidneys' nephrons are not sensitive to ADH (a kidney-related etiology).

Assessment

The child with diabetes insipidus experiences excessive thirst (**polydipsia**) that is relieved only by drinking water, not breast milk or formula, as well as polyuria. The specific gravity of the urine is low (1.001 to 1.005); normal values are more often 1.010 to 1.030. Urine output may reach 4 to 10 L in a 24-hour period (normal range, 1 to 2 L), depending on age.

Signs and symptoms of diabetes insipidus usually appear gradually. Parents may notice the polyuria first as bed-wetting in a toilet-trained child. Weight loss occurs because of the large loss of fluid. If the condition remains untreated, the child will lose such a quantity of water that dehydration and death may result.

Radiography, CT scanning, or ultrasound study of the skull reveals whether a lesion or tumor is present. A further test is the administration of vasopressin (Pitressin) to rule out kidney disease. After the child's urine output has been measured, to establish a baseline, vasopressin is administered. The drug decreases the blood pressure, alerting the kidney to retain more fluid to maintain vascular pressure. If the fault that is causing the dilute urine is with the pituitary, not the kidney, the child's urine output will decrease; if the fault is with the kidney, urine will remain dilute and excessive in amount.

Therapeutic Management

Surgery is the treatment of choice if a tumor is present. If the cause is idiopathic, the condition can be controlled by the administration of desmopressin (DDAVP), an arginine vasopressin. In an emergency, this drug can be given intravenously (IV). For long-term use, it is given intranasally or orally. If desmopressin is given as an intranasal spray, children should use the small tube supplied with the medication to deposit the prescribed dose well into the nose. Nasal irritation may result from intranasal administration, and such administration will not be effective if the child has an upper respiratory tract infection and swollen mucous membranes. Caution children that they will notice an increasing urine output just before the next dose is due (Karch, 2004).

NURSING DIAGNOSES AND RELATED INTERVENTIONS

●——————

Nursing Diagnosis: Risk for deficient fluid volume related to constant, excessive loss of fluid through urination

Outcome Evaluation: Child's blood pressure and pulse are within normal limits for age; specific gravity of urine is between 1.003 and 1.030; skin turgor is good; child states thirst is not excessive.

Teach About Long-Term Therapy. If an IM medication is prescribed, the child and at least one parent must learn the injection technique to ensure adherence. Be sure to explain the difference between diabetes insipidus and diabetes mellitus, the disorder most people think of when they hear the word "diabetes," so that the family is not confused about differences in therapy. Help the family establish a routine to ensure that the child receives adequate fluid to discourage a feeling of thirst and has access to bathroom facilities possibly more frequently than others.

Encourage Communication. Caution parents that, when seeking any type of health care, they should always notify health care providers that the child has diabetes insipidus. For example, surgery poses particular dangers because of the fluid restrictions that accompany most procedures. Encourage children to wear a medical alert tag identifying them as having diabetes insipidus. With the child's and parents' permission, inform school personnel that the child may need to use the bathroom frequently; help the child and family plan frequent bathroom stops and adequate fluid intake on long trips or activity-filled days.

THE THYROID GLAND

The thyroid gland is responsible for controlling the rate of metabolism in the body through production of the hormones thyroxine (T_4) and triiodothyronine (T_3) by its follicular cells.

A third hormone, thyrocalcitonin, is produced by the interstitial cells of the gland. Thyrocalcitonin is released if a high serum calcium level occurs. This hormone inhibits bone resorption, thereby slowing the rate of release of calcium from bone to plasma and resulting in a lowered serum calcium level. It reflects the reverse action of parathyroid hormone, which elevates serum calcium levels.

Assessment of Thyroid Function

Radioimmunoassay of T_4 and T_3 is a specific blood study to determine how much protein-bound iodine (PBI) is present. If a child has recently taken large amounts of cough medicine containing iodide or underwent a study using an iodine-based contrast medium (e.g., urography, bronchography), the PBI level may be abnormally elevated. The small amount of iodine ingested from iodized salt does not affect PBI levels.

Children who have low circulating albumin levels can have abnormally low PBI levels, because iodine is carried bound to protein. Phenytoin (Dilantin), a common anticonvulsant medication prescribed for children with recurrent seizures, may displace thyroxine from binding globulin and further contribute to these low PBI levels.

Another test of thyroid function is a radioactive iodine uptake test. The child is given an oral dose of a solution containing radioactive iodine (^{123}I). The thyroid gland "traps" this iodine, and 24 hours later, after the maximum amount has been trapped, the amount of radioactive iodine present can be determined. It is important in this type of test that the child swallow all the solution. In infants, the solution usually is given as a gavage feeding, so that accuracy of the dose can be ensured.

An uptake of less than 10% of the test dose suggests hypothyroidism. If the child vomits after ingesting the substance, this event should be recorded and called to the attention of the laboratory; it will obviously result in a lower uptake value, because only a part of the actual dose will be available for uptake. Be certain that the child does not receive iodine or thyroid extract in any other form during the test time, because it will compete with uptake of the radioactive iodine and, again, produce a falsely low value.

THYROID GLAND DISORDERS
Congenital Hypothyroidism

Thyroid hypofunction causes reduced production of both T_4 and T_3. Congenital **hypofunction** (reduced or absent function) usually occurs as a result of an absent or nonfunctioning thyroid gland. The condition may not be noticeable initially, because the mother's thyroid hormones maintain adequate levels in the fetus during pregnancy. The symptoms of congenital hypothyroidism become apparent, however, during the first 3 months of life in a formula-fed infant and at about 6 months in a breast-fed infant. The disorder occurs in 1 of every 4,000 live births and about twice as often in girls as in boys (Grimsberg, 2003). Because congenital hypothyroidism causes progressive physical and cognitive challenges, early diagnosis is crucial. In most states, a screening test for hypothyroidism is mandatory at birth (using the same few drops of blood obtained for a Guthrie or phenylketonuria [PKU] test).

Assessment

Parents may report that their child sleeps excessively. The tongue becomes enlarged, causing respiratory difficulty, noisy respirations, or obstruction. The child may suck poorly because of sluggishness or choking. The skin of the extremities usually feels cold, and the overall body temperature may be subnormal because of slowed metabolism. A slow metabolic rate is also revealed by slow pulse and respiratory rates. Prolonged jaundice may be present, due to the immature liver's inability to conjugate bilirubin. Anemia may increase the child's lethargy and fatigue.

The child's neck appears short and thick. The facial expression becomes dull, as the result of being cognitively challenged, and open-mouthed because of the child's attempts to breathe around the enlarged tongue. The extremities appear short and fat, with hypotonic muscles, giving the infant a floppy, rag-doll appearance. Deep tendon reflexes are slower than normal. Generalized obesity usually occurs. Hair is brittle and dry. Dentition is de-

layed, or teeth may be defective when they do erupt. A sonogram reveals a small or absent thyroid gland (Eugster et al., 2004).

The hypotonia affects the intestinal tract as well, so the infant develops chronic constipation; the abdomen enlarges because of intestinal distention and poor muscle tone (Fig. 48.2). Many infants have an umbilical hernia. Overall, the skin is dry and perhaps scaly, and the child does not perspire. Infants have low radioactive iodine uptake levels, low serum T_4 and T_3 levels, and elevated thyroid-stimulating factor. Blood lipids are increased. Radiographs may reveal delayed bone growth.

Therapeutic Management

The treatment for hypothyroidism is oral administration of synthetic thyroid hormone, sodium levothyroxine. A small dose is given at first, and then the dose is gradually increased to therapeutic levels. The child needs to continue taking medication indefinitely to supplement that which the thyroid does not make. Supplemental vitamin D may also be given to prevent the development of rickets when, with the administration of thyroid hormone, rapid bone growth begins.

Further cognitive challenges can be prevented as soon as therapy is started, but any degree of impairment that is already present cannot be reversed.

Helping parents administer medication over a long period is a major nursing role. Be certain that parents know the rules for long-term medication administration with children, particularly the rule about not putting medicine in a large amount of food (thyroxine tablets must be crushed and added to food or a small amount of formula or breast milk) (see Box 48.3). Periodic monitoring of T_4 and T_3 helps to ensure an appropriate medication dosage. If the dose of thyroid hormone is not adequate, the T_4 level will remain low, and there will be few signs of clinical improvement. If the dose is too high, the T_4 level will rise, and the child will show signs of hyperthyroidism: irritability, fever, rapid pulse, and perhaps vomiting, diarrhea, and weight loss.

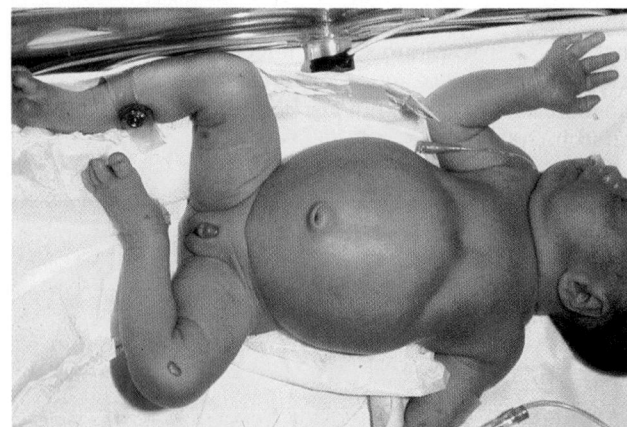

FIGURE 48.2 An infant with congenital hypothyroidism. Notice the short, thick neck and enlarged abdomen. (© David/NMSB/Custom Medical Stock Photo.)

Acquired Hypothyroidism (Hashimoto's Disease)

Hashimoto's disease is the most common form of acquired hypothyroidism in childhood; the age at onset is often 10 to 11 years, and there may be a family history of thyroid disease. It occurs more often in girls than in boys. The decrease in thyroid secretion is caused by the development of an autoimmune phenomenon that interferes with thyroid production. Excretion of thyroid-stimulating hormone (TSH) from the pituitary increases when thyroid hormone production decreases, in an attempt to cause the thyroid to be more effective (Foley, 2004).

Assessment

In response to TSH, hypertrophy of the thyroid gland (goiter) occurs, and body growth is impaired by lack of thyroxine. In infants, congenital goiter can lead to airway obstruction; in children, prominent symptoms are obesity, lethargy, and delayed sexual development.

Antithyroid antibodies will be present in serum if the illness was caused by an autoimmune process. The thyroid not only enlarges but may become nodular in response to the oversecretion of TSH. Although in childhood a nodular thyroid is usually benign, an investigation into the possibility of thyroid malignancy must be considered. For diagnosis, children are administered radioactive iodine. If the nodes are benign, there is generally a rapid uptake of radioactive iodine ("hot nodes"). If there is no uptake ("cold nodes"), carcinoma is a much more likely diagnosis (rare at this age).

Therapeutic Management

Treatment for acquired hypothyroidism is the administration of synthetic thyroid hormone (sodium levothyroxine), the same as for congenital hypothyroidism. With adequate dosage, the obesity diminishes and growth begins again. It is important that the disease be recognized as early as possible so there is time to stimulate growth before the epiphyseal lines close at puberty.

If acquired hypothyroidism exists in a woman during pregnancy, her infant can be born cognitively challenged. Therefore, it is important that girls with this syndrome be identified before they reach childbearing age.

Hyperthyroidism (Graves' Disease)

Hyperthyroidism is oversecretion of thyroid hormones by the thyroid gland. In children, it usually occurs at the time of puberty or during adolescence and is more common in girls than in boys (Gruneiro-Papendieck et al., 2003). Overactivity of the thyroid gland can occur from the gland's being overstimulated by TSH from the pituitary gland due to a pituitary tumor. More frequently, hyperthyroidism in children is caused by an autoimmune reaction that results in production of immunoglobulin G (IgG), which stimulates the thyroid gland to overproduce thyroxine. An exophthalmos-producing pituitary substance causes the prominent-appearing eyes that accompany hyperthyroidism in some children.

Assessment

Graves' disease often follows a viral illness or a period of stress. Some children may have a genetic predisposition to development of the disorder. With overproduction of T_3 and T_4, children gradually experience nervousness, loss of muscle strength, and easy fatigue. Their basal metabolic rate is high; blood pressure and pulse are increased. They perspire freely. They are always hungry, and, although they eat constantly, they do not gain weight and may even lose weight because of the increased basal metabolic rate. On radiography, bone age appears advanced beyond the chronologic age of the child. Unless the condition is treated, the child will not be able to reach normal adult height, because epiphyseal lines of long bones will close before normal height is attained.

The thyroid gland, which usually is not prominent in children, appears as a swelling on the anterior neck (goiter). This enlargement can be confirmed by ultrasound. When the child protrudes the tongue or extends the hands, fine tremors are noticeable. In a few children, the eye globes are prominent (exophthalmos), giving the child a wide-eyed, staring appearance. Laboratory tests show elevated T_4 and T_3 levels and increased radioactive iodine uptake. TSH is low or absent because the thyroid is being stimulated by antibodies, not by the pituitary gland.

Therapeutic Management

Therapy consists first of a course of a beta-adrenergic blocking agent, such as propranolol, to decrease the antibody response. After this, the child is placed on an antithyroid drug, such as propylthiouracil (PTU) or methimazole (Tapazole), to suppress the formation of thyroxine. While the child is taking these drugs, the blood is monitored for leukopenia (decreased white blood cell count) and thrombocytopenia (decreased platelet count), side effects of the drugs. If either of these results, the drug is discontinued until the white blood cell or platelet count returns to normal, so the child does not develop an infection or experience spontaneous bleeding.

Because the thyroid stores considerable thyroid hormone that must be used up first, it takes about 2 weeks for these drugs to have an effect. The child usually has to take the drug for 2 to 3 years before the condition "burns itself out." The exophthalmos may not recede, but it will not become worse after therapy is instituted.

If the child has a toxic reaction to medical management (severely lowered white blood cell count or platelet count) or is noncompliant about taking the medicine, radioiodine ablative therapy with ^{131}I to reduce the size of the thyroid gland can be accomplished (Read et al., 2004). Surgical removal of part or almost all of the thyroid gland, which may be necessary in a young adult, also can be completed safely (Sugino et al., 2004). After both radioiodine ablative therapy and thyroidectomy, supplemental thyroid hormone therapy may be needed indefinitely because the gland is no longer able to produce an adequate amount.

NURSING DIAGNOSES AND RELATED INTERVENTIONS

Nursing Diagnosis: Situational low self-esteem related to lack of coordination and presence of prominent goiter

Outcome Evaluation: Child states positive traits about self and identifies friends and activities enjoyed.

Hyperthyroidism begins gradually and may become fairly involved before it is detected. Suspect children at puberty of having hyperthyroidism if they are losing weight or having behavior problems in school because of hand tremors and tongue tremors that make it hard for them to write or speak. Behavior problems may also arise because of nervousness and inability to sit still during class.

Offer parents support to supervise medication administration, so that they can be certain the child takes the medicine every day. Caution children not to stop taking the medicine abruptly or a thyroxine crisis (sudden onset of extreme symptoms of hyperthyroidism) can occur. Parents may ask if their child can have surgery as a cure so that long-term administration of medicine will not be required. Help them understand that surgery may not dispel the need for medication; if a large portion of the thyroid gland is removed, it may be necessary to give medicine indefinitely to make up for the missing gland. In any event, it is preferable to try a course of medical management before resorting to surgery.

Because the onset of hyperthyroidism is gradual, children may be aware of their difficulties in school before their parents are. Exophthalmos may lead to an appearance about which other children tease them. After therapy, encourage children to return to activities that require fine coordination or social interaction and to think of themselves as well again.

Checkpoint Question 1

Rob's sister developed hyperthyroidism (Graves' disease) at puberty. Which is a typical appearance she would have shown?

a. Slow, lethargic movements.
b. Swollen protuberant abdomen.
c. Jittery, nervous mannerisms.
d. Reduced intellectual processing.

THE ADRENAL GLAND

The two adrenal glands are located retroperitoneally, just above each kidney. (Because of their location, they are also referred to as suprarenal glands.) The adrenal glands are made up of two distinct parts, which differ not only in tissue origin but also in function. The *adrenal medulla* is a small core surrounded by the *adrenal cortex.* Although each of these parts has different functions and releases different hormones, together they protect the body against acute and chronic forms of stress.

Adrenal Hormones

The adrenal cortex produces cortisol (a glucocorticoid), androgen, and aldosterone (a mineralocorticoid)—three hormones that can cause childhood illness. Norepinephrine and epinephrine, hormones important for maintaining blood pressure, are produced by the adrenal medulla.

Cortisol

Cortisol, a glucocorticoid that is necessary for glucose and protein metabolism, is released by the adrenal cortex in response to adrenocorticotropic hormone (ACTH) stimulation from the pituitary gland. ACTH is strongly influenced by biorhythm or circadian rhythms. In the hours just before and after a person awakens, ACTH reaches its highest peak. The level decreases again gradually throughout the day and night. The level of ACTH secretion also increases during periods of emotional stress, leading to increased production of cortisol. Severe trauma, major surgery, hypotension, extreme cold, and acute or chronic illness also increase production of cortisol.

Cortisol is necessary during a time of stress to provide the body with readily available glucose and protein for emergency processes. It elevates serum glucose by increasing the amount of glucose formed by the liver (gluconeogenesis), decreasing use of glucose by tissue, and releasing free fatty acids from tissue stores into the plasma, to make them available for energy. To increase available protein, protein synthesis in cells is halted, which frees up amino acids for liver production of protein.

Cortisol is also important in decreasing an inflammatory response. In the bloodstream, it causes a reduced number of eosinophils and lymphocytes, whereas production of red blood cells and platelets is increased. A drawback of this response is that the decreased number of lymphocytes may allow infection to occur.

Aldosterone

Aldosterone is secreted in response to the renin-angiotensin system, serum potassium, and sodium levels. Renin is released from kidney nephrons in response to a lowered blood pressure; shortly thereafter, it is converted to angiotensin II. In the presence of angiotensin II, aldosterone is released from the adrenal cortex. This causes retention of sodium and water and elevates blood pressure. When angiotensin is decreased, the production of aldosterone stops. When serum potassium levels rise, aldosterone secretion increases. Lowered levels of potassium decrease aldosterone secretion. Sodium influences aldosterone by a reverse process: when sodium levels are low, aldosterone secretion increases; an increased sodium concentration inhibits aldosterone secretion.

The end result of aldosterone secretion is always sodium retention by the body. As sodium is retained, fluid is also retained. Aldosterone plays a direct role in stabilizing blood volume and pressure because of its role in maintaining sodium balance. Infants born with an inability to produce aldosterone quickly become dehydrated, and their lives can be in immediate danger.

Androgen

Androgen is the hormone responsible for muscular development, increase in linear size, growth of body hair, and the increase in sebaceous gland secretions that cause typical acne at puberty (see Chapters 32 and 47).

ADRENAL GLAND DISORDERS

Disorders of the adrenal gland include those related to hypofunction, which can lead to acute or chronic insufficiency, and those related to **hyperfunction** (overactivity), which most often leads to overproduction of androgen or cortisol.

Acute Adrenocortical Insufficiency

Insufficiency (hypofunction) of the adrenal gland may be either acute or chronic. In many adrenal syndromes, only one hormone is involved, and the symptoms are directly related only to that hormone. In acute adrenocortical insufficiency, the function of the entire cortical adrenal gland suddenly becomes insufficient. Usually this occurs in association with severe overwhelming infection, typically involving hemorrhagic destruction of the adrenal glands. It is seen most commonly in meningococcemia. It also can occur when corticosteroid therapy that has been maintained at high levels for long periods is abruptly stopped.

Assessment

The symptoms of acute adrenocortical insufficiency are acute and sudden. The blood pressure drops to extremely low levels; the child appears ashen gray and may be pulseless. Temperature becomes elevated; dehydration and **hypoglycemia** (an abnormally low concentration of blood glucose) are marked. Sodium and chloride blood levels are very low, but serum potassium is elevated, because there is usually an inverse relationship between sodium and potassium values. The child is prostrate, and seizures may occur. Without treatment, death can occur abruptly (Lecamwasam et al., 2004).

Therapeutic Management

Treatment involves the immediate replacement of cortisol (with IV hydrocortisone sodium succinate [Solu-Cortef]); administration of deoxycorticosterone acetate (DOCA), the synthetic equivalent of aldosterone; and IV 5% glucose in normal saline solution to restore blood pressure, sodium, and blood glucose levels. A vasoconstrictor may be necessary to elevate the blood pressure further.

Acute adrenocortical insufficiency is a medical emergency. Although it is seen less often now than in the past, because of the availability of antibiotics that quickly halt the course of infectious disease, it is not an obsolete entity. Now that more conditions are being treated with corticosteroids, the chances that acute adrenocortical insufficiency will occur from sudden withdrawal of high-dose steroids is actually increasing.

Congenital Adrenal Hyperplasia

Congenital adrenal hyperplasia is a syndrome that is inherited as an autosomal recessive trait. The primary defect is an inability of the adrenal glands to synthesize cortisol from its precursors. Because the adrenal gland is unable to produce cortisol, the level of ACTH increases, stimulating the adrenal glands to improve function. Although the adrenals enlarge (hyperplasia), they still cannot produce cortisol, but they overproduce androgen.

Assessment

The excessive androgen production masculinizes the female fetus or increases the size of genital organs in a male fetus (Lajic et al., 2004). Because this process begins as early as fetal life, the female infant is born with a clitoris so enlarged that it appears more like a penis (Fig. 48.3). Internal female organs are usually normal, although a sinus between the urethra and vagina may be present (see discussion of ambiguous genitalia in Chapter 47). Because the labia are typically fused as well, the girl resembles a boy with undescended testes and hypospadias. If the condition is not recognized at birth and the child remains untreated, pubic and axillary hair and acne will appear precociously and a deep masculine voice will develop. The bone age is usually advanced, so the epiphyseal line of the long bones closes early. This closure prevents the child from reaching adult height unless treatment is initiated. At puberty, there will be no breast development or menstruation.

The male child may appear normal at birth, but by 6 months of age signs of sexual precocity appear. By 3 or 4 years of age, these boys have pubic hair and enlargement

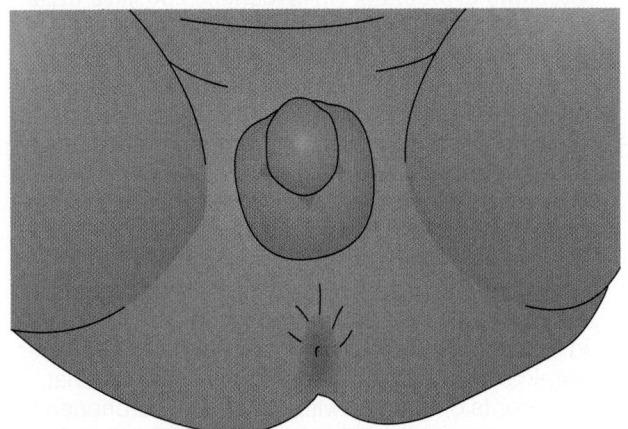

FIGURE 48.3 A female infant with congenital adrenogenital hyperplasia. Note the fused labia and abnormally enlarged clitoris.

of the penis, scrotum, and prostate. They may have acne and a deep, mature voice. The testes do not enlarge, however, and, although they are normal in size, they appear small in relation to the size of the penis. Spermatogenesis does not occur, so the child is infertile.

Children with congenital adrenogenital hyperplasia have increased levels of androgen, an important point for diagnosis. By determining the levels of other adrenal hormones, the exact degree of the metabolic defect in production of cortisol can be measured.

Therapeutic Management

Both male and female infants are given a corticosteroid agent, such as oral hydrocortisone, to replace what they cannot produce naturally. When a corticosteroid is given to the child in this way, stimulation by ACTH decreases, production of androgen returns to normal limits, and no further masculinization occurs. Corticosteroid therapy needs to continue indefinitely. The child needs periodic analysis of serum cortisol levels and growth measurements to estimate the effectiveness of the therapy.

It is possible to identify the fetus with congenital adrenogenital hyperplasia as early as 6 to 8 weeks of pregnancy by means of chorionic villi sampling and at 15 weeks by amniocentesis (see Chapter 7). Treatment of a mother with dexamethasone (a corticosteroid), which crosses the placenta to the fetus, can prevent masculinization in the fetus for the remainder of the pregnancy (Lajic et al., 2004).

NURSING DIAGNOSES AND RELATED INTERVENTIONS

Nursing Diagnosis: Situational low self-esteem related to genital formation at variance with true gender

Outcome Evaluation: Child identifies positive traits about self and describes activities enjoyed with peers; expresses satisfaction with gender identity.

If children with congenital adrenogenital hyperplasia are not closely examined at birth, they can be wrongly identified as boys when chromosomally they are actually girls (Ozbey et al., 2004). Therefore, all newborns require an extensive physical examination at birth. It is sometimes recommended that a girl's enlarged clitoris be reduced by plastic surgery early in life. This treatment is controversial, however, because clitoral reduction can also result in reduced clitoral sensation. Fortunately, with finer surgical techniques, this problem is now minimal.

Parents of females with congenital adrenogenital hyperplasia may need a great deal of support during the first few days of their child's life if they feel that their child is imperfect in an embarrassing, hard-to-explain way. When they are told the results of the chromosome analysis, parents may react with grief for the loss of the son they thought had been born to them. Parents need support from health care personnel who recognize that the child is simply lacking a completely formed hormone but is complete in every other way.

Nursing Diagnosis: Health-seeking behaviors related to lack of knowledge about long-term treatment needed to sustain adequate growth and development

Outcome Evaluation: Parents state plans for incorporating medication administration into the daily routine whether at home or away (e.g., vacation, summer camp).

Parents, and children as they grow older, need to understand the importance of continuing to take the oral medication prescribed. When this condition is first diagnosed, it is easy for parents to remember to give the drug. As the years pass, however, it becomes more difficult to remember medication administration, because the child has no acute symptoms. Cortisol is necessary for glucose and protein metabolism. The body needs adequate levels to allow it to react to physical and emotional stress. When plans are made for summer camp or vacation away from home, special arrangements for regular medicine administration must be made. Children may need to have a routine dose increased when they are undergoing periods of stress, such as surgery or infection. They may need support throughout life if their body image is distorted because of body changes at birth (Berenbaum et al., 2004).

Salt-Losing Form of Congenital Adrenogenital Hyperplasia

If there is a complete blockage of cortisol formation, aldosterone production will also be deficient. Without adequate aldosterone, salt is not retained by the body, so fluid is not retained. Almost immediately after birth, affected infants begin to have vomiting, diarrhea, anorexia, loss of weight, and extreme dehydration. If these symptoms remain untreated, the extreme loss of salt and fluid can lead to collapse and death as early as 48 to 72 hours after birth (Gassner et al., 2004).

About one third of children with congenital adrenogenital hyperplasia are affected by this complete deficiency. Because boys with this syndrome appear normal at birth, the symptoms may be incorrectly diagnosed as pyloric stenosis, intestinal obstruction, or failure to thrive. In girls, because of the ambiguous genitalia, the correct diagnosis can be made more easily.

Assessment

The salt-losing form of congenital adrenogenital hyperplasia must be detected in infants before they reach an irreversible point of salt depletion. Weighing of a newborn at birth and again at 24 hours aids in detecting this condition.

Weighing of infants at each well-child health checkup is also important. In boys, the inability to gain back their birth weight may be the first sign of the syndrome.

Therapeutic Management

Children with the salt-losing form of congenital adrenogenital hyperplasia need to take supplements of hydrocortisone in conjunction with a high amount of salt and DOCA, a synthetic aldosterone, to maintain a balance of fluid and electrolytes. A long-acting form of DOCA can be given once a month IM. Capsules of DOCA can be implanted subcutaneously (SC) as another form of long-acting therapy. As the child grows older, fludrocortisone (Florinef), a mineralocorticoid, may be given orally to aid salt retention.

NURSING DIAGNOSES AND RELATED INTERVENTIONS

Nursing Diagnosis: Risk for deficient fluid volume related to loss of body fluid

Outcome Evaluation: Child's skin turgor remains good; specific gravity of urine is between 1.003 and 1.030.

Teach parents about the body's critical need to balance aldosterone, salt, and water, so that they understand the drastic consequences if their child skips a dose of medication. Help them to set up a schedule as necessary for measuring the child's weight, giving medication, or measuring urine output. Help them to understand that, although salt seems to be an "extra" in their own diet, it is as vital to their child's intake as digitalis is in heart disease or insulin in diabetes.

Cushing Syndrome

Cushing syndrome is caused by overproduction of the adrenal hormone cortisol; this usually results from increased ACTH production due to a pituitary tumor. It may occur from a malignant or benign tumor of the adrenal cortex. The peak age of occurrence is 6 or 7 years, but the syndrome can occur as early as infancy (Simard, 2004). Overproduction of cortisol results in increased glucose production; this causes fat to accumulate on the cheeks, chin, and trunk, causing a moon-faced, stocky appearance. Cortisol is catabolic, so protein wasting occurs. This leads to muscle wasting, making the extremities appear thin. Loss of protein matrix in bones causes osteoporosis (loss of calcium in bones). Cortisol also suppresses the immune system, so humoral immunity is decreased, leaving children susceptible to infection. Additionally, it causes vasoconstriction, so extreme hypertension may occur.

Hyperpigmentation occurs from the melanin-stimulating properties of ACTH. This causes the child's face to be unusually red, especially the cheeks. Signs of abnormal masculinization or feminization may occur from accompanying overproduction of androgen or estrogen. Purple striae resulting from collagen deficit appear on the child's hips, abdomen, and thighs, similar to those seen in pregnancy (Fig. 48.4).

Polyuria develops as the body tries to excrete increased glucose levels. Growth ceases, and, if the condition is not reversed before the epiphyseal lines close, short stature results.

Children who receive high doses of synthetic corticosteroids, such as prednisone, over a long period may develop the same symptoms as those observed in Cushing syndrome. Such children are said to have a *cushingoid appearance.* Cushing syndrome is often suspected as the cause of obesity in children, and some obese children do have elevated levels of plasma corticosteroids, a fact that complicates the diagnosis. However, these elevated levels of corticosteroids are secondary to the obesity; they are not the cause. Children with natural obesity are generally tall; those with Cushing syndrome are short.

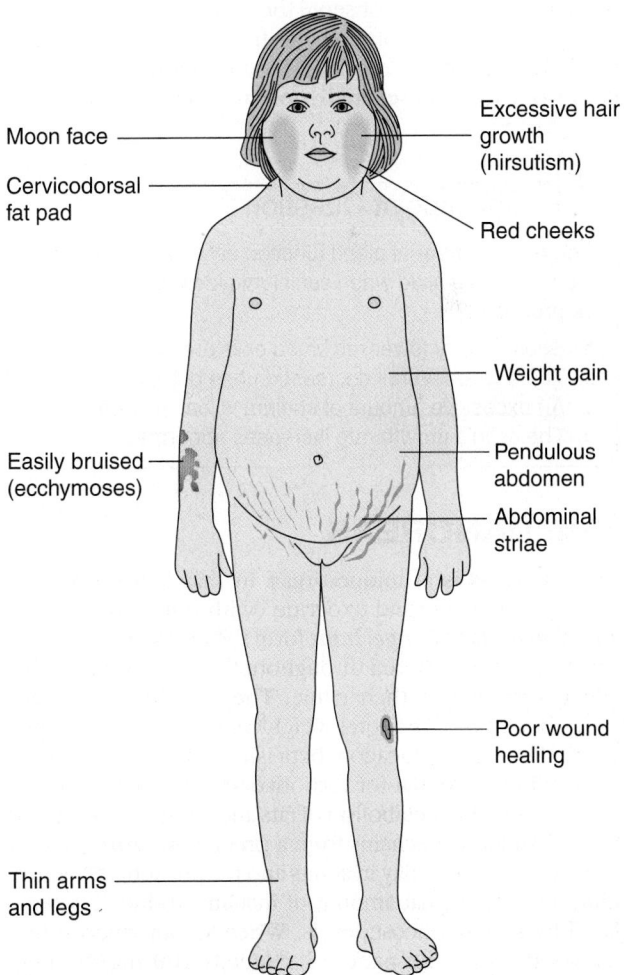

FIGURE 48.4 Signs and symptoms of Cushing syndrome.

Assessment

Children with Cushing syndrome have elevated plasma cortisol and increased urinary free-cortisol levels. A dexamethasone suppression test confirms the diagnosis. If a normal child is given a test dose of dexamethasone (a glucocorticoid), the plasma level of adrenal cortisol will fall. It will not fall in children with adrenocortical tumors, because the tumor continues to stimulate the adrenal glands to oversecretion. If cosyntropin (Cortrosyn), a synthetic corticotropin, or ACTH is administered, plasma cortisol levels will normally rise. In patients with an adrenal tumor, the gland is already functioning at full capacity, so no cortisol elevation occurs. A CT scan or sonogram reveals the enlarged adrenal or pituitary gland, confirming the diagnosis.

Therapeutic Management

Treatment of Cushing syndrome is surgical removal of the causative tumor. The prognosis depends on whether the tumor is benign or malignant; carcinoma of this type tends to metastasize rapidly. If a major part of the adrenal gland is surgically removed, the child will need replacement cortisol therapy indefinitely.

If a major portion of the pituitary gland is removed, replacement of all pituitary hormones may be necessary. After adrenal surgery, observe the child carefully for signs of shock: without epinephrine from the adrenal gland, the body's ability to maintain blood pressure is severely compromised, and severe hypotension can result.

 Checkpoint Question 2

Rob has his adrenal gland function assessed. What is the effect on a child when sufficient aldosterone cannot be produced?

a. Substantially fewer red blood cells are produced.
b. There is an overall decreased urine output.
c. An excessive amount of sodium is lost in urine.
d. The child's growth rate increases abnormally.

THE PANCREAS

The pancreas is a unique organ in that it has both endocrine (ductless) and exocrine (with duct) types of tissue. The *islets of Langerhans* form the endocrine portion; these cells are scattered throughout the exocrine cells like small islets; hence their name. The islet cells represent only about 1% of the total weight of the pancreas. Alpha islet cells secrete glucagon; beta islet cells secrete insulin.

Insulin is essential for carbohydrate metabolism and is important to the metabolism of fats and protein. It is formed by two amino acid chains from a precursor, *proinsulin,* at a rate of 35 to 50 U/day in adults and proportionately less in children. The actual amount of insulin produced is regulated by serum glucose levels. When serum glucose that passes through the pancreas exceeds 100 mg/dL, beta cells immediately increase insulin production. When blood serum levels are lowered, production decreases. Both the ability to secrete additional insulin and the action to decrease production are immediate responses.

Also important in the secretion of insulin is the presence of gastrointestinal hormones, such as gastrin, that rise when the stomach is full, because these also stimulate the pancreas to produce the necessary insulin. Other hormones that stimulate insulin production include glucagon, cortisol, GH, progesterone, and estrogen. In contrast, increasing levels of epinephrine or norepinephrine inhibit the secretion of insulin.

The principal childhood disorders associated with pancreatic dysfunction are type 1 diabetes mellitus and cystic fibrosis. Because the nursing care for children with cystic fibrosis includes many respiratory care procedures, it is discussed in Chapter 40.

Type 1 Diabetes Mellitus

Diabetes is a disorder that involves an absolute or relative deficiency of insulin. There are two main types of diabetes, as shown in Table 48.2. Type 1 diabetes (formerly referred to as juvenile diabetes or insulin-dependent diabetes) most commonly occurs in childhood. The disease affects as many as 1 in 1,500 children before 5 years of age and increases to 1 in 350 by age 16 (Weinzimer, 2003). It apparently results from immunologic damage to insulin-producing cells in susceptible individuals. Environmental effects may be necessary to create the immunologic response. Children with this type of diabetes must take insulin to replace what their pancreas can no longer produce. This is a separate disease from type 2 diabetes (formerly known as non–insulin-dependent diabetes), which is characterized by diminished insulin secretion. Usually individuals with type 2 diabetes do not need daily insulin, because their disease can be managed with diet alone or with diet and oral hypoglycemic agents. Once thought to occur only in older people, type 2 diabetes is also seen in overweight adolescents, termed maturity-onset diabetes of youth (MODY) (Rapaport et al., 2004; Schreiner, 2005).

Etiology

Why autoimmune destruction of islet cells occurs in some children and not in others is unknown, but children with this disorder have a high frequency of certain human leukocyte antigens (HLA), particularly HLA-DR3 and HLA-DR4, located on chromosome 6.

Although specific HLA antigens predispose a child to developing diabetes, they do not always result in the actual disease. An environmental factor, such as a viral infection, must trigger active pancreatic dysfunction through an autoimmune process. Symptoms of the disease usually are not manifested until preschool or school age. The incidence of type 1 diabetes mellitus is equal among girls and boys.

If one child in a family has diabetes, the chance that a sibling will also develop the illness is higher than in other families, because siblings also tend to have one of the specific HLA antigens that lead to the development of the disease. Because no prevention measures are available to stop diabetes from developing, children are not routinely tissue-typed for the disorder, although this may be done experimentally. Administration of immune suppressors to

TABLE 48.2

Comparison of Type 1 and Type 2 Diabetes

Assessment	Type 1	Type 2
Age at onset	5–7 years or at puberty	40–65 years (may occur in adolescents as maturity-onset diabetes of youth [MODY])
Type of onset	Abrupt	Gradual
Weight changes	Marked weight loss often initial sign	Associated with obesity
Other symptoms	Polydipsia	Polydipsia
	Polyuria (often begins as bedwetting)	Polyuria
	Fatigue (marks fall in school)	Fatigue
	Blurred vision (marks fall in school)	Blurred vision
	Glycosuria	Glycosuria
	Polyphagia	
	Pruritus	Pruritus
	Mood changes (may cause behavior problems in school)	Mood changes
Therapy	Hypoglycemia agents never effective; insulin required	Diet, oral hypoglycemic agents, or insulin
	Diet recommended as 55% carbohydrates, 15% protein, and 30% fat; no dietary foods used	Nutrition concentrating on no excess weight gain and balanced intake of carbohydrates, protein, and fat
	Common-sense foot care for growing children	Meticulous skin and foot care necessary
Period of remission	Period of remission for 1–12 months ("honeymoon period") generally after initial diagnosis	Not demonstrable

stop destruction of insulin-secreting cells is a possibility, although the long-term effects of immune suppression, such as development of opportunistic infections, limit the use of these drugs.

Progress of Disease

Insulin can be thought of as a compound that opens the doors to body cells, allowing them to admit the glucose needed to function. It does not play a major role in glucose transport into the brain, erythrocytes, leukocytes, intestinal mucosa, or kidney epithelium. These cells can survive insulin deficiency but not glucose deficiency.

If glucose is unable to enter body cells because of a lack of insulin, it builds up in the bloodstream (**hyperglycemia**), and this underlying defect leads to other metabolic consequences. When the kidneys detect hyperglycemia (greater than the renal threshold of about 160 mg/dL), the kidneys attempt to lower it to normal levels by excreting excess glucose into the urine, causing **glycosuria.** While attempting to excrete this excess glucose, the body also excretes a large amount of fluid (polyuria). Excess fluid loss, in turn, triggers the thirst response (polydipsia).

Because the body cells are unable to use glucose but still need a source of energy, the body begins to break down protein and fat for cell utilization. If large amounts of fat are metabolized in this way, weight loss occurs

and ketone bodies, the acid end-product of fat breakdown, begin to accumulate in the bloodstream and spill into the urine. Because the blood bicarbonate cannot effectively continue to buffer this high an acid level, the pH of the blood becomes acidic, resulting in severe acidosis. The breakdown of fat also leads to increased serum cholesterol levels. Potassium and phosphate, attempting to serve as buffers, pass from body cells into the bloodstream. As they are evacuated, the body loses these important electrolytes.

Untreated diabetic children, therefore, lose weight, are acidotic due to the buildup of ketone bodies in their blood (a state known as **ketoacidosis**), are dehydrated because of the loss of water, and experience an electrolyte imbalance because of the loss of electrolytes in urine. Because large amounts of protein and fat are being used for energy instead of glucose, these children lack the necessary components for growth; they therefore remain short in stature and underweight (Houghton, 2004).

Assessment

Although children may be prediabetic for some time, the onset of symptoms in childhood is usually abrupt. The first symptoms likely to be reported are increased thirst (polydipsia) and increased urination (polyuria). Increased urination may begin as bedwetting (enuresis) in a previously toilet-trained child. In addition, children may have constipation because of the dehydration.

Laboratory Studies.   In some children, diabetes is detected at a routine health screening. For others, although the disease has been progressing internally for some time, outward symptoms have such an abrupt onset that the child is in coma from acidosis and hyperglycemia by the time it is detected. Laboratory studies usually show a random plasma glucose level greater than 200 mg/dL (normal range, 70 to 110 mg/dL fasting, 90 to 180 mg/dL not fasting) and significant glycosuria (Table 48.3).

Two diagnostic tests, the fasting blood glucose test and the random blood glucose test, are used to diagnose diabetes. A diagnosis of diabetes is confirmed based on finding one of the following three criteria on two separate occasions:

- Symptoms of diabetes with a random blood glucose level greater than 200 mg/dL
- Fasting blood glucose level greater than 126 mg/dL
- Two-hour plasma glucose level greater than 200 mg/dL during an oral glucose tolerance test (GTT)

Typically, a GTT, which involves oral ingestion or IV administration of a concentrated glucose solution followed by blood glucose levels drawn at fasting (baseline), after 1 hour, and after 2 hours, is rarely performed in children. This test is difficult for children to undergo, because it requires them to fast and submit to painful, intrusive procedures (routine application of EMLA cream to fingerstick or venipuncture sites and use of intermittent infusion devices greatly reduces this problem). Do not take blood for glucose analysis from functioning IV tubing, because the glucose in the IV solution will cause the serum reading to be abnormally high.

Other Diagnostic Tests.   If diabetes is detected, the diagnostic workup also usually includes analysis of blood samples for pH, partial pressure of carbon dioxide (Pco_2), sodium, and potassium levels; a white blood cell count; and glycosylated hemoglobin (HbA_{1c}) evaluation. Normally, red blood cells carry only a trace of glucose incorporated into the hemoglobin. If the serum glucose is excessive, however, it attaches itself to hemoglobin molecules, causing glycosylated hemoglobin. The higher the serum glucose level, the higher the HbA_{1c} becomes. In nondiabetic children, the usual HbA_{1c} value is 1.8 to 4.0. A value greater than 6.0 reflects an excessive level of serum glucose. Measuring glycosylated hemoglobin provides information about what the child's glucose levels have been during

the preceding 3 to 4 months, because red blood cells have a lifespan of less than 120 days.

If the potassium level of the blood is low, a child may need an electrocardiogram to observe for T-wave abnormalities, the mark of potassium deficiency. The white blood cell count of a child with diabetes may be elevated even though no infection is present, apparently as a response to the ketoacidosis. The presence of infection must always be suspected, however, because it is often a precipitant to a diabetic crisis. For this reason, nose and throat cultures may be obtained as well.

Therapeutic Management

Therapy for children with type 1 diabetes involves five measures: insulin administration; regulation of nutrition and exercise; stress management; and blood glucose and urine ketone monitoring. Children with newly suspected diabetes mellitus may be admitted to the hospital for a few days for diagnosis, regulation of insulin dosage, and education. This may not be necessary if the child's symptoms are minimal. Teaching the parents and the child the techniques of intensive management (frequent insulin injections and adherence to nutritional guidelines with regulation of exercise) produces immediate well-being and reduces the incidence of long-term complications. Allow parents and children time to adjust to this illness, which will require constant vigilance in the months and years to follow.

Initial Regulation of Insulin.   When children are first diagnosed with diabetes, they are usually hyperglycemic and perhaps ketoacidotic. To correct the metabolic imbalance, they are given insulin. This is usually administered IV at a dose of 0.1 to 0.2 U per kilogram of body weight per hour, depending on the severity of the symptoms. This initial IV infusion of insulin is followed by further dose reductions once the blood glucose level is lower than 200 mg/dL. The dosage depends on the change in the acidosis and the degree of glycosemia and ketonuria. Some controversy exists regarding the belief that insulin binds to the plastic IV tubing. Therefore, check your institution's policy and be prepared to change the IV tubing as required. Ideally, within 12 hours, the acidosis is considerably less than when the child was admitted to the hospital, and the serum glucose level is near the normal range. The insulin given for emergency replacement is regular (short-acting) insulin (Humulin-R), because this is the form that takes effect most quickly when administered IV in normal saline. Lispro (Humalog), which is also rapid acting, is another possibility.

It may seem that, in a diabetic child in a state of acidosis, the administration of glucose would not be warranted. Because the child is being given insulin, however, body cells soon become ready to use glucose, and they incorporate and use available glucose quickly. If more is not provided, cells are forced to continue to break down fats and protein, and the acidosis can increase, not decrease. Glucose may be added to the infusion, if necessary, to meet this need.

After 24 hours, as the child begins to improve, oral feedings may replace the IV route. Further management in the

TABLE 48.3

Acceptable Blood Glucose Ranges for Young Children

Timing	Value (mg/dL)
Before a meal	70–110
1 h after a meal	90–180
2 h after a meal	80–150
Between 2 and 4 AM	70–120

days after this first crucial 24-hour period is based on the serum glucose determinations. A child may remain on regular insulin alone (given three or four times a day) for the first 1 or 2 days. Typically, intermediate-acting insulin is started as soon as oral fluids are taken, usually on the second day of therapy.

Insulin Administration. Before insulin was discovered in 1920, few children with diabetes lived to adulthood. Even after its discovery, not all children responded well to insulin administration, because early forms were manufactured from a pork or beef base that caused development of antibodies against insulin, making the therapy less effective than predicted. Today, insulin is manufactured by a recombinant DNA technique to simulate human insulin (Humulin, Novolin), and this has largely eliminated the problem of antibody reaction.

Types of insulin vary as to their time of onset, peak action, and duration of action (Table 48.4). Regular insulin is usually referred to as short-acting insulin; Humulin-L and Humulin-N are examples of intermediate-acting insulins, and Humulin-U is long acting. Children are regulated on a variety of insulin programs, but most receive a dose of 0.4 to 0.7 U per kilogram of body weight daily in two divided doses (one before breakfast and one before dinner); adolescents may need as much as 1.2 U/kg daily. The most common mixture of insulin used with children is a combination of an intermediate-acting insulin and a regular insulin, usually in a 2:1 ratio (i.e., ⅔ U of the intermediate-acting insulin to ⅓ U regular insulin), and given in the same syringe, although this prescription varies for individual children. The morning dose is two thirds of the total daily dose; the evening dose is the remaining one third. The peak effects of the short-acting insulins are at 3 to 4 hours (see Table 48.4). This means that the child who takes insulin before breakfast will notice a peak effect between 10 AM and 12 noon; that is the time of day when hypoglycemia (a reaction to an excessive insulin level) is most likely to occur. The peak effect period of the intermediate-acting insulins is 8 to 14 hours, or late afternoon, just before dinner. This is another prime time for hypoglycemia.

Some children require a program of insulin therapy that includes three injections daily (a short-acting and interme-diate-acting insulin before breakfast, a short-acting insulin before supper, and a bedtime injection of an intermediate-acting insulin). Still others receive an injection of regular or Humalog insulin before each meal, plus a bedtime injection of intermediate-acting insulin (a total of four injections daily). Although a regimen with the fewest injections daily at first seems advantageous, multiple injections allow for greater variation in activity and meal consumption.

In the past, fixed doses of insulin were prescribed, and parents were advised not to vary the dose. Today, parents are educated to be able to vary the dose based on an insulin algorithm or protocol determined by the child's level of activity, the size of meals consumed, and the time of the injection (referred to as "thinking scales"). The time between the insulin injection and a meal is known as "lag time." If a child's premeal blood glucose level is above a target range, parents learn that increasing the lag time will help prevent hyperglycemia. If the blood glucose is low at a premeal test, decreasing the lag time could help prevent hypoglycemia. If it is anticipated that the child will eat an unusually large meal (e.g., a birthday dinner), parents can increase the size of the premeal regular insulin injection. If the child is to participate in a strenuous sport in the afternoon, the regular insulin injection can be decreased. Lantus is a new long-acting insulin that lasts 24 hours. A disadvantage of this insulin is its pH, which is so low that it cannot be mixed in a syringe with other insulins. In some children, glucose levels can be regulated on Lantus plus three doses of Humalog before meals.

Injection Technique. When insulins are mixed in one syringe, the regular or short-acting insulin should be drawn into the syringe first. Then, if mixing accidentally occurs in the bottle, the time of effectiveness of the short-acting insulin (which needs to be kept short-acting for emergency treatment) will not be lengthened by the addition of the intermediate-acting insulin.

Insulin is always injected SC except in emergencies, when half the required dose may be given IV. Children should be encouraged to rotate sites in a pattern based on their planned activity. Absorption is increased if the muscles at the injection site are exercised after the injection, so it is best to choose sites that will not be exercised soon after the injection. SC tissue injection sites include those of the upper outer arms and the outer aspects of the thighs (Fig. 48.5). The abdominal SC tissue injection sites may be preferred for injection, because many children have a greater amount of subcutaneous tissue there. However, most children dislike this site. If a child will be jogging after an injection, the thigh probably should not be used. Similarly, if the child will be playing tennis, the injection probably should not be given in the dominant arm.

Work out a plan of rotation for each child so that everyone who will be working with the child and giving injections knows what injection site should be used next. In the hospital, record the injection site in the child's chart or nursing plan of care, so that each nurse can check it before an injection and not repeat an injection site. If the same injection site is used repeatedly, a great deal of subcutaneous atrophy (lipodystrophy) can occur at the site, causing deep, obvious pockmarks. However, this is less of a problem now that synthetic human insulin is available.

TABLE 48.4

Common Types of Human Insulin

Preparation	Onset (hr)	Peak Effect (hr)	Duration of Effect (hr)
Lispro (Humalog)	Immediate	½–1	3–4
Regular (Humulin-R)	0.5–1.0	2–4	5–7
Lantus	1	5	24
Humulin-N	1–2	4–12	24+
Humulin-L	1–3	6–14	24+
Humulin-U	6	16–18	36+

Karch, A. M. (2004). *Lippincott's nursing drug guide.*
Philadelphia: Lippincott Williams & Wilkins.

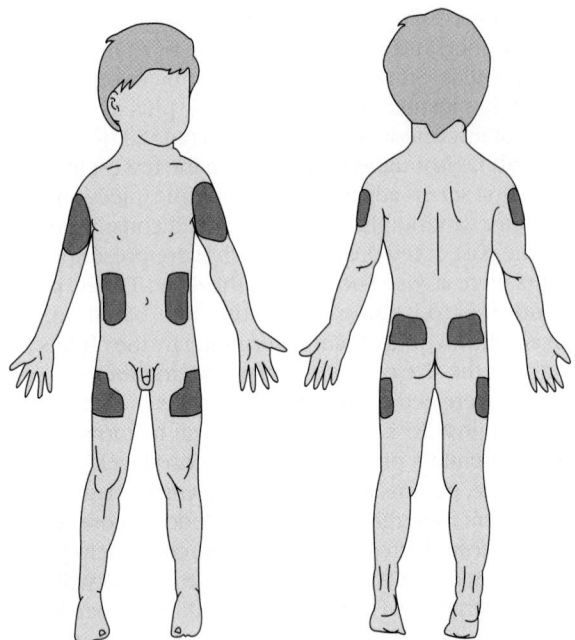

FIGURE 48.5 According to the American Diabetes Association, insulin injection sites in children and adults are the upper outer portions of the arms; the thighs— 4 inches below the hip and 4 inches above the knee (adjusted proportionally for children); and the abdominal area just above and just below the waist. The navel and a circular area just around it are excluded as injection sites. In some children the abdominal area may not be an appropriate injection site.

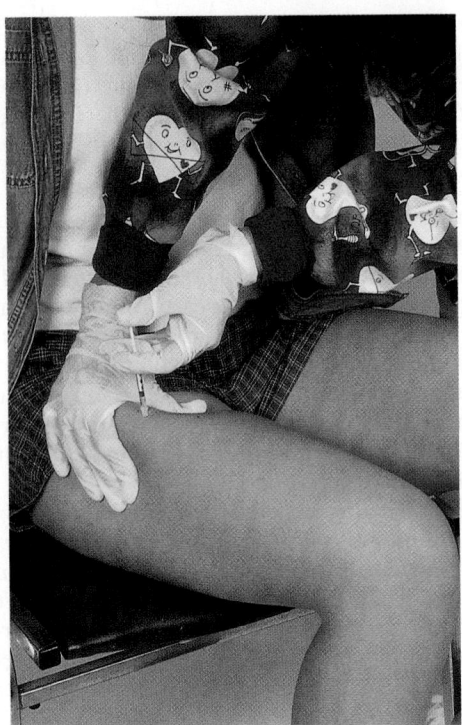

FIGURE 48.6 Insulin is usually injected at a 90-degree angle with a short needle. This angle places the insulin in the subcutaneous space. (© Lesha Photography.)

Children quickly learn that, if they continuously give injections in the same site, scar tissue (lipohypertrophy) forms there, and no pain will be felt on injection. This is a dangerous practice, however, because insulin no longer absorbs well from this site. The dose will have to be increased beyond what the child actually needs for glucose metabolism, because a portion of each dose is "locked" in the tissue. Should the child then inject this larger dose of insulin into a new site, there is a potential for overdose (which would cause hypoglycemia).

Insulin should be given at room temperature. This diminishes subcutaneous atrophy and ensures peak effectiveness. Parents may keep additional bottles in the refrigerator to increase the insulin's shelf life.

If a short needle (less than 0.4 inch) is used, children can administer insulin without bunching skin at the site and can give the injection to themselves at a 90-degree angle, a technique more closely resembling that of IM rather than SC injection. Because the needle is so short, the insulin is deposited in the subcutaneous tissue. This technique is easier for children to learn, because it takes less coordination to administer an injection at a 90-degree angle than at a 45-degree subcutaneous angle (Fig. 48.6). Automatic injection devices, such as pens and jet injectors, are easy for children to use, promote early independence, and can be given with the 90-degree technique (Fig. 48.7).

Insulin Pumps. An insulin pump is an automatic device approximately the size of a transistor radio. It delivers insulin at a constant rate, so it regulates serum glucose levels

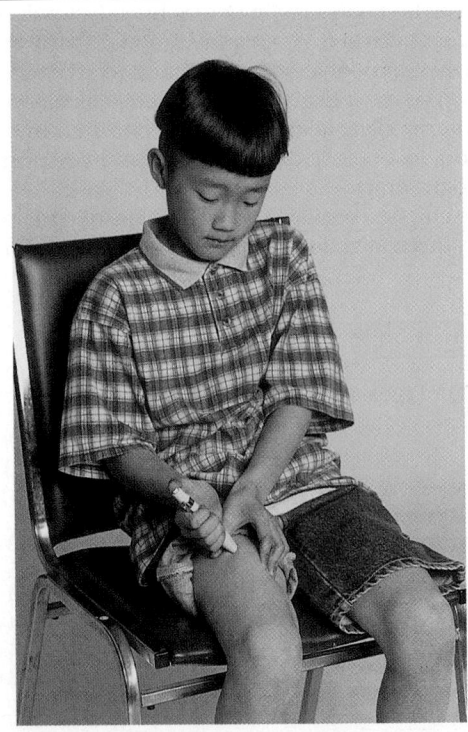

FIGURE 48.7 Injection of insulin by an automatic device. (© Lesha Photography.)

better than periodic injections do. It has the potential to decrease future complications (Deiss et al., 2004). To use a pump, a syringe of regular insulin is placed in the pump chamber; a length of thin polyethylene tubing leads to the child's abdomen, where it is implanted into the subcutaneous tissue by a small-gauge needle. Throughout the day, the pump edges the syringe barrel forward, infusing insulin at a continuous rate into the subcutaneous tissue. Before a snack or meal, the parent or child presses a button on the pump and forces a bolus of insulin forward, thus increasing the amount of insulin injected in order to manage these times of high carbohydrate intake. Children need to inspect the site of the pump insertion to make sure that it is not inflamed; the site is cleaned and changed every 48 to 72 hours to ensure that absorption is still optimal.

Restrictions with pump therapy include keeping it dry: the child must remove the pump (not the syringe and tubing) while showering unless it is a brand that is waterproof or is equipped with a waterproof pouch so it can be taken into a shower or swimming pool. A disadvantage of pump therapy is that the pump is always present. Children usually prefer to wear clothing that hides the pump's outline (it can be held against the abdomen by an over-the-shoulder sling or hung from a belt around the waist). To assess the pump's delivery of insulin, the child must do blood glucose determinations about four times a day. When pump therapy first begins, a parent must wake at 2 AM and test the child's blood glucose level, because this is such a vulnerable time for hypoglycemia (i.e., the pump is delivering insulin, but the child has not eaten since bedtime). Pump therapy is fairly easy to manage (Box 48.6).

Inhalation Insulin. In the future, insulin may be administered by way of inhalation, because it is absorbed well across mucous membranes. This method releases the child from the chore of daily injections. However, if the child develops a cold or allergies that cause edema of the nasal membrane, drug absorption is reduced. Absorption also can be influenced by whether the child is upright or lying down at the time of administration (Karch, 2004).

Nutrition. Children with type 1 diabetes need to consume a diet appropriate for their age in the proportion of 55% carbohydrate, 15% protein, and 30% fat. The meal pattern should include three spaced meals plus a snack in the midmorning, midafternoon, and evening (Weinzimer, 2003).

Urine Testing. Urine testing has the disadvantage of not being as accurate as blood serum testing; it is now used only to test for ketonuria if the child's blood glucose level is above 200 mg/dL. A dipstick technique may be used. Acetone appearing in the urine is a sign that fat is being used for energy; this situation occurs with infection or if not enough food has been ingested.

Self Blood Glucose Monitoring (SBGM). Children as young as early school age can learn the techniques of finger puncture (fingerstick) and reading a computerized monitor. Using a spring-loaded puncture device to obtain the blood sample helps minimize pain, and an automatic readout monitor, such as a Glucometer, simplifies the procedure and gives a more accurate reading than does matching the shade of blood on a test strip to the colors on the test strip container (Fig. 48.8). Some meters measure the

BOX 48.6 FOCUS ON . . .

EVIDENCE-BASED PRACTICE

Can Children as Young as Preschool Age Use Insulin Pumps?

To answer this question, 42 preschool children with type 1 diabetes were divided into either a study group, who received insulin by continuous subcutaneous insulin infusions, or a control group, who received insulin injections. Results showed a significant decrease in HbA1c during the 6-month study period for both groups. No differences were observed between the two groups in premeal blood sugar levels. Children who had pumps had more meter-detected episodes of hypoglycemia than did children in the injection group. No episodes of ketoacidosis occurred in either group, and one hypoglycemic episode occurred in each group.

The researchers concluded that insulin pumps are a safe and effective alternative method for administering insulin to preschool children. Parents and children should be allowed to choose the method of insulin administration that is most satisfactory to their lifestyle.

This is an interesting study for nurses, because it not only documents the effectiveness of insulin pumps for very young children but also confirms that parents can effectively manage pump therapy at home. Because nurses are often the health care practitioners parents ask about a new technology and whether it will be too complicated for them to manage, it is helpful to know that insulin pumps are safe and well tolerated.

DiMeglio, L. A., et al. (2004). A randomized, controlled study of insulin pump therapy in diabetic preschoolers. *Journal of Pediatrics, 145*(3), 380–384.

whole blood value, not the serum glucose level. This means that the result will be about 15% higher than a serum determination (i.e., a blood determination of 115 mg/dL equals 100 mg/dL of serum). However, some newer meters automatically convert the whole blood value to a plasma

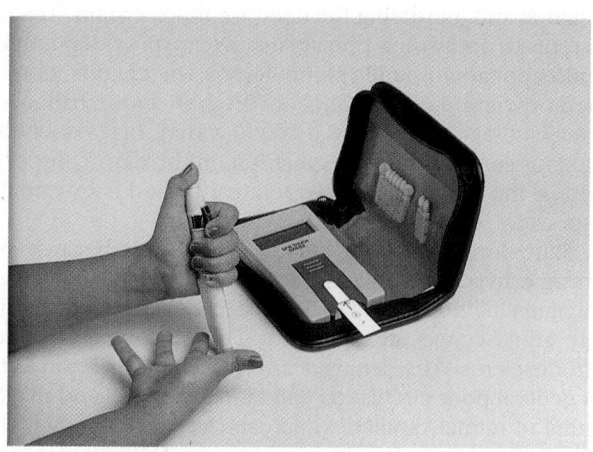

FIGURE 48.8 A child uses an automatic lancet for blood sampling (*left*). Blood glucose level will be determined by the glucometer (*right*). (© Lesha Photography.)

value. Be sure that parents and children understand the type of monitor they are using.

The "Honeymoon" Period. After the child's diagnosis has been confirmed and the blood glucose level has been initially regulated by insulin, a honeymoon period may follow, during which only a minimal amount of insulin, or none at all, is needed for glucose regulation. This apparently occurs because the exogenous insulin stimulates the islet cells to produce natural insulin, as if they are being reminded of their true function. After a month or even up to a year, the islet cells begin to fail once again, and diabetic symptoms recur. This can be upsetting to parents if they began to believe that their child was wrongly diagnosed or that a cure had taken place. Caution both the parents and the child that symptoms will inevitably recur. Sometimes, a child is maintained on a minimum amount of insulin during this period to prevent unrealistic expectations of a cure. This practice may also help to reduce islet cell destruction.

Stress Adjustment. Whenever children with diabetes undergo a stressful situation, either emotionally or physically, they may need increased insulin to maintain glucose homeostasis. When children are seen at health care facilities for periodic checkups, ask them whether they are having any difficulty with blood testing or insulin injection and how things are at home and at school.

Try to interview children separately from their parents, so they can feel free to talk about anything that may be happening or going wrong. There must be cooperation between primary health care personnel and school health care personnel so that conflicts about the child's regimen do not cause problems or tensions at school. Parents may have to meet with schoolteachers to help them view the child as well, not ill, so that they will allow participation in all activities, including sports. Sometimes, children are embarrassed to have to do blood glucose testing in school, especially in the public lavatory. It may be easier for them if they can go to the nurse's office for privacy when testing (Box 48.7).

Complications. If temperature rises and infection occurs, counter-regulatory hormones increase, causing insulin resistance and increasing the need for more insulin. Teach parents to notify their primary health care provider if their child appears to be ill (particularly if the child is nauseated or vomiting) for careful observation and a change in insulin dosage if necessary. If a child with diabetes is scheduled for surgery, careful regulation on the day of surgery and in the immediate postoperative period is essential, especially if oral fluids will be restricted.

Many long-term body changes that occur because of chronic hyperglycemia are not a major part of management in childhood because their onset does not begin until late adolescence or adulthood. These changes include arteriosclerosis (hardening of artery walls), which can lead to general poor circulation and kidney disease, and thickening of retinal capillaries and cataract formation, which ultimately can result in blindness. Some children may notice blurred vision when their disease is not in control, but this should not be confused with the final retinopathy that may result with older age. It is a temporary change in

---

BOX 48.7 FOCUS ON . . .

DIVERSITY OF CARE

The way people view endocrine disorders can be culturally influenced. Because many of these disorders are inherited, they tend to cluster in various populations, so that either the incidence of the condition in family or friends is high, or else people know nothing about the condition. In the past, because many endocrine disorders led to changes in body appearance, particularly overgrowth or undergrowth, and because the reason for these changes was poorly understood, children with these disorders found themselves poorly accepted by peers. Being aware of the way these diseases used to be viewed aids in understanding a parent's anxiety at diagnosis of these disorders and helps with nursing care planning to include reassurance and modern concepts of therapy in education. Also, be sure to ask parents if they are using alternative therapies, because many herbs are advertised to suggest that they increase growth.

---

depth of the eye globe related to hyperglycemia. Because women with diabetes eventually develop some degree of arteriosclerosis in adulthood, women are encouraged not to delay childbearing past 35 years of age. Current research supports the use of low-dose progestin and estrogen combination oral contraceptives (high doses of estrogen can elevate blood glucose). Alternative measures of birth control, such as the diaphragm or vaginal foam along with condoms for their sexual partner, also should be discussed. Care of the woman with diabetes mellitus during pregnancy is discussed in Chapter 14.

Pancreas Transplantation. For children who develop severe kidney disease or retinopathy, pancreas transplantation may be considered. In contrast to other organ transplantation procedures, the original pancreas is not removed entirely. The portion that supplies digestive enzymes is still functioning and is left in place. During surgery, a new pancreas is grafted to the iliac artery and vein, to allow insulin from the new organ to enter the systemic circulation. For this reason, pancreatic replacement is more accurately called grafting. The digestive enzymes of the new pancreas can be diverted into the intestine or bladder, or the pancreatic ducts can be sclerosed so that the digestive enzymes do not leave the transplanted organ. Grafts may be taken from cadavers or from live donors, who can lose up to 45% of their pancreas and still maintain a functioning organ for themselves.

To reduce the child's immune response and protect against graft rejection, drugs such as antilymphocyte globulin, cyclosporine, prednisone, or azathioprine (Imuran) are administered after surgery. If rejection does start to occur, the patient is given monoclonal T-cell antibodies (OKT3).

Pancreatic transplantation is a last-resort solution for children, because the outcome is guarded (about 50% of transplanted organs are rejected) and the outcome—

continuous immunosuppressive medication for life—may not be regarded as a major improvement over the original illness, which would require continuous daily insulin for life (Joseph et al., 2003).

NURSING DIAGNOSES AND RELATED INTERVENTIONS

Nursing Diagnosis: Health-seeking behaviors related to self-administration of insulin, balanced exercise, and hygiene

Outcome Evaluation: Child demonstrates insulin injection technique to nurse, describes steps correctly, and discusses plans for an exercise and hygiene program.

Self-Administration of Insulin. From about 8 years of age, children can be taught to administer their own insulin (Fig. 48.9). Many children younger than this do not have the dexterity to handle a syringe or an understanding of the importance of sterile technique and proper dosage. They may skip injections if they are tired or busy.

Do not underestimate how difficult it is for children to learn to give injections to themselves. Although it may seem like a two-step process (draw up the medication, and give it), in actuality more than 25 steps are involved.

If the child has to mix insulins, the number of steps increases. Besides lacking dexterity and adult-level fine motor skills, children have to face *injecting themselves.* There is no such thing as getting used to injections. Children grow used to the *idea* of self-injection, not to the injections themselves.

Even if children are taught to give their own insulin from the beginning, at least one adult in the family should be taught to give it as well. There will be days when the child refuses to administer his or her own insulin or is not feeling well and needs to have or appreciates having someone do it for them. Parents may have a hard time giving their child a painful injection; teaching them to view it as a helping action helps to alleviate their distress.

Exercise. Exercise is an important component of care, because it uses up carbohydrates and helps reduce hyperglycemia. No type of exercise is restricted for children with diabetes (Box 48.8).

A problem that arises with vigorous exercise, however, is the development of hypoglycemia due to increased absorption of insulin from the injection site and utilization of glucose by active body cells. One way to minimize this effect is to choose the injection site that is least likely to be exercised. Another method is to eat additional carbohydrate or decrease the regular insulin injection according to an established protocol (algorithm) before exercise. Keep in mind that hypoglycemia may be delayed for up to 18 hours after exercise.

Teach children to design a consistent daily exercise program (e.g., briskly walking the dog or 10 minutes of aerobics every day before school). Once a daily program is established, the child needs to continue this type of exercise every day (including weekends) to avoid becoming hyperglycemic on days of no exercise.

Hygiene. Skin care, particularly foot care, is extremely important for adults with diabetes, because arteriosclerosis causes loss of circulation to the feet, and decreased circulation leads to poor healing ability. This is not as important a concern with children, but they (and all children) should be taught to cut their toenails straight across, to prevent ingrown toenails, and to tend to cuts and scrapes promptly so that healing can begin right away. Properly fitting shoes are essential. Girls may need to be reminded of good perineal care to prevent vaginal infection.

Nursing Diagnosis: Parental anxiety related to newly diagnosed diabetes mellitus in a child

Outcome Evaluation: Parents accurately describe their child's illness and treatment and ways in which the disease will affect their lifestyle. They state a specific plan for daily routine child care and identify potential problems in the schedule and ways they can be handled.

Parents whose child is newly diagnosed with diabetes mellitus have a great deal of new responsibility. Ensure that they have the telephone number of the health care facility, liaison, or home care person to call during the first days of home management. During these days, most parents appreciate having someone to consult before they give insulin, for reassurance that they are giving the correct dose.

Encourage Expression of Feelings. Although parents may be aware that other family members have the disease, they may be surprised that it has occurred in

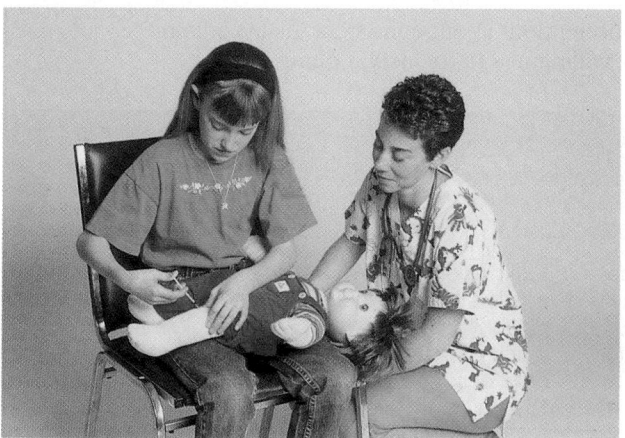

FIGURE 48.9 A school-age child is taught insulin administration using a teaching doll for practice. (© Lesha Photography.)

(text continues on page 1530)

B O X 4 8 . 8 : Focus on Nursing Care Planning

A Multidisciplinary Care Map for An Adolescent with Type 1 Diabetes Mellitus

●

Rob Tebecco is a 16-year-old boy with type 1 diabetes whom you meet in the emergency room, where he was taken after he became comatose while ice skating. His diabetes was diagnosed when he was 7 years old. His records indicate that his disease has generally been under good control over the past years, but in the last 6 months he has "forgotten" to take his insulin at least once a week. When you ask him about this, he tells you that ice skating practice every morning and a new girlfriend have occupied his time and interrupted what used to be a strict schedule of home-cooked meals and a rigid routine.

Family Assessment

Adolescent lives with one younger sister and parents. Father works as Zamboni operator at professional hockey arena. Mother works part time at local post office. Family rates finances as, "We have everything we need."

Client Assessment

Child was skating at local ice rink when he suddenly collapsed. Was brought to emergency room by EMT service, unconscious and breathing deeply. Breath smelled sweet. Blood glucose was 700 mg/dL. Received regular insulin IV. As soon as blood glucose returned to normal, he regained consciousness. Arterial blood gases: pH, 7.20; Pco_2, 10 mm Hg; Hco_3, 10 mEq/mL. Right heel has red and inflamed ulcer.

Currently takes short-acting and intermediate-acting insulin every morning before breakfast and intermediate-acting insulin before dinner. Child self-injects with automatic injection device with some parental supervision. Child performs fingerstick blood glucose levels four times a day. Blood glucose levels normally range between 105 and 115 mg/dL. Dietary history reveals three meals per day with midmorning, afternoon, and bedtime snack. Rob states, "Okay. I'm ready to do better. That was scary to black out."

Nursing Diagnosis

Health-seeking behaviors related to need to follow more conscientious diabetes regimen.

Outcome Evaluation

Child and parents voice intention to be more conscientious about consistent insulin administration and serum glucose testing. Child voices willingness to try insulin pump therapy.

Team Member Responsible	Assessment	Intervention	Rationale	Expected Outcome
		Activities of Daily Living		
Nurse	Explore with child and parents their understanding of the interrelationship of nutrition, exercise, and diabetes.	Review and reinforce the importance of insulin administration, blood glucose monitoring, and exercise.	Exploration and review provide baseline information for identifying teaching needs and developing possible strategies.	Adolescent and parent state they understand new regimen; glucose levels do not fluctuate higher than 126 mg/dL.

(continued)

Team Member Responsible	Assessment	Intervention	Rationale	Expected Outcome
Consultations				
Physician	Assess whether adolescent is candidate for insulin pump therapy to increase adherence.	Consult with diabetic service team to present new method of insulin administration.	Use of an insulin pump offers a continuous supply of insulin; can be advantageous for busy adolescent.	Diabetic service team meets with adolescent and parent to present possibility of using insulin pump.
Procedures/Medications				
Nurse	Assess adolescent's level of understanding about action of insulin with pump therapy.	Demonstrate and observe adolescent draw up, refill insulin syringe, and begin insulin pump infusion.	Adolescent's return demonstration best reveals whether he understands how to maintain insulin pump.	Adolescent demonstrates proper preparation and administration of insulin pump.
Nutrition				
Nutritionist	Assess adolescent's usual meal pattern and determine who prepares food.	Review importance of regular meals plus bedtime snack to keep glucose within consistent levels.	Irregular meal patterns can cause hypoglycemia with pump therapy and inconsistent exercise.	Parents and adolescent state that they will try to arrange a more regular pattern of meals. Will test blood glucose according to set schedule.
Patient/Family Education				
Nurse/ Diabetic Service Team Member	Assess whether adolescent and parents are aware of actions to take if hypoglycemic symptoms should occur with pump therapy.	Review signs and symptoms of hypoglycemia. Review need to always carry a source of carbohydrate.	Having a readily available source of carbohydrate helps raise blood glucose levels quickly should hypoglycemia occur.	Adolescent and parents describe signs of hypoglycemia and action of carbohydrate to prevent this.
Nurse/ Diabetic Service Team Member	Assess whether adolescent and parents are aware of necessity to safeguard feet against trauma.	Review necessity to wear properly fitting shoes and skates and to clean any cuts or scrapes promptly.	Diabetes can result in decreased circulation to the feet and slowed healing, increasing the possibility for infection, which can ultimately affect glucose control.	Adolescent states he will be more conscientious about foot care; acknowledges foot infection may have contributed to his hyperglycemic episode.
Psychosocial/Spiritual/Emotional Needs				
Nurse/Nurse Practitioner	Assess whether child's busy schedule allows for adequate diabetic control.	Encourage parents to discuss adolescent's needs with him and ways he could modify schedule to better accommodate diabetic routine.	Poor medicine adherence may be a way adolescents express identity.	Parents and child plot out a weekly schedule that allows both freedom for new activities and conscientious diabetic care.
Discharge Planning				
Nurse	Assess whether child has experience with keeping a diabetic care journal.	Advise adolescent to keep a written diary of blood glucose levels, dietary intake (including snacks), and any symptoms of hypoglycemia and measures used.	A written diary provides objective evidence for evaluation of the new regimen, indicating the need for possible changes or adjustments.	Adolescent agrees to keep a detailed journal until return to clinic for follow-up visit.

(continued)

Team Member Responsible	Assessment	Intervention	Rationale	Expected Outcome
Discharge Planning				
Nurse	Assess whether adolescent or parents have any additional questions.	Arrange for a follow-up appointment in 1 week. Encourage adolescent and parents to call with any questions or concerns.	Follow-up visit provides a means for evaluating effectiveness of new regimen and child's adaptation.	Adolescent and parents state they understand importance of follow-up visit for regulation of insulin pump therapy.

their child. Both the parents and the child need time to describe their perceptions of diabetes. If there are other family members with the illness, children may have heard many false stories about the disorder and may have been told how difficult it was in the past to achieve insulin control. These misconceptions need to be corrected before the child can begin to accept the diagnosis and view himself or herself as basically well except for faulty insulin release.

What if... Rob wants to try out for soccer on his school team, but the soccer coach thinks diabetic children should be excluded from sports? What information can you give the parents about diabetes that they could share with the coach?

Teach About Disease and Principles of Care. Teaching is one of the main interventions necessary for children newly diagnosed with diabetes. Review general principles of care, including the fact that insulin injections, supervised intake of food, and exercise all decrease the blood glucose level, and increased intake of food increases it. Infection and emotional upset also increase insulin requirements. If this process is not explained, parents may attempt to keep the child relatively quiet, unaware that exercise is actually healthful.

Teach that an episode of hypoglycemia is an extremely serious condition and must be prevented, if possible. Otherwise, parents may view continuous low blood glucose levels as a positive sign rather than a potentially threatening condition that deprives body cells of glucose. If early signs are not recognized and treated, they can lead to coma and seizures. Severe glucose depletion can lead to permanent brain damage with mental and motor impairment, because brain cells need glucose for metabolism.

Be certain that parents have opportunities to practice supervised insulin injection and blood glucose testing so that they can become familiar with these procedures and any accompanying problems. Help them make a fair appraisal of how much care their child will be able to undertake for himself or herself. In the beginning, it is often better to limit the child's share of care to one blood glucose test-

ing session and one self-administered insulin injection per day. This helps parents to avoid expecting too much from their child, and possibly growing frustrated if the child does not meet their expectations. It makes successful management of the child's diabetes a rewarding experience rather than a chore.

Teach parents about the type of insulin their child will be taking. However, avoid giving too much confusing detail about all the different types. If the insulin is changed at a later date, the new form can be described in greater depth at that time. Also, urge the parents or the child to begin keeping a log of blood glucose test results in a permanent notebook so that these numbers can be evaluated for any unusual patterns at periodic checkups.

Establish Mode of Supervision and Support. Children with diabetes need frequent health supervision visits, approximately every 3 months. Those who appear to accept their diagnosis initially may have difficulty later, when their true feelings about their disorder surface. When they reach adolescence and are rebelling against a multitude of things, they may choose to rebel against blood glucose testing and insulin administration. Assess that children with diabetes have supportive friends to help them through "bad days." Sometimes what is needed most from health care personnel is understanding and appreciation of the difficulties encountered by children living with diabetes.

Serving as an active support person for the parents is also necessary. Often, parents are so concerned with learning the techniques of insulin administration and blood glucose testing that they do not think through other problems of everyday living that will arise later. Make sure that the parents can identify support people and others to contact if they have problems or questions.

Nursing Diagnosis: Risk for imbalanced nutrition, less than body requirements, related to decreased insulin level

Outcome Evaluation: Child's growth follows percentile curve on standard growth chart; serum glucose is between 70 and 110 mg/dL fasting; child states that nutrition and exercise program is being followed.

Plan Nutrition Program. At one time, children with diabetes were placed on rigidly specified diets in which each food item had to be weighed. Then followed a period when children were allowed free diets, and any resulting glycosuria was managed by increasing their insulin doses. Today, it is generally accepted that conscientious diet modification is necessary, because chronic hyperglycemia can lead to vascular disease in later years. The American Diabetes Association no longer recommends a food exchange list. Rather, they recommend that children follow a nutrition pattern consistent with their lifestyle and cultural preferences. General guidelines for good nutrition are shown in Box 48.9.

Teach Hypoglycemic Management. Symptoms of hypoglycemia occur when the blood glucose level falls to about 60 mg/dL. At this point, there is no glycosuria. Parents and children, as soon as they

---

BOX 48.9 FOCUS ON . . .

FAMILY TEACHING

Nutritional Guidelines

Q. Rob's mother is concerned that Rob, as an adolescent, doesn't eat well. She asks you, "How can we make sure our child who has diabetes gets adequate nutrition?"

A. Here are some nutritional guidelines to help you:

- Plan well-balanced and appealing meals. Caloric content should be appropriate for your child's age group.
- Provide three meals throughout the day, plus snacks. Total daily caloric intake is divided to provide 20% as breakfast, 20% as lunch, 30% as dinner, and 10% as morning, afternoon, and evening snacks. Distribution of calories should be 55% carbohydrate, 30% fat, and 15% protein.
- Do not use dietetic food. This food is expensive and not necessary.
- Urge your child not to omit meals. Getting him to eat at every meal calls for creative planning so the child likes the foods served and eats readily.
- Maintain a positive outlook by stressing the foods your child is allowed to eat, not those he must avoid.
- Steer clear of concentrated carbohydrate sources, such as candy bars; be sure to include foods with adequate fiber, such as broccoli, because fiber helps prevent hyperglycemia.
- Keep complex carbohydrates available to be eaten before exercise, such as swimming or a softball game, to provide sustained carbohydrate energy sources.
- Teach children about meal planning so they can wisely select what to eat at school or at a friend's home. This teaching will promote independent self-care.

---

are old enough to understand, need to be aware of the reasons for hypoglycemia and what measures they must take to counteract it if it occurs.

Hypoglycemia can result from the administration of too much insulin, excessive exercise (because exercise uses up glucose), or failure to eat enough food. Typically, beginning symptoms include nervousness, weakness, dizziness, sweating, or tremors. In many children, the first signs of hypoglycemia are behavior problems: temper tantrums, stubbornness, silliness, irritability, or simply "not acting like himself." A few children become insensitive to the symptoms of hypoglycemia (termed *hypoglycemia unawareness*) and are then unable to recognize that it is occurring. Such children need more blood glucose determinations built into their routine.

When the signs of hypoglycemia are recognized, the child needs an immediate source of carbohydrate. Fifteen grams of a fast-acting carbohydrate are recommended, such as a half-glass of orange juice or regular soda. It is easy for children always to carry glucose tablets or hard candy such as Lifesavers with them and have them available for these times. If there is no improvement in symptoms and the blood glucose level has not risen by 15 mg/dL after 15 minutes, more carbohydrate (e.g., juice) should be given.

If the child is comatose when first discovered or is too upset or uncooperative to take oral sugar, parents can inject a specified dose of glucagon hydrochloride. This converts the glycogen that is stored in the liver to glucose. Usually, enough glycogen is converted after the drug injection to bring the child out of coma, after which an oral form of glucose can be given. The drug is not effective if the child's supply of glycogen is depleted.

If parents cannot give their child an injection and oral sugar cannot be given, honey, corn syrup, cake icing gel, or glucose can be rubbed onto the gums or inside the cheek (of course, parents should be taught how to prevent aspiration); corn syrup can be given as an enema. As soon as children are out of coma or are cooperative, they must take a source of complex carbohydrate, such as crackers or toast, to prevent further hypoglycemia. The primary health care provider needs to be notified of the incident so that its cause can be determined and steps taken to prevent it from occurring again.

Urge parents to anticipate occasions when hypoglycemia is likely to occur and to take preventive measures. Hypoglycemia is most likely to occur at the peak effective time of the insulins being given (i.e., just before lunch or just before dinner). This means that many children who are attending school need to be scheduled for the first lunch period, not the second, or need a snack before lunch. Encourage the child and parents to discuss lunch times with the physician and dietitian so that appropriate meal planning is coordinated with the child's insulin schedule. Follow-up at 6-month intervals is advised to make adjustments for changes in growth and school schedules. Children also should eat dinner at a regular time or have a snack to tide them over until dinner. Additionally, children need a snack before bedtime, to prevent hypoglycemia from developing during the night.

If children are going to engage in an active sport, such as swimming, tennis, or basketball, they should ingest a source of sugar before participation. This precaution is extremely important before swimming, because a child who suddenly becomes weak in the middle of a pool may be unable to reach the side safely. Although eating before swimming is something that children typically are taught not to do, the child with diabetes must be taught to break this rule—sensibly, of course: before swimming, the child eats a complex carbohydrate, such as crackers, not a full meal. Day and residential camps are available to help children learn more about diabetes and common measures other athletic children use to prevent hypoglycemia.

Occasionally, insulin overuse and persistent hypoglycemia cause a rebound hyperglycemic response; this is referred to as the **Somogyi phenomenon.** This phenomenon is suspected when children have nighttime (2 or 3 AM) hypoglycemia followed by high early-morning hyperglycemia. These children need to be referred to their health care provider, because they actually need less insulin rather than more to correct the problem.

Teach Signs of Ketoacidosis. It is often difficult to distinguish between hypoglycemia (occurring from too much insulin) and hyperglycemia (occurring from too little insulin for the level of glucose present in the bloodstream). Hyperglycemia leads to ketoacidosis, with symptoms of vomiting and abdominal pain and the same kind of behavior changes exhibited with hypoglycemia.

If a parent does not know the cause of the upset, the child should be offered a carbohydrate, as if the problem were hypoglycemia. The added carbohydrate will do no harm if the problem is already hyperglycemia, whereas giving insulin is harmful if the cause is hypoglycemia. Inability to void suggests that the problem is hypoglycemia. With hyperglycemia, urine output is copious—one of the primary signs of diabetes. The real key to differentiating ketoacidosis from hypoglycemia is the blood glucose level. Assessing the blood glucose concentration by fingerstick solves the problem of whether symptoms relate to hypoglycemia or hyperglycemia.

If ketoacidosis is severe, respirations become deep and rapid (Kussmaul breathing) as the body attempts to "blow off" carbon dioxide and lessen the acidotic state. The breath smells sweet because of the presence of ketone bodies, and the pulse rate may be rapid. Children may have signs of dehydration, including dry mucous membranes and skin, sunken eyeballs, and no tears. This may be the picture when children with diabetes are first diagnosed. It is often seen in children with diabetes who develop gastroenteritis and hence eat poorly for a number of meals. Because the child is not eating well, parents

may omit giving insulin. In actuality, because of an increased metabolic rate due to fever, the child may need more insulin and glucose than usual during these times.

A comparison of hypoglycemia and hyperglycemia appears in Table 48.5.

Checkpoint Question 3

When Rob was first diagnosed with diabetes mellitus, he experienced a "honeymoon" period. This means

a. He developed an unnatural craving for sweets.
b. Puberty occurred because of glucose stimulation.
c. His need for injectable insulin was drastically reduced.
d. He became lightheaded or "giddy" every afternoon.

THE PARATHYROID GLANDS

The four parathyroid glands, located posterior and adjacent to the thyroid gland, function to regulate serum levels of calcium in the body; they control the rate of bone metabolism by secretion of parathyroid hormone. This hormone is not under the control of the pituitary gland but is controlled by a negative feedback from the circulating serum levels of calcium. If blood calcium levels fall, parathyroid hormone secretion increases; if blood calcium levels increase, hormone production decreases. Vitamin D is necessary for absorption of calcium from the gastrointestinal tract into the bloodstream, so it also influences parathyroid hormone secretion. Calcitonin (thyrocalcitonin), secreted by the thyroid gland, opposes the action of parathyroid hormone, decreasing blood calcium levels.

Hypocalcemia

Hypocalcemia is a lowered blood calcium level. It occurs to some extent in all newborns before they begin eating well (Hsu & Levine, 2004). Phosphorus and calcium levels are maintained in an inverse proportion to each other in the bloodstream (i.e., if phosphorus levels rise, calcium levels decrease; if calcium levels rise, phosphorus levels decrease). Hypocalcemia, therefore, may be caused by changes in either calcium or phosphorus metabolism.

Assessment

Hypocalcemia tends to occur in infants who experienced birth anoxia (phosphorus is released with anoxia), in immature infants (the parathyroid gland is immature), and in infants of diabetic mothers (it tends to accompany the hypoglycemia that occurs in these infants shortly after birth). It may be caused by the imbalance between phosphorus and calcium in cow's milk; such an imbalance does not exist in breast milk and is modified in commercial formulas.

Latent Tetany. The chief sign of hypocalcemia is neuromuscular irritability, often referred to as **latent tetany.** This occurs if the blood calcium level is less than 7.5 mg/dL.

TABLE 48.5

Comparison of Hypoglycemia and Hyperglycemia

Comparison Factor	Hypoglycemia	Hyperglycemia
Cause	Excessive insulin injection	Inadequate insulin injection
	Excessive exercise	Excessive food intake
	Limited food intake	Stress from infection, surgery, etc.
Symptoms	Hunger	Glycosuria and ketonuria
	Lethargy	Polyuria, polydipsia
	Sensorium changes	Kussmaul respirations
	Pallor	Flushing
	Sweating	Sweet (acetone) breath
	Seizures	Decreased CO_2 combining power
	Coma	Dehydration
		Lowered sodium, potassium, bicarbonate, chloride, and phosphate levels
		Vomiting, abdominal pain
		Coma
Danger	Brain cells need glucose for function and survival	Fatty acids are used and acidosis develops
Major nursing interventions	Administration of source of glucose by oral or IV route	Reestablishment of electrolyte balance and hydration
	Education to prevent recurrences	Education to prevent recurrences

Newborns with latent tetany are jittery when they are handled, or they cry for extended periods.

Four methods can be used to produce the clinical manifestations of tetany for diagnosis of hypocalcemia; these are shown in Table 48.6. These are all useful tests to determine or suggest whether a newborn's jitteriness is a result of hypocalcemia, a central nervous system problem, or some other cause.

If tetany is caused by infant formula, it occurs at about day 7 of life. A community health nurse making a follow-up visit after a home birth might be the one to recognize the problem initially.

Manifest Tetany. If the blood calcium level falls well below 7 mg/dL, **manifest tetany** may result, commonly observed as muscular twitching and carpopedal spasms. A **carpal spasm** (hand spasm) involves abduction of the hand and flexion of the wrist with the thumb positioned across the palm. In **pedal spasm** (foot spasm), the foot is extended, the toes flex, and the sole of the foot cups. Generalized seizures may occur. There may be spasm of the larynx, with the infant emitting a high-pitched, crowing sound on inspiration because of the constricted airway. If the spasm is prolonged, respirations may cease.

Therapeutic Management

Treatment is aimed at increasing the calcium level in the blood above the point of latent tetany. Calcium may be

TABLE 48.6

Detection of Hypocalcemia

Sign	Description
Chvostek's	When skin anterior to external ear (just over sixth cranial nerve) is tapped, facial muscles surrounding eye, nose, and mouth contract unilaterally.
Trousseau's	When upper arm is constricted by tourniquet for 2–3 min and area becomes blanched, carpal spasm is elicited (hand abducts, wrist flexes, thumb is positioned across cupped palm).
Peroneal	When fibular side of leg over peroneal nerve is tapped, foot abducts and dorsiflexes.
Erb's	This test is dramatic to see demonstrated, although it requires a mild galvanic current so is not used routinely. A person with tetany has greater muscular irritability than a person with a normal calcium level; therefore, when a mild current is applied over the peroneal nerve just below the head of the fibula, the foot on that side will abduct and dorsiflex.

administered orally as 10% calcium chloride if the infant can and will suck. It can be given IV as a 10% solution of calcium gluconate if the tetany has so progressed that the child does not have enough muscular coordination to take oral fluid safely. Calcium gluconate should not be given IM or SC, because necrosis may occur at the injection site. Newborns who are having generalized seizures may require anticonvulsant therapy in addition to the calcium gluconate to halt the seizures. Emergency equipment for intubation to relieve laryngospasm should be available.

After immediate therapy to increase the low blood calcium levels, infants are given oral calcium therapy until their calcium level stabilizes at greater than 7.5 mg/dL. Because vitamin D is necessary for absorption of calcium and phosphorus from the gastrointestinal tract, the infant also may be given a vitamin D supplement.

METABOLIC DISORDERS

Earlier in this chapter, ways in which overproduction or underproduction of certain hormones can seriously hinder body metabolism—creating such problems as hypothyroidism, congenital adrenogenital hyperplasia, and type 1 diabetes mellitus—were discussed. There are many causes for hormonal deficiency or excess, most of which are related to the endocrine glands and the highly complex system of feedback and communication between these glands and the hypothalamus. The neuroendocrine regulation of hormonal balance is so sensitive that it is affected by the body's internal and external environments (i.e., injury, stress, and emotional changes).

In addition to endocrine disorders, a group of hereditary biochemical disorders also affect metabolism. These are caused largely by some specific defect in the body biochemistry that disrupts one step of the metabolic process. The term *inborn errors of metabolism* is used to refer to these disorders. Most of them are caused by a lack of or deficiency in a particular enzyme, which seriously impairs the ability of the body to metabolize properly the components of food for energy.

Inborn errors of metabolism affect the metabolism of amino acids and proteins, carbohydrates, and lipids. Many of these disorders are evident at or soon after birth and can cause severe symptoms rapidly. Early detection and treatment are essential to prevent irreversible cognitive challenge and early death. Gene therapy is expected to be available in the future to reverse symptoms of these disorders.

Phenylketonuria

Phenylketonuria (PKU) is a disease of metabolism that is inherited as an autosomal recessive trait. Absence of the liver enzyme phenylalanine hydroxylase prevents conversion of phenylalanine, an essential amino acid, into tyrosine (a precursor of epinephrine, thyroxine, and melanin). As a result, excessive phenylalanine builds up in the bloodstream and tissues, causing permanent damage to brain tissue and leaving children severely cognitively challenged (Kahler & Fahey, 2003).

The metabolite phenylpyruvic acid (a breakdown product of phenylalanine) spills into the urine to give the disorder its name. It causes urine to have a typical musty or "mousy" odor that is so strong it often pervades not only the urine but the entire child.

Tyrosine is necessary for building body pigment and is incorporated into thyroxine. Without it, body pigment fades and the child becomes very fair skinned, light blonde haired, and blue eyed. The child fails to meet average growth standards because of the lack of thyroxine production. Many children develop an accompanying seizure disorder. The skin is prone to eczema (atopic dermatitis). There is such a strong association between these two disorders that all infants with atopic dermatitis need to be rescreened for PKU.

PKU is found in 1 of every 10,000 births in the United States. It occurs rarely in people of African or Jewish ancestry. If the condition remains untreated, the child with PKU usually will have an IQ below 20. In addition, about one third of affected children have recurrent seizures, and about half have muscular hypertonicity and spasticity. PKU cannot be detected by amniocentesis or percutaneous umbilical cord blood sampling as a routine screening measure, because the phenylalanine level does not rise in utero, while the infant is still under the control of the mother's enzyme system. Recombinant DNA techniques can be used for carrier detection and prenatal diagnosis.

Assessment

Early identification of the disorder is essential to prevent the child from becoming severely cognitively challenged. Infants are screened at birth after receiving 2 full days of feedings (at least 120 mL of formula at a concentration of 20 calories per ounce, or the equivalent amount obtained by breast-feeding). The screening is done by pricking the infant's heel with a blood lancet and letting a few drops of blood fall onto a specially prepared filter paper. The filter paper is then analyzed by a bacterial inhibition process for the amount of phenylalanine contained in the infant's blood (the Guthrie test). If an infant is born at home or is discharged from a hospital or birthing center before the second day of life, the parents will need to have the test performed on the second or third day after birth. If there is a question as to whether a breast-fed baby has received only colostrum, a repeated Guthrie test should be performed by the second week of life, during a health care visit.

Some infants demonstrate a benign, transitory, elevated level of phenylalanine shortly after birth, apparently due to immature processing of amino acids. This benign, transitory form needs to be differentiated from the actual disease so that parents are not frightened unnecessarily and the child is not unnecessarily placed on a restricted diet.

Therapeutic Management

Infants in whom this disease is detected during the first few days of life are placed on a formula that is extremely low in phenylalanine, such as Lofenalac. Beginning the diet early helps to keep the child from becoming cognitively challenged. A dietitian may recommend that a small amount of milk be added to the infant's diet every day so the child does receive some phenylalanine (this essential amino acid is necessary for growth and repair of body cells). As a result, a mother who wants to breast-feed may be able to do so on a limited basis.

Parents of children with PKU need a realistic prognosis of their child's potential. If the disorder was detected during the first few days of life and the child's diet is well controlled to avoid any abnormally high level of phenylalanine, the child's IQ will not be adversely affected. On the other hand, if the disorder was not detected until some brain involvement or other symptoms were noticeable, such symptoms cannot be reversed.

Providing nutrition for a child with PKU is a difficult task. There is no natural protein with both a low phenylalanine concentration and normal levels of other essential amino acids. A diet that simply restricted protein would result in restriction of all essential amino acids and would be incompatible with life. Specially manufactured formulas such as Lofenalac are synthetic compounds that have a low phenylalanine concentration but contain enough other essential nutrients so that, with the exception of some additional milk, they are the only food required in early infancy. Unfortunately, amino acid formulas have a rather disagreeable taste. When infants are given these formulas in the first few days of life, however, they do not seem to react to the flavor and will drink them readily into adulthood. These formulas can cause stools to be loose.

As children grow older and have solid foods added to their meals, these foods also must be low in phenylalanine so that the phenylalanine level of the child's blood stays below 8 mg/dL. Foods highest in phenylalanine are those that are rich in protein, such as meats, eggs, and milk. Foods low in phenylalanine include orange juice, bananas, potatoes, lettuce, spinach, and peas. A formula such as Lofenalac can be used to prepare treat foods, such as ice cream, milk shakes, birthday cakes, and puddings (foods that would otherwise be forbidden because they are made with milk). Children need their blood and urine monitored frequently for phenylalanine levels. Hemoglobin levels should also be closely monitored to ensure that the child is not becoming anemic, because iron is found primarily in protein-rich foods, which the child must avoid.

At health visits, offer parents an opportunity to express their feelings about the difficulty of maintaining a young child on such a restricted diet. In addition, assess the child's ability to cope with the illness; by the time they reach adolescence, children grow tired of the constant testing and restrictive diet (Walter & White, 2004).

When to discontinue the diet is controversial because of reports of progressive neurologic deterioration in children who are no longer following a restricted diet. Generally, current advice is for children to follow the diet indefinitely. A woman who has PKU must anticipate when she wants to have children as an adult; if she has not been following her diet conscientiously, she must return to a low-phenylalanine diet for about 3 months before conception and remain on the diet during pregnancy (see Chapter 12). Otherwise, her fetus will be exposed to high levels of phenylalanine during pregnancy and will be born cognitively challenged (Rouse & Azen, 2004).

What if... you are helping at a preschool and notice the teacher urging a little boy with PKU to drink his milk? When you suggest that milk might not be good for him, the teacher says, "Of course it is. Milk is nature's perfect food." How would you respond? What would you do?

Maple Syrup Urine Disease

Maple syrup urine disease is a rare disorder, inherited as an autosomal recessive trait, in which there is a defect in metabolism of the amino acids leucine, isoleucine, and valine that leads to cerebral degeneration similar to that observed in children with PKU.

Assessment

Infants appear well at birth but quickly begin to show signs of feeding difficulty, loss of the Moro reflex, and irregular respirations. The symptoms progress rapidly to *opisthotonos,* generalized muscular rigidity, and seizures. If the condition remains untreated, the child may die of the disease as early as 2 to 4 weeks of age (Nellis et al., 2004).

Although the disorder is rare, it is mentioned here because it is relatively easy to detect. By the first or second day of life, the urine of the child develops the characteristic odor of maple syrup; hence the name of the disease. The odor is caused by the presence of ketoacids, the same phenomenon that makes the breath of diabetic children in severe acidosis smell sweet. Because nurses are most likely to detect the characteristic urine odor in the first few days of life, they should be aware of this disorder so that they do not discount the pleasant urine odor as an innocent finding. Prenatal detection is possible by analyzing cells obtained by amniocentesis.

Therapeutic Management

If maple syrup urine disease is diagnosed during the first day or two of life and the child is placed on a well-controlled diet that is high in thiamine and low in the amino acids leucine, isoleucine, and valine, the cerebral degeneration can be prevented, just as it can be prevented in PKU. Such a diet is extremely difficult to maintain, however, because of its low protein content. Parents need intensive nutritional counseling. Hemodialysis or peritoneal dialysis can be used to temporarily reduce abnormal serum levels at birth or during a childhood infection, when catabolism of cells releases increased amino acid into the bloodstream.

Galactosemia

Galactosemia is a disorder of carbohydrate metabolism that is characterized by abnormal amounts of galactose in the blood (*galactosemia*) and in the urine (*galactosuria*). It occurs in about 1 of every 60,000 births, most often as an inborn error of metabolism, transmitted as an autosomal recessive trait. The child is deficient in the liver enzyme galactose 1-phosphate uridyltransferase (Bosch, 2004).

Lactose (the sugar found in milk) normally is broken down into galactose and glucose; galactose is then further broken down into additional glucose. Without the galactose 1-phosphate uridyltransferase enzyme, this second step, the conversion of galactose into glucose, cannot take place, and galactose builds up in the bloodstream and spills into the urine. When it reaches toxic levels, it destroys body cells.

Assessment

Symptoms appear when the child begins formula feeding or breast-feeding and include lethargy, hypotonia, and perhaps diarrhea and vomiting. Next, the liver enlarges as cirrhosis develops. Jaundice is often present and persistent; bilateral cataracts develop. The symptoms begin abruptly and worsen rapidly. If the condition remains untreated, the child may die by 3 days of age. Untreated children who survive beyond this time may be cognitively challenged or have bilateral cataracts. Because early detection is the key to preventing brain damage, nursing assessment is particularly important in this disorder.

Diagnosis is made by measuring the level of the affected enzyme in the red blood cells. A screening test (the Beutler test) can be used to analyze cord blood if a child is known to be at risk for the disorder.

Therapeutic Management

The treatment of galactosemia consists of placing the infant on a diet that is free of galactose or on a formula made with milk substitutes such as casein hydrolysates (e.g., Nutramigen). Once the child's condition is regulated on this diet, symptoms of the disease do not progress; however, any neurologic or cataract damage that is already present will persist. The duration of the restricted diet is controversial, but probably it should be followed for life.

Glycogen Storage Disease

Glycogen storage disease is actually a group of genetically transmitted disorders that involve altered production and use of glycogen in the body. Twelve of the 13 described types are inherited as autosomal recessive traits; the other is a sex-linked disorder (Mundy et al., 2003).

Glycogen is normally stored in the liver as a reserve supply of glucose. When the body needs glucose for energy, this glycogen is transformed back to glucose. In children with glycogen storage disease, glycogen is deposited normally, but an enzyme deficiency prevents retransformation of the glycogen back to glucose. As a result, children's livers rapidly increase in size from the stored glycogen. Children with this disorder are susceptible to periods of hypoglycemia, because their only source of ready glucose is oral intake.

In one form of this disorder (type II or Pompe's disease), children deposit large stores of glycogen, not only in the liver, but in the muscle and heart as well (Kishnani & Howell, 2004). The muscles begin to feel hard to palpation due to the deposits of glycogen. The heart becomes enlarged, and often an arrhythmia is present. Without therapy, children with this form usually die of heart failure before they reach adulthood.

Assessment

A common sign of glycogen storage disease is liver enlargement, because the liver must store the large supply of glycogen. Consequently, the abdomen protrudes. Over a long period, the child's growth is stunted because there is not enough glucose for any function but immediate energy. If hypoglycemic episodes have been severe, brain damage may result. Many children have a tendency toward epistaxis or hemorrhage and are at risk when having surgery performed because of impaired clotting ability due to decreased platelet adhesiveness.

Therapeutic Management

Children with glycogen storage disease need to be maintained on a high-carbohydrate diet with snacks between meals to prevent hypoglycemia. In addition, a continuous glucose nasogastric or gastrostomy feeding during the night may be necessary to prevent hypoglycemia while sleeping. Therapy with diazoxide (Proglycem), an antihypoglycemic drug that inhibits insulin release, may help regulate the glucose level to provide additional growth. Liver transplantation may be a possibility, but it will not cure the enzyme deficiency (Liu et al., 2003).

Tay-Sachs Disease

Tay-Sachs disease is an autosomal recessively inherited disease in which the infant lacks hexosaminidase A, an enzyme necessary for lipid metabolism. Without this enzyme, lipid deposits accumulate on nerve cells, leading to cognitive challenge due to deposits on brain cells and blindness due to deposits on optic nerve cells (Cohn, 2003).

Tay-Sachs disease is found primarily in the Ashkenazi Jewish population (Eastern European Jewish ancestry). Children generally appear normal in the first few months of life except for an extreme Moro reflex and mild hypotonia. At about 6 months of age, they begin to lose head control and are unable to sit up or roll over without support. On ophthalmoscopic examination, a cherry-red macula is noticeable (caused by lipid deposits). By 1 year of age, children have developed symptoms of spasticity and are unable to perform even simple motor tasks. By 2 years of age, generalized seizures and blindness have occurred. Most children die of cachexia (malnutrition) and pneumonia by 3 to 5 years of age.

There is no cure for Tay-Sachs disease. The disorder may be detected in utero by amniocentesis. Carriers for the disease trait may be identified by hexosaminidase A assay.

Key Points

Endocrine disorders are almost all long-term disorders. Helping parents and children remember to take medicine on a long-term basis is an important nursing responsibility.

Children with endocrine or metabolic disorders often develop height or weight discrepancies. Help children continue to feel high self-esteem by concentrating on the things they are able to do despite a growth lag.

Growth hormone (GH) deficiency, a pituitary disorder, results in short stature. Therapy for children consists of the injection of synthetic GH. Children can experience situational low self-esteem if they do not receive adequate emotional support from significant others.

Other pituitary disorders include GH excess and diabetes insipidus. As the name implies, with GH excess, there is overproduction of GH. With diabetes insipidus, there is decreased release of antidiuretic hormone (ADH). Urine becomes dilute, and large amounts are excreted. Therapy is administration of desmopressin (DDAVP), an arginine vasopressin. Children with this are at high risk for fluid volume deficit.

Congenital hypothyroidism occurs as a result of an absent or nonfunctioning thyroid gland. The condition is discovered by a blood test at birth. The therapy is oral administration of synthetic thyroid hormone.

Acquired hypothyroidism (Hashimoto's disease) is an autoimmune phenomenon that interferes with thyroid gland function. Therapy is administration of synthetic thyroid hormone.

Acute adrenocortical insufficiency can occur in children from causes such as an overwhelming infection in which there is hemorrhagic destruction of the adrenal gland. A more common disease in children is congenital adrenogenital hyperplasia. Girls are born masculinized; either sex may be unable to retain sodium, which results in rapid fluid loss. Therapy is administration of hydrocortisone.

Cushing syndrome is caused by overproduction of cortisol by the adrenal gland. This usually results from a tumor in the gland. Children appear abnormally obese. Therapy is surgical removal of the tumor.

The most frequently occurring pancreatic disorder is type 1 diabetes mellitus. This may be an autoimmune process in which there has been destruction of insulin-producing islet cells. Therapy is a combination of administration of insulin, diet, and exercise.

Hypocalcemia, a parathyroid gland disorder, results in a lowered blood calcium level. In children, tetany develops. Therapy is the administration of calcium.

Various disorders of metabolism that interfere with carbohydrate, amino acid, or fat metabolism occur in children. Representative of these are PKU, galactosemia, and Tay-Sachs disease.

Critical Thinking Exercises

1. Rob is the 16-year-old boy diagnosed as having type 1 diabetes whom you met at the beginning of the chapter. In the last 6 months, he has "forgotten" to take his insulin at least once a week. Is Rob's history unusual for an adolescent? What health teaching do you think will most help him re-establish control?

2. A 12-year-old girl with GH deficiency is only 3 feet tall and has been told she probably will not grow taller than 4 ft, 6 in. Her parents tell you they find her "cute," so they do not want her to receive GH. How would you approach this family? To what extent should the child be able to contribute to this decision?

3. A newborn is diagnosed as having the salt-losing form of congenital adrenal hyperplasia. What would be the most important measure to teach her parents before she is discharged from the hospital? How may having a child with this disorder change this family's life?

4. Examine the National Health Goals related to endocrine or metabolic disorders in children. Most government-sponsored money for nursing research is allotted based on these goals. What would be a possible research topic to explore pertinent to these goals that would be applicable to the Tebecco family and also advance evidence-based practice?

References

Alter, C. A. (2003). Growth hormone deficiency. In Schwartz, M. W. (Ed.) *5-minute pediatric consult* (3rd ed.). Philadelphia: Lippincott Williams & Wilkins.

Berenbaum, S. A., et al. (2004). Psychological adjustment in children and adults with congenital adrenal hyperplasia. *Journal of Pediatrics, 144*(6), 741–746.

Bosch, A. M. (2004). Living with classical galactosemia: Health-related quality of life consequences. *Pediatrics, 113*(5), 423–428.

Carel, J. C., Huet, F., & Chaussain, J. L. (2003). Treatment of growth hormone deficiency in very young children. *Hormone Research, 60*(Suppl 1), 10–17.

Cohn, R. M. (2003). Metabolic disorders with neurologic dysfunction. In Schwartz, M. W. (Ed.), *5-minute pediatric consult* (3rd ed.). Philadelphia: Lippincott Williams & Wilkins.

Deiss, D., et al. (2004). Assessment of glycemic control by continuous glucose monitoring system in 50 children with type 1 diabetes starting on insulin pump therapy. *Pediatric Diabetes, 5*(3), 117–121.

Department of Health and Human Services. (2000). *Healthy people 2010*. Washington, D.C.: DHHS.

DiMeglio, L. A., et al. (2004). A randomized, controlled study of insulin pump therapy in diabetic preschoolers. *Journal of Pediatrics, 145*(3), 380–384.

Eugster, E. A., et al. (2004). Definitive diagnosis in children with congenital hypothyroidism. *Journal of Pediatrics, 144*(5), 643–647.

Foley, T. P., Jr. (2004). Hypothyroidism. *Pediatrics in Review, 25*(3), 94–100.

Gassner, H. L., et al. (2004). Near-miss apparent SIDS from adrenal crisis. *Journal of Pediatrics, 145*(2), 178–183.

Grimsberg, A. (2003). Congenital hypothyroidism. In Schwartz, M. W. (Ed.), *5-minute pediatric consult* (3rd ed.). Philadelphia: Lippincott Williams & Wilkins.

Gruneiro-Papendieck, L., et al. (2003). Pediatric Graves' disease: Outcome and treatment. *Journal of Pediatric Endocrinology, 16*(9), 1249–1255.

Houghton, J. (2004). Diagnosis and management of type 1 diabetes. *Paediatric Nursing, 16*(10), 22–23.

Hsu, S. C., & Levine, M. A. (2004). Perinatal calcium metabolism: Physiology and pathophysiology. *Seminars in Neonatology, 9*(1), 23–36.

Joseph, J. T., et al. (2003). Quality of life after kidney and pancreas transplantation: A review. *American Journal of Kidney Diseases, 42*(3), 431-445.

Kahler, S. G., & Fahey, M. C. (2003). Metabolic disorders and mental retardation. *American Journal of Medical Genetics, 117*(1), 31-41.

Karch, A. M. (2004). *Lippincott's nursing drug guide.* Philadelphia: Lippincott Williams & Wilkins.

Kishnani, P. S., & Howell, R. R. (2004). Pompe disease in infants and children. *Journal of Pediatrics, 144*(5 Suppl), S35-S43.

Krieger, M. D., Couldwell, W. T., & Weiss, M. H. (2003). Assessment of long-term remission of acromegaly following surgery. *Journal of Neurosurgery, 98*(4), 719-724.

Lajic, S., et al. (2004). Prenatal treatment of congenital adrenal hyperplasia. *European Journal of Endocrinology, 151*(Suppl 3), U63-U69.

Lecamwasam, H. S., Baboolal, H. A., & Dunn, P. F. (2004). Acute adrenal insufficiency after large-dose glucocorticoids for spinal cord injury. *Anesthesia and Analgesia, 99*(6), 1813-1814.

Liu, P. P., et al. (2003). Outcome of living donor liver transplantation for glycogen storage disease. *Transplantation Proceedings, 35*(1), 366-368.

Marcus, B. J., & Collins, K. A. (2004). Childhood panhypopituitarism presenting as child abuse: A case report and review of the literature. *American Journal of Forensic Medicine and Pathology, 25*(3), 265-269.

Mundy, H. R., et al. (2003). The regulation of growth in glycogen storage disease type 1. *Clinical Endocrinology, 58*(3), 332-339.

Nellis, M. M., et al. (2004). Relationship of causative genetic mutations in maple syrup urine disease with their clinical expression. *Molecular Genetics and Metabolism, 80*(1-2), 189-195.

Ozbey, H., et al. (2004). Gender assignment in female congenital adrenal hyperplasia: A difficult experience. *BJU International, 94*(3), 388-391.

Rapaport, R., et al. (2004). Type 1 and type 2 diabetes mellitus in childhood in the United States: Practice patterns by pediatric endocrinologists. *Journal of Pediatric Endocrinology, 17*(6), 871-877.

Read, C. H., Jr., Tansey, M. J., & Menda, Y. (2004). A 36-year retrospective analysis of the efficacy and safety of radioactive iodine in treating young Graves' patients. *Journal of Clinical Endocrinology and Metabolism, 89*(9), 4229-4233.

Rouse, B., & Azen, C. (2004). Effect of high maternal blood phenylalanine on offspring congenital anomalies and developmental outcome at ages 4 and 6 years: The importance of strict dietary control preconception and throughout pregnancy. *Journal of Pediatrics, 144*(2), 235-239.

Schreiner, B. (2005). Promoting lifestyle and behavior change in overweight children and adolescents with type 2 diabetes. *Diabetes Spectrum, 18*(1), 9-12.

Simard, M. (2004). The biochemical investigation of Cushing syndrome. *Neurosurgical Focus, 16*(4), E4.

Sugino, K., et al. (2004). Surgical treatment of Graves' disease in children. *Thyroid, 14*(6), 447-452.

Thornton, P. S. (2003). Diabetes insipidus. In Schwartz, M. W. (Ed.), *5-minute pediatric consult* (3rd ed.). Philadelphia: Lippincott Williams & Wilkins.

Walter, J. H., & White, F. J. (2004). Blood phenylalanine control in adolescents with phenylketonuria. *International Journal of Adolescent Medicine and Health, 16*(1), 41-45.

Weinzimer, S. A. (2003). Diabetes mellitus. In Schwartz, M. W. (Ed.), *5-minute pediatric consult* (3rd ed.). Philadelphia: Lippincott Williams & Wilkins.

Suggested Readings

Bramwell, J., Hibbert-Jones, E., & Regan, G. (2005). Developing an education resource pack for children and young people. *Journal of Diabetes Nursing, 9*(1), 21-23.

Durham, E. (2003). Growth hormone deficiency in children: A change in diagnostic approach. *Advances for Nurse Practitioners, 11*(1), 41-42.

Kruse, B., et al. (2004). Congenital adrenal hyperplasia: How to improve the transition from adolescence to adult life. *Experimental and Clinical Endocrinology and Diabetes, 112*(7), 343-355.

Maffei, P., et al. (2003). The cardiac complications of acromegaly. *Journal of Endocrinological Investigation, 26*(8 Suppl.), 20-27.

Pho, L. T., et al. (2004). Attitudes and psychosocial adjustment of unaffected siblings of patients with phenylketonuria. *American Journal of Medical Genetics, 126*(2), 156-160.

Read, C. Y. (2003). The demands of biochemical genetic disorders: A survey of mothers of children with mitochondrial disease of phenylketonuria. *Journal of Pediatric Nursing: Nursing Care of Children and Families, 18*(3), 181-186.

Van Vliet, G., & Czernichow, P. (2004). Screening for neonatal endocrinopathies: Rationale, methods and results. *Seminars in Neonatology, 9*(1), 75-85.

Wagner, J. A., Abbott, G., & Lett, S. (2004). Age related differences in individual quality of life domains in youth with type 1 diabetes. *Health and Quality of Life Outcomes, 2*(1), 54-55.

Waisbren, S. E., et al. (2004). Brief report: Predictors of parenting stress among parents of children with biochemical genetic disorders. *Journal of Pediatric Psychology, 29*(7), 565-570.

Yensel, C. S., Preud'homme, D., & Curry, D. M. (2004). Childhood obesity and insulin-resistant syndrome. *Journal of Pediatric Nursing, 19*(4), 238-246.

CHAPTER 49

Nursing Care of the Child With a Neurologic Disorder

Key Terms

- astereognosis
- automatisms
- autonomic dysreflexia
- central nervous system (CNS)
- cerebrospinal fluid (CSF)
- choreoathetosis
- choreoid
- decerebrate posturing
- decorticate posturing
- diplegia
- dyskinetic
- graphesthesia
- hemiplegia
- infantile spasms
- kinesthesia
- neuron
- paraplegia
- peripheral nervous system (PNS)
- pulse pressure
- quadriplegia
- status epilepticus
- stereognosis

Objectives

After mastering the contents of this chapter, you should be able to:

1. Describe common neurologic disorders in children.
2. Assess a child with a neurologic disorder.
3. Formulate nursing diagnoses for a child with a neurologic disorder.
4. Establish expected outcomes for a child with a neurologic disorder.
5. Plan nursing care for a child with a neurologic disorder.
6. Implement nursing care, such as monitoring medicine effectiveness, for a child with a neurologic disorder.
7. Evaluate expected outcomes for achievement and effectiveness of care.
8. Identify National Health Goals related to neurologic disorders and children that nurses could help the nation achieve.
9. Identify areas related to care of children with neurologic disorders that could benefit from additional nursing research or application of evidence-based practice.
10. Analyze ways in which care of a child with a neurologic disorder can be optimally family centered.
11. Integrate knowledge of neurologic disorders and the nursing process to achieve quality maternal and child health nursing care.

*T*asha is a 2-year-old girl who is brought to an emergency room by her mother because she had a seizure. Her physician suspects she may have meningitis. Her parent is visibly upset. She says, "Does this mean she'll always have seizures? How will she ever be independent?"

The discovery of a neurologic disorder in a child can be devastating to parents. Helping a family deal with the possible long-term and permanent effects of the disorder is essential. Nurses play a key role in providing support and education to the parents and the child to promote the child's optimal level of functioning.

Previous chapters described normal growth and development in children and nursing care of children with disorders of other systems. This chapter adds information about the dramatic changes, both physical and psychosocial, that occur when a child develops a neurologic disorder. This is important information because it builds a base for care and health teaching for children with these disorders.

What education does this parent need about recurrent seizures?

After you've studied this chapter, access the accompanying website. Read the patient scenario and answer the questions to further sharpen your skills, grow more familiar with RN-CLEX types of questions, and reward yourself with how much you have learned.

Neurologic disorders encompass a wide array of problems resulting from congenital disorders, acquired dysfunction, infection, or trauma. Many of these disorders can cause severe illness. Others can result in life-threatening complications. In addition, because neural tissue does not have the regenerative power of other body tissue, any nervous system degeneration is permanent. Whenever possible, prevention must be the highest priority for keeping the nervous system healthy. If degeneration has already occurred, nursing care often focuses on helping the child and family develop strategies for dealing with the associated loss in mental or physical functioning, making the child comfortable, and providing an environment conducive to the child's growth and self-esteem. Two major causes of neurologic dysfunction in children have been addressed by the National Health Goals. These are shown in Box 49.1.

Nursing Process Overview

For Care of a Child With a Neurologic System Disorder

● **Assessment**

Neurologic disorders often manifest with vague symptoms of something being wrong. Parents may indicate that their child "seems to be walking strangely" or is "just not herself." A thorough history and neurologic examination provide the best source of information regarding the cause of the child's problem. Possible findings are highlighted in Box 49.2.

The neurologic examination covers six areas of neurologic functioning, including mental or cognitive processes as well as motor and sensory functioning. If more information is needed, numerous diagnostic laboratory tests may be ordered. The parents and child need considerable support throughout the assessment process. Although the neurologic examination can be made "fun" for a child, other procedures such as a computed tomography (CT) scan or lumbar puncture can be frightening. Additionally, the anxiety of not knowing what is wrong and fearing the worst can make the waiting period for test results especially difficult for the child's parents.

● **Nursing Diagnosis**

Nursing diagnoses for children with neurologic disorders vary according to the child's needs. Initially, the child may need emergency care and constant observation, and the parents may need to discuss their fears about their child's illness. If the child undergoes surgery, nursing diagnoses should address immediate preoperative and postoperative care and long-term care such as rehabilitation and home care, taking into account the child's specific limitations and health care needs. Two nursing diagnoses should be kept in mind throughout these treatment phases:

- Risk for disuse syndrome related to neurologic deficit affecting one area of functioning
- Interrupted family processes related to stress associated with the long-term effects of the neurologic dysfunction

BOX 49.1 FOCUS ON . . .

NATIONAL HEALTH GOALS

Bacterial meningitis and head injuries are major causes of neurologic damage and subsequent disability in children. Three National Health Goals address children with disabilities:

- Reduce the proportion of children and adolescents with disabilities who report being sad, unhappy, or depressed, from a baseline of 31% to a target level of 17%.
- Reduce the number of people 21 years of age and younger with disabilities who are in congregate care facilities, from a baseline of 24,300 to 0.
- Increase the proportion of children and youth with disabilities who spend at least 80% of their time in regular education programs, from 45% to 60% (DHHS, 2000).

Nurses can help the nation achieve these goals through prevention of neurologic injury by educating children and parents about the use of helmets for bicycle and motorcycle safety, by administering and teaching paramedical personnel to administer safe care at accident scenes so that children's heads and necks are protected, and by decreasing the possible spread of bacterial meningitis through good handwashing and infection control precautions in hospitals.

Topics of nursing research that might help prevent neurologic injury or disease and subsequent disability include the following: What kinds of programs can school nurses initiate that would effectively teach bicycle safety? Could serious outcomes of bacterial meningitis be reduced if parents were educated about the symptoms of meningitis and brought children with such symptoms to health care facilities earlier?

Other nursing diagnoses are described along with specific disorders in this chapter.

● **Outcome Identification and Planning**

Be realistic when establishing expected outcomes. Children who have permanent limitations may not be able to achieve in some areas. When neurologic disorders are first diagnosed, parents may be able to focus only on the short term, such as whether the child will survive meningitis or whether the child has stopped convulsing. Later, they may need help to look at the long-term picture: Will they need assistance to care for the child at home? What type of education can be obtained? What type of exercise program will be required?

Before a diagnosis is confirmed, parents may attribute their child's functional deficits to immaturity (she is not walking yet because she is simply too young). They insist that, with age, her ability to function will improve. They are unable to make plans because they have not accepted their child's neurologic deficits. Until this occurs, they will not be ready for specific planning.

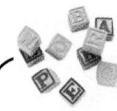

BOX 49.2 ASSESSMENT

Assessing a Child for Signs and Symptoms of a Neurologic Disorder

History
Chief concern: Seizure, loss of consciousness, delay in developmental tasks, headache, clumsiness at motor tasks.
Past medical history: Infection during pregnancy; difficult birth; difficulty with initiating respirations at birth; head injury from fall or accident.
Family medical history: History of seizures or headaches in other family members.

Physical examination

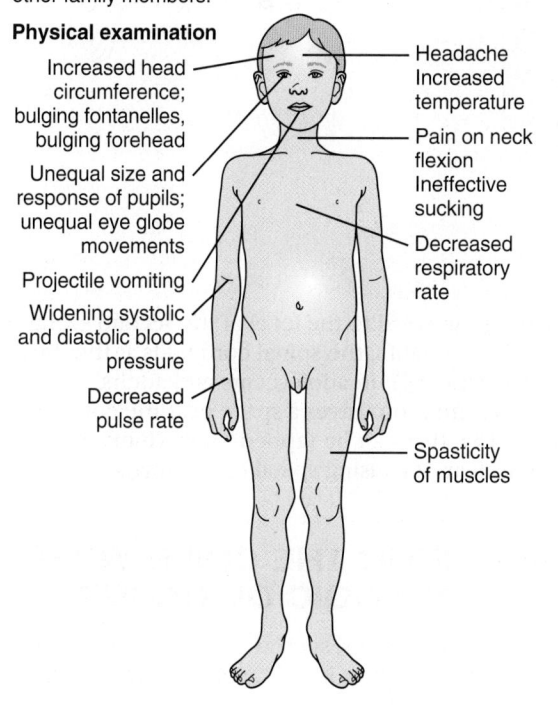

Increased head circumference; bulging fontanelles, bulging forehead

Unequal size and response of pupils; unequal eye globe movements

Projectile vomiting

Widening systolic and diastolic blood pressure

Decreased pulse rate

Headache
Increased temperature

Pain on neck flexion
Ineffective sucking

Decreased respiratory rate

Spasticity of muscles

- Epilepsy Foundation of America (*www.epilepsyfoundation.org*)
- National Information Center for Children and Youth with Disabilities (*www.nichcy.org*)
- National Fibromatosis Foundation (*www.ctf.org*)
- National Spinal Cord Injury Association (*www.spinalcord.org*)
- United Cerebral Palsy Association (*www.ucp.org*)

● *Outcome Evaluation*
Evaluation of the child with a neurologic disorder should address not only the child's progress in regaining physical function but also his or her level of self-esteem. Further planning to increase the child's self-esteem is necessary if the disorder is long-term. Some examples indicating achievement of possible outcomes are the following:

- Child states he is aware of potential for injury related to recurrent seizures.
- Family members state they are able to maintain family cohesiveness yet sustain contact with hospitalized child.
- Child practices exercises daily to reduce possibility of contracture from disuse syndrome.

ANATOMY AND PHYSIOLOGY OF THE NERVOUS SYSTEM

Nerve cells (**neurons**) are unique among body cells in that, instead of being compact, they consist of a cell nucleus and extensions: one axon and several dendrites. The *dendrite* transmits impulses to the cell nucleus; the *axon* transmits impulses away from the cell nucleus to body organs. These cells vary in size, ranging from a few inches to several feet long, reaching from distant body sites such as the feet, through the spinal cord, and to the brain. Although their great length is vital to motor and sensory function, it also makes nerve cells more susceptible than other body cells to injury.

The nervous system continues to mature through the first 12 years of life. It actually consists of two separate systems: the **central nervous system (CNS)** and the **peripheral nervous system (PNS).** The PNS consists of the cranial nerves, the spinal nerves, and the somatic and visceral divisions. The visceral division includes the autonomic system.

The CNS consists of the brain, the spinal cord, and the surrounding membranes or meninges that protect the delicate tissues from normal trauma. These tissues are also protected by the skull, the vertebral column, and the **cerebrospinal fluid (CSF),** the fluid in the subarachnoid space, which serves as a cushion.

The brain is covered by three membranes: the *dura mater* (a fibrous, connective tissue structure containing many blood vessels), the *arachnoid membrane* (a delicate serous membrane), and the *pia mater* (a vascular membrane) (Fig. 49.1).

Four fluid-filled cavities, or ventricles, lie within the brain (Fig. 49.2). CSF forms in the two lateral ventricles in the choroid plexus of the pia mater and flows through the foramens of Monro into the third ventricle, then through

When parents begin to adjust to the new reality, the time is right for support and help in solving problems.

● *Implementation*
Nursing interventions for the child with a neurologic problem must address both short- and long-term needs. For instance, while feeding an infant with increased intracranial pressure (ICP), demonstrate a caring attitude by showing her parents how to handle her gently. For parents of a child with seizures, explain that turning him gently to his side will prevent him from choking. This will help them feel less anxious about future seizures. The child, too, will feel more in control of his illness if he believes that both he and his parents will be able to handle any acute symptoms. Providing nursing care that meets everyone's needs takes a great deal of sensitivity and planning.

Long-term care needs can be a source of stress, physically, emotionally, socially, and financially. Numerous organizations are available for assistance and support. Some organizations concerned with children with neurologic disorders are the following:

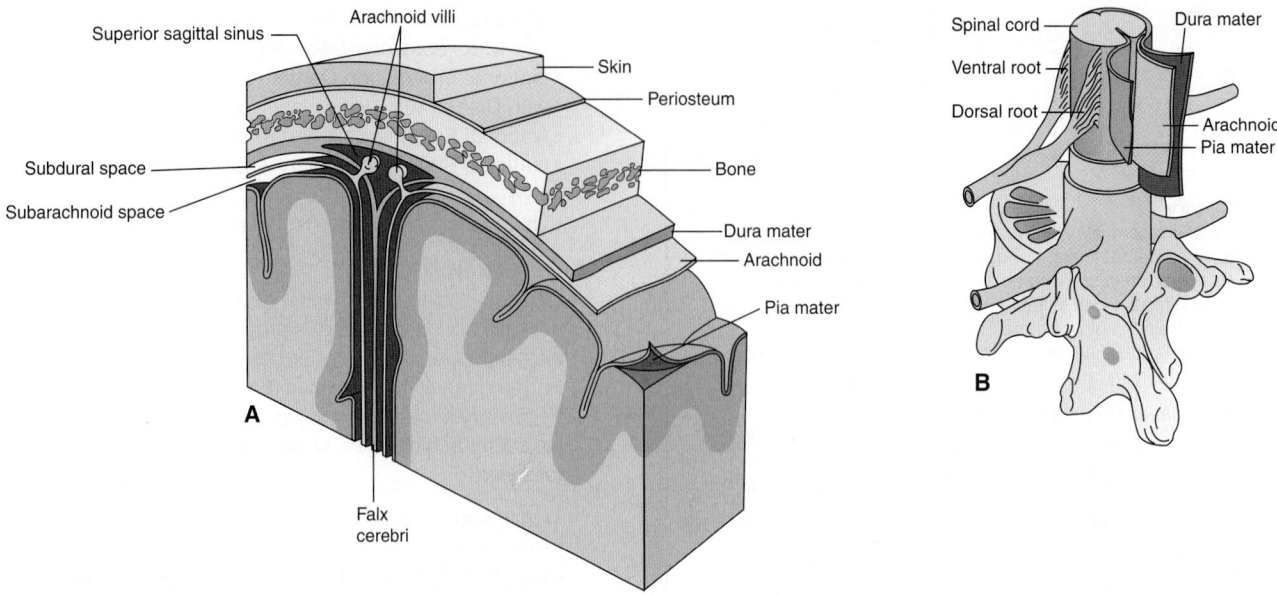

FIGURE 49.1 Meninges of the (**A**) brain and (**B**) spinal cord.

a narrow canal (the aqueduct of Sylvius) to the fourth ventricle. It leaves the fourth ventricle by the foramen of Magendie and the two foramens of Lushka and flows into the cisterna magna, a collection pool at the base of the skull. From the cisterna magna, the fluid circulates to the subarachnoid space of the spinal cord, bathing both the brain and the spinal cord. The fluid is then absorbed by the arachnoid membrane. The time span for replacement is approximately 6 hours.

The properties of CSF are shown in Table 49.1. It is basically a colorless, alkaline fluid with a specific gravity of approximately 1.004 to 1.008, containing traces of protein, glucose, lymphocytes, and body salts. The fluid cir-

culates downward to the level of the second sacral vertebra (S2). In infants, the spinal cord ends at the third lumbar vertebra (L3); in adolescents and adults, at L1 or L2. This configuration leaves a space near the cord base containing CSF that can be tapped safely (lumbar puncture) without fear of causing spinal cord damage.

ASSESSING THE CHILD WITH A NEUROLOGIC DISORDER

Neurologic symptoms, such as headache, an unsteady gait, or lethargy, are often insidious. Both a thorough history

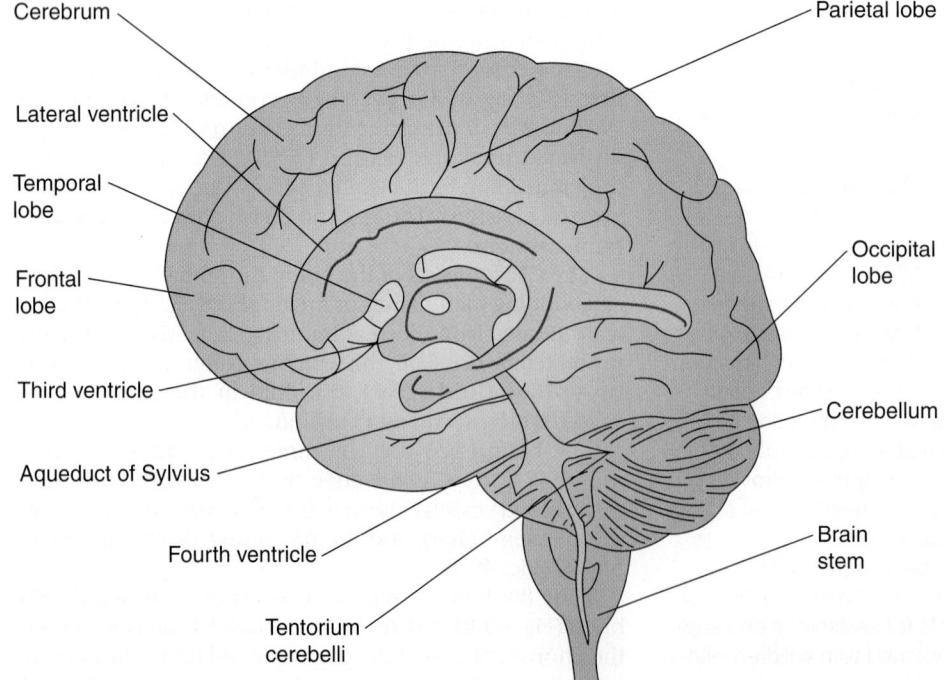

FIGURE 49.2 Ventricles of the brain. Cerebrospinal fluid flows from the lateral ventricles into the third ventricle, then through the narrow aqueduct of Sylvius to the fourth ventricle.

TABLE 49.1

Normal Properties of Cerebrospinal Fluid

Parameter	Normal Finding	Abnormal Finding: Possible Significance
Opening pressure	60–160 cm H_2O	Lowered pressure usually indicates that there is subarachnoid obstruction in the spinal column above the puncture site.
		Elevated pressure suggests intracranial compression, hemorrhage, or infection.
		Pressure increases if a child coughs or pressure is applied to the external jugular vein (Valsalva maneuver).
Appearance	Clear and colorless	If cloudy, indicates possible infection with an increased number of white blood cells (WBCs).
		If reddened, color is probably red blood cells (RBCs).
Cell count	0–8/mm³	Granulocytes suggest CSF infection.
		Lymphocytes suggest meningeal irritation and inflammation.
		A few RBCs and WBCs are normally present in the newborn CSF due to the trauma of birth.
Protein	15–45 mg/100 mL	Elevated count (> 45/100 mL) occurs if RBCs are present.
		If both protein content and RBC count are elevated, meningitis or subarachnoid hemorrhage is suggested.
		If protein content alone is elevated, it more likely suggests a degenerative process such as multiple sclerosis.
Glucose	60%–80% of serum glucose level	Decreased glucose level suggests that a glycolytic process is occurring.
		Bacterial meningitis causes a marked decrease in CSF glucose; invasion of fungi, yeast, tuberculosis, or protozoans into the CSF results in some decrease in glucose level.
		Viral infections do not cause a decrease in CSF glucose and may occasionally cause a slight increase.
Albumin/globulin (A/G)	8:1	Increased level suggests infection or A/G ratio neurologic disorder.

and a neurologic examination are needed to reveal the cause and extent of such symptoms.

Health History

The child's history may be the first clue in assessing a neurologic disorder. Because many neurologic problems result from fetal injury, it is important to obtain the mother's pregnancy history as well.

At primary care visits, ask parents about their child's developmental milestones and ability to perform age-appropriate tasks successfully. A Denver Developmental Screening Test can indicate whether a parent's concern about a preschool child is well founded. The ability to perform well in school is important documentation for an older child.

Neurologic Examination

A complete neurologic examination takes at least 20 minutes. It requires patience and skill to keep a child's attention while observing for possible indications of neurologic disease. For a full examination, six areas are assessed: cerebral, cranial nerve, cerebellar, motor, sensory, and reflex function.

Cerebral Function

Both general and specific cerebral functions are evaluated. General cerebral function is indicated by level of consciousness, orientation, intelligence, performance, mood, and general behavior.

Evaluate the child's level of consciousness through conversation. Note any drowsiness or lethargy and whether the child is oriented to his or her surroundings. Allow the child to answer questions without prompting, and listen carefully that the answer is appropriate to the question.

Orientation refers to whether a child is aware of who he is, where he is, and what day it is (person, place, and time). Be careful to take into account the child's age and development; children younger than 4 years of age may not know both their first and last names. Children may be of school age before they know their address. Children younger than 7 or 8 years of age may have difficulty with the days of the week, confusing "yesterday" with "today" or "tomorrow." Generally, you will be able to sense whether a child is in touch with his or her surroundings and has a clear sense of self.

Intellectual performance can be determined by the child's score on a standard intelligence test. Estimates of intellectual function can be made by asking the child questions on common topics.

Immediate recall is the ability to retain a concept for a short time. Ask the child to repeat numbers after you. A child who is 4 years old can usually repeat three digits. A child older than 6 years can repeat five digits. *Recent memory* covers a slightly longer period. Show the preschool child an object such as a key and ask him to remember it, because later you will ask him to tell you what it was. After about 5 minutes, ask whether he remembers what object you showed him. Ask older children what they ate for breakfast.

Remote memory is long-term recall. Ask preschoolers what they ate for breakfast that morning (to them, it was a long time ago); ask older children the name of their first-grade teacher.

Specific cerebral function can be measured by assessing language, sensory interpretation, and motor integration. When assessing language, listen to the child's ability to articulate. Remember that many preschoolers substitute "w" for "r," saying "west time" instead of "rest time."

Stereognosis refers to the ability to recognize an object by touch and tests sensory interpretation. Ask the child to close her eyes; then place a familiar object, such as a key, a penny, or a bottle cap, in her hand and ask her to identify it. This is something even preschoolers are able to do successfully.

Graphesthesia is the ability to recognize a shape that has been traced on the skin. Ask a preschooler to close his eyes; trace first a circle, then a square, on the back of his hand, and ask him whether the shapes are the same or different. Be sure that the child understands the concept of "different" by first showing him objects such as two keys and a bottle cap and documenting that he is able to identify the keys as being the same and the bottle cap as being different. For older children, trace numbers (8, 3, 0, and 1 work well) and ask the child to identify each one.

Kinesthesia is the ability to distinguish movement. Have the child close her eyes and extend her hands in front of her. Raise one of her fingers and ask her whether it is up or down. Hold the finger by its sides so that your other fingers do not brush against the child's palm or the back of her hand (this will reveal the finger position). Repeat the same movement with a toe on each foot. For preschoolers, first determine whether the child understands the concept of up and down.

Measure motor integration by asking the child to perform a complex motor skill, such as folding a piece of paper and putting it into an envelope. A child of 4 years and older should be able to do this neatly.

Children do best when these tests are presented as a game. Be certain to convey that there are no right or wrong answers. A child who believes that he has failed these tests may not respond well to further testing.

Cranial Nerve Function

Testing for cranial nerve function consists of assessing each pair of cranial nerves separately. Methods of cranial nerve testing are described in Table 49.2.

Cerebellar Function

Tests for cerebellar function are tests for normal balance and coordination. Observe the child walking. Does she do so naturally and freely? (Most children walk self-consciously when being observed.) Ask the child to stand on one foot. A child as young as 4 years should be able to do this for as long as 5 seconds. Ask the child to attempt a tandem walk (walk a straight line, one foot directly in front of the other, heel touching toe) (Fig. 49.3A). A child older than 4 years of age should be able to do this for about four consecutive steps. Ask the child to touch his nose with his finger, then reach and touch your finger with the same hand (held about 1½ feet in front of him) (see Fig. 49.3B). Tell him to repeat this action, and move your finger to a new position each time. The average child rarely reaches past your finger or stops before touching it.

Ask the child to pat one knee with the palm of her hand, then quickly turn the hand over and pat the knee with the back of her hand; repeat over and over. She should be able to do this rapid, coordinated motion without much difficulty. Always ask her to do the motion one hand at a time. Preschoolers will mirror the movement of the actively moving hand by moving the inactive hand as well. Older children should not demonstrate this (or should show only a small amount of movement).

Ask the child to touch each finger on one hand with the thumb of that hand in rapid succession. Ask him to run the heel of one foot down the front of his other leg while he is lying supine (he should be able to do this without "running off" the leg). While he is still lying on the examining table, ask him to close his eyes and to draw a circle or figure 8 in the air with his foot.

Tests of cerebellar function are all fun for children to do, as long as they know that there are no passes or failures. Show approval for effort even if they are having difficulty with a task, so that they have confidence to try another one.

Motor Function

Muscle size, strength, and tone are part of motor function assessment. Compare the size of the extremities on each side. If in doubt about symmetry, measure the circumference of the calves and thighs or upper and lower arms for comparison. Palpate muscles for tone. Move the extremities through passive range of motion; evaluate for symmetry, spasticity, and flaccidity bilaterally. Ask the child to extend her arms in front of her and resist your action as you push down or up on her hands or push them out to the side. Do the same with the lower extremities.

Sensory Function

If children's sensory systems are intact, they should be able to distinguish light touch, pain, vibration, hot, and cold. Have a child close his eyes and then ask him to point to the spot where you touch him with an object. Light touch

TABLE 49.2

Cranial Nerve Function

Cranial Nerve	Function	Assessment
I (olfactory)	Sense of smell	Assess child's ability to recognize common odors (e.g., peanut butter, an orange) while eyes are closed.
II (optic)	Vision	Assess vision fields and visual acuity; examine retinas.
III (oculomotor)	Motor control and sensation for eye muscles and upper eyelid elevation	Assess ability to move eyes to follow an object in all directions. Note nystagmus (jerking motion). Assess pupillary size, equality, and reaction to light. Cranial nerves III, IV, and VI are tested together.
IV (trochlear)	Movement of major eye globe muscles	As for nerve III.
V (trigeminal)	Mastication muscles and some facial sensations	Assess ability to discern light touch to test sensory component; assess symmetry and strength of bite to test motor component.
VI (abducens)	Movement and muscle sense of eye globe	As for nerves III and IV.
VII (facial)	Impulses for hyoid and facial muscles, salivation, and taste	Assess motor strength by asking child to close eyes while you attempt to open them. Note symmetry of facial expression (such as smile) and movement (such as wrinkling forehead). Assess taste by asking child to identify salt or sugar.
VIII (acoustic)	Equilibrium and hearing	Assess hearing by the response to a whispered word or a Weber or Rinne test. Equilibrium is not tested routinely.
IX (glossopharyngeal)	Motor impulses to heart and other organs; sensation from pharynx, thorax, and abdominal organs	Assess gag reflex by pressing on rear of tongue with tongue blade. Note midline uvula (tested together with nerve X).
X (vagus)	Swallowing and gag reflexes	Assess ability to swallow; elicit gag reflex by pressing a tongue blade on posterior tongue.
XI (accessory)	Impulses to striated muscles of pharynx and shoulders	Ask child to turn head to the side; try to turn it to center. Ask the child to elevate shoulders while you press down on them.
XII (hypoglossal)	Motor impulses to tongue and skeletal muscles; sensation from skin and viscera	Ask child to protrude tongue. Assess for tremors. Ask child to press on side of cheek with tongue; assess tongue strength.

is tested by using a wisp of cotton, deep pressure by pressure of your finger, pain by a safety pin, temperature by test tubes filled with hot or cold water. Vibration is tested by touching the child's bony prominences (iliac crest, elbows, knees) with a vibrating tuning fork. Warn the child that on pin testing, he will feel a momentary prick. Otherwise, he may be unwilling to close his eyes again for further testing.

Reflex Testing

Deep tendon reflex testing, which is part of a primary physical assessment (see Chapter 33), is also a basic part of a neurologic assessment. In newborns, reflex testing is especially important, because the infant cannot perform tasks on command to demonstrate the range of neurologic function (see Chapter 24).

Checkpoint Question 1

Tasha has a full neurologic examination after a seizure. What cranial nerve is assessed when you ask a child to raise her shoulders as you push against them?

a. Nerve VII or facial.
b. Nerve VIII or auditory.
c. Nerve XI or accessory.
d. Nerve XII or hypoglossal.

Diagnostic Testing

A variety of diagnostic tests may be ordered to provide more information should any abnormalities be detected

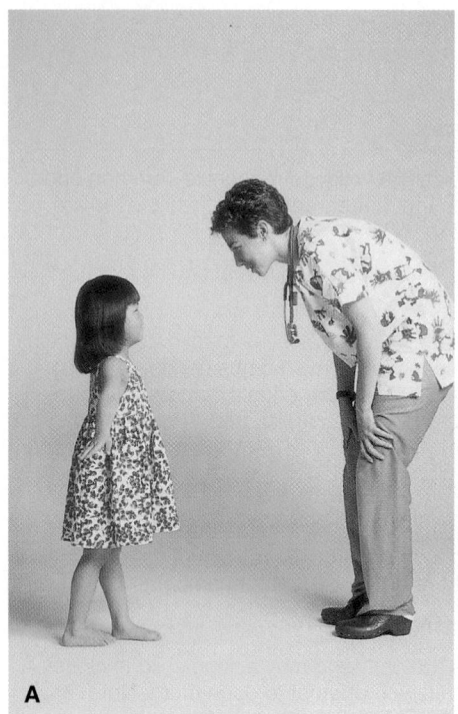
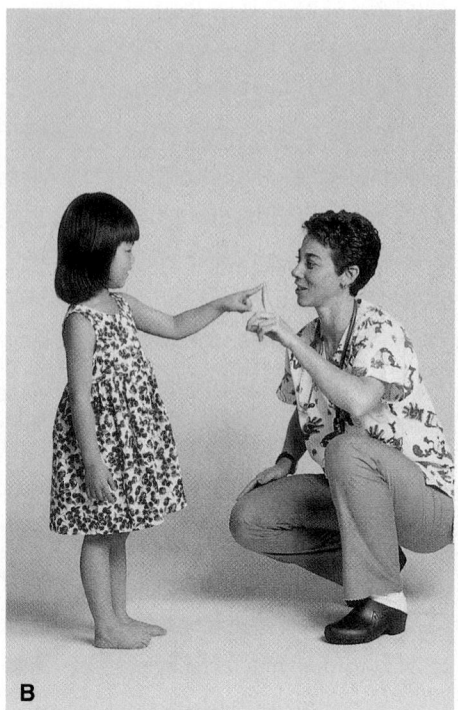

FIGURE 49.3 Cerebellar function tests. (**A**) A child attempting a tandem walk. (**B**) Nose-to-finger test. (© Lesha Photography.)

in the health history, physical examination, or neurologic examination. Many of these tests are invasive, and it is best to try to schedule the least invasive procedures first, before the painful or more frightening procedures are done, to help promote the child's cooperation. Ensuring that the child and the child's family are well prepared for these procedures is an important nursing responsibility. When explaining tests, take into account not only the child's chronologic age but also his or her level of cognitive functioning. Otherwise, explanations may not be well understood. Be sure to provide an explanation that includes a description of all of the sensory experiences the child might undergo—that is, not only what will be done but also how the child might feel, or what he or she might see or hear or even smell or taste (if appropriate).

Lumbar Puncture

Lumbar puncture involves the introduction of a needle into the subarachnoid space (under the arachnoid membrane) at the level of L4 or L5 to withdraw CSF for analysis (Fischbach, 2004). The procedure is used most frequently to diagnose hemorrhage or infection in the CNS or to diagnose an obstruction of CSF flow. Lumbar puncture is contraindicated if the skin over the needle insertion site is infected (to avoid introducing pathogens into the CSF) or if there is a suspected elevation of CSF pressure. In the latter instance, if fluid is removed, the higher pressure in the intracranial space could cause the brainstem to be drawn down into the spinal cord space, compressing the medulla and compromising the action of the cardiac and respiratory centers. EMLA or lidocaine cream can be applied to the puncture site 1 hour before the procedure to reduce pain. Alternatively, the child may receive conscious sedation (see Chapter 38).

For the procedure, the newborn is seated upright with the head bent forward (Fig. 49.4A). The older infant or child is placed on one side on the examining table. The head is flexed forward, the knees are flexed on the abdomen, and the back is arched as much as possible. This position opens the space between the lumbar vertebrae, facilitating needle insertion (see Fig. 49.4B). Children younger than school age need to be held in this position, because they may be so frightened by someone working on their back unseen that they are unable to hold this arched position; they may try to turn over or turn their head to see what is happening. It helps a school-age child or adolescent if you stand by the table facing him and gently rest your hand on the back of his head, keeping it bent forward. This helps to maintain good position without the impression of restraining him.

Children need good preparation for a lumbar puncture, because they cannot see what is happening. Be certain that they know that the health care provider performing the procedure will wash their back with a solution that feels cold and inject a local anesthetic that might sting like a mosquito bite (if an analgesic cream was not applied before the procedure). Caution children that they probably will feel pressure but not pain as the lumbar puncture needle is inserted. Remind them to remain absolutely still throughout the procedure. You might describe the position as "rolling into a ball" or "folding up like an astronaut in a small spaceship." Occasionally during a lumbar puncture, the needle will press against a dorsal nerve root and the child will experience a shooting pain down one leg. If this happens, reassure the child that this feeling passes quickly and does not indicate an injury.

When the insertion stylette is removed and CSF drips from the end of the needle, the procedure has been successful. An initial pressure reading is made, which varies

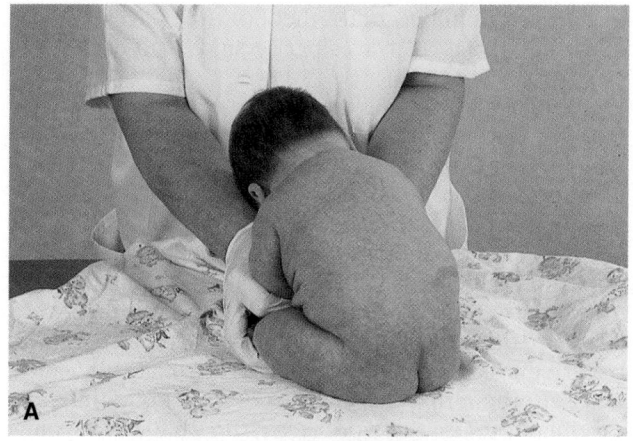

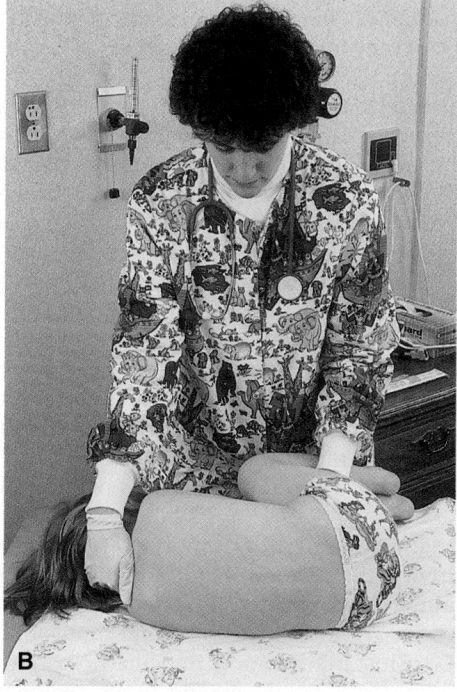

FIGURE 49.4 (A) Positioning an infant for a lumbar puncture. **(B)** Positioning a young child for a lumbar puncture. (© Barbara Proud.)

with the child's age. To confirm that the subarachnoid space in the cord is patent with that in the skull, the examiner may ask a child who is older than 3 years of age to cough, or the examiner may ask you to press on the child's external jugular vein during the procedure. Either of these measures will cause an increase of CSF pressure if fluid is flowing freely through the subarachnoid space. Typically, three tubes of CSF, containing 2 to 3 mL each, are collected, a closing pressure reading is taken, and the needle is withdrawn. Samples are usually sent for culture, sensitivity, glucose level, and presence of red blood cells. Other evaluations are determining whether there is an alteration in the albumin/globulin ratio in the CSF and measuring the gamma globulin level. An increased level of gamma globulin is suggestive of multiple sclerosis or meningitis. The first sample obtained may contain blood or skin pathogens from the puncture, so it should not be

the sample sent for determination of red blood cell content or culture. Throughout the procedure, sterile technique must be strictly observed to ensure that an uncontaminated sample of fluid is sent for culture and also to avoid the introduction of pathogens into the CSF.

Lumbar puncture involves at least momentary pain, so children need to be comforted afterward. A child may develop a headache after a lumbar puncture as a result of the reduction in CSF volume or invasion of a small air pocket during the puncture, although this is rare because of the small needle used. Encouraging the child to lie flat for about 30 minutes and to drink a glass of fluid can help prevent cerebral irritation caused by air rising in the subarachnoid space and helps increase the amount of CSF. Some children have a headache despite these precautions and may need an analgesic for pain relief. Although post–lumbar puncture headache is seen less frequently in young children than in adults, assessing for it is important to reduce the risk of pain for the child.

If a child had minimally increased CSF pressure at the time of the puncture, closely observe the child after the procedure to prevent respiratory and cardiac difficulty from medulla pressure. An increase in blood pressure or a decrease in pulse and respiration is an important sign of increased intracranial compression. Other important signs include a change in consciousness, pupillary changes, and a decrease in motor ability.

Ventricular Tap

In infants, CSF may be obtained by a subdural tap into the ventricle through the coronal suture or anterior fontanelle (Fischbach, 2004). A small space on the scalp over the insertion site is shaved or clipped, and the area is prepared with an antiseptic. The infant's head must be held firmly in a supine position to prevent movement during the procedure, which could cause the needle to strike and lacerate meningeal tissue.

Fluid must be removed from this site slowly, rather than suddenly, to prevent a sudden shift in pressure that could cause intracranial hemorrhage. After the procedure, a pressure dressing is applied to the site, and the infant is placed in a semi-Fowler's position to prevent prolonged drainage from the puncture site. After the procedure, comfort the infant or allow the parents to do so; this both reduces the stress of a painful procedure and prevents the infant from crying excessively, an action that could increase ICP.

Radiographic Techniques

A flat-plate skull radiographic film may be used to obtain information about increased ICP or skull defects such as fracture or craniosynostosis (premature knitting of cranial sutures). Increased ICP is suggested if skull sutures are separated. If the process is chronic, other subtle changes, such as a flattening of the sella turcica or an increase in the convolutions of the inner table of the skull, may be present.

Cerebral Angiography. Cerebral angiography is a radiographic study of cerebral blood vessels that involves the injection of a contrast material into an extracranial artery.

Serial radiographs are taken as the dye flows through the blood vessels of the cerebrum. The injection site chosen is often a femoral artery, although a carotid artery may be used. The study shows any vessel defects or space-occupying lesions that are occluding cranial blood vessels.

Myelography. Myelography is radiographic study of the spinal cord that involves the introduction of a contrast material into the CSF by lumbar puncture. It is used to show the presence of space-occupying lesions of the spinal cord. After the procedure, keep the head of the child's bed elevated to prevent contrast medium from reaching the meninges surrounding the brain.

Computed Tomography. CT involves the use of radiographic images to reveal densities at multiple levels or layers of brain tissue. It is helpful in confirming the presence of a brain tumor or other encroaching lesions. CT is discussed in further detail in Chapter 36. Single photon emission computed tomography (SPECT) is a similar procedure used mainly for blood flow evaluation.

Magnetic Resonance Imaging

Magnetic resonance imaging (MRI) uses magnetic fields to show differences in tissue composition, revealing normal versus abnormal brain tissue very effectively. MRI is discussed in greater detail in Chapter 36.

Nuclear Medicine Studies

Brain Scan. For a brain scan, a radioactive material is injected intravenously (IV), and, after a fixed time during which the injected material is deposited in cerebral tissue, radioactivity levels over the skull are measured. If the blood–brain barrier is not functioning, the radioactive material will accumulate in specific areas, suggesting possible tumor, subdural hematoma, abscess, or encephalitis.

Positron Emission Tomography. The diagnostic technique of positron emission tomography (PET) involves imaging after injection of positron-emitting radiopharmaceuticals into the brain. These radioactive substances accumulate at diseased areas of the brain or spinal cord. PET is extremely accurate in identifying seizure foci.

Echoencephalography

Echoencephalography involves the projection of ultrasound (high-frequency sound waves above the audible range) toward the child's head or spinal cord (a sonogram). Sonography may be used to outline the ventricles of the brain. Because this technique of scanning is noninvasive, produces no discomfort, and has no known complications, it may be repeated frequently to monitor changes in the size of ventricles or an invading lesion.

Electroencephalography

The electroencephalogram (EEG) reflects the electrical patterns of the brain. It summarizes the physical and chemical interactions within the brain at the time of the test. Normally, a tracing indicates four types of waves: delta (1 to 3 waves per second), theta (4 to 7 waves per second), alpha (8 to 12 waves per second), and beta (13 to 20 waves per second).

To reduce extraneous movements of the eyes, head, or muscles that would affect the tracing, the child must be cooperative and quiet during the procedure. Traditionally, parents are asked to keep their child up later than usual the night before so that they will be sleepy (Gilbert et al., 2004). Good preparation and encouragement can be more important in helping a child relax. Caution children that the room will probably be darkened to help them rest. Compare the electrode wires attached to their scalp with adhesive paste to those attached to astronauts in space. Reassure them that these electrodes are not painful. Be careful not to use the word *electrical*. Children as young as 3 years of age know that electrical wires are ordinarily dangerous and can hurt them. They cannot relax if they are worried that they may be shocked or even electrocuted by the procedure.

Children who are unable to lie still and cooperate even after careful explanation may need conscious sedation (Burton & Germann, 2004). However, sedation alters the electrical pattern of the cortex and should be avoided if possible. For example, chloral hydrate, a frequently used sedative for this procedure, may increase the fast activity of brain waves; chlorpromazine (Thorazine) may increase slow activity. Because phenobarbital and phenytoin sodium (diphenylhydantoin [Dilantin]) also cause an increase in fast activity, be sure to inform the person interpreting the recording what medications the child is receiving. Although it is usually unnecessary, be sure parents know if anticonvulsant medications should be withheld on the morning of an EEG to reduce the effect of medications on tracings.

Although EEGs can show important information about brain activity, they are not helpful in all circumstances. For example, approximately 15% of children who are absolutely normal clinically demonstrate some abnormality on an EEG. Most brain tumors in pediatric patients are in the posterior fossa, but the activity of this region does not show up well on an EEG. This limitation means that an EEG may appear normal even if a brain tumor is present, unless the tumor is pressing on more distal brain portions. On inspection of the symmetry of hemispheres, local lesions may be suggested. Where there is a lesion, there will be slower waves, a higher voltage pattern, and an overall more irregular pattern. A subdural lesion (perhaps from a hematoma) can interfere with transmission of the electrical impulses, lowering the voltage pattern.

An EEG is most beneficial in diagnosing absence seizures. The typical pattern with this disorder is discussed later in this chapter.

Visual stimulation, such as having a child look at a whirling disk, may be used in connection with the EEG, because various types of electrical discharges increase with rapid eye movements. In a child who is sensitive to this type of stimulation, the testing may produce a seizure. If this occurs, the child may be very disturbed and disoriented after the procedure. Describe what has happened, letting him know that things are all right to help him relax.

After an EEG, children will be sleepy if they have been sedated. Allow them to sleep as long as needed.

HEALTH PROMOTION AND RISK MANAGEMENT

Health promotion for nervous system health begins prenatally with measures to ensure optimal fetal growth and development and prevention of problems associated with anoxia. It continues throughout childhood with routine health maintenance visits, screening for possible neurologic or developmental problems, and timely immunizations to prevent sequelae of typical childhood infections such as measles or chickenpox. Nurses play a key role in providing education to parents about the importance of obtaining immunizations and completing medication therapy to ensure complete resolution of an infection.

Parents also need anticipatory guidance about safety measures to prevent injury, specifically, head and spinal cord injury. Reinforce the need for seat belts and child restraints while riding in automobiles and use of protective gear, such as helmets, for bicycle and motorcycle riding.

For the child with seizures, parents need instructions to prevent injury during a seizure (see later discussion) and to administer anticonvulsants conscientiously. Guidelines for safe administration of anticonvulsants include the following:

- Caution children to be careful around motor vehicles and electrical equipment, because many anticonvulsants cause drowsiness.
- Advise the child and parents to observe for easy bruising, because several anticonvulsants may suppress bone marrow function.
- Caution the adolescent to avoid alcohol while taking anticonvulsants, because alcohol can potentiate the CNS effects of some anticonvulsants.
- Use caution when administering anticonvulsants to children with liver disease. Because many of these drugs are metabolized by the liver, they may not be fully effective in such children.
- Caution the child and parents not to discontinue anticonvulsant therapy abruptly, because this may lead to uncontrolled seizures.
- Remind parents about the need for follow-up blood tests to evaluate the drug level. Maintaining a therapeutic blood level enhances the drug's effectiveness and minimizes the risk for toxicity.

For the child with a long-term neurologic disorder, rehabilitation and early intervention play a major role in reducing the risk of complications and in promoting the child's and family's optimal level of functioning.

INCREASED INTRACRANIAL PRESSURE

Increased ICP is not a single disorder but a sign that may occur with many neurologic disorders. When caring for a child with a potential neurologic disorder, it is important to observe him or her closely for this sign (Tamburrini et al., 2004).

Increased ICP may occur with an increase in the CSF volume, blood entering the CSF, cerebral edema, or space-occupying lesions such as tumors. Examples of causes of increased ICP include the following:

- Birth trauma or hydrocephalus
- Head trauma from an accident
- Infection
- Brain tumor
- Guillain-Barré syndrome

The rate at which symptoms develop depends on the cause and the ability of the child's skull to expand to accommodate the increased pressure. Children with open fontanelles can withstand more pressure without brain damage than can older children, whose suture lines and fontanelles have already closed.

Assessment

Assessment of neurologic function may involve only a few quick procedures, such as obtaining vital signs, evaluating pupil response, and determining level of consciousness and motor and sensory function, or it may include more elaborate electronic monitoring. Signs and symptoms of ICP are presented in Table 49.3.

With increased ICP, symptoms are often subtle at first. The child may report a headache, irritability, or restlessness. An infant with a headache becomes increasingly fussy or difficult to comfort. Changes in vital signs may be important indicators of ICP. Growing pressure on the brainstem, which controls respiration and cardiac activity, causes pulse and respirations to slow. Compression of cranial vessels leads to a compensatory increase in blood pressure (or **pulse pressure,** the gap between the systolic and diastolic blood pressures). Pressure on the hypothalamus, the temperature-regulating center of the body, causes an increase in temperature. These changes may occur gradually, so a single measurement may not show the extent of the change. Always compare the new information against all recordings taken in the last 24 hours.

Ocular changes may indicate that pressure is increasing posterior to the eye globe. One obvious abnormality is a dilated pupil, which suggests compression of cranial nerve II. Test pupil reactivity by shining a light into each eye. To elicit the most dramatic and sudden response, bring the light to the child's eye from the side or down from the forehead, to make it appear suddenly rather than gradually. Repeat this with the other eye. Each pupil should constrict, and the constriction should be equal bilaterally.

Consensual constriction should also be present. As you shine the light on the right pupil, the left pupil also should constrict, and vice versa.

If the child is alert and able to cooperate, have her follow the light through the six cardinal positions of gaze, and test convergence (ability to follow the light as it approaches closer and closer to the nose). Note any tendency toward strabismus, nystagmus (constant eye movement), "sunset eyes" (white sclera showing over the top of the cornea), or inability to follow the light into any quadrant. Be specific about what you document. "Inability to follow light" is not as informative as "Inability to follow light into left superior field; vertical nystagmus noted as child follows light into other fields."

If a child is lying supine and you turn his head gently but rapidly to the right, the eyes will normally turn toward the left, and vice versa (doll's eye reflex). If a child has

TABLE 49.3

Signs and Symptoms of Increased Intracranial Pressure

Sign or Symptom	Indication of Increased ICP
Increased head circumference	An increase >2 cm/month in first 3 months of life, >1 cm/month in the second 3 months, and >0.5 cm/month for the next 6 months
Fontanelle changes	Anterior fontanelle tense and bulging; closing late
Vomiting	Occurring in the absence of nausea, on awakening in morning or after nap; possibly projectile
Eye changes	Diplopia (double vision) from pressure on abducens nerves; white of sclera evident over pupil (setting sun sign); limited visual fields, papilledema
Vital sign changes	Elevated temperature and blood pressure; decreased pulse and respiration rates
Pain	Headache, often present on awakening and standing
	Increasing with straining at stool (Valsalva maneuver) or holding breath
Mentation	Irritability, altered consciousness such as sleepiness

increased ICP, this phenomenon will be absent. (This test is useful in assessing a comatose child who is unable to cooperate by following a light.) An older child may be able to report symptoms such as diplopia. On funduscopic examination, papilledema may be detected.

Assess the child's level of consciousness. If the child is alert but unable to comprehend surroundings, time, or place, this may be the first indication of increased ICP. As pressure increases, a pseudoawake state may occur, in which the child is awake but unable to follow light or noise. Finally, the child may be comatose, unable to be roused by any stimuli. Levels of coma are rated by a Glasgow coma scale. This is discussed in Chapter 52 in connection with assessment for head injury.

Children, like adults, generally become disoriented about time first, then place, then self. It is useful, therefore, to assess that the child is alert enough to answer these questions. Explain that you will be asking these seemingly simple questions periodically to make sure the child can answer them accurately each time. Otherwise, the child may quickly become annoyed with your questions and may refuse to answer them or make up silly answers instead. Or she may pretend to be asleep to avoid being asked.

Be aware that many children, even when healthy, are groggy when they first wake up; until fully awake, they may not be able to say who or where they are. This happens especially when a child is awakened from a dream. Make sure the child is fully awake before attempting to determine his or her level of consciousness.

Be certain that you ask questions appropriate to a child's age. Preschoolers do not usually know the day of the week or concepts such as *morning* or *night.* They do not necessarily know their whole name. With children of this age, it is often more helpful to identify an area of knowledge with which they are familiar, such as colors. Every half hour or every hour, show them a colored block and ask them its color. Even if they give the wrong answer, it does not matter. Your concern is that they understood your request, not that they actually recognize the colors. Also remind parents

that you are asking these questions to assess their child's level of consciousness, not to quiz for right answers or to be intrusive. Remind them not to answer for the child.

A good way to test an infant's level of consciousness is to determine whether he or she responds to sounds such as a music box or voices or reaches for an attractive object.

Evaluate motor ability by asking a child to perform some simple motor task, such as squeezing your hands. Have her push against your hand with both feet. Have her perform rapid, alternating hand movements, such as turning her hand over and back several times. Evaluate cranial nerves grossly by having her make a face, close her eyes tightly, and show you her teeth. With all these assessments, be sure to evaluate whether the responses are equal and symmetric bilaterally.

Test deep tendon reflexes, because these decrease in intensity with decreased level of consciousness. Carefully observe the child's resting posture. When motor control grows weaker because of loss of cell function, characteristic posturing (primitive reflexes) occurs. Cerebral loss is shown mainly by **decorticate posturing.** The child's arms are adducted and flexed on the chest with wrists flexed, hands fisted. The lower extremities are extended and internally rotated, and the feet are plantar flexed (Fig. 49.5A). **Decerebrate posturing,** which occurs when the midbrain is not functional, is characterized by rigid extension and adduction of arms and pronation of the wrists with the fingers flexed. The legs are extended, and the feet are plantar flexed (see Fig. 49.5B).

Observe the child carefully for any seizure activity. However, keep in mind that this is a late sign of increased ICP.

Intracranial Pressure Monitoring

ICP can be measured by several methods:

- An intraventricular catheter inserted through the anterior fontanelle
- A subarachnoid screw or bolt inserted through a burr hole in the skull

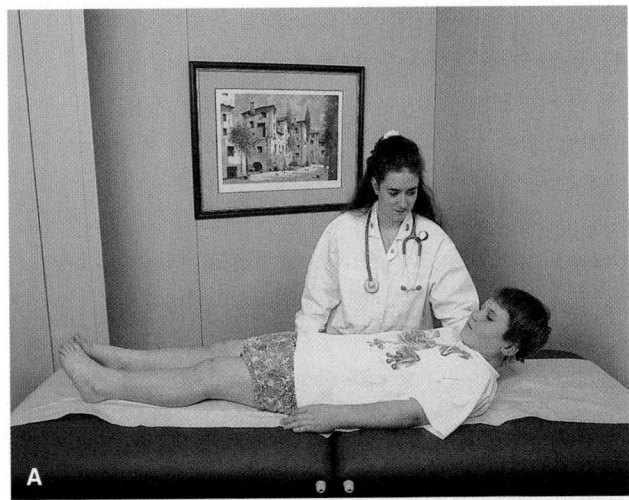
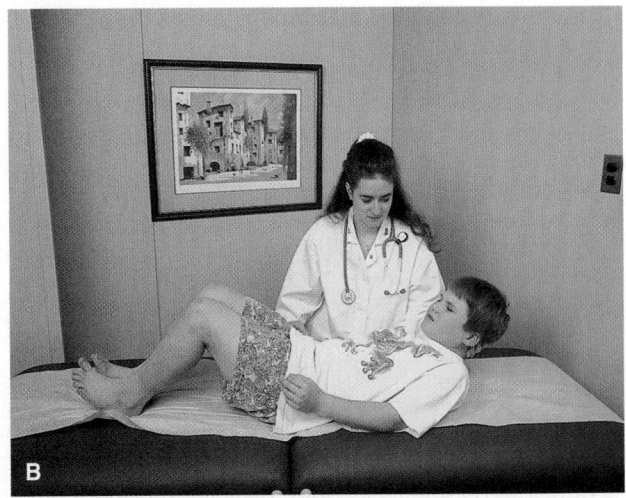
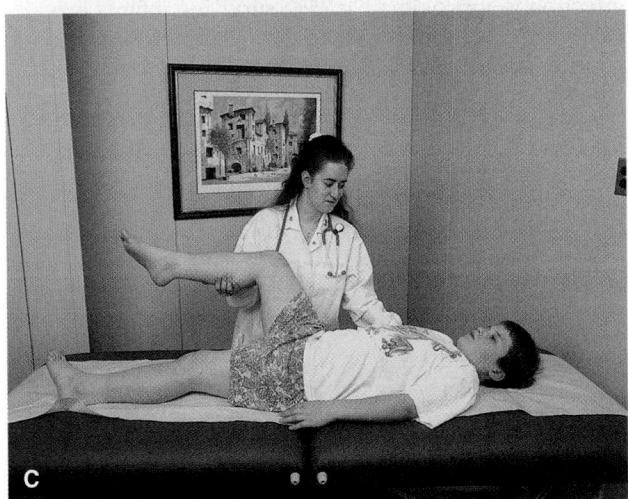
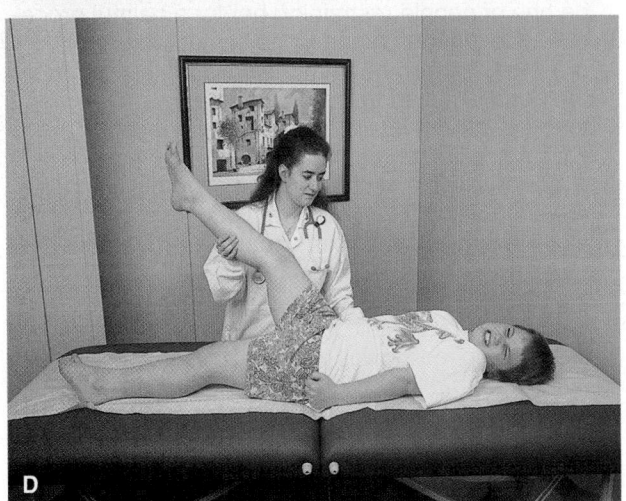

FIGURE 49.10 (A) Brudzinski's sign. The nurse flexes the child's neck forward. (B) Positive response. Bilateral hip, knee, and ankle flexion indicates meningeal irritation. (C) Kernig's sign. The nurse flexes the child's hip and knee, forming a 90-degree angle. (D) Positive response. As the leg is extended, pain, resistance, and spasm are noted, indicating meningeal irritation. (Photos by John Gallagher.)

fluenzae, ampicillin usually is the drug of choice. In other instances, a third-generation cephalosporin, such as cefotaxime (Claforan) or ceftriaxone (Rocephin), may be used for 8 to 10 days. In some children, it takes a month before the CSF cell count returns to normal. A corticosteroid such as dexamethasone or the osmotic diuretic, mannitol, may be administered to reduce ICP and help prevent hearing loss.

In addition to standard precautions, children with meningitis are placed on respiratory precautions for 24 hours after the start of antibiotic therapy to prevent transmission of the infection. Antibiotics also may be prescribed prophylactically for the immediate family members of the ill child or for others who have been in close contact with the child.

Meningitis is always a serious disorder, because it can run a rapid, fulminating, and possibly fatal course. However, if symptoms are recognized early enough and treatment is effective, the child will recover with no sequelae. Neurologic sequelae, such as learning problems, seizures,

hearing and cognitive challenges, and inability to concentrate urine, must be assessed after the infection, because these can be long-term consequences.

NURSING DIAGNOSES AND RELATED INTERVENTIONS

If a child has meningitis, the parents may feel responsible for the illness. They knew the child had a cold, and they wonder whether they could have prevented meningitis if only they had taken the child to a physician as soon as the cold symptoms started. Reassure them that the symptoms of meningitis occur insidiously and that no one could have predicted the full extent of the disease from the first signs.

Encourage parents to care for their child during the illness, both to help make the child more comfortable and to help them manage their own anxiety. Teach them good infection control techniques so that they can perform these tasks safely.

Nursing Diagnosis: Pain related to meningeal irritation

Outcome Evaluation: Child states that pain is tolerable and shows no facial grimacing or other signs of discomfort.

For a child with meningitis, dealing with hospitalization and numerous invasive treatments and procedures is usually difficult. If the child had a lumbar puncture on admission, her initial impression may be one of people restraining her for a painful procedure. Continuous IV infusions contribute to this impression. Remember that the child feels pain when the head is flexed forward and usually is more comfortable without a pillow. Be careful not to flex the child's neck when turning or positioning her.

On admission, a child may be extremely irritable. Although he would benefit from puppet play or drawing, which would help him express how he feels about so many intrusive procedures, frequently he is too uncomfortable to play and is not able to be comforted. This is a result of the disease process, and he cannot help feeling this way. Be aware of this, so as not to interpret the child's withdrawal as unfriendliness and feel hurt when advances are rebuffed. Parents also need to understand that the child's behavior is caused by the disease and not by anything that they did or are doing. The child needs a good explanation of everything that is happening. He needs extra attention from health care personnel consistently, not just when they perform painful procedures. As the child recovers, irritability lessens and the child usually shows more interest in communicating his feelings. Promote rest for the child by keeping stimulation in the room to a minimum.

Nursing Diagnosis: Risk for ineffective tissue perfusion (cerebral), related to increased ICP

Outcome Evaluation: Child's vital signs return to normal; child is alert and oriented; motor, cognitive, and sensory function are within acceptable parameters for the child's age; specific gravity of urine is 1.003 to 1.030.

Observe the child carefully for signs of increased ICP. Carefully monitor the rate of all IV infusions to prevent overhydration. Measure urine specific gravity to detect oversecretion or undersecretion of antidiuretic hormone due to pituitary pressure. Measure the child's head circumference, and weigh him or her daily.

Monitor hearing acuity (reduced if there is compression of the eighth cranial nerve) by asking an older child a question or observing whether an infant listens to a music box or to your voice.

Group B β-Hemolytic Streptococcal Meningitis

A major cause of meningitis in newborns is group B β-hemolytic streptococci. The organism is contracted either in utero or from secretions in the birth canal at birth. It can spread to other newborns if good handwashing technique is not used.

Group-B β-hemolytic streptococci colonization may result in early-onset or late-onset illness. With the early-onset form, symptoms of pneumonia become apparent in the first few hours of life.

The late-onset type often leads to meningitis instead of pneumonia. At approximately 2 weeks of age, the infant may gradually become lethargic, developing a fever and upper respiratory tract symptoms. The fontanelles bulge from increased ICP. Mortality from group B β-streptococcal infection is approximately 25%; surviving infants may develop neurologic consequences such as hydrocephalus or seizures (Bell, 2003). Treatment is with antibiotics, such as ampicillin and cephalosporins, that are effective against group B β-hemolytic streptococcal infections. It can be difficult for parents to understand how their infant suddenly became so ill. They may need considerable support in caring for an infant who is left neurologically challenged.

Checkpoint Question 3

Tasha is diagnosed as having bacterial meningitis. How long should she be placed on respiratory precautions for this condition?

a. Four hours.
b. Twenty-four hours.
c. Ten days.
d. Thirty days.

Encephalitis

Encephalitis is an inflammation of brain tissue and, possibly, the meninges as well (Marra, 2004). It can arise from protozoan, bacterial, fungal, or viral invasion. Enteroviruses are the most frequent cause, followed by arboviruses (e.g., togavirus). A number of encephalitis viruses, such as those that cause St. Louis encephalitis, West Nile encephalitis, and eastern equine encephalitis, are borne by mosquitoes and are seen most often during the summer months. In endemic areas, mosquito repellents are strongly suggested. Encephalitis also can result from direct invasion of the CSF during lumbar puncture. It may occur as a complication of common childhood diseases, such as measles, mumps, or chickenpox. Therefore, it is crucial that children receive immunization against these childhood diseases.

Assessment

Symptoms of encephalitis can begin gradually or suddenly. Symptoms include headache, high temperature, and signs of meningeal irritation, such as nuchal rigidity (positive

Brudzinski's sign and Kernig's sign). Symptoms of ataxia, muscle weakness or paralysis, diplopia, confusion, or irritability also may occur. The child becomes increasingly lethargic and eventually comatose.

The diagnosis is made by the history and physical assessment. CSF evaluation shows an elevated leukocyte count and an elevated protein level. An EEG shows widespread cerebral involvement. A brain biopsy, usually from the temporal lobe, may be done to identify the virus.

Therapeutic Management

Treatment for a child with encephalitis is primarily supportive. An antipyretic is given to control fever. Take and record vital signs frequently, because brainstem involvement can affect cardiac or respiratory rates. Mechanical ventilation may be required to maintain the child's respirations during the acute phase. An antiviral agent, such as acyclovir (Zovirax), is usually prescribed. Anticonvulsants, such as carbamazepine (Tegretol), phenobarbital, or phenytoin (Dilantin), may be prescribed for seizures. A steroid such as dexamethasone or an osmotic diuretic such as mannitol may be prescribed to decrease brain edema and ICP.

Encephalitis is always a serious diagnosis because, although the child may recover from the initial attack, there may be residual neurologic damage, such as seizures or learning disabilities. Parents may find it hard to believe that their child is seriously ill because he or she only seemed tired and had a slight headache. They will find it even harder to accept a diagnosis of permanent impairment, such as a learning disability. Follow-up care after the hospitalization is important for the child's rehabilitation and to help parents deal with their grief, shock, and anger. Although complete recovery is possible, parents may find themselves with a child whose health and abilities have been permanently changed.

Reye's Syndrome

Reye's syndrome is acute encephalitis with accompanying fatty infiltration of the liver, heart, lungs, pancreas, and skeletal muscle. It occurs in children from 1 to 18 years of age regardless of gender (Kamienski, 2003).

The cause is unknown, but it usually occurs after a viral infection such as varicella (chickenpox) or influenza that was treated with a salicylate such as acetylsalicylic acid (aspirin). Anticipatory guidance to parents and children about avoiding the use of aspirin during viral infections has led to almost total prevention of this syndrome.

Assessment

After seeming to recover from an initial viral illness, children become ill again 1 to 3 weeks later, with lethargy, vomiting, agitation, anorexia, confusion, and combativeness. Symptoms in adolescents may be so extreme that they mimic those of drug intoxication. As fatty droplets invade the liver, enzyme abnormalities, hypothrombinemia, hypoglycemia, and elevated blood ammonia levels occur. Although CSF findings remain normal, cerebral symptoms progress from confusion to stupor to deep coma, with seizures and respiratory arrest resulting from pressure on the brainstem.

Laboratory diagnosis of Reye's syndrome is confirmed by elevated liver enzyme levels (alanine aminotransferase [ALT or SGPT] and aspartate aminotransferase [AST or SGOT]), elevated serum ammonia, normal direct bilirubin, delayed prothrombin time and partial thromboplastin time, decreased blood glucose, elevated blood urea nitrogen, elevated serum amylase, elevated short-chain fatty acids, and an elevated white blood count. A lumbar puncture is usually done to rule out other infection. CSF findings are normal, except for slightly elevated opening pressure. A skull CT scan or sonogram will be normal at first. Later, it will show cerebral edema and decreased ventricle size. A liver biopsy shows fatty infiltration, establishing a definitive diagnosis.

Therapeutic Management

Left untreated, Reye's syndrome is rapidly fatal. If it is diagnosed early and promptly treated, the child usually recovers quickly and without any residual neurologic effects.

Reye's syndrome is not infectious. It is categorized by stages of involvement from 1 to 5, depending on the degree of the child's lethargy or coma. In stages 1 and 2, the child responds to stimuli but may exhibit lethargy or delirium and possibly combativeness. In stages 3 through 5, the child is unresponsive to stimuli with a progressively deepening coma. Frequent neurologic assessments are necessary to evaluate the child's status and possible progression to a more serious stage of involvement. Therapy is directed toward supporting respiratory function, controlling hypoglycemia, and reducing brain edema.

Guillain-Barré Syndrome

Guillain-Barré syndrome (inflammatory polyradiculoneuropathy) is a perplexing syndrome that involves both motor and sensory portions of peripheral nerves. It affects both sexes and occurs most often in school-age children and adolescents (Sladky, 2004).

The cause of the condition is unknown, but it is suspected that the reaction is immune mediated, occurring after upper respiratory tract or gastrointestinal illnesses or immunizations. Inflammation of the nerve fibers apparently causes temporary demyelinization of the nerve sheaths.

Assessment

Children experience peripheral neuritis several days after the primary infection. Tendon reflexes are decreased or absent. Muscle paralysis and paresthesia (loss of sensation) begin first in the legs and then spread to involve the arms, trunk, and head. The symmetric nature of the disorder helps to differentiate it from other types of paraplegia. Cranial nerve involvement leads to facial weakness and difficulty in swallowing. As the respiratory muscles become involved, spontaneous respirations are no longer possible. This can lead to respiratory involvement severe enough to warrant mechanical ventilation.

A significant laboratory finding is an elevated CSF protein level. An EEG may show denervation and decreased nerve conduction velocity.

Therapeutic Management

Treatment of Guillain-Barré syndrome is supportive until the process runs its course; paralysis peaks at 3 weeks and is followed by gradual recovery. A course of prednisone to halt the autoimmune response may be tried, but its use is controversial. Plasmapheresis or transfusion of immune serum globulin may shorten the course of the illness.

Care of the child with Guillain-Barré syndrome includes preventing all of the effects of extreme immobility while guarding respiratory function. The child's cardiac and respiratory function must be closely monitored. An indwelling urinary catheter is usually inserted to monitor urine output. Enteral or total parenteral nutrition may be used to support protein and carbohydrate needs. If the child has discomfort from neuritis, adequate analgesia should be administered.

To prevent muscle contractures and effects of immobility, the child should have passive range-of-motion exercises every 4 hours. Turning and repositioning every 2 hours also is important to protect skin integrity. Providing adequate stimulation for the long weeks when the child is unable to perform any care for himself or herself is also important. Most children recover completely, without any residual effects of the syndrome, although they may continue to have minor problems such as residual weakness.

Botulism

Botulism occurs when spores of *Clostridium botulinum* colonize and produce toxins in the immature intestine. The source of the spores is usually unknown, but honey and corn syrup are frequently contaminated and should be avoided in infants. The disease cannot be transmitted from person to person. It usually occurs in infants younger than 6 months of age (Walker, 2004).

In infant botulism, symptoms occur within a few hours after ingestion of contaminated food. Almost immediately, there is generalized weakness, hypotonia, listlessness, a weak cry, and a diminished gag reflex. This is followed by a flaccid paralysis of the bulbar muscles that leads to diminished respiratory function. The organism can be cultured from stools or serum. Electromyography may be helpful to support the diagnosis.

Treatment is supportive care. The antitoxin for botulism is rarely given to infants, because it is made from a horse serum base and can cause a hypersensitivity reaction and because it usually is not necessary for full recovery. Infant botulism may account for some fatalities credited to sudden infant death syndrome.

INFLAMMATORY DISORDERS
Carpal Tunnel Disorders

Carpal tunnel syndrome is nerve compression of the median nerve supplying the hand in the carpal tunnel at the wrist (MacDermid & Wessel, 2004). Compression of the nerve causes numbness and sharp pain and burning in the thumb and the second, third, and fourth fingers. The pain usually occurs at night and is enough to keep a child awake at night. The pain occurs because the nerve becomes inflamed as a result of repetitive motion such as word processing. It occurs more frequently in children who have a rheumatoid process such as arthritis. The usual therapy is application of a splint to the wrist, which holds the wrist in a neutral (not flexed and not extended) position. An oral anti-inflammatory medication and perhaps a corticosteroid injection into the inflamed wrist help to relieve pain. If these therapies are not successful, the stricture at the carpal canal can be relieved surgically. Although carpal tunnel syndrome is still rare in children, it is increasing in incidence as more and more teenagers spend hours in repetitive motion while they play video games, do word processing, or surf and chat on the Internet.

Facial Palsy (Bell's Palsy)

Facial palsy is facial paralysis of the seventh (facial) cranial nerve, the nerve that innervates the muscles of facial expression. The syndrome occurs abruptly, usually after a herpes or Lyme disease infection. It may occur as a result of cold air from skiing or from riding in a convertible. Therapy consists of prednisone to reduce inflammation and acyclovir if the syndrome is herpes related. If the child is unable to close the eye on the affected side, eye drops 3 or 4 times daily will be needed. Although recovery is slow, usually not until 4 months, most children recover without any permanent disability (Chung, 2003).

PAROXYSMAL DISORDERS

A paroxysmal disorder is one that occurs suddenly and recurrently. Seizures, headaches, and breath-holding spells are the most frequent types seen in childhood.

Recurrent Seizures

A *seizure* is an involuntary contraction of muscle caused by abnormal electrical brain discharges. Approximately 2% to 3% of children will have at least one seizure by the time they reach adulthood (Bromfield, 2004). These episodes are always frightening to parents and other children. Although seizures can be idiopathic (without cause), they also can be attributed to infection, trauma, or tumor growth. Familiar or polygenic inheritance may be responsible. Fifty percent of seizures are unexplained. Because they are not so much a disease as a symptom of an underlying disorder, they should be investigated carefully (Box 49.4).

The term *epilepsy* comes from a Greek word meaning "to take hold of" and refers to chronic seizures. The preferred term now is *recurrent seizures,* because epilepsy carries the stigma of cognitive challenge, behavioral disorders, institutionalization, or just unexplainable strangeness.

The types and causes of seizures vary with age. They have been classified into two major categories: partial seizures and generalized seizures (Box 49.5). With partial seizures, only one area of the brain is involved; with generalized seizures, the disturbance involves the entire brain, and loss of consciousness usually occurs. It is important

BOX 49.4 FOCUS ON . . .

DIVERSITY OF CARE

The degree of understanding about the cause of disorders such as recurrent seizures varies in different cultures. Because the cause of recurrent seizures is often unknown (idiopathic), they have, in the past, been attributed to an invasion by evil spirits. Many people today still fear that recurrent seizures will lead to cognitive impairment. Adults with recurrent seizures may be refused jobs because they are viewed as undependable. Being aware of these common misconceptions can help you appreciate parents' anxiety about the diagnosis of recurrent seizures. This anxiety can accentuate the need for parent education and careful planning to maintain self-esteem in the child.

that seizures be differentiated by their degree of severity, so that appropriate management and drug therapy can be instituted.

Seizures in the Newborn Period

Seizure activity in the newborn period may be difficult to recognize because it may consist only of twitching of the head, arms, or eyes; slight cyanosis; and perhaps respiratory difficulty or apnea. Afterward, the infant may appear limp and flaccid. Whereas older children often have seizures of unknown cause, 75% of seizures in neonates have a known cause. Some possible causes are

- Trauma and anoxia (head trauma involved with the birth process, tight maternal cervix, use of forceps, or placenta previa)
- Metabolic disorders, such as hypoglycemia (glucose level less than 40 mg/100 mL in the full-term infant or 20 mg/100 mL in the preterm infant); infants of dia-

betic mothers; hypocalcemia; and lack of pyridoxine (vitamin B_6)
- Neonatal infection (CNS infection or prolonged rupture of membranes before delivery)
- Kernicterus

Because of the nervous system's immaturity, EEGs in the newborn may be normal despite extensive disease. Therefore, a noticeably abnormal EEG generally means a poor prognosis, indicating that the involvement this early in life must be severe. Because almost 20% of all newborns have abnormal CSF values compared with adult standards, lumbar puncture also is not conclusive. Protein is increased, and there may be a few red blood cells from rupture of subarachnoid capillaries with the pressure of birth.

High doses of anticonvulsant medication may be needed to control seizures in newborns because they metabolize drugs more rapidly than older infants. In adults, for example, phenobarbital may be administered in the range of 1.5 mg/kg body weight per day. In newborns, the dose might be as high as 3 to 10 mg/kg per day.

Seizures in the Infant and Toddler Periods

Seizures commonly seen in this age group are **infantile spasms,** a form of generalized seizure ("salaam" or "jack-knife"), or infantile myoclonic seizures. They are characterized by very rapid movements of the trunk with sudden strong contractions of most of the body, including flexion and adduction of the limbs. The infant suddenly slumps forward from a sitting position or falls from a standing position. These episodes may occur singly or in clusters as frequently as 100 times a day. They are most common during the first 6 months of life (Brooks-Kayal, 2003b).

The cause is unknown, but the spasms apparently result from a failure of normal organized electrical activity in the brain. Sometimes, the seizures accompany a pre-existing form of neurologic damage. In approximately 50% of those affected, there is an identifiable cause such as trauma or a metabolic disease such as phenylketonuria. In the other 50%, there may be no identifiable cause. Seizures may develop after invasion by viruses such as herpes or cytomegalovirus. Approximately 90% of these infants are developmentally delayed (Brooks-Kayal, 2003b).

In infants whose development was previously normal, intellectual development appears to halt and even regress after seizures start. Most children with infantile spasms show high-amplitude slow waves and spikes, a chaotic discharge called *hypsarrhythmia,* on an EEG tracing.

The response to treatment with anticonvulsant therapy is poor. Parenteral adrenocorticotropic hormone (ACTH) and pyridoxine (vitamin B_6) therapy is commonly used. High-dose valproic acid or a newer anticonvulsant agent such as topiramate (Topamax) may be used in children who do not respond to usual therapy. The infantile seizure phenomenon seems to "burn itself out" by 2 years of age. The associated cognitive or developmental delay remains, however, so children need follow-up planning and care.

Seizures Caused by Poisoning or Drugs. The possibility of poisoning must be considered in any child who

BOX 49.5

Classification of Seizures

Partial (Focal) Seizures
- Simple partial seizures (no altered level of consciousness)
- Simple partial seizures with motor signs (includes aversive, rolandic, and jacksonian march)
- Simple partial seizures with sensory signs
- Complex partial (psychomotor) seizures (some impairment or alteration in level of consciousness)

Generalized Seizures
- Tonic-clonic seizures (formerly grand mal)
- Tonic
- Clonic
- Absence seizures (formerly petit mal)
- Atonic seizures (formerly "drop attacks")
- Myoclonic seizures
- Infantile spasms

has a first seizure. Although poisoning is most likely between 6 months and 3 years of age, it must be considered again in adolescence, when drugs may be intentionally self-administered. Seizures also can be a late symptom of encephalopathy caused by lead poisoning (see Chapter 52).

Seizures in Children Older Than 3 Years of Age

Febrile Seizures. Seizures associated with high fever (102°F to 104°F [38.9°C to 40.0°C]) are the most common in preschool children (5 months to 5 years), although they can occur as early as 3 months or as late as 7 years of age. The seizure shows an active tonic–clonic pattern, which lasts for 15 to 20 seconds. The EEG tracing usually is normal. There usually is a history of other family members' having had similar seizures. Febrile seizures may occur after immunization because of an accompanying fever.

It is unclear whether this type of seizure is initiated by a consistently high fever or by a sudden spike of temperature. The seizure subsides quickly once the fever is lowered. Such seizures must be taken seriously, however, and investigated for a possible cause, because meningitis often manifests initially with high fever and a seizure (Pantell, 2004).

Prevention of Febrile Seizures. Because these seizures arise with high fever, they are largely preventable. If acetaminophen is given to keep a developing fever below 101°F (38.4°C), seizures rarely occur. They happen most often when the child develops a fever at night, when the parent is not aware of it, or when the parent is reluctant to give acetaminophen in large enough doses to be therapeutic. Although this type of seizure can be prevented by phenobarbital, prophylactic use during an upper respiratory tract infection is not recommended, because phenobarbital takes 2 or 3 days to reach therapeutic blood levels. By this time, the seizures would already have occurred. In addition, phenobarbital is associated with sleepiness, which possibly reduces cognitive function in children. If a second febrile seizure occurs, diazepam (Valium) may be prescribed for the parents to administer the next time the child has a high fever (Brooks-Kayal, 2003a).

Instruct parents that every child who has a febrile seizure must be seen by a health care provider. A good rule of thumb is to assume that the child in this situation has meningitis until it is ruled out by a complete neurologic workup.

Therapeutic Management. Teach parents that, after the seizure subsides, they should sponge the child with tepid water to reduce the fever quickly. Advise them not to put the child in the bathtub, however, because it would be easy for the child to slip under water should a second seizure occur. Applying alcohol or cold water is also not advisable. Extreme cooling causes shock to an immature nervous system; in addition, alcohol can be absorbed by the skin or the fumes can be inhaled in toxic amounts, compounding the child's problems. Parents should not attempt to give oral medications such as acetaminophen, because the child will be in a drowsy, or *postictal,* state after the seizure and might aspirate the medicine. If attempts to reduce the child's temperature by sponging are unsuccessful, advise parents to put cool washcloths on the child's forehead, axillary, and groin areas and transport the child, lightly clothed, to a health care facility for immediate evaluation.

Additional treatment depends on the underlying cause of the fever. A lumbar puncture will be performed to rule out meningitis. Antipyretic drugs to reduce the fever below seizure levels will be administered. Appropriate antibiotic therapy will be started, depending on the type of infection.

Many parents need to be reassured that febrile seizures do not lead to brain damage and that the child is almost always completely well afterward.

What if... Tasha's mother is worried that Tasha will have another febrile convulsion if she develops a cold in the future? She asks if it will be safe to send Tasha to daycare. How would you respond to this parent?

Complex Partial (Psychomotor) Seizures. More than half of children who develop recurrent seizures during school age have an idiopathic type—the cause of the seizures cannot be discovered. Nevertheless, medication can control idiopathic seizures in almost all affected children. Other seizures in this age group occur because of organic causes, usually from focal or diffuse brain injury that has left residual damage. The injury may have been caused by laceration of brain tissue in a car accident or fall, hemorrhage due to a blood dyscrasia, infection (meningitis or encephalitis), anoxia, or toxic conditions such as lead poisoning. The possibility that a growing brain tumor is causing brain irritation also must be considered.

Complex partial (psychomotor) seizures vary greatly in extent and symptoms and tend to be the most difficult type to control. The child may have a slight aura, but it is rarely as definite as that seen with tonic–clonic seizures. Results of a CT or MRI scan and EEG are invariably normal.

This type of seizure may begin with a sudden change in posture, such as an arm dropping suddenly to the side. Other motor, sensory, and behavioral signs may include **automatisms** (complex purposeless movements, such as lip smacking or fumbling hand movements). The child then slumps to the ground, unconscious. Circumoral pallor may develop due to a halt in respirations. The child usually regains consciousness in less than 5 minutes. He or she may feel slightly drowsy afterward but does not have an actual postictal stage as in tonic–clonic seizures.

Common drugs used include carbamazepine (Tegretol) (Box 49.6), valproic acid (Depakene), phenytoin (Dilantin), and phenobarbital. Carbamazepine can lead to neutropenia, so white blood cell counts need to be monitored during therapy. If these drugs are not effective, surgery to remove the epileptogenic focus may be attempted (Bromfield, 2004).

Partial (Focal) Seizures. Partial seizures originate from a specific brain area. A typical partial seizure with motor signs begins in the fingers and spreads to the wrist, arm, and face in a clonic contraction. If the movement remains localized, there will be no loss of consciousness. If the

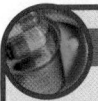

BOX 49.6 FOCUS ON . . .

PHARMACOLOGY

Carbamazepine (Tegretol)

Classification: Carbamazepine is an anticonvulsant.

Action: Exact mechanism of action is unknown. It is believed to inhibit polysynaptic responses and block post-tetanic potentiation (Karch, 2004).

Pregnancy Risk Category: C

Dosage: Initially in children 6 to 12 years of age, 100 mg orally bid on the first day, increased gradually in 100-mg increments at 6- to 8-hour intervals until best response is achieved, or 10 to 30 mg/kg/day in divided doses tid or qid. Not to exceed 1,000 mg/day.

Possible Adverse Effects: Dizziness, drowsiness, behavioral changes, nausea, vomiting, gastrointestinal upset, abnormal liver function tests, bone marrow depression, rash, photosensitivity

Nursing Implications
- Administer the drug with food to minimize gastrointestinal upset. Instruct parents to do the same.
- Obtain serum drug levels as ordered to monitor for effectiveness and to prevent possible toxicity. Keep in mind that the therapeutic range is 4 to 12 µg/mL.
- Monitor liver function studies and blood counts periodically.
- Inform parents about the need for follow-up laboratory tests.
- Suggest that the parents obtain a medical alert bracelet and have the child wear it in case of an emergency.
- Instruct parents and child to avoid alcohol and sleep-inducing or over-the-counter drugs, which could cause dangerous synergistic effects.
- Caution parents not to discontinue the drug abruptly or change the dose unless ordered by the health care provider.
- Instruct parents to notify the health care provider if the child develops bruising, bleeding, or signs of infection. These are signs of possible depression of bone marrow function.

spread is extensive, the seizure may become generalized and then is impossible to differentiate from a tonic–clonic seizure. Therefore, it is important to observe children carefully as a seizure begins. A partial seizure with sensory signs may include numbness, tingling, paresthesia, or pain originating in one area and spreading to other parts of the body. These types of seizures may be caused by a rapidly growing brain tumor. Documenting the spread can help localize the spot where the seizure first began.

Absence Seizures. Absence seizures, formerly known as *petit mal seizures,* are classified as generalized seizures. They usually consist of a staring spell that lasts for a few seconds. A child might be reciting in class when he pauses and stares for 1 to 5 seconds before continuing the recita-

tion; he is unaware that time has passed. Rhythmic blinking and twitching of the mouth or an extremity may accompany the staring. Absence seizures can occur up to 100 times per day. An EEG usually shows a typical 3-Hz wave and slow-wave discharge. Such seizures tend to occur more frequently in girls than in boys. The usual age of occurrence is 6 to 7 years (Posner et al., 2005).

Children with absence episodes may be accused of daydreaming in school and may be referred to the school nurse for behavior problems. These children usually have normal intelligence; however, if they have frequent episodes, they may be doing poorly in school because they are missing instructional content.

Absence seizures can usually be demonstrated in children by asking them to hyperventilate and count out loud. If they are susceptible to such seizures, they will breathe in and out deeply, possibly 10 times, stop and stare for 3 seconds, then continue to hyperventilate and count, unaware that they paused.

No first aid measures are necessary for absence seizures. Downplaying the importance of these episodes helps children maintain a positive self-image.

Absence seizures can be controlled by ethosuximide (Zarontin) or by valproic acid. If seizures are fully controlled by medication, children can participate in normal school activities and ride a bicycle. If seizures cannot be controlled fully, parents need to anticipate potentially hazardous situations during the child's day, such as crossing a busy street on the way to school or learning to drive. This is crucial for adolescents who are eager to get a driver's license, to protect their own safety and that of others.

Approximately one third to one half of all children with absence seizures "outgrow" them by adulthood. This does not mean that treatment is not necessary during childhood. Absence seizures usually occur independently of tonic–clonic seizures, although it is possible for a child to manifest both types. Some children's seizure pattern changes from absence involvement to tonic–clonic involvement as they approach adulthood.

Tonic–Clonic Seizures. Typical tonic–clonic seizures (formerly termed *grand mal seizures*) are generalized seizures consisting of four stages. There may be a *prodromal* period of hours or days; an *aura,* or warning, immediately before the seizure; the tonic–clonic stage; and, finally, a postictal stage. Not all four stages occur with every seizure.

The prodromal period may consist of drowsiness, dizziness, malaise, lack of coordination, or tension. Parents may observe simply that the child is "not himself." As the child reaches school age, he may be able to predict from these vague preliminary feelings when he is going to have a seizure.

The aura, or second phase, may reflect the portion of the brain in which the seizure originates. Smelling unpleasant odors (often reported as feces) denotes activity in the medial portion of the temporal lobe. Seeing flashing lights suggests the occipital area; repeated hallucinations arise from the temporal lobe; numbness of an extremity relates to the opposite parietal lobe; and a "Cheshire-cat grin" relates to the frontal lobe. Young children, unable to describe or understand an aura, may scream in fright or run to their parent with its onset. Note exactly what symptoms the child experiences during this time, because this may help to localize the involved brain portion.

The third phase is the tonic stage. All muscles of the body contract, and the child falls to the ground. Extremities stiffen; the face distorts. Although this phase lasts only about 20 seconds, the respiratory muscles are contracted, so the child may experience hypoxia and turn cyanotic. Contraction of the throat prevents swallowing, so saliva collects in the mouth. The child may bite the tongue when the jaws contract. As the chest muscles contract initially, air is pushed through the glottis, producing a guttural cry.

The seizure then enters a clonic stage, in which muscles of the body rapidly contract and relax, producing quick, jerky motions. The child may blow bubbles or foamy saliva and, if he bit his tongue when his jaw spasmed shut, he may have blood in his mouth. He may be incontinent of stool and urine. This phase usually lasts 20 to 30 seconds.

After the tonic–clonic period, the child falls into a sound sleep, called the *postictal period.* He will sleep soundly for 1 to 4 hours and will rouse only to painful stimuli during this time. When he awakens, he often experiences a severe headache. He has no memory of the seizure.

Seizures may occur only at night. The child wakes in the morning with a bitten tongue, blood on the pillow, or a bed wet with urine. In the child with persistent bedwetting, the possibility of nocturnal seizures must be considered.

Children with this type of seizure usually, although not always, have an abnormal EEG pattern. Other family members may have similarly abnormal EEG patterns without any symptoms.

Therapy usually includes the daily administration of anticonvulsants such as valproic acid (Depakene) and carbamazepine (Tegretol). Phenobarbital has the advantage of being an inexpensive anticonvulsant (Box 49.7). However, drowsiness and sleepiness may interfere with the child's ability to perform in school. Phenobarbital dosages should be tapered, never stopped suddenly, because the body becomes dependent on it. Rapid withdrawal may precipitate a seizure.

Children with tonic–clonic seizures also may be given phenytoin sodium (Dilantin) for control (Box 49.8). One nontoxic side effect of phenytoin is painless hypertrophy of the gums. Unless the gum hypertrophy is extensive, it is not sufficient reason to discontinue the drug. Medications are usually continued until the child has been seizure free for 2 to 3 years.

Some children are prescribed a ketogenic diet. This diet is high in fat and low in protein and carbohydrate. It causes the child to have a high level of ketones, which is believed to decrease myoclonic or tonic–clonic seizure activity. Because a ketogenic diet is monotonous for children and difficult for parents to prepare, however, it is hard to maintain for very long (Brooks-Kayal, 2003b).

BOX 49.7 FOCUS ON . . .

PHARMACOLOGY

Phenobarbital

Classification: Phenobarbital is a central nervous system (CNS) depressant.

Action: Acts as an anticonvulsant by lowering the seizure threshold (Karch, 2004).

Pregnancy Risk Category: D

Dosage: 3 to 6 mg/kg/day orally, or 4 to 6 mg/kg/day parenterally, for 7 to 10 days until a blood level of 10 to 15 µg/mL is achieved, or 10 to 15 mg/kg/day IV or IM. In status epilepticus, 15 to 20 mg/kg IV administered over 10 to 15 min.

Possible Adverse Effects: Somnolence, sedation, confusion, ataxia, lethargy, hangover, paradoxic excitement, nausea, vomiting, constipation, diarrhea, epigastric pain, bradycardia, hypotension, syncope, hypoventilation, respiratory depression, pain or tissue necrosis at the injection site.

Nursing Implications

- When giving phenobarbital parenterally, administer IV doses slowly, directly into tubing or running infusion. Inject a partial dose and assess the response before continuing. If giving phenobarbital IM, administer it deeply into a large muscle.
- Monitor the IV site carefully for signs of irritation or extravasation.

- Assess vital signs closely—especially pulse, blood pressure, and respiratory rate—during IV administration.
- Administer the oral form of the drug with food to minimize gastrointestinal upset. Instruct parents to do the same.
- Caution the parents and child that the drug will make the child drowsy. Advise the child to change positions slowly and to sit at the edge of the bed for a few minutes before arising. Assist parents with safety measures to protect the child from injury.
- Monitor laboratory tests for liver and renal function and blood counts if the child is on long-term therapy.
- Inform parents about the possible need for follow-up laboratory tests.
- Suggest that the parents obtain a medical alert bracelet and have the child wear it in case of an emergency.
- Instruct parents and child to avoid alcohol and sleep-inducing or over-the-counter drugs, which could cause increased CNS depression.
- Warn parents not to discontinue the drug abruptly or change the dose unless ordered by the health care provider.
- Instruct parents to notify the health care provider if the child develops severe dizziness, weakness, or drowsiness that persists.

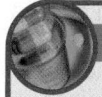

BOX 49.8 FOCUS ON . . .

PHARMACOLOGY

Phenytoin (Dilantin)

Classification: Phenytoin is an anticonvulsant.

Action: Stabilizes neuronal membranes, prevents hyperexcitability caused by excessive stimulation, and limits the spread of seizure activity without causing general central nervous system depression (Karch, 2004)

Pregnancy Risk Category: D

Dosage: Initially, 5 mg/kg/day in two to three equally divided doses up to a maximum of 300 mg/day with a maintenance dose of 4 to 8 mg/kg/day.

Possible Adverse Effects: Nystagmus, ataxia, slurred speech, confusion, fatigue, irritability, nausea, gingival hyperplasia, liver damage, and blood dyscrasias

Nursing Implications

* Administer the drug with food to minimize gastrointestinal upset and enhance absorption. Instruct parents to do the same.
* Advise parents to have the prescription filled each time with the same brand of drug, because differences in bioavailability have been reported.
* Obtain serum drug levels as ordered to monitor for effectiveness and to prevent possible toxicity. Keep in mind that the therapeutic range is 10 to 20 μg/mL.
* Monitor liver function studies and blood counts periodically.
* Inform parents about the need for follow-up laboratory tests.
* Instruct the child and parents about oral hygiene measures to prevent gum problems. Encourage frequent dental checkups.
* Suggest that the parents obtain a medical alert bracelet and have the child wear it in case of an emergency.
* Caution parents not to discontinue the drug abruptly or change the dose unless ordered by the health care provider.
* Instruct parents to notify the health care provider if the child develops nystagmus, ataxia, or diminished mental capacity. These are signs of possible toxicity.

Status Epilepticus. **Status epilepticus** refers to a seizure that lasts continuously for longer than 30 minutes or a series of seizures from which the child does not return to his or her previous level of consciousness (Chin et al., 2005). This is an emergency situation requiring immediate treatment. Otherwise, exhaustion, respiratory failure, permanent brain injury, or death may occur. Oxygen may be necessary to relieve cyanosis. An IV benzodiazepine such as diazepam (Valium) or lorazepam (Ativan) halts seizures dramatically. This may be followed by IV phenobarbital or phenytoin (Dilantin). Diazepam must be administered with

extreme caution, because the drug is incompatible with many other medications, and any accidental infiltration into subcutaneous tissue causes extensive tissue sloughing. Parents may administer diazepam by enema at home. Lorazepam (Ativan), a long-acting benzodiazepine used for children older than 2 years of age, provides a longer duration of action and also less respiratory depression.

Assessment of the Child With Seizures

A thorough pregnancy history must be obtained for a child with seizures. Events that occurred immediately before the seizure and an accurate description of the seizure itself also should be recorded. Investigate the child's overall behavior in the last few weeks. Is the child an A student who has been getting Ds lately? Has the parent noticed bedwetting? These might be signs of absence or nocturnal seizures.

A complete physical and neurologic examination and blood studies are necessary to rule out metabolic or infectious processes. Prepare the child for a lumbar puncture to rule out meningitis or bleeding into the CSF. A CT scan, MRI, skull radiograph, or EEG may be obtained if indicated. During the EEG, the child may be stimulated with rhythm patterns or flashing lights or asked to hyperventilate to see whether a seizure can be provoked.

NURSING DIAGNOSES AND RELATED INTERVENTIONS

Nursing Diagnosis: Risk for injury related to tonic–clonic seizure

Outcome Evaluation: Child exhibits no signs of aspiration or traumatic injury.

Protecting the child from hurting herself during a tonic–clonic seizure is crucial (Box 49.9). Restraining the child's thrashing extremities is not advisable, because it is difficult for an adult to do and could result in injury to the parent or child because of the amount of force needed to keep the child still. In early school-aged children, it is particularly important to avoid inserting a tongue blade between the teeth, because these children often have loose anterior teeth that are on the verge of falling out. Such teeth could be loosened and aspirated.

Remaining calm is also important; be aware that people are frightened by the sight of a child having a seizure because the action is so forceful and violent. It is reassuring for them to see someone calm and in control of the situation and to know that there is no reason to be afraid. If the child passes rapidly from one seizure into another (status epilepticus), be prepared to provide supplemental oxygen and administer anticonvulsant therapy as needed.

BOX 49.9 FOCUS ON . . .

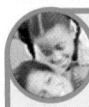

FAMILY TEACHING

Safety During Seizures

Q. Tasha's mother asks you, "What can we do to make sure she doesn't get hurt during a seizure?"

A. When your daughter has a seizure, here are some tips to help keep her safe:

- Remain calm.
- Move away furniture or any sharp object.
- Turn your child gently on her side, or on her abdomen with her head turned to the side, to prevent aspiration of unswallowed mouth secretions.
- Don't restrain her other than to keep her head turned to the side so that mouth secretions continue to drain. Restraining a child could result in injury because of the amount of force necessary.
- Do not attempt to place a stick or padded tongue blade between the child's teeth. Trying to force a tongue blade into the mouth this way could break the tongue blade or loosen teeth.
- Try to keep onlookers from crowding the area. A convulsing child is an abnormal sight and always attracts a crowd. Ask people who are only interested spectators to move away.
- Be aware that a child having this type of seizure may have some slight cyanosis during the tonic and clonic stages, but these stages are so short that administering oxygen is not needed.
- After any seizure, telephone your primary care provider and notify him or her of the seizure so arrangements for any necessary follow-up care can be made.
- If your child should pass rapidly from one seizure into another (status epilepticus), she may need supplemental oxygen or medicine to stop the seizure. If this happens, telephone your emergency medical service number.

Nursing Diagnosis: Interrupted family processes related to diagnosis of long-term illness in child

Outcome Evaluation: Child, parents, and other family members express fears and questions about disease to health care team; parents discuss ways to accommodate the illness in their daily life, such as medication schedules, school accommodations, sports activities, plans for vacation, and discipline.

As soon as the diagnosis of a seizure disorder is made, parents and children need to be told that it is likely to signify a long-term disease. Although the seizures can be controlled with medication, the disease is not cured. If children neglect their medication, seizures are apt to recur (Box 49.10). Most children are given tablets rather than liquid medication, because the latter tends to settle at the bottom of the bottle, resulting in overdiluted or overconcen-

trated doses that might allow seizures to break through. Parents need instruction to plan on always having an adequate supply of medications, especially for a trip away from home or for summer camp. Abrupt discontinuation of seizure medications (particularly phenobarbital) may result in severe seizures.

The child needs to be monitored frequently during childhood to be certain that the medication dosage is adequate. He or she will need periodic blood sampling to ascertain whether therapeutic blood levels of the medication are being maintained.

Provide parents with as much information as possible about the cause of their child's seizures. This helps them feel that they are dealing with a known disease, not an unexplainable and unpredictable illness. If the cause of the seizures is unknown, parents can be reassured that the treatment is known. Many new anticonvulsant medications are available today and are being introduced into therapy. These drugs include topiramate (Topamax), lamotrigine (Lamictal), and tiagabine (Gabitril) (Karch, 2004).

Although it may be difficult, parents need to treat children with seizures as normal members of the family. Alert them that scolding children, asking them to do household chores, or insisting that they do their homework will not cause seizures. A few children with absence seizures can initiate them by hyperventilating and may try to manipulate those around them by doing this to gain sympathy. The few children who use this extreme form of manipulation may need to be referred for counseling.

Assure parents that occasional seizures in children are not harmful. Unless status epilepticus occurs and the child becomes anoxic, the chance that their child will be injured during a seizure is remote. Knowing this helps parents not to worry about the child's becoming cognitively challenged or other misconceptions about seizures. Although some children who have seizures are cognitively challenged, this and the seizures were caused by the same event; the seizures did not cause the impairment. At every health care visit, be certain that parents have time to ask questions about their child's care and to express any concerns they have (Deonna, 2005). There are so many "scare stories" about seizures that every parent is likely to believe some of these stories unless counseled otherwise (Box 49.11).

As a rule, children with seizures should attend regular school and participate in physical education classes and active sports (with possible exceptions such as scuba or sky diving or rock climbing). Many teachers are concerned about the responsibility of having a child with seizures assigned to their classes. Help them learn about the success of modern seizure control. State regulations differ, but most states allow teenagers to apply for a driver's license after they have been seizure free for 1 year.

In many children, seizures increase at puberty. This may be the result of glandular changes or of

BOX 49.10: Focus on Nursing Care Planning

A Multidisciplinary Care Map for
A Child with Recurrent Seizures

●

Tasha is a 2-year-old girl who was brought to the emergency room by her mother because she had a seizure. Her physician suspects she may have meningitis. Her parent is visibly upset. She says, "Does this mean she'll always have seizures? How will she ever be independent?"

Family Assessment
Parents are divorced. No siblings. Child lives in a 2-bedroom apartment with mother; attends preschool daily 9–3 PM. Neighbor watches her from 3 to 6 PM, when mother returns from work as a research librarian.

Client Assessment
Well-proportioned preschooler sleeping soundly on left side since admission. A second seizure occurred approximately 1 hour ago. Vital signs within age-appropriate parameters. Reacts to painful stimuli only. Deep tendon reflexes depressed. "She was watching television this morning. Suddenly, she just fell to the floor and started shaking. I called 911, and they brought her here." Temperature 103°F. Pain on forward flexion of the neck. Lumbar puncture performed; pressures within normal limits; specimens sent for cell count, glucose, and culture.

Nursing Diagnosis
Risk for injury related to diminished level of consciousness resulting from seizure episode

Outcome Evaluation
Child is conscious within the hour. Exhibits no signs of aspiration or traumatic injury.

Team Member Responsible	Assessment	Intervention	Rationale	Expected Outcome
Activities of Daily Living				
Nurse	Assess whether mother was aware child's temperature was elevated. Ask if she has a thermometer for future fevers.	Keep child on side to help ensure an open airway until alert and responsive.	Side-lying position reduces risk for aspiration.	Mother states she understands importance of taking temperature in the future.
Nurse	Assess whether child has continued pain on dorsiflexion of neck.	Determine whether mother feels child is exceptionally irritable.	Pain on dorsiflexion of neck and irritability are symptoms of meningitis.	Mother rates child's emotional state. Unable to assess pain because child is unconscious.
Consultations				
Physician	Assess in light of this second seizure and spinal tap results whether neurologic service should be consulted.	Consult with neurologic service, if indicated, about management of child.	A second febrile seizure suggests this may be more than a simple febrile seizure.	Neurologic service meets with mother and child as appropriate based on findings.

(continued)

Team Member Responsible	Assessment	Intervention	Rationale	Expected Outcome
Procedures/Medications				
Nurse	Assess whether child has had a spinal tap before.	Assist with spinal tap and specimen collection.	Spinal tap is a frightening procedure for both child and parent.	Mother states she understands reason for procedure and gives consent.
Nurse	Assess whether child has prior experience with intravenous administration.	Begin IV fluid administration as prescribed.	IV line supplies a route for emergency medicine should it be needed for seizure control or treatment of infection.	IV line is established and safeguarded with board for unresponsive child.
Nurse	Assess whether mother understands why respiratory precautions are necessary.	Obtain equipment for respiratory precautions as needed.	Meningitis is contagious by contact with nasal secretions.	Mother states she understands the importance of precautions. Respiratory precautions are readied.
Nutrition				
Nurse	Assess child's level of consciousness using a Glasgow coma scale.	Do not give anything by mouth until the child is fully awake, alert, and oriented and the gag reflex is intact.	Giving oral fluids too early increases risk for aspiration.	Child receives no oral fluid until she is awake and aware.
Patient/Family Education				
Nurse/Nurse Practitioner	Assess what mother knows about febrile seizures and meningitis.	Teach that a febrile seizure is more of a symptom of fever than a long-term condition. A meningeal infection could be very serious.	Understanding the basis for febrile seizures and meningitis can help the parent understand the responsibility she needs to take for future care.	Mother states she understands child's current status and possible future implications.
Psychosocial/Spiritual/Emotional Needs				
Nurse	Assess whether mother needs to contact a support person if her child's diagnosis is serious.	Help mother contact a support person if she feels this would be helpful.	A support person can be vital to help a parent withstand an ominous diagnosis.	Mother contacts support person as needed.
Discharge Planning				
Nurse	Assess whether parent has any further questions about child's condition before transfer to pediatric intensive care unit.	Answer any remaining questions to make transfer as comfortable for parent and child as possible.	Parents gain confidence in emergency department staff and may find it difficult to change to new health care providers.	Mother states she understands that if meningitis is diagnosed, her child needs further intensive care.

sudden growth and the need for an increased medicine dosage. It may result in part from adolescent rebellion against following prescribed medication routines. Respect the adolescent's feelings and need for independence, but assist the adolescent with channeling feelings to a more positive area.

All anticonvulsant medications are potentially teratogenic to a fetus. Be certain that adolescent girls are made aware of this so they can choose to delay childbearing until later in life, when their medication can be reduced or even discontinued.

BOX 49.11 FOCUS ON . . .

COMMUNICATION

Tasha, 2 years old, had a febrile seizure and was diagnosed as having meningitis. You talk to her mother about the seizure.

Less Effective Communication

Nurse: Mrs. Jarman, can you describe what happened?

Mrs. Jarman: She just started shaking all over. It was really frightening.

Nurse: Did she voice any symptoms before the seizure?

Mrs. Jarman: No, she just started shaking.

Nurse: That must have been frightening.

Mrs. Jarman: Thinking about what it did to her is scarier.

Nurse: Well, lucky thing she's fine now.

More Effective Communication

Nurse: Mrs. Jarman, can you describe what happened?

Mrs. Jarman: She just started shaking all over. It was really frightening.

Nurse: Did she voice any symptoms before the seizure?

Mrs. Jarman: No, she just started shaking.

Nurse: That must have been frightening.

Mrs. Jarman: Thinking about what it did to her is scarier.

Nurse: Did to her?

Mrs. Jarman: I know seizures cause mental retardation. Our neighbor's son has them, and he's severely retarded.

Nurse: Mrs. Jarman, let's talk about this a little more.

In the first scenario, although the nurse responds with a therapeutic statement ("That must have been frightening"), she fails to identify a misconception verbalized by the mother. In the second scenario, the nurse identifies the concern and attempts to clarify it, providing an opportunity for teaching.

✔ Checkpoint Question 4

Tasha had a generalized or tonic-clonic seizure. What is the usual description of this type seizure?

a. A momentary halt of about ten seconds in respirations.
b. Stiffening of the extremities, then shaking of the body.
c. Extreme pain and twitching of one of the extremities.
d. Rapid blinking, then foaming of the mouth.

Breath Holding

Breath holding is a phenomenon that occurs in young children when they are stressed or angry. The child breathes in and, because he is upset, does not breathe out again or

else breathes out and then does not inhale again (Anderson & Bluestone, 2004). As brain cells become anoxic, the child becomes cyanotic and slumps to the floor, momentarily unconscious. With loss of consciousness, the child begins breathing again. The child's color returns to normal, and he awakens. Breath holding is frightening but represents the immaturity of the child's neurologic control. This differs from a temper tantrum, in which a child deliberately attempts to hold his breath and pass out (see Chapter 29). The child needs no therapy except reassurance that he is all right.

Headache

Headache in children younger than school age is rare, although children may report "headache" in imitation of their parents. Preschoolers may have headache with a fever because of increased ICP caused by increased cerebral blood flow. As the child reaches school age, headaches may occur as a result of conditions as simple as eyestrain and sinusitis or as serious as a brain tumor (Box 49.12). Headache pain results from meningeal or vascular irritation. The brain itself is insensitive to pain, so a cerebral tumor can be present for a long time before meningeal irritation occurs and pain symptoms become apparent. With a brain tumor, pain becomes evident on changing body position, so a young child who reports a headache after getting up should be carefully evaluated. Pain from a brain tumor is also usually occipital, so asking the child to indicate where it hurts helps determine whether a tumor could be the cause.

Tension or Stress Headache

When children are studying intently or taking a test, contraction of their neck muscles from tension can cause temporary ischemia. This is experienced as a dull, steady

BOX 49.12 FOCUS ON . . .

EVIDENCE-BASED PRACTICE

How Frequently Do Teenagers Experience Headaches?

To answer this question, researchers examined self-administered questionnaires of 2,090 adolescents, aged 12 to 13 years, to determine how often they had had a headache in the previous 6 months. Twenty-six percent of students reported that they experienced headaches about once a week. Headaches were related to school or home or mental health causes.

This is an important study for nurses because it reveals how often headaches (once thought to be an adult phenomenon) occur in young adolescents. Knowing this, nurses can respect students' reports of pain and alert them that therapy is available for frequent headaches.

Source: Gordon, K. E., Dooley, J. M., & Wood, E. P. (2004). Self-reported headache frequency and features associated with frequent headaches in Canadian young adolescents. *Headache, 44*(6), 555–561.

pain in the head. Children with these symptoms should have their vision tested, because poor eyesight may be causing them to hunch over their books. Tension or stress is relieved by simple analgesics, such as acetaminophen, or by sleep or application of a cool compress.

Sinus Headache

Sinus headache usually accompanies sinusitis and is associated with inflammation and possible obstruction of the sinuses. Sinusitis is discussed in Chapter 40.

Migraine Headache

Migraine headache refers to a specific type of headache that may or may not begin with an aura or visual disturbance such as diplopia or a zigzag pattern across the visual field. The pain that follows is usually unilateral and extremely intense, with throbbing that is moderate to severe. The headache is aggravated by routine physical activity and may be compounded by nausea and vomiting and intolerance to bright lights and noise (Gladstone et al., 2004).

The cause of migraine headache in any age group is not well understood. It probably results from abnormal constriction of intracranial arteries that temporarily reduces cerebral blood supply. This is followed by compensating overdistention of cranial blood vessels. The aura accompanying such headaches is the result of the temporary ischemia, whereas the headache is the result of the overdistention. Some children who have migraine headaches have an abnormal EEG.

Most children with migraine headache have a positive family history. This syndrome may be inherited as a dominant trait.

Assessment. To help assess the cause of a headache, obtain a thorough history, including the following information:

- When the headache usually occurs
- The events preceding it (to detect an aura)
- Its duration, frequency, intensity, description, and associated symptoms
- Any actions taken to treat the headache

The child needs a thorough physical examination, including funduscopic examination, to rule out papilledema. Blood pressure must be measured to rule out hypertension. If an aura is documented, an EEG will be ordered.

Therapeutic Management. A drug commonly prescribed for migraine headache in children is ergotamine tartrate (Cafergot), which constricts cerebral arteries. Propranolol and flunarizine may also be helpful (Victor & Ryan, 2005). Beta-blockers or calcium channel blockers that result in vasodilation may be prescribed prophylactically. At the time of the headache, sleep or lying down may be necessary to relieve the pain and vomiting. Frequent headaches interfere with a child's ability to achieve in school. Children need to be reassured that migraine headaches are benign, although painful and incapacitating, and they are not signs of a developing brain tumor. Follow-up visits are necessary to confirm that there is no progressive disease.

If other family members have migraine headaches, counsel them on how their reactions to their headaches influence their child's reaction to his or her own headaches. If the mother goes to bed for the day when she has a migraine headache, she cannot expect her child to go to school when he has one.

ATAXIC DISORDERS

Ataxia is failure of muscular coordination or irregularity of muscle action. Ataxic disorders are often manifested by an awkward gait or lack of coordination. Causes of ataxia differ, but degeneration of cerebellar or vestibular function is always involved.

Ataxia-Telangiectasia

Ataxia-telangiectasia, transmitted as an autosomal recessive trait attributable to a defect of chromosome 11, is a primary immunodeficiency disorder that results in progressive cerebellar degeneration. This is a multisystem disease with neurologic and immunologic aspects. In addition, endocrine abnormalities may occur, and there is an increased risk of cancer, particularly brain tumor. Telangiectasia (red vascular markings) appear on the conjunctiva and skin at the flexor creases (Sudarsky, 2004).

Both immunologic and neurologic symptoms of this disorder vary in severity and onset. Serum immunoglobulin A (IgA) and IgE levels may be low, and there is often evidence of reduced T-cell function. Children develop frequent infections (primarily sinopulmonary) because of the immunologic deficits. Tonsillar tissue in the pharynx is scant.

Neurologic symptoms caused by the degeneration process can usually be detected in early infancy when developmental milestones are not met. Children develop an awkward gait when they begin to walk. **Choreoathetosis** (rapid, purposeless movements), nystagmus, an intention tremor, or scoliosis may develop. Children may be unable to move their eyes on demand or follow movement through visual fields. Eye changes (conjunctival telangiectasia) develop by 5 years of age. There is no effective treatment. Children with this disorder often die in late adolescence of infection, respiratory failure, or a malignant brain tumor.

Friedreich's Ataxia

Friedreich's ataxia, which is carried on the short arm of chromosome 9 as an autosomal recessive trait, involves a variety of degenerative symptoms. Symptoms such as progressive cerebellar and spinal cord dysfunction occur in late adolescence. Teenagers develop a progressive gait disturbance or a lack of coordinated arm movements. They also develop a high-arched foot (pes cavus), hammer toes, and scoliosis. The combined symptoms of a positive Babinski reflex, absence of deep tendon reflexes in the ankle, and ataxia are strongly diagnostic. Neurologic examination shows difficulty in recognizing foot position (whether the foot is moved up or down). The cause of the neurologic injury appears to be excess iron deposits in cells. If the ataxia remains untreated, death occurs in young adulthood from myocardial failure. Antioxidant therapy may help to delay this outcome (Pandolfo, 2003).

SPINAL CORD INJURY

Because of the resilience of their vertebrae, children have fewer spinal cord injuries than adults do. However, the incidence among adolescents is increasing, because more adolescents are involved in motor vehicle accidents, particularly motorcycle accidents (Tator, 2004). Another major cause of spinal cord injury is diving into too-shallow water. Any child with multiple traumatic injuries should be assessed for spinal cord damage. Spinal cord injury without radiographic abnormality (SCIWRA syndrome) may occur. Stabilizing the neck is the best protection against further injury in these children (Henderson, 2004).

Recovery Phases

Spinal injuries result when the spinal cord becomes compressed or severed by the vertebrae; further cord damage can be caused by hemorrhage, edema, or inflammation at the injury site as the blood supply becomes impeded. Table 49.5 summarizes functional ability after spinal cord injury. The first questions asked by the parents or the child after the injury are, How much damage is there? and

Will our child be able to walk again? Predictions of useful body function cannot be made at the time of the accident, however. Three phases of recovery must first take place.

First Recovery Phase

Immediately after the injury, the child experiences spinal shock syndrome or loss of autonomic nervous system function (anterior nerve fibers traveling through the anterior horn of the spinal canal). This leads to loss of motor function, sensation, and reflex activity, as well as flaccid paralysis in body areas below the level of the injury. If a cervical injury is present, there is loss of respiratory function attributable to flaccidity of the diaphragm. In high thoracic lesions, use of accessory muscles of the chest is lost, so the child has difficulty maintaining effective respirations. The child has no ability to sweat or shiver to change body temperature below the level of the lesion because of loss of autonomic nerve control; therefore, hypothermia or hyperthermia becomes a threat. Blood vessels below the level of the injury are no longer able to constrict, so blood tends to pool in the lower body, leading to hypotension, especially if the upper body is elevated. Loss of bladder control occurs (when flaccid, the bladder overdistends and continually empties). The bowel becomes equally distended, and bowel sounds are absent.

TABLE 49.5

Functional Ability After Spinal Cord Injury

Injury Site	Highest Key Functions Still Present	Effects and Possible Interventions
C1–3	Head and neck muscles intact	Respiratory paralysis from loss of phrenic nerve innervation; will need ventilatory assistance
		No voluntary motion below chin; possibly able to learn to use mouth to control pen for writing and mouthstick to reach objects
C4	Diaphragm intact	Loss of motor function of upper and lower extremities and trunk; able to learn to use abdominal muscles to breathe independently
C5	Shoulder control; biceps, deltoid function	Able to feed self and operate wheelchair if fitted with self-care aids
C6	Forearm pronation; wrist extension	Use of upper extremities for self-care. Can transfer to wheelchair and so have increased independence
C7	Triceps function	Able to transfer to wheelchair readily; increasing independence
C8	Thumb and finger function	Able to do fine motor tasks; increases self-care ability
T1–7	Intercostal muscles (able to breathe with chest, not abdominal, muscles)	Full use of upper extremities but is still dependent on wheelchair
		Possibly able to drive car with hand controls
		Possibly able to have high leg braces fitted for standing
T10–12	Abdominal muscles	Use of long leg braces and four-point crutch to ambulate
L2–4	Hip flexion	Use of long or short leg braces to ambulate
	Leg extension	
L5–S1	Gluteus maximus muscle function	Walking without aids
S4	Bladder and anal sphincter control	Controlling bladder and bowel function
		Penile erection and ejaculation possible

This phase of spinal cord injury lasts from 1 to 6 weeks. As a rule, the shorter the phase of spinal shock, the better the final outcome.

Administration of a corticosteroid helps to reduce edema and possibly protects function of the spinal cord during this phase. A vasopressor agent such as dopamine may be prescribed to maintain blood pressure and perfusion to the cord.

Second Recovery Phase

During the second phase of recovery, the flaccid paralysis of the shock phase is replaced by spastic paralysis. Normally, motor impulses begin in the brain cortex and are transmitted to the medulla, where they cross to the opposite side of the cord; they then travel down the descending motor tracts of the spinal cord. They synapse in the anterior horn of the spinal cord and travel by way of the spinal and peripheral nerves to the designated muscle group, which they set in motion. The nerve pathways of the brain and the descending tracts are termed *upper motor neurons.* Those in the anterior horn cells and the spinal and peripheral nerves are termed *lower motor neurons.* Whether a motor neuron has upper or lower function, therefore, does not depend on its height in the spinal tract but rather on its position in relation to an anterior horn: between the brain and the anterior horn, it is an upper motor neuron; between the anterior horn and the point of innervation, it is a lower motor neuron (Fig. 49.11).

Spasticity in the second phase is caused by the loss of upper level control or transmission of meaningful innervation to the lower muscles. Lacking upper motor neuron function because of a severed cord, the lower motor neurons or reflex arcs cause the muscles to contract and remain that way. Parents and children are quick to interpret the sudden spastic movement of a lower extremity as meaningful activity. This is particularly easy to believe with an infant, who cannot tell you that she has no control over her leg movement. Differences between upper and lower neuron damage are listed in Table 49.6. If the injury is very low in the spinal tract, affecting mostly lower motor neurons, the muscles will remain flaccid, because the lower motor neurons cannot send impulses for contraction.

During this phase, if the child's bladder is allowed to fill, the resultant sensory stimulation relayed to the damaged cord will initiate a powerful sympathetic reflex reaction (**autonomic dysreflexia**), and the child will show signs of hypertension, tachycardia, flushed face, and severe occipital headache. This is an emergency situation; if the severe hypertension is not relieved, cerebral vascular accident can result (McCance & Huether, 2004). Assess that the child's urinary catheter is not obstructed, so urine can flow freely and reduce the sensory stimulation.

What if... you are caring for a child with a spinal cord injury and he suddenly develops hypertension, tachycardia, diaphoresis, and headache? What would you initially assess for? How would you intervene?

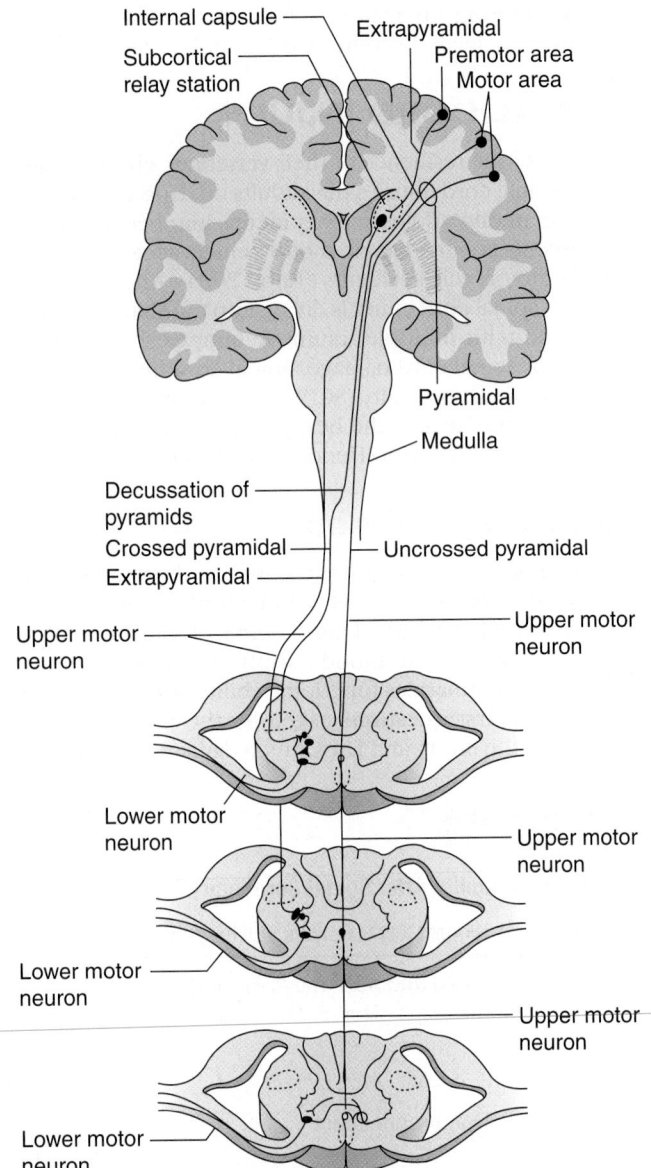

FIGURE 49.11 Diagram of motor pathways between the cerebral cortex, one of the subcortical relay stations, and lower motor neurons in the spinal cord. Decussation (crossing of fibers) means that each side of the brain controls skeletal muscles on the opposite side of the body.

Third Recovery Phase

The third phase of recovery from spinal cord injury is the final outcome, or permanent limitation of motor and sensory function. If the compression of the spinal cord is caused by edema that is then relieved, no permanent motor and sensory disability will occur.

Assessment of Spinal Cord Injury

Spinal cord injury should be suspected whenever a child has sustained a forceful trauma of any kind. The signs of spinal cord injury vary according to the level of the injury.

TABLE 49.6

Characteristics of Upper and Lower Motor Nerve Lesions After Spinal Shock Phase

Finding	Upper Motor Lesion	Lower Motor Lesion
Spasticity	Present	Absent (flaccidity present)
Clonus	Present, increased	Absent
Tendon reflexes	Increased	Absent
Babinski reflexes	Present	Absent
Reflexes below level of lesion	Present	Absent
Reflex at level of lesion	Absent	Absent
Atrophy of muscles	Absent or present only to slight degree	Present (muscle fasciculations may be present)

The cervical and thoracolumbar areas of the spine are the ones most likely to sustain injury.

Do not move a child with suspected spinal cord injury until the back and head can be supported in a straight line to prevent further injury to the spinal column from twisting or bending. In the emergency department, do not attempt to move the child from the stretcher to an examining table until spinal radiographic films have been obtained. This reduces any unnecessary movement. When moving the child onto the x-ray table, use a gentle log-rolling technique to avoid additional injury. If resuscitation is necessary, maintain the head in a neutral position; do not hyperextend it. To keep the neck immobilized, do not remove a child's football or motorcycle helmet or neck brace.

The child will need a thorough neurologic assessment to determine the level of injury. Help maintain spinal immobilization during procedures.

NURSING DIAGNOSES AND RELATED INTERVENTIONS

———●———

During the first phase of recovery, the child's major problems are those resulting from almost complete immobility: pressure ulcers on bony prominences; loss of appetite and subsequent poor nutrition from depression or being in the supine position; urinary calculi caused by excessive calcium loss from bones; atrophy of flaccid muscle groups; and urinary retention and bladder infection. These effects of immobility are presented in Figure 49.12.

Nursing Diagnosis: Impaired physical mobility related to effects of spinal cord injury

Outcome Evaluation: Child demonstrates movement of all extremities with a minimum of artificial support and equipment; participates in exercise program within limitations; exhibits ability to move about environment within limitations.

To relieve edema at the injury site and prevent further injury, IV corticosteroids will be administered. Children may be placed in cervical traction with Crutchfield tongs and a traction belt (Fig. 49.13) or with halo traction (see Chapter 51). Having tongs inserted into the skull is a very frightening procedure for children. They are afraid that the tongs will burrow into their skull and strike their brain. Children need someone they know and trust to help them lie still during the procedure.

To promote circulation and prevent loss of calcium that results from inactivity, full range-of-motion exercises must be done approximately three times per day. These are time-consuming but important in maintaining joint function.

During the second phase of recovery, when spasticity of muscle groups occurs, preventing contractures becomes an important nursing responsibility. Specialized splints, boots, or even hightop sneakers may be used to prevent footdrop (Fig. 49.14). If children have upper extremity mobility but will be left with lower extremity paralysis, exercises to strengthen the upper extremity muscle groups will be started. Strengthening the arms helps children be able to lift themselves from bed to a wheelchair or raise themselves with a trapeze over the bed when changing positions. Holding legs and arms at the joints while moving them helps reduce muscle spasms.

One major problem of ambulation after spinal cord injury is helping a child's body readjust to a vertical position after being maintained in the supine position for so long. When the child's head is raised, blood tends to pool in dilated blood vessels below the level of the lesion. This pooling of blood results in pseudohypovolemia and hypotension, and the child may faint. Gradually increasing the angle of the bed helps the child become acclimated to the upright position without experiencing vascular pooling.

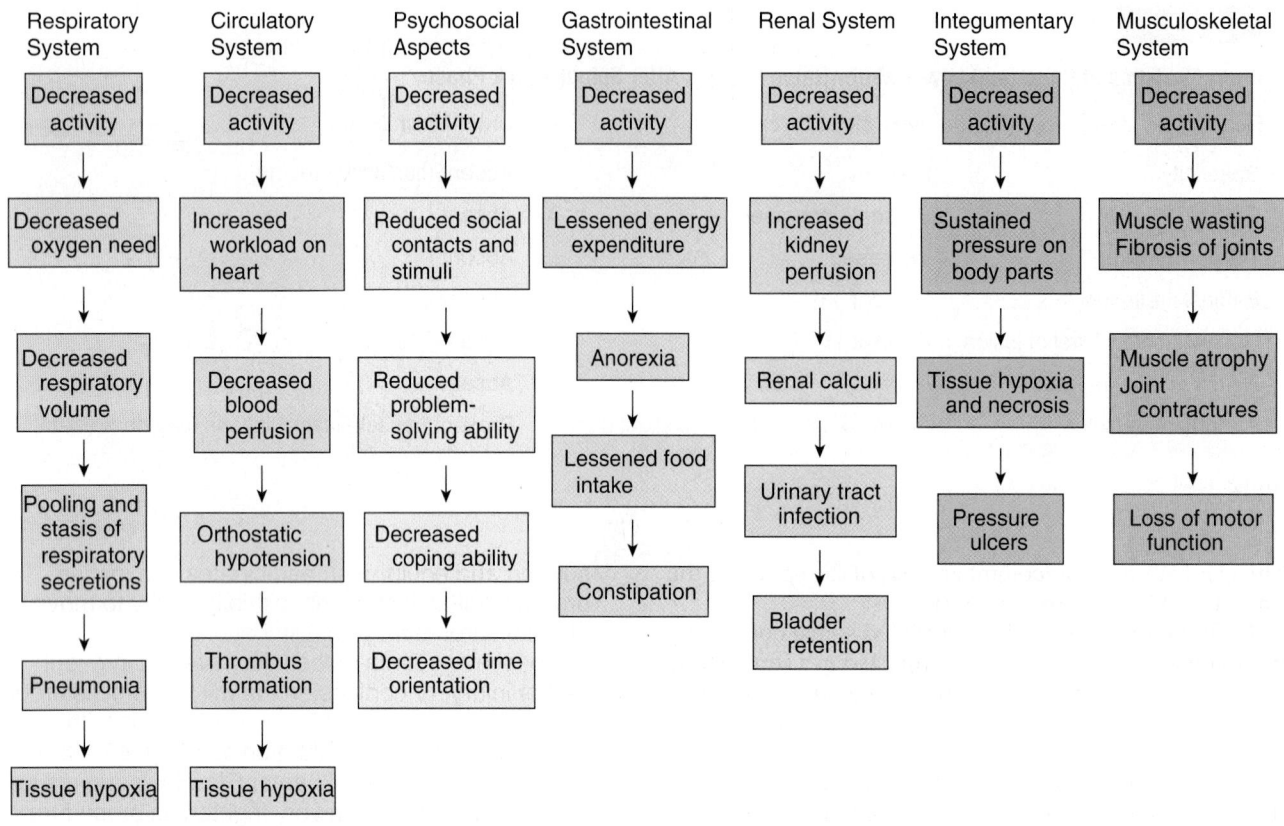

FIGURE 49.12 Effects of immobilization.

Nursing Diagnosis: Self-care deficit related to spinal cord injury

Outcome Evaluation: Child states intention of taking over self-care; practices using equipment for eating, bathing, and toileting; participates in one new aspect of self-care each week.

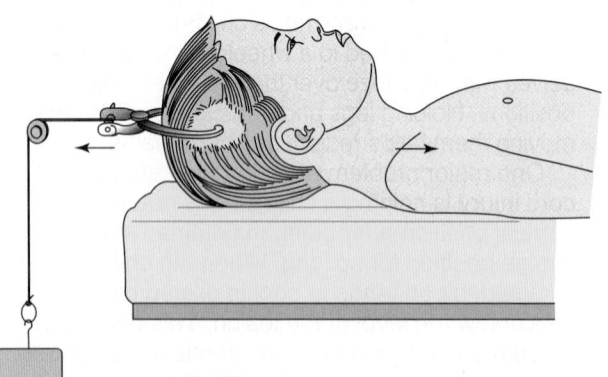

FIGURE 49.13 Crutchfield tongs used to create spinal traction.

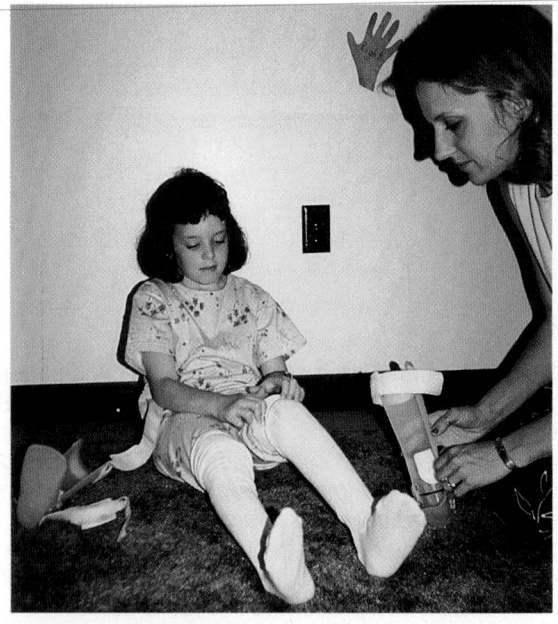

FIGURE 49.14 Specialized splints are used for a child with a low spinal cord injury to prevent contractures and foot drop. Here the physical therapist prepares to apply the splint to the child's leg. (Photo courtesy of Sue Moses.)

As soon as possible, children should be introduced to self-help methods for activities of daily living. Most parents need to be encouraged to allow the child to become as self-sufficient as possible and not to take over complete care. The child may well outlive them and will some day need to be able to function as independently as possible.

With autonomic nervous system dysfunction, the child is unable to sweat and becomes hyperthermic if covered too warmly; if not covered warmly enough, the capillaries dilate, and the child loses considerable heat into the environment. If the room temperature cools at night, be careful to dress the child appropriately for sleeping.

Specific measures for bowel evacuation may be necessary, depending on the level of the injury. A bowel program incorporating the use of stool softeners, suppositories, and bowel retraining may be required. The child and parents need support and instructions in accomplishing this task and gaining independence.

For some children and parents, the first day of using a wheelchair is exciting (proof that the child can be partially ambulatory). For others, it is the day on which they must face the reality that they cannot undo the results of the accident and are faced with a lifelong disability. For some parents who have almost overcome their grief and accepted their child's disability, the introduction of a symbol of disability such as a wheelchair or long-leg braces may bring new grieving and a sense of loss.

When the child reaches sexual maturity, limitations in this area may become apparent. If a male has had an upper motor neuron injury, he will not be able to achieve spontaneous erection or ejaculation. However, with manual stimulation of the penis (stimulation of lower motor neuron function), he may be able to achieve an erection and engage in coitus. Ejaculation and fertility remain limited. At the time of injury, lack of lower extremity motor control may seem to be the greatest loss. In adolescence, loss of normal sexual function may become even more disturbing. With most spinal cord injuries, a female is not able to experience orgasm but is able to conceive and bear children.

The limitations caused by a spinal cord injury become especially evident to the child (and the parents) when choosing a vocation and selecting an appropriate school program. (Children cannot be denied normal schooling by federal law in the United States, even with a severe physical disability.)

Counseling and rehabilitation are crucial aspects to achieve an optimal level of functioning and independence.

Nursing Diagnosis: Risk for impaired gas exchange related to spinal cord injury

Outcome Evaluation: Respiratory rate is within acceptable parameters; lungs are clear; airway is patent.

If the cervical level of the cord is involved, the child will need ventilatory assistance. She may be intubated at first, but orotracheal or nasotracheal intubation is only a temporary measure to maintain a patent airway. A tracheostomy may be done for long-term airway management and to prevent sloughing of pharyngeal tissue from the pressure of the intubation tube. If this is required, the parents will need instruction about caring for the tracheostomy and working with a mechanical ventilator. A phrenic nerve pacemaker may be used to stimulate the diaphragm to contract and initiate respirations. If the child has a thoracic level injury (which is rare because the rib cage gives extra strength to thoracic vertebrae), she will be able to breathe on her own but will have reduced vital capacity. Periodic positive-pressure breathing treatments may be necessary to encourage increased lung filling. Be careful when positioning the child not to compromise chest movement with equipment or other restricting objects. Other respiratory care measures, such as suctioning and chest physiotherapy, are also important.

Nursing Diagnosis: Risk for impaired skin integrity related to immobility

Outcome Evaluation: Child's skin remains clean, dry, and intact without signs of erythema or ulceration.

To prevent skin breakdown, a child should be turned about every 2 hours (always be sure to log-roll or maintain immobilization with a striker frame or a continuously moving, automatically controlled bed). The use of an alternating-pressure mattress may be helpful. With loss of sensation in body parts, the child is unable to report skin irritation from a wrinkled sheet or wet clothing. If the child is incontinent, the bedding must be changed immediately to prevent skin breakdown. Once children begin to be ambulatory, their legs and buttocks should be checked regularly to prevent pressure ulcers caused by sitting in a wheelchair or using leg braces.

Nursing Diagnosis: Risk for impaired urinary elimination related to spinal cord injury

Outcome Evaluation: Child's urine output is adequate for intake; child identifies measures to assist with voiding; child demonstrates procedure for self-catheterization.

To prevent urinary retention during the first phase of recovery, a Foley catheter is inserted, or the bladder can be emptied by periodic suprapubic aspiration or intermittent catheterization. Second-stage spasticity causes periodic reflex emptying. This rarely empties the bladder completely, however, so the same problems of stasis and infection continue. To live independently, the child will need to learn self-catheterization to empty the bladder.

Nursing Diagnosis: Anticipatory grieving related to loss of function secondary to spinal cord injury

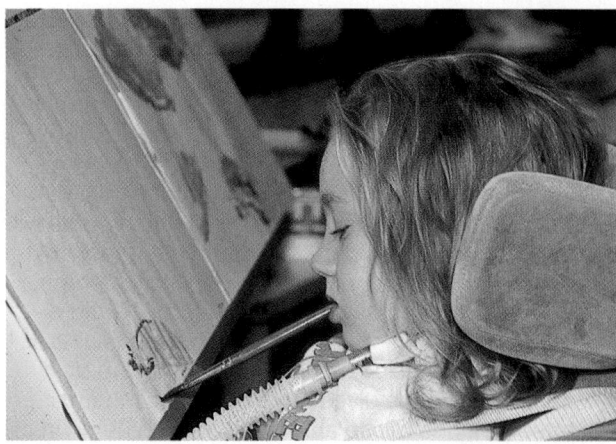

FIGURE 49.15 A 6-year-old girl with a cervical spine injury adapts to her disability by using her mouth to hold a paintbrush and participate in age-appropriate activities. (© Elisa Peterson/Stock Boston.)

Outcome Evaluation: Child and parents openly discuss their feelings about the injury and its effect on their lives.

The second recovery phase is the time for parents and children to begin thinking about what this degree of disability will mean to them and to face its full extent. Children and parents typically react to the initial diagnosis with grief. They may still be in denial or shock when the second phase begins. With no sudden miracle cure in sight, they may begin to move through stages of anger, bargaining, depression, and then acceptance (the accident happened; we must go on from this point). They need assistance and support to work through these feelings. Both the parents and the child may need counseling to reach acceptance. Incorporation of a rehabilitation program can help in maximizing the child's potential despite the limitations imposed by the injury (Fig. 49.15).

Checkpoint Question 5

Spinal cord injuries occur from accidents. Which is the most common type of injury in adolescents?

a. Cervical fracture from a diving accident.
b. Sacral fracture from a bicycle accident.
c. Thoracic fracture from a bullet injury.
d. Thoracic/sacral injury from lifting weights.

Key Points

Nerve cells are unique in that they do not regenerate if damaged. This makes neurologic disease a long-term type of illness. Parents and children alike need support from health care providers to cope with problems that continue to occur over a long period.

Increased ICP arises from an increase in the volume of CSF or from blood accumulation, cerebral edema, or space-occupying lesions. Neurologic changes, such as increased temperature and blood pressure and decreased pulse and respirations, that occur with increased ICP are subtle. Always compare assessments with previous levels to detect that a consistent, although minor, change is occurring.

Cerebral palsy (CP) is a nonprogressive disorder of upper motor neurons. The exact cause is usually unknown, but the condition is associated with anoxia occurring before, during, or shortly after birth. Four major types are identified: spastic (excessive tone in the voluntary muscles), dyskinetic or athetoid (abnormal involuntary movement), atonic (decreased muscle tone), and mixed (symptoms of both spasticity and athetoid movements).

Meningitis is infection of the cerebral meninges. It is caused most frequently by bacterial invasion. Children need follow-up afterward to monitor for hearing acuity and impaired secretion of antidiuretic hormone.

Encephalitis is inflammation of brain tissue. This is always a serious diagnosis, because the child may be left with residual neurologic damage, such as seizures or learning disabilities.

Reye's syndrome is acute encephalitis with accompanying fatty infiltration of the liver, heart, and lungs; it is associated with the administration of aspirin to children with a viral infection. Its incidence is declining.

Guillain-Barré syndrome is inflammation of motor and sensory nerves. The reaction may be immune mediated, occurring after an upper respiratory tract illness. Temporary demyelinization of the nerve sheaths causes loss of function.

Botulism occurs when spores of *C. botulinum* produce toxins in the intestine. Because honey and corn syrup can be sources of the organism, they should not be given to infants.

Recurrent seizures are involuntary contractions of muscle caused by abnormal electrical brain discharges. Common types seen in children include febrile seizures, infantile spasms, partial (focal) seizures, absence seizures, and tonic–clonic seizures. Therapy is administration of anticonvulsant drugs.

Spinal cord injury is occurring at increased rates in children involved in sports and motor vehicle accidents. Children pass through a first, second, and third recovery phase after the injury.

Critical Thinking Exercises

1. Tasha is the 2-year-old girl you met at the beginning of the chapter, who was diagnosed with bacterial

meningitis after a febrile seizure. Her parent is concerned about long-term problems. Would you encourage her to concentrate on these problems or on more short-term concerns?

2. Tasha is diagnosed with bacterial meningitis. She has severe neck pain when she is moved. Her mother asks you not to worry so much about measuring intake and output, so her daughter can rest. How would you answer her? Suppose you call the child's name and she does not answer you? Why is this a particular cause of concern in a child with meningitis?

4. A spinal cord injury can cause severe disability in adolescents. If you were designing a program to teach measures to prevent spinal cord injury, what topics would you include in your presentation?

5. Examine the National Health Goals related to neurologic disorders in children. Most government-sponsored money for nursing research is allotted based on these goals. What would be a possible research topic to explore pertinent to these goals that would be applicable to Tasha's family and also advance evidence-based practice?

References

Anderson, J. E., & Bluestone, D. (2004). Breath-holding spells in children: Scary but not serious. *Patient Care for the Nurse Practitioner, 1*(2), 1-9.

Bell, L. M. (2003). Meningitis. In Schwartz, M. W. (Ed.), *5-minute pediatric consult* (3rd ed.). Philadelphia: Lippincott Williams & Wilkins.

Bromfield, E. B. (2004). Epilepsy. In Samuels, M. A. *Manual of neurologic therapeutics* (7th ed.). Philadelphia: Lippincott Williams & Wilkins.

Brooks-Kayal, A. R. (2003a). Seizures—febrile. In Schwartz, M. W. (Ed.), *5-minute pediatric consult* (3rd ed.). Philadelphia: Lippincott Williams & Wilkins.

Brooks-Kayal, A. R. (2003b). Seizures—partial and generalized. In Schwartz, M. W. (Ed.), *5-minute pediatric consult* (3rd ed.). Philadelphia: Lippincott Williams & Wilkins.

Burke, L. (2003). Neurofibromatosis. In Schwartz, M. W. (Ed.), *5-minute pediatric consult* (3rd ed.). Philadelphia: Lippincott Williams & Wilkins.

Burton, J. H., & Germann, C. A. (2004). Guide to procedural sedation and analgesia. *Emergency Medicine, 36*(7), 43-46.

Chin, R. F., Neville, B. G., & Scott, R. C. (2005). Meningitis is a common cause of convulsive status epilepticus with fever. *Archives of Disease in Childhood, 90*(1), 66-69.

Chung, S. S. (2003). Bell palsy. In Schwartz, M. W. (Ed.), *5-minute pediatric consult* (3rd ed.). Philadelphia: Lippincott Williams & Wilkins.

Deonna, T. (2005). Management of epilepsy. *Archives of Disease in Childhood, 90*(1), 5-9.

Department of Health and Human Services. (2000). *Healthy people 2010.* Washington, D.C.: DHHS.

Fischbach, F. T. (2004). *Manual of laboratory and diagnostic tests* (7th ed.). Philadelphia: Lippincott Williams & Wilkins.

Gilbert, D. L., DeRoos, S., & Bare, M. A. (2004). Does sleep or sleep deprivation increase epileptiform discharges in pediatric electroencephalograms? *Pediatrics, 114*(3), 658-662.

Gladstone, J. P., Eross, E. J., & Dodick, D. W. (2004). Symposium on migraine. Migraine in special populations: Treatment strategies for children and adolescents, pregnant women, and the elderly. *Postgraduate Medicine, 115*(4), 39-44.

Gordon, K. E., Dooley, J. M., & Wood, E. P. (2004). Self-reported headache frequency and features associated with frequent headaches in Canadian young adolescents. *Headache, 44*(6), 555-561.

Griffin, H. C., Fitch, C. L., & Griffin, L. W. (2004). The causal pathway model and cerebral palsy. *Neonatal Network: The Journal of Neonatal Nursing, 23*(6), 43-47.

Henderson, G. V. (2004). Coma, head trauma, and spinal cord injury. In Samuels, M. A. *Manual of neurologic therapeutics* (7th ed.). Philadelphia: Lippincott Williams & Wilkins.

Kamienski, M. C. (2003). Emergency. Reye syndrome: Patients don't always have a history of taking aspirin or display obvious symptoms. *American Journal of Nursing, 103*(7), 54-57.

Karch, A. M. (2004). *Lippincott's nursing drug guide.* Philadelphia: Lippincott Williams & Wilkins.

MacDermid, J. C., & Wessel, J. (2004). Clinical diagnosis of carpal tunnel syndrome: A systematic review. *Journal of Hand Therapy, 17*(2), 309-319.

Marra, C. M. (2004). Infections of the central nervous system. In Samuels, M. A. *Manual of neurologic therapeutics* (7th ed.). Philadelphia: Lippincott Williams & Wilkins.

Mason, J. D., & Sadalla, J. K. (2003). Avoiding the pitfalls of bacterial meningitis. *Emergency Medicine, 35*(12), 36-37.

McCance, K. L., & Huether, S. E. (2004). *Understanding pathophysiology* (3rd ed.). St. Louis: Mosby.

Mitchell, R. M. (2003). Cerebral palsy. In Schwartz, M. W. (Ed.), *5-minute pediatric consult* (3rd ed.). Philadelphia: Lippincott Williams & Wilkins.

Morton, R. E., Hankinson, J., & Nicholson, J. (2004). Botulinum toxin for cerebral palsy: Where are we now? *Archives of Disease in Childhood, 89*(12), 1133-1137.

Muniz, A. E. (2004). Sturge-Weber syndrome presenting as an acute life-threatening event. *Pediatric Emergency Care, 20*(9), 610-612.

Orliaguet, G. A. (2004). Cerebral monitoring in children. *Paediatric Anaesthesia, 14*(5), 407-411.

Pandolfo, M. (2003). Friedreich ataxia. *Seminars in Pediatric Neurology, 10*(3), 163-172.

Pantell, R. H., et al. (2004). Management and outcomes of care of fever in early infancy. *Journal of the American Medical Association, 29*(10), 1203-1212.

Posner, E. B., Mohamed, K., & Marson, A. G. (2005). Ethosuximide, sodium valproate or lamotrigine for absence seizures in children and adolescents. *The Cochrane Library (Oxford) (4)* (CD003032).

Rawlins, P. K. (2004). Intrathecal baclofen therapy over 10 years. *Journal of Neuroscience Nursing, 36*(6), 322-327.

Shevell, M. I. (2004). The "Bermuda triangle" of neonatal neurology: Cerebral palsy, neonatal encephalopathy, and intrapartum asphyxia. *Seminars in Pediatric Neurology, 11*(1), 24-30.

Sladky, J. T. (2004). Guillain-Barré syndrome in children. *Journal of Child Neurology, 19*(3), 191-200.

Sudarsky, L. R. (2004). Movement disorders, In Samuels, M. A. *Manual of neurologic therapeutics* (7th ed.). Philadelphia: Lippincott Williams & Wilkins.

Tamburrini, G., et al. (2004). Prolonged intracranial pressure (ICP) monitoring in non-traumatic pediatric neurosurgical diseases. *Medical Science Monitor, 10*(4), 53-63.

Tator, C. H. (2004). Current primary to tertiary prevention of spinal cord injury. *Topics in Spinal Cord Injury Rehabilitation, 10*(1), 1-14.

Towers, R. (2004). The physical and psychological implications of neurofibromatosis. *Nursing Times, 100*(27), 34-36.

Victor, S., & Ryan, S. W. (2005). Drugs for preventing migraine headaches in children. *The Cochrane Library (Oxford) (4)* (CD002761).

Walker, B. W. (2004). Combating infection. Beating botulism. *Nursing, 34*(6), 74.

Welch, S. B., & Nadel, S. (2003). Treatment of meningococcal infection. *Archives of Disease in Childhood, 88*(7), 608-614.

Suggested Readings

Fleener, V. S., & Holloway, B. (2004). Migraines: Not just an adult problem. *Nurse Practitioner: American Journal of Primary Health Care, 29*(11), 27-28.

Gibbs, M., Miles, H., & Lloyd, J. (2005). Improving outcomes in children with disability. *Paediatric Nursing, 17*(1), 21-23.

Hickey, K. J., & Hickey, E. M. (2004). Pediatric perspectives. Educating children, adolescents, and their families following spinal cord injury. *SCI Nursing, 21*(3), 168-171.

Ketcham, E. M., & Gomez, H. F. (2003). Pediatric perspective. Infant botulism: A diagnostic and management challenge. *Air Medical Journal, 22*(5), 6-11.

Kilic, R., et al. (2003). A case presentation of bilateral simultaneous Bell's palsy. *American Journal of Otolaryngology, 24*(4), 271-273.

Page, T. Z., & Franklin, J. (2004). Neurofibromatosis type 1. *School Nurse News, 21*(4), 22-24.

Roberts, G., Palfrey, J., & Bridgemohan, C. (2004). A rational approach to the medical evaluation of a child with developmental delay. *Patient Care for the Nurse Practitioner, 1*(5), 21.

Sanger, T. D., et al. (2003). Classification and definitions of disorders causing hypertonia in childhood. *Pediatrics, 111*(1), 89-97.

Warschausky, S., et al. (2004). Associations between family and child adjustment following traumatic injury of brain versus spine. *SCI Psychosocial Process, 17*(2), 97-105.

Yamamoto, L., Olaes, E., & Lopez, A. (2004). Challenges in seizure management: Neurologic versus cardiac emergencies. *Topics in Emergency Medicine, 26*(3), 212-224.

CHAPTER 50

Nursing Care of the Child With a Disorder of the Eyes or Ears

Key Terms

accommodation
amblyopia
astigmatism
diplopia
enucleation
fovea centralis
goniotomy
hyperopia
light refraction
myopia
nystagmus
orthoptics
photophobia
ptosis
stereopsis
strabismus
tympanocentesis

Objectives

After mastering the contents of this chapter, you should be able to:

1. Describe the structure and function of the eyes and ears and disorders of these organs that affect children.
2. Assess a child who has a disorder of vision or hearing.
3. Formulate nursing diagnoses related to a child with a disorder of vision or hearing.
4. Establish expected outcomes for a child with a disorder of vision or hearing.
5. Plan nursing interventions for a child with a disorder of vision or hearing, such as educating parents about otitis media.
6. Implement nursing care to meet the specific needs of a child who has a disorder of the eyes or ears.
7. Evaluate expected outcomes for achievement and effectiveness of care.
8. Identify National Health Goals related to vision and hearing disorders of children that nurses could help the nation achieve.
9. Identify areas related to care of children with vision or hearing disorders that could benefit from additional nursing research or application of evidence-based practice.
10. Use critical thinking to analyze ways that nursing care of children with a disorder of vision or hearing could be more family centered.
11. Integrate knowledge of childhood disorders of the eyes or ears with the nursing process to achieve quality maternal and child health nursing care.

*C*arla Vander, a 4-year-old child, is brought to a pediatric clinic for evaluation. Her mother states, "She's always had a lot of problems. She had strabismus as a baby. Now, I think she has another ear infection. It started out as a head cold but now she's pulling at her ear. Why does she get so many of these?"

Previous chapters discussed the growth and development of well children. This chapter adds information about the changes, physical and psychosocial, that occur when a child develops a disorder of the eyes (vision) or ears (hearing). This is important information because it builds a base for care and health teaching.

How would you answer Ms. Vander?
What information does she need to know about ear infections?

After you've studied this chapter, access the accompanying website. Read the patient scenario and answer the questions to further sharpen your skills, grow more familiar with RN-CLEX types of questions, and reward yourself with how much you have learned.

Any interference with vision or hearing poses a threat to normal growth and development, because so much of what and how a child learns about the world is achieved through these sensory organs. Infants first learn how to interact with others by watching their parents' faces. They learn to speak by listening to words spoken to them. They continue to depend on sensory input for stimulation throughout life.

Eye and ear disorders may be transitory. However, they always have the potential for becoming long-term illnesses if they permanently affect vision and hearing. This is an area in which health promotion, illness prevention, and health rehabilitation are important aspects of nursing care. Because of the importance of vision and hearing, National Health Goals have been established in relation to them (Box 50.1).

Nursing Process Overview

For Care of a Child with a Vision or Hearing Disorder

● *Assessment*

All newborns should be assessed for their ability to focus on or see an examiner's face and to follow an object from the periphery to midline. Observe the infant closely to ensure that the newborn's interest is evoked by sight, not sound. Newborn vision can be further tested by optokinetic nystagmus testing (the infant is shown alternating black and white stripes), visual-evoked potential testing (similar, but checkerboard-appearing pictures are shown), and forced-choice preferential looking testing (the infant is shown a pattern and a plain picture; the seeing child focuses on the pattern).

Assessing newborn infants for hearing loss is an equally important part of newborn care. Newborns should quiet to the sound of a soothing voice. (For this, you need to stay out of sight so you are certain the infant is not quieting to your face.) Many hospitals routinely test newborn hearing with an audible sound before the newborn is discharged from the facility.

Throughout childhood, children should be assessed by history for vision problems and hearing loss: Is a parent or teacher concerned about vision? Does a parent worry that the child may not be hearing well? Is the child having any difficulty in school? Vision should also be assessed by inspection: Do the child's eyes follow a moving light into all six fields of vision? Is a red reflex present? Do the child's eyes appear to be in straight alignment? Hearing acuity should be checked periodically at well-child visits. In addition, children also should be assessed for their ability to speak clearly and appropriately for their age, because language development is influenced by hearing. Detailed vision and hearing assessments are discussed in Chapter 33 (Box 50.2).

● *Nursing Diagnosis*

Teaching health promotion measures to safeguard vision and hearing is one of the most important roles in nursing. Examples of nursing diagnoses in this area are the following:

- Health-seeking behaviors related to prevention of trauma to eyes or ears
- Deficient knowledge related to importance of early diagnosis and treatment of eye infection

Nursing diagnoses for a child with a vision or hearing disorder should focus on the child's and the parents' responses to the loss of sight or hearing, not on the deficit itself (Carpenito, 2004). Such nursing diagnoses may include the following:

- Self-care deficit related to impaired visual acuity
- Risk for injury related to hearing loss
- Risk for situational low self-esteem related to long-term vision deficit
- Impaired verbal communication related to congenital hearing deficit
- Social isolation related to effects of hearing loss
- Dysfunctional grieving related to child's loss of sight

BOX 50.1 FOCUS ON . . .

NATIONAL HEALTH GOALS

Adequate vision and hearing ability are necessary for normal growth and development. Four National Health Goals address these areas:

- Reduce the rate of otitis media in children and adolescents, from 344 health care visits yearly per 1000 children to 294 visits yearly.
- Reduce the prevalence of blindness and vision disorders in children and adolescents aged 17 years and under, from a baseline of 24 per 1,000 to 20 per 1,000 children.
- Reduce the incidence of noise-induced hearing loss in children and adolescents aged 17 years and younger.
- Increase the proportion of preschool children who receive vision screening (DHHS, 2000).

Nurses can help the nation achieve these goals by screening for vision and hearing at all well-child assessments, paying particular attention to those children who had low birth weight, were cared for in neonatal intensive care units, or were excessively exposed to loud noises such as loud music. Nursing research questions that might yield helpful information include the following: Can infants who are prone to hearing and vision disorders be better identified before discharge from a neonatal intensive care unit? What are effective techniques for teaching adolescents to avoid excessive sound levels, such as those associated with loud music? What are effective ways to teach school-age children to avoid eye injury?

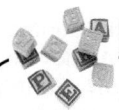

BOX 50.2 ASSESSMENT

Assessing a Child for Vision or Hearing Disorders

History
Chief concern: Are symptoms of vision or hearing difficulty present—blurriness of vision, squinting, turning head, leaning toward speaker, ignoring instructions?
Past health history: Has child had any exposure to loud noises? Eye trauma? Ear infection?
Family medical history: Do any family members have a hearing disorder? What is the vision level of parents?

Physical assessment

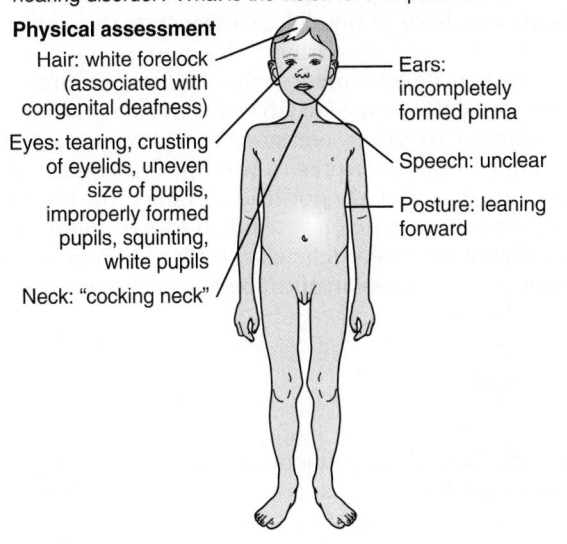

Hair: white forelock (associated with congenital deafness)

Eyes: tearing, crusting of eyelids, uneven size of pupils, improperly formed pupils, squinting, white pupils

Neck: "cocking neck"

Ears: incompletely formed pinna

Speech: unclear

Posture: leaning forward

• Readiness for enhanced family coping related to child's traumatic injury and subsequent loss of vision in one eye

● *Outcome Identification and Planning*
Be certain that expected outcomes established are realistic and address areas in which treatments can have some impact. By listening attentively to parents' concerns and providing useful anticipatory guidance, you can help to increase a child's ability to function effectively. Because many eye and ear disorders cause pain, helping parents reduce pain is a major nursing responsibility. Expected outcomes should address preventive aspects of care in all areas of daily living.

When parents learn that a child has a vision or hearing disorder, they usually need help in planning for schooling and activities such as toilet training and self-care. Discuss with them the importance of talking to and touching their infant and the importance of teaching their child how to communicate and learn about the world through touch as well as through other functioning senses.

Children with sensory disorders benefit from very early preschool education programs. This exposes them to interesting and stimulating tasks while their initiative is strongest, allowing them to accomplish learning tasks despite their sensory disorder. It may be difficult for parents to relinquish their children to such programs during the day, especially at an early age. It takes careful planning to enable parents to accept this separation.

Parents of children with hearing disorders may need to be encouraged to talk to their children, even in infancy. Although the infant may not be able to hear what the parents are saying, observing the facial expressions and spontaneous body movements that accompany verbal speech helps the child learn important aspects of communication. For example, although an older child may not be able to hear her mother say, "I'm so proud of you," the child can see the positive reaction displayed on her mother's face.

● *Implementation*
Nursing interventions for a child with a disorder of the eyes or ears range from providing anticipatory guidance and teaching children and parents measures to promote eye and ear health to preparing a child for surgery. Nursing interventions also include helping a child and parents adjust to aids that are used to improve hearing, speech, or sight. Referrals to organizations that can provide information and support to parents of children with vision or hearing impairment can be particularly useful, especially if the impairment will be long term. Some of the organizations concerned with sensory impairment are the following:

• Alexander Graham Bell Association for the Deaf and Hard of Hearing (*www.agbell.org*)
• American Foundation for the Blind (*www.afb.org*)
• American Speech-Language-Hearing Association (*www.asha.org*)
• National Association for Visually Handicapped (*www.navh.org*)
• National Federation of the Blind, Deaf-Blind Division (*www.nfb-db.org*)
• Recording for the Blind and Dyslexic (*www.rfbd.org*)
• National Association of the Deaf (*www.nad.org*)

● *Outcome Evaluation*
As stated earlier, a disorder of the eyes or ears can range from an acute, one-time illness to a chronic and developmentally debilitating condition if steps are not taken to treat the initial problem quickly and completely. However, even the most rigorous preventive care and attention cannot avert the occurrence of some serious disorders affecting vision and hearing. Nursing care must then focus on helping the child and parents adjust to the condition, ensuring that the child receives the stimulation needed to grow and develop on a normal continuum.

Continued follow-up is essential. Self-esteem is an important factor to be evaluated. Does the child see himself as well or ill, as a person able to do things or as helpless? Plans to promote self-esteem may have to be devised. Some parents may require help with their own feelings of worth. (Feeling inferior to other parents is common among parents of children with disabilities.) They may need help in letting go as their children begin school. The growth of parents in allowing their child to be independent is just as important to evaluate as the child's own progress toward independence (Robinson & Lieberman, 2004).

Examples of expected outcomes are the following:

- Parent states that she understands antibiotics are no longer prescribed for simple otitis media.
- Parents state concrete plans for enrolling child in preschool program.
- Child wears corrective lenses for major portion of each day.
- Child with hearing disorder communicates effectively with health care providers by lip reading or writing out needs.

HEALTH PROMOTION AND RISK MANAGEMENT

All children should be screened routinely for vision and hearing problems, so that these problems can be detected as early in life as possible (Elliman et al., 2004). A history and physical examination performed at each health maintenance visit can provide important clues to possible problems and need for further evaluation. Pay special attention to any questions or concerns voiced by the parents at these visits, because children's needs change as they grow. As the child grows older and attends school, often the school nurse assumes a major responsibility for vision and hearing testing. General guidelines for evaluation are listed in Table 50.1.

Providing anticipatory guidance to parents about safety measures to prevent accidental injury is another major nursing responsibility. Box 50.3 summarizes safety measures for preventing eye injuries and hearing loss in children.

If a child has a vision or hearing impairment, safety measures take on even greater importance. Assist the parents with measures to adapt the child's environment to meet his needs while promoting growth and development and independence as much as possible. Supplement verbal explanations with tactile and visual aids as appropriate, and allow the child to use drawings, writing, or gestures to respond and communicate. Encourage the use of specialized devices, such as a talking picture board or e-mail, if the child is hearing impaired with limited speech. Assess whether parents are interested in investigating cochlear implants for a hearing-impaired child (Box 50.4). Provide ample time for interaction, and incorporate the use of therapeutic play. Children with vision or hearing disorders need to attend regular classrooms in school, if possible, so that they can have contact with seeing and hearing children to promote normal growth and development. School nurses or preschool nurse consultants need to advocate for such placements. In addition to safety measures, parents may need instruction about measures to prevent eye and ear infections, so that they do not lead to long-term problems. Mild vitamin A deficiency leads to loss of night vision, and severe vitamin A deficiency leads to blindness (keratomalacia), so assessing nutrition is also important (Colev et al., 2004).

VISION

Vision occurs because light rays reflect from an object through the corneas, aqueous humors, lenses, and vitreous humors to the retinas (Fig. 50.1). If any of these structures have defects, light rays may not be able to reach the retinas or focus correctly there, resulting in a vision disturbance. The retinas are studded with rods, which are instrumental for night vision and movement in the visual

TABLE 50.1

Health Promotion Guidelines

Age	Vision Assessment Parameters	Hearing Assessment Parameters
Infant	Ability to follow objects	Startle reflex (at birth)
	Corneal reflex	Ability to track sounds (3–6 mo)
	Ability to turn to light stimuli	Ability to recognize sounds (6–8 mo)
		Ability to locate sounds (8–12 mo)
Toddler	Corneal light reflex	Ability to react to soft sounds (whispers)
	Cover test	Ability to track source of sounds
	Smooth ocular movements	Ability to form a noun–verb sentence by 2 yr
	Hand–eye coordination	Ability to follow simple directions
		Awareness of pitch and tone
Preschooler	Corneal light reflex	Pure tone audiometry (starting at age 4 yr)
	Cover test	Understandable language with increasing vocabulary
	Snellen E chart (or modification)	
School age	Visual acuity testing every 1–2 yr	Pure tone audiometry at ages 6, 8, and 11 yr
Adolescent	Visual acuity testing every 1–2 yr	Pure tone audiometry at ages 14 and 18 yr

BOX 50.3 FOCUS ON . . .

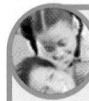

FAMILY TEACHING

Protecting Vision and Hearing

Q. Carla's mother says to you, "What can we do to protect our children from having problems with their eyes and ears?"

A. Here are some helpful tips to protect your children's vision and hearing:

To protect vision:

- Place infants and small children in a car seat (for older children, use a seat belt) when in a car to keep them from hitting the dashboard or front seat in case of an accident.
- Do not allow infants to hold sharp objects. If an infant is holding such an object in his hand, there is the danger that the object could strike his eye as he brings his fist to his mouth to suck his thumb.
- Do not allow toddlers to carry sharp objects such as lollipop sticks in their hands while walking. They fall readily because of their unsteady gait.
- Do not allow older children to run with sharp objects in their hands, because they can fall while running and puncture an eye.
- Caution older children to use eye-protection measures, such as goggles, when working with projects, such as soldering metal, in school.
- Encourage the use of face masks for hockey players.
- Teach children not to place any medication in their eyes that is not prescribed by a health care provider;

do not use outdated eye medication, because it may become contaminated with bacteria or may change in composition with time.
- Caution children that chemicals can cause burns to the eye; alert them to the emergency shower installations in science rooms that are used to wash away any spilled chemical from their eyes. Chemical burns may be worse in children who have contact lenses in place, because chemicals can flow under the lens and remain in contact with the cornea longer.
- Teach children not to wear contact lenses for longer intervals than recommended by the manufacturer, to prevent drying and lack of oxygen supply to the cornea.

To prevent hearing loss:

- Teach children to avoid chronic exposure to loud noises, such as can occur with radios and earphones.
- Secure prompt treatment for pharyngitis (fever and sore throat), because this condition can lead to otitis media (middle ear infection).
- Caution children not to put anything in their ear canals, because they could puncture their eardrums.
- Be certain children's immunizations are up to date, because illnesses such as parotitis (mumps) or bacterial meningitis can lead to hearing loss.

---

field, and cones, which register daylight and color vision. Rods and cones join in a major network to register at the optic nerve. The **fovea centralis** (the center of the macula) is an area of closely packed cones on the retinas where color is best perceived.

Each eye globe must develop good central and peripheral vision. However, in addition, *fusion* must occur—that is, both eyes together must interpret a visual image as one image, fusing visual perception into a single image. This is called *single binocular vision.* Infants with poor eye

BOX 50.4 FOCUS ON . . .

EVIDENCE-BASED PRACTICE

Do Nonhearing Parents Want Their Nonhearing Children to Have Cochlear Implants?

When cochlear implants first became a reality, they met unexpected resistance in the deaf community, because hearing-challenged parents wanted to raise their children in their world, not the hearing one. To determine whether attitudes are changing, researchers analyzed questionnaires from 439 parents and interviews with 56 additional parents of children with cochlear implants. Results of the study showed that opposition to pediatric cochlear implantation within the deaf community is giving way to the perception that it is one of a continuum of possibilities for parents to consider. This change is related to the desire

to have their children welcomed into both deaf and hearing societies; many children with cochlear implants can be included in regular school classrooms. Most parents interviewed wished their children could have received their implant earlier in life, so that their spoken language could be optimal.

This is an interesting study for nurses, because it accentuates how therapy and schooling for nonhearing children are changing. Being aware of these changes is important so that you can discuss trends with parents and children to help them understand their options.

Source: Christiansen, J. B. & Leigh, I. W. (2004). Children with cochlear implants: Changing parent and deaf community perspectives. *Archives of Otolaryngology—Head & Neck Surgery, 130*(5), 673–677.

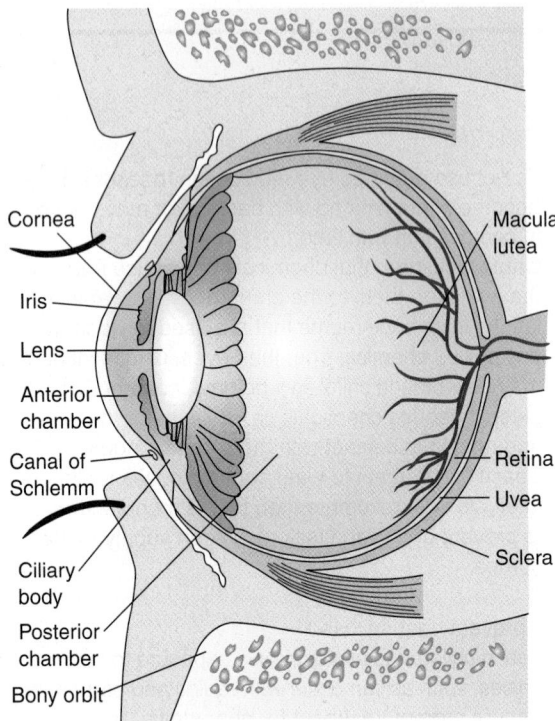

FIGURE 50.1 Anatomy of the eye.

alignment cannot establish single binocular vision but have **diplopia,** or double vision.

Stereopsis

Stereopsis is depth perception, or the ability to locate an object in space relative to other objects. The right eye sees more of the right side of an object, whereas the left eye sees more of the left side. This makes the object appear to be three-dimensional. Children with vision loss in one eye do not develop stereopsis and, consequently, tend to reach farther than or closer than the actual distance to an object when attempting to grasp it. They have difficulty learning to ride a bicycle and have great difficulty driving a car safely. Children without stereopsis do not realize that their sight is different from that of other people. The *Stereo-Fly* or random dot test, a simple test for depth perception, is a specially constructed picture of a large fly made of colored dots. When asked to touch the fly's wings, a child with good depth perception touches them accurately. A child with poor depth perception touches a spot 2 or 3 inches above the pattern.

Accommodation

Accommodation is the adjustment the eye makes when focusing on a close image. To focus on a close object, the ciliary bodies of the eye contract, changing the curvature of the lens. The action of the ciliary body allows accommodation but also causes the eye to converge (look medially) and the pupil to constrict. To test accommodation, ask a child to follow a penlight as it moves in toward the nose. Children should be able to do this by 6 months of age. Actually, convergence is what is demonstrated with this test,

but because convergence does not occur without accommodation, the test indirectly measures accommodation. Children who cannot accommodate have double vision (diplopia) or are unable to focus on objects near their eyes.

DISORDERS THAT INTERFERE WITH VISION

Eye disease in children is always potentially serious. If permanent vision impairment occurs, a child's functioning at many everyday tasks can be severely compromised.

Refractive Errors

The largest category of vision defects in children is refractive errors (Mills, 2003). **Light refraction** refers to the manner in which light is bent as it passes through the lens. Normally, this bending causes a ray of light to fall directly on the retina (Fig. 50.2*A*). Because the depth of the eye globe in infants and children increases with age, the light rays do not always focus onto the retina accurately, but at a point behind the retina. This results in **hyperopia** (farsightedness), in which vision is blurry at a close range and clear at a far range. The normal hyperopia of a preschooler needs no correction. It is important to keep this in mind when performing vision screening with children of this age. At about 5 years of age, as a result of developmental changes, hyperopia begins to diminish. Some children, however, remain hyperopic. Focusing on close objects requires such strong accommodation that these children often have headaches or dizziness after completing schoolwork. A finding of hyperopia in a school-age child is cause for referral so that the child can get a prescription for glasses with a convex lens.

Approximately 10% of school-age children have eye changes that result in **myopia** (nearsightedness), meaning that the light rays focus at a point in front of the retina (Mills, 2003). These children can read a book or a computer screen immediately in front of them but are unable to read the blackboard clearly in a classroom. They have difficulty reading signs across the street or playing baseball. Once myopia begins, it often progresses into the teen years, when it plateaus. Children with myopia need corrective (concave) lenses to enable them to see at a distance.

Myopia tends to be familial. If both parents are myopic, their children should be screened yearly during the early school years. Children with myopia try to focus on objects by squinting and rubbing their eyes, which changes the shape of the eye globe. Any child who reports difficulty seeing or who shows mannerisms suggestive of refraction errors—rubbing the eyes, tearing, red-rimmed eyes, blinking, squinting, or pressing on the eyes—should be screened for visual difficulty.

In the past, the only correction for refractive errors of vision was by eyeglasses or contact lenses (Fig. 50.2*B,C*). Today, adolescents can have laser surgery (LASIK) to permanently change the depth of the eye globe and correct refractive vision errors.

Although wearing glasses is more acceptable today, children still may encounter name calling. Encourage them to give glasses a fair try. In most instances, glasses improve vision to such an extent that after trying them children

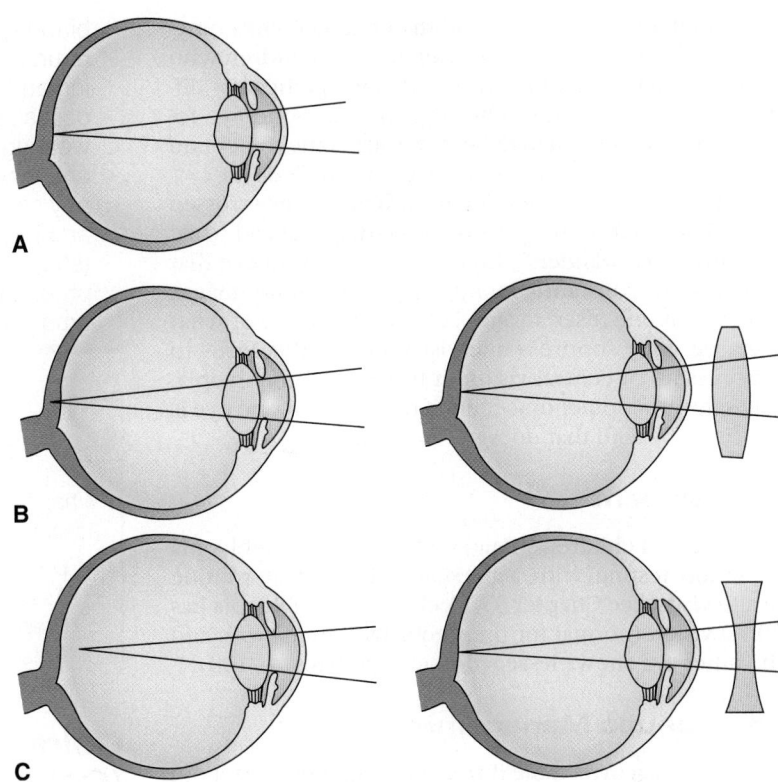

FIGURE 50.2 Corrective lenses for refractive errors of vision. (**A**) Normal vision. (**B**) Convex lens for hyperopia (farsightedness). (**C**) Concave lens for myopia (nearsightedness).

will continue to wear them. However, throughout their development, they may need continued encouragement to keep wearing the glasses.

If parents are going to purchase eyeglasses, advise them to choose frames fitted with plastic or safety glass (shatterproof) lenses so that, if the lenses accidentally break, the child's eye will not be injured. It is possible for contact lenses to be fitted for even young infants. Children as young as 5 years of age are capable of putting them in and taking them out if taught properly. Contact lenses are a big responsibility, however; they require conscientious cleaning or changing to prevent eye irritation or infection. Children are usually about 12 years of age before they can be relied on to take appropriate care of contact lenses independently.

Laser in Situ Keratomileusis (LASIK)

Laser in situ keratomileusis (LASIK) is laser surgery for correction of myopia. It involves making an incision under the cornea to change the contour of the eye globe so that light rays fall more accurately on the retina. Because having the procedure carried out before the child's eye globe has reached its adult size would require that the surgery be repeated with maturity, the youngest age at which LASIK therapy is appropriate is controversial. As the technique improves, it will become a major method of correcting refractive vision errors in children (Phillips et al., 2004).

Astigmatism

Astigmatism is congenital or acquired unevenness of the curvature of the cornea (Kunimoto et al., 2004). Light rays coming to the retina are not all refracted in the same way;

the result is an uneven quality of vision. When children with astigmatism look at the letter T, for example, they may see the crossbar but not the letter stem. If they focus on the stem, they cannot see the crossbar. On any given page of print, therefore, they may see only half the letters. For this reason, they will have difficulty reading or following written instructions. They may report headache and vertigo after doing close work. Their vision may appear deceptively normal on vision screening tests because they are able to see all of the numbers on a chart by tilting their head. These children need to be referred to an ophthalmologist, however, on the basis of their other problems (i.e., vertigo, headaches, and difficulty with reading). Corrective lenses for close work relieve the symptoms and restore functional vision. Contact lenses may be even more helpful, because they actually smooth out the curvature of the cornea.

Nystagmus

Nystagmus is rapid, irregular eye movement, either vertically or horizontally. It is not a disease in itself but rather a symptom of an underlying disease condition. Ocular nystagmus is seen in children with vision-impairing lesions such as congenital cataracts. It also occurs as a neurologic sign if there is a lesion of the cerebellum or brainstem. Children with nystagmus must be referred to a physician so that the underlying cause of the symptom can be determined.

Amblyopia

Amblyopia is "lazy eye," or subnormal vision in one eye; the child may be using only one eye for vision while "resting" the other eye. If this process continues too long, central vision fails to develop (or the central vision that had developed fades), and the child becomes functionally blind in one eye. This can occur in children who have a refractive error in one eye that is significantly different from that of the other eye. Because one eye focuses more readily than the other, they come to depend on only the easily focused eye (Gold et al., 2004).

Amblyopia can also develop from **strabismus** (crossed eyes). With strabismus, one eye looks straight ahead while the other eye "wanders." Children who have an eye that wanders are constantly looking at two separate images rather than one fused image. To make sense out of what they see, they suppress one visual image; this leads to suppression of central vision in that eye, or amblyopia. The same phenomenon occurs if the vision in one eye is obscured by a lid that does not open fully (ptosis).

Assessment

All preschool children should be screened for amblyopia by vision testing with a preschool E chart at routine health visits (see Chapter 33). A child with amblyopia has 20/50 vision (normal for preschool age) in one eye, and the other eye shows lessened vision (perhaps 20/100).

Therapeutic Management

Amblyopia is correctable if treated during the preschool period. Although there are reports of success with older children and adolescents (Mohan et al., 2004), the prognosis for correction is considerably diminished after 6 years of age. For treatment, the good eye is covered by a patch held firmly in place. This forces the child to use the poor eye, thus developing vision in that eye. Usually, the child has some difficulty initially adjusting to the patch; being unable to see well from the unpatched eye, he or she may develop headaches or dizziness. Only constant attempts to see with the poor eye, however, can improve binocular vision. The patch is removed for 1 hour each day to prevent amblyopia from developing in the nonamblyopic eye. Administration of levodopa in addition to occlusion therapy may also be prescribed. Atropine, which causes pupil dilation, may be another solution.

NURSING DIAGNOSES AND RELATED INTERVENTIONS

Nursing Diagnosis: Deficient knowledge deficit related to need for consistent wearing of patch

Outcome Evaluation: Parents state that the reason their child must wear a patch over the functioning eye is to improve vision in the poorly functioning eye. Child wears patch over functioning eye for all but 1 hour per day.

Parents need support to be firm with their child about keeping the patch in place. A child may beg to remove the patch for special occasions, such as a birthday party or a family wedding, or just for an hour, because she or he finds the patch embarrassing and uncomfortable. Soon, however, the "special occasions" become so frequent that the child is wearing the patch only half the time. Remind parents how important it is to adhere to occlusion therapy so that their child will achieve good vision. If amblyopia occurs secondary to another disorder (strabismus, ptosis, or refraction error), the primary problem also needs to be corrected. Otherwise, the amblyopia will recur after the patching is completed.

Checkpoint Question 1

What if Carla had amblyopia? What is a common assessment for amblyopia?

a. Doing a cover test.
b. Assessing for a red reflex.
c. Preschool E chart testing.
d. Pressing for tenseness.

Color Vision Deficit (Color Blindness)

Color deficit is the inability to perceive color correctly. It occurs because one of the sets of cones of the retina that perceive red, green, or blue is absent. It is inherited as a sex-linked disorder and occurs in about 8% of boys. There is a high incidence of color vision deficit in children with hemophilia, congenital nystagmus, or glucose-6-phosphate dehydrogenase deficiency. It may be associated with exposure to occupational solvents during pregnancy (Dick et al., 2004).

The vision problem may involve the inability to distinguish red from green or blue from yellow. A small proportion of children are unable to see any colors. Color plates or discs may be used to detect color deficit in children as young as preschool age. Children with normal vision see numbers or patterns on these plates, whereas children with a color vision deficit see only a jumble of dots or unclear images.

There is no therapy for color vision deficit, but the condition should be detected early so the child is not asked to complete color identification assignments in school and so can be educated about traffic signals and other color-dependent signs necessary for safety.

Some children associate color blindness with total "blindness" and fear that they will eventually lose their eyesight. Reassure them that, although color blindness means that they have a loss of color discrimination, their loss will be limited to that one area.

STRUCTURAL PROBLEMS OF THE EYE

Coloboma

A *coloboma* is a congenital incomplete closure of the facial cleft. The incomplete closure may involve only the

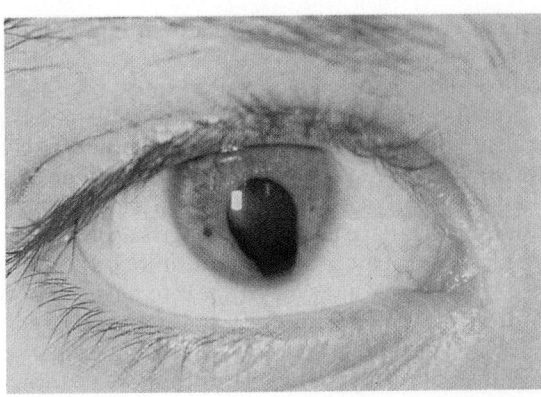

FIGURE 50.3 Coloboma involving the iris, showing a "keyhole" appearance. (From Tasman, W., & Jaeger, E. A. [1996], *Willis Eye Hospital atlas of clinical ophthalmology*. Philadelphia: Lippincott-Raven Publishers.)

lower eyelid (there is a notch in the lid); it may involve the iris, giving it the shape of a keyhole, rather than a circle (Fig. 50.3). It may involve the ciliary body, the lens, the choroid, the retina, and the optic nerve. Children with any degree of coloboma should be referred to an ophthalmologist for further investigation to determine the extent of the condition. Children with retina and optic nerve coloboma will have some vision impairment in the affected eye.

Hypertelorism

Hypertelorism is a congenital condition involving abnormally wide-spaced eyes. Children with wide epicanthal folds by the inner canthus may appear to have wide-spaced eyes, but, when the distance between the pupils is measured and compared with standards for the child's age, the true condition is revealed. Detecting true hypertelorism in children is important, because this condition is associated with chromosomal abnormalities, most notably Waardenburg's syndrome, which also involves congenital hearing impairment. These children also have a white forelock of hair, different-colored irises, and eyebrows that tend to grow together in the center line. These signs may not be noticeable in newborns. Therefore, wide-spaced eyes, because of a broad-bridged nose, are the chief clue in the newborn that the child can hear no sound and will need close follow-up to determine whether cochlear implants or hearing aids can provide ability to hear.

Ptosis

Ptosis is the inability to raise the upper eyelid normally. The eyelid always remains slightly closed. The condition may be congenital (frequently hereditary and bilateral) or acquired (usually unilateral). It may be a result of injury to the third cranial nerve (neurogenic) or to the lid or levator muscle. Usually, with injury to the third cranial nerve, paralysis of one or more of the other muscles supplied by that nerve is also present. In addition, children may exhibit the following:

- Dilated pupil
- Inability to rotate the eye globe upward, medially, or downward
- Weakness of accommodation (looking at near objects)

Myasthenia gravis, which produces generalized muscle weakness, must always be ruled out as a cause of bilateral ptosis.

Children with ptosis tend to wrinkle their forehead and raise their eyebrows more than usual in an attempt to lift the eyelid further. Also, they may cock their heads back to see under the lowered lid.

After careful investigation of the cause has been completed, ptosis is corrected surgically. The correction is usually important to the child from a cosmetic standpoint. More importantly, if the lid obstructs vision, early surgery is necessary to prevent the development of amblyopia (from lack of use of the eye). Be sure that parents understand the importance of surgical correction. Otherwise, they may insist on delaying a corrective procedure "until the child is older." When the child is older, although the ptosis can be corrected, the amblyopia cannot.

Strabismus

The movement of each eye globe is controlled by extraocular muscles. These can be compared in movement to the handling of reins of a horse (Fig. 50.4). Strabismus is unequally aligned eyes (cross-eyes) caused by unbalanced muscle control. Approximately 1% to 2% of children have some degree of strabismus. The condition occurs without regard to gender, social status, or geographic area. Approximately 30% of children with strabismus have a history of a similar strabismus in the family. If there is a family

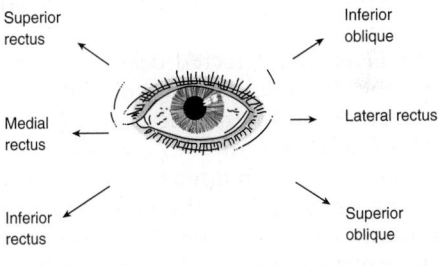

Eye muscle	Action	Innervation
Superior rectus	Turns eye up and medially	Oculomotor (third cranial) nerve
Medial rectus	Turns eye inward	Oculomotor (third cranial) nerve
Inferior rectus	Turns eye down and medially	Oculomotor (third cranial) nerve
Lateral rectus	Turns eye out	Abducens (sixth cranial) nerve
Superior oblique	Turns eye down and laterally	Trochlear (fourth cranial) nerve
Inferior oblique	Turns eye up and laterally	Oculomotor (third cranial) nerve

FIGURE 50.4 Extraocular eye muscles.

history of strabismus, the child needs to be observed and examined yearly for this problem (Govindan et al., 2005).

Normally, with good eye alignment, the resting position of the eyes is straight, largely as a result of neuromuscular influences the child cannot control. In strabismus, the resting position of one eye may be *divergent* (turned out) or *convergent* (turned in). One pupil may be higher than the other (vertical strabismus). The strabismus may be monocular, in which the same eye deviates constantly, or it may be an alternating strabismus, in which one eye and then the other deviates.

Both the resting position of eyes and the amount of turning necessary to read small print depend on the eyes' ability to fuse and see only one image. This ability is minimal in infancy but becomes stronger with practice. In adulthood, it is automatic. If children cannot fuse vision effectively early in life because of strabismus, they may be unable to achieve fusion later on or be unable to maintain good eye position.

Assessment

Infants' eyes may cross occasionally until 6 weeks of age. If infants demonstrate strabismus past this age, they should be referred for diagnosis and treatment. Infants who demonstrate a constant strabismus before 6 weeks of age need referral right away.

Definite deviations are obvious (Fig. 50.5). These can be *exotropia* (eye turning out), *esotropia* (eye turning in), or *hypertropia* (eye turning up). If the deviation is not so obvious and occurs only when the child is fatigued or ill and, therefore, less able to maintain fixation, the terms used are *exophoria, esophoria,* and *hyperphoria.* If the parents report that the deviation occurs only when the child is tired or sick, you should attempt to assess the strabismus at such a time, because then the deviation will be most striking.

Strabismus may be detected best when children examine a nearby object. It takes muscular effort to look medially (turn an eye in toward the nose). When children read small print, they turn both eyes medially, or *converge,* to focus at the short distance. If they are farsighted in one eye, they will have to turn the affected eye in more than the other, causing strabismus. If one eye is nearsighted, they will not need to turn that eye in as far as the other one; this results in divergence of the nearsighted eye. Although these children have good eye alignment at

rest, they "cross their eyes" when attempting to focus at a reading distance.

Some children have a latent strabismus, but, because they are able to maintain fusion, the strabismus is not overt. They maintain this fusion at the expense of eyestrain, however. They may experience headaches; tired, irritated eyes; and perhaps even nausea and vomiting.

Children who have flat, broad-bridged noses, a narrow interpupillary distance, and an epicanthal fold or oval-shaped palpebral fissures may appear to have strabismus when they truly do not (pseudostrabismus). These children have less white sclera visible in the inner margin of the eye than normally, so the eye appears to be turned in (*pseudoesotropia*). A cover test reveals the true condition. If pseudostrabismus is present, the covered eye will not move after being uncovered. It only appears to be turned medially because of the obscured sclera at the inner canthus. Hirshberg's test is another method of detecting strabismus (see Chapter 33).

Once strabismus is detected, it is important to attempt to discern whether it is concomitant (measures the same in all directions of gaze) or nonconcomitant (greater in one direction than another; often called *paralytic strabismus*).

Concomitant (nonparalytic) strabismus is the most usual type found in children. All the muscles of the eye are capable of function, but they are not functioning together. The deviation is equally apparent in all directions of gaze.

Paralytic strabismus is caused by paralysis of a muscle or nerve, perhaps from an injury, such as a birth injury, or an invading lesion. The eyes appear straight except when they are moved in the direction of the paralyzed muscle. Then double vision occurs, and the crossed eye is evident. Such children often close one eye or tilt their head to decrease the double vision. They may tilt their head so much they appear to have a torticollis, or "wry neck"— an orthopedic rather than an eye problem. They are often fussy or clumsy because of the diplopia. They cannot see well and may be too young to describe what is happening to them through any means other than fussiness.

Therapeutic Management

The therapy for strabismus depends on the cause of the problem. If the fusion mechanism is weak, eye exercises (**orthoptics**) may be necessary. If eyes are diverging with attempted convergence because of farsightedness or nearsightedness, the child needs glasses to correct the basic visual defect. If the misalignment is caused by unequal muscle strength, eye-muscle surgery usually is necessary to correct the problem, although injection of botulinum toxin into the eye muscle may be tried first as temporary therapy or as an adjunct to surgery (Ruiz et al., 2004). This paralyzes the muscle, temporarily aligning vision.

Because strabismus causes the eyes to be viewing two different fields of vision, diplopia occurs. To prevent this, the child suppresses the vision in one eye or looks with one eye (amblyopia). Even if diplopia is not present, the lack of fusion leads to the same consequence. For this reason, eye correction for strabismus must be done early in life, before 6 years of age. Some children whose eyes are crossing because of an accommodation problem caused by hyperopia in one eye outgrow the condition as the

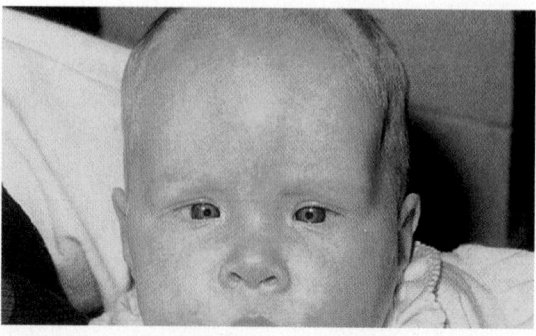

FIGURE 50.5 Strabismus (esotropia) in an infant.

however, deciding to remove the injured eye is extremely difficult for parents. Fortunately, immediate treatment with corticosteroids and antibiotics has significantly reduced the incidence of this complication.

Contusion Injuries

Many eye injuries happen not from a sharp object striking the eye but from blunt trauma such as being hit in the eye by a baseball, a fist, a soccer ball, or an automobile dashboard. With this type of injury, the eyelid and the surrounding tissue, including the intraorbital tissue, may hemorrhage and become edematous.

The simplest form of contusion injury is a "black eye." After this occurs, inspect the eye globe (including a funduscopic examination) and assess vision in the eye. If a vision chart is not available, vision can be assessed by having children tell you how many fingers they can count at a distance of about 6 feet (assuming they are old enough to count accurately) or by having them read a printed page at reading distance (assuming they are old enough to read). Ask children if they are having any difficulty seeing. Evaluate extraocular eye movements for adequate function. Children should be able to look up and down, left and right, upward obliquely, and downward obliquely—the six cardinal positions of gaze (Nucci et al., 2004).

If there is no apparent eye injury, ocular movement is good, and vision is normal (for that child), the only treatment necessary is an ice pack applied to the eye to minimize swelling (20 minutes on, 20 minutes off, and repeat). Reabsorption of hemorrhage in the tissue surrounding the eye will take place over the next 1 to 3 weeks. Often, tissue hemorrhage extends across the nose and surrounds the other eye the day after the injury. Assure both parents and child that this is not a worsening of the condition but mainly evidence of the severity of the initial blow.

Limited eye movement or reports of diplopia (double vision) are strong evidence that a "blow out" fracture of the floor of the orbit (the maxillary bone) has occurred. This fracture line is trapping intraorbital tissue and preventing the eye globe from moving freely. Refer these children to an ophthalmologist. Surgery is needed to free the entrapped tissue, prevent interference with vascular flow, and restore normal eye movements (Nucci et al., 2004).

After a blunt contusion to the eye globe, a number of serious findings in addition to limited motion may be present. These include disturbances of the pupil, such as a dilated, fixed, or cloudy pupil; cloudy lens or cornea; loss of vision in the eye; and visible blood in the anterior chamber (hyphema). These conditions may indicate dislocation of the lens or retinal detachment requiring evaluation by an ophthalmologist.

Eyelid Injuries

Eyelid injuries may accompany eye globe injuries, or they may be the only finding present after a foreign body has struck the eye. Although such injuries appear to be trivial, they should not be dismissed lightly. Refer the child to an ophthalmologist for care. A deep laceration of the eyelid can cause a permanent ptosis. A laceration to the inner canthal area can disrupt the lacrimal drainage system (dacryostenosis).

What if... Carla's father tells you he always buys fireworks to celebrate the 4th of July and sets them off in his back yard? What type of safety teaching does he need?

INNER EYE CONDITIONS

Congenital Glaucoma

Glaucoma is increased intraocular pressure (IOP) in the eye globe caused by inadequate or blocked drainage of aqueous humor. Aqueous humor, produced by the ciliary body, flows from the posterior chamber through the pupil to the anterior chamber and is excreted through the canal of Schlemm at the lateral angle into the venous circulation (Fig. 50.7). In congenital glaucoma, a developmental anomaly in the angle of the anterior chamber prevents proper drainage at the canal. Later in life, glaucoma occurs when the canal becomes blocked. The increased fluid content causes the globe of the eye to increase in size. After it has increased in size to the extent that it can, the pressure in the eye globe continues to rise, compressing and ultimately destroying the optic nerve. Glaucoma (meaning "gray") gets its name from the color of the retina or red reflex (which appears gray to green) in the eye after the sight has been lost (Khaw et al., 2004). The condition occurs in as many as 1 in every 10,000 live births.

Assessment

Although congenital glaucoma is a rare disease, all infants must be assessed for it because the disease accounts for vision disorders in 5% to 13% of children in schools for the visually impaired. In most infants, the condition is bilateral and is caused by inheritance of a recessive gene. In

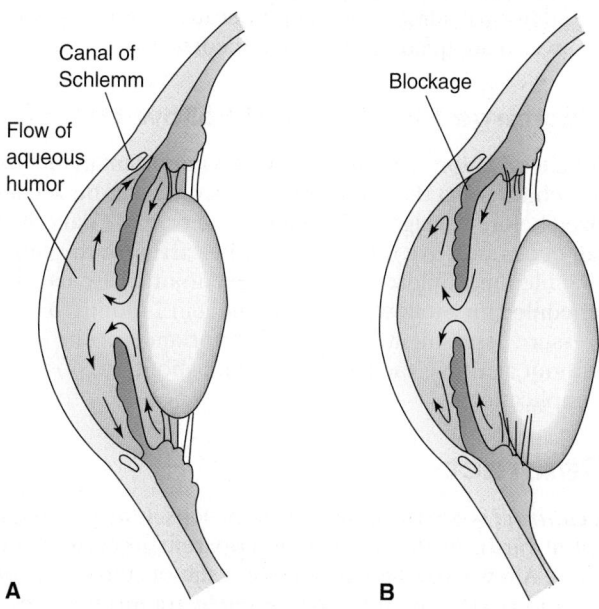

FIGURE 50.7 (A) Circulation of aqueous humor. **(B)** Blockage of canal of Schlemm in congenital glaucoma.

most children with this condition, symptoms are noticeable shortly after birth; in almost all affected children, glaucoma is apparent at 1 year of age. It occurs more often in females than in males (Khaw et al., 2004).

The cornea, which appears enlarged, may be edematous and hazy. In addition, there may be tearing, pain, and **photophobia** (sensitivity to light), all difficult to identify in a newborn. The eye globe may feel tense to finger palpation.

Eye pressure is measured by means of a *tonometer*, a pressure-sensitive device that is placed against the anterior eye globe and measures eye pressure by a beam of light directed toward the eye. Tension greater than the normal range of 12 to 20 mm Hg is suggestive of glaucoma. If local anesthesia is needed for tonometry, caution parents to avoid allowing children to rub their eyes after the procedure (an infant's arms may need to be gently restrained to prevent eye rubbing for about 4 hours after such an examination). Otherwise, corneal abrasions may occur because of the cornea's lack of sensitivity.

Therapeutic Management

Immediate surgery—a **goniotomy,** or trabeculotomy, in which a new opening to the canal of Schlemm is constructed—is scheduled for the infant. A drug such as acetazolamide (Diamox), a carbonic anhydrase inhibitor that suppresses the formation of aqueous humor, may be used temporarily to reduce eye pressure before the surgery can be scheduled. Newer surgical techniques include laser therapy (Quinn, 2003).

Before surgery, the infant should not receive any drug, such as atropine sulfate, that dilates the pupil, because it will further occlude the canal of Schlemm. After surgery, rough play activities should be restricted for 1 week.

Surgery may need to be repeated before the new opening for drainage of fluid is adequate to keep eye globe tension at a normal level. Inform parents of this possibility when surgery is first proposed, so that they will not think the additional surgery is needed because the first operation was inadequate or was done incorrectly.

Discharge Planning and Follow-Up

Eye examination at regular intervals is important in infants and children so that congenital glaucoma can be recognized before damage to the optic nerve occurs. Glaucoma can occur after eye trauma if there is scarring at the canal of Schlemm. Children who have eye injuries are usually scheduled for a follow-up appointment in 1 month for eye pressure assessment. Stress the importance of this visit without alarming the parents or child about the possible complication.

Cataract

A *cataract* is a marked opacity of the lens. It may be present at birth, or it may become apparent in early childhood. A few cases may occur as a result of steroid use or radiation exposure. It can be caused by trauma to the eye if the lens is injured. Some children have cataracts as a dominantly inherited condition. They also can be caused

by galactosemia, or inability to metabolize the lactose in milk (Leslie, 2003). If the opacity is on the anterior surface of the lens, the cause is thought to be birth injury or possibly contact between the lens and the cornea during intrauterine life. If the opacity is located at the edge of the lens, it may be a result of nutritional deficiency during intrauterine life, such as rickets or hypocalcemia. Infants who contract rubella prenatally may develop opacity throughout the lens (Forbes, 2003).

Assessment

When you inspect the pupil of a child with a cataract, the pupil opening appears to be white (leukocoria). The red reflex elicited by shining a light into the pupil appears white. Older children may report blurred vision due to cataract formation. In the infant, this can be detected by lack of response to a smile or inability to reach and grasp a nearby object. The infant may also demonstrate nystagmus, being unable to focus the eye on objects. A few other conditions, such as retinoblastoma, retinopathy of prematurity, or an abscess of the posterior chamber, simulate this appearance. In congenital glaucoma, the lens may be opaque due to edema. This can be differentiated from simple cataract by the accompanying enlargement of the eye and pupil opening.

Therapeutic Management

Treatment of childhood cataract is surgical removal of the cloudy lens, followed by insertion of an internal intraocular lens. If the total lens is involved, this may be done as early as 3 months of age. If this is not done before 6 months of age, amblyopia may result.

With modern surgical techniques, the incision is so small that eye patching is not necessary. Infants may be given a sedative to help them rest for 24 hours. Introduce fluids cautiously after eye surgery so nausea and vomiting do not occur. Vomiting increases IOP, which could injure the suture line. Encourage parents to stay with the infant, helping with care so that the infant does not cry after surgery, because crying also increases eye pressure. Infants can be expected to have some discomfort but, in general, they should not have acute eye pain after surgery. If they are unusually restless, fussy, or crying and seem to be in pain, notify the physician immediately. Although this could be unrelated to the surgery, it may be a sign of increased IOP from hemorrhage or from occlusion of the canal of Schlemm, causing a developing glaucoma.

As a rule, children will be given a mydriatic agent to dilate the pupil and steroids to prevent postoperative development of pupillary adhesions. If the eye that had the cataract is now amblyopic, patching of the normal eye (as with usual amblyopia correction) may be necessary to restore vision.

Parents of children with congenital cataracts need support to carry out the procedures necessary and to give the long-term medication and corrective measures needed. Outcome evaluation should include the child's current vision status and also how the child views himself or herself in light of this early life problem.

THE CHILD UNDERGOING EYE SURGERY

Surgery to treat cataracts or glaucoma in childhood is usually performed on infants. Preparation for this surgery primarily consists of helping the baby to adjust to the strange environment and encouraging parents or a primary care person to spend as much time with the infant as possible. This is particularly important if the eyes will be patched after surgery. Surgery for strabismus is often done during the preschool period. The operation can be explained to the preschooler through the use of puppets or dolls. As with all surgical procedures, you should talk about the child's affected parts (in this case, the eyes) being "fixed" or "made better," never "cut." Even a very young child knows how important his or her eyes are and will agree to having them made better, but not cut.

NURSING DIAGNOSES AND RELATED INTERVENTIONS

Nursing Diagnosis: Anxiety related to lack of knowledge about eye surgery and postoperative experience

Outcome Evaluation: Child asks questions and expresses fears about surgery; child states plans for postoperative period and practices putting on eye patches, if appropriate.

Most eye surgery is completed as ambulatory surgery. A major nursing role is preparing the parents to support the child through the procedure.

If the child's eyes are going to be patched after surgery, it is helpful to allow the child to become accustomed to the feeling of the patches beforehand. Even when only one eye is going to be operated on, it is not unusual for both eyes to be patched, because the eyes move conjugately (i.e., when the right eye looks to the right, so does the left eye). The repaired eye, therefore, will stay immobile under a bandage only if both eyes are patched.

Parents could show the child a doll with eye patches, and let the child practice wearing them. They could play a game such as "pin the tail on the donkey" or "blindman's bluff" to adjust to the sensation of the eyes being covered. Another helpful game is to have the child pull out familiar objects from a paper bag—a key, an orange, a spoon, and a penny—and, with eyes covered, try to guess what they are.

When you meet the child before surgery, be certain to speak with the child so he or she will be able to recognize your voice afterward. Practice having the child identify his or her parent's voice by covering the eyes and then guessing whether you or the parent is speaking.

Postoperatively, check that the young child's favorite toy is within reach if his or her eyes are patched. If the child will require arm restraints to prevent him from pressing on his eyes or removing the patches, urge the parents to introduce these preoperatively as well. Children who awaken from conscious sedation and find their arms tied down can be extremely frightened or believe they are being punished.

Checkpoint Question 2

After cataract surgery, why should vomiting be prevented if at all possible?

a. Vomitus could be splashed into the eye.
b. Loss of sodium discolors the new lens.
c. Vomiting increases intraocular pressure.
d. Loss of fluid causes the globe to shrink.

THE HOSPITALIZED CHILD WITH A VISION DISORDER

Like other children, those with vision disorders experience diseases such as appendicitis or pneumonia that may require hospitalization. Severe vision impairment or blindness can cause increased difficulty adjusting to a hospital environment. The World Health Organization defines severe vision impairment as testing 20/60 to 20/200 in the better eye on a standard eye examination. Blindness is defined as vision less than 20/200 or peripheral vision less than 10°. It occurs for a multitude of reasons, including vitamin A deficiency, inadequately treated eye infections, and corneal scarring. It is more common in developing countries than in industrialized ones (Gilbert & Awan, 2003).

NURSING DIAGNOSES AND RELATED INTERVENTIONS

Nursing Diagnosis: Powerlessness related to difficulty adjusting to strange environment, secondary to vision disorder

Outcome Evaluation: Child identifies specific fears and concerns; child is able to make age-appropriate decisions regarding self-care

Vision problems can range from very mild disorders to total blindness. Assess children carefully for the degree of their vision impairment to better gauge their abilities, helping them neither too much nor not enough (Shapiro et al., 2005). Children who are blind need to feel secure in a strange hospital environment. Be sure to thoroughly orient them to the experience and their surroundings. Remember that they may think a parent has left them when the parent has only moved a few feet away. Some children with severe vision disorders rock back and forth excessively, an action that apparently gives them additional stimulation (McHugh & Lieberman, 2003). Also, keep in mind that severe vision disorders can lead to chronic depression as a child grows older and realizes more and more the many ways that lack of vision affects his or her life.

Before you approach a child who is blind, speak first to avoid startling her. The child who is blind is very aware of another person's presence in the room and may be frightened if you slip in quietly to straighten another child's bed or pick up some equipment without speaking to her.

Remember that the sounds of a hospital are strange sounds to any child. The whirring noise of a floor-polishing machine or another child's oxygen administration, the hissing of a ventilator, and the clanking of waste baskets being emptied can be frightening sounds if you do not know what they are. Stand by the child's bed and explain the sounds you both hear. Sound is a major way in which visually impaired children experience their environment.

Children who are blind need to learn self-care like other children; they can be taught to bathe themselves, brush their teeth, brush their hair, and put on their clothes like other children their age. Toilet training may come later, because they cannot see the excretions that parents are asking them to dispose of in a special place. They must be able to understand cognitively what is expected of them.

Blind children often want to be told what is on their food tray when it is first presented to them. Name the foods so that they can identify tastes with names. Do not hesitate to use food colors: "Those are green beans; this is an orange; those are red beets." These words are names as well as colors. Visually impaired preschoolers enjoy the same finger foods as sighted children do. Children with severe vision disorders have difficulty getting food from spoons or forks to their mouths neatly. However, they should not be spoon-fed just because it is neater and faster: eating is an important self-care skill that the blind child must learn to be independent as an adult.

Be certain to offer frequent descriptions of what is happening or planned for these children. They cannot see their surgical dressing, for example, so encourage them to feel it. They cannot see the intravenous infusion, but they can feel the tubing and the arm board that is holding their arm in place.

Parents of a severely visually impaired child usually plan to room-in with their child during a hospitalization experience. Demonstrate competence and consistency when caring for their child by using good techniques and by relating to the child warmly. Ask the parents about their child's routines at mealtime and bedtime, his or her favorite toy, what word is used for voiding, and so on, and pass this information on to the entire nursing staff. Only when parents have confidence in you and the other staff members will they be able to leave their child to meet their own needs, such as eating.

STRUCTURE AND FUNCTION OF THE EARS

Ear anatomy is shown in Figure 50.8. Most ear disease in children involves the external and middle portions.

Physiology of Hearing Loss

Hearing loss is termed a *conduction loss* if there is interference with sound reaching the inner ear (difficulty with the external canal, the tympanic membrane, or the ossicles). It is termed *nerve* or *sensorineural loss* if the inner ear or the eighth cranial nerve is affected. Conduction loss can occur if the external canal is obstructed with cerumen (wax) or a foreign object, if the tympanic membrane is damaged or immobile, or if the middle ear is filled with fluid, as occurs in *serous otitis media*. Sensorineural loss results from disease that affects the transmission of sound sensation to the cerebral cortex or from a pathologic condition of the cochlea. In children, this condition is usually congenital, although it can occur after drug therapy or an infection such as meningitis. It also can occur from exposure to loud sound.

Hearing Impairment

Hearing impairment occurs in many different degrees and can be rated by level of severity. Usual classifications are shown in Table 50.3. Approximately 1 in 1,000 children in the United States are profoundly hearing impaired; 17 in 1,000 children have a moderate to severe hearing impairment. Congenital sensorineural hearing loss occurs in 2 to 3 of every 1,000 live births (National Institute on Deafness and Other Communication Disorders, 2005). Prenatal rubella infection accounts for another large percentage. Treacher Collins syndrome, otosclerosis, osteogenesis imperfecta, and Waardenburg's syndrome, all transmitted by autosomal dominant inheritance, are examples of disorders that result in congenital deafness. Causes of slight hearing impairment include serous otitis media, trauma, and untreated acute otitis media with rupture of the tympanic

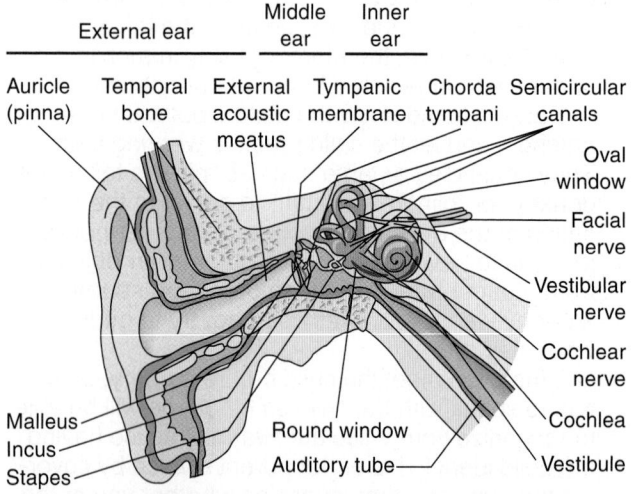

FIGURE 50.8 Structures of the ear.

TABLE 50.3

Levels of Hearing Impairment

Decibel Level	Hearing Level Present
Slight (<30)	Unable to hear whispered words or faint speech
	No speech impairment present
	May not be aware of hearing difficulty
	Achieves well in school and home by compensating (e.g., leaning forward, speaking loudly)
Mild (30–50)	Beginning speech impairment may be present
	Difficulty hearing if not facing speaker; some difficulty with normal conversation
Moderate (55–70)	Speech impairment present; may require speech therapy
	Difficulty with normal conversation
Severe (70–90)	Difficulty with any but nearby loud voice
	Hears vowels more easily than consonants
	Requires speech therapy for clear speech
	May still hear loud sounds, such as jets or train whistles
Profound (>90)	Hears almost no sound

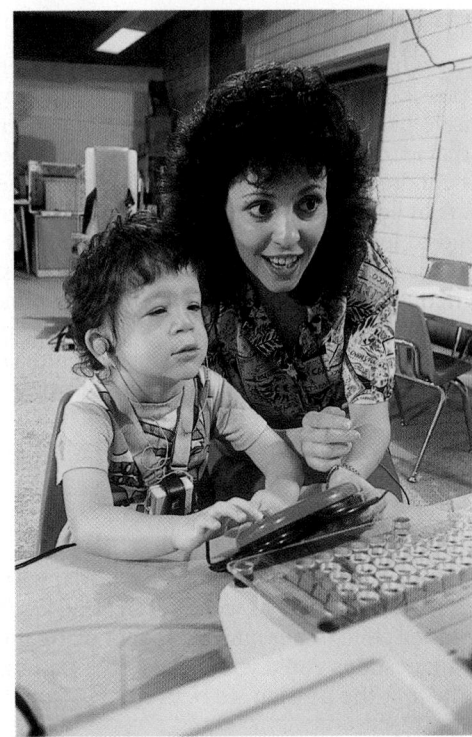

FIGURE 50.9 A hearing-challenged young girl learning to use the computer with the aid of a speech therapist. (© Bob Daemmrich/ Stock Boston.)

membrane. Activated airbags can also cause ruptured eardrums and hearing loss (Chao & Pomerantz, 2004).

Children with congenital hearing impairment should be enrolled in special programs for hearing-challenged children as soon as the hearing loss is discovered. This early exposure is necessary so that the child can learn effective speech (Fig. 50.9). For children who have conductive losses, an improvement in hearing usually can be achieved by use of a hearing aid (which intensifies the level of sound waves). Children who have inner ear or nerve deafness cannot expect this kind of improvement. Parents of children with neural deafness need an explanation of the difference so that they do not continue to search for a "cure" for their child or spend a great deal of money for hearing aids, hoping that a different brand or model will help their child. Acupuncture, often recommended to parents by friends as therapy for nerve deafness, has no documented effect.

Cochlear implants are available to replace a nonfunctioning inner ear that has sustained nerve damage (Ramsden, 2004). After implantation, hearing is often reported as "muffled" but adequate. Hearing-challenged adults may be reluctant to consent to a cochlear implant in their child, believing that the change from hearing-impaired to non–hearing-challenged status will remove the child

from their deaf culture (see Box 50.4). Children who spoke with an impediment before implantation usually need speech therapy afterward to improve their speech pattern.

Because the diseases that lead to inherited hearing challenge tend to be autosomal dominant, there is a strong chance that they will occur in future siblings of the hearing-challenged child. Genetic counseling can aid in increasing parental awareness.

Hearing Aids

Hearing aids pick up sound through a microphone, convert the sound waves into electrical impulses, and amplify them across the tympanic membrane. They are powered by batteries that must be changed periodically.

Hearing aids are designed to be as inconspicuous as possible so that children will not feel self-conscious wearing them. The receiver of the hearing aid may be incorporated into eyeglasses, molded into a plastic form that fits behind or in the ear, or housed in a small box (resembling a small transistor radio) that children wear on a cord around their neck or carry in a blouse or shirt pocket. Teach children to remove hearing aids before washing their hair, showering, or swimming. Hearing aids should be turned off when removed, to preserve the life of the batteries.

Children with a hearing impairment may grow self-conscious about wearing a hearing aid during school years. Encourage such children to view themselves as whole persons despite their need for their device, rather than as someone with something to hide.

Speech Therapy

If children who are hearing-challenged are to interact as fully as possible with the world around them, they need an intensive program of speech therapy. Some therapists believe that learning sign language early is helpful because it allows children to express their needs early. Others believe that, by learning sign language, children decrease their need to learn to articulate speech sounds or to lip read and, for this reason, learning sign language should not be encouraged. It is true that, for real independence and to perform in regular school classes, children need to communicate by means other than sign language. For children with a profound impairment, however, learning speech sounds may be a long-term process, making sign language necessary for contact with the world around them until they learn to speak.

What if... you discover that Carla, who is hearing impaired, refuses to wear her hearing aid because another child in her nursery school made fun of it? What suggestions could you make to her parents to help her accept the hearing aid better?

DISORDERS OF THE EAR

Ear disorders are always serious in children, because hearing is such an important function for the growing child. Assessment of hearing is discussed in Chapter 33.

External Otitis

External otitis (otitis externa) is inflammation of the external ear canal. Although external ear inflammation rarely threatens hearing or causes permanent damage, it does cause discomfort in the form of itching and sometimes extreme pain.

Assessment

The history of children with external otitis usually indicates that they have recently been swimming, which is why this condition is popularly called *swimmer's ear*. It also can occur if a young child pushes a foreign object, such as a peanut, into the ear canal. Unlike middle ear infection (otitis media), there is no history of a recent respiratory infection. Children first notice itching of the canal, then pain. When the external ear is touched, the pain becomes acute. The moisture in the canal left from swimming has caused inflammation; a secondary infection may occur in the closed space. *Pseudomonas* and *Candida* are agents frequently involved in these infections. Otoscopic examination may indicate only the sharply localized, tender swelling of a furuncle, or the entire canal may be swollen shut and tender to the touch. If a fungal infection is present, the entire canal may appear brown or black. If the inflammation is from a foreign body, such as a peanut or the tip of a cotton applicator, white or gray debris may surround the object; the skin under the object will be moist, red, and eroded.

In otitis externa, the tympanic membrane must be visualized to ensure that there is no extension of the external otitis into the middle ear (Atkinson, 2003). In some instances, the eardrum is so inflamed from the external infectious process that it is difficult to tell whether the middle ear is free of disease. Before the tympanic membrane can be visualized, it is often necessary to remove superficial debris from the canal. A Weber test (discussed in Chapter 33) should show that hearing is equal in both ears. A tuning fork vibration that sounds louder in the affected ear suggests that otitis media (middle ear infection) is present.

Removal of debris from an infected external canal requires patience and skill. Foreign material should not be irrigated until it is shown that the tympanic membrane is intact. Otherwise, infected material could be washed through a rupture into the middle ear. Material should be removed by an ear curette using extremely gentle pressure. Children must be securely restrained for the procedure to prevent them from suddenly turning their head, causing the curette to puncture the tympanic membrane. If the debris is hard and difficult to remove, it can be softened and loosened by touching it with a hydrogen peroxide–soaked, soft, cotton applicator; alternatively, 2% acetic acid can be instilled into the canal and allowed to stand for a few minutes.

Therapeutic Management

The treatment of otitis externa differs according to the organism causing the infection. If the canal is so swollen that ear drops cannot flow back into the canal, a cotton wick moistened with Burow's solution may be threaded into the canal. The cotton extending out into the auricle is kept moistened by rewetting it for 24 hours with Burow's solution. This usually reduces the swelling of the canal to a point that further treatment can be initiated.

The parents are then instructed to use ear drops containing hydrocortisone and an antibiotic or an antifungal mixture. Hydrocortisone reduces inflammation; the antibiotic or antifungal preparation reduces the infection. Some ear drops have an additional alcohol base, which serves to dry the external canal further. If ear pain is present, an analgesic, such as acetaminophen or ibuprofen, may be necessary to control discomfort. Children must keep the ear canal dry, avoiding swimming and hair washing during this time. If they shower, they should first insert ear plugs into the external meatus, to keep the moisture out.

NURSING DIAGNOSES AND RELATED INTERVENTIONS

Nursing Diagnosis: Deficient knowledge related to technique for ear drop instillation and preventive care measures

Outcome Evaluation: Parents demonstrate proper instillation of ear drops; parents state the importance of continuing prescribed treatment to completion.

Administering ear drops can be a challenging task. Show parents how this is done (see Chapter 37) before they leave the health care facility. Encourage them to give the medication for the full time prescribed. Otherwise, because the drops are difficult to administer, they may give them only until the pain subsides (24 to 48 hours). As a result, the infection may recur a week later. Caution parents not to put anything but the ear drops into their child's ear.

Follow-Up

Evaluation after external otitis should include not only whether the inflammation and pain have decreased but also whether the child and the parents are aware of how to prevent the condition in the future. This includes knowing not to put any object into the ear canal and using ear plugs during swimming. Instillation of a dilute alcohol or acetic acid solution by dropper after swimming is a prophylactic measure that helps keep the ear canal dry. This is often recommended for children who swim competitively or spend a great deal of time in water.

Impacted Cerumen

Cerumen (ear wax) serves the important function of cleansing the external ear canal as it gradually moves outward, bringing with it shed epithelial cells and any foreign objects. Parents are often concerned that ear wax will lead to loss of hearing (or they view it as dirty) and ask to have it removed. Wax accumulation rarely is extensive enough to interfere with hearing. Cerumen serves a protective function and should not be removed routinely. Caution parents not to clean the child's ears with cotton-tipped applicators as a regular practice, because they may scratch the ear canal, causing an invasion site for a secondary infection. This practice may also push accumulated cerumen farther into the ear canal, causing a true plugging of wax.

Commercial softeners are available if cerumen accumulates to such an extent that hearing is affected. Some physicians advise a dilute solution of hydrogen peroxide to dissolve cerumen. This may be done once in a while but, again, should not be done regularly because this will keep the ear canal constantly moist, an environment that leads to external otitis. For most children, the basic rule of thumb—never put anything smaller than an elbow in a child's ear—is the best rule.

Acute Otitis Media

Inflammation of the middle ear (otitis media) is the most prevalent disease of childhood after respiratory tract infections. It occurs most often in children 6 to 36 months of age and again at 4 to 6 years. It is seen most frequently in males, in Alaskan and Native American children, and in children with cleft palate. There is a higher incidence of otitis media in formula-fed infants than those who are breast-fed, because formula-fed infants are held in a more slanted position while feeding, and this allows milk to enter the eustachian tube. Otitis media is also associated with constant pacifier use. The incidence of otitis media is highest in the winter and spring and is higher in homes in which a parent smokes cigarettes (Graessle, 2003).

Otitis media is an extremely serious disease of childhood, because permanent damage can occur to middle ear structures, leading to hearing impairment.

Assessment

Acute otitis media usually occurs after a respiratory tract infection. Children have a "cold," rhinitis, and perhaps a low-grade fever for a number of days. Suddenly, they have a fever of about 102°F (38°C) and a sharp, constant pain in one or both ears. Older children can verbalize reports of pain. Infants become extremely irritable and frequently pull or tug at the affected ear in an attempt to gain relief from pain. The external canal is usually free of wax because the warmth of the inflammation and fever melts the wax and moves it more readily out of the canal. In contrast to an external ear canal infection, the discomfort does not increase on manipulation of the auricle. The mastoid process behind the ear should not be tender to touch. If it is, the infection probably has spread out of the middle ear into the mastoid cells, a very serious complication.

The appearance of a normal eardrum shows the outline of the malleus (see Chapter 33). With infection, the tympanic membrane appears inflamed or reddened on otoscopic examination. It may be seen bulging into the external canal. The light reflex of the otoscope will not be as definite as usual because of the convex shape of the eardrum. The landmarks of the tympanic membrane, the malleus and incus, can be visualized only poorly or not at all. There is decreased mobility on pneumatic examination. A **tympanocentesis** (withdrawal of fluid from the middle ear through the tympanic membrane) may be performed by a physician to obtain fluid for culture at the time of assessment.

Therapeutic Management

Most middle ear infections are caused by *Streptococcus pneumoniae*, *Haemophilus influenzae* (especially in children younger than 5 years of age), or group A β-hemolytic streptococci. Most otitis media infections resolve spontaneously without therapy, but, to avoid the possibility of complications, most children in the past were prescribed an antibiotic such as ampicillin or amoxicillin (antibiotics that eliminate *H. influenzae* organisms). Today, it is recognized that antibiotic therapy is unnecessary and may add to bacterial resistance, so it is no longer routinely prescribed (Glasziou et al., 2005).

Children need an analgesic and antipyretic such as acetaminophen (Tylenol). Some health care providers may prescribe decongestant nose drops to open the eustachian tubes and allow air to be admitted to the middle ear. Although not proven, this may be helpful in preventing the infection from becoming a serous or long-term otitis media. Nasal decongestant drops usually are given for only 3 days. If they are given longer, a rebound effect may occur, causing edema and a subsequent increase in mucous membrane size.

During the course of otitis media, most children have a conductive hearing loss; this may last up to 6 months after an acute infection. Caution parents about this fact, so they will not think the infection is growing worse if they first notice the impairment after they arrive home from the health care facility. They also need to know about the hearing loss so that, if the child is routinely screened for hearing in school during the next 6 months, they can account for the loss. If a child still has a conductive hearing loss after 6 months (or has other symptoms), he or she should be examined again to see whether a new infection or serous otitis media is present (Box 50.6).

Chronic or persistent otitis media may be caused by *Staphylococcus*, which would require treatment with an antibiotic, such as a cephalosporin, that is effective against *Staphylococcus*.

Otitis Media With Effusion

Otitis media with effusion is a result of chronic otitis media. Normally, the middle ear is an air-filled cavity, air being supplied to it by the eustachian tube. The tube

BOX 50.6: Focus on Nursing Care Planning

A Multidisciplinary Care Map for A Child With Otitis Media

•

Carla Vander, a 4-year-old child, is brought to a pediatric clinic for evaluation. Her mother states, "She's always had a lot of problems. She had strabismus as a baby. Now, I'm sure she has an ear infection. Can you get me the antibiotic prescription in a hurry, before the drug store closes?" How would you answer Ms. Vander? What information does she need about ear infections?

Family Assessment
Child lives with parents and 7-year-old brother in three-bedroom suburban cottage. Father works as a travel agent; mother is a grade school librarian. Father describes finances as "Middle class."

Client Assessment
Child has had two previous ear infections in the past 8 months. Child had a clear, watery nasal discharge and slight cough for 2 days. Now, thick, purulent, white nasal drainage is noted from both nostrils. Last evening, she developed a fever of 102.2°F (39.0°C). Temperature now 100.8°F (38.2°C). Observed tugging vigorously on right ear. On examination, right tympanic membrane erythematous and bulging, with poor mobility on pneumoscopy. Left ear examination unremarkable. Child is diagnosed with otitis media of the right ear.

Nursing Diagnosis
Pain related to inflammation and erythema secondary to ear infection

Outcome Evaluation
Child no longer tugs at right ear; tympanic membrane no longer reddened or bulging; child rates pain as no higher than 2 on a FACES pain scale.

Team Member Responsible	Assessment	Intervention	Rationale	Expected Outcome
		Activities of Daily Living		
Nurse	Assess whether child is able to sleep or wakes with pain.	Suggest mother give antihistamine at bedtime. Urge child to sleep with affected ear up.	Antihistamines can make children sleepy. Sleeping on affected ear can put pressure on eustachian tube and increase pain.	Mother reports child is able to sleep through the night.

(continued)

Team Member Responsible	Assessment	Intervention	Rationale	Expected Outcome
Consultations				
Physician	Assess whether child has susceptibility to ear infections or whether this could be reoccurrence of a former infection.	Meet with ear, nose, and throat service to consult on cause of frequent otitis media.	Otitis media can be so persistent it needs an antibiotic to cure it.	Consultant meets with mother to discuss cause of frequent ear infections.
Procedures/Medications				
Nurse	Assess whether child has experience with taking oral medicine. Rate child's level of pain by FACES pain scale.	Instruct the mother to administer acetaminophen q4h or ibuprofen q8h.	Acetaminophen and ibuprofen are effective analgesics and antipyretics for this degree of pain.	Child is able to take oral medicine cooperatively. Rates pain level as not above 2 on FACES pain scale.
Nurse	Assess whether child has ever had nasal medicine administered and whether mother knows technique.	Instruct mother in use of saline nose drops or nasal spray as prescribed.	Saline nose drops or nasal spray helps to relieve nasal inflammation and subsequent pressure on the eustachian tube.	Child cooperates with administration of nose drops or spray.
Nutrition				
Nurse	Assess what soft foods and fluids child likes to eat.	Encourage mother to offer liquids and soft foods.	Movement of the eustachian tube, such as with chewing, may increase pain.	Child names some foods and fluid she is willing to eat. Eats less than usual, but adequate amount.
Patient/Family Education				
Nurse	Assess how much mother and child understand about the cause of otitis media and the newer, no-antibiotic approach to treatment.	Educate the mother about the common characteristics of otitis media. Reassure mother that the infection will resolve without an antibiotic.	Education promotes better understanding of the problem, alleviating some of the stress and anxiety associated with it.	Mother states her prime goal is to get child well again. Will follow clinic physician's recommendation for care.
Psychosocial/Spiritual/Emotional Needs				
Nurse	Assess how much experience mother has with care of ill child.	Praise the mother for her ability to recognize signs and symptoms and seek treatment.	Praise enhances mother's self-esteem, helping to promote feelings of control.	Mother states she feels capable of caring for child with acute otitis media without antibiotic prescription.
Discharge Planning				
Nurse	Assess whether child or parents have any questions about care that they still need answered.	Instruct the mother to contact the clinic or health care provider if there is no improvement within 24 to 48 hr or if the child exhibits increased pain or a sudden relief of pain.	Lack of improvement within 24 to 48 hr indicates the need for further evaluation. Increased pain may indicate excessive fluid accumulation, which could lead to tympanic rupture, evidenced by a sudden relief of pain.	Mother states she feels prepared to care for child at home. Has clinic telephone number. Will telephone if symptoms of complications occur.

opens with swallowing, yawning, or chewing. If this source of air to the middle ear is shut off, the epithelial cells of the middle ear change in function, becoming secretory cells. The middle ear fills with these secretions. Over time, the fluid becomes so thick and tenacious that it is described as "gluelike." Some children notice a feeling of fullness or the sound of popping or ringing in their ears. There may be a drop in hearing of 20 to 40 dB because of the fluid content. Because the loss is gradual, parents and children may not be aware of it until it is noticed on a routine hearing screening. Involvement is usually bilateral. The condition occurs most frequently in children 3 to 10 years of age (Atkinson, 2003).

Assessment

The child experiences muffled hearing and a feeling of pressure in the ear. Examination of the ears may show a level of fluid behind the tympanic membrane. However, a fluid line will be visible only if there is also a quantity of air in the middle ear to contrast with it. As the collected fluid becomes thick, it tends to retract the eardrum. This makes the malleus more prominent and perhaps displaced to a horizontal angle as the membrane is retracted around it; the light reflex from the otoscope light becomes distorted. If a pneumatic otoscope is used, gentle introduction of air against the eardrum produces no movement of the tympanic membrane (as there would be normally).

Therapeutic Management

Therapy for otitis media with effusion may be long-term. If the condition appears to be intensified by inflammation from an allergy, measures to control the allergy must be instituted. These may include avoidance of the allergen, hyposensitization, or pharmacologic alteration of the allergic response. Treatment of children with allergies is discussed in Chapter 42.

Definitive medical treatment is aimed at supplying air to the middle ear. For mild involvement, the daily administration of an antihistamine or a nasal decongestant to shrink the mucous membrane of the eustachian tube may be enough to achieve an air supply. In a few children, the eustachian tube is blocked by enlarged adenoids, and their removal is indicated. Fluid from the middle ear can be removed by tympanocentesis (needle inserted through the tympanic membrane); it usually returns, however, unless some intervention to introduce air to the middle ear (tubal myringotomy) is undertaken.

Tubal Myringotomy. A source of air can be supplied to the middle ear by the insertion of small plastic (Teflon) tubes through the tympanic membrane (tympanostomy). The insertion of such tubes is done after a myringotomy at a point in the tympanic membrane that is not instrumental for hearing, so as not to interfere with this function (Fig. 50.10). Myringotomy tubes can be placed in one or both ears as an ambulatory procedure after the local injection of lidocaine (Xylocaine). Tubes tend to be extruded after 6 to 12 months. For many

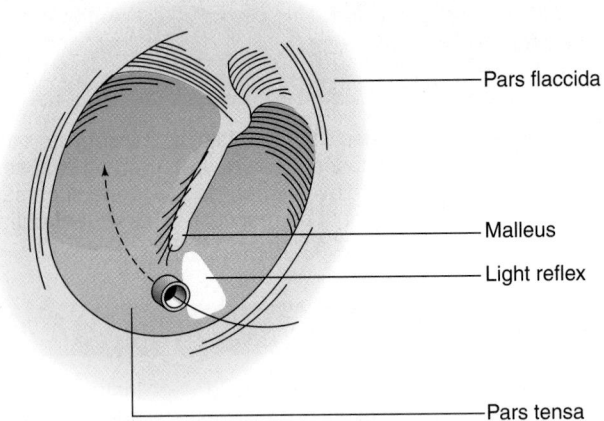

FIGURE 50.10 A myringotomy tube provides air to the middle ear to prevent otitis media with effusion.

children, this period is long enough to halt the secretory process of the middle ear. In others, tubes must be reinserted to continue the aeration.

When myringotomy tubes are in place, water should not be allowed to enter the child's ears. Most physicians prefer children to bathe rather than shower, but showering may be allowed if ear plugs are used. Hair washing should be done with ear plugs in place. Similarly, swimming is either contraindicated or allowed only with ear plugs in place.

Otitis media with effusion runs a long-term course in many children. Teach parents to continue giving medications as prescribed. They often need a great deal of support to accept the insertion of myringotomy tubes. They are afraid that cutting of the eardrum will do more harm than if they just leave the situation alone. Because the course of the process is long, the hearing impairment associated with it may also be long-term. Urge parents to notify the school nurse of the problem. Children may need to be changed to a front seat in a classroom so they do not miss important class content or discussion. They need support through this puzzling and annoying condition.

Cholesteatoma

Cholesteatoma is a lesion of the pars flaccida or upper portion of the tympanic membrane. A retraction cyst forms, and there is necrosis of the pars flaccida with foul-smelling drainage from the ear. If the retraction cyst is not discovered and surgically removed at this point, it grows gradually deeper and deeper, until it eventually invades the mastoid cells. It can progress to mastoiditis, meningitis, and possibly facial nerve paralysis if it is not surgically removed.

Any child with foul-smelling drainage from the ear should be referred to a primary care provider for further investigation to rule out this problem. If you are inspecting children's tympanic membranes during health maintenance visits, be certain to inspect the pars flaccida and pars tensa to detect cholesteatoma (Rash, 2004).

Checkpoint Question 3

Carla has an acute otitis media. How does this differ from otitis externa?

a. Otitis media manifests as a sudden disease; externa tends to be a chronic disease.
b. Otitis media is infection of the middle ear; externa is infection of the outer canal.
c. Otitis media occurs on the inner surface of the eardrum; externa occurs on the cochlear nerve.
d. Otitis media is treated with antibiotics; externa is treated with antifungal agents.

THE HOSPITALIZED CHILD WITH A HEARING IMPAIRMENT

A hearing loss greater than 49 dB is sufficient enough to interfere with hearing normal conversation and developing language. Like visually challenged children, children with hearing loss may be hospitalized for other health problems. It can be difficult for parents to prepare children who cannot hear for hospitalization. Words such as *surgery, tonsils, hurts, operating room,* and *recovery room* are new to them. Showing the child a book with good pictures demonstrating what is going to happen is helpful. Allowing children time to play with dolls or puppets can help them understand hospital routine. Because children who are hearing challenged may not be as well prepared for hospitalization as those without a hearing impairment, make an extra effort on admission to ensure that they receive such instruction.

Always allow hearing-challenged children to see you before you touch them. They will not find this nearly as intrusive as being touched without warning. If children are sleeping when you approach them, use a light touch to waken them gently. Some children turn off their hearing aid or remove it while they sleep. You may need to turn it on before you call them to wake them, or they may need to replace the hearing aid as soon as they awaken. Children as young as 2 years of age are effective lip readers as long as you are facing them. Position yourself at eye level, so the child can view your face. In a group, help the child follow conversation by directing him to the person who is speaking. Assign consistent staff members to decrease the number of people with whom the child must attempt to communicate. Have a staff person accompany the child and stay with him or her in all departments to help with communication.

Do not underestimate the intelligence level of hearing-challenged children. Because they do not speak clearly, others may assume that hearing-challenged children are cognitively challenged. As a result, they may not be given information that the average hearing child receives, such as explanations of how things work. On a hospital unit, hearing-challenged children, locked in a silent world, are unable to express how they feel about procedures. They need help from health care personnel who understand this and take more than the usual amount of time to offer them explanations and support.

Ask parents of children who are hearing challenged to draw pictures or demonstrate the sign language symbols their children use for important words such as *pain, drink,* and *bathroom.* Encourage children to use or draw pictures of what they want if they are still too young to write words and you cannot understand what they are saying.

Hearing-challenged children have the right to be provided with an interpreter during care. Advocate for this, especially if the parents will not be present during care.

Key Points

Teaching preventive measures to avoid eye and hearing injuries (using proper eye protection during sports or play and wearing goggles or ear protection as appropriate) and screening children for sensory impairments are important nursing roles.

Refractive errors of vision such as myopia and hyperopia are the most common eye disorders in children. Amblyopia (lazy eye) is subnormal vision in one eye. Children with these disorders need correction at the time the disorder is recognized to prevent further vision distortion.

Coloboma is congenital incomplete closure of the pupil or lower eyelid. Ptosis is the inability to open the upper eyelid normally. Ptosis needs correction to avoid development of amblyopia. Strabismus is unequally aligned eyes. Like ptosis, it can lead to amblyopia if not corrected.

Infections of the lids, such as styes or chalazions, can occur in children. Conjunctivitis (inflammation of the conjunctiva) often manifests with acute symptoms. An antibiotic is necessary for therapy.

Eye injuries such as penetration by a foreign body need follow-up after treatment to be certain that vision remains adequate.

Children who are either vision or hearing challenged need special preparation and orientation for a hospital or ambulatory health visit, so that they can fully understand what is going to happen during the visit.

Help children who are vision challenged to work through new experiences by letting them feel equipment as much as possible. Guide their hands through the steps of a new procedure you are teaching them.

Otitis media (middle ear infection) is a common childhood illness. Some children who have otitis media with effusion have myringotomy tubes inserted to relieve pressure and supply air access to the middle ear.

Use photographs, drawings, or demonstration with hearing-challenged children to help them learn new skills. Contact a signing interpreter as appropriate to be certain that children understand instructions.

Critical Thinking Exercises

1. Carla is the 4-year-old girl with an ear infection whom you met at the beginning of the chapter. Her mother states, "She's always had a lot of problems. She had strabismus as a baby. Now, I think she has another ear infection. It started out as a head cold but now she's pulling at her ear. Why does she get so many of these?" How would you answer Ms. Vander? What information does she need to know about ear infections?

2. Carla will be having surgery to remove a chalazion from her eyelid. What special steps do you want to take to prepare her for this surgery? Is she old enough to appreciate the importance of seeing?

3. You are going to teach a first-grade class on ways to prevent eye and hearing injuries. What would you include in your class? How would your teaching plan be different if the class was for 16-year-old students?

4. Examine the National Health Goals related to sensory disorders in children. Most government-sponsored money for nursing research is allotted based on these goals. What would be a possible research topic to explore pertinent to these goals that would be applicable to the Vander family and also advance evidence-based practice?

References

Atkinson, L. R. (2003). Otitis externa. In Schwartz, M. W. (Ed.), *5-minute pediatric consult* (3rd ed.). Philadelphia: Lippincott Williams & Wilkins.

Carpenito, L. J. (2004). *Handbook of nursing diagnosis* (9th ed.). Philadelphia: Lippincott Williams & Wilkins.

Centers for Disease Control and Prevention. (2004). Injuries associated with homemade fireworks—Selected states, 1993–2004. *MMWR: Morbidity Mortality Weekly Report, 53*(25), 562–563.

Chao, N., & Pomerantz, W. J. (2004). Acute hearing loss after airbag deployment. *Pediatric Emergency Care, 20*(10), 683–686.

Christiansen, J. B., & Leigh, I. W. (2004). Children with cochlear implants: Changing parent and deaf community perspectives. *Archives of Otolaryngology—Head and Neck Surgery, 130*(5), 673–677.

Colev, M., et al. (2004). Vegan diet and vitamin A deficiency. *Clinical Pediatrics, 43*(1), 107–109.

Department of Health and Human Services. (2000). *Healthy people 2010*. Washington, D.C.: DHHS.

Dick, F., et al. (2004). Is colour vision impairment associated with cognitive impairment in solvent exposed workers? *Occupational and Environmental Medicine, 61*(1), 76–78.

Elliman, D., Bedford, H., & Hugman, J. (2004). Newborn and childhood screening programmes. *Community Practitioner, 77*(2), 41–43.

Forbes, B. J. R. (2003). Cataract. In Schwartz, M. W. (Ed.), *5-minute pediatric consult* (3rd ed.). Philadelphia: Lippincott Williams & Wilkins.

Gilbert, C., & Awan, H. (2003). Blindness in children. *British Medical Journal, 327*(7418), 760–761.

Glasziou, P. P., et al. (2005). Antibiotics for acute otitis media in children. *The Cochrane Library (Oxford) (4)* (CD000219).

Gold, R. S., et al. (2004). Round table. Amblyopia studies changing pediatric ophthalmic practice patterns. *Ocular Surgery News, 22*(20), 80–83.

Govindan, M., et al. (2005). Incidence and types of childhood exotropia: A population-based study. *Ophthalmology, 112*(1), 104–108.

Graessle, W. R. (2003). Otitis media. In Schwartz, M. W. (Ed.), *5-minute pediatric consult* (3rd ed.). Philadelphia: Lippincott Williams & Wilkins.

Ho, V. H., et al. (2004). Retained intraorbital metallic foreign bodies. *Ophthalmic Plastic and Reconstructive Surgery, 20*(3), 232–236.

Khaw, P. T., Shah, P., & Elkington, A. R. (2004). Glaucoma: Diagnosis. *British Medical Journal, 328*(7431), 97–99.

Kunimoto, D. Y., et al. (Eds.). (2004). Cornea. In Kunimoto, D. Y., et al. (Eds.). *Wills eye manual: Office and emergency room diagnosis and treatment of eye disease.* Philadelphia: Lippincott Williams & Wilkins.

Leslie, N. D. (2003). Insights into the pathogenesis of galactosemia. *Annual Review of Nutrition, 23*(1), 59–80.

McHugh, E., & Lieberman, L. (2003). The impact of developmental factors on stereotypic rocking of children with visual impairments. *Journal of Visual Impairment & Blindness, 97*(8), 453–474.

Mills, M. (2003). Refractive error. In Schwartz, M. W. (Ed.), *5-minute pediatric consult* (3rd ed.). Philadelphia: Lippincott Williams & Wilkins.

Mohan, K., Saroha, V., & Sharma, A. (2004). Occlusion therapy for amblyopia successful in older children. *Ocular Surgery News, 22*(10), 61–66.

National Institute on Deafness and Other Communication Disorders (NIDCD). (2005). *Statistics about hearing disorders, ear infections, and deafness.* Hyattsville, Md.: National Center for Health Statistics.

Nucci, P., et al. (2004). Restrictive strabismus after blow-out orbital fracture in children: Is the muscle involved? *Journal of Trauma: Injury, Infection, and Critical Care, 56*(1), 209–210.

Phillips, C. B., et al. (2004). Laser in situ keratomileusis for high hyperopia in awake, autofixating pediatric and adolescent patients with fully or partially accommodative esotropia. *Journal of Cataract and Refractive Surgery, 30*(10), 2124–2129.

Poppovich, D. M., & McAlhany, A. (2004). Practitioner care and screening guidelines for infants born to chlamydia-positive mothers. *Newborn and Infant Nursing Reviews, 4*(1), 51–55.

Quinn, G. E. (2003). Glaucoma—congenital. In Schwartz, M. W. (Ed.), *5-minute pediatric consult* (3rd ed.). Philadelphia: Lippincott Williams & Wilkins.

Ramsden, R. T. (2004). Prognosis after cochlear implantation. *British Medical Journal, 328*(7437), 419–420.

Rash, E. M. (2004). Recognize cholesteatomas early. *Nurse Practitioner: American Journal of Primary Health Care, 29*(2), 24–29.

Robinson, B. L., & Lieberman, L. J. (2004). Effects of visual impairment, gender, and age on self-determination. *Journal of Visual Impairment and Blindness, 98*(6), 351–366.

Ruiz, M. F., et al. (2004). Surgery and botulinum toxin in congenital esotropia. *Canadian Journal of Ophthalmology, 39*(6), 639–649.

Shapiro, D. R., et al. (2005). Perceived competence of children with visual impairments. *Journal of Visual Impairment and Blindness, 99*(1), 15–25.

A B C
X Y Z

Suggested Readings

Brennan, R. A. (2004). A nurse-managed universal newborn hearing screen program. *The American Journal of Maternal/Child Nursing, 29*(5), 320–325.

Jindal-Snape, D. (2004). Generalization and maintenance of social skills of children with visual impairments: Self-evaluation and the role of feedback. *Journal of Visual Impairment and Blindness, 98*(8), 470–483.

Knoors, H., Meuleman, J., & Klatter-Folmer, J. (2003). Parents' and teachers' evaluations of the communicative abilities of deaf children. *American Annals of the Deaf, 148*(4), 287–294.

Levy, Y., & Zadok, D. (2004). Systemic side effects of ophthalmic drops. *Clinical Pediatrics, 43*(1), 99–101.

Lieberman, L. J., & MacVicar, J. M. (2003). Play and recreational habits of youths who are deaf-blind. *Journal of Visual Impairment and Blindness, 97*(12), 755–768.

Loots, G., Devise, I., & Sermijn, J. (2003). The interaction between mothers and their visually impaired infants: An intersubjective developmental perspective. *Journal of Visual Impairment and Blindness, 97*(7), 403–417.

Monsen, R. B. (2003). The child in the community: Nursing makes a difference. Children hearing. *Journal of Pediatric Nursing: Nursing Care of Children and Families, 18*(6), 421–422.

Powell, C., Wedner, S., & Richardson, S. (2005). Screening for correctable visual acuity deficits in school-age children and adolescents. *The Cochrane Library (Oxford) (1)* (CD005023).

Reed, M. J., Kraft, S. P., & Buncic, R. (2004). Parents' observations of the academic and nonacademic performance of children with strabismus. *Journal of Visual Impairment and Blindness, 98*(5), 276–288.

Wake, M., & Poulakis, Z. (2004). Slight and mild hearing loss in primary school children. *Journal of Paediatrics and Child Health, 40*(1–2), 11–13.

CHAPTER 51

Nursing Care of the Child With a Musculoskeletal Disorder

Key Terms

apposition
arthroscopy
cartilage
compartment syndrome
diaphysis
distraction
epiphyseal plate
epiphysis
fracture
malleoli
metaphysis
myopathy
periosteum
remodeling
resorption
sequestrum
sprain
strain
traction

Objectives

After mastering the contents of this chapter, you should be able to:

1. Describe common musculoskeletal disorders in children.
2. Assess a child with a musculoskeletal disorder.
3. Formulate nursing diagnoses related to a child with a musculoskeletal disorder.
4. Establish expected outcomes for a child with a musculoskeletal disorder.
5. Plan nursing care, such as age-appropriate diversional activities, for a child with a musculoskeletal disorder.
6. Implement nursing care for a child with a musculoskeletal disorder.
7. Evaluate expected outcomes for achievement and effectiveness of care.
8. Identify National Health Goals related to musculoskeletal disorders and children that nurses can help the nation achieve.
9. Identify areas related to care of a child with a musculoskeletal disorder that could benefit from additional nursing research or application of evidence-based practice.
10. Use critical thinking to analyze ways that care of a child with a musculoskeletal disorder can be more family centered.
11. Integrate knowledge of musculoskeletal disorders with nursing process to achieve quality maternal and child health nursing care.

Jeffrey, 13 years old, is a boy with scoliosis. He is brought to a clinic today because he has pain in his left lower leg. He has a fever, and his leg is warm to the touch and edematous. His mother tells you he had an infected mosquito bite in that area 2 weeks ago. After further evaluation, Jeffrey is diagnosed with osteomyelitis. His mother asks, "How could he get an infection all the way into his bone from such a simple thing? I thought he was just having growing pains."

Previous chapters described the growth and development of well children and the nursing care of children with a disorder of other body systems. This chapter adds information about the dramatic changes, both physical and psychosocial, that occur when a child develops a musculoskeletal disorder. This is important information because it builds a base for care and health teaching.

What does Jeffrey's mother need to know about bone infections?
How would you explain what has happened?

After you've studied this chapter, access the accompanying website. Read the patient scenario and answer the questions to further sharpen your skills, grow more familiar with RN-CLEX types of questions, and reward yourself with how much you have learned.

The skeletal system, composed of more than 200 bones connected by the joints and tendons, provides a structural casing or protective armor for the internal organs of the body. Skeletal muscles, which are attached to the bones by connective tissue, tendons, and ligaments, allow for voluntary movement, including gross motor activity, such as running, and fine motor activity, such as writing. Together, the skeletal and muscular systems support the body and make coordinated movement possible.

Because their bones and muscles are still growing, children suffer from disorders of the musculoskeletal system more frequently than do adults. On the other hand, because bones are still growing, fractures heal much more quickly in children than in adults. However, if a growth plate is injured (which can result in halting of bone growth), an injury that might be simple in an adult becomes serious in a child. Because many musculoskeletal system disorders lead to problems with locomotion and possibly limitations of activity, they can threaten a child's ability to develop optimally in other ways. Some problems of locomotion are slight and self-limiting, whereas others are extensive and incapacitating. In either instance, because children gain much of their knowledge by interacting with people and exploring the environment around them, a problem of locomotion can be a serious impairment during childhood. Nurses play a key role in teaching parents ways to expose their children to the same sorts of stimuli that might be experienced if the child were able to move around independently.

Maintenance of musculoskeletal function is addressed by the National Health Goals. These are shown in Box 51.1.

Nursing Process Overview

For Care of the Child With a Musculoskeletal Disorder

● *Assessment*

Unlike many other diseases in children, disorders of the skeletal system usually manifest with specific, localized symptoms. Parents usually bring children to health care facilities early in the course of such illnesses. On the other hand, disorders of the muscles or joints such as juvenile rheumatoid arthritis (JA) may manifest insidiously; when the disorder is diagnosed, parents may feel guilty for not having sought health care earlier.

One condition whose seriousness parents may underestimate is a childhood limp. A limp is never normal, and it may be the first manifestation of a serious hip or knee problem. When weighing or measuring a child, take the opportunity to assess gait (whether the child walks naturally or stiffly, on tiptoes or on the whole foot; whether the feet are in good alignment; whether the back is held straight). Such assessments may detect that a child brought to a health care center because of an upper respiratory condition has another, perhaps more important, musculoskeletal problem requiring evaluation (Box 51.2). Because scoliosis is a common spinal deformity requiring early detection, school nurses have direct responsibility for instituting scoliosis screening programs in their schools.

BOX 51.1 FOCUS ON . . .

NATIONAL HEALTH GOALS

To maintain a healthy musculoskeletal system, proper exercise is necessary. Several National Health Goals address this issue:

- Increase the proportion of the nation's public and private schools that require daily physical education for all students, from 17% to 25%.
- Increase the proportion of adolescents who participate in moderate physical activity for at least 30 minutes on 5 of 7 days, from a baseline of 27% to at least 30%.
- Increase the proportion of adolescents who view television 2 or fewer hours on a school day, from 57% to 75%.
- Increase the proportion of trips that children and adolescents make by walking, from 31% to 50% (DHHS, 2000).

Nurses can help the nation achieve these goals by educating children about the importance of physical activity, serving as consultants for school systems in designing physical education programs, and being certain to ask children about their usual activity level at health maintenance visits.

Nursing research that would help add to nursing knowledge includes investigating whether children sustain interest longer in group or single-person exercise programs; whether adolescents are accurate in reporting the time and intensity of exercise in which they engage; and whether designing exercise programs for well children and for those with chronic illness can be a nursing role.

Because skeletal injuries can be a sign of abuse, careful history taking is necessary to rule out this possibility.

● *Nursing Diagnosis*

The nursing diagnoses most frequently identified for children with musculoskeletal disorders include those that deal with pain, lack of mobility, and, because of immobilization, a need for diversional activities. Children, especially adolescents, who require a walker or other equipment to aid in skeletal support or locomotion may encounter problems with self-concept. Examples of some typical nursing diagnoses are the following:

- Pain related to chronic inflammation of joints
- Impaired physical mobility related to cast on leg
- Deficient diversional activity related to need for imposed activity restriction for 4 weeks
- Situational low self-esteem related to continuous use of body brace

● *Outcome Identification and Planning*

Many musculoskeletal problems in children require long-term care. Despite current therapies, some disorders may leave a child with a permanent disability. Before a child is discharged from an ambulatory or

BOX 51.2 ASSESSMENT

Assessing a Child for Possible Signs and Symptoms of a Musculoskeletal Disorder

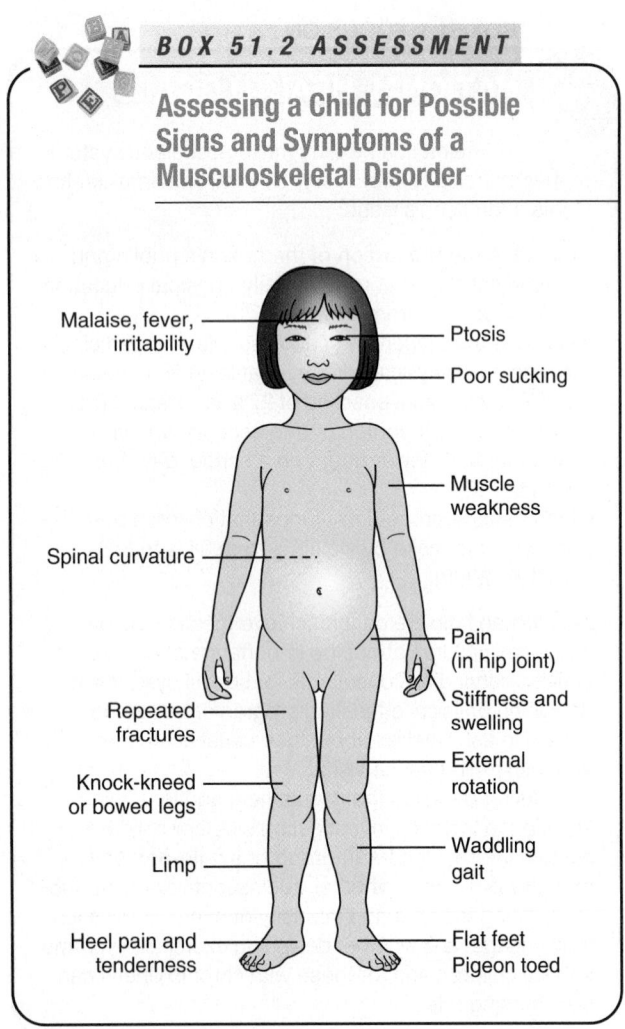

Malaise, fever, irritability

Ptosis

Poor sucking

Muscle weakness

Spinal curvature

Pain (in hip joint)

Repeated fractures

Stiffness and swelling

External rotation

Knock-kneed or bowed legs

Waddling gait

Limp

Flat feet Pigeon toed

Heel pain and tenderness

---

traction or teaching about common concerns, such as posture or children's shoes. Parents and children who are kept well informed in these matters are much more likely to be able to cope with changing circumstances. Referrals to appropriate organizations may be helpful. Organizations that can be used for referral include the following:

- Arthritis Foundation (*www.arthritis.org*)
- Muscular Dystrophy Association of America, Inc. (*www.mdausa.org*)
- National Institutes of Health, Osteoporosis and Related Bone Diseases—National Resource Center (*www.osteo.org*)
- Osteogenesis Imperfecta Foundation, Inc. (*www.oif.org*)

● *Outcome Evaluation*

Children with musculoskeletal disorders invariably need follow-up care after discharge from an ambulatory visit or inpatient care, because bone healing is a slow process. Parents may ask to have x-ray studies done frequently to evaluate healing progress. They may need to be reminded that radiographs are never taken on children unless there is a documented need for them, because excessive radiation at epiphyseal plates can lead to uneven growth. Although controversial, extensive radiation of bones has also been associated with the development of leukemia in children (Berrington de Gonzalez & Darby, 2004).

Both parents and children may need support at reevaluation visits when learning that a cast or brace must stay on longer or that they must continue exercises. Praise for their management thus far is an effective intervention for helping parents realize that they can cope with the situation in the future.

During reevaluation visits, spend time assessing the child's body image and self-esteem. Does the child view himself or herself as a basically well person who has, for example, a right leg shorter than the left leg, or as a deformed person who is inferior to others? Success of treatment is incomplete if a child's self-concept is diminished.

Some examples indicating achievement of outcomes are the following:

- Child states he feels no pain or numbness in extremity after application of a cast.
- Child demonstrates allowable weight-bearing activities with casted lower extremity.
- Parents accurately state child's care needs to be met both in and out of the hospital.
- Child states positive aspects of self, participates in activities, establishes friendships with peers.

---

inpatient setting, help the parents plan how they will care for the child at home. At first, a cast on an arm seems exciting to a school-age child: It is something to show off, an injury to describe, an excuse not to write in school. After a few days, the cast may become more frustrating than enjoyable. Take the time to review what wearing the cast will mean to the child in everyday situations. For example, the cast may not fit through shirts with tight cuffs. In this instance, dressing for school might be a problem. Planning transportation may be a problem if the child has a large cast and is not able to fit in a car seat. If the child must stay home from school, plans for tutoring need to be made. If both parents work, child care may be necessary.

Depending on the child's and family's circumstances, the answers to these problems differ. However, taking the time to sit down with the parents and asking them whether these concerns will pose problems initiates problem solving. Doing so helps parents plan and prepare solutions with a concerned person rather than by themselves at home.

● *Implementation*

Many nursing interventions for children with musculoskeletal disorders involve care of a child in a cast or in

THE MUSCULOSKELETAL SYSTEM

Bones and Bone Growth

Bones are generally classified by their shape as long, short, flat, or irregular. Long bones are the bones of the extremities, including the fingers and toes, in which most childhood bone disorders are found. The short bones are those found in the ankle and wrist. Flat bones are found in the skull, ribs, scapula, and clavicle. Irregular bones are found in the vertebrae, the pelvis, and the facial bones of the skull.

Long bones are composed of a long central shaft (the **diaphysis**), a rounded end portion (the **epiphysis**), and a thin area between them (the **metaphysis**) (Fig. 51.1). Increase in the length of long bones occurs at the cartilage segment (the **epiphyseal plate**), between the epiphysis and the metaphysis. As **cartilage** (connective tissue) cells grow away from the shaft, they are replaced by bone, thereby increasing bone length. Injury to this area in a growing child is always potentially serious, because it may halt growth, stimulate abnormal growth, or cause irregular or erratic growth. The central shafts of long bones are covered by an outer sensitive layer of **periosteum.** Bone width increases by growth at the inner surface of the periosteum. Injury to the periosteum, such as may occur with osteomyelitis, can also threaten bone growth.

Although it is easy to think of bones as rigid, solid structures, they are, in fact, living tissue, to which nutrients must be supplied for growth. Calcium, one of the main components of bone, is an important element for bone formation, **remodeling** (replacement of old by new bone tissue), and **resorption** (bone breakdown). These processes are influenced by parathyroid hormone, calcitonin, vitamin D, other minerals, nutrients, and enzymes. "Bone age" can be determined by a radiograph of the wrists that shows the ossification level of the bones. The inner core of long bones is filled with yellow and red marrow and is responsible for the formation of platelets, red blood cells, white blood cells, and adipose cells. Red marrow is primarily involved in blood component production, whereas yellow marrow is chiefly involved in adipose cell formation. The blood supply to bones is abundant, so that the marrow can actively supply enough blood components for the body. As with other tissues, if the blood supply is cut off, bone cells die.

The bones of children tend to be more resilient than those of adults. This means that accidents that might result in severe breaks to adult bones are apt to result in lesser breaks or only torsional twists in children. Because bones heal more quickly in children than in adults, children usually are incapacitated for a shorter time after an injury.

Muscle

The skeletal muscular system is composed of one type of muscle, called striated muscle, which is the predominant muscle in the body (differentiated from smooth muscle, which is responsible for, among other things, gastrointestinal peristalsis). Activation of skeletal muscle occurs with innervation from a motor nerve and is under voluntary control. **Myopathy,** or disease of the muscular system, can be inherited (as in muscular dystrophy) or acquired (as in myasthenia gravis).

ASSESSMENT OF MUSCULOSKELETAL FUNCTION

In addition to a history and physical examination, diagnostic tests frequently are necessary to detect musculoskeletal dysfunction in children. These may include radiography and bone scans, bone and muscle biopsies, electromyography, and arthroscopy. Ultrasound and magnetic resonance imaging (MRI) studies are used to reveal soft tissue disease.

Radiography

Because bones are opaque, they outline well on radiographs. X-ray studies provide information about a specific bone, groups of bones, or a joint. They can also provide information about soft tissue structure, swelling, or calcification around bones. However, other tests are indicated to confirm problems with cartilage, tendons, and ligaments.

Bone Scan

A bone scan is a study of the uptake of intravenously (IV) injected radioactive substances by bone. The distribution and concentration of the substance are evaluated to determine the problem. For example, areas of increased metabolic activity cause the substance to concentrate in that area. A bone scan provides information on very early stages of bone disease and healing, often before they are visible on radiographs.

Electromyography

Electromyography studies the electrical activity of skeletal muscle and nerve conduction. It can determine the location and cause of disorders such as myasthenia gravis, muscular dystrophy, and lower motor neuron and peripheral nerve disorders.

For the test, needle electrodes are inserted into muscle masses; the electrical activity of the muscle at rest and in motion is detected by audioamplification and recorded on an oscilloscope. Normally, resting muscle is quiet. If defects such as fasciculations are present, abnormal noises or oscilloscope spikes will be observed.

Although the needle electrodes are small, the test may be frightening for children because they are pricked by needles. They need support from someone they know during the procedure. Before and after the procedure, provide

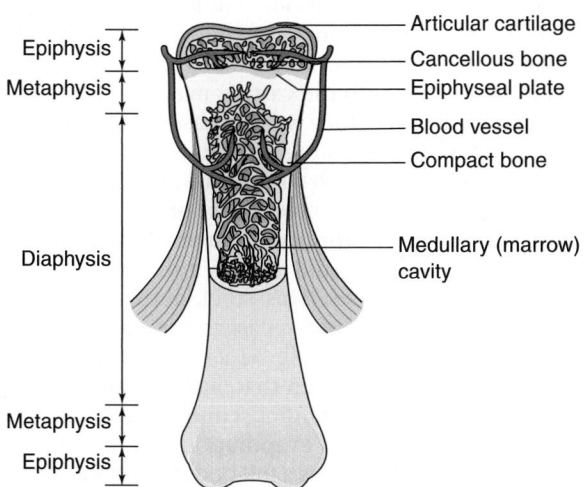

Epiphysis — Articular cartilage
— Cancellous bone
Metaphysis — Epiphyseal plate
— Blood vessel
— Compact bone

— Medullary (marrow) cavity
Diaphysis

Metaphysis
Epiphysis

FIGURE 51.1 Structure of a bone.

opportunities for therapeutic play so the child can express his or her anxiety and feelings.

Muscle or Bone Biopsy

A muscle or bone biopsy involves removal of a tissue sample for examination of its microscopic structure. It can provide evidence about infection, malignant bone growth, inflammation, or atrophy of the area. Either type may be done during surgery or as an ambulatory procedure.

Muscle biopsy is usually done using conscious sedation and a local anesthetic. If local anesthesia is used, caution children that they will feel the initial prick of an anesthetizing needle; as the actual biopsy needle enters the muscle mass, they will feel an additional momentary pressure. They can be assured that the amount of tissue taken from them is no larger than the inner bore of the biopsy needle, comparable to the size of the lead in a pencil.

Arthroscopy

Arthroscopy involves direct visualization of a joint with a fiberoptic instrument. It is usually done under local anesthesia in an ambulatory care setting. Arthroscopy allows a joint, most commonly the knee, but also the hip, shoulder, elbow, or wrist, to be examined without a large incision. It is most often used to diagnose athletic injuries and to differentiate between acute and chronic joint disorders (Kimura et al., 2004).

HEALTH PROMOTION AND RISK MANAGEMENT

Health promotion focuses on thorough assessment at all health maintenance visits. A child's ability to achieve developmental milestones, specifically gross and fine motor abilities, provides important information about his or her musculoskeletal function. The ability of a child to be fully mobile directly influences the child's exploration of the environment and exposure to stimuli. If mobility is impaired, it can interfere with growth and development to a high degree. Screening for musculoskeletal disorders, such as for scoliosis in the prepubescent child and adolescent, is an extremely important health promotion measure.

Safety is paramount for any child to prevent injury. Anticipatory guidance for parents is essential to minimize the risk of injury, specifically to the extremities, in all aspects of everyday life. As a child grows and becomes active in sports, parental and child education about the importance of using face masks for hockey, batting helmets for baseball, and mouth guards for football takes on an even greater role.

Nutrition education is important to ensure adequate calcium intake for bone growth and healing. However, if a child requires bed rest, calcium intake should be moderated to reduce the risk of renal calculi formation resulting from immobilization. The teenage years are an important time for both males and females to build calcium stores to protect against osteoporosis later in life (Flynn, 2003).

If a child experiences a musculoskeletal disorder, education helps to prevent complications, maximize the child's ability to function, and minimize the risk of residual impaired physical mobility. Parents and children need instruction about all aspects of treatment and follow-up—for example, caring for a child who requires a cast, traction, a body brace, or drug therapy (e.g., antibiotics for osteomyelitis, nonsteroidal anti-inflammatory drugs [NSAIDs] for juvenile arthritis). Teaching provides a basis for maximizing the effectiveness of treatment and minimizing the possible long-term risk for complications.

THERAPEUTIC MANAGEMENT OF MUSCULOSKELETAL DISORDERS IN CHILDREN

Various methods may be used as therapy for a child with a musculoskeletal disorder, including casts, traction, distraction, and open reduction. Amputation is discussed in Chapter 53.

Casting

Casts may be used to treat a variety of musculoskeletal system disorders, from simple fractures in the extremities to correction of congenital structural bone disorders (see Chapter 39 for a discussion of the latter).

Cast Application

Casts are created from either plaster of Paris or fiberglass. Fiberglass is an attractive material to use for children's casts because it is light; comes in colors; and, when a special waterproof liner is used, can be immersed in water. Unfortunately, it is more expensive and may not be practical for casts that need frequent changing, such as those used to correct talipes disorders.

Children need an explanation of what to expect with casting. To maintain alignment of body parts, a physician gently exerts a pull on the body part being casted during the cast application. If a large body cast is being applied, children may be positioned on a special cast table with traction apparatus at the chin and pelvis. These are stark, steel tables and may resemble torture racks children have seen in horror movies. Allow a support person to accompany the child to the cast room to hold his hand or talk to him during the application. Most children (and adults) are unaware that casts are formed from strips or rolls of material impregnated with the casting material. The normal curiosity of children as they watch a cast grow and mold to their body part makes casting a pleasant procedure. Some children look forward to having a cast applied. It may be a badge of courage or a conversation piece.

Before the cast is applied, a tube of stockinette is stretched over the area, and a soft cotton sheet is placed over bony prominences. This stockinette is pulled up and over the raw edges of the cast as it is applied to form a smooth, padded surface (Fig. 51.2). If a plaster cast is to be applied, caution children that, at first, the wet strips of plaster of Paris feel cool. Almost immediately, the strips begin to generate heat as evaporation begins, and body parts feel warm. If the cast is a full-body cast, children may become uncomfortably warm, with perspiration possibly

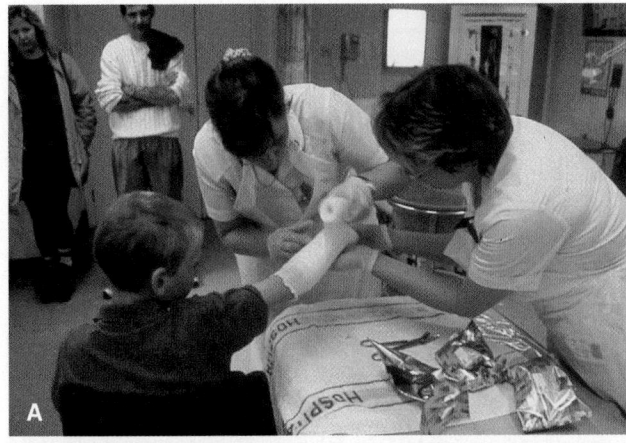

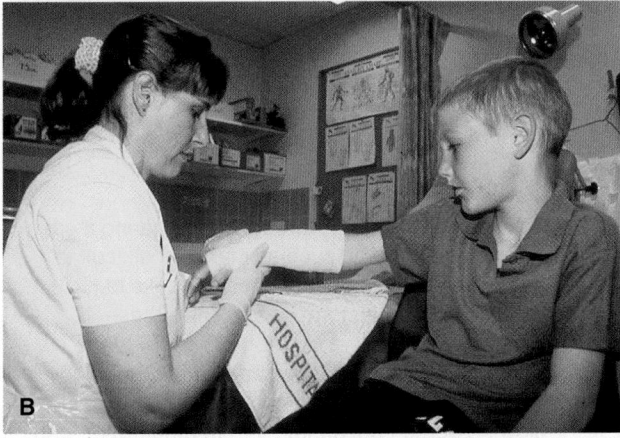

FIGURE 51.2 Cast application. (**A**) A fiberglass cast is applied to a young boy's arm over a stockinette already in place. (**B**) Casts do not cover the fingers so these can be assessed for color and warmth. (© Shout Pictures/Custom Medical Stock Photo.)

running from their forehead. Assure them that this feeling of warmth is transient and is never enough to cause a burn.

A plaster cast takes 10 to 72 hours to dry, depending on its size. Fiberglass casts usually dry within 5 to 30 minutes. A window may be placed in a cast if an infection is suspected, so that the area can be observed. A window also may be used with an open fracture, to permit observation and care of the wound site. If the child has a body or hip spica cast, windowing may prevent uncomfortable abdominal distention.

Compartment syndrome is a phenomenon that occurs when a cast or tight constrictive dressing puts pressure on an enclosed space such as the forearm. This pressure results in severely decreased blood flow that potentially threatens damage to and necrosis of surrounding soft tissue or nerves. The child develops sharp pain on passive stretching of the fingers. Assess fingers or toes carefully after application of a cast to be certain a compartment syndrome is not developing. If signs of compartment syndrome are present, the cast needs to be released immediately to prevent permanent damage.

NURSING DIAGNOSES AND RELATED INTERVENTIONS

Nursing Diagnosis: Risk for ineffective peripheral tissue perfusion related to pressure from cast

Outcome Evaluation: Child states she feels no pain or numbness in extremity; distal nail bed blanches and refills in less than 5 seconds; pedal pulses are palpable.

If an extremity has been casted, keep it elevated to prevent edema in the part. Check circulation frequently, such as every 15 minutes during the first hour, hourly for the first 24 hours, and then every 4 hours thereafter. Assess for color, warmth, presence of pedal pulses, and sensations of numbness or tingling. Signs of impaired neurovascular function include pallor (including blueness or coldness of a distal part), pulselessness, pain in the casted part, paresthesia (such as numbness or tingling in the part, as if it were "asleep"), and paralysis. Keep in mind that children younger than 6 or 7 years of age have difficulty describing paresthesia; however, they may whine or cry with the discomfort of the sensation. Edema that does not improve with elevation is also an important sign. Any of these symptoms requires immediate attention, because neurovascular impairment can lead to nerve ischemia and destruction, possibly causing permanent paralysis of an extremity.

Preventing the flow of urine under the edges of a cast can be a problem with full body or high leg casts. If a cast surrounds the genital area of a non–toilet-trained child, cover the edges of the cast with plastic or waterproof material. Keeping children in a semi-Fowler's position by using pillows or raising the head of the bed helps to direct urine and feces downward. Because a cast is heavy, an infant tends to slip down in bed a great deal, so he or she needs frequent repositioning to remain in the raised position.

Make certain that children who are being fed or feeding themselves have a bib or cover over the top edge of their cast so that crumbs and fluid cannot be spilled inside. Toys should be chosen carefully for the same reason. A piece of food inside a cast will mold and macerate the skin; a small part of a toy dropped inside a cast can cause irritation and a pressure ulcer. If a child spills food on the outside of a cast or the cast becomes soiled, it can be cleaned with a damp cloth.

Nursing Diagnosis: Parental health-seeking behaviors related to care of child with cast at home

Outcome Evaluation: Parents state plans for adapting home environment and lifestyle to accommodate child with cast; parents demonstrate measures to check neurovascular status.

If the child has an upper-extremity cast, be sure the parents understand how to position the extremity properly, such as with a sling. If the cast is on a lower extremity, instruct the child and parents on the amount of weight bearing allowed to the affected extremity and the use of crutches, if prescribed.

Handling a child in a large cast is a major task for parents. For many, it seems so overwhelming that they do not see how they will be able to care for the child at home. Assure them that the child is quite comfortable in the cast, despite its awkward, constricting appearance. Role-model moving the child and positioning him or her to give them direction. Be sure to caution them that, if an abduction bar is used with a cast, it must never be used as a handle for lifting the cast. Such use can break the bar from the cast or weaken its support.

A body cast is heavy, so caution parents to use good body mechanics (e.g., lift with the thighs instead of the back) when turning or positioning the child. If a cast is bulky, parents often appreciate suggestions on ways to help move the child from room to room, such as using a toy wagon with a flat board on top or using a skateboard for the child to propel herself forward. It is important to point out that all children thrive on being touched. Children in a large body cast need their head and arms stroked (or any areas of the body that are not covered by a cast). Demonstrate how even a child in a large hip spica cast can be held, cuddled, and supported for feeding. Otherwise, parents may neglect this aspect of care.

Many children report a sensation of itching inside a cast at about the end of the first week. If the area is immediately under the edge of the cast, the itching is probably the result of dry skin caused by the drying effect of the cast. Reaching a hand under the edge of the cast and massaging the area usually relieves the itching. Applying hand lotion may relieve the dryness. If the area is unreachable, blowing cool air through the cast with a fan, a hair dryer set on cool air, or a vacuum cleaner attachment may relieve the uncomfortable feeling. Caution the child and parents not to use implements such as a coat hanger or knitting needle to scratch the area. These can injure the skin, causing infection under the cast (Box 51.3).

Transporting the child in a car, particularly fitting a bulky cast into an infant car seat, can be a major problem. Before a child is discharged from the health care facility, give parents a telephone number to call if they have any questions about their child's care or condition.

Cast Removal

Most casts remain in place for 4 to 8 weeks and are then removed, using an electric cast cutter with a rapidly vibrating, circular disk (Fig. 51.3). Cast cutters are frightening,

---

BOX 51.3 FOCUS ON . . .

FAMILY TEACHING

Cast Care at Home

Q. Jeffrey's sister has a fiberglass cast on her arm. Her parents ask you, "How do we care for this?"

A. Here are some helpful tips to care for your child's cast at home:

- Keep the casted body part elevated on a pillow for the first day, to decrease swelling.
- Observe the hands and fingers (the body part distal to the cast) for swelling or blueness, and ask your child to move the part about every 4 hours for the first 24 hours. If she is unable to move distal parts or if swelling, blueness, or pain is present, telephone your health care provider. These signs could mean the cast is pressing on a nerve or constricting a blood vessel.
- Monitor strenuous activities, such as rough-housing, while the cast is in place, but urge usual activities, so your child remains active.
- Ask your child to think through how wearing a cast will change her day, such as making it difficult to eat in the school cafeteria or carry books to classes, and brainstorm how to solve these problems.
- Be certain your child knows not to put anything inside the cast. If itching occurs inside the cast, blowing some cool air into it from a hair dryer can be comforting.
- Be sure that your child keeps the cast dry (cover it with a plastic bag to shower); no swimming is allowed. Remind her that autographs are not allowed, because fiberglass is a porous material.
- Be certain to keep your return appointment for follow-up care. Because children grow so quickly, they can outgrow a cast rapidly. Outgrowing the cast could put pressure on nerves and lead to permanent disability.

---

because the disk makes a very loud noise as it cuts through the cast material and also generates heat. To the child, the disk appears capable of cutting through not only the plaster but an arm or leg as well. The person removing the cast usually demonstrates that the disk does not cut skin by touching a thumb to the edge of it. Not all children are totally convinced by the demonstration, however, and they may require additional support while the disk moves from one end of a cast to the other, such as saying, "It's all right to cry; I know this looks scary" or by holding your hands over the child's ears to lessen the noise.

The skin of the child's extremity looks macerated and dirty after a cast is removed; a good bath usually washes away most of this. If an arm has been casted in flexion, the elbow may feel stiff and even sore as the child is asked to extend it for the first time. Children often use extremities with caution after a cast has been removed. Advise parents

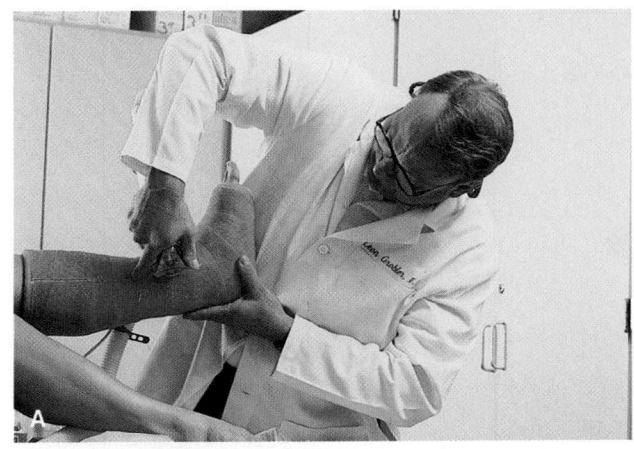

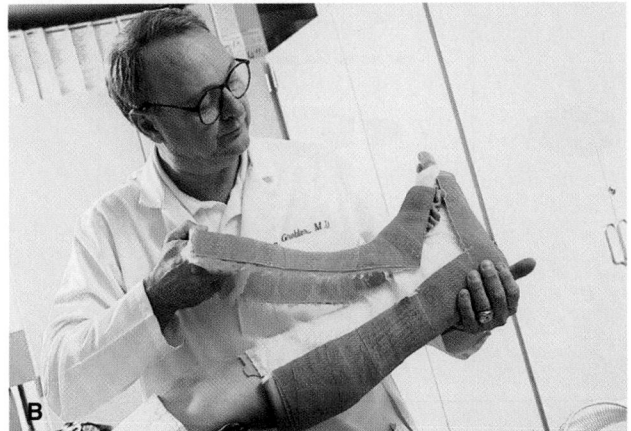

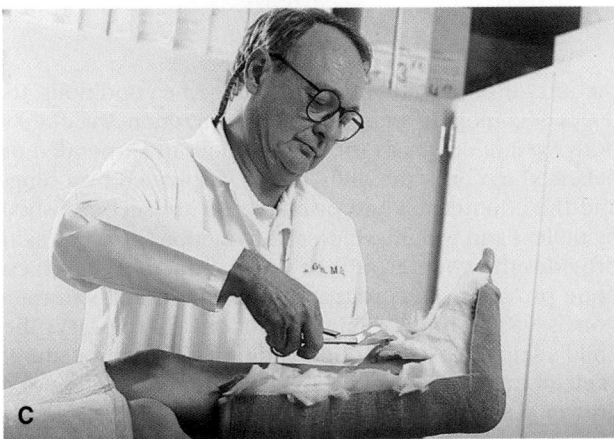

FIGURE 51.3 Cast removal. **(A)** A cast cutter is used to begin the removal of a fiberglass cast on an adolescent's leg. **(B)** The fiberglass cast is lifted off the leg. **(C)** Underlying stockinette and padding are removed. (© Will and Deni McIntyre/Science Source/Photo Researchers.)

to allow the child to begin using the extremity again at his or her own pace. As children naturally play and reach for objects, they gradually forget to favor the arm or leg, and full function then returns. Once healing has taken place, the extremity is as strong as it was before the fracture. The child does not need to continue to favor the extremity to protect it from a second fracture.

Crutches

Crutches are prescribed for children for one of three reasons: to keep weight off one or both legs, to support weakened legs, or to maintain balance. Usually, a physical therapist measures crutch length and gives beginning instruction in crutch walking. Be familiar with measuring and supervising crutch walking, so that you can offer emotional support to children as they learn to use crutches and can assess progress at follow-up visits.

Fit and Adjustment

If crutches are properly fitted, there should be a space of 1 to 1½ inches between the axilla crutch pad and the child's axilla. When the child stands upright and places his hands on the hand rests of the crutches, the elbows should flex about 20 degrees. This degree of flexion ensures that, when the child bears weight on the crutch, the body weight will be borne by the arm, not the axilla. Pressure of a crutch against the axilla could lead to compression and damage of the brachial nerve plexus crossing the axilla, resulting in permanent nerve palsy. Teach children not to rest with the crutch pad pressing on the axilla but always to support their weight at the hand grip.

Always assess the tips of crutches to see that the rubber tip is intact and not worn through. The tip prevents the crutch from slipping when it is in place. Be certain that the child is walking with the crutches placed about 6 inches to the side of the foot. This distance furnishes a wide, balanced base for support.

Explore with children any problems crutches may cause with their daily activities. If they carry books to school, for example, they may prefer to wear a backpack until they are free of crutches so their hands are free for the hand rests. Caution parents to clear articles such as throw rugs and small footstools out of the paths at home. If there are small children at home, the parents will need to keep traffic areas free of toys to prevent an accident.

Crutch Walking

Two main crutch-walking patterns are used (Fig. 51.4). A two-point gait is used when a child needs support for weakened muscles or balance but may bear weight on both lower extremities. The child places the right crutch and left foot forward, then left crutch and right foot forward, and so on. Using the crutch opposite a foot provides a wider base of support than using the crutch next to the foot. Caution children to take small steps until they feel confident.

A three-point swing-through gait is used when no weight bearing is allowed on one foot. For this, the crutches are both brought forward. The weight of the body is then shifted forward as both legs are swung through the crutches. The child bears weight on the unaffected (good) leg and moves the crutches forward again. It takes strong arm support to bear full weight on crutches this way. Be certain the child is bearing weight on the hands and not on the axillae when swinging through. Some children use a swing-through gait rather recklessly and need to be advised to slow their pace to a safer one.

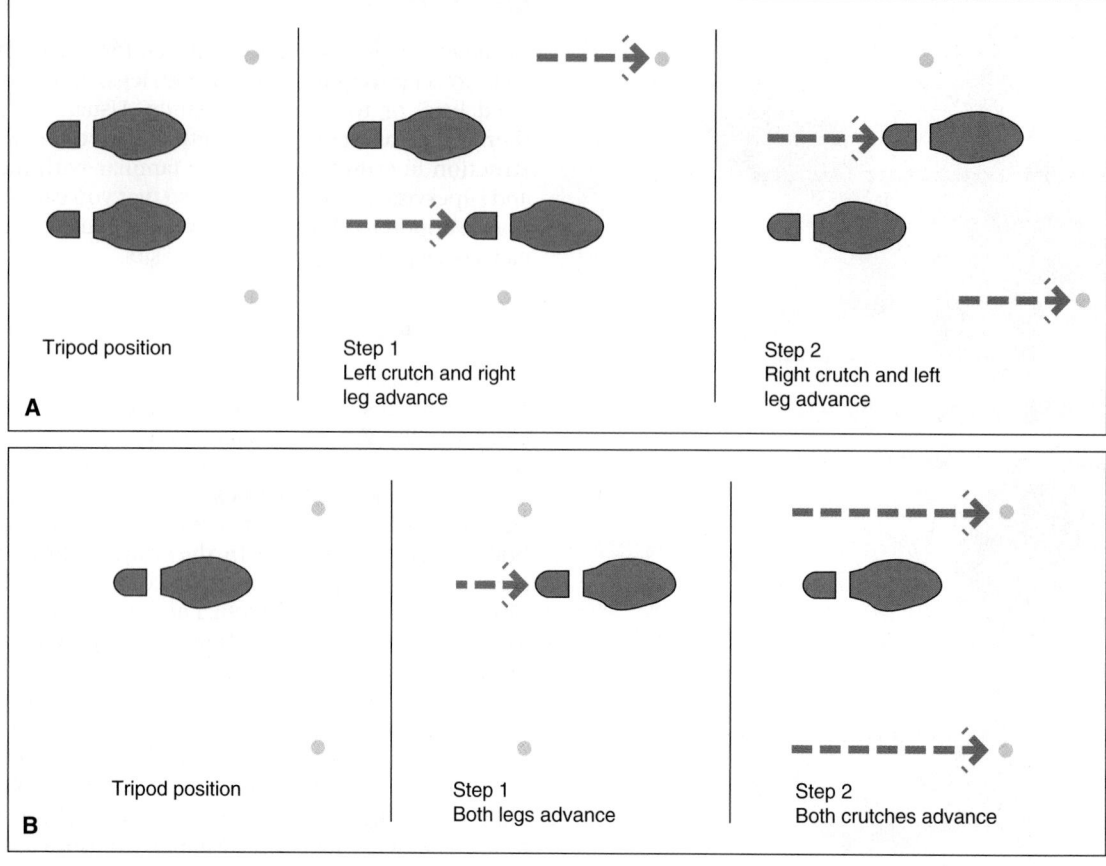

FIGURE 51.4 Crutch-walking patterns. (**A**) Two-point gait. (**B**) Swing-through gait.

To walk downstairs using a swing-through gait, children place their crutches on the lower step, then swing the unaffected (good) foot forward and down to that step. To go upstairs, they place their unaffected (good) foot on the elevated step, then raise the crutches onto the step and lift themselves up. To help children remember this pattern, a saying—"angels" (the good foot) go up; "devils" (the bad foot with the crutches) go down—is traditionally used.

Checkpoint Question 1

You are teaching a child to walk with crutches. Which is the best instruction?

a. He should bear weight on his armpits to keep stress off his arms.
b. He should lean forward at a 45° angle while walking.
c. He should bear weight on his arms to avoid pressure on his axilla.
d. It is unsafe to walk downstairs with crutches; upstairs is all right.

Traction

Traction, which is used to reduce dislocations and immobilize fractures, involves pulling on a body part in one direction against a counterpull exerted in the opposite direction. Although still necessary for some conditions, its use is declining. In straight (running) traction, the child's body weight serves as the counterpull. In suspended or balanced traction, the body part is suspended by a sling, and the counterpull and primary pull are accomplished by pulleys and weights. Either skin traction (in which skin provides the counterpull) or skeletal traction (in which bone provides the counterpull) may be used. Skin traction is used if only minimal traction is necessary; the child's skin must be in good condition for this procedure. Skeletal traction is used if a longer period of traction or a greater strength of traction pull is needed. Types of traction are illustrated in Figure 51.5. Use of traction in the home shortens hospital stays and enables the child to interact with family members, so it should be encouraged.

Skin Traction

Bryant's traction, used for fractured femurs in children younger than 2 years of age, is an example of skin traction (Fig. 51.6). It also may be used in preparation for surgical repair of congenital developmental disorders, such as developmental hip dysplasia (see Chapter 39). This type of traction is used less frequently now because the elevation of the extremities causes blood to pool at the hips. This and the possible tourniquet effect of the traction strips, bandages, and traction itself increase the risk for vasospasm and avascular hip necrosis.

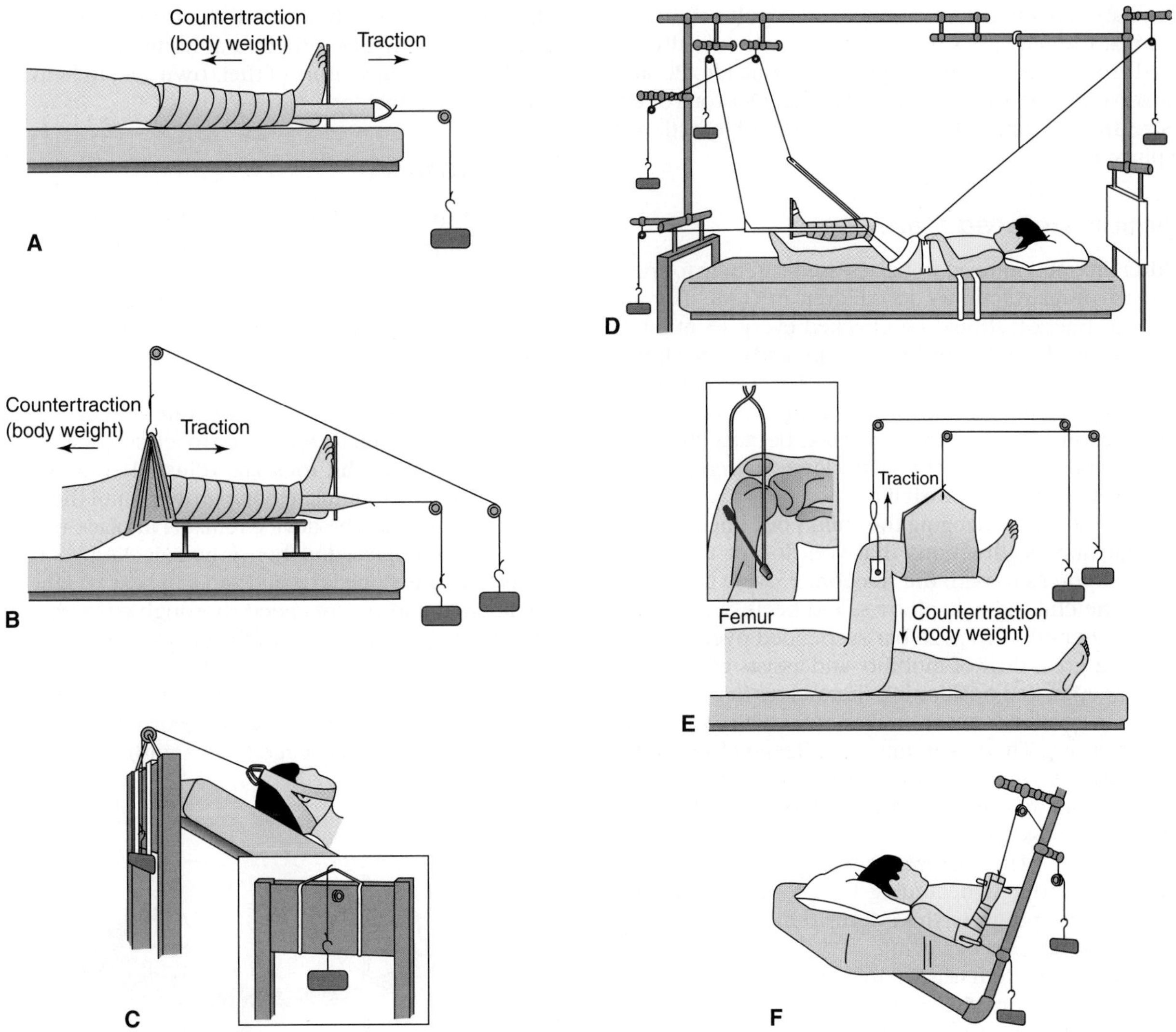

FIGURE 51.5 Types of skin traction: (**A**) Buck's extension, (**B**) Russell, (**C**) Cervical skin traction. Types of skeletal traction: (**D**) Balanced suspension, (**E**) 90-degree, (**F**) Dunlop's traction with pin insertion.

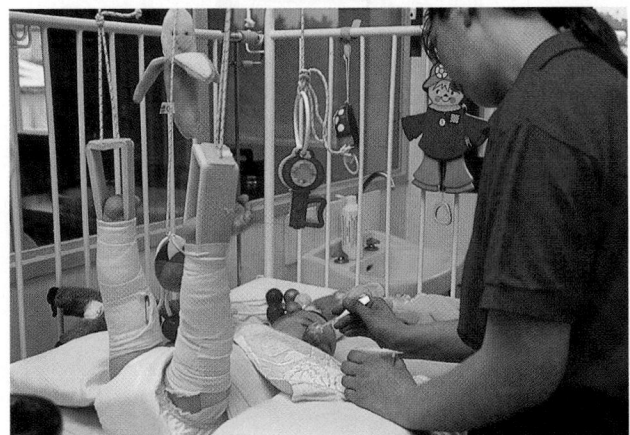

FIGURE 51.6 An infant in Bryant's traction. Here, the father feeds the infant while the infant is maintained in traction. (© BSIP/Custom Medical Stock Photo.)

Buck's extension is an example of skin traction used for immobilizing lower-extremity fractures in older children. Dunlop's traction is used to immobilize an upper extremity. This can be by skin traction or by skeletal traction if a wire or pin is used to immobilize. Cervical skin traction may be used to decrease muscle spasms in the back. This type of traction uses a halter-type device attached to weights. With this type of traction, the head of the bed is elevated to provide some countertraction.

Skeletal Traction

Skeletal traction involves the use of a pin, such as a Steinmann pin, or a wire, such as a Kirschner wire, that is passed through the skin into the end of a long bone. The pin or wire can be inserted in an emergency department under local anesthesia if the child can hold absolutely still, but usually it is done under general anesthesia in the operating room. With skeletal traction, ropes strung over pulleys and attached to weights exert a pull on the extremity at the pin site. Cotton gauze squares usually are placed around the ends of the pin on the outside. Be sure to observe the pin sites daily for drainage. Odorous or excessive drainage or erythema may be a sign of infection at the pin site.

Traction-Related Care

Children in traction need to be assessed carefully for neurovascular impairment, as do children in casts. The extremity in traction should be checked every 15 minutes during the first hour, hourly for 24 hours, and every 4 hours thereafter for signs of pallor (or blueness), lack of warmth (coldness), tingling, absent peripheral pulse, edema, or pain. Traction can lead to hypertension because the head typically is positioned lower than the lower extremities. Assess once a day for this possibility.

Be careful when changing the child's bed linens or carrying out nursing functions that you do not move the weights or interfere with the traction. Provide good skin care on the child's back, elbows, and heels, which may become irritated. A trapeze bar suspended over the bed provides a great deal of mobility and assists children in using a bedpan and positioning themselves in bed.

Being in traction is not as dramatic for children as being placed in a cast. There is an unspoken feeling from other children that "if what you have is really serious, you'd have a cast." Explain to children why this type of treatment is best for them. Keep them informed of radiographic assessments (e.g., "The fracture is being held in just the right position; the bone is beginning to re-form."), Although they cannot see progress, this information can help assure them that progress is occurring.

Children in traction usually are not "ill" children. They feel well except for the leg or arm being held in correct position. Therefore, they have the energy and the need for stimulation of well children. Keeping them occupied and exposed to activities appropriate to their age group is a major part of nursing care (Fig. 51.7).

Help children to maintain contact with their school friends through cards, letters, or tape-recorded messages. If hospitalized, their bed should be located so that they can see unit activities. Whether at home or in the hospital, allow frequent visitors of their own age, to help maintain peer relationships.

Distraction

Distraction involves the use of an external device to separate opposing bones, which encourages new bone growth. It can be used to lengthen a bone if one limb is shorter than the other. It also can be used to immobilize fractures or correct defects if the bone is rotated or angled.

A device such as the Ilizarov external fixator is used to achieve distraction (Fig. 51.8). It consists of wires that are inserted through the bone. The wires are attached to either full or half rings, which are secured to telescoping rods. For bone lengthening, the rods are adjusted approximately 1 mm each day to stimulate bone growth until the desired length is achieved. The device remains in place until consolidation is complete and there is no pain, limp, or edema. At this time, the bone is healed and can bear weight.

The child and parents need thorough preparation for the surgery and application of the device. Because the device is external, large, and awkward, they need to be prepared for its appearance and the reactions of others to it. Provide suggestions for ways to minimize the device's appearance, such as wide-legged pants with adjustable clo-

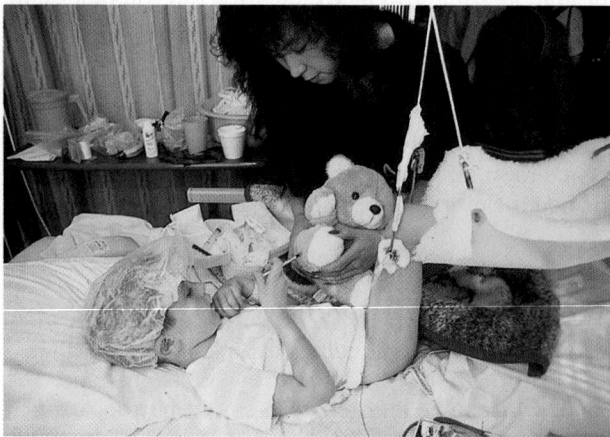

FIGURE 51.7 A child in skeletal traction engages in play. (© Gary Wagner/Stock Boston.)

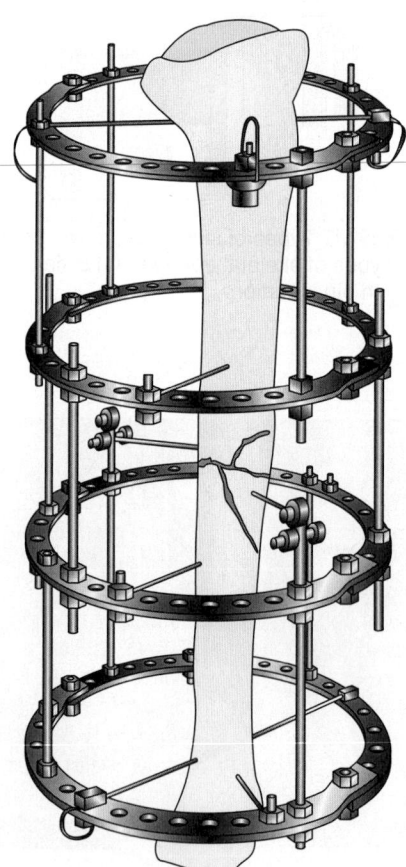

FIGURE 51.8 Ilizarov device in place to treat comminuted fracture.

sures. Parents also need instructions about adjusting the telescoping rods, if ordered; providing care to the wire insertion sites; assessing for signs and symptoms of infection; and instituting activity restrictions. Follow-up care is essential to ensure the optimal outcome for the child.

Open Reduction

Open reduction is a surgical technique that is used to align and repair bone. If there is a spinal fracture or both bones of a forearm or lower leg are fractured, open reduction may be necessary to stabilize the bones. Internal fixation, such as the use of rods or screws, is rarely used with children except in cases of scoliosis.

Once an open reduction is completed, the area usually is casted to provide support. Invariably, serosanguineous fluid oozes from an open-reduction site. Outline with a ballpoint pen any stain on the cast that suggests oozing from a surgical incision, so that an increase in the size of the mark can be detected. Do not use a magic marker for this, because the fluid tends to penetrate through the cast. Noting the time at which you make the pen mark on the cast allows you to tell how rapidly the spot is increasing. Children with an open-reduction incision are prone to incision infection, as is any child after a surgical incision. Be aware of systemic symptoms (increased pulse, increased temperature, lethargy) and local signs (edema, pain, tingling, blueness or coolness of the distal extremity) of infection.

DISORDERS OF BONE DEVELOPMENT

Flat Feet (Pes Planus)

The term *flat feet* refers to relaxation of the longitudinal arch of the foot. Although it is rare, many parents worry that their children have this problem. Parents become concerned because a newborn's foot is normally flatter and proportionately wider than an adult's. A transverse arch rarely is visible. A longitudinal arch may not be present until the child has been walking for months. Parents notice that when their child walks in the sand or makes wet tracks on the bathroom floor, he or she makes an impression of a "flat foot."

Evaluate children's feet by having them stand on tiptoe. In this position, a longitudinal arch should be visible. If they can stand on their heels with the soles of the feet off the ground, the feet probably are normal. Examine the ankle joint to be certain a full range of motion is present and to demonstrate that the Achilles tendon is not shortened. Tarsal and metatarsal joints should normally show a full range of motion.

Some children experience foot pain at the end of the day. This probably occurs not from lack of a longitudinal arch, but from poor arch development. The arch can be strengthened and the pain usually can be eliminated if the child walks on tiptoe for 5 to 10 minutes daily or practices picking up marbles with the toes. For an older child, standing pigeon toed (toes pointed in) and throwing the weight forward onto the lateral aspect of the feet tends to strengthen arches.

Teach parents that children do not need a hightop or rigid shoe for foot development. If the child notices leg pain from poor arch support, a sports shoe is usually adequate to correct the problem.

Bowlegs (Genu Varum)

Genu varum is lateral bowing of the tibia. If genu varum is present, the **malleoli** (rounded prominence on either side of the ankles) will be touching and the medial surfaces of the knees will be more than 2 in (5 cm) apart (Fig. 51.9*A*). Children may develop this condition as part of normal development; it is seen most commonly in 2-year-olds. Record the extent of the bowing at health maintenance visits by approximating the medial malleoli of the ankles and measuring the distance between the patellas (knees) for changes.

Genu varum gradually corrects itself by about 3 years of age or, at the latest, by school age. If the problem is unilateral, is becoming rapidly worse, or persists beyond this time, the child needs referral to an orthopedist for further evaluation.

Blount's Disease (Tibia Vara)

Blount's disease is retardation of growth of the epiphyseal line on the medial side of the proximal tibia (inside of the knee) that results in bowed legs. Unlike the normal developmental aspect of genu varum, Blount's disease is a serious disturbance in bone growth that requires treatment (Ramachandran et al., 2003).

Because it is not possible to rule out Blount's disease by appearance alone, almost all children with bowed legs have an initial radiograph. In those with Blount's disease, the medial aspect of the proximal tibia will show a sharp, beaklike appearance on the radiograph.

Bracing or osteotomy may be necessary to correct this deformity or prevent it from becoming more severe. Explain to the parents why their child requires treatment or

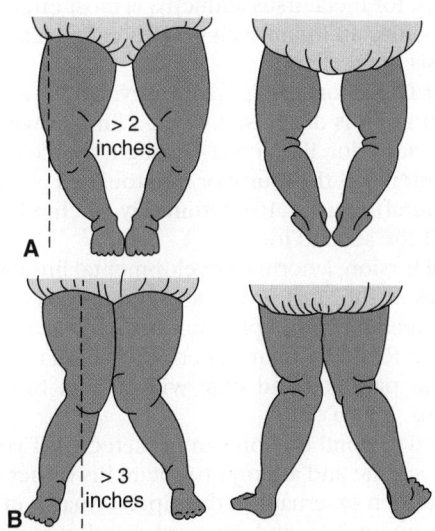

FIGURE 51.9 (A) Genu varum. **(B)** Genu valgum.

surgery when another child on the block with a similar appearance (developmental genu varum) is expected to outgrow the problem.

Knock Knees (Genu Valgum)

Genu valgum, or knock knee, appears as the opposite of genu varum. The medial surfaces of the knees touch, and the medial surfaces of the ankle malleoli are separated by more than 3 inches (7.5 cm) (see Fig. 51.9*B*).

This is seen most commonly in children 3 to 4 years old. No treatment is necessary for genu valgum. The problem tends to correct itself as the child grows. By school age, few children continue to have the problem. Those who do, and those in whom the abnormality is unilateral or becoming more pronounced, need a referral to an orthopedist for further evaluation. The severity of the deformity can be measured at regular health maintenance visits by approximating the medial aspects of the knees and measuring the distance between the medial malleoli of the ankles.

Toeing-In

Toeing-in (pigeon toe) in children may occur as a result of foot, tibial, femoral, or hip displacement. Assess for these conditions if parents describe their child as "always falling over his feet" or "awkward."

Metatarsus adductus is turning in of the forefoot. The heel is in good alignment; only the forefoot is turned in. This condition may develop or become more pronounced in infants who sleep prone with the feet adducted and in older children who watch television by kneeling, resting on their feet, and turning their feet in. If you stand the child on a copying machine and make a print, the turning in of the foot can be well demonstrated.

Most instances of metatarsus adductus resolve without therapy. Those that persist beyond 1 year can be corrected by passive stretching exercises.

A few infants with extremely rigid, incorrect foot posture may require casts or splints for correction. Early detection of these extreme instances is important, because treatment for metatarsus adductus is most effective if it is begun before an infant walks. With early treatment, the prognosis is excellent.

Inward tibial torsion also may be evidenced as toeing-in. This condition is diagnosed when a line drawn from the anterior superior iliac crest through the center of the patella intersects the fourth or fifth toe (or a position even more lateral) (Fig. 51.10). Ordinarily, such a line should intersect the second toe.

Tibial torsion, a normal developmental finding, usually improves as the tibia grows and requires no treatment. Parents need a good explanation of why no treatment is necessary. Reassure them at periodic health maintenance visits that patience and time will correct tibial torsion (Dormans, 2003a).

Inward femoral torsion can be detected if you have a child lie supine and attempt to rotate his or her leg internally and then externally at the hip. Normally, internal rotation is about 30°, and outward rotation is about 90°. With inward femoral torsion, the internal rotation is closer to 90°. In some children, the femur rotates so far that the

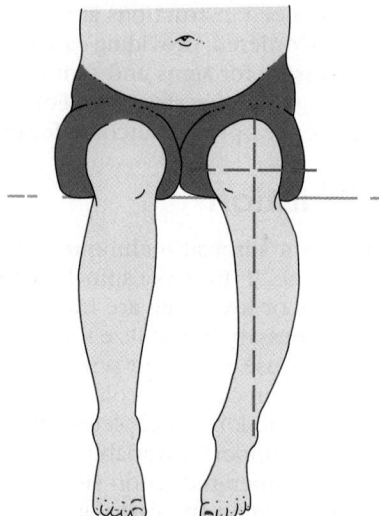

FIGURE 51.10 Toeing-in caused by inward tibial torsion. In good alignment, a line drawn from the antero-superior iliac crest through the patella should intersect the second toe.

patellar bones face each other. As with tibial torsion, no treatment is necessary. Inward femoral rotation will not correct itself, but a compensating tibial torsion will develop and make feet appear straight.

A fourth cause of toeing-in may be improper hip placement or developmental hip dysplasia, a problem that is very serious and needs early therapy for correction (see Chapter 39).

Limps

Observation of a child's gait is part of health assessment at any health maintenance visit. Gait is a variable characteristic; however, limping is never normal. Although limping may reflect a simple problem (e.g., a recently stubbed toe, a shin splint from excessive running), it may also reflect serious bone or muscle involvement, such as occurs with osteomyelitis or cerebral palsy.

History is important in determining the cause of a limp. When children have pain in a lower extremity, they protect the extremity by limping—stepping gingerly and quickly on the affected leg. Although children may seem to be favoring an ankle or a knee, ask them specifically what hurts. Because a hip hurts, they may be walking gingerly on the leg and causing pain in a knee (Hamer, 2004).

The lower extremities need careful, thoughtful examination, including inspection, measurement of leg length, range of motion, palpation, and a neurologic examination. Radiography or bone scan may be necessary to rule out a pathologic process.

Growing Pains

Listen to parents carefully when they state that their child has "growing pains." What they are reporting may be symptoms indicative of rheumatic fever or juvenile arthritis rather than a simple, transient phenomenon. Growing pains occur most frequently in the muscle of the calf, never in a joint. They occur in preschool and school-age children, who wake at night because of the pain (Evans & Scutter, 2004). Such cramping usually is associated with a day of vigorous activity or wearing new shoes with a heel of a different height than before. Children with genu varum (bowlegs) tend to have more of such pain than do other children. Some children reported to have growing pains may have restless leg syndrome (Rajaram et al., 2004).

Osteogenesis Imperfecta

Osteogenesis imperfecta is a connective tissue disorder in which fragile bone formation leads to recurring (pathologic) fractures (Engelbert. et al., 2004). It occurs in two main forms: a severe autosomal dominant form that is recognized at birth (osteogenesis imperfecta type 1) and an autosomal recessive form that occurs later in life (osteogenesis imperfecta type 3).

Children with type 1 disease are born with countless fractures already present from the force of birth. They develop many more fractures during childhood. Radiographs reveal a particular ribbon-like or mosaic pattern in bones, which aids in diagnosis. The sclera of the eye is unusually blue because of poor connective tissue formation. Children with the type 3 form may have associated deafness and dental deformities. In both instances, the major clinical manifestation is a tendency for bones to fracture easily because of poor collagen formation. In some children, the bones are so fragile that fracture results not only from trauma, such as a fall, but from simple walking.

As the child grows older, the multiple breaks tend to cause limb and spinal column deformities, interfering with alignment or growth. A number of therapies, such as growth hormone to stimulate growth, calcitonin to aid bone healing, and bisphosphonates (e.g., pamidronate) to increase bone mass, may be prescribed, although no therapy is curative (Robinson et al., 2004). Parents need to protect children from trauma; fractures need to be aligned and casted; and children need to be educated about a lifestyle that is productive yet minimizes the risk of trauma. Lightweight leg braces or intermedullary rods may be effective to strengthen bones.

Always be careful when caring for a child with this disorder. Be sure to raise side rails on cribs or beds. Keep floors dry, and remove objects that could cause falls. Always lift children gently and avoid lifting them by a single arm or leg, to avoid placing strain on a bone.

Legg-Calvé-Perthes Disease (Coxa Plana)

Legg-Calvé-Perthes disease is avascular necrosis of the proximal femoral epiphysis. Although the cause is not proven, the condition is associated with incomplete clotting factors (Balasa et al., 2004). The disorder occurs more often in boys than in girls and has a peak incidence between 4 and 8 years of age. It usually occurs unilaterally but may occur bilaterally.

The child notices pain in the hip joint accompanied by spasm and limited motion. Radiographic studies are used to distinguish between Legg-Calvé-Perthes disease and simple synovitis (inflammation of the hip joint), which begins with the same symptoms. Radiographic changes may not be apparent when a child is first seen, but they appear after about 3 weeks. For this reason, most children seen for synovitis of the hip joint are asked to return in 3 weeks for a repeat film.

Children with Legg-Calvé-Perthes disease pass through four stages. First is the synovitis stage, or period of painful inflammation. Next is a necrotic stage, during which bone in the femur head becomes smaller and shows increased density on radiography. This stage lasts 6 to 12 months. The third stage is a fragmentation stage; resorption of dead bone occurs over a 1- to 2-year period. The fourth stage, a reconstruction stage, marks final healing, with deposition of new bone.

Treatment for Legg-Calvé-Perthes disease focuses on pain reduction with NSAIDs and on keeping the head of the femur within the acetabulum, which acts as a mold to preserve the shape of the femoral head and maintain range of motion.

Initially, rest is used to reduce inflammation and restore motion. To keep the head of the femur correctly positioned within the acetabulum, "containment" devices, such as abduction braces, casts, or leather harness slings, or weight-bearing devices, such as abduction ambulation braces or casts (after bed rest and traction), may be used.

A reconstructive surgery technique (an osteotomy to center the femur head in the acetabulum followed by cast application) also may be used. This technique returns the child to normal activity within 3 to 4 months (Herring et al., 2004).

Parents and children need thorough education about treatment and care, because most of it occurs on an ambulatory basis. Be sure parents understand the need for a containment device. Without the apparatus, the femur head tends to remold in a mushroom shape, making the hip unstable thereafter. Because this shape does not conform well to the acetabulum, degenerative changes may occur later in life, leading to chronic pain, reduced mobility of the hip joint, and possibly permanent disability.

It can be difficult for children to accept the extended treatment period involved with this disorder. Be certain that parents and children both understand the long-term consequences. In addition, parents may need assistance with devising appropriate activities for the child during treatment, because of the presence of the device and the limited weight bearing allowed.

Osgood-Schlatter Disease

Osgood-Schlatter disease is thickening and enlargement of the tibial tuberosity resulting from microtrauma. Children notice pain and swelling over the tibia tubercle. The pain is aggravated by running and squatting. This tends to occur in early adolescence or preadolescence in children who are athletic, probably because of rapid growth at these times (Bloom & Mackler, 2004).

Therapy depends on the extent of the bone changes. Administration of NSAIDs, ice, and limiting strenuous physical exercise may be all that is necessary. Occasionally, immobilization of the leg in a walking cast or immobilizer for about 6 weeks may be required.

Slipped Capital Femoral Epiphysis

Slipped epiphysis (coxa vera) is, as the name implies, a slipping of the femur head in relation to the neck of the femur at the epiphyseal line. The proximal femoral head displaces posteriorly and inferiorly. The cartilage covering the femur head may be destroyed by necrosis, resulting in permanent loss of motion of the femoral head. An avascular necrosis similar to that observed in Legg-Calvé-Perthes disease may occur. With both complications, surgical reconstruction of the hip joint is necessary.

This disorder occurs most frequently in preadolescence. It is twice as frequent in young African Americans as in children of other races, and twice as frequent in boys as in girls. It is more common in obese or rapidly growing children. This suggests that it occurs due to the influence of growth hormone and excessive weight bearing in the preadolescent child.

The onset of symptoms is gradual. On inspection, children often are observed to be limping and holding their leg externally rotated to relieve stress and pain in the hip joint. They may report pain first in the knee, because favoring the hip joint puts abnormal stress on the knee. On physical examination, internal rotation of the hip is difficult and painful. Radiographs reveal the slipped epiphysis at the femoral head.

Early detection is important, because correction is easiest if it is attempted before the condition has progressed to epiphyseal destruction. Surgery with pinning or external fixation, such as with skeletal traction, is used to stabilize the femur head. After surgery, the child may have activity restrictions or be confined to bed. Because the disease is most common in preadolescence, these children need continued support. Help them to understand the potential seriousness of the condition. Although they may not like being restricted or confined in this way, supportive communication and education can help them accept this treatment as necessary to maintain good healing and function of the hip joint. Encourage frequent visits and telephone calls with friends to provide optimal growth and development.

Although this condition usually is unilateral, a number of affected children later develop the same condition in the opposite hip. All children with a slipped epiphysis, therefore, need follow-up care, with careful attention to the condition of the opposite hip.

What if... Jeffrey's parents report that he has been waking up at night because of "growing pains"? Is there such a thing?

INFECTIOUS AND INFLAMMATORY DISORDERS OF THE BONES AND JOINTS

All bone infections are potentially dangerous because bones have rich blood supplies, so infection can easily spread and become septicemia.

Osteomyelitis

Osteomyelitis is infection of the bone. It is most often caused by *Staphylococcus aureus* in older children and by *Streptococcus pyogenes* in younger children. Children with sickle cell anemia have a special susceptibility to *Salmonella* invasion in long bones. Organisms are carried to the bone site by septicemia (blood infection). Osteomyelitis may occur after extensive impetigo, burns, or something as simple as a furuncle (skin abscess). It also may occur directly by outside invasion from a penetrating wound, open fracture, or contamination during surgery (Chalom, 2003).

Osteomyelitis begins typically as a metaphyseal infection, because the blood supply is sluggish in that portion of the bone. An abscess forms and spreads along the shaft of the bone under the periosteum, possibly extending to and penetrating the bone marrow. Sinuses may form between the marrow and the periosteum, or between the infected bone and the skin above. If the epiphyseal plate is infected, altered bone growth may result.

Assessment

Osteomyelitis usually begins with acute symptoms. Children show systemic malaise, fever, and irritability. They may have sharp pain at the bone metaphysis. By the second day, the area of skin over the infected bone feels warm to the touch; edema is present. Edema reduces the blood supply to vast expanses of bone, causing death of bone tissue. This dead bone tissue, which appears dense on radiographs, is called **sequestrum.**

Blood studies reveal an increased white blood cell count, C-reactive protein level, and sedimentation rate; blood culture results usually are positive. Radiographs may not reveal bone changes (formation of sequestrum) until 5 to 10 days after the beginning of the infection. Computed tomography may demonstrate early-stage bone changes. Some children with osteomyelitis are not seen at health care facilities as soon as they should be, because parents account for the pain as "growing pains." Children with systemic symptoms, such as fever, malaise, and joint pain, must be evaluated carefully so that developing osteomyelitis, if present, can be detected early.

Therapeutic Management

Medical therapy includes limitation of weight bearing on the affected part, bed rest, immobilization, and administration of an IV antibiotic such as oxacillin (Bactocill), as indicated by the blood culture. This therapy is usually initiated in the hospital and then continued at home for as long as 2 weeks; often an intermittent infusion device or peripherally inserted central catheter is used. After this, the child will be prescribed an oral antibiotic for 3 to 4 more weeks.

If pus forms under the periosteum, it may be aspirated using a technique similar to bone marrow aspiration. After the procedure, a tube may be inserted into the area for instillation of an antibiotic solution. A drainage tube may be inserted and attached to suction to evacuate the subperiosteum area.

For a child younger than 2 years of age, Bryant's traction is used (see Figure 51.6). For the older child with a fractured femur, skeletal traction with a pin through the distal femur is used. After muscle spasm has been reduced enough to allow close approximation of the bone edges and callus formation is good (7 to 14 days), the child is removed from traction and placed in a hip spica cast. A young child will remain in the cast for an additional 3 to 4 weeks. For older children, healing of a fractured femur requires an extended time. In a child who is 12 years old, firm union of the bone fragments takes about 12 weeks. Help the child and family identify ways for the child to continue school work and contact with friends if he or she is unable to attend school because of the large cast during this time.

Dislocation of the Radial Head

If a small child is lifted by one hand, as happens when a parent pulls on one arm to lift the child over a curb or up a step, the head of the radius may escape the ligament surrounding it and become dislocated (nursemaid's elbow). The child holds the arm flexed at the elbow with the forearm pronated. The child winces with pain when the radial head is palpated.

A simple dislocation of the radial head can be reduced by a physician, using gentle pressure on the radial head while the arm is flexed and supinated. Relief of pain is immediate, and the child begins to use the arm again.

Reassure the parent that this is a common injury in small children. Parents feel guilty because they caused this dislocation. They rarely need to be cautioned that lifting a child in this manner is not wise. Be aware, however, that a dislocation of the radial head can occur from extremely rough handling, as is seen in child abuse. Investigate the circumstances of the injury closely.

Checkpoint Question 5

Why is casting an elbow a potentially dangerous type of cast application?

a. It prevents the ulna and radius from continuing to grow.
b. Edema at the elbow can cause permanent nerve damage.
c. Holding the arm bent at the elbow causes low-grade pain.
d. These casts get dirty and so lead to humeral osteomyelitis.

Athletic Injuries

Although participating in athletics promotes growth and development, it can also lead to injury. Playing on backyard trampolines, in particular, is a dangerous sport for children (Black & Amadeo, 2003). Strategies to prevent sports injuries include preparticipation health examinations; medical coverage at sporting events; proper coaching; adequate hydration; proper officiating; and proper equipment and field or surface playing conditions (Adirim & Cheng, 2003).

Knee Injuries

Participation in sports such as football, skiing, soccer, and track are frequent causes of knee injuries in children. These injuries usually involve the ligaments surrounding the knee—the medial, lateral, posterior, or cruciate ligaments (figure-eight ligaments that stabilize the knee). After the injury, the child has severe pain in the knee with localized edema. A radiograph will be taken to rule out fracture.

If the injury is mild (only a few torn fibers), bed rest with ice applied to the knee is often the only therapy needed. Local infiltration of an anesthetic may be necessary to minimize pain. After 24 hours, heat is applied to the knee to hasten healing.

If the injury is more severe, the knee joint may fill with fluid. The child will need bed rest and ice applied to the joint. The abnormal synovial fluid will be aspirated, and a compression dressing will be applied to discourage accumulation of further fluid. After 24 hours, heat treatments will be started to hasten healing.

If the injury is severe, a cast may be applied for complete immobilization. It takes as long for a severe ligament injury to heal as it does for a bone fracture, so the cast will remain in place for about 8 weeks. Arthroscopy may be done to visualize and surgically repair the knee ligaments. Arthroscopic surgery makes repair of ligaments or cartilage a minor procedure and limits the necessity for immobilization and a cast.

A severe twisting motion to the knee can cause a dislocation of the kneecap (it moves to the posterior surface of the knee). The knee appears deformed, and the child is in acute pain (Fithian et al., 2004). Immediate treatment for a dislocated kneecap is to slide it again to the front of the knee. After this realignment, the child usually has to use a leg immobilizer for 1 week. If the problem is chronic or occurs frequently, surgery to strengthen the ligaments may be necessary. Quadriceps exercises (straight-leg raising) are important to prevent the dislocation from occurring again.

Throwing Injuries

Throwing places repeated stress on an upper extremity, particularly the elbow joint. The injury tends to occur during the forward motion of the arm or during the follow-through. After the injury, the child is unable to extend the elbow completely because of minute tears and fibrous contractures in the muscle. The child notices pain and tenderness and has loss of complete elbow extension for 24 to 48 hours after the injury. Resting the arm and applying ice packs for 15 to 20 minutes three times a day relieves the pain. An anti-inflammatory agent may be helpful. A limited number of cortisone injections into the elbow musculature may be helpful. Exercises to strengthen flexor muscles help to prevent this type of injury.

"Little Leaguer's elbow" is epiphysitis of the medial epicondylar epiphysis. Throwing curve balls and breaking pitches increases the stress in this area because of the forceful flexion and pronation required. A radiograph of the elbow may reveal increased growth, separation, and fragmentation of the medial epicondylar epiphysis. Children usually need extra protection against injury until the epiphyseal growth centers at the elbow have fused at 14 to 17 years of age (Hutchinson & Wynn, 2004).

Children who participate in Little League sports need time for proper warm-up. They should be encouraged to refrain from throwing curve balls or breaking pitches and should be limited to pitching about six innings per week with a 3-day rest between games. Treatment for Little Leaguer's elbow is rest and immobilization until pain, tenderness, and limitation of movement have passed. If the injury is not treated adequately, permanent damage to the epiphyseal line and elbow deformity can occur.

Strains and Sprains

A **strain** is a muscle-tendon injury. A **sprain** is a ligament injury. Strained or sprained ankles are common but difficult childhood injuries. The joint is painful and swollen. They are typical injuries that occur with inline skating or snow- or skateboarding. When the radiograph reveals no fracture, the child may feel as though someone has said that the injury is not serious but "just a sprain." He or she finds the extent of the swelling and pain baffling. Some children may be accused by parents of "putting on" pain, because the injury is "only a sprain."

Help the child and parents to understand that strains and sprains are truly painful. Because a cast is not used and the ankle is not immobilized completely, strains and sprains can be more painful than fractures, which are casted.

If the injury is recent, an ice pack should be applied for approximately 20 minutes at a time to reduce edema at the site. An elastic bandage may be applied for firm support. The child may be given crutches to limit weight bearing for the next 3 or 4 days. Make certain that the parents of the child understand how the elastic bandage is applied so that it can be rewrapped if it loosens, and be sure that the child is using the crutches properly before being discharged from the emergency department.

Key Points

Bone and muscle disorders tend to be long-term disorders. Help children and their families to think about how the disorder will affect tasks of daily living, to help a child better adjust to interventions such as a cast or brace. Help children plan self-diversional activities as necessary, so they continue to grow developmentally while confined to a cast or traction.

As a rule, children with a broken bone need additional calcium in their diet to aid bone healing. If they are on strict bed rest, however, this should only be a moderate addition to their diet, to prevent renal calculi from forming.

Many children have casts applied to allow broken bones to heal. If broken bones are not easily aligned, children are placed in traction.

Developmental disorders that occur in children include flat feet (pronation), genu varum (bowlegs), and genu valgum (knock knees). The majority of these disorders are corrected naturally by normal growth.

Slipped epiphysis is slipping of the femur head in relation to the neck of the femur at the epiphyseal line. It occurs most frequently in obese or rapidly growing boys.

Osteomyelitis is infection of the bone. It can result in extensive destruction of the bone. Antibiotic therapy is necessary to combat the infection.

Scoliosis is a lateral curvature of the spine. It is treated by bracing or surgery.

Juvenile arthritis (JA) occurs in a number of different forms: polyarticular, pauciarticular, and systemic onset. Therapy includes exercise, heat application, and administration of medications such as NSAIDs or methotrexate.

Myasthenia gravis can occur in three types: neonatal transient myasthenia, congenital myasthenia, and juvenile myasthenia. Anticholinesterase drugs (e.g., neostigmine), which prolong acetylcholine action, are used.

Muscular dystrophies are a group of disorders that lead to progressive degeneration of skeletal muscles. Different types can occur, including congenital myotonic, facioscapulohumeral, and pseudohypertrophic. Children and parents need support throughout this long-term illness.

A fracture or bruise of soft tissue can result from any trauma, including child abuse. Be certain to secure a detailed history of an injury, to be sure that the history is consistent with the degree of injury.

Volkmann's ischemic contracture is a complication that occurs when an arm is casted in a bent position and the radial artery and nerve are compressed at the elbow. Frequent assessments of finger color and warmth are safeguards to prevent this from occurring.

Critical Thinking Exercises

1. Jeffrey is the 13-year-old boy with osteomyelitis you met at the beginning of the chapter. How would you explain to his mother what has happened to him?
2. Jeffrey is required to wear a brace 23 hours a day for treatment of scoliosis. During the last month, he dropped out of the school band and the one after-school club to which he belonged. He tells you he is dropping activities "to have more time to study." Would you be concerned about him? What areas would you need to assess, and how would you intervene?
3. Jeffrey's sister has juvenile arthritis. You notice when she returns for a follow-up visit to the arthritis clinic that the inflammation in her joints is worse than at

her last visit, and she says she has more pain. Her mother tells you she has been giving her acetaminophen instead of her prescribed NSAID because she read that NSAIDs cause stomach irritation and heart disease. Was she wise to substitute another medication this way? How would you suggest she proceed at this point?

4. Examine the National Health Goals related to musculoskeletal disorders in children. Most government-sponsored money for nursing research is allotted based on these goals. What would be a possible research topic to explore pertinent to these goals that would be applicable to Jeffrey's family and also advance evidence-based practice?

References

Abi Daoud, M. S., Dooley, J. M., & Gordon, K. E. (2004). Depression in parents of children with Duchenne muscular dystrophy. *Pediatric Neurology, 31*(1), 16–19.

Adirim, T. A., & Cheng, T. L. (2003). Overview of injuries in the young athlete. *Sports Medicine, 33*(1), 75–81.

Amato, A. A. (2004). Neuromuscular junction disorders and myopathies. In Samuels, M. A., *Manual of neurologic therapeutics* (7th ed.). Philadelphia: Lippincott Williams & Wilkins.

Andrews, P. I. (2004). Autoimmune myasthenia gravis in childhood. *Seminars in Neurology, 24*(1), 101–110.

Auh, J. S., Binns, H. J., & Katz, B. Z. (2004). Retrospective assessment of subacute or chronic osteomyelitis in children and young adults. *Clinical Pediatrics, 43*(6), 549–555.

Balasa, V. V., et al. (2004). Legg-Calve-Perthes disease and thrombophilia. *Journal of Bone and Joint Surgery, 86A*(12), 2642–2647.

Berrington de Gonzalez, A., & Darby, S. (2004). Risk of cancer from diagnostic X-rays: Estimates for the UK and 14 other countries. *Lancet, 363*(9406), 345–351.

Betz, R. R., et al. (2004). Acute evaluation and management of pediatric spinal cord injury. *Journal of Spinal Cord Medicine, 27*(Suppl. 1), S11–S15.

Black, G. B., & Amadeo, R. (2003). Orthopedic injuries associated with backyard trampoline use in children. *Canadian Journal of Surgery, 46*(3), 199–201.

Bloom, O. J., & Mackler, L. (2004). What is the best treatment for Osgood-Schlatter disease? *The Journal of Family Practice, 53*(2), 153–156.

Chalom, E. C. (2003). Osteomyelitis. In Schwartz, M. W. (Ed.), *5-minute pediatric consult* (3rd ed.). Philadelphia: Lippincott Williams & Wilkins.

Chen, C. S., Roberton, D., & Hammerton, M. E. (2004). Juvenile arthritis-associated uveitis: Visual outcomes and prognosis. *Canadian Journal of Ophthalmology, 39*(6), 614–620.

Christian, C. W. (2003). Child abuse—physical. In Schwartz, M. W. (Ed.), *5-minute pediatric consult* (3rd ed.). Philadelphia: Lippincott Williams & Wilkins.

Cron, R. Q. (2003). Synovitis—transient. In Schwartz, M. W. (Ed.), *5-minute pediatric consult* (3rd ed.). Philadelphia: Lippincott Williams & Wilkins.

Department of Health and Human Services. (2000). *Healthy people 2010.* Washington, D.C.: DHHS.

Dormans, J. P. (2003a). Intoeing—tibial torsion. In Schwartz, M. W. (Ed.), *5-minute pediatric consult* (3rd ed.). Philadelphia: Lippincott Williams & Wilkins.

Dormans, J. P. (2003b). Scoliosis. In Schwartz, M. W. (Ed.), *5-minute pediatric consult* (3rd ed.). Philadelphia: Lippincott Williams & Wilkins.

Dudek, S. G. (2005). *Nutrition handbook for nursing practice* (5th ed.). Philadelphia: Lippincott Williams & Wilkins.

Engelbert, R. H., et al. (2004). Osteogenesis imperfecta in childhood: Impairment and disability. *Archives of Physical Medicine and Rehabilitation, 85*(5), 772–778.

Evans, A. M., & Scutter, S. D. (2004). Prevalence of "growing pains" in young children. *Journal of Pediatrics, 145*(2), 255–258.

Fithian, D. C., et al. (2004). Epidemiology and natural history of acute patellar dislocation. *American Journal of Sports Medicine, 32*(5), 1114–1121.

Flynn, A. (2003). The role of dietary calcium in bone health. *Proceedings of the Nutrition Society, 62*(4), 851–858.

Flynn, J. M., & Schwend, R. M. (2004). Management of pediatric femoral shaft fractures. *Journal of the American Academy of Orthopaedic Surgeons, 12*(5), 347–359.

Gajdos, P., Chevret, S., & Toyka, K. (2005). Intravenous immunoglobulin for myasthenia gravis. *The Cochrane Library (Oxford) (2)* (CD002277).

Hamer, A. J. (2004). ABCs of rheumatology: pain in the hip and knee. *British Medical Journal, 328*(7447), 1067–1069.

Herring, J. A., Kim, H. T., & Browne, R. (2004). Legg-Calve-Perthes disease: Prospective multicenter study of the effect of treatment on outcome. *Journal of Bone and Joint Surgery, 86A*(10), 2121–2134.

Hutchinson, M. R., & Wynn, S. (2004). Biomechanics and development of the elbow in the young throwing athlete. *Clinics in Sports Medicine, 23*(4), 531–544.

Karch, A. M. (2004). *Lippincott's nursing drug guide.* Philadelphia: Lippincott Williams & Wilkins.

Kimura, M., et al. (2004). Eight- to 14-year followup of arthroscopic meniscal repair. *Clinical Orthopaedics and Related Research, 421*(4), 175–180.

Lehman, T. J., et al. (2004). Thalidomide for severe systemic onset juvenile rheumatoid arthritis: A multicenter study. *Journal of Pediatrics, 145*(6), 856–857.

Lovell, D. (2004). Biologic agents for the treatment of juvenile rheumatoid arthritis: Current status. *Paediatric Drugs, 6*(3), 137–146.

Luhmann, S. J., et al. (2004). Differentiation between septic arthritis and transient synovitis of the hip in children with clinical prediction algorithms. *Journal of Bone and Joint Surgery, 86A*(5), 956–962.

Mehta, J. A., & Bain, G. I. (2004). Elbow dislocations in adults and children. *Clinics in Sports Medicine, 23*(4), 609–627.

Rajaram, S. S., et al. (2004). Some children with growing pains may actually have restless legs syndrome. *Sleep, 27*(4), 767–773.

Ramachandran, M., Utukuri, M., & Hill, R. (2003). Spot the diagnosis. Recurrent Blount's disease. *Journal of Postgraduate Medicine, 49*(4), 324–327.

Robinson, R. E., et al. (2004). Effectiveness of pretreatment in decreasing adverse events associated with pamidronate in children and adolescents. *Pharmacotherapy, 24*(2), 195–197.

Thorarensen, O. (2003). Muscular dystrophies. In Schwartz, M. W. (Ed.), *5-minute pediatric consult* (3rd ed.). Philadelphia: Lippincott Williams & Wilkins.

Ugwonali, O. F., et al. (2004). Effect of bracing on the quality of life of adolescents with idiopathic scoliosis. *Spine Journal: Official Journal of the North American Spine Society, 4*(3), 254–260.

Wazeka, A. N., DiMaio, M. F., & Boachie-Adjei, O. (2004). Outcome of pediatric patients with severe restrictive lung disease following reconstructive spine surgery. *Spine, 29*(5), 528–534.

Wise, C. M. (2004). Polymyositis/dermatomyositis. In Dambro, M. R. (Ed.). *Griffith's 5-minute clinical consult.* Philadelphia: Lippincott Williams & Wilkins.

Suggested Readings

Brown, J. C., et al. (2003). Emergency department analgesia for fracture pain. *Annals of Emergency Medicine, 42*(2), 197–205.

Cain, E. L., Jr., et al. (2003). Elbow injuries in throwing athletes: a current concepts review. *American Journal of Sports Medicine, 31*(4), 621–635.

Calmbach, W. L., & Hutchens, M. (2003). Evaluation of patients presenting with knee pain: Differential diagnosis. *American Family Physician, 68*(5), 917–922.

Duffy, C. M. (2004). Health outcomes in pediatric rheumatic diseases. *Current Opinion in Rheumatology, 16*(2), 102–108.

LaMontagne, L. L., et al. (2004). Adolescents' coping with surgery for scoliosis: Effects on recovery outcomes over time. *Research in Nursing and Health, 27*(4), 237–253.

Palermo, T. M., et al. (2004). Juvenile idiopathic arthritis: Parent-child discrepancy on reports of pain and disability. *Journal of Rheumatology, 31*(9), 1840–1846.

Powell, E. C., & Tanz, R. R. (2004). Incidence and description of scooter-related injuries among children. *Ambulatory Pediatrics, 4*(6), 495–499.

Simon, T. D., Bublitz, C., & Hambidge, S. J. (2004). External causes of pediatric injury-related emergency department visits in the United States. *Academic Emergency Medicine, 11*(10), 1042–1048.

Stuart, M. J. (2005). Managing and preventing ice hockey injuries. *Journal of Musculoskeletal Medicine, 22*(1), 37–44.

Taitz, J., Moran, K., & O'Meara, M. (2004). Long bone fractures in children under 3 years of age: Is abuse being missed in Emergency Department presentations? *Journal of Paediatrics and Child Health, 40*(4), 170–174.

CHAPTER 52

Nursing Care of the Child With a Traumatic Injury

Key Terms

allografting
autografting
contrecoup injury
débridement
drowning
escharotomy
heterografts
homografting
near drowning
otorrhea
plumbism
rhinorrhea
stupor

Objectives

After mastering the contents of this chapter, you should be able to:

1. Describe the causes and consequences of common accidents and injuries in childhood and measures to prevent them.
2. Assess a child who is traumatically injured from an accident.
3. Formulate nursing diagnoses related to a traumatically injured child.
4. Establish expected outcomes for a traumatically injured child.
5. Plan nursing care related to a traumatically injured child.
6. Implement nursing care for a child with a traumatic injury, such as providing pain relief.
7. Evaluate expected outcomes for achievement and effectiveness of nursing care.
8. Identify National Health Goals related to children who have experienced trauma that nurses can help the nation achieve.
9. Identify areas related to care of children with traumatic injuries that could benefit from additional nursing research or application of evidence-based practice.
10. Use critical thinking to analyze ways that care of children with traumatic injuries can be more family centered.
11. Integrate knowledge of traumatic injuries in childhood with nursing process to achieve quality maternal and child health care.

Jason, a 5-year-old boy, is seen in the emergency room after an automobile accident. He is crying and upset, although the only visible signs of trauma are a reddened and edematous area on the middle of his forehead. Vital signs reveal the following: temperature, 99.4°F (37.5°C); respirations, 18 breaths/ minute; pulse, 62 bpm; and blood pressure, 110/62 mm Hg. His left pupil is more dilated than his right; it reacts sluggishly to light. His Glasgow Coma score is 10. His mother tells you, "I'm sure he's not injured badly. He was wearing his seat belt."

Previous chapters described the growth and development of well children and care of children with disorders of specific body systems. This chapter adds information about the characteristic changes, both physical and psychosocial, that occur when children experience a traumatic injury. This is important information because it provides a base for care and health teaching.

You are the triage nurse. Would you rate Jason as a child to be seen immediately, or could he be given second priority?

After you've studied this chapter, access the accompanying website. Read the patient scenario and answer the questions to further sharpen your skills, grow more familiar with RN-CLEX types of questions, and reward yourself with how much you have learned.

Accidents, such as those involving motor vehicles, falls, burns, and water immersions, cause more deaths in the 1- to 4-year age group than the next six most prevalent causes combined. In the 15- to 24-year age group, they cause more deaths than all other combined causes (Gassner et al., 2004). If unintentional injuries could be prevented, therefore, a major cause of childhood morbidity and mortality would be eliminated. However, total accident elimination may not be possible. Children commonly believe that accidents will not happen to them and, as a result, fail to take sensible precautions against them. Some parents may predispose their children to accidents by overestimating their development and giving them responsibility beyond their capabilities.

The frequency of various types of accidents varies according to age group (Table 52.1). Because the anatomy and physiology of children are different from those of adults, they are not only involved in different types of accidents than adults, but they are affected by accidents differently.

Family stress plays a large role in childhood poisoning accidents because these types of accidents tend to occur when parents are preoccupied. Many accidental poisoning ingestions occur on the same day that the medicine was purchased, implying that the stress of family illness plays a major role. Eliminating accidents in children, therefore, is not a simple procedure, because it involves reducing family stress as well. National Health Goals related to children and trauma are shown in Box 52.1.

Nursing Process Overview

For Care of a Child With a Traumatic Injury

● *Assessment*

When children are seen at health care facilities because of traumatic injuries, neither they nor their parents may

BOX 52.1 FOCUS ON . . .

NATIONAL HEALTH GOALS

Because prevention of unintentional injuries could have immediate and long-term effects on the nation's health, a number of National Health Goals are concerned with preventing accidents and traumatic injuries in children:

- Reduce the number of drownings each year, from a baseline of 1.6/100,000 to 0.9/100,000.
- Reduce the rate of firearm-related deaths, from 11.3/100,000 to 4.1/100,000.
- Reduce the number of nonfatal poisonings, from 348/100,000 to 292/100,000.
- Reduce the number of deaths caused by suffocation, from 4/100,000 to 3/100,000.
- Reduce the rate of deaths caused by unintentional injury, from 36/100,000 to 17.5/100,000.
- Reduce the number of deaths caused by motor vehicle crashes, from 15.6/100,000 to 9.2/100,000.
- Increase the use of child safety restraints, from 92% to 100%.
- Increase the use of helmets by bicyclists.
- Reduce the number of residential fire deaths, from 1.2/100,000 to 0.2/100,000 (DHHS, 2000).

Nurses can help the nation achieve these goals by providing counseling on safety precautions to parents and children. Additional nursing research in these areas would be helpful: What are effective ways to communicate safety information to parents at well-child visits when time is at a premium? In what ways should safety teaching given after an accident to prevent a further accident be different from that given as primary prevention? Is there an association between children setting fires and their exposure to fire experiences with fireplaces or candles?

TABLE 52.1

Most Common Accidents in Children by Age Group

Age (yr)	Type of Accident
0–1	Falls, inhalation of foreign objects, poisoning, burns, drowning
2–4	Falls, drowning, motor vehicles, poisoning, burns
5–9	Motor vehicles, bicycle accidents, drowning, burns, firearms
10–14	Motor vehicles, drowning, burns, firearms, falls, bicycle accidents
15–18	Motor vehicles, drowning, firearms

National Center for Health Statistics. (2005). *Trends in the Health of Americans.* Hyattsville, MD: NCHS.

be functioning at their optimal level because of the stress of the situation. Both may be apprehensive and frightened not only about what *has* happened, but also about what could have happened. Children often feel guilty and fear that they will be scolded or punished. Their parents may feel equally guilty; for example, they may feel that if they were really "good" parents, they would have been watching more closely. They may feel defensive because they are worried about being criticized. People under stress do not hear well and may not perceive the information given to them correctly. Information they receive in the emergency department may be grossly misinterpreted or not heard at all.

Children are likely to be in pain. They are frightened not just from the pain of the injury but also from the circumstance of the injury. Children count on their parents to keep them safe, yet they have been hurt. The trust is broken momentarily. How can they be safe here if their parents no longer are protecting them?

Because the emergency department nurse is often the first person who sees a child after an injury, be ready to make a preliminary assessment of the extent of the child's injuries before a physician arrives. Remember that children may be seriously hurt but not crying because they are in shock. They may be hemorrhaging, but, if they are bleeding internally, the blood may not be visibly evident. Accidents become fatal when lung, heart, or brain function becomes inadequate. These three body systems, therefore, must be evaluated first. Table 52.2 lists signs and symptoms to assess when determining the respiratory, cardiovascular, and neurologic status of an injured child.

While conducting a preliminary assessment of a child's major body systems, take a brief history of the accident. What happened? How long ago did it happen? What have the parents done? If the child fell, how far did he or she fall? On what body part did the child land? (A head injury is more likely to be serious than an ankle injury, although a child may be in more pain and may have more obvious symptoms with the lesser injury.) Ask the parents what they think are their child's major injuries. Children may report one body part hurts at first, but then a small cut elsewhere begins to bleed, and they focus on the minor bleeding as their major injury. If parents say, "At first, he acted as if his stomach hurt," this may be the first suggestion that he has a serious abdominal injury such as splenic rupture.

Evaluating children in an emergency department is difficult, because they are so frightened that they cannot stop crying to report which body parts are painful or to indicate which parts should be assessed first. Spend a few minutes attempting to calm children and get them past this initial fright, unless symptoms of major body system disturbances require that you direct your immediate efforts elsewhere. Parents need frequent explanations of care given or planned, because as long as they are worried and tense, children cannot be calmed easily.

A proportion of traumatic injuries in children result from child abuse. Ask yourself if this could be a possibility (see Chapter 55).

● **Nursing Diagnosis**

The nursing diagnosis used most frequently with injured children is Pain. Depending on the particular injury, a number of other nursing diagnoses are relevant, as are those that relate to the suffering that parents experience when their child is injured. Examples of possible nursing diagnoses are the following:

- Ineffective airway clearance related to burned esophageal tissue
- Impaired physical mobility related to severe burn injury
- Disturbed body image related to change in physical appearance with thermal burns
- Parental fear related to outcome after head injury in child
- Interrupted family processes related to child's unintentional injury
- Anxiety related to apprehension and lack of knowledge regarding medical treatment of child

● **Outcome Identification and Planning**

Parents in an emergency department are rarely ready for long-term planning. They have great difficulty in coming up with answers even to the most straightforward questions. Therefore, long-term planning may have to be delayed until the immediate concern of the injury has passed.

On discharge from the emergency department, parents need printed instructions about the child's care at home and the name and number of the person to call if they have questions about care or progress. They also need an appointment (or the number to call for a return appointment) for follow-up care. If the child is admitted to the hospital from the emergency department, it is helpful if the nurse who cared for the child in the emergency department can accompany him or her to the hospital unit. The first person who cares for a child after an injury become very important to the child and parents, because that person was the first one to recognize their distress. Parents have difficulty letting them go and accepting new caregivers. A transition period, a "passing on of care," helps a parent to accept

---

TABLE 52.2

Important Assessments on Initial Examination of an Injured Child

Body System	Assessment
Respiratory system	Quality of respirations
	Rate of respirations
	Sound of obstruction (wheezing, stridor, retractions, coughing?)
	Color (cyanotic?)
	Oxygen hunger (restlessness, inability to lie flat?)
Cardiovascular system	Color (pallor from hemorrhage or cardiovascular collapse?)
	Gross bleeding
	Pulse rate (increases with hemorrhage)
	Blood pressure (decreases with hemorrhage)
	Feeling of apprehension from altered vascular pressure
Nervous system	Level of consciousness (child answers questions coherently, infant attunes to parent's voice?)
	Pupils (equal and reacting to light?)
	Bumps or bruises on head or spinal column
	Loss of motion or sensory function in a body part

the child's new caregivers as being as dependable and trustworthy as the emergency department staff.

● *Implementation*

The extent of a child's injury depends on the injuring agent, the part of the body that was injured, and often the immediate care, including both physical and psychological management, that the child received.

The diameter of the airway in children is smaller than in adults, so an injury to this body area almost always results in a greater danger of airway closure than in adults. This could happen from the child's inhaling a substance, such as water, that directly obstructs the airway or from inhaling toxic fumes that cause inflammation along the lining of the airway, resulting in obstruction. A blow to the neck can result in edema of surrounding tissues, causing the airway to close.

Most injuries involve some blood loss. Fortunately, a child's circulatory system is capable of rapid compensation for blood loss by vasoconstriction. Because the total volume of blood in a child is reduced, however, blood loss in children is always potentially serious.

Often, in the emergency department, large portions of the child's body must be exposed to view so that care can be given easily. This means that rapid cooling can occur. Because of the large body surface area of children in relation to weight, always be conscious of body temperature and take active measures to decrease cooling by keeping the child covered as much as possible during examination times.

Standard precautions are maintained in emergency situations, the same as at any other time. Parental consent must be obtained for treatment procedures even in an emergency, except for life-saving actions, such as cardiopulmonary resuscitation procedures. In these instances, action can and should be taken to save the child's life with or without parental permission (it is assumed that parents would consent to life-saving procedures). Delaying emergency procedures until parents can be located may result in permanent disability or death.

A key component of nursing intervention in an emergency department is to help parents understand why an injury happened and plan ways to make their immediate or community environment safe for children. An organization that might be appropriate for referral is the American Association of Poison Control Centers (*www.aapcc.org*).

● *Outcome Evaluation*

After an injury, children need follow-up care to be certain that the immediate interventions were adequate and that healing is taking place. Evaluation visits are also the time to determine whether the child's environment has been changed and is safer now than at the time of the accident (if applicable). At the time of the accident, parents may have been too anxious to hear health supervision information. Now, with the accident behind them, they are ready for such information and prepared to make changes.

If an injury could not have been anticipated, parents appreciate hearing one more time that such an accident could not have been avoided and that they are good parents. This helps them maintain adequate self-esteem to continue to function well as parents.

Examples of expected outcomes suggesting achievement are the following:

• Child swallows fluids without distress after esophageal burns.
• Child states pain is at tolerable level within 30 minutes.
• Child demonstrates full range of motion in hand after thermal injury.

HEALTH PROMOTION AND RISK MANAGEMENT

In every care setting, nurses have the unique opportunity among health care professionals to provide child and family teaching concerning the prevention of accidents. Even in the acute care setting when an accident has already occurred, nurses can provide valuable instruction to families about safeguarding their children against future accidents. In a community setting, nurses have a great opportunity for assessment of the unique threats that are present in particular environments (e.g., lead-based paint or kerosene heaters in older homes, risk of drowning in a home with an unfenced swimming pool, the danger for children riding in the back of pickup trucks). Nurses need to be knowledgeable about the interventions to be used and the measures to prevent injury.

Poisoning is an important cause of serious injuries in children younger than 6 years of age; more than 1 million episodes occur every year (Demorest et al., 2004). Common household agents are often the cause. Since passage of the Poison Prevention Packaging Act of 1970, potentially hazardous products must be sold in child-resistant containers. Passage of this act initiated a decrease in the incidence of childhood poisonings from common medicines.

The home environment may still contain products that can be hazardous and poisonous to children if handled improperly. Plants, cosmetics, and cleaning products can be dangerous to children if ingested or absorbed through the skin. Teach parents to be aware of these dangers and of strategies for maintaining a safe home environment, including learning basic first aid procedures.

Measures for a safe home environment include actions such as installing child-resistant locks on low cabinets where household products are stored, moving plants to a higher surface or removing them from the home until the child is older, keeping matches in safe places, and teaching street safety. In addition, parents should anticipate that, even in the safest environment, a child can be injured. Along with knowledge of basic first aid, the phone number of the local poison control center should be posted by the phone.

HEAD TRAUMA

Children receive head injuries when they are involved in multiple-trauma accidents, such as automobile accidents.

Falls from swing sets, porches, and bunk beds also cause many head injuries. Other children are injured by being struck on the head by an object, such as a baseball, rock, or hockey puck, or by falling from a bicycle (Adelson et al., 2003).

Head injuries are serious not only because they cause an immediate threat to the life of the child, but also because a number of complications may follow. With a depressed skull fracture, for example, recurrent seizures can occur. Many of these children show focal abnormalities on an electroencephalogram (EEG) due to scar tissue formation. A number of children with seizure involvement have normal EEGs, however, so, by itself, the EEG is of limited value in predicting whether posttraumatic seizures will occur.

Some children experience memory deficits or minor personality changes after head injury (Thompson & Irby, 2003). Symptoms such as headache, irritability, and postural vertigo (sensation of faintness or an inability to maintain normal balance—also known as posttrauma syndrome) also may occur. Behavioral manifestations may include aggressiveness or poor school performance. It often is difficult to determine whether these symptoms are organic or the result of being treated differently than usual by anxious parents.

Immediate Assessment

All children with head trauma require a neurologic assessment as soon as they are seen and again at frequent intervals to detect signs and symptoms of increased intracranial pressure (ICP). Increasing pressure puts stress on the respiratory, cardiac, and temperature centers, causing dysfunction in these areas. With increased pressure, the pupils become slow or unable to react immediately. Level of consciousness and motor ability decrease, pulse and respiratory rates decrease, and temperature and pulse pressure increase.

Assess vital signs to detect these changes and observe children's pupils to be certain that they are equal and react to light. Assess children's level of consciousness and motor function. Stabilize the neck with a brace until cervical trauma has been ruled out.

Immediate Management

After a head injury, brain edema is likely because fluid rushes into the inflamed and bruised area. Both central venous and central arterial lines may be inserted. ICP monitoring may be initiated (see Chapter 49). A computed tomography (CT) scan or magnetic resonance imaging (MRI) will be ordered to determine areas of edema or bleeding. An attempt may be made to decrease brain edema by intravenous (IV) administration of a hypertonic solution, such as mannitol. This will increase intravascular pressure and shift the edema fluid back into the blood vessels. Steroids such as dexamethasone may be added to decrease inflammation and edema. Keeping the head elevated is also effective in reducing ICP.

NURSING DIAGNOSES AND RELATED INTERVENTIONS

Nursing Diagnosis: Risk for excess fluid volume related to administration of hypertonic solution

Outcome Evaluation: The child's respiratory rate remains between 16 to 24 breaths/minute; specific gravity of urine is between 1.003 and 1.030; pulse remains between 60 to 100 bpm; blood pressure remains consistent for age group; lungs are clear to auscultation.

When hypertonic solutions are being infused into children, assess vital signs frequently to be certain that the fluid load being pulled into the intravascular system does not overtax it. This fluid must be excreted by the kidneys to keep the vascular system from becoming overloaded. Keep accurate intake and output records to ensure that the kidneys are functioning, and test the specific gravity of urine to detect the development of pituitary compression and resultant overproduction or underproduction of antidiuretic hormone from the posterior pituitary.

Nursing Diagnosis: Risk for delayed growth and development related to late sequelae of head injury

Outcome Evaluation: Child shows no evidence of any alteration in thought processes, seizure activity, or memory at follow-up visits. Cognitive and physical development are appropriate for age.

Helping care for a child with a head injury can be difficult for parents because they are so worried. Offer information on the child's progress as it becomes available to you. Urge parents to help care for the child to increase their sense of control.

During the acute phase of illness, ensure that parents are informed about the dangers of increased ICP. If they ask about the possibility that personality changes or seizures will develop later in life, their questions should be answered truthfully. At the same time, do not give unnecessary warnings about observing the child carefully in the months to come. Head injuries by themselves are worrisome enough to parents and children without adding to their burden.

Skull Fracture

A skull fracture is a crack in the bone of the skull (Gassner et al., 2004). Recognizing skull fractures in children is important, because associated cerebral injury often occurs under the fracture. Many skull fractures are simple linear types, most often involving the parietal bones. In some children, the skull does not fracture, but the suture lines

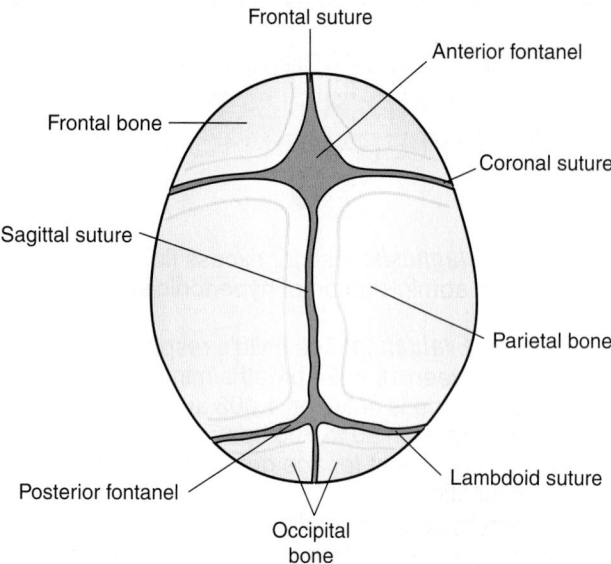

FIGURE 52.1 Location of suture lines of the skull.

separate. This occurs more commonly in the lambdoid suture line; a coronal suture separation is rare and, if present, indicates severe trauma (Fig. 52.1).

Assessment

If the base of the skull is fractured, a child usually exhibits orbital or postauricular ecchymosis. **Rhinorrhea** or **otorrhea** (clear fluid draining from the nose or ear, respectively) may be present. This is escaping cerebrospinal fluid (CSF)—a serious finding, because it means that the child's central nervous system is open to infection. Test the fluid discharge with a glucose reagent strip if there is doubt about the source of the drainage. CSF will test positive for glucose, whereas the clear, watery drainage from an upper respiratory tract infection will not.

Skull fractures are confirmed by skull radiography. Take a careful history of the accident, so that the strength of the blow to the head can be judged. Shock with hypotension rarely occurs with an isolated head injury. If a child is in shock, investigate for bleeding points other than the head injury.

If a skull fracture is linear with no underlying pathology, no treatment except observation and prescription of an analgesic is necessary. In about 3 weeks, a repeat radiograph will be needed to confirm that healing has taken place. Parents can be reassured that a second radiograph this soon is not harmful but necessary.

If a fracture is depressed (a bone fragment is pressing inward) or compounded (bone is broken into pieces), surgery will be necessary to remove or repair broken fragments. Cranial surgery is discussed in Chapter 49.

Therapeutic Management

If CSF is draining from the nose, the child will be admitted for observation. Keep him in a semi-Fowler's position so that fluid drains out, not inward, to reduce the possibility of introducing infection. Make certain that children do not attempt to hold their nose or pack their nostrils with some-

thing to halt the drainage. Because coughing and sneezing may allow air to enter the meningeal space, coughing may be suppressed by medication. If the drainage is excoriating to the upper lip, coat the space with petrolatum. Children may be prescribed a prophylactic antibiotic to reduce the risk for meningitis. If the drainage does not stop within a few days, surgery will be necessary to repair the fracture and reduce the danger of meningitis. Air that enters intracranial spaces usually is absorbed rapidly. If radiographs at 72 hours still show air in the cerebral spaces, it implies that a skull defect remains, and surgery may be indicated to close the defect.

Potential Complications

A long-term complication of even a linear fracture may be a *leptomeningeal cyst.* This results from projection of the arachnoid membrane into the fracture site. With the interfering tissue, bone cannot heal and actually erodes, so that the fracture site becomes progressively larger, not smaller. This becomes evident on a follow-up radiograph. It may be suspected if a child develops focal seizures or symptoms of increased ICP. The defect may be palpated on the skull as an underlying indentation. Surgical resection is necessary to remove the cyst.

Subdural Hematoma

Subdural hematoma is venous bleeding into the space between the dura and the arachnoid membrane (Fig. 52.2*A*). It occurs when head trauma lacerates minute veins in this area (Whitby et al., 2004). The collection of blood is usually bilateral.

Subdural hematomas tend to occur in infants more often than in older children. Symptoms may occur within 3 days or as late as 20 days after trauma. Infants usually have symptoms of increased ICP. Seizures, vomiting, hyperirritability, and enlargement of the head may occur. Anemia caused by the substantial blood loss is a prominent sign. Angiography or sonography reveals the extent of the hematoma.

In infants, accumulated subdural blood may be removed by a subdural puncture through the lateral aspect of a patent anterior fontanelle. The procedure is similar to a lumbar puncture. Infants receive conscious sedation or must be held extremely still during the procedure so that they do not move and cause the aspiration needle to be inserted incorrectly. Without conscious sedation, half of the success of subdural puncture depends on the ability to hold the child still.

Subdural punctures may need to be repeated daily to empty the subdural space. Once the space is empty, expanding brain tissue will naturally occlude it. If the space has not been occluded after 2 weeks of daily punctures, active bleeding is still present, and surgery usually is necessary to reduce the space and halt bleeding.

In older children, surgery usually is necessary, because the anterior fontanelle is closed and the space cannot be reached by puncture.

Epidural Hematoma

Epidural hematoma is bleeding into the space between the dura and the skull (Fig. 52.2*B*). This happens when head

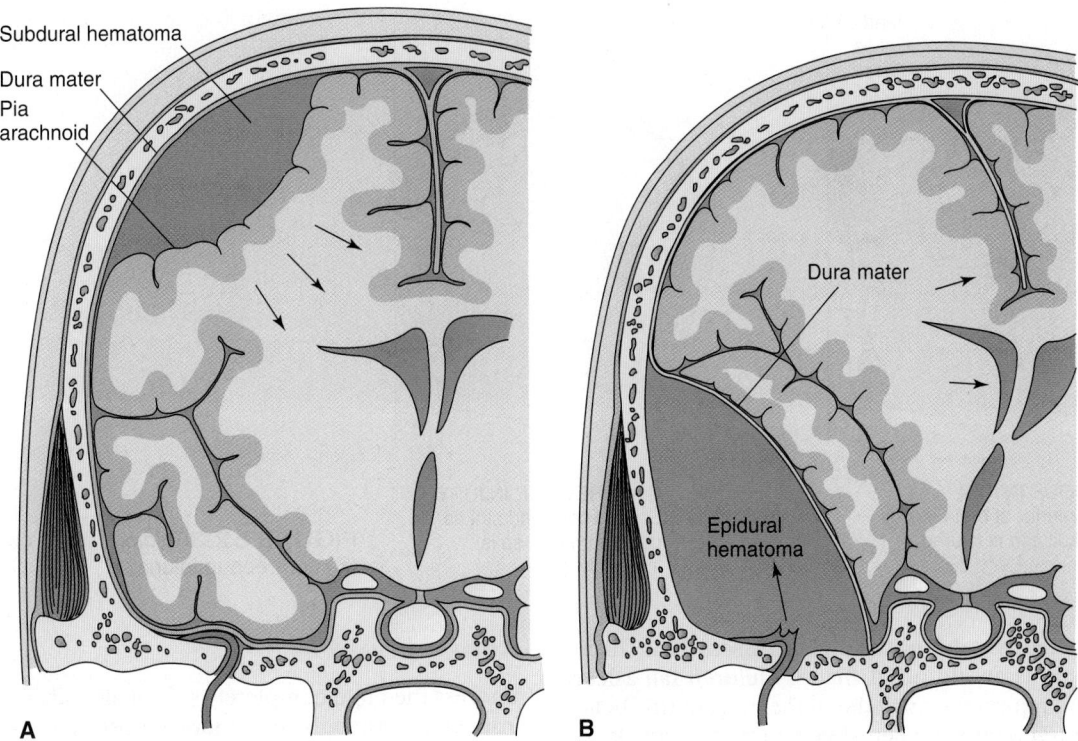

FIGURE 52.2 (A) Subdural hematoma. The dark area in the upper left area of the drawing is the hematoma. Note the shift of structures. **(B)** Epidural hematoma. The dark area in the lower left area of the drawing is the hematoma. Note the broken blood vessel and the shift of midline structures.

trauma is severe. Subdural hemorrhage is usually venous bleeding, but epidural hemorrhage is usually a result of rupture of the middle meningeal artery and is, therefore, arterial bleeding. It usually is intense and causes rapid brain compression.

At the time of the injury, children become momentarily unconscious. They then regain consciousness and, to the untrained eye, appear to be well for minutes or hours. Then signs of cortical compression—vomiting, loss of consciousness, headache, seizures, or hemiparesis (paralysis on one side)—are observed. On physical examination, unequal dilation or constriction of the pupils may be present. Decorticate posturing (see Chapter 49) may be seen, indicating extreme pressure on upper cortical centers. If the pressure is allowed to continue unchecked, cortical compression may be so great that brainstem, respiratory, or cardiovascular function is impaired.

As a rule, the closer to the time of the injury that symptoms of compression occur, the more extreme is the amount of blood loss. The treatment is surgical removal of the accumulated blood and cauterization or ligation of the torn artery. The earlier the process is recognized and treated, the less the chance of residual damage from extreme pressure or anoxia to the involved portion of the brain.

Concussion

Concussion is defined as temporary and immediate impairment of neurologic function caused by a hard, jarring shock (Willer et al., 2004). It may occur on the side of the skull that was struck (a *coup injury*) or on the opposite side of the brain (a **contrecoup injury;** Fig. 52.3). As the brain recoils from the force of the blow and strikes the posterior surface of the skull, this second injury occurs. Children have at least a transient loss of consciousness at the time of the injury. They may vomit and may show irritability after regaining consciousness. They typically have no memory (amnesia) of the events leading up to the injury or of the injury itself. For some children, being asked questions about the accident is extremely upsetting because they do not remember anything that happened and feel a frightening loss of control. The child requires a skull radiograph, to rule out skull fracture, and observation for 24 hours, to rule out severe brain trauma, edema, or laceration. The child usually can be observed at home by the parents, who are instructed to rouse him or her every 1 to 2 hours while awake to check the level of consciousness. Parents usually are instructed not to keep waking children during the night, because multiple wakings are disorienting and can be confused with unconsciousness. Parents should wake the child at least once during the night, however, and assess that the pulse rate is greater than 60 bpm.

To be certain that children are alert, parents can ask them to name a familiar object, such as a favorite toy, or to name the color of some object shown to them. Telling parents their name or where they live is equally revealing.

Give parents the telephone number to call if they have any questions about their child's care. Advise them to call if their child's behavior changes in any way that makes them suspicious. Many parents need to set an alarm clock

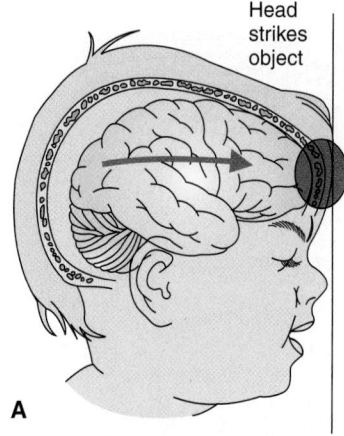

A

COUP INJURY
Anterior of brain strikes
skull and is injured

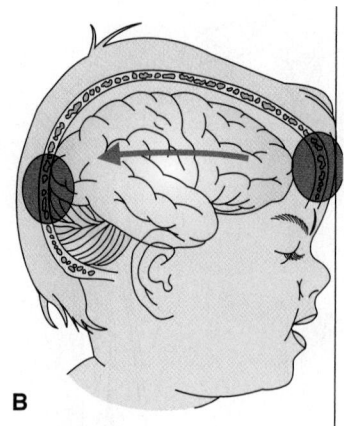

B

CONTRECOUP INJURY
Brain recoils and strikes
posterior skull, so is
injured twice

FIGURE 52.3 Etiology of (**A**) coup and (**B**) contrecoup injuries.

to wake themselves during the night to assess their child's status. There is an old belief that, if children fall asleep after a head injury, they will die in their sleep; this belief causes some parents to keep shaking children awake or making them walk continually. Be certain they understand that it is all right for children to sleep, but they must wake them at least once to assess their status (Box 52.2).

Contusion

A brain contusion occurs when there is tearing or laceration of brain tissue (Fig. 52.4). The symptoms are the same as for concussion but more severe. In addition, there are specific symptoms related to the lacerated brain area (e.g., focal seizure, eye deviation, loss of speech). Surgery may be necessary to halt bleeding. The child's prognosis depends on the extent of the injury and effectiveness of therapy.

What if... In the emergency room, Jason's parents state that since his head injury he has been vomiting? Is it more likely that the vomiting is a result of the head injury, or that he has contracted a gastrointestinal infection?

Coma

Coma (unconsciousness from which a child cannot be roused) or **stupor** (grogginess from which a child can be roused) may be present in children after severe head trauma. Coma and stupor are both symptoms of underlying disorders; a history of the injury must be obtained so that treatment can be directed specifically toward the cause (Jay & Cowell, 2003).

Obtain a history to determine the circumstances immediately before the time the child became comatose. Assess children in coma carefully and completely, so that the cause of the decreased consciousness can quickly be determined.

Assessment

Undress the child completely so that all body parts can be inspected. Although head injury is most likely to be the underlying cause of coma or seizure, metabolic disturbances such as diabetes mellitus, dehydration, severe hemorrhage, or drug ingestion, also must be considered as possible causes. Count respirations and pulse and measure blood pressure to establish baseline values, because changes in these values often provide good clues. A child with increased ICP will show decreased pulse and respiratory rates and increased blood pressure. Diabetes leads to increased respirations. Hemorrhage leads to an increased pulse rate and decreased blood pressure. Drug ingestion may lead to increased or decreased measurements, depending on the drug ingested.

If bulbar (brainstem) compression is present, the child cannot swallow effectively or safely. If this is suspected, turn the child on one side to prevent aspiration. Observe the eyes for signs of increased ICP. If both pupils are dilated, irreversible brainstem damage is suggested, although such a finding may also be present with poisoning from an atropine-like drug. Pinpoint pupils suggest barbiturate or opiate intoxication. One pupil dilated more than the other suggests third cranial nerve compression. The eye may be deviated downward and laterally as well. This also may be caused by a tentorial tear (laceration of the membrane between the cerebellum and cerebrum) and herniation of the temporal lobe into the torn membrane. This situation requires immediate surgery to correct temporal compression.

The retina of the eye should be examined for papilledema, which will be present if increased pressure is longstanding (more than 24 to 48 hours). Lack of a doll's eye reflex suggests that compression of the oculomotor nerves (third, fourth, or sixth) or of the brainstem is involved. Observe for posturing, such as decerebrate posturing, which suggests cerebral compression and dysfunction.

Many laboratory studies are helpful in determining the cause of coma. Blood glucose, blood electrolytes, blood urea nitrogen (BUN), liver function tests, blood gas stud-

A Multidisciplinary Care Map for
A Child With a Concussion

●

Jason, a 5-year-old boy, is seen in the emergency room after an auto-mobile accident. His family is here on vacation. Child is crying and upset, although the only visible signs of trauma are a reddened and edematous area on the middle of his forehead. His twin sister, in a car seat beside him, was not injured. His mother tells you, "I'm sure he's not injured badly. He was wearing his seat belt."

Family Assessment

Child is staying with twin sister and two parents in motel room while on 10-day vacation. Father normally works as a salesman. Mother clerks in department store. Father describes finances as "good." Father concerned because rented car was totally destroyed in accident and his insurance may not cover this.

Client Assessment

Five-year-old male visibly upset and crying. Height and weight at 75th percentile for age. Child unable to report or recall anything about the incident. Mother reports he was restrained by a seat belt but not a car seat. Head hit side window when a car struck their vehicle.

Vital signs: temperature, 99.4°F (37.5°C); respirations, 18 breaths/minute; pulse, 62 bpm; and blood pressure, 110/62 mm Hg. Left pupil is more dilated than his right; it reacts sluggishly to light. Glasgow Coma score is 10. Alert enough to name toy racing car brought in with him. Pupils equal, round, reactive to light and accommodation bilaterally. 1.5-cm raised area noted on forehead. Skin intact without evidence of bleeding. Child cries when area is touched. Negative otorrhea or rhinorrhea. Small 2-cm abrasion noted on right knee; 3-cm abrasion noted on right hand. No other injuries noted. Able to move all extremities through range of motion.

A diagnosis of mild contrecoup concussion is made, and child is to be discharged to motel in parents' care.

Nursing Diagnosis

Risk for injury related to effects of concussion

Outcome Criteria

Child remains alert and oriented; easily arousable. Pupils equal, round, react to light and accommodation; vital signs within age-acceptable parameters; exhibits no signs or symptoms of neurologic dysfunction.

Team Member Responsible	Assessment	Intervention	Rationale	Expected Outcome
Activities of Daily Living				
Nurse	Take history of accident, speed car was traveling, and position of child in vehicle.	Assess child's vital signs, level of consciousness, and neurologic function initially, and then every 30 min until discharge.	Changes in vital signs, level of consciousness, or neurologic function indicate a worsening of the child's condition and possibly increasing intracranial pressure.	Parent describes accident and reactions of child since accident.

(continued)

Team Member Responsible	Assessment	Intervention	Rationale	Expected Outcome
Consultations				
N/A	N/A	N/A	N/A	N/A
Procedures/Medications				
Physician/ Nurse	Assess whether child's demeanor (crying) is from fright or pain.	Institute measures to calm the child. Encourage the parents to hold and reassure him.	Crying increases intracranial pressure. Involving the parents provides them with a concrete activity, helping to provide some sense of control over the situation.	Parents are able to calm child to allow for better evaluation of condition.
Physician/ Nurse	Assess whether child has had experience with x-ray examination.	Schedule a skull radiograph or other diagnostic tests as ordered, such as CT scan or MRI.	Skull radiograph rules out a possible skull fracture secondary to the trauma. CT scan or MRI helps determine any areas of bleeding or edema if present.	Child cooperates with diagnostic procedures; results are available for physician review.
Nutrition				
Nurse	Assess whether child has vomited since head injury.	If not NPO, feed small amount of a favorite food to be certain child does not have vomiting.	Vomiting is a symptom of increased intracranial pressure.	Child eats some food without vomiting.
Patient/Family Education				
Nurse	Assess what parents understand about concussion in children.	Teach parents how contrecoup injuries occur and symptoms they cause.	A contrecoup injury causes injury or edema to the posterior brain.	Parents state they understand why their child has posterior (eye control) cranial symptoms, such as unequal pupils.
Psychosocial/Spiritual/Emotional Needs				
Nurse	Assess whether child or parents have any questions about care.	Orient the child to his surroundings. Offer explanations about any treatments or procedures that are to come.	Children often have no memory of events with concussion. Parents are in strange community. Orientation and explanation help to minimize a child's fear of the unknown and of his situation.	Parents and child state they understand procedures being carried out. Voice confidence in new situation.
Nurse	Attempt to identify the meaning and effect of the child's accident for the parents (e.g., father upset over rent-a-car liability).	Encourage parents to express their feelings about themselves as parents and their role in the child's accident.	Identification of the meaning and effect of the child's accident assists in determining the degree to which the situation is affecting the parents.	Parents state they were not responsible for accident, or at least did everything possible to avoid their child's injury.

(continued)

Team Member Responsible	Assessment	Intervention	Rationale	Expected Outcome
Discharge Planning				
Nurse/ Physician	Assess whether parents will be staying in city or traveling back home during next 24 hr.	Instruct parents to rouse the child approximately every 2 hr during day-time hours and at least once during the night, asking the child to name a familiar object or color.	Frequent waking can be disorienting to a child and can be confused with altered levels of consciousness, but occasional waking is a good way to assess whether complications are occurring.	Parents state they will remain in motel for 24 hr, rather than fly home immediately, so they can observe child.
Nurse	Assess whether parents will be able to keep a follow-up appointment for additional care.	Schedule a return appointment to clinic for 24-hr follow-up visit. Supply clinic telephone number if needed before then.	A follow-up visit is necessary to be certain child can travel safely.	Parents state they understand importance of follow-up visit and will keep appointment with child.

ies, lumbar puncture, and toxicology tests may be ordered to rule out possible causes such as bacterial meningitis or hemorrhage.

Coma is usually graded according to a standard scale so that changes can be evaluated accurately. Figure 52.5 shows the Glasgow Coma Scale, a commonly used evaluation system (Jay & Cowell, 2003). Because this system was devised to be an adult assessment scale, it must be modified for use with children or infants (Worrall, 2004). Such a modification is shown in Box 52.3.

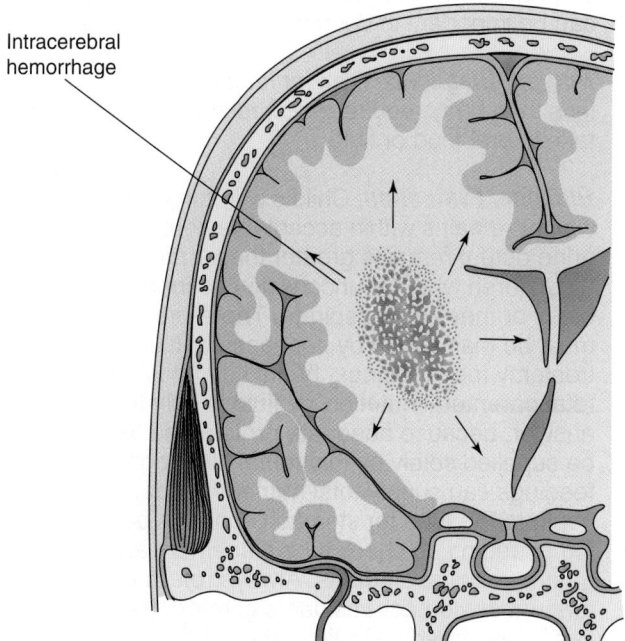

FIGURE 52.4 Intracerebral hemorrhage. The central large dark area represents the hemorrhage. Note the midline shift.

Intracerebral hemorrhage

A score of 3 to 8 suggests severe trauma (less than 5 carries a very severe prognosis); a score of 9 to 12, moderate trauma; and 13 to 15, slight trauma.

Therapeutic Management

If children are unconscious for longer than a transient period, they usually are admitted to an observation unit for further assessment. As a general rule, place a child who is comatose on the side to reduce the risk of aspiration. Oral suctioning to remove mucus from the mouth and pharynx may be necessary. If the child has acute signs of respiratory difficulty, endotracheal intubation or tracheostomy may be necessary to ensure respiratory function.

An IV route is established so that, when specific measures are needed (e.g., blood replacement, electrolyte replacement, fluid replacement), a route for immediate administration will be available. Blood will be drawn for a complete blood count, electrolyte determination, toxicology tests, and cross-matching. If the cause of the coma is unknown, a lumbar puncture and EEG may be done. Skull radiography, CT scan, or MRI may be done.

Lumbar puncture has little value at first in predicting the severity of a head injury, because any degree of cerebral contusion usually leads to increased CSF pressure. Lumbar puncture is contraindicated if increased ICP is present. Otherwise, brainstem compression can result. Obtain the child's vital signs and assess neurologic status, such as state of consciousness and the ability of pupils to react to light, every 15 to 20 minutes or as ordered. Accurately and carefully record this information so that a picture of gradual change will become apparent.

A child's prognosis after coma depends on the initial cause of the coma. If the increased ICP can be relieved before any permanent brain damage results, the effects of the coma will be transient. Prognosis is always guarded, however, because coma reflects a major health problem for a child.

Glasgow Coma Scale			A.M.			P.M.				A.M.					
Assessment	Reaction	Score	8	10	12	2	4	6	8	10	12	2	4	6	8
Eye Opening	Spontaneously	4	X						X	X	X	X	X		
Response	To speech	3		X				X							
	To pain	2			X	X	X								
	No response	1													
Motor Response	Obeys verbal command	6	X						X	X	X	X	X		
	Localizes pain	5		X	X										
	Flexion withdrawal	4				X		X							
	Flexion	3					X								
	Extension	2													
	No response	1													
Verbal Response	Oriented x3	5	X						X	X	X	X	X		
	Conversation confused	4		X				X							
	Inappropriate speech	3			X										
	Incomprehensible sounds	2				X	X								
	No response	1													

FIGURE 52.5 Glasgow Coma Scale scoring for a child. A score of 3 to 8 denotes severe trauma; 9 to 12, moderate trauma; 13 to 15, slight trauma. Notice the gradual improvement from coma in this example.

NURSING DIAGNOSES AND RELATED INTERVENTIONS

●

Care of the child in coma is directed toward maintaining body function in an optimal state until the child reawakens.

Nursing Diagnosis: Risk for ineffective airway clearance related to brainstem pressure

Outcome Evaluation: Child's respiratory rate remains between 16 and 20 breaths/minute; there are no retractions or signs of obstruction.

Some children who are comatose require endotracheal intubation or tracheostomy to ensure an open airway. Some are placed on mechanical ventilation. Oxygen may be prescribed if arterial blood gases reveal poor oxygenation of body cells (oxygen tension [Po_2] lower than 80 mm Hg). Endotracheal tubes are replaced with a tracheostomy after 3 or 4 days to prevent necrosis of the pharynx from pressure of the tube.

Nursing Diagnosis: Risk for impaired skin integrity related to lack of mobility

Outcome Evaluation: Child exhibits no areas of broken or irritated skin.

Bathe children who are comatose daily to stimulate skin circulation. Include the hair as part of the bath about every 3 days. Change their position at least every 2 hours to prevent pressure ulcer formation and development of hydrostatic pneumonia from pooled secretions. When turning, assess skin for reddened points. Keep linen dry and free from wrinkles. Perform thorough passive range-of-motion exercises to maintain muscle tone and prevent contractures. Use of a sheepskin, an egg-carton foam, or an alternating pressure or water mattress also can be important in decreasing pressure to the skin.

Nursing Diagnosis: Risk for imbalanced nutrition, less than body requirements, related to inability to take in oral food or fluid

Outcome Evaluation: Child's skin turgor is normal; weight remains within acceptable percentile; hourly urine output remains greater than 1 mL/kg.

Children who are unconscious cannot be fed orally or they might aspirate. Therefore, nutrition must be maintained by nasogastric (NG) or gastrostomy tube feedings, IV fluid administration, or total parenteral nutrition. IV fluid is only a short-term answer, because adequate protein and fat cannot be supplied solely by this route. NG or gastrostomy feedings can supply total nutrient needs. Always aspirate the tube for stomach contents before giving a feeding, to check tube placement and assess gastric residual amounts. Always return any amount of stomach residue aspirated, because if this is discarded each time, the child will lose a large amount of stomach acid, possibly leading to alkalosis. Check whether the amount of the feeding should be reduced by the amount of fluid remaining in the stomach before feeding the full amount of prescribed formula.

BOX 52.3

Scoring for Glasgow Coma Scale

Eye Opening

4. Child opens his or her eyes spontaneously when you approach.
3. Child opens his or her eyes in response to speech (spoken or shouted).
2. Child opens his or her eyes only in response to painful stimuli, such as pressure on a nail bed.
1. Child does not open his or her eyes in response to painful stimuli.

Motor Response

6. Child can obey a simple command such as "hand me a toy" (infant smiles or attunes).
5. Child moves an extremity to locate a painful stimulus applied to the head or trunk and attempts to remove the source.
4. Child attempts to withdraw from the source of pain.
3. Child flexes his or her arms at the elbows and wrists in response to painful stimuli to the nail beds (decorticate rigidity).
2. Child extends his or her arms (straightens the elbows) in response to painful stimuli (cerebrate rigidity).
1. Child has no motor response to pain on any extremity.

Verbal Response

5. Child is oriented to time, place, and person (child > 4 yr knows name, date, and where he or she is; infant appears to recognize parent).
4. Child is able to converse, although not oriented to time, place, or person (does not know who or where he or she is; infant says words but does not appear to differentiate parents from others).
3. Child speaks only in words or phrases that make little or no sense ("I want frazzle no"; infant's vocabulary is less than it is normally).
2. Child responds with incomprehensible sounds, such as groans.
1. Child does not respond verbally at all.

Modified from Teasdale, G., & Bennett, B. (1974). Assessment of coma and impaired consciousness: A practical scale. *Lancet, 2*(7872), 81–84.

Give mouth care at least twice daily with clear water and a padded tongue blade. Coat lips with petrolatum to prevent drying and cracking. If the child's eyes tend to dry, close them to prevent corneal ulceration. Artificial tears (methylcellulose) may be prescribed to keep eyes from drying until the child regains consciousness.

ABDOMINAL TRAUMA

When children are brought to a health care facility after suffering a multiple-injury trauma, several medical special-ists may be required: a neurosurgeon for consultation about a head injury; an orthopedic physician for consul-tation about a fractured extremity; and a thoracic surgeon to intubate or investigate lung trauma. A nurse may serve the important function of being the person who is best able to observe a total child and recognize subtle signs such as abdominal trauma.

Assessment

Abdominal trauma can result from any object striking the abdomen, such as a baseball bat or a seat belt drawing tight in a motor vehicle crash (Davies, 2004) (Box 52.4). Assess vital signs frequently until they are stable. Hypotension (less than 80 mm Hg systolic pressure in an older child; less than 60 mm Hg in an infant) usually suggests hemorrhage, which may be hidden abdominal bleeding. In addition, children may have increasing pallor and rapid respirations. If internal bleeding is present, blood pressure will show little improvement when IV fluid is administered.

If abdominal trauma is suspected, an NG tube is passed and stomach contents are aspirated to be checked visu-ally for blood and to test for occult blood. Attach the tube to low intermittent suction if the presence of blood is es-tablished. An indwelling urinary (Foley) catheter is also inserted to evaluate urine for blood and urine output. Evi-dence of blood in the urine or decreased output may in-dicate accompanying kidney or bladder trauma. If the urine contains blood, an emergency IV pyelogram may be

BOX 52.4 FOCUS ON . . .

EVIDENCE-BASED PRACTICE

When Children Use Seatbelts in Cars, Are They Still Ejected during Automobile Accidents?

To study this problem, a study was conducted of chil-dren who had been involved in severe car crashes in Canada. The results of the study showed that only 0.2% of 5.5 million children involved in crashes experi-enced ejection, but of the 6,570 child fatalities resulting from these crashes, 1,924 (29%) involved ejections. The researchers concluded that ejection from the vehi-cle is more common (29%) among fatally injured chil-dren than is usually believed. Shoulder straps alone (as found in T-shield or overhead shield child seats) may not prevent toddlers from being ejected from child safety seats during rollover accidents.

This is an important study for nurses, because it documents how seriously hurt children can be in auto-mobile accidents even with safety restraints in place. Many accidents happen within a 5-mile radius from home or occur while parents drive for short-term errands. Teaching parents to drive responsibly and not be distracted by children in the car could help avoid this type of accident.

Source: Howard, A., et al. (2003). Ejections of young children in motor vehicle crashes. *Journal of Trauma: Injury, Infection, and Critical Care, 55*(1), 126–129.

ordered. Be aware that having NG tubes or catheters passed is always frightening for a child (unsure of their anatomy, children have no clear idea where the tubes are going). After an accident, when they are already frightened, they and their parents need a great deal of support to accept these procedures (Box 52.5).

An abdominal radiograph or sonogram may be ordered to rule out a fractured pelvis, a condition that could contribute to blood loss. Air under the diaphragm on the radiograph suggests gastric or intestinal rupture with escape of air from these organs into the peritoneal cavity. Free fluid in the abdomen, shown on the radiograph when the child is turned on the side, suggests leakage of bowel fluid or splenic rupture and pooling of blood. If the radiograph does not suggest the source of the fluid, an abdominal paracentesis may be done. This procedure is very frightening to children, not only because it is intrusive, but also because their abdomen is likely to be tender. Parents may be so frightened by the sight of the procedure that they are unable to remain with their child while it is done. A nurse, therefore, needs to be present to offer support.

For a paracentesis, children are placed in a sitting or side-lying position; their abdomen is cleaned with an antiseptic and covered with a sterile drape. Caution children that they will feel a pinprick as a local anesthetic is inserted into their abdominal wall and pressure as the paracentesis needle is inserted. Appreciate children's concern. It is almost impossible for them to lie or sit still while the procedure is being done. Comments such as "Don't cry; be a good boy" are not therapeutic. "It's all right to cry; I know this is scary" is much more comforting and achieves better results, because it lets children know that you understand what you are asking of them.

Parents often find it difficult to appreciate the seriousness of abdominal trauma, because the signs are not as dramatic or obvious as those of fractured extremities or lacerations. Some parents may not bring their child to an emergency department immediately after abdominal trauma, because they are unaware that serious injury can result to this part of the body. Without frightening them, explain that an injury need not be obvious at first glance to be serious and need care. They may ask why an x-ray is necessary. When their child is asked to turn on the x-ray table so that an abdominal fluid level can be revealed, they may perceive this as unnecessary manipulation of an injured child.

NURSING DIAGNOSES AND RELATED INTERVENTIONS

———◆———

Nursing Diagnosis: Pain related to abdominal injury

Outcome Evaluation: Child states that level of pain is tolerable; child does not grimace when body parts are touched.

Routinely, analgesics are not administered to most children after abdominal trauma unless their

---

BOX 52.5 FOCUS ON . . .

COMMUNICATION

Jason, a 5-year-old boy, is brought to the emergency room after an automobile accident. He is being assessed for multiple trauma.

Less Effective Communication

Mr. Varton: Why are you looking at his belly? He didn't hurt that.

Nurse: We need to assess his entire body just to make sure that there aren't any problems. He's had major trauma. You need to sign a consent form so he can have a central intravenous line and indwelling urinary catheter inserted and a CT scan to rule out any problems.

Mr. Varton: I don't want to put him through any more. What if something else goes wrong?

Nurse: If you don't consent to these tests and treatments, we cannot take care of your child.

Mr. Varton: OK. Do what you have to. But I'm still not sure.

Nurse: Good. Sign this consent for me.

More Effective Communication

Mr. Varton: Why are you looking at his belly? He didn't hurt that.

Nurse: We need to assess his entire body just to make sure that there aren't any problems. He's had major trauma. You need to sign a consent form so he can have a central intravenous line and indwelling urinary catheter inserted and a CT scan to rule out any problems.

Mr. Varton: I don't want to put him through any more. What if something else goes wrong?

Nurse: I know it's difficult for you to see your child in such pain. Are you worried about anything specific?

Mr. Varton: Is he going to die?

Nurse: The things we're doing are aimed to prevent that very thing. Let me explain a little more about what we're doing and why these things are necessary. I want you to feel comfortable signing the consent form.

In the first scenario, the nurse focuses on obtaining the parent's consent but fails to recognize the fear and apprehension in the parent. In the second scenario, the nurse recognizes and attends to the fears of the parent. By doing so, she helps to establish a sense of support and trust in addition to obtaining consent for procedures.

pain is severe, to avoid masking the pain, so that the location of the pain can help identify which organs may be injured. If parents did not recognize that the child was injured, guilt and fear on their part may compound the problem. Goal setting is usually concerned with the immediate diagnostic procedures or anticipated surgery. Interventions differ according to the specific injury present.

Splenic Rupture

In children, the spleen is the most frequently injured organ in abdominal trauma, because it is usually palpable under the lower left ribs (Mooney & Forbes, 2004). It is frequently injured by inappropriately applied seat belts in automobiles and by handlebar injuries in bicycle accidents. Children with splenic injury have tenderness in the left upper quadrant, especially on deep inspiration, when the diaphragm moves down and touches the spleen. They may hold their left shoulder elevated, so that the diaphragm is raised on the left side, to keep this from happening. Occasionally, a child notices radiated left shoulder pain while lying in a supine position (Kehr's sign). A radiograph will show little about the spleen itself but may reveal a broken rib over the spleen, suggesting the extent of the trauma to that area. Fluid in the abdomen suggests bleeding from some source. Obtaining blood on abdominal paracentesis strongly suggests splenic rupture.

An IV line is started immediately for fluid replacement, and an IV pyelogram or MRI will be done to rule out damage to the left kidney, which, because of its location in that area, may also have suffered trauma. A complete blood count is done to estimate the extent of the blood loss. Blood is typed and cross-matched, so that blood for replacement can be readied if necessary. The child will be admitted to an observation unit if the blood loss from rupture appears to be mild. If bleeding is severe, immediate surgery, such as a partial or total splenectomy, may be necessary to halt bleeding and save the child's life.

After a splenectomy, children are very susceptible to infection, particularly pneumococcal infections. Therefore, a large percentage of children are managed expectantly to see if the bleeding will halt without spleen removal (Mooney & Forbes, 2004).

Liver Rupture

Livers are also more prone to rupture in children than in adults, because the liver, like the spleen, is not completely sheltered by the rib cage in children (Chun, 2003). Children with liver rupture or laceration usually have severe abdominal pain that is most marked on inspiration, when the diaphragm descends and touches the liver. They show symptoms of blood loss, including tachycardia, hypotension, anxiety, and pallor. The hematocrit will be low or falling. Such children need to be prepared for immediate surgery, because the liver is a highly vascular organ, and blood loss from it is acute and possibly life-threatening.

Occasionally, a communication between an artery and the bile duct occurs at the time of trauma. In this situation, symptoms are not immediate, but gastrointestinal (GI) bleeding, such as hematemesis or melena, may occur in a few days. The child may have colicky upper abdominal pain that is relieved by emesis. Liver studies, such as a liver arteriogram, are necessary to reveal the extent of the problem.

After either liver or spleen surgery, children need careful observation for return of bowel function, assessment for the possibility that peritonitis may develop, and careful reintroduction of oral nutrition.

DENTAL TRAUMA

Injuries to teeth occur most often from falls in which the child strikes the upper front incisors or from blows to the face by objects such as baseball bats or hockey sticks. They are always potentially serious, because they can lead to aspiration of the injured teeth or malalignment of future teeth. If a tooth is knocked out, parents should rinse the tooth in water, drop it in a salt solution or milk, and bring it to the emergency department with them (Corwell, 2003). If permanent teeth that have been knocked out recently can be washed with saline in the emergency department and replaced, there is a good chance that they will reimplant successfully. Some dentists advocate immersing the tooth in an antiseptic and then in an antibiotic solution before replacing it. If a tooth is replaced, it usually is wired into place to hold it in good alignment. The child receives a course of oral antibiotics, such as penicillin, to prevent infection. Only soft food must be eaten until the tooth has firmly adhered (approximately 2 weeks).

If a blow to a child's teeth was extensive, a radiograph may be taken to rule out a mandibular or maxillary fracture. If a portion of a tooth cannot be located, the possibility of aspiration must be considered and confirmed or ruled out by a chest radiograph. In young children, often a tooth is not knocked out but is pushed back up into the gum. These teeth gradually regrow, and, although they may darken in color, they usually are healthy. If the affected tooth is a deciduous tooth, the permanent tooth is rarely injured even though it is already formed in the gum. At the appropriate time, the permanent tooth will erupt normally.

NEAR DROWNING

Drowning is defined as death due to suffocation from submersion in liquid. Inhaled water fills the lungs and therefore blocks the exchange of oxygen in the alveoli. More than 3,500 children die from drowning annually. It is the second most common cause of death by unintentional injury among children (Turner, 2004). The term **near drowning** is used to describe the child with a submersion injury who requires emergency treatment and who survives the first 24 hours after injury.

Most infant drownings occur in bathtubs; 1- to 4-year-old children most frequently drown in artificial pools; older children most frequently drown in bodies of fresh water. The majority of drowning accidents that take place outside the home occur in the summer months, when more children are swimming and boating. Particularly at risk are male adolescents, because they may take dares to swim farther than their ability allows or may swim under the influence of alcohol, which impairs their decision-making ability and their physical coordination.

Pathophysiology of Drowning

When children's heads are submerged and they first inhale water, they cough violently from the irritation of the water in their nose and throat. If they cannot get their head out of water at this point, water will enter the larynx. This causes the larynx to spasm, preventing any further water but also air from entering the trachea, so asphyxia results. If a child is ventilated at this point, treatment usually is very effective because there is little water in the lungs. The condition more closely simulates asphyxia that occurs with croup or when a foreign body, such as a nut, lodges in the larynx and stops air flow.

If treatment is not given at this point, the larynx relaxes from the asphyxia and water enters the lungs. Oxygen can no longer be exchanged, because the alveoli fill with water. Hypoxia deepens, and cardiac arrest occurs.

Additional changes that occur when water enters the lungs depend on whether the water is fresh or salt. Salt water is hypertonic, causing fluid to osmose from the bloodstream and enter the alveoli, increasing the amount of fluid in the lung tissue and increasing hypoxia. Tachycardia and decreased blood pressure from hypovolemia result. Blood viscosity increases (increased hematocrit level).

Fresh water is hypotonic, so fluid in the lungs shifts into the bloodstream due to changes in osmotic pressure. This may lead to hemolysis of red blood cells, a dilution of plasma, and possibly hypervolemia with tachycardia and increased blood pressure. If the release of potassium from destroyed red blood cells is great enough with freshwater drowning, cardiac arrhythmias may occur. In both instances, loss of surfactant from the lung alveoli, caused by introduction of water, can lead to alveolar collapse (Shaw, 2003).

Parents should advocate for neighborhood pools to be fenced (Turner, 2004). Hyperventilating before swimming should be discouraged. When children blow off carbon dioxide this way, during an extended period of underwater swimming, carbon dioxide levels rise, but not adequately enough to cause them to experience distress. This results in decreased oxygen levels with drowsiness and listlessness (children drown without struggling or realizing their danger).

Very young children display a mammalian diving reflex when they plunge under cold water. Immediately, a life-saving bradycardia and shunting of blood away from the periphery of the body to the brain and heart occur. This is triggered when water is 70°F (21°C) or less and the face is submerged first. This explains why very young children can survive better than older children after being submerged in water that is very cold (32°F to 60°F [0°C to 15°C]).

Emergency Management

When a child is pulled from the water after near drowning, mouth-to-mouth resuscitation should be started at once. If cardiac arrest has occurred from hypoxia, simultaneous measures to initiate cardiac action must be taken. The technique of cardiopulmonary resuscitation for infants and children is discussed in Chapter 41.

Assuming that cardiopulmonary resuscitation is effective, the child needs follow-up care at a health care facility, because he or she is certain to be acidotic from accumulated carbon dioxide and hypoxia (resulting from lack of oxygen because of the water in the alveoli) and is at risk for respiratory infection from contaminants in the water.

Follow-up care aims to increase the child's oxygen and carbon dioxide exchange capacity, using the lung areas that are not filled with water. Typically, the child is intubated with a cuffed intratracheal tube; mechanical ventilation with positive end-expiratory pressure may be necessary to force air into the alveoli. Because water has been swallowed, vomiting usually occurs as the child is revived. The cuff of the intratracheal tube prevents vomitus from being aspirated. The child is given 100% oxygen so that as much space as possible in the available lung alveoli can be used. An NG tube is inserted to decompress the stomach, prevent vomiting, and free up breathing space. Usually, albuterol is administered by aerosol to prevent bronchospasm and, again, to allow the child to make maximum use of the oxygen administered. If the child aspirated salt water, plasma may be administered to replace protein being lost into the lungs and prevent hypovolemia.

If the child's body temperature is very low, gradual warming (not using a warming blanket) is advised so that the metabolic requirement does not rise sharply before alveolar space is ready to accommodate this need. Extracorporeal membrane oxygenation may be used.

Unfortunately, neurologic damage occurs in as many as 21% of near-drowning incidents. If the child is awake or only lethargic at the scene of the accident and immediately afterward in the hospital, the prognosis is greatly improved over that of the child who is comatose.

NURSING DIAGNOSES AND RELATED INTERVENTIONS

Nursing Diagnosis: Risk for infection related to foreign substance in respiratory tract

Outcome Evaluation: Child's temperature remains within normal parameters orally; rales are absent on lung auscultation; respiratory rate is within age-acceptable parameters.

The child may be prescribed prophylactic antibiotic therapy to prevent pneumonia and additional airway interference. Assess vital signs and auscultate lung sounds for adventitious sounds, such as rales or fine rhonchi. Turning the child every 2 hours if on bed rest and encouraging deep breathing and incentive spirometry every hour help to aerate the lungs fully and prevent the accumulation of fluid, which promotes infection.

Nursing Diagnosis: Fear related to near-drowning experience

Outcome Evaluation: Child discusses fears; child states that she understands that, although frightening, the experience is over, and she is now safe.

Children may be admitted to an observation unit for monitoring of blood gases until water from the alveoli is absorbed and they once again can ventilate effectively on their own. Children may wake at night from a nightmare that they are drowning. They need their parents to reassure them that they are now safe and definitely out of the water. Near drowning is a thoroughly frightening experience. Encourage children to verbalize this fright. They need support from parents before they engage in an activity such as swimming again after such a frightening experience.

POISONING

Poisoning occurs most commonly in children between the ages of 2 and 3 years and in all socioeconomic groups. Common agents in childhood poisoning include soaps, cosmetics, detergents or cleaners, and plants. Poisoning can occur from over-the-counter drugs, such as vitamins, iron compounds, aspirin, or acetaminophen, or from prescription drugs, such as antidepressants. Poisoning is entirely preventable. Parents need education about the high risk for poisoning and strategies for maintaining a home environment that is safe for children of all ages. Be aware that when poisoning occurs in an older child, it may be a suicide attempt.

NURSING DIAGNOSES AND RELATED INTERVENTIONS

Nursing Diagnosis: Risk for injury related to maturational age of child and presence of poisons

Outcome Evaluation: Parents identify poisonous and toxic items in the home and describe how they are stored safely; parents state local poison control center number; parents describe measures to seek help immediately if poisoning occurs.

Emergency Management of Poisoning at Home

The American Academy of Pediatrics (AAP) no longer recommends that parents keep syrup of ipecac on hand to administer if poisoning should occur (AAP, 2004). Instead, they should telephone their local poison control center to ask for advice. Information parents need to provide includes the following:

- Child's name, telephone number, address, weight, and age and what the child swallowed
- How long ago the poisoning occurred

- The route of poisoning (oral, inhaled, sprayed on skin)
- How much of the poison the child took. (This may be difficult for parents to judge if they do not know how much was in a bottle. If they just answer, "a whole bottle," ask them to read from the bottle how much that is.)
- If the poison was in pill form, whether there are pills scattered under a chair or if they are all missing and presumed swallowed
- What was swallowed; if the name of a medicine is not known, what it was prescribed for and a description of it (color, size, shape of pills)
- The child's present condition (e.g., sleepy, hyperactive, comatose)

If one child has swallowed a poison, parents should investigate whether other children have also poisoned themselves. A preschooler often gives a younger sibling some of the "candy" he or she has been eating. Ask if parents have transportation to the health care facility or if they need an ambulance.

Emergency Management of Poisoning at the Health Care Facility

In the emergency department, the best method to deactivate a poison is the administration of activated charcoal, either orally or by way of an NG tube.

Activated charcoal is supplied as a fine black powder that is mixed with water for administration. A sweet syrup may be added to the mixture to make it more palatable. As the charcoal is excreted through the bowel over the next 3 days, stools will appear black (Box 52.6).

BOX 52.6 FOCUS ON . . .

PHARMACOLOGY

Activated Charcoal

Classification: Activated charcoal is an antidote for poisoning.

Action: Absorbs toxic substances that have been swallowed to prevent them from being absorbed from the stomach (Karch, 2004)

Pregnancy Risk Category: C

Dosage: Provided as a powder that must be mixed with water and administered orally or by way of nasogastric (NG) tube.

Possible Adverse Effects: Vomiting, diarrhea, black stools

Nursing Implications
- Administer orally to conscious victims only.
- Give the drug as soon as possible after poisoning.
- Store the drug in a closed container, because it absorbs gases from the air and is inactivated.
- Know that the solution feels gritty and tastes disagreeable, so young children have difficulty swallowing the drug. May have to be administered by NG tube.
- Caution child or parent that stools will be black for several days after administration.

Always follow emergency measures to neutralize a poison with an education program for the family to prevent poisoning from happening again. Specific measures for each age group are discussed in previous chapters, along with problems and concerns of the age group.

Acetaminophen Poisoning

Acetaminophen (Tylenol) is the drug most frequently involved in childhood poisoning today, because parents use acetaminophen to treat childhood fevers. Told that acetaminophen is safer than aspirin, parents may not be as careful about putting this substance away as they were with aspirin. If their child swallows acetaminophen, they may delay bringing the child for help, thinking it is a harmless drug.

Acetaminophen in large doses, however, is not an innocent drug; it can cause extreme liver destruction (Losek, 2004). Immediately after ingestion, the child will experience anorexia, nausea, and vomiting. Soon, serum aspartate transaminase (AST [SGOT]) and serum alanine transaminase (ALT [SGPT]) liver enzymes become elevated. The liver may be tender as liver toxicity occurs.

Parents should call their local poison control center. In the emergency department, activated charcoal or acetylcysteine, the specific antidote for acetaminophen poisoning, will be administered. Acetylcysteine prevents hepatotoxicity by binding with the breakdown product of acetaminophen so that it will not bind to liver cells. Unfortunately, acetylcysteine has an offensive odor and taste. Administer it in a carbonated beverage to help the child swallow it. For small children, it is administered directly into an NG tube to avoid this difficulty. If the child is admitted to an observation unit, continue to observe for jaundice and tenderness over the liver; assess ALT and AST levels as ordered.

NURSING DIAGNOSES AND RELATED INTERVENTIONS

Nursing Diagnosis: Situational low self-esteem related to child's poisoning

Outcome Evaluation: Parents state guidelines for continued assessment of child at home; parents state ways they can improve "childproofing."

After the child is stabilized, take some time to talk with the parents about how they feel about this event. Remember that poisoning tends to happen in homes where there is stress. If stress was already present, how has this poisoning added to it?

Before a child is discharged from a health care facility, be certain the parents are comfortable with any further assessment measures they will need to continue at home, such as temperature taking and urging a high fluid intake. Talk with the parents about childproofing their home.

Checkpoint Question 1

You see Jason's sister in the emergency department after acetaminophen poisoning. Which of the following would be an appropriate action to take?

a. Advise the parents that their child must never receive acetaminophen again.
b. Counsel the parents about not taking medications in front of children.
c. Question an order to give activated charcoal to neutralize the drug.
d. Sympathize with parents, but reassure them this poisoning is not serious.

Caustic Poisoning

Ingestion of a strong alkali, such as lye, which is often contained in toilet bowl cleaners or hair care products, may cause burns and tissue necrosis in the mouth, esophagus, and stomach. It is important that the parents do not try to make a child vomit after ingestion of these substances, because they can cause additional burning as they are vomited (LoVecchio, 2003).

Assessment

After a caustic ingestion, the child has immediate pain in the mouth and throat and drools saliva because of oral edema and an inability to swallow. The mouth turns white immediately from the burn. Later, the mouth turns brown as edema and ulceration occur. There may be such marked edema of the lips and mouth that it is difficult to examine them. The child may immediately vomit blood, mucus, and necrotic tissue. The loss of blood from the denuded, burned surface may lead to systemic signs of tachycardia, tachypnea, pallor, and hypotension.

A chest radiograph may be ordered to determine whether pulmonary involvement has occurred from any aspirated poison or whether an esophageal perforation has allowed poison to seep into the mediastinum. An esophagoscopy under conscious sedation may be done to assess the esophagus, although this test may be omitted because of the possibility that an esophagoscope might perforate the burned esophagus. After 2 weeks, a barium swallow may be ordered to reveal the final extent of the esophageal burns.

Therapeutic Management

When parents whose child has ingested a caustic substance call a poison control center to ask for advice on how to proceed, they will be advised to immediately take the child to a health care facility for treatment.

There is a high possibility that pharyngeal edema will be severe enough to obstruct the child's airway by even 20 minutes after the burn. Intubation may be necessary to provide a patent airway.

To detect respiratory interference, assess vital signs closely, especially the respiratory rate. In infants, increasing restlessness is an important accompanying sign of oxygen want. Assess the child for the degree of pain involved. A strong analgesic, such as morphine, may need to be ordered and administered to achieve pain relief.

NURSING DIAGNOSES AND RELATED INTERVENTIONS

———•———

Nursing Diagnosis: Risk for ineffective airway clearance related to burns of esophagus and mouth

Outcome Evaluation: Child's respiration rate will remain within 16 to 20 breaths/minute.

Starting therapy immediately with a steroid such as dexamethasone (Decadron) and continuing it for about 4 weeks may be prescribed to reduce the chance of permanent esophageal scarring. In addition, children may be prescribed a prophylactic antibiotic to reduce the possibility of infection and additional inflammation in the denuded mouth and esophageal area.

Children who respond well to steroid therapy usually recover with no important sequelae. Children who do not receive steroid therapy for some reason may be left with scarring of the esophagus, resulting in complete obstruction. To correct complete obstruction, repeated surgical procedures are necessary. Sometimes transplantation of intestinal tissue or a synthetic graft is required to replace stenosed esophageal tissue.

Nursing Diagnosis: Risk for imbalanced nutrition, less than body requirements, related to esophageal stricture from burn scarring

Outcome Evaluation: Child's diet meets recommended daily allowance requirements for age.

Oral intake commonly will be a problem for the first week because of soreness in the child's mouth. Observe the child carefully the first time he drinks to observe for signs, such as coughing, choking, and cyanosis, that are indicative of esophageal stenosis or perforation. IV fluid may be needed as a supplement. If the child is totally unable to swallow, gastrostomy feedings or total parenteral nutrition may be necessary. After the child is able to take food, he should begin with a liquid diet. Liquid passing through the burned and scarring esophagus tends to maintain esophageal patency, so it is therapeutic for the burn as well as nutritious for the child.

Hydrocarbon Ingestion

Hydrocarbons are substances contained in products such as kerosene and furniture polish. Because these substances are volatile, fumes rise from them, and their major effect is respiratory irritation (see Chapter 40).

Iron Poisoning

Iron is frequently swallowed by small children because it is an ingredient in vitamin preparations, particularly pregnancy vitamins. When it is ingested, it is corrosive to the gastric mucosa and leads to the signs and symptoms of gastric irritation (Black & Zenel, 2003). The immediate effects include nausea and vomiting, diarrhea, and abdominal pain. After 6 hours, these symptoms fade, and the child's condition appears to improve. By this time, however, hemorrhagic necrosis of the lining of the GI tract has occurred. By 12 hours, melena (blood in stool) and hematemesis (blood in emesis) are present. Lethargy and coma, cyanosis, and vasomotor collapse may occur. Coagulation defects may occur, and hepatic injury also can result. Shock resulting from an increase in peripheral vascular resistance and decreased cardiac output can occur. Long-term effects can include gastric scarring from fibrotic tissue formation.

Assessment

It is difficult to estimate the amount of iron a child has swallowed, because parents can only guess at the number of pills in the bottle. In addition, the amount of elemental iron in compounds varies. The child's serum iron level should be measured to establish a baseline.

Therapeutic Management

Parents should contact their poison control center. In the emergency room, stomach lavage will be done to remove any pills not yet absorbed. A cathartic may be given to help the child pass enteric-coated iron pills. Activated charcoal is not given, because it is not effective at neutralizing iron.

A child who has ingested a potentially toxic dose will be given a chelating agent, such as IV or intramuscular (IM) deferoxamine. Chelating agents combine with metals and allow them to be excreted from the body. Deferoxamine causes urine to turn orange as iron is excreted.

An exchange transfusion is another way that excess iron can be removed from the body. An upper GI radiographic series and liver studies may be ordered 1 week after the ingestion to screen for long-term effects. The hope is that the iron load was removed from the stomach in time so that not all of it was absorbed.

Assist with emergency measures, such as gastric lavage, and administer chelating agents as ordered. Parents may be asked to test any stool passed for the next 3 days for occult blood, to assess for stomach irritation and subsequent GI bleeding. Be certain that parents understand how to do this accurately.

NURSING DIAGNOSES AND RELATED INTERVENTIONS

———•———

Nursing Diagnosis: Deficient parental knowledge related to the danger of iron as a poison

Outcome Evaluation: Parents state ways they have safeguarded their child from future iron exposure.

Iron poisoning occurs frequently because parents do not think of iron pills or vitamins containing iron as real medicine. Additionally, because many children's vitamins are manufactured in the shapes of familiar television or cartoon characters, children often think of vitamins as candy.

When you instruct parents to use an iron supplement for themselves or their children, stress that overdoses can be fatal to small children. Teach them to think of iron as they would any other medicine and keep it out of the reach of small children.

Lead Poisoning

Lead in the body interferes with red blood cell function by blocking the incorporation of iron into the protoporphyrin compound that makes up the heme portion of hemoglobin in red blood cells (Feingold & Anderson, 2004). This leads to a hypochromic, microcytic anemia. Kidney destruction may occur, causing excess excretion of amino acids, glucose, and phosphates in the urine. The most serious effect, however, is lead encephalitis: inflammation of brain cells due to the toxic lead content. Lead poisoning (**plumbism**), like all forms of poisoning in children, tends to occur most often in the toddler or preschool child. (See Chapter 29 for measures to prevent lead poisoning.)

Assessment

The usual sources of ingested lead are paint chips or paint dust, home-glazed pottery, or fumes from burning or swallowed batteries (Bekhof et al., 2004). Paint tastes sweet, and a child will repeatedly pick chips up off the floor or off the walls. If a crib rail is painted with lead paint, a child will ingest it as he or she teethes on the rail. Chewing on windowsills is also common. In fishing communities, swallowing lead sinkers can be a common source. Restoring an older home saturates the air with lead dust. In such homes, lead plumbing also may contaminate the drinking water.

The most widely used method of screening for lead levels is the blood lead determination (serum ferritin). Unfortunately, this test requires the use of atomic absorption spectrophotometry, which is a costly procedure. The free erythrocyte protoporphyrin test is a simple screening procedure that involves only a fingerstick. Because protoporphyrin is blocked from entering heme by the lead, it will be elevated in a child with lead poisoning.

Many children with fairly high blood lead levels are asymptomatic. Others show insidious symptoms of anorexia and abdominal pain caused by the presence of lead in the stomach. Children with encephalopathy usually have beginning symptoms of lethargy, impulsiveness, and learning difficulties. As the child's blood level of lead increases,

severe encephalopathy with seizures and permanent neurologic damage will result.

Basophilic stippling (an odd striation of basophils) may be apparent on a blood smear. A radiograph of the abdomen may reveal paint chips in the intestinal tract (Fig. 52.6*A*). "Lead lines" (areas of increased density) may be present near the epiphyseal line of long bones (see Fig. 52.6*B*). The thickness of the line shows the length of time lead ingestion has been occurring (Gandhi et al., 2003). Damage to the kidney nephrons from the presence of lead leads to proteinuria, ketonuria, and glycosuria. The CSF may have an increased protein level. Lead poisoning is usually said to be present when the child has two successive blood lead levels greater than

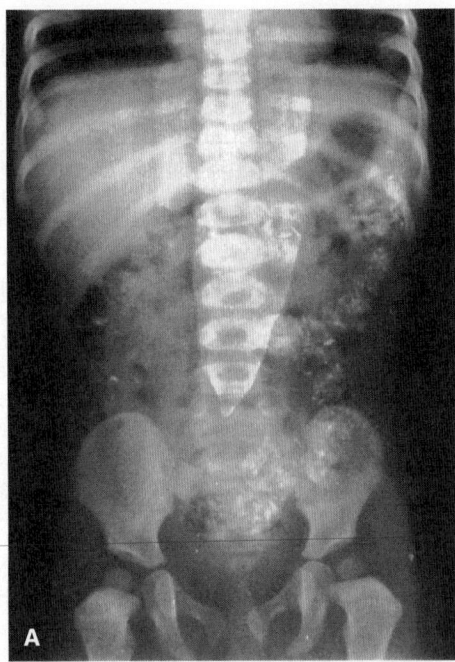

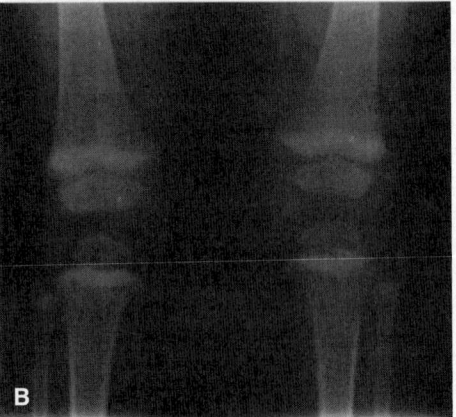

FIGURE 52.6 (A) Ingested paint chips (white crescents) in the intestinal tract. **(B)** A radiograph of the long bones of a child with chronic lead ingestion showing the characteristic "lead line" or white marking at the epiphyseal line. (Radiographs courtesy of Dr. Jerald P. Kuhn, Children's Hospital, Buffalo, NY.)

TABLE 52.3

TABLE 52.3

Classification of Lead Poisoning Risk

Class	Lead Blood Level Concentration (μg/dL)	Recommended Action
Class I (low risk)	< 9	Retest at 24 mo for children age 6–35 mo who are considered low risk; retest every 6 mo for ages 6–35 mo who are considered high risk
Class IIa (rescreen)	10–14	Retest yearly; continue retesting yearly for children > 36 mo until age 6 yr
Class IIb (moderate risk)	15–19	Retest every 3–4 mo for children age 6–35 mo
Class III (high risk)	20–44	Retest every 3–4 mo; begin home abatement program
Class IV (urgent risk)	45–69	Initiate chelating therapy and environmental remediation
Class V (urgent risk)	> 70	Immediately treat with a chelating agent

Centers for Disease Control and Prevention. (2005). *Preventing lead poisoning in young children.* Washington, DC: U.S. Department of Health and Human Services, Public Health Service.

10 μg/dL. A classification of levels of lead poisoning is shown in Table 52.3.

Therapeutic Management

A child with a blood lead level between 10 and 14 μg/dL needs to be rescreened to confirm the level. If the lead level is 15 μg/dL or higher, the child needs active interventions to prevent further lead exposure. These interventions may include removal of the child from the environment containing the lead source or removal of the source of lead from the child's environment. Removal of the lead source can be difficult. If the family lives in a rented apartment, the landlord may be legally obligated to remove the lead. Simple repainting or wallpapering does not remove a source of peeling paint adequately. After some months, the new paint will begin to peel because of the defective paint underneath. The walls must therefore be covered by paneling or Masonite. All children with lead levels greater than 20 μg/100 mL may be prescribed an oral chelating agent such as succimer (Box 52.7).

Children with blood lead levels of greater than 45 μg/100 mL may be admitted to the hospital for chelation therapy with agents such as dimercaprol (BAL) or edetate calcium disodium (CaEDTA) (Neblett & Irizarry, 2003).

Chelating agents remove the lead from soft tissue and bone (although not from red blood cells), allowing it to be eliminated in the urine. Injections of EDTA, which must be given IM into a large muscle mass, are painful and may be combined with 0.5 mL of procaine. EDTA also removes calcium from the body; therefore, serum calcium must be measured periodically to determine whether it is at a safe level. Measure intake and output to ensure that kidney function is adequate to handle the lead being excreted. BUN, serum creatinine, and protein in urine may also be assessed. If kidney function is not adequate, EDTA may lead to nephrotoxicity or kidney damage.

BAL has the advantage of removing lead from red blood cells, but, because of severe toxicity, it is used only for children who have severe forms of lead intoxication.

Penicillamine (Cuprimine) is another drug used for lead poisoning. It is given orally after BAL or EDTA. Weekly complete blood cell counts and renal and liver function tests accompany the administration of penicillamine. It may be given for as long as 3 to 6 months.

BOX 52.7 FOCUS ON . . .

PHARMACOLOGY

Succimer (Chemet)

Classification: Succimer is a chelating agent.

Action: Forms water-soluble chelates with lead, leading to increased urinary excretion of lead (Karch, 2004)

Pregnancy Risk Category: C

Dosage: Orally, starting with 10 mg/kg or 350 mg/m^2 every 8 hours orally for 5 days, then reducing dosage to 10 mg/kg or 350 mg/m^2 every 12 hours for 2 weeks. The drug is taken for a total of 19 days.

Possible Adverse Effects: Nausea; vomiting; loss of appetite; back, stomach, flank, head, or rib pain; chills; flulike symptoms

Nursing Implications

- Obtain serum lead levels before beginning therapy and again at the close of therapy.
- Instruct parents and child about the need to take the full 19-day course for optimal effectiveness.
- If the child has difficulty swallowing capsules, encourage parents to open capsules and mix capsule contents with a small amount of soft food or administer capsule contents on a spoon followed by a fruit drink.
- Urge the child to drink increased amount of fluid to provide enough urine for removing the chelated lead from the body.
- Ensure that a lead abatement program is instituted concurrently to reduce the amount of lead to which the child is exposed.

NURSING DIAGNOSES AND RELATED INTERVENTIONS

Planning can be difficult because parents are upset at learning their child has been exposed to lead. They may experience a loss of self-esteem and a sense of powerlessness when realizing that their financial circumstances or lifestyle has hurt their child.

Nursing Diagnosis: Deficient knowledge related to the dangers of lead ingestion

Outcome Evaluation: Parents state ways they have safeguarded their child against further lead ingestion; parents identify measures to reduce lead in the environment.

Parental education about the risk of lead poisoning is crucial. Teach parents to keep toddlers away from windowsills and other common sources of lead paint. Placing the television or an overstuffed chair against the windowsill may be effective as a temporary measure. As a rule, children's cribs should be placed about 3 feet away from walls in older homes to reduce the risk of children's picking at loose wallpaper when they first wake in the morning or before they fall asleep at night. (Plaster, which contains lead, clings to the wallpaper.) All children with elevated lead levels need careful follow-up care to determine the seriousness of their condition and to ensure that they are kept from a lead source. Because children who recover from symptomatic lead poisoning have a high incidence of permanent neurologic damage, all children with elevated blood lead levels need appropriate follow-up care to evaluate development and intelligence (Centers for Disease Control and Prevention, 2005).

Insecticide Poisoning

Insecticide poisoning can occur by accidental ingestion or through skin or respiratory tract contact when children play in an area that has recently been sprayed. Long-term exposure may result from exposure to a parent's clothing if he or she comes home covered with insecticide spray. Although insecticide poisoning was once thought to be only a rural problem, the increase in the use of lawn sprays by commercial companies now makes this a suburban problem as well.

Many insecticides have an organophosphate base that causes acetylcholine to accumulate at neuromuscular junctions; this accumulation leads to muscle paralysis. Within a few minutes to 2 hours after exposure, children develop nausea and vomiting, diarrhea, excessive salivation, weakness of respiratory muscles, confusion, depressed reflexes, and possibly seizures.

In the emergency department, activated charcoal may be administered if the insecticide was swallowed. If clothing is contaminated, remove it and wash the child's skin and hair. To prevent coming in contact with the insecticide yourself, wear gloves while bathing the child.

IV atropine and a cholinesterase reactivator, pralidoxime (Protopam Chloride) are effective antidotes to reverse symptoms. To avoid mosquitoes and exposure to West Nile virus infection, diethyltoluamide (DEET)-based insecticides appear to be safe if used as recommended (Koren et al., 2003).

Plant Poisoning

Plant poisoning (ingestion of a growing plant) occurs because parents commonly do not think of plants as being poisonous. Common plants to which children may be exposed and the effects of ingestion are shown in Box 52.8.

Poisoning by Drugs of Abuse

Adolescents and even grade-school children are brought to health care facilities by parents or friends because of a drug overdose or a "bad trip" caused by an unusual reaction or the effect of an unfortunate combination of drugs (Enevoldson, 2004). Typical drugs involved include codeine and antidepressant drugs.

Children are often extremely disoriented after this form of ingestion. They may be having hallucinations. Obtaining a history may be difficult because children may have

---

BOX 52.8 FOCUS ON . . .

FAMILY TEACHING

Identifying Poisonous Plants

Q. Jason's father says to you, "We never realized plants could be poisonous to our children. Which ones should we be aware of?"

A. A number of common plants can lead to poisoning in children. Here are some and the symptoms they produce:

English ivy: Nausea, vomiting, excess salivation, diarrhea, abdominal pain
Holly (berries): Vomiting, diarrhea, abdominal pain
Hydrangea: Nausea, vomiting, muscular weakness, seizures, dyspnea
Lily of the valley: Vomiting, abdominal pain, diarrhea, cardiac disturbances
Mistletoe: Vomiting, diarrhea, bradycardia
Morning glory (seeds): Nausea, diarrhea, hallucinations
Philodendron: Swelling of the tongue, lips, irritation of mouth
Poinsettia: Nausea, vomiting
Rhubarb (leaves): Irritant action on gastrointestinal tract
Rhododendron: Nausea, vomiting, abdominal pain, seizures, limb paralysis

no idea what they took except that it was a red or a yellow capsule. They may know but may be reluctant to name a drug if it was obtained illegally.

Assessment

Although the child may not appear to hear well or may not seem coherent, try to elicit a history from him or her. Avoid shouting or aggravating, because children who are having a paranoid reaction will be unable to cope rationally with this approach. If friends accompany an ill child, point out that your role is not that of a law enforcer. Your role is to help the child, and you cannot do that effectively unless the drug is identified. Approaching a child's friends in this way is more likely to result in their naming the drug. If a child is brought in by parents who have no idea what drug could possibly have been taken, ask them to have someone at home check the child's bedroom for drugs (provided the child became ill while at home).

Try to determine whether the ingestion was an accident (e.g., the child was unaware that two drugs would react this way or took a wrong dose) or whether the child was actually attempting suicide. In the first instance, the child will need counseling to avoid drug use or about which drugs do not mix. If the incident was an attempted suicide, the child will need observation and counseling toward more effective coping mechanisms in self-care. All poisonings or drug ingestions in children older than 7 years of age should be considered potential suicides until established otherwise.

Expect to obtain blood specimens for electrolyte levels and a toxicology screen. If the child is vomiting, save any vomitus for analysis.

Therapeutic Management

Children need supportive measures for their specific symptoms, including oxygen administration, electrolyte replacement (particularly if there is accompanying nausea and vomiting), and perhaps IV fluid administration in an attempt to dilute the drug.

Children who have swallowed a drug of abuse need immediate treatment followed by empathic investigation into the events leading to the poisoning. This potentially lethal ingestion may act as a turning point in the child's life, possibly alerting the child and family to a drug problem and the need for help. Factors such as reduction of fear and anxiety, increased coping mechanisms, knowledge of the effects of drug use, and availability of referral sources for a drug problem are important areas to address. (See Chapter 32 for more information related to adolescents and drug use.)

Checkpoint Question 2

Suppose Jason's older brother had lead poisoning. What is the most common source of lead poisoning in young children?

a. Smelling lead fumes from cooking utensils.
b. Chewing on batteries that fall out of toys.
c. Drinking lead-contaminated drinking water.
d. Chewing on chips of lead-based outdoor paint.

FOREIGN BODY OBSTRUCTION

Foreign bodies can become lodged in children's throats or other body openings, causing stasis of secretions and infection. Direct obstruction or laceration of the mucous membrane may also result, leading to serious consequences.

Whether a foreign substance is inhaled or embedded elsewhere, nursing interventions will focus first on comforting the child and aiding in removal of the substance, and then on teaching the child and parents ways to avoid such occurrences in the future.

Foreign Bodies in the Ear

Any child with a history of draining exudate from the ear canal needs an otoscopic examination to establish the reason for the drainage. In toddlers and preschoolers, the drainage often is the result of a foreign body in the ear canal. The object might be a small piece of a toy, a piece of paper, a small battery, or food, such as a peanut (Nasci & Pollack, 2003).

Removal of a foreign body from the ear is difficult because children are afraid that the instrument used will hurt them, so they have difficulty lying still for the procedure. If there is reason to think that the tympanic membrane is intact, irrigating the object from the ear canal with a syringe and normal saline may be possible. This should not be done if the object is a substance that will swell when wet, such as a peanut. If it is possible that the tympanic membrane is ruptured, the ear canal must not be irrigated or fluid will be forced into the middle ear, possibly introducing infection (otitis media).

Often, it is better to wait for an otolaryngologist to care for the child, because trauma to the ear canal during an attempt to remove a foreign body will increase the edema and make removal even more difficult.

Foreign Bodies in the Nose

Foreign objects stuffed into the nose eventually cause inflammation and purulent discharge from the nares. The odor accompanying such impaction is often the first sign noticed by a parent. Objects pushed into the nose usually can be removed with forceps. A local antibiotic might be necessary after removal if ulceration resulted from the local irritation (Blackburn, 2003).

Foreign Bodies in the Esophagus

Children tend not to chew food well and to swallow portions that are too big to pass safely through the esophagus. Pieces of candy, such as Lifesavers, are common objects caught in the esophagus in young children; coins may be swallowed by adolescents (Lukens, 2003). Orthodontic appliances may become dislodged and swallowed. Intense pain at the site where the object is lodged will result. If it is an object that will dissolve, such as a Lifesaver or a piece of digestible meat, offer the child fluid to drink to help flush the object into the stomach. Even after the object dissolves or passes into the stomach, the child will feel transient pain at the original site of the obstruction.

Objects, such as a part of a toy or a chicken bone, that will not dissolve and should not be passed, are removed by esophagoscopy (Ozguner, 2004). Small coins, such as pennies and dimes, usually pass by themselves without difficulty.

Parents (or children themselves if adolescents) should observe stools over the next several days to determine when the coin passes through the GI tract (about 48 hours after ingestion). Without frightening them, caution parents to observe for signs of bowel perforation or obstruction, such as vomiting or abdominal pain, until the object has passed. If there is any doubt, a radiograph taken 3 to 7 days after ingestion will establish whether the object has been evacuated from the body.

Subcutaneous Objects

Children receive many wood splinters in the hands and feet. These usually are removed easily by a probing needle and tweezers after cleaning with an antiseptic solution. If the penetrating object is metal, such as a sewing needle or nail, its presence can be detected radiographically. If the object is one that would have been in contact with soil, such as a rusty nail, the child may need tetanus prophylaxis after extraction of the object.

What if... You received a call from your neighbor stating that her 2-year-old son has swallowed a penny? What interventions would you expect to be necessary? What signs and symptoms would suggest obstruction?

TRAUMA RELATED TO ENVIRONMENTAL EXPOSURE

Frostbite

Frostbite is tissue injury caused by freezing cold. Cold exposure leads to peripheral vasoconstriction, cutting off the oxygen supply to surrounding cells. In children, the body parts involved usually are the fingers or toes (Arnold, 2003). Cells at the site are so injured that they actually die.

Assessment

The affected part appears white or erythematous with edema and feels numb. Degrees of frostbite are summarized in Table 52.4. Explore the cause of frostbite by careful history taking. It occurs most frequently in children who have been skiing or snowmobiling for long periods. If parents failed to provide adequate clothing because they underestimated the degree of cold outside, the possibility of neglect or child abuse must be ruled out as a cause. Frostbite also can occur from sucking on popsicles and from inhalant abuse.

Therapeutic Management

Always warm frostbitten areas gradually. Sudden warming will increase the metabolic rate of cells; without ade-

TABLE 52.4

Degrees of Frostbite

Degree	Description
First	Mild freezing of epidermis; appears erythematous with edema
Second	Partial- or full-thickness injury; appears erythematous with blisters and pain occurring after rewarming
Third	Full-thickness injury (epidermis, dermis, and subcutaneous tissue); appears white
Fourth	Complete necrosis with gangrene and possible ultimate loss of body part

quate blood flow to the area because of still-present vasoconstriction, additional damage can occur. Administration of a vasodilator and use of hyperbaric oxygen also may help.

NURSING DIAGNOSES AND RELATED INTERVENTIONS

Nursing Diagnosis: Pain related to frostbite damage to cells

Outcome Evaluation: Child states that pain is controlled at a tolerable level.

As soon as warming begins, the area becomes extremely painful because the cells that are injured but not destroyed register their anoxic state. Children need an analgesic for pain, such as IV morphine. Morphine administered epidurally can be used for pain relief in lower body areas.

During the next few days after severe frostbite, necrosis of destroyed tissue occurs, and the affected tissue sloughs away. Apply dressings as necessary to avoid secondary bacterial contamination of a necrotic injury site. Assess body temperature conscientiously to detect early symptoms of infection.

BITES

Mammalian Bites

Dog bites account for approximately 90% of all bites inflicted on humans, and children and adolescents are involved in one third to one half of reported incidents. The dog is usually one owned by the child's family. Cat bites, wild animal bites, and human bites also constitute a threat, although they are less common in children. All of these bites can cause abrasions, puncture wounds, lacerations, and crushing injuries related to the size of the animal and the location of the bite (Wu, 2003). The biggest concerns associated with animal bites are the possibility of long-term scarring and disfigurement and the possibility of infection, especially rabies, from the presence of microorganisms in the animal's mouth. This latter subject is discussed in Chapter 43.

Snakebite

In the United States, snakebites tend to occur during the warm months of the year, from April to October. Most fatal snakebites (envenomations) in the United States are copperhead or rattlesnake bites. (Copperheads are found in eastern and southern states, and rattlesnakes in almost every state.) A few bites occur from cottonmouth moccasins or coral snakes (both found in southeastern states). The effect of the bite of a rattlesnake, copperhead, or cottonmouth moccasin (all pit vipers) is a failure of the blood coagulation system (Black & Erickson, 2003). Coral snakes are known for the small coral, yellow, and black rings encircling their body. Fortunately, they are shy and seldom bite. However, the venom injected through the bite of these snakes leads to neuromuscular paralysis.

Assessment

Reaction to a pit viper bite is almost immediate. A white wheal forms at the site, showing the puncture marks, accompanied by excruciating pain at the site. Purplish erythema and edema begin to extend rapidly from the site.

By the time a child is seen at a health care facility, sanguineous fluid may be oozing from the bite. Systemic symptoms, such as dizziness, vomiting, perspiration, and weakness, may be present. Because snake venom interferes with blood coagulation, the child may have hematemesis or bleeding from the nose, intestines, or bladder due to subcutaneous or internal hemorrhage. The pupils may be dilated, showing the potent effect on cerebral centers. If the envenomation is not treated, seizures, coma, and death may result.

Emergency Management at the Scene

At the scene of a snakebite, apply a cold compress to the bite, in the hope of slowing the spread of the venom and to reduce edema formation. Urge the child to lie quietly, to slow circulation. Keep the bitten extremity dependent, again to slow venous circulation. Commercial snakebite kits have rubber suction cups in them for suctioning out venom. If these are available, they should be used at the site where the bite occurred. Excising the bite with a knife and sucking out the venom orally (often shown in old western movies) is of questionable value and contradicts rules of standard precautions. If the person administering the treatment has open mouth lesions, such as carious teeth, the procedure could be dangerous to that person (venom is not dangerous when swallowed, only when absorbed through open lesions). Excising the bite also may lead to secondary infection and, if done too vigorously, may injure tendon or muscle. No time should be wasted

before the child is transported to a health care facility for treatment.

Emergency Management at the Health Facility

In the emergency facility, ask the child or a person who was with the child to describe the snake. In areas where snakebites are frequent, keep available photographs of the venomous snakes commonly found. Even a preschooler may be able to identify the snake by pointing to a photograph. Specific antivenin is then administered. Because rattlesnakes, copperheads, and cottonmouth moccasins are all one type of snake (pit vipers), one form of antivenin acts against all of these bites. Specific antivenin is prepared for coral snake or cobra bites and is kept at most zoos. If the child receives antivenin promptly after a bite, the prognosis for full recovery is good. Tetanus prophylaxis is instituted if the child's immunization status is unknown or if it has been more than 10 years since a tetanus immunization was given.

Antivenin may contain a horse-serum base. Therefore, before the serum is injected IM or IV, a skin test may need to be performed to prevent a possible anaphylactic reaction to the horse serum. If the serum is given IM, do not inject it into an edematous body part, because medication absorption will be poor. Giving antivenin in the limb opposite the bitten limb is just as effective as administering it into the bitten limb.

NURSING DIAGNOSES AND RELATED INTERVENTIONS

Nursing Diagnosis: Fear related to seriousness of child's condition

Outcome Evaluation: Parents and child state that they are able to cope with the degree of fear present.

Children with snakebites are extremely frightened. Their parents who have seen old western movies showing the agony of snakebite also are thoroughly frightened. Children need a great deal of support from health care personnel, because their parents may be too frightened to offer adequate support.

As a final care measure, teach children safety rules for avoiding snakebites:

• Look for snakes before stepping into underbrush.
• Do not lift up rocks without looking at what could be under them.
• Listen for the telltale sound of a rattlesnake.
• Be aware that snakes sun on rocks.
• Know the markings of poisonous snakes.

BURN TRAUMA

A burn is injury to body tissue caused by excessive heat (heat greater than 104°F [40°C]). Such injuries commonly occur in children of all ages after infancy. They are the second greatest cause of unintentional injury in children 1 to 4 years of age and the third greatest cause in children age 5 to 14 years (Fuchs, 2003). Toddlers are often burned by pulling pans of scalding water or grease off the stove and onto themselves (Allen & Kagan, 2004). They can bite into electrical cords. Older children are more apt to suffer burns from flames when they move too close to a campfire, heater, or fireplace; touch a hot curling iron; or play with matches or lighted candles. Some burns (particularly scalding) can be caused by child abuse (Greenbaum et al., 2004). Any thermal burn tends to be more serious in children than in adults, because the same size burn covers a larger surface of a child's body. As many as 50% of burns could be prevented with improved parent and child education.

Assessment

When children are brought to a health care facility with a thermal injury, the first questions must be, "Where is the burn and what is its extent and depth?" Burns are classified according to the criteria of the American Burn Association as major, moderate, or minor burns (McCance & Huether, 2004). These classifications are shown in Table 52.5. Along with the size and depth, be certain to assess and document the location of the burn. Face and throat burns are particularly hazardous because there may be unseen burns in the respiratory tract. Resulting edema could lead to respiratory tract obstruction. Hand burns are also hazardous because, if the fingers and thumb are not positioned properly during healing, adhesions will inhibit full range of motion in the future. Burns of the feet and genitalia carry a high risk for secondary infection. Genital burns are also hazardous because edema of the urinary meatus may prevent a child from voiding.

With adults, the "rule of nines" is a quick method of estimating the extent of a burn. For example, each upper extremity represents 9% of the total body surface; each

lower extremity represents two 9s, or 18%, and the head and neck represent 9%. Because the body proportions of children are different from those of adults, this rule does not always apply and is misleading in the very young child. Data for determining the extent of burns in children are shown in Figure 52.7. Computer analysis is now available to rapidly assess the extent of burns.

Depth of Burn

Assessing the depth of burns can be difficult on initial inspection. Descriptions of tissue at various burn depths appear in Table 52.6 and are illustrated in Figure 52.8. *Partial-thickness* burns include first- and second-degree burns. A first-degree burn involves only the superficial epidermis. The area appears erythematous. It is painful to touch and blanches on pressure (Fig. 52.9*A*). Scalds and sunburn are examples of first-degree burns. Such burns heal by simple regeneration and take only 1 to 10 days to heal.

A second-degree burn involves the entire epidermis. Sweat glands and hair follicles are left intact. The area appears very erythematous, blistered, and moist from exudate. It is extremely painful. Scalds can cause second-degree burns (see Fig. 52.9*B*). Such burns heal by regeneration of tissue but take 2 to 6 weeks to heal.

A third-degree burn is a full-thickness burn involving both skin layers, epidermis and dermis. It may also involve adipose tissue, fascia, muscle, and bone. The burn area appears either white or black (Fig. 52.10). Because the nerves, sweat glands, and hair follicles have been burned, third-degree burns are not painful. Flames are a common cause of third-degree burns. Such burns cannot heal by regeneration because the underlying layers of skin are destroyed. Skin grafting is usually necessary, and healing takes months. Scar tissue will cover the final healed site. When estimating the depth of a burn, use the appearance of the burn and the sensitivity of the area to pain as criteria. Many burns are compound, involving first-, second-, and third-degree burns. There may be a central white area that is insensitive to pain (third degree), surrounded by an area of erythematous blisters (second degree), surrounded by another area that is erythematous only (first degree).

Undress children with burns completely so the entire body can be inspected. A first-degree burn is painful, whereas a third-degree burn is not. Therefore, a child may be crying from a superficial burn that is obvious on the arm, although the condition needing the most immediate attention is a third-degree burn on the chest, which is covered by a jacket.

Be certain to ask what caused the burn, because different materials cause different degrees of burn. Hot water, for example, causes scalding, a generally lesser degree of burn than one caused by flaming clothing. Ask where the fire happened. Fires in closed spaces are apt to cause more respiratory involvement than fires in open areas.

Ask whether the child has any secondary health problem. In their anxiety over the present burn, parents may forget to report important facts, such as that the child has diabetes or is allergic to a common drug. After a fire, parents may pick up the burned child and bring him or her to a health care facility, leaving other children unprotected at home. Ask about other children and where they

TABLE 52.5

Classification of Burns

Classification	Description
Minor	First-degree burn or second-degree burn < 10% of body surface or third-degree burn < 2% of body surface; no area of the face, feet, hands, or genitalia burned
Moderate	Second-degree burn between 10% to 20% or on the face, hands, feet, or genitalia or third-degree burn < 10% of body surface or if smoke inhalation has occurred
Severe	Second-degree burn > 20% of body surface or third-degree burn > 10% of body surface

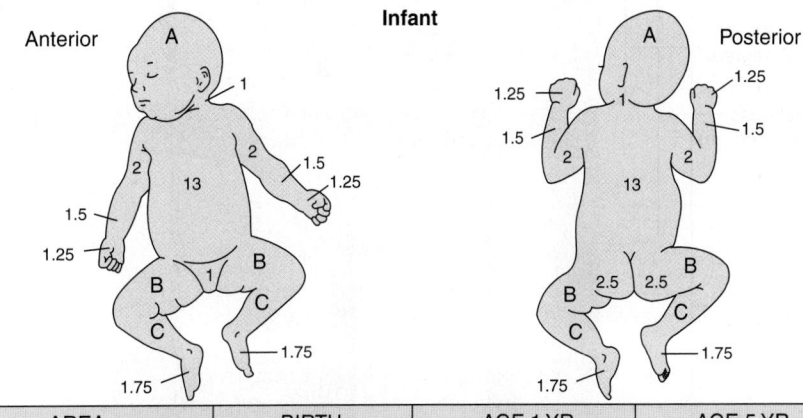

AREA	BIRTH	AGE 1 YR	AGE 5 YR
A = 1/2 of head	9 1/2	8 1/2	6 1/2
B = 1/2 of one thigh	2 3/4	3 1/4	4
C = 1/2 of one leg	2 1/2	2 1/2	2 3/4

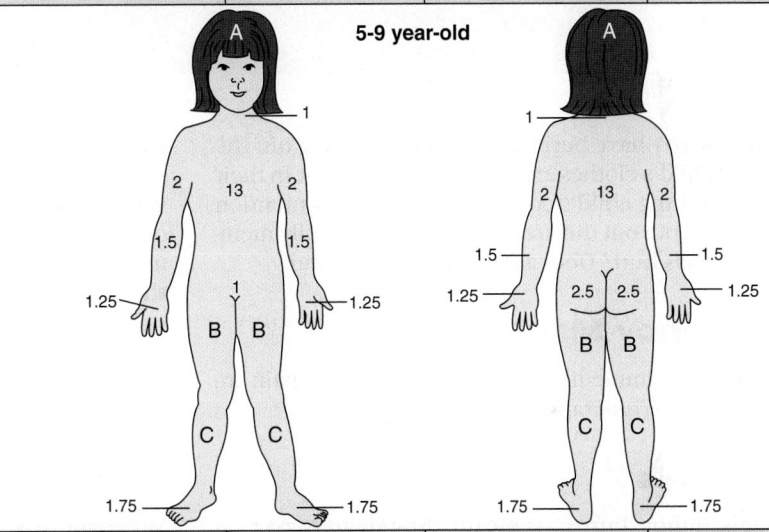

AREA	AGE 10 YR	AGE 15 YR	ADULT
A = 1/2 of head	5 1/2	4 1/2	3 1/2
B = 1/2 of one thigh	4 1/2	4 1/2	4 3/4
C = 1/2 of one leg	3	3 1/4	3 1/2

FIGURE 52.7 Determination of extent of burns in children.

TABLE 52.6

Characteristics of Burns

Severity	Depth of Tissue Involved	Appearance	Example
First degree (partial thickness)	Epidermis	Erythematous, dry, painful	Sunburn
Second degree (partial thickness)	Epidermis Portion of dermis	Blistered, erythematous to white	Scalds
Third degree (full thickness)	Entire skin, including nerves and blood vessels in skin	Leathery; black or white; not sensitive to pain (nerve endings destroyed)	Flame

Depths of burns

Skin grafts

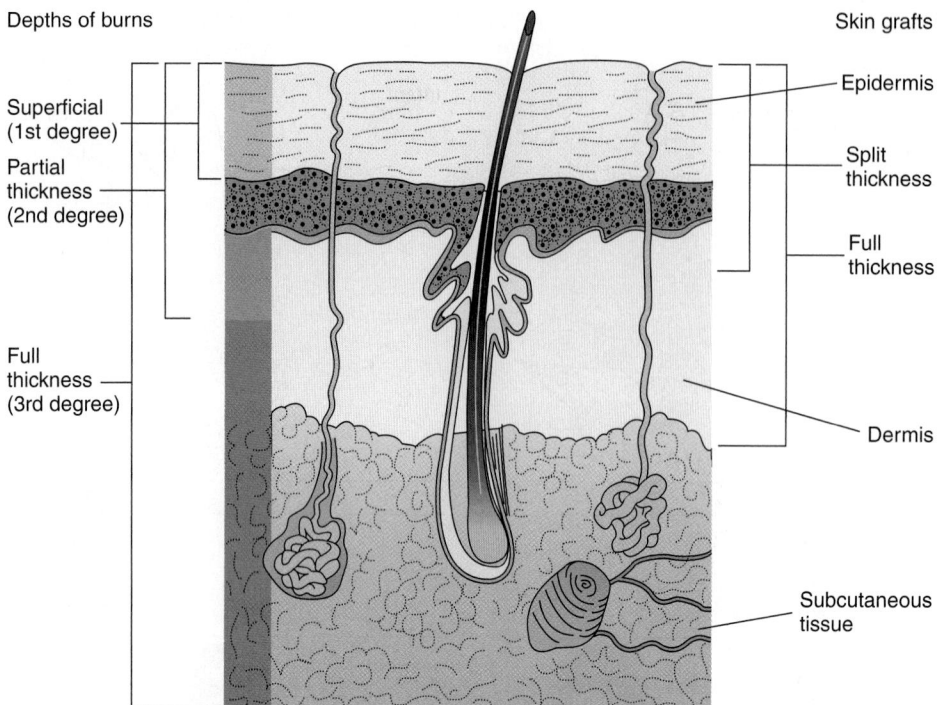

Superficial
(1st degree)

Partial
thickness
(2nd degree)

Full
thickness
(3rd degree)

Epidermis

Split
thickness

Full
thickness

Dermis

Subcutaneous
tissue

FIGURE 52.8 Depths of burns.

are. Parents may have burned hands from putting out the fire on the child's clothes and need equal care, but in their anxiety about the child's condition, they do not mention this. Ask who put out the fire. Were any other family members or animals hurt? Does anyone else need care?

Emergency Management

All burns need immediate care because of the pain involved (Reed & Pomerantz, 2005).

Minor Burns

Although minor burns (typically first-degree partial-thickness burns) are the simplest type of burn, they involve pain and death of skin cells, so they must be treated seriously. Immediately apply ice to cool the skin and prevent further burning. Application of an analgesic–antibiotic ointment and a gauze bandage to prevent infection is usually the only additional treatment required. The child should have a follow-up visit in 2 days to have the area inspected for a secondary infection and to have the dressing changed. Caution parents to keep the dressing dry (no swimming or getting the area wet while bathing for 1 week). A first-degree burn heals in about that time.

Moderate Burns

Moderate or second-degree burns may have blisters. Do not rupture them, because doing so invites infection. Bro-

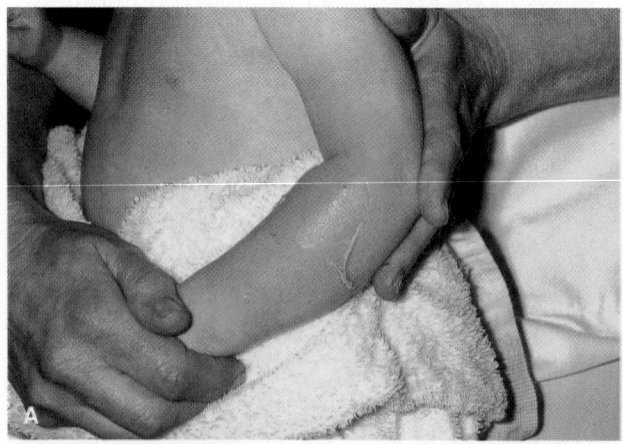

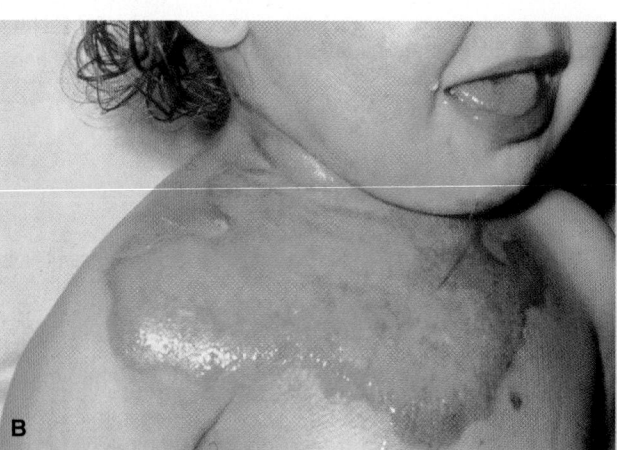

FIGURE 52.9 Partial-thickness burns. **(A)** An infant with a first-degree burn on the arm and chest caused by scalding with hot water. **(B)** A toddler with a second-degree burn caused by scalding. The area appears severely reddened and moist with some blistering. (**A,** © Dr. P. Marazzi/SPL/Science Source/Photo Researchers. **B,** © NMSB/Custom Medical Stock Photo.)

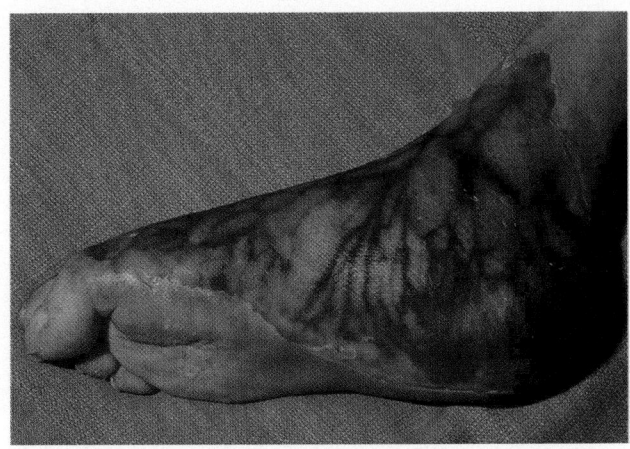

FIGURE 52.10 Full-thickness (third-degree) burn of the foot. Both layers of skin are involved with this type of burn. (© Dr. Michael English/Custom Medical Stock Photo.)

ken blisters may be débrided (cut away) to remove possible necrotic tissue. The burn will be covered with a topical antibiotic such as silver sulfadiazine and a bulky dressing to prevent damage to the denuded skin. The child usually is asked to return in 24 hours to assess that pain control is adequate and there are no signs and symptoms of infection.

Severe Burns

The child with a severe burn is critically injured and needs swift, sure care, including fluid therapy, systemic antibiotic therapy, pain management, and physical therapy, to survive the injury without a disability caused by scarring, infection, or contracture.

NURSING DIAGNOSES AND RELATED INTERVENTIONS

───●───

Nursing Diagnosis: Pain related to trauma to body cells

Outcome Evaluation: Child states that pain is at a tolerable level.

Children who experience smoke inhalation may be unconscious from brain anoxia immediately after a burn. Most children, however, are awake and very aware of the pain and treatments involved. Therefore, a priority need is immediate pain relief. After the first week following a major burn, some children develop symptoms of delirium, seizures, and coma that result from toxic breakdown of damaged cells, sensory deprivation, isolation, and lack of sleep. Nursing care aimed at reducing unnecessary stimuli and providing adequate pain relief helps to prevent these late symptoms from occurring.

A child needs a potent analgesic to relieve pain. Morphine sulfate is commonly the agent of choice. It can be administered IM, but, because circulation is impaired in children with shock, IV or epidural administration is most effective. Use of patient-controlled analgesia before performing any burn care such as débridement is also effective. Be sure to assess after administration that pain relief was adequate.

In addition to the pain from the burn, children may be required to remain in awkward positions to keep joints overextended for most of every day. Doing so helps to prevent formation of contractures from scar tissue (Fig. 52.11). If the anterior throat is burned, for example, the head will be hyperextended to keep scar tissue that forms on the anterior neck from pulling the chin down against the chest in a contracture. It is difficult for children to watch television in this position or even to view activities on the unit. If they have burns at extremity joints, they may have

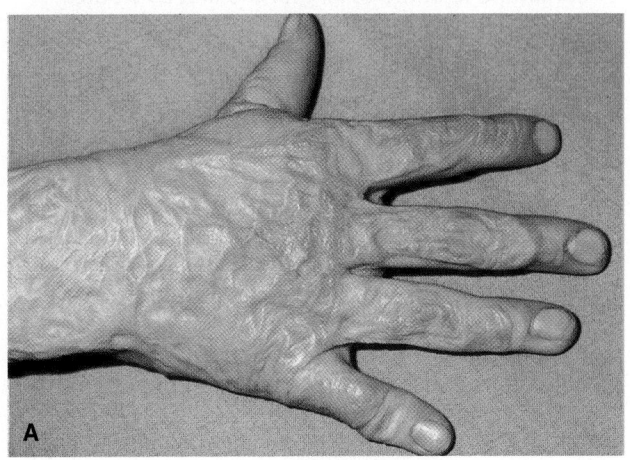

A

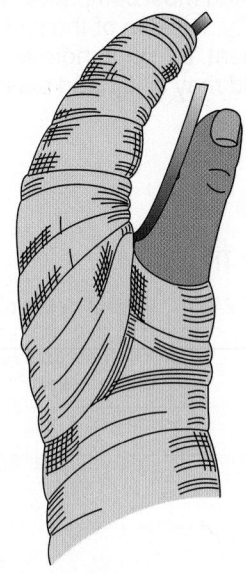

B

FIGURE 52.11 (A) An adolescent's hand scarred from third-degree burns. Note the proper extension and alignment of the hand and fingers, which were maintained by the use of splints (B) during healing. (A, © Dr. P. Marazzi/SPL/ Science Source/Photo Researchers.)

splints applied over burn dressings to maintain the joints in extension. Again, this makes activities very difficult and adds to their stress if they do not have adequate pain relief.

Nursing Diagnosis: Deficient fluid volume related to fluid shifts from severe thermal burn

Outcome Evaluation: Skin turgor remains good; hourly urine output is greater than 1 mL/kg, with specific gravity between 1.003 and 1.030; vital signs are within acceptable parameters.

Immediately after a severe burn, the child's circulatory system becomes hypovolemic, due to a loss of plasma, which oozes from the vascular system into the burn site and then sequesters in edematous tissue surrounding the site. This outpouring of plasma is caused by an increased permeability of capillaries (or damage to capillaries). It is most marked during the first 6 hours after a burn. It continues to some extent for the first 24 hours.

A primary response of the myocardium to the shock of thermal injury and hypovolemia can lead to a marked reduction in cardiac output and decreased blood pressure. Therefore, even with relatively minor burns, monitor vital signs closely to allow early detection of this event. A child may be severely anemic because of injury to red blood cells caused by heat and loss of blood at the wound site, and he or she may have severe electrolyte abnormalities as a result of fluid shifts (Table 52.7). The large amount of sodium lost with the edematous burn fluid and the release of potassium from damaged cells can lead to an immediate hyponatremia and hyperkalemia.

Lactated Ringer's solution is the commercially available solution most compatible with extracellular fluid. Usually, it is one of the first fluids begun for fluid replacement, although normal saline may be used. The child may also need plasma replacement

and additional fluid, such as 5% dextrose in water. Do not administer potassium immediately after a burn until kidney function is evaluated, to be certain that extra potassium can be eliminated. IV fluid is usually administered by the most convenient venous access, so that morphine sulfate can be administered to relieve pain. A more stable fluid line may then be inserted. The amount of fluid necessary is calculated carefully, based on predicted insensible fluid loss and loss due to the burn. The Parkland formula is commonly used to calculate the amount of fluid needed for the first 24 hours: 4 mL/kg for each 1% of body surface area burned.

This fluid is administered rapidly for the first 8 hours (half of the 24-hour load), then more slowly for the next 16 hours (the second half). It is important that administration be continued beyond the time of increased capillary permeability (at least the first 24 hours). The administration site, therefore, must be protected to prevent infiltration. A central venous pressure or pulmonary artery catheter may be inserted to determine hemodynamic and fluid volume status and evaluate that the child is receiving adequate fluid.

About 48 hours after the burn, as inflammation decreases, the extracellular fluid at the burn site begins to be reabsorbed into the bloodstream. Edema begins to subside; the child has diuresis and loses weight. The heart rate increases because of temporary hypervolemia. The hematocrit level is low because red blood cells are diluted. The child needs frequent evaluation of electrolyte levels to determine fluid balance during this period. Potassium supplements may be necessary to maintain normal heart function, because, although potassium was released into the serum from destroyed cells, it is rapidly excreted by the kidneys. If the child needs continued electrolyte replacement at this time, carefully monitor the rate of flow so the blood volume does not exceed the child's tolerance. If many red blood cells were destroyed at the burn site, the child may need packed red blood cells to maintain an adequate hemoglobin level.

Nursing Diagnosis: Risk for ineffective tissue perfusion related to cardiovascular adjustments after thermal injury

Outcome Evaluation: Child's vital signs stay within normal limits; hourly urine output remains greater than 1 mL/kg.

Take height, weight, and vital signs on admission, and continue to take vital signs every 15 minutes until they are stable. Once vital signs are stabilized, record pulse, blood pressure, and central venous pressure hourly until the child passes the immediate danger of shock (at least 24 hours). Another important period occurs at 48 hours after the injury, when fluid is returning to the bloodstream. Remember that gradual but persistent changes in blood pressure may be as informative as sudden changes.

TABLE 52.7

Fluid Shifts After Thermal Injury

Fluid Shifts in First 24 Hr	Remobilization of Fluid After 48 Hr
Burn	Edematous tissue surrounding burn area
↓	↓
Increased capillary permeability	Intravascular compartment
↓	↓
Hypoproteinemia	
Hyponatremia	Hypervolemia
Hyperkalemia	Hypernatremia
Hypovolemia	Hypokalemia

A complete blood cell count, blood typing and cross-matching, electrolyte and BUN determinations, and blood gas studies to ascertain blood levels of oxygen and carbon dioxide are important to obtain.

Nursing Diagnosis: Risk for ineffective breathing patterns related to respiratory edema from thermal injury

Outcome Evaluation: Child's respiratory rate remains within 16 to 20 breaths/minute; lung auscultation reveals no rales.

If the child inhaled smoke from a fire, the injury from the smoke inhalation can be more serious than the skin surface burns. Smoke coming from a fire is at the temperature of the fire. Inhaling smoke, therefore, is the same as exposing the upper respiratory tract to open flame. In addition, toxic substances and soot given off by the fire cause even more irritation to the respiratory tract. If carbon monoxide is inhaled with the smoke, it enters red blood cells in place of oxygen, shutting off the oxygen supply to body cells. If this is extensive, it can lead to loss of consciousness due to cerebral anoxia. If the trachea is burned, edema fluid will pass into the injured bronchioles and trachea, causing pulmonary edema or obstruction limiting air inflow. This can lead to dyspnea and stridor. About 1 week after the smoke inhalation, the child is at risk for the development of pneumonia because of denuded tracheal and bronchial tract areas. The fact that inhalation of smoke or flame from a fire can be more serious than the skin burns the child suffers may be difficult for parents to understand. They are relieved if they learn that the child has suffered only smoke inhalation. They may need an explanation of the physiologic consequences that can result from pulmonary injury.

To help rule out smoke inhalation, obtain a history to assess whether the fire occurred in a closed space, such as a garage. Assess for burns of the face, neck, or chest, which would indicate that the fire was near the nose and respiratory tract. Assess the quality of the child's voice (it will be hoarse if the throat is irritated from smoke). Carefully, monitor the respiratory rate of all burned children, because the respiratory rate increases with respiratory obstruction. A child also may become restless and thrash about because of lack of oxygen. Measurement of blood gases will demonstrate the degree of hypoxia present from carbon monoxide intoxication. Administration of 100% oxygen is the best therapy for displacing carbon monoxide and providing adequate oxygenation to body cells. The child may need endotracheal intubation or a tracheostomy with assisted ventilation to ensure adequate oxygenation. Intubation is best, because tracheostomies can lead to infection, and this child is at a much higher risk for pneumonia than the average child.

Symptoms of smoke inhalation may not occur immediately but only 8 to 24 hours after the burn.

A chest radiograph taken at this time will reveal collecting edematous fluid and decreased aeration. Continue to assess the child's temperature every 4 hours for the first week after the injury, to assess that lung infection is not developing. Bronchodilators and antibiotics may be prescribed. High-frequency ventilation may be helpful to keep alveoli functioning. Some children need extracorporeal membrane oxygenation (ECMO) support because smoke inhalation has compromised their lung function to such a great extent.

Nursing Diagnosis: Risk for impaired urinary elimination related to thermal trauma

Outcome Evaluation: Child's urine output is greater than 1 mL/kg of body weight per hour.

Because the child's blood volume decreases immediately after a burn, renal function is threatened by kidney ischemia just when it is needed to rid the body of breakdown products from burned cells. If the child is burned over more than 10% of his or her body surface, urinary output may decrease immediately. Blood volume must be maintained by IV fluid administration to establish good urinary output once more. Urine output should be 1 mL/kg of body weight per hour. The specific gravity of urine also should be monitored to determine whether the kidneys can concentrate the urine to conserve body fluid (failing kidneys lose this ability rapidly). In the days after the burn, because products of necrotic tissue and toxic substances must be evacuated by the kidney and antidiuretic hormone and aldosterone levels are increased in response to low blood pressure, kidney function may fail again. If free hemoglobin from destroyed red blood cells plugs kidney tubules (acute tubular necrosis), urine color will be red to black due to the hemoglobin present.

An indwelling urinary (Foley) catheter should be inserted in the emergency department, and an immediate urine specimen should be obtained for analysis. A diuretic, such as mannitol, may be administered to flush hemoglobin from the kidneys. If this is effective, the urine returns to its usual straw color. Throughout the child's hospital stay, observing urinary output is a major nursing responsibility. An hourly urine output of less than 1 mL/kg/hr suggests renal insufficiency.

Nursing Diagnosis: Risk for imbalanced nutrition, less than body requirements, related to thermal trauma

Outcome Evaluation: Child's weight remains within normal age-appropriate growth percentiles; skin turgor remains normal; urine specific gravity remains between 1.003 and 1.030.

After burns, the metabolic rate increases in children as the body begins to pool its resources to adjust to the insult. If the child does not receive enough calories in IV fluid, he or she will begin to break down protein. This is particularly dangerous because the child needs protein now for burn healing. Additionally, breakdown of protein can lead to acidosis.

After a severe burn, some children are nauseated from the systemic shock. An NG tube may be inserted and attached to low, intermittent suction as prophylactic therapy to prevent aspiration of vomitus. The tube must remain in place until bowel sounds are detected. This usually occurs within 24 hours but may take as long as 72 hours in severely burned children. Fluid suctioned from an NG tube may be blood-tinged (coffee-ground fluid) due to bleeding caused by stomach vessel congestion. Closely observe this drainage for a change to fresh bleeding, which can be caused by a stress ulcer (Curling's ulcer). This type of ulcer can be prevented by administering a histamine-2 receptor antagonist, such as cimetidine (Tagamet) or a proton pump inhibitor such as omeprazole (Prilosec) in an attempt to reduce gastric acidity and ulcer formation.

If a bleeding ulcer occurs, gastric lavage with iced saline may be necessary. Blood for transfusion should be readily available, because the blood loss from a GI ulcer can be rapid and severe.

If a child has burns over more than 30% of the body surface, paralytic ileus may occur. Symptoms of intestinal obstruction, such as vomiting, abdominal distention, and colicky pain, will appear within hours of the burn.

Children with severe burns usually are allowed nothing by mouth for 24 hours because of the danger of vomiting or paralytic ileus. After this, most children are able to eat, so oral feedings are begun as soon as possible. To supply adequate calories for increased metabolic needs and spare protein for repair of cells, the diet is high in calories and protein (1,800 cal/m^2 plus 22 cal/m^2 of burned area per 24 hours). Children may also need vitamin (particularly B and C) and iron supplements. High-protein drinks may be necessary between meals to ensure an adequate protein intake (Dudek, 2005).

Because adequate nutrition is important, it may be necessary to supplement the child's diet with IV or parenteral nutrition solutions or NG tube feeding. As additional methods of stimulating interest in eating, encourage school-age children to help add intake and output columns, help the dietitian add a calorie-count list, or keep track of their own daily weight (taken at the same time each day in the same clothing). It may be helpful to make contracts with older children for a good nutritional intake.

Nursing Diagnosis: Risk for injury related to effects of burn, denuded skin surfaces, and lowered resistance to infection with thermal injury

Outcome Evaluation: Child's temperature remains at 98.6°F (37°C); skin areas surrounding burned areas show no signs of erythema or warmth.

There appears to be some defect in the ability of neutrophils to phagocytize bacteria after thermal injury. The formation of immunoglobulin G antibodies

also apparently fails. For these reasons, the child has reduced protection against infection. *Staphylococcus aureus* and group A β-hemolytic streptococci are the gram-positive organisms, and *Pseudomonas aeruginosa* is the gram-negative organism, that commonly invade burn tissue. Children are usually prescribed parenteral penicillin to prevent group A β-hemolytic streptococcal infection and tetanus toxoid to prevent tetanus. In addition to bacteria, fungi also may invade burns. *Candida* species are the most frequently seen (Fuchs, 2003).

Bacteria and fungi can penetrate the burn eschar readily, so this tissue offers little protection from infection. Fortunately, granulation tissue, which forms under the eschar 3 to 4 weeks after the burn, is resistant to microbial invasion.

Nose, throat, and wound cultures may be done immediately and then daily to detect offending organisms. Until granulation tissue forms, the child has lost the integumentary defense against infection. Therefore, prophylactic treatment is important to prevent infection. Systemic antibiotics are not very effective in controlling burn-wound infection, probably because the burned and constricted capillaries around the burn site cannot carry the antibiotic to the area. For this reason, any equipment used with the child must be sterile, to avoid introducing infection. Children are placed on a sterile sheet on the examining table. Personnel caring for the severely burned child should wear caps, masks, gowns, and gloves, even for emergency care.

Although their burns may be covered by gauze dressings, children usually are cared for in private rooms. Helping children maintain their self-esteem and keeping them from withdrawing from social contacts are commonly difficult when infection control precautions are required.

Checkpoint Question 3

If Jason spilled scalding hot water on his hand, which of the following would be the best emergency action?

a. Apply an ice compress to his hand.
b. Pour vegetable oil over his hand.
c. Cover his hand with a gauze dressing.
d. Apply hand lotion to keep the area moist.

Therapy for Burns

Second- and third-degree burns may receive open treatment, leaving the burned area exposed to the air, or a closed treatment, in which the burned area is covered with an antibacterial cream and many layers of gauze. These two methods are compared in Table 52.8. A synthetic skin covering (Biobrane) or artificial skin (Integra) can be used to help decrease infection and protect granulation tissue. As a rule, burn dressings are applied loosely for the first 24 hours to prevent interference with circu-

TABLE 52.8

Comparing Open and Closed Burn Therapy

Method	Description	Advantages	Disadvantages
Open	Burn is exposed to air; used for superficial burns or body parts that are prone to infection, such as perineum	Allows frequent inspection of site; allows child to follow healing process	Requires strict isolation to prevent infection; area may scrape and bleed easily and impede healing
Closed	Burn is covered with nonadherent gauze; used for moderate and severe burns	Provides better protection from injury; is easier to turn and position child; allows child more freedom to play	Requires dressing changes that are painful; possibility of infection may increase because of dark, moist environment

lation as edema forms. Be certain not to allow two burned body surfaces, such as the sides of fingers or the back of the ears and the scalp, to touch, because, as healing takes place, a webbing will form between these surfaces. Do not use adhesive tape to anchor dressings to the skin; it is painful to remove and can leave excoriated areas, which provide additional entry for infection. Netting is useful to hold dressings in place, because it expands easily and needs no additional tape.

Topical Therapy

Silver sulfadiazine (Silvadene) is the drug of choice for burn therapy to limit infection at the burn site for children. It is applied as a paste to the burn, and the area is covered with a few layers of mesh gauze. Silver sulfadiazine is an effective agent against both gram-negative and gram-positive organisms and even against secondary infectious agents, such as *Candida*. It is soothing when applied and tends to keep the burn eschar soft, making débridement easier. It does not penetrate the eschar well, which is its one drawback.

Antiseptic solutions, such as povidone-iodine (Betadine), may be used to inhibit bacterial and fungal growth. Unfortunately, iodine stings as it is applied and stains skin and clothing brown. Dressings must be kept continually wet to keep them from clinging to and disrupting the healing tissue.

If *Pseudomonas* is detected in cultures, nitrofurazone (Furacin) cream may be applied. If a topical cream is not effective against invading organisms in the deeper tissue under the eschar, daily injections of specific antibiotics to the deeper layers of the burned area may be necessary.

If a burned area, such as the female genitalia, cannot be readily dressed, it can be left exposed. The danger of this method is the potential invasion of pathogens.

Escharotomy

An eschar is the tough, leathery scab that forms over moderately or severely burned areas. Fluid accumulates rapidly under eschars, putting pressure on underlying blood vessels and nerves. If an extremity or the trunk has been burned so that both anterior and posterior surfaces have eschar formation, a tight band may form around the extremity or trunk, cutting off circulation to the distal body portions. Distal parts feel cool to the touch and appear pale. The child notices tingling or numbness. Pulses are difficult to palpate, and capillary refill is slow (longer than 5 seconds). To alleviate this problem, an **escharotomy** (cut into the eschar) is performed (Black & Miller, 2004). Some bleeding will occur after escharotomy. Packing the wound and applying pressure usually relieves this.

Débridement

Débridement is the removal of necrotic tissue from a burned area. Débridement reduces the possibility of infection, because it reduces the amount of dead tissue present on which microorganisms could thrive. Children usually have 20 minutes of hydrotherapy before débridement to soften and loosen eschar, which then can be gently removed with forceps and scissors. Débridement is painful, and some bleeding occurs with it. Premedicate the child with a prescribed analgesic, and help the child use a distraction technique during the procedure to reduce the level of pain. Transcutaneous electrical nerve stimulation (TENS) therapy or patient-controlled analgesia may be helpful. Praise any degree of cooperation. Plan an enjoyable activity afterward to aid in pain relief and also to help reestablish some sense of control over the situation.

Children need to have a "helping" person with them, to hold their hand, to stroke their head, and to offer some verbal comfort during débridement: "It's all right to cry; we know that hurts. We don't like to do this, but it's one of the things that makes burns heal" (Fig. 52.12). Nursing personnel need a great deal of talk time to voice their feelings about assisting with or doing débridement procedures. Be careful when serving as the "helping" person that you do not project yourself as the healer and comforter and a fellow nurse as the hurter or "bad guy." It helps if people alternate this chore so that, on alternate days, each serves as the protector and the comforter.

If eschar tissue is débrided in this manner day after day, granulation tissue forms underneath. When a full bed of granulation tissue is present (about 2 weeks after the injury), the area is ready for skin grafting. In some burn centers, this waiting period is avoided by immediate surgical excision of eschar and placement of skin grafts. Another

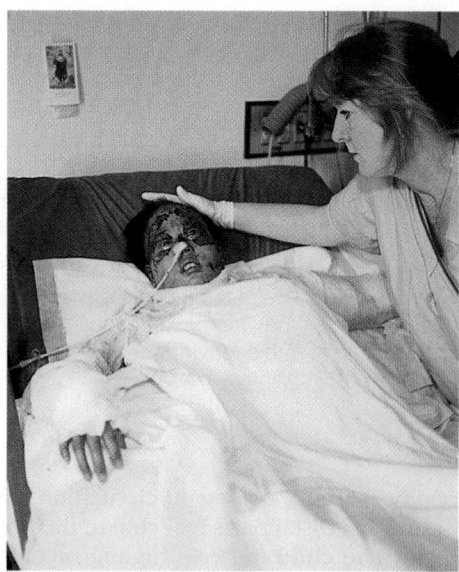

FIGURE 52.12 A nurse provides comfort and support to a child before débridement. (© Kathy Sloane/Science Source/Photo Researchers.)

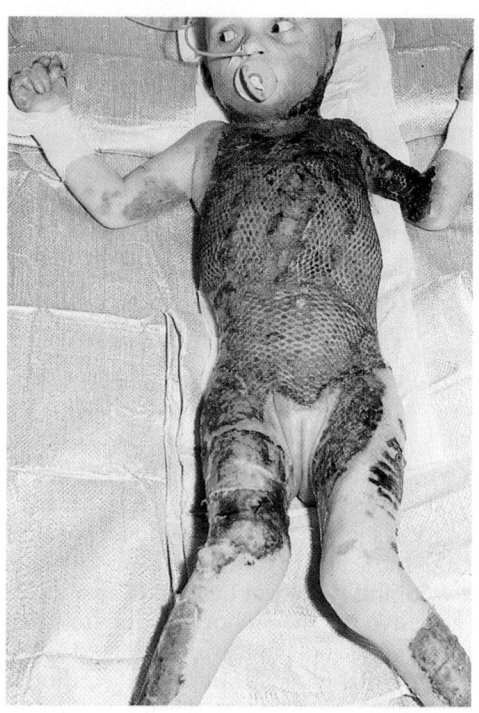

FIGURE 52.13 Mesh grafting is necessary to cover large areas of the body such as in this young child with third-degree burns. (© CC Studio/SPL/Photo Researchers Inc.)

trend in débridement is the use of collagenase (Santyl), an enzyme that can dissolve devitalized tissue.

Grafting

Homografting (also called **allografting**) is the placement of skin (sterilized and frozen) from cadavers or a donor on the cleaned burn site. These grafts do not grow but provide a protective covering for the area. In small children, **heterografts** (also called *xenografts*) from other sources, such as porcine (pig) skin, may be used. **Autografting** is a process in which a layer of skin of both epidermis and a part of the dermis (called a *split-thickness graft*) is removed from a distal, unburned portion of the child's body and placed at the prepared burn site, where it will grow and replace the burned skin (Thourani et al., 2003). Cultured epithelium is derived from a full-thickness skin biopsy. This can be grown into a coherent sheet or supply an unlimited source for autografts. Larger areas may require mesh grafts (a strip of partial-thickness skin that is slit at intervals so that it can be stretched to cover a larger area; Fig. 52.13). The advantage of grafting is that it reduces fluid and electrolyte loss, pain, and the chance of infection (Merz, 2003).

After the grafting procedure, the area is covered by a bulky dressing. So that the growth of the newly adhering cells will not be disrupted, this should not be removed or changed. The donor site on the child's body (often the anterior thigh or buttocks) is also covered by a gauze dressing. Both donor and graft dressings should be observed for fluid drainage and odor. Observe the child to determine whether he or she has pain at either site, which might indicate infection. Monitor the child's temperature every 4 hours. A rise in systemic temperature may be the first indication that there is infection at the

graft or donor site. Autograft sites can be reused every 7 to 10 days, so any one site can provide a great deal of skin for grafting.

NURSING DIAGNOSES AND RELATED INTERVENTIONS

Nursing Diagnosis: Social isolation related to infection control precautions necessary to control spread of microorganisms

Outcome Evaluation: Child states that he understands the reason for infection control precautions; child accepts it as a necessary part of therapy.

Infection control measures involved in the care of children with major burns consist of more than just placing the child in a private room. Aseptic technique and appropriate barriers are necessary to reduce the risk of exposing the child to infection. Health care facilities differ in their policies for preventing infection in a child with a burn. Check your agency's policy. In some agencies, all the people who come into the room must wear gowns, masks, caps, and sterile gloves. The child is doubly isolated—by distance and by never being touched directly.

It is easy for children with burns (who were told measures such as not to play with matches or go too close to the fireplace) to interpret confinement in a room as punishment. Make every effort to make the child's environment as warm and comforting as possible, despite the infection control procedures. Place children's beds so they can see as much unit activity as possible. Decorate walls in front of them with cards they receive or with a changing gallery of pictures drawn by staff members of things in which the child appears interested.

Provide time for children to discuss their feelings about being kept in a room by themselves. A question such as, "It's hard to understand a lot of things about a hospital; do you understand why your bed is in this special room?" gives children a chance to express their feelings.

Show parents how to put on gowns, gloves, and masks (depending on agency policy), so they can participate in the child's care as much as possible. Parents often do not ask to do these things spontaneously when their children are severely burned. They are in a state of grief, so they do not react in a normal manner. They may believe the bulky dressings will make it impossible for them to hold the child. Actually, the closed bulky dressings on the burned area make it *possible* for the child to be held. If it is not possible for the child to be held, help the parents to see that stroking their child's face or touching a hand (even with gloves in place) gives the child a feeling of still being loved.

Nursing Diagnosis: Interrupted family processes related to the effects of severe burns in family member

Outcome Evaluation: Family members state that they are able to cope effectively with the degree of stress to which they are subjected; family demonstrates positive coping mechanisms.

Children with severe burns always have a difficult hospitalization because of the pain, restrictions, and (at some point) awareness of the disfigurement that accompanies major burns.

Some parents grieve so deeply over the child's condition or are so concerned with other upsetting factors in their lives (many burns happen because of situational crises in the family) that their interaction with the child seems to falter or proves very difficult for them. They may avoid visiting because the sound of the child's crying when they leave is more than they can endure. At the same time, they may have lost their home and possessions to fire. They may need help in establishing priorities. It may be important that they wait at home one morning for an insurance inspector to make an estimate on damage to their house or furniture caused by the fire. Other tasks, such as shopping or house cleaning, could possibly be done by relatives or neighbors, leaving them time to visit their child.

Nursing Diagnosis: Deficient diversional activity related to restricted mobility after severe burn

Outcome Evaluation: Child expresses interest in obtaining school homework; child communicates with friends and relatives by way of telephone, letters, or e-mail.

Remember that, even if a child's chest, abdomen, and hands are burned, he does not stop thinking. Children need stimulation in their environment. A television set is good for passing time but should not be the child's main communication with the outside world. Listening to favorite tapes, having stories read to them, talking about what is going on at home or what they normally do at school, and doing schoolwork are also important.

It is important to make toys and play materials available. Make certain to visit the child just to talk to him or come to play a game at times other than procedure or treatment times. The child may be hospitalized for a long time. He needs to view the nursing staff as friends and caregivers. Frequent visits convey that he is not alone and that others are aware of important needs.

Nursing Diagnosis: Disturbed body image related to changes in physical appearance with thermal injury

Outcome Evaluation: Child expresses fears about physical appearance; demonstrates desire to resume age-appropriate activities.

Children with burns are often forced to become extremely dependent on the nursing staff because of the position in which they must lie and because the bulky dressings that cover their arms or hands prevent them from feeding themselves. They respond to this forced dependence at first with gratitude. They are hurt, and someone is taking care of them. After a period, however, the response may become less healthy. The young school-age child or preschooler may revert to bedwetting or baby talk. Older children respond by becoming openly aggressive to counteract their feelings of helplessness. They attempt to reestablish independence in the ways that they can, often by refusing to eat or to lie in a position that is best for them. Although good nutrition is vitally important for rapid healing, it may suffer because of children's need to assert their independence. Make certain to allow independent decision-making whenever possible. Children must take their 10 o'clock medicine, but they can choose the fluid they want to swallow after it. They must be fed meals because of the bulky dressings over their hands, but they can decide which food they will eat first. They must have their dressings changed, but they can choose the story you will read them afterward.

Be careful not to give choices when there really are none to give. Inappropriate questions include, "Can I change your dressing now?" "Do you want dinner now?" "Will you swallow this pill?"

Immediately after a severe burn, children (if they are old enough to understand), parents, and probably the hospital staff are most concerned with whether the child will live. After body systems have stabilized and it seems appropriate to reassure the parents that their child will live, thoughts turn to the child's cosmetic appearance. At first, it is easy for children and parents to ignore this problem, because the burned areas are covered by dressings. Even when the dressings are removed for débridement or whirlpool therapy, it is easy for children to assume that the appearance of the burned area is only temporary and that the area will eventually heal and have a good appearance. They have probably never seen anyone with a scar from a second- or third-degree burn and have no reason to worry about it (Fig. 52.14).

When children see others on the unit with burn scars, they begin to realize what healing will look like. Depending on the extent and the site of the burn, parents and children have varying degrees of difficulty accepting this reality. It can cause them to lose confidence in health care personnel.

Parents and children need time to talk about their feelings. A girl may be extremely concerned if her chest is burned because she is worried that breast tissue will not develop (a very real concern, depending on the extent of the burn). Her parents may be most concerned because they can see that, although a blouse can cover her chest, her right hand will not have full function. Do not assume that your biggest concern is the same as the child's or the parents' biggest concern. A father who dreamed that his son would be a great track star may be most concerned about a leg scar; the child may be most concerned about a facial burn.

Children watch you as you care for them to see if you find them unattractive. As dressings are removed, children may expose parts of their body seemingly inappropriately, to see if you are shocked or revolted by them. It is easy to think that you will not react this way, but, for everyone, the first sight of a severe burn is a shock and it is difficult not to react accordingly. Imagining how the child feels, realizing that this mutilated skin is his or hers, helps health care providers maintain a professional attitude.

Returning to school can be difficult for children who have been hospitalized or have been receiving home care for a long time. Their old friends have new friends, so they may feel cut out of school activities. They look different if they have burn scars. The appearance of scar formation can be improved by the application of pressure dressings that the child wears 24 hours a day. If the child has facial burns, facing friends with a compression bandage in place may be difficult. They need a great deal of support from health care personnel to be able to endure this. Some children need referral for formal counseling. Some parents need formal counseling also, to help them accept their child's changed appearance.

Electrical Burns of the Mouth

If a child puts the prongs of a plugged-in extension cord into her mouth or chews on an electric cord, the mouth will be burned severely (Doucette, 2003). Electrical current from the plug is conducted for a distance through the skin and underlying tissue, so a tissue area much larger than where the prongs or cord actually touched is involved.

Tissue will be destroyed at the entry site, leaving an angry-looking ulcer. If blood vessels were burned, active bleeding will be present. The immediate treatment for electrical burns is to unplug the electric cord and control bleeding. Pressure applied to the site with gauze is usually effective. Most children are admitted to a hospital for at least 24 hours in an observation unit after electrical burns of the mouth, because edema in the mouth can lead to airway obstruction.

Supply adequate pain relief. Clean the wound about four times a day with an antiseptic solution, such as half-strength hydrogen peroxide, to reduce the possibility of infection (a real danger in this area, because bacteria are always present in the mouth).

Eating will be a problem for the child because her mouth is so sore. She may be able to drink fluids from a cup best. Bland fluids, such as artificial fruit drinks or flat ginger ale, are best.

Electrical burns of the mouth turn black as local tissue necrosis begins. They heal with white, fibrous scar tissue, possibly causing a deformity of the lip and cheeks with healing. This can be minimized by the use of a mouth appliance, which helps maintain lip contour. Some children have difficulty with speech sounds because of resulting lip scarring. They need follow-up care by a plastic surgeon to restore their lip contour and function again. Obviously,

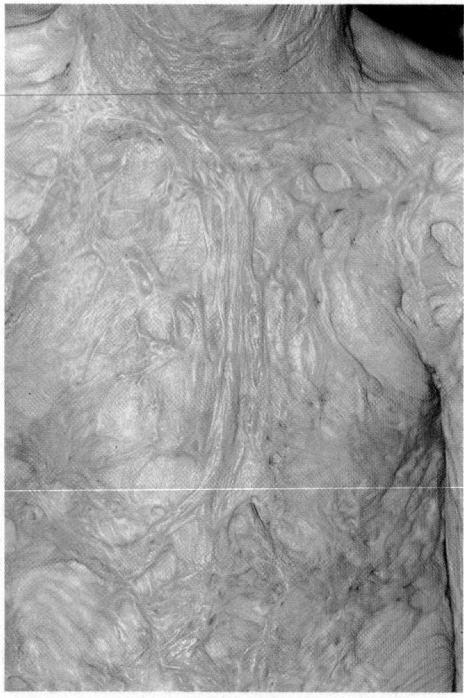

FIGURE 52.14 Extensive scarring on the chest of a 9-year-old boy with third-degree burns. The child and his family will need much support to help them deal with his appearance. (© Dr. P. Marazzi/SPL/Science Source/Photo Researchers.)

you need to review with parents the importance of not leaving "live" electrical cords where young children can reach them.

Key Points

Children need total body assessment after a traumatic injury, because they may be unable to describe other injuries besides the primary one they have suffered. Be aware that some trauma in children occurs as a result of child abuse. Screen for this by history and physical examination. Use aseptic technique when caring for trauma victims, so that the child does not develop an additional unnecessary infection.

Head injuries are always potentially serious in children. Skull fractures, subdural hematomas, epidural hematomas, concussions, and contusions can occur. Coma (unconsciousness from which a child cannot be roused) may be present after severe head trauma.

Abdominal trauma resulting in rupture of the spleen or liver may occur in connection with multiple trauma.

Near drowning can occur in salt or fresh water. The physiologic basis for complications after drowning differs depending on the type of water.

Common substances children swallow that result in poisoning include acetaminophen (Tylenol), caustic substances, and hydrocarbons. Teach parents to keep the number of the local poison control center next to their telephone and always to call first before administering an antidote for poisoning.

Lead poisoning most frequently occurs from the ingestion of lead chips in older housing units. Preventing this is a major nursing responsibility.

Burns are classified as mild, moderate, and severe and can be divided into three types—first, second, and third degree—depending on the depth of the burn. Burns produce systemic body reactions and require long-term nursing care.

Critical Thinking Exercises

1. Jason, a 5-year-old boy, is seen in the emergency room after an automobile accident. He is crying and upset, although the only visible signs of trauma are a reddened and edematous area on the middle of his forehead. Vital signs reveal the following: temperature, 99.4°F (37.5°C); respirations, 18 breaths/minute; pulse, 62 bpm; and blood pressure, 110/62 mm Hg. His left pupil is more dilated than his right; it reacts sluggishly to light. His Glasgow Coma score is 10. His mother tells you, "I'm sure he's not injured badly. He was wearing his seat belt." You are the triage nurse. Would you rate Jason as a child to be seen immediately, or could he be given second priority?

2. Jason's twin sister was seen in the emergency room for acetaminophen poisoning last month. Her father tells you they normally lock all medicine away carefully. His wife left acetaminophen on the counter because she had a bad headache. Would you want to discuss the necessity of poisoning prevention with these parents, or should they have learned from this experience that their actions were not safe?

3. A 10-year-old girl has third-degree burns on her legs from lighting a fire to burn leaves. She will probably have a lengthy hospitalization and may need skin grafts to improve healing. What precautions does this child need to prevent infection until healing is complete? What areas of care would you plan to address during the hospitalization?

4. Examine the National Health Goals related to trauma and children. Most government-sponsored money for nursing research is allotted based on these goals. What would be a possible research topic to explore pertinent to these goals that would be applicable to Jason's family and also advance evidence-based practice?

References

American Academy of Pediatrics, Committee on Injury, Violence, and Poison Prevention. (2004). *Poison treatment in the home.* Evanston, IL: AAP.

Adelson, P. D., et al. (2003). Guidelines for the acute medical management of severe traumatic brain injury in infants, children, and adolescents. *Pediatric Critical Care Medicine, 4*(3 Suppl), S72–S75.

Allen, S. R., & Kagan, R. J. (2004). Grease fryers: A significant danger to children. *Journal of Burn Care and Rehabilitation, 25*(5), 456–460.

Arnold, P. (2003). Frostbite. In Schraider, J., et al. (Eds.), *Rosen and Barkin's 5-minute emergency medicine consult* (2nd ed.). Philadelphia: Lippincott Williams & Wilkins.

Bekhof, J., et al. (2004). Clinical picture: Babies and batteries. *Lancet, 364*(9435), 708.

Black, A., & Erickson, T. (2003). Snake envenomation. In Schraider J., et al. (Eds.), *Rosen and Barkin's 5-minute emergency medicine consult* (2nd ed.). Philadelphia: Lippincott Williams & Wilkins.

Black, J., & Zenel, J. A. (2003). Child abuse by intentional iron poisoning presenting as shock and persistent acidosis. *Pediatrics, 111*(1), 197–199.

Black, T. L., & Miller, J. P. (2004). Burns. In Dambro, M. R. (Ed.), *Griffith's 5-minute clinical consult.* Philadelphia: Lippincott Williams & Wilkins.

Blackburn, P. (2003). Foreign body, nasal. In Schraider J., et al. (Eds.), *Rosen and Barkin's 5-minute emergency medicine consult* (2nd ed.). Philadelphia: Lippincott Williams & Wilkins.

Centers for Disease Control and Prevention. (2005). *Preventing lead poisoning in young children.* Washington, DC: Author.

Chun, T. H. (2003). Pediatric trauma. In Schraider J., et al. (Eds.), *Rosen and Barkin's 5-minute emergency medicine consult* (2nd ed.). Philadelphia: Lippincott Williams & Wilkins.

Corwell, B. (2003). Dental trauma. In Schraider J., et al. (Eds.), *Rosen and Barkin's 5-minute emergency medicine consult* (2nd ed.). Philadelphia: Lippincott Williams & Wilkins.

Davies, K. L. (2004). Issues in pediatrics. Buckled-up children: Understanding the mechanism, injuries, management, and prevention of seat belt related injuries. *Journal of Trauma Nursing, 11*(1), 16-24.

Demorest, R. A., et al. (2004). Poisoning prevention education during emergency department visits for childhood poisoning. *Pediatric Emergency Care, 20*(5), 281-284.

Department of Health and Human Services. (2000). *Healthy people 2010*. Washington, DC: DHHS.

Doucette, M. (2003). Electrical injury. In Schraider J., et al. (Eds.), *Rosen and Barkin's 5-minute emergency medicine consult* (2nd ed.). Philadelphia: Lippincott Williams & Wilkins.

Dudek, S. G. (2005). *Nutrition handbook for nursing practice* (5th ed.). Philadelphia: Lippincott Williams & Wilkins.

Enevoldson, T. P. (2004). Recreational drugs and their neurological consequences. *Neurology in Practice, 75*(S3), 9-15.

Feingold, M., & Anderson, R. L. (2004). Lessons and tactics to lead the charge against lead poisoning. *Contemporary Pediatrics, 21*(4), 49-54.

Fuchs, M. A. (2003). Burns. In Schraider J., et al. (Eds.), *Rosen and Barkin's 5-minute emergency medicine consult* (2nd ed.). Philadelphia: Lippincott Williams & Wilkins.

Gandhi, D., Shanbag, P., & Vaidya, M. (2003). Clinical picture: Lead lines. *Lancet, 362*(9379), 197.

Gassner, R., et al. (2004). Craniomaxillofacial trauma in children: A review of 3,385 cases with 6,060 injuries in 10 years. *Journal of Oral and Maxillofacial Surgery, 62*(4), 399-407.

Greenbaum, A. R., et al. (2004). Intentional burn injury: An evidence-based, clinical and forensic review. *Burns, 30*(7), 628-642.

Howard, A., et al. (2003). Ejections of young children in motor vehicle crashes. *Journal of Trauma: Injury, Infection, and Critical Care, 55*(1), 126-129.

Jay, G. D., & Cowell, L. C. (2003). Coma. In Schraider J., et al. (Eds.), *Rosen and Barkin's 5-minute emergency medicine consult* (2nd ed.). Philadelphia: Lippincott Williams & Wilkins.

Karch, A. (2004). *Lippincott's nursing drug guide*. Philadelphia: Lippincott Williams & Wilkins.

Koren, G., Matsui, D., & Bailey, B. (2003). DEET-based insect repellents: Safety implications for children and pregnant and lactating women. *CMAJ-JAMC: Canadian Medical Association Journal, 169*(3), 209-212.

Losek, J. D. (2004). Acetaminophen dose accuracy and pediatric emergency care. *Pediatric Emergency Care, 20*(5), 285-288.

LoVecchio, F. (2003). Poisoning, gastric decontamination. In Schraider J., et al. (Eds.), *Rosen and Barkin's 5-minute emergency medicine consult* (2nd ed.). Philadelphia: Lippincott Williams & Wilkins.

Lukens, T. W. (2003). Foreign body, esophageal. In Schraider J., et al. (Eds.), *Rosen and Barkin's 5-minute emergency medicine consult* (2nd ed.). Philadelphia: Lippincott Williams & Wilkins.

McCance, K. L., & Huether, S. E. (2004). *Understanding pathophysiology* (3rd ed.). St. Louis: Mosby.

Merz, J., et al. (2003). Wound care of the pediatric burn patient. *AACN Clinical Issues: Advanced Practice in Acute and Critical Care, 14*(4), 429-441.

Mooney, D. P., & Forbes, P. W. (2004). Variation in the management of pediatric splenic injuries in New England. *Journal of Trauma: Injury, Infection, and Critical Care, 56*(2), 328-333.

Nasci, K., & Pollack, C. (2003). Foreign body, ear. In Schraider J., et al. (Eds.), *Rosen and Barkin's 5-minute emergency medicine consult* (2nd ed.). Philadelphia: Lippincott Williams & Wilkins.

National Center for Health Statistics. (2005). *Trends in the health of Americans*. Hyattsville, MD: NCHS.

Neblett, M., & Irizarry, L. (2003). Lead poisoning. In Schraider J., et al. (Eds.), *Rosen and Barkin's 5-minute emergency medicine consult* (2nd ed.). Philadelphia: Lippincott Williams & Wilkins.

Ozguner, I. F., et al. (2004). Clinical experience of removing aerodigestive tract foreign bodies with rigid endoscopy in children. *Pediatric Emergency Care, 20*(10), 671-673.

Reed, J. L., & Pomerantz, W. J. (2005). Emergency management of pediatric burns. *Pediatric Emergency Care, 12*(2), 118-129.

Shaw, K. N. (2003). Near drowning. In Schwartz, M. W. (Ed.), *5-minute pediatric consult*. (3rd ed.). Philadelphia: Lippincott Williams & Wilkins.

Teasdale, G., & Bennett, B. (1974). Assessment of coma and impaired consciousness: A practical scale. *Lancet, 2*(7872), 81-84.

Thompson, M. D., & Irby, J. W., Jr. (2003). Recovery from mild head injury in pediatric populations. *Seminars in Pediatric Neurology, 10*(2), 130-139.

Thourani, V. H., Ingram, W. L., & Feliciano, D. V. (2003). Factors affecting success of split-thickness skin grafts in the modern burn unit. *Journal of Trauma: Injury, Infection, and Critical Care, 54*(3), 562-568.

Turner, J. (2004). Prevention of drowning in infants and children. *DCCN: Dimensions of Critical Care Nursing, 23*(5), 191-193.

Willer, B., et al. (2004). A population based investigation of head injuries and symptoms of concussion of children and adolescents in schools. *Injury Prevention, 10*(3), 144-148.

Whitby, E. H., et al. (2004). Frequency and natural history of subdural hemorrhages in babies and relation to obstetric factors. *Lancet, 362*(3), 846-851.

Worrall, K. (2004). Use of the Glasgow coma scale in infants. *Paediatric Nursing, 16*(4), 45-49.

Wu, D. (2003). Bite, mammal. In Schraider J., et al. (Eds.), *Rosen and Barkin's 5-minute emergency medicine consult* (2nd ed.). Philadelphia: Lippincott Williams & Wilkins.

Suggested Readings

Chen, L. E., et al. (2004). Trauma stat and trauma minor: Are we making the call appropriately? *Pediatric Emergency Care, 20*(7), 421-425.

Dowd, M. D. (2004). Motor vehicle injury prevention: Current recommendations for child passenger safety. *Pediatric Emergency Care, 20*(11), 778-785.

Lubit, R., et al. (2003). Impact of trauma on children. *Journal of Psychiatric Practice, 9*(2), 128-138.

Gurses, D., et al. (2003). Cost factors in pediatric trauma. *Canadian Journal of Surgery, 46*(6), 441-445.

Lyons, R. A., et al. (2005). Modification of the home environment for the reduction of injuries. *The Cochrane Library (Oxford) (1)* (CD003600).

Maconochie, I. (2003). Accident prevention. *Archives of Disease in Childhood, 88*(4), 275-277.

Percy, M. S. (2004). Pediatric NPs help families cope with trauma. *Sourcebook for Advanced Practice Nurses, 1*(1), 21-22.

Rzucidlo, S. E., & Shirk, B. J. (2004). Trauma nursing: Pediatric patients. *RN, 67*(6), 36-42.

Skokan, E. G., Junkins, E. P., Jr., & Kadish, H. (2003). Serious winter sport injuries in children and adolescents requiring hospitalization. *American Journal of Emergency Medicine, 21*(2), 95-99.

Zengerle-Levy, K. (2004). Practices that facilitate critically burned children's holistic healing. *Qualitative Health Research, 14*(9), 1255-1275.

CHAPTER 53

Nursing Care of the Child With Cancer

Key Terms

biopsy
chemotherapeutic agent
Ewing's sarcoma
leukemia
lymphoma
metastasis
neoplasm
nephroblastoma
neuroblastoma
oncogenic virus
osteogenic sarcoma
rhabdomyosarcoma
sarcoma
tumor staging

Objectives

After mastering the contents of this chapter, you should be able to:

1. Define terms related to tumor growth, such as neoplasm, benign, malignant, sarcoma, and carcinoma.
2. Describe normal cellular growth and theories that explain how cells alter to become cancerous in children.
3. Assess a child with a cancerous process, such as a rhabdomyosarcoma, neuroblastoma, nephroblastoma, and leukemia.
4. Formulate nursing diagnoses related to a child with cancer.
5. Establish expected outcomes for a child with cancer.
6. Plan nursing care specific to a child with cancer.
7. Implement nursing care for a child receiving cancer therapy.
8. Evaluate expected outcomes for a child with cancer.
9. Identify National Health Goals related to the care of the child with cancer that nurses can help the nation to achieve.
10. Identify areas related to care of children with cancer that could benefit from additional nursing research or application of evidence-based practice.
11. Use critical thinking to propose ways that nursing care for the child with cancer can be more family centered.
12. Integrate knowledge of abnormal cell growth in children with the nursing process to achieve quality maternal and child health nursing care.

*G*eri is a 6-year-old boy you meet at a health maintenance organization clinic. He is there for a well-child checkup. His mother tells you that Geri wakes up every morning with a headache and then vomits. Immediately after that, he is fine. The problem began just after he started a new school in the fall, so she is certain it is related to this. His teacher has suggested that Geri needs an eye examination because he cocks his head to see the chalkboard. You notice that he has lost weight. "What do I do for school phobia?" his mother asks you.

Previous chapters described the growth and development of well children and disorders associated with specific body systems. This chapter adds information about the dramatic changes, both physical and psychosocial, that occur when children develop cancer, a phenomenon that can present in any body system. This is important information because it forms a base for care and health teaching.

Is Geri's mother describing school phobia?
What additional questions would you want to ask her to help discover whether this is something more serious?

After you've studied this chapter, access the accompanying website. Read the patient scenario and answer the questions to further sharpen your skills, grow more familiar with RN-CLEX types of questions, and reward yourself with how much you have learned.

The terms *malignant* and *cancerous* describe cells that are growing and proliferating in a disorderly, chaotic fashion. In adults, cancer usually occurs in the form of a solid tumor. In children, the most frequent type of cancer is that of an immature blood cell overgrowth, or leukemia (McCance & Huether, 2004).

Many parents assume that a diagnosis of cancer means that their child's life will be very limited. Because of the tremendous advances in cancer research and treatment over the last 20 years, however, the prognosis for children and the chances for a cure improve daily. To help parents and children adjust to this illness, however, nursing support is necessary from the time of diagnosis throughout the long-term therapy required. National Health Goals related to cancer and children are shown in Box 53.1.

Nursing Process Overview

For the Child With Cancer

● *Assessment*

The symptoms of cancer in children are often insidious and difficult to define. Headaches or pain at a particular body site can often be explained away by other factors, such as sports injuries or fatigue. Weight loss, however, is a common symptom of cancer and is never normal in healthy children. Therefore, at every health care visit, plot and analyze a child's height and weight to document evidence of this important finding. Be sure to refer children with swelling or pain of major joints to their primary health care provider for further assessment so that bone tumors will not go undetected (Box 53.2).

● *Nursing Diagnosis*

Selected nursing diagnoses established for the child with cancer address specific symptoms caused by the cancer, side effects of the cancer therapy, or coping abilities of the child and family. Examples are the following:

- Pain related to neoplastic process in bone
- Imbalanced nutrition, less than body requirements, related to stomatitis from radiation therapy
- Risk for infection related to immunosuppressive effects of chemotherapy
- Disturbed body image related to loss of hair after radiation treatment
- Compromised family coping, related to long-term chemotherapy program

● *Outcome Identification and Planning*

When a neoplasm is first diagnosed in their child, parents may be able to deal only with short-term out-

BOX 53.1 FOCUS ON . . .

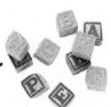

NATIONAL HEALTH GOALS

A number of National Health Goals concern cancer prevention and children:
- Reduce the overall cancer death rate in children from a baseline of 202/100,000 of the population to 159/100,000.
- Increase the proportion of adolescents in grades 9 through 12 who follow protective measures that may reduce the risk of skin cancer.
- Reduce the rate of melanoma cancer deaths, from a baseline of 2.8/100,000 of the population to a target level of 2.5/100,000 (DHHS, 2000).

Nurses can help the nation achieve these goals by careful history taking at health assessments to reveal the symptoms of cancer, which are often subtle in children, and by active teaching of self-screening measures, such as testicular examination and preventive measures such as avoiding excessive sun exposure.

Areas that could benefit from additional nursing research are effective ways to teach young clients about the dangers of tanning booths and excessive sun exposure; reasons adolescents give for avoiding self-examination; and reasons parents give for delaying health care consultation after discovering an abnormal growth, unexplainable bruising, or weight loss.

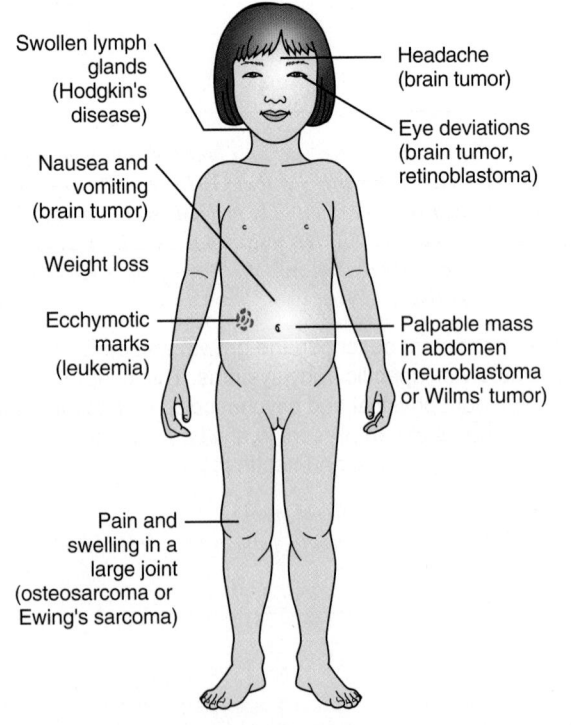

BOX 53.2 ASSESSMENT

Assessing a Child For Signs of Cancer

History
Chief concern: Weight loss, loss of appetite, easy bruising, swelling in a body part, headache, eye deviations.
Past medical history: Family member with a history of cancer.

Physical examination

Swollen lymph glands (Hodgkin's disease)

Headache (brain tumor)

Eye deviations (brain tumor, retinoblastoma)

Nausea and vomiting (brain tumor)

Weight loss

Ecchymotic marks (leukemia)

Palpable mass in abdomen (neuroblastoma or Wilms' tumor)

Pain and swelling in a large joint (osteosarcoma or Ewing's sarcoma)

comes and plans. They may concentrate on learning about the effect or toxic properties of a particular chemotherapeutic drug given their child, or they may ask how long the child's surgical incision will be. Dealing with such specifics helps them to control their anxiety because it prevents them from dealing with the overall picture or prognosis—that their child has a potentially lethal condition.

The family of a child with cancer needs support beginning with the diagnosis. When planning, sit down with the parents and discuss the treatment protocol. Explain measures they will need to take to make their child more comfortable during therapy (e.g., not forcing food if the child is nauseated, playing games or reading stories while an intravenous [IV] chemotherapy agent is administered).

Parents are usually eager for results of diagnostic tests. They may need support while waiting until all the findings have been assembled for an accurate assessment of staging and prognosis. Establishing a primary relationship with both the child and the parents is important so that, no matter how many hospitalizations are necessary, they know a support person is waiting to help them through this long-term illness. Long-term therapy can be expensive, so consider the family's financial capabilities, helping them make any necessary financial arrangements for care. The siblings of a child with cancer should be included in planning care, not only because the illness is serious but also because the treatment may last for an extended period, further stressing the family (Box 53.3).

BOX 53.3 FOCUS ON . . .

EVIDENCE-BASED PRACTICE

What Aspects of Care Are Important for Siblings of Children Treated for Cancer, So The Siblings Can Feel Well Cared For?

To answer this question, nurse researchers interviewed 97 parents and 105 nurses about the care measures they thought siblings of cancer patients need and the help, if any, they need outside the hospital. Care measures that were identified were amusement, emotional support, participation in family life, information, and normal lifestyle. Needed assistance identified most often included emotional support, fair attention, and practical and school support. Overall, parents tended to mention that siblings need information more often than nurses mentioned this fact.

This is an important study for nurses, because it documents the needs of siblings of children with cancer and illustrates how caring for children with cancer is family nursing. It is an alert for nurses that although identifying needs is helpful, recognizing what assistance is needed to meet those needs is also important.

Source: von Essen, L., & Enskar, K. (2003). Important aspects of care and assistance for siblings of children treated for cancer: a parent and nurse perspective. *Cancer Nursing, 26*(3), 203–210.

Parents hear of many questionable cancer cures from newspapers or friends during the course of their child's illness. Help them to voice their hopes and concerns for these cures as they hear them. Open discussion helps parents keep such cures in perspective without putting any more emphasis on them than they warrant. If these questionable cures cannot be discussed with health care personnel, they appear to grow in importance, and parents may turn to them in preference to established therapy.

Parents can be expected to experience grief if they learn their child's prognosis is poor. They move slowly through stages of denial, anger, bargaining, depression, and acceptance. When planning with parents, be certain to take into account their current stage of grief (see Chapter 56).

● **Implementation**

Nursing interventions for a child with cancer include supporting the child and parents from the time of diagnosis through procedures such as surgery, radiation therapy, chemotherapy, and continued health supervision. This is a stressful and long-term process, because chemotherapy may be continued for 2 to 3 years after diagnosis. Increasingly, cancer treatment is offered on an ambulatory basis to keep hospitalization to a minimum, so many interventions include teaching the parents how to give care or monitor for recurring signs.

Keep in mind that the stress of long-term treatment may put the child and family at risk for developmental or family coping problems. You can be a positive force in encouraging healthy adaptation to the demands of the child's illness and in reassessing the situation periodically during therapy to be certain the child is receiving appropriate stimulation for developmental growth. Providing comfort and alleviating pain are often primary concerns in oncology nursing. Measures for pain relief are discussed in Chapter 38.

Organizations that may be helpful in supplying information to parents include the following:

- American Cancer Society (*www.cancer.org*)
- National Cancer Institute (*www.cancer.gov*)
- Children's Oncology Group (*www.childrensoncologygroup.org*)
- Candlelighters Childhood Cancer Foundation (*www.candlelighters.org*)
- The Leukemia and Lymphoma Society (*www.leukemia-lymphoma.org*)

● **Outcome Evaluation**

Because cancer therapy includes long-term care, children must be evaluated periodically to be certain that outcomes are being met and are still current. Some examples indicating outcome achievement are the following:

- Child keeps all appointments for chemotherapy treatments.
- Child maintains passing grades in school despite interruptions for therapy.
- Parents state that they can keep anxiety at an acceptable level between clinic appointments.

Children with cancer need the same well-child maintenance care that all children do, with one exception. While they are undergoing chemotherapy, which causes a decreased immune response, they should not receive live-virus vaccines.

Returning for health care follow-up visits causes anxiety. The child seems well, but parents may be apprehensive while the health care practitioner palpates the child's abdomen or blood specimens are obtained. Some parents may find the strain of returning for follow-up visits too great and miss appointments (not to know seems better than to be told bad news). Such parents need help in understanding that initial remissions can be maintained, and second remissions can be achieved, so maintenance therapy must be continued. Because a child with a tumor such as retinoblastoma and children who receive chemotherapy or radiation are more prone than others to develop a second cancer later in life, follow-up is an essential detection measure (Bottomley & Kassner, 2003).

Parents of a child with cancer may seek health maintenance care or evaluation for their other children more often than other parents would. This is because they are worried that what seems just a minor symptom is actually a sign of cancer in that child also. They need greater amounts of reassurance that their other children are well than the average parent does.

Most children with cancer, even if no cure is possible, will be cared for at home rather than being hospitalized. Their parents may need extensive preparation for home care (see Chapter 35). Help them to maintain close contact with health care personnel to prevent feeling abandoned. If the child dies, the parents may feel a need to return to their primary caregiver for support. This provides an opportunity to evaluate their adjustment to the child's death and offer support if needed. Being with a child who dies at home appears to make death a more understandable phenomenon for siblings and, in many instances, can be advocated. Care in a separate hospice setting is another option for the child in whom a remission cannot be achieved (see Chapter 56).

NEOPLASIA

All body tissue undergoes growth necessary to develop into that specific type of tissue. Normally, the body is able to maintain the proliferation necessary to replace old cells that die while also sustaining physical growth needs. However, cancerous, or malignant, tissue is unable to maintain this balance and begins to proliferate in disorderly, chaotic ways.

The word **neoplasm** means new growth; it usually refers to a new *abnormal* growth that does not respond to normal growth-control mechanisms. Whether this process is one that produces a solid tumor or one that involves blood-forming elements, growth begins insidiously. The process may have been ongoing for some time before the parents or child realize that it is present. Even after they are aware that a change exists, some time may pass before they realize that it is serious enough to require health care, particularly if it is not well defined.

Although cancer in children is rare, it is the leading cause of death from disease among children younger than 15 years of age. Approximately 8,000 new cases of cancer occur in children in the United States each year, and approximately 1,700 deaths occur annually from this cause. Fortunately, the overall survival rate for children with cancer today has improved dramatically (National Cancer Institute, 2005). Knowing the processes involved in cell growth—both normal and abnormal—is essential to help parents understand what is happening to their child and why specific treatment measures are necessary at various stages of cell growth.

Cell Growth

The normal cell cycle consists of two main divisions: an interphase (resting) phase and a mitosis (dividing) phase. The interphase has four periods: G0, G1, S, and G2. Activity during these periods is summarized in Table 53.1. The time span of a cell's life cycle varies. A bone cell cycle is short—about 10 hours; a nerve cell cycle is long—the lifetime of the person. The rate of the cycle is slowed or increased by outside stimuli, such as hypoxia, genetic and immunologic factors, and physical and chemical agents. Normally, both resting and active cells are always present.

Body cells apparently have the ability to recognize their own type, possibly by recognizing surface enzymes or glucose particles on cell membranes. Normally, cells of like type do not migrate away from each other because they

TABLE 53.1

Phases of the Cell Cycle

Phase	Activity
G	Gap, or the phase between mitosis and synthesis.
G0	Cell at rest. Cells remain in this state until some stimulant, such as death of surrounding cells, triggers the cell to enter an active phase; it is difficult to destroy cells in this resting state.
G1	Period until DNA stabilization is complete; it remains difficult to destroy cells in this phase.
S (synthesis)	Period (6–8 hr) during which DNA and chromosomes are duplicated or a cell readies itself for division into two daughter cells.
G2	Cell doubling in size as preparation for dividing into two daughter cells; if protein synthesis can be stopped at this point so that the cell cannot reach a "critical mass," mitosis (cell division) cannot take place.
M (mitosis)	Period of cell division into two like daughter cells.

recognize and adhere to each other to form a solid mass. In neoplastic cells, the ability to keep together is defective (they are autonomous). This may be related to decreased calcium in the cell membrane or to an increased negative charge that repels other cells rather than bonding them together.

Normally, like cells appear to be able to recognize when they are being crowded for the space they must occupy, and they apparently communicate with one another to halt growth when they touch or become crowded. Neoplastic cells do not respond to this communication or cannot receive it, so, despite how crowded they are, they continue to grow. By the time a tumor mass is detected by palpation, it is probably about 30 times the size of its original aberrant cell. In many instances, it may be necessary to kill as many as a billion cells to destroy the entire mass (McCance & Huether, 2004).

Neoplastic Growth

Neoplasms can be either *benign* (growth is limited) or *malignant* (cancerous). Even when a tumor is benign, however, it may not be completely harmless. It can cause damage by pressing on adjacent tissue. For example, brain tumors in children are often benign, but they can cause extensive respiratory depression from increasing pressure on the respiratory center.

Causes of Neoplastic Growth

The exact origin of neoplastic growth is unknown, and any growth may actually involve more than one cause. As more and more research is accomplished on the nature of genes, specific markers in tumors that fail to suppress, or stimulate, cancer-causing genes are being identified (Eberhart et al., 2004). In adults, tumors may grow because normal cell growth has been altered by environmental irritation, such as chronic exposure to chemical irritants or cigarette smoke. Tumors of the skin, bladder, lung, and intestines involve organs exposed to such outside influences and irritation. In children, tumors most frequently occur in organs unexposed to the environment (e.g., leukemia of the bloodstream, nephroblastoma of the kidney, brain tumors, neuroblastoma in the abdomen). Because many tumors occur in children younger than 5 years of age, exposure to environmental carcinogens is limited, so this cause of tumors is probably not a great influence in childhood cancer. Exposure to harmful substances in utero may be a cause (Mueller et al., 2004). Two substances that lead to lung cancer and to which children may be exposed are secondary smoke and asbestos. Asbestos is a particular problem if a child's school or home is insulated with this material or a parent works in asbestos removal and brings home particles on his or her clothing.

A child who has survived one cancer appears to be at higher than normal risk for the development of a second cancer. Radiation exposure used to treat the first malignancy may be responsible for this. In addition, there may be a predisposition to cancer in some families (Codori et al., 2003).

Another common theory of why neoplasms grow is the cell mutation theory. This suggests that carcinogenic agents and hereditary susceptibility combine to alter the nature of cells, leading to abnormal growth. A first stage of initiation may mark the cells for abnormal growth. A second stage of promotion actually begins the abnormal growth. Carcinogens can be living (viral), physical (radiation), or chemical. Radiation during intrauterine life is a documented cause of leukemia. Radiation of the thyroid in infancy can cause thyroid cancer later in life. Use of androgenic steroids may lead to hepatocellular cancer.

This theory explains why the growth of neoplastic cells is irreversible (the cells cannot return to a normal state because they are intrinsically changed) and why neoplasms occur in some people but not in others (both an intrinsic and an extrinsic factor, or an inherited tendency and an environmental insult, must be present). It is difficult to document this process because it stipulates that two separate steps are necessary for a cell to become cancerous. If there is a lengthy time span between these steps, the cause-and-effect relationship is difficult to trace (McCance & Huether, 2004).

Yet another theory is that oncogenic (cancer-causing) viruses are responsible for tumor growth. According to the viral theory, **oncogenic viruses** have the ability to change the structure of DNA or RNA in cells. C-type RNA viruses may be implicated in leukemia. Epstein-Barr virus, a DNA virus, may be associated with Burkitt's lymphoma. This theory is supported by the fact that an immunodeficient state increases the risk for development of a neoplastic growth. Both viral surveillance and removal of abnormal cells are lost; therefore, virus invasion and abnormal cell growth begin. Still another theory is that tumor suppressor cells exist in some individuals and not in others. Retinoblastoma is an example of a cancer that may occur when such cells are not present.

HEALTH PROMOTION AND RISK MANAGEMENT

Because childhood cancers do not seem to arise from environmental contaminants as much as adult cancers do, methods to reduce the risk are not as well defined. Urging parents to reduce children's exposure to secondary cigarette smoke and urging adolescents not to begin smoking can help reduce the incidence of lung cancer when they reach adulthood. Applying sunscreen and reducing the overall time of sun exposure for children can help reduce the development of skin cancer in later life. Children who receive chemotherapy or radiation for one cancer have a higher incidence of developing another cancer later in life. Therefore, urging these children to continue health appointments so that any additional tumor development can be discovered is another important preventive measure. A vaccine against human papilloma virus (HPV), which leads to cervical cancer, will soon be available (Cohen, 2005).

ASSESSING CHILDREN WITH CANCER

The incidence of various types of childhood cancers is shown in Figure 53.1. Because these cancers involve different body systems, signs and symptoms can vary greatly.

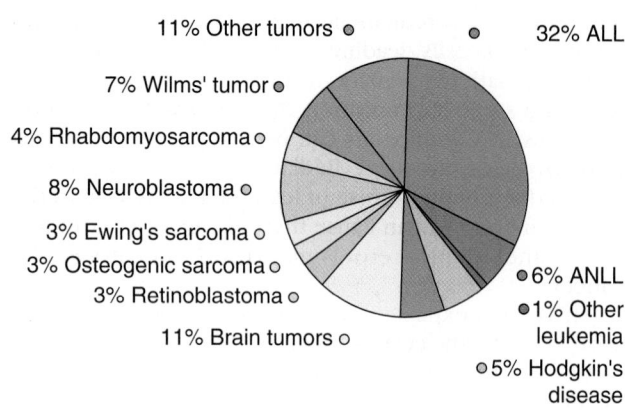

FIGURE 53.1 Approximate incidence of common childhood cancers.

History

Many cancers in children have been developing for some time before the child is brought for care because the symptoms (bruising, nosebleeds, pain in a knee, constipation) are not perceived as important by the parents. Thorough history taking at health care visits can help reveal these symptoms, so that a child can be further evaluated and a cancer discovered early in its growth. For example, symptoms of obstruction (e.g., constipation) or pressure (e.g., headache) may be revealed first by this method. As malignant tumors grow, they tend to cause systemic effects in the child. Cachexia (loss of weight, anorexia) occurs if the tumor is growing so rapidly that it takes nutrients from normal cells. Excessive hormone production (overproduction of antidiuretic, thyroid, or adrenocorticotropic hormone) may occur because of tumor growth in a specific body area that leads to systemic symptoms. Although the warning signs of cancer listed by the American Cancer Society (Box 53.4) apply primarily to cancers in adults, they should also be kept in mind as general guidelines when assessing children (Box 53.5).

Physical and Laboratory Examination

Any suspicion of a malignancy requires a thorough physical examination. Assessing height and weight of children is an important component. To confirm a diagnosis, a number of diagnostic procedures may be used, including radiography, sonography, magnetic resonance imaging (MRI), blood analysis, and biopsy.

Biopsy

A **biopsy** is the surgical removal of tissue cells for laboratory analysis. Most children with a possible diagnosis of cancer will have a biopsy performed to confirm their initial diagnosis. Although biopsies are classified as minor surgery and usually are done on an ambulatory basis, do not treat them lightly. They carry a definite surgical risk if

BOX 53.4

Warning Symptoms and Signs of Cancer

General Symptoms
1. Unexplained weight loss
2. Fever
3. Fatigue
4. Pain
5. Skin changes (itching, darkening, reddening, hairiness)

General Signs
1. A change in bowel or bladder habits
2. A nonhealing sore
3. Unusual bleeding or discharge
4. A thickening or lump in the breast or other body part
5. Indigestion or difficulty swallowing
6. An obvious change in a wart or mole
7. A nagging cough or persistent hoarseness

The American Cancer Society. (2005). *Seven signs of cancer.* Atlanta: Author.

conscious sedation or general anesthesia is used. Moreover, they are an anxiety-producing procedure for the parents and the child. Up to this point, parents can convince themselves that their child has something innocent. A biopsy clouds this hope, because the word "biopsy" implies that cancer is at least a possibility. For this reason, parents and children need thorough preparation for the biopsy procedure and the care the child will need after the procedure. Anxious parents do not "hear" well and may need to have postoperative instructions repeated. Bone marrow aspiration is a frequent type of biopsy used with children. Although this can be done with only local anesthesia, it is equally frightening (see Chapter 44).

BOX 53.5 FOCUS ON . . .

DIVERSITY OF CARE

People in various cultures have differing beliefs as to what causes cancer, ranging from evil spirits or evil past lives to totally environmental or psychological causes. Talking with the parents and the child, if old enough, about what they think is the cause of cancer can add understanding to parents' actions; it can make explanations of therapy more meaningful to parents, because explanations can be geared to fit within their beliefs.

Additionally, many parents ask whether complementary therapies such as herbal medications or special diets will help cure their child. Provide time to discuss these therapies, because they offer parents a sense of control in an otherwise possibly bewildering environment of medical treatments.

Staging

Tumor staging is a procedure by which a malignant tumor's extent and progress are documented. Knowing the stage of the tumor helps the health care team design an effective treatment program, establish an accurate prognosis, and evaluate the progress or regression of the disease. In general staging, stage I refers to a tumor that can be completely removed surgically. Stage II refers to a tumor that cannot be completely removed surgically. Stages III and IV designate tumors that have extended beyond the original site or have spread systemically (**metastasis**). There are various staging systems, but one of the most common is known as the TNM system; it describes the tumor's size (T), its presence in the lymph nodes (N), and its metastasis (M) or spread to other organs, if any. A TNM system is most applicable to carcinomas (tumors of the epithelial tissue). Because most childhood tumors are sarcomas (tumors derived from connective tissue), the system is not as useful for childhood cancers as it is for adult cancers.

OVERVIEW OF CANCER TREATMENT MEASURES USED WITH CHILDREN

The treatment of a child with cancer focuses on devising ways to kill the growth of the abnormal cells while protecting normal surrounding cells. This is done by a combination of surgery, radiation, chemotherapy, bone marrow transplantation, immunotherapy (biologic response modifiers), and general health measures. Bone marrow transplantation is discussed in Chapter 44 as part of the discussion of common blood disorders.

Radiation Therapy

Radiation therapy changes the DNA component of a cell nucleus to a point at which the cell cannot replicate DNA material and thereby inhibits further cell division and growth. Radiation is not effective on cells that have a low oxygen content (a proportion of cells in every tumor mass), nor is it effective at the time of cell division (mitosis). Therefore, radiation schedules are designed so that therapy occurs over a period of 1 to 6 weeks. In this way, cells that are not in a susceptible stage on one day will be in a susceptible stage on another. Tumors that require such a massive dose of radiation that normal tissue through which the radiation must pass to penetrate the tumor would be destroyed in the process are said to be radioresistant.

Immediate Side Effects

Radiation has both systemic and localized effects. Radiation sickness (anorexia, nausea, vomiting) is the most frequently encountered systemic effect. This occurs if the gastrointestinal (GI) tract is irradiated. It also can occur to a lesser degree as a result of the release of toxic substances from destroyed tumor cells. A child may need to receive an antiemetic before each procedure to counter nausea and vomiting. Extreme fatigue is also very common. Skin reactions, such as erythema and tenderness, are typical local effects.

Long-Term Side Effects

The long-term side effects of radiation are becoming more apparent as increasing numbers of children who have undergone intense radiation therapy survive. Because radiation damages all cells in its path to some extent, any body tissue can be affected by radiation therapy.

Effects on Bone. Asymmetric growth of bones, easy fracturing, scoliosis, kyphosis, or spinal shortening can occur. Bones are most vulnerable during times of rapid growth, such as during the first year of life or during a prepubertal growth spurt. Scoliosis and kyphosis can be avoided if an entire vertebra is irradiated rather than only one side or the other; this means that a larger area of bone may be irradiated than formerly, so that both sides of the vertebra are in the radiation path.

Effects on Hormones. Radiation to the head and neck can result in long-term thyroid, hypothalamic, and pituitary gland dysfunction. This may result in growth hormone deficiency or hypothalamic-pituitary stimulation to the thyroid gland. Children's growth and thyroid function should be evaluated every 6 months for the next 3 years to detect these changes. Both hypothyroidism and hypopituitary growth failure can be treated with hormone replacement in coming years. Radiation to ovaries or testes can result in infertility. In girls, normal estrogen production may lag or fail, preventing the development of secondary sexual changes. In boys, testosterone production rarely fails. However, pretreatment sperm banking may be advocated for a boy past puberty before he undergoes radiation to the testes.

Effects on the Nervous System. Long-term effects of radiation to the nervous system are demyelination and necrosis of the white matter of the brain. This can result in symptoms of lethargy, sleepiness, and seizures. Effects on the gray matter can result in learning disabilities. There may be abnormal electroencephalograph tracings; the child may have low-intensity headaches, cataracts, salivary gland damage, and a chronic change in or loss of taste.

Effects on the Organs of the Chest and Abdomen. Radiation to the lungs may result in a chronic pneumonitis and pulmonary fibrosis or thickening. Heart effects may include pericardial thickening and reduced heart expandability. Radiation to the GI system can result in chronic malabsorption from changes in intestinal villi. Hepatic fibrosis can result in reduced liver function. Radiation to the kidney and bladder can result in nephritis and chronic cystitis.

The possibility of these long-term effects of radiation should be explained to parents when radiation is initially discussed, as a part of obtaining informed consent. At the early stage of diagnosis, however, parents rarely are concerned with these long-term effects. Their thoughts are understandably filled with such short-term outcomes as the achievement of a remission or destruction of the tumor.

NURSING DIAGNOSES AND RELATED INTERVENTIONS

———•———

Nursing Diagnosis: Parental and child anxiety related to radiation procedure

Outcome Evaluation: Parents state that they understand necessity of therapy and can help support child during therapy.

Before Treatment. The points where radiation therapy will be directed are marked on the child's skin, usually in indelible ink. As a rule, no cream or lotion should be applied to radiation areas until the treatment series is complete. If a cream contains any metal, it could distort or interfere with the entrance of radiation. If the head will be irradiated, a dental consultation may be suggested. This is because radiation therapy can slow healing if a tooth extraction is necessary.

During Treatment. Most children have previously had x-ray films taken by the time that radiation therapy is begun, so they are not frightened by the procedure. However, because the procedure requires them to lie still for a period of time, possibly on an uncomfortable table in a room away from personnel or their parents, they may experience extreme fear. Reassure the parents and the child that during the treatment, just as there is no sensation from x-ray exposure, the child will experience no sensation from radiation exposure. Infants are usually prescribed a sedative or conscious sedation before therapy to ensure that they lie still during the procedure. To make this approach effective, keep the child fairly active early in the day and introduce calming activities after the sedative is administered. The child will be sleepy and may fall asleep during irradiation. An older child may want to plan an activity to think about during irradiation, such as selecting 10 people to take on a camping trip (and why), or choosing 10 places to visit next year—mental activities that require no movement.

After Treatment. If the head area is involved in therapy, alopecia (hair loss) may result. Moreover, radiation to the head may reduce salivary gland function, leading to a constantly dry mouth. Tooth growth may be halted due to root atrophy. Radiation to bone marrow may depress the production of white blood cells (WBCs) and platelets. Children undergoing radiation therapy need their leukocyte and platelet counts monitored periodically for changes. Teaching points for parents to maintain skin integrity are summarized in Box 53.6.

Chemotherapy

A **chemotherapeutic agent** is one that is capable of destroying malignant cells. In most instances, several chemotherapeutic agents are used to cause multiple damage to cells and thereby increase the chance that the cells will no longer be able to reproduce. Like radiation, chemotherapy is scheduled over a period of time so that all cells can eventually be destroyed (i.e., cells that are not susceptible on one day because they are undergoing meiosis will be susceptible on the next day).

Types of Chemotherapeutic Agents

Several categories of chemotherapeutic agents are available. Typically, all agents that need mixing are prepared under a specialized hood in the pharmacy to prevent airborne drug residue. When administering such agents, wear gloves and wash your hands well afterward to prevent skin exposure and absorption of the drug.

Alkylating Agents. Alkylating agents interfere with DNA synthesis. They are cell-cycle specific (i.e., they are most effective against cells in the G1 and S phases of growth). Alkylating agents commonly used with children are cyclophosphamide (Cytoxan) and chlorambucil (Leukeran).

Antimetabolites. Antimetabolites are drugs that so closely resemble natural products that a cell incorporates them into its structure. However, they are not the natural product, so the cell cannot function or replicate with them in its structure and will die. They act only in the S (synthesis) phase of the cell cycle. Methotrexate (Folex PFS), a folic acid antagonist, is an example.

Plant Alkaloids. Plant alkaloids interfere with cell mitosis (M phase). Two commonly used plant alkaloids are vincristine (Oncovin) and vinblastine (Velban).

Antibiotics. A number of antibiotics are effective in destroying malignant cells by impairing DNA synthesis. These are not cell-cycle specific, which means that they can be effective at any cell phase (resting or dividing). Dactinomycin (Cosmegen) and doxorubicin (Adriamycin) are examples.

Nitrosoureas. Nitrosoureas disrupt protein synthesis, thereby interfering with DNA synthesis. Because these drugs cross the blood–brain barrier, they are effective as chemotherapy agents in brain tumor therapy. A common example is carmustine (BCNU).

Enzymes. Body cells need a ready supply of L-asparagine (an essential amino acid) to grow. L-Asparaginase (Elspar), a chemotherapeutic agent, is an enzyme that converts L-asparagine into L-aspartic acid, thereby making L-asparagine unavailable for leukemia cell growth.

Steroids. A corticosteroid, most frequently prednisone, binds to DNA to inhibit mitosis and probably RNA synthesis in cells. When it is added to therapy, the formation of new cells is prevented.

Immunotherapy. Immunotherapy is the stimulation of the body's immune system to attempt destruction of

BOX 53.6 FOCUS ON . . .

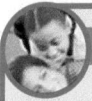

FAMILY TEACHING

Caring for the Child Receiving Radiation Therapy

Q. Geri's mother asks you, "What sorts of things do we need to do when Geri begins receiving radiation therapy?"

A. In addition to preventing infection, you need to take some special actions to meet your child's needs. Here are some tips designed to promote radiation's therapeutic benefits and minimize its adverse effects:

Skin Care
- Expose irradiated area to air but not to direct heat or sunlight.
- Avoid lengthy soaks in bath water or swimming pools.
- If the head is irradiated, use mild shampoo on hair and rinse gently with water. Air dry or pat excess moisture gently. Avoid rough towels and hair dryers.
- Supply a soft toothbrush to protect gums and oral mucous membranes. Keep the mouth moist by offering frequent sips of water—particularly if radiation decreases salivary gland secretions.
- Encourage clothing that fits loosely over irradiated areas.
- Because some skin preparations are drying and some interfere with radiation, do not apply creams or lotions unless prescribed.

Nutrition
- To promote retention of nutrients, administer antiemetics as prescribed.
- Encourage high-calorie meals when child is least likely to be nauseated. Praise the child's efforts to eat. Strive for peaceful and pleasant meal and snack times.
- Provide foods identified by child as special favorites. Serve easy-to-swallow foods at tolerable temperatures.

Hydration
- Reduce amounts of fresh fruit and veggies rich in cellulose, and eliminate apple juice from the child's diet, because these may contribute to diarrhea and subsequent fluid loss.
- If diarrhea occurs, administer antidiarrheal medication as prescribed.

Activity
- Provide adequate rest periods. Schedule activities to avoid waking the child frequently at night.
- Structure the child's activities to be stimulating but not physically tiring.
- Recommend mild activity that does not stress bones that may be weakened by radiation and, therefore, easily fractured.

Instruction and Distraction
- Prepare the child for the effects of radiation therapy, particularly hair loss. Some comfort measures may include wearing a wig or special cap; introducing play things, such as dolls without hair; and stressing that people like people for themselves, not for their appearance.
- Schedule a tour of the radiation department. As possible, let the child play-act and become familiar with the equipment. Provide ample time to answer questions.
- Encourage active games before the procedure and quiet games afterward.
- Help the child devise "mind games" to play during the procedure (e.g., listing 10 friends to take camping, 10 activities to do, or 10 favorite games to play).

---

foreign or malignant cells. The administration of bacille Calmette-Guérin vaccine (the vaccine for tuberculosis) is an example of this type of therapy. The tuberculin antigen stimulates the immune system to identify and destroy an antigen, with the hope that the system will "recognize" foreign tumor cells and act against them as well. Interferon is an antiviral agent that prevents growth of viruses; stimulation of interferon or interferon therapy may be used to attempt to halt malignant cell growth.

Neuroblastoma is an example of a childhood cancer that appears to respond to antibody-based therapy (Kushner et al., 2003).

Immune therapy is limited if the immune system has been so altered by the malignant process that it cannot respond when stimulated. It is also possible that the immune response to malignant cells is so different from the response to invading microorganisms that specific types of immunotherapy are necessary to stimulate it.

Chemotherapy Protocols

Chemotherapy is scheduled for children at set times and days and by various predetermined routes. At first, children may remain in the hospital for a few days of treatment; later, they may report on a specific day for therapy, or parents may administer the designated therapy at home. Parents must learn about the child's treatment protocol so that they know which drug the child will be receiving each day and on which day each drug must be administered. Knowing the protocol and the specific drug therapy helps parents begin to prepare the child for it, such as increasing fiber in the child's diet for a few days before the beginning of a constipation-causing drug like vincristine. An example of such a protocol is shown in Table 53.2. Chemotherapy for acute lymphocytic leukemia (ALL), the most common cancer in children, is given first in a remission phase, next in a sanctuary or prophylactic phase, then in a delayed intensification

TABLE 53.2

Sample Protocol for Treating Acute Lymphocytic Leukemia

	Remission Phase						Sanctuary (or Consolidation) Phase							
Day	1	8	15	22	29	36	43	50	57	64	71	78	85	92
Week	1	2	3	4	5	6	7	8	9	10	11	12	13	14
	V	V	V	V	L	L	M		M		V	M		
							M'+			M'+				
	P	P	P	P	P	P								

V, vincristine; P, prednisone; M, intrathecal methotrexate; L, L-asparaginase; M', methotrexate IV; +, leucovorin.

phase, and finally in a maintenance phase for up to 3 years (Cagen & Franco, 2003).

While children are receiving chemotherapy, parents should not give them aspirin. In addition to increasing the child's susceptibility to Reye's syndrome, aspirin may interfere with blood coagulation, a problem that is already present because of lowered thrombocyte levels. Instead, they should use acetaminophen (Tylenol) or ibuprofen (Motrin) to relieve a headache or to reduce fever. A parent who wants to give a child vitamins should be certain that the vitamin preparation will not interfere with a chemotherapeutic agent. For example, administration of a vitamin that contains folic acid could interfere with the effectiveness of methotrexate, a folic acid antagonist.

Live-virus vaccines should not be given. The child's immune mechanism is so deficient that these vaccines could cause widespread viral disease. The child is particularly susceptible to infections and should be kept away from people with known infections. Zoster immune globulin will be needed if the child has not been immunized against varicella and is exposed to chickenpox during chemotherapy.

Side Effects and Toxic Reactions

All chemotherapeutic agents have side effects and toxic effects. Table 53.3 lists commonly used chemotherapeutic agents, their specific side effects, and their potential toxic effects. Malnutrition, nausea and vomiting, hair loss, stomatitis, constipation, diarrhea, cushingoid effects, and susceptibility to infection are side effects common to almost all of these agents. Nursing diagnoses and related interventions associated with these side effects are described in the following paragraphs.

If an IV infusion of a chemotherapeutic agent that is a vesicant infiltrates into the subcutaneous tissue, there is apt to be extensive tissue sloughing and damage. Monitor IV infusions of chemotherapeutic vesicants carefully to prevent extravasation. Discontinue the infusion if it occurs. Then, apply an ice pack to the site, to cause vasoconstriction and prevent further spread of the toxic solution. Hyaluronidase is an example of a drug that may be injected into the site to speed absorption. After this, application of warm compresses hastens absorption and clearance of the solution from subcutaneous tissue.

NURSING DIAGNOSES AND RELATED INTERVENTIONS

Nursing Diagnosis: Imbalanced nutrition, less than body requirements, related to nausea, vomiting, or anorexia resulting from chemotherapy

Outcome Evaluation: Child is able to eat frequent, small meals; calorie intake is adequate for age and size.

It is easy for the child with cancer to become malnourished. The fast-growing malignant cells take more than their share of nutrients from normal cells. Nausea and vomiting resulting from chemotherapy make it difficult to maintain an adequate oral intake. If stomatitis occurs as a result of chemotherapy, eating becomes difficult due to mouth pain (Chen et al., 2004). Stomach and intestinal ulcers can interfere with absorption. Changes in fatty acid metabolism may alter the responsiveness of body cells to insulin metabolism. Unable to use glucose effectively, cells cannot function at an optimum level. This may account for the sense of fatigue that children with cancer frequently report (Erickson, 2004). Anorexia may occur from a factor produced by the tumor that acts directly on the center for hunger in the hypothalamus, reducing appetite and altering taste perception. Cyclophosphamide, a commonly used chemotherapeutic agent, is associated with taste changes. Many children report that foods taste bitter; they do not describe foods as sweet until they are very sweet. Because of these taste changes, foods the child used to enjoy are no longer enjoyable. Unwilling to try new foods, the child decreases his or her oral intake.

To counteract these taste changes, you may need to suggest different foods or methods of food preparation or include a dietitian as a major health team member. Chicken, for example, often tastes less bitter than beef or pork. Sprinkling brown sugar

Diarrhea may occur from effects of chemotherapeutic agents on the absorptive surfaces of the intestine. Keep careful records of the number and consistency of bowel movements in children receiving chemotherapy. If diarrhea is present, IV fluid will usually be administered to supplement fluid loss; an antidiarrheal agent may be prescribed for older children. Be certain to change infants' diapers frequently to prevent excoriation of the skin from the acid stool content. Diarrhea is frightening for children because of the loss of control they experience. Offer support and comfort for this annoying side effect of their primary therapy.

Nursing Diagnosis: Risk for deficient diversional activity related to neuropathy resulting from chemotherapy

Outcome Evaluation: Child identifies activities in which he can participate that do not require fine motor skills while neuropathy is present.

Almost all children receiving chemotherapy experience fatigue and are unable to participate in their usual activities. If they develop neutropenia, they may require temporary seclusion from other children to prevent exposure to and subsequent development of infection. Help children who are restricted in these ways to find an activity they enjoy, such as drawing, coloring, or playing handheld video games, so they can remain active.

Vincristine therapy results in specific neurologic symptoms, such as weakness, tingling, and numbing of the extremities and sometimes an inability to walk. These symptoms subside after the medication is discontinued. Children may be unable to hold a pen or pencil or maneuver small parts of toys because their fingers are so affected. Think of games they can accomplish until the numbness in the hands fades. Children on bed rest may develop foot drop with vincristine. In some children, physical therapy may be needed along with special braces or boots to prevent foot drop.

Nursing Diagnosis: Risk for infection related to therapy-induced depression of immune system

Outcome Evaluation: Child's temperature remains lower than 98.6°F (37.0°C); no areas of erythema or other signs or symptoms of infection are present.

Children with cancer are very susceptible to infection, not only because their immune system is depressed by chemotherapy but also because they develop a degree of malnutrition that decreases the effectiveness of macrophage and phagocytosis functions, and possibly the production of interferon, which is important for destroying viral invaders. A malignant process in the body decreases the body's overall ability to recognize foreign invaders and respond with the usual efficient rejection process. Frequent insertion of IV devices, the development of dry and cracking mucous membranes, and ulcer formation throughout the GI tract provide ready sites for the entrance of microorganisms.

When infection occurs, it may be difficult to recognize because common findings such as local erythema, swelling, systemic fever, and swollen lymph glands may not be present or may be reduced in relation to the degree of infection present.

Although not well studied in children, administration of colony-stimulating factors such as filgrastim (Neupogen) can help the body quickly begin replacing damaged WBCs (Karch, 2004). Even with the use of this agent, bacterial infections are common. Gram-negative bacteria such as *Escherichia coli, Pseudomonas aeruginosa,* and *Klebsiella pneumoniae,* and gram-positive bacteria such as *Staphylococcus aureus* and streptococci, are common organisms responsible for causing infections. Viral infections such as varicella (chickenpox), varicella zoster (shingles), herpes simplex, viral hepatitis, and cytomegalovirus also are common invaders.

Treating bacterial infections with antibiotics can cause overgrowth of fungal infections such as candidiasis or aspergillosis. When children are treated with immunosuppressive drugs, protozoal infections, such as *Pneumocystis carinii* pneumonia (normally a very rare pneumonia), may occur.

If infection is discovered in a child with cancer, the causative agent is identified by culture. Specific antibiotics are then prescribed. The most important nursing role in caring for children with cancer is to prevent infection. Box 53.9 identifies interventions to reduce the possibility of infection in a child with neutropenia (lowered WBC count).

What if... Geri's mother tells you that she does not want her child to have an antiemetic drug before chemotherapy, because she sees the nausea and vomiting as proof that the chemotherapy is working? Would you give the drug?

Bone Marrow Transplantation

Transplantation of bone marrow that was previously harvested from a child with cancer or transplantation of marrow from a well person to a child with cancer has become a frequently used treatment for children. This can allow higher doses of chemotherapy and radiation to be used because, in the event of severe bone marrow depression, the child can have healthy marrow restored. Immune cells in the transplanted marrow may actually help to kill remaining cancer cells in the child's circulation.

If the child's own marrow is used, the procedure is called *autologous* transfusion. Bone marrow may be donated by someone who is histocompatible (immune compatible) with the child; this is an *allogeneic* transplant. A *syngeneic* transplant is one between twins.

Before transplantation, the child receives a chemotherapy agent, such as cyclophosphamide, and total-body irradiation to kill as many marrow cells as possible, suppress

BOX 53.9 FOCUS ON . . .

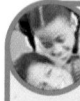

FAMILY TEACHING

Preventing Infection in the Child With Neutropenia

Q. Geri's mother asks you, "What special things should I do to help prevent my child from developing an infection until his white blood cell count returns to normal?"

A. Here are some suggestions to help prevent infections:

- Arrange for your child to sleep in a single bed and room, if possible, to avoid close contact with other family members who may be developing upper respiratory tract infections.
- Limit the child's exposure to large crowds, such as those at movie theaters.
- Screen and prohibit visitors who have signs of infection (e.g., runny nose, oral herpes, rashes); who have been exposed to a communicable disease, such as chickenpox; or who have recently been vaccinated.
- Wash your hands frequently before child care and after handling potentially contaminated items (e.g., tissues, diapers, other containers of body secretions or fluids).
- Urge the child to wash hands well after using a bathroom and before eating.
- Keep child's immediate surroundings free of plants, flowers, and goldfish, all of which could harbor mold spores.
- Be sure the child has a daily bath or shower. Clean mouth with soft toothbrush to reduce opportunity for bacteria, always present in the mouth, to invade.
- Inspect mouth daily for breaks in the tissue, bleeding, or white patches that suggest oral thrush (*Monilia*) infection. Apply a moisturizing and protective barrier, such as KY Jelly, to the lips to help prevent them from cracking.

- Take pulse and respiratory rate and temperature daily. Avoid taking rectal temperatures, to protect against injuring rectal tissue.
- Inspect all skin surfaces daily for scratches that could become entrances for infection. Include IV or IM injection sites, venous access device insertion sites, and the diaper area.
- Administer stool softeners, if prescribed, to promote soft stools and bowel movements and avoid rectal tears.
- Provide high-calorie, high-protein foods and food supplements to help rebuild white blood cells. Do not serve the child fresh fruits and vegetables, because they have more potential to harbor infectious organisms than cooked foods do.
- Assess for respiratory tract infection by listening for cough and throat clearing; inspect throat for redness and nasal passage for discharge. Keep child active and moving (e.g., playing games, such as "Simon Says," that encourage deep breathing).
- Assess for possible genitourinary tract infections. Note the color, clarity, frequency, and concentration of urine. If necessary, obtain a urine specimen using a clean-catch method for testing. Promote increased fluid intake to keep urine flowing. Advise girls to wipe from front to back after voiding or defecating, to avoid bringing organisms forward to the urethra. If a girl is menstruating, sanitary napkins do not have the potential to harbor as many germs as tampons do; urge her to change pads frequently (every 4 hr).
- Question the administration of any vaccine made with a live virus until the child's white blood cell count returns to normal.

the child's immune response to the transplanted tissue, and create space in the bone marrow to allow the newly transplanted cells a place to grow.

Bone marrow is aspirated from the child and treated to reduce the number of abnormal cells present (called purging), or stem cells are removed from the circulating blood of a designated donor or donated placenta. Bone marrow or stem cells are then processed and transfused into the child intravenously. The new marrow migrates to the bone marrow in about 3 weeks. Until this time, the child is at extreme risk for infection. Everyone coming in contact with the child must wash their hands well, and specific infection control precautions must be maintained. Transfusion of blood products may be necessary to maintain functional blood components until the transplanted marrow begins to function.

Not all medical centers perform bone marrow transplantation, so a family may have to travel a distance for the therapy. Complications of bone marrow transplantation are discussed in Chapter 44, because this technique also is used for children with blood dyscrasias. Previously

used only with children with leukemia, it is now being used in children with other cancers, such as neuroblastoma and Hodgkin's disease (Stoneham, 2004).

Pain Assessment

Because growing tumors displace cells, causing anoxia to those cells, pain is a common symptom experienced by children with cancer. Methods to assess pain and interventions to help children deal with pain are discussed in Chapter 38.

THE LEUKEMIAS

Acute Lymphocytic (Lymphoblastic) Leukemia

Leukemia is the distorted and uncontrolled proliferation of WBCs (leukocytes). It is the most frequently occurring type of cancer in children. The most frequent type of leukemia in children, ALL, accounts for 75% of leukemias

(Colby-Graham & Chordas, 2003). The malignant cell involved is the lymphoblast, an immature lymphocyte. With the rapid proliferation of lymphocytes, the production of red blood cells (RBCs) and platelets falls, and invasion of body organs by the rapidly increasing WBC elements begins. Because the abnormally proliferating cells are so immature, they may be identifiable only at the immature "blast cell" or "stem cell" stage.

The highest incidence of ALL is in children between 2 and 6 years of age. The prognosis in children younger than 1 year or older than 10 years at the time of first occurrence is not as good as in those between 2 and 10 years of age. The prognosis in children who have a WBC count higher than 50,000/mm³ or who have more than 10% L2 cells (see classification of cells, described later) in bone marrow at the time of diagnosis is not as good as in those with a lower WBC count and fewer L2 cells at first diagnosis. The incidence of ALL is slightly higher in boys than in girls, and the disease is seen more often in white children than in children of other races (Brown, 2003).

Although it can be shown that leukemia in mice and cats is of viral origin, the cause of leukemia in children is unknown. Radiation, exposure to chemicals, or genetic factors may have some influence on the occurrence. Children with Down syndrome or Fanconi's syndrome are more likely to develop leukemia than are other children (Ravindranath, 2005). If a twin has leukemia, his or her twin (as opposed to a non-twin sibling) is more likely to develop it as well. Bone irradiation may be implicated, so children should be submitted to as few x-rays as possible, including while in utero. An association between magnetic fields or power lines and leukemia is disputed (Brain et al., 2003).

Assessment

With ALL, bone marrow overproduces lymphocytes and therefore is unable to continue normal production of other blood components. The first symptoms of ALL in children usually are pallor, low-grade fever, and lethargy (symptoms of anemia caused by decreased RBC production). A child may have petechiae and bleeding from oral mucous membranes and may bruise easily because of a low thrombocyte count. As the spleen and liver begin to enlarge from infiltration of abnormal cells, abdominal pain, vomiting, and anorexia occur. As abnormal lymphocytes invade the bone periosteum, the child experiences bone and joint pain. Central nervous system (CNS) invasion leads to symptoms such as headache or unsteady gait.

Physical assessment reveals painless, generalized lymphadenopathy, especially of the submaxillary or cervical nodes. Laboratory studies reveal a variable leukocyte count. In some children, the leukocyte count is normal or even slightly decreased but includes the very immature blast cells; in other children, there is a marked leukocytosis of the blast cells. The platelet count and hematocrit are low, but the RBCs that are present are normocytic and normochromic (of normal size and color).

A bone marrow aspiration is done to identify the type of WBC involved or to document the type of leukemia. If there are more than 25% blast cells present, a leukemia diagnosis is established. In children, bone marrow is aspirated at the iliac crest rather than the sternum, both because this is less frightening and because it yields more marrow. Radiographs of the long bones may reveal lesions caused by the invasion of abnormal cells. A lumbar puncture may show evidence of blast cells in the cerebrospinal fluid (CSF).

Checkpoint Question 1

Parents are often unaware that their child is developing leukemia. What are the first signs commonly seen in a child with acute lymphocytic leukemia (ALL)?

a. Nodules and pink rash.
b. Headaches and sleepiness.
c. Fatigue and purpura.
d. Joint pain and coughing.

Therapeutic Management

Up to 95% of children will have a first remission. If a child experiences a relapse, the chances of long-term survival are reduced to approximately 70%. Although remission can be reinduced, the length of each subsequent remission tends to be shorter and less effective (Brown, 2003).

Disease Classification and Prognosis. Leukemia is classified to define subgroups of cells and to predict the usual response to treatment. Blasts with B-lymphocyte cell characteristics can be recognized by the presence of immunoglobulin and antigen–antibody receptors on their surfaces. B-lymphocyte cell types account for 85% of cases of ALL. A specific antigen found on cell surfaces has been named CALLA, and cells are labeled as CALLA positive or CALLA negative. About 15% to 20% of children have T-lymphocyte cell involvement. T lymphocytes are also categorized as CALLA positive or negative.

Cure as Goal. The goal of therapy for leukemia is complete cure, based on the use of chemotherapeutic agents. A chemotherapy program is aimed at, first, achieving a complete remission or absence of leukemia cells (induction phase); second, preventing leukemia cells from invading or growing in the CNS (sanctuary or consolidation phase); third, administering delayed intensive therapy; and fourth, maintaining the original remission (maintenance phase).

Chemotherapy in children is often administered by means of a central venous catheter or port, because administration into a major vessel helps prevent irritation to the vessel walls. These access devices have the secondary advantage of being able to be clamped or "trapped" so that the child can be ambulatory between treatments.

Drugs frequently used to initiate a remission include vincristine, prednisone, L-asparaginase, doxorubicin, and methotrexate. These are given over a period of about 1 month. Because so many cells are destroyed by chemotherapy, a high level of uric acid is excreted during treatment. This can lead to plugging of kidney glomeruli and loss of kidney function. To prevent this, a drug such as allopurinol is often administered with chemotherapy, to reduce the formation of uric acid. Keeping a child well hydrated also helps maintain safe uric acid excretion.

Because many chemotherapy drugs do not cross the blood–brain barrier in effective concentrations, leukemic cells in the CNS continue to flourish even with remission chemotherapy. A combination of intrathecal administration (injection of drugs into the CSF by lumbar puncture) of a drug such as methotrexate and oral administration of 6-mercaptopurine, is next instituted to eradicate this source of leukemic cells. (This is called a *consolidation* or *sanctuary phase,* because no "sanctuary" is given to malignant cells.) Cranial radiation, once used extensively for this purpose, is less used today than previously because, over the long-term, minimal learning disorders may result.

The third phase of therapy intensifies the assault against leukemic cells using chemotherapeutic agents such as vincristine, prednisone, L-asparaginase, doxorubicin, cyclophosphamide, cytosine arabinoside (ARA-C), or 6-thioguanine.

Maintenance and Monitoring. Maintenance chemotherapy aims to eliminate completely any remaining leukemic cells, so that the child's immune system can complete the eradication. Standard maintenance therapy includes a combination of daily 6-mercaptopurine, weekly methotrexate, and sporadic vincristine and prednisone, and intrathecal methotrexate. This is continued for 2 to 3 years. A drug such as leucovorin is usually given after systemic methotrexate, to neutralize its action and protect normal cells from the effect of the drug. During the maintenance phase, the child's blood values must be monitored at least monthly. If there is serious bone marrow depression, medication levels may be reduced or a transfusion may be necessary.

If a bone marrow study during the maintenance phase shows that leukemic cells are again evident, a new induction phase will be initiated, followed by a new sanctuary, intensification, and maintenance phase. Children who are free of disease for 4 years are considered cured, and their maintenance therapy can then be stopped. Bone marrow transplantation or immunotherapy may be used with children who do not respond well to standard therapy. Newer drugs are constantly being investigated to use for relapse therapy. Help parents evaluate the use of nonapproved drugs and the safety of using them with chemotherapeutic agents (Box 53.10).

Complications

Throughout therapy, the health care team and family need to be alert for complications of therapy. Among these problems are CNS, renal, and reproductive system disorders.

Central Nervous System Involvement. If CNS involvement occurs, it can be severe and intense. Blindness, hydrocephalus, and recurrent seizures are possible. The meninges and the sixth and seventh cranial nerves are the structures most often affected. With meningeal involvement, the child develops nuchal rigidity, headache, irritability, and perhaps vomiting and papilledema. A lumbar puncture reveals the presence of blast cells in the CSF. If these are discovered, the child will be treated with intrathecal injections of methotrexate. Always check that a child is not prescribed oral or IV methotrexate at the same time, because some of the dose of intrathecal methotrex-

---

BOX 53.10 FOCUS ON . . .

COMMUNICATION

Geri, a 6-year-old boy, was diagnosed with a brain tumor 3 months ago. His mother brings him into the emergency room because of a severe nosebleed. While you are putting pressure on his nose, you notice that one eye seems to have poor alignment.

Less Effective Communication

Nurse: Is Geri still having chemotherapy, Mrs. Miller?
Mrs. Miller: No. He's in remission.
Nurse: Is he taking anything that would lower his platelet count or clotting factors?
Mrs. Miller: All he takes is asparagus powder we get from Mexico.
Nurse: From Mexico?
Mrs. Miller: It's a new treatment that's not legal here.
Nurse: Has he been back to clinic here for a checkup or follow-up?
Mrs. Miller: No. Asparagus powder is a kind of chemotherapy.
Nurse: Well, let's focus right now on getting this bleeding stopped.

More Effective Communication

Nurse: Is Geri still having chemotherapy, Mrs. Miller?
Mrs. Miller: No. He's in remission.

Nurse: Is he taking anything that would lower his platelet count or clotting factors?
Mrs. Miller: All he takes is asparagus powder we get from Mexico.
Nurse: From Mexico?
Mrs. Miller: It's a new treatment that's not legal here.
Nurse: Are you worried that he still has so many new black and blue marks?
Mrs. Miller: No, asparagus powder is a kind of chemotherapy.
Nurse: Well, let's get this nosebleed stopped. Then we can take a minute to talk about what chemotherapy means.

Of all known diseases, no other disease has as many false "cures" as cancer. When talking with parents, see if they are using any of these unproven methods. Some of them do no harm, so parents can continue to give them along with proven therapies. Others actually interfere with the action of a chemotherapy drug and are contraindicated. In the above scenario, the parent has chosen an unproven regimen. Ignoring the possibility that this choice may be an unhelpful one and denying a potential recurrence of cancer or other problem is not therapeutic and could be detrimental in the long term.

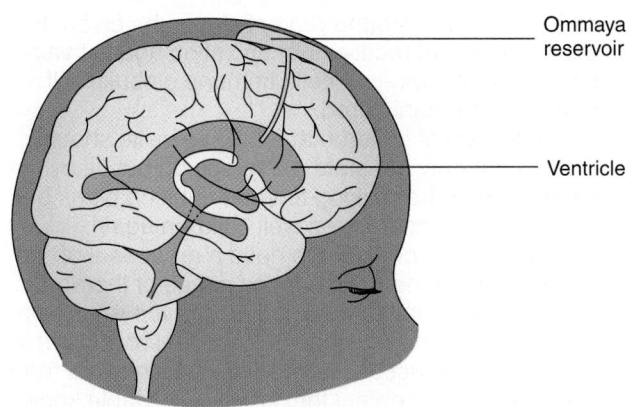

Ommaya
reservoir

Ventricle

FIGURE 53.4 An Ommaya reservoir. Medication injected into the reservoir flows down to the ventricle and enters the cerebrospinal fluid.

ate is absorbed systemically and could lead to a toxic reaction. Inserting silicon tubing into a cerebral ventricle and threading it under the scalp (an Ommaya reservoir) provides easy access to the CSF for sampling or injection without the need for lumbar punctures (Fig. 53.4).

Renal Involvement. Kidney involvement, resulting from invasion of leukemia cells, is a second serious complication. The kidneys may enlarge, and their function will be impaired. If uric acid levels rise as a result of the breakdown of leukemic cells during chemotherapy, plugging of renal tubules with uric acid crystals and kidney failure may result. Renal involvement may limit the use of chemotherapeutic agents, because they cannot be excreted effectively due to the kidney damage.

Testicular Invasion. In boys, leukemic cells tend to invade the testes. Unless this problem is specifically addressed, these cells will not be destroyed by chemotherapy. As a result, once chemotherapy is halted, the leukemic cells may grow and proliferate again. In most boys, therefore, the testes will be irradiated to destroy this sanctuary site for cells. This treatment leads to sterilization later in life. If a boy is past puberty and is forming sperm, sperm banking might be suggested before chemotherapy and radiation to preserve sperm for reproduction later in life.

NURSING DIAGNOSES AND RELATED INTERVENTIONS

Nursing Diagnosis: Risk for infection related to nonfunctioning WBCs and immunosuppressive effects of therapy

Outcome Evaluation: Child's temperature remains lower than 98.6°F (37.0°C); no areas of erythema or drainage are present on skin.

Because the number of functioning WBCs is reduced and the drugs used for treatment are

immunosuppressive, children with leukemia are at an extremely high risk for infection during chemotherapy. Most deaths in children result from infections, such as septicemia, pneumonia, or meningitis. *Pseudomonas* is commonly an invading organism.

While children are receiving care at home, parents must learn to observe them carefully and to promptly report any indication of infection, such as low-grade fever or behavior that does not seem typical of the child. The sooner the symptoms are reported, the sooner antiinfective therapy can begin.

To increase the functioning leukocyte count, leukocytes may be transfused. Symptoms of fever and chills from leukocyte transfusion tend to be more common than with RBC transfusion. This is not a true transfusion reaction and usually is not a reason to stop the transfusion.

Children may be prescribed prophylactic antibiotics to reduce the possibility of infection. Parents may be advised to limit visitors, especially anyone with an infection, until the child's functioning WBC improves.

Nursing Diagnosis: Risk for deficient fluid volume related to increased chance of hemorrhage from poor platelet production

Outcome Evaluation: No evidence of hemorrhage is present (no epistaxis, hematuria, hematemesis); pulse rate and blood pressure remain normal for age group.

Because the platelet count is low due to poor platelet production and the effect of chemotherapy, children with leukemia also are extremely prone to massive hemorrhage. Epistaxis (nosebleed) is the most common kind of bleeding; GI, renal, or CNS bleeding also may occur.

Digital pressure is usually effective to stop epistaxis. The application of Gelfoam soaked in topical thrombin may be necessary. In some children, postnasal packing is necessary. Children may need a transfusion to replace the lost blood volume. Platelet-rich plasma or a concentrated preparation of platelets will be ordered to improve the platelet count. Because the lifespan of transfused platelets is short (1 to 3 days), frequent platelet transfusion may be necessary. After an intramuscular (IM) injection or the removal of an IV needle, apply firm pressure to the injection site to prevent bleeding.

Because children with leukemia have blood samples drawn frequently, receive transfusions, and have IV chemotherapeutic drugs administered, they need the opportunity for therapeutic play with needles and syringes or IV tubing so they can work through some feelings about these intrusive, hurtful procedures. Advocate for intermittent infusion devices such as heparin locks or multilumen central venous catheters that minimize the need for repeated venipunctures.

Nursing Diagnosis: Pain related to invasion of leukocytes

Outcome Evaluation: Child states that pain is tolerable (if infant, not crying).

Children with acute leukemia experience pain because of the vast number of WBCs that invade the periosteum of the bones. Assess pain using a standard scale for accuracy. Handle legs and arms gently to minimize pain. Use of an alternating mattress device underneath body joints helps to reduce skin irritation caused by always resting in the same position. Give analgesia as needed.

Nursing Diagnosis: Ineffective health maintenance related to long-term therapy for leukemia

Outcome Evaluation: Parents and child state importance of regular health maintenance visits; child continues chemotherapy regimen at home and keeps all ambulatory appointments.

During the maintenance phase of therapy, children are allowed normal activity and should attend regular school. Encourage parents to continue to report promptly any sign of infection, so antibiotic therapy can be started early. Because chickenpox can be fatal to a child who is immunosuppressed, have parents ask the child's school to notify them if any other child in the school develops chickenpox,

so appropriate immune protection can be given. If the child did not receive immunization against varicella (chickenpox), varicella immune globulin will need to be administered.

Evaluation of children at follow-up visits should include not only the state of their blood but also whether they are making forward-thinking plans or thinking of themselves as well children again.

Parents may continue to need a great deal of support during the maintenance phase of therapy. They live from day to day, hoping that the remission will not end, and they need a great deal of support if a relapse does occur. Parents who are told that their child has a heart defect that is not correctable know from the beginning that the child will die. In contrast, parents of a child with leukemia constantly hope that a remission is permanent, that their child will be one who is cured. In a sense, the child dies many times—at diagnosis and again if a relapse occurs. If death does occur, the reality of what has happened may be extremely difficult for the parents to accept. They may return to the hospital for visits weeks or months after the child's death in an effort to accept reality and work through their grief. Box 53.11 summarizes care for the child with leukemia.

BOX 53.11: Focus on Nursing Care Planning

A Multidisciplinary Care Map for A Child Receiving Chemotherapy

•

Geri, 6 years old, has had surgery to remove a brain tumor. He is now on ambulatory care receiving additional chemotherapy postoperatively. His father states, "He's nauseated all the time. He says he's never going back to school because he looks so funny. This cure is worse than the disease."

Family Assessment
Child lives with parents and two older sisters (ages 10 and 12 yr) in four-bedroom first-floor flat. Father is manager of a local computer store. Mother used to work as a manicurist. Is stay-at-home-mom since Geri was diagnosed with cancer. Father rates finances as, "Okay. If nothing unexpected happens."

Client Assessment
Sad and pale-appearing school-age child with bald head and recent surgical scar. Weight decreased 5 lb in last 2 weeks. Skin turgor sluggish. Oral mucous membranes red and irritated. Two ulcers noted on inner aspect of left cheek at gum line. Child states, "I look like an old man."

Nursing Diagnosis
Disturbed body image related to hair loss and nausea secondary to the effects of chemotherapy

Outcome Criteria
Child states effect of hair loss and nausea on appearance and feelings; verbalizes measures to cope with hair loss and nausea; reports continued participation in age-appropriate activities.

(continued)

Team Member Responsible	Assessment	Intervention	Rationale	Expected Outcome
Activities of Daily Living				
Nurse	Assess whether child is capable of self-care in light of changes that have occurred with chemotherapy.	Encourage child to perform as many self-care activities as he did before becoming ill.	Maintaining self-care activities is a way of maintaining self esteem and competence.	Child states that although he doesn't feel well, he will try to do self-care.
Consultations				
Nurse	Assess whether parents would like an oncology nurse to discuss nutritional side effects of chemotherapy with them.	Contact oncology nurse if desired to review problems with nutrition during chemotherapy.	An expert can help parents to determine more effective strategies to combat and accept the nausea and appearance caused by chemotherapy.	An oncology nurse speaks with the parents if indicated.
Procedures/Medications				
Nurse	Assess oral mucous membrane to detect and document oral lesions.	Instruct child and parent in oral care. Advise using a soft toothbrush or swabs to cleanse teeth.	Good oral care is essential to prevent further ulceration.	Child is able to maintain nutrition despite oral lesions.
Physician/ Nurse	Assess whether topical anesthetic solution would help to decrease pain from mouth ulcers.	Teach parent to apply topical anesthetic to the ulcers as appropriate.	Topical anesthetics may decrease the discomfort of the ulcers and improve nutrition.	Child states he would like to try topical therapy to see if it can reduce ulcer pain.
Nutrition				
Nurse	Assess whether child has had any relief from prescribed antiemetics.	Administer prescribed antiemetic approximately 30 min before initiating chemotherapy.	Antiemetics administered before chemotherapy help to prevent nausea and vomiting.	Child agrees to administration of antiemetic before chemotherapy to help reduce nausea.
Nurse/ nutritionist	Assess child's intake by a 24-hr recall history.	Encourage parent to offer food early in the day before chemotherapy. Suggest frequent, high-calorie snacks, such as high-energy snack bars.	Eating before chemotherapy enhances nutrition because the child is less likely to be nauseated at this time.	Parent states she will try to have child eat highly nutritious snacks during times he is not nauseated, to optimize nutrition intake.
Patient/Family Education				
Nurse	Assess parents' and child's understanding of the action of chemotherapy.	Teach parents about the type of medications child is receiving and their usual actions and side effects.	Understanding that side effects are expected, not unique, can help parents and child accept the appearance changes that occur.	Parents/child state they understand what changes to expect and they understand these are temporary.
Psychosocial/Spiritual/Emotional Needs				
Nurse	Assess the child's understanding of hair loss and its cause.	Review the structure and function of the hair and explain why hair loss develops.	Understanding that this appearance change, although dramatic, is not permanent can help the child to accept it.	Child states he understands his hair will grow back.

(continued)

Team Member Responsible	Assessment	Intervention	Rationale	Expected Outcome
Psychosocial/Spiritual/Emotional Needs				
Nurse	Assess whether child can devise any measures that would make him feel better about his changed appearance.	Brainstorm with child and parents about measures such as wearing a scarf or cap or modeling an action figure.	Fostering a positive outlook can help child accept changed appearance as a mark signifying he is managing a stressful time of life very well.	Child states he will try to view hair loss as a positive feature, not a detrimental one.
Discharge Planning				
Nurse	Assess whether parents or child have any further questions before discharge about nutrition or appearance.	Urge parent to contact clinic if child develops further ulcerations or experiences continued weight loss or an increase in nausea and vomiting.	Continued nausea and vomiting, weight loss, or development of more ulcers requires further evaluation and follow-up to minimize the risk of additional problems for the child.	Parents and child state they feel confident in managing nutrition adequately during remainder of chemotherapy.
Nurse	Assess whether parents are aware of continuous pattern of chemotherapy and need to return for further therapy.	Review the chemotherapy protocol with parents and child so they know the dates of therapy.	When chemotherapy is administered on an ambulatory basis it can better keep a family intact.	Parents/child state they understand the importance of return appointments and will keep them.

Acute Myeloid Leukemia

Acute myeloid leukemia (AML) involves the overproliferation of granulocytes. It accounts for about 20% of all childhood leukemias (Lange et al., 2005). The frequency of the disorder increases in late adolescence. In its chronic form, it is the most common type of leukemia in adulthood.

With AML, granulocytes grow so rapidly that they often are forced out into the bloodstream while still in the blast stage. As with ALL, the overproliferation of granulocytes limits the production of RBCs and platelets.

Assessment

Children with AML have the same symptoms as those with ALL. Because they do not have mature granulocytes, they are susceptible to infection and may have noticed many recent upper respiratory tract infections before the time of diagnosis.

Therapeutic Management

The diagnosis is established by bone marrow aspiration and biopsy. Cells are typed (M1 to M6) to establish prognosis. After diagnosis, chemotherapy to effect remission begins. Doxorubicin and cytosine arabinoside (ARA-C) are two drugs commonly used for therapy. It may take 1 to 2 months to reach a full remission.

During the maintenance phase, additional chemotherapeutic agents in common use are cyclophosphamide and 6-thioguanine. Maintenance therapy is continued for 6 to 9 months (Kang, 2003).

Remission is more difficult to achieve in children with AML than in those with ALL, and if one is achieved, it may be brief. Bone marrow transplantation may be attempted after the initial remission to ensure new growth of normal granulocytes.

THE LYMPHOMAS

Lymphomas are malignancies of the lymph or reticuloendothelial system; they account for about 15% of all malignancies and are categorized as Hodgkin's or non-Hodgkin's lymphomas. Although Hodgkin's disease is better known, non-Hodgkin's lymphomas are more common worldwide in children (about 60% versus 40%). They both occur more frequently in males than in females (Ginsberg, 2003).

Hodgkin's Disease

With Hodgkin's disease, lymphocytes proliferate, and special *Reed-Sternberg cells* (large, multinucleated cells that are probably nonfunctioning monocyte-macrophage cells) are found. Although these lymphocytes are capable of DNA synthesis and mitotic division, they are abnormal because they lack both B- and T-lymphocyte surface markers and cannot produce immunoglobulins (Max et al., 2003).

As with all neoplastic diseases, the etiology of Hodgkin's disease is unknown, but both genetic and environmental factors probably play a part. It is rarely seen in children younger than 7 years of age. The incidence increases greatly during adolescence and young adulthood. Metastasis is through lymphatic channels. Late in the disease, spread to lung, liver, and bone marrow occurs.

Assessment

Symptoms of Hodgkin's disease usually begin with only one painless, enlarged, rubbery-feeling lymph node, usually a cervical node. Other nodes then become involved, along with the liver, spleen, bone marrow, and, eventually, the CNS. The child usually has accompanying symptoms of anorexia, malaise, night sweats, and loss of weight. Fever may be present. The sedimentation rate is elevated; anemia is usually present as a result of reduced RBC survival.

Hodgkin's disease is confirmed by biopsy of the lymph nodes. Further studies (bone marrow analysis, liver function tests, chest and abdominal computed tomography [CT] scans, lymphangiography, and abdominal biopsy) are done to classify the clinical stage of the disorder. Chest radiography reveals enlarged mediastinal nodes; the abdominal CT reveals enlarged lymph nodes of the abdomen.

A lymphangiogram, performed by injecting dye into the hand or foot, allows visualization of the lymphatic system. A catheter is inserted into a lymph vessel, and radiopaque dye is added, as in angiography. Lymphatic channels can be visualized on x-ray films. The lymph system does not eradicate opaque dye readily; in some children, lymph chains will still be outlined on x-ray films for up to 1 year. The original dye injected into the skin to visualize the lymph vessels stains the skin a bluish green. This dye will remain as a skin stain for about 1 year. Nodes opacified by lymphangiogram dye can be used as markers of disease progress on plain, flat-plate x-ray films for 6 to 12 months.

Therapeutic Management

Four subcategories of Hodgkin's disease can be documented: lymphocyte predominant, nodular sclerosing, mixed cellularity, and lymphocyte depletion. The most frequently occurring types in children are nodular sclerosing and lymphocyte predominant.

The disease is staged according to regional involvement (Table 53.4). Such staging may be determined by a CT scan followed by multiple lymph node and bone marrow biopsies.

Treatment depends on the clinical stage of the disease at the time of diagnosis. Although Hodgkin's disease once was treated mainly with radiation therapy, children today in all stages receive chemotherapy. Common agents include mechlorethamine (nitrogen mustard), vincristine (Oncovin), procarbazine, and prednisone, a protocol commonly called MOPP therapy. Other drugs used include cyclophosphamide and cytarabine. Current therapy results in a 90% 5-year survival rate for children with stage I or stage II disease, and 60% to 90% for more advanced disease. If a relapse occurs, additional chemotherapy, radiation, or bone marrow transplantation will be scheduled.

Children need conscientious follow-up for symptoms of Hodgkin's disease relapse during adult life. A relapse is often retreatable, using a chemotherapy course different from that used initially.

TABLE 53.4	
Stages of Hodgkin's Disease	
Stage	**Extent of Disease**
I	Disease affects single lymph node or single extralymphatic organ or site.
II	Disease affects two or more lymph node regions on the same side of the diaphragm, or there is localized involvement of an extralymphatic organ or site.
III	Disease affects lymph node regions on both sides of the diaphragm, or there is localized involvement of an extralymphatic organ or site.
IV	There is diffuse or disseminated involvement of extralymphatic organs with or without associated lymph node involvement.

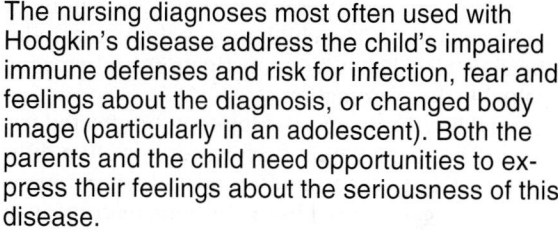

NURSING DIAGNOSES AND RELATED INTERVENTIONS

The nursing diagnoses most often used with Hodgkin's disease address the child's impaired immune defenses and risk for infection, fear and feelings about the diagnosis, or changed body image (particularly in an adolescent). Both the parents and the child need opportunities to express their feelings about the seriousness of this disease.

Nursing Diagnosis: Risk for powerlessness related to constant possibility of disease recurrence

Outcome Evaluation: Child states that he feels healthy during remission, participates in school and extracurricular activities, and voices confidence in health care team to treat symptoms if they recur.

The course of treatment for Hodgkin's disease is long. Some adolescents, in whom the disease is most prevalent, live from day to day wondering whether symptoms will recur.

Encourage adolescents to attend regular school during periods of remission, so that they can lead as normal a life as possible. Keep them informed about the disease and their progress. Some adolescents want to know exactly what stage they are in; others prefer not to be told, so they can continue to believe that a cure will be possible. Both adolescents and their parents need continued support from health care personnel during the long course of therapy.

Non-Hodgkin's Lymphoma

Non-Hodgkin's lymphomas are malignant disorders of the lymphocytes (Ginsberg, 2003). They involve stem cells and lymphocytes in varying degrees of differentiation. In the pediatric population, diffuse lymphoblastic, undifferentiated, and large-cell lymphomas are commonly seen. Unlike Hodgkin's disease, spread is through the bloodstream rather than directly by lymph flow. The course of the disease is therefore unpredictable. Metastatic spread to the CNS tends to occur early in the disease. The most common age at occurrence is 5 to 15 years.

The cause of non-Hodgkin's lymphomas may be an oncogenic virus, because they occur with increased frequency in children with agammaglobulinemia or acquired immunodeficiency syndrome (AIDS) and in those who are receiving long-term immunosuppressive therapy, such as would be given after organ transplantation. Such immunosuppressed states may reduce the body's ability to recognize and destroy oncogenic viruses or malignant cells.

Assessment

Non-Hodgkin's lymphomas of the lymphoblastic type involve the lymph glands of the neck and chest most commonly, although axillary, abdominal, or inguinal nodes may be the first involved. If mediastinal lymph glands are swollen, the child may first notice a cough or chest "tightness." If mediastinal nodes press on the veins returning blood from the head, edema of the face may result. Diffuse, undifferentiated types manifest most commonly with an abdominal mass. The child notices abdominal pain; he or she may have diarrhea or constipation, and a mass may be palpable on examination.

To establish the diagnosis, biopsy of the affected lymph nodes and bone marrow is performed. It is often difficult to distinguish between undifferentiated lymphoma cells and ALL. This can be established by bone marrow analysis (if a bone marrow biopsy shows more than 25% blasts, the diagnosis is acute leukemia). Areas of metastases are identified by chest radiography; lymphangiography; gallium, liver-spleen, and CT scans; and bone marrow aspiration.

Therapeutic Management

Non-Hodgkin's lymphomas are treated with systemic chemotherapy, similar to that used for ALL. The initial phase of therapy is an induction phase (a time during which the child is put into remission, or no tumor can be detected by clinical means); this is followed by a maintenance phase up to 2 years long. Common drugs used are cyclophosphamide, vincristine, methotrexate, and prednisone (COMP therapy) and a multiple-agent program that includes cytosine arabinoside, cyclophosphamide, daunorubicin, vincristine, prednisone, L-asparaginase, thioguanine, and methotrexate. Intrathecal chemotherapy may be included because of the tendency for non-Hodgkin's lymphoma to metastasize to the CNS (Ginsberg, 2003). Because the breakdown of cells is so rapid with chemotherapy, assess for hyperkalemia and hyperphosphatemia. Anticipate that allopurinol will be added to the therapy to prevent uric acid accumulation in the kidney. A granulocyte colony-stimulating factor may be given to prevent neutropenia.

Autologous bone marrow transfusion (using bone marrow removed at diagnosis, before the disease has spread to the marrow, and then replaced after blood components have been destroyed by chemotherapy) allows more aggressive chemotherapy to be used than formerly.

Between 80% and 90% of children with non-Hodgkin's lymphoma with minimal symptoms achieve remission.

Burkitt's Lymphoma

Burkitt's lymphoma (a non-Hodgkin's lymphoma) is a specifically named but rare form of cancer in the United States; it is more commonly seen in Africa. When this lymphoma does occur, however, it tends to affect children. Children 2 to 14 years of age have the highest incidence, with a peak at 7 years (Lones et al., 2004).

An association between Burkitt's lymphoma and Epstein-Barr virus, which causes infectious mononucleosis, exists. That is not to say that the virus causes the lymphoma, only that the virus is present at the same time as Burkitt's lymphoma.

The first indication of disease is an enlarged lymph node of the neck or abdomen. It is usually painless unless it blocks some body system.

A Burkitt's lymphoma is a rapidly growing tumor; the cell mass may double in size in 24 hours. Surgery is used to remove the primary tumor. This is followed by chemotherapy; cyclophosphamide, methotrexate, doxorubicin, vincristine, and prednisone are commonly used agents. To prevent CNS involvement, intrathecal methotrexate may be given.

Because Burkitt's lymphomas are such rapidly growing tumors, they respond dramatically to chemotherapy (the cells are almost always in a susceptible state). As with other lymphomas, tissue breakdown may be so voluminous that the uric acid level of the urine may cause renal tubule plugging unless the child is kept well hydrated and a drug such as allopurinol is administered concurrently.

NEOPLASMS OF THE BRAIN

Brain tumor is the second most common form of cancer in children and the most common solid tumor form. Tumors tend to occur between 1 and 10 years of age, with 5 years being the peak age of incidence. In children, brain tumors tend to occur at the midline in the brainstem or cerebellum, located beneath the tentorial membrane; in contrast, they usually are lateral and above the tentorial membrane in adults. This feature makes them particularly difficult to remove in children without damage to normal brain tissue (Fine, 2005).

Types of Brain Tumors

Common sites for brain tumors in children are shown in Figure 53.5. The most common brain tumors are cerebellar astrocytomas, medulloblastomas, and brainstem tumors.

Astrocytomas are slow-growing, cystic tumors that arise from the glial or support tissue of neural cells. They account for about one fourth of all brain tumors in children. The peak age of incidence is 5 to 8 years.

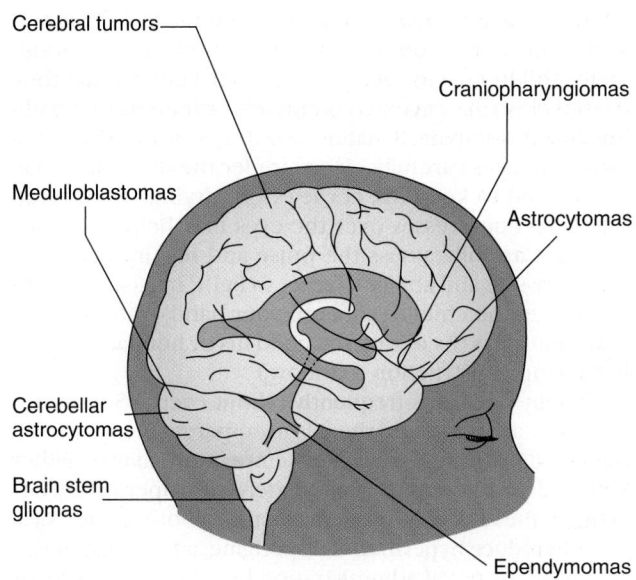

Cerebral tumors

Craniopharyngiomas

Medulloblastomas

Astrocytomas

Cerebellar
astrocytomas

Brain stem
gliomas

Ependymomas

FIGURE 53.5 Common sites for brain tumors in children.

Medulloblastomas are fast-growing tumors found most commonly in the cerebellum. The peak age of incidence is 5 to 10 years. Usually found at the midline, they cause fourth-ventricle compression and disturbances in the flow of CSF.

Brainstem tumors arise from the support tissue of the neural cells. They often cause paralysis of the fifth, sixth, seventh, ninth, and tenth cranial nerves. They may produce symptoms of ataxia, nystagmus, and changes in respiratory and pulse findings due to pressure on these centers.

Assessment

Children with brain tumor develop symptoms of increased intracranial pressure: headache, vision changes, vomiting, an enlarging head circumference, or papilledema. Lethargy, projectile vomiting, and coma are late signs.

The headache associated with brain tumor usually occurs on arising in the morning. It may be intermittent because of pressure changes related to position and the ability of the cranium to expand to some degree and temporarily relieve the associated pressure. It becomes intense on straining, such as occurs with coughing or bowel movements. A parent may report these symptoms in an increasingly irritable young child who is constipated because of reluctance to strain to pass stool. With some tumors, the pain is occipital. This is an important finding, because this is an unusual location for a headache from any other cause.

Vomiting, like headache, more commonly occurs on arising. Unlike the child who vomits because of GI distress, the child with a brain tumor is not usually nauseated and will eat immediately afterward. The vomiting pattern occurs morning after morning. It eventually become projectile after a long time, but projectile vomiting is not an initial symptom. Vomiting in this pattern may be discounted by parents as school phobia (reluctance to attend school), because the child is able to eat again immediately and seems to recover about half an hour after getting out of bed (at the same time the school bus leaves).

Diplopia due to sixth cranial nerve involvement or strabismus due to suppression of vision in one eye is usually noted. Children with strabismus may tend to tilt the head to the side or partially close one eye when viewing objects to compensate for the suppression and strabismus. The child may develop a torticollis (wry neck) or ptosis (lag of the eyelid). Papilledema (swelling of the optic nerve) may be evident on funduscopic examination.

Apart from these generalized symptoms of increased intracranial pressure, a growing tumor produces specific localized signs, such as nystagmus (constant horizontal movement of the eye), cranial nerve paralysis, or visual field defects. Tumors of the cerebellum tend to cause a definite head tilt due to vision suppression. As tumor growth continues, symptoms of ataxia, personality change (emotional lability, irritability), and seizures may occur.

Four to 6 months may pass from the time of initial symptoms until symptoms become localized enough to arouse suspicion of a brain tumor. When this suspicion arises, the child needs a thorough neurologic examination; skull films, a bone scan, a sonogram or MRI, cerebral angiography, or a CT scan will be performed as needed. Myelography may be done to identify tumors that have spread into the spinal column. Lumbar puncture must be done cautiously, because the release of CSF can cause the brainstem (under pressure from the tumor) to herniate into the spinal cord, interfering with respiratory and cardiac function.

Therapeutic Management

Therapy for brain tumors includes a combination of surgery, radiotherapy, and chemotherapy, depending on the location and extent of the tumor. Because they are located so deeply, most tumors cannot be completely removed in children; this makes radiotherapy and chemotherapy increasingly important. Radiation therapy may be intense because, if tumor tissue is not rapidly proliferating, cells are not easily destroyed. Chemotherapy is limited because many chemotherapeutic agents do not cross the blood–brain barrier. Lomustine (CCNU) and vincristine are two drugs that do cross the barrier and so are used. Administration of the drug directly into the ventricular system via a reservoir (Ommaya) may increase drug effectiveness. Research is revealing special gene activating factors found in children's brain tumors that will serve as a basis for future therapy (Boon et al., 2004).

The diagnosis of brain tumor at any age is always a serious one and a stress for parents (Freeman et al., 2004). Closely observe a child who is admitted to the hospital for a possible diagnosis of brain tumor, to detect signs of increased intracranial pressure or new localizing signs as they occur. Record pulse rate, blood pressure, and respiratory rate with extreme accuracy, so that subtle changes become apparent. Note and document episodes of irritability, drowsiness, speech difficulty, and eye involvement. Statements such as, "Child says he sees two forks when I show him one" or "Child is unable to see objects held in her left field of vision" are much more meaningful to a neurosurgeon than "Child has difficulty seeing." Completely describe any seizure activity observed, particularly the beginning movements of the seizure, because these may help to localize the point of maximum brain pressure. Side rails should be in place for protection if a seizure occurs while the child is in bed.

Preoperative Care

Before brain surgery, the child may receive a stool softener to prevent straining with bowel movements. Usually no preoperative enema is given, because expelling an enema increases intracranial pressure.

Dexamethasone (Decadron) may be prescribed to reduce edema. An anticonvulsant such as phenytoin (Dilantin) will be ordered if the child is experiencing seizures or if surgery is apt to induce seizures. Also before surgery, a portion of the child's head is shaved. Prepare the child for this in a positive way by emphasizing that hair grows back very rapidly (Fig. 53.6).

If the child will go to an intensive care unit (ICU) for the first few days after surgery, a preoperative visit to meet the ICU staff should be made.

Postoperative Care

If laser surgery techniques were used for surgery, the postoperative course is simplified and shortened. Position the child as the surgeon prescribes. The position depends on the location of the tumor and the extent of surgery, but in general a child is positioned on the side opposite the incision. Keep the bed flat or only slightly elevated. Do not lower the head of the bed, because this would increase intracranial pressure from accumulation of increased blood in the area. Note carefully how much movement of the child's neck is allowed. If surgery was in the low occipital area, the surgeon may want the child to be moved as though the head and neck were a single body part. A neck brace or cast can be applied to stabilize the head and neck and prevent movement.

You can expect the child to be comatose or extremely lethargic for a number of days after surgery due to brain irritation and edema. In addition, the child may require mechanical ventilation because of pressure on the respiratory center. Unless they are being ventilated, comatose

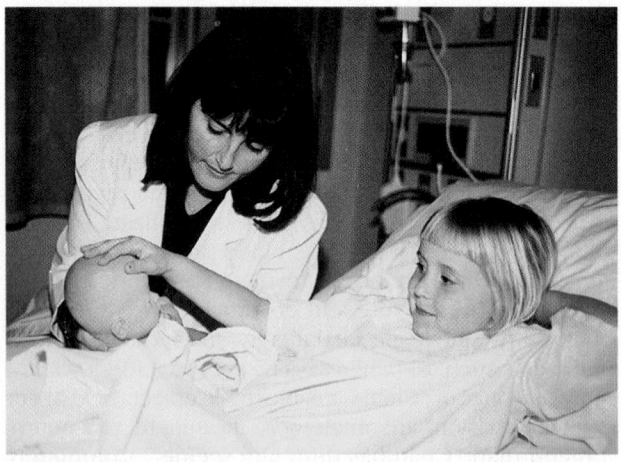

FIGURE 53.6 A nurse uses a doll to help prepare a child for shaving her head for brain surgery. (© Caroline Brown, RNC, MS, DEd.)

children need to be positioned on their side so that oral secretions drain from the mouth, to prevent aspiration. Many children have such extreme facial edema that they cannot close their eyelids completely or their nasal breathing space is impaired. Saline eye drops or eye dressings (with the eyes carefully closed under the dressings) may be ordered to keep the cornea from drying and ulcerating. Cool compresses over the eyes may help to reduce edema. Carefully assess the pulse and respiratory rates, pupillary size and ability to react to light, muscle strength (by asking the child to squeeze your hands), and level of consciousness (by asking the child his or her name or giving a simple instruction to follow).

Obtain vital signs frequently (about every 15 minutes) until they are stable and there is no apparent increase in intracranial pressure. The child's temperature may be either elevated or decreased immediately postoperatively because of the effect of the edema on the hypothalamus. Measures to reduce hyperthermia (sponging, antipyretics given by gavage or rectal administration because of lethargy or coma, or a hypothermia blanket) may be necessary to reduce the temperature to less than 101°F (38.4°C).

Regulate the rate of IV fluid infusion carefully. An increase in the infusion rate will increase intracranial pressure. Children may receive solutions of mannitol or hypertonic dextrose to aid in evacuating the cerebral hemispheres of edematous fluid. As the child regains consciousness, small amounts of oral fluid may be started. Make certain, when introducing fluid, that the child is free of nausea from the anesthetic, because vomiting increases intracranial pressure.

Observe head dressings carefully for serosanguineous drainage. A wet dressing is no longer a sterile dressing, because pathologic organisms may filter through its folds to reach the meninges and cause meningitis. Place a sterile towel under a wet dressing or reinforce the dressing with sterile compresses. Report signs of drainage, and estimate the extent of the seepage so that you can tell later whether seepage has increased.

Children regaining consciousness after brain surgery usually are confused as to time and place; they may have difficulty performing simple tasks that they could do easily before. As the cerebral edema subsides and children begin to regain consciousness, they may need to be restrained to stop them from touching their head dressing or IV line. Use as few restraints as possible because fighting restraints causes intracranial pressure to increase. Help the child gradually regain independence in self-care.

After the child is discharged from the hospital, parents should allow the child as near-normal activity as possible. Some children may need a football helmet to protect their head if a section of skull was removed or is not yet firmly closed. When the bulky head dressing is removed, the child may become aware of baldness for the first time. Some children need support to return to school because they are aware that other children will treat them differently now, having heard from their parents that they are dying or "had to have their head fixed." Urge parents to make the school administration aware of what has happened to the child; the school nurse should be encouraged to take an active role in helping the child readjust to school after a long absence.

Late effects may occur in children who survive a malignant brain tumor. Long-term neurologic and pituitary dysfunction (especially lack of growth hormone) and cognitive challenge are not unusual in survivors of pediatric brain tumor, especially if they received high doses of cranial radiation at a very young age.

Checkpoint Question 2

Geri is going to have surgery for a brain tumor. Why may children be prescribed a stool softener before this type of surgery?

a. Constipation stimulates the release of hypopituitary hormones.

b. Straining with bowel movements increases intra-cranial pressure.

c. Constipation can lead to anal fissures and a source of infection.

d. Children in Trendelenburg positions cannot evacuate bowels well.

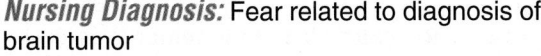

NURSING DIAGNOSES AND RELATED INTERVENTIONS

Nursing Diagnosis: Fear related to diagnosis of brain tumor

Outcome Evaluation: Parents and child continue to maintain function as a family, visit in hospital, and plan appropriately for discharge and continued care.

Parents of children with brain tumors usually are not prepared for the severity of their child's diagnosis. They bring the child to a health care facility because of insidious symptoms—vomiting, headache, strabismus. They may think that the child has a mild GI upset or needs eyeglasses. They are shocked to learn that such benign symptoms are signs of a condition that may be fatal. This can cause such distress at the time of the initial diagnosis that they cannot think of questions to ask. In the hours or days after the diagnosis, they often have a great need to talk to people who are familiar with the care of children with brain tumors and to ask questions of the neurosurgeon.

Most parents want to hear a definite statement about prognosis—for example, "All of the tumor can be removed; your child will be as good as new" or "Your child's chances are 1 in 4 of surviving surgery (or of having permanent effects)." Because the type of tumor, its exact location, and its extent are not fully known until the surgery, these predictions cannot be made with more than an informed guess. Reassure parents that it is normal in these instances for a surgeon not to give more definitive information.

Otherwise, they may interpret a surgeon's unwillingness to give them definite figures as incompetence or lack of interest. Help assure parents that earlier diagnosis would not have made a difference in the outcome. This makes it possible for them to live with themselves afterward and not be overwhelmed by the guilt, thinking that they could have prevented a bad outcome by recognizing symptoms earlier. Symptoms of brain tumor *are* insidious when they first begin, and the average parent cannot be expected to recognize them as important.

Help parents understand that, because of the importance of brain tissue, brain surgery is never minor surgery. Inform them how their child will appear after surgery: Their child will have a large, bulky head dressing; be drowsy or unresponsive; and have possible facial edema. Still, even parents who are well prepared are likely to be shocked at the actual sight of their child. Before you take them to the child's room after surgery, review with them once more that the child has a bulky dressing and is unconscious.

Some parents may not "hear" the full extent of their child's diagnosis before surgery. They cannot believe that the surgeon will not be able to remove the entire tumor and cure their child. After surgery, when they are told that the entire tumor could not be removed, a very genuine grief reaction occurs. As a result, they may be unable to sit and hold the child's hand, read to the child, and talk to him or her, because their minds have already jumped ahead to the time when the child might die. The child may have difficulty relating to them because they are no longer acting like the parents he or she knew before surgery (more like two strangers). Parents need a great deal of support from the time a child is first seen until the surgery, through discharge and readmissions, to the last hospital admission, when the child finally dies.

Children as young as 5 years old are aware that the head and the brain are important parts of the body. They are very aware of the feeling tone they detect in the words of parents and health care personnel. Because they undergo a number of diagnostic studies, followed by surgery and prolonged therapy, provide children with opportunities to express their feelings about intrusive procedures through play with puppets or hospital equipment. Remember that, when a patient becomes unconscious, hearing is often the last sense lost. Although children do not appear to respond after surgery, they may be able to hear everything that is said.

BONE TUMORS

Tumors derived from connective tissue, such as bone and cartilage, muscle, blood vessels, or lymphoid tissue, are called **sarcomas.** They are the second most frequently occurring neoplasms in adolescents (only lymphomas occur more frequently). Bone tumors may arise during adolescence because rapid bone growth is occurring at this time. Because girls have a puberty growth spurt earlier than boys, bone tumors tend to occur slightly earlier in girls

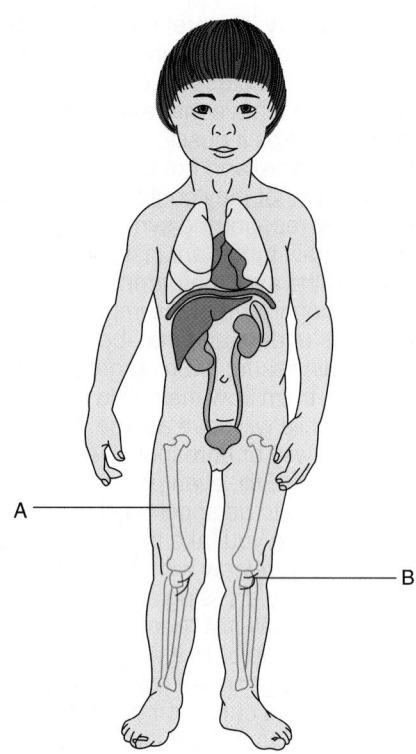

FIGURE 53.7 (A) The diaphysis (midshaft) is one of the most frequent sites of Ewing's sarcoma. **(B)** The epiphysis of a bone is a common site of osteogenic sarcoma.

than in boys (13 compared with 14 or 15 years of age). The two most frequently occurring types are osteogenic sarcoma and Ewing's sarcoma (Fig. 53.7).

Osteogenic Sarcoma

An **osteogenic sarcoma** is a malignant tumor of long bone involving rapidly growing bone tissue (mesenchymal-matrix forming cells). It tends to occur more commonly in boys than in girls. The most common sites of occurrence are the distal femur (40% to 50%), the proximal tibia (20%), and the proximal humerus (10% to 15%). Osteogenic sarcoma can occur in children who have had radiation for other malignancies as a later life effect. Children with retinoblastoma have a higher incidence than normal of osteosarcoma, so a hereditary influence may be present.

Although bones do not have a lymphatic system, metastasis occurs early because of the extensive vascular system in bones (Malawer et al., 2005). Metastasis to the lungs is the most common site; as many as 25% of adolescents have lung metastasis already by the time of initial diagnosis. When this is present, the adolescent usually has a chronic cough, dyspnea, chest pain, and leg pain (if the tumor originates in the leg). Other common sites of metastasis are brain and other bone tissue.

Assessment

Children with osteogenic sarcoma often are taller than average, indicating rapid bone growth. They notice pain and swelling at the tumor site. Often, they report a history of recent trauma to the site (e.g., they fell playing basketball and bumped their knee) and attribute pain in the knee to this injury for some time. All adolescents with extremity pain and swelling, particularly near the knee, require evaluation because of the possibility that a malignant process may be at work. It is important that both adolescents and their parents understand that trauma did not cause the process; it merely called attention to the leg or arm where a malignant process was at work. This prevents adolescents from thinking that they caused the tumor.

The area may be inflamed and feel warm, because tumors are highly vascular and therefore call increased blood into the area. As the tumor invades and weakens bone tissue, a pathologic fracture of the bone can occur.

For diagnosis, a biopsy is done of the area under suspicion. Bone cells produce alkaline phosphatase, and rapidly growing bone cells raise the serum level of this enzyme markedly, so serum analysis for alkaline phosphatase will be obtained. To determine metastasis, a complete blood cell count, urinalysis, chest radiograph, chest CT scan, and bone scans will be done. Caution children not to bear weight on an affected appendage while waiting for tests or surgery. The bone may be so weakened by the growing tumor that weight bearing results in a fracture at the tumor site.

Therapeutic Management

If the tumor is in the leg and is small at the time of diagnosis, and if the child has reached adult height, the single bone involved may be surgically removed and replaced with an internally placed bone or metal prosthesis. This will preserve the child's leg. If the tumor is extensive at the time of diagnosis, the leg may be amputated at the joint above the tumor (this usually involves a total hip amputation). If the cancer has spread to the lung, metastases can usually be removed by thoracotomy.

An adolescent may have chemotherapy to shrink the tumor before surgery. Parents may be very concerned with the delay before surgery. Then need an explanation that, with bone tumor, this is an accepted and helpful intervention before surgery. Common treatment drugs include methotrexate, cisplatin, doxorubicin, and ifosfamide.

Only a few years ago, a diagnosis of osteogenic sarcoma was ominous; few children survived into adulthood. Today, 60% to 65% of adolescents in whom the diagnosis is made early and who are treated rigorously can be cured.

NURSING DIAGNOSES AND RELATED INTERVENTIONS

Diagnosis of malignant bone tumor is a shock to both parents and children. The symptoms begin so insidiously that the diagnosis seems unreal. Parents can be reassured that any delay in seeking treatment would not have had a marked effect on the chances for a cure. Neither the adolescent nor the parents could have been expected to seek medical attention any earlier. This is important preparation, because guilt-ridden parents cannot function effectively to help a child through this extensive illness.

Be certain that outcomes established are realistic. It is not realistic, for example, for an adolescent to accept with understanding leg surgery that could compromise an athletic career. The highest achievable outcome might be that the adolescent realizes surgery is necessary to save her life.

Nursing Diagnosis: Risk for injury related to surgery and bone prosthesis

Outcome Evaluation: Extremity distal to surgical incision remains warm to touch; capillary filling is less than 5 seconds; adolescent reports no tingling or numbness in distal extremity.

The major danger associated with surgery for excising osteosarcoma and placement of a bone prosthesis (limb salvage surgery) is that the swelling that occurs during surgery or immediately afterward can disrupt neurologic or circulatory function. Therefore, position and handle the leg carefully to prevent further disruption. Assess frequently for signs that the neurologic and circulatory systems are intact distal to the surgery (toes are warm and pink; capillary filling is less than 5 seconds; client reports no numbness or tingling).

Adolescents who had pain in the leg before surgery may continue to feel this pain even after the involved bone has been removed. This is known as phantom pain, and it occurs because nerve tracts continue to report pain for a time after the pain has been relieved. Although you might think that phantom limb pain could be simply explained away, this is not true. The pain is very real. The adolescent may need an analgesic to control it.

Ewing's Sarcoma

Ewing's sarcoma is a malignant tumor occurring most often in the bone marrow of the diaphyseal area (midshaft) of long bones. It spreads longitudinally through the bone (see Fig. 53.7). Ewing's sarcoma occurs primarily in young adolescents and older school-age children; it is slightly more common in boys than in girls. It almost never occurs in African-Americans. Metastasis is usually present at the time of diagnosis; the lungs and bones are the most common sites. Eventually, CNS and lymph node sites become involved (Krasin et al., 2004).

Assessment

Most children have had pain at the site of the tumor for some time before seeing a physician. At first, the pain is intermittent, and the child attributes it to an injury (a friend punched her leg; she bumped it against a foot-

stool). Finally, the pain becomes constant and so severe that the child cannot sleep at night. Because of this delay, multiple areas of involvement are often found at the time of diagnosis.

Radiography reveals an unusual "onion-skin" reaction (fine lines disclosed on the x-ray film) surrounding the invading tumor cells. A bone scan, bone marrow aspiration and biopsy, CT scan of the lungs, and IV pyelogram or kidney MRI will probably be done to determine whether metastasis to the lung, bone, kidney, or lymph nodes has occurred. A biopsy of the tumor site will be done for a definite diagnosis. During tests, urge the child to avoid bearing weight on the affected extremity, because this could cause a pathologic fracture at the site.

Therapeutic Management

With Ewing's sarcoma, therapy consists of a combination of surgery to remove the primary tumor, radiotherapy, and chemotherapy. Drugs often used are vincristine, dactinomycin, cyclophosphamide, doxorubicin, etoposide, and ifosfamide. Irradiation of the entire involved bone may be scheduled.

About 50% of children survive for at least 5 years; older children have a better survival rate than younger children. Caution adolescents to continue to be careful about stress on a leg that has received extensive radiation (e.g., no football, no weight lifting with pressure on that leg) because it may not be as strong as normal afterward.

What if... a parent tells you his son developed an osteosarcoma from falling while playing basketball? Is that a possible cause of bone cancer?

OTHER CHILDHOOD NEOPLASMS
Neuroblastoma

Neuroblastomas are tumors that arise from the cells of the sympathetic nervous system; cells are highly undifferentiated and invasive, occurring most frequently in the abdomen near the adrenal gland or spinal ganglia. They are the most common abdominal tumor in childhood (Kushner et al., 2003). Neuroblastoma occurs primarily in infants and preschool children; it is slightly more common in boys than in girls. These tumors may occur so early in life that they are detected by fetal sonography or at birth. There may be an association between the development of neuroblastomas and fetal alcohol syndrome or cigarette or marijuana smoking by parents. Common sites of metastasis include the bone marrow, liver, and subcutaneous tissue.

Assessment

The growing tumor is most often discovered on abdominal palpation as an abdominal mass (Ebb, 2005). The general symptoms of weight loss and anorexia may be present. Pressure on the adrenal gland from the tumor may cause excessive sweating, flushed face, and hypertension.

Abdominal pain and constipation may be present. Compression on the spinal nerves or invasion into the intervertebral foramina may cause loss of motor function in lower extremities.

If the primary lesion is in the upper chest, children will report dyspnea; swallowing may be difficult, and neck and facial edema may occur from compression on the vena cava. If liver metastasis is present, children may have jaundice. If metastasis to the skin has occurred, blue or purplish nodules (prominent raised areas) on arms or legs may be seen.

The extent of the tumor and any metastases present are identified by an IV pyelogram (a mass growing on the adrenal gland just above the kidney will demonstrate kidney compression); an arteriogram (neuroblastomas are vascular tumors and incorporate veins and arteries into their structure as they grow); a sonogram, CT or MRI scan of the chest, abdomen, and pelvis; a gallium bone scan; or bone marrow aspiration and biopsy. If an adrenal tumor is present, it will stimulate production of adrenal gland hormones or catecholamines. To detect these substances, a urine sample will be tested for the presence of catecholamines or vanillylmandelic acid and homovanillic acid (the breakdown products of catecholamines). Children who have a high level of serum ferritin have a poorer prognosis than do those with a low level.

A biopsy of the tumor site will be planned so the tumor can be definitely identified and staged (Table 53.5).

Therapeutic Management

If the tumor is localized (stage I), therapy will consist of surgical removal of the primary tumor. If the tumor is stage II to IV, surgery will be followed by chemotherapy using agents such as doxorubicin, cyclophosphamide, etoposide, vincristine, ifosfamide, cisplatin, and carboplatin. A "second look" surgical procedure may be scheduled within several months to determine the effectiveness of therapy and to attempt the possible removal of further tumor. If aggressive chemotherapy is not effective, bone marrow transplantation to restore functioning bone marrow may be scheduled. Administration of cis-retinoic acid, a growth-inhibiting agent, improves eradication of resid-

ual disease. Immunotherapy is another possibility to eliminate residual disease after chemotherapy.

Stage IV disease is a unique form because it has a high rate of spontaneous regression. This occurs because the tumor either spontaneously degenerates or undergoes differentiation to normal tissue (Stern, 2003).

Overall, children with neuroblastoma have a 5-year survival rate of 70% to 90%. Although most children have a positive initial response to therapy, recurrence is common within the first year. The prognosis is better in children diagnosed before 1 year of age (Ebb, 2005).

Rhabdomyosarcoma

A **rhabdomyosarcoma** is a tumor of striated muscle. It arises from the embryonic mesenchyme tissue that forms muscle, connective, and vascular tissue (Ebb, 2005). The peak age of incidence of these tumors is 2 to 6 years, with a second peak occurring during puberty. Common sites of occurrence include the eye orbit, paranasal sinuses, uterus, prostate, bladder, retroperitoneum, arms, and legs. CNS invasion occurs from direct tumor extension. This results in cranial nerve palsy, nuchal rigidity, bradycardia, or bradypnea (due to brainstem compromise). Distant metastasis most commonly occurs in lungs, bone, or bone marrow.

Assessment

The symptoms relate to the site of the tumor (Table 53.6). A biopsy specimen of the tumor is taken and examined

---

TABLE 53.5

Staging Neuroblastoma

Stage	Extent of Disease
I	Tumor is well encapsulated and completely removed by surgery.
II	Tumor cannot be completely removed by surgery or disease extends to lymph nodes.
III	Tumor extends beyond the midline; regional lymph nodes may be involved bilaterally.
IV	Distant metastases; bone, eyes, or liver involved.
IVs	Metastasis is present in child <1yr old.

TABLE 53.6

Common Sites and Associated Symptoms of Rhabdomyosarcoma

Site of Tumor	Symptoms
Orbit	Proptosis (extruding eye); visible and palpable conjunctival or eyelid mass
Neck	Hoarseness, dysphagia; visible and palpable mass in neck
Nasopharynx	Airway obstruction, epistaxis, dysphagia, visible mass in nasal or nasopharyngeal passages
Paranasal sinuses	Swelling, pain, nasal discharge, epistaxis
Middle ear	Pain, chronic otitis media, hearing loss, facial nerve palsy, mass protruding into external ear canal
Bladder and prostate	Dysuria, urinary retention, hematuria, constipation, palpable lower abdominal mass
Vagina	Mass protruding from uterus or cervix into vagina, abnormal vaginal bleeding
Trunk, extremities	Visible and palpable soft-tissue mass
Testicles	Visible and palpable soft-tissue mass

for tissue identification. Metastasis is ruled out by bone scan, chest radiography, CT scanning, MRI, and bone marrow aspiration.

Therapeutic Management

The primary treatment is surgical removal of the tumor, followed by chemotherapy with agents such as vincristine, dactinomycin, cyclophosphamide, doxorubicin, etoposide, and ifosfamide. The child receives chemotherapy every 3 or 4 weeks for 18 to 24 months. If CNS extension has occurred, intrathecal chemotherapy may be included in the regimen.

A child's prognosis depends on the size of the tumor and whether metastasis was present at the time of initial diagnosis. If all of the tumor was removed and no lymph node metastasis has occurred, the chances are as high as 80% that the tumor will not recur. If some of the tumor had to be left because of its size or location, the chance of recurrence rises to about 50%. If metastasis to the lungs or bone was present at the time of the initial diagnosis, the prognosis drops still further; about 20% of children in this situation have long-term survival. Among children who do survive, long-term complications such as cardiomyopathy and infertility may occur from the side effects of chemotherapy (Kelly, 2003).

Nephroblastoma (Wilms' Tumor)

Nephroblastoma (Wilms' tumor) is a malignant tumor that rises from the metanephric mesoderm cells of the upper pole of the kidney (Ebb, 2005). It accounts for 20% of solid tumors in childhood; there is no increased incidence based on sex or race. It occurs in association with congenital anomalies such as aniridia (lack of color in the iris), cryptorchidism, hypospadias, pseudohermaphroditism, cystic kidneys, hemangioma, and talipes disorders. Some children with the disorder have a deletion on chromosome 11. Metastatic spread by the bloodstream is most often to the lungs, regional lymph nodes, liver, bone, and, eventually, brain (Kang, 2003).

Assessment

A nephroblastoma is usually discovered early in life (6 months to 5 years; peak at 3 to 4 years), although it apparently arises from an embryonic structure present in the child before birth. Nephroblastomas distort the kidney anteriorly so that the tumor is felt as a firm, nontender abdominal mass. Parents sometimes are aware that their infant has a mass in the abdomen but bring him or her to a physician thinking that it is hard stool from chronic constipation. Fathers often discover the tumor when they toss a baby in the air, catch him or her by the abdomen, and feel the abdominal mass. Parents often report that the mass seemed to appear overnight. This actually can happen, because tumors can hemorrhage into themselves, doubling their size in a matter of hours. Nephroblastoma may manifest with hematuria and a low-grade fever. Although hypertension may also occur because of excessive renin production, blood pressure is not taken routinely in children of this age, so the tumor is rarely discovered by this method. The child

may be anemic from lack of erythropoietin formation by the diseased kidney.

A CT scan or sonogram reveals the primary tumor and any points of metastasis. Kidney function studies, such as glomerular filtration rate or blood urea nitrogen, will be done to assess function of the kidneys before surgery. Little time, however, can be allotted for preoperative testing, because these tumors metastasize rapidly as a result of the large blood supply to the kidneys and adrenal glands.

It is important that the child's abdomen not be palpated any more than is necessary for diagnosis, because handling appears to aid metastasis. Place a sign reading "No Abdominal Palpation" over the child's crib to prevent this.

Therapeutic Management

Nephroblastomas are staged according to the criteria of the National Wilms' Tumor Study Group (Table 53.7) to predict therapy and prognosis. The tumor will be removed by nephrectomy (excision of the affected kidney). This is usually followed immediately by radiation therapy (omitted in stage I tumors) and by chemotherapy with dactinomycin, doxorubicin, or vincristine. The chemotherapy may be given at varying intervals for as long as 15 months. A second surgical procedure may be scheduled after 2 or 3 months to remove any remaining tumor.

If tumor involvement is bilateral, the operative decisions obviously become more complex. If the tumors are small, both can be removed, leaving functioning kidney cells intact. Or only the kidney with the larger tumor may be removed. Tumor sites are then treated with both radiation and chemotherapy.

Complications can occur from nephroblastoma therapy. Both small bowel obstruction from fibrotic scarring and hepatic damage from radiation to the lesion can occur. Nephritis in the kidney also is a possibility. In girls, radiation-related damage to the ovaries may result in sterility. Radiation to the lungs may result in interstitial pneumonia; spine radiation can result in scoliosis.

Therapy for nephroblastoma is so effective that about 90% of children who had no metastatic spread at diagnosis survive for at least 5 years (Kang, 2003).

TABLE 53.7

Staging Nephroblastoma (Wilms' Tumor)

Stage	Description
I	Tumor confined to the kidney and completely removed surgically
II	Tumor extending beyond the kidney but completely removed surgically
III	Regional spread of disease beyond the kidney with residual abdominal disease postoperatively
IV	Metastases to lung, liver, bone, distant lymph nodes, or other distant sites
V	Bilateral disease

Checkpoint Question 3

What is an important intervention to take for a child with nephroblastoma (Wilms' tumor)?

a. Post a sign over the crib: "No Abdominal Palpation."
b. Alert the mother that her child will be infertile after surgery.
c. Be certain the child eats no red vegetables before surgery.
d. Record a head circumference in the nursing care plan.

Retinoblastoma

Retinoblastoma is a malignant tumor of the retina of the eye (Ebb, 2005). A rare tumor, it accounts for only 1% to 3% of childhood malignancies. In about 10% of the cases, these tumors develop because of an inherited autosomal dominant pattern that causes an alteration of chromosome 13. Parents who have one child with retinoblastoma have about a 4% chance of having a second child with a similar tumor. If two or more children have the tumor, the parents are probably carriers, and it can be predicted that up to 50% of their children will be affected. Because of the dominant pattern of inheritance, a person who survives retinoblastoma has a 90% chance of having a child with a similar tumor. Parents who may be carriers, or the parent who has survived the disease, need genetic counseling so that they are aware of the risk to their children. Because the 5-year survival rate for children with retinoblastoma is good (at least 90%), this will become a very important counseling role in the future.

Retinoblastoma occurs most often, however, as spontaneous development, not the inherited type. Children with the inherited type tend to develop bilateral disease; those with the spontaneous type may or may not have the tumor in both eyes.

Assessment

Retinoblastoma occurs early in life, from about 6 weeks of age through the preschool period. It occurs equally in boys and girls, and there is no preference for either the right or the left eye. One tumor or many individual tumors may be present. They are located on the retina or in the vitreous fluid or extend backward into the choroid, the optic nerve, and the subarachnoid space.

On examination, the child's pupil appears white (the red reflex is absent) or is described as a typical "cat's eye." The child develops strabismus as the eye becomes nonfunctional. This tumor metastasizes readily along the course of the optic nerve to the subarachnoid space and brain; it quickly involves the second eye. Metastasis to distant body sites, such as bone marrow and liver, occurs because of the rich blood supply to the brain.

Children with a family history should be examined at least three times yearly until they reach 5 years of age. If a tumor is suspected, an examination under general anesthesia or conscious sedation is scheduled, because children this age cannot cooperate well with eye examinations. CT scanning and sonography may be ordered to detect intraocular calcification or the presence of tumor. The possibility of distant metastasis is evaluated by lumbar puncture, liver and skeletal survey, MRI, or bone marrow biopsy.

Therapeutic Management

Retinoblastomas are serious tumors involving the retina of the eye; they cause blindness. If the tumor is very small at the time of diagnosis, it may be treated with cryosurgery (freezing the tumor to destroy local cells). This will preserve partial vision in the eye. Photocoagulation using laser surgery to destroy the blood vessels supplying the tumor may be used. Localized radioactive applicators or plaques sutured to the sclera over the tumor may be used. Such plaques remain in place for 4 to 7 days. The child may also receive radiation treatment and chemotherapy (nitrogen mustard, vincristine, and cyclophosphamide are commonly used) if the tumor has metastasized.

If the tumor is large when first discovered, enucleation of the eye may be necessary. After enucleation, the child has a large pressure dressing applied to the empty socket. Observe for bleeding on the dressing and assess vital signs frequently. To keep young children from tugging at the dressing and removing it, they may need to be restrained if a parent cannot be with them constantly. After about 48 hours, the pressure dressing is removed (usually by the surgeon), and a small eye patch is applied. Irrigation of the empty socket with normal saline solution or application of an antibiotic ointment may be prescribed with future dressing changes.

An eye prosthesis is fitted about 3 weeks after surgery. Prostheses in children do not need to be removed and cleaned daily, and, in children this young, leaving the prosthesis in place prevents the child from playing with it (an interesting, colorful, round ball).

As discussed earlier, the long-term survival rate for children with retinoblastoma is as high as 90% (Hogarty, 2003). Evaluation of the child after retinoblastoma must include not only whether metastasis can be detected but whether the child is adjusting to the loss of sight in one or both eyes. Children who do not have binocular vision this early in life usually do not have difficulty adjusting. They notice it most at school age when they are unable to compete in sports that require three-dimensional sight, such as baseball. They may be restricted from obtaining a driver's license. If radiation was used for therapy, cataracts may develop several years later. The high incidence of osteogenic and soft-tissue sarcomas that occurs with retinoblastomas may not be related to therapy as much as to a tendency for tumor growth.

NURSING DIAGNOSES AND RELATED INTERVENTIONS

Nursing Diagnosis: Decisional conflict related to approval of eye removal to save child's life

Outcome Evaluation: Parents and child state that they can accept removal of eye to save child's life.

With the diagnosis of retinoblastoma, parents may be asked to make a most difficult decision. To save their child's life, they must agree to the removal of an eye. Even after this procedure, the second eye may become involved or distant metastasis may occur. Parents need support in the decision they make. If there is metastasis at a later date, they may feel guilty that they agreed to enucleation, thinking they have put the child through the surgery for nothing. They may feel guilty that they did not notice that the child's eye was abnormal before metastasis occurred. They may have noticed that the eye was abnormal but thought nothing more than that the child needed glasses and so delayed seeking health care. Be certain that parents understand fully what surgery will entail (i.e., loss of the eye). Provide time for discussion to help them work through this very emotional time in their life.

Skin Cancer

One in five people develop skin cancer in their lifetime (Aasi & Leffell, 2005). Three types are involved: basal cell carcinoma (a surface epithelial growth that manifests as a small ulcer that does not heal), squamous cell carcinoma (a tumor of the epidermis that manifests as a white scaly lesion), and malignant melanoma (a tumor originating in melanocytes or nevi) that manifests as a mole that changes in appearance. All three types of skin cancer are increasing in incidence and, although the symptoms usually do not appear until adulthood, the chief cause (excessive sun exposure) begins in childhood (McCance & Huether, 2004). Nurses can play a major role in helping to reduce the incidence of skin cancer by teaching parents and adolescents ways to better protect against excessive sun exposure, including the following measures:

- Applying a sunscreen or wearing protective clothing if a child will be out in the sun for longer than 20 minutes
- Using tanning beds or ultraviolet light with the same precautions as sunlight
- Avoiding sunburn, because there is a direct association between two or more episodes of sunburn in adolescence and the development of malignant melanoma in young adulthood

Key Points

After a diagnosis of cancer, parents and children need help to change their thinking from an older concept of cancer as being an always painful, fatal disease to a newer concept of cancer as a condition for which there is therapy and hope.

Because the therapy for cancer involves so many health care visits and so much parental concern, the siblings of children with cancer may begin to feel left out of family activities. Remind parents to incorporate the entire family into activities whenever possible, to help them grow as a family during the course of therapy.

Radiation is an important treatment modality in cancer therapy. Immediate side effects include anorexia, nausea, vomiting, and hair loss if radiation is to the head. Long-term effects may include growth retardation or learning disabilities.

A chemotherapeutic agent is one that is capable of destroying malignant cells. Common side effects are the same as those for radiation therapy. Help children to use time during chemotherapy treatments in constructive ways, such as playing a game, to keep them mentally stimulated yet quiet.

Be aware of the need to use gloves, and mix preparations under a hood when preparing a chemotherapy drug, to protect yourself from adverse effects of the medication.

Leukemia is the distorted and uncontrolled proliferation of WBCs and is the most frequently occurring type of cancer in children. About 90% of children with an initially good prognosis now have long-term survival.

Hodgkin's disease and non-Hodgkin's lymphomas are malignancies of the lymphatic system. Hodgkin's disease occurs most often in adolescents; the initial symptom is often one painless, enlarged lymph node. Therapy is radiation and chemotherapy.

Brain tumors are the most common solid tumors occurring in childhood. Beginning symptoms are usually those of increased intracranial pressure. Therapy may include a combination of surgery followed by radiation and chemotherapy.

Bone tumors occur in two main forms: osteogenic sarcoma and Ewing's sarcoma. These tumors tend to be fast growing because of the ready blood supply to bone. Therapy consists of surgery followed by radiation and chemotherapy.

Neuroblastomas are tumors that arise from the cells of the sympathetic nervous system. They are the most common abdominal tumor in childhood. Therapy is surgery and chemotherapy.

Rhabdomyosarcomas are tumors of striated muscle. The peak age of incidence is 2 to 6 years. Therapy is surgery and chemotherapy.

Nephroblastoma (Wilms' tumor) is a malignancy that arises from the metanephric mesoderm cells of the kidney. It is usually discovered early in life. Therapy is surgery followed by radiation and chemotherapy.

Retinoblastoma is a malignant tumor of the retina of the eye. It may be inherited as an autosomal dominant pattern. Therapy involves surgery, radiation, chemotherapy, and possibly enucleation if the tumor is large.

Skin cancer is a type of malignancy that begins in childhood. Cautioning children about sensible sun exposure can be an important health promotion role for nurses.

Critical Thinking Exercises

1. Geri is the 6-year-old boy you met at the beginning of the chapter. His mother told you that he wakes up every morning with a headache and then vomits. She says this pattern began just after school started, so she is certain it is related to school. His teacher has suggested that Geri have an eye examination. What are some additional questions you would want to ask to determine whether you should pursue this problem further?

2. A 2-year-old child is going to be receiving chemotherapy after surgery for a neuroblastoma. How would you prepare the child for chemotherapy? What activities would you propose to keep the child occupied while an IV solution is infusing?

3. An adolescent has been diagnosed as having Hodgkin's disease. How would you explain this disease to him? He is active in a school sports program and works part-time in a supermarket. How will you answer if he asks you whether he should stop these activities?

4. Examine the National Health Goals related to neoplasms and children. Most government-sponsored money for nursing research is allotted based on these goals. What would be a possible research topic to explore pertinent to these goals that would be applicable to Geri's family and also advance evidence-based practice?

References

Aasi, S. Z., & Leffell, D. J. (2005). Cancer of the skin. In DeVita, V. T., Hellman, S., & Rosenberg, S. A. (Eds.), *Cancer: Principles and practice of oncology* (7th ed.). Philadelphia: Lippincott Williams & Wilkins.

American Cancer Society. (2005). *Seven signs of cancer*. Atlanta: Author.

Boon, K., et al. (2004). Identification of astrocytoma associated genes including cell surface markers. *BMC Cancer Journal, 4*(1), 39–40.

Bottomley, S. J., & Kassner, E. (2003). Late effects of childhood cancer therapy. *Journal of Pediatric Nursing: Nursing Care of Children and Families, 18*(2), 126–133.

Brain, J. D., et al. (2003). Childhood leukemia: Electric and magnetic fields as possible risk factors. *Environmental Health Perspectives, 111*(7), 962–970.

Brown, V. I. (2003). Acute lymphoblastic leukemia. In Schwartz, M. W. (Ed.), *5-Minute pediatric consult* (3rd ed.). Philadelphia: Lippincott Williams & Wilkins.

Cagen, D., & Franco, M. (2003). Acute lymphoblastic leukemia in children. *Clinical Journal of Oncology Nursing, 7*(5.1), 604–606.

Chen, C., et al. (2004). Assessment of chemotherapy-induced oral complications in children with cancer. *Journal of Pediatric Oncology Nursing, 21*(1), 33–39.

Codori, A. M., et al. (2003). Genetic testing for hereditary colorectal cancer in children: Long-term psychological effects. *American Journal of Medical Genetics, 116*(2), 117–128.

Cohen, J. (2005). Public health. High hopes and dilemmas for a cervical cancer vaccine. *Science, 308*(5722), 618–621.

Colby-Graham, M. F., & Chordas, C. (2003). The childhood leukemias. *Journal of Pediatric Nursing: Nursing Care of Children and Families, 18*(2), 87–95.

Department of Health and Human Services. (2000). *Healthy people 2010.* Washington, DC: DHHS.

Ebb, E. H. (2005). Solid tumors of childhood. In DeVita, V. T., Hellman, S., & Rosenberg, S. A. (Eds.), *Cancer: Principles and practice of oncology* (7th ed.). Philadelphia: Lippincott Williams & Wilkins.

Eberhart, C. G., et al. (2004). Histopathological and molecular prognostic markers in medulloblastoma: c-myc, N-myc, TrkC, and anaplasia. *Journal of Neuropathology and Experimental Neurology, 63*(5), 441–449.

Erickson, J. M. (2004). Fatigue in adolescents with cancer: A review of the literature. *Clinical Journal of Oncology Nursing, 8*(2), 139–145.

Fine, H. A. (2005). Neoplasms of the central nervous system. In DeVita, V. T., Hellman, S., & Rosenberg, S. A. (Eds.), *Cancer: Principles and practice of oncology* (7th ed.). Philadelphia: Lippincott Williams & Wilkins.

Freeman, K., O'Dell, C., & Meola, C. (2004). Childhood brain tumors: Parental concerns and stressors by phase of illness. *Journal of Pediatric Oncology Nursing, 21*(2), 87–97.

Ginsberg, J. P. (2003). Non-Hodgkin lymphoma. In Schwartz, M. W. (Ed.), *5-Minute pediatric consult* (3rd ed.). Philadelphia: Lippincott Williams & Wilkins.

Hogarty, M. D. (2003). Retinoblastoma. In Schwartz, M. W. (Ed.), *5-Minute pediatric consult* (3rd ed.). Philadelphia: Lippincott Williams & Wilkins.

Houtzager, B. A., et al. (2005). One month after diagnosis: Quality of life, coping and previous functioning in siblings of children with cancer. *Child: Care, Health, and Development, 31*(1), 75–87.

Kang, T. I. (2003). Wilms' tumor. In Schwartz, M. W. (Ed.), *5-Minute pediatric consult* (3rd ed.). Philadelphia: Lippincott Williams & Wilkins.

Karch, A. (2004). *Lippincott's nursing drug guide.* Philadelphia: Lippincott Williams & Wilkins.

Kelly, K. M. (2003). Rhabdomyosarcoma. In Schwartz, M. W. (Ed.), *5-Minute pediatric consult* (3rd ed.). Philadelphia: Lippincott Williams & Wilkins.

Krasin, M. J., et al. (2004). Efficacy of combined surgery and irradiation for localized Ewing's sarcoma family of tumors. *Pediatric Blood and Cancer, 43*(3), 229–236.

Kushner, B. H., et al. (2003). Neuroblastoma in adolescents and adults: The Memorial Sloan-Kettering experience. *Medical and Pediatric Oncology, 41*(6), 508–515.

Lange, B. J., et al. (2005). Mortality in overweight and underweight children with acute myeloid leukemia. *JAMA: Journal of the American Medical Association, 293*(2), 203–211.

Lones, M. A., et al. (2004). Chromosome abnormalities may correlate with prognosis in Burkitt/Burkitt-like lymphomas of children and adolescents: A report from Children's Cancer Group Study CCG-E08. *Journal of Pediatric Hematology/Oncology, 26*(3), 169–178.

Max, A., et al. (2003). Developing nursing care guidelines for children with Hodgkin's disease. *European Journal of Oncology Nursing, 7*(4), 253–258.

Malawer, M. M., Helman, L. J., & O'Sullivan, B. (2005). Sarcomas of bone. In DeVita, V. T., Hellman, S., & Rosenberg, S. A. (Eds.), *Cancer: Principles and practice of oncology* (7th ed.). Philadelphia: Lippincott Williams & Wilkins.

McCance, K. L. & Huether, S. E. (2004). *Pathophysiology.* St. Louis: Mosby.

Mueller, B. A., et al. (2004). Household water source and the risk of childhood brain tumours: Results of the SEARCH International Brain Tumor Study. *International Journal of Epidemiology, 33*(6), 1209-1216.

National Cancer Institute. (2005). *Annual report to the nation.* Rockwell, MD: National Institutes of Health.

Ravindranath, Y. (2005). Down syndrome and leukemia: New insights into the epidemiology, pathogenesis, and treatment. *Pediatric Blood and Cancer, 44*(1), 1-7.

Stern, J. W. (2003). Neuroblastoma. In Schwartz, M. W. (Ed.), *5-Minute pediatric consult* (3rd ed.). Philadelphia: Lippincott Williams & Wilkins.

Stoneham, S., et al. (2004). Outcome after autologous hemopoietic stem cell transplantation in relapsed or refractory childhood Hodgkin disease. *Journal of Pediatric Hematology/Oncology, 26*(11), 740-745.

von Essen, L., & Enskar, K. (2003). Important aspects of care and assistance for siblings of children treated for cancer: A parent and nurse perspective. *Cancer Nursing, 26*(3), 203-210.

Suggested Readings

Brady, G. (2003). Retinoblastoma: Care and support of the pediatric patient and family. *Insight: The Journal of the American Society of Ophthalmic Registered Nurses, 28*(3), 67-69.

Bryant, R. (2003). Managing side effects of childhood cancer treatment. *Journal of Pediatric Nursing: Nursing Care of Children and Families, 18*(2), 113-125.

Frierdich, S., Goes, C., & Dadd, G. (2003). Community and home care services provided to children with cancer. *Journal of Pediatric Oncology Nursing, 20*(5), 252-259.

Hilton, L. (2004). "Back to school" after cancer. *Nursing Spectrum, 16*(4), 11-12.

Hudson, M. M., et al. (2004). A model of care for childhood cancer survivors that facilitates research. *Journal of Pediatric Oncology Nursing, 21*(3), 170-174.

Lin, Y. (2003). Early recognition of infant malignancy: The five most common infant cancers. *Neonatal Network: The Journal of Neonatal Nursing, 22*(5), 11-19.

Linnard-Palmer, L., & Kools, S. (2005). Parents' refusal of medical treatment for cultural or religious beliefs: An ethnographic study of health care professionals' experiences. *Journal of Pediatric Oncology Nursing, 22*(1), 48-57.

Pengelly, T. (2003). Research and commentary: Communicating with young people with life-threatening conditions. *Paediatric Nursing, 15*(4), 12-13.

Sheppard, L., Eiser, C., & Kingston, J. (2005). Mothers' perceptions of children's quality of life following early diagnosis and treatment for retinoblastoma (Rb). *Child: Care, Health, and Development, 31*(2), 137-142.

Tunn, P. U., et al. (2004). Osteosarcoma in children: Long-term functional analysis. *Clinical Orthopaedics and Related Research, 1*(421), 212-217.

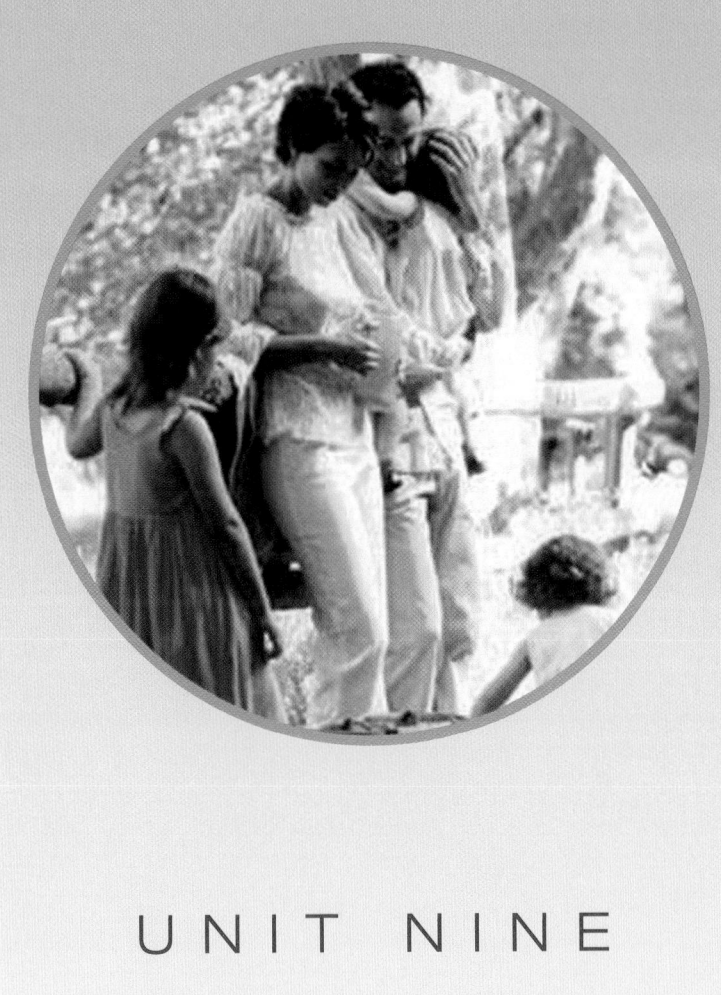

UNIT NINE

The Nursing Role in Restoring and Maintaining the Health of Children and Families With Mental Health Disorders

CHAPTER 54

Nursing Care of the Child With a Cognitive or Mental Health Disorder

Key Terms

anhedonia
binge eating
catatonia
choreiform movements
complex vocal tics
coprolalia
dyslexia
echolalia
flat affect
graphesthesia
hyperactivity
labile mood
motor tics
palilalia
purging
stereognosis
vocal tics

Objectives

After mastering the contents of this chapter, you should be able to:

1. Describe common cognitive and mental health disorders in children.
2. Assess a child for a cognitive or mental health disorder.
3. Formulate nursing diagnoses related to the cognitive or mental health disorders of childhood.
4. Establish expected outcomes for a child with a cognitive or mental health disorder.
5. Plan nursing care for a child with a cognitive or mental health disorder.
6. Implement nursing care for a child with a cognitive or mental health disorder, such as helping a parent reduce environmental stimuli.
7. Evaluate expected outcomes for achievement and effectiveness of care.
8. Identify National Health Goals related to cognitive or mental health disorders nurses can be instrumental in helping the nation achieve.
9. Identify areas related to cognitive or mental health that could benefit from additional nursing research or application of evidence-based practice.
10. Analyze ways that care of a child with a cognitive or mental health disorder can be more family centered.
11. Integrate knowledge of childhood cognitive and mental health disorders and nursing process to achieve quality maternal and child health nursing care.

You are working as a school nurse and meet Todd, a second grader who was diagnosed with attention-deficit hyperactivity disorder (ADHD) approximately 6 months ago. You observe Todd coloring; running to the window; running to the door, opening and closing the door; and then throwing pamphlets out of an information rack. His mother tells you she is "at her wits' end" because Todd's attention span is so short and his behavior so disruptive. His father tells you he's proud that his son is "all boy."

Previous chapters described the growth and development of well children and the care of children with physiologic disorders. This chapter adds information about the dramatic changes that occur when children demonstrate a cognitive or mental health disorder. This is important information because it builds a base for care and health teaching.

How can you help Todd's family?
What additional education do they need?

After you've studied this chapter, access the accompanying website. Read the patient scenario and answer the questions to further sharpen your skills, grow more familiar with RN-CLEX types of questions, and reward yourself with how much you have learned.

A child who is mentally healthy successfully masters the tasks of each developmental phase, develops the ability to trust adults, and possesses a positive self-concept and sense of contentment within his or her own limits. In addition, there is a good emotional relationship between the parents and the child and a sense of safety and security in the home environment. Promoting healthy family functioning during health care visits, providing anticipatory guidance for parents about developmental milestones and needs, and listening carefully to both children *and* parents are important in fostering both the physical and mental health of children.

Mental health implies that a child is able to use adaptive coping mechanisms appropriately to meet the normal stressors of life. Often, these stressors provide growth-producing challenges in life or help a child achieve the tasks of each developmental phase, such as establishing a sense of trust or independence. This is one of the reasons why providing age-appropriate stimulation is an essential nursing responsibility. Some stressors in life, however, go beyond what is considered "the norm." Acute illness and hospitalization are examples of increased stress. Chronic illness may provide an even greater stress, as the acute phase fades into recognition of long-term disability or an ultimately fatal prognosis. Nurses must be able to recognize the effects of illness and hospitalization on children and their families and to provide interventions to prevent maladaptive coping mechanisms. Being aware of the potential emotional responses a child might have to a particular illness and the implications for family functioning is essential to this ability.

Children can develop the same mental health disorders that affect the adult population, such as depression or schizophrenia. In addition, a number of disorders (e.g., pervasive developmental disorders such as autistic disorder) appear to begin in childhood. Some problems, such as separation anxiety, may consist of behavior that is considered normal at one stage of development (infancy) but pathologic at another (adolescence). Current research attributes some of these disorders to genetic vulnerability and others to disruption in family life, temperament, or inadequate parent–child bonding and attachment difficulties. Children with mental illness, whatever the cause, must be evaluated and treated by specialists in the mental health field as early in their disease process as possible. The child health nurse is often the first to become aware of such problems and can be instrumental, through appropriate referrals, in helping the child and family adjust to the disorder.

Cognitive and mental health disorders addressed by National Health Goals are shown in Box 54.1.

Nursing Process Overview

For Care of a Child With a Cognitive Challenge or Mental Illness

● *Assessment*
Both personality and mental growth potential in a child are influenced by a number of factors, including ge-

---

BOX 54.1 FOCUS ON . . .

NATIONAL HEALTH GOALS

Cognitive and mental health disorders in children produce major costs to the nation, as well as to individual families, because these disorders have the potential to reduce the earning power and contributions of future citizens. Two National Health Goals directly address this issue:

- Increase the proportion of children with mental health problems who receive treatment.
- Reduce the proportion of children and adolescents with disabilities who are reported to be sad, unhappy, or depressed, from a baseline of 31% to a target level of 17% (DHHS, 2000).

Nurses can help the nation achieve these goals by educating parents to seek prenatal care, so that low birth weight and the threat of physical challenges can be reduced; educating about ways to reduce stress in families; and identifying children in school and health care agency settings who demonstrate a high level of stress or other symptoms of mental illness.

Additional nursing research questions for this area could include the following: What are the questions on a health history that would best reveal mental stress? Can nurses successfully identify adolescents who are at high risk for eating disorders? What support measures are most helpful to families of a child with mental illness or cognitive challenge?

---

netic makeup, cultural background, family environment, and community resources. All of these need to be taken into account when assessing a child's cognitive or mental health. Assess children for emotional as well as physical problems at regular health maintenance visits. If an emotional problem has been identified or is suspected, obtain a detailed history of the presenting problem, the presumed reason for its appearance, relevant past history, the child's school and social history, the child's developmental history, the family history, and the current pattern of family functioning.

Table 54.1 lists some helpful observational and interview data for assessing these areas.

● *Nursing Diagnosis*
Nursing diagnoses established for ill children often address mental health or the response of children and their families to their condition or treatment. Examples of these diagnoses are the following:

- Anxiety related to surgical experience
- Deficient diversional activity related to lack of appropriate play materials for hospitalized child
- Fear related to potential loss of independence secondary to traumatic injury
- Situational low self-esteem related to disfiguring scars after accident
- Impaired social interactions related to hearing deficit

TABLE 54.1

Guidelines for the Mental Health Interview of a Child

Observational Data

General appearance	Height, weight, grooming and hygiene, nutrition, physical health, distinguishing features (deformities, tics), maturity level
Motor behaviors	Fine and gross balance, bizarre motor activity
Speech and language	Receptive, expressive; content, tone, and articulation
Affect	Range of emotion, predominant emotion (depressed, angry, anxious, happy, irritable, labile), emotional reactions to process and/or content of interview (appropriate, inappropriate)
Thought process	Estimated intellectual level via language and knowledge base (organization and thought content), orientation (to person, place, time), perceptual distortions (hallucinations, illusions, tangentiality, obsessions, delusions), attention span, learning disabilities
Ability to relate to evaluator	Eye contact, attitude toward interviewer (negative, positive, shy, suspicious, withdrawn, friendly, self-centered)
Behaviors displayed during interview	Impulsivity, aggression, inhibition, distractibility, low frustration tolerance, ability to have fun, sense of humor, creativity

Interview Data

Interpersonal relationships	Attitudes toward and perceptions of family, siblings, peers, transitional objects (inanimate objects used to allay anxiety), pets; social skills with peers, best friend; relationships with family, siblings, and peers; conflicts; behavior problems; adjustment to changes in routine or new situations
Self-concept and image	Self-appraisal (does child like self?), comparison of self with others (siblings, peers), what does child like most about self? What would he or she like to change about self? Sense of pride in accomplishments, sex role, and gender identity
Conscience	Understands right and wrong, is able to express common judgments or values.

- Powerlessness related to loss of independence and control in hospital environment
- Decisional conflict related to lack of relevant information
- Hopelessness related to prolonged caretaking responsibilities for chronically ill child
- Compromised family coping related to overwhelming number of stressors placed on family at one time

Additional nursing diagnoses are appropriate if a problem of cognitive or mental health is present:

- Risk for self-directed violence related to impulsivity
- Impaired social interaction related to short attention span and distractibility
- Interrupted family processes related to inability of child to follow instructions
- Disturbed thought processes related to the effects of schizophrenia
- Impaired verbal communication related to depression and withdrawn behavior
- Ineffective health maintenance related to inattention to food or hygiene needs
- Situational low self-esteem related to lack of successful coping strategies
- Disturbed sleep pattern related to hallucinations
- Social isolation related to low self-esteem
- Compromised family coping related to chronic mental health problems in child

● *Outcome Identification and Planning*

Although the diagnosis of a mental health disorder or referral to a child guidance or psychiatric clinic does not carry the stigma it once did, many parents still believe that such a referral is a mark of inadequacy or a sign of failure for themselves as parents. Help parents to see that this type of referral is no different from one to a cardiologist or orthopedist for a purely physical reason.

Parents can be reminded that everyone recognizes the many pressures and stresses on children today that cannot be controlled or guarded against completely. Many parents find it reassuring to be told that their contact with a child guidance clinic, psychologist, or psychiatrist will be kept confidential. They also feel reassured by knowing that the health care personnel making the referral will continue to offer episodic or health maintenance care—that they are not being "transferred out" but asked to seek additional help only in this one area.

● *Implementation*

Often what parents and children need most when a cognitive or mental health disorder is identified is an empathic but uninvolved person to listen to their story objectively and to provide support for them as they try to resolve and manage the situation to a satisfactory conclusion. Recognizing when you are the person best able to serve this function requires professional judgment. Serving in this capacity can be important and can provide a source of personal satisfaction.

Additionally, outside organizations may be a source of support and education for the family. Organizations that might be helpful for referral include the following:

• Anorexia Nervosa and Related Eating Disorders, Inc. (*www.anred.com*)
• Autism Society of America (*www.autism-society.org*)
• Tourette Syndrome Association, Inc. (*www.tsa-usa.org*)
• National Association for Down Syndrome (*www.nads.org*)
• National Mental Health Association (*www.nmha.org*)

● *Outcome Evaluation*

Children who have a cognitive or mental health disorder need ongoing evaluation by health care personnel at routine visits, because these disorders are long term. In addition, it is important to determine whether any circumstances that might have led to a temporary problem have truly been corrected or only superficially changed, which could lead to the problem's resurfacing. On the whole, if the circumstances surrounding the child remain the same, the child's problem may return or be manifested later in another way.

Examples suggesting achievement of expected outcomes are the following:

• Child does not injure himself during the coming month.
• Parents state they are able to cope with child's disruptive behavior since prescription of antipsychotic drug.
• Child ingests a minimum of 500 calories daily with no binge eating.
• Parents state that they accept that their child is cognitively challenged.

HEALTH PROMOTION AND RISK MANAGEMENT

Nurses play a key role in assessing and promoting the mental and cognitive health of children and their families. A working knowledge of the typical growth and development of a child provides the basis for assessment. This knowledge also helps in developing appropriate educational strategies for parents so that they can better identify problems early on. Like adults, children and adolescents are exposed to stress; however, they cope with these stresses differently. Nurses can help parents better understand how children respond to and cope with stress, which also aids in early identification should a problem arise. Acting as educator, facilitator, and advocate, nurses can assist children and families to identify their needs and implement measures to meet them.

Various factors have been associated with an increased risk for mental health disorders in children, including the following:

• Trauma or neglect
• Difficult temperament
• Attachment problems
• Experience of major losses
• Negative sibling relationships

• Medical problems and illnesses
• Exposure to high-risk activities, such as drug abuse
• Poverty and homelessness
• Parental substance abuse

A thorough assessment of the child and family can provide clues to the existence of such possible risk factors and suggest strategies to reduce their impact.

If a child develops a cognitive or mental health disorder, nurses can act as advocates to obtain referrals to support services and early intervention programs, helping to minimize the overall effects of the disorder on the child and family.

CLASSIFICATION OF MENTAL HEALTH DISORDERS

For many years, psychopathology in children was not classified according to a standard system; as a result, conditions were not clearly defined or described. Today, after several revisions, the *Diagnostic and Statistical Manual of Mental Disorders—Text Revised,* fourth edition (DSM-IV-TR; 2000), published by the American Psychiatric Association (APA), provides a standardized classification system that can be used by all members of the mental health care team.

DEVELOPMENTAL DISORDERS

Developmental disorders, although not related by etiology, typically share a common feature in that there is a delay in one or more areas of development. These areas include attention, cognition, language, affect, and social and moral behavior. Because these behaviors are interrelated, a delay in one area may interfere with development in another area. Developmental disorders include cognitive challenge, pervasive developmental disorders, and specific developmental disorders such as learning disorders, motor skills disorders (developmental coordination disorders), and communication disorders.

Cognitive Challenge

The DSM-IV-TR defines cognitive challenge (mental retardation) on the basis of two criteria: significantly subaverage general intellectual functioning—an intelligence quotient (IQ) of 70 or lower with onset before 18 years of age—and concurrent deficits in adaptive functioning (APA, 2000). For infants, because available intelligence tests do not yield numerical values, a clinical judgment of significant subaverage intellectual function must be made.

Approximately 2% of children in the United States are cognitively challenged. This is not the result of a single cause but of conditions such as genetic abnormalities (e.g., fragile X syndrome, Down syndrome [trisomy 21]) and metabolic disorders (e.g., phenylketonuria). In addition, an interplay of several genes with environmental factors (polyfactorial causes) has been identified as a possible cause in some children (Box 54.2).

Children who are cognitively challenged are seen in health care settings for diagnosis, and they come to health settings throughout their lives for the same reasons as other children do—for well-child care at ambulatory health

---

BOX 54.2

Common Causes of Cognitive Challenge

Chromosomal abnormalities such as Down syndrome and fragile X syndrome

Infection in utero, such as rubella or cytomegalic inclusion disease

Anoxia at birth from such causes as umbilical cord compression

Fetal alcohol syndrome

Inherited metabolic disorders such as phenylketonuria

Head trauma

Lead poisoning

Hypothyroidism

Brain malformations such as anencephaly

Very low birth weight

Infections such as measles encephalitis

---

maintenance visits; for treatment of lacerations or poisoning in emergency departments; or for treatment of illnesses such as pneumonia or appendicitis in in-service units. For these reasons, child health nurses need to be skilled in meeting the needs of cognitively challenged children.

Classification

Assessing children who are cognitively challenged for physical disorders is difficult because they cannot relate symptoms as well as other children (Roberts et al., 2004). It is unfair to categorize children only according to the results of intelligence tests, because children do not always perform well in testing situations. Commonly, cognitive challenge is classified as mild, moderate, severe, or profound according to IQ. The IQ level of 70 was chosen as the upper limit of cognitive challenge because most children with IQs below this level are so limited in their functioning that they require special services, protection, and schooling. IQ tests are considered to have an error of measurement of about 5 points. Therefore, many children with an IQ of 75 are included in special schooling programs.

Mild Cognitive Challenge. About 85% of children who are cognitively challenged fall into this category (APA, 2000). In this group, a child's IQ is between 50 and 70. The category is equivalent to the educational category "educable." During early years, these children learn social and communication skills and are often not distinguishable from average children. They are able to learn academic skills up to about the sixth-grade level. As adults, they can usually achieve social and vocational skills adequate for minimum self-support. They can live independently but need guidance and assistance when faced with new situations or unusual stress.

Moderate Cognitive Challenge. Children in this category have an IQ between 35 and 49. About 10% of cognitively challenged children fall into this category (APA, 2000). During preschool years, these children learn to talk and communicate, but they have only poor awareness of social conventions. They can learn some vocational skills

during adolescence or young adulthood and can learn to take care of themselves with moderate supervision. They are unlikely to progress beyond the second-grade level in academic subjects. As adults, they may be able to contribute to their own support by performing unskilled or semiskilled work under close supervision in a sheltered workshop setting. They may learn to travel alone to familiar places. They need supervision and guidance when in stressful settings.

Severe Cognitive Challenge. Children in this group have an IQ between 20 and 34. About 4% of cognitively challenged children fall into this category (APA, 2000). During the preschool period, these children develop only minimal speech and little or no communicative speech. They usually have accompanying poor motor development. During school years, they may learn to talk and can be trained in basic hygiene and dressing skills. As adults, they may be able to perform simple work tasks under close supervision, but as a group they do not profit from vocational training. They need constant supervision for safety.

Profound Cognitive Challenge. The IQ of children in this group is less than 20. Fewer than 1% of cognitively challenged children fall into this group (APA, 2000). During the preschool period, these children show only minimal capacity for sensorimotor functioning. They need a highly structured environment and a constant level of help and supervision. Some children respond to training in minimal self-care, such as toothbrushing, but only very limited self-care is possible.

Assessment

Assessment as to whether a child is cognitively challenged is done by history taking and IQ testing. Early assessment is key and should be done as soon as parents become aware that their child is experiencing problems with development. This helps to prevent the parents from developing unrealistic expectations of the child or punishing the child for doing things that he or she doesn't understand not to do. Assessment also allows parents to look at the things the child can do and to see where they can be of most help (King et al., 2005).

Intelligence is routinely measured with standardized tests, such as the Stanford-Binet test. Adaptive behavioral functioning, which may vary in different environments, is judged according to several methods, including standardized instruments for assessing social maturity and adaptive skills. A composite picture of life functioning is drawn from these multiple sources.

Parents may react to the diagnosis of cognitive challenge in the same way as parents who have been told that their child has a chronic or fatal illness—with a grief reaction. This may be manifested as disbelief, anger, or extreme sorrow. The grief may become chronic—always present, always waiting to strike a parent especially hard at times when the child would have reached milestones in his or her life, such as the first day of school or high school graduation. Work with the family to develop plans that are realistic. A child cannot achieve more than his or her individual disability will allow, but you can help parents better accept the child's limited capabilities (Box 54.3).

BOX 54.3 FOCUS ON . . .

DIVERSITY OF CARE

Cognitive and mental health disorders have always been perplexing to people, so the history of acceptance for children with such disorders is poor. In ancient civilizations, physicians bored holes in children's heads to let out what they perceived to be evil spirits; modern television programs or movies still show distorted perceptions of behaviors associated with people who are cognitively challenged or have a mental illness. Such misperceptions make it difficult for parents or siblings to accept these diagnoses. Taking time to talk with them about modern management of these disorders and the ways that children who are mentally ill or cognitively challenged can be integrated into a family can be a major intervention in helping families adjust to and grow with these disorders.

Therapeutic Management

To aid in planning, parents need a realistic prognosis for their child. This may be difficult to offer in early life, because infant intelligence tests are not accurate and more sophisticated tests are difficult to administer until the preschool years. Because prediction based on these early tests involves some subjective input, a child's potential may be overrated or underrated by them. Once parents have a realistic expectation based on the best judgment possible, however, they are ready, with guidance, to help their children achieve their full potential.

NURSING DIAGNOSES AND RELATED INTERVENTIONS

———●———

Nursing Diagnosis: Health-seeking behaviors related to increasing knowledge of care needs of a cognitively challenged child

Outcome Evaluation: Parents identify their particular options; identify child's care needs; demonstrate measures to care for child.

Parents of children who are cognitively challenged have a number of important decisions to make concerning care of their child.

Institutional Care Versus Home Care. At one time, if a child was born with a disorder such as Down syndrome, parents were advised to place the child in an institution immediately. Today, very few institutions of this type are available. Parents are encouraged to keep children at home and to maintain a home and school environment for them that is as near normal as possible. This plan has definite advantages

for children who are only mildly or moderately delayed. The give-and-take of a home environment improves their ability to relate to other people. Because a small group of people cares for them, stimulation and desire to achieve are increased.

Parents shoulder a great deal of responsibility to provide constant watchful care, especially for a child with problems affecting judgment. This responsibility increases as both the child and the parents grow older. The parents' freedom to go on vacation or to have an adult life apart from the child is restricted. They may spend so much time with the child that other children in the family feel left out, unloved, or burdensome.

If parents are unable to care for a child at home, a suitable foster home placement may be possible, offering the child the advantage of a family setting. Halfway houses or group homes (6 to 12 children living in a home with assigned counselors) can provide a care setting with a home atmosphere and community experiences.

Before giving advice to any family about where a child should be raised, consider the individual circumstances of the family. Every family has its own coping mechanisms, and individual parents may be at different stages of coping, especially during the first year after the birth of a child with a severe disability. Be certain to consider the feelings of each family member and how adequately they are coping.

Health Maintenance Needs. Children who are cognitively challenged need the same health maintenance supervision as other children do. At health care visits, parents may need reinforcement and review of precautions against accidents. Remind them to treat children according to their intellectual age, not their chronologic age. All 2-year-old children would turn on the burners of the stove to see the flame if they could reach them. Most do not, however, because they cannot reach that high. The mother of a 6-year-old child who thinks like a 2-year-old must be exceedingly careful: her child can reach the same dangerous areas as any 6-year-old child can but may explore and touch them with a 2-year-old child's judgment.

Illness. It may be more difficult to detect illness in a child who is cognitively challenged because he or she may not be able to describe the problem. For example, children experiencing pain may respond to it by generalized crying, as infants do. Parents must observe their child closely for symptoms such as tugging at an ear, refusing to swallow food, rapid breathing, or limping, because these symptoms will help to localize the discomfort. When they call health care personnel, parents may be apologetic about their lack of ability to judge their child. Help parents to become advocates for their child. They know their child better than anyone else. The parents may not know exactly what is wrong, but they do know that something is wrong. Reassure the parents that they have done the correct thing by calling to check out the problem.

When children with a cognitive challenge are seen in an emergency department or an ambulatory setting for care, they need simple explanations of what will happen. The average 6-year-old child sees you with a thermometer in your hand and thinks, "She's going to take my temperature." Your explanation that you are going to do that only confirms what the child has already guessed. A child who is cognitively challenged may be unable to make this association between the thermometer and what you are going to do. Your explanation, therefore, is the first introduction to the event. Make certain that it is adequate.

When children are admitted to the hospital, nursing care must meet the needs of their intellectual age, not their chronologic one. For example, whether safety precautions such as side rails or possibly restraints will be necessary must be judged according to intellectual age. The explanations and preparations for procedures also must be geared to intellectual age.

When cognitively challenged children are discharged from a hospital, parents need careful explanations of signs and symptoms to look for to ensure continued good health in the child. Remember that such signs may be more difficult to elicit, depending on the degree of the child's cognitive delay. Be sure parents have a telephone number they can call to seek further information or advice if they are unsure of their own observations in the period immediately after discharge.

Education. Most children who are cognitively challenged do well in preschool programs, possibly giving them a head start in learning to socialize with peers and to develop fine and gross motor coordination.

The school chosen for the child depends on the degree of intellectual delay and on the school situations available in the community. Children should be included in regular classes as much as possible (Fig. 54.1). These classes offer children a great deal of stimulation and help them reach their best potential. They also help them learn to work and socialize with people, something they will need to do for the rest of their lives. Advocating for school placement of a child in an inclusive program may be necessary. By federal law, children have the right to be educated in the least restrictive environment possible. Children who are cognitively challenged need an individualized education plan (IEP) developed based on the child's individual learning style and projected capabilities. In addition, they need safety instructions such as how to locate the correct bus for the trip home from school. If they walk to school, they need appropriate supervision to ensure safety when crossing streets.

Nursing Diagnosis: Delayed growth and development related to cognitive impairment

Outcome Evaluation: Child performs self-care within limits of disorder; exhibits feelings of satisfaction with accomplishments.

Self-Care Activities. Children who are cognitively challenged need to learn the maximum amount of self-care possible. Doing so provides them with a sense of control and accomplishment. Carefully assess whether children need special aids to achieve such skills as brushing teeth, combing hair, taking a bath, and eating. Even after children learn how to perform these skills, they may need continued reminders to do them, because they are unaware of the reason for or importance of the skill. If you perform these skills for children, such as during a period of hospitalization, they can forget how to perform them and need to be retaught after they return home (Box 54.4).

Play. Children with intellectual delays enjoy play like any child. Guide parents to choose toys that are appropriate for their child's developmental, not chronologic, age. Toys that cover a wide age range, such as music boxes or tape players, are good choices. Because children who are cognitively challenged may be older and stronger than the age stated for a toy, toys that are developmentally correct still may not be appropriate because they break too easily to be safe.

Social Relationships. The ability to communicate may be delayed in children who are cognitively challenged, because the ability to develop language is often delayed. Speech therapy may be necessary to help them articulate correct sounds. Talking picture boards (boards with pictures on them, available commercially or made by parents), to which children can point if they want something, can help speed communication.

Teaching early social behavior, such as saying "thank you" and "excuse me," shaking hands, and taking turns, is important to help children relate to other children and adults. Cognitively challenged children imitate this type of behavior the same as other children do. Providing good role models is an effective way of teaching social behavior.

Encourage parents to enroll children in preschool programs to help them learn to be comfortable with other children at the earliest time possible. Many programs enroll children as early as 1 year of age to begin education. For a school-age child, participating in organized groups such as Girl Scouts or Special Olympics is an important way to learn to interact with others and feel successful.

Preparation for Adulthood. As children who are cognitively challenged reach adolescence, they benefit from orientation to sexual responsibility, the same as all children do. Girls can understand a simple explanation of menstruation and necessary menstrual hygiene. Both boys and girls need explanations of how pregnancy occurs and the measures they need to take to prevent this. Help them understand socially acceptable sexual activities.

If a girl is going to use a contraceptive and lives with a responsible adult, she can be given an oral

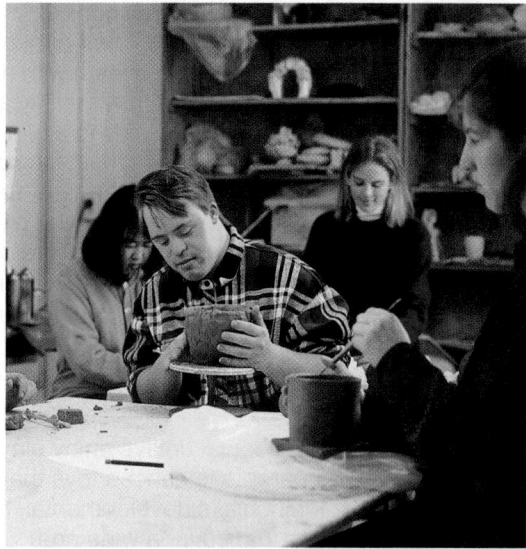

FIGURE 54.1 A teenage boy with Down syndrome participates in a high school art class. (© Richard Hutchings/Science Source/Photo Researchers.)

contraceptive daily by that adult. Longer-acting contraceptives, such as Depo-Provera and Norplant, which do not require daily administration, also are available. Sterilization is not recommended, because it is difficult for a cognitively challenged adolescent to understand fully the implications of the procedure, so their consent is not fully informed. If pregnancy should occur, an adolescent who is cognitively challenged can be counseled but not forced to have an abortion. If the adolescent decides to continue the pregnancy, assist her through the pregnancy and planning safe care for her child.

What if... a 15-year-old girl who is mildly cognitively challenged, comes to your school office. During your conversation, she asks you if she should have a baby. How would you respond?

Pervasive Developmental Disorders: Autistic Disorder

As a category, pervasive developmental disorders are characterized by impairment in social and communication skills and the display of stereotypical behaviors (APA, 2000). Autistic disorder is marked by severe deficits in language, perceptual, and motor development; defective reality testing; and an inability to function in social settings. There often is a lack of responsiveness to other people, gross impairment in communication skills, and bizarre responses to various aspects of the environment, all developing within the first 30 months of age. It is a rare condition, occurring in only 2 to 10 of every 10,000 children, although its incidence may be increasing. A former concern that immunization may precede or cause the dis-

BOX 54.4 FOCUS ON...

FAMILY TEACHING

Teaching Guidelines for the Cognitively Challenged Child

Q. The mother of a child who is cognitively challenged says to you, "How can we make sure our son can learn as much as he is able?"

A. Here are some guidelines for teaching:

- Teach one step at a time. Short-term memory is often possible, whereas long-term memory is not. This means a child can learn only one step of a skill at a time (remembering three consecutive steps requires long-term memory).
- Introduce motivators for learning, such as generous praise. Learning may not be rewarding all by itself when intelligence is impaired.
- Reduce the number of extra stimuli present. Faced with too many stimuli, a child cannot focus attention on the task to learn (or realize that the task is more important than surrounding stimuli).
- Demonstrate the skill to be learned. Seeing a skill performed is generally better than just hearing it explained.
- Keep things simple. Cognitively challenged children may have difficulty with learning principles or abstractions. They may be able to learn to wash their hands, for example, but not why they should wash them (other than that it pleases you).
- Give praise accordingly. Remember that accomplishing even the most simple skill may be very difficult for your child. Learning to tie shoes may take the same effort as another child spends learning mathematics. Learning to cross streets safely may be equivalent to earning a high school diploma.

order has now been ruled out as a cause (Jack, 2004). Autism occurs more often in boys than in girls. As many as 50% of children with the disorder are also cognitively challenged (APA, 2000).

Assessment

Common symptoms of autistic disorder are summarized in Box 54.5. Because of the lack of responsiveness to people that is part of the syndrome, normal attachment behavior does not develop. Although autism often is not diagnosed until the child is 2 to 3 years of age, parents report that they were worried much earlier because their infant failed to cuddle, make eye contact, or exhibit facial responsiveness. Infants may not reach to be picked up. They are unable to play cooperatively or make friendships. Parents may first bring a child to a health care facility thinking that he or she is deaf because of this inability to establish normal relationships.

The impairment in communication is shown in both verbal and nonverbal skills. Language may be totally ab-

BOX 54.5

BOX 54.5

Common Symptoms in the Child With Autistic Disorder

Failure to develop social relations
Stereotyped behaviors such as hand gestures
Extreme resistance to change in routine
Abnormal responses to sensory stimuli
Decreased sensitivity to pain
Inappropriate or decreased emotional expressions
Specific, limited intellectual problem solving abilities
Stereotyped or repetitive use of language
Impaired ability to initiate or sustain a conversation

sent. If a child does speak, grammatical structure may be impaired, such as the use of "you" when "I" is intended. There is inability to name objects (nominal aphasia) and abnormal speech melody, such as question-like rises at the end of statements. **Echolalia** (repetition of words or phrases spoken by others) and concrete interpretation also may be present.

Bizarre responses to the environment may include intense reactions to minor changes in the environment (e.g., screaming if a toy box is moved across the room) and attachment to odd objects (e.g., always carrying a string or a shoe). Repetitive hand movements, rocking, and rhythmic body movements are often observed. Children are intensely preoccupied by objects that move, such as a fan, the swirling water in the toilet bowl, or a spinning top. Music often holds a special interest for them. Hitting, head banging, and biting also may be present.

Children with autistic disorder have a **labile mood** (e.g., crying occurs suddenly and is followed immediately by giggling or laughing). They may react with overresponsiveness to sensory stimuli, such as light or sound, but then be unaware of a major event in the room, such as the sounding of a fire alarm.

In contrast to these mannerisms, long-term memory and "savant" skills may be excellent (Volkmar et al., 2005). Autistic children may be able to recall dates and spoken words from conversations that took place years before. This excellent memory previously led to the belief that most of these children have normal intelligence. Actually, the majority of children with autistic disorder have an IQ of less than 70 (APA, 2000). Intelligence testing is difficult, however, because children with autistic disorder do not respond well to test situations, and they score poorly on the verbal parts of these tests. Tasks requiring manipulative or visual skills or immediate memory may be performed at above-normal levels.

Therapeutic Management

Autistic disorder is a perplexing condition. Parents need a great deal of support so that they do not reject their child because he or she seems to be rejecting them. Behavior modification therapy may be effective in controlling some of the bizarre mannerisms that accompany autism, but, because the basic cause of the disorder is not known, therapy will not always succeed. Although various medications such as tranquilizers or antidepressants have been tried,

no medications specific for autism are available (Volkmar et al., 2005).

As children mature, they develop greater awareness of and attachment to parents and other familiar adults. A day care program can help to promote social awareness. Some children may eventually reach a point where they can become passively involved in loosely structured play groups. Some children may be able to lead independent lives, although social ineptness and awkwardness may remain, especially if accompanied by cognitive challenges.

Checkpoint Question 1

Suppose Todd had symptoms of autism. Which of these symptoms is common in autism?

a. Lack of short-term memory
b. Hallucinations of voices talking
c. Whirling and whirling around in a circle
d. Severe depression or feelings of sadness

Specific Developmental Disorders

Specific developmental disorders may be characterized by the more narrowed area of development involved with the delay. Typically, these include learning disorders, communication disorders, and motor skills disorders.

Learning disorders occur in approximately 5% of the children in the United States. Although the degree may vary, these disorders involve a discrepancy between actual achievement and what is expected based on the child's age and intelligence. Learning disorders may involve reading (e.g., **dyslexia** [reading reversal]), mathematics, or writing. Children may develop accompanying low self-esteem and deficits in social skills (APA, 2000). Children need individualized educational plans to help them achieve at the highest level possible.

Communication disorders involve problems of speech (motor aspect) or language (formulation and comprehension of verbal communication). Examples include expressive disorders, phonologic disorders, and stuttering. Like learning disorders, these conditions can lead to a lack of self-esteem unless a child receives support and encouragement from parents, teachers, and health care providers. Speech therapy can effectively improve these disorders and allow children to achieve sufficiently to become successful adults.

ATTENTION-DEFICIT AND DISRUPTIVE BEHAVIOR DISORDERS

Attention-deficit disorder and the disruptive behavior disorders may begin with behavior problems that are not so different from what most families experience. For this reason, parents may be unaware of the need for intervention initially. By the time they do seek help, they may already be extremely distressed about the seeming unmanageability of their child.

These disorders need to be diagnosed as early as possible, before the child's behavior leads to a deteriorating level of self-esteem, compromised social skills, and social and legal complications in family functioning. The home environment may be the most important factor in determining whether a disorder turns into a more complicated psychopathologic process or can be channeled into purposeful, productive activity.

Attention-Deficit Hyperactivity Disorder

Attention-deficit hyperactivity disorder (ADHD) is a persistent pattern of inattention and/or hyperactivity-impulsiveness revealed before the age of 7 years (APA, 2000). It is estimated to occur in about 3% to 7% of school-age children in the United States. Boys are affected more frequently than girls. Although the cause is unknown, it occurs more frequently among some families than in the general population, indicating a possible genetic etiologic component. ADHD has also been associated with child neglect, lead poisoning, and drug exposure in utero (APA, 2000). Both drug and behavior modification treatment methods have been used with success, a fact that may support the theory of varying causes.

The disorder is characterized by three major behaviors: inattention, impulsiveness, and hyperactivity (Hechtman, 2005). Inattention makes children unable to complete tasks effectively. They become easily distracted and often may not seem to listen. Impulsiveness causes them to act before they think and therefore to have difficulty with such tasks as awaiting turns at games. With hyperactivity, children may shift excessively from one activity to another, exhibiting excessive or exaggerated muscular activity, such as excessive climbing onto objects, constant fidgeting, or aimless or haphazard running.

Assessment

The disorder is diagnosable by 36 months of age, although parents may excuse the behavior as "active" or "always on the go" until school age, when it is apparent that the child cannot sit still in school or concentrate on problem solving for longer periods. When the disorder is first suspected, a thorough initial history to reveal the extent of the problem must be obtained. The history is important, because some children have enough control in a one-to-one situation that their extremes of behavior are not apparent in an ambulatory health care setting.

Review the pregnancy and birth history, the child's ability to meet developmental milestones, and a typical day for the child. The term **hyperactivity,** or excessive movement, is commonly carelessly used by parents to describe any active child. Have the parent give an exact description of what the child is unable to do, such as sitting still long enough to finish a full meal or running to the window 10 times in 15 minutes, to document that hyperactivity truly exists.

Assess for activity that is not only excessive but also disorganized. For example, in school, children with ADHD may run from the back of the room to the front of the room, to the window, to the teacher's desk, to their own desk throughout class. They perform repetitive activities such as pencil tapping, arm swinging, and finger tapping. At home, they may leave a project they are working on or a television program they are watching intently and run to the window or open the refrigerator door, unaware of why they are running. This is driven or compulsive behavior.

Variability is another important symptom. Everyone has days when they perform at their peak and days when their performance is less than optimum. Children with ADHD may have behavior so variable that they have good and bad *moments.* This type of variability causes them to lose track of systems and methods, not just answers, so school performance may falter. When asked to add, for example, a child might add 4 and 3 correctly, but then lose track of the system and add 2 and 3 as 23 or 32.

A high level of impulsiveness can cause children to make statements without thinking, to touch objects they have just been told not to touch, or to speak or act before they have time to think about what they want to say or do. When angered, they may shout, strike out, or bite before they can be offered an explanation. They may be unable to wait in line for a drink of water—their impulsiveness tells them that they must have their drink immediately.

Usually, average children can filter out stimuli that are not important to them at that moment. Children with ADHD seem to have an "all-or-none" reaction to stimuli. They may block out all incoming stimuli and, as a result, do not hear their parents or a teacher calling them. They may be disciplined at school for something such as not answering a fire drill (unaware that a bell was ringing and that children around them were moving toward the exit). At other times, they may be unable to suppress any incoming stimuli. They mean to concentrate on a desk assignment in school, but, outside the window, they hear a bird singing; next to them, they smell a girl's perfume; they feel their watch on their wrist—so they cannot concentrate on the problem at hand. This may be reported by parents or teachers as an exceedingly short attention span.

Children with ADHD may also have difficulty with concepts such as *right* and *left, before* and *after, in front of, in back of,* and *yesterday* and *tomorrow,* because these concepts call for sequencing, the process of relating things to one another in time or space. If children cannot tell the difference between left and right, they can have difficulty forming common letters such as *b* and *d,* which vary only in the direction of the bottom loop. They can have difficulty with common tasks such as washing their hands, because they never know which way to turn a faucet. Turning door knobs and keys, tying shoe laces, and screwing on bottle caps are all complex tasks for a child who has difficulty with sequencing. They may show awkward motor movements and cannot work all muscles gracefully in proper sequence. These children may reach beyond an object, possibly spilling a glass of milk at the table at every meal.

Long after the average child is speaking in fluent sentences, children with ADHD may have difficulty using conjunctions or prepositions correctly (sequencing of words). They may have difficulty learning to read. To read words of more than one syllable, they must sound the first syllable, then retain that sound in their mind while they sound the second syllable. If they have difficulty retaining the first syllable long enough to connect it with the second, they cannot construct the word. Similarly, they can have difficulty with arithmetic, because they may be unable to retain the sum of two numbers long enough to add a third. Spelling may be equally difficult. Not only are they unable to sequence the letters in a word correctly, but they also cannot retain memory rules such as "i before e" to help them.

As a rule, children with ADHD do not have a deficit in intelligence, although they may seem to because of their impulsive behavior. They may be unaware that their behavior is upsetting to family, friends, and teachers and therefore are not anxious about their inability to conform to society's rules.

On physical assessment, these children often show many "soft" neurologic signs, such as inability to use a pencil or scissors well. A thorough neurologic examination often is difficult because their attention span is so short. On such an examination, they often have difficulty performing tests such as a finger-to-nose test or rapid hand movements (e.g., touching one finger after another with the thumb). They tend to show "mirroring" with this movement (the second hand imitates what the first hand attempts to do). Cerebellar difficulty may be evidenced further by inability to perform a tandem walk or a heel-to-shin test. They may be able to identify one touch but not two simultaneous touches on their body. They may not show the normal responses of **graphesthesia** (ability to recognize a shape that has been traced on the skin) or **stereognosis** (ability to recognize an object by touch). When asked to stand with arms outstretched, **choreiform movements** (aimless movements) and rising of the fingers are often present. More definite neurologic signs, such as a unilateral Babinski reflex or strabismus, may also be present. Testing children through the use of games may be necessary so that their attention is maintained long enough to complete the assessment.

IQ testing is used to document a child's intelligence. The Wechsler Intelligence Scale for Children (WISC), the test most often chosen, consists of two portions: a verbal scale and a performance scale. A child is given three final scores: verbal IQ, performance IQ, and combination or full-scale IQ. The child with perceptual and motor deficits tends to do poorly on the performance scale but average or better on the verbal scale. Children with language difficulty typically do poorly on the verbal scale but average or greater on the performance scale. Children with ADHD show a "scatter" pattern on both performance and verbal portions, doing well on some portions and poorly on others.

Children who have difficulty filtering out stimuli do poorly on group-administered intelligence tests because they are too distracted by those around them. For this reason, such children should take IQ tests individually. Neurologic examinations also should be performed in rooms that are free of distractions such as attractive toys.

Children with ADHD are often referred to a health care facility because they have had difficulty achieving in school. Parents may have been reassured on previous occasions that, although their child had difficulty settling down to tasks, this was because he was "all boy" or "every child is different." They may need time to accept that their child has a condition that interferes with learning. Active listening is essential. This is a difficult situation that may have persisted for a long time. The parents may be unaware

themselves of the strain that has been produced until they start to describe it.

Therapeutic Management

A variety of treatment methods are used, often in combination, in the management of ADHD.

Environment. Construction of a stable learning environment is crucial for children with ADHD. This may include special instruction, free from the distractions of an entire class. Parents may have difficulty accepting the fact that their child needs special schooling (the intelligence test, after all, said that he or she was above average). They may need help in seeing that their child's condition interferes with intellectual functioning and that a special program must be constructed for the child to succeed.

Parents at home need to construct an environment that is as free of stimulating distractions as possible. Exposure to the soothing influence of green may reduce behavior symptoms (Kuo & Taylor, 2004). Parents having difficulty at home with discipline and management often appreciate support and advice. Encourage them to be fair but firm and to set consistent limits. Although every child has the right to an opinion, many decisions that the average child enjoys making for himself or herself must be made for a child with ADHD. "Do you want to wear your red or your blue shirt today?" is less effective than "Here is your blue shirt to wear today."

Children who are easily distracted have difficulty completing chores or picking up their toys. They can be assigned age-appropriate chores with the understanding that a parent must give many reminders to them to get the job completed. Teach parents to give instructions slowly and to make certain that they have their child's attention before beginning instructions. Breaking down a chore into several steps may help (get the toy box is one step; pick up toys is a second). This helps to avoid confrontation that may arise later if children do not hear or do not process what is said to them.

All children like to participate in dinner conversation or discussions about their day. Children with ADHD often have difficulty telling a story or repeating a joke told to them (a sequencing problem). Suggest that parents help them by asking questions such as "Why?" "Where?" or "Who?" to reach the point of the story. Also encourage parents to be sure, when they correct behavior, that their anger is about something the child has deliberately done wrong, not about some incident that happened because of the child's inability to sequence, filter, or integrate concepts. Punishment should follow an offense quickly, because a child with ADHD quickly forgets what he or she did. As with all children, parents should make sure the child understands that the parent is angry at the behavior, not the child. Children with ADHD commonly develop poor self-esteem because, although they are intelligent, they cannot succeed. Help parents to build, not hinder, the development of self-esteem at every stage possible.

Medication. A number of medications are helpful in controlling the excessive activity of the child with ADHD and in lengthening the attention span or decreasing the distractibility so that he or she can function in a normal classroom. All of these medications have advantages and disadvantages.

Methylphenidate hydrochloride (Ritalin, Concerta [extended-release form]) is frequently prescribed for this disorder (Box 54.6). It works by stimulating dopamine receptors to achieve a more regular nerve transmission. Insomnia and anorexia are side effects. The insomnia may be relieved by administering the drug early in the day. The extended-release form is advantageous in that it needs to be administered only once a day. Children receiving the drug for extended periods of time need careful height and weight assessment to evaluate that long-term anorexia is

not causing weight loss. Caution parents that Ritalin gives a "high" to children who do *not* have ADHD, so their child must be careful that his medication is not stolen to be used by other children for its drug euphoria effect (Williams et al., 2004). Other medications that may be useful are atomoxetine, norepinephrine reuptake inhibitors, and tricyclic antidepressants (Hectman, 2005).

Family Support. Parents of a child with ADHD often need frequent health care visits while their child is growing up. A responsive, listening ear is crucial to their ability to handle the challenge of raising a child with these symptoms. Any parents can grow short-tempered and irritable at times with a child who does not seem to hear them or follow what they say. They may need reminders at intervals that their child does not act this way on purpose. Help them to understand that, because of a very complex and as yet ill-understood syndrome, the behavior is the best their child can achieve. Children with ADHD have an increased number of childhood accidents such as burns, so they need close parental supervision to avoid injury (Mangus et al., 2004). (See Box 54.7.)

Although hyperactivity fades, some children with ADHD continue to experience problems with impulsivity and inattention into adulthood. They achieve best if they can find careers that allow them to cope with these behaviors.

Oppositional Defiant Disorders

Oppositional defiant disorders consist of hostile, negativistic, or defiant behaviors that result in disturbed functioning in academic and social domains and last for longer than 6 months. Children typically have difficulty controlling their temper; their anger is often directed at an authority figure (APA, 2000).

The disorder develops most frequently in late preschool or early school age. The cause may be a combination of temperament, inheritance, and adverse social factors. Therapy must be individually designed to meet the needs of the child and includes such techniques as family therapy and anger management.

Conduct Disorders

Conduct disorders are persistent antisocial acts that involve violations of personal rights or societal rules, such as disobedience, stealing, fighting, destruction of property, fire setting, and early sexual behavior (APA, 2000). Symptoms can be clustered as involving aggression toward people and animals, destruction of property, deceitfulness and theft, and serious violations of rules. Many teenage runaways may fall into this category. The incidence is about 5% of children (Thomas, 2005).

Children seem to develop an increasing loss of self-regulation or an inability to know when to stop an action.

Conduct disorders are seen more frequently in males than in females, particularly if property or violent crimes are involved; however, the prevalence of conduct disorders in girls is increasing, which may reduce the male predominance over time. A number of etiologic factors have been described for this disorder, including genetic predisposition, neurologic deficit correlates, and sociologic factors related to poverty and cultural disadvantage. In ad-

---

BOX 54.6 FOCUS ON . . .

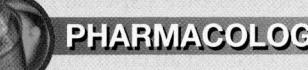
PHARMACOLOGY

Methylphenidate Hydrochloride (Ritalin, Concerta)

Classification: Methylphenidate is a central nervous system stimulant.

Action: Acts paradoxically in children with ADHD, possibly by stimulating dopamine receptors to calm rather than simulate activity (Karch, 2004).

Pregnancy Risk Category: C

Dosage: Initially, 5 mg orally before breakfast and lunch, gradually increased in 5- to 10-mg increments weekly, not to exceed 60 mg/day. The extended-release form (Concerta) is administered once daily; dosage is determined by weight and symptoms.

Possible Adverse Effects: Nervousness, insomnia, anorexia, pulse rate changes, hypertension or hypotension, tachycardia, leukopenia, anemia, and growth suppression.

Nursing Implications
- Administer the drug exactly as prescribed, and instruct parents to do the same. Reinforce proper administration of once-daily extended-release form; instruct parents to have child swallow extended-release tablets whole and to refrain from chewing or crushing them.
- Instruct the parents to administer the drug before 6 PM to prevent interference with sleep.
- Advise the parents and child to avoid over-the-counter drugs, such as cold remedies and cough syrups that contain alcohol.
- Obtain baseline vital signs and monitor on follow-up visits for changes.
- Arrange for follow-up laboratory tests, including complete blood count for children on long-term therapy.
- Stress the need for adequate nutrition in light of possible anorexia. Monitor child's weight closely for changes.
- Assess child's growth on subsequent visits for possible growth suppression.
- Keep in mind that the safety of using methylphenidate for children younger than 6 years of age has not been established.

A Multidisciplinary Care Map for A School-age Child With Attention Deficit Hyperactivity Disorder (ADHD)

•

Todd, a second grader, is admitted to the 1-day surgery unit to have plaque removed from his teeth under conscious sedation. He was diagnosed with attention-deficit hyperactivity disorder (ADHD) approximately 6 months ago; he has had symptoms since he was 6 months old. You observe Todd coloring; running to the window; running to the door, opening and closing the door; and then throwing pamphlets out of an information rack. His mother tells you she is "at her wits' end" because Todd's attention span is so short and his behavior so disruptive. His father tells you he's proud that his son is "all boy."

Family Assessment

Child lives with two parents in two-bedroom condominium. Father works as a sail maker; mother woks part-time in local fish market. Father rates finances as "Not good. My wife wants to work more, but we can't find anyone to watch Todd, he's such a handful."

Client Assessment

7-year-old, slightly overweight male. Child observed holding toy dog tightly. Mother states, "He talks to the dog about what he wants to do." Some difficulty interacting and talking with others. He often repeats himself, asking "What's your name?" and "What do you like to do?" Mother feeds him mainly fast food meals because his attention span is so short. Toilet trained but sometimes has accidents as he "forgets" to go. Needs supervision dressing because he loses track of task at hand. Refuses to let mother brush teeth. Mother says, "He gets upset and cries easily if his routine changes." Attends special class in public school, as he was too disruptive in regular classroom.

Nursing Diagnosis

Impaired social interaction related to short attention span and distractibility

Outcome Criteria

Child states he understands purpose of dental procedure; cooperates to extent possible with IV therapy and bed rest after conscious sedation.

Team Member Responsible	Assessment	Intervention	Rationale	Expected Outcome
Activities of Daily Living				
Nurse	Assess what self-care activities child typically does for himself.	Allow child to change to hospital gown; supervise bathroom use.	Self-care can offer a sense of control unless it becomes frustrating.	Child cooperates to help with self-care to the extent a short attention span will allow.
Consultations				
Nurse	Assess whether child care specialist is available for consultation.	Consult with child care specialist about what games, toys would be best for child with short attention span.	Games can become frustrating if they can't be completed in a short period.	Child care specialist visits with child and mother and suggests at least two activities for period before surgery.

(continued)

Team Member Responsible	Assessment	Intervention	Rationale	Expected Outcome
Procedures/Medications				
Nurse	Assess whether child has past experience with IV therapy.	Begin IV line in non-dominant hand.	Use of non-dominant hand allows child to complete small, frequent tasks.	Child states he understands purpose of IV line. Does not try to remove it.
Nurse	Assess whether child took his daily methylphenidate hydrochloride pill before admittance.	Check with physician and dental surgeon to determine whether child should receive medicine if it was not taken before procedure.	Methylphenidate hydrochloride can substantially reduce behavior symptoms of ADHD.	Mother reports whether morning medication was taken.
Nutrition				
Nurse/ Nutritionist	Assess what mother means by "fast food" meals.	Discuss a diet with child that doesn't involve so many fatty foods, if appropriate.	Child is overweight, a finding that can be caused by eating fat-heavy fast food meals.	Mother states she understands that even though child eats in a hurry, his meals can still be nutritious.
Patient/Family Education				
Nurse	Assess what parent understands about good tooth care.	Talk to mother about techniques to make toothbrushing a game, not a chore.	Plaque will form again on teeth if they are not brushed after this procedure.	Mother suggests two different ways, such as Simon Says, that she could interest child in toothbrushing.
Nurse/ Physician	Assess what parents understand about ADHD.	Educate parents that ADHD is a disorder, not normal boyish behavior.	As long as one parent continues to think of child's behavior as within normal limits, it will be difficult for them to be consistent in care.	Mother and father state they understand that their son's condition is one that needs therapy.
Psychosocial/Spiritual/Emotional Needs				
Nurse	Assess what mother means by "at wit's end"; whether she feels she has adequate support to care for a child with extreme behaviors.	If appropriate, talk with mother about "respite" time to give her relief; perhaps contact a local school of nursing to find a trusted baby-sitter.	A child's activity level with ADHD can easily exhaust a parent if the parent cannot fit in some time for self.	Mother states whether she feels she needs additional outside support or whether her husband can provide this.
Nurse	Assess whether child can take favorite toy to operating room.	Respect that toy dog is favorite toy and important to child.	Children can find comfort and security in a favorite toy.	Toy is respected by unit and surgery personnel.
Discharge Planning				
Nurse	Assess whether parents have any questions about care at home after dental procedure.	Discuss that child will be sleepy for remainder of day after conscious sedation.	Conscious sedation is necessary because of child's resistance to new procedures.	Mother repeats care needed for next 24 hrs to safeguard still sleepy child.

dition, the home environment is frequently characterized by rejection, frustration, and harsh and inconsistent discipline. Parents may have marital conflicts or substance abuse problems, or children may have had a series of inconsistent caretaking by stepparents or foster parents.

Therapy for children with conduct disorders focuses on modifying the home environment and training the child in social and problem-solving skills. Social skills training teaches the child to recognize how his or her behavior affects others. Problem-solving skills training teaches the child to generate alternative solutions to situations, sharpen thinking about the consequences of choices, and evaluate his or her responses. Parental education is also important but can be difficult until the parents realize that this is a family problem. Removing the child from the home to a structured day care environment may be necessary. Unfortunately, the child may interpret this as more rejection, further compounding the problem. Any new environment that is created must be consistent and loving, not institutional, to be effective.

Numerous medications such as carbamazepine (Tegretol), propranolol (Inderal), and lithium carbonate may reduce the aggressive behavior. Long-term therapy with an agent such as buspirone (BuSpar) may be effective in helping children control temper or explosive outbursts.

Checkpoint Question 2

Children like Todd, with ADHD, have difficulty with concepts such as *before* and *after*. This difficulty reflects which underlying problem?

a. Not being able to sequence.
b. Not hearing equally in both ears.
c. Feeling chronically depressed.
d. Being too hyperactive to care.

ANXIETY DISORDERS OF CHILDHOOD OR ADOLESCENCE

Because anxiety is considered a normal part of certain phases of development (e.g., stranger anxiety in the 6- to 8-month-old child, separation anxiety in the toddler, fear of mutilation and fear of the dark in the preschooler, and performance anxiety or school avoidance in the school-age child or adolescent), genuine anxiety disorders in children may often be overlooked. If these disorders are left untreated, children may cope with fear by becoming overdependent on others for support or by turning away from the problem and withdrawing into themselves. This can leave a child socially immature and unable to achieve in school. The DSM-IV-TR identifies separation anxiety disorder and anxiety-based school refusal as anxiety disorders in children (APA, 2000). School refusal is discussed with other concerns of the school-age child (see Chapter 31).

Posttraumatic Stress Disorder

Posttraumatic stress disorder is a condition that occurs in children who have survived an experience that is more traumatic than usual, such as child abuse, domestic vio-

lence, a natural disaster such as a flood, a harrowing accident such as a house fire, a home robbery, or a near-fatal illness. Children continue to have recurring recollections or dreams of the event or demonstrate intense psychological symptoms if a reminder of the initiating event occurs. They may feel guilt that they survived the event if a close family member or friend did not.

Absence of effective support people may contribute to symptoms. Therapy consists of counseling with psychological debriefing to help the child rework the event and reduce the feeling of threat. Play therapy may be helpful (Cohen, 2005).

Separation Anxiety

Separation anxiety, a normal phase of development in the infant (see Chapter 28), is considered a disorder when an older child shows excessive anxiety about separation or the possibility of separation from those to whom the child is attached (Bernstein & Layne, 2005). Children may worry when apart from parents that their parents will have an accident or become ill. They may be so worried that they have difficulty falling asleep at night or insist on sleeping with their parents or just outside their parents' bedroom door. They experience acute distress, frequent nightmares about separation, and reluctance and refusal to separate. Repeated reports of physical symptoms during separations or when separation is anticipated are also possible. Such a degree of anxiety can be incapacitating to children; it may prevent them from visiting at friends' houses, enjoying a camp experience, or actively participating in school.

Separation anxiety tends to run in families and occurs slightly more frequently in girls than in boys. Unresolved internal conflicts, uncertainty about one's caregiver, and parent-induced anxious attachment are psychodynamic factors attributed to this disorder. Temperament may also be a contributing factor.

Treatment for separation anxiety includes individual counseling sessions combined with antidepressant medication. In addition, family therapy may be helpful in allowing the family to gain greater insight into the dynamics of the problem and aiding the child to gain more confidence in his or her ability to function independently. Remind parents that when children take antidepressant medication, it may lead to thoughts of suicide (Culpepper et al., 2004).

EATING DISORDERS

Eating disorders in young children consist of pica, rumination, and feeding disorders. In older children, eating disorders include anorexia nervosa and bulimia (APA, 2000).

Pica

Children who persistently eat nonfood substances such as dirt, clay, paint chips, crayons, yarn, or paper are said to have pica (Chatoor, 2005). *Pica* is the Latin word for magpie (a bird that is an indiscriminate eater). The primary danger lies in the possibility of accidental poisoning. Other complications include constipation, gastrointestinal malabsorption, fecal impaction, and intestinal obstruction.

The disorder is seen predominantly between the ages of 2 and 6 years, although it may be present into adolescence. Often, it is not diagnosed until the child presents with a pica-induced complication, such as lead poisoning (see Chapter 52).

The incidence of pica increases in children who are cognitively challenged, possibly because of their inability to distinguish edible from inedible substances as early as other children can. It is highly associated with iron deficiency anemia, and it occurs with a high incidence in pregnant teenage girls (who also may be iron deficient). In these children, correcting the anemia also corrects the pica. An individualized therapy plan needs to be devised to meet the child's needs until the phenomenon fades. Keeping the child safe from ingesting inedible substances is a major responsibility until then.

Rumination Disorder of Infancy

The term *rumination* comes from the Latin word for "chewing the cud" (as cattle do). It is the act of regurgitating and then reswallowing previously ingested food. It is a rare disorder that usually affects infants between the ages of 3 and 12 months. It is seen most often in children who are cognitively challenged and appears to be pleasurable (Chatoor, 2005). Both organic and environmental theories have been explored to explain the disorder. In some children, an accompanying gastroesophageal reflux disorder has been implicated. It has also been postulated that rumination is a form of self-stimulation by the infant, similar to actions such as head banging and body rocking. It may be related to an understimulating environment, but attempts to implicate the role of the primary caregiver in contributing to the disorder have failed.

A parent may report that a child is constantly "spitting up" or vomiting or that the child's breath smells sour. Children can lose a great deal of fluid and electrolytes through this process if they do not reswallow the regurgitated fluid, and they may show signs of failure to thrive. (Failure to thrive as a distinct problem is discussed in Chapter 55.) Distracting infants by holding, rocking, and talking to them tends to decrease rumination. Thickening formula with cereal occasionally is effective because this is more difficult to regurgitate. Attachment between the child and the parents may be at risk because of the anxiety the parents suffer from their infant's constant regurgitation of food and lack of growth. Parents may need support, reassurance, and education to help them maintain or reestablish this bond.

Food Refusal or Aversion

Food refusal or aversion is a persistent failure to eat adequately that results in significant failure to gain weight or actual weight loss when no medical reason or lack of food is present. The disorder begins in infancy and is usually seen in children younger than 6 years of age. Meal time becomes a battlefield as parents insist on the child's eating and the child persistently refuses food or exhibits extremely faddish or bizarre food preferences. As many as 35% of children may demonstrate some degree of this disorder.

Therapy is a combination of counseling for the parents, to help them appreciate that food refusal used this way can be a potent controlling measure, and therapy for the child, to learn to recognize hunger as a stimulant to eating rather than using food refusal as a controlling or attention-getting mechanism (Chatoor, 2005).

Anorexia Nervosa

Anorexia nervosa is a disorder characterized by refusal to maintain a minimally normal body weight because of a disturbance in perception of the size or appearance of the body (APA, 2000). It includes three separate features: a self-induced starvation to a significant degree; a relentless drive for thinness, a morbid fear of fatness, or both; and medical signs and symptoms resulting from starvation (Anderson & Yager, 2005).

Specific characteristics of anorexia nervosa include the following:

- Body mass index (BMI) less than 17.5 or less than 85% of expected weight
- Intense fear of gaining weight or becoming fat even though underweight
- Severely distorted body image
- Refusal to acknowledge seriousness of weight loss
- Amenorrhea (in girls)

Anorexia nervosa occurs most often in girls (90%), usually at puberty or during adolescence, between 13 and 20 years of age. It is more common among sisters and daughters of mothers who also had the disorder. It may be preceded by a traumatic event such as a rape (APA, 2000).

The disorder may be manifested as severe weight restriction controlled by limiting food intake, by excessive exercise, or by **binge eating** or **purging**—episodes of uncontrollable intake of large amounts of food over a specified period of time (binge eating) followed by self-induced vomiting or the use of laxatives, enemas, or diuretics (purging).

Children who develop this disorder tend to have a poor self-image (they cannot live up to their own expectations). Excessive dieting gives them a sense of control over their own body.

Lack of nutrition becomes so extreme that it causes delayed psychosexual development. With a lean, almost starved appearance, girls do not appear as sexually developed or as old as they are. They may have significant symptoms of dehydration and acidosis due to starvation.

Assessment

Because of an intense fear of becoming obese, children with anorexia come to perceive food as revolting and nauseating, and refuse to eat or else vomit food immediately after eating. Refusal to eat may be accompanied by the use of laxatives or diuretics and extensive exercising to further lose weight. Girls may ingest ipecac to induce vomiting. These measures lead eventually to excessive weight loss, acidosis, dependent edema, hypotension, hypothermia, bradycardia, and the formation of lanugo (fine, neonatal-like hair). Compulsive mannerisms such as handwashing may develop. If the process is allowed to continue without therapy, it can lead to starvation and death. The use of ipecac can be exceptionally damaging and possibly cardiotoxic.

Therapeutic Management

By the time most children are seen at health care facilities, they are often already extremely underweight, pale, and lethargic. Amenorrhea is commonly present. Often, the child's parents have tried various methods of getting the child to eat, such as threatening, coaxing, and punishing; as a result, parent–child relationships may be strained. Parents may feel guilty for insisting their child lose weight if the girl was once overweight.

Planning and outcome identification need to be realistic. A girl who grows nauseated just looking at food cannot quickly begin to ingest a large amount of it. When caring for children with anorexia nervosa, remember that, although the condition began as a psychosocial problem, by the time a girl is seen for care, physical starvation and its effects are a second important component. For therapy, typically, oral foods are withheld and total parenteral nutrition is initiated to supply needed fat, protein, and calories. Children usually accept total parenteral nutrition well because they view it as medicine, not as food. Enteral feedings may also be accepted and used to restore weight.

In addition, establishing trust and effective communication are crucial to help the child resolve any interpersonal issues that are present (Box 54.8). Other therapeutic interventions include the following:

BOX 54.8 FOCUS ON . . .

COMMUNICATION

Brenda is a 15-year-old female who is diagnosed with anorexia nervosa. She is 5 ft 8 in tall and weighs 95 lb.

Less Effective Communication

Nurse: Let's talk about your weight, Brenda.
Brenda: I'm fat. Look at this belly of mine.
Nurse: You need to eat at least three good meals a day.
Brenda: I do. I eat a lot.
Nurse: You should have a healthy breakfast. After all, it is the most important meal of the day.
Brenda: I eat huge breakfasts. I'm just so active, I don't gain weight.

More Effective Communication

Nurse: Let's talk about your weight, Brenda.
Brenda: I'm fat. Look at this belly of mine.
Nurse: You feel fat?
Brenda: Yes, just look at me.
Nurse: Tell me what you eat for a typical breakfast.
Brenda: A lot. I pig out for breakfast.
Nurse: Pig out? What did you eat this morning?
Brenda: A quarter piece of toast.
Nurse: Anything else? Tell me more about what it is that you eat.

In the first scenario the nurse is intent on getting the client to eat. In the second scenario, the nurse is attempting to obtain more information about the client, her image of herself, and her diet.

BOX 54.9

What Family Members and Friends Can Do to Help Those With Eating Disorders

- Tell the person that you are concerned, that you care and would like to help. Suggest that the person seek professional help.
- If the person refuses to seek help, encourage reaching out to an adult such as a teacher, school nurse, or counselor.
- Do not discuss weight, the number of calories being consumed, or particular eating habits. Try to talk about things other than food, weight, counting calories, or exercise.
- Avoid making comments about the person's appearance. Concern about weight loss may be interpreted as a compliment; comments about weight gain may be interpreted as criticism.
- Offer support but keep in mind that, ultimately, the responsibility for accepting help and deciding to change belongs to the person.
- Read and educate yourself about these disorders.

White, J. H., and Marshall, L. (2005). Eating disorders. In Boyd, M. & Nihart, M. *Psychiatric nursing: Contemporary practice* (3rd ed.). Philadelphia: Lippincott Williams & Wilkins.

- Medications such as antidepressants
- Identification of emotional triggers
- Self-monitoring (awareness training)
- Education about normal nutritional needs

Gradual weight gain is recommended, because rapid gain of weight can cause a child to begin dieting to reduce this weight gain. Weighing once a week is better than every day, to reduce the focus on weight. Box 54.9 describes common strategies for assisting family and friends to help a child with anorexia.

Children who have had anorexia nervosa need continued follow-up after weight is regained, to be certain that they do not revert to their former dieting pattern (Fig. 54.2). Counseling may need to be continued for 2 to 3 years to be certain that self-image is maintained. With adequate counseling, most girls achieve full recovery with adulthood.

Bulimia Nervosa

Bulimia refers to recurrent and episodic binge eating and purging, accompanied by an awareness that the eating pattern is abnormal but not being able to stop (APA, 2000). A period of depression or guilt usually follows the period of bingeing. Like anorexia nervosa, bulimia typically is seen in adolescence or early adult life and predominantly in girls. The disorder may last for months or years. Periods of normal eating may be interspersed, or the girl may constantly move from bingeing to fasting. Food consumed during a binge often has a high caloric content and a texture that facilitates rapid eating. It may be eaten secretly, such as late at night or in the privacy of a bedroom. After ingestion of this food, the girl notices abdominal pain; she vomits to decrease the physical pain of abdominal distention and to improve self-concept (she feels more in control).

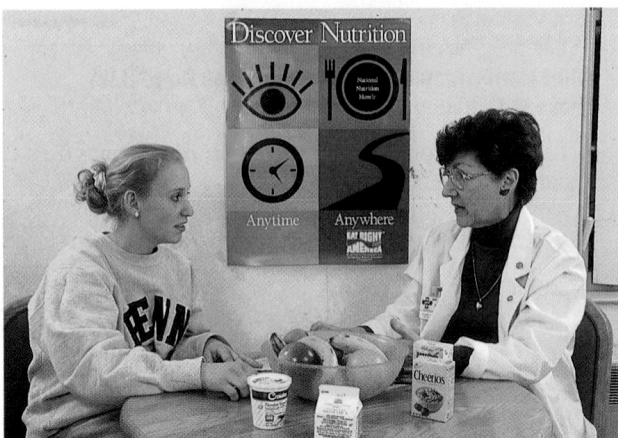

FIGURE 54.2 This anorexic teen, who is in the later stages of treatment, continues to meet with the counselor to discuss her food choices, exercise program, and overall well-being. (© Barbara Proud.)

Children with bulimia may abuse purgatives, laxatives, and diuretics to aid in weight control (Le Grange et al., 2004). The combination of frequent vomiting and use of these drugs can result in serious physical complications, notably electrolyte abnormalities, which can ultimately lead to changes as severe as cardiac arrest. People with bulimia may develop severe erosion of their teeth because of the constant exposure to acidic gastrointestinal juices from vomiting. Esophageal tears may also result (Anderson & Yager, 2005).

Like adolescents with anorexia nervosa, these children exhibit great concern about their weight and overall body image and appearance. In contrast to children with anorexia, most of those with bulimia are only slightly underweight or are of average weight and therefore may be discounted as merely slim unless a thorough history is obtained. As with anorexia nervosa, counseling is aimed at increasing the child's self-esteem and sense of control (APA, 2000).

 Checkpoint Question 3

Which child is most apt to have anorexia nervosa?

a. Jake, a 7-year-old boy whose parents are divorced.
b. Mary, a 15-year-old girl who has a poor self-image.
c. Odom, a 14-year-old boy who plays varsity sports.
d. Jenny, a 13-year-old girl who is overweight.

TIC DISORDERS

Tic disorders are abnormalities of semi-involuntary movement that are thought to result from dysfunction in the basal ganglia. *Tics* are rapid, repetitive muscle movements, such as rapid eye blinking or facial twitching. They usually become more pronounced during periods of stress and diminish during sleep. **Motor tics** include eye blinking, neck jerking, and facial grimacing. Simple **vocal tics** include coughing, throat clearing, snorting, and barking. Complex

motor tics include facial gestures, grooming behaviors, jumping, touching, and smelling objects.

Children are most prone to these disorders between the ages of 9 and 13 years. They occur more frequently in boys than in girls, and more frequently in children who demonstrate obsessive–compulsive behavior. Some instances tend to be familial, possibly due to dopamine receptor inhibition. Tic disorders are subclassified into Tourette's syndrome, chronic motor or vocal tic disorder, and transient tic disorder. They occur so frequently that as many as 15% of children experience some form of transient tic disorder (APA, 2000). Because transient tics are associated with high stress, treatment usually focuses on reducing areas of stress in the child's life. Pointing out the mannerism to the child is not usually helpful and may intensify the manifestation if it increases stress. Behavior modification may be successful in eliminating a particular tic. If the stress is not removed, however, the child may substitute another compulsive mechanism for the original tic.

Tourette's Syndrome

Tourette's syndrome is an inherited syndrome of motor and phonic vocal tics (Scahill & Leckman, 2005). It occurs three times more frequently in boys than in girls. Often, there is some other form of tic in other family members. **Complex vocal tics** include the repeated use of words or phrases out of context—specifically, **coprolalia** (use of socially unacceptable words, usually obscenities), **palilalia** (repeating one's own words), and echolalia (repeating others' words). Some children with this syndrome have nonspecific electroencephalographic abnormalities and soft neurologic signs. Typically, the age of onset is around 7 years, with motor tics usually occurring before vocal tics. Although most children can suppress their tics for short periods, the syndrome lasts a lifetime. Children with Tourette's syndrome can develop low self-esteem because of their uncontrollable actions before the syndrome is fully diagnosed. Fortunately, this syndrome responds to administration of neuroleptic agents such as haloperidol (Haldol) or pimozide (Orap).

ELIMINATION DISORDERS

Elimination disorders include functional enuresis (involuntary loss of urine) and encopresis (involuntary loss of feces). Developmental enuresis is discussed in Chapter 30 with the development of the preschooler.

Encopresis

Loss of feces is *encopresis* if there is repeated passage of feces at least once a month in places not culturally appropriate for that purpose. It is considered primary if the child was never fully toilet trained and secondary if the problem began after effective training. Encopresis is considered to exist only after medical causes such as lactase deficiency, thyroid disease, hypercalcemia, Hirschsprung's disease, and infectious diarrhea have been ruled out. It is more common in boys than in girls (Mikkelsen, 2005).

Isolated occurrences of encopresis may happen when a sibling is born (as part of an overall regression reaction) or when a child is visiting a strange house or new school and is too shy to ask for the bathroom. It can occur in school because a teacher does not allow children to use a bathroom when they wish or because a school bathroom is occupied by a school gang.

Encopresis is a distressing condition for children, because other children in school can detect the odor of a bowel movement on their clothing. In a few instances, encopresis occurs because of extreme constipation. Hard bowel movements cause anal fissures. Because it hurts to move the bowels, children avoid bowel movements, leading to chronically distended rectums. They are then no longer able to sense when they need to defecate, so involuntary or overflow defecation occurs.

Assessment

To document encopresis, take a careful history of the condition, including usual bowel evacuation habits, the number of bowel accidents, and the times at which they occur. Investigate any recent changes or stress factors in the child's environment. A physical examination that includes a rectal examination should be done to establish whether there is proper anal sphincter control.

Therapeutic Management

Therapy is based on the apparent cause. Arranging to have children attempt to evacuate their bowels about two times daily (in the morning and after dinner) may create "habit" periods for them. Allowing children adequate time to sit on the toilet or encouraging them to take the time to do so may be helpful. If children evacuate their bowels before they leave for school in the morning, they are less likely to experience encopresis and embarrassment in school. The administration of 1 to 6 tablespoons of mineral oil daily for 2 or 3 months often softens stools so that bowel movements are not painful. Children receiving long-term mineral oil therapy usually are given water-soluble forms of vitamins A, D, and K, because these vitamins tend to be removed from the gastrointestinal tract with the mineral oil. Imipramine (Tofranil), a tricyclic antidepressant, may be helpful in reducing encopresis, just as it is effective for enuresis.

Emphasize to parents that children should not be punished for encopresis. Encourage them to pay as little attention as possible to bowel accidents and to give praise for days when encopresis does not occur. Box 54.10 highlights appropriate outcomes and interventions using the terminology identified by the Nursing Outcomes Classification (NOC) and Nursing Interventions Classification (NIC) for encopresis.

Enuresis

Enuresis is defined as repeated involuntary or intentional urination during the day or at night after an age at which the child has attained or should have attained control over bladder function, when no organic cause for the problem can be found (APA, 2000). Although stress may be a factor in occurrences of enuresis, its primary cause is unknown. Most children outgrow the problem by adolescence. As

---

BOX 54.10

Nursing Outcomes Classification (NOC) and Nursing Interventions Classification (NIC)

Encopresis

NOC: Bowel Elimination

Bowel elimination is defined as the ability of the gastrointestinal tract to form and evacuate stool effectively (Johnson, Maas, & Moorhead, 2000). Some specific indicators suggesting that this outcome has been achieved include the following:

- Elimination patterns within expected range
- Stool color, odor, and fat within normal range with amount appropriate for diet
- Stool soft and firm
- Absence of bloating, painful cramping, discomfort with stool passage, constipation, diarrhea, and blood or mucus in stool
- Uncompromised sphincter control and muscle tone
- Ingestion of adequate fluids and fiber
- Uncompromised control of bowel movements

NIC: Bowel Incontinence Care, Encopresis

Bowel incontinence care, encopresis is defined as the promotion of bowel continence in children

(McCloskey & Bulechek, 2000). Some important activities involved when implementing this intervention include the following:

- Obtaining information about child's toilet training history, duration of encopresis, and measures tried to control the problem
- Attempting to determine the cause of incontinence as appropriate
- Recommending dietary changes or behavioral therapy as indicated
- Conducting family psychosocial assessment
- Using play therapy to assist child in working through feelings
- Investigating family communication patterns, strengths, and coping abilities
- Encouraging parents to foster security and demonstrate love and acceptance at home
- Discussing the psychosocial dynamics of encopresis with the family
- Referring for family therapy as appropriate

with encopresis, the most serious result of enuresis is related to the child's feelings of failure with each occurrence and associated rejection by peers, parents, or other caregivers. All this contributes to a lowered sense of self-esteem. The problem and associated nursing diagnoses are described in more detail in Chapter 46.

OTHER PSYCHIATRIC DISORDERS AFFECTING CHILDREN

Childhood Depressive Episodes

Children and adolescents both have depressive episodes similar to those experienced by adults. The incidence ranges from 1% to 3% before puberty and 3% to 6% among adolescents (Shaffer, 2005). Depression is becoming an increasing concern in our society, because the escalating suicide rate among children and adolescents that arises from depression has become a major societal problem. A child is considered to be depressed when symptoms such as loss of interest or pleasure, significant weight loss or gain, depressed mood, insomnia, psychomotor agitation, feelings of worthlessness or excessive or inappropriate guilt, diminished concentration, recurrent thoughts of death, and suicidal ideation exist for 2 weeks or longer (APA, 2000). Because these symptoms are easily missed, a history should be taken from the child as well as from the parents (Box 54.11). Depression can be differentiated from "normal" sadness when children report they cannot remember the last time they felt happy or had a good time (**anhedonia**) (Fig. 54.3).

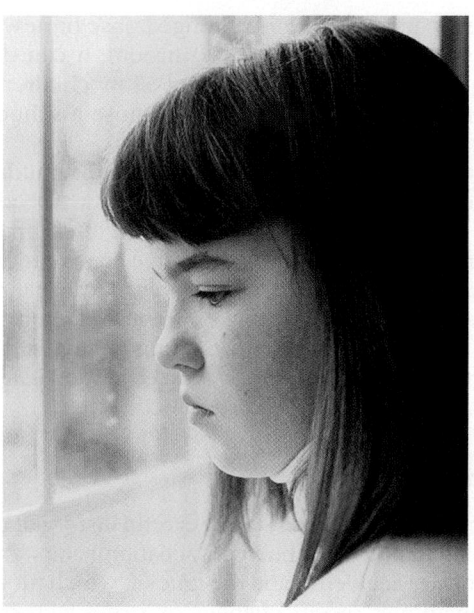

FIGURE 54.3 Symptoms of depression are easily missed in school-aged children unless history taking is thorough. (© Caroline Brown, RNC, MS, DEd.)

Children who are depressed need treatment to prevent their depression from worsening. Counseling to discuss problems is necessary. Many children require antidepressant therapy, such as a selective serotonin reuptake inhibitor, to relieve the symptoms. In addition to the pharmacologic approach, family or individual counseling may be necessary to help the child regain self-esteem and the family to understand the level of depression that has occurred. Few antidepressants are approved for children, and when adolescents have been prescribed these drugs, attempts at suicide have been noticed to rise dramatically (Culpepper et al., 2004)—possibly because, at the point at which the child feels less depressed, increased ability to act makes a suicide attempt possible. Observe any child who is prescribed an antidepressant carefully to detect presuicidal behavior. Adolescent suicide as a result of depression is discussed in Chapter 32 with concerns of the adolescent.

What if... during a routine health maintenance visit, you notice that an adolescent boy has lost 20 lb in the last 6 months? His mother states, "He's the perfect son, always getting straight As in school." How would you respond?

Childhood Schizophrenia

Schizophrenia is actually a group of disorders of thought processes characterized by the gradual disintegration of mental functioning; it occurs in about 2 out of every 10,000 children (APA, 2000). It is a devastating mental illness that usually strikes in adolescence or young adulthood. Symptoms during childhood may be undifferentiated or ill defined.

BOX 54.11 FOCUS ON . . .

EVIDENCE-BASED PRACTICE

Are Children With Type 1 Diabetes More Apt to Feel Depressed Than Others?

To investigate this problem, researchers asked 32 children diagnosed with type 1 diabetes and 32 children without a medical diagnosis, matched for age and gender, to fill out several questionnaires designed to detect depression, social anxiety, and loneliness. Results of the study revealed that children with diabetes reported they were more often the victim of bullies than other children. They were also less apt to receive emotional and social support from their peers than those without diabetes. The bullying and poor support were positively linked with increased feelings of depression, social anxiety, and loneliness.

This is an important study for nurses, because it accentuates how medical conditions can be compounded when emotional support is lacking. It is an alert that frank talking may be needed with children about how much emotional support they are receiving and whether their illness is affecting their mental health.

Source: Storch, E. A., et al. (2004). Peer victimization and psychosocial adjustment in children with type 1 diabetes. *Clinical Pediatrics, 43*(5), 467–471.

Over the years, there has been a great deal of debate about the cause of schizophrenia. For a long time, it was hypothesized that schizophrenia resulted solely from an impaired parent–child relationship. Current research, however, indicates that there is as much a genetic as an environmental basis for this disorder (Sawa & Kamiya, 2003). Magnetic resonance imaging has shown that cerebral involvement, such as enlarged ventricles or decreased blood to the frontal lobe, may be present (APA, 2000). Neurochemical mediators may influence or prolong the disorder.

Children with schizophrenia experience hallucinations (hear or see people or objects that other people cannot). They display rambling or illogical speech patterns. They may not be responsive (have a **flat affect**), or they may withdraw so completely that they are stuporous (**catatonia**). They may be extremely suspicious that others want to harm them (paranoia). Although schizophrenic manifestations may occur suddenly after a major stress in a child's life (such as rejection by a boyfriend or girlfriend), subtle signs of mental illness have usually been present for some time (McClellan, 2005).

The diagnosis of a psychotic disorder of this extent is a shock to parents. Fortunately, therapy with modern antipsychotic drugs such as haloperidol (Haldol), a neuroleptic, is effective in reducing children's hallucinations and bizarre thinking. Parents need help to support a child during a long period of therapy. Many children who are diagnosed as having schizophrenia in childhood continue to have mental illness as adults. Continuing support and long-term follow-up are essential (McClellan, 2005).

Key Points

Both cognitive and mental health disorders pose long-term care concerns for children and their families.

For children who are cognitively challenged, a stigma still may be present in many communities, although less so than previously. Parents may have a more difficult time accepting this diagnosis in their child than they would a physical illness. Help parents to gain the insight that cognitive challenges occur in a proportion of infants in every population and that having a child with this problem merely reflects a chance occurrence.

Mental health disorders often begin subtly in children and are often first manifested as behavior problems in school. Assess thoroughly any child who is referred for disruptive behavior in class for the possibility that he or she has a serious mental health problem.

Autistic disorder is a pervasive developmental disorder that has a syndrome of behaviors, including fascination with movement, impairment of communication skills, and insensitivity to pain.

Attention-deficit and disruptive behavior disorders, such as oppositional defiant and conduct disorders, may occur in childhood. Children with ADHD may be treated with methylphenidate hydrochloride (Ritalin, Concerta) to reduce the hyperactivity and allow them to achieve better in school and interact better at home.

Eating disorders seen in childhood include pica, rumination, anorexia nervosa, and bulimia. All of these disorders can lead to loss of weight and electrolyte imbalances if left unrecognized and untreated.

Tic disorders (e.g., Tourette's syndrome) are abnormalities of semi-involuntary movement that are thought to result from dysfunction of the basal ganglia or distorted dopamine reception.

Encopresis is the repeated passage of feces in places not culturally appropriate for that purpose. Therapy is both physiologic and psychological.

Children who are depressed are at high risk for committing suicide. They need thorough assessment and close observation to be certain that this does not happen. Schizophrenia may occur in childhood. This usually presents as disorganized behavior. Long-term therapy is necessary.

Critical Thinking Exercises

1. Todd is the second grader diagnosed with ADHD whom you met at the beginning of the chapter. His mother feels "at her wits' end" because his attention span is so short and his behavior so disruptive. His father is proud of his behavior. What suggestions could you make to his parents to help them adjust better to a child with ADHD?

2. A 3-year-old child in your school's preschool program who is cognitively challenged is critically ill with pneumonia. It is difficult to believe that her mother did not recognize how ill the child was becoming and bring her in sooner for care. What reasons might explain a parent's reacting this way?

3. The parents of an adolescent tell you that he seems increasingly depressed, so much so that he sleeps almost all day on weekends. Does this adolescent need a referral, or is he simply demonstrating usual adolescent behavior? What questions would you want to ask to be able to tell?

4. Examine the National Health Goals related to mental health disorders in children. Most government-sponsored money for nursing research is allotted based on these goals. What would be a possible research topic to explore pertinent to these goals that would be applicable to Todd's family and also advance evidence-based practice?

References

American Psychiatric Association. (2000). *Diagnostic and statistical manual of mental disorders, text revised (DSM IV-TR)* (4th ed.). Washington, DC: American Psychiatric Association.

Anderson, A. E., & Yager, J. (2005). Eating disorders. In Sadock, B. J., & Sadock, V. A. (Eds.), *Kaplan and Sadock's comprehensive textbook of psychiatry.* Philadelphia: Lippincott Williams & Wilkins.

Bernstein, G. A., & Layne, A. E. (2005). Separation anxiety disorder and other anxiety disorders. In Sadock, B. J., & Sadock, V. A. (Eds.), *Kaplan and Sadock's comprehensive textbook of psychiatry.* Philadelphia: Lippincott Williams & Wilkins.

Chatoor, I. (2005). Feeding and eating disorders of infancy and early childhood. In Sadock, B. J., & Sadock, V. A. (Eds.), *Kaplan and Sadock's comprehensive textbook of psychiatry.* Philadelphia: Lippincott Williams & Wilkins.

Cohen, J. A. (2005). Posttraumatic stress disorder in children and adolescents. In Sadock, B. J., & Sadock, V. A. (Eds.), *Kaplan and Sadock's comprehensive textbook of psychiatry.* Philadelphia: Lippincott Williams & Wilkins.

Culpepper, L., et al. (2004). Suicidality as a possible side effect of antidepressant treatment. *Journal of Clinical Psychiatry, 65*(6), 742-749.

Department of Health and Human Services. (2000). *Healthy people 2010.* Washington, DC: DHHS.

Hechtman, L. (2005). Attention-deficit/hyperactivity disorder. In Sadock, B. J., & Sadock, V. A. (Eds.), *Kaplan and Sadock's comprehensive textbook of psychiatry.* Philadelphia: Lippincott Williams & Wilkins.

Jack, S. (2004). Review: Existing epidemiological evidence does not show an association between mumps, measles, and rubella vaccination and autism. *Evidence-Based Nursing, 7*(1), 25-26.

Johnson, M., Maas, M., & Moorhead, S. (2000). *Nursing outcomes classification* (2nd ed.). St. Louis: Mosby.

Karch, A. M. (2004). *Lippincott's nursing drug guide.* Philadelphia: Lippincott Williams & Wilkins.

King, B. H., Hodapp, R. M., & Dykens, E. M. (2005). Mental retardation. In Sadock, B. J., & Sadock, V. A. (Eds.), *Kaplan and Sadock's comprehensive textbook of psychiatry.* Philadelphia: Lippincott Williams & Wilkins.

Kuo, F. E., & Taylor, A. F. (2004). A potential natural treatment for attention-deficit/hyperactivity disorder: evidence from a national study. *American Journal of Public Health, 94*(9), 1580-1586.

Le Grange, D., et al. (2004). Bulimia nervosa in adolescents: A disorder in evolution? *Archives of Pediatrics and Adolescent Medicine, 158*(5), 478-482.

Mangus, R. S., et al. (2004). Burn injuries in children with attention-deficit/hyperactivity disorder. *Burns, 30*(2), 148-150.

McClellan, J. M. (2005). Early-onset schizophrenia. In Sadock, B. J., & Sadock, V. A. (Eds.), *Kaplan and Sadock's comprehensive textbook of psychiatry.* Philadelphia: Lippincott Williams & Wilkins.

McCloskey, J., & Bulechek, G. (2000). *Nursing interventions classification* (3rd ed.). St. Louis: Mosby.

Mikkelsen, E. J. (2005). Elimination disorders. In Sadock, B. J., & Sadock, V. A. (Eds.), *Kaplan and Sadock's comprehensive textbook of psychiatry.* Philadelphia: Lippincott Williams & Wilkins.

Roberts, G., Palfrey, J., & Bridgemohan, C. (2004). A rational approach to the medical evaluation of a child with developmental delay. *Contemporary Pediatrics, 21*(3), 76-78.

Sawa, A., & Kamiya, A. (2003). Elucidating the pathogenesis of schizophrenia. *BMJ: British Medical Journal, 327*(7416), 632-633.

Scahill, L., & Leckman, J. F. (2005). Tic disorders. In Sadock, B. J., & Sadock, V. A. (Eds.), *Kaplan and Sadock's comprehensive textbook of psychiatry.* Philadelphia: Lippincott Williams & Wilkins.

Shaffer, D. (2005). Depressive disorders and suicide in children and adolescents. In Sadock, B. J., & Sadock, V. A. (Eds.), *Kaplan and Sadock's comprehensive textbook of psychiatry.* Philadelphia: Lippincott Williams & Wilkins.

Storch, E. A., et al. (2004). Peer victimization and psychosocial adjustment in children with type 1 diabetes. *Clinical Pediatrics, 43*(5), 467-471.

Thomas, C. R. (2005). Disruptive behavior disorders. In Sadock, B. J., & Sadock, V. A. (Eds.), *Kaplan and Sadock's comprehensive textbook of psychiatry.* Philadelphia: Lippincott Williams & Wilkins.

Volkmar, F. R., Klin, A., & Schultz, R. T. (2005). Pervasive developmental disorders. In Sadock, B. J., & Sadock, V. A. (Eds.), *Kaplan and Sadock's comprehensive textbook of psychiatry.* Philadelphia: Lippincott Williams & Wilkins.

White, J. H., and Marshall, L. (2004). Eating disorders. In Boyd, M., & Nihart, M. *Psychiatric nursing: Contemporary practice* (2nd ed.). Philadelphia: Lippincott Williams and Wilkins.

Williams, R. J., et al. (2004). Methylphenidate and dextroamphetamine abuse in substance-abusing adolescents. *American Journal on Addictions, 13*(4), 381-389.

Suggested Readings

Arcia, E., et al. (2004). Modes of entry into services for young children with disruptive behaviors. *Qualitative Health Research, 14*(9), 1211-1226.

Armstrong, M. B., & Nettleton, S. K. (2004). Attention deficit hyperactivity disorder and preschool children. *Seminars in Speech and Language, 25*(3), 225-232.

Dalle Grave, R. (2003). School-based prevention programs for eating disorders: Achievements and opportunities. *Disease Management and Health Outcomes, 11*(9), 579-593.

Demonet, J., Taylor, M. J., & Chaix, Y. (2004). Developmental dyslexia. *Lancet, 363*(9419), 1451-1460.

Luther, E. H., Canham, D. L., & Cureton, V. Y. (2005). Coping and social support for parents of children with autism. *Journal of School Nursing, 21*(1), 40-47.

Ransby, M. J., & Swanson, H. L. (2003). Reading comprehension skills of young adults with childhood diagnoses of dyslexia. *Journal of Learning Disabilities, 36*(6), 538-555.

Rau, J. D. (2004). Is it autism? *Contemporary Pediatrics, 20*(4), 54-56.

Schowalter, J. E. (2003). Special report. Child and adolescent psychiatry: A history of child and adolescent psychiatry in the United States. *Psychiatric Times, 20*(9), 43-47.

Waslick, B., Schoenholz, D., & Pizzaro, R. (2003). Diagnosis and treatment of chronic depression in children and adolescents. *Journal of Psychiatric Practice, 9*(5), 354-366.

Zinner, S. H. (2004). Tourette syndrome. Much more than tics: Management tailored to the entire patient. *Contemporary Pediatrics, 21*(8), 38-41.

CHAPTER 55

Nursing Care of the Family in Crisis: Abuse and Violence in the Family

Key Terms

abuse
disorganization phase
failure to thrive
incest
intimate partner abuse
learned helplessness
mandatory reporters
molestation
Munchausen syndrome by proxy
pedophile
permissive reporters
rape trauma syndrome
reorganization phase
shaken baby syndrome
silent rape syndrome

Objectives

After mastering the contents of this chapter, you should be able to:

1. Discuss the types of abuse seen in families and the theories explaining their occurrence.
2. Assess a family that is physically or emotionally abused.
3. Formulate nursing diagnoses related to an abused family.
4. Develop expected outcomes for an abused family.
5. Plan nursing care for an abused family, such as ways to role-model better parenting.
6. Implement nursing care for a family in which abuse has occurred.
7. Evaluate expected outcomes for effectiveness and achievement of care.
8. Identify National Health Goals related to an abused family that nurses can help the nation achieve.
9. Identify areas related to care of the abused family that could benefit from additional nursing research or application of evidence-based practice.
10. Analyze ways that nurses can help make care more family centered and ideally help to prevent family abuse.
11. Integrate knowledge of family abuse with nursing process to achieve quality maternal and child health nursing care.

Hillary is a 3-year-old you see in an emergency room. Her mother tells you Hillary fell off a swing in the back yard. Hillary has a broken forearm, a broken rib, and multiple bruises on her chest and back. You notice in her chart Hillary was seen in the same emergency room a month ago for a burn on the palm of her hand. When you mention to her mother that Hillary's injuries seem extreme for a simple fall, her mother says, "Hillary isn't very pretty. I guess she's also clumsy."

Previous chapters described the normal growth and development of children and care of the child with disorders of specific body systems. This chapter adds information about the effect on children when abuse occurs in a family. This is important information because it builds a base for care and for preventing further abuse.

You suspect that Hillary may be a victim of child abuse. What additional questions would you want to ask to help determine whether this is so?

After you've studied this chapter, access the accompanying website. Read the patient scenario and answer the questions to further sharpen your skills, grow more familiar with RN-CLEX types of questions, and reward yourself with how much you have learned.

Child abuse occurs at an incidence of about 250,000 cases per year in the United States. It accounts for 2,000 deaths per year (DHHS, 2000). Abuse is associated with stress and has been linked to inability of a family to handle external and internal stressors. Accordingly, abuse in a family is rarely an isolated event but rather an indication of how much the family needs care overall.

Abuse, defined as the "willful injury by one person of another" by the researchers who first identified the phenomenon (Helfer & Kempe, 1987), takes many forms: child abuse, which can be physical or emotional and includes neglect and sexual abuse; intimate partner abuse; and maltreatment of the elderly. Maternity, child health, and family care nurses need to be especially observant for signs of possible abuse in a family and prepared to handle this highly emotional and complex problem objectively. The victim's safety is paramount, but ensuring this safety must be done with sensitivity to the importance of maintaining and improving overall family functioning.

Abuse has long-term consequences, because as many as 30% of children from abusive families become abusive parents themselves (Christian, 2003). It also may lead to a posttraumatic stress disorder with long-term effects (Carr, 2004). National Health Goals related to child abuse are shown in Box 55.1.

Nursing Process Overview

For Care of a Family That Experiences Abuse

● *Assessment*

Commonly, nurses are the first individuals to identify symptoms of possible abuse in a family, because they are often the first to see a child undressed at a health care visit and recognize significant bruising, and they are often the person in whom a pregnant woman or child confides about the problem (Box 55.2). If abuse in any form is suspected, it is essential to get as full a picture as possible. If child abuse is suspected, talk with the parents first, without the child, and then interview the child to help to uncover any inconsistencies in the parents' explanations.

● *Nursing Diagnosis*

Nursing diagnoses associated with abuse should address both the physical and the emotional results of abuse. Some examples are the following:

• Pain related to burn on hand
• Risk for injury related to previous abuse
• Risk for other-directed violence related to admitted poor self-control
• Impaired parenting related to high level of stress
• Compromised family coping as manifested by child abuse related to alcohol use by father
• Disturbed self-esteem related to rape

● *Outcome Identification and Planning*

Planning must center first on ensuring the safety of the abused family member and minimizing the effects of trauma. Long-term planning includes helping an abused family member find safe refuge and re-establishing self-esteem through a self-help or advocacy program.

BOX 55.1 FOCUS ON . . .

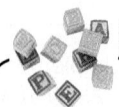

NATIONAL HEALTH GOALS

Abuse of children is a national health disgrace and so is rated as a national health concern. One National Health Goal specifically addresses this issue:

• Reduce the rate of maltreatment of children younger than 18 years of age, from a baseline of 12.9/1,000 to a target level of 10.3/1,000 (DHHS, 2000).

Nurses can help the nation achieve this goal by educating parents about how to parent more effectively and by identifying children in school or health care agency settings who have been abused or neglected.

Additional nursing research would be helpful to answer the following questions: Can potentially abusing parents be identified on postpartum units and helped to avoid this behavior? What counseling is necessary for adolescents who have been abused to help them be successful parents? What are the most helpful nursing interventions to use with parents when a child who has been abused is admitted to the hospital?

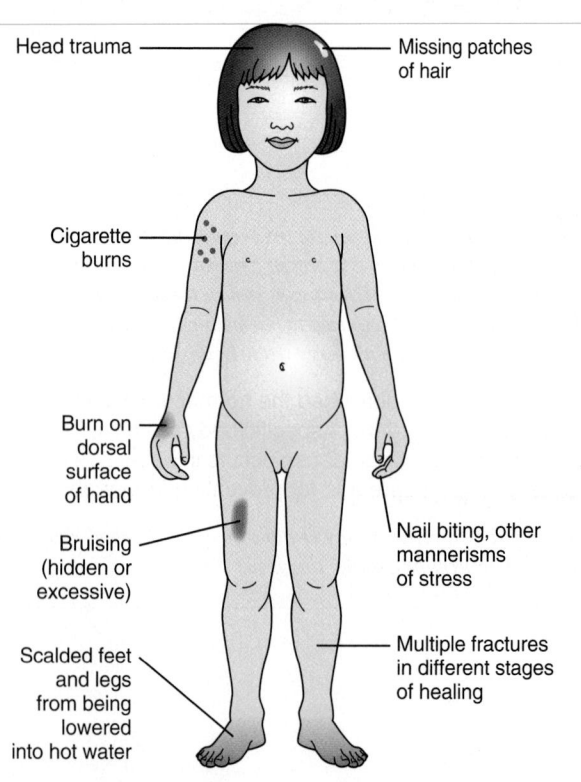

BOX 55.2 ASSESSMENT

Assessing a Child for Signs of Abuse

Head trauma — Missing patches of hair

Cigarette burns

Burn on dorsal surface of hand

Bruising (hidden or excessive)

Scalded feet and legs from being lowered into hot water

Nail biting, other mannerisms of stress

Multiple fractures in different stages of healing

Teaching empowerment, or the ability to take charge of one's life, is particularly important for older children and women in abusive families. In addition, the abuser needs a program of therapy to help prevent future abuse.

● *Implementation*

The most important intervention related to family abuse is prevention. Nurses can do much in all settings through serving as a role model or providing education to promote healthy patterns of childrearing and optimal ways of handling family stress. They can be particularly observant for families who seem to be at risk for abusive behavior. When instances of abuse are uncovered, appropriate reporting is required. Further education is an intervention that can help parents who may be ignorant about their children's needs or normal child behavior. Lecturing is not a useful intervention, but supportive education can be extremely valuable.

The following organizations are helpful for referral:

- Parents Anonymous (*www.parentsanonymous.org*)
- Child Abuse Prevention Network (*www.child-abuse.com*)
- National Coalition Against Domestic Violence (*www.ncadv.org*)
- Victims of Child Abuse Laws (VOCAL) (*http://www.menweb.org/throop/mitch/vocal2.html*)
- Women Organized Against Rape (WOAR) (*www.WOAR.org*)

● *Outcome Evaluation*

Nurses are mandated by law to report child abuse; identifying and reporting this problem are important nursing actions. Expected outcomes should focus on specific measures of improved interaction, such as the following:

- Parent holds baby in a caring manner and maintains good eye contact.
- Parent admits to losing control with children at home and voices desire to undergo counseling for problem.
- Parent states she has the Crisis Center telephone number by the telephone and will call for help if she feels under threat by partner.
- Adolescent states she can still think of herself with high self-esteem despite rape by stepbrother.
- Parent attends monthly meetings of Parents Anonymous.

CHILD ABUSE

Because parenting is not an easy task and good parenting is not an automatic or truly instinctive ability, children in every community are injured because of abuse. Abuse may be physical (the child is beaten or burned), or it may be neglect (the child is not fed, clothed, supervised properly, or offered medical care or educational opportunities). Abuse may also be psychological or emotional. In some instances, women who threatened the health of their fetus by drug abuse have been viewed by the courts as child abusers (Bernet, 2005).

Abuse not only places a child at immediate risk but can also lead to long-term effects. For example, physically abused children are found to be more angry, noncompli-

ant, and hyperactive than others; they may demonstrate poor self-control and low self-esteem. Children whose parents do not interact with them (emotional abuse) are apt to be more withdrawn and to have a flatter affect than others. Because the abusive family is a disrupted one, children often have undiagnosed medical problems, such as anemia, otitis media, lead poisoning, or sexually transmitted infections. Children who suffer sexual abuse can have long-term effects of depression, guilt, and difficulty enjoying sexual relations (Mezey et al., 2005).

In addition, when children reach adulthood and begin parenting, they tend to rear their children in basically the same way as they were reared. Parents who themselves received little love or were abused as children may never form a basic sense of trust; they tend to grow into nonloving and abusing parents unless there is effective intervention.

Theories of Child Abuse

The most commonly accepted theory as to why child abuse occurs is that a special triad of circumstances is present (Helfer & Kempe, 1987):

- A parent has the potential to abuse a child (special parent).
- A child is seen as "different" in some way by the parent (special child).
- An event or circumstance brings about the abuse (special circumstance).

Special Parent: Parents Who Abuse

Parents who abuse seem, on the surface, little different from others. Only a small fraction of them (probably less than 10%) have a history of mental illness. Many of these parents, however, were abused as children. Such parents may have less self-control than other parents. They may be unfamiliar with the normal growth and development of children and so have unrealistic expectations of a child. These parents may be socially isolated, with no support people readily available, and so can become overwhelmed by childrearing. The isolation may be by distance (e.g., a parent separated from other people in a farmhouse miles from neighbors), or it may be the type that exists in communities or apartment houses where neighbors do not routinely speak to one another. Abuse is strongly associated with excessive parental use of alcohol, a substance that removes inhibitions and self-control (Christian, 2003).

Special Child: Children Who Are Abused

Abused children are viewed as somehow "different" by their parents. They may be more or less intelligent than other children in the family; they may have been unplanned. They may have a birth defect; they may have an attention span deficit. Because the child is perceived as different, a good parent–child relationship does not develop. A category of children who are at high risk includes those who are born prematurely or who have an illness at birth, because they are kept from parents or separated from them by special nurseries or equipment for the first weeks of life, which is when normal bonding occurs.

Special Circumstance: Stress

A third factor in child abuse is stress, which may be a response to an event that would not necessarily be stressful for an average parent. It might be something as common as a blocked toilet, an illness in the family, a lost job, a landlord asking for the rent, or a rainstorm that cancels a planned activity. Child abuse crosses all socioeconomic levels because stress occurs at all levels. Stress generally has a greater impact on individuals who do not have strong support people around them. Families whose internal support system is faulty or who have not formed outside support systems are apt to have a higher incidence of abuse.

During a health crisis, parents who are unable to deal with stress may not show the usual degree of compassion for their child's pain or offer to comfort him or her. They may appear more concerned with how the injury affects them than how it affects the child: "Don't cry. You'll make me look like a bad parent," not "It's okay to cry. I know that it hurts."

To prevent abuse, a child may assume a role reversal with the parent or become the comforting, solacing person. These children recognize very early in life that when a parent is upset, they will be hurt. They learn to comfort the parent and reduce the parent's stress and anxiety, thereby avoiding the hurt. It is important to assess who is comforting whom during a child health crisis.

Reporting Suspected Child Abuse

State laws typically identify two types of responsibility in reporting child abuse: **mandatory reporters** and **permissive reporters.** Nurses are included in the mandatory category in most states; this means they *must* report suspected child abuse when they identify it. Failure to do so can result in a fine or possible loss of nursing licensure. The fact that the information was given in a confidential interview does not free a nurse from this responsibility.

All health care institutions and agencies have protocols on how the reporting of child abuse should be handled. It is important to learn the protocol required by your particular agency, community, and state. After an official report of child abuse has been made to a child protection agency, a health care agency has the right, in most instances, to hold the child for 72 hours for protection, to give an appointed caseworker time to investigate whether abuse has occurred. After the 72 hours, a court proceeding will determine whether the child should be returned to the parents' care or kept in a safer location. Because child abuse is a crime, the health care record of the child can be subpoenaed and displayed in court. Be certain when charting information related to child abuse that you make specific and factual notes (observations, not interpretations), such as "Parent spoke loudly and slurred his words," rather than "Parent was intoxicated," or "Mother stated 'This child is nothing but trouble,'" not "I think this mother dislikes this child." Record conversations with parents using exact quotations if possible. Photographs of physical abuse enhance the strength of the testimony of abuse, so these are usually ordered.

A second provision in state laws is protection from having a lawsuit brought against a health care provider for reporting suspected abuse that is then proved false. In other words, it is better to err on the side of reporting suspected abuse rather than not reporting it, from both a child safety standpoint and from a legal perspective. When abuse is officially reported, parents should be told that child abuse is suspected, because open lines of communication with parents are important to protect the child and to arrange counseling for the parents.

Physical Abuse

Physical abuse is the action of a caregiver that causes injury to a child. It is commonly revealed by burns or by injuries to the head or hands (Box 55.3).

Assessment

Interview. Always ask parents to account for any injury to a child's body. Remember, however, that most childhood injuries are the result of unintentional accidents caused by the child's inability to distinguish safe situations from dangerous ones, or by parents' overestimating their child's ability to do such things as lighting a fire to burn trash or using a saw in a wood project. Most toddlers have a number of ecchymotic spots on their legs from bumping into tables or chairs during normal toddler walking. Some childhood diseases, such as leukemia or purpura, begin with easy bruising. Children with osteogenesis imperfecta have frequent broken bones as a natural consequence of their disease. Because of inadequate fact-finding in these instances, false reports do occur. This can lead to severe stress on a family that has been falsely accused and can interfere with the relationship between the parents of an ill child and the health care personnel who will then give care to the child (Box 55.4).

If a child has been physically abused, the injury is usually out of proportion to the history of the injury given by the parent (Fig. 55.1). The parent may report, for example, that the child was playing underneath the coffee table when he reared up quickly and hit his head, sustaining a large hematoma and temporary loss of consciousness, or that an infant "rolled off the couch" and now has two broken arms. In other instances, the parents may give conflicting stories (e.g., the mother says that the child fell, but the father says that the child broke his arm throwing a baseball), or they may give no reason for the injury ("He woke up from his nap and couldn't move his arm; I don't know what could be wrong").

When questioned about the injury, abused children often repeat the parent's story; this loyalty to parents seems misplaced, but they may fear further beatings or simply believe that living with such parents is better than not having anyone. Ask about behavior problems in school, because the constant stress under which these children live can result in disruptive school behavior.

It is often difficult to remain emotionally uninvolved and not grow angry when talking to the parents of an abused child. Emotional involvement is not constructive, however; it rarely helps the parents to change, and it may cause them to avoid seeking health care in the future, leaving the child totally unprotected.

Always assume that the parents have done the best they could under the circumstances in which they found

BOX 55.3: Focus on Nursing Care Planning

A Multidisciplinary Care Map for A Child Who Has Been Abused
•

Hillary is a 3-year-old you see in an emergency room. Her mother tells you Hillary fell off a swing in the back yard. She has a broken forearm, a broken rib, and multiple bruises on her chest and back. You notice in her chart that Hillary was seen in the same emergency room a month ago for a burn on the palm of her hand. When you mention to her mother that Hillary's injuries seem extreme for a simple fall, her mother says, "Hillary isn't very pretty. I guess she's also clumsy." You suspect Hillary may be a victim of child abuse.

Family Assessment
Mother divorced. Boyfriend lives with mother and child in one-bedroom apartment. Mother works as a waitress in a local restaurant from approximately 4 PM to midnight four nights a week. Finances rated as "not good." When physician suggested the child may have been beaten and abused, she stated, "What can I do? I need my boyfriend to watch her while I work."

Client Assessment
3-year-old girl dressed in wool coat and cap carried in by mother. Outside temperature 80°F. Mother's boyfriend present and protesting removal of the child's clothing for examination: "It's too cold in here for that." Odor of alcohol noted on boyfriend's breath. On examination, child's right forearm is misaligned and swollen; 3 × 4-inch bruise on right side of anterior ribs. Further examination reveals four ½-inch-diameter circular lesions on right arm; large 4-cm ecchymotic area on both buttocks and anterior left thigh. Sharp, pointed, triangular blistering and inflamed area noted on back of left hand. Mother states circular lesions are "mosquito bites;" mark on hand is a "birthmark." Child remained passive while being examined but drew back when mother's boyfriend approached.

Nursing Diagnosis
Fear related to repeated episodes of abuse

Outcome Criteria
Child expresses fears verbally and through play; interacts with caregivers appropriately; demonstrates positive age-appropriate coping behaviors.

Team Member Responsible	Assessment	Intervention	Rationale	Expected Outcome
Activities of Daily Living				
Nurse	Assess what self-care activities child is able to complete after right arm is casted.	Assist child as necessary with self-care.	Abused children may lack self-esteem; allowing them to do as much self-care as able can help improve self-esteem.	Child names tasks she thinks she can do herself; asks for appropriate help for others.

(continued)

Team Member Responsible	Assessment	Intervention	Rationale	Expected Outcome
Consultations				
Physician	Assess physical and history findings to establish suspicion of abuse.	Contact hospital Child Abuse Team and alert them to suspicious findings.	Child health care providers have an obligation to report abuse to the proper authorities.	Physician files report with Child Abuse Team. Police and social service are contacted.
Procedures/Medications				
Nurse/Nurse Practitioner	Assess whether child has ever had a full physical and anogenital examination before.	Perform or assist with a complete physical and anogenital examination. Reassure and sooth child as much as possible.	Physical examinations, especially an anogenital examination, are frightening and refresh memories of the abuse.	Child has physical and anogenital examination completed within acceptable stress limits.
Nurse	Assess whether child has ever had photographs of her whole body taken before.	Accompany child to photography to have her injuries photographed.	Photographs are necessary to document the extent and type of injuries.	Child cooperates with photographer; photographs are obtained.
Nutrition				
Nurse	Assess whether child is able to manage fork and spoon with cast in place.	Offer help with eating as necessary.	Eating is a self-care activity that can increase self-esteem.	Child demonstrates ability to eat satisfactorily with cast in place.
Patient/Family Education				
Nurse/ Physician	Assess whether parent understands the seriousness of the diagnosis of child abuse.	Explain the reporting procedures and actions that accompany a child abuse report.	Child abuse is not a simple problem, so the parent's cooperation is essential to a successful outcome.	Mother states she understands what are the next steps to be taken; will cooperate with procedures.
Nurse	Assess whether child understands need for hospitalization.	Explain all procedures and treatments in language the child can understand.	Explanations in the child's terms help to alleviate additional stress and anxiety associated with the experience.	Child states she understands she will be in hospital at least overnight.
Psychosocial/Spiritual/Emotional Needs				
Nurse	Assess which nurse would be the best primary care provider for the child.	Provide a primary care provider; assure child she is now in safe hands.	Removing the child from the threatening environment and providing a primary caretaker can help reduce fear.	Child states she feels safe in the hospital; discusses; participates in therapeutic play.
Discharge Planning				
Nurse	Assess whether parent would like a referral to Parents Anonymous.	Make a referral as appropriate for support people for mother. Refrain from blaming.	Not having adequate support people may be one reason mother relied on unsafe caregiver for her child.	Mother states she will attend at least one parents' group meeting.
Physician/ Nurse	Assess whether mother understands child will not be safe with boyfriend in the future.	If boyfriend is not incarcerated, urge mother to obtain a restraining order against him for future.	A parent may believe an abuser can easily correct behavior and can be allowed to return as child caregiver in the future.	Mother states she understands she has placed her trust in an unsafe care provider; will not allow boyfriend into her or child's life in the future.

BOX 55.4 FOCUS ON . . .

DIVERSITY OF CARE

Some health practices can be confused with child abuse. For example, coin-rolling, a type of massage to draw illness out of the body used by some Asian cultures, leaves bruises on the back similar to those that would appear on a child who has been struck. Coin-rolling involves heating a coin and then vigorously rubbing it over the body, leaving red welts. Being aware of a practice such as coin-rolling aids understanding of the meaning of illness to parents and prevents false reports of child abuse.

themselves. The fact that they have brought the child for care means they are seeking help; this may be their way of saying, "Help me; I don't want this to happen again." Child abuse is rarely an isolated phenomenon. Often a parent is also a victim and needs as much help and protection as the child.

Physical Examination. When children are examined at a well-child visit or because of illness, be certain that they are fully undressed (including removing all bandages and Band-Aids) so that the entire body can be observed. Plot height and weight on a standard growth chart. Delays in growth may suggest neglect.

A number of injuries in children clearly signal child abuse. Children who are beaten with electrical cords, belts, or clotheslines have peculiar circular and linear lesions (Fig. 55.2). Children who are beaten with a belt buckle have additional curved lacerations from the imprint of the buckle; few other weapons produce such contusions. Abrasions or ecchymotic areas on the wrists or ankles may be present if the child was tied to a bed or against a wall. Most parents protect their children's hands carefully; children who are abused have a higher incidence of hand injury than others.

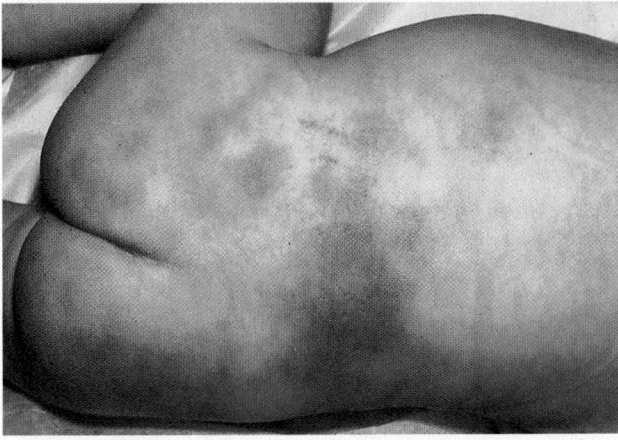

FIGURE 55.1 Large bruises on a child's body. With this type of injury, carefully assessing the history of the traumatic event would be essential. (© Biophoto Associates/Photo Researchers.)

Burns or scalds are frequent injuries in abused children. The peak age at which children accidentally burn themselves is 2 years; that of burns related to abuse is closer to 3 years. When children burn their hand by accident, they usually burn the palm; burns from abuse are often on the dorsal surface. Scalding with hot water may be seen. A child who was placed in a tub of hot water buttocks first may have no burn in the center of the buttocks because they touched the tub; the result is a ring of burns causing a "doughnut-hole" effect. Young children do accidentally step into bathtubs containing water that is hot enough to burn. When this happens, however, the child usually falls forward and so also has burns on the hands and splash marks on the chest or face. If a child is lowered into scalding water as punishment, only the feet and the skin up to the knees are scalded.

Cigarette burns are another common finding on the bodies of physically abused children. A fresh cigarette burn causes a blister that resembles the scab of impetigo; differentiation at this stage is often difficult. Impetigo lesions, however, heal without scarring. Cigarette burns heal with a definite circular scar.

Human bites or chunks of hair pulled off the scalp may be present. Head injury is common.

Broken bones are another frequent finding. Children who are preschool age and younger usually do not fall far enough in normal accidents to break bones; a broken bone at this age suggests the child was thrown or struck so hard that the bone broke. Common findings include multiple fractures in different stages of healing, a single fracture with multiple bruises, rib or occipital fractures, and metaphyseal-epiphyseal injuries. Bones are not always broken if a child is shaken roughly, but the periosteum may be torn, so that the radiograph reveals a strange haziness along both sides of the bone shaft. Tibial torsion (twisting) is often seen (Fig. 55.3).

Deliberate poisoning is yet another form of child abuse; this usually occurs in a child younger than 2.5 years. Bruises on a child who is too young to walk also are highly suspicious (Maguire et al., 2005).

Listen to children while they are being examined. If they did not hear the parent's explanation of the accident, they may say something that is inconsistent with the parent's explanation. They may cry little in response to a painful procedure, such as an injection, because they are not used to receiving comfort for pain. They may draw back from an examiner more than the average child would because they are afraid of adults. These are very subjective observations, however, because children react in different ways to the fear produced by a recent injury or a health examination.

 Checkpoint Question 1

Which finding in Hillary's background is a typical finding of child abuse?

a. Hillary's mother describes her as "not pretty."
b. Hillary's birthday is in the fall of the year.
c. Hillary's mother works part-time for low pay.
d. Hillary's father smokes a pack of cigarettes a day.

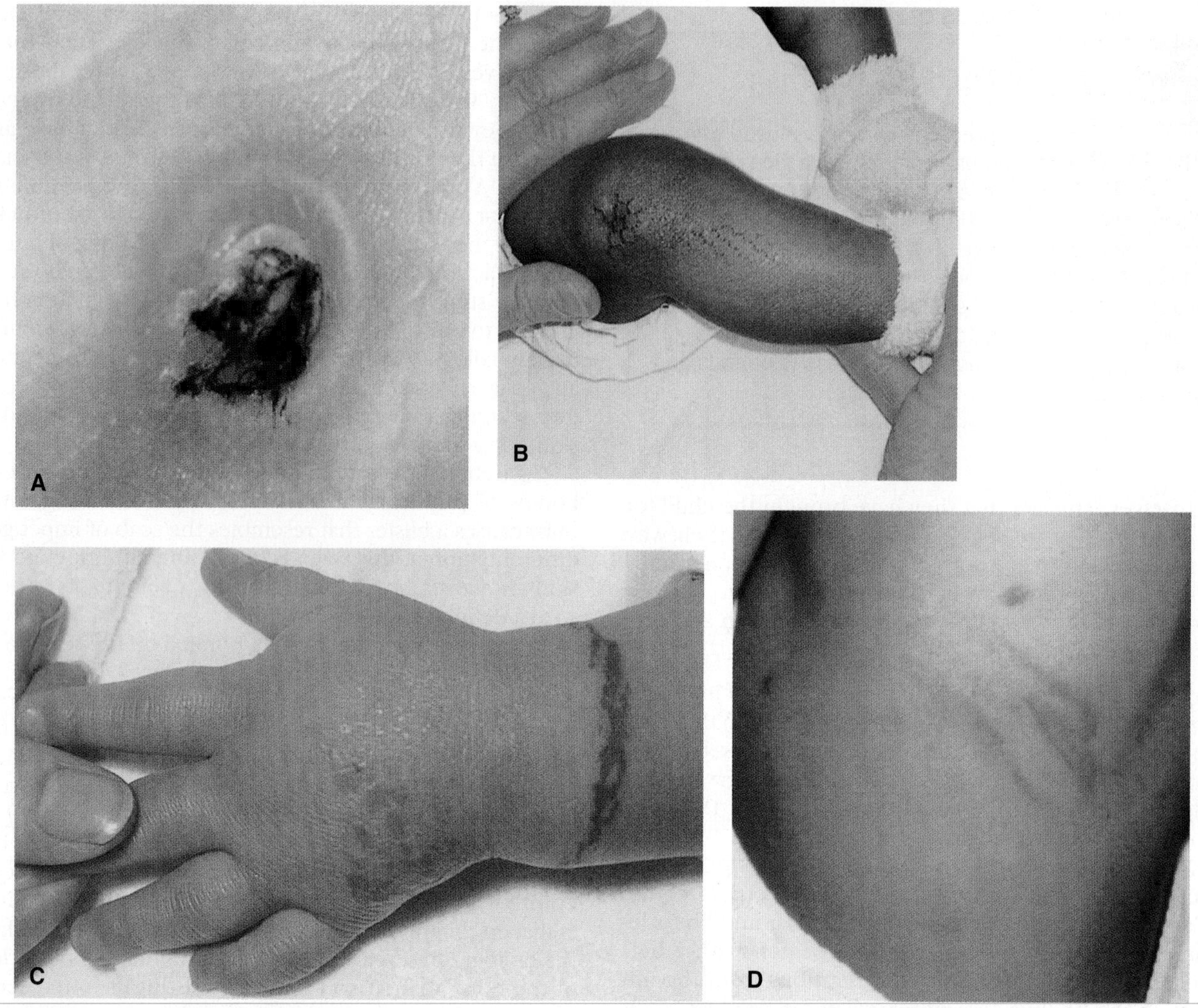

FIGURE 55.2 (A) Cigarette burn on child's foot. **(B)** Branding injury showing imprint of radiator cover. **(C)** Rope burn with edema and skin breakdown from being tied to crib rails. **(D)** Imprint marks from beating with a looped electrical cord. (Zitelli, B. J. & Davis, H. W. [1997]. *Atlas of pediatric physical diagnosis* [3rd ed.]. St. Louis: Mosby-Year Book, Inc.)

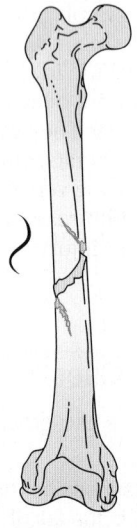

FIGURE 55.3 A spiral fracture around the bone is caused by a wrenching force and is frequently associated with child abuse.

NURSING DIAGNOSES AND RELATED INTERVENTIONS

Nursing Diagnosis: Risk for injury related to documented abuse by parent

Outcome Evaluation: Child has no further physical injuries identifiable as being inflicted by abusing parent.

Prevent Further Abuse. When child abuse is discovered, it would be ideal if the abuser's behavior could be changed and the family kept intact. In reality, once child abuse has been discovered, the child must usually be removed from the home so that no more abuse occurs. Even so, it is impossible to reverse the damage that has been done to the child's sense of trust and self-esteem. Therefore, prevention must be the goal of health care providers in cases of child abuse (Box 55.5). Because many child abusers were abused themselves, stopping child abuse in any one generation helps prevent it in the next.

Identifying parents who are potential abusers is a necessary step in prevention. Some parents can be identified as potential abusers during pregnancy. Listen carefully to the way pregnant women or their partners talk about the child they are expecting. A parent who is overly concerned about the physical appearance or sex of the child ("This had better be a girl" or "He'd better not have his father's nose") may have difficulty accepting a child who does not meet these expectations. Listen for a parent who is concerned about "not letting children get the upper hand" or who says a child "had better be good." This parent may be conveying worry about how he or she will act when the child is "bad."

A parent may also be identified as a potential child abuser during the early postpartum period. Not all parents immediately bond or react warmly to their newborns. They may tentatively touch or pick up their infant. Be aware of parents who do not touch their infant within 24 hours and those who make disparaging remarks about the child's appearance. Risk factors during pregnancy and the early postpartum period are shown in Box 55.6.

Parents may also be identified as potential abusers during health maintenance visits for the infant. By the time a

---

BOX 55.6

Characteristics of Women at High Risk for Child Abuse or Neglect

1. Frequent changes of address in the year before child's birth
2. Past or present psychiatric treatment
3. Emotional problems
4. Lack of intellectual ability
5. Unrealistic expectations of the new baby
6. Changed decision about adoption
7. Abuse or neglect of a previous child
8. History of parental violence or neglect in childhood
9. Low self-esteem
10. Unable to earn independent income

---

baby is brought to a health care agency for an initial health maintenance visit, a good parent–child interaction should have begun. Listen for parents who say the baby is "nothing but trouble," "cries all the time," or "is bad." Ask new parents how it feels to be a new parent. "I'm enjoying it" is a different answer from "not what I expected" or "it's not much fun." Specific observations to make during postpartum and pediatric health care checkups are summarized in Box 55.7.

Helping parents to seek assistance from support people is another necessary step in prevention. Home visits and organizations for parents who abuse, such as Parents Anonymous, can be highly effective in encouraging parents to reach out for help in times of crisis. Interventions that appear promising include home visits, family counseling, and therapy.

Another nursing responsibility aimed at preventing child abuse is helping young parents learn about normal growth and development of children and how to be better parents (Fig. 55.4). Courses in high school that describe sound parenting and review normal growth and development and the responsibilities involved in parenting are important measures in preventing child abuse. Classes conducted in high-risk prenatal settings might also have an impact.

Provide Consistent Care and Support for the Abused Child. A major nursing role is supplying a consistent, caring adult presence for the abused child or furnishing a relationship that the child has never enjoyed.

Use a primary or case management type of nursing care assignment with abused children, to offer them consistency and the security of a one-to-one relationship. Many abused children are not used to playing for their own enjoyment but only to the point at which a parent wants to play a game; this means that they may watch you carefully for signs that you approve of their behavior. They may not be used to activities such as rocking or talking. Be careful when asking questions not to imply that any one answer is the correct one, or they will supply what they think you want to hear rather than the truth. (A question such as, "That feels better, doesn't it?" may be followed by an instant "yes" even though the child feels no improvement in symptoms.)

Evaluate and Promote Family Health. Nurses can help evaluate whether a child would be safe in the parents'

BOX 55.5

Measures to Prevent Child Abuse

1. Advocate for high school courses on parenting and growth and development of children.
2. Help children learn problem-solving techniques so they are not overwhelmed by mounting problems as adults.
3. Foster high self-esteem in children so they are not dependent on others but are assertive (they will not become passive observers to abuse).
4. Help parents with responsible reproductive planning, so children are desired.
5. Help parents locate support people in their community, such as Parents of Retarded Citizens or church or social contacts.
6. Teach children to verbalize their problems and to seek help for problems so they do not mount to overwhelming proportions.
7. Role-model caring behaviors with children for parents.
8. Identify children who may be viewed as special in some way by parents (e.g., those separated from the family at birth, premature, physically challenged).
9. Identify parents who were abused as children, and offer specific help to them to break the chain of child abuse.
10. Suggest that potential abusers join Parents Anonymous, an effective support group.

BOX 55.7

Questions to Ask to Detect the Potential for Child Abuse in New Parents

1. Does the parent have fun with the baby?
2. Does the parent establish eye contact (direct *en face* position) with the baby?
3. How does the parent talk to the baby? Is everything expressed as a demand?
4. Are most of the verbalizations about the child negative?
5. Does the parent remain disappointed about the child's sex?
6. Was the child named immediately? Does the name have meaning for the family?
7. Are the parent's expectations for the child's development far beyond the child's capabilities?
8. Is the parent very bothered by the baby's crying?
9. Does the parent see the baby as too demanding during feedings? Does she or he ignore the baby's demands to be fed?
10. What is the parent's reaction to the task of changing diapers? Is the parent repulsed by the messiness?
11. When the baby cries, does the parent or can the parent comfort the child?
12. Are the parents receiving adequate support?
13. Is sibling rivalry a problem?
14. Is the husband jealous of the baby's claim on the mother's time and affection?
15. When a parent brings the child to the physician's office, does the parent become involved and take control over the baby's needs and what is going to happen (during the examination and while in the waiting room)? Or does the parent relinquish control to the physician or nurse (e.g., undressing the child, holding him or her, allowing the child to express fears)?
16. Can attention be focused on the child in the parent's presence? Can the parent see something positive in that focus?
17. Does the parent report nonexistent symptoms in the baby? Describe the child in terms that you do not recognize at all? Call with strange stories, such as the child has stopped breathing, changed color, or is doing something "on purpose" to aggravate the parent?
18. Does the parent make emergency calls to health care providers for very small things?

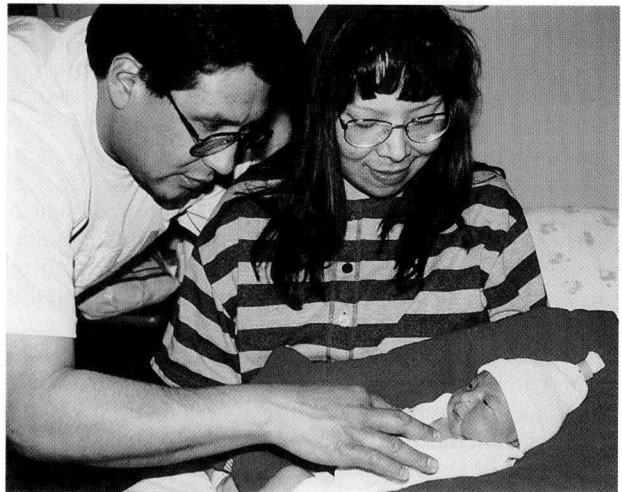

FIGURE 55.4 Teaching that all children have unique characteristics helps to prevent child abuse. Here, new parents explore the already noticeable unique aspects of their newborn. (© Caroline Brown, RNC, MS, DEd.)

cause lack of knowledge of normal growth and development may have contributed to the abuse.

For many parents, the response to a charge of child abuse is anger. For others, it is relief; now an unwanted child will be taken away from them. In some families, one of the parents is the abuser and the other is a victim also. The diagnosis of abuse may force the passive partner to make some important decisions about whether he or she wants to continue a marriage or relationship with the abusive partner. These are not easy decisions to make; if decision making of any kind were easy for this parent, the circumstances probably would never have reached the point at which child abuse occurred.

Praise abusing parents for the things they do well; take time to talk to them away from the child, so that your total attention is focused on them. Be certain they are referred for counseling.

Sometimes an abused child is removed temporarily from a home and then returned later, after the stress that led to the abuse has been removed. Such children need careful follow-up, because parents may revert to an abusive pattern if stress occurs again.

If a child was injured seriously enough to be hospitalized so has had to be removed permanently from the parents' care, the foster family should visit before discharge from the hospital to make the change less frightening for the child. Children who are being removed from their parents in this way can feel an acute sense of loss and may grieve for the nonabusing parent or siblings very much. An abused child may also grieve for the abusing parent, especially if the child is convinced that he or she was responsible for the abuse and that the parent really was not to blame.

Outcome evaluation for abused children must include not only whether they are physically safe but also whether they are developing self-esteem, so that they can become adults who do not need role reversal with their children. It should include whether the abuser received counseling and changed his or her behavior.

care in the future. When parents who are suspected child abusers visit the health care facility, be certain they are given the same welcome and orientation to the facility and procedures as are other parents. When caring for a child, point out positive characteristics about the child, as well as growth and development markers that he or she has reached and realistic expectations of the child's age, be-

What if... Hillary keeps telling her mother that everything is all right and she knows her fall wasn't her mother's fault, even though the mother reported that she wasn't watching Hillary? Is this a typical sign of abuse?

Shaken Baby Syndrome

Shaken baby syndrome is caused by repetitive, violent shaking of a small infant by the arms or shoulders, which causes a whiplash injury to the neck, edema to the brainstem, and distinct retinal hemorrhages. In extreme instances, the infant may suffer brain hemorrhage and die (Lowenstein, 2004). This is a particularly insidious form of child abuse, because the damage inflicted on the infant is not readily apparent. Increased use of computed tomography scans and magnetic resonance imaging is helping to detect children with these internal symptoms. Parents have used covert camcorders ("Nanny cams") to reveal that a caregiver shook a baby this way.

Ritual Abuse

Ritual abuse is cult based or religiously, spiritually, or satanically motivated. It can involve physical, sexual, or psychological abuse with bizarre or ceremonial activities. With this type of abuse, multiple perpetrators may abuse multiple victims over an extended period (Bernet, 2005).

Physical Neglect

Physical neglect is a more subtle form of abuse than physical abuse, but it can be just as damaging to a child's welfare. A neglected child may appear unwashed, thin, and malnourished or be dressed inappropriately, such as without mittens, a coat, or shoes in cold weather. In some families, no one has a warm coat to wear or receives enough food because there is no money for these things; that is different from the family in which parents do have these things, but the children or this particular child does not. This type of abuse may be overlooked because, if you never see the other members of the family, it is easy to believe that all are dressed poorly.

Failing to bring a child for immunizations and failing to seek early medical care for an infection are other signs of neglect. Not requiring a child to attend school, deliberately keeping a child out of school without setting up a home school program, or allowing a child to go unsupervised after school may also be interpreted as neglect.

Neglect may be willful, or it may occur if parents simply do not realize the normal needs of a child. Such parents need guidance from health care personnel to understand their child's needs.

Psychological Abuse

Psychological abuse includes constant belittling or threatening, rejecting, isolating, or exploiting the child. Psychological neglect is the absence of positive parenting. Children who are psychologically abused are likely to have difficulty becoming emotionally confident adults. This type of abuse is the most difficult form of abuse to detect because it may occur only in the home, and its effects, although severe, may be subtle. However, it can be every bit as damaging to the child's ability to achieve as is physical abuse.

The parent who uses only negative terms to describe a child may be psychologically abusing the child. Be sure to include enough growth and development questions during a health assessment to reveal this, and observe the parent–child interaction to determine whether it is positive and healthy or negative and potentially unhealthy.

Munchausen Syndrome by Proxy

Munchausen syndrome by proxy refers to a parent who repeatedly brings a child to a health care facility and reports symptoms of illness when, in fact, the child is well (Yonge & Haase, 2004). For example, a parent might report symptoms such as seizures, excessive sleepiness, or abdominal pain in the child. The reporting of these symptoms causes the child to undergo needless diagnostic procedures or therapeutic regimens. The parent may deliberately inflict injury on the child (e.g., giving a laxative to induce diarrhea or slowly poisoning the child with a prescription drug). Two classic findings of the syndrome are always present: first, the symptoms are not easily detected by physical examination, only by history; second, the symptoms are present only when the abuser is providing care and disappear when care is provided by another person. The parent usually has some degree of medical or child care knowledge; this knowledge may have been obtained through formal education, reading, or Internet browsing. The parent tends to stay with the child constantly, offering to give the majority of care. This can be very deceptive because wanting to stay and give care is also the hallmark of a very conscientious and caring parent. To diagnose this disorder, covert video surveillance may be necessary. Because this syndrome reveals distorted perceptions on the part of the parent, it is almost always necessary to remove the child from the home to protect him or her, even if the parent receives counseling.

> **Checkpoint Question 2**
>
> If Hillary had been abused as an infant, she might have experienced "shaken baby" syndrome. Which of the following is a usual finding with this syndrome?
>
> a. A baby is fearful of strangers.
> b. Retinal hemorrhages develop.
> c. A baby develops Crohn's disease.
> d. A major bone, such as a femur, is broken.

Failure to Thrive (Reactive Attachment Disorder)

Failure to thrive is a unique syndrome in which an infant falls below the 5th percentile for weight and height on a standard growth chart or is falling in percentiles on a growth chart. This condition can be divided into two categories: syndromes with organic causes, such as cardiac disease; and syndromes with nonorganic causes that occur because of a disturbance in the parent–child relationship, resulting in maternal role insufficiency. Sometimes both physical and emotional factors play a role in failure to thrive (Krugman & Dubowitz, 2003).

The nonorganic type can be considered a form of child neglect, although this represents a very complex interplay between parent and child. In many instances, the parent feels little emotional attachment to the child and may have a history of frequent moves and little family support. The parent may not be offering enough food (the parent may not be aware of the hunger cues the infant is offering, or the parent does not have enough concern for the child to offer food regularly). Some infants are offered sufficient food, but the emotional deprivation they sense makes them so lethargic that they do not eat enough. A child may contribute to the poor parenting interaction by being an irritable, fussy, colicky, or "difficult" child. In some instances, the child has neurologic dysfunction resulting from a birth injury and does not respond as a normal child would. The mother may have interpreted this lethargic behavior as lack of response to her and so did not carry out her half of the interaction adequately. Failure to thrive must be taken seriously, because it can lead to cognitive impairment in the child and even death if allowed to continue.

Assessment

Weigh all children at routine health assessments, and plot and compare their weight with standard growth curves so that children who are failing to thrive can be identified. Because of a lack of parent–child interaction, accompanying motor and social developmental delays also may be present.

Take a detailed pregnancy history, because in many instances a breakdown in the development of parenting began in the prenatal period. A pregnancy that was unplanned or not accepted; a boyfriend or husband who left during the pregnancy; the death of a close friend or parent; an economic catastrophe, such as loss of a job; or a long-distance move during pregnancy are all situations that can cause inadequate parenting after the child is born.

On physical examination, these infants usually demonstrate some typical characteristics, such as the following:

- Lethargy with poor muscle tone, a loss of subcutaneous fat, or skin breakdown (Fig. 55.5)
- Lack of resistance to the examiner's manipulation, unlike the response of the average infant
- Rocking on all fours excessively, as if seeking stimulation, if emotionally deprived
- Possibly a greater reluctance to reach for toys or initiate human contact than is demonstrated by the average infant
- Staring hungrily at people who approach them as if they are starved for human contact. Some health care personnel have an uneasy feeling when caring for these infants because this eye contact is so intense.
- Little cuddling or conforming to being held by the second month of life

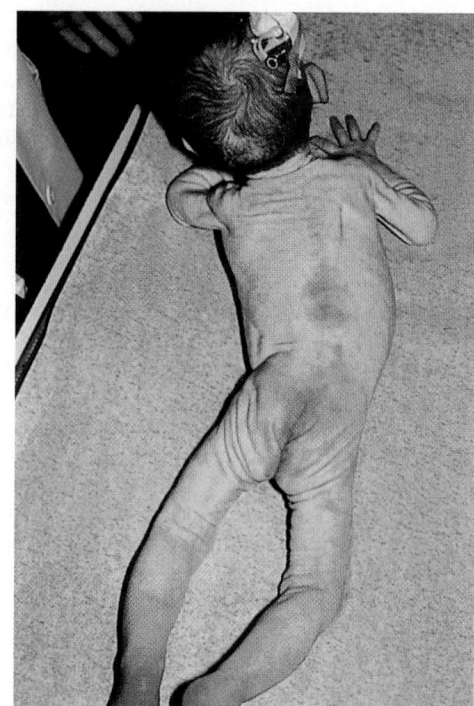

FIGURE 55.5 The child with failure to thrive experiences a loss of subcutaneous fat, muscle wasting, and skin breakdown. (Zitelli, B. J. & Davis, H. W. [1997]. *Atlas of pediatric physical diagnosis* [3rd ed.]. St. Louis: Mosby-Year Book, Inc.)

- Achievement of developmental milestones in the prone position (e.g., lifting the head and chest and following an object with the eyes) by the third or fourth month, but delays in other behaviors that should appear in later months (e.g., sitting erect, pulling to a standing position, crawling, and walking) because the child spends so much time alone
- Markedly delayed or absent speech because of the lack of interaction
- Diminished or nonexistent crying

With advanced failure to thrive, the child's physical condition may be extremely poor; he or she may be nearing acidosis from starvation. If an upper respiratory tract infection develops, the child's resistance to infection may be so low that it could result in pneumonia.

Therapeutic Management

With rare exceptions, children with failure to thrive need to be removed from the parents' care for evaluation and therapy. If they are admitted to a hospital, studies other than routine admission blood work and urinalysis are usually delayed, to avoid submitting these understimulated children to needless pain.

Severe failure to thrive in the early months must be treated rigorously, or it may lead to permanent neurologic damage or leave a child cognitively challenged because of protein deficits and interference with brain metabolism. Infants are placed on a diet appropriate for their ideal

Emergency Care

Although most large city police forces have special officers assigned to investigate rape charges, victims can be confused and further traumatized by police officers who imply that they provoked the attack or could have at least done more to resist or prevent it. This increases the victim's feelings of shame and degradation. It may be especially harmful to adolescents, because people they have been taught to respect have no concept of the degree of fright they have experienced or the strength of their attacker. Health care providers usually are the second group of people victims see after an attack, so they need to be extremely cautious that they do not show this type of callous behavior.

Most health care agencies where many rape victims are seen have a rape trauma team with specially educated counselors to talk to victims immediately after a rape and to offer long-term counseling as needed. Nurses serve as important members of such teams and may provide primary care after a rape. Any nurse should be able to offer emergency support, however, because it might be a long time before a specifically designated staff member arrives, and such services are not available in every community.

Because rape is a crime, the hospital chart of a rape victim is often displayed as part of a court procedure. For the victim to bring charges against the attacker, information concerning the victim's appearance and history needs to be detailed in the hospital chart. Therefore, statements in a chart must be accurate and unbiased. When recording a history, quote the victim's exact words whenever possible. Describe the victim's physical appearance carefully, including the presence and location of injuries, such as bruises, lacerations, teeth marks, or abrasions, and the condition of clothing. Ask whether the victim bathed or washed before coming for care, because this can obscure evidence and obliterate the presence of sperm or DNA material. Ask whether the woman was menstruating or using a tampon. The force of penis penetration with rape can cause a tampon to tear through the posterior vaginal wall into the abdominal cavity, causing an extreme loss of blood internally. Photographs should be taken as necessary to document the extent of injuries. Any clothing that is ripped or stained should be considered as evidence of violent assault and secured according to hospital policy.

After this preliminary observation, a gynecologic or anal examination will be done to evaluate the physical condition of the victim and to document that rape occurred. This is done by recording the existence of any vaginal or perineal lacerations and aspirating sperm or acid phosphate from the vagina or rectum. Acid phosphate, a component of prostatic fluid, is a substance that is not normally present in vaginal or rectal secretions but is present in semen. The presence of acid phosphate is extremely important if the attacker is infertile or sterile, making DNA analysis difficult. Its presence may be the best evidence that rape occurred. Vaginal and anal cultures are taken for gonorrhea, and a Pap test is also performed. Blood is drawn for a pregnancy test and a VDRL test for syphilis. Prophylactic administration of antibiotics against gonorrhea and syphilis is given. If the woman is not menstruating, she may be given oral contraceptives to avoid pregnancy. Victims may have a baseline blood sample drawn for human immunodeficiency virus (HIV) status.

Be certain during emergency care to provide privacy. Many people may want to ask the victim questions, including police officers or detectives, the victim's family, a rape trauma team, and the examining physician or nurse practitioner. Describing the experience is good, but lack of privacy during a perineal examination demonstrates little concern for the victim's self-esteem. Many female victims are uncomfortable with a male physician examining them after rape, because they are temporarily fearful of men. Having a female nurse remain with the victim during this time may be helpful. A male nurse can be equally supportive, because it is not the male–female contrast that a victim is seeking so much as a contrast between aggression and caring. Table 55.1 summarizes common tests and procedures for emergency care of rape victims.

Legal Considerations

Nurses working in emergency departments may be asked to testify in court about the victim's appearance after the assault, although the documentation in the chart is usually all that is necessary. Many victims, especially adolescents, do not press charges against their assailants because they were too frightened or unable at the time to observe the assailant's appearance and therefore cannot identify him later. They may fear that if they name him in court, he will return and kill them. Whether victims follow through with a legal action or not is their choice, but the incidence of rape might be reduced if rapists were aware that they are not apt to escape without a penalty for their crime. Taking the rapist to court may be an opportunity and appropriate time for victims to "fight back" and therefore not be as helpless as they were during the attack.

Checkpoint Question 3

Which description most accurately describes rape?

a. It is a crime of deep passion.
b. It is associated with poverty.
c. It occurs in mentally ill adults.
d. It is a crime of violence.

NURSING DIAGNOSES AND RELATED INTERVENTIONS

Nursing Diagnosis: Rape trauma syndrome related to recent rape

Outcome Evaluation: Victim is able to discuss what happened and voice intense feelings about the crime; victim states ability to go forward with life.

TABLE 55.1

Common Specimen Procedures After Rape*

Procedure	Purpose
Oral washing	Client rinses mouth with 5 mL sterile water, which is then collected in test tube. Analyzed for blood group antigens, or sperm or DNA of attacker.
Fingernail scraping	Scraping under all of client's fingernails is done, and scrapings are placed in envelope. Analyzed for blood, skin, DNA, and clothing fibers of attacker.
Blood VDRL, HIV, and HbsAg	Blood is drawn for antibody titer for syphilis, HIV, and hepatitis B.
Blood typing	Blood is drawn for typing to differentiate it from attacker's type.
Pregnancy test	Either blood or urine specimen is collected; complete vaginal examination before woman voids.
Hair samples	Both scalp and pubic hairs of client (about 10) are removed for comparison with attacker's and placed in envelope.
Vaginal smear for sperm and DNA	Vagina is swabbed with dry applicator and smeared onto slide. Allow to dry. Sperm and DNA analysis performed.
Gonococcus smear	Cervix, vagina, rectum are cultured (also throat is cultured if oral coitus was attempted).
Vaginal washing	5 mL of sterile saline is placed in vagina and aspirated. Analyzed to detect sperm, DNA, and acid phosphate.
Skin washings	Any dried stain of blood or semen on skin or clothing is touched with a moistened cotton swab, which is then dropped into test tube. Analyzed for attacker's blood, semen, or DNA.
Clothing	Any clothing stained or torn is placed into a paper bag. Evidence of violent attack.

* Label all specimens carefully, indicating where they were obtained, to aid medical therapy and provide legal evidence.

One of the major needs of any victim after a violent act is to talk about what happened. A person who can describe an incident begins to "put a fence around" or contain the event. This process brings the event down from "something terrible has happened," a situation that leaves a person with a continuing high anxiety level, to "this specific thing has happened," a situation that allows the traumatic event to be examined and handled. Something that is concrete and describable is rarely as frightening as "something out there."

Ask the victim to describe the incident to you with an introduction such as, "Most people find that it helps to talk about what happened to them." Table 55.2 lists areas to explore with victims to help them reduce the incident to a size they can begin to handle.

Victims should be given the number of a counseling service to telephone before they leave the emergency department. Because genital bruising may not be apparent until 24 hours after the rape, they may be asked to return for a re-examination the next day so this can be documented. Syphilis will not be apparent for up to 6 weeks in serum, so they should return for a repeat VDRL at that time. They may be advised to return in 6 weeks for HIV testing also. Be certain that victims have a support person to accompany them home. Be sure they know that, if their distress becomes acute, they can return as needed to the health care facility for additional care or counseling. Inform them about any local support groups that provide follow-up counseling for victims of rape. One such organization, Women Organized Against Rape, is active in many communities.

Nursing Diagnosis: Disabling family coping related to recent rape of family member

Outcome Evaluation: Partner or other family members express feelings about the rape to health care provider; states confidence in ability to support rape victim.

In many instances, the victim's usual sexual partner has difficulty being a support person to her after a rape because he has as much difficulty dealing with the rape as she does. Not infrequently, a relationship that was meaningful before the rape deteriorates because the partner now sees the victim as "soiled" or mistakenly believes she was somehow responsible for the trauma or actually enjoyed the experience. In other instances, the partner may become so overprotective (not allowing the victim to go out alone; checking on her constantly) that she is not free to maintain her identity. The man may be so filled with vengefulness and anger that he cannot relate to her without his anger surfacing toward her as well

TABLE 55.2

Areas to Explore in Rape Counseling

Area	Considerations
The event	Where did the attack occur? What was happening at the time? This information is important for the victim to discuss and work through; otherwise, any time she is in similar circumstances again, she may have uncontrollable fears related to the attack. Walking home from school or waiting for an elevator in a public building are everyday actions that she will repeat often during her life. If she was raped in such circumstances, she can be reassured that she was acting sensibly and that the rape was not her fault.
The assailant	Allowing the victim to review the description of the rapist may help her to realize that she may react in negative ways in the future to a man with the same build or description. For example, the man may have approached her with a simple gesture, such as a hand on her shoulder. Others will perform this gesture again. She must work through her revulsion to handle it when it occurs in friendly circumstances.
The conversation	Describing the conversation with the rapist helps the victim to accept that she did not provoke the attack.
Details of the assault	Describing the actual assault is extremely difficult for most victims, but doing so allows them to work through it. Until they can describe the attack or the sexual act to which they had to submit, they may have difficulty in performing similar acts with persons of their choice.
Resistance to the assault	Many victims do not struggle during an assault because they realize that it could result in further harm to them. If someone asks them what they did to try to fight off the assailant, they may feel again that they provoked or agreed to the attack. Reassure them that no action was probably the best action and the reason they are still alive. To improve self-esteem, counsel victims that rape is a violent crime and that usually the strength of an attacker is far too great for any woman to resist effectively.

as toward the attacker. Parents of a young adolescent may feel the same way. Counseling for the victim's partner or family may help them to be truly supportive (Box 55.11).

What if... a stepbrother rapes his younger step-sibling? Because they are not blood relatives, would this be considered incest?

INTIMATE PARTNER ABUSE

Intimate partner abuse is abuse by a family member against other individuals living in the household, such as a spouse, child, parent, or grandparent (Magnussen et al., 2004). The fact that spouse abuse and child abuse may both exist in a family strengthens the importance of providing family-centered nursing care so that both these situations can be identified and halted. Abuse occurs at a higher rate during pregnancy than other times (Lipsky et al., 2004). Methods of assessing and caring for pregnant victims of intimate partner abuse are discussed in Chapter 14.

Intimate partner abuse can be destructive to children, because they learn that violence is an acceptable method of managing aggression. This conditioning perpetuates abuse into the next generation.

Children who are exposed to intimate partner abuse may demonstrate conduct problems, noncompliance, and aggression. They may develop low levels of empathy, or they may display distress behaviors such as clinging, crying, abdominal pain, or sleeping disorders. They may regress in language or social developmental milestones. Effects may be long term if the abuse causes teenage girls to shy away from relationships with boys, afraid that they will be exposed to abuse in the same way as their mother was, or if they develop a lack of respect for the abused parent because they blame that person for the abuse.

Like child abuse, intimate partner abuse affects all ethnic and social groups. If it appears to be more prevalent in the lower socioeconomic classes, it is because families at this level are more visible to service organizations and law enforcement officials. When it occurs in middle-class or upper-class houses, wives are often too embarrassed to let people know and tend to keep the violence hidden longer.

Theories About Intimate Partner Abuse

Violent family situations can be divided into two groups: those in which violence preceded the relationship or children and those in which the violence developed after the relationship was established or children were born.

In the first situation, which is more common, violence is usually brought into the family by a man with a history of violence (although the woman may be the offender). His violence-prone characteristics usually erupt early in the courtship and grow progressively worse. He uses violence to handle even small conflicts and provokes a

BOX 55.11

Goals of Crisis Intervention for Families of Rape Victims

Help the family to express openly their immediate feelings in response to a rape as a shared life crisis.

Help the family to be supportive of and reassuring to the victim.

Help the family work through immediate practical matters and initiate problem-solving techniques.

Help the family develop cognitive understanding of what the rape experience actually means to the victim and to the family.

Explain the possibility of future psychological and somatic symptoms that characterize a rape trauma syndrome and what the family can do to minimize these symptoms.

Activate qualities characteristic of healthy family functioning during the impact and resolution phases of the shared crisis.

Educate the family about rape as a *violent crime,* not a sexually motivated act, and eliminate focus on the victim's guilt or responsibility.

Eliminate the family's sense of guilt for not protecting the victim by assuring them that they could not have anticipated or prevented the rape.

Discourage violent, destructive, or irrational retribution toward the rapist (under the guise of being on the victim's behalf) by encouraging sharing of feelings of helplessness, sadness, hurt, and anger.

Encourage discussion of the sexual relationship between partners; suggest that the victim's partner let her know (a) that his feelings have not changed (if this is true) and that he still sexually desires her, (b) that he will wait for her to approach him, and (c) that sex therapy is available if they have persistent difficulties and want assistance in re-establishing normal sexual relations.

Explain the possibility of sexually transmitted disease and pregnancy that may result from a rape, the preventive care necessary for the victim and spouse or boyfriend, and the follow-up care indicated.

Explain that early crisis intervention often prevents long-term problems in resolving the crisis, and that to seek counseling at this time does not imply inadequacy (specify that crisis intervention usually lasts for 3–6 hr during the first few weeks after the rape).

Refer the family for direct counseling if members' shared responses to the crisis interfere with their ability to cope adaptively.

Provide factual data, resource lists for counseling, and follow-up care *in writing* (because highly stressed persons do not hear or recall information verbally communicated).

Let families know that some decisions, such as whether to prosecute the rapist or move to a safer residence, can be postponed while more immediate needs, such as medical care, are taken care of. (This action helps the family set priorities and organize decisions about what has to be done now and gain emotional distance from the urgency and confusion felt during a crisis state to permit sound decision-making later.)

Identify how the family has handled crises in the past, and encourage members to use adaptive coping mechanisms for this crisis.

Encourage contact with persons identified as supportive to the family, and offer to contact such persons.

Assign a primary nurse to spend time talking with the family in the emergency department waiting room while the victim receives medical care.

Allow time for thoughts and feelings in the decision-making process.

Use empathetic listening to convey understanding of the family's feelings and concerns.

Ask if you can check back with the family the next day to see how they are getting along and answer any questions they may have.

---

pervasive feeling of powerlessness in the people around him. Such men usually have a history of early and prolonged exposure to family violence as children; alcohol is frequently associated with the expression of violence.

Intimate partner abuse often follows a cycle of violence that includes three phases: tension-building, acute violence, and a "honeymoon" or tranquil, loving phase. During the first phase, the abuser displays actions such as anger, arguing, and blaming the victim for external problems or for provoking the abuse. The acute violence phase can be triggered by an internal response in the abuser or by an external crisis. It can result in extreme physical harm to the victim. The tranquil, loving phase, characterized by kind and contrite behavior, follows the violence, lulling the victim into forgiveness and a wish to continue the relationship. Without intervention, however, this phase ends

at some point, and the cycle of violence repeats (Willis & Porche, 2004).

Partners react to the situation in three phases (Table 55.3). During the impact phase (stage I), a light level of abuse, the victim uses denial as a defense mechanism. If she does not end the relationship at this point, the abuse grows more frequent and more violent; by not stopping it, she is indirectly giving the offender permission to continue. During the second stage, the victim can no longer deny that the violence is occurring. At the same time, she cannot stop it because she does not provoke the violence; she is only a convenient recipient of poorly controlled violent behavior. She is forced to use coping mechanisms such as becoming very obedient and cooperative and doing everything her abuser asks in a desperate effort to reduce the violence. This phase is termed psychological

TABLE 55.3

Levels of Intimate Partner Abuse

Level	Description
I	Abuse is occasional; consists of slapping, punching, kicking, verbal abuse. Contusions occur.
II	Abuse is becoming more frequent; beatings are sustained and cause fractures, such as a broken jaw or rib fracture.
III	Abuse is even more frequent, perhaps daily. A weapon, such as a gun, baseball bat, or broom handle, may be used. Permanent disability or death from injuries, such as intracranial hemorrhage or concussion, may occur.

infantilism or **learned helplessness.** The level of abuse can continue until the woman is being almost constantly physically abused (stage III). A fetus is in danger if abuse of a pregnant woman occurs at this stage. During this stage, the woman is forced to become isolated; she sinks into hopelessness and depression. She has difficulty seeking help because she is unable to believe that outside people might want to help her.

In the second type of violent family, in which violence begins late in a relationship, violence occurs as a last resort after all other attempts at communication have failed. The behavior of one partner threatens the psychological defenses of the other, and each projects his or her feelings and shortcomings onto the other. Such a situation, however, is not typical of intimate partner abuse: in most instances, one partner brings violence into the family.

Assessment

When any type of abuse against an individual family member is identified, it is important to investigate further for evidence of abuse against other family members. Asking about the possibility of abuse should be a priority with any woman seen for trauma. As many as 20% to 25% of women seen in emergency departments for trauma received their wounds from abuse. Common injuries suffered by abused women include burns, lacerations, bruises, and head injuries. Asking all women at physical examinations to account for any bruise they have helps detect physical abuse. Asking them whether they are ever concerned about their safety or well-being helps detect emotional abuse. In addition, screening for intimate partner abuse is important when parents bring children for health care visits.

Therapeutic Management

It may be difficult to understand how adults can tolerate abuse against themselves or their children. It is important, however, not to blame the victims. Hopelessness and powerlessness are consequences of continual abuse. Bat-

tered and emotionally abused individuals are often immobilized by a sense of guilt: they believe that if they were better people, their partners would not resort to beatings or verbal badgering. Because victims may have no access to money and no skills to earn any, they need a great deal of support to be able to leave their partners. Even if they have a skill and have supported themselves in the past, their self-esteem may be so low that they no longer believe they can put the skill to use. As the abuse becomes more violent, they may be afraid that their abusers will follow and kill them and their children if they leave. Other extended family members may be unwilling to shelter the victims for fear of being included in the violence. An important role for nurses is helping an abused family find a shelter where they can feel safe. Treatment for abusers needs to be scheduled, but safety is the first priority.

Key Points

Child abuse can exist in many forms. It may be physical, emotional, or sexual and may encompass neglect and abuse.

A high suspicion for child abuse should be present if burns, head injury, or rib fractures are present or if the history of the accident seems out of context for the injury.

Shaken baby syndrome involves repetitive, violent shaking of a small infant by the arms or shoulders, causing a whiplash injury to the neck, edema to the brainstem, and distinct retinal hemorrhages.

A triad of "special parent, special child, special circumstance" is characteristic of the family in which child abuse occurs.

Failure to thrive is a syndrome in which an infant falls below the 5th percentile for weight and height on a standard growth chart. It is associated with a disturbance in the parent–child relationship.

Children who comfort parents in emergency settings may just be sensitive children, or they may be demonstrating role reversal, a behavior characteristic of abused children.

In families in which a child is abused, a parent may also be a victim of abuse. Ask enough questions at health care visits to be certain that this problem does not exist as well.

Child abuse is reportable by law. Nurses can initiate reporting as an independent action or through their health agency's referral network.

Methods to prevent abuse in which nurses can actively participate include teaching about the expected growth and development of children, educating teenage parents for parenting roles, and teaching empowerment, or a sense that children and adults have control of their own lives.

Sexual abuse of children can be prevented by teaching children to recognize abnormal advances and to know it is right to speak out about wrongs against them.

Abuse is a family problem, not an individual problem. Therapy must include all family members to be effective.

Rape is a crime of violence, not of sexual intent. Rape victims need both short-term and long-term counseling.

Critical Thinking Exercises

1. Hillary is the 3-year-old you met at the beginning of the chapter. Although her mother told you that Hillary fell from a swing, Hillary has a broken forearm, a broken rib, and multiple bruises on her chest and back. Her mother tells you, "Hillary isn't pretty. I guess she's also clumsy." What additional questions would you want to ask to determine whether Hillary has been abused?

2. You weigh a baby at a well-child conference and discover that the infant's weight is below the 2nd percentile on a standardized growth chart. What questions would you want to ask the mother to see if you can account for this? What particular areas would you want to assess on a physical examination?

3. Physical examination determines that a 4-year-old has a purulent vulvovaginitis. A culture reveals this infection is gonorrhea. What questions would you want to ask her to determine how she contracted this infection? Suppose her parents are influential people in your community. Would this fact influence what questions you ask?

4. Examine the National Health Goals related to family violence. Most government-sponsored money for nursing research is allotted based on these goals. What would be a possible research topic to explore pertinent to these goals that would be applicable to Hillary's family and also advance evidence-based practice?

References

Bernet, W. (2005). Child maltreatment. In Sadock, B. J., & Sadock, V. A. (Eds.), *Kaplan and Sadock's comprehensive textbook of psychiatry* (8th ed.). Philadelphia: Lippincott Williams & Wilkins.

Beveridge, K., & Cheung, M. (2004). A spiritual framework in incest survivors treatment. *Journal of Child Sexual Abuse, 13*(2), 105–120.

Brilleslijper-Kater, S. N., Friedrich, W. N., & Corwin, D. L. (2004). Sexual knowledge and emotional reaction as indicators of sexual abuse in young children: Theory and research challenges. *Child Abuse and Neglect, 28*(10), 1007–1017.

Carr, A. (2004). Interventions for post-traumatic stress disorder in children and adolescents. *Pediatric Rehabilitation, 7*(4), 231–244.

Christian, C. W. (2003). Child abuse: Physical. In Schwartz, M. W. (Ed.), *5-Minute pediatric consult* (3rd ed.). Philadelphia: Lippincott Williams & Wilkins.

Department of Health and Human Services (2000). *Healthy people 2010.* Washington, DC: DHHS.

Duncan, M. K., & Sanger, M. (2004). Coping with the pediatric anogenital exam. *Journal of Child and Adolescent Psychiatric Nursing, 17*(3), 126–136.

Gahlinger, P. M. (2004). Club drugs: MDMA, gamma-hydroxybutyrate (GHB), Rohypnol, and ketamine. *American Family Physician, 69*(11), 2619–2626.

Helfer, R. E., & Kempe, R. S. (1987). *The battered child.* Chicago: University of Chicago Press.

Krugman, S. D., & Dubowitz, H. (2003). Failure to thrive. *American Family Physician, 68*(5), 879–884.

Levenson, J. S. (2003). Policy interventions designed to combat sexual violence: Community notification and civil commitment. *Journal of Child Sexual Abuse, 12*(3/4), 17–52.

Lipsky, S., et al. (2004). Police-reported intimate partner violence during pregnancy and the risk of antenatal hospitalization. *Maternal and Child Health Journal, 8*(2), 55–63.

Lowenstein, L. F. (2004). Recent research and views on shaking baby syndrome. *International Journal of Psychiatry in Medicine, 34*(2), 131–141.

Magnussen, L., et al. (2004). Intimate-partner violence: a retrospective review of records in primary care settings. *Journal of the American Academy of Nurse Practitioners, 16*(11), 502–512.

Maguire, S., et al. (2005). Are there patterns of bruising in childhood which are diagnostic or suggestive of abuse? A systematic review. *Archives of Disease in Childhood, 90*(2), 182–186.

Mezey, G., et al. (2005). Domestic violence, lifetime trauma and psychological health of childbearing women. *BJOG: An International Journal of Obstetrics & Gynaecology, 112*(2), 197–201.

Person, E. S. (2005). Paraphilias. In Sadock, B. J., & Sadock, V. A. (Eds.), *Kaplan and Sadock's comprehensive textbook of psychiatry* (8th ed.). Philadelphia: Lippincott Williams & Wilkins.

Saewyc, E. M., Pettingell, S., & Magee, L. L. (2003). The prevalence of sexual abuse among adolescents in school. *Journal of School Nursing, 19*(5), 266–272.

Schelble, D. T. (2004). Rape crisis syndrome. In Dambro, M. R. (Ed.), *Griffith's 5-minute clinical consult.* Philadelphia: Lippincott Williams & Wilkins.

Testa, M. (2004). The role of substance use in male-to-female physical and sexual violence: A brief review and recommendations for future research. *Journal of Interpersonal Violence, 19*(12), 1494–1505.

Valente, S. M. (2005). Sexual abuse of boys. *Journal of Child and Adolescent Psychiatric Nursing, 18*(1), 10–16.

Willis, D. G., & Porche, D. J. (2004). Male battering of intimate partners: Theoretical underpinnings, intervention approaches, and implications. *Nursing Clinics of North America, 39*(2), 271–282.

Yonge, O., & Haase, M. (2004). Munchausen syndrome and Munchausen syndrome by proxy in a student nurse. *Nurse Educator, 29*(4), 166–169.

Suggested Readings

Bosch, K., & Schumm, W. R. (2004). Accessibility to resources: helping rural women in abusive partner relationships become free from abuse. *Journal of Sex and Marital Therapy, 30*(5), 357–370.

Ettaro, L., Berger, R. P., & Songer, T. (2004). Abusive head trauma in young children: Characteristics and medical charges in a hospitalized population. *Child Abuse and Neglect, 28*(10), 1099-1111.

Howe, M. L., et al. (2004). True and false memories in maltreated children. *Child Development, 75*(5), 1402-1417.

Jones, J. G., & Worthington, T. (2005). Management of sexually abused children by non-forensic sexual abuse examiners. *Journal of the Arkansas Medical Society, 101*(7), 224-226.

Kimball, C., & Golding, J. (2004). Adolescent maltreatment: An overview of the research. *School Nurse News, 21*(5), 36-39.

Polaschek, D. L., & Gannon, T. A. (2004). The implicit theories of rapists: What convicted offenders tell us. *Sexual Abuse: Journal of Research and Treatment, 16*(4), 299-314.

Schaaf, H. S. (2004). Forensic medicine: Child abuse: management of physical abuse (children 0-13 years of age). *SADJ, 59*(9), 379-380.

Sibert, J. (2004). Bruising, coagulation disorder, and physical child abuse. *Blood Coagulation and Fibrinolysis, 15*(Suppl. 1), S33-S39.

Straus, M. A., & Kantor, G. K. (2005). Definition and measurement of neglectful behavior: Some principles and guidelines. *Child Abuse and Neglect, 29*(1), 19-29.

Thomas, K. (2003). Munchausen syndrome by proxy: Identification and diagnosis. *Journal of Pediatric Nursing: Nursing Care of Children and Families, 18*(3), 174-180.

CHAPTER 56

Nursing Care of the Family Coping With a Child's Long-Term or Terminal Illness

Key Terms

anticipatory grief
death
grief process
vulnerable children

Objectives

After mastering the contents of this chapter, you should be able to:

1. Describe common concerns of parents of children with a long-term or terminal illness.
2. Assess adjustment of a child or family to a long-term or terminal illness.
3. Formulate nursing diagnoses for a child with a long-term or terminal illness.
4. Identify expected outcomes for a child with a long-term or terminal illness.
5. Plan nursing care for a child with a long-term or terminal illness, such as helping parents with time management.
6. Implement nursing care for a child with a long-term or terminal illness.
7. Evaluate expected outcomes for effectiveness and achievement of care.

8. Identify National Health Goals related to children with long-term or terminal illnesses that nurses could help the nation achieve.
9. Identify areas related to the care of children with long-term or terminal illnesses that could benefit from additional nursing research or application of evidence-based practice.
10. Use critical thinking to analyze ways that nursing care of a child with a long-term or terminal illness can be more family-centered.
11. Integrate knowledge of long-term and terminal illness in children with nursing process to achieve quality maternal and child health nursing care.

Charlie is a 3-year-old who has had a relapse after 18 months of chemotherapy for leukemia. You meet him in the emergency department because he has developed a severe cough and high fever. He is diagnosed as having pneumonia. "He's been so sick for so long," his mother tells you. "We're all so tired, and he's been through so much. How could he develop something else?"

Previous chapters described the growth and development of well children and the care of children with specific disorders. This chapter adds information about the care of chronically and terminally ill children. This is important information because it builds a base for care and health teaching and support for the parents and child.

How could you best help these parents?
What would be important topics to talk to them about?

After you've studied this chapter, access the accompanying website. Read the patient scenario and answer the questions to further sharpen your skills, grow more familiar with RN-CLEX types of questions, and reward yourself with how much you have learned.

W hen children have acute illnesses, both they and their parents may be frightened by the sudden onset and severity of symptoms. Because human beings have a great capacity for coping with stress, however, they can usually adjust to the strain of disrupted daily routines, hospital visits, and home care as long as they are given adequate support.

When a child's illness becomes long term or is one that can be projected to have a terminal outcome, a family's capacity to cope can become stretched beyond its limits. Support is essential for such a family if it is to survive under this level of pressure and stress.

People cope with situations depending on their perception of the event, the type and kind of support they receive from people around them, and the ways that they have found to be successful in coping with stressful situations in the past. When working with parents of a child with a long-term or terminal illness, discovering how the parents perceive the problem, what resources they have available, and how they plan to use these resources are crucial in planning nursing care.

Whether the medical diagnosis involves a permanent disability or impending death, a parent's first response will be grief. The parent has either lost the "perfect" child imagined during pregnancy or the well child he or she had up to the time of diagnosis. Depending on their age and maturity, children may also experience a grief response. National Health Goals related to the care of children with a long-term or terminal illness are shown in Box 56.1.

Nursing Process Overview

For Care of the Family Coping With a Long-Term or Terminal Illness

● *Assessment*

Because a family's coping abilities are best assessed gradually, over a period of many contacts, nurses' assessments of the degree of a family's coping are often the most thorough and meaningful of all health care providers.

Observing children at home, where they are most comfortable, or at school in a familiar atmosphere, often reveals a great deal more about their present disease status or coping potential than does a formal test situation. Often a toy offered by a parent, sister, or brother will be grasped and manipulated by a child with a chronic disability, whereas the same toy offered by a stranger will not be accepted. Children with a long-term illness, on the whole, have probably been through many tests and procedures in the diagnosis of their disorder; they may have reason to think of health care providers as hurting people, not people for whom they wish to achieve. It may be possible to change their perception by maintaining a reassuring, gentle manner during assessment and subsequent care procedures.

● *Nursing Diagnosis*

Long-term illness takes many forms. A condition that requires daily attention, such as diabetes (insulin injec-

BOX 56.1 FOCUS ON . . .

NATIONAL HEALTH GOALS

Long-term illness or early death in children is a major cost to the nation and individual families because it has the potential to reduce the earning power and contribution of future citizens. A number of National Health Goals address this:

- Reduce the proportion of children and adolescents with disabilities who are reported to be sad, unhappy, or depressed, from 31% to 17%.
- Increase the proportion of children and youth with disabilities who spend at least 80% of their time in regular education programs, from 45% to 60%.
- Reduce the rate of infant deaths, from a baseline of 7.2/100,000 to a target rate of 4.5/100,000.
- Reduce the death rate for children 1 to 4 years of age, from a baseline of 34.6/100,000 to no more than 18.6/100,000 children, and for children aged 5 to 9 years, from a baseline of 17.7/100,000 to 12.3/100,000.
- Reduce the death rate for children 10 to 14 years of age, from a baseline of 22/100,000 to no more than 16.8/100,000, and the death rate for adolescents 15 to 19 years of age, from a baseline of 70.6/100,000 to 39.8/100,000 (DHHS, 2000).

Nurses can help the nation achieve these goals by educating women to seek care during pregnancy so that congenital anomalies, a common cause of infant morbidity and mortality, are less frequent and to seek immunizations for their children so that diseases that can lead to long-term illness, such as rubeola and meningitis, can be prevented. Nursing research on the following areas would further these goals: What are special techniques for preparing children who are physically challenged to be more independent? How can children who use a wheelchair maintain a high sense of self-esteem? What specific measures are most helpful to parents when they learn their child has a terminal illness?

tions), but that is stabilized may not be as stressful to parents as an illness, such as muscular dystrophy, that slowly progresses in severity. In the former, although the child and family must adjust their lifestyle to incorporate the child's daily needs, they feel they have some control over the course of the illness and the child's overall health. In the latter, the child and family can feel powerless, lacking any ability to alter the course of the disease; they must simply wait for the next acute crisis to develop. Nursing diagnoses for children with long-term or terminal illnesses should address both the child and the family as a whole. Some examples of nursing diagnoses when a long-term illness is present are the following:

- Interrupted family processes related to recent diagnosis of long-term or chronic illness in oldest child
- Compromised family coping related to child's disability

- Disabling family coping related to parents' inability to accept child's long-term illness
- Anticipatory grieving related to chronicity of the child's illness
- Risk for delayed growth and development related to lack of age-appropriate stimulation because of disability

New issues develop when the child's disorder is considered terminal. The family must learn to accept not only the child's illness, but also its eventual outcome. Some examples of nursing diagnoses when a terminal illness is present are the following:

- Hopelessness related to steady progression of child's disease
- Anticipatory grieving related to child's terminal illness
- Powerlessness related to inability to prolong child's life
- Decisional conflict related to treatment options and choice of setting for child's final care

● *Outcome Identification and Planning*

Be certain when planning care that outcomes established are realistic. You probably cannot alter the course of a child's illness, but you can help parents cope with the illness or the impending death and its aftermath.

Parents who have not yet accepted the seriousness of their child's illness may make plans that the child cannot possibly accomplish. These parents are holding on to the hope that their child will eventually be cured or restored to full health. Sometimes this level of denial is essential to the parents' ability to cope with the child's daily needs and the needs of the rest of the family. They may believe that they must shield the child or other family members from the truth. Focusing on hopeful but realistic outcomes, such as the desire that the child will go through the day without experiencing pain or that the child will learn how to move about independently in a wheelchair, are helpful in moving a family forward toward final, realistic acceptance of a child's illness.

● *Implementation*

When children have a long-term or terminal illness, parents may begin to overprotect them so much that they neglect to encourage their growth. They may forget to provide play materials or other stimulation appropriate for their age. Helping parents to look at their child's capabilities and arranging appropriate activities for the child are ways in which nurses can facilitate parents' acceptance of the diagnosis and the road ahead. Suggestions for helping children achieve developmental milestones are discussed for each age group in previous chapters.

Helping parents to learn better coping strategies and teaching them ways to remember to give medication for a number of years, ways to maintain quality care without becoming exhausted, and the importance of maintaining a lifestyle of their own are other important measures.

The following organizations are helpful for referral:

- Candlelighters Childhood Cancer Foundation (*www.candlelighters.org*)
- The Compassionate Friends (*www.compassionatefriends.org*)
- National Association of School Psychologists (*www.nasponline.org*)
- Centers for Loss in Multiple Births (CLIMB) (*www.climb-support.org*)

● *Outcome Evaluation*

Children with a long-term or terminal illness need periodic follow-up care, because plans made for a newborn may no longer be suitable as soon as the child becomes a toddler. Plans made in the early school years may need to be modified by the time the child is 12 years old, and they must change again with adolescence. In addition to follow-up of specific therapy by a specialty clinic, children also need routine health maintenance care. Otherwise, children will be well protected from the complications of a special illness but unprotected from common childhood illnesses that could be even more devastating.

Evaluation of whether expected outcomes for the family of a child who died were met helps to strengthen your planning with the next dying child you care for, improve your self-esteem, and build confidence in your ability to care for dying children. Evaluation reveals discrepancies between the wish and the reality of care, identifying areas you need to strengthen to grow as a health care provider. Some examples suggesting achievement of outcomes are the following:

- Parents state realistic plans for their child regarding school placement.
- Parents state they have been able to deal with their grief over child's diagnosis to maintain normal family functioning.
- Parents state they are able to cope with present stressors.
- Child states he or she is aware the illness is chronic (long-term) but thinks of himself or herself as a person who is able to accomplish many things in life.

THE CHILD WITH A LONG-TERM ILLNESS

Because families have different resources and everyone reacts to situations differently, each child with a long-term illness and his or her family need to be assessed for their potential to cope with the illness and provide necessary care. Through such assessment, appropriate interventions to help the family adapt can be started early in the course of the illness (Boling, 2005).

The Parents' Adjustment

Children have difficulty adjusting to events without good role-modeling from their parents. Therefore, assessment begins with a look at how well the parents are responding to the diagnosis of a long-term illness (Hopia et al., 2004).

Grief Response

Parents can be expected to experience a **grief process,** or regulated steps in grieving, when they are told their child will be physically or cognitively challenged or is terminally ill. The most commonly accepted steps or stages of grief are those outlined by Kübler-Ross (1969). Table 56.1 summarizes these stages. Most parents with a child who is physically or cognitively challenged never arrive at the final stage of acceptance; for parents with a terminally ill child, this may come only with the child's death.

During the first stage of grief (shock or denial), parents are unable to plan past immediate or short-term actions (learning to change a dressing or which pills to give each day). Trying to establish long-term outcomes at this point (what type of school the child will attend, the vocations that are open to him or her) is rarely productive, because this must all be done again when parents are truly ready to look this far ahead. During the second stage, anger, parents may be unwilling to learn (the whole thing is so unfair; planning is asking too much of them; how can they trust you? If you were really helpful, you would cure their child). This becomes a time of waiting also, so be sure to refrain from giving advice. During the bargaining stage of grief, parents are still not ready for planning. If their bargain is fulfilled (let their child be able to walk, and they will spend the rest of their life doing good), the plans they make now (such as purchasing a wheelchair) will have to be modified later, after the child's condition improves.

During the next stage of grief, depression, parents are ready to make plans but need a great deal of help in planning because they feel so fatigued. Be careful in working with people who are depressed that you do not totally plan *for* them rather than *with* them. Many parents of children who are physically or cognitively challenged have low self-esteem (they believe that if they were really good people they would have had a normal child). This makes them feel that your suggestions must be better than any they could make. After they return home, however, they are the ones who must live with these plans, so they should participate in making them.

Even after they reach the final stage of grief—acceptance—some parents need guidance in making plans to avoid becoming so self-sacrificing that the needs and wishes of the spouse and other children are ignored. For example, parents may spend every waking moment with their ill child. Being a martyr is a way of easing guilt, a part of grief bargaining, a way of proving that they are equal to others—perhaps even the best parents in the entire world. These parents need time to talk about possible reasons why they feel they must push themselves in this manner. Perhaps they can find a middle-of-the-road approach to a child's care that allows time for all family members. Helping them to plan a respite from the care of a sick child, such as an evening out while a babysitter cares for the child, is a part of this approach.

By the time a child who is physically or cognitively challenged is of school age, parents should begin to make some concrete plans as to who will care for the child after they die. This is very difficult for parents; it asks them to contemplate their own mortality (something that people rarely want to do) as well as the vulnerability of their children when it occurs. They might consult with family members about guardianship and with a lawyer to help them write a will that will provide future caretaking and economic support for the child.

Factors Influencing Parental Adjustment

Certain circumstances appear to increase parents' difficulty in adjusting to a disabling or long-term illness in their child. These include the degree and timing of the illness, the experience of the parents, the availability of support people, and the ability to make long term plans (Goble, 2004).

Degree of Illness. The seriousness of an illness obviously affects the ability of parents to adjust. A child who needs total care will require a much more radical readjustment of the parents' lives than will a child who only needs additional speech therapy for an hour a day. In most instances, the parents' perception of the child's illness is as important as the child's condition itself (Fig. 56.1). For example, a parent who envisioned a son as someday becoming an Olympic runner may perceive a son with developmental hip dysplasia as having a serious physical challenge; a parent whose mental image of the child was that of a lawyer doing mainly desk work may not view the hip problem as a serious illness.

TABLE 56.1

Stages of Grief

Stage	Parents' Reaction	Description
1	Denial	Parents have difficulty realizing what has occurred. They ask, "How could this have happened?"
2	Anger	Parents react to the injustice of being singled out this way. They say, "It isn't fair this is happening."
3	Bargaining	Parents attempt to work out a "deal" to buy their way out of the situation. They say, "If my child gets well, I'll devote the rest of my life to doing good."
4	Depression	Parents begin to face what is happening. They feel sad and unprotected.
5	Acceptance	Acceptance is being able to say, "Yes, this is happening, and it is all right that it is happening." With a child with long-term illness, parents may never reach this stage but will always remain in the chronic sorrow of the depression stage.

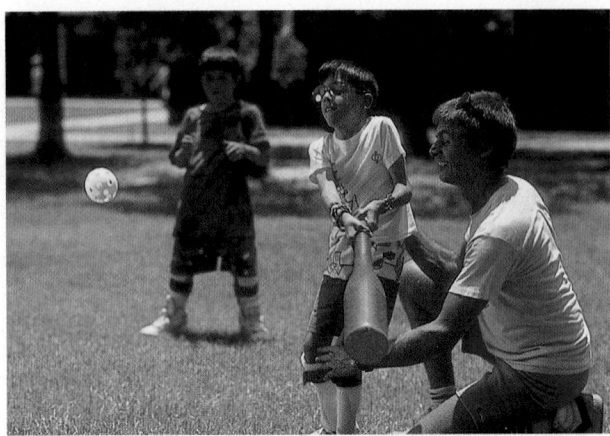

FIGURE 56.1 A parent's perception of a child's disability is important to how well the family adjusts. Often it is easier to accept a disability that allows for greater functioning in everyday activities. (© Bachman/Science Source/Photo Researchers.)

Many parents are not aware of the mental image that they carry of their child, an image that began to form the moment the woman realized she was pregnant. Hidden desires are often revealed if you ask parents, "If things could have been different, what kind of person would you have liked your child to be?" A parent who answers, "a kind person" can still have that wish fulfilled, no matter what the degree of illness. A parent who says, "I always assumed my child would take over my business some day" may have some major mental readjustments to make.

Whether an illness is noticeable (spastic cerebral palsy) or not noticeable (controlled seizures) also can make a difference in how parents adjust to the illness. A mother who takes her child with cerebral palsy shopping (a child who walks unsteadily and knocks over a display) may hear other shoppers say, "Wouldn't you think a mother would watch her child more carefully?" On days that her child uses a wheelchair, however, shoppers' comments are more apt to be, "Poor little thing. Isn't it wonderful that his mother brings him shopping with her?" She is happy to have a signal (the wheelchair) that announces that her child is different and cannot be held to the same standards as other children. Other parents might be more grateful that a child's illness is not a visible one: it makes the illness seem lesser in extent, and therefore easier for them to accept.

Onset of the Illness. Whether a condition is apparent at birth (e.g., a myelomeningocele) or occurs at a later time (the child is struck by a car at school age) may make a difference in the parents' ability to adjust. For some parents, never having had a well child can make the child's illness easier to accept. In any event, the need for long-term care of a child can totally change the parents' lifestyle. They may no longer be able to live in a high-rise apartment because it is not wheelchair accessible; a parent may have to reduce work hours or give up a career to devote full time to the child's care (Loprest & Davidoff, 2004).

Effect of Parental Experience. First-time parents may have more difficulty caring for a child with a long-term illness than older, more experienced parents do, because

all phases of parenting are more difficult for them. They might have difficulty evaluating how much activity a child needs or what toys are appropriate, for example. On the other hand, first-time parents, because they have no preconceived opinions, may be more flexible than other parents. A young parent who has just this one child may have more time to spend in a daily exercise program than does a parent with five children.

Availability of Support People. A family that has few close friends and lives some distance from relatives is apt to have more difficulty adjusting to illness in a child than a family that has close support people. People who have secondary support systems in the community, such as an organization for parents of children who are physically or cognitively challenged or a local church or synagogue, usually do better than parents who are without these resources. People who are able to use health care resources effectively adjust more easily than those who cannot do so. The ability to use health care resources depends on a number of factors, including the following:

- Transportation (it is difficult to take a child in a 50-lb cast on a bus)
- Language barriers (it is frustrating to go for care and be unable to make your needs known)
- Finances and insurance coverage (it is frustrating to be told that you need to see a specialist when you have no money or your health coverage does not pay for one)
- Past experience with health care providers (if the best advice that has been given to the parents up to this point has been, "Take your baby home and treat him as near normally as possible," the parents may not see health care providers as a source of useful information or help)

Life Events. A child's illness usually appears to be more acute at times when the child would normally reach developmental milestones: at 12 months, when the baby should be taking his or her first step and is not; 6 years, when the child should begin school; first communion or bar mitzvah; time for a driver's license; or voting age. When the child does not reach these milestones, parents are reminded of the illness in a particularly painful way.

Factors that indicate that a family will probably be able to adjust to caring for a child with a long-term illness are summarized in Table 56.2.

The Child's Adjustment

A child's reaction to being physically or cognitively challenged or having a long-term illness is strongly influenced by the family's reaction to the illness (Box 56.2). Family reactions may range from overprotectiveness to rejection and from denial to acceptance. The child's adjustment may also be influenced by peers and other support people, such as school personnel or health care providers. Whether a child can take medicine during school hours can make a big difference in adjustment (Weller et al., 2004). Social exclusion, discrimination, and physical barriers make it difficult for a child to adjust to a physical challenge or long-term illness. On the other hand, inclusion in school and social activities, acceptance by peers and support people, and the ability to function as normally as possible help the child adjust.

TABLE 56.2

Factors That Ease Parental Adjustment to a Child's Long-Term Illness

Factor	Rationale
Support people are available.	Caring for a child is a series of crises during which support people become very important.
A strong marital bond exists between the parents.	A marriage partner can serve as the strongest support person.
A good relationship exists between the child's parents and their parents.	The parents (because they had good care) have a firm sense of trust and the ability to give care to another.
The child is other than the first-born.	The parents have had practice parenting.
The family lives close to shopping, schools, and transportation.	The family is not isolated.
The family has a strong religious faith.	Secondary support systems are important in times of stress.
The parents are told of the child's disability as soon as possible.	A handicap is easier to accept if the parents never thought of the child as totally well.

Checkpoint Question 1

What factor is most apt to help parents accept long-term illness in their child?

a. The parents are isolated so cannot compare their child to others.
b. The parents have good relationships with their own parents.
c. The parents are wealthy so have few worries other than the child.
d. Parents believe in alternative therapies so have many options.

A child's ability to cope is further influenced by his or her personal attitude and temperament, self-concept, age and development, understanding of the condition, and degree of the disorder. As the child grows and life situations change, his or her ability to cope may improve or worsen. For example, an adolescent who is physically challenged may become more optimistic about her condition because she is successfully working at her first job; another adolescent may become angered by his deteriorating condition because he is suddenly confined to a wheelchair.

Nursing interventions to help a child better adjust to a chronic condition include encouraging optimal growth and development (see Chapters 28 to 32), promoting self-care activities, enhancing self-esteem, preventing social isolation, providing health teaching, and aiding the child and family in accepting the child's condition.

Siblings' Adjustment

Siblings' reactions to a child with a long-term or terminal illness may be influenced by a number of factors; how-

BOX 56.2 FOCUS ON . . .

EVIDENCE-BASED PRACTICE

Do Mothers of Critically Ill Children Follow Health Promotion Measures for Themselves?

The caregivers of critically ill children can find their time completely consumed by caring for their child. To see whether such caregivers also have time to look out for their own health, researchers administered a Personal Lifestyle Questionnaire to 38 female caregivers whose children were on ventilator-assisted care. The questionnaire assessed, in addition to the child's functional status, the effect of the illness on the family, family coping ability, and the social support they received. Findings of the study revealed that mothers scored low on personal health promotion measures such as following good nutrition patterns, receiving adequate exercise and relaxation, and participating in preventive health measures such as yearly health examinations. Inadequate personal health promotion was most evident when both the child's functional score and family coping scores were low. The researchers concluded that nurses could help mothers better maintain their own health during their children's illnesses by teaching better coping skills.

This is an important study for nurses, because it accentuates how time-consuming the care of chronically ill children is for parents. It is an alert that parents may need counseling to maintain a life for themselves even as they give that care.

Source: Kuster, P. A., et al. (2004). Factors influencing health promoting activities of mothers caring for ventilator-assisted children. *Journal of Pediatric Nursing: Nursing Care of Children and Families*, *19*(4), 276–287.

ever, their reactions are most profoundly affected by the reactions and perceptions of the parents. Without counseling, they may react with jealousy, anger, hostility, resentment, competition, guilt, or withdrawal. They may feel that they take second place to the child who needs more care. These reactions are common when parents focus most of their attention on the ill child, allow the health problem and its treatment to disrupt family life significantly, or grant the ill child special privileges and minimal discipline.

With counseling and support, siblings can develop acceptance, care, concern, and cooperation (Guite et al., 2004). Such reactions are common when parents make it a point to set aside time each day for special activities with the well siblings (e.g., playing a table game, walking in the park, teaching a child to swim), carefully explain the condition and the necessity for special care, include siblings in the care of the ill child, provide siblings with respite from care if needed, and establish realistic rules for all family members.

At any one time, the siblings may experience a mixture of feelings. For example, if a boy's parents must take his sister for chemotherapy during his swim meet, the boy may feel both resentment that his parents missed the meet and sadness that his sister could not compete in that meet or in any others.

The Nurse and the Ill Child

Caring for children with long-term illnesses can be a stressful role for nurses (Hopia et al., 2004). To help the parents and child with a long-term illness, learn specific aspects of the child's condition and the possible complications that could occur. Over a period of years, parents become experts on the care of a child with a particular condition (Box 56.3). This can make them grow impatient with health care providers who appear to be unaware of things that they know well. When young children are seen at an ambulatory care setting or admitted to a hospital for care, review with the parents their typical way of carrying out a procedure so that you can continue to care for their child in the same way. As the child grows older, do this same review with the child. On the other hand, be available to show a parent or a child an easier way to do something if it seems appropriate. Frankly admitting to parents, "You're more familiar with Jennifer's care than I am; you'll have to teach me some things" is a refreshing approach; it not only allows parents to feel confidence in you (you are honest), but it also increases their self-esteem (they are knowledgeable people).

Also, you should be familiar with the community resources that are available for children with long-term illnesses. Advising parents to see a dentist who specializes in caring for children with cerebral palsy when there is no one of that description less than 200 miles away, for example, is not only unhelpful but is actually destructive. It raises expectations in parents that cannot be met—accentuating, not solving, a problem.

Sometimes parents of children with long-term illnesses do not adhere well to instructions or do not keep health care appointments consistently. This inability to adhere usually is related to their adjustment to the illness. As long

---

BOX 56.3 FOCUS ON . . .

COMMUNICATION

Charlie is admitted to the hospital and intravenous therapy is started. You notice that his skin where the adhesive tape was removed is unusually reddened. He cries when you touch the irritated skin.

Less Effective Communication

Nurse: Look at Charlie's skin. It looks really red and sore.

Mrs. Circuso: That's from the adhesive tape.

Nurse: Oh, I don't think so. I tape this way all the time.

Mrs. Circuso: I never use it, even on myself.

Nurse: Well, it usually works really well. I'll ask the doctor what she recommends.

More Effective Communication

Nurse: Look at Charlie's skin. It looks so red and sore.

Mrs. Circuso: That's from the adhesive tape.

Nurse: Oh, has Charlie had this type of reaction before?

Mrs. Circuso: All the time. That's why I never use it, even on myself.

Nurse: I should have asked you how you usually do things for Charlie. You've been caring for him longer than I have.

It is easy to believe that a fellow nurse who has spent a great deal of time caring for a child has become an expert in a child's care. It is often more difficult to remember that a parent can easily become this type of expert also. Asking parents of children with long-term illness for their input not only can simplify care but also adds to the parents' feeling of self-esteem, improving their parenting.

---

as denial, anger, bargaining, or depression is functioning (and there is rarely a parent who has successfully moved completely through these stages of grief to acceptance), coming in for health care or evaluation is a major demand. Each visit is more a reminder of the child's illness than a time of reassuring health assessment.

Developmental Tasks

Children with long-term illnesses often do not meet developmental milestones on schedule; achieving developmental tasks can be very difficult. When you are helping parents teach a child who is physically or cognitively challenged a developmental task, such as toilet training or using a spoon, help them to break the task down into its component parts (e.g., reach for the spoon; grasp it; move it toward you; push it under the chosen food; lift it toward the mouth). This allows parents to appreciate that they are asking the child to do a task that, although it looks easy, actually encompasses 20 or more coordinated motions. Helping them learn this technique enables them to be patient in teaching all tasks in future years (Ygge & Arnetz, 2004).

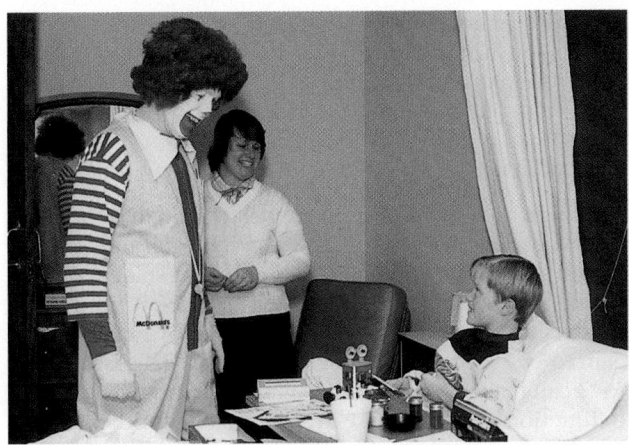

FIGURE 56.2 Ronald McDonald, a familiar face to many children, visits a young boy with a long-term illness. This interaction helps him keep active and in touch with usual events during hospitalization. (© Bob Kramer.)

Ways to help children who are physically challenged achieve developmental tasks are discussed in Chapters 28 to 32. These include exposing them to normal events during a hospital stay or an ambulatory health care visit (Fig. 56.2).

Education

Children with a long-term illness often need special education programs or at least separate hours of individualized instruction to achieve in school. Most of these children benefit from preschool programs; these programs offer them a head start on school adjustment and learning. Children with a long-term illness tend to miss school more often than do their healthier classmates because of health care visits, and exacerbations of the illness can easily cause them to fall behind in school unless individualized plans to keep them with their school group are made. By federal law (Public Law 99-457, Education of the Handicapped Amendment), a school system must provide educational opportunities in the least structured setting possible for physically and cognitively challenged children, beginning with preschool. You may have to be a strong child advocate to see that the best educational program available is being provided for an individual child.

Home Care

Most children with a long-term illness receive care at home today (Frierdich et al., 2003). Planning for this care is discussed in Chapter 35. Important aspects to consider include the best school setting (home or away?), ways to involve the family in community activities, ways to include the child in a play group (children as young as preschool age may not choose an ill child as a playmate), how much self-care the child can achieve, and future plans, such as preparing a child for puberty or college.

Many parents today seek complementary or alternative therapies for children with long-term illnesses. Ask what therapies and medications they are using, to document the full extent of treatment that the child is receiving.

What If... You arrange for Charlie's mother to spend an afternoon shopping so she can have some respite time away from her ill child, and she spends the time cleaning her kitchen cupboards instead? How would you respond? Would you consider this a good use of respite time?

THE CHILD WHO IS TERMINALLY ILL

Death comes suddenly to some families, such as when an adolescent commits suicide or is killed in an automobile accident, providing no time for parents to prepare for the death (Kalischuk & Hayes, 2003–2004). Most children die after a terminal illness, however, so steps can be taken to help prepare parents for the coming death. This is one of the hardest tasks in nursing. Most people are raised to accept the fact that elderly people die, but they have also lived a long life. Most people can accept the death of middle-aged people with the same philosophy—they experienced at least a portion of their life. It is often more difficult to accept the death of children because they have had so little opportunity to live. This can make it so difficult to work though your own feelings about a child's dying that you can find it hard to care for the child or support the parents.

Parental Grief Responses

Although reactions to learning that a child has a terminal illness are strongly culturally influenced, each family reacts in a unique way. Being aware of the usual grief response that occurs in anticipation of a child's death helps in recognizing a response as grief and supporting a family through this very difficult period.

Denial

A parent's usual response to the diagnosis of a terminal illness in a child is denial, the first stage of grief (see Table 56.1). Although people are aware that children die, most proceed through life thinking, "It won't happen to my child." When it does, they respond with disbelief or denial. The likelihood of this response is enhanced by the fact that many terminal illnesses, such as brain tumor or leukemia, begin insidiously ("How can a few black-and-blue marks on her arms be the symptoms of a potentially terminal disease?").

How the parents handle this initial disbelief has a great deal to do with their relationship with health care personnel. If they have trusted health care personnel up to this point, they may be able to accept the diagnosis without questioning any further. If they do not have this relationship, they may feel the need to obtain a second opinion. This often involves considerable expense, but for many parents it is a necessary step in moving past this first reaction. Parents who feel a need for a third, fourth, or fifth opinion may be having an unusually difficult time resolving a "Surely not me" response. They need a factual explanation of why it is certain that their child has this disease, such as a copy of the blood report or the pathologist's biopsy report. They need time to talk about how they feel. Only after people can grasp that the illness is definitely present can they begin to accept that the disease will ultimately prove fatal.

During this stage of denial, parents' actions may be inappropriate to the child's condition. They may talk of an "upset stomach from the flu" when the child is vomiting blood or "his cold" when the child has cystic fibrosis. It is easy to view such denial as a step that should be hurried, because parents cannot begin to deal with the problem as long as they deny that there is a problem. This is true, but neither can they deal with a problem when it hurts as much as this does. Denial is a temporary pain-relief measure that is a necessary step on the way to acceptance.

Anger

Parents can be expected to enter a stage of anger soon—a change from "Surely not me" to "It's not right that this is happening to me." When parents are angry about a diagnosis, they may be unable to direct their anger appropriately. They may find themselves angry with the child (scolding him or her for crying during a painful procedure). One parent may be angry with the other parent (criticizing him or her for reckless driving or for eating a fattening food for lunch). They may be angry with you (for not answering the child's call light immediately). They may be angry with the medical, radiography, laboratory, and dietary staff or with the entire health care system. It can be difficult to react to this kind of angry attack, because it seems unjustified (after all, you came as soon as you could). Be certain that your first reaction is not to be angry in return. This could result in your avoiding the child's room for the rest of the day, so as not to undergo that kind of unfair criticism again, and therefore not meeting the child's basic need to have support people around him or her.

A more therapeutic reaction is to accept this angry response as the stage of grief that it is and respond accordingly: "I'm sorry it seemed to take me so long to answer your call bell, but you seem angry about more than just the light. Would it help to talk about it?"

Parents may "shop" for another health care provider during the stage of anger, although their reaction will depend to a great extent on their experience with death in the past and the meaning this child has to them. Because grandparents live longer today, for some parents fatal illness in a child is their first contact with death. Another influential factor is that different children mean different things to parents. A child born to them at a happy time can represent all that is good and happy in their life, so loss of that child could also mean loss of all the joy the child represents.

When you ask grieving parents to talk, therefore, they may talk not about the child, but about how they felt when a parent died, how hard their job is for them, or how they feel their marriage is failing. This is part of grief: gathering resources, reworking stress from the past, and arming themselves to face stress in the near future. Parents often receive support from other parents on the hospital unit whose children also are terminally ill. They are helped by seeing parents of other children adjusting to approaching death—or, if not adjusting, at least functioning in what passes for a normal manner.

Bargaining

Although not everyone progresses through a grief response in a linear fashion, instead going back and forth between stages, bargaining is often the next stage to occur. Bargaining is an intermediate step in grief, a time when parents try to correct what is happening by making a bargain to be better people (a change from "This isn't right" to "I can make it right"). They vow to be better people or to function in a different way in exchange for their child's life. When parents realize that bargaining is ineffective, they are at a very low point: they have been let down not only by health care providers, but also by the superior power with whom they tried to bargain. They may need more support after bargaining fails than at any other point.

Depression

When parents have passed through stages of denial, anger, and bargaining, a further step occurs: developing awareness of the true meaning of what is happening, with accompanying depression. This is a change from "I can make it not happen" to "It is happening." Behavior such as crying is the most common sign that this stage has been reached. Parents may ask more questions about care, procedures, or medications than before. Be careful that you do not interpret this questioning as criticism. Parents are asking why a child must have continuous dialysis not to criticize care, but because this is the first time they are fully aware of its serious implication.

Parents may work through the expected loss of a child by talking about their plans for the child, the kind of child he or she was, or how the child was doing in school. They may suddenly shower him or her with expensive gifts or trips. They may have a great deal of difficulty leaving the child after visiting hours. On the surface, this reaction appears to be a step backward (they were accepting the diagnosis so well; now they seem demanding and overwhelmed by it). Actually, this is the first time they have actually begun to appreciate the diagnosis and what it means.

At about this stage, parents need to think about preparing other children in the family for the death of the ill child. If the ill child is hospitalized and siblings are not allowed to visit, they may interpret this as meaning that death is such a horrible sight that they are not allowed to be exposed to it, rather than that visiting is against the hospital rules. You may need to advocate for sibling visitation to overcome this concern.

Some siblings feel responsible for the death of the ill child. They may have wished the child dead, for example, so that they could have a room all by themselves or so that they could have the child's bicycle. They were told not to wrestle with the ill sibling, and they did anyway. These children need reassurance that wishing for something does not make it come true, and that the sibling's death is uncontrollable: it will happen no matter what they or their parents did or will do.

Acceptance

The acceptance stage of the grief process is resolution that the child will die (a change from "This is happening" to "It's all right that this is happening"). Few parents reach this stage by the time of the child's death; grief work will need to continue for years past the time of the death until this stage is reached.

Checkpoint Question 2

Charlie's parents are starting to grieve because they fear he will not survive this reoccurrence of his illness. During which stage of grief do parents usually feel saddest?

a. The first stage, because everything is such a shock.
b. The last stage, because they fully accept the death.
c. The fourth stage, as they realize death is happening.
d. The stage at which the child talks about death.

Parental Coping Responses

Throughout the stages of grieving, parents are developing important coping mechanisms to see them through this crisis. They may have already learned to cope positively with their child's illness and treatment measures, but the determination that the illness is terminal requires additional adjustments. Promoting the development of positive coping strategies while being sensitive to the unique needs of each family member is an important nursing responsibility. It may be difficult to determine when a coping strategy is truly helpful and when it has become maladaptive. For instance, seeking information, such as surfing the Internet and asking to have medical library access, is generally a very useful strategy for parents with ill children: knowing what to expect reduces anxiety. Some parents, however, continue these seeking procedures past the point at which information is helpful to them. They may believe that if they look hard enough, they'll discover a way to cure their child (prolonged denial), or they may "overintellectualize" their child's illness and impending death to block feelings of sadness.

Problem-solving is always an effective coping strategy as long as the parents are realistic about which problems they can solve. Seeking the support of others, including health care providers and families with similar needs, is another positive strategy to encourage; providing the names of support groups or individual families (with their permission) who have gone through similar experiences can be a helpful nursing action. Nurses may also need to help parents who are not comfortable accepting the help of others learn how to do so or simply learn how to feel comfortable expressing their feelings to others.

Assuring parents that their child will be kept comfortable and will not die in pain can be extremely comforting. Parents may also be able to cope by searching for the meaning of their child's impending death in philosophical, spiritual, or religious terms. For these parents, body organ donation may be a meaningful way to give themselves some solace that their child will in some way continue to live and contribute to others.

Anticipatory Grief

Parents who have some warning that death is expected can begin a preparatory or **anticipatory grief** phase in which they gradually incorporate the reality of their child's fate into their thoughts. Such anticipatory mourning prepares parents for their child's death and spares them the abrupt, devastating, intolerable grief reaction that comes to parents whose child dies suddenly from trauma, such as a car accident, or from sudden infant death syndrome (Box 56.4).

Although anticipatory grief does not shield the parents from experiencing renewed grief once their child has died, it can be a very useful process for them. A danger of anticipatory grief is that a parent may reach the acceptance stage of the grief process too far in advance of the child's death. If this happens, parents may accept the child's death so thoroughly that they begin to treat the child as if he or she had already died. They stop visiting, or when they do visit, they spend most of their time visiting other children on the unit or sitting in the waiting room talking to other parents. When once they spent time comforting their child, now they may fail to rock or touch the child as much. They may clean out the child's room and throw out or give away toys. Gradually they are drawing back from emotional attachment, to shield themselves from the abrupt, stabbing pain that death will bring.

Children need a great deal of support if this happens, just as they did during the initial denial stage. Parents cannot help that the grief process did not time itself to coincide exactly with the child's death. They need understanding and not criticism for this reaction.

For some parents, when the child actually dies, the event seems anticlimactic. They have anticipated death so long that, when it does occur, they cannot believe that it has actually happened. They may be so used to thinking constantly about their child's needs and having their child dependent on them that they do not know what to do. Some parents are reluctant to leave the hospital this final time. Leaving with the child's possessions is the step that will make the death real.

The Vulnerable or Fragile Child Syndrome

When anticipatory grief proceeds so effectively that parents begin to think of a youngster as already dead and then the child does not die, parents may find that their grief reaction was so complete that they are unable to reverse it; they cannot view the child as they did before. They begin to treat him or her in a cold and unfeeling way, as if the child were not really there but actually did die. Such children are termed **vulnerable** or fragile **children** (Allen et al., 2004). They may develop behavior problems as they grow older (acting-out behavior, such as temper tantrums, stealing in school, shoplifting as adolescents) as if to say, "Notice me! I'm not dead!" They require skilled counseling

BOX 56.4: Focus on Nursing Care Planning

A Multidisciplinary Care Map for The Family of a Child Who is Dying

●

Charlie is a 3-year-old who has had a relapse after 18 months of chemotherapy for leukemia. His parents have arranged for hospice care for him at home. They state, "He's been through so much already. We just want him to die at home, close to us."

Family Assessment
Child lives with parents on their llama ranch. Two older siblings (ages 20 and 26 years) have left home. Parents report finances as "tight." They have no health insurance because they are self-employed.

Client Assessment
Child cachexic. Physiologic parameters deteriorating. Skin cool, damp, and mottled. Pulse rate, 62 bpm and weak; respirations, 8 breaths/min. Rattling sounds noted from chest. Responsive only to deep pain stimuli. Parents at bedside; older siblings (20-year-old brother and 26-year-old sister) absent.

Nursing Diagnosis
Anticipatory grieving related to impending death of child

Outcome Criteria
Parents express feelings about anticipated death; demonstrate positive coping mechanisms.

Team Member Responsible	Assessment	Intervention	Rationale	Expected Outcome
Activities of Daily Living				
Nurse	Assess whether parents have any concerns about child's final days of care.	Stay with the family and sit with them quietly if they prefer not to talk; allow them to cry.	Staying with the family demonstrates caring and concern for their well-being and wishes and offers support.	Parents discuss any concerns they have with care.
Consultations				
Nurse	Assess whether parents would like a final visit from their clergy.	Arrange for visit by clergy if desired.	A visit by clergy provides the family with spiritual support.	Parents state whether a clergy visit would be helpful to them.
Procedures/Medications				
Nurse	Assess whether child appears comfortable.	Provide for the child's comfort, including positioning, turning, changing linen, applying lotion, and alleviating pain.	Providing comfort to the child is comforting to the family.	Parents state they feel child is comfortable.

(continued)

Team Member Responsible	Assessment	Intervention	Rationale	Expected Outcome
Procedures/Medications				
Nurse	Ask whether parents would like to provide final care.	Allow family members to provide care as desired without forcing them.	Allowing family participation in care provides them with some sense of control over the situation, decreasing their feelings of powerlessness.	Parents state they feel they have had a voice in and are satisfied with child's care.
Nutrition				
Nurse	Assess whether child could be hungry.	Child is too comatose for oral feeding. IV fluid prescribed only as maintenance.	Hunger is an uncomfortable sensation.	Parents agree they feel child is comfortable.
Patient/Family Education				
Nurse	Assess whether parents have any questions about what actions they should take when the child dies.	Inform the family about what to expect. Explore their expectations and clarify any misconceptions.	Providing information helps to ease the family's fears and anxiety about the unknown.	Parents state they feel comfortable caring for child in final minutes and immediately afterward.
Psychosocial/Spiritual/Emotional Needs				
Nurse	Assess whether parents need any type of additional emotional support. Question why older siblings are not present.	Explore as far as parents are willing whether support from their other children would be helpful.	Close family members can supply the most meaningful type of emotional support.	Parents state that their other children do not support hospice care and that, although they are disappointed, they are managing well.
Nurse	Ask whether parents have begun "grief work" such as reviewing and preserving memories of child.	Provide the family with opportunities to review special memories or experiences with the child.	Reviewing memories and special experiences provides a positive method for coping with grief.	Parents report they have begun a scrapbook of favorite photos they anticipate will give them solace in years to come.
Discharge Planning				
Nurse	Assess whether parents have made final arrangements for child's burial; responsibility for reporting death to hospice group.	Assist family with making arrangements for what to do when the child dies.	Assistance with planning provides support and aids in grieving, allowing time to be spent with the child rather than on arrangements.	Parents state that they understand obligations for reporting death; have good relationship with hospice group to answer questions.
Nurse	Assess whether parents have contacted a community support group other than hospice group.	If not already accomplished, initiate referral to community organizations as appropriate.	Community organizations can supply long-term support for after child dies.	Parents state they have the name of a community support group and will contact group if they feel need in future.

so that they can feel secure and learn to react effectively with others.

Checkpoint Question 3

Suppose parents are told their child will die, but then the child doesn't die. What is an unexpected consequence of anticipatory grieving?

a. It has no effect, because the child doesn't die.
b. It can disrupt the parent–child relationship.
c. It teaches the child that parents can be wrong.
d. It breaks parents' confidence in their religion.

Children's Reactions to Impending Death

Children's reactions to death are strongly influenced by their previous experiences, the family's attitudes, and their developmental level. If children have little or no exposure to death, it can be a strange and frightening phenomenon. This is often the case when children are reared without pets or older relatives, forbidden to visit a dying relative, excluded from the rites of death, or discouraged from discussing the death of a loved one. To help ease the fear of death, encourage parents to maintain an open attitude, even if it is painful or uncomfortable. Children's reactions to death are also influenced by their stage of development and cognitive ability. Children's ability to understand death and the steps families can take to help their children cope with death are shown in Box 56.5.

Infants and Toddlers

Infants and toddlers are certainly too young to appreciate that their own death is about to occur. If the person who cared for them dies, they experience deep loss and a void in their life. If such a loss interferes with the development of a sense of trust, its implications for the child's ability to achieve warm, close relationships could last a lifetime.

Preschoolers

Preschoolers usually learn about the concept of death when a pet dies or they discover a dead bird or mouse. They envision death as temporary, however, and appear to have little of adults' fear of it. This casualness toward death is sometimes interpreted as callousness. For example, the first response of a child who is told that his brother has just been killed in an automobile accident may be to ask if he can have his brother's radio. This happens because he thinks of his brother as being gone for only a short time, making this a chance to take advantage of his property. This concept is strengthened by children's cartoons, in which characters frequently are killed and then immediately revive and go on with the story.

Because preschoolers fear separation greatly, they are stunned by the death of a parent. If children grasp the concept that they are dying, their major worry might be that they will be alone and separated. These children may need

BOX 56.5 FOCUS ON . . .

FAMILY TEACHING

Guidelines to Help Children Cope With Death

Q. Charlie's mother asks you, "Suppose Charlie doesn't get better? How can we help him cope with dying?"
A. Here are some helpful guidelines for each age level:

- Infants have no understanding of their impending death. Important points for caring for an infant who is dying are to keep him or her comfortable and secure and to remain nearby to prevent loneliness and insecurity.
- Toddlers, likewise, do not understand death. Even though a close relative or friend may have died, they are unable to relate this to what is about to happen to them. Toddlers like routine, so allowing them opportunities to make choices and providing consistent care are the most important measures for them.
- Preschool children probably envision death as a long sleep. This way of understanding death makes them fear separation much more than the thought of dying. Urge parents or family members to spend time with them.
- Early school-age children understand death as separation but tend to view the separation as temporary. After 9 years of age, children are able to realize that death is final. They still are not as fearful of death, however, as they are sad at the thought of being away from their parents and frightened as to how they will manage without their parents. Answer questions about death honestly (no one knows what it is really like, but because it happens to everyone, it must not be anything to be fearful of). It is important to praise children for accomplishments to help them maintain their self-esteem so they can face this coming change.
- Adolescents have adult concerns and understanding of death. They may ask if it will be painful; they may feel angry about all that they will miss in life by dying. They may be concerned that they will need to answer for past ill deeds after death. Providing time and opportunities for them to ask and talk about death is important to help them work through the coming change. Allowing them to continue their usual activities as much as possible helps them maintain self-esteem.

someone to stay with them constantly to reassure them that they are not alone.

School-Age Children

School-age children begin to have additional experience with death, so their knowledge of it as a final measure increases. They may think of it, however, as something that

BOX 56.6

Books About Death for Children

Bradbury, M. T. (2004). *My friend Christopher is dead.* Frederick, MD: Publish America Incorporated.

Breebaart, J., & Breebaart, P. (1993). *When I die, will I get better?* New York: P. Bedrick Books.

Brown, L. K. (1996). *When dinosaurs die: A guide to understanding death.* Boston: Little, Brown.

Davis, C. (1997). *For every dog an angel.* Portland, OR: Lighthearted Press.

Isherwood, S., & Isherwood, K. (2000). *Remembering Grandad.* London: Oxford Press.

Liss-Levenson, N. (1995). *When a grandparent dies: A kid's own remembering.* Woodstock, VT: Jewish Lights.

Millis, J. C. (2003). *Gentle Willow: A story for children about dying.* Warminster, PA: Marco Publishers.

Mundy, M., & Alley, R. W. (1998). *Sad isn't bad: A good grief guidebook for kids dealing with a loss.* Meinard, IN: Abbey Press.

Tott-Rizzuti, K. (1992). *Mommy, what does dying mean?* Pittsburgh: Dorrance.

Weitzman, E. (1996). *Let's talk about when a parent dies.* New York: Rosen Group.

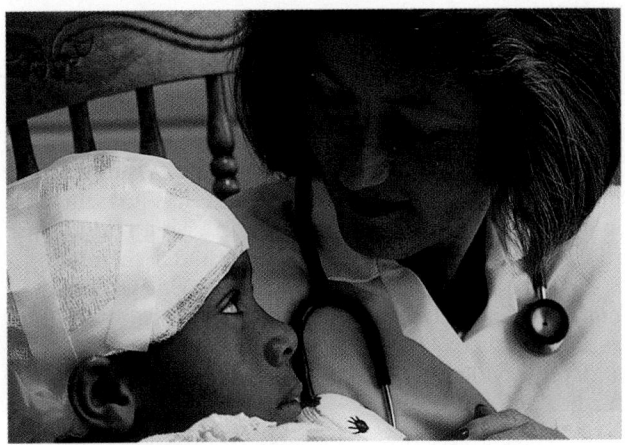

FIGURE 56.3 A one-to-one nursing relationship helps children with long-term illnesses not to feel deserted.

happens only to adults. Children's books tend to deal only shallowly with the subject, although many books that deal specifically with death are available for children (Box 56.6). As children near 8 or 9 years of age, they begin to appreciate that death is permanent. It is the same feeling they experienced when their parents left them at camp or went away for a weekend, but this time the separation will be permanent.

Most children of school age are aware of what is happening to them when their disorder has a fatal prognosis. They may learn from other children on the unit ("Are you the kid who's dying?"), from their parents' strange responses to questions, or from overhearing snatches of conversation about reports or physical findings. Children, however, are accustomed to meeting new situations—starting school, visiting a museum for the first time, boarding an airplane for the first time—and they cope with these experiences very well, as long as they know that someone they care about will be there to support them. Dying can be viewed in this same light, as another new experience for them. They are able to cope with it well if they know that there will be someone with them. If the parents become unable to relate to a child this age because of their grief, a nurse may need to fill the gap (Fig. 56.3).

Many children associate death with sleep (perhaps that was the explanation they were given for a grandparent's death), so they may be afraid to fall asleep without someone near them. They may need to have you sit with them while they fall asleep. The child may need the light left on because he or she may associate death with darkness, not with nap time. Often a child who is dying is moved to the end of the hallway, away from the nurses' station. This move frees the nearby room for a child who needs frequent procedures (a justifiable move in terms of efficiency). However, it further isolates both a child who needs support and the child's parents, who also need your support and your presence nearby. Advocate as necessary for continued interaction with a child who is dying.

Adolescents

Although adolescents have an adult concept of death, they also may feel immune to death. Risky activities such as driving at high speeds reflect this judgment. They may deny symptoms for longer than usual because they believe it is impossible that anything serious could be happening to them. They appreciate time provided for discussion of how they view death and the ways they have contributed to their family even though they are dying young. Continuing to participate in typical activities helps them maintain a sense of control.

Environment for Death

The environment in which children die can influence their acceptance and their family's acceptance of death.

The Hospital

A few children who need a great deal of physical care (have a new tracheotomy, need lung ventilation) may remain in a hospital for care because their family does not have the skill, energy, or money to care for them at home. In a hospital setting, be certain that visiting hours are extended to parents and other family members so that a child is not left alone when he or she needs people around the most. Be certain the child has opportunities to maintain contact with peers.

The Home

Today, most children are not kept in the hospital past the time when it is determined that therapy is no longer effective. Many families prefer that a child die at home, surrounded by family and familiar possessions, rather than in a hospital. Time spent talking about arrangements—such as whom they should contact if the child suddenly becomes more ill than usual, how they will manage periodic checkups, or how they will purchase medicine or supplies—is important preparation for home care. Assess how the family will schedule its time to have some leisure periods free so they can balance the care of the ill child in their lives.

Home care can be an extremely satisfying experience, both for the child who is dying and for the family, as long as safeguards exist for protecting the caregivers' health and for providing good care for the child. This is discussed further in Chapter 35.

The Hospice

In 1967, St. Christopher's Hospice in London opened as a facility for people who wanted to die in a homelike setting while still receiving skilled professional health care. Most large communities today have similar hospice settings, although places specifically for children are still not available in many communities (Hain, 2004). In a hospice, friends and family are allowed unlimited visiting; and younger children and pets are allowed to visit. Children are invited to bring possessions that are important to them. They are urged to choose the degree of pain relief they want. Strong analgesia is often used to make a child pain-free (a criticism of hospice care is that this level of analgesia slows the respiratory rate and actually hastens death).

A basic philosophy of hospice care is that death is an extension or part of life, not a separate entity; therefore, it can be accepted not with separate or awkward rituals but with the same warm concern as other situations in everyday life. For many children, hospice care is furnished as part of home care, so that they are not separated from their families.

Preparation for a Nursing Role With Dying Children and Their Families

Caring for dying clients can be an emotionally draining experience for health care providers as well as family members (Maytum et al., 2004). Although it is best that nursing assignments be consistent so that the child has meaningful support, for everyone there is a point at which he or she may need a respite from caring for a certain child or help in offering support for the parents. This is not admitting weakness but recognizing humanness and a sense of compassion that interferes with client need.

Self-Awareness

Before you can offer support to children in any circumstance, you need to be aware of your own reactions and feelings. To offer support to a child who is dying, examine how you feel about caring for someone who is dying.

Fear. Fear is a natural response to death, because the phenomenon is new and strange. To overcome this fear, put it into perspective. In nursing, you care for many people who have illnesses and experiences you will never have; so, caring for people with experiences beyond your own is not really strange but almost routine in nursing.

People who have never seen someone die are often afraid that the moment of death will be terrifying to watch. Death usually occurs gently, however, with body functioning gradually lessening until it stops in a pain-free, quiet manner. People who have been declared dead and were then resuscitated by heroic measures report that death was not frightening but involved a feeling of exceptional calm and comfort; a number of people have said afterward that they wished they had been allowed to die rather than being called back to their body, because death seemed so appealing (Childers, 2004).

Failure. Some health care professionals find themselves drawing back from caring for dying children because death symbolizes failure to them. This can make children feel as if they have failed—they have not been able to keep their body from dying despite everyone's best efforts.

Remind yourself that death is the ultimate outcome for everyone. At the point that death becomes unpreventable, the only failure that can exist is the failure of health care professionals to help a child achieve death with dignity and consideration, free of guilt that he or she has failed caregivers (Andreson et al., 2004).

Grief

Nursing care is so intense that the relationship formed may be closer than you realize until a child is diagnosed as having a terminal illness or dies; only then do you feel the depth of the relationship. Because nurses and staff can develop such close bonds with terminally ill children, they may experience profound grief when a child dies or no longer requires their care. The grief that accompanies caring for dying children can be broken down into the same stages of grief experienced by the children themselves when they learn that they are dying.

Denial. There is a danger that a nurse who is in a stage of denial may care for children without mentioning that they have more than a simple illness. This includes omitting the use of such common expressions as, "How are you this morning?" to avoid having to hear the answer. Denial may be so extensive that you avoid going into a child's room unless an important procedure must be done. This is confusing and lonely for children, because they miss the normal exchange of conversation and contact.

Nurses sometimes change professions after the death of a child to whom they felt close, because they are unwilling to submit themselves to that level of hurt again.

Anger. Anger may be intense when a young child dies, because the death seems so unfair. Nurses who are angry have difficulty offering effective care: they may perceive themselves as giving thorough, comforting care, but actually they inflict discomfort with sharp, abrupt movements. Anger clouds a nurse's judgment, such as which analgesic would be best to administer. Dying children cannot approach angry caregivers or ask questions; they are left alone and perhaps feeling guilty that they have caused this anger.

Bargaining. Caregivers begin to bargain for life just as children do. A statement such as, "If Tommy just makes it through the weekend while I'm off, I'll spend all my extra time with him next week" is a bargaining statement. Statements of this kind are easy to overlook in your coworkers or yourself. Listening for them helps you to evaluate when a fellow worker is having difficulty caring for a particular patient and perhaps needs to change assignments. Hearing yourself say them should alert you that you are more involved with a child than you perhaps have realized. You need to talk to someone about your feelings or ask for help. Remember that when bargaining fails, people reach their lowest point in grief. Recognizing bargaining statements in yourself helps you to be prepared for the depression that will follow.

Depression. Nurses who enter this phase may be ineffective caregivers, because depressed people are poor problem-solvers (everything becomes a crisis). Nurses may make unwise decisions in their personal lives (e.g., drop out of a night school course, file for divorce) because they cannot solve problems effectively.

Depression is doubly destructive because when you are depressed, your reasoning processes are so distorted that you lose the ability to recognize that depression is the problem. When caring for a child who is expected to die, monitor your usual behavior to see if you are following your usual pattern. If irregularities occur (sleeping a great deal, not sleeping, loss of appetite), assess whether depression has overwhelmed you. When depressed, try to make no major decisions for at least a week, to give your perspective time to change, or you may find later that you have made an unwise, irreversible decision.

Acceptance. The average person can reach a stage of acceptance in grief because he or she is subjected to few true losses in a lifetime. As a nurse on a unit where many terminally ill children come for care, you may find yourself facing loss or death repeatedly. Therefore, a stage of acceptance may never be reached. A caregiver who cannot reach a stage of acceptance is left in a stage of depression and cannot function.

To achieve a stage of acceptance, you may need to modify what it is you are accepting. You cannot accept the unfairness of death in children, but you can accept your ability to offer care that gives death dignity and compassion. Do not compensate for being unable to feel good by not feeling. This is a dangerous attitude, because it also blocks your ability to feel happiness, love, and trust. You may need to ask for a temporary change of assignment to re-establish your perspective. You may need to concentrate on self-esteem therapy for yourself (doing something special for yourself, such as taking an evening to do nothing but meet your own needs).

What If... While caring for Charlie for an extended period, you notice yourself making poor judgments in your personal life (e.g., not following through on projects, spontaneous buying)? Could this be an expression of grief?

Caring for the Dying Child

A child may live for days, weeks, or even months in a "dying phase." Attentive physical and emotional care is essential to the child's maintaining a sense of security and positive self-esteem during this time. It is also essential to the grieving process for both the child and the child's family. Frequent and substantive communication is a major part of providing this care. Children, like their parents, need the opportunity to talk about their fears and feelings about death. Practicing good communication skills when providing any care (e.g., when administering pain medication, starting intravenous lines, or providing basic comfort measures such as a bath) will help to establish a trusting relationship with the child, making the child feel more comfortable about sharing feelings with you (Fig. 56.4). Box 56.7 provides some specific guidelines about communicating with a child who is dying.

The Child's Family

For many children, terminal illness involves a series of hospital admissions interspersed with ambulatory care or home visits. Parents need time during these visits to talk about the problems they are having, not only with physical care (Should the child attend regular school? Could he come on vacation? How many times a day are they supposed to give the immunosuppressant?) but also about how it feels to live with a child who is dying (Are they having any difficulty answering the child's or siblings' questions?). Although many parents are reluctant to tell a child that he is dying, this is probably the soundest course once the child can see that his condition is deteriorating. There is often less anxiety in knowing what is happening than in hearing people whispering or spelling out words around you.

If a child experiences an exacerbation of the disease, parents may again begin an anticipatory grief reaction: anger, bargaining, depression, acceptance. The process will be cut short by improvement, only to begin again at the next exacerbation. For this reason, the parents of a child who is being admitted to the hospital for the 12th time for

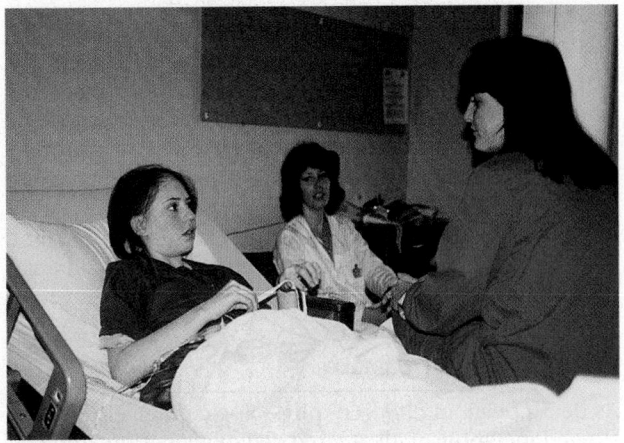

FIGURE 56.4 Good communication skills help build a trusting relationship, allowing a child to share feelings about being terminally ill. (© Caroline Brown, RNC, MS, DEd.)

BOX 56.7

Approaches to Communicating With Dying Children

1. Continue active conversation. Children who are dying need to receive stimulation in as near normal a way as possible.
2. Use moments of silence therapeutically. Such moments occur normally just as speech occurs normally. Do not feel you have to chatter to fill quiet intervals.
3. Use the words *death* and *dying* as appropriate in conversation. Trying to avoid a word makes interchanges awkward. Statements such as, "These flowers are dying," "That's a dead-end job," or "I'm dying to try that" may make it acceptable for the child you are caring for to voice for the first time what is happening to him or her—"I'm dying, too; let me tell you about dead-ending."
4. Preserve dying children's defenses. If they are using denial or bargaining, do not try to push them to the next step of grieving by confrontation. Children will move on to the next step when they are psychologically ready.
5. Remember that many children assume that they will die at night. Therefore, night is "owned" by the dying. A child may talk more freely at night about fears or an unfulfilled life ambition than during the day. Children may also be more frightened at night and enjoy having someone sit beside them until they fall asleep.
6. Be supportive, not trite. A statement such as "All of us are dying" is true but not helpful. A supportive statement such as, "This must be hard for you" is better.
7. Be aware that not all people's beliefs are the same as yours. A statement such as, "God works in mysterious ways" may explain death for you but can be little comfort to a family who does not envision that as true. A statement such as, "I believe God made some children die early to teach us to appreciate life" may evoke an angry response such as, "Who could believe in a God like that?" rather than be comforting.

---

leukemia may be in the same stage of grief as the parents of a child with newly diagnosed leukemia.

During health supervision visits, ask parents how other children in the family are managing. The parents may need to be reminded that, although the dying child does need a lot of their time, other children find this illness in a sibling even more baffling than do the parents. When the ill child dies, siblings need active support to help them grieve.

The Onset of Death

As death nears in children, physiologic changes, such as slowed metabolism, decreased cell oxygenation, and cell dysfunction, begin to occur.

Stroke volume of the heart decreases, so the power to circulate blood is reduced. The child's skin feels cool and appears mottled or cyanotic because blood can no longer be pushed to distal sites. Just before death, blood will begin to pool in the dependent body parts, making them appear purple. As circulation fails, absorption of a drug from a muscle becomes virtually impossible; an emergency drug would need to be administered intravenously to have an effect.

As peripheral circulation fails, less heat is lost from the body, and the temperature rises. The child's body may compensate for this by increased perspiration to increase heat loss through evaporation. This makes the child's skin feel cool and damp. You may need to change linens frequently because of the increased moisture on the skin. Because perfusion of distal body parts is impaired, turn the child slowly to allow the circulatory system to accommodate to the change in position.

Slowed respiration leads to increased secretions in the lungs and the appearance of rales, the sound of air being pulled through fluid in the alveoli. To compensate for a few minutes of very slow respirations, a child may take a number of quick or extremely deep inhalations periodically. Be certain the child's chest is not compressed, so that he or she has optimal lung expansion to do this.

A decrease in muscular function leads to severe weakness and fatigue. More and more, the child maintains the exact position into which he or she was placed. As the throat muscles become lax, the possibility of aspiration increases. Assess a child carefully for an intact gag reflex before offering oral fluid. If the gag or swallowing reflex is impaired, position the child on the side to allow saliva to drain from the mouth, to prevent aspiration. An often-noticed phenomenon is constant hand movement—picking at bedclothes, for example—which probably represents the loss of upper centers of voluntary muscular control. Neurologically, deep reflexes, such as the Achilles tendon reflex, begin to fade.

As children grow closer and closer death, they begin to demonstrate a lessened level of consciousness, although they may remain perfectly alert until seconds before death. Vision apparently blurs, because children tend to turn toward a light. Touch seems to remain intact, because children often quiet to a gentle stroking of the arm or shoulder; they grasp your hand meaningfully, as if touch is appreciated and felt. Hearing remains intact; remind family members and, on occasion, other health care personnel of this. Continue to explain procedures to unconscious children as if they were conscious, because they undoubtedly do hear you. Never make any comment in their presence that you would not make if they were alert. Continue to use the same gentle touch and nonverbal communication motions, such as holding a hand or brushing hair from the forehead, as if children were fully conscious. They may be fully aware of your actions even though they can give no indication of it.

Digestion slows as total body metabolism slows. Constipation due to poor bowel tone and decreased peristaltic action will occur. The abdomen may become distended from intestinal flatus. Dehydration with dry mucous membranes and conjunctivae will occur unless intravenous fluid replacement is initiated. Mouth dryness will lead to cracking and secondary infection and pain; prevent this by frequent cleaning of the mucous membrane with clear water and applications of petroleum jelly to the lips. If the conjunctivae appear dry, ask a physician to prescribe moistening eye drops; keep any crusting at the eyelids washed away so that optimal vision is possible.

Keep skin surfaces from rubbing against one another by using supportive pillows and good positioning. Keep the skin free of urine or feces from incontinence; this prevents the development of painful ulcers. (These are normally not a major concern in children, but they are a concern here because of the lessened peripheral blood perfusion.) Assess for pain (thrashing or moaning), and provide relief with appropriate comfort measures.

Documentation of Death

Defining when death occurs is controversial and involves both legal and ethical issues. Signs of death in a child not receiving ventilatory or mechanical assistance are the same as in adults:

- Absence of respirations
- No audible heart sounds by stethoscope
- No pulse by palpation
- No apparent blood pressure
- Absence of body movement or reflexes
- Dilated, fixed pupils

Death is officially determined by unreceptivity and unresponsivity; no spontaneous muscular movement or breath; no reflex response; and a flat electroencephalogram—again, the same as in adults. Emergency medical technicians make a preliminary assessment in the home or hospice setting, and then death is confirmed by a physician.

Organ Donation

Parents may be asked by their physician or by a specifically designated transplantation team before a child's death to grant permission for body organs to be transplanted after death occurs. This is particularly important for liver and kidney transplants, because it is difficult to transplant adult-size organs into children. If parents decide to allow organ donation, mark this information on the child's plan of care in a conspicuous place, and alert the physician about the decision. When death does occur, the child's body will be maintained by a life-support system to ensure that the organ remains perfused until it can be removed. The donation of body organs may help parents accept their child's death more easily, because they can feel their child has helped another person live. On the other hand, if parents are reluctant to agree to organ donation, you may need to advocate for them. Donating their child's organs is not a practice everyone wants to follow (McCunn et al., 2003).

Aftercare

Before beginning any aftercare for a child who has died in a health care facility or at home, check with family members to see if they want to spend a few minutes with the child or if there are any religious rites they want to complete before the body is transported to the morgue. Some parents need this time to comprehend that death has really occurred. Some people have special prayers they want

to say; others want to say a final, private goodbye. In the hospital, check that the child's bed and room look neat and clean before you ask family whether they would like to spend some time in the room, particularly if a final resuscitation attempt resulted in blood-soaked sponges or scattered equipment.

Remain in the room with the family in case they need your support, but be unobtrusive. Some parents fear touching a child's body after death, but touch is a strong and intimate communication technique that a family member may appreciate being shown how to use. Role-model touching by holding the child's hand or brushing hair away from the forehead as if the child were still alive. Some parents may seem unable to leave the room or to let go of the child's hand. You may need gradually to separate their hands, saying something such as, "I'll always remember Molly the way she was when I first met her—so full of life and always laughing. I'm sure that's how you'll always remember her, too." This helps parents begin to accept the fact that, in more than a physical sense, it is time to let go.

As a rule, crying is helpful for parents. You may need to tell them that it is all right to cry. On the other hand, do not interpret a lack of tears as a lack of feeling, because crying is not everyone's response to death. It is not unprofessional for nurses to cry when a child dies. A parent's warmest memory of a hospital experience may be that a nurse cried as she said goodbye to their child—the implication being that the child made an impact on people other than family.

Autopsy Permission

If a child's death is a result of homicide, suicide, death within 24 hours after a hospital admission, suspected harmful death (foul play), or death in an institution or home where the child was not under a physician's care, an autopsy is required by law; parents have no input as to whether this is done. In other instances, it would be helpful to medical process or to research if an autopsy could be done, but parents must give permission for it. Parents may refuse to allow an autopsy for a child, believing that doing so will protect the child from any more hurt, or out of religious convictions (Box 56.8). Autopsies advance

---

BOX 56.8 FOCUS ON . . .

DIVERSITY OF CARE

The way that death is viewed and the manner in which people express grief differ greatly across cultures. Some people are very expressive with grief; some are very restrained. The manner in which a child's body is handled after death also differs. Some religions, for example, forbid organ donations or transplants. Autopsies are not approved because it is important that children be buried quickly after death. Cremation is not permitted. Being aware that people have different expectations for final care and that grief is expressed differently by different cultures enables better understanding of parents' concerns and reactions during a child's terminal illness and when death occurs.

medical science, so they should be done if at all possible; on the other hand, parents have every right to refuse permission without being made to feel guilty for their actions. You may need to advocate for them.

Key Points

Children with long-term illnesses need continual reassessment because, like all children, their needs change as they grow older. Larger doses of medicine will become necessary; care such as additional muscle-strengthening exercises may be necessary.

Factors that make it easier for parents to accept a long-term illness in a child include having support people present and being told about the child's condition as early as possible.

Long-term illness in a child is often most difficult for parents to accept at times when the child would have been achieving specific milestones of development. Extra support for both the parents and the child may be necessary at these times.

Help children to do as much care for themselves as possible within the limits of their illnesses. Self-care empowers them to be as independent as possible.

Children are about 9 years old before they are able to understand the meaning of death and that it is permanent. A child and parents can be expected to move through the stages of grief (denial, anger, bargaining, depression, and acceptance).

Children and parents are apt to need help to face a terminal diagnosis in a child. Urge the parents and the child to ask for help to see them through this very difficult time in their lives.

Critical Thinking Exercises

1. Charlie is the 3-year-old boy with leukemia you met at the beginning of the chapter. His parents tell you that Charlie's disease has put them through a great deal of strain. What would be important topics to discuss with these parents?
2. Charlie's parents are both 50 years old and live on a ranch; finances are tight, and they have no health insurance. Two grown children have expressed resentment at their parents for spending so much time and money trying to find a cure for Charlie. Does this family have risk factors that might make adjusting to a child with a long-term illness more difficult than usual?
3. You notice Charlie's parents in the waiting room of the hospital comforting parents whose child was just hit by a car and killed instantly; you hear them say that losing a child suddenly is better than what they are experiencing. Why do you think these parents feel this way? What stage of grief could they be experiencing? How could you help them with their feelings?

4. Examine the National Health Goals related to long-term or terminal care of children. Most government-sponsored money for nursing research is allotted based on these goals. What would be a possible research topic to explore pertinent to these goals that would be applicable to Charlie's family and also advance evidence-based practice?

References

Allen, E. C., et al. (2004). Perception of child vulnerability among mothers of former premature infants. *Pediatrics, 113*(2), 267–273.

Andresen, E. M., Seecharan, G. A., & Toce, S. (2004). Provider perceptions of child deaths. *Archives of Pediatrics and Adolescent Medicine, 158*(5), 430–435.

Boling, W. (2005). The health of chronically ill children: Lessons learned from assessing family caregiver quality of life. *Family Community Health, 28*(2), 176–183.

Childers, L. (2004). Death's door, ajar: Nurses who research near-death experiences encourage colleagues to keep an open mind about patients who believe they have returned from the brink. *NurseWeek California, 17*(4), 33–37.

Department of Health and Human Services. (2000). *Healthy people 2010.* Washington, DC: DHHS.

Frierdich, S., Goes, C., & Dadd, G. (2003). Community and home care services provided to children with cancer. *Journal of Pediatric Oncology Nursing, 20*(5), 252–259.

Goble, L. A. (2004). The impact of a child's chronic illness on fathers. *Issues in Comprehensive Pediatric Nursing, 27*(3), 153–162.

Guite, J., et al. (2004). Discordance between sibling and parent reports of the impact of chronic illness and disability on siblings. *Children's Health Care, 33*(1), 77–92.

Hain, R. D. W. (2004). Paediatric palliative medicine: a unique challenge. *Pediatric Rehabilitation, 7*(2), 79–84.

Hopia, H., Paavilainen, E., & Astedt-Kurki, P. (2004). Promoting health for families of children with chronic conditions. *Journal of Advanced Nursing, 48*(6), 575–583.

Kalischuk, R. G., & Hayes, V. E. (2003–2004). Grieving, mourning, and healing following youth suicide: A focus on health and well being in families. *Omega: Journal of Death and Dying, 48*(1), 45–67.

Kübler-Ross, E. (1969). *On death and dying.* New York: Macmillan.

Kuster, P. A., et al. (2004). Factors influencing health-promoting activities of mothers caring for ventilator-assisted children. *Journal of Pediatric Nursing: Nursing Care of Children and Families, 19*(4), 276–287.

Loprest, P., & Davidoff, A. (2004). How children with special health care needs affect the employment decisions of low-income parents. *Maternal and Child Health Journal, 8*(3), 171–182.

Maytum, J. C., Heiman, M. B., & Garwick, A. W. (2004). Compassion fatigue and burnout in nurses who work with children with chronic conditions and their families. *Journal of Pediatric Health Care, 18*(4), 171–179.

McCunn, M., et al. (2003). Impact of culture and policy on organ donation: A comparison between two urban trauma centers in developed nations. *Journal of Trauma: Injury, Infection, and Critical Care, 54*(5), 995–999.

Weller, L., et al. (2004). Chronic disease medication administration rates in a public school system. *Journal of School Health, 74*(5), 161–165.

Ygge, B. M., & Arnetz, J. E. (2004). A study of parental involvement in pediatric hospital care: Implications for clinical practice. *Journal of Pediatric Nursing: Nursing Care of Children and Families, 19*(3), 217–223.

Suggested Readings

Bonifazi, W. L. (2004). When a child dies. *Nursing Spectrum, 14*(18), 24–25.

Ethier, A. M. (2005). Death-related sensory experiences. *Journal of Pediatric Oncology Nursing, 22*(2), 104–111.

Farmer, J. E., Clark, M. J., & Marien, W. E. (2003). Building systems of care for children with chronic health conditions. *Rehabilitation Psychology, 48*(4), 242–249.

Finnegan, A. (2004). Sexual health and chronic illness in childhood. *Paediatric Nursing, 16*(7), 32–36.

Janzen, L., Cadell, S., & Westhues, A. (2003–2004). From death notification through the funeral: Bereaved parents' experiences and their advice to professionals. *Omega: Journal of Death and Dying, 48*(2), 149–164.

Kessler, D. (2004). In memoriam. The extraordinary ordinary death of Elisabeth Kübler-Ross. *American Journal of Hospice and Palliative Medicine, 21*(6), 415–416.

Lang, A., Goulet, C., & Amsel, R. (2004). Explanatory model of health in bereaved parents post-fetal/infant death. *International Journal of Nursing Studies, 41*(8), 869–880.

McMenamy, J. M., & Perrin, E. C. (2004). Filling the GAPS: Description and evaluation of a primary care intervention for children with chronic health conditions. *Ambulatory Pediatrics, 4*(3), 249–256.

Pector, E. A. (2004). Views of bereaved multiple-birth parents on life support decisions, the dying process, and discussions surrounding death. *Journal of Perinatology, 24*(1), 4–10.

Waldrop, D. P., et al. (2004). Life and death decisions: Using school-based health education to facilitate family discussion about organ and tissue donation. *Death Studies, 28*(7), 643–657.

The Rights of Children and Childbearing Women

THE RIGHTS OF CHILDBEARING WOMEN

We must ensure that all childbearing women have access to information and care that is based on the best scientific evidence now available, and that they understand and have opportunities to exercise their right to make health care decisions. Women whose rights are violated need access to legal or other recourse to address their grievances.

Every Woman's Rights

Consideration and respect for every woman under all circumstances is the foundation of this statement of rights.

1. Every woman has the right to health care before, during, and after pregnancy and childbirth.
2. Every woman and infant has the right to receive care that is consistent with current scientific evidence about benefits and risks.* Practices that have been found to be safe and beneficial should be used when indicated. Harmful, ineffective, or unnecessary practices should be avoided. Unproven interventions should be used only in the context of research to evaluate their effects.
3. Every woman has the right to choose a midwife or a physician as her maternity care provider. Both caregivers skilled in normal childbearing and caregivers skilled in complications are needed to ensure quality care for all.
4. Every woman has the right to choose her birth setting from the full range of safe options available in her community, on the basis of complete, objective information about benefits, risks and costs of these options.*
5. Every woman has the right to receive all or most of her maternity care from a single caregiver or a small group of caregivers, with whom she can establish a relationship. Every woman has the right to leave her maternity caregiver and select another if she becomes dissatisfied with her care.* (Only second sentence is a legal right.)
6. Every woman has the right to information about the professional identity and qualifications of those involved with her care, and to know when those involved are trainees.*
7. Every woman has the right to communicate with caregivers and receive all care in privacy, which may involve excluding nonessential personnel. She also has the right to have all personal information treated according to standards of confidentiality.*
8. Every woman has the right to receive maternity care that identifies and addresses social and behavioral factors that affect her health and that of her baby.** She should receive information to help her take the best care of herself and her baby and have access to social services and behavioral change programs that could contribute to their health.
9. Every woman has the right to full and clear information about benefits, risks, and costs of the procedures, drugs, tests and treatments offered to her, and of all other reasonable options, including no intervention.* She should receive this information about all interventions that are likely to be offered during labor and birth well before the onset of labor.
10. Every woman has the right to accept or refuse procedures, drugs, tests and treatments, and to have her choices honored. She has the right to change her mind.* (Please note that this established legal right has been challenged in a number of recent cases.)
11. Every woman has the right to be informed if her caregivers wish to enroll her or her infant in a research study. She should receive full information about all known and possible benefits and risks of participation, and she has the right to decide whether to participate, free from coercion and without negative consequences.*
12. Every woman has the right to unrestricted access to all available records about her pregnancy, her labor, and her infant; to obtain a full copy of these records; and to receive help in understanding them, if necessary.*
13. Every woman has the right to receive maternity care that is appropriate to her cultural and religious background, and to receive information in a language in which she can communicate.*
14. Every woman has the right to have family members and friends of her choice present during all aspects of her maternity care.**
15. Every woman has the right to receive continuous social, emotional, and physical support during labor and birth from a caregiver who has been trained in labor support.**
16. Every woman has the right to receive full advance information about risks and benefits of all reasonably available methods for relieving pain during labor and birth, including methods that do not require the use of drugs. She has the right to choose which methods will be used and to change her mind at any time.*

(At this time in the United States, childbearing women are legally entitled to those rights marked with *. The legal system would probably uphold those rights marked with **.)

Maternity Center Association. (2004.) *The rights of childbearing women.* New York: MCA.

17. Every woman has the right to freedom of movement during labor, unencumbered by tubes, wires, or other apparatus. She also has the right to give birth in the position of her choice.*
18. Every woman has the right to virtually uninterrupted contact with her newborn from the moment of birth, as long as she and her baby are healthy and do not need care that requires separation.**
19. Every woman has the right to receive complete information about the benefits of breastfeeding well in advance of labor, to refuse supplemental bottles and other actions that interfere with breastfeeding, and to have access to skilled lactation support for as long as she chooses to breastfeed.**
20. Every woman has the right to decide collaboratively with caregivers when she and her baby will leave the birth site for home, based on their condition and circumstances.**

UNITED NATIONS DECLARATION OF THE RIGHTS OF THE CHILD†

Preamble

Whereas the peoples of the United Nations have, in the Charter, reaffirmed their faith in fundamental human rights, and in the dignity and worth of the human person, and have determined to promote social progress and better standards of life in larger freedom,

Whereas the United Nations has, in the Universal Declaration of Human Rights, proclaimed that everyone is entitled to all the rights and freedoms set forth therein, without distinction of any kind, such as race, color, sex, language, religion, political or other opinion, national or social origin, property, birth, or other status,

Whereas the child, by reason of his physical and mental immaturity, needs special safeguards and care, including appropriate legal protection, before as well as after birth,

Whereas the need for such special safeguards has been stated in the Geneva Declaration of the Rights of the Child of 1924, and recognized in the universal Declaration of Human Rights and in the statutes of specialized agencies and international organizations concerned with the welfare of children,

Whereas mankind owes to the child the best it has to give.

Now therefore the general assembly proclaims

This Declaration of the Rights of the Child to the end that he may have a happy childhood and enjoy for his own good and for the good of society and rights and freedoms herein set forth, and calls upon parents, upon men and women as individuals, and upon voluntary organizations, local authorities, and national governments to recognize these rights and strive for their observance by legislative and other measures progressively taken in accordance with the following principles:

†United Nations. (1959). *Declaration of the rights of the child.* Geneva: The United Nations. Reaffirmed by the Universal Declaration of Human Rights, 2004.

Principle 1
The child shall enjoy all the rights set forth in this Declaration. All children, without any exception whatsoever, shall be entitled to these rights, without distinction or discrimination on account of race, color, sex, language, religion, political or other opinion, national or social origin, property, birth, or other status, whether of himself or of his family.

Principle 2
The child shall enjoy special protection, and shall be given opportunities and facilities, by law and by other means, to enable him to develop physically, mentally, morally, spiritually, and socially in a healthy and normal manner and in conditions of freedom and dignity. In the enactment of laws for this purpose, the best interests of the child shall be the paramount consideration.

Principle 3
The child shall be entitled from his birth to a name and a nationality.

Principle 4
The child shall enjoy the benefits of social security. He shall be entitled to grow and develop in health; to this end special care and protection shall be provided both to him and to his mother, including adequate prenatal care. The child shall have the right to adequate nutrition, housing, recreation, and medical services.

Principle 5
The child who is physically, mentally, or socially handicapped shall be given the special treatment, education, and care required by his particular condition.

Principle 6
The child, for the full and harmonious development of his personality, needs love and understanding. He shall, wherever possible, grow up in the care and under the responsibility of his parents, and in any case in an atmosphere of affection and of moral and maternal security; a child of tender years shall not, save in exceptional circumstances, be separated from his mother. Society and the public authorities shall have the duty to extend particular care to children without a family and to those without adequate means of support. Payment of state and other assistance toward the maintenance of children of large families is desirable.

Principle 7
The child is entitled to receive education, which shall be free and compulsory, at least in the elementary stages. He shall be given an education that will promote his general culture and enable him on a basis of equal opportunity to develop his abilities, his individual judgment, and his sense of moral and social responsibility and to become a useful member of society.

The best interests of the child shall be the guiding principle of those responsible for his education and guidance; that responsibility lies in the first place with his parents.

The child shall have full opportunity for play and recreation, which shall be directed to the same purposes as education; society and the public authorities shall endeavor to promote the employment of this right.

Principle 8

The child shall in all circumstances be among the first to receive protection and relief.

Principle 9

The child shall be protected against all forms of neglect, cruelty, and exploitation. He shall not be the subject of traffic, in any form.

The child shall not be admitted to employment before an appropriate minimum age; he shall in no case be caused or permitted to engage in any occupation or employment that would prejudice his health or education, or interfere with his physical, mental, or moral development.

Principle 10

The child shall be protected from practices that may foster racial, religious, and any other form of discrimination. He shall be brought up in a spirit of understanding, tolerance, friendship among peoples, peace, and universal brotherhood and in full consciousness that his energy and talents should be devoted to the service of his fellow men.

APPENDIX B

Composition and Ingredients of Infant Formulas

	Calories					
Formula	(Per oz)	(Per mL)	Protein	Fat	Carbohydrate	Comments
Cow's milk	20	.67	80% casein, 20% whey	Butterfat	Lactose	
Enfamil 20[†]	20	.67	40% casein, 60% whey	45% soy, 55% coconut oils	Lactose	
Enfamil premature	20	.67	40% casein, 60% whey	40% medium-chain triglyceride (MCT) oil, soy and coconut oil	Corn syrup solids, lactose	Premature infants
Human milk	21	.70	40% casein, 60% whey	Human milk, fat	Lactose	
Isomil	20	.67	Soy protein	Coconut and soy oils	Corn syrup solids and sucrose	For cow's milk protein or lactose intolerance
Isomil SF	20	.67	Soy protein	Coconut and soy oils	Corn syrup solids	For cow's milk protein, lactose, or sucrose intolerance
Lofenalac	20	.67	Casein hydro-lysate processed to remove most of the phenylalanine	Corn oil	Corn syrup solids and modified tapioca starch	For phenylketonuria (PKU); low in phenylalanine
MJ 3232A[‡]	20	.67	Casein hydrolysate	MCT oil	Tapioca starch, mono- and disaccharide free	Management of disaccharidase deficiencies
Nursoy	20	.67	Soy protein	Coconut, safflower, and soybean oils	Sucrose	For cow's milk protein or lactose intolerance
Nutramigen	20	.67	Casein hydrolysate	Corn oil	Corn syrup solids, modified corn starch	Use for sensitivity to intact milk protein, or for lactose intolerance
Portagen	20	.67	Sodium caseinate	88% MCT oil, 12% corn oil	Corn syrup sucrose	Use in fat mal-absorption states, lactose intolerance (liver disease)
Pregestimil	20	.67	Casein hydro-lysate with added L-cystine, L-tyrosine, L-tryptophan	60% corn oil, 40% MCT oil	Corn syrup solids, modified tapioca starch	Suitable for many malabsorption syndromes

(continued)

Formula	Calories (Per oz)	(Per mL)	Protein	Fat	Carbohydrate	Comments
Prosobee	20	.67	Soy protein isolate and L-methionine	Soy oil, coconut oil	100% corn syrup solids (glucose polymers)	Use for lactose and cow's milk protein intolerance; sucrose intolerance; galactosemia
RCF (Ross Carbohydrate-Free)	20	.67	Soy protein isolate	Coconut and soy oils	None	Contains no carbohydrates; used for seizure management
Similac 20[†]	20[§]	.67	Nonfat cow's milk	Coconut and soy oils	Lactose	
Similac 24LLBW	24	.80	Nonfat cow's milk	MCT oil, coconut and soy oils	Lactose and corn syrup solids	Dilute initial feedings. For premature infants with fluid intolerance
Similac PM 60/40	20	.67	Casein and whey (60/40 ratio whey/casein)	Coconut and soy oil	Lactose	(Ca:P=2:1) For infants predisposed to hypocalcemia; low salt content
Similac special care	20	.67	60% whey, 40% casein	MCT oil, soy oil, coconut oil	50% lactose, 50% corn syrup solids	Premature infants Ca:P-2:1
Similac whey plus iron	20	.67	60% whey, 40% casein	Coconut and soy oils	Lactose	
SMA 20	20	.67	Nonfat cow's milk, demineralized whey	Coconut, safflower, and soybean oils	Lactose	Low salt content
SMA Preemie	24	.80	60% whey, 40% casein	MCT, coconut, and soy oils	Lactose and glucose polymers	Premature infants

* Percentage of calories supplied
† Also comes with iron (12 mg/L)
‡ Mixed as 81 g diet powder plus 59 g added carbohydrate per quart
§ Varies with amount of carbohydrate added
Nechyba, C. & Gunn, V. L. (2003). *The Harriet Lane handbook* (16th ed.). St Louis: Mosby.
Values listed were provided by manufacturers except where indicated otherwise.

Drug Effects in Lactation

Women who are breast feeding should ask their health care providers about the safety of any medicine or alternative therapy during breast feeding.

Drug Effects in Lactation	
Adrenergics	Parenteral *epinephrine* (Adrenalin) is excreted in breast milk; the status of other adrenergic bronchodilators is not known. *Albuterol* (Proventil, Ventolin) has tumorigenic effects in animals; if considered necessary, breast-feeding should be discontinued. Oral drugs used as nasal decongestants (e.g., *pseudoephedrine* [Sudafed], others) are contraindicated in nursing mothers because of higher than usual risks to infants from sympathomimetic drugs.
Analgesics	*Most nonsteroidal anti-inflammatory drugs, such as ibuprofen (Motrin, Advil), are excreted in breast milk, and nursing is not recommended. However, occasional use of therapeutic doses is probably acceptable. Acetaminophen* (Tylenol) is excreted in breast milk in low concentrations. No adverse effects have been reported, and it is probably the analgesic-antipyretic drug of choice for nursing mothers. Salicylates (e.g., *aspirin*) are excreted in breast milk in small amounts. Adverse effects on nursing infants have not been reported but are a potential risk. Narcotic analgesics such as *meperidine* (Demerol) are excreted in breast milk, but amounts may not be enough to cause adverse effects in the nursing infant. Some authorities recommend waiting 4 to 6 h after a dose before nursing. *Alfentanil* (Alfenta) should probably not be given. Significant amounts have been found in breast milk 4 h after a dose.
Angiotensin-converting enzyme (ACE) inhibitors	*Captopril* (Capoten) is excreted in breast milk, but effects on the infant are unknown. It is not known whether *enalapril* (Vasotec) or *lisinopril* (Prinivil, Zestril) is excreted in breast milk. In general, nursing is not recommended while taking these drugs.
Antianginal agents (nitrates)	Safety for use in the nursing mother has not been established.
Antianxiety and sedative-hypnotic agents (benzodiazepines)	*Diazepam* (Valium) and other benzodiazepines should generally be avoided. They are excreted in breast milk and may cause lethargy and weight loss in the infant. The drugs and their metabolites may accumulate to toxic levels in neonates because of slow drug metabolism.
Antiarrhythmics	When these agents are required for a nursing mother, breast-feeding should generally be discontinued. *Quinidine* (Quinaglute), *disopyramide* (Norpace), and *mexiletine* (Mexitil) are excreted in breast milk; it is unknown whether *procainamide* (Pronestyl, Procan), *lidocaine* (Xylocaine), and *flecainide* (Tambocor) are excreted. Potential exists for serious adverse effects in infants.
Antibiotics	Read the labeling on all antibiotics, antifungals, and antivirals to be certain they are safe for lactating women and infants. Examples of those commonly prescribed for women are:
	Penicillins are excreted in breast milk in low concentrations and may cause diarrhea, candidiasis, or allergic responses in nursing infants. *Cephalosporins* are excreted in small amounts and may alter bowel flora, cause pharmacologic effects, and interfere with interpretation of culture reports with fever or infection. *Aztreonam* (Azactam) is excreted in small amounts; discontinuing breast-feeding temporarily is probably indicated. It is unknown whether *imipenem/cilastatin* (Primaxin) is excreted. The aminoglycosides *netilmicin* (Netromycin) and *streptomycin* are excreted in small amounts. Because these drugs are nephrotoxic and ototoxic, the immature kidney function of neonates and infants should be considered. *Tetracyclines* are excreted in breast milk and should be avoided. *Sulfonamides* are excreted and generally contraindicated. They may cause kernicterus in the neonate and diarrhea and skin rash in the nursing infant. *Erythromycin* is excreted and may become concentrated in breast milk. No adverse effects on nursing infants have been reported.

(continued)

Drug Effects in Lactation

However, the potential exists for alteration in bowel flora, pharmacologic effects, and interference with fever workup. *Nitrofurantoin* (Macrodantin) is excreted in very small amounts. However, safety for use in nursing mothers has not been established, and infants with glucose-6-phosphate dehydrogenase (G-6-PD) deficiency may be adversely affected. *Clindamycin* (Cleocin) is excreted. Breast-feeding is probably best discontinued if the drug is necessary, to avoid potential problems in the infant. *Cinoxacin* (Cinobac) and *norfloxacin* (Noroxin) are probably excreted, and there is a potential for severe adverse effects in nursing infants. Depending on the mother's need for the drug, either the drug or breast-feeding should be discontinued. *Isoniazid* (INH) and *rifampin* (Rifadin) are excreted in breast milk, and nursing infants should be observed for adverse drug effects. *Trimethoprim* (Proloprim, Bactrim) is excreted and may interfere with folic acid metabolism in the infant.

Anticholinergics	*Atropine* and others are excreted and may cause infant toxicity or decreased breast milk production. Safety for use is not established.
Anticoagulants	*Heparin* is not excreted in breast milk; *warfarin* (Coumadin) is excreted, but some evidence suggests no harm to the nursing infant. More data are needed, and heparin is preferred if anticoagulant therapy is required.
Anticonvulsants	*Phenytoin* (Dilantin) and other hydantoins are excreted and may cause serious adverse effects in nursing infants. The drug or breast-feeding should be discontinued. *Phenobarbital* is excreted in small amounts and may cause drowsiness in the infant.
Antidepressants	Tricyclic antidepressants such as *amitriptyline* (Elavil) and others are excreted in small amounts; effects on nursing infants are not known. Other antidepressants have not been established as safe for use.
Antidiabetic drugs	*Insulin* does not enter breast milk and is not known to affect the nursing infant. However, insulin requirements of the mother may be decreased while breast-feeding. Oral agents *chlorpropamide* (Diabinese) and *tolbutamide* (Orinase) are excreted in breast milk; the status of other sulfonylureas is unknown. There is a potential for hypoglycemia in nursing infants.
Antidiarrheals	*Diphenoxylate* (Lomotil) and *loperamide* (Imodium) should be used cautiously during lactation; effects on the nursing infant are unknown.
Antiemetics	Although information is limited, most of the drugs (e.g., phenothiazines such as *promethazine* [Phenergan] and antihistamines such as *dimenhydrinate* [Dramamine]) are apparently excreted in breast milk and may cause drowsiness and possibly other effects in nursing infants. Antihistamines used for antiemetic effects also may inhibit lactation. *Metoclopramide* (Reglan) is excreted and concentrated in breast milk; it should be used cautiously, if at all.
Antihistamines	Histamine$_1$ receptor antagonists such as *diphenhydramine* (Benadryl) may inhibit lactation by their drying effects and may cause drowsiness in nursing infants. For most of the commonly used drugs, including over-the-counter allergy and cold remedies, little information is available about excretion in breast milk or effects on nursing infants. Histamine$_2$ receptor antagonists such as *cimetidine* (Tagamet) and *ranitidine* (Zantac) are excreted in breast milk. *Famotidine* (Pepcid) is excreted in animals, but it is not known whether it is excreted in human breast milk. It is generally recommended that either the drug or nursing be discontinued.
Antihypertensives	Beta-adrenergic blocking agents should generally be avoided by nursing mothers. *Propranolol* (Inderal) and *metoprolol* (Lopressor) are excreted in low concentrations; *acebutolol* (Sectral) and its major metabolite are excreted; it is unknown whether *nadolol* (Corgard) and *timolol* (Blocadren) are excreted. *Methyldopa* (Aldomet) is excreted; effects on nursing infants are unknown. It is unknown whether *hydralazine* (Apresoline) is excreted; safety for use is not established. *Captopril* (Capoten), *clonidine* (Catapres), *guanabenz* (Wytensin), and *guanfacine* (Tenex) are not generally recommended, because information about effects on nursing infants is limited. Calcium channel blocking drugs should not be given to nursing mothers. *Verapamil* (Calan) and *diltiazem* (Cardizem) are excreted in breast milk.
Antimanic agent	*Lithium* is excreted in breast milk and reaches about 40% of the mother's serum level. Infant serum and milk levels are about equal. If the drug is required, nursing should be discontinued.
Antipsychotic drugs	Little information is available considering the extensive use of these drugs. *Chlorpromazine* (Thorazine) and *haloperidol* (Haldol) have been detected in breast milk in small amounts. Safety has not been established.
Antithyroid drugs	Nursing is contraindicated for clients on the antithyroid drugs *propylthiouracil* and *methimazole* (Tapazole).

Drug Effects in Lactation

Beta-adrenergic blocking agents	See **Antihypertensives.**
Bronchodilators (Xanthine)	*Theophylline* (Theo-Dur) enters breast milk readily; use with caution.
Calcium channel blocking agents	See **Antihypertensives.**
Corticosteroids	*Prednisone* (Deltasone), *dexamethasone* (Decadron), and others appear in breast milk and could suppress growth, interfere with endogenous corticosteroid production, or cause other adverse effects in nursing infants. Advise mothers taking pharmacologic doses not to breast-feed.
Digitalis	*Digoxin* (Lanoxin) is excreted. However, infants receive very small amounts, and no adverse effects have been reported.
Diuretics	If diuretic drug therapy is required, nursing mothers should discontinue breast-feeding. Thiazide diuretics such as *hydrochlorothiazide* (HydroDIURIL) and the loop diuretic *furosemide* (Lasix) are excreted in breast milk. It is unknown whether *bumetanide* (Bumex) and ethacrynic acid (Edecrin) are excreted. Little information is available about potassium-sparing diuretics, such as *amiloride* (Midamor), *triamterene* (Dyrenium, Dyazide, Maxide), and *spironolactone* (Aldactone). They are not recommended for use.
Laxatives	*Cascara sagrada* is excreted in breast milk and may cause diarrhea in the nursing infant. It is not known whether *docusate* (Colace) is excreted.
Nonsteroidal anti-inflammatory drugs	See **Analgesics.**
Thyroid hormones	Small amounts are excreted in breast milk. The drugs are not associated with adverse effects on nursing infants but should be used with caution in nursing mothers.

From: Karch, A. M. (2004). *Lippincott's nursing drug guide.* Philadelphia: Lippincott Williams & Wilkins.

Temperature and Weight Conversion Charts

CONVERSION OF POUNDS AND OUNCES TO KILOGRAMS

Pounds	Ounces									
	0	1	2	3	4	5	6	7	8	9
0	—	0.45	0.90	1.36	1.81	2.26	2.72	3.17	3.62	4.08
10	4.53	4.98	5.44	5.89	6.35	6.80	7.25	7.71	8.16	8.61
20	9.07	9.52	9.97	10.43	10.88	11.34	11.79	12.24	12.70	13.15
30	13.60	14.06	14.51	14.96	15.42	15.87	16.32	16.78	17.23	17.69
40	18.14	18.59	19.05	19.50	19.95	20.41	20.86	21.31	21.77	22.22
50	22.68	23.13	23.58	24.04	24.49	24.94	25.40	25.85	26.30	26.76
60	27.21	27.66	28.12	28.57	29.03	29.48	29.93	30.39	30.84	31.29
70	31.75	32.20	32.65	33.11	33.56	34.02	34.47	34.92	35.38	35.83
80	36.28	36.74	37.19	37.64	38.10	38.55	39.00	39.46	39.91	40.37
90	40.82	41.27	41.73	42.18	42.63	43.09	43.54	43.99	44.45	44.90
100	45.36	45.81	46.26	46.72	47.17	47.62	48.08	48.53	48.98	49.44
110	49.89	50.34	50.80	51.25	51.71	52.16	52.61	53.07	53.52	53.97
120	54.43	54.88	55.33	55.79	56.24	56.70	57.15	57.60	58.06	58.51
130	58.96	59.42	59.87	60.32	60.78	61.23	61.68	62.14	62.59	63.05
140	63.50	63.95	64.41	64.86	65.31	65.77	66.22	66.67	67.13	67.58
150	68.04	68.49	68.94	69.40	69.85	70.30	70.76	71.21	71.66	72.12
160	72.57	73.02	73.48	73.93	74.39	74.84	75.29	75.75	76.20	76.65
170	77.11	77.56	78.01	78.47	78.92	79.38	79.83	80.28	80.74	81.19
180	81.64	82.10	82.55	83.00	83.46	83.91	84.36	84.82	85.27	85.73
190	86.18	86.68	87.09	87.54	87.99	88.45	88.90	89.35	89.81	90.26
200	90.72	91.17	91.62	92.08	92.53	92.98	93.44	93.89	94.34	94.80

To use this chart: Find weight in pounds in the left-hand column; find weight in ounces in the top row. Where they intersect is weight in kilograms. For example, 10 lbs, 3 oz = 5.89 kg.

CONVERSION OF POUNDS AND OUNCES TO GRAMS FOR NEWBORN WEIGHTS

Pounds	Ounces															
	0	1	2	3	4	5	6	7	8	9	10	11	12	13	14	15
0	—	28	57	85	113	142	170	198	227	255	283	312	430	369	397	425
1	454	482	510	539	567	595	624	652	680	709	737	765	794	822	850	879
2	907	936	964	992	1021	1049	1077	1106	1134	1162	1191	1219	1247	1276	1304	1332
3	1361	1389	1417	1446	1474	1503	1531	1559	1588	1616	1644	1673	1701	1729	1758	1786
4	1814	1843	1871	1899	1928	1956	1984	2013	2041	2070	2098	2126	2155	2183	2211	2240
5	2268	2296	2325	2353	2381	2410	2438	2466	2495	2523	2551	2580	2608	2637	2665	2693
6	2722	2750	2778	2807	2835	2863	2892	2920	2948	2977	3005	3033	3062	3090	3118	3147
7	3175	3203	3232	3260	3289	3317	3345	3374	3402	3430	3459	3487	3515	3544	3572	3600
8	3629	3657	3685	3714	3742	3770	3799	3827	3856	3884	3912	3941	3969	3997	4026	4054
9	4082	4111	4139	4167	4196	4224	4252	4281	4309	4337	4366	4394	4423	4451	4479	4508
10	4536	4564	4593	4621	4649	4678	4706	4734	4763	4791	4819	4848	4876	4904	4933	4961
11	4990	5018	5046	5075	5103	5131	5160	5188	5216	5245	5273	5301	5330	5358	5386	5415
12	5443	5471	5500	5528	5557	5585	5613	5642	5670	5698	5727	5755	5783	5812	5840	5868
13	5897	5925	5953	5982	6010	6038	6067	6095	6123	6152	6180	6209	6237	6265	6294	6322
14	6350	6379	6407	6435	6464	6492	6520	6549	6577	6605	6634	6662	6690	6719	6747	6776
15	6804	6832	6860	6889	6917	6945	6973	7002	7030	7059	7087	7115	7144	7172	7201	7228

To use this chart: Find weight in pounds in the left-hand column; find weight in ounces in the top row. Where they intersect is weight in grams. For example, 1 lb, 4 oz = 567 g.

CONVERSION OF FAHRENHEIT TO CELSIUS

Celsius	Fahrenheit	Celsius	Fahrenheit	Celsius	Fahrenheit
34.0	93.2	37.0	98.6	40.0	104.0
34.2	93.6	37.2	99.0	40.2	104.4
34.4	93.9	37.4	99.3	40.4	104.7
34.6	94.3	37.6	99.7	40.6	105.2
34.8	94.6	37.8	100.0	40.8	105.4
35.0	95.0	38.0	100.4	41.0	105.9
35.2	95.4	38.2	100.8	41.2	106.1
35.4	95.7	38.4	101.1	41.4	106.5
35.6	96.1	38.6	101.5	41.6	106.8
35.8	96.4	38.8	101.8	41.8	107.2
36.0	96.8	39.0	102.2	42.0	107.6
36.2	97.2	39.2	102.6	42.2	108.0
36.4	97.5	39.4	102.9	42.4	108.3
36.6	97.9	39.6	103.3	42.6	108.7
36.8	98.2	39.8	103.6	42.8	109.0

$(°C) \times (9/5) + 32 = °F$
$(°F - 32) \times (5/9) = °C$

Growth Charts

Birth to 36 months: Boys
Length-for-age and Weight-for-age percentiles

NAME _____

RECORD # _____

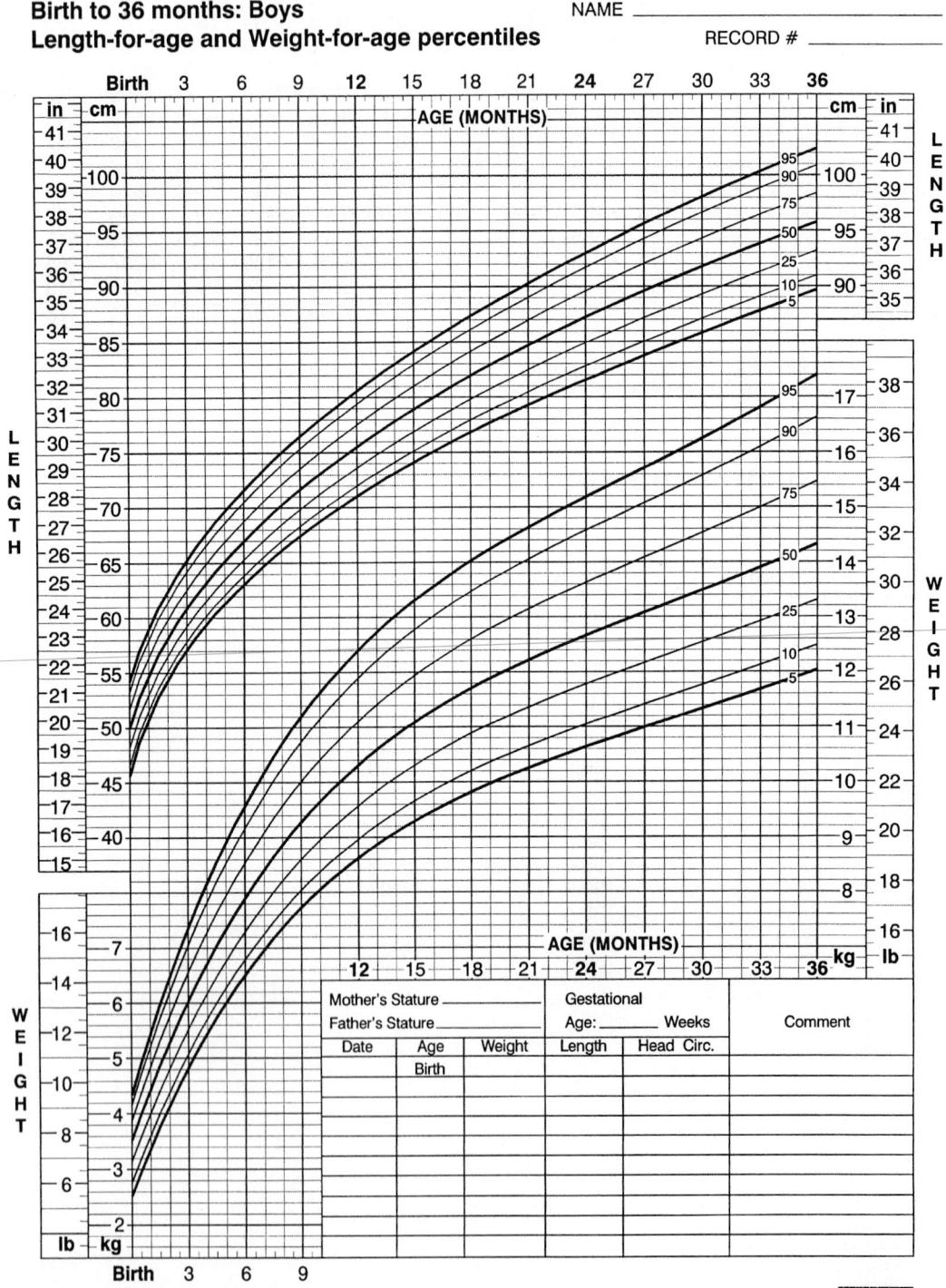

Published May 30, 2000 (modified 4/20/01).
SOURCE: Developed by the National Center for Health Statistics in collaboration with
the National Center for Chronic Disease Prevention and Health Promotion (2000).
http://www.cdc.gov/growthcharts

CDC
SAFER • HEALTHIER • PEOPLE™

Birth to 36 months: Boys
Head circumference-for-age and
Weight-for-length percentiles

NAME _____

RECORD # _____

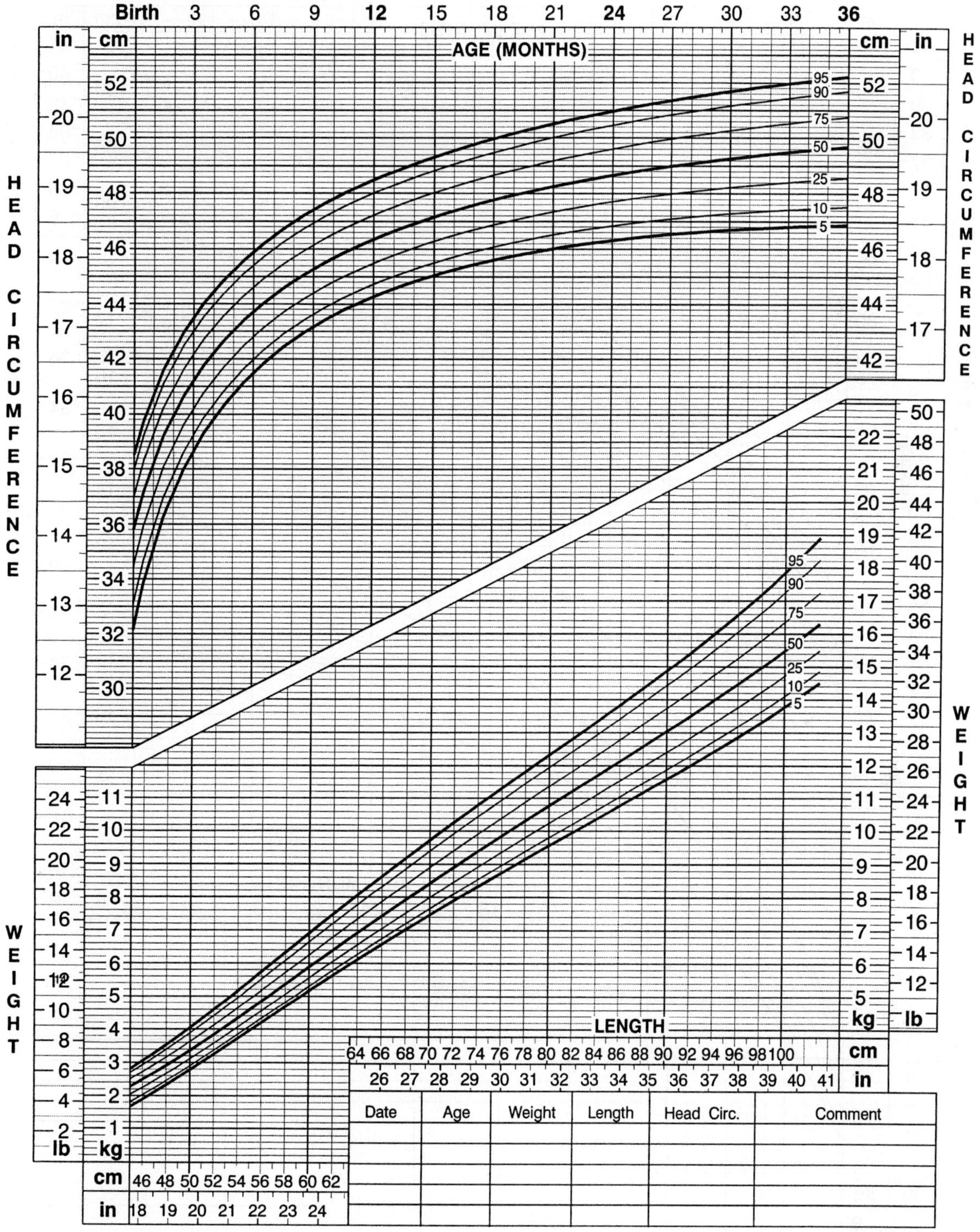

AGE (MONTHS)

Birth 3 6 9 12 15 18 21 24 27 30 33 36

HEAD CIRCUMFERENCE

in / cm ... cm / in

95
90
75
50
25
10
5

LENGTH

cm: 64 66 68 70 72 74 76 78 80 82 84 86 88 90 92 94 96 98 100
in: 26 27 28 29 30 31 32 33 34 35 36 37 38 39 40 41

95
90
75
50
25
10
5

WEIGHT

kg / lb

Date	Age	Weight	Length	Head Circ.	Comment

cm: 46 48 50 52 54 56 58 60 62
in: 18 19 20 21 22 23 24

Published May 30, 2000 (modified 10/16/00).
SOURCE: Developed by the National Center for Health Statistics in collaboration with
the National Center for Chronic Disease Prevention and Health Promotion (2000).
http://www.cdc.gov/growthcharts

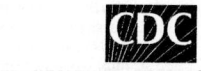

SAFER · HEALTHIER · PEOPLE™

Birth to 36 months: Girls
Length-for-age and Weight-for-age percentiles

NAME ______________________

RECORD # ____________

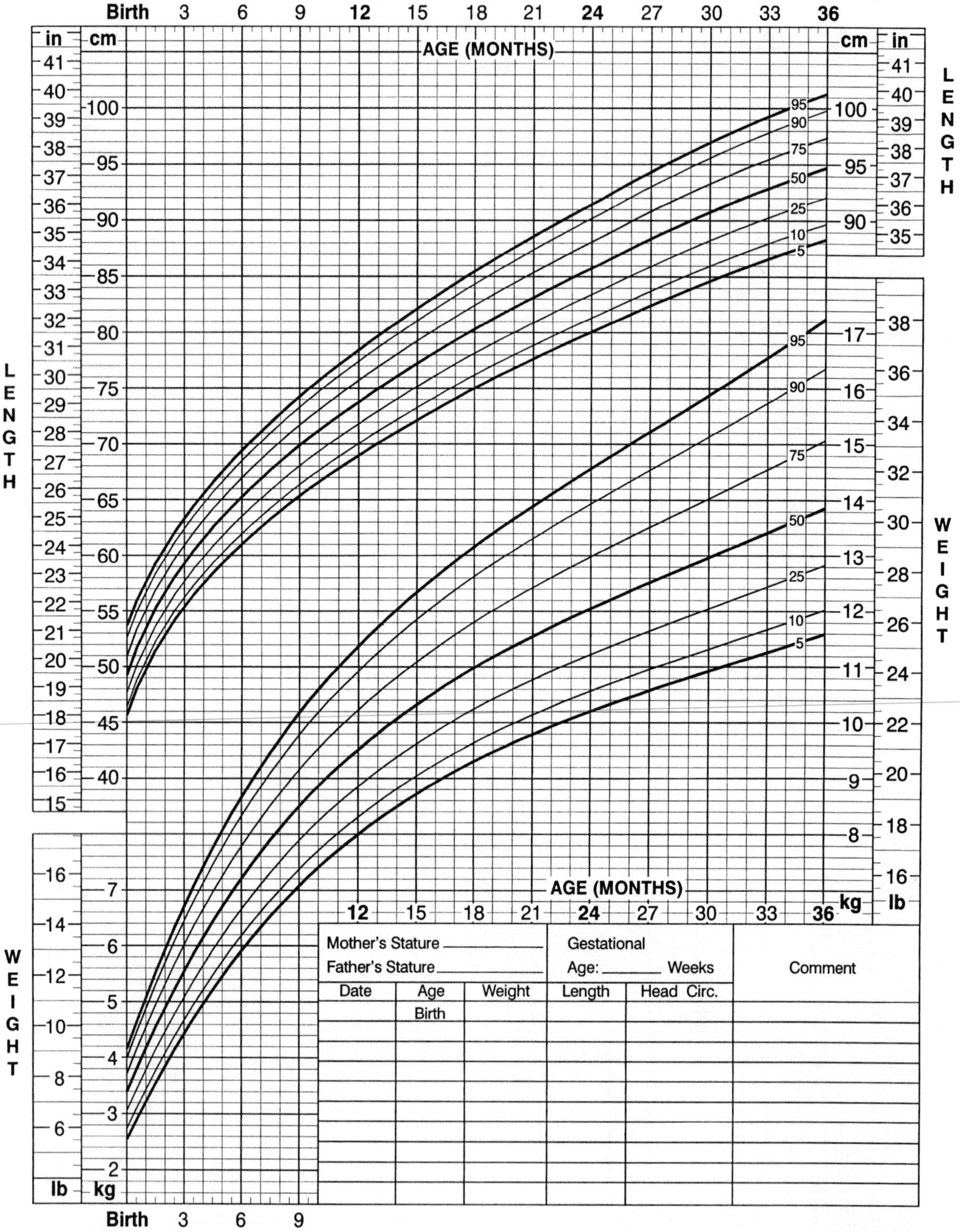

Mother's Stature ______			Gestational		Comment
Father's Stature ______			Age: ______ Weeks		
Date	Age	Weight	Length	Head Circ.	
	Birth				

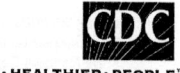

Published May 30, 2000 (modified 4/20/01).

SOURCE: Developed by the National Center for Health Statistics in collaboration with the National Center for Chronic Disease Prevention and Health Promotion (2000).

http://www.cdc.gov/growthcharts

SAFER • HEALTHIER • PEOPLE™

Birth to 36 months: Girls
Head circumference-for-age and Weight-for-length percentiles

NAME ______________________

RECORD # ______________

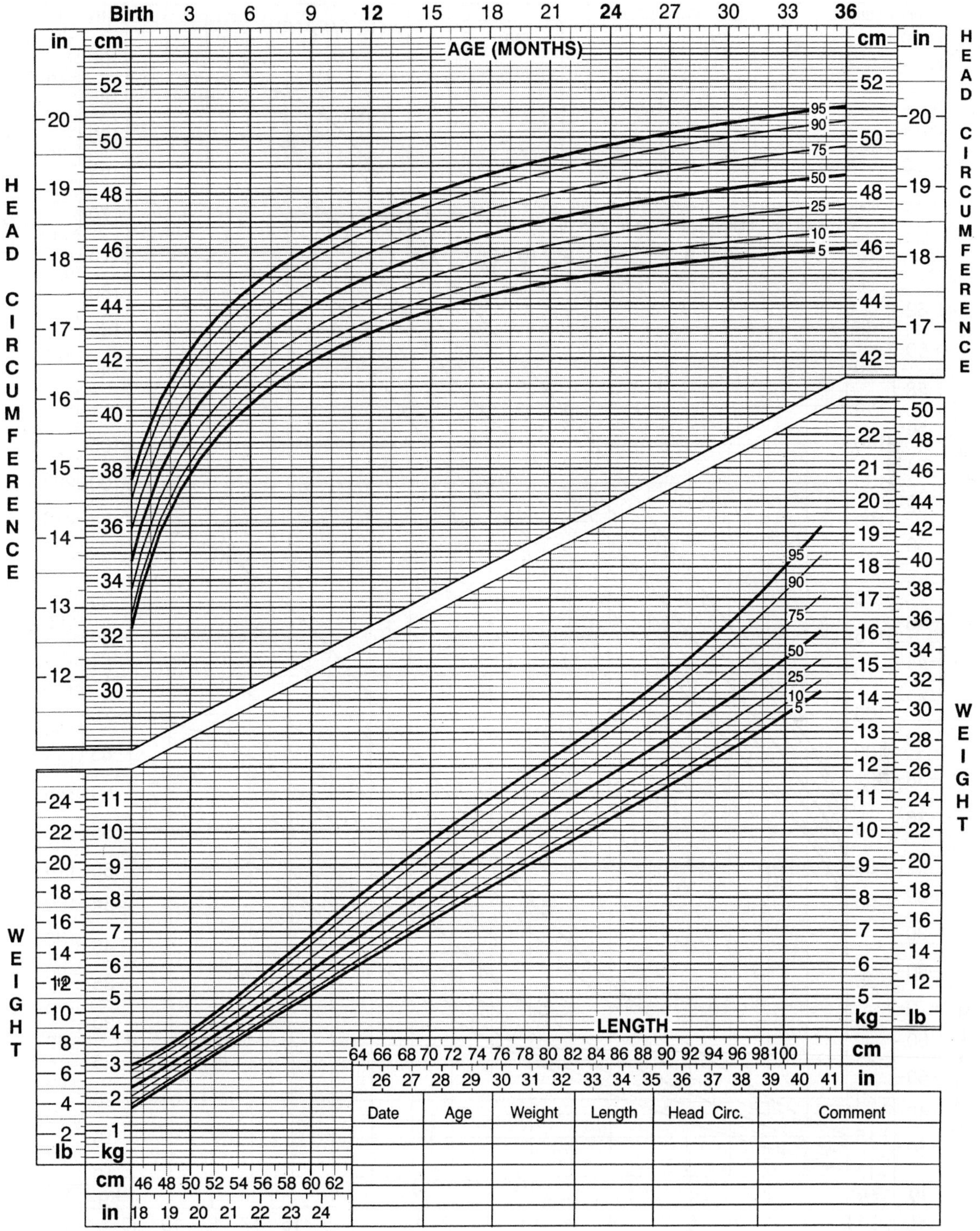

Date	Age	Weight	Length	Head Circ.	Comment

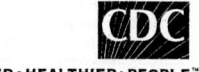

Published May 30, 2000 (modified 10/16/00).
SOURCE: Developed by the National Center for Health Statistics in collaboration with the National Center for Chronic Disease Prevention and Health Promotion (2000).
http://www.cdc.gov/growthcharts

CDC
SAFER · HEALTHIER · PEOPLE™

2 to 20 years: Boys
Stature-for-age and Weight-for-age percentiles

NAME _____

RECORD # _____

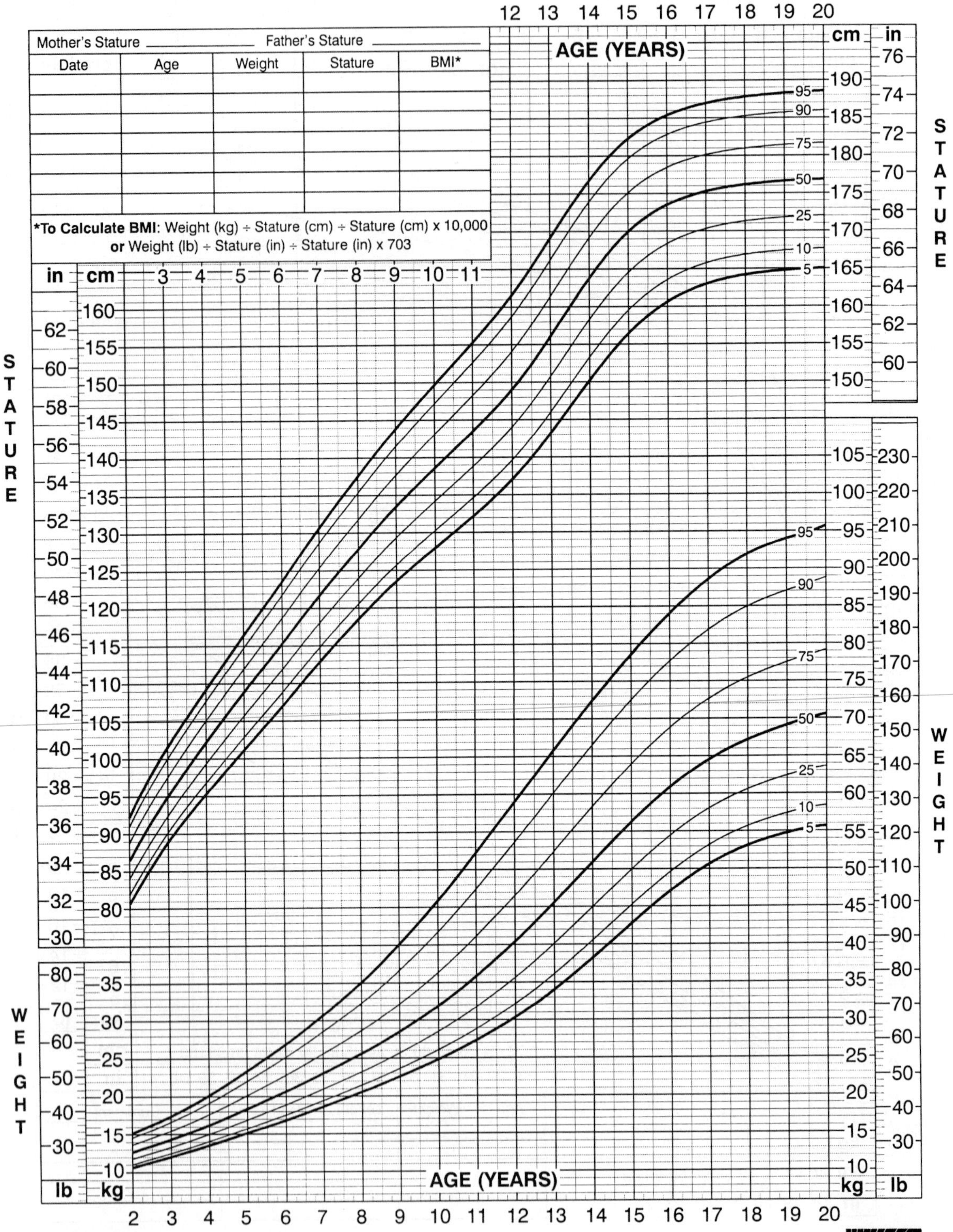

Mother's Stature _____ Father's Stature _____

Date	Age	Weight	Stature	BMI*

*To Calculate BMI: Weight (kg) ÷ Stature (cm) ÷ Stature (cm) x 10,000
or Weight (lb) ÷ Stature (in) ÷ Stature (in) x 703

AGE (YEARS)

12 13 14 15 16 17 18 19 20

STATURE

STATURE

WEIGHT

WEIGHT

AGE (YEARS)

2 3 4 5 6 7 8 9 10 11 12 13 14 15 16 17 18 19 20

Published May 30, 2000 (modified 11/21/00).

SOURCE: Developed by the National Center for Health Statistics in collaboration with
the National Center for Chronic Disease Prevention and Health Promotion (2000).
http://www.cdc.gov/growthcharts

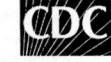

SAFER · HEALTHIER · PEOPLE

2 to 20 years: Boys
Body mass index-for-age percentiles

NAME _____

RECORD # _____

Date	Age	Weight	Stature	BMI*	Comments

*To Calculate BMI: Weight (kg) ÷ Stature (cm) ÷ Stature (cm) x 10,000
or Weight (lb) ÷ Stature (in) ÷ Stature (in) x 703

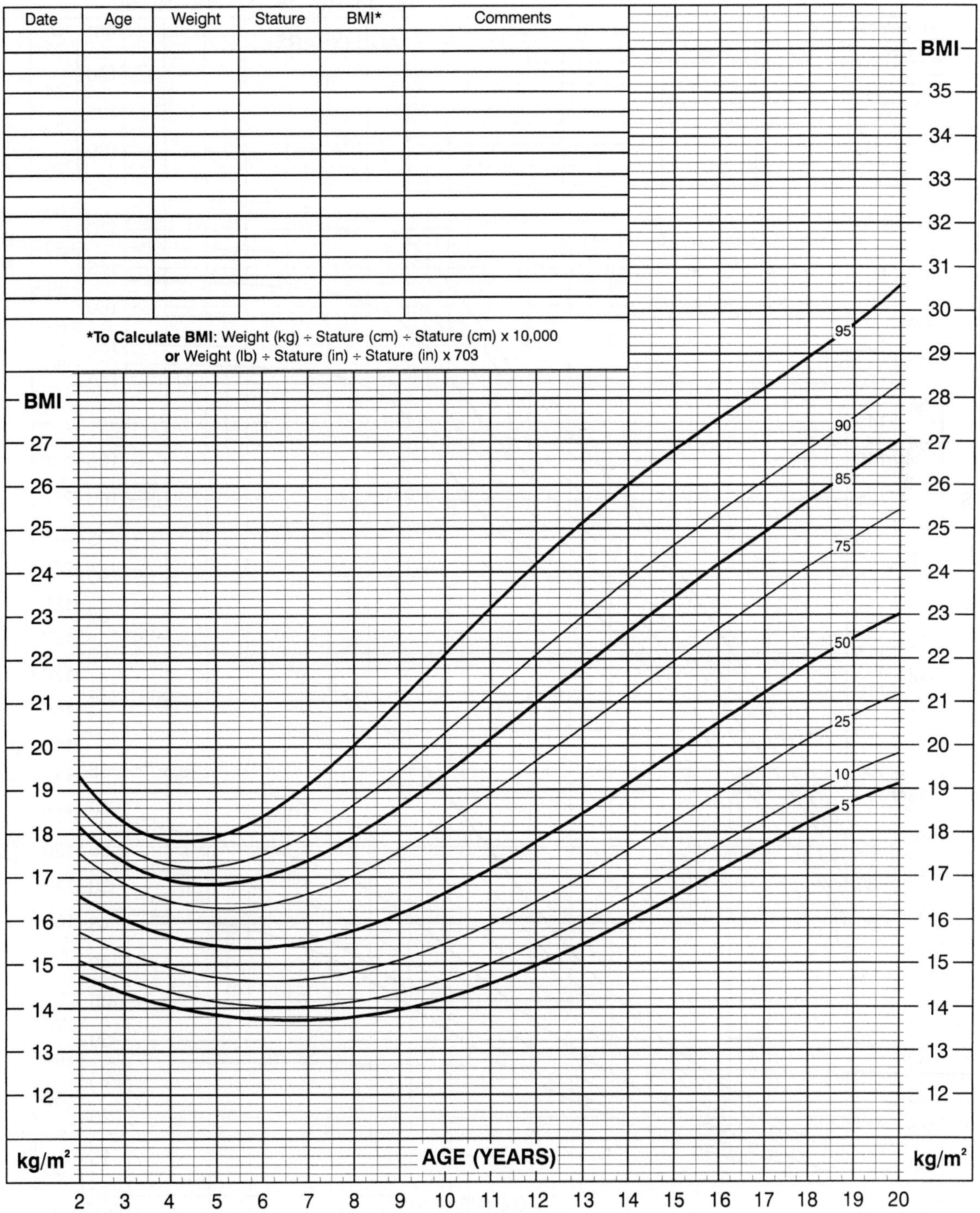

BMI

AGE (YEARS)

kg/m²

Percentile lines: 95, 90, 85, 75, 50, 25, 10, 5

SOURCE: Developed by the National Center for Health Statistics in collaboration with
the National Center for Chronic Disease Prevention and Health Promotion (2000).
http://www.cdc.gov/growthcharts

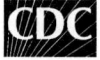

2 to 20 years: Girls
Stature-for-age and Weight-for-age percentiles

NAME _____

RECORD # _____

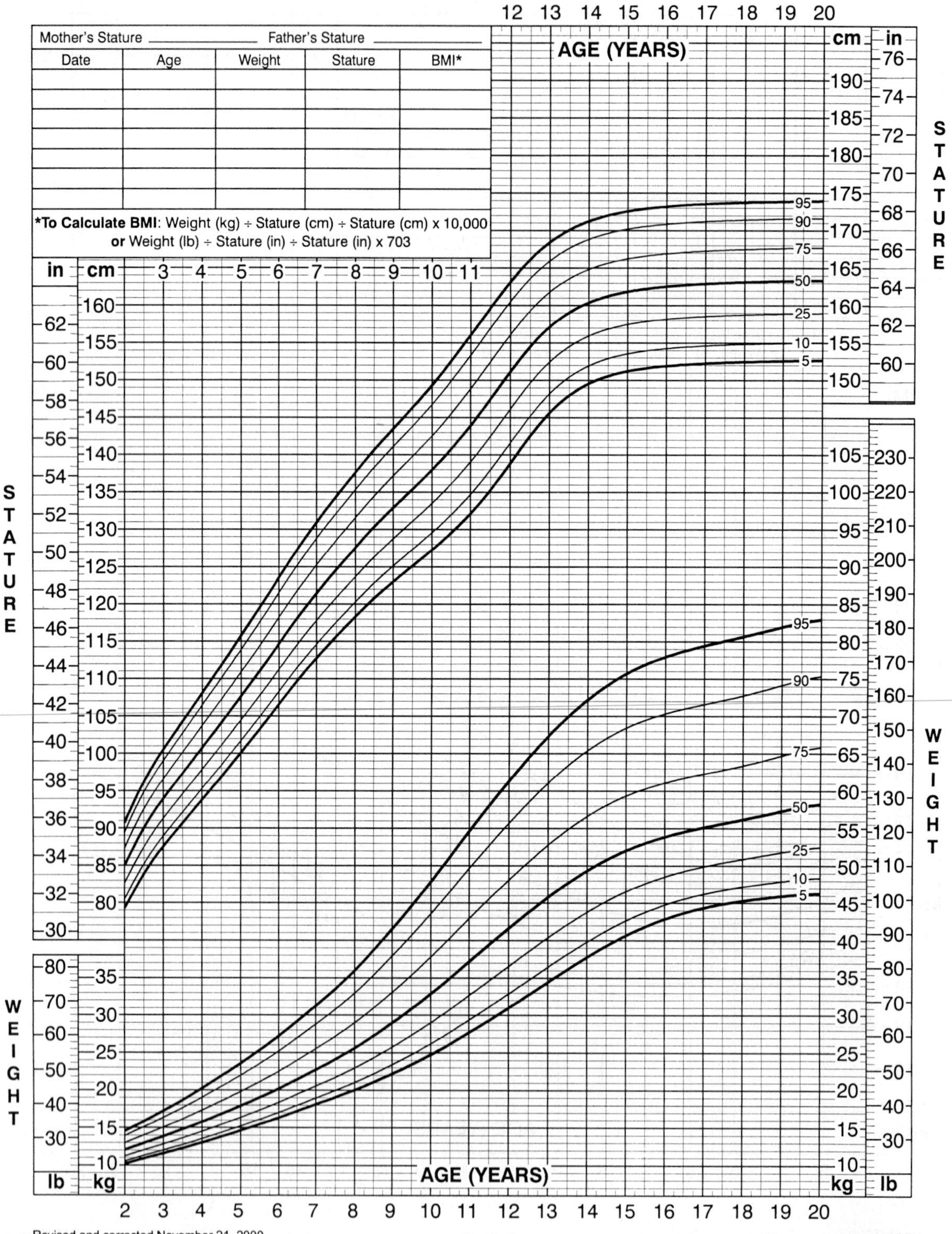

Mother's Stature _____		Father's Stature _____		
Date	Age	Weight	Stature	BMI*

*To Calculate BMI: Weight (kg) ÷ Stature (cm) ÷ Stature (cm) x 10,000
or Weight (lb) ÷ Stature (in) ÷ Stature (in) x 703

AGE (YEARS)

12 13 14 15 16 17 18 19 20

STATURE

cm in
190 — 76
185 — 74
180 — 72
175 — 70
95 — 68
90 — 170
75 — 66
165 — 64
50 — 160
25 — 62
155 — 60
10 — 150
5

in cm 3 4 5 6 7 8 9 10 11
160
62 — 155
60 — 150
58 — 145
56 — 140
54 — 135
52 — 130
50 — 125
48 — 120
46 — 115
44 — 110
42 — 105
40 — 100
38 — 95
36 — 90
34 — 85
32 — 80
30

STATURE

95 — 80 — 180
90 — 75 — 170
160
75 — 65 — 150
140
60 — 130
50 — 55 — 120
25 — 50 — 110
10 — 100
5 — 45

WEIGHT

cm — 105 — 230
100 — 220
95 — 210
90 — 200
85 — 190

lb kg
80 — 35
70 — 30
60 — 25
50 — 20
40 — 15
30
10

WEIGHT

35 — 80
30 — 70
60
25 — 50
20 — 40
15 — 30
10

kg lb

AGE (YEARS)

2 3 4 5 6 7 8 9 10 11 12 13 14 15 16 17 18 19 20

Revised and corrected November 21, 2000.
SOURCE: Developed by the National Center for Health Statistics in collaboration with
the National Center for Chronic Disease Prevention and Health Promotion (2000).
http://www.cdc.gov/growthcharts

2 to 20 years: Girls
Body mass index-for-age percentiles

NAME _____

RECORD # _____

Date	Age	Weight	Stature	BMI*	Comments

*To Calculate BMI: Weight (kg) ÷ Stature (cm) ÷ Stature (cm) x 10,000
or Weight (lb) ÷ Stature (in) ÷ Stature (in) x 703

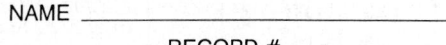

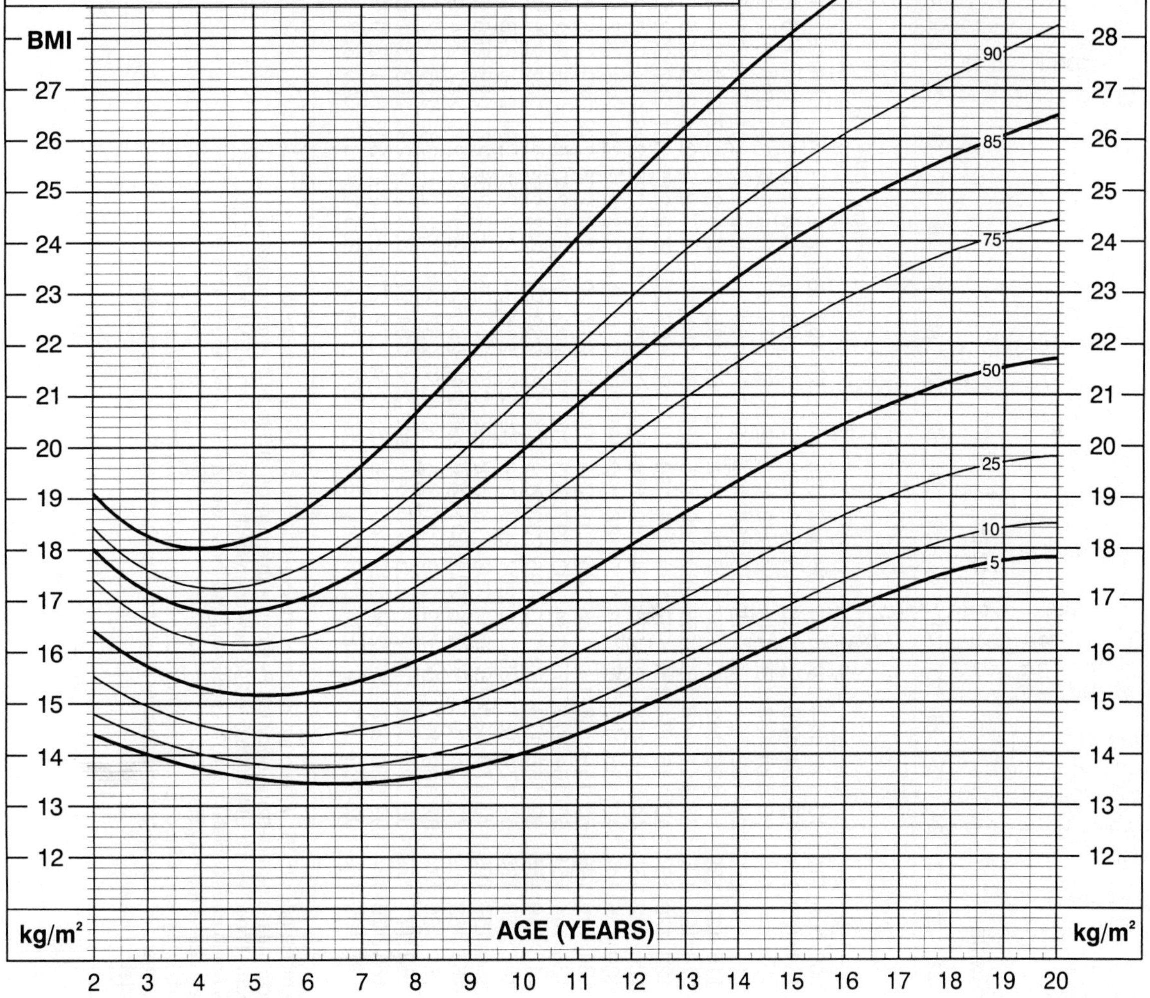

SOURCE: Developed by the National Center for Health Statistics in collaboration with
the National Center for Chronic Disease Prevention and Health Promotion (2000).
http://www.cdc.gov/growthcharts

Body Mass Index Table

BMI	19	20	21	22	23	24	25	26	27	28	29	30	31	32	33	34	35	36	37	38	39	40	41	42	43	44	45	46	47	48	49	50	51	52	53	54
Height (inches)																		Body weight (pounds)																		
58	91	96	100	105	110	115	119	124	129	134	138	143	148	153	158	162	167	172	177	181	186	191	196	201	205	210	215	220	224	229	234	239	244	248	253	258
59	94	99	104	109	114	119	124	128	133	138	143	148	153	158	163	168	173	178	183	188	193	198	203	208	212	217	222	227	232	237	242	247	252	257	262	267
60	97	102	107	112	118	123	128	133	138	143	148	153	158	163	168	174	179	184	189	194	199	204	209	215	220	225	230	235	240	245	250	255	261	266	271	276
61	100	106	111	116	122	127	132	137	143	148	153	158	164	169	174	180	185	190	195	201	206	211	217	222	227	232	238	243	248	254	259	264	269	275	280	285
62	104	109	115	120	126	131	136	142	147	153	158	164	169	175	180	186	191	196	202	207	213	218	224	229	235	240	246	251	256	262	267	273	278	284	289	295
63	107	113	118	124	130	135	141	146	152	158	163	169	175	180	186	191	197	203	208	214	220	225	231	237	242	248	254	259	265	270	278	282	287	293	299	304
64	110	116	122	128	134	140	145	151	157	163	169	174	180	186	192	197	204	209	215	221	227	232	238	244	250	256	262	267	273	279	285	291	296	302	308	314
65	114	120	126	132	138	144	150	156	162	168	174	180	186	192	198	204	210	216	222	228	234	240	246	252	258	264	270	276	282	288	294	300	306	312	318	324
66	118	124	130	136	142	148	155	161	167	173	179	186	192	198	204	210	216	223	229	235	241	247	253	260	266	272	278	284	291	297	303	309	315	322	328	334
67	121	127	134	140	146	153	159	166	172	178	185	191	198	204	211	217	223	230	236	242	249	255	261	268	274	280	287	293	299	306	312	319	325	331	338	344
68	125	131	138	144	151	158	164	171	177	184	190	197	203	210	216	223	230	236	243	249	256	262	269	276	282	289	295	302	308	315	322	328	335	341	348	354
69	128	135	142	149	155	162	169	176	182	189	196	203	209	216	223	230	236	243	250	257	263	270	277	284	291	297	304	311	318	324	331	338	345	351	358	365
70	132	139	146	153	160	167	174	181	188	195	202	209	216	222	229	236	243	250	257	264	271	278	285	292	299	306	313	320	327	334	341	348	355	362	369	376
71	136	143	150	157	165	172	179	186	193	200	208	215	222	229	236	243	250	257	265	272	279	286	293	301	308	315	322	329	338	343	351	358	365	372	379	386
72	140	147	154	162	169	177	184	191	199	206	213	221	228	235	242	250	258	265	272	279	287	294	302	309	316	324	331	338	346	353	361	368	375	383	390	397
73	144	151	159	166	174	182	189	197	204	212	219	227	235	242	250	257	265	272	280	288	295	302	310	318	325	333	340	348	355	363	371	378	386	393	401	408
74	148	155	163	171	179	186	194	202	210	218	225	233	241	249	256	264	272	280	287	295	303	311	319	326	334	342	350	358	365	373	381	389	396	404	412	420
75	152	160	168	176	184	192	200	208	216	224	232	240	248	256	264	272	279	287	295	303	311	319	327	335	343	351	359	367	375	383	391	399	407	415	423	431
76	156	164	172	180	189	197	205	213	221	230	238	246	254	263	271	279	287	295	304	312	320	328	336	344	353	361	369	377	385	394	402	410	418	426	435	443

Calculation of body mass index (BMI) is recommended by the National Heart, Lung, and Blood Institute as a practical means of assessing body fat. Persons with a BMI of 18.5 to 24.9 are considered to be of normal weight. Those with a BMI of 25.0 to 29.9 are overweight. Patients with a BMI of 30.0 to 34.9 or 35.0 to 39.9 are in obesity class I or II, respectively; and those with a BMI of 40 and over are considered extremely obese (obesity class III).

From National Heart, Lung, and Blood Institute (2005). *Clinical guidelines on the identification, evaluation, and treatment of overweight and obesity in adults: The Evidence Report.* Bethesda, MD: National Institutes of Health.

Standard Laboratory Values

PREGNANT AND NONPREGNANT WOMEN

Values	Nonpregnant	Pregnant
Hematologic		
Complete Blood Count (CBC)		
Hemoglobin, g/dL	12–16*	11.5–14*
Hematocrit, PCV, %	37–47	32–42
Red cell volume, mL	1600	1900
Plasma volume, mL	2400	3700
Red blood cell count, million/mm³	4–5.5	3.75–5.0
White blood cells, total per mm³	4500–10,000	5000–15,000
Polymorphonuclear cells, %	54–62	60–85
Lymphocytes, %	38–46	15–40
Erythrocyte sedimentation rate, mm/h	≤0–20	30–90
MCHC, g/dL packed RBCs (mean corpuscular hemoglobin concentration)	30–36	No change
MCH (mean corpuscular hemoglobin per picogram)	29–32	No change
MCV/μm³ (mean corpuscular volume per cubic micrometer)	82–96	No change
Blood Coagulation and Fibrinolytic Activity†		
Factors VII, VIII, IX, X		Increase in pregnancy, return to normal in early puerperium; factor VIII increases during and immediately after delivery
Factors XI, XIII		Decrease in pregnancy
Prothrombin time (protime)	60–70 sec	Slight decrease in pregnancy
Partial thromboplastin time (PTT)	12–14 sec	Slight decrease in pregnancy and again decrease during second and third stage of labor (indicates clotting at placental site)
Bleeding time	1–3 min (Duke) 2–4 min (Ivy)	No appreciable change
Coagulation time	6–10 min (Lee/White)	No appreciable change
Platelets	150,000 to 350,000/mm³	No significant change until 3–5 days after delivery, then marked increase (may predispose woman to thrombosis) and gradual return to normal
Fibrinolytic activity		Decreases in pregnancy, then abrupt return to normal (protection against thromboembolism)
Fibrinogen	250 mg/dL	400 mg/dL
Mineral and Vitamin Concentrations		
Serum iron, μg	75–150	65–120
Total iron-binding capacity, μg	250–450	300–500

(continued)

Values	Nonpregnant	Pregnant
Iron saturation, %	30–40	15–30
Vitamin B_{12}, folic acid, ascorbic acid	Normal	Moderate decrease
Serum protein		
Total, g/dL	6.7–8.3	5.5–7.5
Albumin, g/dL	3.5–5.5	3.0–5.0
Globulin, total, g/dL	2.3–3.5	3.0–4.0
Blood sugar		
Fasting, mg/dL	70–80	65
2-hour postprandial, mg/dL	60–110	Under 140 after a 100-g carbohydrate meal is considered normal
Cardiovascular		
Blood pressure, mm Hg	120/80‡	114/65
Peripheral resistance, dyne/s · cm^{-5}	120	100
Venous pressure, cm H_2O		
Femoral	9	24
Antecubital	8	8
Pulse, rate/min	70	80
Stroke volume, mL	65	75
Cardiac output, L/min	4.5	6
Circulation time (arm-tongue), sec	15–16	12–14
Blood volume, mL		
Whole blood	4000	5600
Plasma	2400	3700
Red blood cells	1600	1900
Plasma renin, units/L	3–10	10–80
Chest x-ray studies		
Transverse diameter of heart	—	1–2 cm increase
Left border of heart	—	Straightened
Cardiac volume	—	70-mL increase
Electrocardiogram	—	15° left axis deviation
V_1 and V_2	—	Inverted T-wave
kV_4	—	Low T
III	—	Q + inverted T
aVr	—	Small Q
Hepatic		
Bilirubin total	Not more than 1 mg/dL	Unchanged
Cephalin flocculation	Up to 2+ in 48 h	Positive in 10%
Serum cholesterol	110–300 mg/dL	↑ 60% from 16–32 weeks of pregnancy; remains at this level until after delivery
Thymol turbidity	0–4 units	Positive in 15%
Serum alkaline phosphatase	2–4.5 units (Bodansky)	↑ from week 12 of pregnancy to 6 weeks after delivery
Serum lactate dehydrogenase		Unchanged
Serum glutamic-oxaloacetic transaminase		Unchanged
Serum globulin albumin	1.5–3.0 g/dL	↑ slight
	4.5–5.3 g/dL	↓ 3.0 g by late pregnancy
A/G ratio		Decreased
α_2-globulin		Increased
β-globulin		Increased
Serum cholinesterase		Decreased
Leucine aminopeptidase		Increased
Sulfobromophthalein (5 mg/kg)	5% dye or less in 45 min	Somewhat decreased

Values	Nonpregnant	Pregnant
Renal		
Bladder capacity	1300 mL	1500 mL
Renal plasma flow (RPF), mL/min	490–700	Increase by 25%, to 612–875
Glomerular filtration rate (GFR), mL/min	105–132	Increase by 50%, to 160–198
Nonprotein nitrogen (NPN), mg/dL	25–40	Decreases
Blood urea nitrogen (BUN), mg/dL	20–25	Decreases
Serum creatinine, mg/kg/24 hr	20–22	Decreases
Serum uric acid, mg/kg/24 hr	257–750	Decreases
Urine glucose	Negative	Present in 20% of gravidas
Intravenous pyelogram (IVP)	Normal	Slight to moderate hydroureter and hydro-nephrosis; right kidney larger than left kidney
Miscellaneous		
Total thyroxine concentration	5–12 µg/dL thyroxine	↑ 9–16 µg/dL thyroxine (however, unbound thyroxine not greatly increased)
Ionized calcium		Relatively unchanged
Aldosterone		↑ 1 mg/24 hr by third trimester
Dehydroisoandrosterone	Plasma clearance 6–8 L/24 hr	↑ plasma clearance tenfold to twentyfold

* At sea level. Permanent residents of higher levels (e.g., Denver) require higher levels of hemoglobin.
From Scott, J. R., et al. (2003). *Danforth's obstetrics and gynecology.* Philadelphia: Lippincott Williams & Wilkins.
† Pregnancy represents a hypercoagulable state.
‡ For the woman about 20 years of age.
10 years of age: 103/70.
30 years of age: 123/82.
40 years of age: 126/84.

INFANTS AND CHILDREN

The following reference values for laboratory tests represent guidelines only, since the reference range from one institution to the next will vary, depending on the laboratory method used. To simplify the interpretation of laboratory results reported in International System (SI) units, conversion factors (from SI to conventional units) are provided. SI base units are the gram (g), the liter (L), and the mole (mol). Other abbreviations used throughout this table are listed below.

SI Prefixes

Factor	Prefix	Symbol
10^3	kilo	k
10^{-1}	deci	d
10^{-2}	centi	c
10^{-3}	milli	m
10^{-6}	micro	µ
10^{-9}	nano	n
10^{-12}	pico	p
10^{-15}	femto	f

Abbreviations

CI	confidence interval
d	day
F	female
h	hour
Hb	hemoglobin
M	male
MCHC	mean corpuscular hemoglobin concentration
MCV	mean corpuscular value
mEq	milliequivalent
min	minute
RBC	red blood cell
s	second
SD	standard deviation
U	unit
WBC	white blood cell
yr	year

Blood

Test	SI Reference Range	Conversion Factor	Conventional Units Reference Range
Adrenocorticotropic hormone (ACTH)	Cord: 130–160 ng/L 1st week: 100–140 Adult 0800 h: 25–100 　　　1800 h: <50		Cord: 130-160 pg/mL 1st week: 100–140 Adult 0800 h: 25–100 　　　1800 h: <50
Alanine aminotransferase (ALT)	<1 yr: 5–28 U/L >1 yr: 820		Same as SI
Albumin	35–50 g/L		3.5–5.0 g/dL
Aldolase	Newborn: <32 U/L Child: <16 Adult: <8		Same as SI
Aldosterone	Newborn: 0.14–1.66 nmol/L 1 wk–1 yr: 0.03–4.43 1–3 yr: 0.14–1.66 3–5 yr: <0.14–2.22 5–7 yr: <0.14–1.39 7–11 yr: 0.14–1.94 11–15 yr: <0.14–1.39	nmol/L × 36.1 = ng/dL	Newborn: 5–60 ng/dL 1 wk–1 yr: 1–160 ng/dL 1–3 yr: 5–60 ng/dL 3–5 yr: <5–80 5–7 yr: <5–50 7–11 yr: 5–70 11–15 yr: <5–50
Alkaline phosphatase	Infant: 150–400 U/L 2–10 yr: 100–300 11–18 yr (M): 50–375 11–18 yr (F): 30–300 Adult: 30–100		Same as SI
α_1–antitrypsin	2–4 g/L		200–400 mg/dL
α–fetoprotein	Fetal: peak of 2–4 g/L Cord: <0.05 g/L >1 yr: <30 µg/L		Fetal: 200–400 mg/dL Cord: <5 >1 yr: <30
Ammonia nitrogen	9–34 µmol/L	µmol/L × 1.4 = µg/dL	13–48 µg/dL
Amylase	Newborn: 5–65 U/L >1 yr: 25–125		Same as SI
Androstenedione	Child: 0.17–1.7 nmol/L Adult (M): 2.4–5.2 Adult (F): 2.7–8.0	nmol/L × 28.7 = ng/dL	Child: 5–50 ng/dL Adult (M): 70–150 Adult (F): 76–228
Angiotensin–converting enzyme	<670 nmol · L^{-1} · S^{-1}	nmol · L^{-1} · S^{-1} × 0.06 = nmol/mL/min	<40 nmol/mL/min
Anion gap [Na – (Cl + HCO$_3$)]	7–14 mmol/L		7–14 mEq/L
Aspartate aminotransferase (AST)	<1 yr: 15–60 U/L >1 yr: ≤20 U/L		Same as SI
Bicarbonate	<2 yrs: 20–25 mmol/L >2 yrs: 22–26 mmol/L		<2 yrs: 20–25 mEq/L >2 yrs: 22–26

Bilirubin (total)	*Preterm*	*Full term*		*Preterm*	*Full term*
	Cord: 　　<34 0–1 d: 　<137 1–2 d: 　<205 3–5 d: 　<274 Thereafter: <34	<34 µmol/L <103 <137 <205 <17	µmol/L × 0.05848 = mg/dL	Cord: 　　<2 0–1 d: 　<8 1–2 d: 　<12 3–5 d: 　<16 Thereafter: <2	<2 mg/dL <6 <8 <12 <1

Test	SI Reference Range	Conversion Factor	Conventional Units Reference Range
Bilirubin (conjugated)	0–3.4 µmol/L	µmol/L × 0.05848 = mg/dL	0–0.2 mg/dL
Calcium (ionized)	1.12–1.23 mmol/L	mmol/L × 4 = mg/dL	4.48–4.92 mg/dL
Calcium (total)	Preterm <1 wk: 1.5–2.5 mmol/L Term: <1 wk: 1.75–3 Child: 2–2.6 Adult: 2.1–2.6		6–10 mg/dL 7–12 8–10.5 8.5–10.5

Test	SI Reference Range	Conversion Factor	Conventional Units Reference Range
Carbon dioxide (CO_2 content)	22–26 mmol/L		22–26 mEq/L
Carbon monoxide (carboxyhemoglobin)	*% total HB*		*Fraction of HB sat*
	Nonsmokers: <0.02 Smokers: <0.01 Toxic: >0.20		Nonsmokers: <2 Smokers: <10 Toxic: >20
Carotene	Infant: 0.37–1.30 µmol/L Child: 0.74–2.42 Adult: 1.12–3.72	µmol/L × 53.7 = µg/dL	Infant: 20–70 µg/dL Child: 40–130 Adult: 60–200
Ceruloplasmin	1–12 yr: 300–650 mg/L >12 yr: 150–600 mg/L		1–12 yr: 30–65 mg/dL >12 yr: 15–60
Chloride	94–106 mmol/L		94–106 mEq/L
Cholesterol	Infant: 1.81–4.53 mmol/L Child: 3.11–5.18 Adolescent: 3.11–5.44 Adult: 3.63–6.48	mmol/L × 38.61 = mg/dL	Infant: 53–135 mg/dL Child: 70–175 Adolescent: 140–250 Adult: 140–250
Complement, C_3	1 mo: 0.61–1.30 g/L 6 mo: 0.87–1.36 Adult: 1.11–1.71		1 mo: 61–130 mg/dL 6 mo: 87–136 Adult: 111–171
Complement, C_4	Newborn: 0.16–0.39 g/L Adult: 0.15–0.45 g/L		Newborn: 16–39 mg/dL Adult: 15–45
Complement, total hemolytic (CH 50)	75–160 U/mL		75–160 U/mL
Copper	0–6 mo: 3.1–11 mmol/L 6 yr: 14–30 12 yr: 12.5–25 Adult (M): 11–22 Adult (F): 12.6–24	µmol × 6.353 = µg/dL	0–6 mo: 20–70 µg/dL 6 yr: 90–190 12 yr: 80–160 Adult (M): 70–140 Adult (F): 80–155
Cortisol	0800 h (or pre–ACTH): 225–505 nmol/L Post–ACTH: twice pre–ACTH value	nmol/L × 0.0362 = µg/dL	0800 h (or pre–ACTH): 8–18 µg/dL Post–ACTH: twice pre–ACTH value
Creatine kinase	Newborn: 76–600 U/L Adult (M): 38–174 Adult (F): 96–140		Same as SI
Creatine kinase isoenzymes	*Fraction of total activity*		*% Activity*
	CK-BB (CK-1): absent or trace CK-MB (CK-2): 0.04–0.06 CK-MM (CK-3): 0.94–0.96		CK-BB (CK-1): absent or trace CK-MB (CK-2): 4%–6% CK-MM (CK-3): 94%–96%
Creatinine	Newborn: 27–88 µmol/L Infant: 18–35 Child: 27–62 Adolescent: 44–88 Adult (M): 53–106 Adult (F): 44–97	µmol/L × 0.0113 = mg/dL	Newborn: 0.3–1.0 mg/dL Infant: 0.2–0.4 Child: 0.3–0.7 Adolescent: 0.5–1.0 Adult (M): 0.6–1.2 Adult (F): 0.5–1.1
Dehydroepiandrosterone (DHEA)	Child: 3–10 nmol/L Adult (M): 6–15 Adult (F): 7–18	nmol/L × 0.2884 = µg/L	Child: 1–3 µg/L Adult (M): 1.7–4.2 Adult (F): 2–5.2
Dehydroepiandrosterone sulfate (DHEA–S)	1–4 days: <52 µmol/L Child: 1.6–6.6	µmol/L × 0.37 = µg/mL	1–4 days: <20 µg/mL Child: 0.6–2.54

(continued)

Test	SI Reference Range	Conversion Factor	Conventional Units Reference Range
	Males		

Estradiol	Pubertal stage I: 7–29 pmol/L
	                II: 40
	                III: >73
	Adult: 29–132
		pmol/L × 0.2723 = pg/mL	2–8 pg/mL
			11
			>20
			8–36

	Females		

	Pubertal stage I: 0–84 pmol/L
	                II: 0–242
	                III: 0–385
	                IV: 73–1101
	Follicular: 37–330
	Midcycle: 367–1835
	Luteal: 184–881
			0–23 pg/mL
			0–66
			0–105
			20–300
			10–90
			100–500
			50–240

Free fatty acids	Child: <1.10 mmol/L Adult: 0.3–0.9	mmol/L × 28.25 = mg/dL	Child: <31 mg/dL Adult: 8–25
Ferritin	Child: 7–144 µg/L Adult (M): 30–265 Adult (F): 10–110		Child: 7–144 ng/mL Adult (M): 30–265 Adult (F): 10–110
Fibrinogen	2–4 g/L		200–400 mg/dL
Folate	4–20 nmol/L	nmol/L × 0.4413 = ng/mL	1.8–9.0 ng/mL
Folate (RBCs)	340–1020 nmol/L packed cells	nmol/L × 0.4413 = ng/mL	150–450 ng/mL
Follicle-stimulating hormone (FSH)	Prepubertal: <5 IU/L Adult (M): 1.5–16 Adult (F): 2–17.2		Prepubertal: <5 mIU/mL Adult (M): 1.5–16 Adult (F): 2–17.2
Fructose	55–330 µmol/L	µmol/L × 0.018 = mg/dL	1–6 mg/dL
Galactose	Newborn: 0–1.11 mmol/L Thereafter: <0.28	mmol/L × 18.02 = mg/dL	Newborn: 0–20 mg/dL Thereafter: <5
Gamma glutamyl transferase (GGT)	0–3 wk: 0–130 U/L 3 wk–3 mo: 4–120 3 mo–1 yr (M): 5–65 3 mo–1 yr (F): 5–35 1–15 yr: 0–23 Adult: 0–35		Same as SI
Gastrin	<100 ng/L		<100 pg/mL
Glucagon	50–100 ng/L		50–100 pg/mL
Glucose	Preterm: 1.1–3.6 mmol/L Full term: 1.1–6.1 1 wk–16 yr: 3.3–5.8 >16 yr: 3.9–6.4	mmol/L × 18.02 = mg/dL	Preterm: 20–65 mg/dL Full term: 20–100 1 wk–16 yr: 60–105 >16 yr: 70–115
Haptoglobin	0.4–1.8 g/L		40–180 mg/dL
Hemoglobin A_{1c}	0.039–0.077 fraction of total Hb		3.9%–7.7% of total HB
β-Hydroxybutyrate	<100 µmol/L	µmol/L × 0.01041 = mg/dL	<1 mg/dL

17-Hydroxyprogesterone	Prepubertal (M): 0.3–0.91 nmol/L
	Prepubertal (F): 0.61–1.52
	Adult (M): 0.61–5.45
	Adult (F):
	  Follicular: 0.61–2.42
	  Luteal: 2.42–9.10
		nmol/L × 0.33 = ng/mL	Prepubertal (M): 0.1–0.3 ng/mL
			Prepubertal (F): 0.2–0.5
			Adult (M): 0.2–1.8
			Adult (F):
			  Follicular: 0.2–0.8
			  Luteal: 0.8–3.0

Test	SI Reference Range	Conversion Factor	Conventional Units Reference Range
Immunoglobulins A, G, M	*IgA*	*IgG*	*IgM*
	Newborn: 0–0.05 g/L	6.4–16 g/L	0.06–0.24 g/L
	1–3 mo: 0.03–0.66	3.0–10.0	0.15–1.50
	3–6 mo: 0.04–0.90	1.4–10.0	0.15–1.10
	6–12 mo: 0.45–2.25	4.0–11.5	0.43–2.25
	1–2 yr: 0.35–2.40	3.5–12.0	0.36–2.40
	2–6 yr: 0.40–1.90	5.0–13.0	0.50–1.99
	6–12 yr: 0.40–2.70	7.0–16.5	0.50–2.60
	12–16 yr: 0.50–2.32	7.0–15.5	0.45–2.40
	Adult: 0.70–3.90	6.5–15.0	0.40–3.4
Immunoglobulin E	Newborn: 0–24 µg/L		Newborn: 0–10 U/mL
	6–12 yr: 0–480		6–12 yr: 0–200
	Adult: 0–960		Adult: 0–400
Insulin, fasting	3–23 mU/L		3–23 µU/mL
Iron	Newborn: 20–48 µmol/L	µmol/L × 5.587 = µg/dL	Newborn: 110–270 µg/dL
	4–10 mo: 5.4–12.5		4–10 mo: 30–70
	3–19 yr: 9.5–27.0		3–10 yr: 53–119
	Adult: 13.0–33.0		Adult: 72–186
Iron–binding capacity	Newborn: 10.6–31.3 µmol/L	µmol/L × 5.587 = µg/dL	Newborn: 59–175 µg/dL
	Thereafter: 45–72		Thereafter: 250–400
Lactate	Venous: 0.5–2.0 mmol/L	mmol/L × 9.01 = mg/dL	Venous: 5–18 mg/dL
	Arterial: 0.3–0.8		Arterial: 3–7
Lactate dehydrogenase	Newborn: 160–1500 U/L		Same as SI units
	Infant: 150–360		
	Child: 150–300		
	Adult: 100–250		
Lactate dehydrogenase isoenzymes		*Fraction of total*	
		LD 1 (heart): 0.24–0.34	
		LD 2 (heart, RBCs): 0.35–0.45	
		LD 3 (muscle): 0.15–0.25	
		LD 4 (liver, muscle): 0.04–0.10	
		LD 5 (liver, muscle): 0.01–0.09	
Lead	<1.16 µmol/L	µmol/L × 20.7 = mgm/dL	<24 gmg/dL

Lipids

	95th %ile values—mmol/L (mg/dL)				5th %ile values—mmol/L (mg/dL)	
	VLDL (Cholesterol)		*LDL (Cholesterol)*		*HDL (Cholesterol)*	
	M	*F*	*M*	*F*	*M*	*F*
5–9 yr:	0.47 (18)	0.62 (24)	3.34 (129)	3.62 (140)	0.98 (38)	0.93 (36)
10–14 yr:	0.57 (22)	0.59 (23)	3.41 (132)	3.52 (136)	0.96 (37)	0.91 (35)
15–19 yr:	0.67 (26)	0.62 (24)	3.36 (130)	3.49 (135)	0.80 (31)	0.91 (35)

Test	SI Reference Range	Conversion Factor	Conventional Units Reference Range
Luteinizing hormone	Prepubertal: <5 IU/L	mmol/L × 38.61 = mg/dL	Prepubertal: <5 mIU/L
	Adult (M): 3.9–18		Adult (M): 3.9–18
	Adult (F): 2.0–22.6		Adult (F): 2.0–22.6
Magnesium	0.75–1.0 mmol/L	mmol/L × 2 = mEq/L	1.5–2.0 mEq/L
Methemoglobin	<46 mmol/L	µmol/L × 0.0065 = g/dL	<0.3 gdL
Osmolality	285–295 mmol/kg		285–295 mOsm/kg
Phosphorus	Newborn: 1.36–2.91 mmol/L	mmol/L × 3.097 = mg/dL	Newborn: 4.2–9.0 mg/dL
	1 yr: 1.23–2.00		1 yr: 3.8–6.2
	2–5 yr: 1.13–2.20		2–5 yr: 3.5–6.8
	Adult: 0.97–1.45		Adult: 3.0–4.5
Phytanic acid	<0.003 fraction of total serum fatty acids		<0.3% of total serum fatty acids

(continued)

Test	SI Reference Range	Conversion Factor	Conventional Units Reference Range
Potassium	<10 days: 3.5–6.0 mmol/L >10 days: 3.5–5.0		<10 days: 3.5–6.0 mEq/L >10 days: 3.5–5.0
Progesterone	**Males**		
	Prepubertal: 0.35–0.83 nmol/L Adult: 0.38–0.95	nmol/L × 0.314 = ng/mL	0.11–0.26 ng/mL 0.12–0.30
	Females		

	Prepubertal: <0.95
	Pubertal stage II: <1.46
	                     III: <1.91
	                     IV: 0.16–41.34
			≤0.30
			≤0.46
			≤0.60
			0.05–13.0

	Follicular: 0.06–2.86 Luteal: 19.08–95.40		0.02–0.9 6.0–30.0
Prolactin	Newborn: <200 μg/L Adult: <20 μg/L		Newborn: <200 ng/mL Adult: <20 ng/mL
Protein, total	Preterm: 40–70 g/L Term newborn: 50–71 1–3 mo: 47–74 3–12 mo: 50–75 1–15 yr: 65–86		Preterm: 4.0–7.0 g/dL Term newborn: 5.0–7.1 1–3 mo: 4.7–7.4 3–12 mo: 5.0–7.5 1–15 yr: 6.5–8.6
Pyruvate	0.03–0.10 mmol/L	mmol/L × 8.81 = mg/dL	0.3–0.9 mg/dL
Renin	Adults: 0.30–1.14 ng · L^{-1} · S^{-1}	ng · L^{-1} · S^{-1} × 3.6 = ng/mL/h	Adults: 1.1–4.1 ng/mL/h
Sodium	135–145 mmol/L		135–145 mEq/L
Somatomedin C	0–2 yr: 220–1000 IU/L 3–5 yr: 270–1600 6–10 yr: 370–2100 11–12 yr: 450–2800 13–14 yr: 1100–4000 15–17 yr: 1000–2900 Thereafter: 460–1500		0–2 yr: 0.22–1.00 U/mL 3–5 yr: 0.27–1.60 6–10 yr: 0.37–2.10 11–12 yr: 0.45–2.80 13–14 yr: 1.10–4.00 15–17 yr: 1.00–2.90 Thereafter: 0.46–1.50
Testosterone, free	Prepubertal: 2.08–13.19 pmol/L Adult (M): 48.6–201 Adult (F): 6.94–25		Prepubertal: 0.06–0.38 ng/dL Adult (M): 1.40–5.79 Adult (F): 0.20–0.73
Testosterone, total	Prepubertal: 0.35–0.70 nmol/L Adult (F): 0.8–2.6 Adult (M): 9.5–30		Prepubertal: 10–20 ng/dL Adult (F): 23–75 Adult (M): 275–875
Thyroid-stimulating hormone (TSH)	Cord 0–17.4 μU/L 1–3 days: 0–13.3 Thereafter: 0–5.5		Cord: 0–17.4 mIU/mL 1–3 days: 0–13.3 Thereafter: 0–5.5
Thyroxine (T$_4$), total	Cord: 95–168 nmol/L <1 mo: 90–292 1 mo–1 yr: 93–213 1–5 yr: 94–194 5–10 yr: 83–172 10–15 yr: 72–151 Adult: 55–161	nmol/L × 0.0775 = μg/dL	Cord: 7.4–13.0 μg/dL <1 mo: 7.0–22.6 1 mo–1 yr: 7.2–16.5 1–5 yr: 7.3–15.0 5–10 yr: 6.4–13.3 10–15 yr: 5.6–11.7 Adult: 4.3–12.5
Thyroxine (T$_4$), free	9–22 pmol/L	pmol/L × 0.0777 = ng/dL	0.7–1.7 ng/dL
Transferrin	Newborn: 1.30–2.75 g/L Adult: 2.20–4.00		Newborn: 130–275 mg/dL Adult: 220–440
Triglycerides	**Normal Upper Limits—mmol/L (mg/dL)**		
	Male	**Female**	
	0–4 yr: 1.12 (99) 5–9 yr: 1.14 (101) 10–15 yr: 1.41 (125) 15–19 yr: 1.67 (148)	1.26 (112) 1.19 (105) 1.48 (131) 1.40 (124) mmol/L × 88.55 = mg/dL	

Test	SI Reference Range	Conversion Factor	Conventional Units Reference Range
Triiodothyronine (T$_3$)	Cord: 0.23–1.16 nmol/L <1 mo: 0.49–3.70 1 mo–1 yr: 1.70–4.31 1–5 yr: 1.62–4.14 5–10 yr: 1.45–3.71 10–15 yr: 1.28–3.31 Adult: 1.08–3.14	nmol/L × 65.1 = ng/dL	Cord: 15–75 ng/dL <1 mo: 32–240 1 mo–1 yr: 110–280 1–5 yr: 105–269 5–10 yr: 94–241 10–15 yr: 83–215 Adult: 70–204
Triiodothyronine resin uptake	0.25–0.35		25%–35%
Urea nitrogen	2–7 µmol/L	mmol/L × 28 = mg/dL	5–20 mg/dL
Uric acid	120–420 µmol/L	µmol/L × 0.0169 = mg/dL	2–7 mg/dL
Vitamin A	Newborn: 1.22–2.62 µmol/L Child: 1.05–2.79 Adult: 1.05–2.27	µmol/L × 28.65 = mg/dL	Newborn: 35–75 µg/dL Child: 30–80 Adult: 30–65
Vitamin B$_6$	14.6–72.8 nmol/L	nmol/L × 0.247 = ng/mL	3.6–18 ng/mL
Vitamin B$_{12}$	96–579 pmol/L	pmol/L × 1.355 = pg/mL	130–785 pg/mL
Vitamin C	11.4–113.6 µmol/L	µmol/L × 0.176 = mg/dL	0.2–2.0 mg/dL
Vitamin D$_3$ (1,25 dihydroxy)	60–108 pmol/L	pmol/L × 0.417 = pg/mL	25–45 pg/mL
Vitamin E	11.6–46.4 µmol/L	µmol/L × 0.043 = mg/dL	0.5–2.0 mg/dL
Zinc	10.7–22.9 µmol/L	µmol/L × 6.54 = µg/dL	70–150 µg/dL

Hematology

Age	HB (g/dL) Mean	HB (g/dL) −2 SD	Hematocrit (%) Mean	Hematocrit (%) −2 SD	MCV (fL) Mean	MCV (fL) −2 SD	MCHC (g/dL RBC) Mean	MCHC (g/dL RBC) −2 SD	Reticulocyte %	WBC (1,000/mm³) Mean	WBC (1,000/mm³) 95% CI	Platelets (1,000/mm³) Mean (Range)
Term (cord blood)	16.5	13.5	51	42	108	98	33.0	30.0	3.0–7.0	18.1	9.0–30.0	290
1–3 days	18.5	14.5	56	45	108	95	33.0	29.0	1.8–4.6	18.9	9.4–34.0	192
2 weeks	16.6	13.4	53	41	105	88	31.4	28.1		11.4	5.0–20.0	252
1 month	13.9	10.7	44	33	101	91	31.8	28.1	0.1–1.7	10.8	5.0–19.5	
2 months	11.2	9.4	35	28	95	84	31.8	28.3				
6 months	12.6	11.1	36	31	76	68	35.0	32.7	0.7–2.3	11.9	6.0–17.5	
6–24 months	12.0	10.5	36	33	78	70	33.0	30.0		10.6	6.0–17.0	(150–300)
2–6 years	12.5	11.5	37	34	81	75	34.0	31.0	0.5–1.0	8.5	5.0–15.5	(150–300)
6–12 years	13.5	11.5	50	35	86	77	34.0	31.0	0.5–1.0	8.1	4.5–13.5	(150–300)
12–18 years (M)	14.5	13.0	43	36	88	78	34.0	31.0	0.5–1.0	7.8	4.5–13.5	(150–300)
12–18 years (F)	14.0	12.0	41	37	90	78	34.0	31.0	0.5–1.0	7.8	4.5–13.5	(150–300)

Urine

Test	SI Reference Range	Conversion Factor	Conventional Units Reference Range
Aminolevulinic acid	8–53 µmol/d	µmol/d × 0.131 = mg/d	1–7 mg/d
Calcium	<0.1 mmol/kg/d	mmol/d × 40 = mg/d	<4 mg/kg/d
Copper	<0.6 µmol/d	µmol/d × 63.7 = gmg/d	<40 µg/d
Coproporphyrin	<300 nmol/d	nmol/d × 1.527 = µg/d	<200 µg/d
Cortisol, free	70–340 nmol/d	nmol/d × 0.362 = µg/d	25–125 µg/d
Creatinine	Infant: 71–177 µmol/kg/d Child: 71–194 Adolescent: 71–265	µmol/kg/d × 0.113 = mg/kg/d	Infant: 8–20 mg/kg/d Child: 8–22 Adolescent: 8–30
Cystine	40–260 µmol/d	µmol/d × 0.12 = mg/d	5–31 mg/d
Dehydroepiandrosterone (DHEA)	<5 yr: <0.3 µmol/d 6–9 yr: <0.7 10–15 yr: <1.4 Adult (M): <8.0 Adult (F): <4.2	µmol/d × 0.288 = mg/d	<5 yr: <0.1 mg/d 6–9 yr: <0.2 10–15 yr: <0.4 Adult (M): <2.3 Adult (F): <1.2
Epinephrine	<55 nmol/d	nmol/d × 0.183 = µg/d	<10 µg/d
Fluoride	<50 µmol/d	µmol/d × 0.019 = mg/d	<1 mg/d
Homovanillic acid (HVA)	*mmol/mol/creatinine* 1–12 mo: 0.75–21.7 1–2 yr: 2.5–14.3 2–5 yr: 0.43–8.4 5–10 yr: 0.31–5.6 10–15 yr: 0.15–7.4 15–18 yr: 0.31–1.24	mmol/mol/creatinine × 1.61 = µg/mg creatinine	*µg/mg creatinine* 1–12 mo: 1.2–35.0 1–2 yr: 4.0–23.0 2–5 yr: 0.7–13.5 5–10 yr: 0.5–9.0 10–15 yr: 0.25–12.0 15–18 yr: 0.5–2.0
Metanephrines	*mmol/mol/creatinine* <1 yr: 0.001–2.64 1–2 yr: 0.15–3.09 2–5 yr: 0.20–1.72 5–10 yr: 0.25–1.55 10–15 yr: 0.001–0.38 15–18 yr: 0.03–0.69	mmol/mol creatinine × 1.74 = µg/mg creatinine	*µg/mg creatinine* <1 yr: 0.001–4.6 1–2 yr: 0.27–5.38 2–5 yr: 0.35–2.99 5–10 yr: 0.43–2.70 10–15 yr: 0.001–1.87 15–18 yr: 0.001–0.67
Norepinephrine	<590 nmol/d	nmol/d × 0.169 = µg/d	<100 mg/d
Osmolality	50–1200 µgmol/kg		50–1200 mOsm/kg
Oxalate	110–440 µmol/d	µmol/d × 0.088 = mg/d	10–40 mg/d
Porphobilinogen	0–8.8 µmol/d	µmol/d × 0.226 = mg/d	0–2 mg/d
Potassium	25–125 mmol/d (varies with diet)		25–125 mEq/d
Pregnanetriol	<7.4 µmol/d	µmol/d × 0.3365 = mg/d	<2.5 mg/d
Protein	10–140 mg/L		1–14 mg/dL
Steroids: 17-hydroxycorticosteroid	Prepubertal: 2.76–15.5 µmol/d Adult (M): 11–33 Adult (F): 11–22	µmol/d × 0.3625 = mg/d	Prepubertal: 1–5.6 mg/d Adult (M): 4–12 Adult (F): 4–8
Steroids: 17-ketosteroids	<1 mo: ≤6.9 µmol/d 1 mo–5 yr: <1.73 6–8 yr: 3.47–6.9 Adult (M): 21–62 Adult (F): 14–45	µmol/d × 0.2884 = mg/d	<1 mo: <2 mg/d 1 mo–5 yr: <0.5 6–8 yr: 1–2 Adult (M): 6–18 Adult (F): 4–13
Uric acid	1.48–4.43 mmol/d	mmol/d × 169 = mg/d	250–750 mg/d
Vanilylmandelic acid (VMA)	*mmol/mol/creatinine* 1–6 mo: 1.71–9.71 6–12 mo: 1.14–8.57 1–5 yr: 1.14–5.71 5–10 yr: 0.86–4.00 10–15 yr: 0.57–3.43 >15 yr: 0.57–3.43	mmol/mol creatinine × 1.75 = µg/mg	*µg/mg creatinine* 1–6 mo: 3–7 6–12 mo: 2–15 1–5 yr: 2–10 5–10 yr: 1.5–7 10–15 yr: 1–6 >15 yr: 1–6

Cerebrospinal Fluid

Cell Count Range

Preterm: 0–25 WBC $\times$ 10^6 cells/L (57% polymorphonuclears)
Term: 0–22 WBC $\times$ 10^6 cells/L (61% polymorphonuclears)
Child: 0–7 WBC $\times$ 10^6 cells/L (0% polymorphonuclears)

Cell Count Percentiles

	Total WBC			*Polymorphonuclears*			*Monocytes*		
	25%	*50%*	*75%*	*25%*	*50%*	*75%*	*25%*	*50%*	*75%*
<6 wk	0.50	2.57	5.16	0	0	2.42	0	0.83	2.71
6 wk–3 mo	0.34	1.86	3.75	0	0	0.66	0	0.96	2.78
3–6 mo	0.00	1.11	2.31	0	0	0.40	0	0.43	1.64
6–12 mo	0.41	1.47	3.25	0	0	0.52	0.03	0.93	2.32
>12 mo	0.00	0.68	1.82	0	0	0	0	0.25	1.45

Test	SI Reference Range	Conventional Units Reference Range
Glucose	Preterm: 1.3–3.5 mmol/L Term: 1.9–6.6 Child: 2.2–4.4	Preterm: 24–63 mg/dL Term: 34–119 Child: 40–80
Protein	Preterm: 0.65–1.50 g/L Term: 0.20–1.70 Child: 0.05–0.40	Preterm: 65–150 mg/dL Term: 20–170 Child: 5–40
Pressure	<200 mm H_2O	<200 mm H_2O

(Crocetti, M. [2004]. Laboratory values. In M. Crocetti, M. A. Barone, & F. A. Oski [Eds.] *Oski's essential pediatrics* [2nd ed.]. Philadelphia: Lippincott Williams & Wilkins.)

Pulse, Respiration, and Blood Pressure Values

Pulse Rate (bpm) at Various Ages

Age	Range	Average
Newborn	70–170	120
1–11 months	80–160	120
2 years	80–130	110
4 years	80–120	100
6 years	75–115	100
8 years	70–110	90
10 years	70–100	90

	Girls		Boys	
	Range	*Average*	*Range*	*Average*
12 years	70–110	90	65–105	85
14 years	65–105	85	60–100	80
16 years	60–100	80	55–95	75
18 years	55–95	75	50–90	70

Variations in Respirations with Age

Age	Rate Per Minute
Newborn	40–90
1 year	20–40
2 years	20–30
3 years	20–30
5 years	20–25
10 years	17–22
15 years	15–20
20 years	15–20

Average Blood Pressure in Adult American Females

		White Women		Black Women	
	Age	*Average (mm Hg)*	*SD*	*Average (mm Hg)*	*SD*
Systolic	Under 20	111.0	13.7	112.7	13.2
	20–29	116.9	13.8	119.1	14.7
	30–39	121.4	16.3	128.1	20.2
	40–49	129.3	19.6	138.3	22.8
Diastolic	Under 20	69.3	9.8	70.0	10.1
	20–29	73.7	7.2	75.4	9.7
	30–39	76.9	10.7	82.0	13.0
	40–49	80.6	11.6	86.9	13.9

SD = standard deviation.
(Adapted from Stamler, J, et al. [1976]. Hypertension screening of one million Americans. *Journal of the American Medical Association,* 235, 2299. Copyright © 1976, American Medical Association.)

Normal Blood Pressure (mm Hg) for Various Ages

Age	Systolic (Mean ± 2 SD)	Diastolic (Mean ± 2 SD)
Newborn	80 ± 16	46 ± 16
6 months–1 year	89 ± 29	60 ± 10*
1 year	96 ± 30	66 ± 25*
2 years	99 ± 25	64 ± 25*
3 years	100 ± 25	67 ± 23*
4 years	99 ± 20	65 ± 20*
5–6 years	94 ± 14	55 ± 9
6–7 years	100 ± 15	56 ± 8
8–9 years	105 ± 16	57 ± 9
9–10 years	107 ± 16	57 ± 9
10–11 years	111 ± 17	58 ± 10
11–12 years	113 ± 18	59 ± 10
12–13 years	115 ± 19	59 ± 10
13–14 years	118 ± 19	60 ± 10

*The point of muffling is shown as the diastolic pressure.

Denver II

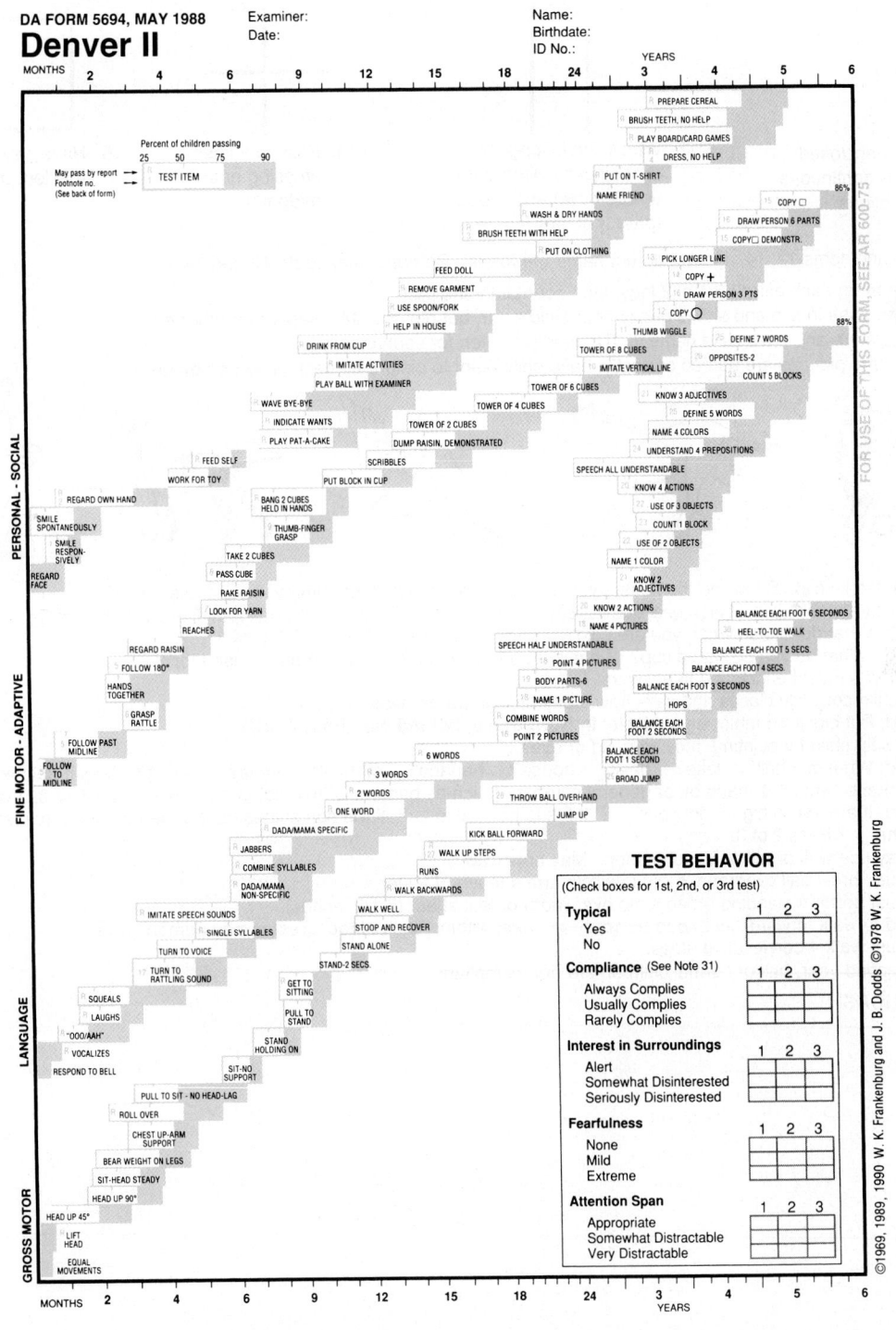

DIRECTIONS FOR ADMINISTRATION

1. Try to get child to smile by smiling, talking or waving. Do not touch him/her.
2. Child must stare at hand several seconds.
3. Parent may help guide toothbrush and put toothpaste on brush.
4. Child does not have to be able to tie shoes or button/zip in the back.
5. Move yarn slowly in an arc from one side to the other, about 8" above child's face.
6. Pass if child grasps rattle when it is touched to the backs or tips of fingers.
7. Pass if child tries to see where yarn went. Yarn should be dropped quickly from sight from tester's hand without arm movement.
8. Child must transfer cube from hand to hand without help of body, mouth, or table.
9. Pass if child picks up raisin with any part of thumb and finger.
10. Line can vary only 30 degrees or less from tester's line. |/
11. Make a fist with thumb pointing upward and wiggle only the thumb. Pass if child imitates and does not move any fingers other than the thumb.

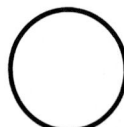 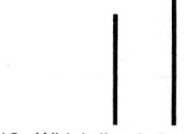 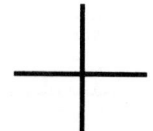 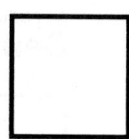

12. Pass any enclosed form. Fail continuous round motions.
13. Which line is longer? (Not bigger.) Turn paper upside down and repeat. (pass 3 of 3 or 5 of 6)
14. Pass any lines crossing near midpoint.
15. Have child copy first. If failed, demonstrate.

When giving items 12, 14, and 15, do not name the forms. Do not demonstrate 12 and 14.

16. When scoring, each pair (2 arms, 2 legs, etc.) counts as one part.
17. Place one cube in cup and shake gently near child's ear, but out of sight. Repeat for other ear.
18. Point to picture and have child name it. (No credit is given for sounds only.)
    If less than 4 pictures are named correctly, have child point to picture as each is named by tester.

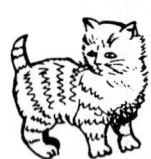 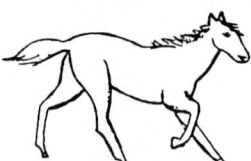 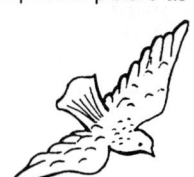 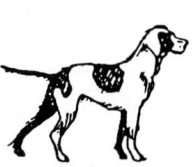 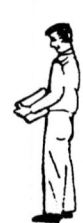

19. Using doll, tell child: Show me the nose, eyes, ears, mouth, hands, feet, tummy, hair. Pass 6 of 8.
20. Using pictures, ask child: Which one flies?... says meow?... talks?... barks?... gallops? Pass 2 of 5, 4 of 5.
21. Ask child: What do you do when you are cold?... tired?... hungry? Pass 2 of 3, 3 of 3.
22. Ask child: What do you do with a cup? What is a chair used for? What is a pencil used for? Action words must be included in answers.
23. Pass if child correctly places <u>and</u> says how many blocks are on paper. (1, 5).
24. Tell child: Put block **on** table; **under** table; **in front of** me, **behind** me. Pass 4 of 4. (Do not help child by pointing, moving head or eyes.)
25. Ask child: What is a ball?... lake?... desk?... house?... banana?... curtain?... fence?... ceiling? Pass if defined in terms of use, shape, what it is made of, or general category (such as banana is fruit, not just yellow). Pass 5 of 8, 7 of 8.
26. Ask child: If a horse is big, a mouse is __? If fire is hot, ice is __? If the sun shines during the day, the moon shines during the __? Pass 2 of 3.
27. Child may use wall or rail only, not person. May not crawl.
28. Child must throw ball overhand 3 feet to within arm's reach of tester.
29. Child must perform standing broad jump over width of test sheet (8 1/2 inches).
30. Tell child to walk forward, ∞∞∞➤ heel within 1 inch of toe. Tester may demonstrate. Child must walk 4 consecutive steps.
31. In the second year, half of normal children are non-compliant.

OBSERVATIONS:

APPENDIX I

Standard Precautions

Standard precautions are specific steps to prevent the transmission of infectious agents. Use Standard Precautions, or the equivalent, for the care of all patients.

A. Handwashing
   (1) Wash hands after touching blood, body fluids, secretions, excretions, and contaminated items, whether or not gloves are worn. Wash hands immediately after gloves are removed, between patient contacts, and when otherwise indicated to avoid transfer of micro-organisms to other patients or environments. It may be necessary to wash hands between tasks and procedures on the same patient to prevent cross-contamination of different body sites.
   (2) Use a plain (nonantimicrobial) soap for routine handwashing.
   (3) Use an antimicrobial agent or a waterless antiseptic agent for specific circumstances (e.g., control of outbreaks or hyperendemic infections), as defined by the infection control program.

B. Gloves
   Wear gloves (clean, nonsterile gloves are adequate) when touching blood, body fluids, secretions, excretions, and contaminated items. Put on clean gloves just before touching mucous membranes and nonintact skin. Change gloves between tasks and procedures on the same patient after contact with material that may contain a high concentration of microorganisms. Remove gloves promptly after use, before touching noncontaminated items and environmental surfaces, and before going to another patient, and wash hands immediately to avoid transfer of micro-organisms to other patients or environments.

C. Mask, Eye Protection, Face Shield
   Wear a mask and eye protection or a face shield to protect mucous membranes of the eyes, nose, and mouth during procedures and patient-care activities that are likely to generate splashes or sprays of blood, body fluids, secretions, and excretions.

D. Gown
   Wear a gown (a clean, nonsterile gown is adequate) to protect skin and to prevent soiling of clothing during procedures and patient-care activities that are likely to generate splashes or sprays of blood, body fluids, secretions, or excretions. Select a gown that is appropriate for the activity and amount of fluid likely to be encountered. Remove a soiled gown as promptly as possible, and wash hands to avoid transfer of micro-organisms to other patients or environments.

E. Patient-Care Equipment
   Handle used patient-care equipment soiled with blood, body fluids, secretions, and excretions in a manner that prevents skin and mucous membrane exposures, contamination of clothing, and transfer of micro-organisms to other patients and environments. Ensure that reusable equipment is not used for the care of another patient until it has been cleaned and reprocessed appropriately. Ensure that single-use items are discarded properly.

F. Environmental Control
   Ensure that the hospital has adequate procedures for the routine care, cleaning, and disinfection of environmental surfaces, beds, bedrails, bedside equipment, and other frequently touched surfaces, and ensure that these procedures are being followed.

G. Linen
   Handle, transport, and process used linen soiled with blood, body fluids, secretions, and excretions in a manner that prevents skin and mucous membrane exposures and contamination of clothing, and that avoids transfer of microorganisms to other patients and environments.

H. Occupational Health and Bloodborne Pathogens
   (1) Take care to prevent injuries when using needles, scalpels, and other sharp instruments or devices; when handling sharp instruments after procedures; when cleaning used instruments; and when disposing of used needles. Never recap used needles, or otherwise manipulate them using both hands, or use any other technique that involves directing the point of a needle toward any part of the body; rather, use either a one-handed "scoop" technique or a mechanical device designed for holding the needle sheath. Do not remove used needles from disposable syringes by hand, and do not bend, break, or otherwise manipulate used needles by hand. Place used disposable syringes and needles, scalpel blades, and other sharp items in appropriate puncture-resistant containers, which are located as close as practical to the area in which the items were used, and place reusable syringes and needles in a puncture-resistant container for transport to the reprocessing area.
   (2) Use mouthpieces, resuscitation bags, or other ventilation devices as an alternative to mouth-to-mouth

(From Guideline for isolation precautions in hospitals developed by the Centers for Disease Control and Prevention and the Hospital Infection Control Practices Advisory Committee [HICPAC], update 2004.)

resuscitation methods in areas where the need for resuscitation is predictable.

I. Patient Placement

Place a patient who contaminates the environment or who does not (or cannot be expected to) assist in maintaining appropriate hygiene or environmental control in a private room. If a private room is not available, consult with infection control professionals regarding patient placement or other alternatives.

Recommended Childhood and Adolescent Immunization Schedule, United States, 2005

Recommended Childhood and Adolescent Immunization Schedule, United States, 2005

Vaccine ▶	Birth	1 month	2 months	4 months	6 months	12 months	15 months	18 months	24 months	4–6 years	11–12 years	13–18 years
Hepatitis B[1]	HepB #1	HepB #2			HepB #3						HepB Series	
Diphtheria, Tetanus, Pertussis[2]			DTaP	DTaP	DTaP		DTaP	DTaP		DTaP	Td	Td
Haemophilus influenzae type b[3]			Hib	Hib	Hib	Hib	Hib					
Inactivated Poliovirus			IPV	IPV	IPV					IPV		
Measles, Mumps, Rubella[4]						MMR #1	MMR #1			MMR #2	MMR #2	MMR #2
Varicella[5]						Varicella		Varicella			Varicella	Varicella
Pneumococcal Conjugate[6]			PCV	PCV	PCV	PCV	PCV		PCV	PCV / PPV	PPV	
Influenza[7]						Influenza (Yearly)	Influenza (Yearly)			Influenza (Yearly)	Influenza (Yearly)	
Hepatitis A[8]										Hepatitis A Series	Hepatitis A Series	

------ Vaccines below red line are for selected populations ------

Legend:
- Range of recommended ages
- Preadolescent assessment
- Only if mother HBsAg(–)
- Catch-up immunization

This schedule indicates the recommended ages for routine administration of currently licensed childhood vaccines, as of December 1, 2004, for children through age 18 years. Any dose not given at the recommended age should be given at any subsequent visit when indicated and feasible. ▨ Indicates age groups that warrant special effort to administer those vaccines not previously given. Licensed combination vaccines may be used whenever any components of the combination are indicated and the vaccine's other components are not contraindicated. Providers should consult the manufacturers' package inserts for detailed recommendations. Clinically significant adverse events that follow immunization should be reported to the Vaccine Adverse Event Reporting System (VAERS). Guidance about how to obtain and complete a VAERS form can be found on the Internet: www.vaers.org or by calling 800-822-7967.

1. **Hepatitis B (HepB) vaccine.** All infants should receive the first dose of hepatitis B vaccine soon after birth and before hospital discharge; the first dose may also be given by age 2 months if the infant's mother is hepatitis B surface antigen (HBsAg) negative. Only monovalent HepB can be used for the birth dose. Monovalent or combination vaccine containing HepB may be used to complete the series. Four doses of vaccine may be administered when a birth dose is given. The second dose should be given at least 4 weeks after the first dose, except for combination vaccines which cannot be administered before age 6 weeks. The third dose should be given at least 16 weeks after the first dose and at least 8 weeks after the second dose. The last dose in the vaccination series (third or fourth dose) should not be administered before age 24 weeks.

   Infants born to HBsAg-positive mothers should receive HepB and 0.5 mL of Hepatitis B Immune Globulin (HBIG) within 12 hours of birth at separate sites. The second dose is recommended at age 1–2 months. The last dose in the immunization series should not be administered before age 24 weeks. These infants should be tested for HBsAg and antibody to HBsAg (anti-HBs) at age 9–15 months.

   Infants born to mothers whose HBsAg status is unknown should receive the first dose of the HepB series within 12 hours of birth. Maternal blood should be drawn as soon as possible to determine the mother's HBsAg status; if the HBsAg test is positive, the infant should receive HBIG as soon as possible (no later than age 1 week). The second dose is recommended at age 1–2 months. The last dose in the immunization series should not be administered before age 24 weeks.

2. **Diphtheria and tetanus toxoids and acellular pertussis (DTaP) vaccine.** The fourth dose of DTaP may be administered as early as age 12 months, provided 6 months have elapsed since the third dose and the child is unlikely to return at age 15–18 months. The final dose in the series should be given at age ≥4 years. **Tetanus and diphtheria toxoids (Td)** is recommended at age 11–12 years if at least 5 years have elapsed since the last dose of tetanus and diphtheria toxoid-containing vaccine. Subsequent routine Td boosters are recommended every 10 years.

3. **Haemophilus influenzae type b (Hib) conjugate vaccine.** Three Hib conjugate vaccines are licensed for infant use. If PRP-OMP (PedvaxHIB or ComVax [Merck]) is administered at ages 2 and 4 months, a dose at age 6 months is not required. DTaP/Hib combination products should not be used for primary immunization in infants at ages 2, 4 or 6 months but can be used as boosters following any Hib vaccine. The final dose in the series should be given at age ≥12 months.

4. **Measles, mumps, and rubella vaccine (MMR).** The second dose of MMR is recommended routinely at age 4–6 years but may be administered during any visit, provided at least 4 weeks have elapsed since the first dose and both doses are administered beginning at or after age 12 months. Those who have not previously received the second dose should complete the schedule by the visit at age 11–12 years.

5. **Varicella vaccine.** Varicella vaccine is recommended at any visit at or after age 12 months for susceptible children (i.e., those who lack a reliable history of chickenpox). Susceptible persons aged ≥13 years should receive 2 doses, given at least 4 weeks apart.

6. **Pneumococcal vaccine.** The heptavalent **pneumococcal conjugate vaccine (PCV)** is recommended for all children aged 2–23 months. It is also recommended for certain children aged 24–59 months. The final dose in the series should be given at age ≥12 months. **Pneumococcal polysaccharide vaccine (PPV)** is recommended in addition to PCV for certain high-risk groups. See *MMWR* 2000;49(RR-9):1–35.

7. **Influenza vaccine.** Influenza vaccine is recommended annually for children aged ≥6 months with certain risk factors (including but not limited to asthma, cardiac disease, sickle cell disease, HIV, and diabetes), healthcare workers, and other persons (including household members) in close contact with persons in groups at high risk (see *MMWR* 2004;53[RR-6]:1–40) and can be administered to all others wishing to obtain immunity. In addition, healthy children aged 6–23 months and close contacts of healthy children aged 0–23 months are recommended to receive influenza vaccine, because children in this age group are at substantially increased risk for influenza-related hospitalizations. For healthy persons aged 5–49 years, the intranasally administered live, attenuated influenza vaccine (LAIV) is an acceptable alternative to the intramuscular trivalent inactivated influenza vaccine (TIV). See *MMWR* 2004;53(RR-6):1–40. Children aged ≤8 years who are receiving influenza vaccine for the first time should receive 2 doses (separated by at least 4 weeks for TIV and at least 6 weeks for LAIV).

8. **Hepatitis A vaccine.** Hepatitis A vaccine is recommended for children and adolescents in selected states and regions and for certain high-risk groups; consult your local public health authority. Children and adolescents in these states, regions, and high-risk groups who have not been immunized against hepatitis A can begin the hepatitis A immunization series during any visit. The 2 doses in the series should be administered at least 6 months apart. See *MMWR* 1999;48(RR-12):1–37.

From Department of Health and Human Services, Centers for Disease Control and Prevention.

The Childhood and Adolescent Immunization Schedule is approved by:

Advisory Committee on Immunization Practices www.cdc.gov/nip/acip

American Academy of Pediatrics www.aap.org

American Academy of Family Physicians www.aafp.org

Food Guide Pyramid

(U.S. Department of Agriculture, Center for Nutrition Policy and Promotion, 2005. Washington, D.C.: USDA.)

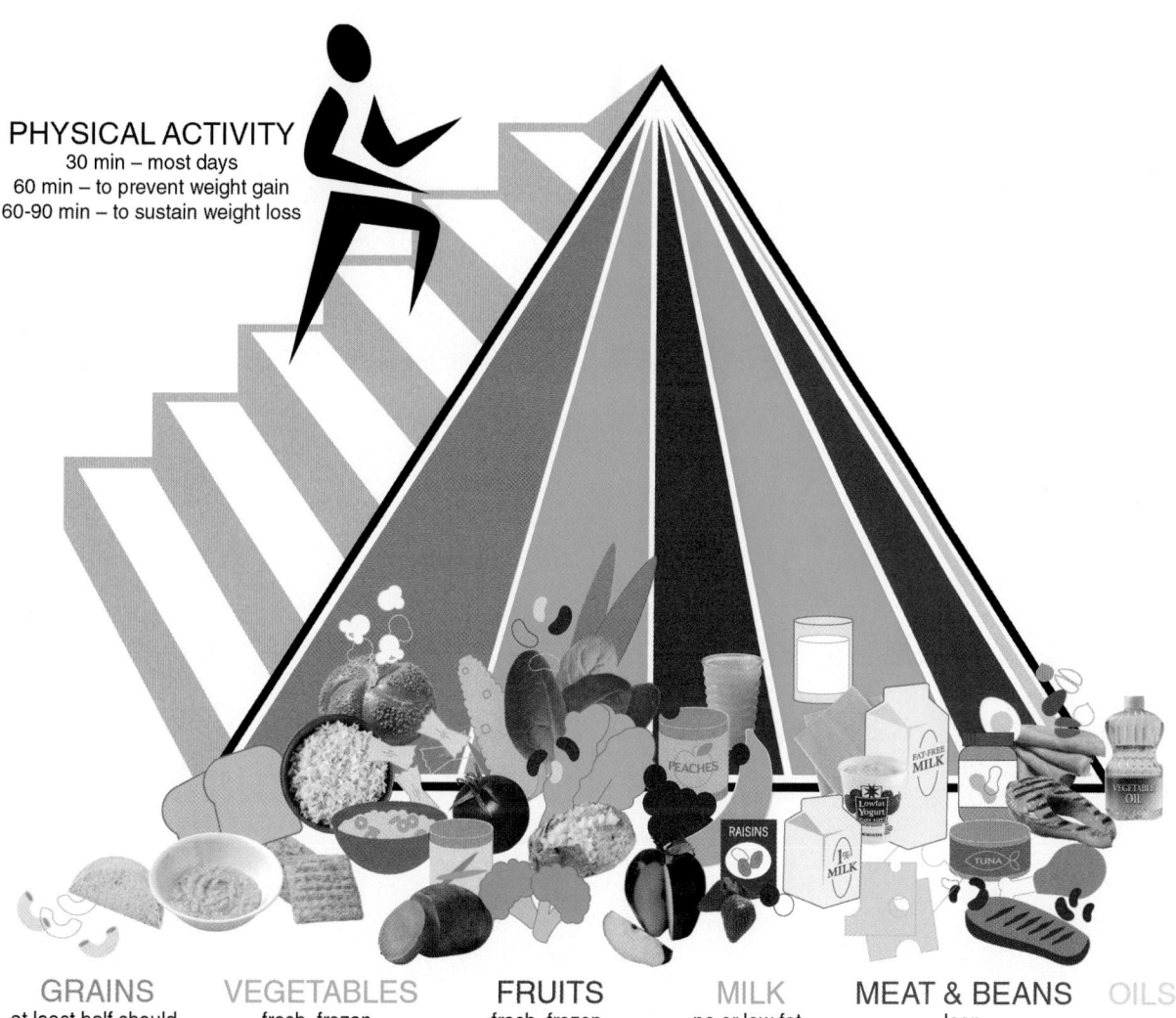

PHYSICAL ACTIVITY
30 min – most days
60 min – to prevent weight gain
60-90 min – to sustain weight loss

GRAINS	VEGETABLES	FRUITS	MILK	MEAT & BEANS	OILS
at least half should be whole grain	fresh, frozen, canned, dried	fresh, frozen, canned, dried	no or low fat, calcium rich	lean	

GRAINS Make half your grains whole	VEGETABLES Vary your veggies	FRUITS Focus on fruits	MILK Get your calcium-rich foods	MEAT & BEANS Go lean with protein
Eat at least 3 oz. of whole-grain cereals, breads, crackers, rice, or pasta every day 1 oz. is about 1 slice of bread, about 1 cup of breakfast cereal, or 1/2 cup of cooked rice, cereal, or pasta	Eat more dark-green veggies like broccoli, spinach, and other dark leafy greens Eat more orange vegetables like carrots and sweetpotatoes Eat more dry beans and peas like pinto beans, kidney beans, and lentils	Eat a variety of fruit Choose fresh, frozen, canned, or dried fruit Go easy on fruit juices	Go low-fat or fat-free when you choose milk, yogurt, and other milk products If you don't or can't consume milk, choose lactose-free products or other calcium sources such as fortified foods and beverages	Choose low-fat or lean meats and poultry Bake it, broil it, or grill it Vary your protein routine — choose more fish, beans, peas, nuts, and seeds

For a 2,000-calorie diet, you need the amounts below from each food group. To find the amounts that are right for you, go to MyPyramid.gov.

Eat 6 oz. every day	Eat 2 1/2 cups every day	Eat 2 cups every day	Get 3 cups every day; for kids aged 2 to 8, it's 2	Eat 5 1/2 oz. every day

Find your balance between food and physical activity
- Be sure to stay within your daily calorie needs.
- Be physically active for at least 30 minutes most days of the week.
- About 60 minutes a day of physical activity may be needed to prevent weight gain.
- For sustaining weight loss, at least 60 to 90 minutes a day of physical activity may be required.
- Children and teenagers should be physically active for 60 minutes every day, or most days.

Know the limits on fats, sugars, and salt (sodium)
- Make most of your fat sources from fish, nuts, and vegetable oils.
- Limit solid fats like butter, margarine, shortening, and lard, as well as foods that contain these.
- Check the Nutrition Facts label to keep saturated fats, *trans* fats, and sodium low.
- Choose food and beverages low in added sugars. Added sugars contribute calories with few, if any, nutrients.

GLOSSARY

abortion any interruption of a pregnancy before the fetus is viable (a stage of development that will enable the fetus to survive outside the uterus if born at that time)

absorption transfer of a drug from its point of entry in the body into the bloodstream

abstinence refraining from sexual intercourse

abstract thought final stage in cognitive thought processes; allows problem solving and creating hypotheses

abuse willful injury by one person of another

accommodation adjustment of the eye to focus on a close image (ophthalmology); the ability to adapt thought processes to fit what is perceived (Piaget)

acculturation the process of losing cultural beliefs and values to those of a dominant society

achalasia inability of a muscle to relax, particularly the cardiac sphincter

acrocyanosis cyanosis (blue color) in the feet and hands

acute pain sharp pain, generally occurring abruptly after an injury

acute transplant rejection reaction to a transplanted organ, usually occurring within the first 3 months after transplantation

acyanotic heart disorders heart or circulatory anomalies that involve either a stricture to the flow of blood or a shunt that moves blood from the arterial to the venous system (oxygenated to unoxygenated blood, or **left-to-right shunts**)

adaptability the ability to change one's reaction to stimuli over time

adolescence the time period between 13 years and 18 to 20 years

adrenarche the hormonal changes that occur with puberty

adventitious sounds extra or abnormal breathing sounds

affective learning learning that involves a change in attitude

afterload the resistance against which the cardiac ventricles must pump

afterpains intermittent cramping due to uterine contraction during involution in the postpartal period

aganglionic megacolon (Hirschsprung's disease) absence of ganglionic innervation to the muscle of a section of the bowel

age of viability the earliest age at which fetuses could survive if they were born at that time; generally accepted as 24 weeks, or fetuses weighing more than 400 g

agranulocytes white blood cells without granules in the cell cytoplasm

alleles two like genes

allergen antigen that causes the release of mediating substances causing tissue injury and allergic symptoms

allogeneic transplantation transfer of body tissues from an immune-compatible (histocompatible) donor

allografting transfer of body tissue between two genetically dissimilar individuals

Alport's syndrome a progressive chronic glomerulonephritis inherited as an autosomal dominant disorder

alternative birthing center a setting for birth separate from a hospital

amblyopia reduced vision in one eye; "lazy eye"

amenorrhea absence of a menstrual flow

amniocentesis the withdrawal of amniotic fluid from the uterus by means of introduction of a needle through the abdominal and uterine wall

amnioinfusion enlarging the amount of amniotic fluid by administration of normal saline or lactated Ringer's solution intravaginally into the uterus

amniotic cavity the space in the developing conceptus from which the ectodermal cells develop

amniotic fluid embolism condition in which amniotic fluid is forced into maternal circulation and travels to the lungs as small emboli

amniotic membrane the innermost membrane surrounding the fetus; it secretes amniotic fluid

analgesia a medication that reduces or decreases awareness of pain

anaphylaxis acute hypersensitivity (type I) reaction characterized by extreme vasodilation that leads to circulatory shock and extreme bronchoconstriction that decreases the airway lumens

andrology the branch of medicine that treats the male and diseases specific to the male sex

anesthesia a medication that causes partial or complete loss of sensation

angioedema edema of the skin and subcutaneous tissue

anhedonia inability to remember the last time when a person felt happy or had a good time

ankle clonus continued motion of the foot

ankyloglossia an abnormal restriction of the tongue caused by an abnormally tight frenulum

anovulation faulty or inadequate production of ova

anteflexion a uterus that is bent forward just above the cervix

anteversion a uterus that is tipped abnormally forward including the cervix

anticipatory grief preparatory phase in which people gradually incorporate the reality of impending death into their thoughts

antigen any foreign substance (molecule) capable of stimulating an immune response

antitoxins antibodies against toxin-producing bacteria

aplastic anemias depression of hematopoietic activity in bone marrow affecting all blood cells

apnea pause in respirations longer than 20 seconds with accompanying bradycardia

apparent life-threatening event (ALTE) infant who is cyanotic and limp in bed but survives after mouth-to-mouth resuscitation

appendicitis inflammation of the appendix

apposition the amount of end-to-end contact of bone fragments

approach a child's response on initial contact with a new stimulus

appropriate for gestational age (AGA) newborn who falls between the 10th and 90th percentile of weight for age regardless of gestational age

areola the pigmented circle surrounding the nipple

arthroscopy direct visualization of a joint with a fiber-optic instrument

aspermia absence of sperm

aspiration inhalation of a foreign object into the airway

aspiration studies studies involving the removal of body fluids by such techniques as lumbar puncture or bone marrow aspiration

assimilation changing a situation or one's perception of it to fit one's thoughts

astereognosis difficulty identifying objects placed in the hand when the eyes are closed

astigmatism congenital or acquired unevenness of the curvature of the cornea

atelectasis collapse of alveoli

atresia complete closure of a body opening

attention span the time interval a person can maintain interest in a topic or object

attitude the degree of head flexion a fetus assumes during labor, or the relation of the fetal parts to each other

audiogram a test to measure hearing

augmentation of labor assisting labor that has started spontaneously to be more effective

auscultation listening with the aid of a stethoscope

autografting transplantation of tissue from one part of the body to another in the same individual

autoimmunity an inability to distinguish self from non-self, causing the immune system to carry out immune responses against normal cells and tissue

autologous transplantation transplantation using the person's own previously removed tissue

automatisms complex purposeless movements, such as lip smacking or fumbling hand movements

autonomic dysreflexia a powerful sympathetic reflex reaction that causes signs of hypertension, tachycardia, flushed face, and severe occipital headache

autonomy independence

azotemia accumulation of nitrogen waste in the bloodstream

B lymphocytes lymphocytes formed in the bone marrow; responsible for antibody formation

baby-bottle syndrome decay of all the upper teeth and the lower posterior teeth, usually due to putting an infant to bed with a bottle

balloon angioplasty procedure usually by way of cardiac catheterization in which a catheter with an un-inflated balloon at its tip is inserted and passed through the heart into a stenosed valve. As the balloon is inflated, it breaks valve adhesions and may relieve the stenosis.

ballottement the sensation of an object rebounding after being pushed by an examining hand; used for pregnancy diagnosis

barium contrast studies x-ray involving the use of barium, a radiopaque substance to outline the gastrointestinal tract

barrier method a method of reproductive life planning in which sperm are prevented from entering the cervix

basal body temperature method a method of natural family planning based on the use of the body temperature on arising

battledore placenta a placenta with the cord inserted marginally rather than centrally

behavior modification a system of rewarding a person for desired behavior and ignoring or punishing the person for undesired behavior

beriberi deficiency of vitamin B_1 involving tingling and numbness of extremities, heart palpitations, and exhaustion

bicornuate uterus a uterus that has two fundal horns; it may have an accompanying septum

bifidus factor specific growth-promoting factor for the bacteria *Lactobacillus bifidus* whose presence in breast milk interferes with colonization of pathogenic bacteria in the gastrointestinal tract

binge eating episodes of uncontrollable intake of large amounts of food over a specified period of time

binocular vision ability to fuse two images into one

biologic gender a person's chromosomal sexual designation of being male (XY) or female (XX)

biopsy surgical removal of tissue cells for laboratory analysis

birthing bed a bed specifically prepared for birth

birthing chair a chair used in labor and birth

birthing room a specifically prepared room for aiding comfort, safety, and conduct of birth

blastocyst a hollow sphere of cells that forms in early fetal development

blood dyscrasias hematologic disorders

blood plasma liquid portion containing proteins, hormones, enzymes, and electrolytes

body mass index determination of body weight by comparing height to weight (weight divided by height squared)

Bowman's capsule double-walled chamber enclosing the glomerulus of the kidney

Braxton Hicks contractions painless, erratic uterine contractions that occur toward the end of pregnancy. They ready the cervix for labor, but cervical dilation does not occur with them.

breech presentation fetal presentation in which either the buttocks or feet are the first body parts to contact the cervix

broken fluency repetition and prolongation of sounds, syllables, and words

bronchoscopy a procedure in which a bronchoscope, a specially designed tube, is passed through the nose or mouth to observe the larynx, trachea, bronchi, and alveoli

brown fat the special tissue present in newborns to maintain body temperature

bruit a swishing or blowing sound that occurs with turbulent blood flow, such as if there is an outpouching of the aorta

bruxism grinding the teeth during sleep

calendar method a method of natural family planning based on the determination of fertile and nonfertile days each month

calorie counting counting the number of calories that a person ingests in 1 day

caput succedaneum edema of the scalp at the presenting part of the head

cardiac catheterization a procedure in which a small radiopaque catheter is passed through a major vein in the arm, leg, or neck into the heart to secure blood samples or inject dye, to evaluate cardiac function

cardinal movements of labor position changes to keep the smallest diameter of the fetal head (in cephalic presentations) always presenting to the smallest diameter of the birth canal (descent, flexion, internal rotation, extension, external rotation, and expulsion)

caries dental cavities

carpal spasm hand spasm involving abduction of the hand and flexion of the wrist with the thumb positioned across the palm

cartilage connective tissue

case management nursing one nurse being in charge of a patient's care from admission to discharge

catarrhal stage inflammation of the nose and throat during infectious diseases

catatonia immobility

caudal regression syndrome hypoplasia of the lower extremities occurring primarily in infants of diabetic mothers

cavernous hemangioma type of birthmark evidenced as a dilated vascular space

celiac disease sensitivity or immunologic response to protein, particularly the gluten factor of protein found in grains—wheat, rye, oats, and barley

cell-mediated immunity type of immune response due to T-lymphocyte activity

centering focusing on only one aspect of an object or situation

central cyanosis cyanosis of the trunk

central nervous system (CNS) the brain, the spinal cord, and the surrounding membranes or meninges that protect the delicate tissues from normal trauma

cephalhematoma a collection of blood under the periosteum of the skull bone

cephalic presentation fetal presentation in which the head is the body part that first contacts the cervix

cephalocaudal relating to head and tail; progression of development in a fetus and child

cephalopelvic disproportion inability of the fetal head to pass through the maternal pelvis due to a discrepancy in size

cerebrospinal fluid (CSF) the fluid in the subarachnoid space, which serves as a cushion to the spinal cord

cervical cap a latex barrier method of contraception that fits over the uterine cervix

cervical cerclage suturing of the cervix to maintain a pregnancy to prevent premature cervical dilatation

cervical ripening change in cervical consistency from firm to soft

cesarean birth birth accomplished through an abdominal incision into the uterus

Chadwick's sign discolorization of vaginal walls from pink to violet

chain of infection method by which organisms are spread and enter a new individual to cause disease

chemotaxis "calling" leukocytes into the area

chemotherapeutic agent one that is capable of destroying malignant cells

chief concern the reason the parents or patient has come to the health care agency

chloasma extra pigment on the face

choreiform movements aimless movements

choreoathetosis rapid, purposeless movements

choreoid irregular and jerking movements

chorioamnionitis infection of the fetal membranes and amniotic fluid

chorionic membrane the outer fetal membrane

chorionic villi projections of the trophoblast that produce human chorionic gonadotropin and begin osmosis of nutrients to the embryo

chromosome the structure that weaves genes into strands in the nucleus of all body cells

chronic pain pain that lasts for a prolonged period of time (often defined as 6 months' time)

clarifying repeating statements others have made so that you and they can be certain that you understood

class inclusion the ability to understand that objects can belong to more than one classification

classic cesarean incision an incision that is made vertically through both the abdominal skin and the uterus

clean-catch specimen urine specimen obtained after the urinary meatus has been cleaned

cleansing breath a deep breath taken at the beginning and end of breathing exercises during labor that helps prevent hyperventilation

cleft lip failure of the maxillary and median nasal processes to fuse normally

cleft palate an opening of the palate

clinical nurse specialist a nurse prepared at the master's degree level who is capable of acting as a consultant in an area of expertise, as well as serving as a role model, researcher, and teacher of quality nursing care

clubbing a change in the angle between the fingernail and nailbed because of increased capillary growth in the fingertips; a response to hypoxia

coelocentesis the transvaginal aspiration of fluid collected in the extraembryonic cavity early in pregnancy for analysis

cognitive development the acquisition of the ability to think and reason

cognitive learning learning that involves a change in the individual's level of understanding or knowledge

coitus interruptus a method of contraception in which the penis is withdrawn from the vagina before ejaculation

colonoscopy a procedure in which a colonoscope, a specially designed tube, is passed through the anus to examine the rectum or colon

colostrum a thin, watery, yellow fluid composed of protein, sugar, fat, water, minerals, vitamins, and maternal antibodies that precedes breast milk

comedones the lesions of acne vulgaris; "blackheads"

communication the exchange of ideas between two or more persons

community a limited geographic area in which the residents relate to and interact among themselves

complement a special body protein that is capable of lysing cells; comprised of 20 different proteins that are normally nonfunctional molecules but become active with the immune response

complete miscarriage the entire products of conception (fetus, membranes, and placenta) are expelled spontaneously without any assistance

complete protein a protein that supplies all of the essential amino acids

complex vocal tics repeated use of words or phrases out of context

computed tomography (CT) x-ray procedure in which many views of an organ or body part are made to represent what the organ would look like if it were cut into thin slices

concrete operational thought typical thought pattern of school-age children, preceding abstract thought

conditioned reflex a reflex to respond to a specific stimulus developed by training

condom a latex barrier method of contraception worn on the penis (a male condom) or inserted vaginally (a female condom); provides some protection against STIs as well

conduction transfer of body heat to a cooler solid object in contact with the body

congestive heart failure a condition in which the myocardium of the heart cannot pump and circulate enough blood to supply oxygen and nutrients to body cells

conjugate vera true conjugate; measurement between the anterior surface of the sacral prominence and the posterior surface of the inferior margin of the symphysis pubis

conjunctivitis commonly called "pink eye" by parents; an infection of the conjunctiva that covers the eye

conscious relaxation deliberate relaxation

conscious sedation a state of depressed consciousness obtained by IV analgesia therapy

consciously controlled breathing deliberately spaced breathing to achieve a desired rate

conservation property of an object that a change in form does not equate to a change in size or amount

constriction ring a simple type of contraction ring that occurs at any point in the myometrium and at any time during labor

contact dermatitis example of a delayed or type IV hypersensitivity response; it is a reaction to skin contact with an allergen (a substance irritating only to the person with prior sensitization)

contraceptive a method or device to prevent the fertilization of the human ovum

contractility the ability of the ventricles to stretch; refers to the force of contraction generated by the myocardial muscle

contraction a rhythmic tightening of the uterus that aids in achieving cervical dilatation and effacement

contrecoup injury an injury resulting from a blow to one side of the skull that causes the brain to rebound and then injure the opposite side

convalescent period interval between when infectious symptoms begin to fade and the child returns to full wellness

convection flow of heat from the body surface to cooler surrounding air

conventional development adult level of moral development (Kohlberg)

coordination of secondary schema stage associated with infant's development of object permanence (Piaget)

coprolalia use of socially unacceptable words, usually obscenities

corona radiata the crown-like grouping of cells that surrounds the ovum immediately after ovulation

cotyledons subdivisions of the maternal surface of the placenta; filled with maternal blood to allow for osmosis of nutrients to the fetal placental villi

couvade syndrome somatic symptoms experienced by the father during pregnancy simulating those of the pregnant mother

couvelaire uterus uteroplacental apoplexy due to blood entering the uterine musculature

crackles the sound of rales

Crohn's disease inflammation of segments of the intestine, affecting any part of the gastrointestinal tract, but most commonly the terminal ileum

crowning the appearance of the fetal head at the perineum just before birth

cryptorchidism failure of one or both testes to descend from the abdominal cavity to the scrotum

culdoscopy the introduction of an endoscope through the posterior vaginal wall to view the pelvic organs

cultural values beliefs generally held by the majority of people in a community or society

culture the learned way of life of a community or society

cutaneous pain pain that arises from superficial structures such as the skin and mucous membrane

cyanosis a blue tinge to the skin indicating hypoxia

cyanotic heart disease cardiac anomaly when blood is shunted from the venous to the arterial system as a result of abnormal communication between the two (deoxygenated blood to oxygenated blood; **right-to-left shunt**)

cystocele a pouching of the bladder into the anterior vaginal wall

cytomegalovirus a member of the herpes virus family; teratogen that can cause extensive damage to a fetus yet causes few symptoms in the woman

cytotoxic (cell-destroying) **response** cells are detected as foreign and immunoglobulins directly attack and destroy the cells without harming surrounding tissue

cytotoxic (killer) **T cells** T lymphocytes that have the specific feature of binding to the surface of antigens and directly destroying the cell membrane and therefore the cell

death end of life; officially determined by unreceptivity and unresponsivity; no spontaneous muscular movement or breath; no reflex response; and a flat electroencephalogram

debridement the removal of foreign material from a burn or wound

decenter to project the self into other peoples' situations and see the world from their viewpoint

decerebrate posturing typical posture occurring when the midbrain is not functional; characterized by rigid extension and adduction of arms and pronation of the wrists with the fingers flexed; legs extended and the feet plantar flexed

decidua basalis the endometrium portion under the implanted blastocyst

decidua capsularis the endometrium portion that covers the blastocyst

decidua vera the endometrium portion that covers the nonimplanted portion of the uterus

deciduous teeth temporary teeth that are replaced by permanent teeth at around age 6 to 7 years

decorticate posturing a child's arms adducted and flexed on the chest with wrists flexed, hands fisted; lower extremities extended and internally rotated; feet plantar flexed; denotes brainstem involvement

deep tendon reflexes neurologic reflexes such as triceps, biceps, patellar, and Achilles reflexes

deep vein thrombosis (DVT) formation of thrombus (blood clot) in the deep veins secondary to stasis, vessel damage, and hypercoagulation

deferred imitation ability to remember an action and imitate it later

dehiscence the separation of a muscle or surgical incision

dehydration an excessive loss of body water

delayed hypersensitivity T-lymphocyte activity occurring solely without an accompanying humoral response

demonstration the showing of a procedure to stimulate learning

dermatoglyphics the study of surface markings of the skin

development an increase in ability (a qualitative change)

developmental care care designed to meet the specific needs of each infant

developmental hip dysplasia (often referred to as *congenital hip dysplasia*) improper formation and function of the hip socket

developmental milestone major marker of normal development

developmental task a skill or a growth responsibility arising at a particular time, the successful achievement of which will provide a foundation for the accomplishment of future tasks

diagonal conjugate distance between the anterior surface of the sacral prominence and the anterior surface of the inferior margin of the symphysis pubis

dialysis separation and removal of solutes from body fluid by diffusion through a semipermeable membrane

diaphragm a mechanical barrier contraceptive device fitted over the cervix in the woman

diaphragmatic excursion distance the diaphragm moves as measured from inspiration to expiration

diaphysis central shaft of a long bone

diastasis recti overstretching and separation of the abdominal musculature

diastole relaxation of the heart chambers

dilatation widening of the opening of the cervix in labor

diplegia (paraplegia); paralysis of the lower extremities

diplopia double vision

direct bilirubin water-soluble end breakdown product of heme that is combined and excreted in bile

direct care a nurse remains in continual attendance or visits frequently and actually administers care

discipline setting rules so people know what is expected

disorganization phase first phase of rape trauma syndrome in which victims feel a combination of humiliation, shame and guilt, embarrassment, anger, and vengefulness

distractibility the ability to shift concentration from one focus to another

distraction (a) a technique that allows the cells of the brain stem that register an impulse as pain to be preoccupied with other stimuli so the pain impulse cannot register; (b) use of an external device to separate opposing bones, thus encouraging new bone growth

distribution movement of a drug through the bloodstream to the specific site of action

dominant gene expressed in preference to the other genes

doula a person without professional experience who guides and assists a woman in labor

drowning asphyxiation because of submersion in a liquid

ductus arteriosus a blood vessel joining the pulmonary artery and aorta in fetal life; closes at birth

ductus venosus a blood vessel joining the umbilical vein and the inferior vena cava in fetal life; closes at birth

dysfunctional labor previously termed *inertia;* occurrence of sluggishness of contractions, or the force of labor

dyskinetic disordered muscle tone

dyslexia reading impairment disorder in which letters or words are reversed

dysmature newborn who is before term or post-term or is under- or overweight for gestational age

dysmenorrhea painful menstruation

dyspareunia pain on sexual intercourse

dystocia difficult labor

echocardiography ultrasound involving the use of high-frequency sound waves to locate and study the movement and dimensions of the cardiac structures

echolalia repetitive words or phrases spoken by others

eclampsia development of a seizure from hypertension of pregnancy

ecomap a diagram of the family's interactions within the community

ectoderm one of the layers of primary germ cell tissue in the embryo

ectomorphic having a slim body build

ectopic pregnancy one in which implantation occurs outside the uterine cavity

effacement thinning of the cervix in labor

effleurage light massage done by the fingertips

egocentrism perceiving that one's thoughts and needs are better or more important than those of others

eighth-month anxiety fear of strangers that peaks during the eighth month

elective termination of pregnancy termination of a pregnancy by medical intervention

Electra complex strong emotional attachment of a preschool girl to her father (Freud)

electrical impulse studies those that include electrical conduction

electrocardiogram (ECG) written record of the electrical voltages generated by the contracting heart

emancipated minor a person before the age of majority who is free from the custody, care, and control of his or her parents and is capable of health care decisions; a pregnant adolescent

embryo the intrauterine growth period from the time following implantation until organogenesis is complete (tenth day to 5 to 8 weeks)

empathy the ability to put yourself in another's place and experience a feeling as that person does

en face position a position in which a caregiver's face and an infant's face look directly at each other

enanthem rash on the mucous membrane

endocervix the inner surface of the cervix

endometriosis abnormal growth of extrauterine endometrial cells, often in the cul-de-sac of the peritoneal cavity, the uterine ligaments, and the ovaries

endometritis an infection of the endometrium, the lining of the uterus

endometrium the inner layer of the uterus that is shed with menstruation

endomorphic having a large body build

endorphins naturally occurring opiate-like substances in the body

endoscopy a procedure in which an endoscope, a specially designed tube, is passed through the mouth to examine the gastrointestinal tract

engagement settling of the fetal head into the pelvis during labor

engorgement breast distention with swelling caused by vascular and lymphatic congestion arising from an increase in the blood and lymph supply to the breasts

engrossment staring at the newborn in the en face position for long intervals

entoderm one of the layers of primary germ cells in the embryo

enucleation eye removal

enuresis involuntary passage of urine past the age when a child should be expected to have attained bladder control

environmental control as many common allergens as possible are removed from the environment

epidural analgesia injection of an analgesic agent into the epidural space just outside the spinal canal, to provide analgesia to the lower body for 12 to 24 hours

epiphyseal plate area where the increase in the length of long bones occurs

epiphysis rounded end portion of a long bone

episiotomy surgical incision of the perineum to prevent tearing and to release pressure on the fetal head with birth

epispadias opening of the urinary meatus on the dorsal or superior surface of the penis

erectile dysfunction impotence; the inability to achieve erection in order to complete a sex act

erosion inflammation of the epithelium of the cervical canal spreading onto the area surrounding the os, giving the cervix a reddened appearance

erythema toxicum newborn rash that usually appears in the 1st to 4th day of life; sometimes called a flea-bite rash

erythroblastosis fetalis see *hemolytic disease of the newborn*

erythroblasts large, nucleated early red blood cells

erythrocytes red blood cells

erythropoietin a hormone produced by the kidneys that stimulates red blood cell development

escharotomy a surgical incision into the hard crust that forms over a burn

esotropia condition in which the eye is always turning in

estimated date of birth the predicted date on which a baby will be born (also estimated date of confinement or EDC)

ethnicity the cultural group into which a person is born

ethnocentrism the belief that one's own values or beliefs are superior to others

evaporation loss of heat through conversion of a liquid to a vapor

evidence-based practice the use of research or controlled investigation of a problem using a scientific method in conjunction with clinical expertise as acquired through experience and practice as a foundation for action

Ewing's sarcoma malignant tumor occurring most often in the bone marrow of the diaphyseal area (mid-shaft) of long bones

exanthem a skin rash

excretion elimination of raw drug or drug metabolites, a process that largely prevents properly administered drugs from becoming toxic

exophthalmos protrusion of the eyeballs

exotoxins poisons produced by some bacteria

exotropia condition in which the eye is always turning outward

expected date of birth calculated date on which birth can be predicted to occur (EDB)

expiration carbon dioxide-filled air discharged to the outside

exstrophy of the bladder midline closure defect occurring during the embryonic period of gestation (first 8 weeks) and resulting in the bladder lying open and exposed on the abdomen

external cephalic version turning of a fetus from a breech to a cephalic position before birth

extracorporeal membrane oxygenation (ECMO) mechanical means of oxygenating blood

extremely-very-low-birth-weight (EVLBW) infant an infant weighing 500 to 1000 g

extrusion reflex a tongue reflex in infants that expels solid objects from the mouth; fades at 4 months

failure to thrive also called reactive attachment disorder; unique syndrome in which an infant falls below the fifth percentile for weight and height on a standard growth chart or is falling in percentiles on a growth chart

family two or more people who live in the same household (usually), share a common emotional bond, and perform certain interrelated social tasks

family nurse practitioner nurse who provides health care not only to women but all persons throughout the age span; in conjunction with a physician, an FNP can provide prenatal care for the woman with an uncomplicated pregnancy

family nursing the concept that clients do not exist outside a family; the family rather than an individual is considered the client

family of orientation one's birth family: oneself, mother, father, and siblings

family of procreation one's marriage family: oneself, spouse, and children

family theory a way of analyzing problems or concerns from a family's point of view

feedback a reply to communication indicating that the message has been received and interpreted

fertility awareness a method of contraception based on analyzing the consistency of vaginal secretions

fertility rate the proportion of women who could have babies who are having them

fertilization the union of the sperm and ovum

fetal alcohol syndrome condition associated with an infant born to a woman who uses alcohol during pregnancy; infant typically is small for gestational age, cognitively challenged, and has a characteristic craniofacial deformity including short palpebral fissures, thin upper lip, and upturned nose

fetal descent sinking of the fetus in the birth canal just prior to birth (one of six cardinal movements of labor)

fetoscopy the visualization of the fetus by inspection through a fetoscope

fetus the developing structure from the eighth week postfertilization until birth

fibrocystic breast disease benign multiple cysts in the breasts

fine motor development ability to accomplish smaller, more defined body movement; measured by observing or testing prehensile ability

fistula abnormal opening

flat affect not revealing feelings

fluoroscopy a radiologic serial-images technique

focusing helping a person to center on a subject

fomites inanimate objects, such as soil, food, water, bedding, towels, combs, or drinking glasses, that provide a means of infection transmission

foramen ovale an opening between the atria of the heart during intrauterine life

forceps birth birth using forceps (steel double-bladed instruments used to prevent pressure on the fetal head); forceps outlet procedure when the forceps are applied after the fetal head reaches the perineum

foremilk constantly forming breast milk

formal operational thought final stage of cognitive development, involving the ability to think in abstract terms and use the scientific method to arrive at conclusions

fovea centralis (the center of the macula); an area of closely packed cones on the retinas where color is best perceived

fracture break in the continuity or structure of bone

frenulum the membrane attached to the lower anterior tip of the tongue

gamma globulin serum obtained from the pooled blood of many people; rich in antibodies

gastroesophageal reflux (commonly called achalasia in infants) a neuromuscular disturbance in which the gastroesophageal (cardiac) sphincter and the lower portion of the esophagus are lax, allowing easy regurgitation of gastric contents into the esophagus

gate control theory a theory of how pain impulses can be interrupted before they travel between a site of injury and the brain where the impulse is actually registered as pain

gavage feedings nasogastric tube feedings given to an infant

gender identity the inner sense of being male or female, which may be the same as or different from biologic gender

gender role the behavior a person conveys about being male or female

genes basic units of heredity that determine both the physical and mental characteristics of people

genetics study of how and why chromosomal disorders occur; the science of heredity

genogram a diagram of family structure depicting essential family relationships; the interactive roles that exist in a family

genome complete set of genes present

genotype actual gene composition

genu valgus knock-knees

geographic tongue term for the rough-appearing tongue surface that often accompanies general symptoms of illness such as fever

gestational age number of weeks fetus remained in utero

gestational trophoblastic disease proliferation and degeneration of the trophoblastic villi

glomerular filtration rate rate at which substances are filtered from the blood to the urine

glomerulonephritis inflammation of the glomeruli of the kidney

glucose tolerance test a test of the body's ability to metabolize carbohydrate by measuring the serum glucose level after ingestion of a fixed amount of glucose

glycogen loading depleting, then replenishing glycogen stores by altering carbohydrate intake, to store extra glycogen for the purpose of sustaining energy through an athletic event

glycosuria excess glucose in the urine

glycosylated hemoglobin measure of the amount of glucose attached to hemoglobin

gonad a sex gland; an ovary in the female; a testis in the male

goniotomy surgical procedure used to treat congenital glaucoma

Goodell's sign softening of the cervix; a probable sign of pregnancy

granulocytes white blood cells with granules in the cell cytoplasm

graphesthesia ability to recognize a shape that has been traced on the skin

gravida number of times a woman has been pregnant, including the present pregnancy; a pregnant woman

grief process regulated steps in grieving

gross motor development ability to accomplish large body movements

growth an increase in size; a quantitative change

gynecology the study of the female reproductive organs and female disorders

gynecomastia enlargement of the breasts; excess development of male breast tissue; a transient occurrence in normal adolescence

hand regard infants holding their hands in front of their face and studying their fingers for long periods of time

hapten formation process whereby a substance, not antigenic in itself, becomes antigenic when combined with a higher-weight molecule, usually a protein

Hawthorne effect an improvement in behavior because of being studied

health fair a display to teach healthful behaviors

Hegar's sign softening of the lower uterine segment; a probable sign of pregnancy

Heinz bodies oddly shaped particles in red blood cells

HELLP syndrome a variation of hypertension of pregnancy named for the common symptoms that occur: *h*emolysis, *e*levated *l*iver enzymes, and *l*ow *p*latelets

helper T cells lymphocytes that stimulate B lymphocytes to divide and mature into plasma cells and begin secretion of immunoglobulins

hemangioma vascular tumor of the skin

hemiplegia paralysis of both extremities on one side

hemochromatosis deposition of iron in body tissues from destruction of red blood cells

hemoglobin a complex protein that is the oxygen-carrying component of red blood cells

hemolysis destruction of red blood cells

hemolytic disease of the newborn condition involving red blood cell destruction in the fetus who is Rh positive and whose mother is Rh negative

hemorrhagic disease of the newborn newborn bleeding disorder resulting from a deficiency of vitamin K

hemosiderosis deposition of iron in body tissues

hepatitis inflammation and infection of the liver

hermaphrodite having both ovaries and testes

heterograft tissue from another species (such as a pig) used as a temporary skin covering

heterosexual an individual whose sexual relations are with persons of the opposite sex

heterozygous trait having two different or unlike genes for a designated characteristic

hiatal hernia intermittent protrusion of the stomach up through the esophageal opening in the diaphragm

high-risk pregnancy one in which a concurrent disorder, pregnancy-related complication, or external factor jeopardizes the health of the mother and/or fetus

hind milk new breast milk formed after the let-down reflex

Homans' sign pain in the calf on dorsiflexion of the foot

home care care of people in their own home, provided by or supervised through a certified home health care or community health care agency

homosexual an individual whose sexual relations are with persons of his or her own sex

homozygous trait having two like genes for a designated characteristic

hordeolum an infection of an eyelash

hormones chemicals produced by ductless glands of the endocrine system

hospice care care of the person with a terminal disease; can be cared for at home

humoral immunity immunity created by antibody production or B-lymphocyte involvement

hydramnios an excessive amount of amniotic fluid (generally over 2,000 mL)

hydrocele collection of fluid in the scrotal sac

hydrocephalus an excess of cerebrospinal fluid (CSF) in the ventricles and subarachnoid spaces of the brain

hydronephrosis enlargement of the pelvis of the kidney with urine as a result of back-pressure in the ureter

hydrops fetalis old term for the appearance of a severely involved infant with Rh incompatibility at birth

hyperactivity excess movement

hyperbilirubinemia increased serum bilirubin

hypercholesterolemia greater than usual levels of cholesterol in the blood

hyperfunction overfunction of a gland or organ

hyperglycemia increased blood glucose level

hyperopia farsightedness

hyperplasia an increase in the number of cells of a body part

hyperptyalism excessive secretion of saliva

hypersensitivity response excessive antigen-antibody response when the invading organism is an allergen rather than a simple immunogen

hypertension elevated blood pressure

hypertonic uterine contractions contractions with an increase in resting tone to more than 15 mm Hg

hypertrophy an increase in the size of an organ because the cells have increased in size rather than number

hypocalcemia decreased serum calcium level

hypodermoclysis subcutaneous infusion

hypofunction underfunction of a gland or organ leading to acute or chronic insufficiency

hypoglycemia decreased blood glucose level

hyposensitization immunotherapy; a process to diminish an allergic response

hypospadias urethral defect in which the urethral opening is not at the end of the penis but on the ventral (lower) aspect of the penis

hypothalamus an organ located in the center of the brain that is the regulator of the autonomic nervous system

hypotonic uterine contractions the number of contractions are low or infrequent (not increasing beyond two or three in a 10-minute period) or ineffective

hypoxemia deficient oxygenation of the blood

hypoxia inadequate oxygenation of body tissue

identity developmental task of adolescence; determining who one is

imminent or inevitable miscarriage a threatened miscarriage accompanied by uterine contractions and cervical dilation

immune response body's action plan devised to combat invading organisms or substances by leukocyte and antibody activity

immune serum serum that provides passive immunity

immunity the ability to destroy invading antigens

immunocompetent cells cells capable of resisting foreign invaders

immunogen substance (antigen) that can be readily destroyed by an immune response

immunoglobulins antibodies that bind to and destroy specific antigens

implantation nidation; the attachment of the zygote to the uterine endometrium

imprinting differential expression of genetic material that allows researchers to identify whether the chromosomal material has come from the male or female parent

incest sexual activity between family members

inclusion children with physical or cognitive challenges attending regular schools and classes

incompetent cervix a cervix that dilates and causes birth of a fetus before term

incomplete miscarriage part of the conceptus (usually the fetus) is expelled, but the membranes or placenta is retained in the uterus

incomplete protein a protein that does not contain all of the essential amino acids

incubation period time between the invasion of an organism and the onset of symptoms of infection

indirect care the nurse plans and supervises care given by others, such as home health care aides or parents

induction of labor labor that is artificially started

industry the developmental task of the school-age child, according to Erikson; to learn how to do things well

infant mortality rate percent of infants who die during the first year of life per 1000 births

infantile spasms a form of generalized seizures—"salaam" and "jackknife"—or infantile myoclonic seizures, characterized by very rapid movements

infertility the inability to produce children

inguinal hernia protrusion of a section of the bowel into the inguinal ring

initiative the developmental task of the preschooler, according to Erikson; to learn how to do things

innocent heart murmur heart murmur of no significance; also called insignificant or functional heart murmur

insensible fluid loss fluid loss occurring as a result of evaporation from skin and lungs and from saliva

inspection visual observation to determine health

inspiration delivery of warmed moistened air via the respiratory system to the alveoli

insulin pump an automatic pump about the size of a transistor radio used to deliver insulin continuously

intelligence ability to think abstractly, to adjust to new situations, and to profit from experience

intercostal spaces spaces between the ribs

interferon a protein that protects against viruses

intermittent infusion devices (heparin locks) devices that maintain open venous access for medicine administration, yet allow patients to be free of intravenous tubing so that they can be out of bed and more active

intimate partner abuse abuse by a significant other

intracath a slim, pliable catheter threaded into a vein

intrauterine device (IUD) a contraceptive device inserted into the uterine cavity

intrauterine growth restriction or retardation (IUGR) failure to grow at the expected rate in utero

intuitive thought a stage of preschool thinking in which children can only see one characteristic of an object (centering)

intussusception invagination of one portion of the intestine into another

involution the process whereby the reproductive organs return to their nonpregnant state

irritable bowel syndrome presence of either intermittent episodes of loose and normal stools or recurrent abdominal pain

ischial tuberosity diameter distance between the ischial tuberosities, or the transverse diameter of the outlet (the narrowest diameter at that level or the one most apt to cause a misfit)

isoimmunization production of antibodies against Rh-positive blood in a fetus by a woman's immunologic system

jaundice yellowing of the skin

kangaroo care placing a newborn against a parent's skin to transfer heat from the parent to the newborn, thus conserving body heat

karyotype a visual presentation of chromosomes

keratomalacia necrosis of the cornea with perforation, loss of ocular fluid, and blindness

kernicterus permanent brain cell damage secondary to elevated bilirubin levels

ketoacidosis a lowered serum pH resulting from accumulation of ketones

kinesthesia ability to distinguish movement

Koplik's spots, small, irregular, bright red spots with a blue-white center point, appearing on the buccal membrane with measles

kwashiorkor disease caused by protein deficiency

labile mood sudden mood changes (e.g., crying occurs, followed immediately by giggling or laughing)

labor-delivery-recovery room a hospital room specifically designed to accommodate labor and birth so that a separate delivery room is not needed

labor-delivery-recovery-postpartum room a specifically designed room that serves as the location not only for labor and birth but also for the post-partum recovery period

lactase the enzyme that converts lactose to glucose and galactose

lactiferous sinuses reservoirs for milk located behind the breast nipple

lactoferrin iron-binding protein in breast milk that interferes with growth of pathogenic bacteria

Lamaze method of childbirth a method of childbirth based on conditioned reflexes using paced breathing and relaxation techniques

Landau reflex develops at 3 months; when held in ventral suspension, the infant's head, legs, and spine extend. When the head is depressed, the hips, knees, and elbows flex

lanugo fine, downy hair that covers a newborn's shoulders, back, and upper arms

laparoscopy examination of the abdominal cavity and organs by insertion of a surgical instrument through the anterior abdominal wall

large-for-gestational-age (LGA) infant an infant who falls above the 90th percentile in weight

latchkey child a child who is without adult supervision for a part of each weekday

latent tetany neuromuscular irritability associated with hypocalcemia

learned helplessness psychological infantilism; phase of intimate partner violence in which the partner is forced to use coping mechanisms such as becoming very obedient and cooperative in a desperate effort to reduce the violence

LeBoyer method a birth method encouraging a quiet, darkened room and maternal-infant bonding

left-to-right shunts heart or circulatory anomalies that involve blood movement from the arterial to the venous system (oxygenated to unoxygenated blood)

Leopold's maneuvers a method of observation and palpation to determine fetal presentation and position

lesbian a female homosexual

let-down reflex collecting sinuses of the mammary glands contract, forcing milk forward through the nipples, thus making it available for the baby

letting-go phase the third phase of the postpartal period in which the woman redefines her new role

leukemia distorted and uncontrolled proliferation of white blood cells (leukocytes)

leukocytes white blood cells

leukopenia a decrease in the number of white blood cells

leukorrhea a whitish, viscous vaginal discharge or an increase in the amount of normal vaginal secretions

libido sexual nature

lie the relationship between the long axis of the fetus and the long axis of the mother

light refraction manner that light is bent as it passes through the lens of the eye

lightening descent of the fetus into the pelvis at about 2 weeks prior to birth; also called engagement

lithotomy position a position with a woman on her back with her thighs flexed and her feet resting in the examining table stirrups

liver transplantation surgical replacement of a malfunctioning liver by a donor liver

lochia uterine flow, consisting of blood, fragments of decidua, white blood cells, mucus, and some bacteria following childbirth

lochia alba colorless or white vaginal discharge occurring about the 10th postpartal day

lochia rubra vaginal discharge consisting almost entirely of blood with only small particles of decidua and mucus, occurring from days 1 to 3 of the postpartal period

lochia serosa pink or brownish vaginal discharge beginning at about the 4th postpartal day

lordosis forward curve of the spine

low segment incision an incision made horizontally across the abdomen just over the symphysis pubis and also horizontally across the uterus just over the cervix

low-birth-weight infant an infant weighing under 2500 g

lymphokine a substance that contains or prevents migration of antigens

lymphoma malignancy of the lymph or reticuloendothelial system

lysis killing

lysozyme enzyme found in breast milk that apparently actively destroys bacteria by lysing (dissolving) their cell membranes, possibly increasing the effectiveness of antibodies

macronutrient mineral with a daily requirement greater than 100 mg

macrophages mature white blood cells

macrosomia birth weight above the 90th percentile on an intrauterine growth chart for that gestational age

magnetic resonance imaging (MRI) combination of a magnetic field, radio frequency, and computer technology to produce diagnostic images

malleoli rounded prominence on either side of the ankles

malocclusion deviation from normal teeth positioning

mandatory reporters persons who are required to report suspected child abuse when they identify it

manifest tetany muscular twitching and carpopedal spasms from hypocalcemia

mastitis infection of the breast

maternal and child health nursing the full scope of nursing that deals with families during childbearing and childrearing periods

maturation reaching adulthood

McBurney's point one third of the way between the anterior superior iliac crest and the umbilicus; location of the appendix

McDonald's Rule the fundus-to-symphysis distance in cm is equal to the week of gestation between the 20th to 31st week of pregnancy

means of transmission method of spread of pathogens that cause infectious disease

Meckel's diverticulum the remains of a small pouch of the omphalomesenteric (vitelline) duct off the ileum, approximately 18 inches from the ileum-colon junction

meconium a sticky, tarlike, blackish-green, odorless material formed from mucus, vernix, lanugo, hormones, and carbohydrates that accumulates during intrauterine life in the intestine

meconium plug extremely hard portion of meconium that completely obstructs the intestinal lumen, causing bowel obstruction

megakaryocytes immature thrombocytes

megaloblastic anemia enlarged red blood cells

meiosis type of cell division in which the number of chromosomes in the cell is reduced to the haploid (half) number for reproduction (23 rather than 46 chromosomes)

melasma excessive body pigment on the face that occurs during pregnancy

memory cells B lymphocytes that are responsible for retaining the formula or ability to produce specific immunoglobulins

menarche the first menstrual period

menopause the cessation of ovarian function

menorrhagia an abnormally heavy menstrual flow

mesoderm one of the layers of primary germ cell tissue in the embryo

metabolism conversion of a drug into an active form (biotransformation) or an inactive form (inactivation)

metaphysis thin area between the diaphysis and epiphysis in long bones

metastasis tumors that have extended beyond the original site or have spread systemically

metrorrhagia bleeding between menstrual periods

micronutrient mineral with a daily requirement less than 100 mg

milia pinpoint white papule (a plugged or unopened sebaceous gland) that can be found on the cheek or across the bridge of the nose of newborns

missed miscarriage now more commonly referred to as early pregnancy failure; the fetus dies in utero but is not expelled

mittelschmerz abdominal pain during ovulation from the release of accompanying prostaglandins

molding change in shape of the fetal skull owing to the force of uterine contractions pressing the vertex against the not-yet-dilated cervix

molestation vague term that includes "indecent liberties," such as oral-genital contact, genital fondling and viewing, and masturbation

Mongolian spot collection of pigment cells (melanocytes); slate-gray patches across the sacrum or buttocks and possibly the arms and legs of newborns

monophasic oral contraceptive birth control pills that contain the same amount of estrogen and progestin content in each pill throughout the cycle

Montgomery's tubercles sebaceous glands of the areola of the breast

mood quality a person's usual emotional state

mores customs generally accepted as right to follow by a community or society

mortality rate the number of deaths per 1000 persons

morula the developing blastomere structure as it multiplies rapidly and forms a bumpy surface

motor tics eye blinking, neck jerking, and facial grimacing

multigravida woman who has been pregnant more than once

multipara a woman who has given birth to more than one child past the age of viability

mumps orchitis testicular inflammation and scarring due to the mumps virus

Munchausen syndrome by proxy parent who repeatedly brings a child to a health care facility, reporting symptoms of illness when in fact the child is well

myometrium the muscle layer of the uterus

myopathy disease of the muscular system

myopia nearsightedness

natal teeth teeth present at birth

natural family planning contraception involving no medical devices or chemicals

near drowning a state in which a person has survived drowning

neck righting reflex turning of shoulders, trunk, and pelvis in the same direction when the infant turns the head to the side

necrotizing enterocolitis (NEC) development of necrotic patches in the bowel, interfering with digestion and possibly leading to a paralytic ileus; seen in infants in intensive care nurseries

neonatal nurse practitioner nurse skilled in the care of the newborn, both well and ill

neonatal period the interval from birth to 28 days of age

neonatal teeth teeth erupting in the first 4 weeks of life

neonate a baby in the neonatal period, the first 28 days of life

neoplasm new growth, usually referring to new *abnormal* growth that does not respond to normal growth-control mechanisms

nephrosis altered glomeruli permeability due to fusion of the glomeruli membrane surfaces causing abnormal loss of protein in urine

neural plate the embryonic structure from which the nervous system develops

neuroblastomas tumors that arise from the cells of the sympathetic nervous system

neurons nerve cells

nevus flammeus a macular purple or dark red lesion (sometimes called a *port-wine stain* because of its deep color) that is present at birth

nociceptors specialized group of sensory receptors for pain

nocturnal emissions ejaculation during sleep

nondisjunction uneven cell division that leads to abnormal chromosome divisions

non–rapid-eye movement (NREM) sleep first stage of sleep; type of sleep that occurs in up to 80% of total sleep time

nonstress test an assessment of fetal well-being determined from examination of the fetal heart rate in relationship to fetal activity

nontherapeutic communication communication that lacks deliberate purpose (e.g., socializing)

normoblast a developmental stage of RBC after erythroblasts

norms customs generally accepted as right to follow by a community or society

nulligravida woman who is not or never has been pregnant

nurse-midwife nurse who assists women with pregnancy and childbearing either independently or in association with an obstetrician; can assume full responsibility for the care and management of women with uncomplicated pregnancies

nursing research controlled investigation of problems that have implications for nursing practice

nutritional marasmus disease caused by deficiency of all food groups, basically a form of starvation

nystagmus rapid, irregular eye movement

obese a body mass index over 30.0 or, in a child, a weight over the 90th percentile on a weight chart

object permanence awareness that an object exists even when it is out of sight

Oedipus complex strong emotional attachment of a preschool boy to his mother (Freud)

oligohydramnios a decreased amount of amniotic fluid

omphalocele protrusion of abdominal contents through the abdominal wall at the point of the junction of the umbilical cord and abdomen

oncogenic viruses viruses associated with causing cancer due to their ability to change the structure of DNA or RNA

oocyte an immature ovum

operculum the mucous plug formed in the cervical canal during pregnancy

ophthalmia neonatorum eye infection at birth or during the first month, most commonly caused by *Neisseria gonorrhoeae* or *Chlamydia trachomatis*

orchiectomy removal of the testis

orchiopexy surgery to repair undescended testes

orchitis inflammation of the testes

organic heart murmur murmur occurring as the result of heart disease or a congenital defect

organogenesis organ formation

orthopnea position with the head and chest elevated to ease breathing

orthoptics eye exercises

osteogenic sarcoma malignant tumor of long bone involving rapidly growing bone tissue (mesenchymal-matrix forming cells)

otorrhea discharge from the external ear

overhydration excess body fluid, usually extracellular fluid

overweight a body mass index between 25.0 and 29.9

oxytocin a pituitary hormone that initiates or sustains uterine contractions

pain an unpleasant sensation caused by pressure, injury, or tissue anoxia; whatever the person experiencing it says it is, and existing whenever he or she says it does

pain threshold the point at which the individual reports that a stimulus is painful

pain tolerance the point at which an individual withdraws from a stimulus or seeks relief

palilalia repeating one's own words

palpation an assessment technique that yields information on warmth and edema through touching

pancytopenia reduction of all blood cell components

para number of children above the age of viability a woman has previously birthed

parachute reaction arm extension seen in 6- to 9-month-old infants who are suddenly lowered toward an examining table from ventral suspension, as if to protect themselves from falling

parallel play playing alongside, not with, other children; characteristic of toddlers

paraphrasing restating what a person has said not only to assure the person that you have heard correctly (as in clarifying), but to help explain what the person was trying to say

paraplegia (diplegia) paralysis of the lower extremities

paroxysmal coughing series of expiratory coughs after a deep inspiration

paroxysmal nocturnal dyspnea suddenly waking at night short of breath

passage the birth canal

passenger the fetus

patent urachus failure of the urachus (narrow tube that joins the bladder to the umbilicus in utero) to close properly during embryologic development, leading to the development of a fistula between the bladder and umbilicus

pathologic retraction ring (Bandl's ring) a type of contraction ring that occurs at the juncture of the upper and lower uterine segments; a warning sign that severe dysfunctional labor is occurring

patient-controlled analgesia (PCA) form of administration that allows self-administration of IV boluses of medication, usually opioids, with a medication pump

pedal (foot) spasm foot spasm manifested as the foot is extended, the toes are flexed, and the sole of the foot is cupped

pediatric nurse practitioner an advanced nursing role that specializes in the well care of children

pedophile adult who seeks out children for sexual gratification

pellagra deficiency of niacin involving dermatitis and resembling a sunburn

pelvic inflammatory disease (PID) infection of the pelvic organs: the uterus, fallopian tubes, ovaries, and their supporting structures

peptic ulcer shallow excavation formed in the mucosal wall of the stomach, the pylorus, or the duodenum

perception checking documenting a feeling or emotion

percussion a chest physiotherapy technique that uses a cupped or curved palm against the chest; an assessment technique that helps determine the consistency of tissue beneath the surface area

perimetrium the outer coat of the uterus

perinatal home care health care at home during pregnancy or the neonatal period

periodic respirations irregular breathing pattern typically seen in newborns

periosteum outside sensitive layer covering of central shafts of long bones

peripartal cardiomyopathy myocardial failure apparently due to the effect of the pregnancy on the circulatory system

peripheral nervous system (PNS) the cranial nerves, the spinal nerves, and the somatic and visceral divisions

peritonitis infection of the peritoneal cavity

periventricular leukomalacia (PVL) abnormal formation of the white matter of the brain

permanence the awareness that objects exist when out of sight

permissive reporters people who may, but are not legally required to, report child abuse

petechiae pinpoint, macular, purplish-red spots caused by intradermal or submucous hemorrhage

phagocytosis destruction of invading substances

pharmacokinetics the way a drug is absorbed, distributed throughout the body, metabolized, inactivated, and excreted

phenotype outward appearance or the expression of the genes

phonocardiogram diagram of heart sounds translated into electrical energy by a microphone placed on the chest and then recorded as a diagrammatic representation of heart sounds

photophobia sensitivity to light

physiologic jaundice yellowing of the skin occurring on the 2nd or 3rd day of life as a result of the breakdown of fetal red blood cells

physiologic retraction ring ridge on the inner uterine surface marking the boundary between the upper and lower segments of the uterus during labor

physiologic splitting term to denote closure of the pulmonary valve slightly later than the aortic valve

pica indiscriminate eating of non-food substances

pincer grasp ability to bring the thumb and first finger together to pick up small objects

placenta accreta an unusually deep attachment of the placenta to the uterine myometrium

placenta circumvallata the fetal side of the placenta is covered with chorion membrane

placenta marginata the fold of chorion reaches just to the edge of the placenta

placenta previa low implantation of the placenta

placenta succenturiata one or more accessory lobes connected to the main placenta by blood vessels

plasma cells B lymphocytes that secrete large quantities of immunoglobulins

play therapy a psychoanalytic technique used by psychiatrists to help children better understand their feelings and thoughts and motivations

plethora marked reddened appearance of the skin

plumbism lead poisoning

pneumothorax the presence of atmospheric air in the pleural space

poikilocytic irregular in shape

point of maximum impulse (PMI) the point on the chest where the apical heartbeat can be heard best

polycystic kidney large, fluid-filled cysts forming in place of normal kidney tissue

polycythemia an increase in the number of red blood cells that results as a compensatory response to insufficient oxygenation of the blood

polydactyly presence of one or more additional fingers

polydipsia excessive thirst

polyuria excessive urination

portal of entry means by which a pathogen can enter a person's body

portal of exit method by which organisms leave an infected person's body to be spread to others

position the relationship of a specific fetal part to the maternal pelvis

positive reinforcement rewarding someone for demonstrating desired behavior

positive signs of pregnancy findings that definitely indicate a pregnancy is present

positron emission tomography (PET) CT scan involving the use of an injectable radioactive contrast medium

postcardiac surgery syndrome febrile illness with pericarditis and pleurisy that appears to be a benign inflammatory response to a surgical procedure, developing at the end of the first postoperative week

postconventional development the mature form of moral reasoning in which standards of conduct are internalized (Kohlberg)

postpartal depression overall feeling of sadness in a woman accompanied by extreme fatigue, an inability to stop crying, increased anxiety about her own or her infant's health, insecurity (unwilling to be left alone or unable to make decisions), psychosomatic symptoms, and either depressive or manic mood fluctuations during the first year following birth

postpartal psychosis psychiatric illness occurring during the postpartum period

postperfusion syndrome a complication after cardiac surgery manifested by fever, splenomegaly, general malaise, maculopapular rash, hepatomegaly, and leukocytosis

post-term infant infant born after the onset of week 43 of pregnancy

post-term pregnancy a pregnancy that exceeds the limit of 42 weeks

post-term syndrome infant who stays in utero past week 42 of pregnancy and demonstrates the characteristics of malnourishment

postural proteinuria also called postural albuminuria; condition in which albumin spills into the urine when children stand upright for an extended period and decreases when resting in the supine position

powers of labor labor contractions

precipitate labor uterine contractions so strong that the woman gives birth with only a few rapidly occurring contractions

preconventional reasoning stage of moral development centering on "niceness" or "fairness"

preeclampsia in pregnancy-induced hypertension, the phase before the pregnant woman experiences a seizure

prehensile ability ability to coordinate hand movements

preload volume of blood in the ventricles at the end of diastole (the point just before contraction)

premature cervical dilatation previously termed an incompetent cervix; refers to a cervix that dilates prematurely and therefore cannot hold a fetus until term

premature ejaculation deposition of sperm before vaginal penetration or the full enjoyment of the sexual partner

premature separation of the placenta also called abruptio placentae; separation of the placenta before birth of the fetus

premenstrual dysphoric disorder (PDD) condition occurring in the luteal phase of the menstrual cycle and relieved by the onset of menses that has both behavioral and physiologic symptoms

preoperational thought period of cognitive development at the end of the toddler stage; the child begins to use assimilation (Piaget)

prereligious stage the infant period of moral reasoning, according to Kohlberg

pressure anesthesia a natural yet simplest form of pain relief for birth that results from the fetal head pressing against the stretched perineum

presumptive signs of pregnancy findings, largely subjective in nature, that suggest but do not confirm that a pregnancy is present

preterm infant infant born before term (less than the full 37th week of pregnancy)

preterm labor labor that occurs before the end of week 37 of gestation

preterm rupture of membranes rupture of fetal membranes with loss of amniotic fluid during pregnancy

priapism persistent, painful erection

primary apnea period of halted respirations during the first few seconds of life

primary circular reaction infant's exploration of objects by grasping them with the hands or by mouthing them

primary engorgement feeling of tension in the breasts on the 3rd or 4th day postpartum

primary infertility no previous conceptions have occurred

primary nursing a nursing pattern in which one nurse assumes complete responsibility for the care of a patient

primigravida a woman during her first pregnancy

primipara a woman who has given birth to one viable infant

probable signs of pregnancy findings, largely objective in nature, that suggest but do not confirm that a pregnancy is present

prodromal period a time between the beginning of nonspecific symptoms and specific infectious symptoms

prolactin an anterior pituitary hormone that acts on the acinar cells of the mammary glands to stimulate the production of milk

proteinuria protein in the urine

prune belly syndrome severe urinary tract dilation that develops as early as intrauterine life from an unknown cause

pseudoanemia the apparent anemia that occurs early in pregnancy due to rapid expansion of blood volume

pseudocyesis false pregnancy

pseudohermaphrodite a child with some external features of both sexes, although only either ovaries or testes (or neither) are present

pseudomenstruation mucous vaginal secretion in female newborns, which is sometimes blood-tinged

psychomotor learning learning that requires a change in an individual's ability to perform a skill

psychoprophylactic method the Lamaze method of childbirth

ptosis drooping of the eyelid

puberty the stage at which a person first becomes capable of sexual reproduction

pudendal nerve block the injection of a local anesthetic near the right and left pudendal nerves at the level of the ischial spine

puerperium the first 6 weeks following childbirth

pulse pressure the gap between systolic and diastolic blood pressure

punishment a consequence that results from a breakdown in discipline (disregarding the rules)

purging self-induced vomiting or the use of laxatives, enemas, or diuretics

purpura hemorrhagic rash or small hemorrhages occurring in the superficial layer of skin

pyloric stenosis hypertrophy or hyperplasia of the muscle surrounding the pyloric sphincter (opening between the lower portion of the stomach and the beginning portion of the intestine, the duodenum), making it difficult for the stomach to empty

pyrosis heartburn

quadriplegia paralysis of all four extremities

quickening the first movement of the fetus perceived by the mother

radiation transfer of body heat to a cooler solid object not in contact with the baby

radiopharmaceuticals radioactive-combined substances that, when given orally or by injection, flow to designated body organs

rales fine crackling lung sound; denotes fluid in alveoli

rape trauma syndrome a form of post-traumatic stress syndrome consisting of two phases: disorganization and reorganization

rapid eye movement (REM) last stage of sleep lasting 10 to 30 minutes in which eyes move in rapid, involuntary motions and respirations are irregular; body turnings, movements, and penile erections may occur

recessive gene gene that is not dominant

rectocele a herniation of the rectum into the posterior vaginal wall

recurrent pregnancy loss having three spontaneous miscarriages that occurred at the same gestation age in three pregnancies

redemonstration returning a demonstration to show competency of the skill

referred pain pain that is perceived at a site distant from its point of origin

reflecting technique for therapeutic communication that involves restating the last word or phrase a person has said

remodeling new bone tissue replacing old bone tissue

reorganization phase second phase of rape trauma syndrome that may last for months or years; rape victims possibly continue to report recurring nightmares, perhaps sexual dysfunction, and continuing inability to relate to men or face new and surprising situations. They may continue to have a great deal of difficulty discussing the rape

reproductive life planning planning to space children or prevent children from being conceived

reservoir container or place in which organisms grow and reproduce

resorption the breakdown of bone cells

reticulocyte a developmental stage of red blood cells prior to the formation of mature RBCs

retinopathy of prematurity (ROP) an acquired ocular disease that leads to partial or total blindness in children, due to vasoconstriction of immature retinal blood vessels; commonly caused by use of too-high oxygen levels

retractions indentation of intercostal spaces reflecting difficulty breathing

retractors long, metal, curved instruments used to aid birth

retroflexion a uterus that is bent backward just above the cervix

retroversion a uterus that is tipped abnormally backwards

reversibility the ability to retrace steps

review of systems summary of body symptoms as the last step in a health interview

Rh incompatibility an Rh-negative mother (one negative for a D antigen or one with a dd genotype) is carrying a fetus with an Rh-positive blood type (DD or Dd genotype)

rhabdomyosarcoma tumor of striated muscle

rhinorrhea discharge from the nose

rhythmicity a regular rhythm in physiologic functions

rickets deficiency of vitamin D involving poor bone formation

right-to-left shunt cardiac anomaly when blood is shunted from the venous to the arterial system as a result of abnormal communication between the two (deoxygenated blood to oxygenated blood)

ripening softening of the cervix with the approach of labor

role confusion characteristic of people who do not develop a sense of identity; uncertainty about what kind of person one is

role fantasy a method of thinking that changes perceptions to how the child would like things to turn out (magical thinking)

rooming-in a hospital pattern in which infant stays in the room with the mother

sarcomas tumors derived from connective tissue, such as bone and cartilage, muscle, blood vessels, or lymphoid tissue

schemas the means by which thoughts are organized (Piaget)

scope of practice range of activity

scurvy vitamin C deficiency involving muscle tenderness and petechiae

seborrhea a scaly scalp condition, often called cradle cap

secondary apnea weakening of a newborn's respiratory effort after attempts to initiate respirations with a few strong gasps after 1 to 2 minutes of apnea

secondary circular reaction infant's ability to realize that his or her actions can initiate pleasurable sensations

secondary infertility a couple is unable to conceive at present although they have had a previous viable pregnancy

secondary stuttering stuttering that develops after a child learns to speak without stuttering

sella turcica a depression of the sphenoid bone

sensorimotor stage the period from birth to 2 years of age (Piaget)

sensory deprivation loss of environmental stimuli

sensory overload receiving more stimulation than can be tolerated or processed

septicemia pathogenic organisms in the blood stream

sequestrum dead bone tissue detached from adjoining healthy bone

sexually transmitted infections (STIs) those spread through sexual contact with an infected partner

shaken baby syndrome repetitive, violent shaking of a small infant by the arms or shoulders causing a whiplash injury to the neck, edema to the brain stem, and distinct retinal hemorrhages

shoulder dystocia an infant's wide shoulders are unable to pass through the outlet of the pelvis

sickle-cell crisis term used to denote a sudden, severe onset of sickling with sickle-cell anemia

sickle-cell trait the existence of hemoglobin AS (normal hemoglobin and abnormal hemoglobin S); a disease carrier

silent rape syndrome long-term effects in victims who do not report rape and receive no counseling

Sims' position turned to the left side with the weight of the uterus resting on the bed

single photon emission computerized tomography (SPECT) CT scan involving the use of an injectable iodine-based contrast medium

sinus arrhythmia a marked heart rate increase occurring as the child inspires and a marked decrease in heart rate as the child expires

sitz bath small, portable basin that fits on a toilet seat to provide a constant supply of water to the perineal area. It soothes healing tissue and decreases inflammation by vasodilation to the area

skilled home care care that includes physician-prescribed procedures such as dressing changes, administration of drugs, health teaching, and observation of the client's progress

sleep deprivation lack of adequate amount of sleep leading to difficulty in concentrating and episodes of disorientation and misperception

small-for-gestational-age (SGA) infant an infant who falls below the 10th percentile of weight for age

social smile a definite response (smiling) to an interaction occurring at about 6 weeks of age

somatic pain pain that originates from deep body structures such as muscles or blood vessels

Somogyi phenomenon rebound hyperglycemic response, typically manifested with nighttime hypoglycemia and early morning hyperglycemia

speculum a metal or plastic instrument with movable flat blades used for pelvic examinations

sperm count the number of sperm present in a measured amount of semen

sperm motility whether sperm are seen to be active

spermatogenesis production of sperm cells

spina bifida Latin for "divided spine"; most often used as a collective term for all spinal cord disorders

spontaneous miscarriage pregnancy interruption due to natural causes

stalking repetitive, intrusive, and unwanted actions directed at an individual to gain the individual's attention or evoke fear

station the relationship of the presenting part of the fetus to the level of the ischial spines

status epilepticus a seizure that lasts continuously for more than 30 minutes or a series of seizures from which the child does not return to his or her previous level of consciousness

steatorrhea large, bulky, greasy stools

stenosis narrowing

stereognosis the ability to recognize an object by touch

stereopsis depth perception; the ability to locate an object in space relative to another object

stereotyping applying a fixed conception

strabismus crossed eye

strawberry hemangioma a type of birthmark identified as an elevated area formed by immature capillaries and endothelial cells

striae gravidarum reddish steaks appearing on the abdominal wall during pregnancy

stridor a harsh, strident breath sound on inspiration

stupor lethargy and unresponsiveness

subconjunctival hemorrhage rupture of a conjunctival capillary appearing as a red spot on the sclera, frequently seen in newborns

substance abuse the use of chemicals to improve a mental state or induce euphoria

substance dependent when a person has withdrawal symptoms following discontinuation of the substance, and such activities as abandonment of important activities, spending increased time in activities related to substance use, using substances for a longer time than planned, and continued use despite the existence of worsening problems due to substance use

substitution of meaning also called guided imagery; distraction technique to help a person place another meaning (a non-painful one) on a painful procedure

suppressor T cells T cells that reduce the production of immunoglobulins against a specific antigen and prevent their overproduction

surfactant a lipoprotein secreted by the alveoli cells to reduce surface tension in alveoli

susceptible host individual more prone to infection than others

syndactyly fusing of the fingers

synergeneic transplantation transplantation between a donor and recipient who are genetically identical (i.e., identical twins)

systole contraction of the heart chambers

T lymphocytes lymphocytes that are produced by the bone marrow but mature under the influence of the thymus gland (hence the term *T cells*)

taboos actions that are prohibited in a specific culture

tachypnea an increased respiratory rate

taking-hold phase the second phase of the postpartal period where the woman begins to initiate action

taking-in phase the first phase of the postpartal period experienced when the woman is reflective and plays a largely passive role

teaching plan a design of content to be taught and the teaching–learning techniques to be used

temperament a child's innate behavioral characteristics such as activity level, rhythmicity, tendency to approach or withdraw, and adaptability to situations

teratogen substance that causes fetal harm

teratogenicity capable of causing fetal harm

term infant an infant born after the beginning of week 38 and before week 42 of pregnancy

tertiary circular reaction stage a stage of development in which the child discovers new properties of objects (Piaget)

thelarche breast development changes at puberty

theory a systematic statement of principles that provides a framework for explaining some phenomenon

therapeutic communication an interaction between two people that is planned, has structure, and is helpful and constructive

therapeutic play play technique that can be used by nurses to better understand children's feelings and thoughts and relieve their anxiety

thought stopping technique whereby children are taught to stop anxious thoughts by substituting a positive or relaxing thought

threatened miscarriage pregnancy interruption manifested by vaginal bleeding, initially beginning as scant bleeding, and usually bright red in color

threshold of response the intensity level of stimulation that is necessary to evoke a reaction

threshold sensation the amount of stimulus that results in pain

thrombocytes platelets

thrombocytopenia decreased platelet count

thrombophlebitis inflammation of the lining of a blood vessel with the formation of blood clots

thrush a *Candida* infection that usually appears on the tongue and sides of the cheeks as white or gray patches

thumb opposition ability to bring the thumb and fingers together

tocolytic agent a drug to halt labor

tolerance a state of not responding to an allergen

total parenteral nutrition (TPN) concentrated hypertonic solutions of intravenous fluid containing glucose, vitamins, electrolytes, trace minerals, fat, and protein to meet all of the child's nutritional needs

toxic shock syndrome (TSS) an infection usually caused by toxin-producing strains of *Staphylococcus aureus* organisms

toxoid extract of a toxin with reduced virulence

toxoplasmosis a protozoan infection spread most commonly through contact with uncooked meat; also contracted through handling cat stool in soil or cat litter

tracheostomy an opening into the trachea to create an artificial airway

tracheotomy procedure to create an airway

traction pulling on a body part in one direction against a counterpull exerted in the opposite direction to reduce dislocations and immobilize fractures

transcultural nursing a philosophy of nursing that focuses on the unique cultural beliefs of people

transcutaneous electrical nerve stimulation (TENS) pain relief measure that achieves its effect by counterirritation on nociceptors by use of a light electric current

transillumination holding a bright light such as a flashlight or a specialized light—a Chun gun—against a body part to reveal fluid inside

transition the end of the first stage of labor, just before the woman experiences pushing sensations

transitional stool green and loose stool passed on the 2nd to 3rd day of the newborn's life

transsexual a person of one sex whose perceived identity is of the opposite sex

transvestite a person who engages in the practice of dressing in the clothes of the opposite sex for sexual gratification

triphasic oral contraceptives birth control pills in which the estrogen and progestin content varies throughout the cycle

trophoblast the outer layer of the blastocyst

true conjugate conjugate vera; measurement between the anterior surface of the sacral prominence and the posterior surface of the inferior margin of the symphysis pubis

trust the developmental task of the infant, according to Erikson; learning to love and be loved

tubal ligation a method of contraception in which the fallopian tubes are cauterized, tied, or clamped to prevent sperm from reaching the discharged oocyte

tumor staging procedure by which a malignant tumor's extent and progress are determined

turgor skin characteristic reflecting the amount of fluid in body tissue

tympanocentesis withdrawal of fluid from the middle ear through the tympanic membrane

ulcerative colitis inflammation of continuous intestinal segments, typically the colon and rectum, with the distal colon and rectum most severely affected

ultrasound painless diagnostic procedure in which pictures of internal tissue and organs are produced by high-frequency sound waves

umbilical cord the structure composed of two veins and one artery that connects the placenta to the fetus

umbilical cord prolapse a loop of the umbilical cord slipping down in front of the presenting fetal part

underweight a body mass index under 18.5

urticaria swelling and itching caused by capillary dilatation

uterine atony relaxation of the uterus in the postpartal period

uterine inversion a rare phenomenon in which the uterus turns inside out

vacuum extraction birth of a fetus by means of vacuum pressure

vaginal birth after cesarean birth (VBAC) a birth in a woman who previously had a child by cesarean birth

vaginismus painful, involuntary spasms of the vagina

varicocele abnormal dilation of the veins of the spermatic cord

vascular access port (VAP) small device (infusion port) implanted under the skin, usually on the anterior chest just under the clavicle to allow for circulatory access

vasculitis inflammation of blood vessels

vasectomy a surgical ligation of the vas deferens that results in male sterility

ventral suspension infant's appearance when held in midair on a horizontal plane, supported by a hand under the abdomen

vernix caseosa a white, cream cheese-like substance that serves as a skin lubricant; usually noticeable on a newborn's skin at birth in a term neonate

very-low-birth-weight infant infant weighing less than 1500 g

vesicoureteral reflux retrograde flow of urine from the bladder into the ureters

vibration a chest physiotherapy technique that involves pressing a vibrating hand against a child's chest during exhalation to loosen and raise mucus

visceral pain involves sensations that arise from internal organs such as intestines

vocal tics coughing, throat clearing, snorting, and barking

volvulus a twisting of the bowel causing obstruction

voyeurism the practice of obtaining sexual pleasure by looking at the nude body of another

vulnerable or fragile children children whose parents were told they would die, but who lived and are treated in a cold and unfeeling way—as if they actually did die

vulvovaginitis inflammation of the vulva or vagina

Wharton's jelly the gelatinous substance that gives bulk to the umbilical cord

wheezing whistling expiratory sound

women's health nurse practitioner an advanced practice nurse who specializes in the health care of women

xerophthalmia dry and lusterless conjunctivae caused by vitamin A deficiency

yolk sac the space in the blastocyst from which the hemopoietic system develops

zona pellucida a layer of fluid that surrounds the ovum at ovulation

zygote a fertilized ovum

Answers to Checkpoint Questions

Chapter 1

1. **B.** One of the hallmarks of a profession is that members utilize a unique body of knowledge.
2. **C.** Technology has contributed greatly to making nursing care more complex. Children still need immunizations; pregnant women still need prenatal care.
3. **C.** An advantage of family nurse practitioners is that they can care for people of all ages.

Chapter 2

1. **B.** Because women earn less than men, and single-parent families are usually headed by women, finances are a common problem.
2. **B.** The person who allows information in or out of a family is a gatekeeper.
3. **C.** The oldest child marks the stage, so the Hanovans are a Schoolage family.

Chapter 3

1. **A.** Ethnocentrism means believing that what you think or your lifestyle is better than others' thoughts or lifestyles.
2. **B.** Stereotyping is categorizing all people together, rather than respecting individual characteristics.

Chapter 4

1. **C.** Adrenarche is the development of body hair; menarche is the first menstrual period.
2. **B.** As the vas deferens is easy to locate, it is the organ blocked for a vasectomy.
3. **D.** A cystocele is herniation of the bladder into the vagina.
4. **D.** Ovulation followed by conception usually occurs on the 14th day from the end of the menstrual cycle, or in this case, on the 20th day.
5. **A.** Women who have sex with women are termed lesbian. Men who have sex with men are called gay.

Chapter 5

1. **B.** Cervical mucus is thin and watery at ovulation.
2. **D.** Migraine headaches are a contraindication to COCs.
3. **C.** Subcutaneous implants are effective for 5 years.
4. **B.** Female condoms should not be reused; they already contain a spermicide.
5. **A.** A tubal ligation seals fallopian tubes to prevent the passage of sperm.

Chapter 6

1. **A.** Lack of a uterus would be sterility. Six months is too short a time.
2. **D.** With endometriosis, endometrium regurgitates into fallopian tubes.
3. **A.** A hysterosalpingogram is an X-ray study of the uterus and tubes, using radio-opaque dye.
4. **B.** Donor insemination is injection of donated sperm into the cervix or uterus.
5. **A.** With GIFT, sperm and ova are introduced into a fallopian tube.

Chapter 7

1. **D.** Phenotype is outward appearance; genotype is the actual chromosome makeup.

2. **C.** Amy has a 21 chromosome attached to another chromosome, so with meiosis or cell division, there is a greater than usual chance a child will inherit an extra chromosome. It is not sex related.
3. **D.** Genetic counseling is confidential, so it can't be shared with family members indiscriminately. Health care providers shouldn't inject their own values into counseling.
4. **B.** The loose skin at the back of the neck is so apparent it can be revealed by sonogram during pregnancy. Babies tend to be hypotonic, not hypertonic. Sole creases are an indication of any mature fetus.

Chapter 8

1. **D.** The baby is called an embryo during the period between implantation and 5 to 8 weeks. After that, it is called a fetus.
2. **B.** A normal cord has 1 vein and 2 arteries. Other patterns suggest a cardiac disorder.
3. **A.** Surfactant decreases alveolar surface tension on expiration.
4. **C.** A full bladder, from drinking fluid, improves the scan. There is no pain.
5. **A.** Reducing bladder size helps keep it out of the puncture field.

Chapter 9

1. **B.** Ensuring safe passage for the fetus consists of accepting the pregnancy (1st trimester), accepting the coming baby (2nd trimester), and preparing for parenthood (3rd trimester).
2. **B.** Narcissism refers to interest in yourself in contrast to interest in others.
3. **D.** The three positive signs of pregnancy are: fetal heart beat heard by examiner or seen on sonogram and fetal movement felt by examiner.
4. **D.** Chadwick's sign is a color change in the vagina from pink to purple because of increased formation of blood vessels.
5. **A.** With insulin ineffective, glucose levels rise, serving to safeguard the fetus from hypoglycemia. Maternal insulin does not cross the placenta.

Chapter 10

1. **C.** Prenatal care is a prime time for health education, which is why nurses play such an important role in effective prenatal care.
2. **B.** Surgery such as an appendectomy can leave adhesions, which then interfere with uterine growth.
3. **D.** Palmar erythema can occur from increasing estrogen levels.
4. **D.** Relaxation is important to reduce pain with a pelvic exam. Holding the breath or pushing down on the diaphragm does not relax abdominal muscles.
5. **C.** The ischial tuberosity diameter should be greater than 11 cms to allow the fetal head to be born.

Chapter 11

1. **C.** Julberry can still contact a sexually transmitted infection, so she still needs to use precautions against them.
2. **A.** Jogging is not recommended during pregnancy, because the extra weight of the pregnancy can cause knee injuries.
3. **D.** Witch hazel feels cool and may shrink hemorrhoids. Mineral oil is contraindicated as it prevents absorption of vitamin A; fiber is helpful to prevent constipation; she can't lie on her stomach, as she is pregnant.
4. **C.** Ankle edema occurs from increased pressure on lower extremity veins.
5. **C.** Pregnant women should check with their health care provider before taking medicine during pregnancy. All over-the-counter medicine is not safe; measles vaccine is a live virus so is contraindicated during pregnancy.

Chapter 12

1. **C.** A typical recommended weight gain in pregnancy is 25 to 30 pounds.
2. **D.** Iron is absorbed best from an acid medium.
3. **C.** A 24-hour recall history usually secures the most accurate nutrition pattern.
4. **A.** Pica is the ingestion of nonfood substances.
5. **D.** Vitamin B_{12} is found only in animal sources.

Chapter 13

1. **B.** Tightening and relaxing perineal muscles (Kegel exercises) best strengthens them.
2. **A.** Lamaze is based on the Gating Theory of pain relief, which says pain sensations can be interrupted.
3. **C.** All settings are designed to make birth safe for both mother and baby. The other options describe additional features of specific types of birth settings.

Chapter 14

1. **D.** Changes in vagina flora with gestational diabetes can cause candida organisms to thrive.
2. **C.** Heparin can be given safely in pregnancy because it does not cross the placenta.
3. **C.** Women with sickle-cell anemia don't take iron pills during pregnancy because sickle cells are unable to incorporate as much iron in their structure as normal red cells can.
4. **A.** Because the fetus requires calcium to build bones, calcium-surrounded lesions can be activated if a woman doesn't ingest adequate calcium.
5. **A.** Salicylates decrease platelet formation so can cause increased bleeding with birth.
6. **B.** Women should typically eat a snack before bedtime, to prevent fetal hypoglycemia from ingesting little food during the night.
7. **B.** Leg veins are under more pressure than usual because of uterine pressure on veins returning to the vena cava.

Chapter 15

1. **C.** Women should not discard clots, as they may need to be inspected for the possibility of a hydatidiform mole, rather than a simple miscarriage. A woman should not use a tampon; early miscarriages do happen all the time, but this sounds heartless.
2. **D.** Ectopic pregnancy does not usually come to completion. It can be treated either with surgery or a drug such as methotrexate or mifepristone.
3. **B.** Because a low-lying placenta has to spread further to establish a good blood supply, she has a larger denuded placental site than usual so is more prone to bleeding than others.
4. **B.** Walking could increase contractions; good hydration may help halt preterm labor.
5. **A.** Magnesium sulfate is the drug of choice for preventing eclamptic seizures.
6. **B.** HELLP syndrome includes a low platelet count, so the person is prone to poor blood coagulation.
7. **D.** RhIG is passive Rh (D) antibodies that can prevent an Rh-negative mother from forming permanent antibodies against an Rh-positive fetus.

Chapter 16

1. **B.** First home visits are typically made within 24 hours, a time interval that allows small problems to be identified before they become large problems.
2. **D.** Always call for help if you feel that you are in danger. Leaving the home would leave your client still in danger. Changing the locks would not solve the immediate problem. It is difficult to reason with angry people.
3. **C.** Fiber helps prevent constipation; milk is not high fiber. Walking is contraindicated, as Lee is on bed rest. An adequate fluid intake helps prevent constipation.

Chapter 17

1. **A.** Erikson's four tasks of adolescence are: establish a value system, gain independence from parents, choose a vocation, and accept their changed body image.
2. **B.** Reticulocytes are immature red blood cells, which will start to grow rapidly if sufficient iron is available.
3. **D.** Pregnancy-induced hypertension is caused by marked vasospasm. This is more acute if blood vessels have limited elasticity.
4. **C.** Autonomic dysreflexia causes extreme hypertension. A hypotensive agent is frequently prescribed to reduce this high blood pressure.
5. **B.** A fetus receives about 50% of the drug dose of the mother.

Chapter 18

1. **D.** For the mucus plug to be loosened, cervical dilatation must be occurring.
2. **A.** An occiptoanterior position means the lie is cephalic, the back of the baby's head is facing the right anterior quadrant of the mother's pelvis; full flexion means the smallest diameter of the fetal head presents to the cervix.
3. **B.** Seventy seconds is so long it can compromise fetal oxygenation.
4. **B.** A late deceleration means the fetal heart rate decreases as a contraction ends, rather than at the beginning of a contraction, as is usual.
5. **C.** With rupture of the membranes, the fetal cord may prolapse and compromise the fetal oxygen supply. FHR would detect this is happening.

Chapter 19

1. **C.** A doula is a second support person in labor. She doesn't replace a woman's partner.
2. **B.** Warm water is comforting during labor; it may be contraindicated if membranes are ruptured, because of the increased risk of infection.
3. **A.** Peripheral relaxation can lead to systemic hypotension; slowed second stage of labor also may occur.
4. **C.** A drug to increase gastric emptying helps to avoid vomiting.
5. **A.** Walking, sitting, or standing helps gravity put pressure on the cervix and may increase the strength of contractions.

Chapter 20

1. **D.** Women may lose almost twice as much blood with cesarean as with vaginal birth.
2. **B.** A urinary catheter reduces the size of the bladder and removes it from the surgical field.
3. **C.** Modern c-birth incisions are made into the lower uterine segment, so they barely show above the pubic hair line.

Chapter 21

1. **A.** If a fetal head is too large, it will have difficulty navigating the pelvis.
2. **C.** Removing the placenta or maneuvering the uterus could increase blood loss. An oxytocin would increase uterine tension, making the uterus more difficult to replace.
3. **B.** Common symptoms of water intoxication are vomiting and headache.

Chapter 22

1. **C.** The taking hold phase means a woman is interested in actively caring for her baby.
2. **A.** An "en face" position suggests she is interested in becoming acquainted with the newborn.
3. **B.** A uterine fundus sinks below the pelvic bone at about 10 days after birth.

Chapter 23

1. **C.** HCG is produced by the placenta so will be present as long as placenta is present.
2. **B.** An upright position prevents pooling of infected lochia.
3. **B.** Postpartum psychosis means a woman has separated from reality.

Chapter 24

1. **D.** Conduction is the transfer of body heat to a cold object that touches the infant.
2. **B.** This action best initiates a Moro reflex. Making a noise or shaking a crib are less effective ways to test the reflex.
3. **C.** Milia are immature sebaceous glands, which will open and drain without therapy.
4. **A.** These five areas are used to assess newborn well-being.
5. **C.** A week is an average time for a dried cord to detach.

Chapter 25

1. **B.** Because newborns carry so much extracellular water, they can become dehydrated more quickly than adults.
2. **C.** An advantage of breast milk is it contains maternal antibodies.
3. **C.** Breastfeeding women should increase their calorie intake by 500 cal/day, being sure to use protein-rich foods, not empty calories.

Chapter 26

1. **D.** Naloxone acts to reverse the effects of common opioid drugs such as morphine and meperidine.
2. **C.** Small for gestation age infants have not thrived in utero so typically do not have fat stores for insulation.
3. **B.** If alveoli do not collapse on expiration, they open easily with the next breath.
4. **B.** Bile is incorporated into meconium so is evacuated with early feedings. Bilirubin lights is a second possibility.
5. **B.** Because of increased insulin production, infants of diabetic mothers need protection against hypoglycemia.

Chapter 27

1. **B.** The lymphatic system reaches such a peak in early school-age children that their throats are "all tonsils."
2. **D.** A sense of industry is the ability to do things well or bring tasks to completion.
3. **A.** This is magical thinking: giving human properties to inanimate objects.

Chapter 28

1. **C.** Although many infants sit steadily by 6 months, the milestone for sitting is 8 months.
2. **A.** Twelve-month-old infants use about four words.
3. **A.** Understanding object permanence means an infant knows an object still exists while it is out of sight.
4. **D.** Aspiration of small objects and falls from tables or counters are the most common type of accident in infants.
5. **C.** Baby bottle syndrome refers to caries in teeth that occur from a baby drinking from a bottle before falling asleep.

Chapter 29

1. **B.** Two year olds should speak with two-word, noun-verb sentences.
2. **C.** Reducing the number of questions asked reduces the number of time a toddler can say no. Reasoning with toddlers or mimicking behavior is rarely effective.
3. **A.** This seems like a short time, but for a 2 year old, sitting still for 2 minutes is a long time.

Chapter 30

1. **C.** Although this is variable, preschoolers typically ask 300–400 questions a day.
2. **C.** Preschoolers need to be moved to new beds because they are growing up, not because they are being replaced.
3. **C.** Masturbation is a normal phenomenon of the period as children learn more about their bodies.

Chapter 31

1. **C.** Clubs for 9-year-olds typically include children of only one gender, have a secret code or password, and are designed to exclude a certain child.
2. **B.** Candy that dissolves rapidly remains in contact with teeth for the shortest time.
3. **C.** Aerosolized cooking oils can produce a "high" because of the ingredient that creates the aerosol.

Chapter 32

1. **B.** Apocrine glands, found predominantly in the axilla and groin, are responsible for body odor.
2. **A.** Formal operational thought means children are able to use scientific reasoning.
3. **D.** Sniffing cocaine can cause loss of nasal hair.

Chapter 33

1. **B.** Parents may be unwilling to discuss a chief concern until they feel comfortable with an interviewer.
2. **C.** Blood pressure is routinely assessed beginning at 3 years.
3. **B.** Gagging a child who has a swollen epiglottis can cause it to obstruct breathing.
4. **C.** Sinus arrhythmia is a normally increased heart rate because of increased chest pressure on inspiration.
5. **A.** Varicella (chickenpox) vaccine is typically administered at 12 to 18 months. Nonimmunized children older than this could receive it at any time.

Chapter 34

1. **C.** Paraphrasing is repeating a statement to help you better understand it.
2. **B.** Cognitive learning is learning facts or increasing knowledge. A and D are affective learning; C is skill learning.
3. **C.** Ten years is about the first age children have enough ego development they can lose in a competitive game without feeling a loss of self esteem.

Chapter 35

1. **B.** Because so much fluid is held as extracellular fluid, this is easily lost with vomiting or diarrhea.
2. **A.** Protest, the first stage of separation anxiety, is marked by loud, intense crying.
3. **B.** School children do best with small tasks and a feeling of reward.
4. **C.** Any item smaller than the internal roll on toilet paper is a dangerous size to be aspirated.
5. **B.** Therapeutic play materials are best if they are most relevant to a child's condition or procedures.

Chapter 36

1. **C.** Try to restrain only the minimum amount necessary. Parents should not be asked to restrain for painful procedures.
2. **A.** Timing from the discard urine helps ensure it is a 24 hour specimen.
3. **A.** The glucose solution is hypertonic so is evacuated by the kidneys.

Chapter 37

1. **C.** With no I.D. band in place, a parent's identification is the next best verification.
2. **D.** Keeping the head still helps the drops flow all the way into the ear canal. Ear drops are never given cold. The ear should be pulled up and back in an 8 year old.
3. **A.** Activities that require Terry to use her hand are more apt to dislodge the infusion needle.

Chapter 38

1. **C.** Imagery requires a child to be able to replace a painful image with a nonpainful one.
2. **A.** Some children will avoid asking for pain medication if they know it will be injected.
3. **D.** This is a comforting explanation. A. Try never to say, "put to sleep," because the child may misinterpret this expression. C is too technical for a 3 year old.

Chapter 39

1. **D.** Keeping the intestine moist can help prevent the membrane from drying. Ice would lower body temperature.
2. **D.** Sitting the infant upright could help reduce the amount of intestine in the chest.
3. **C.** Increased intracranial pressure causes increased temperature and blood pressure, decreased pulse and respirations.
4. **A.** Stretching the neck helps to restore full neck function.
5. **B.** Muscles in a Down syndrome infant are so flaccid they can touch their toes to their nose.

Chapter 40

1. **B.** Choanal atresia is blockage of the posterior nares in newborns.
2. **C.** Beta A hemolytic streptococcus can lead to glomerulonephritis or rheumatic fever.
3. **D.** Dark red blood is old blood; suctioning or coughing could initiate new bleeding. A Heimlich maneuver is not needed.
4. **D.** Michael could have epiglottitis. Eliciting a gag reflex with this could result in obstruction of the airway.
5. **C.** Capsules should be opened but not added to hot foods or large amounts of foods.

Chapter 41

1. **C.** Murmurs that occur from a diseased heart are organic. Those that are caused by normal fluctuations are functional or innocent.
2. **C.** As the catheter is inserted it can touch the electrical conduction system of the heart.
3. **A.** Stress causes excess aldosterone and antidiuretic hormone production.
4. **A.** Because blood pressure is stronger in the left than right heart, blood will shunt from the left to the right side of the heart.
5. **A.** A one to five ratio is necessary for circulation in an infant. Two to fifteen may be used with older children.

Chapter 42

1. **C.** Mother to fetal transmission is the usual route of HIV transfer to children.
2. **B.** Epinephrine causes bronchodilation, so it can quickly enlarge the constricted airway.
3. **C.** Many children are developing allergies to latex.

Chapter 43

1. **A.** Chickenpox lesions typically move through all 4 stages. All stages may be present at the same time.
2. **C.** The parotid gland is above the jaw line in front of the ear.

3. **B.** The swollen spleen could rupture easily from pressure.
4. **A.** Scarlet fever has an unusual pattern: the rash appears on both skin and mucous membrane.
5. **B.** Pinworms migrate to the anal skin at night and deposit eggs; movement of the worms causes itchiness.

Chapter 44

1. **B.** To prevent infection, children are usually restricted from eating raw fruit until their white cell count returns to normal. Bone marrow is infused intravenously, not into the hip bones. A child will need at least one follow-up bone marrow aspiration.
2. **A.** Iron chelation therapy removes excess iron from the body to prevent hemosiderosis.
3. **B.** Blood thickens with dehydration and sickled cells clump together, shutting off circulation to distal body parts.
4. **D.** With autoimmune acquired hemolytic anemia, antibodies attach to red cells and destroy them. The phenomenon frequently follows a viral infection.
5. **C.** DIC is both abnormal coagulation and hemorrhage. Heparin frees up blood coagulation components to halt bleeding.

Chapter 45

1. **C.** As potassium ions are excreted in exchange for H+ ions, a low potassium level occurs.
2. **B.** Salmonella is easily spread by raw chicken or raw egg.
3. **A.** Because the pyloric valve does not allow milk to enter the duodenum, vomiting occurs immediately after a feeding.
4. **B.** Hepatitis A is spread by fecal contamination and contaminated water, so shellfish can be affected.
5. **C.** Kwashiorkor is a deficiency of quality protein.

Chapter 46

1. **C.** As preschoolers have recently been taught voiding is a private activity, voiding while an x-ray is taken may feel uncomfortable.
2. **A.** A hypospadias means the urinary meatus is patent, but misplaced.
3. **B.** Old blood occurs from kidney inflammation and bleeding.
4. **C.** A major concern with nephrotic syndrome is that protein is lost in urine.
5. **A.** Transplanted kidneys are placed in the abdomen to be certain there is adequate space. Children shouldn't eat raw eggs, because they may carry infection, and children are immunosuppressed after transplantation.

Chapter 47

1. **C.** Undescended testes may be more susceptible to developing cancer.
2. **D.** Some adolescents feel a heightened sense of self-esteem following breast augmentation, and it has no long-term risky side effects.
3. **C.** Candidal vaginal infections usually cause a thick, pruritic, white vaginal discharge.

Chapter 48

1. **C.** Hyperthyroidism increases metabolism, so it leads to rapid movements.
2. **C.** A function of aldosterone is to retain sodium in the body.
3. **C.** When children first begin injections of insulin, it reminds their pancreas to produce insulin, so this added amount reduces the child's need for injected insulin.

Chapter 49

1. **C.** The eleventh nerve innervates the neck and shoulder muscles
2. **C.** As the child needs fine motor control to achieve at writing or ambulating, the loss of function may seem more acute.

3. **B.** Respiratory precautions are necessary for at least 24 hours following the beginning of antibiotic therapy.
4. **B.** A generalized convulsion involves the total body.
5. **A.** Cervical injuries are common as are diving accidents.

Chapter 50

1. **A.** Covering the eye, removing the cover, and assessing whether the eye shifts position is a test for misalignment or strabismus.
2. **C.** Increased intraocular pressure from vomiting could disrupt the suture line.
3. **B.** Otitis media is an infection of the middle ear; otitis externa is infection of the ear canal.

Chapter 51

1. **C.** Crutches should not press on the axilla, as pressure can cause axillar nerve damage.
2. **A.** Children need antibiotics to cure the infection. Weight bearing is restricted.
3. **D.** As JA is probably an autoimmune process, anti-inflammatory drugs help reduce the symptoms.
4. **B.** Children who become obese are not able to ambulate as long as others. They need activities daily for intellectual stimulation.
5. **B.** Compression of the radial artery or nerve can lead to impaired nerve function.

Chapter 52

1. **B.** Preschoolers often imitate adults, so they can poison themselves if they imitate adults taking medicine. Activated charcoal is an effective drug to neutralize the poison.
2. **D.** Paint chips taste sweet, so children enjoy their taste.
3. **A.** Applying ice will reduce the temperature of his skin and stop the burning as well as reduce the pain.

Chapter 53

1. **C.** As so many white blood cells are produced, red blood cell and platelet numbers fall, leading to fatigue and bleeding disorders.
2. **B.** Straining causes increased intracranial pressure, which is already elevated from edema from surgery. A Trendelenburg position would rarely be used, as this position would increase ICP.
3. **A.** If nephroblastomas are palpated, they appear to metastasize faster than if not palpated.

Chapter 54

1. **C.** Repetitive movements are a common symptom of autism.
2. **A.** Sequencing depends on being able to recognize the way that events are related to one another in time.
3. **B.** Anorexia nervosa usually occurs in girls who have a poor self image.

Chapter 55

1. **A.** A triad of factors that lead to child abuse are special child, special parent, special circumstance. As the average parent does not make disparaging remarks about her child, Hillary may be viewed as a special child.
2. **B.** Shaking a baby causes small hemorrhages in the retina of the eye as well as more serious injuries such as subdural hematoma.
3. **D.** Rape is a crime of violence.

Chapter 56

1. **B.** As with any crisis, support people can offer help and guidance.
2. **C.** The fourth stage of grief is depression or the stage when parents start to realize death will happen.
3. **B.** Anticipatory grieving can make it hard for parents to relate to their child, as they have already grieved as if the child were dead.

Answers to What If Questions

Chapter 1

1. Because the first days of life are the time when bonding between parents and children first begins, it's advantageous to have mothers and babies cared for in the same facility. Unfortunately, if a baby must be transported for critical care, this isn't possible. Helping the new parents keep in contact with their infant through such actions as taking an instant photo of the baby before transport or reserving time for them to talk on the telephone with the baby's primary care nurse are important nursing actions.
2. This is not a simple problem because a lot of factors could be playing into it. The first responsibility, therefore, would be to discover the parent's motivation for wanting the child in the hospital. Does she understand that with current antibiotics, the care of children with this disease has been completely modified? Does she feel too insecure to care for a sick child? Does her health insurance cover only in-hospital care? Once these questions are answered, the task is not simply advocating for hospitalization (or not) but attacking the more basic problem.

Chapter 2

1. When both parents work, so that medication supervision isn't available at the usual times for medicine administration, the times should be adjusted to enable medication when supervision is possible. The parents could ask a responsible adult neighbor or relative to supervise the medicine or give it before breakfast, at lunch, after school, or before bedtime.

2. As a rule, families with many connections to their community have a ready source of support if a crisis should occur. A family with few connections in the community often requires more discharge planning.

Chapter 3

1. This situation calls for assessing why the father is saying he wants no role. If the answer is that he knows nothing about what to do, then teaching him how to be a part of an activity, such as timing contractions, would be helpful. If he does not want to be part of the process because he sees that action as culturally inappropriate, allowing him to sit quietly would be more appropriate. For many women in labor, the fact that their support person is there is the important consideration, not that the person is actively doing any particular thing.
2. In every situation, you want to respect cultural beliefs. Educating Anna about bicycle and street safety could be done without disrespecting beliefs, however.

Chapter 4

1. Observing women for urine output following uterine or fallopian tube surgery is more important than usual because the ureters pass just beneath the fallopian tubes. This means that they can be accidentally injured in surgery or, because they are so near the surgery site, be obstructed by local edema.

2. Fetishes such as this one are not unusual. Choosing to respect patient privacy in relation to the suitcase's findings is the best course of action.

Chapter 5

1. Adolescents need good explanations that sexual aids, such as diaphragms, can spread sexually transmitted diseases so should not be shared. Diaphragms also can not be shared because they must be individually fitted to provide adequate protection against pregnancy.
2. Oral contraceptives can reduce dysmenorrhea because they decrease the likelihood of endometriosis, which is a common cause of dysmenorrhea; they also reduce the length of menses. They carry a risk, however, because estrogen use can cause blood clots. A better solution for simple pain relief is an anti-inflammatory such as ibuprofen (Motrin or Advil).

Chapter 6

1. This is a very practical problem, as many women today work different shifts and exist without long periods of sustained sleep. In order to detect a pattern for a baseline, this woman probably needs to take her temperature twice a day for several days: once on arising in the morning and again on arising after her longest period of sustained sleep in the afternoon. Whichever of these times shows the most constant temperature would be her baseline temperature.
2. Ownership of cryopreserved sperm is a legal quandary not yet clearly answered in court. Before couples agree to store sperm in this way, they need to discuss their feelings about this problem, so that misunderstanding about their desires does not arise later in life.

Chapter 7

1. X-linked recessive inherited illnesses are carried by the mother on an X chromosome, but the symptoms of these diseases are apparent in male offspring. Having only boys, therefore, would increase the chance a child would have the disease, not decrease it.
2. This is a true ethical question, so the answer depends on many factors. A major thing to consider would be the length of the pregnancy, as the risk to the second child increases with duration of pregnancy. Other values to weigh would be the value of this pregnancy to the parents, their personal beliefs about abortion, and their philosophy about raising a child who is cognitively challenged. Making certain this mother was aware of all her options would be important.

Chapter 8

1. Nagele's rule is: subtract three months and add seven days from the first day of the last menstrual period. Based on this rule, the EDB would be December 20th.
2. The important rule for Liz is to count them three times a day. Counting after she has eaten has an advantage, in that a fetus may be more active at this time because the maternal blood glucose level is higher. Perhaps a bigger question to ask is why she reports that she snacks constantly rather than eating meals. Is she eating nutritious food or "snack" foods at all these times?

Chapter 9

1. You don't really have enough information to draw any conclusion here. It's doubtful this is couvade syndrome, though, because this man's wife is probably no longer experiencing nausea and vomiting of pregnancy at this point; this symptom typically disappears after the first 3 months of pregnancy.
2. Good advice for women who are having morning sickness is to be certain to eat well in the afternoon and evening after their feelings of nausea have passed. The answer to fatigue is for women to rest more. Both of these instructions may be meaningless for a homeless woman, as she doesn't have access to ready sources of food

(only at the time it is served at a nearby shelter) or a place to rest except at night in the shelter. "Walking through" such a woman's day helps you to identify opportunities to better adapt her lifestyle for pregnancy.

Chapter 10

1. If a woman knows nothing about the diseases she had as a child, asking her to question other family members about their memories can be of some help. In reality, the only truly important fact to know is whether she had German measles (rubella), because this illness can cause fetal damage if it is contracted during pregnancy. If she doesn't know whether she's had rubella, she can have a serum titer drawn, which will confirm whether she has immunity against the illness.
2. Tables in examining rooms should face away from the door, to avoid this problem. It is also important that women meet the person performing a pelvic examination before they are placed in a lithotomy position on a table, so that they meet the person at eye level, not from a lesser, vulnerable position.

Chapter 11

1. Train travel could be a helpful way to travel. Questions to ask might be whether she will be able to obtain a nutritious snack while traveling and cautioning her not to spend long time periods sitting in one position. Sitting with her knees sharply bent can lead to severe stasis of her lower extremities.
2. Your evaluation should begin with additional assessment. Urinary tract infections generally have additional symptoms: pain on urination, and possibly blood in urine or a low grade systemic fever. Asking about the type and amount of vaginal discharge would also be important, as this is a symptom of a normal change in pregnancy but also could be a STI symptom. Alerting the woman's primary care provider to her concerns is important, to be certain a clean catch urine or a vaginal swab for culture is not needed.

Chapter 12

1. Breaking a "coffee habit" is hard, partly because of the caffeine intake and partly because drinking coffee is associated with good conversation and "breaks" from work. Helping a woman see that "coffee breaks" don't have to include drinking coffee, but could include a fruit or milk drink, helps. Helping her select a restaurant for lunch other than one featuring coffee also helps.
2. The three desserts will probably add pounds. Her action needs to be considered in light of everything else she is eating, however, to be meaningful. It's important for women to understand that a good diet during pregnancy means eating better, not necessarily eating more.

Chapter 13

1. Most women appreciate having someone whom they know well with them during labor to both support them and share this very personal experience with them. You might suggest that Julia ask a close family member or friend to fill this role. For women who are alone in labor, a nurse can fill this role.
2. The most important criteria for choosing a place for birth should be choosing a setting that will be safe for mother and baby. Secondary considerations should be enjoyment, ability to actively participate, and cost. Choosing an alternative birth center could be a compromise, as this setting could supply safety plus a less structured environment.

Chapter 14

1. Angelina needs to check with her primary care provider for additional guidance. This is a common finding with women who are taking medication for a chronic illness such as heart disease. They

abruptly stop taking the medicine when they become pregnant, following the guideline, "Take no medicine during pregnancy." It is one of the reasons that obtaining a thorough health history at a pregnancy's beginning is so important.
2. Angelina needs to check with her primary care provider. Unless she was restricted in salt use before pregnancy, salt limitation is not recommended during pregnancy. Salt is necessary to regulate and maintain fluid balance, and a large circulatory volume is necessary during pregnancy to supply nutrients to the fetus.

Chapter 15

1. This is a difficult problem, because a woman needs to avoid becoming pregnant again until it is clear that all remnants of the hydatidiform mole have been removed and she is free of the possibility of developing choriocarcinoma. The first step in problem solving would be not to give her advice but to explore with her what she understands about her condition and risks. When she appreciates there are serious health risks involved for her (birth control is being advised for her not to prevent pregnancy, but to help prevent a malignancy), her attitude toward using birth control will likely improve.
2. Heparin cannot be administered orally, as it is destroyed by gastrointestinal secretions. Because heparin does not cross the placenta, the newborn should have no more tendency for a blood coagulation disorder at birth than any other infant. You should be able to answer this question, because it is often asked by women who are prescribed heparin.

Chapter 16

1. This is a situation that is occurring more and more frequently. The biggest physical problem of caring for women in these situations is that all the accommodations of a home environment (nearby kitchen, bathroom, sense of privacy, etc.) are not necessarily present. A woman may also be at the location only temporarily, so good follow-up care will need to be planned. The biggest psychosocial problem is often that a woman is not the best problem-solver, or she wouldn't be homeless. This lengthens the time spent in nursing care planning to promote optimal outcomes.
2. Mice in the house of a newborn baby is a problem that must be dealt with, because mice can carry the potentially deadly hanta virus. Rats in a home can be large enough that they will actually attack a sleeping newborn. The family, therefore, needs to deal with the problem (contacting an exterminator; setting traps, etc.) Working with them to understand the importance of these actions is the nursing responsibility.

Chapter 17

1. This diet seems to be almost totally lacking in two important food groups: fruits and vegetables. Unless the liquid drink is high in protein, it probably also lacks this important nutrient component as well. Many adolescents follow this type of diet because they simply do not know a better nutrient pattern. Help for the adolescent would start by assessing what she knows about pregnancy nutrition, then building on her food likes to construct a diet higher in essential pregnancy nutrition.
2. Most women who are drug dependent are able to discuss their dependency with health care providers, because they want to know the effect, if any, a drug will have on fetal health. Discovering evidence that possibly reveals drug use, therefore, presents an opportunity for frank discussion, and probably referral for help, for a woman so she can break free of her dependency. Ignoring the packets would serve no function and would also leave a woman uninformed about possible fetal risk.

Chapter 18

1. Most people recommend that women lie on their sides during labor, as this frees up the vena cava, ensuring a good blood supply to the uterus and fetus. Occasionally, a woman will lie on her back after monitors are attached, because she believes they will come

loose if she turns on her side or not record accurately in that position. As a rule, urge women in labor to assume a side lying position and assure them that fetal and uterine monitors record accurately in any position.
2. One of the difficulties with having more than one support person in labor is that differences in opinion can arise. In this instance, the person to consult is neither the doula nor the mother, but Celeste herself, as pain is a subjective sensation, which can be evaluated only by the person experiencing it.

Chapter 19

1. This is an individual choice. Most women today receive an epidural injection, which offers total pain relief. Gripping a hand tightly can trigger an acupressure point, thereby reducing pain. This also could be a distraction technique.
2. Naloxone hydrochloride is a narcotic antagonist that counteracts the effect of narcotic analgesics. If no narcotic is present when it is given, naloxone acts as a narcotic and will cause respiratory depression. Because the mother did not receive any narcotic during labor, administering naloxone to the newborn would be inappropriate. Asking the mother if she has recently used a recreational drug would be appropriate in order to help discover the reason for the newborn's sleepiness.

Chapter 20

1. Women receiving an epidural anesthesia are not unconscious; therefore, there is little reason that they have to remove contact lenses for anesthesia (although removing contact lenses would be important if general anesthesia was anticipated). As seeing her newborn and holding him at birth is important for bonding, advocating for this woman—and also investigating whether this routine policy should be changed—would be important.
2. Women are concerned that palpation of their fundal height will cause pain (and if they do not have adequate pain management, they are right). To reduce discomfort, be certain the woman is receiving optimal pain relief. Explain why the assessment is important and use a gentle touch.

Chapter 21

1. It's unsafe for anyone to be administered a general anesthetic when they have been eating, as vomiting and fatal aspiration can occur. You need to report she has been eating, therefore, so the anesthesiologist knows. Most important here is determining why a woman would be so opposed to cooperating with a procedure that could save her infant's life. What about general anesthesia does she think would be so intolerable?
2. A precipitous birth in a sister doesn't mean that Roseann will have one. Roseann should take a copy of her health record with her and be sure there is a medical facility nearby in case her labor does progress faster than she anticipates.

Chapter 22

1. These are normal assessment findings for a woman 12 hours postpartum. The first nursing action, therefore, would be to assure Ms. Cooper that these are normal findings. In addition, she needs guidance to rest to relieve the fatigue and measures to make her comfortable in the face of diaphoresis.
2. As a rule of thumb, saturating more than one pad an hour is more than a normal amount of lochia flow. The fact that Ms. Cooper is also passing large clots suggests her uterus is not as contracted as it could be. Assessing her fundal height and consistency would be the first assessment needed.

Chapter 23

1. This assessment certainly suggests the woman has signs of infection (the elevated temperature, the foul smelling lochia, the tender

abdomen). A referral to her primary care provider would be the next step in care.

2. Diuresis begins almost immediately following birth, so by 7 hours post birth, most women's bladders are full. A woman may not be aware of the usual sensation of filling, however, because of edema from the birth. Assessing for bladder distention by palpation and percussion would reveal the full bladder. Urging the woman to walk to the bathroom to void would be a second step. If she is unable to void by 8 hours post birth and her bladder is distended, most primary care providers advocate bladder catheterization to relieve bladder pressure.

Chapter 24

1. This mother is describing acrocyanosis, a normal finding in newborns because peripheral circulation is not functioning at an optimal level. Assuring her that this is normal in newborns would be helpful.

2. The American Academy of Pediatrics suggests all newborns receive eye prophylaxis, as there is a danger organisms can enter the amniotic fluid during labor making infants born by cesarean birth also susceptible to eye infection at birth.

Chapter 25

1. Breastfeeding an infant is a very personal experience, so whether to breastfeed is the mother's choice to make. As a rule, it is helpful to urge all mothers to at least try breastfeeding. Some who insist they will not like it are surprised to find how enjoyable and convenient it is. Equally important with this mother would be a discussion of total baby care and other areas she and her husband need to resolve before they can operate as a parental unit.

2. A number of questions come to mind. Where is the baby going to be cared for that is so remote there is not access to a refrigerator? If no refrigeration is available, could she keep the bottle in an ice chest or a cool sandwich bag? Milk, left unrefrigerated, spoils easily because warmth encourages the growth of bacteria.

Chapter 26

1. Holding a very small newborn can be frightening, as the infant seems so delicate. Discussing with a parent how important human contact is for even immature newborns can help her take the first step toward parenting or beginning interaction with her newborn.

2. If power fails while an infant is receiving pancuronium, you would want to initiate respirations immediately by means of a resuscitation bag, as the infant cannot do this on his own. A second step would be to ready the antidote for pancuronium (an anticholinesterase such as neostigmine) and administer it if prescribed.

Chapter 27

1. This is a common problem as families struggle to match paychecks to the increasing cost of food. Referral to a dietician would probably be helpful to this mother. Helping her understand that protein is important for growth, and that although meat is the best source of protein, she can also obtain protein from combinations of grains and legumes, would be helpful as she looks at her week's menus.

2. Preschoolers thrive on free form play, the type that doesn't necessarily fit well into an orderly household. Suggestions might be for these preschoolers to have one spot in the house that is their "messy spot" where they can finger paint, etc. Another might be for them to have a play space outdoors where their activities don't have to be so restricted. Urging the father to solve this problem in conjunction with his daughters is important because it is only one of many they will need to solve together in the years to come.

Chapter 28

1. If a 10-month-old infant can pick up a small marble, it probably means he has developed a pincer grasp (opposes the thumb and finger). This is a big developmental step, as it means cephalocaudal development has progressed to fine motor control. It also means that an infant can pick up and swallow (and possibly choke on) small objects so needs to be supervised closely for safety.

2. Always cleaning a plate can lead to overeating in children. A better rule is usually to serve a smaller portion and then allow the child to ask for seconds. Even young children have food preferences and will generally select a balanced diet over a week's time.

Chapter 29

1. Toddlers can be very literal-minded. Jason may have been told that the only place he should urinate is in the toilet at home. Suggesting to his mother that she tell him he can use any toilet, not specifically the one at home, would be important.

2. Again, this is a typical toddler response. If the policy of ignoring temper tantrums is to be effective, then ignoring them no matter where they happen is important. Assuming that the child will not be physically harmed by the number of people passing by in the hallway, ignoring the tantrum would be good advice.

Chapter 30

1. Because preschoolers are very concrete in their thinking, they do not generalize well. A child who knows the first rule, therefore, might not know the second statement is actually the same rule.

2. This is a good area to explore, because Cathy's concept of "stranger" is someone who looks "strange." When a good-looking man or woman approaches her, therefore, she may go with them willingly. Clarifying that the word "stranger" means anyone her parents have not said she can go with solves the problem.

Chapter 31

1. The child who does not understand accommodation can make this kind of mistake (because a first action one day led to a second action, he assumes the same action will lead to the same action on a second day).

2. School-age children have a great deal of difficulty with this concept, which is why shoplifting is so common with this age child. Frank discussion that the principle is the same helps children understand that stealing is always wrong, no matter who is involved.

Chapter 32

1. Being happy after a time of unhappiness is a possible warning sign of suicidal intent, but it could also be an innocent finding that an adolescent is having a good day. You would want to assess thoroughly to be certain you identify the reason for this change in mood.

2. Many parents are able to find another family member or family friend who can care for an adolescent when the relationship between a teenager and parents becomes unbearable. Other families need referral to a social agency to help them solve this problem. The fact that a family is asking for help is a major forward step that indicates a workable solution can be found.

Chapter 33

1. Ninety-three lbs at 13 years puts this girl's weight in the 10th percentile; a year ago her weight reached the 50th percentile. Growing children, as a rule, never go backward in growth, so the information that this girl has lost 17 lbs in 6 months needs investigation. She may have been dieting vigorously or have developed an eating disorder such as bulimia. Such a drastic weight loss may also signal the onset of illness such as diabetes mellitus, hyperthyroidism or cancer.

2. Because many families are so mobile today, this is a common situation. As a rule, immunization series are not completely started over; they are picked up at the point most practical (if this father knew his child had vaccines at 2 months, for example, the child would

start with a second DtaP and IPV). An important nursing intervention is to be certain parents receive a record of their child's immunizations, with an explanation of what the immunization was and that this is important information for parents to know.

Chapter 34

1. The answer to this question is ideally "all family members, including the adolescent." It is an example of the way that health teaching affects an entire family, not just the one member receiving the primary instructions.
2. This is an interesting quandary because you want to support the preschooler's action (Don't speak to strangers) but at the same time, you need the child to talk to you to evaluate if his pain is growing less or not. A good start would be to talk to the parent and have the parent introduce you to the child and say it's all right to talk to you. That way, you're not a stranger (strangers are not strange; they are people your parents do not know).

Chapter 35

1. Children often play with nontypical "toys" such as pots and pans from the cupboard; soft toys such as teddy bears often have missing arms or legs. The purpose of bringing a toy to the hospital is so the child has a familiar, comforting object with him or her. You can assure parents, therefore, that a worn toy is probably the most comforting as it is one well loved.
2. As you have no information on what colors this child had to draw with or what she was trying to draw, all by itself the drawing isn't remarkable. Many preschoolers cannot draw a person with more body parts than this. "Centering" often makes them concentrate on one aspect of a drawing (the body parts) but not the color. You'd need more information to evaluate the drawing.

Chapter 36

1. Many adolescents try to cover their fear of the unknown by projecting a pseudo-sophisticated attitude. To counteract this, it is often helpful to introduce procedures to teenagers with a statement such as, "You probably already know this, but let me review it with you." This approach allows adolescents to maintain a pretense of knowing everything, but still receive the information they need about procedures. It is important that adolescents do understand procedures before they are carried out; doing otherwise violates the principle of informed consent.
2. As eating in a restaurant offers more experience than simply the consumption of food, parents should be encouraged to include this type of experience in a child's activities even if the child is not going to eat in the setting. Such an experience builds vocabulary (words like menu, waiter, or waitress), encourages conversational skills, and exposes children to such skills as taking turns while they wait to be served.

Chapter 37

1. This parent may have a misunderstanding of what "no drugs" means, so advising her to meet with the school nurse to discuss the problem would be appropriate. In many instances, the "no drug" rule applies only to self-administration of medicine, not nurse-administered drugs. Even if the child cannot be given medicine in school, most medicines are not prescribed more than three times a day, so the schedule for most medicines can be arranged so that the child takes the medicine before school, immediately after returning home, and again at bedtime. These time periods do not fall into exactly even time periods but may be necessary if school rules restrict drug administration during school hours.
2. When instructions with a medicine advise that the medication is taken with a meal, it generally means that the medication is irritating to the stomach lining and taking it with a meal will help reduce the irritation. The point, though, is to be sure that the child eats something with the medicine, not necessarily a full meal. Drinking

a glass of milk or eating a snack would both furnish enough food to allow her to take the medicine safely.

Chapter 38

1. A child who colors in the entire figure has most likely not understood the directions and is using the figure drawing as a coloring activity, not a pain assessment tool. Some adolescents will do this because they consider the tool "too babyish" for them and respond by using it as a "babyish" coloring activity rather than using it to assess their pain.
2. It takes a minimum of an hour for EMLA cream to work. Doing the procedure early, therefore, will cause the child unnecessary pain. Advocating to ask the technician to respect the hour's time needed for pain relief would be an important nursing role.

Chapter 39

1. One of the problems of detecting bowel obstruction in a newborn who also had meconium staining is that bile-stained vomitus and meconium stained mucus look a great deal alike. Assessing the infant for other signs of bowel obstruction such as a distended abdomen would help reveal the problem.
2. Most authorities believe the child's rights are paramount. The decision varies with each individual child, however, depending on the extent of the defect present and the quality of life that can be anticipated. This is a family that needs referral to the agency's committee on ethical concerns.

Chapter 40

1. If a child has respiratory secretions in the airway, coughing occurs as a reflex to clear these secretions. You can help initiate this reflex by asking the child to take several deep breaths. This causes the secretions to move and trigger the reflex. Playing "Simon Says" with the child and having Simon say, "Take two deep breaths" also accomplishes this.
2. This is a common mistake made by new nurses (assuming the lack of sound shows improvement, when it actually means the child's condition is worsening). The second problem here (not enough air is entering the airway to make the sound of stridor) is the major concern. To rule this out, assess his lungs. If good air exchange is present, then the first conclusion (the child's condition is improving) can be made.

Chapter 41

1. This could just be a habitual position Megan uses, but it must be investigated, as it is a way for a child to trap blood in the lower extremities, the way that younger children use squatting or a knee-chest position. It suggests she is experiencing shortness of breath from poor heart function.
2. Ibuprofen has anti-inflammatory action in addition to analgesic action. In a child with Kawasaki disease, the drug is being used for its anti-inflammatory action as well as for pain relief, so it should be continued.

Chapter 42

1. This is a typical description of a leather allergy to a wallet, carried in the back pants pocket.
2. Itch-scratch cycles are often associated with times of stress. Final examinations, which occur at these times of the year, are often the "triggers" for this.

Chapter 43

1. The first four diseases are rubella (German measles), rubeola (regular measles), varicella (chickenpox) and scarlet fever.
2. Adolescents with pertussis cough so forcefully and long (paroxysmal coughing) that they can vomit, not from nausea, but from the

force of the coughing. They can eat again immediately, because no nausea is present.

Chapter 44

1. This is a problem that can arise because of the magical thinking of children (they believe that what they wish will come true). The fact that all transplantations are not successful should be addressed the first time the topic of transplantation arises, so both the donor and the recipient know this may happen. This helps prevent the donor child from feeling that he or she has failed (and possibly done something wrong to cause this failure); it helps to keep the recipient child from feeling that he has been let down (or possibly done something wrong).
2. Children with sickle-cell anemia need to be kept well hydrated, so this solution to bedwetting may not be the best one for this particular child. Reducing, but not eliminating, fluid intake in the evening would be a better program. Urging the parent to talk to the primary care provider about the problem and possibly beginning the child on a specific medication for nocturnal enuresis would be important.

Chapter 45

1. This question sounds as if a parent has taken a care instruction literally and not as intended. You might want to explain to the parent that "force fluids" doesn't mean she should literally force fluids but was intended to mean she should offer fluids frequently. Once the parent is clear on the instruction, then it's time to talk about what amount and types she should offer.
2. This is a practical problem because parents do "drop everything" to rush a child to the hospital for appendicitis. Good questions to ask are: Did you leave anything cooking on the stove? Do your other children have safe child care? Did you park your car or leave it by the emergency entrance? Helping the parent look at particular problems this way helps them reduce this happening from "something terrible is happening to me" to a situation they can handle with support.

Chapter 46

1. A child who is voiding black urine needs to be seen by a primary care provider as the color is undoubtedly being caused by the addition of old blood. Testing urine by a test strip procedure is the quickest method to determine if blood is present. The urine could also be examined under a microscope for the presence of red blood cells.
2. Dependent edema means that fluid is collecting in lower body parts. Edematous tissue tends to trap and store medicine, so injecting into lower body parts in this child would not be ideal. Giving an injection in the deltoid muscle, therefore, would be better, as, high on the body, it would be less effected by edema.

Chapter 47

1. All breast tissue, even that under accessory nipples, is susceptible to breast cancer. The answer to this question, therefore, is yes. If the tissue is extensive, having it removed would offer her both protection against breast cancer and probably an improved cosmetic appearance.
2. Many adolescents are not aware of exactly what immunizations they have had, so they feel confident that they have been immunized against all infectious diseases. They need to be educated that STIs, with the exception of hepatitis B, cannot be immunized against, so they can not only contract these infections but can contract them more than once.

Chapter 48

1. Because many people do not understand the great forward strides that have been made in diabetes control, it is not unusual to discover a person who still thinks of people with diabetes as disabled

or at least handicapped enough not to be able to participate actively in a sports program. Frank discussion with the coach (with the child's permission) would go a long way toward informing him about modern management. Most school systems maintain a board that specifically investigates and advocates for children with illness within the system. Informing the parents how to contact this board and that participation on a sports team is their child's right would make them better informed parents.
2. Although milk may be nutritious for the average child, it is high in phenylalanine, so it is contraindicated for the child with PKU. Investigating why the school wasn't informed of the child's special diet would be in order. Supplying the school with the needed nutritional information would also be helpful.

Chapter 49

1. This is a common problem for children who are away from home for part of every day. It's important for the mother to keep Tasha safe but also not to shelter her unnecessarily. You might talk to the mother about being certain the child's caretakers have equipment to assess her temperature and a telephone number to reach the parent if the child should develop another high temperature.
2. These are classic symptoms of autonomic dysreflexia that most often occurs because of a full bladder. Assessing to see if an indwelling catheter is free flowing would be a crucial first step.

Chapter 50

1. Explosions from fireworks are a frequent cause of loss of vision and hearing in children. You'd want to be certain this father knows to keep children a distance from the explosions, so debris doesn't strike a child's eye or the noise rupture an eardrum.
2. Many children are self-conscious about hearing aids. Some common suggestions: She could wear her hair long so the hearing aid is covered as much as possible. If the aid is a type with a large battery, it can be worn under a scarf around her neck. A better solution, though, is to help the child understand that no one is perfect. Help her learn to accept she has a hearing loss and succeed in life nevertheless.

Chapter 51

1. Children who have exercised in a different way than usual can have pain in muscles, the same as adults. An important assessment would be that the pain is truly in the muscle and not in a joint, as joint pain is much more apt to be serious.
2. Most children with scoliosis will have a good outcome as they reach adulthood. Assessing the child's current image of himself (why he thinks of himself as a cripple) would be important.

Chapter 52

1. The first priority here is to obtain a complete health history, as these symptoms are vague enough that they could be occurring from a number of reasons. Vomiting is a sign of increased intracranial pressure, so this symptom could mean that ICP is increased.
2. Small coins do pass readily in children, so usually no intervention needs to be carried out for swallowed pennies. Signs that the obstruction has occurred would be abdominal pain, abdominal distention, and failure to pass stool.

Chapter 53

1. This situation calls for increased education to help the parent understand that although nausea and vomiting imply that the drug is attacking rapidly forming cells, they are extremely uncomfortable sensations and wearying for the child. Helping the parent to see that there are better ways to evaluate chemotherapy effects, such as examining the white blood count, would also be helpful. Being certain that the parent receives information in a timely and helpful manner would be another nursing responsibility.

2. This is a typical way in which cancer can be discovered: a physician examines a body part after some trauma. The exam only revealed an already present condition, though; the trauma did not cause it.

Chapter 54

1. This is an interesting question because it makes you wonder why the girl is asking. Is she worried she is pregnant? Is she seeking sex education information on where babies come from? Does she need contraceptive information? Did she simply watch a television show last night in which there was a cute baby? Once the unvoiced question (why is she asking) is answered, the answer to the actual question will differ depending on the reason it was raised.

2. Weight loss in children always should be investigated, as normally children never lose weight. Exploring whether this boy has been dieting or has any additional symptoms would be important. Whether he could be depressed and his stress level—from trying to maintain all those As and be a perfect son—also needs to be explored.

Chapter 55

1. This type of "role reversal"—a child comforting a parent—is very typical of child abuse. Listen for it in emergency rooms. It is not diagnostic because some children who are well loved and cared for are so sensitive to their parent's emotions that they also respond this way.

2. This is a legal question depending on how "family" is interpreted. It is usually regarded as incest, however, and is definitely rape.

Chapter 56

1. Respite time means time spent doing activities that the parent enjoys. In this example, if cleaning cupboards was what the mother enjoyed and found relaxing, it was an appropriate activity. When helping parents plan for respite time, it is important the activities they choose are those they would enjoy, not necessarily those the health care provider would prefer.

2. These are typical signs of anger that can occur as an expression of grief. Recognizing these in yourself allows you to reassess how involved you are with a patient and seek respite care for yourself.

INDEX

Note: Page numbers followed by *b, f,* or *t* indicate boxes, figures, and tables, respectively.

A

AAP. *See* American Academy of Pediatrics

Abandonment
  fear of, in preschoolers, 897–899
  maternal feelings of, in postpartal period, 627

ABC. *See* Alternative birthing centers

Abciximab, for Kawasaki disease, 1313

ABCX system, for family assessment, 41, 41*f*

Abdomen
  assessment of
    in child, 1006–1008
    in six-week postpartal examination, 651*t*
  in cystic fibrosis, 1270
  of newborn, 698–699
    congenital anomaly and, 705*t*
  organs of, radiation therapy and, 1687
  palpation of, to determine fetal presentation, 513–514, 515*b*–516*b*
  quadrants of, 1006, 1007*f*
  skin changes, in pregnancy, 229, 230*f*

Abdominal breathing exercises, in postpartal period, 646*t*

Abdominal circumference, in child health assessment, 994

Abdominal contour, in labor, abnormal, 512

Abdominal crunches, in postpartal period, 646*t*

Abdominal discomfort, in pregnancy, 283–284, 286

Abdominal exercises, in labor preparation, 329–331

Abdominal massage, in labor and birth, 334–335

Abdominal muscle contractions, in childbirth preparation, 331

Abdominal pain, chronic recurrent, in children, 1445–1446

Abdominal pregnancy, 410

Abdominal reflexes, assessment of, 1010

Abdominal trauma
  blunt, in pregnancy, 389
  in children, 1655–1657

Abducens (VI) nerve, 1545*t*

ABGs. *See* Arterial blood gases

ABO incompatibility, 785–788

Abortion
  definition of, 252, 402, 1825
  induced, 125–130
  medically induced, 125–127
    complications of, 126, 127*t*
  NOC/NIC for, 126*b*
  psychological aspects of, 130
  septic, 407
  spontaneous. *See* Spontaneous abortion/miscarriage
  surgically induced, 127–129

Abruptio placentae, 401*t*, 415–417, 415*f*, 416*t*.
    See also Placenta, premature separation of

Abscess
  breast, postpartal, 670
  retropharyngeal, 1247–1248

Absence seizures, 1565

Absorption
  definition of, 1825
  of medications, in children, 1141

Abstinence, 105
  definition of, 1825
  promoting, 109*b*

Abstract thought
  in cognitive development theory, 819*t*, 820
  definition of, 1825

Abuse
  child. *See* Child abuse
  definition of, 1742, 1825
  domestic, 39
  in family, 1741–1762
  family that experiences
    nursing process for, 1742–1743
    support groups for, 1743
  intimate partner. *See* Intimate partner abuse
  in pregnancy, 254
  reduction of, National Health Goals for, 27*b*, 1742, 1742*b*
  sexual. *See* Sexual abuse
  signs of, 1742, 1742*b*

Acarus scabiei, 1375*t*

Acceleration(s)
  of active phase of labor, 505, 506*f*
  of fetal heart rate, 525

Acceptance, in grief response, 1715*t*
  in nurses caring for child with terminal illness, 1779
  in parents of child with terminal illness, 1773

Accessory (XI) nerve, 1545*t*

Accessory nipples, 1495–1496, 1496*f*

Accident(s). *See also* Traumatic injury
  childhood, 1643–1679
    health promotion and risk management for, 1646
    National Health Goals for, 1160*b*, 1644*b*
    types of, by age group, 1644*t*
  child injured in, nursing process for, 1644–1646
  prevention of. *See also* Safety
    for adolescents, 950
    for infants, 839, 841*t*
    in pregnancy, 384, 384*b*
    for toddlers, 869*t*, 870*b*

Accolate. *See* Zafirlukast

Accommodation
  cognitive, 819*t*, 820, 919
  definition of, 1825
  visual, 1586

Acculturation, definition of, 52, 1825

Accutane. *See* Isotretinoin

Acebutolol (Sectral), effects in lactation, 1790

ACE inhibitors. *See* Angiotensin-converting enzyme inhibitors

Acetaminophen (Tylenol)
  for afterpains, 637
  for backache, 284
  effects in lactation, 1789
  for exanthem subitum, 1357
  for fever, in children, 1136, 1246, 1257
  for headache, 285
  for influenza, 367
  for muscle aches, 637
  oral contraceptives and, 113
  for pain management in children, 1174
  for pain with scoliosis bracing, 1627
  pharmacology of, 1136*b*
  poisoning with, 1660
  for pruritus of infectious diseases, 1355
  for rubella, 1358
  for sickle-cell anemia, 1397
  for sinusitis pain, 1250
  for stem cell transplantation, 1387
  for teething, 851
  for urinary tract infection, 673, 1464

Acetazolamide (Diamox), for hydrocephalus, 1200

Acetylcholine (ACh), in myasthenia gravis, 1633

Acetylcholinesterase inhibitors, for myasthenia gravis, 1634

Acetylcysteine (Mucomyst)
  for acetaminophen poisoning, 1660
  for cystic fibrosis, 1272
  for meconium plug syndrome, 1194

Acetylsalicylic acid (aspirin)
  allergy to, 1344
  anticoagulants and, interactions of, 668
  for artificial (heart) valve replacement, 1295
  for children, 1174
  contraindications to, 577, 639, 1690
    in children, 1136
  for dysmenorrhea, 1491
  for fever, in children, 1246
  for juvenile rheumatoid arthritis, 370
  for Kawasaki disease, 1313
  for pregnancy-induced hypertension, in adolescent pregnancy, 471
  and Reye's syndrome, 1561
  teratogenicity of, 291*t*

Achalasia. *See also* Gastroesophageal reflux
  definition of, 1825
  in infants, 1423

Achilles reflex, assessment of, 1010, 1013*f*

Achondroplasia, 700, 1213

Acid-base balance. *See also* Acidosis; Alkalosis
  of fetus, assessment of, 527
  in respiratory disorders in children, 1229*t*, 1230*t*, 1231*b*

Acid-base imbalance, 1417–1418

Acid, definition of, 1417

Acidosis
  metabolic, 1417
    in pregnancy, 220*t*

Prepare your students for the challenges of maternity and pediatric nursing With two exciting video series that make complex concepts easy to grasp.

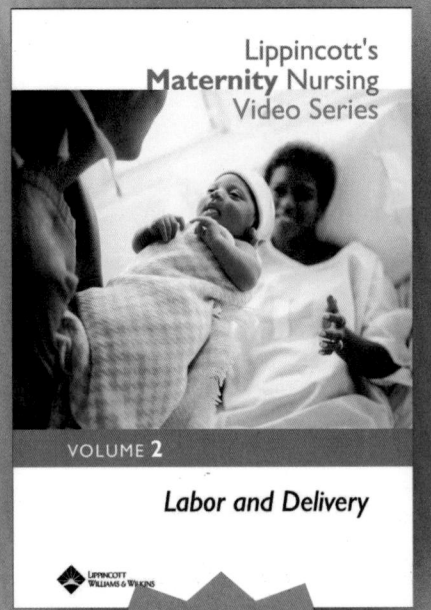

VOLUME 2

Labor and Delivery

Ideal for today's visual learners, these outstanding documentary-style videos let viewers explore first-hand the critical elements of nursing care for pregnant women, infants, children, and families—developing the clinical and communication skills required for safe, effective practice.

Maternity Nursing Videos

The full series covers several pregnancy experiences, types of labors and deliveries, and postpartum experiences-highlighted by nurse, patient, and family interviews.

Explore every phase of care…in high-quality visual detail!

- **Volume 1: Prenatal Care** addresses family adaptations to pregnancy, ways to promote a healthy pregnancy, and nursing management of at-risk pregnancies.
  VHS: ISBN: 0-7817-8250-3 • DVD: ISBN: 0-7817-9778-0
- **Volume 2: Labor and Delivery** begins from the moment of admission and addresses the nurse's role in assessment, monitoring, pain management, emotional support, stabilization of the newborn, and maternal-neonatal bonding.
  VHS: ISBN: 0-7817-7590-6 • DVD: ISBN: 0-7817-9547-8
- **Volume 3: Cesarean Delivery** covers several labor scenarios, including nursing care during an emergency C-section, and planned C-section.
  VHS: ISBN: 0-7817-9532-X • DVD: ISBN: 0-7817-6599-4
- **Volume 4: Postpartum Care** presents three normal range cases, from 12 hours to 6 weeks postpartum, with emphasis on maternal and newborn assessment, pain management, and family teaching.
  VHS: ISBN: 0-7817-7511-6 • DVD: ISBN: 0-7817-6545-5

2006 • Set of 4 VHS tapes: ISBN: 0-7817-6071-2 • Set of 4 DVDs: ISBN: 0-7817-8626-6

NEW!

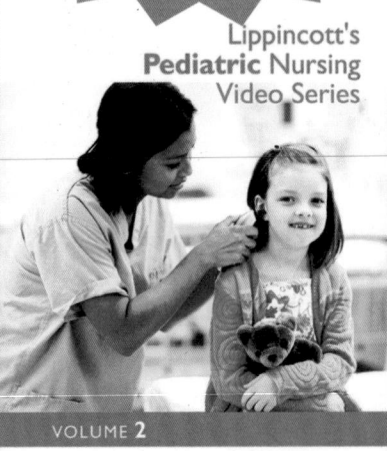

VOLUME 2

Communicating with Children and Families

Pediatric Nursing Videos

Be sure your students are ready to meet the challenges of pediatric nursing with confidence. Each video in dynamic series addresses a critical element of pediatric nursing care, and focuses on issues specific to five age groups—Infancy (28 days to 1 year); Toddler (1-3 years); Pre-School (3-6 years); School Age (6-12 years and Adolescencet (12-18 years). Nurse, patient, and family interviews highlight each program.

Give your students the visual guidance they need for safe, effective practice

- **Volume 1: Growth and Development** addresses normal physical, psychosocial, and cognitive development from infancy through adolescence.
  VHS: ISBN: 0-7817-8949-4 • DVD: ISBN: 0-7817-8714-9
- **Volume 2: Communicating with Children and Families** provides viewers with effective communication techniques specific to each age group.
  VHS: ISBN: 0-7817-7890-5 • DVD: ISBN: 0-7817-9231-2
- **Volume 3: Care Of The Hospitalized Child** examines the role of family caregivers, play, safety, pain management, and medication in the hospital setting.
  VHS: ISBN: 0-7817-6352-5 • DVD: ISBN: 0-7817-7975-8

2006 • Set of 3 VHS tapes: ISBN: 0-7817-6110-7 • Set of 3 DVDs: ISBN: 0-7817-9172-3

Add these skill-building videos to your curriculum…
ORDER TODAY!
Call TOLL FREE 1-800-638-3030
Visit us on the Web at <u>LWW.com/nursing</u> or <u>nursingcenter.com</u>
or visit your local health science bookstore

D5G3127